DEVELOPMENTAL-BEHAVIORAL
Pediatrics

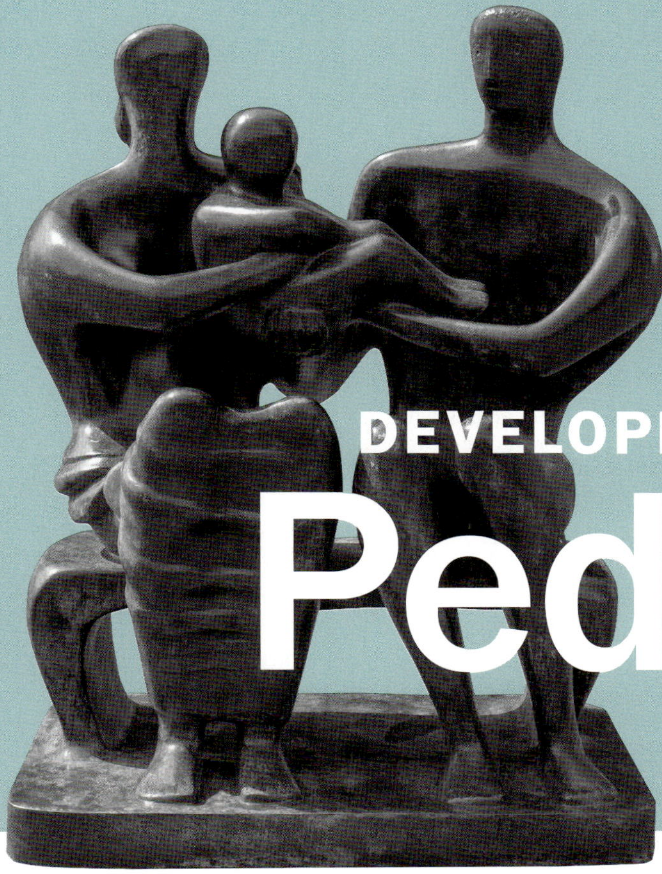

FIFTH EDITION

DEVELOPMENTAL-BEHAVIORAL Pediatrics

Heidi M. Feldman
Ballinger-Swindells Professor of Developmental and Behavioral Pediatrics
Chief, Division of Developmental-Behavioral Pediatrics
Stanford University School of Medicine
Stanford California
Service Chief, Developmental-Behavioral Pediatrics,
Stanford Childrens Health
Palo Alto, California

Ellen Roy Elias
Director, Special Care Clinic
Children's Hospital Colorado
Professor of Pediatrics and Genetics
University of Colorado School of Medicine
Aurora, Colorado

Nathan J. Blum
W.T. Grant Professor of Pediatrics
Perelman School of Medicine
University of Pennsylvania
Chief, Division of Developmental and Behavioral Pediatrics
Children's Hospital of Philadelphia
Philadelphia, Pennsylvania

Manuel E. Jimenez
Associate Professor of Pediatrics and Family Medicine and Community Health
Rutgers Robert Wood Johnson Medical School
Attending Developmental and Behavioral Pediatrician
Children's Specialized Hospital
New Brunswick, New Jersey

Terry Stancin
Chief of Psychology
Director, Child & Adolescent Psychiatry & Psychology
The MetroHealth System
Professor, Departments of Psychiatry
Pediatrics & Psychological Sciences
Case Western Reserve University
Cleveland, OH

ELSEVIER

Elsevier
1600 John F. Kennedy Blvd.
Ste 1800
Philadelphia, PA 19103-2899

Developmental-Behavioral Pediatrics,
FIFTH EDITION

ISBN: 978-0-323-80972-6

ISBN: 9780323809726

Content Strategist: Sarah Barth
Content Development Specialist: Rishi Arora
Publishing Services Manager: Shereen Jameel
Project Manager: Nadhiya Sekar
Design Direction: Brain Salisbury

Printed in India

Last digit is the print number: 9 8 7 6 5 4 3 2 1

CONTRIBUTORS

May V. Albee, BS
Clinical Research Coordinator
Division of Oncology
Children's Hospital of Philadelphia
Philadelphia, Pennsylvania

Kathleen Angkustsiri, MD
Associate Professor of Clinical Pediatrics
Developmental-Behavioral Pediatrician
MIND Institute
University of California–Davis
Davis, California

Arash Anoshiravani, MD, MPH
Division of Adolescent Medicine
Department of Pediatrics
Stanford University
Palo Alto, California

David Alan Ansel, MD
Clinical Associate Professor of Pediatrics
Division of Developmental-Behavioral Pediatrics
Stanford University School of Medicine
Lucille Packard Children's Hospital
Palo Alto, California

Tanni L. Anthony, PhD
Director of Access, Learning, and Literacy
Colorado Department of Education
Denver, Colorado

Melissa Armstrong-Brine, PhD
MetroHealth Medical Center
Center Case Western Reserve University
Cleveland, Ohio

Jenna Arruda, MD, MPH
Pediatric Integrative Medicine
The Sutcliffe Clinic
Los Altos, California
Pediatric Hospitalist
Central Maine Medical Center
Lewiston, Maine

Joan Rosenbaum Asarnow, PhD
Professor, Psychiatry and Biobehavioral Sciences
Semel Institute for Neuroscience and Human Behavior
David Geffen School of Medicine
University of California Los Angeles
Los Angeles, California

Marilyn Augustyn, MD
Professor of Pediatrics
Boston University School of Medicine
Director of Developmental-Behavioral Pediatrics BMC
Boston, Massachusetts

Peter Baker II, MD
Associate Professor of Pediatrics and Clinical Genetics & Metabolism
Department of Pediatrics
University of Colorado
Children's Hospital Colorado
Aurora, Colorado

Linda G. Bandini, PhD
Healthy Weight Research Network
E.K. Shriver Center
UMass Chan Medical School
Boston, Massachusetts

William J. Barbaresi, MD
Chief, Division of Developmental Medicine
Boston Children's Hospital
Division of Developmental Medicine
Boston Children's Hospital & Harvard Medical School
T. Berry Brazelton Professor of Pediatrics
Harvard Medical School
Boston, Massachusetts

W. Steven Barnett, PhD
Graduate School of Education
The State University of New Jersey
Rutgers University
New Brunswick, New Jersey

Brenda Bassingthwaite, PhD, BCBA
Associate Professor
Munroe-Meyer Institute
University of Nebraska Medical Center
Omaha, Nebraska

Brittany S. Bassitt, MD
General Pediatrician
Kaiser Permanent Northwest
Hillsboro, Oregon

Courtney E. Batt, MD
Assistant Professor of Pediatrics
Section of Adolescent Medicine
University of Colorado School of Medicine
Children's Hospital of Colorado
Aurora, Colorado

Rebecca A. Baum, MD
Clinical Professor of Pediatrics
University of North Carolina School of Medicine
Developmental Behavioral Pediatrician
UNC Health
Chapel Hill, North Carolina

Fiona M. Baumer, MD
Assistant Professor of Neurology and of Pediatrics
Stanford University School of Medicine
Palo Alto, California

Ronald E. Becker, MD
Assistant Professor of Pediatrics
Harvard Medical School
Assistant in Pediatrics
Boston Children's Hospital
Boston, Massachusetts

Anna Malia Beckwith, MD
Assistant Professor of Pediatrics
Rutgers Robert Wood Johnson Medical School
Section Chief of Developmental Behavioral Pediatrics
Children's Specialized Hospital
New Brunswick, New Jersey

Nathaniel S. Beers, MD, MPA
Children's National Hospital
HSC Health Care System
Washington, District of Columbia

David C. Bellinger, PhD, MSc
Professor of Neurology
Harvard Medical School
Boston Children's Hospital
Boston, Massachusetts

Amanda E. Bennett, MD, MPH
The Children's Hospital of Philadelphia
Division of Developmental and Behavioral Pediatrics
Philadelphia, Pennsylvania

Kelly Blankenship, DO
Associate Chief Medical Officer for Behavioral Health
Dayton Children's Hospital
Dayton, Ohio

Nathan J. Blum, MD
W.T. Grant Professor of Pediatrics
Perelman School of Medicine
University of Pennsylvania
Chief, Division of Developmental and Behavioral Pediatrics
Children's Hospital of Philadelphia
Philadelphia, Pennsylvania

Kristen Boog, MA
School of Psychological and Behavioral Sciences
Southern Illinois University
Carbondale, Illinois

Renée Boynton-Jarrett, MD, ScD
Department of Pediatrics
Boston University School of Medicine
Vital Village Community Engagement Network
Boston, Massachusetts

Nicholas J. K. Breitborde, PhD, ABPP
Department of Psychiatry and Behavioral Health
The Ohio State University
Columbus, Ohio

Zoe Brennan-Krohn
Staff Attorney
Disability Rights Program of the American Civil Liberties Union
San Francisco, California

Annelise Brochier, MPH
Research Project Manager
Boston Medical Center
Department of Pediatrics
Boston, Massachusetts

Shalonda Brooks, PhD
Nationwide Children's Hospital
Ohio State University
Child Development Center
Westerville, Ohio

Mariah Brown, BA
Pediatric Endocrinology
Children's Hospital Colorado
University of Colorado School of Medicine
Aurora, Colorado

Michelle R. Brown, PhD
Clinical Professor of Psychiatry
Department of Psychiatry and Behavioral Sciences
Division of Child and Adolescent Psychiatry
Stanford Children's Health
Stanford University School of Medicine
Stanford, California

Sophie Brunt, M Ed
Doctoral Student
Department of Human Services
School of Education and Human Development
University of Virginia
Charlottesville, Virginia

Kimberly Burkhart, PhD
Clinical Psychologist
Associate Professor of Pediatrics and Psychiatry
Case Western Reserve University School of Medicine
Rainbow Babies and Children's Hospital
Division of Developmental-Behavioral Pediatrics and Psychology
Cleveland, Ohio

Nicole R. Bush, PhD
University of California (UCSF)
Department of Pediatrics
Division of Developmental Medicine
San Francisco, California

Eric M. Butter, PhD
Nationwide Children's Hospital
Department of Pediatric Psychology and Neuropsychology
Ohio State University
Columbus, Ohio

Eliza Buyers, MD
Assistant Professor
Department of Obstetrics and Gynecology
University of Colorado
Anschutz Campus
Pediatric and Adolescent Gynecology
Children's Hospital Colorado
Aurora, Colorado

Caitlin F. Canfield, PhD
Division of Developmental and Behavioral Pediatrics
Department of Pediatrics
NYU Grossman School of Medicine
New York, New York

Laura Arnstein Carpenter, PhD
Medical University of South Carolina
Charleston, South Carolina

Kaitlyn Cavanaugh, MS, OTR/L, CLC
Occupational Therapist & Certified Lactation Counselor
Children's Hospital Colorado
Highlands Ranch, Colorado

Philip B. Cawkwell, MD
Child and Adolescent Psychiatrist
Bay Area Clinical Associates
Stanford University
Palo Alto, California

Diane Chen, PhD
Potocsnak Family Division of Adolescent and Young Adult Medicine
Pritzker Department of Psychiatry and Behavioral Health
Ann & Robert H. Lurie Children's Hospital of Chicago
Department of Psychiatry and Behavioral Sciences
Department of Pediatrics
Northwestern University Feinberg School of Medicine
Chicago, Illinois

Gayle Chesley, PhD
Children's Hospital of Philadelphia
Perelman School of Medicine
University of Pennsylvania
Philadelphia, Pennsylvania

Marie A. Clark, MD, MPH
Assistant Professor of Pediatrics
Case Western Reserve University School of Medicine
Rainbow Babies and Children's Hospital
Division of Developmental-Behavioral Pediatrics and Psychology
Cleveland, Ohio

Elizabeth Coan, PsyD
Psychologist
Developmental Pediatrics
Denver Fragile X Clinic
Children's Hospital Colorado
University of Colorado School of Medicine
Aurora, Colorado

Shereen J. Cohen, PhD
Postdoctoral Fellow
MIND Institute
University of California–Davis
Davis, California

Cara Coleman, JD, MPH
Director of Public Policy and Advocacy
Family Voices
Lexington, Massachusetts

Sean T. Corbett, MD
Associate Professor
Department of Urology
University of Virginia School of Medicine
Charlottesville, Virginia

DePorres Cormier II, MD
Division of Developmental Pediatrics
Department of Pediatrics
Saint Louis University School of Medicine
SSM Cardinal Glennon Children's Hospital
Knights of Columbus Developmental Center
St. Louis, Missouri

Claire A. Coyne, PhD
Potocsnak Family Division of Adolescent and Young Adult Medicine
Pritzker Department of Psychiatry and Behavioral Health
Ann & Robert H. Lurie Children's Hospital of Chicago
Department of Psychiatry and Behavioral Sciences
Northwestern University Feinberg School of Medicine
Chicago, Illinois

Catherine Crouse, MM, MT-BC, NICU-MT, NMT
Master of Music in Music Therapy
Music Therapist-Board Certified
Neonatal Intensive Care Music Therapist
Neurologic Music Therapist
Lucile Packard Children's Hospital
Palo Alto, California

Carol Curtin, PhD
Healthy Weight Research Network
E.K. Shriver Center
UMass Chan Medical School
Worcester, Massachusetts

Beth Ellen Davis, MD, MPH
Professor of Pediatrics
Division of Neurodevelopmental and Behavioral Pediatrics
University of Virginia
Charlottesville, Virginia

Katie Davis, MSN, RN, PHNA-BC
Population Health Innovation Institute
Institute for H.O.P.E.
The MetroHealth System
Cleveland, Ohio

Shanlee Davis, MD
Pediatric Endocrinology
University of Colorado School of Medicine
Aurora, Colorado

Thomas P. Demaria, PhD
Consultant and Advisor
National Center for School Crisis and Bereavement
Children's Hospital Los Angeles
Los Angeles, California

Allison G. Dempsey, PhD
Department of Psychiatry
University of Colorado School of Medicine
Aurora, Colorado

Katie A. Devine, PhD, MPH
Rutgers Cancer Institute of New Jersey
New Brunswick, New Jersey

Mary Beth DeWitt, PhD
Chief, Division of Child Psychology
Dayton Children's Hospital
Dayton, Ohio

Liliane Diab, MD
Assistant Professor
Department of Pediatrics, Section of Nutrition
University of Colorado School of Medicine
Clinical Director
Clinical Nutrition: Growth and Parenting
Lifestyle Medicine Clinics
Aurora, Colorado

Irene Cihon Dietz, MD
Division of Comprehensive Care Pediatrics
MetroHealth Medical Center
Case Western Reserve University School of Medicine
Cleveland, Ohio

Elizabeth Dubow, MD
Assistant Professor, Pediatrics-Neurology
Children's Hospital Colorado
University of Colorado
Aurora, Colorado

Sarah E. Dubner, MD
Instructor
Division of Developmental-Behavioral Pediatrics
Stanford University School of Medicine
Stanford, California

John C. Duby, MD, CPE
Wright State University Boonshoft School of Medicine
Dayton Children's Hospital
Dayton, Ohio

Jessica Duis, MD, MS
Assistant Professor of Pediatrics and Genetics
Director, Chromosome 15 clinics
Children's Hospital Colorado
University of Colorado Anschutz Medical Campus
Aurora, Colorado

Mei Elansary, MD, MPhil
Assistant Professor of Pediatrics
Boston University School of Medicine
Attending Physician BMC
Boston, Massachusetts

Ellen Roy Elias, MD
Director, Special Care Clinic
Children's Hospital Colorado
Professor of Pediatrics and Genetics
University of Colorado School of Medicine
Aurora, Colorado

Janice Enriquez, PhD
Associate Clinical Professor of Pediatrics
MIND Institute
UC Davis Health
Davis, California

Robert W. Enzenauer, MD, MPH/MSPH
Professor of Ophthalmology
University of Colorado School of Medicine
Aurora, Colorado

Shannon Erisman, PhD
Assistant Professor of Psychiatry and Human Behavior Clinician Educator
Alpert Medical School at Brown University Clinical Director
Postpartum Day Hospital
Women & Infants Hospital
Providence, Rhode Island

Krista Eschbach, MD
Assistant Professor, Pediatrics-Neurology
Children's Hospital Colorado
University of Colorado
Aurora, Colorado

Jordan Ezell Klein, PhD
Medical University of South Carolina
Charleston, South Carolina

Karla K. Fehr, PhD
School of Psychological and Behavioral Sciences
Southern Illinois University
Carbondale, Illinois

Heidi M. Feldman, MD, PhD
Ballinger-Swindells Professor of Developmental and Behavioral Pediatrics
Chief, Division of Developmental-Behavioral Pediatrics
Stanford University School of Medicine
Stanford California
Service Chief, Developmental-Behavioral Pediatrics
Stanford Childrens Health
Palo Alto, California

Lauren B. Fishbein, PhD
Department of Child and Adolescent Psychiatry and Behavioral Sciences
The Children's Hospital of Philadelphia
Philadelphia, Pennsylvania

Jason M. Fogler, PhD
Senior Staff Psychologist
Co-Director: ADHD Program
Training Director: Leadership Education in Neurodevelopmental & related Disabilities (LEND)
Division of Developmental Medicine, Boston Children's Hospital
Assistant Professor of Pediatrics & Psychology, Harvard Medical School
Boston, Massachusetts

Deborah A. Frank, MD
Founder
Grow Clinic for Children Boston Medical Center
Founder and Principal Investigator
Children's Health Watch
Professor of Child Health and Well-Being
Boston University School of Medicine
Boston, Massachusetts

Sandra L. Friedman, MD, MPH
Professor of Pediatrics
University of Colorado School of Medicine
Section Head, Developmental Pediatrics
Children's Hospital Colorado
Aurora, Colorado

Sarah L. Friedman, PhD
Research Professor
Department of Psychological and Brain Sciences
The George Washington University
Washington, District of Columbia

Mary A. Fristad, PhD, ABPP
Division of Child & Family Psychiatry
Big Lots Behavioral Health Services
Nationwide Children's Hospital
Columbus, Ohio

Nadine Gaab, PhD
Associate Professor of Education
Harvard Graduate School of Education and
Associate Professor of Pediatrics
Harvard Medical School
Boston, Massachusetts

Rachel Lee Gilgoff, MD
Senior Clinical and Science Advisor
ACEs Aware Initiative
Office of the California Surgeon General
Aurrera Health Group
Sacramento, California

R. Emily Gonzalez, PhD
Department of Pediatrics
University of Virginia School of Medicine
Charlottesville, Virginia

Julie Good, MD
Clinical Associate Professor
Pediatric Pain Management and Pediatric Palliative Care
Department of Anesthesiology, Perioperative and Pain Medicine (by courtesy, Pediatrics)
Stanford Children's Health
Stanford University School of Medicine
Center for Academic Medicine
Stanford, California

Susan Hayden Gray, MD
Associate Professor of Pediatrics
Medical Director of UVA Teen and Young Adult Health Center
University of Virginia
Charlottesville, Virginia

A. Dawn Greathouse, PhD, BCBA
Pediatric Neurodevelopmental Psychologist
Child Development Center
Nationwide Children's Hospital
Assistant Professor
The Ohio State University
Columbus, Ohio

Randi Hagerman, MD
Developmental Pediatrics
University of California–Davis MIND Institute
Sacramento, California

Eleanore M. Hall, PsyD
Department of Psychiatry
University of Colorado School of Medicine
Aurora, Colorado

Howard Hall, PhD, PsyD, BCB
Professor of Pediatrics, Psychiatry, and Psychological Sciences
Rainbow Babies & Children's Hospital
University Hospitals Cleveland Medical Center
Division of Developmental/Behavioral Pediatrics & Psychology
Cleveland, Ohio

Bonnie Halpern-Felsher, PhD
Professor of Pediatrics, Epdemiology and Population Health, and Psychiatry and Behavioral Sciences
Division of Adolescent Medicine
Department of Pediatrics
Stanford University
Palo Alto, California

Sarah A. Hamilton, MD
Department of Psychiatry and Behavioral Health
The Ohio State University
Columbus, Ohio

Robin L. Hansen, MD
Professor of Pediatrics Emerita
MIND Institute
University of California
Davis School of Medicine
Davis, California

Sandra G. Hassink, MD, MSc
Healthy Weight Research Network
Emeritus Associate Professor of Pediatrics
Nemours Children's Hospital
Wilmington, Delaware

Marissa Hauptman, MD, MPH
Associate Director
Pediatric Environmental Health Center and Region 1 New England Pediatric Environmental Health Specialty Unit (PEHSU)
Boston Children's Hospital
Boston, Massachusetts
Assistant Professor, Harvard Medical School
Boston, Massachusetts

Katheleen Hawes, PhD, PMH-CNS, BC
Assistant Professor of Pediatrics, Clinician Educator
Alpert Medical School at Brown University
Women & Infants Hospital
Providence, Rhode Island

Rebecca A. Hazen, PhD
Division of Developmental and Behavioral Pediatrics & Psychology
Rainbow Babies and Children's Hospital
University Hospitals
Cleveland Medical Center
Department of Pediatrics
Case Western Reserve University
Cleveland, Ohio

Albert Hergenroeder, MD
Professor of Pediatrics
Pediatrics-Adolescent Medicine and Sports Medicine
Chief, Adolescent Medicine and Sports Medicine
Baylor College of Medicine
Texas Children's Hospital
Houston, Texas

Jenniffer Herrera, MD
Assistant Professor of Pediatrics
Division of Neurodevelopmental and Behavioral Pediatrics
University of Virginia
Charlottesville, Virginia

Francis Hickey, MD
Children's Hospital Colorado
Aurora, Colorado

Pamela High, MD
Professor of Pediatrics, Clinician Educator
Alpert Medical School at Brown University
Director, Developmental Behavioral Pediatrics
Hasbro Children's Hospital
Providence, Rhode Island

Matthew C. Hocking, PhD
Pediatric Psychologist
Division of Oncology
Children's Hospital of Philadelphia
Department of Psychiatry
Perelman School of Medicine
University of Pennsylvania
Philadelphia, Pennsylvania

Cody A. Hostutler, PhD
Clinical Assistant Professor of Pediatrics
The Ohio State University
Pediatric Psychologist
Nationwide Children's Hospital
Columbus, Ohio

Susan Howell, MS, CGC
Genetic Counselor
Developmental Pediatrics
Denver Fragile X Clinic
Children's Hospital Colorado
University of Colorado School of Medicine
Aurora, Colorado

Lynne C. Huffman, MD
Professor of Pediatrics
Division of Developmental-Behavioral Pediatrics
Stanford University School of Medicine
Stanford, California

Abby Hughes-Scalise, PhD
Clinical Psychology PsyD Program
Augsburg University
Minneapolis, Minnesota

Susan L. Hyman, MD
Healthy Weight Research Network
University of Rochester Medical Center
Rochester, New York

Kida Ingram, PhD
Psychologist
Development Medicine Center
Instructor
Harvard Medical School
Boston, Massachusetts

Sandhyaa Iyengar, MD MPH
Practice-Based Scholar
The Center for Violence Prevention
Children's Hospital of Philadelphia
The Perelman School of Medicine
The University of Pennsylvania
Philadelphia, Pennsylvania

Carissa R. Jackel, MD
Assistant Professor of Clinical Pediatrics
Perelman School of Medicine
University of Pennsylvania
Associate Fellowship Program Director
Children's Hospital of Philadelphia
Philadelphia, Pennsylvania

Bayan Jalalizadeh, MD
Child, Adolescent, and Adult Psychiatrist
Children's Health Council
Palo Alto, California

Manuel E. Jimenez, MD, MS
Associate Professor of Pediatrics and Family Medicine and Community Health
Rutgers Robert Wood Johnson Medical School
Attending Developmental and Behavioral Pediatrician
Children's Specialized Hospital
New Brunswick, New Jersey

Megan M. Julian, PhD
Department of Psychiatry
University of Michigan
Ann Arbor, Michigan

Colleen Kahn, MA-MFT-AT, MA-ATR-BC
Marriage and Family Therapy and Art Therapy Board Certified Art Therapist
Lucile Packard Children's Hospital
Palo Alto, California

Robert D. Keder, MD
Connecticut Children's Medical Center
University of Connecticut School of Medicine
Farmington, Connecticut

Brooks Keeshin, MD
University of Utah
Salt Lake City, Utah

M. Kathleen Kelly, PhD, PT
Associate Professor
University of Pittsburgh
School of Health & Rehabilitation Sciences
Pittsburgh, Pennsylvania

Karen Kelminson, MD
Children's Hospital Colorado
Aurora, Colorado

Mary A. Khetani, ScD, OTR/L
Departments of Occupational Therapy and Disability and Human Development
University of Illinois
Chicago, Illinois

Bridget Kiley, MSc, LMCH
Arlington Youth Counseling Center
Cambridge, Massachusetts

Judy Lu Kim, MD
Assistant Professor
Section of Transition Medicine
Department of Medicine
Department of Family and Community Medicine
Baylor College of Medicine
Houston, Texas

Patricia A. Kinser, PhD, WHNP-BC, RN
Professor
Virginia Commonwealth University
School of Nursing
Richmond, Virginia

Michael W. Kirkwood, PhD, ABPP-CN
Director
Rehabilitation Psychology & Neuropsychology
Department of Rehabilitation
Children's Hospital Colorado
Professor, Department of Physical Medicine & Rehabilitation
University of Colorado School of Medicine
Aurora, Colorado

John R. Knight, Jr., MD
Founder and Director Emeritus
Center for Adolescent Substance Use & Addiction Research (CeASAR)
Department of Pediatrics
Boston Children's Hospital
Boston, Massachusetts
Associate Professor Pediatrics (Ret.)
Harvard Medical School
Boston, Massachusetts

Holly Knotowicz, MS, CCC-SLP
Speech Language Pathologist
Picky Eaters Anonymous, LLC
Portland, Maine

Aaina Kochhar, MD
Assistant Professor
Section of Genetics & Metabolism
Department of Pediatrics
University of Colorado Anschutz Medical Campus
Aurora, Colorado

Anson J. Koshy, MD, MBE
Associate Professor
McGovern Center for Humanities and Ethics
McGovern Medical School
Houston, Texas

Mary C. Kral, PhD
Professor of Pediatrics
Medical University of South Carolina
Charleston, South Carolina

Nancy F. Krebs, MD, MS
Professor of Pediatrics Head
Section of Nutrition
Associate Vice Chairman, Academic Affairs, Department of Pediatrics
University of Colorado School of Medicine
Aurora, Colorado

Casey E. Krueger, PhD
Clinical Assistant Professor (Affiliated)
Division of Developmental-Behavioral Pediatrics
Department of Pediatrics
Stanford University School of Medicine
Palo Alto, California

Jeremy Kruger, MD
Department of Psychiatry and Behavioral Sciences
University of Washington
Seattle, Washington

Sara Kupzyk, PhD, LP, BCBA-D
Assistant Professor
University of Nebraska at Omaha
Omaha, Nebraska

Gary Kwok, PhD
Rutgers Cancer Institute of New Jersey
New Brunswick, New Jersey

Philip J. Landrigan, MD, MSc
Director
Program for Global Public Health and the Common Good
Boston College
Chestnut Hill, Massachusetts

Austin Larson, MD
Assistant Professor of Pediatrics and Clinical Genetics & Metabolism
Department of Pediatrics, Section of Clinical Genetics and Metabolism
University of Colorado
Children's Hospital Colorado
Aurora, Colorado

Adrienne Lazaro, MS
Department of Pediatrics
Division of Adolescent Medicine
Stanford University
Palo Alto, California

Michele Ledesma, MD
Assistant Professor of Pediatrics
New York Medical College
Developmental & Behavioral Pediatrics
Boston Children's Health Physicians
Maria Fareri Children's Hospital
Valhalla, New York

Stephen S. Leff, PhD
Co-Director
The Center for Violence Prevention
Children's Hospital of Philadelphia
The Perelman School of Medicine
The University of Pennsylvania
Philadelphia, Pennsylvania

John E. Leikauf, MD
Clinical Assistant Professor
Child and Adolescent Psychiatry and Child Development
Psychiatry and Behavioral Sciences
Stanford University
Palo Alto, California

Mary L. O'Connor Leppert, MB BCH
Kennedy Krieger Institute
Johns Hopkins University School of Medicine
Baltimore, Maryland

Bethany Leraas, MA
School of Psychological and Behavioral Sciences
Southern Illinois University
Carbondale, Illinois

Irene M. Loe, MD
Division of Developmental-Behavioral Pediatrics
Department of Pediatrics
Stanford University School of Medicine
Stanford, California

Julie C. Lumeng, MD
Department of Pediatrics
University of Michigan
Ann Arbor, Michigan

Michelle M. Macias, MD
Division of Developmental-Behavioral Pediatrics
Department of Pediatrics
Medical University of South Carolina
Charleston, South Carolina

Dawn M. Magnusson, PT, PhD
Department of Physical Medicine and Rehabilitation
University of Colorado Anschutz Medical Campus
Aurora, Colorado

Fatima Malik, MD
Clinical Assistant Professor
Department of Pediatrics
University Hospitals Connor Whole Health
Rainbow Babies and Children's Hospital
Cleveland, Ohio

Kathryn Mancini, PhD
MetroHealth Medical Center
Department of Psychiatry
Case Western Reserve University School of Medicine
Cleveland, Ohio

Kilby Mann, MD
Department of Physical Medicine and Rehabilitation
University of Colorado
Children's Hospital Colorado
Aurora, Colorado

Melissa Marquardt, PhD
Licensed Psychologist
Independent Practice
Oregon Health Sciences University
Portland, Oregon

Raman Marwaha, MD
Child/Adolescent Psychiatrist
MetroHealth System
Director
MetroHealth Psychiatry Residency Program
Assistant Professor of Psychiatry
Case Western Reserve University School of Medicine
Cleveland, Ohio

Micah Mazurek, PhD
Professor
Department of Human Services
School of Education and Human Development
University of Virginia
Charlottesville, Virginia

Susan H. McDaniel, PhD
Dr. Laurie Sands Distinguished Professor of Families & Health
Departments of Psychiatry & Family Medicine
University of Rochester School of Medicine & Dentistry
Rochester, New York

Eric McDonald, MD
Child and Adolescent Psychiatry
The Permanente Medical Group
Santa Clara, California

Laura Joan McGuinn, MD
Professor of Pediatrics
Thomas Lowder Chair in Developmental-Behavioral Pediatrics
Division of Developmental-Behavioral Pediatrics
Department of Pediatrics
The University of Alabama School of Medicine
Birmingham, Alabama

Naomi J.L. Meeks, MD
Assistant Professor
Section of Genetics & Metabolism
Department of Pediatrics
University of Colorado Anschutz Medical Campus
Aurora, Colorado

Robyn Mehlenbeck, PhD, ABPP
George Mason University
Center for Psychological Services
Fairfax, Virginia

Alan L. Mendelsohn, MD
Professor of Pediatrics and Population Health
Division of Developmental and Behavioral Pediatrics
Department of Pediatrics
NYU Grossman School of Medicine
New York, New York

Cheryl Messick, PhD
Department of Communication Science and Disorders
School of Health and Rehabilitation Sciences
University of Pittsburgh
Pittsburgh, Pennsylvania

Jonathan W. Mink, MD, PhD
Endowed Professor in Pediatric Neurology
Professor of Neurology, Neuroscience, and Pediatrics
University of Rochester School of Medicine & Dentistry
Rochester, New York

Laura J. Mintz, MD, PhD
Assistant Professor
CWRU School of Medicine
MetroHealth Medical Center
Cleveland, Ohio

Susan Mizner
Director
Disability Rights Program of the American Civil Liberties Union
San Francisco, California

Sonia A. Monteiro, MD
Department of Pediatrics
Section of Developmental Pediatrics
Baylor College of Medicine
Meyer Center for Developmental Pediatrics & Autism
Texas Children's Hospital
Houston, Texas

Deborah Mood, PhD
Department of Pediatrics
University of Colorado Denver
Aurora, Colorado

Jessica Moore, PhD
Assistant Professor
Departments of Pediatrics and Psychiatry
University of Rochester School of Medicine & Dentistry
Rochester, New York

Sara W. Moyer, RN, BS
Virginia Commonwealth University
School of Nursing
Richmond, Virginia

Claudia M. Mueller, MD, PhD
Associate Professor
Department of Surgery
Stanford University
Stanford, California

Christina Mulé, PhD, NCSP
Assistant Professor
Division of Developmental and Behavioral Pediatrics
Department of Pediatrics, University of Rochester School of Medicine & Dentistry
Assistant Professor, Division of Developmental and Behavioral Pediatrics
Department of Pediatrics
Tufts University School of Medicine
Boston, Massachusetts

Tiffany Munzer, MD
Department of Pediatrics
University of Michigan
Ann Arbor, Michigan

Nancy Murphy, MD
Department of Pediatrics
School of Medicine
University of Utah
Salt Lake City, Utah

Caitlin B. Murray, PhD
Department of Anesthesiology and Pain Medicine
University of Washington School of Medicine & Seattle Children's Hospital
Seattle, Washington

Marsheena Murray, PhD, ABPP
MetroHealth Medical Center
Cleveland, Ohio

Brittany R. Myers, PhD
Pediatric Psychologist
MetroHealth System
Assistant Professor of Psychiatry
Case Western Reserve University School of Medicine
Cleveland, Ohio

Cy Nadler, PhD
Director of Autism Services
Division of Developmental and Behavioral Health
Children's Mercy Kansas City
Associate Professor of Pediatrics
University of Missouri-Kansas City School of Medicine
Kansas City, Missouri

Robert Needlman, MD
MetroHealth Medical Center
Department of Pediatrics
Case Western Reserve University School of Medicine
Cleveland, Ohio

Jeffrey Okamoto, MD
John A. Burns School of Medicine
University of Hawaii–Manoa
Kapiolani Medical Center for Women and Children
Honolulu, Hawaii

Joyce Oleszek, MD
Department of Physical Medicine and Rehabilitation
University of Colorado
Children's Hospital Colorado
Aurora, Colorado

Sara O'Rourke, MOT, OTR/L, BCP
Outpatient Occupational Therapy Program Manager
Nationwide Children's Hospital
Columbus, Ohio

Judith A. Owens, MD, MPH
Professor of Neurology
Harvard Medical School
Co-Director of Sleep Medicine
Boston Children's Hospital
Waltham, Massachusetts

Padmini Palat, MD, MPH
Associate Professor
University of Colorado
Department of Pediatrics
Section of Neurology
Children's Hospital Colorado
Aurora, Colorado

Tonya M. Palermo, PhD
Department of Anesthesiology and Pain Medicine
University of Washington School of Medicine
Seattle Children's Research Institute
Seattle, Washington

Craig J. Parris, MS, APRN, PMHNP-BC, FNP-C
Department of Psychiatry and Behavioral Health
The Ohio State University
Columbus, Ohio

Jessica Patel, PhD
Clinical Assistant Professor (Affiliated)
Division of Developmental-Behavioral Pediatrics
Department of Pediatrics
Stanford University School of Medicine
Palo Alto, California

Silvia Pereira-Smith, MD
Division of Developmental-Behavioral Pediatrics
Department of Pediatrics
Medical University of South Carolina
Charleston, South Carolina

Hannah Perrin, MD
University of California (UCSF)
Department of Pediatrics
Division of Developmental Medicine
San Francisco, California

Megan Honor Pesch, MD, MS
Division of Developmental and Behavioral Pediatrics
Department of Pediatrics
University of Michigan Medical School
Ann Arbor, Michigan

Jaime W. Peterson, MD, MPH
Department of Pediatrics
Oregon Health and Science University
Portland, Oregon

Randall Phelps, MD, PhD
Developmental and Behavioral Pediatrician
Associate Professor of Pediatrics
Child Development and Rehabilitation Center
Institute on Development and Disability
Oregon Health and Science University
Eugene, Oregon

Laura Pickler, MD, MPH
Associate Professor
University of Colorado
Aurora, Colorado

Aaron Powell, MD
Pediatric Physiatrist
Department of Rehabilitation
Children's Hospital Colorado
Assistant Professor
Department of Physical Medicine and Rehabilitation
University of Colorado School of Medicine
Aurora, Colorado

Lisa Prock, MD, MPH
Director
Developmental Medicine Center
Boston Children's Hospital Boston
Assistant Professor
Harvard Medical School
Boston, Massachusetts

Michael A. Puente, MD
Assistant Professor of Ophthalmology
University of Colorado School of Medicine
Aurora, Colorado

Marianne Pugatch, PhD, LICSW
Postdoctoral Fellow
Clifford Attkisson Clinical Services Research Training Program (T-32)
Division of Adolescent and Young Adult Medicine
Department of Pediatrics
Benioff Children's Hospital
University of California, San Francisco
Department of Psychiatry and Behavioral Sciences
Weill Institute for Neurosciences
University of California
San Francisco, California

Jamie T. Rabot, MD
Child Development and Rehabilitation Center
Institute on Development and Disability
Oregon Health and Science University
Eugene, Oregon

Lisa Ramirez, PhD, ABPP
Department of Child and Adolescent Psychiatry and Psychology,
The MetroHealth System
Department of Psychiatry
Case Western Reserve University School of Medicine
Cleveland, Ohio

Leonard A. Rappaport, MD, MS
Emeritus Chief
Division of Developmental Medicine
Boston Children's Hospital
Mary Deming Scott Professor of Pediatrics
Harvard Medical School
Boston, Massachusetts

Jennifer M. Rathbun, MD, MA
Clinical Assistant in Psychiatry
Supervisor, Child & Adolescent Psychiatry Training Program
Massachusetts General Hospital
Clinical Instructor in Psychiatry
Harvard Medical School
Boston, Massachusetts

Karen Ratliff-Schaub, MD, MBOE
Children's Hospital, Prisma Health System
Clinical Associate Professor of Pediatrics
University of South Carolina
College of Medicine, Greenville
Greenville, South Carolina

Shelly Reggiani, EdD
North Clackamas School District Equity and Instructional Services
Clackamas, Oregon
Lewis and Clark College
Graduate School of Education & Counseling
Portland, Oregon

Marie Reilly, MD
Developmental Behavioral Pediatrician
Developmental Medicine Center
Boston Children's Hospital
Boston, Massachusetts

Dillon Reitmeyer, MSW
Rutgers School of Social Work
New Brunswick, New Jersey

Bibiana Restrepo, MD
Associate Clinical Professor of Pediatrics
MIND Institute
UC Davis Health
Davis, California

Luis A. Rivas Vazquez, BS
Research Assistant II
Department of Pediatrics (Division of General Pediatrics)
Oregon Health & Science University
Portland, Oregon

Paul M. Robins, PhD
Children's Hospital of Philadelphia
Perelman School of Medicine
University of Pennsylvania
Philadelphia, Pennsylvania

Erin Roby, PhD
Division of Developmental and Behavioral Pediatrics
Department of Pediatrics
NYU Grossman School of Medicine
New York, New York

Nancy J. Roizen, MD
Professor of Pediatrics
Case Western Reserve University School of Medicine
Rainbow Babies and Children's Hospital
Division of Developmental-Behavioral Pediatrics and Psychology
Cleveland, Ohio

Rosmary Ros-DeMarize, PhD
Division of Developmental-Behavioral Pediatrics
Department of Pediatrics
Medical University of South Carolina
Charleston, South Carolina

Erica Fornaris Rouch, PhD
Assistant Professor
Department of Human Services
School of Education and Human Development
University of Virginia
Charlottesville, Virginia

Suzanne Cushwa Rusnak, MEd, MSSA, LSW
Mindfulness Coordinator
Connor Whole Health
University Hospitals Independent Mindfulness Teacher, Coach Consultant
Cleveland, Ohio

Afiya Sajwani, BA
Potocsnak Family Division of Adolescent and Young Adult Medicine
Ann & Robert H. Lurie Children's Hospital of Chicago
Chicago, Illinois

Amy L. Salisbury, PhD, RN, PMH-CNS, BC
Professor and Associate Dean for Research, Scholarship, and Innovation
Clinical Nurse Specialist, Child & Family Psychiatry
Virginia Commonwealth University, School of Nursing
Richmond, Virginia

Benjamin W. Sanders, MD, MSPH, MS
Department of Pediatrics (Division of General Pediatrics)
Oregon Health & Science University
Portland, Oregon

Ishani Sandesara, MD
Division of Hospitalist, Pediatrics Hospice, and Palliative Medicine
Internal Medicine and Pediatrics
University of Michigan School of Medicine
Ann Arbor, Michigan

Kourtney Santucci, MD
Assistant Professor
Department of Pediatrics
University of Colorado School of Medicine
Aurora, Colorado

Ellin K. Scholnick, Ph.D
Professor Emerita
University of Maryland
College Park, Maryland

David J. Schonfeld, MD
Director
National Center for School Crisis and Bereavement
Children's Hospital Los Angeles
Professor of Clinical Pediatrics
Keck School of Medicine
University of Southern California
Los Angeles, California

Alison Schonwald, MD
Department of Pediatrics
Cambridge Health Alliance
Associate Professor
Harvard Medical School
Cofounder
Touchstone Neurodevelopmental Center
Woburn, Massachusetts

Justin Charles Schwartz, MD
Developmental-Behavioral Pediatrician
Associate Professor of Pediatrics
Division of Developmental-Behavioral Pediatrics
Department of Pediatrics
The University of Alabama School of Medicine
Birmingham, Alabama

Brittany L. Schwarz, MD
Johns Hopkins University School of Medicine
Kennedy Krieger Institute
Bloomberg Children's Center
Baltimore, Maryland

Tina Scott-Mordhorst, MD
Clinical Professor
University of Nebraska Medical Center
Omaha, Nebraska

Kylie M.L. Seeley, MD, MPH
Stanford School of Medicine
Palo Alto, California

Emily K. Shabason, MD
Attending Physician
Division of Developmental and Behavioral Pediatrics
Children's Hospital of Philadelphia
Philadelphia, Pennsylvania

Laura A. Shaffer, PhD, ABPP
Department of Pediatrics
University of Virginia School of Medicine
Charlottesville, Virginia

Jeffrey D. Shahidullah, PhD
Assistant Professor of Psychiatry and Behavioral Sciences
Dell Medical School
University of Texas–Austin
Pediatric Psychologist
Developmental and Behavioral Pediatrics
Dell Children's Medical Center
Austin, Texas

Emily Shelkowitz, MD
Fellow in Clinical Genetics & Metabolism
Department of Pediatrics
Section of Clinical Genetics and Metabolism
Children's Hospital Colorado
University of Colorado
Aurora, Colorado

Jaclyn A. Shepard, PsyD
Associate Professor
University of Virginia School of Medicine
Behavioral Medicine Center
Department of Psychiatry & Neurobehavioral Sciences
Charlottesville, Virginia

Kevin M. Simon, MD
Attending Psychiatrist, Department of Psychiatry & Behavioral Science
Adolescent Substance Use & Addiction Program (ASAP)
Developmental Medicine Center, Boston Children's Hospital
Brookline, Massachusetts
Instructor in Psychiatry
Harvard Medical School
Boston, Massachusetts

Kristen Slaymaker, DO
Developmental Pediatrics
Children's Hospital Colorado
University of Colorado School of Medicine
Aurora, Colorado

Peter J. Smith, MD, MA
Associate Professor of Pediatrics
Section of Developmental and Behavioral Pediatrics
University of Chicago
Chicago, Illinois

Barbara Sourkes, PhD
Professor
Department of Pediatrics
Stanford University School of Medicine
John A. Kriewall and Elizabeth A. Haehl Director, Palliative Care Program
Lucile Packard Children's Hospital Stanford
Palo Alto, California

Leslie Speer, PhD, BCBA, NCSP
MetroHealth Medical Center
Center Case Western Reserve University
Cleveland, Ohio

Emily M. Spelbrink, MD, PhD
Stanford University School of Medicine
Palo Alto, California

Adiaha Spinks-Franklin, MD, MPH
Division of Developmental Pediatrics
Department of Pediatrics
Baylor College of Medicine
Houston, Texas

Deborah M. Spitalnik, PhD
The Boggs Center on Developmental Disabilities
Professor of Pediatrics and Family Medicine and Community Health
Rutgers Robert Wood Johnson Medical School
New Brunswick, New Jersey

Margaret Stager, MD
Professor
CWRU School of Medicine
MetroHealth Medical Center
Cleveland, Ohio

Terry Stancin, PhD, ABPP
Chief of Psychology
Director, Child & Adolescent Psychiatry & Psychology
The MetroHealth System
Professor, Departments of Psychiatry
Pediatrics, & Psychological Sciences
Case Western Reserve University
Cleveland, Ohio

Meg Stanger, MS, PT, PCS
Manager of Occupational Therapy and Physical Therapy
UPMC Children's Hospital of Pittsburgh
Pittsburgh, Pennsylvania

Walter H. Stearns, MD
Department of Psychiatry and Behavioral Health
The Ohio State University
Columbus, Ohio

Terri Stillwell, MD, MPH
Division of Pediatric Infectious Diseases
Department of Pediatrics
University of Michigan Medical School
Ann Arbor, Michigan

Stephanie K. Takamatsu, PhD
Department of Psychiatry
University of Colorado School of Medicine
Aurora, Colorado

Nicole Tartaglia, MD
Developmental Pediatrics
Denver Fragile X Clinic
Children's Hospital Colorado
University of Colorado School of Medicine
Aurora, Colorado

Talia Thompson, PhD
Developmental Pediatrics
Children's Hospital Colorado
University of Colorado School of Medicine
Aurora, Colorado

Sarah J. Tlustos, PhD, ABPP-CN
Pediatric Neuropsychologist
Department of Rehabilitation
Children's Hospital Colorado
Assistant Professor
Department of Physical Medicine and Rehabilitation
University of Colorado School of Medicine
Aurora, Colorado

Eric Tridas, MD
Medical Director (retired) of the Tridas Center for Child Development
Tampa, Florida

Paige J. Trojanowski, PhD
George Mason University
Center for Psychological Services
Fairfax, Virginia

Elizabeth Troy, MD
Assistant Professor
University of Colorado
Department of Pediatrics
Section of Neurology
Children's Hospital Colorado
Aurora, Colorado

Megan E. Tudor, PhD
Assistant Clinical Professor of Pediatrics
Licensed Clinical Psychologist
MIND Institute
University of California–Davis
Davis, California

Doris Valenzuela-Araujo, MD
Department of Pediatrics
Oregon Health and Science University
Portland, Oregon

Amanda Van Scoyoc
Community Faculty Member
Yale Child Study Center
New Haven, Connecticut

Douglas L. Vanderbilt, MD
Professor of Clinical Pediatrics (Educational Scholar)
Keck School of Medicine of University of Southern California
Children's Hospital of Los Angeles
Los Angeles, California

Jessica VanOrmer Simpson, PhD
MetroHealth Medical Center
Case Western Reserve University
Cleveland, Ohio

Robert G. Voigt, MD
Department of Pediatrics
Section of Developmental Pediatrics
Baylor College of Medicine
Meyer Center for Developmental Pediatrics & Autism
Texas Children's Hospital
Houston, Texas

Christine Waanders, PhD
Practice-Based Scholar
The Center for Violence Prevention
Children's Hospital of Philadelphia
Philadelphia, Pennsylvania

Kate E. Wallis, MD, MPH
Division of Developmental-Behavioral Pediatrics
Children's Hospital of Philadelphia
Department of Pediatrics
Perelman School of Medicine at the University of Pennsylvania
Philadelphia, Pennsylvania

Laura Weissman, MD
Assistant Professor in Pediatrics
Harvard Medical School
Attending Physician
Division of Developmental Medicine
Boston Children's Hospital
Boston, Massachusetts

Carol Weitzman, MD
Co-Director
Autism Spectrum Center
Boston Children's Hospital
Boston, Massachusetts

Kristen Wigby, MD
Genetics, Rady Children's Hospital
San Diego, California

Breanna M. Winder-Patel, PhD
Assistant Clinical Professor of Pediatrics
Licensed Clinical Psychologist
MIND Institute
University of California–Davis
Davis, California

Larry Wissow, MD
Department of Psychiatry and Behavioral Sciences
University of Washington
Seattle, Washington

Kara K. Wright, MD, MPH
Associate Clinical Professor
Volunteer, Department of Pediatrics
University of California–San Francisco
Pediatrician/Consultant
Tenderloin Community School
Bay Area Women's and Children's Center
San Francisco, California

Michele Yang, MD
Associate Professor, Department of Pediatrics and Neurology
University of Colorado Denver
Children's Hospital Colorado
Aurora, Colorado

Angela Yarnell Bonino, PhD, CCC-A
University of Colorado Boulder
Department of Speech, Language, and Hearing Sciences
Boulder, Colorado

Mary Yarus, M Ed, LDT, CALT
Dyslexia Specialist
Region 4 Education Service Center
Houston, Texas

Ann Ming Yeh, MD
Clinical Associate Professor
Department of Pediatrics
Division of of Gastroenterology, Hepatology, and Nutrition
School of Medicine, Stanford University
Palo Alto, California

Musa Yilanli, MD
Division of Child & Family Psychiatry
Big Lots Behavioral Health Services
Nationwide Children's Hospital
Columbus, Ohio

Samuel H. Zinner, MD
Professor of Pediatrics
University of Washington School of Medicine
Developmental-Behavioral Pediatrician
Seattle Children's Hospital
Seattle, Washington

Marcia Zorrilla, DrPH, MPH
Division of Adolescent Medicine
Department of Pediatrics
Stanford University
Palo Alto, California

Barry Zuckerman, MD
Professor and Chair Emeritus of Pediatrics
Boston University School of Medicine
Boston, Massachusetts

Katharine E. Zuckerman, MD, MPH
Department of Pediatrics (Division of General Pediatrics)
Oregon Health & Science University
Portland, Oregon

Lucas Zullo, PhD
University of California–Los Angeles
Los Angeles, California

PREFACE

Welcome to the fifth edition of *Developmental-Behavioral Pediatrics*. As editors, we have attempted to ensure that the new version maintains the high standards of the previous four editions. We are humbled as we recognize that, for the first time, none of the editors of this textbook served as editors for the first edition of *Developmental-Behavioral Pediatrics*, published in 1983. We recognize and thank all the previous editors and authors whose fine contributions to earlier versions helped to create and define the field of developmental-behavioral pediatrics.

In the almost 40 years since the first edition of this textbook was published, developmental-behavioral pediatrics has evolved with enhanced theories, important scientific discoveries, increasing prevalence of developmental and behavioral conditions, new interventions, and our improved understanding of important influences on outcomes. We sought to reflect these profound changes with a new organization and new chapters in the book. The book begins with a new section on the theoretical foundations of developmental-behavioral pediatrics care and research. The section on life stages has a new chapter on important considerations for the transition to adulthood for all adolescents. The sections on environmental and on biologic influences have been expanded and updated to include more information on parenting, adverse childhood experiences, genetics, and brain injury and to address racism and bias in healthcare settings. The coverage of developmental, behavioral, and emotional conditions and the developmental and behavioral outcomes of physical health conditions has been expanded to include new chapters on suicide and self-harm, stress disorders, movement disorders, brain tumors, and sexuality in children with developmental disabilities. We open each chapter with a pithy vignette, designed to excite the reader's interest and to humanize the conditions and issues we address.

Throughout the book, we have highlighted the interprofessional care required to optimize outcomes for children with developmental and behavioral conditions and their families. An interprofessional focus is reflected in our editor group that now includes Terry Stancin PhD, a leading psychologist in the field of developmental-behavioral pediatrics, complementing the two returning editors, Heidi Feldman MD, PhD and Ellen Elias MD, and the other two new editors, Nathan Blum MD and Manuel Jimenez MD, MS. Where appropriate, the chapters are authored by individuals from more than one professional discipline. With an interprofessional focus, we also greatly expanded the section on assessment and measurement to include chapters on evaluation of children who are minimally verbal, evaluation of emotions and behaviors, neuropsychological assessment, and assessment of adaptive functioning. Another new chapter discusses approaches to integrating data across different assessments and managing uncertainty. Similar expansion has occurred in the management section with new chapters on counseling and readiness to change, a common factors approach to counseling, applied behavior analysis, rehabilitation services, community-based interventions, and endocrine and gynecological care for youth with severe disabilities. As in the previous edition, we end with a section on systems issues, and in the final chapter we, the editors, reflect on implications of the right to belong and the right to be different for interprofessional care for children with developmental and behavioral conditions.

Given the emphasis on interprofessional care throughout the book, we hope that this volume will meet the needs of a varied and interprofessional readership. For the specialist in developmental-behavioral pediatrics providing clinical care or in-training, it should provide a reliable resource for the best information available in this broad and complex field. For clinicians in primary care, psychology, psychiatry, education, nursing, rehabilitation therapies, social work, and other professions, the book offers comprehensive coverage of the wide spectrum of developmental, behavioral, emotional, physical, and psychosocial challenges clinicians assess and manage when they care for children, youth, young adults, and their families. For researchers, the book provides a summary of the current state of knowledge and identifies gaps where our knowledge needs to be expanded and improved.

This book came together with the contributions of many. We thank the outstanding returning and new authors whose contributions allowed us to achieve our ambitious goals for this book. Our publisher has provided tremendous enthusiasm, guidance, and support, critical to completing this project. In addition, we gratefully acknowledge the multitude of ways in which the US Department of Health and Human Services, Health Resources and Services Administration (HRSA), Maternal Child Health Bureau (MCHB) has supported the field of developmental and behavioral pediatrics and interprofessional education. Children and families, faculty, and trainees in multiple disciplines, many authors and readers of the book, and the editors have benefited from HRSA-supported programs, including the Leadership Education in Developmental-Behavioral Pediatrics training program, the Leadership Education in Neurodevelopmental and Related Disabilities (LEND) training program, and a variety of research networks focused on the care of children with autism and on the practice of developmental and behavioral pediatrics. Finally, we thank the children and families we care for, our colleagues, and our own families. All of you inspire us every day.

The previous editions of the book have all ended the Preface with poems or quotes from famous authors. In recognition of the importance of history and tradition, and previous editors of the book, we humbly continue that tradition. We appreciate the sentiments of this poem, though we might have chosen different pronouns for this current era.

CHILDREN LEARN WHAT THEY LIVE

If a child lives with criticism, He learns to condemn.
If a child lives with hostility, He learns to fight.
If a child lives with ridicule, He learns to be shy.
If a child lives with shame, He learns to feel guilty.
If a child lives with tolerance, He learns to be patient.
If a child lives with encouragement, He learns confidence.
If a child lives with praise, He learns to appreciate.
If a child lives with fairness, He learns justice.
If a child lives with security, He learns to have faith.
If a child lives with approval, He learns to like himself.
If a child lives with acceptance and friendship, He learns to find love in the world.

Dorothy Lew Nolte

The Editors

CONTENTS

SECTION 11 Societal and Legal Contexts of Developmental-Behavioral Pediatrics

SECTION 12 Conclusion

Color versions of the figure are available in the online version

1

An Introduction to the Field of Developmental-Behavioral Pediatrics

Douglas L. Vanderbilt and Heidi M. Feldman

For additional material related to the content of this chapter, please see Chapters 2, 3, 113, 117, and 120.

VIGNETTE

A group of medical students from the Pediatric Interest Group approach you seeking career guidance. You probe their interests and goals. They desire that their career be built on a solid molecular and biomedical foundation yet tempered with an understanding of the social context and psychological contributors to health and illness. They want to keep open the possibility of working not only in clinical care, teaching, and research but also in systems-level policy and advocacy. They want to address important clinical and societal needs and prefer to do so in innovative, collaborative partnerships that empower families, primary care colleagues, and interdisciplinary teams. They find thinking both at macro- and microsystems levels to be exciting and understand that important outcomes of medical care include not only disease-free survival but maybe also optimal functional outcomes for individuals and populations. Finally, they want to follow children and families over time with a life-course lens. The students want to know what area of medicine you would recommend for them to consider for a rewarding career.

This chapter provides an orientation to developmental-behavioral pediatrics (DBP), a young and yet maturing subspecialty of pediatrics. In this chapter we explore the origins of DBP; its emergence from historical, medical, and social imperatives; its current challenges; and opportunities for further growth.

RATIONALE FOR THE FIELD OF DBP

The field of DBP emerged from the need to increase the capacity of pediatrics to understand, evaluate, treat, and manage children with developmental disabilities, mental health disorders, and those at risk for these disorders based on the presence of medical conditions or adverse social and psychological environments. These children represent a large swath of the population in the United States and across the globe. In the United States 26% of children are at moderate or high risk for developmental-behavioral (DB) problems. Among the 18% of US children with a special health care need, over half have one or more emotional or behavioral health difficulties. Internationally, almost 53 million children under age 5 years are estimated to have a developmental, behavioral, or emotional disorder (Global Research on Developmental Disabilities Collaborators, 2018). DBP is a distinctive subspecialty developed to help address these needs.

Definition of DBP

The field of DBP was defined in an application to the American Board of Pediatrics (ABP) for subspecialty certification that was approved in 1998. DBP was conceived as a pediatric subspecialty with goals of research, teaching, advocacy, and clinical work in the domains of human development and behavior. All aspects of development—cognitive, social, emotional, and physical development—were acknowledged and seen as linked to contexts of family, school, and larger communities. Although the scope of practice may overlap with child neurology, child psychiatry, and child psychology, DBP was distinct because it retained its foundation in pediatrics, maintaining interest in high-prevalence, lower-severity conditions and typical developmental trajectories as well as in children with low-prevalence, high-severity conditions. Importantly, DBP is an interdisciplinary field. The interdisciplinary perspective can be seen, for example, in the authorship of the chapters in this book; clinical practices that use interdisciplinary teams; and membership of the primary professional organization, the Society for Developmental & Behavioral Pediatrics (SDBP), that includes physicians, psychologists, nurses, and others.

Key Perspectives and Values

DBP conceptualizes development and behavior as arising from biopsychosocial-ecological transactions (see Chapter 2) along a life-course timeframe (see Chapter 3). The life-course frame emphasizes that prevention and early intervention may substantially affect the developmental trajectory. DBP acknowledges that neurobiology shapes developmental outcomes, and the social context and developmental changes shape neurobiology (see Chapter 2).

DBP care is person centered and strengths based; it engages individuals in their own care, to the extent possible, recognizing their unique strengths as well as their needs. DBP clinical practice is family centered, utilizing shared decision making with families in the diagnostic and management phases. The contextual understanding recognizes the important role of culture (see Chapter 20) in the manifestations and understanding of illness and disability and in decisions about the acceptability of approaches to treatment. Cultural humility brings respect to different cultures and acknowledges socially embedded disparities in equity, diversity, and inclusion. DBP care necessitates close collaboration of the health care system with community resources and services. Many DBPs take on advocacy roles through engagement with practice associations, health systems, community-based organizations, or policymakers at local, state, and national levels. What is definitional about DBP is its unique perspective and not a set of organ systems, diagnoses, or practice settings (Schonfeld, 2008).

HISTORICAL GROUNDING FOR DBP PERSPECTIVE

The DBP subspecialty emerged from the confluence of five historical trends: (1) changing concepts about children, (2) the emergence of pediatrics, (3) evolving concepts about disability, (4) evolving concepts about mental health, and (5) the development of public policy and public systems of care.

Changing Concepts of Children in Society

The term *child* comes from the Latin *infans*, which means “the one who does not speak.” Throughout history and across cultures, childhood has been an evolving concept. Childhood was defined as the period from birth to age 7 years in the Roman world and birth to age 18 years in the modern era. Table 1.1 demonstrates that child rearing has shifted perspectives over time with the rationales for the practices in Table 1.2 based on changing constructs about childhood (Haring, Sorin, & Caltabiano, 2019).

Agrarian cultures typically emphasized utilitarian functions for children (i.e., their ability to work). Urbanization led to changes in the state of childhood. As women in cities went to work to support their families, the children required childcare, nutritional infant formulas, and education. Yet, community-wide resources for women and children were limited due to their lack of political power, limitations on property ownership, excessive taxation, political injustice, and corruption.

In the late 17th and early 18th centuries the Enlightenment marked a change in the concept of the child. Philosophers such as John Locke (1632–1704) and Jean-Jacques Rousseau (1712–1778) emphasized the impact of experience on the developing child. This conceptualization accentuated the need to provide children with nurturing environments, education, and growth-enhancing experiences.

In the last century the concept of child agency gradually has taken hold, allowing for legal strategies to promote child welfare. An early instantiation was found in 17th-century France, where children were granted “minor rights” to education, among other areas. In 1908 the New York City Health Department founded the Bureau of Child Hygiene to address child health, including prenatal care, infant mortality, school inspections, and child labor laws. The League of Nations adopted the Declaration of the Rights of the Child in 1924, the first international treaty giving specific rights to children and responsibilities to adults. The United Nations (UN) Fund for Urgency for the Children was created in 1947 to

TABLE 1.1 Evolving Views of Child Rearing

Psychogenic Mode	Time in History	Description
1. Infanticidal	Prehistory to 4th century CE	Children worked to support the family; suffered child abuse, infanticide, and emotional abandonment.
2. Abandoning	4th century to 13th century	Physical and sexual abuse of children continued; children revered people of authority to avoid being abandoned (to monasteries, service to nobility).
3. Ambivalent	13th century to 17th century	Laws were developed to protect children; schools were established. Child still "bad." Shaming and blaming used as discipline. Love-hate relationships between parents and child.
4. Intrusive	18th century	Parents increased love and care to their children; punishment used for bad behavior.
5. Socialization	19th century to mid-20th century	Parents offered increasing respect to their children's wishes, even though beating and shaming discipline methods continued to socialize children.
6. Helping	Mid-20th century to present	Parents began to help their children to achieve their own goals in adult life.
7. Emotionally literate	Early 21st century	Parents raise children aware of their own emotional reactions, responsible for their own life and society.

Adapted from Haring, U., Sorin, R. & Caltabiano, N. J. (2019). Reflecting on childhood and child agency in history. *Palgrave Communications, 5*, 52. https://doi.org/10.1057/s41599-019-0259-0

TABLE 1.2 Typology of Concept of Children

Concept	Description
Innocent child, born pure	Child requires the care and protection of adults and has no agency.
Evil child due to original sin	Child was inherently evil, and severe beatings could put a child on the right path to maturity.
Snowballing child	Child takes power from the adult in an uneven relationship where tired parents give in to the child's demands.
Out-of-control child	Child has lost control, and the adult feels powerless to express agency.
Noble/savior child	Child takes on responsibility to protect others, and adults might depend on child because of illness or substance abuse.
Miniature adult	Child as a small adult with no distinction between childhood and adulthood, so society uses child as laborer, soldier, or other occupation.
Adult-in-training	Child has "human becomings," not as "human beings"; view is favored by developmental psychologists such as Piaget, Erikson, and Freud.
Commodified child	Child has no voice, is open to exploitation by adults.
Child as victim	Child is living in wartimes and crime, is powerless, and often not noticed as adults can only appeal to charities for help.
Agentic child	Child has support of loving adults to help guide and achieve goals; the child's voice is respected and considered, so child acts collaboratively with adults.

Adapted from Haring, U., Sorin, R. & Caltabiano, N. J. (2019). Reflecting on childhood and child agency in history. *Palgrave Communications, 5,* 52. https://doi.org/10.1057/s41599-019-0259-0

promote humanitarianism and development aid and later became UNICEF (UN Children's Fund). In 1959 the General Assembly of the UN adopted the Declaration of the Rights of the Child, which led to the International Charter of the Child Rights. All but one of the 195 UN members signed the document, and 192 ratified it. The United States signed but has not ratified it.

The Emergence of Pediatrics

During ancient history, health care for children had been the province of families and midwives. Physicians avoided the care of children because of prevailing social beliefs, limited medical training about children's health, and the poor prognosis of many childhood diseases. Health care specifically for children emerged in the late 18th and 19th centuries. The first dispensary for children in London, England, was established in 1769. The first children's hospital, L'hôpital des Enfants-Malades, was founded in Paris in 1802. The first children's hospitals in the United States were established in 1855 in Philadelphia and New York City (American Academy of Pediatrics [AAP], 2001). Abraham Jacobi (1830–1919), often considered the father of American pediatrics (Strain, 2004), organized the first children's clinic at the New York Medical College in 1860. He also organized the pediatric subsections for the American Medical Association (AMA) in 1880. He collaborated on public health efforts such as providing safe milk for poor infants in New York (Mahnke, 2000).

Evidence of the crystallization of the field of pediatrics was the launch of *Archives of Pediatrics*, the first US journal to be devoted exclusively to children, in 1884 and the first professional society, the American Pediatric Society, in 1888. Pediatricians recognized that treating childhood diseases required public health as well as clinical interventions. In 1926 the Section on the Diseases of Children of the AMA voted in support of the reauthorization of the Sheppard-Towner Act, a modest federal maternal and child health program, on the same day that the AMA House of Delegates passed a resolution condemning the act. The conflict that followed ultimately led to the creation of the AAP in 1930 and subsequently the ABP. Public health advances promoted by pediatrics, such as sewage treatment, clean water, breastfeeding, and free medical care, all substantially reduced infant mortality and improved the health of children (Mahnke, 2000).

Pediatrics has thrived since the 20th century in medical schools and children's hospitals. With the advent of vaccines and antibiotics, the clinical focus of pediatrics is shifting away from infectious diseases to the management of chronic illnesses, including developmental disabilities, recognition of poverty and environmental causes of disease, and addressing the psychosocial determinants of health (Brosco, 2011).

Evolving Conceptualization of Disability

From antiquity through the Middle Ages in Europe, disabilities were interpreted metaphysically as punishment for sin or the work of evil, as opposed to biomedically (Kanner, 1964). A major shift began when a physician, Jean-Marc-Gaspard Itard (1775–1835), undertook the education of Victor, the Wild Boy of Aveyron, an abandoned and disabled child. He applied Enlightenment principles to educate the child but achieved only incremental success (Kanner, 1964). Itard's student, Eduard Séguin (1812–1880), known as the father of special education, further popularized this concept of a comprehensive individualized educational program for children with disabilities. Maria Montessori (1870–1952), a child psychiatrist and first woman physician in Italy, based her educational philosophy on Séguin's contributions. Center-based habilitation programs emerged, but in the second half of the 19th century they devolved into primarily custodial institutions with poor living conditions—some even practicing sterilization and euthanasia (Kanner, 1964).

After World War II, families championed the cause of disabilities through the establishment of advocacy organizations (Kanner, 1964). Formed in 1950, the National Association of Parents and Friends of Mentally Retarded Children, now known as The Arc, advocated for equal rights, improved education and health care for people with disabilities, taught skills that are important for independence and employment to individuals with disabilities, and encouraged research in the area of disability (Segal, 1974). These efforts dovetailed with a changing legal landscape in public policy and education. A disability-oriented civil rights movement of the 1960s formulated a political agenda, focusing on overcoming the oppression, promoting independence and self-sufficiency, and advocating for social change. The social model of disability conceptualizes the cause of disability not as a health condition but as social, physical, and attitudinal barriers to participation in community life.

Evolving Concepts of Mental Health Disorders

Mental illness was at various times attributed to environmental causes such as loss of status or money, physiologic causes, astrologic alterations, possession by the devil, moral weakness, or divine punishment. Metaphysical treatments sought to correct the individual, such as inducing catharsis, submerging patients in ice baths, inducing vomiting, or bloodletting. Social exclusion and incarceration were other approaches that continue to this day as currently over 35% of prison inmates have a history of a mental health condition.

The Enlightenment dramatically altered the care of individuals with mental health disorders. Philippe Pinel (1745–1826), regarded as the father of modern psychiatry, promoted the method of moral management. The method included intense observation and conversation with individuals affected with mental disorders, supportive care such as hypnosis and relaxation, treatment in home-like settings, and work programs (Weiner, 1992). Attractive asylums were built that promised humane and effective treatments (Weiner, 1992). The institutions became overcrowded and returned to the use of restraints and shock therapies. The institutionalized population remained very high and conditions deplorable until the National Mental Health Foundation exposed the abuses in such institutions as the Byberry Hospital in Philadelphia in the 1940s (Sareyan, 1994). In 1963 President John F. Kennedy proposed the development of comprehensive community mental health centers to reduce the number of individuals in custodial care and support the full spectrum of services from diagnosis through emergency care. Deinstitutionalization gained momentum; however, homelessness and crime are visible indications of the limitations of investment in these community-based programs.

The Development of Psychology

With changing concepts in mental health emerged the field of psychology. Table 1.3 includes several notable psychologists who pioneered psychometrics and developmental assessment. These assessments allowed clinicians to characterize individual differences in development and cognitive skill. Unfortunately, the work on intelligence served as a rationalization of the eugenics movement that claimed the superiority of the white race (Kanner, 1964). While the defeat of the Nazis in World War II discredited the eugenics movement, vestiges of this thinking sadly persist to the present.

Another area of psychology theorized about the origins of emotion. Sigmond Freud (1856–1939), the founder of psychoanalysis, proposed that unconscious conflicts, often thought to be related to psychosexual development, caused emotional disorders (see Chapter 3). Despite its empiric and conceptual limitations, this theory continues to hold a potent basis within psychology. Erik Erikson (1902–1994) later reconceptualized Freudian stages in psychosocial rather than psychosexual terms, which define the major tasks that children face at various points in development. This theory has heuristic value in current conceptualizations (see Chapter 3).

TABLE 1.3 Pioneers in the Psychological Assessment

Individual	Dates	Contributions
Charles Darwin	1809–1882	• Introduced the study of human behavioral development in "A Biographical Sketch of an Infant," a treatise on the development of movement, vision, emotions (anger, fear, and pleasure), reasoning, moral sense, and communication in his infant son.
Francis Galton	1822–1911	• Described the variations of development in human intelligence.
Alfred Binet Theodore Simon	1857–1911 1873–1961	• Designed a carefully constructed Binet-Simon test in 1905 for differentiating children with typical development vs. those needing special education.
Lewis Terman	1877–1956	• Standardized the Binet-Simon on a large sample of US children to create the Stanford-Binet test of intelligence.
Arnold Gesell	1880–1961	• Described the typical developmental milestones in "An Atlas of Infant Behavior" and advocated for the field of developmental pediatrics.

The roots of developmental psychology can also be traced to Charles Darwin (see Table 1.3). James Mark Baldwin (1861–1934) contributed experimental work on infant development in the area of sensation and perception. He strongly influenced Jean Piaget (1896–1980), whose intense observation of his three children formed the foundation of an integrated theory of cognitive development that proposed that development occurred in stages, in which knowledge was acquired through assimilation of environmental experiences and accommodations to those experiences (see Chapter 3).

In the realm of behavior, the 19th-century physiologist, psychologist, and physician, Ivan Pavlov (1849–1936), described the "conditioned reflex" as the pairing of a neutral stimulus, such as a bell, with a motivating stimulus, such as food, to cause a physiologic reaction, such as salivation (see Chapter 4). These concepts are still used to explain the causes of phobias and design treatments. James B. Watson (1878–1958) and B.F. Skinner (1904–1990) described the ability of a reinforcing stimulus to change the probability of behaviors (operant conditioning). As described in Chapters 4, 93, and 94, operant conditioning plays a central role in behavior management of children developing typically and children with disabilities.

The Development of Psychiatry

Early psychiatrists, such as Emil Kraepelin (1856–1926), offered biologic explanations and treatments for mental disorders. He brought together the tradition of the phrenologists, such as Johann Spurzheim (1776–1832), with their organic neurologic basis for behavior, and the public health advocates, such as Anthony Ashley Cooper (1801–1885), who used institutions for the care of the mentally ill. Child psychiatry has turned those concepts to child mental illness with founders such as Moritz Tramer (1882–1963) and later Leo Kanner (1894–1981). The field has been influential in the deinstitutionalization movement and in the pivot to considering both context and biology in treatment.

The discovery of psychoactive medications revolutionized the practice of psychiatry. In 1952 Henri Laborit (1914–1995) discovered that chlorpromazine could calm patients with mental and emotional disorders without completely sedating them. Publication of the *Diagnostic and Statistical Manual of Mental Disorders* (DSM) in 1952 clarified diagnostic criteria for mental and emotional disorders. The first edition had only one pediatric diagnosis, adjustment reaction of childhood/adolescence. Changes up to the fifth edition in 2013 have resulted in an increased number of pediatric diagnoses and increased prevalence of childhood diagnoses. While improving the quality of research, the symptom-based, atheoretic, and nondevelopmental approach of the DSM limits understanding of the complex interactions of biologic predispositions and environmental forces and the changing nature of disorders with development (Jensen & Mrazek, 2006).

Development of Public Policy and Public Systems

Advances in public policy and systems have greatly influenced DBP (see Section 10).

Education

Until the 19th century, formal education was available only to the wealthy. The US public school movement began in the mid-19th century and conceptualized education as a means to integrate poor, immigrant children and former slaves into the American culture by emphasizing moral education and industry (Kanner, 1964). Influential leaders, such as Horace Mann (1796–1859), promoted public education, which encouraged many states to pass mandatory school attendance laws.

A critical legislative landmark was the Education for All Handicapped Children Act (P.L. 94–142) of 1975, which mandated a free and appropriate public education (FAPE) for all children as befitting their needs. The law also required that the education take place in the least restrictive environment, a provision specifically designed to combat institutionalization (see Chapter 114). The law has been reauthorized on several occasions and is now known as the Individuals with Disabilities Education Act (IDEA). The 1986 revision provided grants to states to develop early intervention programs for children birth to 3 years of age.

Health

Due to poor health outcomes of women and children, Theodore Roosevelt convened a White House conference in 1909 that resulted in the establishment of the US Children's Bureau in 1912. The bureau evolved into the Maternal and Child Health Bureau (MCHB), included in the Social Security Act of 1935. One of its first programs was Crippled Children Services, recognition of the high prevalence and unfavorable outcomes of paralytic polio (see Chapters 115 and 116). Eventually, MCHB migrated to Health Resources and Services Administration, reflecting the shift from conceptualizing child health strictly as social service issues to public health and medical issues (Brosco, 2012). MCHB is a critical funder of DBP training and research programs.

Poverty and Social Risk

The post–World War II economic expansion brought an emphasis on addressing children living in poverty and experiencing other social adversities. In the 1960s Julius Richmond (1916–2008) (Fig. 1.1), a pediatrician, became the head of the Office of Employment Opportunities and launched Project Head Start, which offered free, community-based preschool programs for children from low-income families. The objectives of Head Start were to meet the emotional, developmental, health, social, and nutritional needs of the children and to stimulate employment and empowerment of the communities in which these children lived. Positive and long-lasting impacts of high-quality early education have been documented in school-aged children (Lee, Brooks-Gunn, Schnur, & Liaw, 1990) to young adults (Campbell, Ramey, Pungello, Joseph Sparling, & Miller-Johnson, 2002). Dr. Richmond was later US Surgeon General (see Fig. 1.1), during which time he established benchmarks for public health, including for pregnancy outcomes, child growth, and child development.

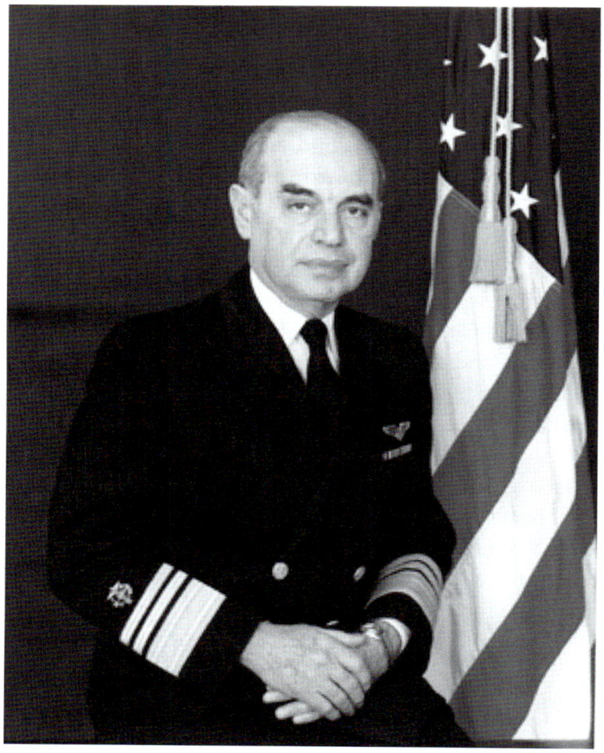

Fig. 1.1 Julius Richmond, MD stimulated the evolution of the field of DBP and went on to serve as Surgeon General of the United States. (From profiles.nlm.nih.gov/NN/B/D/B/K/_/nnbdbk_.jpg)

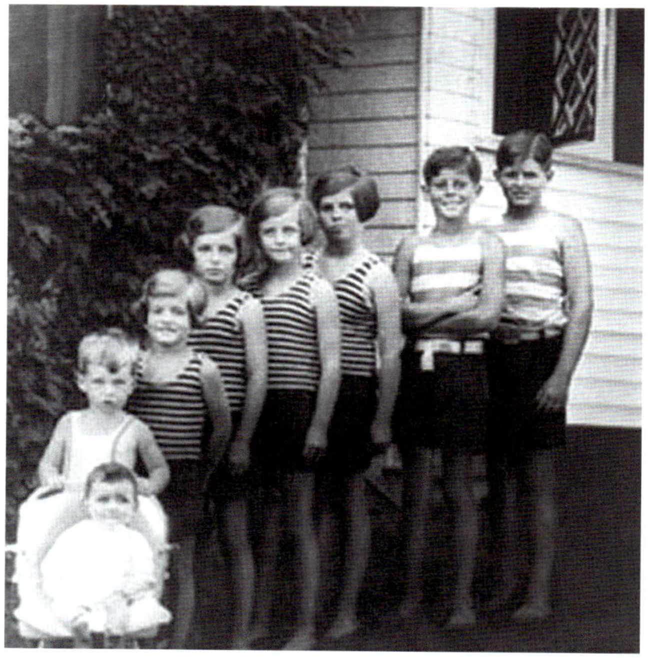

Fig. 1.2 John F. Kennedy and his siblings as children, including his older sister, with developmental and mental health conditions. It was his sister's life experiences that informed his policies regarding facilities and training for professionals to work with individuals with developmental disabilities and mental health disorders. (From www.john-f-kennedy.net/jfksiblings.jpg)

Other important programs addressing poverty-associated risks to child development include childcare supports and home visiting. In 1990 and reauthorized in 2014, the Childcare and Development Block Grant (CCDBG) from the Administration for Children and Families provides federal support through the states to low-income families to support access to high-quality childcare for over 1 million children. The Maternal, Infant, and Early Childhood Home Visiting Program was established in 2010 to provide evidence-based parenting support to over 150,000 at-risk families as of 2019.

Disability

In 1958 voluntary building standards were developed, including reserved parking spaces proximal to buildings and accessible elevators and toilet stalls, which were formalized into the Architectural Barriers Act of 1968. The Rehabilitation Act of 1973 was designed to provide job opportunities and training to adults with disabilities. Section 504 prohibited discrimination based on a disability in service availability, accessibility, or delivery in organizations that receive federal funding. This law prohibits schools from denying public education based on a student's disability and requires accommodations in general education.

The Americans with Disabilities Act of 1990 (ADA) expanded Section 504 to facilitate access to the workforce, education systems, and public domain for individuals with disabilities. In 1999 the US Supreme Court in the landmark *Olmstead* case held that unjustified segregation of persons with disabilities constitutes discrimination violating the ADA. The ruling required public entities to provide community-based services to persons with disabilities if those services are appropriate and could be accommodated in the community.

Professional Training and Research

The DBP field owes much of the current infrastructure for training and research to President John F. Kennedy (Wolraich & Bennett, 2003). Kennedy's oldest sister, Rosemary (Fig. 1.2), had a cognitive impairment and behavioral disorder, worsened by a therapeutic lobotomy, which was chronicled in the *Saturday Evening Post* in 1962 by a sister, Eunice Kennedy Shriver (Shriver, 1962). In 1963 President Kennedy convened the President's Panel on Mental Retardation, highlighting the lack of programs training professionals to work with children and adults with what we then called mental retardation. The panel proposed the development of university-affiliated faculties (UAFs) designed to support training research and clinical services to benefit individuals with disability. Initial federal funding supported 18 UAFs and 12 research centers associated with major universities. After their construction, the UAFs continued as university-affiliated programs (UAPs). A UAP's mission included moving research and technology forward, improving government policies, measuring outcomes, developing and evaluating social and community programs for individuals with disability, training clinicians and researchers involved in disability care and science, and communicating with the community to determine needs.

The programs continue to provide a platform for interdisciplinary collaboration for training and research.

The current UAPs funded through the Administration for Community Living are now known as University Centers for Excellence for Developmental Disabilities (UCEDD). Others funded by the MCHB and the Autism CARES Act are now known as Leadership Education in Neurodevelopmental and Related Disabilities (LEND) programs. Together these programs serve to train professionals to work with individuals with disabilities and promote collaboration with community-based systems, individuals with disabilities, and their family members to ensure that services are responsive to the needs of individuals with disabilities. Additionally, Intellectual and Developmental Disabilities Research Centers (IDDRC) are funded by the National Institute of Child Health and Human Development and are charged with using basic, clinical, and translational research to understand the causes and provide treatments for disabilities. All of these programs are members of the Association of University Centers on Disability, an advocacy network for disabilities and the programs themselves.

EMERGENCE OF THE DBP FIELD

Rise of DBP

Increasing Prevalence

The prevalence of disabilities and mental health conditions rose rapidly in the second half of the 20th century. Advances in medical science and technology simultaneously reduced the impact of infectious diseases and nutritional deficiencies, increased the survival of once fatal developmental conditions, and led to a higher prevalence of disability. For example, because of advances in neonatal intensive care unit (NICU) technology from 1960 to 2000, the limits of viability dropped from 28 weeks to 24 weeks and survival of 1-kg birthweight infants rose from 5% to 95% (Philip, 2005). However, survivors remain at high risk for multiple developmental and behavioral disorders. Similarly, advances in cardiac surgery have increased life expectancy for individuals with Down syndrome from 10 years in 1960 to 47 years in 2007 (Presson et al., 2013).

Increased Awareness

The second half of the 20th century witnessed a substantial increase in the number of families bringing behavioral and academic concerns to pediatricians (Haggerty & Friedman, 2003). Factors included increased parental awareness in the baby boomer generation, changes in family structure, and increasing expectations for children (Haggerty & Friedman, 2003). Higher education became critical to occupational attainment and financial success in life. In the 1900s rates of high school graduation were near 25%, but in 2016 they were greater than 90%.

Evolving Pediatric Practice

In 1972 the AAP issued a policy statement emphasizing the pediatrician's role in promoting optimal growth and development through family support and developmental and behavioral surveillance and screening (AAP, 1972). Practicing pediatricians reported that they did not have the necessary skills to fulfill this recommendation (Dworkin, Leviton, & Levine, 1979; Shonkoff, Dworkin, Leviton, & Levine, 1979). In 1978 and again in 2000 the AAP Task Force on Pediatric Education raised concerns that medical education in the United States was not providing sufficient teaching and training around biopsychosocial aspects of child health and child development to support future roles for pediatricians in managing emotional disorders, learning problems, and chronic conditions (Future of Pediatric Education II, 2000; Haggerty & Friedman, 2003). Recommendations included an improved pediatrics curriculum to raise the capacity for developmental and behavioral assessment.

Establishment of Training Programs

The AAP established the Section on Mental Health in 1949, which became the Section for Child Developmental in 1960 (Haggerty & Friedman, 2003). The only universities offering fellowship training in the 1950s were the Yale Child Study Center, the University of Syracuse, Johns Hopkins University, and Children's Hospital of Philadelphia. Several of the major university centers subsequently began fellowship training in the next decade (Table 1.4). Beginning in 1959, the William T. Grant Foundation provided grant support for behavioral pediatrics training programs in Baltimore and Philadelphia and expanded in the 1970s to 11 programs across the country (Carey, 2003). The MCHB provided financial support for DBP training through the UAPs and later directly through DBP training grants. In 1988 the AAP Section on Child Development became the Section on Developmental and Behavioral Pediatrics.

An early contentious issue was whether training in behavioral pediatrics should most appropriately fall under child psychiatrists or pediatricians (Haggerty & Friedman, 2003). The emerging consensus was that pediatrics, rather than child psychiatry, was more suitable for this training for many reasons: its emphasis on the full range of issues from normal function to severe disorder, the ability to understand and intervene in the complex interplay of psychosocial factors and physical health, and the potential for pediatrics to coordinate the care of psychosocial issues and behavioral health with routine health supervision and treatment of physical disorders (Haggerty & Friedman, 2003). In 1997 the Residency Review Committee of the Accreditation Council of Graduate Medical Education (ACGME) required general pediatric residencies to have 1-month dedicated rotation and a longitudinal component, the equivalent of a second month, spread throughout residency.

A second contentious issue was the balance between a focus on development and in particular developmental disabilities versus behavior. One subgroup, centered at the John F. Kennedy Institute, now called Kennedy-Krieger Institute, emphasized developmental disabilities. This group founded the SDBP in 1978, focusing on the issues of children with developmental disorders. The society created a Section on Children with Disabilities within the AAP in 1990.

TABLE 1.4 Early Centers for DBP in 1960–1970

University Center	Contributions and Features
University of California–San Francisco	• Pediatric residents trained in mental health issues. • Early fellowship training program that emphasized the importance of family in child development.
Harvard University	• Julius Richmond, who was an architect of Head Start and who became US Surgeon General, encouraged pediatricians to establish expertise in development and behavior. • Pioneers included Melvin D. Levine and Allen Crocker, editors of previous editions of this textbook.
Rochester University	• Robert Haggerty and Stanford Friedman began training fellows in behavioral pediatrics and adolescent medicine.
Yale University	• Arnold Gesell founded Yale Child Study Center. • Milton Senn and Albert Solnit brought psychoanalytic focus.
Children's Hospital of Philadelphia	• Henry Cecil began program in psychological pediatrics, funded by William T. Grant Foundation. William B. Carey, editor of previous editions of this textbook, was first fellow.
Johns Hopkins University	• Leo Kanner and Leon Eisenberg began fellowship training through Department of Psychiatry. • Kennedy Center focused on children with disabilities. Arnold Capute was the first fellow.

Establishment of a Journal and DBP Society

The *Journal of Developmental and Behavioral Pediatrics* (JDBP) was established in 1980 and has provided a prominent forum to present research and commentary on topics related to the field. The SDBP was first established in 1982 as the Society of Behavioral Pediatrics (SBP) but was restricted in name by the other society. In 1994 it changed its name to the present form (Society for Developmental and Behavioral Pediatrics [SDBP]) in recognition of the substantial overlap of developmental and behavioral issues in childhood and the scope of practice of its members. Shortly after its formation, the new organization applied for and was granted editorial sponsorship of *JDBP*. The hyphenated term *developmental-behavioral pediatrics* was chosen for use in the title to represent the first comprehensive textbook in the field, published in 1983, to recognize the integral and interacting nature of those two parts (Hansen, 2010; Levine, Carey, Crocker, & Gross, 1983).

Path to Board Certification

Within pediatrics, board certification for DBP was a priority to provide recognition of its distinctive scope of practice and to assure the public about the quality of legitimate practitioners (Haggerty & Friedman, 2003; Perrin, 2000). The two professional societies, with overlapping interests reflective of the tension between a focus on developmental disabilities versus DBP, chose to follow disparate paths for certification through the American Board of Medical Specialties (ABMS).

The SDBP made the first application for subspecialty board certification. Separately, the Society for Behavioral Pediatrics Executive Council voted to pursue board certification in 1991. Efforts to combine these two applications into a single application, given the overlapping scope of practice of the two groups failed. The ABP was initially hesitant to support a subspecialty in DBP because of concerns that the new specialty would overlap with the practice of general pediatrics and thereby reduce the responsibilities of general pediatricians. However, the ABP heard strong support from the AAP Section on DBP and from numerous academic and community pediatricians. Many general pediatricians supported the training of subspecialists who would teach, train, study, and practice child development and behavior. In 1994 the ABP declared that they would support the creation of the DBP subspecialty. However, the concept encountered resistance from the American Board of Psychiatry and Neurology (ABPN) because of concerns that the role of the developmental-behavioral pediatrician was not sufficiently distinct from that of the child psychiatrist. The ABP stipulated that a subspecialty must improve upon the care of children, supplement the role of the general pediatrician, and teach the subspecialty field to trainees and other professionals before it could be considered for subspecialty status (Stockman, 2000). The SDBP addressed the ABPN concerns in a subsequent application. Training in child neurology and child psychiatry was integrated into the training requirements at the time that DBP was recognized as a distinct subspecialty. Participation of psychologists in training was also required to demonstrate the commitment to an interdisciplinary field. In 1999 DBP was approved as a subspecialty by the ABMS. Board certification in DBP was first granted in 2002.

The SDBP subspecialty ultimately sought primary certification from the ABPN, calling its field "neurodevelopmental disabilities (NDD)." The ABP supported the application and cosponsored subspecialty certification during the initial years. NDD was also recognized as a subspecialty by ABMS in 1999. Training in child neurology is required for preparation for board certification in NDD. Board certification for NDD was first granted in 2001.

As of 2019, 904 individuals had been certified in DBP in the United States. In 2020 117 fellows were in training within 43 programs. As of 2019, 55 individuals had been board certified by the ABPN in NDD. In 2020 26 fellows were in training in 8 NDD training programs. By way of contrast, in 2020 941 trainees in child psychiatry were enrolled in 141 programs.

FUTURE OPPORTUNITIES AND CHALLENGES

As DBP moves forward, the field is confronting several challenges. First is sustainability. DBP clinical work requires extensive data gathering and integration, resulting in high levels of uncompensated time and service (Bridgemohan et al., 2018). Results include long wait times for new appointments and high levels of clinician burnout. Revenue models for DBP that share population risk, reimburse time, partner with cross-sector service systems (e.g., schools or disability system), or capture value through interdisciplinary teams all hold potential for improving reimbursements.

Attracting new professionals is critical to strengthening the field. Filling available pediatric training spots has been challenging (Macy, 2021). Many efforts are underway to attract trainees to the field by increasing awareness of the field among undergraduate and medical students, supporting interested trainees to attend professional meetings, and assigning mentors as soon as a trainee declares an interest. If the workforce remains limited, then reimagining how the limited supply is utilized may be required. Possibilities include focusing subspecialty practice on children with high complexity, reducing follow-up to initial consultations, collaborating with general pediatricians to identify and manage children with low severity conditions, and teaming with interdisciplinary partners to reapportion aspects of diagnosis and management (Stein, 2015; Weyand, 2020).

The field is challenged to produce distinctive scholarship. Currently only a small number of DBP faculty seek research career development and study grants from intramural, foundation, SDBP, or National Institutes of Health sources. In 2011 the MCHB funded the multisite DBP Research Network to further collaborative field research. Senior faculty support fellows and junior faculty in settings such as the SDBP Research Scholars Symposium started in 2014. In 2020 the complex attention-deficit/hyperactivity disorder guidelines were the first evidence-based practice effort originating from within the DBP field (Barbaresi et al., 2020). Future research must refine diagnosis and treatment and define the value of the DBP perspective in clinical and academic work (Sandler, 2019).

Finally, DBP must broaden the diversity of providers to improve health equity nationally and internationally. MCHB values diversity in trainee recruitment and training. The International Special Interest Group of SDBP, started in 2011, promotes optimal child development and care for children with disabilities both internationally and among international immigrants, refugees, and adoptees. SDBP and MCHB have supported efforts to develop collaborative educational efforts across low, middle, and high resourced countries, called international Collaborative Office Rounds (iCOR) (Kiing et al., 2021). Many cross-cultural academic collaborations have been fostered through engagement in the International Developmental Pediatrics Association, which had its first meeting in Turkey in 2015. To foster diversity in the United States, the SDBP has developed the Diversity Equity and Inclusion Committee in 2020 to prioritize antiracism and social justice for the field. These efforts integrate the field's equity advocacy orientation into actual diverse DBP membership with skill transformation to create a more just future.

CONCLUSION

DBP is a dynamic and multifaceted pediatric subspecialty that would be an ideal career choice for the medical students described in the opening vignette. DBP has become a unique and impactful field within pediatrics that makes a difference for children, families, and society. A rich experience awaits you, the reader, as you progress through this text, whether you are interested in clinical care, teaching, scholarship, advocacy, or program administration. We invite you to explore further what this field can contribute to your own career path in the following chapters.

REFERENCES

American Academy of Pediatrics (1972). *Bulletin of pediatric practice*. American Academy of Pediatrics.

American Academy of Pediatrics Historical Archives Advisory Committee. (2001). Committee report: American pediatrics: Milestones at the millennium. *Pediatrics, 107*(6), 1482–1491.

Barbaresi, W., Campbell, L., Diekroger, E. Froehlich, T. E., Liu, Y. H., O'Malley, E., Pelham, W. E. Jr., Power, T. J., Zinner, S. H., & Chan, E. (2020). Society for Developmental and Behavioral Pediatrics clinical practice guideline for the assessment and treatment of children and adolescents with complex attention-deficit/hyperactivity disorder. *Journal of Developmental and Behavioral Pediatrics, 41*(Suppl 2S), S35–S57. https://doi.org/10.1097/DBP.0000000000000770. PMID: 31996577.

Bridgemohan, C., Bauer, N. S., Nielsen, B. A., et al. (2018). A workforce study on developmental-behavioral pediatrics. *Pediatrics, 141*(3), e20172164.

Brosco, J. P. (2011). Classics in pediatrics: A 100-year history of pediatrics in the United States. *Archives of Pediatrics and Adolescent Medicine, 165*(12), 1064–1065. https://doi.org/10.1001/archpediatrics.2011.1070. PMID: 22147773.

Brosco, J. P. (2012). Navigating the future through the past: The enduring historical legacy of federal children's health programs in the United States. *American Journal of Public Health, 102*(10), 1848–1857.

Campbell, F. A., Ramey, C. T., Pungello, E., Joseph Sparling, J., & Miller-Johnson, S. (2002). Early childhood education: Young adult outcomes from the abecedarian project. *Applied Developmental Science, 6*(1), 42–57.

Carey, W. B. (2003). History of developmental-behavioral pediatrics. *Journal of Developmental and Behavioral Pediatrics, 24*(3), 215.

Dworkin, P. H. S., Leviton, A., & Levine, M. D. (1979). Training in developmental pediatrics. How practitioners perceive the gap. *American Journal of Diseases of Children, 133*, 709–712.

Future of Pediatric Education II. (2000). Organizing pediatric education to meet the needs of infants, children, adolescents, and young adults in the 21st century. *Pediatrics, 105*(1), S163–S212.

Global Research on Developmental Disabilities Collaborators (2018). Developmental disabilities among children younger than 5 years in 195 countries and territories, 1990–2016: A systematic analysis for the Global Burden of Disease Study 2016. *The*

Lancet. Global Health, 6(10), e1100–e1121. doi: 10.1016/S2214-109X(18)30309-7. Epub 2018 Aug 29. Erratum in: *The Lancet. Global Health*, 2018 6(12), e1287. PMID: 30172774; PMCID: PMC6139259.

Haggerty, R. J., & Friedman, S. B. (2003). History of developmental-behavioral pediatrics. *Journal of Developmental and Behavioral Pediatrics, 24*(1), S1–S18.

Hansen, R. L. (2010). Magical history tour of the Society for Developmental and Behavioral Pediatrics: Reflections on deletions, slashes, hyphens, and developmental context. *Journal of Developmental and Behavioral Pediatrics, 31*(5), 441–448. https://doi.org/10.1097/DBP.0b013e3181e04722. PMID: 20535082.

Haring, U., Sorin, R., & Caltabiano, N. J. (2019). Reflecting on childhood and child agency in history. *Palgrave Communications, 5*, 52. https://doi.org/10.1057/s41599-019-0259-0.

Jensen, P. S., & Mrazek, D. A. (2006). Introduction. In P. S. Pensen, P. Knapp, & D. A. Mrazek (Eds.), *Toward a new diagnostic system for child psychopathology: Moving beyond the DSM* (pp. 1–10). Guilford Publications.

Kanner, L. (1964). *A history of the care and study of the mentally retarded*. C.C. Thomas.

Kiing, J. S. H., Feldman, H. M., Ladish, C., Srinivasan, R., Donnelly, C. L., Chong, S. C., & Weitzman, C. C. (2021). International Interprofessional Collaborative Office Rounds: Addressing childen's developmental, behavioral, and emotional health using distance technology. *Frontiers in Child Health*. In press.

Lee, V. E., Brooks-Gunn, J., Schnur, E., & Liaw, F. -R. (1990). Are head start effects sustained? A longitudinal follow-up comparison of disadvantaged children attending head start, no preschool, and other preschool programs. *Child Development, 81*(2, Special Issue on Minority Children), 495–507.

Levine, M. D., Carey, W. B., Crocker, A. C., & Gross, R. T. (Eds.), (1983). *Developmental-behavioral pediatrics*. W.B. Saunders Co. ISBN 10:0721657443/ISBN 13:9780721657448.

Macy, M. L., Leslie, L. K., Turner, A., & Gary, L. F. (2021). Growth and changes in the pediatric medical subspecialty workforce pipeline. *Pediatric Research*, 89, 1297–1303. https://doi.org/10.1038/s41390-020-01311-7.

Mahnke, C. B. (2000). The growth and development of a specialty: The history of pediatrics. *Clinical Pediatrics, 39*(12), 705–714.

Perrin, E. C., Bennett, F. C., & Wolraich, M. L. (2000). Subspecialty certification in developmental-behavioral pediatrics: Past and present challenges. *Journal of Developmental & Behavioral Pediatrics, 21*(2), 130–132.

Philip, A. (2005). The evolution of neonatology. *Pediatric Research, 58*, 799–815. https://doi.org/10.1203/01.PDR.0000151693.46655.66.

Presson, A. P., Partyka, G., Jensen, K. M., Devine, O. J., Rasmussen, S. A., McCabe, L. L., & McCabe, E. R. (2013). Current estimate of Down syndrome population prevalence in the United States. *Journal of Pediatrics, 163*(4), 1163–1168. https://doi.org/10.1016/j.jpeds.2013.06.013. Epub 2013 Jul 23. PMID: 23885965; PMCID: PMC4445685.

Sandler, A. D. (2019). Value-driven care in developmental-behavioral pediatrics, part 2: Measuring quality and meeting the challenge. *Journal of Developmental and Behavioral Pediatrics, 40*(6), 479–488. https://doi.org/10.1097/DBP.0000000000000686. PMID: 31107770.

Sareyan, A. (1994). *The turning point: How persons of conscience brought major change in the care of America's mentally ill*. Herald Press.

Schonfeld, D. J. (2008). Back to the future: A constructivist perspective of developmental-behavioral pediatrics. *Journal of Developmental and Behavioral Pediatrics, 29*(1), 69–71. https://doi.org/10.1097/DBP.0b013e31816b21a3. PMID: 18301322.

Segal, R. (1974). The national association for retarded citizens. 2007. http://www.thearc.org/history/segal.htm

Shonkoff, J. P., Dworkin, P. H., Leviton, A., & Levine, M. D. (1979). Primary care approaches to developmental disabilities. *Pediatrics, 64*, 506–514.

Shriver, E. K. (1962). Hope for retarded children. *Saturday Evening Post, 234*, 71.

Stein, R. E. (2015). Are we on the right track? Examining the role of developmental behavioral pediatrics. *Pediatrics, 135*(4), 589–591. https://doi.org/10.1542/peds.2014-3274. Epub 2015 Mar 16. PMID: 25780072.

Stockman, J. A. 3rd. (2000). Developmental-behavioral pediatrics: The American Board of Pediatrics' perspective. *Journal of Developmental and Behavioral Pediatrics, 21*(2), 133–135. doi: 10.1097/00004703-200004000-00008. PMID: 10791482.

Strain, J. E. (2004). Celebrating 75 years founding members laid strong foundation for academy. *AAP News*, 180.

Weiner, D. B. (1992). Philippe Pinel's "memoir on madness" of December 11, 1794: A fundamental text of modern psychiatry. *American Journal of Psychiatry, 149*(6), 725–732.

Weyand, A. C., & Freed, G. L. (2020). Pediatric subspecialty workforce: Undersupply or over-demand? *Pediatric Research, 88*(3), 369–371. https://doi.org/10.1038/s41390-020-0766-0. Epub 2020 Jan 20. PMID: 31958801.

Wolraich, M. L., & Bennett, F. C. (2003). History of developmental-behavioral pediatrics [comment]. *Journal of Developmental and Behavioral Pediatrics, 24*(3), 215–216. author reply 216.

WEBSITE REFERENCES

https://www.aucd.org/template/page.cfm?id=156

https://thearc.org/about-us/history/

https://www.humanium.org/en/childrens-rights-history/

http://www.eunicekennedyshriver.org/articles/article/148

www.childhealthdata.org: Child and Adolescent Health Measurement Initiative. 2013. Risk of Developmental or Behavioral Problems State Ranking Map.

Kidsdata.org 1: Population Reference Bureau, analysis of data from the National Survey of Children's Health and the American Community Survey (Jan. 2021).

Kidsdata.org 2: Data Resource Center for Child and Adolescent Health, National Survey of Children with Special Health Care Needs (Dec. 2012)

2

The Biopsychosocial Model: Understanding Multiple, Interactive Influences on Child Development and Behavior

Megan M. Julian and Julie C. Lumeng

For additional material related to the content of this chapter, please see Chapters 3, 5, 15, and 24.

VIGNETTE

Justin, a 6-year-old boy, and his mother, Cynthia, come into the office for a new-patient appointment. Upon reviewing his chart, you see that Justin was born at 34 weeks of gestation and had exposure to nicotine in utero. As soon as you enter the room, tension is clear; Justin appears withdrawn and ashamed, and Cynthia appears overwhelmed and frustrated. You ask, "What brings you to the clinic today?" Cynthia says harshly, "Justin is out of control. If he doesn't get his way, he hits and yells. I don't know what to do with him. His school calls me a few times a week to pick him up because of his behavior. I can't keep doing this—I'm going to lose my job if I keep having to call off because of him." Justin sits quietly, looking down to the floor as you talk. You learn that Justin has been struggling for about 3 years. Cynthia's social support is limited—she is a single mother, following a contentious separation from Justin's father 2 years ago. Justin's father has not been in regular contact. Cynthia becomes more emotional as you ask about the circumstances of their separation. She shares that her relationship with Justin's father became abusive. Justin had witnessed many physical and verbal altercations between them.

OVERVIEW

Children's behavior and development is impacted by a plethora of biologic, psychological, and social factors. As our understanding of the brain and the biology of behavior advances, so too does the window through which we understand clinical scenarios such as that of Cynthia and Justin in the opening vignette. The early years—from pregnancy through early childhood—are characterized by rapid development, with many neural structures being built and organized during this time. In these years, experience is most able to "get under the skin" to shape a child's later development. Processes such as neural pruning and DNA methylation (see Chapter 24) allow experience to alter a child's developing brain, such that brain architecture itself is built through the dynamic interaction of biology and environment. In this chapter we review how nature and nurture interact in meaningful ways for a range of important outcomes and the implications for clinical care.

MAJOR THEORIES

Biology influences behavior and environment, and behavior and environment influence biology throughout development. Children are directly and indirectly influenced by both their proximal context (e.g., relationships with their caregivers) and broader societal factors (e.g., neighborhood violence, community-wide belief systems). Children's development is the product of the accumulation of everyday interactions and experiences as well as the broader community and cultural context in which they are raised. While major events (e.g., changes in family structure) and circumstances (e.g., family resources) are important to children's development, so too are the minute interactions that make up day-to-day life. The multilevel and transactional influences on children's development have been described in two key theoretical models.

Bronfenbrenner's Ecological Systems Theory

Urie Bronfenbrenner's ecological systems theory (Bronfenbrenner, 1979) proposes there are multiple levels of influence on a child's development, spanning from relationships with caregivers to systems such as schools and workplaces, to events in the broader society (Fig. 2.1). The microsystem describes the direct relationships and interactions children have, such as with caregivers, siblings, and peers. These individuals directly influence the child by scaffolding development, providing opportunities to play and learn, and providing emotional support to children. The microsystem also contains structures with which the child interacts, such as school, neighborhood, childcare settings, and family. Children both influence and are influenced by these relationships and structures (e.g., a child's temperament may contribute to setting the tone of a classroom). The mesosystem describes interaction among the structures that are in the microsystem (e.g., bidirectional influences between neighborhoods and schools). The exosystem consists of larger social systems that impact structures in the microsystem (e.g., community-based family resources or parental work schedules). Children do not directly interact with the exosystem, but they experience the impact of changes in these social systems. The macrosystem is the outermost layer of a child's environment and is defined by cultural values, customs, and laws that influence the ways that the inner layers function. The chronosystem captures the influence of time on children's development, reflecting both developmental processes that take place over time and the

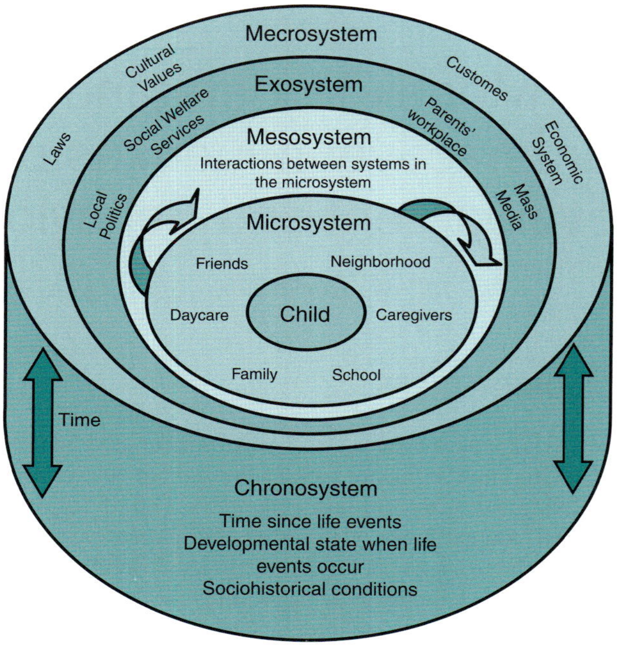

Fig. 2.1 Bronfenbrenner's ecological systems theory describes the multiple interacting levels of analyses that impact the child at any given time and over the course of development.

changing influence of events (e.g., a traumatic event) based on their duration and the developmental stage in which they occur.

Sameroff's Transactional Model

Arnold Sameroff's transactional model builds on Bronfenbrenner's ideas about the bidirectionality of effects on children's development. It discusses the processes that take place between parents and children in everyday interactions and over time (Sameroff, 2009). This model grew out of observations that many risks, such as premature birth or birth complications, were associated with observable developmental problems only for some children—most often those children with additional social risks (e.g., low socioeconomic status). In other words, children's environments moderate the effect of early biologic risks on children's development. Nature and nurture are viewed as inherently inextricable; genes are expressed dependent on one's environment, and parents respond differently to children based on the child's inherent biologic characteristics.

An illustration of this cascading effect in a mother-child dyad is shown in Fig. 2.2A. A child's characteristics impact parenting, and parenting impacts children's development; these bidirectional cascades of influences continue over time across development. Critically, parents' behaviors in response to children are driven by their interpretations and the meaning they make from the behavior. For instance, a parent's anxious handling may arise because of her perception about the child's birth complications (e.g., "He's fragile and I might hurt him by accident"); a parent may disengage from a child with a difficult temperament because of the meaning she attaches to the child's fussy behavior (e.g., "Nothing I do settles him, he must not want me").

Understanding these processes provides several potential ports of entry for intervention in the parent-child relationship (i.e., the three *R*s: remediation, redefinition, reeducation); changing any of these ports of entry has the potential to change the sequelae that follow (see Fig. 2.2B). Remediation refers to directly changing the child. If a child has gastroesophageal reflux that contributes to a difficult temperament, treating the reflux might reduce the child's fussiness, and in turn, the parent may show more warmth and sensitivity with the child. Such treatment would be indicated when the child's condition can be effectively treated. However, it is not always feasible to offer treatment, such as when the child's condition is nonmodifiable or when there are no target symptoms that can be identified in the child that could be changed (e.g., with medical treatment or developmental therapies). Redefinition is changing a parent's interpretations of, attitudes toward, or beliefs about the child. A clinician may help parents to think about what their child is thinking and feeling during a challenging moment, help parents to reinterpret their child's behavior (e.g., aggressive behavior might reflect a child's inability to put words to strong feelings), or reinterpret their role in an interaction with their child (e.g., being a supportive and warm presence can be helpful to your child, even if he doesn't stop crying right away). This work often happens through parent-child psychotherapy, but modest redefinition can also occur through brief clinician visits. Reeducation refers to directly changing the parents' skills or knowledge and is most effective when parents' attitudes and beliefs about the child are healthy, but their parenting approach could be improved (e.g., by providing information about how to position a baby with a physical disability). Remediation, redefinition, and reeducation are inherently intertwined due to the dynamic nature of bidirectional influences in children's development; a change in one domain will likely have cascading effects in other domains.

DEVELOPMENT OF BEHAVIORAL PROBLEMS AND PSYCHOPATHOLOGY

A combination of biologic and environmental factors contributes to the development of behavioral problems and psychopathology. For conditions such as attention-deficit/hyperactivity disorder (ADHD; see Chapter 48), heritability estimates are 50% or higher, though genetic influences typically interact with environmental influences in predicting outcomes. Early in infancy, children show differences in temperament, which are based on biology and can be considered the early roots of eventual psychiatric diagnoses. The dopamine D4 receptor *(DRD4)* and the serotonin transporter receptor *(5-HTTLPR)* are linked to aspects of temperament, including attention, novelty seeking, approach, and inhibition; but the effects of genes are dependent on environmental factors such as social-emotional experience (e.g., less sensitive parenting, child maltreatment). Thus even

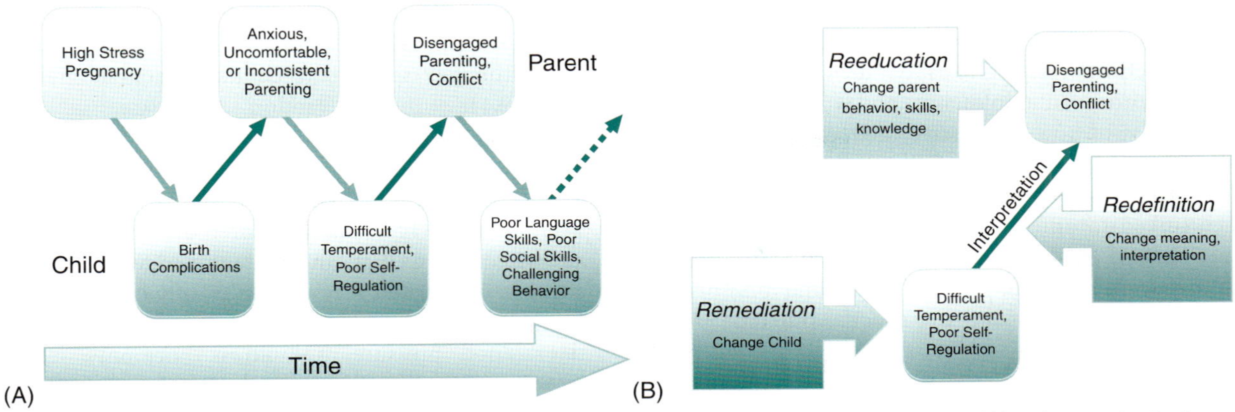

Fig. 2.2 Sameroff's transactional model shows the example of interacting forces impacting the child over time (A) and strategies for intervention to change the course of development (B).

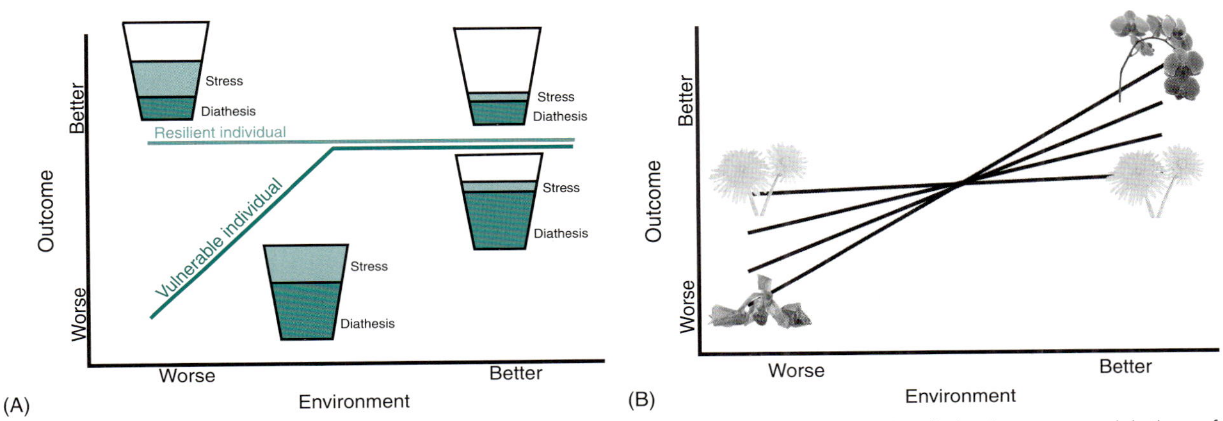

Fig. 2.3 Contrasting the diathesis-stress model (A) and the differential susceptibility model (B). In the diathesis-stress model, the unfavorable environment impacts vulnerable children only. In the differential susceptibility model, environmental quality impacts all children and the orchids more noticeably than the dandelions.

when the underlying risk is predominantly biologic, parenting and other environmental influences can either mitigate or amplify that risk. Children who are more vulnerable—whether from their genetic risk or temperament—are likely to be influenced more than the less vulnerable by both positive and negative experiences (Slagt et al., 2016). Abusive or neglectful parenting, poverty, premature birth, and parental psychopathology all place children at a higher risk for behavioral problems and psychiatric diagnoses, with higher risk for those children who experience multiple risk factors (Evans et al., 2013). Neural plasticity, neural pruning, and epigenetic processes drive these environmental effects on children's later outcomes. Two prominent theories have been developed to account for the ways that genetic and environmental factors interact.

Diathesis-Stress Model

This model suggests that some individuals are more vulnerable to the impacts of stress than others (Zuckerman, 1999) (Fig. 2.3A). Diatheses—hereditary or constitutional predispositions—might include biologic, genetic, temperament-related, or cognitive factors that predispose a child to being vulnerable to the influences of stress. Stresses might include discrete life events (e.g., divorce), chronic stresses (e.g., financial strain), or an accumulation of more minor daily stresses (e.g., school assignments). In a developmentally supportive environment, this model suggests that both resilient and vulnerable individuals are likely to do well. In a challenging environment, resilient individuals would do well, whereas vulnerable individuals would not. Those who have greater predispositions to psychopathology may be overwhelmed by a small to moderate environmental stress, whereas individuals with lower predispositions may withstand higher levels of environmental stress without apparent effects on their functioning.

Differential Susceptibility Theory

This theory posits that individuals vary in their plasticity, or their level of susceptibility to environmental influences (Belsky et al., 2007) (see Fig. 2.3B). Differential susceptibility can contribute to positive and negative outcomes. Some children, sometimes referred to as "orchids," are very sensitive to their environment. When they are in an environment that is highly supportive of their development and well-being, they thrive; however, when they are in an environment that is unsupportive of their development, they struggle. Other children, sometimes referred to as "dandelions," are less susceptible to environmental influences and will do roughly the same regardless of how supportive their environment and relationships are. Children can fall anywhere on the spectrum between these two extremes. This degree of plasticity has been linked to differences in genetic markers, including *5-HTTLPR*, *DRD4*, and *BDNF* (Belsky et al., in press). A child's susceptibility may differ depending on specific environmental influences and the specific outcome being considered.

CAREGIVER-CHILD RELATIONSHIPS

Primary caregivers impact a child's biology through their interactions with the child. The interactions a child has with, or supported by, the caregiver leave a lasting mark on the child's genome (see Chapter 24) and brain structure. Through neural pruning, a child's neural connections are either reinforced or pruned based on their experiences. Epigenetic effects, including those related to the experience of early caretaking behavior, are also active during this developmental period (Roth & Sweatt, 2011).

Caregivers scaffold infants' cognitive, social, behavioral, emotional, and physical development. Young children are not developmentally capable of self-regulation, so caregivers play a crucial role in helping children cope with negative affect by reading their cues, anticipating transitions, redirecting their attention, and responding promptly to their needs. As children gain experience with their caregivers coregulating their emotions, they begin to internalize these regulation strategies and gradually develop the ability to regulate independently. Sensitive and responsive parenting promotes positive child outcomes in domains, including attachment, cognitive development, social skills, and emotion regulation. A sensitive and responsive caregiver is tuned into the child's feelings and needs, and responds promptly with actions that are in tune with the child's feelings and needs throughout everyday activities (e.g., feeding, play, bathing, changing diapers or clothes).

Attachment theory (see Chapter 3) posits that internal working models, which are mental representations of relationships, serve as the foundation of attachment relationships (Bowlby, 1969). Parents come into the role of parents with a long history of experiences in caregiving relationships, which could include the experience of sensitive parenting, maltreatment, dismissive caregivers, or separation and loss. As parents, our own upbringing forms our cognitive schemas for parenting and the interpretations we make with regard to children's behavior, so we are likely to recapitulate the style of parenting that we experienced. For instance, when a child is crying, a parent who experienced sensitive and responsive parenting as a child might interpret that the child is having a hard time and needs help, whereas a parent who experienced emotionally dismissive parenting as a child might interpret the same behavior as reflective of the child "being dramatic." Parents' interpretations and attributions guide their parenting behavior, which then shapes the child's interactions and behavior with the parents and ultimately shapes the child's own attachment quality (Table 2.1).

CHILD STRESS AND TRAUMA

Even at young ages, many children are exposed to levels of stress and trauma that can impact their development. Positive stress is considered a normal part of healthy development (e.g., starting at a new daycare, medical procedure). Heart rate, blood pressure, and stress hormones temporarily increase. Tolerable stress involves greater stress response activations, but stress elevations are still time limited with recovery once the acute stressor passes; events such as disasters, the death of a loved one, or divorce could be tolerable stressors. Caregiving relationships are key in buffering the effect of these stressors, making stressors more manageable and biologic stress responses subside. Toxic stress involves strong, frequent, and prolonged stress system elevations that can cause lasting changes in neurobiologic systems, having a detrimental effect on later physical and mental health (see Chapter 15). Children who have experienced trauma commonly have aggressive behavior, irritability, and emotional withdrawal. Many children will reenact the trauma they have experienced or witnessed either in vivo (e.g., toward their caregiver or peers) or through play. Often these stresses happen in the context of caregiving relationships (e.g., child abuse or neglect, caregiver mental illness or substance use disorder), which both magnifies the felt experience of stress and lessens the potential for buffering of the stress through relationships. When stressors are more intense, prolonged, repeated, and unaddressed, they are likely to become toxic. When they occur in the context of supportive social-emotional relationships, early detection, and effective intervention, it is likely that these stressors will be tolerable.

Social determinants of health are key contributors to stressors and traumas that might lead to chronic elevations in their biologic stress response systems and impact children's development. Families who experience structural racism, discrimination, or economic oppression often experience chronic elevations in their biologic stress response systems that may contribute to a pervasive sense of lack of safety and security. Parents who are experiencing these stressors may understandably have less psychological capacity to support their children, as it is exponentially harder to help a child feel safe and secure when you as a parent do not feel safe and secure.

A child's relationship with a caregiver serves a particularly critical role when the child is experiencing stress. When children have a relationship with a caregiver that is secure, supportive, and attuned, the caregiver's ability to coregulate them supports their ability to withstand stress. On a biologic level, the presence of such a caregiver modulates a child's behavioral and biologic response to stress, including an endocrine stress response (i.e., hypothalamic-pituitary-adrenal [HPA] axis activity; Gunnar & Quevedo, 2007). Prior

TABLE 2.1 **Psychological and Behavioral Sequelae of Secure and Insecure Attachment Relationships**

Secure Attachment Relationship		Insecure Attachment Relationship
• Accepting of their children • Recognize concerns but not overwhelmed • In tune with their child's mindset • Able to reflect on child's internal state and motivations • Able to share memories and examples about their child	Parenting mindset	• Emotionally distant or overly emotionally activated • Unable to imagine child's internal state and motivations • Descriptions of their child are very brief and unelaborated, or confusing and hard to follow • Themes of role reversal or parental-self focus
• Sensitive • Attentive and responsive to child's needs	Parenting behaviors	• Insensitive • Unpredictable • Harsh
• Seek comfort and support from caregiver • Able to settle with support from caregiver	Child behavior	• Unable to be comforted by their caregiver • Appear undisturbed by their caregiver's departure
• Presence of caregiver helps to modulate physiologic and behavioral responses to stressors • Effects of stress are buffered by the caregiver-child relationship • Physiologic stress response remains within the "tolerable" range	During times of stress	• Elevated physiologic stress response (i.e., HPA axis activity); stress levels remain high for longer • Biologic stress response is not brought down by the presence of a caregiver • Physiologic stress response can become "toxic" resulting in changes to brain architecture • Lasting negative effects on physical, mental health
• Better peer relationships • Better emotion regulation, self-reliance • Fewer externalizing or internalizing problems	Child Outcomes	• Poorer peer relationships • Poorer emotion regulation and self-reliance • More externalizing and internalizing problems

HPA, Hypothalamic-pituitary-adrenal.

work with rodents suggests that highly responsive maternal behavior contributes to offspring developing a neurobiologic stress system that is less reactive and can better cope with challenges. These changes to the neurobiologic stress system are linked to changes to DNA that relate to the expression of glucocorticoid receptors, supporting the view that maternal behavior produces lasting changes to the neurobiologic stress system.

For children who don't have a secure attachment relationship, the biologic stress response (e.g., HPA axis activity) may be pronounced; stress hormones spike to higher levels and remain high for a longer period of time. In the shorter term, the biologic stress response is adaptive, helping individuals to face challenges in the environment. Persistent activation of the stress response system without adequate recovery, however, is linked to lasting neurobiologic changes such as reduced neuroplasticity and neurogenesis. These neurobiologic changes are linked to lasting deleterious effects on an individual's mental and physical health. Parenting is the most influential environmental factor that shapes individual differences in stress neurobiology due to the role parents can play in coregulating children and the stress that children experience when relationships are disrupted or insufficient to meet children's needs. Further, experience early in life is formative in the development of endocrine systems, so early experience tends to have more significant and lasting effects on children's later development and functioning.

INTERGENERATIONAL TRANSMISSION OF RISK

Children depend on their caregivers to help them regulate in the context of stress. A regulated, calm, and connected caregiver is able to settle a child more effectively, and these calming effects on children are seen both behaviorally and on a biologic level. However, when a caregiver experiences significant distress, such as that due to trauma, depression, or a substance use disorder, parenting behavior and child outcomes are negatively affected (Julian & Muzik, 2020). Importantly, many of these behavioral changes in both caregivers and children have been linked to biologic changes.

Cynthia describes a recent incident at home. She picked up Justin from school after his principal reported that he had shoved another child on the playground. When they got home, Cynthia yelled at Justin for his behavior. As she recounts the incident, she becomes heated. When Cynthia yelled at him, Justin began yelling, kicking, and hitting. They both continued to get more and more upset until Cynthia closed herself into the bathroom to get some space. Eventually, Justin settled. Cynthia hadn't brought up this event with him since then for fear that he would get upset again.

You appreciate that Cynthia has several chronic stresses, stemming from uncertainty about job stability, her history of domestic violence, and stressful experiences in her own childhood. Epigenetic changes resulting from her own childhood trauma likely have altered her neurobiologic response to the stresses of parenting, and she struggles to regulate her own emotions. Justin became upset at school after another child mocked him; mocking has been a trigger for him, given his dad's frequent mocking and aggression years before. Justin also meets diagnostic criteria for attention-deficit/hyperactivity disorder—a diagnosis his father also had. His impulsivity in responding to the other child's mocking may also be reflective of an ADHD diagnosis.

Parental Trauma Exposure

Intimate partner violence (IPV) and sexual abuse are strong risk factors for posttraumatic stress disorder (PTSD); those who are diagnosed with PTSD are at greater risk of again developing PTSD after a new trauma (e.g., childbirth trauma). Trauma symptoms, such as intrusive thoughts or flashbacks, are often associated with intense or prolonged psychological distress and may make it challenging for a caregiver to be emotionally present to a child's experience.

For many parents who have experienced abuse (e.g., IPV), their child's aggressive behavior can serve as a trauma trigger, a reminder that brings back the memories and physiologic responses of previous traumatic events. When Justin is aggressive toward Cynthia, this behavior is a reminder for Cynthia of the trauma she has experienced, and she becomes flooded with negative emotions that she had previously experienced. Cynthia's emotional distress limits her ability to see the situation from Justin's perspective, so she responds to him in anger. Justin does not yet have the capacity to regulate his emotions on his own, and requires a caregiver's support to settle down. His mother's anger only serves to escalate him—and may also be a reminder for him of the trauma he has witnessed and experienced. Justin's physiologic response to this stress involves persistent elevations in stress hormones that can be neurotoxic. Interactions like Justin and Cynthia's are common in trauma-exposed families. Parents who have PTSD have been reported to perceive a poorer relationship with their children, are less emotionally available to their child, and show more aggression toward their children. Their parenting behavior tends to be less sensitive and responsive, and more controlling, avoidant, overprotective, intrusive, and hostile.

Parents who experience trauma have changes in the HPA axis and autonomic nervous system, and these changes relate to negative parenting. Epigenetic changes in genes related to cortisol and serotonin are related to parents' trauma-related psychopathology. These biologic changes in the stress regulation system precede parenting difficulties. Findings are mixed with regard to whether parents with PTSD parent differently than non–trauma-exposed parents; it may be that mothers with PTSD show impaired parenting when their trauma reactions are activated, but parenting is unaffected when trauma responses are dormant.

Effects of parental PTSD on child outcomes can be mediated by parents' psychological distress or by parenting behavior. Children whose parent has severe PTSD tend to have more sleep difficulty (disruptions in sleep, separation anxiety around bedtime) and a more difficult temperament than those whose parent does not have PTSD. These children develop internalizing and externalizing problems as they grow older and tend to show aggression, attentional bias to danger and distress, and conflict avoidance.

Parental Depression

Parental depression is a common childbirth complication (see Chapter 5) and can impact parenting behavior and interactions with one's child, both during an episode of depression and when depression is in remission. Depressed parents tend to show less positivity with their children, more negativity and disengagement, and may be less attuned to their infant's cues, and thus less likely to respond in a sensitive and responsive way. These parenting behaviors may be driven by a depressed parent's difficulty in taking the child's perspective or other cognitive and affective changes related to depression.

Children of mothers who have depression are more likely to be born preterm, have low birth weight, be more irritabile, show fewer facial expressions, and be less active and attentive than children of nondepressed mothers. As they grow older, they show lower levels of oxytocin and have less flexibility in the HPA axis. They are more likely to develop insecure attachment relationships, have higher rates of psychopathology, experience peer relationship problems and social withdrawal, and tend to show more negative affect and less positive affect than children of nondepressed mothers. Effects of parental depression on children are most pronounced when a parent is depressed during a child's earliest years.

Parental Substance Use Disorders

Substance abuse commonly occurs in the context of other psychosocial risks, such as a history of childhood maltreatment and comorbid psychopathology (see Chapter 53). Those who abuse substances have altered dopaminergic systems. Dopamine is released in the context of positive parent-child interactions and contributes to these interactions feeling rewarding. Substance abusing parents may not experience the same sense of reward and motivation as non–substance abusing mothers experience.

Parents who abuse substances have more authoritarian and harsh disciplinary styles and show less attentiveness and engagement when interacting with their children. Parents' affect dysregulation can interfere with their ability to tune in to their child's thoughts and feelings. Substance abusing parents are three to four times as likely to abuse or neglect their children, and the majority of children removed from their home by child welfare services are removed related to neglect from a parent with a substance use disorder. Substance abuse often leads to incarceration, so children with a parent who abuses substances may experience myriad consequences related to this (e.g., separation from a parent, change in living arrangements and/or caregivers, emotional stress, financial stress, housing instability). Children exposed to substances in utero experience many biologic and behavioral consequences, including stunted development, more unpredictable temperament, and later risk for depression, anxiety, and social problems (see Chapter 37).

Interacting Parental Influences on Children's Behavior

Parents' personal experiences and mental state impact their own biology and the ways they think about and interact with their children. Caregiver-child relationships play a key role in determining children's outcomes. In several cases, research has demonstrated that biologic changes in the parent precede changes to parenting. Children who experience parenting from a caregiver who has mental illness or a substance use disorder often experience harsh or insensitive parenting, social and familial stressors, and even abuse and neglect. All of these risk factors on the child's level predispose the child to adverse outcomes, including developmental delays, physical health problems, low educational and occupational attainment, and later criminality and psychopathology. These adverse outcomes point to the importance of supporting caregivers and caregiver-child relationships throughout our clinical work with families. As children grow and develop, they eventually become parents themselves, and the intergenerational transmission of risk continues. The transmission of risk across generations may be interrupted by promoting secure, supportive caregiver-child relationships.

APPLICATIONS OF THEORIES IN THE PRACTICE OF DEVELOPMENTAL-BEHAVIORAL PEDIATRICS

In the practice of developmental-behavioral pediatrics, clinicians cannot care for the child without also caring for the parents. In the case of Cynthia and Justin it is important to comprehensively evaluate Justin for conditions, including ADHD, language delay, or learning disabilities, which may become increasingly evident at early school age. If Justin meets the criteria for any of these diagnoses, remediation (as described in Sameroff's transactional model) will be an important approach. Remediation may involve treatment for Justin with medical management, educational intervention, and behavioral therapy. Reeducation will also be an essential component of treatment for this dyad. Via the strategy of reeducation, an improved understanding of how ADHD and any coexisting developmental delays or learning difficulties are contributing to Justin's behavior may help Cynthia to be better equipped to manage his behavior. Gaining skills in parenting strategies, connecting effectively with his school to align behavior management, and learning about options for ADHD management will be important for Cynthia and likely increase her sense of parenting efficacy as she becomes more of "an expert" in Justin and his behavior and development. Finally, through redefinition the clinician can convey to Cynthia the range of factors contributing to Justin's externalizing behavior—and to reframe the situation in a manner that puts her in the position of being competent and capable in supporting Justin's developmental and behavioral needs. Treatment of his ADHD symptoms with medication or with parent behavior management may be one critical strategy that can alter the cascading interactions in the parent-child relationship and potentially shift the trajectory in a more positive direction. As Justin is able to better regulate his own emotion and behavior, he will experience more success at school and will elicit less frustration from Cynthia. As Cynthia experiences more success in parenting Justin, her view of Justin will grow to be more positive, and more sensitive interactions may begin to predominate. An ongoing relationship with a mental health clinician who can support and guide the dyad as their relationship evolves will be essential. A list of questions you might consider including in a clinical interview to understand the multiple, interacting forces on a child and family are in Box 2.1.

Supporting Parent-Child Relationships in Clinic

While a core goal of clinical interviews is to understand the problem at hand to guide recommendations for intervention approaches, the interview can also serve as an intervention in itself (e.g., through redefinition or reeducation). In the context of an appointment, be attentive to anything parents are doing—even if it is small—that is helpful to their child's well-being and positive development, and highlight and encourage these behaviors. When caregivers are very upset by their child's behavior, their upset can be reframed as a sign of their care and concern about their child and their awareness of the potential consequences if things don't change. The goal in highlighting caregivers' developmentally supportive behavior and feelings is to motivate a shift in their behavior and cognitions. In reconnecting with the care and concern that might underlie the parent's frustration, caregivers are likely to engage in more of this positive behavior in the future.

During an appointment there is sometimes opportunity to highlight how a child is positively responding to something a caregiver is doing. For instance, a caregiver may have a softer tone of voice, or listen more, or express care and concern for the child, and a child might display a relaxed body posture or lean into the caregiver. What happens in the office between children and their caregivers is often a microcosm of what their relationship looks like at home in their everyday lives. If you see small interactions that are helpful—things you want to see more of—highlighting it increases the likelihood that it will happen again and can cue caregivers in to the role they have in dynamics that may feel automatic or unavoidable. While it can often be tempting to point out the reverse, too (e.g., the negative effect that a caregiver's behavior can have on a child), it is generally not recommended and can be counterproductive.

BOX 2.1 Recommended Interview Questions for Understanding the Multiple, Interactive Forces Impacting Child Development and Behavior

Learn About the Problem

- When did these problems begin? Any ideas about why these problems began?
- What was going on in the family at the time these problems began (or became worse)?
- Has anything worked to make the problems better? What makes them worse?
- Are the problems different in different settings (home, daycare, school)? Are the problems different with different people (mother, father, grandparents, babysitters, peers)?
- What is it like for you [parent/caregiver] when these problems happen?
- How do you [parent/caregiver] typically respond to your child when this problem happens?

Learn About the Family

- Who lives in the home? How is your child's relationship with parents/siblings/others in the household?
- What is a typical day like for your child?
- Why do family and friends think your child is having this problem?
- Who helps you in parenting your child?
- Are you connected to any community supports that are helpful to you (e.g., social services, church)?
- Has anyone else in the family had problems similar to your child?

Learn About Stress and Trauma

- Has your child ever experienced or witnessed anything stressful, scary, or traumatic (e.g., people fighting or a scary medical procedure)? Has your child ever been separated from a parent or caregiver?
- Have there been any changes in the family (e.g., change in who lives in the home, new sibling born, parent relationship changes, moving homes, moving schools)?
- What has your child said or done that might indicate remembrance of parts of the traumatic/stressful events?
- How did your child's emotions or behaviors change after the trauma/stress?
- What was the traumatic/stressful experience like for you [parent/caregiver]?

Learn About the Caregiver-Child Relationship

- Tell me three words/phrases to describe your child's personality. Tell an example/memory to illustrate each trait.
- Tell me three words/phrases to describe your relationship with your child. Tell an example/memory for each one.
- Who does your child remind you of?

Recognizing Your Own Reactions to Patients

Working with families who experience significant challenges can be emotionally draining as a clinician. Reframing our own interpretations of the situation may help us understand our patients and support them. When encountering particularly challenging clinical situations, we might ask ourselves, "What has happened to this family to make them respond in this way?" Typically when we wonder about someone's experiences, we show empathy, and when we attempt to understand the reasons for a patient's behaviors, we are able to respond in sensitive and helpful ways.

CONCLUSION

Developmental and behavioral pediatric clinicians are well positioned to integrate biology and environment in their conceptualization of both the child's behavior and development, and the parent-child relationship. The clinician should integrate the biopsychosocial complexity of development into their understanding of the child and development of a treatment plan and avoid erroneously attributing children's outcomes to a failure of parenting. A biopsychosocial framing provides the foundation for even greater empathy for the parent and child in the therapeutic relationship.

REFERENCES

Belsky, J., Bakermans-Kranenburg, M. J., & Van Ijzendoorn, M. H. (2007). For better and for worse: Differential susceptibility to environmental influences. *Current Directions in Psychological Science*, *16*(6), 300–304.

Belsky, J., Zhang, X., & Sayler, K. (in press). Differential susceptibility 2.0: Are the same children affected by different experiences and exposures? *Development and Psychopathology*, 1–9. https://doi.org/10.1017/S0954579420002205. Epub ahead of print. PMID: 33634774.

Bowlby. J. (1969). *Attachment and loss: Attachment*. Basic Books.

Bronfenbrenner. U. (1979). *The ecology of human development: Experiments in nature and design*. Harvard University Press.

Evans, G. W., Li, D., & Whipple, S. S. (2013). Cumulative risk and child development. *Psychological Bulletin*, *139*(6), 1342–1396. https://doi.org/10.1037/a0031808.

Gunnar, M. R., & Quevedo, K. (2007). The neurobiology of stress and development. *Annual Review of Psychology*, *58*, 145–173.

Julian, M. M., & Muzik, M. (2020). Interventions to enhance mother-infant attachment in the context of trauma, depression, and substance abuse. In P. S. Chandra, H. Herrman, J. Fisher, & A. Riecher-Rössler (Eds.), *Mental health and illness of women* (pp. 403–421). Singapore: Springer.

Roth, T. L., & Sweatt, J. D. (2011). Annual research review: Epigenetic mechanisms and environmental shaping of the brain during sensitive periods of development. *Journal of Child Psychology and Psychiatry and Allied Disciplines*, *52*(4), 398–408.

Sameroff. A. (2009). The transactional model. In A. Sameroff (Ed.), *The transactional model of development: How children and contexts shape each other* (pp. 3–21). American Psychological Association.

Slagt, M., Semon, J., Deković, M., & van Aken, M. A. G. (2016). Differences in sensitivity to parenting depending on child temperament: A meta-analysis. *Psychological Bulletin*, *142*(10), 1068–1110.

Zuckerman. M. (1999). *Vulnerability to psychopathology: A biosocial model*. American Psychological Association.

3

Theories of Human Development[1]

Sarah L. Friedman and Ellin K. Scholnick

For additional material related to the content of this chapter, please see Chapters 2, 4, and 15.

VIGNETTE

The Browns were a family of four: mother, Ann; father, Ben; early adolescent, James; and toddler, David. Before the COVID-19 pandemic, both parents were in the workforce, James was in middle school and in after-school programs, and David was in a full-day center-based early care and education arrangement. When the pandemic hit, they all needed to shelter at home full time. Initially, both parents worked from home, but they did not have separate rooms to work from or bandwidth for multiple wireless connections. The family was physically isolated from their extended family, friends, coworkers, and teachers. Ann and Ben were highly concerned about their future, including lost wages, mounting bills, and financial independence. James began online education, but he struggled to stay engaged without the stimulation of hands-on activities in challenging classes, such as science, and rewards of socializing with his close buddies. David was enrolled in an online preschool, but he did not attend well or learn from the experience. Ann quit work to care for David and to support James. Ann set aside time each morning for learning activities with David, who seemed to thrive cognitively and socially with the increased attention of his mother. Ben also set aside time each afternoon for reviewing the day's lessons and assignments with James. When James returned to school, he willingly wore a mask every day because he recognized it was the agreed-upon solution to maintaining his social connection with peers.

OVERVIEW

Theories of development grow out of keen observations, insights, and preliminary research. They offer a narrative of changes associated with growth/maturation and a network of contemporaneous connections among a selective set of behaviors and processes. They attempt to explain what is behind observed behaviors. They address the roles of nature and nurture and stimulate further scientific research to validate the theories (see Miller, 2002, for a comprehensive discussion). The theories and the scientific evidence to validate them provide ways of thinking that parents, clinicians, educators, and even public officials have understood and used in their daily life and practice. In this chapter we review several influential theories of child development. To demonstrate their heuristic value, we discuss how these theories can help us figure out the effects of living through the time of COVID-19 on children's functioning and development.

The chapter describes three different theoretical perspectives on children's development. Stage theories (Freud, Erikson, Piaget, Kohlberg, Bowlby) tell us what develops. These theories, which stress universal patterns of change, launched important research and clinical traditions. They have become less influential recently due to the rise of sociocultural theories (Vygotsky, Feuerstein, Bronfenbrenner, and Masten) that focus on how variations in social and environmental factors influence development. A third most recent perspective, dynamic systems theory (DST), focuses on the probabilistic nature of phase transitions that depend on the interactions among tiny changes in multiple systems rather than on predetermined plans. This last perspective is well aligned with other interdisciplinary approaches that study the relationship of biologic processes, environmental influences, and behavior.

STAGE THEORIES OF UNIVERSAL DEVELOPMENTAL CHANGE

Sigmund Freud: Psychosexual Development

Freudian Stages

Sigmund Freud (1856–1939) posited that behavior was motivated by a life force—the libido—that at different developmental stages was primarily expressed in different parts of the body. In the first year of life the child focuses on oral sensations such as sucking, focusing primarily on relations with the mother. Freud called the unbridled quest for need satisfaction that begins at birth and continues through life the "id."

Libidinal energy then shifts to anal needs (roughly age 1–3 years). These sensations metaphorically relate to issues of control: of holding on and resistance to letting go. Toilet training occurs during this period. To cope with the pressures to regulate these needs, the child develops the "ego." The ego provides the means of self-control to mediate between the child's id and the demands of external reality. When the conflict between the id and the ego cannot be resolved, the

[1]Note: We thank Flavia De Campos Dutra for assisting with the bibliographic research for this chapter during the time of COVID-19.

ego resorts to solutions acceptable to the id, termed "defense mechanisms." Examples of defense mechanisms include regression, where the child retreats to more infantile ways of behaving and projection, where the child blames another person for feelings the child cannot accept in oneself.

Children then move to the phallic stage (ages 3–5 years). The child is driven by sexual attraction to the parent of the opposite sex and wishes to harm the parent of the same sex. There are strong strictures against fulfilling these desires. This tension is resolved by identifying with the parent of the same sex. This resolution is achieved by developing the "superego," which serves both as a conscience and a codebook of socially acceptable behavior. Difficulties in the phallic stage are thought to influence the lifelong expression of sexuality and the individual's moral standards.

Next the child enters the latency period, in which Freud conceptualized minimal tension (see Chapter 8). That stage ends when the hormonal changes of puberty manifest themselves and start the genital stage (adolescence). Many of the battles of childhood arise again and need to be refought. The results shape the pattern of subsequent development and the strength of the ego and the superego.

Limitations

Freud's theory was based on interviewing his adult patients about their dreams and their childhood memories, not based on observations of children. Freud's emphasis was on the development of boys and on heterosexual identity and relationships. Freud's depiction, particularly of the phallic stage, has been very controversial as society has changed its norms for sex role and sexuality.

Erik Erikson: Psychosocial Development

Erik Erikson (1902–1994) revised and expanded Freudian theory in 1963. Erikson called attention to the growth of cognitive and muscular skills such as talking and walking (i.e., ego skills) that pose developmental challenges because they bring to the child's attention new aspects of the world. The attempt to master these challenges shapes the child's developmental trajectory. For example, walking enables exploration of the environment and presents the child with new opportunities and dangers. Erikson took into account the cultural influences on the growing child's attempts at mastery. Blending multiple sources of growth (drives, ego skills, and culture), Erikson described the life span with eight specific stages, each a dynamic tension between two opposing forces.

Eriksonian Stages

The first stage (infancy) represents the tension between basic trust and mistrust. It embeds Freudian analyses of the oral stage in a broader interplay between parent and child. Reliable, sensitive child rearing builds the child's sense of trust in the parent, whereas negligent care builds a sense of mistrust. These interactions lead to the individual's proclivity to give or not to give to others. Additionally, the child must find a balance between safety and danger. The outcome of judging situations to be safe rather than dangerous produces a sense of hope, which is pervasive throughout life.

The second stage (age 2–3 years) represents the tension between autonomy and shame and doubt. Children's growing language and muscular control provide opportunities both for independence and for going beyond permissible boundaries. Parents place limits on their children, and children must learn to inhibit urges and practice self-control without feeling shame or losing self-esteem when they fail. Arriving at the delicate balance between control of the self and control by others generalizes to the child's attitudes toward law and order.

The third stage (age 4–5 years) represents the tension between initiative and guilt. Like Freud, Erikson characterizes the third stage in terms of the acquisition of sex role and a functioning superego; however, Erikson notes that emerging phallic concerns create in boys the male modality of intrusion and in girls the female modality of receptivity. These tendencies prompt the child to search for the gender-appropriate models and identify with them. Males thrust themselves into social interactions, whereas females are receptive to others' wishes. The phallic analogy of intrusion is extended to ego skills that enable children to create their own projects and purposes. These are fostered by the capacity for imaginative play. But imaginative activities and children's plans can lead into taboo territory. Children must learn to discern for themselves, not just from parental directives, when they have crossed the line into unacceptable thoughts, feelings, and actions. This tension is the origin of the superego and guilt. Attempts to find the appropriate balance of personal initiatives with moral strictures shape the child's sense of purpose.

The fourth stage (age 6–12 years) represents the tension between industry and inferiority. Erikson drew attention to the role of schooling and its demands for mastery of the technological order. This stage lays the groundwork for children's sense of competence.

The fifth stage (adolescence) represents the tension between identity and role confusion. The teen years are marked by physical changes and hormonal surges that seem unpredictable and uncontrollable to teenagers. The demands of adulthood are beginning to become apparent. Therefore, teenagers need to test and gain acceptance for who they are, particularly with their peers. Identity refers not only to sexuality but also to their fit in the structure of society, in school, in their peer groups, and in the ethos of the culture such as presented by the media.

Erikson was a pioneer in describing development throughout the life span. For Erikson the healthy, mature adult was productive at work and was in a mutually satisfying relationship. The latter stages of development were steps toward achieving these endpoints.

The sixth stage (young adulthood) represents the tension between intimacy and isolation. This period is often when adults form committed relationships and begin families. Erikson extended the challenge of forging relationships with significant others to friends and colleagues and to building a collaborative style of interaction.

The seventh stage (middle adulthood) represents the tension between generativity and stagnation. Erikson's definition of healthy relationships requires shared responsibilities and fostering a new generation both in the family and at work. The eighth and final stage of development (old age) represents the tension between integrity and despair. Many cultures value elder wisdom; however, if persons did not achieve their goals in relationships or work, then they may be left with a sense of disappointment. Erikson's wife, Joan, added a different perspective to this stage, focusing on the challenges of dealing with declining abilities while retaining self-esteem and dignity.

Limitations

Erikson's stages remain tied to Freudian constructs. Empirical support for the stages is limited. However, as a heuristic and framework, the stages prove very powerful.

Jean Piaget: Cognitive Development

Jean Piaget (1896–1980) focused his theory of development (Gruber & Voneche, 1977) on how the child develops a logical and scientific framework for understanding the physical world. He posited that children's understanding goes through a series of age-linked qualitative changes or stages. Each stage is a filter that selects and organizes what the child perceives and understands. Each stage is a framework that provides the building blocks for the next, thus there is a definite order in which understanding emerges. Development occurs when children discover a discrepancy between their current understanding of reality (assimilation) and the features of the world that don't mesh with that understanding (accommodation). To resolve the mismatch, children modify their framework. The novel framework may open up new challenges that are more complicated and far reaching.

Sensorimotor Stage

During the sensorimotor stage, which unfolds over the first 24 months of life, a child's body is the source of experiences. The child is born with a set of rigid motor activities (reflexes), such as sucking or grasping. Initially the reflexive acts are performed separately and directed toward specific objects. Gradually the child begins to adapt these reflexes to different objects, such as sucking differently on a nipple than on one's fingers. Later the infant combines these reflexes as in grasping the object that is sucked. This experimentation leads to a better understanding of the external objects to which the child is trying to adapt. The ability to use more than one action simultaneously enables the child to construct sequences that facilitate the creation of sequential goal-directed behavior. In the second year of life these reflexes become internalized. For example, Piaget's infant daughter first opened up her mouth while figuring out how to get into a drawer. Opening her mouth represented the act of opening the drawer. The child's ability to represent leads to language learning since language is representational (see Chapter 44). The first words, however, may be idiosyncratic. One child called dogs "voo-voos," based on the barking sound of dogs. Representational thought further enables the toddler to infer that objects that disappear from view and are outside the range of action nevertheless exist. By the end of the sensorimotor period the child is able to conceptualize a world that exists independent of one's actions upon it (object permanence), and consequently the child can play hide and seek. Representational thought also enables the child to watch someone perform a novel behavior and then carry out the same behavior later (deferred imitation).

Preoperational Stage

By the end of the sensorimotor period toddlers are able to keep in mind objects and events that they cannot see, but those early representational skills are limited and continue to develop during the preoperational period, which lasts up to 6 to 7 years of age. During this period the child slowly starts to use words that have shared conventional meaning for all users of the language. Private speech, based on words that remind the child of objects, is displaced by arbitrary words such as "dog." But the child struggles with understanding that different people who observe the same object from different perspectives gain different information.

Preoperational children think that their own point of view is shared universally. They also tend to center their attention on one salient aspect of an object or event and ignore less salient aspects. When milk is poured from a wide cup into a tall, thin glass, the child does not recognize that although the level of milk has changed, the amount of milk has not changed but is merely redistributed. The child focuses on the initial and final states, not on the transformation. Likewise, the preoperational child judges the moral value of an act (its being good or bad) by the amount of damage, not the intentions of the perpetrator.

Concrete Operations Stage

Concrete operations, which arise between 7 and 11 years of age, enable overcoming egocentrism and failures of conservation by constructing logical frameworks or sets of rules that can be coordinated with one another. This kind of understanding is fostered by formal education. The child understands that liquid poured from one container into the next can be poured back to its exact original state; that is, change in the level of the liquid is reversible. Reversible relations underlie arithmetic (e.g., addition and subtraction) and categorization (class inclusion and class subdivision) and can be used to calculate changes in perspective. The deployment of these relations or operational thinking enables the child to develop a more accurate understanding of space, time, and morality. For example, the child now makes moral evaluations by examining the intentions of the actor.

Formal Operations Stage

Operations are lifted to a higher, more abstract and integrated level during the final stage of cognitive development, which starts at 11 to 12 years of age. The child in the concrete operations stage deals with problems through induction, making generalizations based on a few encountered instances. However, the teenager in the formal operational stage can make hypotheses based on imagined possibilities and can test their current and future validity (deduction) using propositional logic.

Limitations

Stage theory assumes developmental timetables and a universal order of cognitive development; the theory is an idealization of development. The rules of conservation theoretically apply whether the content is number or weight or volume, but children do not master them simultaneously. Similarly, although perspective taking, conservation, and construction of class hierarchies are all purported to be accomplishments of the concrete operational stage, they are not mastered simultaneously. Familiarity with content makes deductive reasoning easier, and even with familiar material errors can be made. Piaget's theory also characterizes the child as a solitary scientist who constructs intellectual tools during the course of problem solving. This characterization ignores the sociocultural world in which the child lives. The contexts of children's development vary in terms of the tools, experiences, and mentors available to the child and consequently affect the trajectory of children's development.

Lawrence Kohlberg: Moral Development

Lawrence Kohlberg's (1927–1987) theory of moral reasoning is one of the best known applications of Piaget's theory. Kohlberg asserted that there was an invariant and unidirectional sequence of moral developmental stages reflecting changes in how the individual conceptualizes the world. In all cultures the direction of development is toward greater scope and hierarchic integration of reasoning. Based on interviews in which he presented children with moral dilemmas, Kohlberg identified six stages of moral decision making (Kohlberg & Hersh, 1977).

Stages

Stage 1 focuses on punishment and obedience. The preoperational child obeys rules that are set by figures in power to avoid being punished. They believe that the larger the damage caused by ignoring directions, the greater the punishment that is deserved.

Stage 2, instrumental relativist orientation, begins the process of taking into account purposes and desires. Children judge morality by its personal benefits but also recognize that others have needs, too. Human relationships and morality associated with it are viewed as exchanges of favors.

Stage 3 emerges when thinking broadens the perspective beyond one's own needs to thinking about pleasing others and acting in ways that would be approved by them. This stage is often labeled "good-boy, nice-girl" morality. The adolescent judges behavior in terms of what people will think about the person who violates social norms.

Stage 4, described as law and order morality, ties social norms to the maintenance of the formalized social order.

Stage 5 describes the social contract, legalistic orientation such as practiced in democratic societies where decisions are the product of open debates. There is awareness of the relativism of personal values and opinions and an emphasis on the need for rules for reaching consensus.

Stage 6 refers to a universal-ethical-principle orientation. Right is defined by decisions based on self-chosen ethical principles appealing to logical comprehensiveness, universality, and consistency. These are universal principles of justice, reciprocity, equality of human rights, and respect for the dignity of human beings. Kohlberg's research shows that the use of the first two stages decreases with age, the next two stages increase until age 13, and the use of the last two stages increases until age 16.

Limitations

Other scholars have presented conceptualizations of moral judgment and its development. Following the leads of Freud and Émile Durkheim (1858–1917), an influential French social scientist, most social scientists viewed moral development as a process of internalizing culturally given rules through rewards, punishment, or identification. Most recently, Gilligan (1982) challenged Kohlberg and argued that the development of female moral reasoning is rooted in concerns for the care of others rather than in developing toward the ideal of abstract legalistic principles.

John Bowlby: Attachment

John Bowlby (1907–1990) believed that the early relationships between children and their parents are critical and have a far-reaching impact on the trajectory and outcomes of human development (Cassidy & Shaver, 2018). Unlike Freud who built his theories of early development on adult recollections of childhood, Bowlby built his attachment theory on ideas from the fields of evolutionary biology, ethology, developmental psychology, cognitive science and control system theory, and observations of actual behaviors of children during their interactions with the most significant people in their lives.

The survival of human infants depends on the existence of caregivers (primarily the mother) who are competent, responsive, and sensitive to their needs. As a result of sensitive caring, the baby not only survives but begins to create an emotional bond with the caregivers (attachment). The manifestations of attachment change from a need for physical proximity to other forms of connection as the young child becomes more competent.

The theory suggests that infants form attachments to the people who interact with them on a consistent basis and primarily to the person who is most available to respond to their needs. In most cases the mother becomes the primary attachment figure, but infants also may form attachments with others (e.g., fathers). Attachment of infants to their caregivers can be secure or insecure. When the attachment is secure, infants are confident that their caregiver is available and is responsive to their needs; when not available, the caregiver will return. Securely attached infants feel free to get away from the secure base provided by the caregiver and explore the world around them. When insecure, the infant is likely to be fearful of abandonment and less free to explore the surroundings. Bowlby asserted that these patterns of interaction were a product of both biologically driven parenting behavior aimed at caring and protecting the infant and learned behaviors derived from childhood experience.

Stages

As described by Marvin and Brittner (1999), Bowlby proposed four phases in the development of the attachment behavioral system. In the first phase (birth through 2–3 months of age) the infant elicits caregiving behavior and responds equally to caregiving regardless of the person who provides it. This phase can last longer under unfavorable conditions in which the infant's needs are not taken care of in an appropriate and responsive manner.

In the second phase (age 4–6 months) the infant orients and signals to one or more discriminated individuals. During this period the infant learns to respond in avoidant or resistant ways as a response to parental behaviors that are not responsive to their needs. At this phase, infants know who their caregivers are but don't yet conceive of them as attachment figures with separate existences beyond the infant's own experiences.

In the third phase (beginning between age 6 and 9 months) there are gains in motor, cognitive, and communicative behaviors as well as in coordination. The infant consolidates attachment to specific caregivers and maintains proximity to those caregivers by locomotion and signals. Locomotion allows the infant to control proximity to the attachment figure, to move away so as to explore and to follow the caregiver when in distress. During this phase the infant shows differential clinging to the attachment figure when alarmed, ill, or distressed and differential burying of the face after an excursion away from the attachment figure. In the second phase the infant has an internal image of an end state that the infant would like to achieve, such as physical contact with the attachment figure. In the third phase infants are capable of selecting behaviors that will allow them to achieve the goal and alter the plan if necessary. During the third phase, the infant creates separate working models of caregiver(s) and the self. These are organized in a hierarchy of images and plans that the infant can mentally operate on to fit goals. However, at this phase the caregiver is not understood as an agent with behaviors and goals that are independent of the infant.

The fourth phase is characterized as "goal corrected partnership." Around the age of 4 years, children require less physical proximity and contact with their attachment figures to maintain a sense of security. They have a well-cemented internal model of attachment. Consequently they are increasingly fine with spending time in the company of unfamiliar peers and adults and will later build expectations about all relationships based on their attachment history.

Implications and Limitations

Bowlby's theory evoked great concern about the effects of long separations between infants and their mothers. Many worried that when mothers join the workforce, child-mother attachment would suffer. This concern led to research about the effects of nonmaternal childcare on attachment. The most comprehensive study found that attachment was not linked to individual aspects of nonmaternal care (the age at which it was started, its quantity, stability, type, or quality). However, infants were less likely to be securely attached when nonmaternal care of poor quality was combined with low maternal sensitivity/responsiveness, more than one care arrangement, or more than minimal amounts of nonmaternal care (Friedman & Boyle, 2008). These findings seem to contradict expectations based on attachment theory. However, the theory does not specify how much maternal care is sufficient for the establishment of attachment.

While attachment theory is used in court cases pertaining to child custody, assessments of attachment are not sensitive enough to be used as diagnostic tools for assessment of individual families (Forslund et al., 2021).

General Implications for Stage Theories During the COVID-19 Pandemic

Each of the stage theories suggests challenges that might arise in an era in which all aspects of life are disrupted. Freudian theory sensitizes us to be attentive to the rise of defense mechanisms, particularly around the developmental challenges of each stage (e.g., young children may regress in toilet training). In Eriksonian terms the stresses in relationships may allow a shift from the positive to the negative pole of any of the stages (e.g., if parents become highly stressed, their child may tend toward mistrust over trust or develop a sense of shame rather than autonomy). Piaget would say that the stresses of the pandemic might affect the progression of cognitive acquisition in part based on the lack of availability of learning environments with hands-on exploration and manipulation. For that reason, in the vignette, David, still a toddler, could not learn from online education. James, in the transition from concrete to formal operational stage of development, had variable success with exclusive online education. Kohlberg's theory helps us understand the extent to which children of different ages can understand public health rules of behavior during a pandemic. It also informs the justifications that adults can offer to children to gain their cooperation with new obligations, such as wearing masks. Young children may respond to simple inducements to be a good child and do as the parents ask. School-aged children may be convinced to obey the law. Adolescents like James (in the vignette) and adults who are capable of a social contract, legalistic orientation may appreciate the relativism of personal values and opinions and therefore may agree with the need for rules for reaching consensus. They may also respond to appeals to statements of universal principles, such as the importance of saving the life of others over the insistence on personal preference. Bowlby's theory can help parents understand shifts in their relationships with their children and do their best to mitigate the pandemic's effects. As in the vignette, during the pandemic, parents and children spent a lot of time together due to the disruption of work, childcare, and school. Being together may support the development and strengthening of their attachment if parents remain calm and behave in a sensitive and responsive manner, as did Ann in the vignette. However, in other cases, the stress experienced by children due to the disruption of their childcare or school may make them more needy of attention than usual. The stresses experienced by parents due to the loss of a job or working from home may make them more impatient and less sensitive to the needs of their children. These changes may threaten the attachment of parent and child.

SOCIOCULTURAL THEORIES

Lev Vygotsky: Environmental Influences on Language and Thought

Like Piaget, Lev Vygotsky (1896–1934) was interested in the origin of knowledge and of reasoning skills, and like Bowlby he was interested in the effects of human relationships on development. From Vygotsky's perspective (Vygotsky, 1978) all aspects of human development are the result of interactions with more experienced others. Those interactions reflect cultural practices. In some cultures very little speech is directed toward young children, whereas in other cultures children are expected to take part in a conversation.

Learning through interaction with more experienced others (e.g., a parent, an older sibling, a teacher, a friend) starts in infancy and continues throughout development. The more experienced other helps a child to construct memories, solve a problem, notice aspects of the environment, or elaborate on verbal communication. To be effective, however, those acts of collaborative exchanges, which Vygotsky names "scaffolding," must be sensitive to what the child would find useful, given the child's abilities and interests. They must be in what Vygotsky termed "the zone of proximal development." The input contributes to the child's understanding only if the child can absorb the information and incorporate it into the repertoire of knowledge. When the child can do so, the child is said to have internalized the knowledge that was not available to the child before. These acts of internalizing new knowledge also occur without the help of others through living as part of a specific culture and observing others as they live their lives, and express the value they place on different activities and goals. But Vygotsky chose to focus primarily on the social interchanges that promote development.

Another important focus of Vygotsky's theory pertains to the role of language in shaping the child's thinking. While thought and language emerge as independent human abilities, language, which expresses thoughts, comes to regulate first through its external expression but later through its becoming internalized and expressed in the child's mind. Early language is social but later is also internalized for self-regulation: In the course of conversations, others may issue directives such as "Don't" or "Get the ball." Eventually the child, tempted to engage in prohibited acts, may say to oneself, "Don't." This external, spoken speech later becomes the basis for representational thought. The speed with which this change from social speech to egocentric spoken speech to inner speech occurs depends on having conversational partners more mature than the child. They provide strategies and instruments for learning and problem solving; they also encourage vocabulary growth.

Reuven Feuerstein: Social Mediation of Cognition

Reuven Feuerstein's (1921–2014) theory and applied work focus on the malleability of children's cognition and intelligence at every developmental stage. Feuerstein et al. (1980) theorized that cognitive development is the product of two modalities of interaction between the organism and the environment. The first is the individual's direct exposure to the environment. This exposure produces changes in the person's behavioral repertoire and cognition, which in turn affects how the individual will interact with the environment. This modality of learning is consistent with the formulations of Piaget and of learning theorists. The second modality is mediated learning experience (MLE), which refers to how environmental stimuli are transformed by a "mediating" agent—usually a parent, a sibling, or a caregiver. The mediating agent's actions are guided by personal intentions, culture, and emotional investment. The mediator highlights for the recipient of MLE (usually a child) stimuli that the mediator thinks of as most important and appropriate. The mediator frames, filters, and schedules their presentation. Thus the mediator influences what the child attends to and gets from the environment. As a result of mediation, the child acquires behavior patterns and learning sets that influence what the child learns through direct exposure. Feuerstein argues that the more and the earlier a child is subjected to MLE, the greater will be the child's capacity to efficiently use and be affected by direct exposure to the environment. MLE is the ingredient that determines differential cognitive development in similarly endowed individuals even when they live in similar environments. Through MLE children learn approaches to mentally organizing, manipulating, and acting upon information gained from external and internal sources.

Feuerstein distinguishes between two groups of determinants of differential cognitive development. The first group of determinants includes genetic factors, the level of environmental stimulation, emotional relationships between child and the mediators, and socioeconomic status. Under unfavorable conditions these determinants interfere with cognitive development. The second group of determinants consists of either lack of or reduced exposure to MLE. Such reduction interferes with cognitive development because the guidance that mediating agents provide regarding the relative importance of sources of information, the classification of stimuli, or their organization is lost. Feuerstein argues that determinants associated with the first group may affect the availability or quality of MLE. When they do, they indirectly affect the child's opportunity to develop cognitive skills. Determinants from the first group may trigger the second group determinants and lead to cognitive developmental issues. However, if the barriers obstructing mediation are removed or bypassed, then it is possible to avert the expected course of impeded development and to restore a typical pattern of cognitive growth. Consequently,

Feuerstein developed a successful intervention program designed to teach children cognitive skills that will enable them to be effective learners and problem solvers.

Urie Bronfenbrenner: Direct and Indirect Environmental Influences

Urie Bronfenbrenner (1917–2005) expanded on the description of the environment that the growing child experiences both directly and indirectly (Bronfenbrenner & Morris, 2006). He postulated five levels of environmental influences. The most immediate is the microsystem, consisting of social environments that the child experiences directly, such as the family, peers, and school. The microsystem is embedded in the mesosystem, the interlinked system of microsystems in which a person participates (e.g., the parent-teacher association, which links the family and school). The next level is the exosystem, which includes neighbors, social and mass media, social services, industry, and local politics. These influence the people who influence the child. Further out is the macrosystem, the attitudes and beliefs of the culture. All these systems are embedded in a historical context called the chronosystem. These levels of the environment form a network of connections, and the individual is at its center potentially influencing children as they actively seek to adapt to their world.

Ann Masten: Resilience in Adverse Environmental Circumstances

Recent ideas about human positive adaptation to adversity explicate the processes and developmental consequences of the intricate interdependence of individual characteristics and environmental conditions. Psychologists have been intrigued that some children who grow under adverse conditions manage to thrive (see Chapter 2). It was initially believed that these children were invulnerable and that understanding their success will help with interventions for other children who were adversely affected by their challenging circumstances. However, accumulating research by Ann Masten (1951-) revealed that resilience only partly resides in the individual (2001). One cannot understand resilience without considering the characteristics of both the individual and the circumstances in which the individual develops. Consequently, understanding resilience requires examining both the individual's response to adversity and the nature of the adversity itself. The adversity may be acute (e.g., death or natural disaster) or chronic (e.g., abuse, poverty, or separation from a parent). Adversity can also vary in scope or scale (affecting an individual, a family unit, or a community). Individuals will differ in the extent to which they are exposed to or protected from the adverse experience. Finally, adverse experiences may have both biologic and behavioral effects.

The effects of adverse experiences can be evaluated with respect to expected achievements or developmental tasks for children of different ages or stages of development. Some of these achievements are considered universal, such as walking, talking, or reaching cognitive stages (defined by Piaget) or moral stages (defined by Kohlberg). Other achievements are culture specific, such as learning to weave in Mayan culture.

Masten argues that resilience is "ordinary magic" that develops under most circumstances and involves the coming together of internal and external strengths. Children's resilience develops in multiple contexts, including the individual, family, school, and culture. The predictors of resilience that are embedded in the child and are closely related to the family context include secure attachment relationships, social skills, self-regulation, mastery motivation, cognitive abilities, hopefulness, and meaning making (National Academies of Sciences, Engineering, and Medicine, 2019). Self-regulation (the ability to monitor one's behavior, attention, thought, and emotions) is an important element of resilience. Children who are good at self-regulating have less emotional and behavioral problems and are better at adapting to the demands of school. Mastery motivation is another key element of resilience. Feelings of mastery develop as a consequence of successful interaction with one's environment. This adaptational system is associated with the development of self-efficacy and possibly persistence. Higher cognitive ability is believed to be linked to flexible problem solving, the ability to navigate in novel situations, and to succeed in school. Consequently cognitive abilities are considered both promotive and protective resilience factors in childhood and adolescence. Finally, based on observations of resilient children and anecdotal accounts, hopefulness and positive meaning making may also be associated with resilience.

The environmental conditions associated with resilience are conceptualized in terms of being either positive assets or challenges or risks. Examples of parental positive assets are sensitive, responsive, loving, predictable, and protective parenting and caregiving. These are linked to the development of secure attachment and indirectly to resilience. Likewise, effective parents who teach social skills, provide safety, set limits, establish routines, monitor children's behavior, and help children make meaning are also supporting resilience in their children. When parents are not supportive in the abovementioned ways, their children's resilience and development may be impeded, especially when no other people in the child's environment step in to support the child. Given the multiplicity of factors that influence resilience, recent research has focused on identifying different patterns over time of reacting to adversity, some more rapid and some more successful than others.

General Implications of Sociocultural Theories During the COVID-19 Pandemic

The theories discussed in this section alone and in combination offer insights into the profound impact of the COVID-19 pandemic. The pandemic impacted microsystems, mesosystems, and exosystems of children and their families. In the vignette recognizing the interacting threats, parents Ann and Ben reassigned roles and responsibilities, thereby resetting the microsystem. Their willingness and ability to support the children led to positive impacts, particularly on David when Ann quit work to better meet his needs. The theories can help parents, educators, and clinicians understand that to thrive physically, emotionally, cognitively, and socially, children depend on supportive individuals, institutions, and culture to make challenges comprehensible and manageable.

MULTISYSTEM PROBABILISTIC PHASE TRANSITIONS

Dynamic Systems Theory

One of the newest approaches to development is the dynamic systems theory. In their analysis of DST Newman and Newman (2020) highlight the theoretical claim that the processes that may account for behavioral change (e.g., genetic potential, neurologic processes, physical characteristics, family structure, personal goals and motives) are intertwined, not independent causal factors. Development is the outcome of interaction of processes at many levels and many systems. Development is shaped by forces within and outside the person, merging and influencing each other to produce new capacities and behaviors. Development emerges as a result of moment-by-moment actions at many levels at once and does not follow a set universal plan.

DST has roots in several fields, including mathematics, astronomy, physics, meteorology, and biology. In the field of human development DST has been applied to the analysis of the development of infant stepping and walking, cognitive development, executive function, infant language, emotion and personality development, moral development, temperament, and developmental psychopathology. These applications are based on the expectation that DST can lead to an accurate and detailed analysis of points or periods in development when there is change. DST also provides the methods for discovering the individual characteristics that are especially sensitive to particular environmental features that result in the emergence of new and enhanced capacities for adaptation.

The core of the theory rests on the definition of systems. All systems (biologic and social) are composed of interdependent elements that share interrelated functions, boundaries, goals, and identity. A dynamic system continuously changes to carry out its functions in a way that maintains the smooth interaction among its components, thereby preserving equilibrium. The elements influence each other and change one another over time. Understanding development requires considering moment-by-moment events and their interplay with changing individual characteristics. It requires tracing a pathway from one point in time to a later point when a new, more mature behavior emerges. This requires a detailed analysis of multiple aspects of behavior and an investigation of the process of reorganization and growth. The theory helps specify the properties of systems that are in flux (open systems) and how feedback acts to regulate change.

In DST developmental changes are referred to as phase transitions. A prerequisite for such transitions is the presence of natural variability in the system, caused by changes in the environment and growth within the individual. Variability within systems or subsystems occurs all the time and can be observed on different timelines, from the fastest and most frequent at the neural and cellular level to the slowest processes required, such as for the maturing of effective decision making. The emergence of new pathways or patterns is possible only when the system's variability already includes the potential for change. Phase transitions are usually preceded by a temporary increase in variability, which allows old patterns to be modified or replaced. Developmental changes cannot be fully predicted because the emergence of some patterns rather than others depends on many factors. Human beings are always in interaction with a changing environment. Moment-by-moment interactions with the environment are influenced by concurrent events and memories of what occurred previously on the motor, sensory, spatial, or communication level. Humans have a variety of strategies for obtaining information about the environment at different experiential levels so that the emergence of qualitatively new behavior is the result of all interactions over time. Small differences in the early phases of an emergent process can have consequences that result in later large differences or effects. Any small change causes changes throughout the system. The accumulation of small quantitative changes can lead to qualitative change (emergence) as one or a number of related skills pass a threshold and contribute to the integration of what seems to be a qualitatively different skill. For that reason, DST considers developmental processes as probabilistic rather than predetermined.

Systems engage in a process of adaptive self-organization. When a system cannot assimilate new information or buffer its subsystems from changes in the environment, new subsystem relationships or functions emerge. These interactions help us to understand developmental change. For most humans, the result of self-organization is an increasingly flexible, efficient way of functioning. However, the new organization may not be effective because, for example, it cannot be sustained by lower-level components and it requires more energy or resources than available. When that occurs, the system may interfere with the functioning and interaction among other systems or subsystems. That in turn may interfere with daily life or social functioning.

Implications of the COVID-10 Pandemic

DST suggests that we are limited in our ability to determine in advance how the challenges of growing up during the COVID-19 pandemic will affect different children of different ages who live in distinctive family environments and communities, which are differentially supportive. However, the theory suggests that developmental progress will inevitably be changed by such a profound environmental factor. Understanding of the effects of the pandemic, therefore, depends on multiple elements and the nature of their interactions. This theoretical approach calls attention to the need to examine how each individual and the institutions in one's specific environment respond to change and what forces reestablish equilibrium.

In the initial vignette after the pandemic disrupted the family, the parents' willingness to shift roles and responsibilities allowed the family to return to a new state of equilibrium.

CONCLUSION

In this chapter we introduced the reader to selected influential theories of human development that have guided research and informed public opinion, interventions, and policies pertaining to human development. We discussed these theories in relation to the COVID-19 pandemic to demonstrate the potential of the theories to inform, explain, and guide during the period of profound environmental stress. These theories have made major contributions to other societal issues. Bowlby's theory of human attachment initially powered the public debate about the nature of childcare. In the period from 2016 to 2021 this same theory provided a theoretical underpinning for the public outcry about the separation of migrant children from their parents among families who entered the United States illegally. Vygotsky's and Feuerstein's theories of the mediation of cognitive development have served as a foundation for educational reform, stimulating the use social and language interventions to improve the education of children. Masten's theory of resilience is particularly relevant for parents, pediatricians, and educators who wish to help children cope successfully with the COVID-19 pandemic. In our vignette we saw how parents Ann and Ben changed their approach to create positive assets to counteract the challenges of social isolation and online education. We hope that this discussion of developmental theories will assist parents, educators, clinicians, public health officers, and public officials to confront new challenges that arise in the future.

REFERENCES

Bronfenbrenner, U., & Morris, P. A. (2006). The bioecological model of human development. In W. Damon & R. M. Lerner (Eds.), *Handbook of child psychology: Vol. 1. Theoretical models of human development* (6th ed., pp. 793–828). Wiley.

Cassidy, J., & Shaver, P. R. (2018). *Handbook of attachment: Theory, research, and clinical applications* (3rd ed.). Guilford Press.

Feuerstein, R., Hoffman, M. B., & Miller, R. (1980). *Instrumental enrichment: An intervention program for cognitive modifiability*. University Park Press.

Forslund, T., Granqvist, P., Van IJzendoorn, M. H., Sagi-Schwartz, A., Glaser, D., Steele, M., & Duschinsky, R. (2021). Attachment goes to court: Child protection and custody issues. *Attachment & Human Development*, 1–52. https://doi.org/10.1080/14616734.2020.1840762.

Friedman, S. L., & Boyle, D. E. (2008). Attachment in U.S. children experiencing nonmaternal care in the early 1990s. *Attachment and Human Development*, *10*(3), 225–261.

Gilligan. C. (1982). *In a different voice: Psychological theory and women's development*. Harvard University Press.

Gruber, H. E., & Voneche, J. J. (1977). *The essential Piaget*. Basic Books Inc.

Kohlberg, L., & Hersh, R. H. (1977). *Moral development: A review of the theory*. Taylor & Francis.

Marvin, R. S., & Brittner, P. A. (1999). Normative development: The ontogeny of attachment. In J. Cassidy & P. R. Shaver (Eds.), *Handbook of attachment: Theory, research and clinical applications* (2nd ed., pp. 44–67). Guildford Press.

Masten. A. S. (2001). Ordinary magic: Resilience processes in development. *American Psychologist*, *56*(3), 227–238. https://doi.org/10.1037/0003-066X.56.3.227.

Miller. P. H. (2002). *Theories of developmental psychology* (5th ed.). Worth Publishers.

National Academies of Sciences, Engineering, and Medicine. (2019). *Strengthening the military family readiness system for a changing American society*. National Academies Press. https://doi.org/10.17226/25380.

Newman, B. M., & Newman, P. R. (2020). *Theories of adolescent development*. Elsevier Inc. https://doi.org/10.1016/C2017-0-03324-4.

Vygotsky. L. S. (1978). *Mind in society: The development of higher psychological processes*. Harvard University Press.

4

Theories of Learning and Behavior Change

Cy Nadler and A. Dawn Greathouse

For additional material related to the content of this chapter, please see Chapters 3 and 94.

VIGNETTE

Emma is a 3-year-old female with developmental delays who presents with her parents in primary care for her annual well-visit. The parents have ongoing concerns regarding her slow language development, coupled with frequent tantrums and rigidness. Emma continues to rely primarily on single words to communicate. When she is calm, she is social, affectionate, and engaging. Some days she is engaged in her speech and special educational programming, but frequently she refuses to sit. She cries, scratches, and falls to the floor when prompted to engage. Similar behavior problems occur at home during most daily routines. Today, the parents express frustration, discouragement, worry, and confusion: "Why isn't Emma making progress? How can we parent a child who isn't learning? Will she ever catch up?"

INTRODUCTION

Learning and behavior change are at the very heart of developmental and behavioral pediatrics. Whether clinicians are supporting children like Emma in the opening vignette, treating older youth with autism or mental health concerns, or managing any other challenge with implications for child health and wellbeing, clinicians from a wide range of disciplines and an even wider array of work settings are directly engaged in helping children develop skills, reach milestones, and move from relying on behaviors that are maladaptive to healthy interaction patterns. Pediatricians, psychologists, speech therapists, occupational therapists, educators, behavior analysts, social workers, and other clinicians are all in the "business of behavior change," though they likely conceptualize their methods quite differently. Individual children (and their parents, who are learning right along with them) require individualized applications of methods drawn from across the continuum of learning paradigms.

This chapter discusses how the major theoretical foundations conceptualize learning and behavior change, and how these paradigms directly inform the ways that clinicians facilitate prosocial development in children. Following the introduction of key concepts from each of the most relevant theoretical areas, we will return periodically to Emma and her family to explore how theories link directly to clinical application. Interventions mentioned in this chapter are described in more detail elsewhere in the volume, but embedding applied ideas here is intended to demonstrate to the reader that these concepts are in play at all times in pediatric clinical contexts whether we attend to them or not. We propose that having a strong foundational understanding of learning and behavior change will improve your practice, help you to adjust and expand intervention approaches, and inevitably improve the outcomes of the children and families you serve.

CLASSICAL CONDITIONING

Behavioral learning theory began with Pavlov's famous work describing *classical conditioning* processes (Michael, 2004). He demonstrated that biologically driven unconditioned responses (or reflexes; UR), such as pupillary dilation and the salivary reflex are naturally elicited by unconditioned stimuli (US) in the environment, and that these relationships can be extended through repeated pairings to a previously neutral stimulus (NS) that does not yet elicit any type of response (Fig. 4.1). This associative learning mechanism (also sometimes referred to as respondent or Pavlovian conditioning) is considered a foundational learning process. Extensions of classical conditioning proposed later by John Watson suggested that emotions, speech, thoughts, and even personalities might be conceptualized as the result of interrelated stimuli and responses unique to an individual's learning history. His work also laid the foundation for understanding how psychopathology might develop through disadvantageous pairings. His infamous "Little Albert" experiment paired a loud noise (US) with a white rabbit (NS) to yield a conditioned response (CR) of crying that serves as an experimental model for the development of childhood phobias.

Ensuing empirical work identified that not all stimuli pairings are created equal. Learning through associations is impacted by several parameters. Stimulus contiguity describes the latency between the presentation of the NS and the US; the shorter the interstimulus interval, the stronger the ensuing association. Of note, stimuli can be paired simultaneously, with slight delays, and even in different orders (e.g., NS followed by US, or US followed by NS) to yield an association. Contingency is also relevant to the development and strength of association, such that the probability of the occurrence of one stimulus is high given the occurrence of the other *prior*

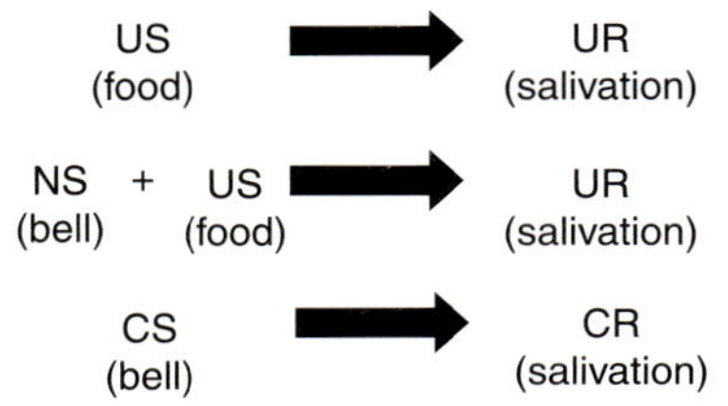

Fig. 4.1 Classical conditioning is the process of pairing an unconditional stimulus (*US*, which produces an unconditioned response *[UR]*) with a neutral stimulus *(NS)* that ultimately elicits a conditioned response *(CR)*. *CS*, Conditioned stimulus. Adapted from Cooper et al. (2007). *Applied behavior analysis* (2nd ed.). Pearson.

to the emission of the UR (i.e., a loud noise will not be successfully paired with a light cue if the rat's fear response occurs before the light turns on). Preparedness also impacts association, where biologic readiness facilitates some associations more than others (e.g., it is evolutionarily adaptive for a single pairing of a novel food with nausea to generate an association). Associations learned through classical conditioning can be unpaired through a learning process called extinction (note that a distinct process also called extinction occurs in the operant learning paradigm described later). If the conditioned stimulus (CS) or US is repeatedly presented alone, the strength of their relationship decreases, and the strength of the CS in eliciting the CR decreases. Spontaneous recovery is the reemergence of a CR after extinction has occurred and might be observed intermittently despite the lack of continued association between the US and CS.

Research on classical conditioning focuses primarily on very specific (and at times reductionist) demonstrations that can be experimentally tested. The extent to which the paradigm can be used to explain complex human learning is less clear, but the processes of classical conditioning absolutely serve as a foundation for essentially all the learning theories that follow.

Emma's parents report that she cries whenever they try to bring her into a public restroom. Upon discussion, her mother notes that on a few occasions Emma has been quite startled by the loud automatic flush of a toilet in these settings. A few pairings of the loud flush (US) with the public bathroom (NS) were enough to generate a conditioned fear response. The family is reluctant to attempt to extinguish her conditioned response because it will require frequent trips to public bathrooms; brainstorming with the family might generate strategies such as using noise-canceling headphones during trips to ensure she is not exposed to the full volume of the flush or providing access to an electronic tablet during the trip (creating a new, positive association) and afterwards (creating an operant contingency, described later).

OPERANT CONDITIONING

Operant conditioning, based on seminal work by B.F. Skinner, expands on the classical conditioning models described earlier by providing a paradigm to describe much broader interrelationships between behavior and environmental events, as well as how to predict and alter these relationships. Operant conditioning is the process by which contingencies between stimuli in the environment (antecedents), behaviors, and subsequent effects (consequences) are learned, as evidenced by the subsequent change in likelihood that those behaviors occur under similar circumstances in the future (Cooper, Heron, & Heward, 2007). These relationships are conceptualized as a three-term contingency (as well as the antecedent-behavio-consequence [ABC]) model. Antecedents set the stage and conditions, and even trigger behavioral sequences; operant models then describe the antecedent as a discriminative stimulus because it specifically signals the presence of the previously learned behavioral contingency. As an example from an experimental paradigm, a pigeon might learn that when the cage light turns on, pecking the lever will release a food pellet. Since the lever does nothing when the light is off and the pigeon only pecks it when the light turns on, the pecking behavior is under the stimulus control of the light. The consequence in the ABC model simply implies that this stimulus is an effect of the behavior, and it does not imply whether the consequence is favorable or not. As indicated in Fig. 4.2, consequences that increase the probability of that behavior being emitted again under the same antecedent conditions are said to have reinforced that behavior, and consequences that decrease the probability of the behavior occurring are said to have punished that behavior. Modifiers of positive and negative (which also carry no implication of the consequence being favorable or not) describe whether the consequence involved the addition or removal of a stimulus. Parents, teachers, and even doctoral level clinicians all routinely misuse these terms when discussing operant processes; in applied contexts it is far more important to emphasize whether the intention is to make a behavior happen more often (e.g., compliance, correct responses on a math worksheet, urinating in the toilet) or less often (e.g., aggression, self-injury, school truancy). Extended discussion of punishment is beyond the scope of this chapter because learning (the increase of a behavior or skill) is, by definition, a reinforcement-based process.

From an operant perspective, questions about how to provide reinforcement for a behavior are central to learning. Four broad categories of reinforcement encompass all possible consequences delivered following a behavior: attention (e.g., praise, affection, and other forms of social interaction), tangibles (e.g., access to toys, foods, activities, privileges), escape/avoidance (the avoidance and delay of work or academic demands, pain/discomfort, and other undesired experiences),

	Positive *(added)*	Negative *(removed)*
Reinforcement *(increases behavior)*	*Providing* something desired following a behavior *increases* the likelihood of the behavior happening again.	*Removing* something aversive following a behavior *increases* the likelihood of the behavior happening again.
Punishment *(decreases behavior)*	*Providing* something aversive following a behavior *decreases* the likelihood of the behavior happening again.	*Removing* something aversive following a behavior *increases* the likelihood of the behavior happening again.

Fig. 4.2 Definitions of reinforcement and punishment in operant conditioning.

and automatic (including internal sensory experiences and other outcomes that are not mediated by other people). Note that simply delivering praise or tablet following a child's successful demonstration of a new skill may or may not reinforce that behavior (increase the likelihood that the behavior occurs again); whether or not the stimulus functions as a reinforcer depends on many factors, including individual preferences as well as fluctuating and relative reinforcer values (much like commodities in the stock market).

Presuming that a high-value reinforcer is available, when and how often reinforcement is delivered following a target behavior will directly impact the rate and frequency that the behavior occurs in the future. *Reinforcement schedules* describe these parameters. Continuous reinforcement describes a schedule where reinforcement is delivered following each instance of the desired behavior, and this consistency is ideal for supporting the development of a skill; that said, it is quite arduous to maintain. Noncontinuous schedules are described as intermittent reinforcement. Fig. 4.3 presents how four variations on these schedules of reinforcement delivery (denoted by the black tick marks) affect the rate of behavioral response. Fixed-ratio schedules describe reinforcement delivery following a set number of responses (e.g., "once you have done 5 math problems, you can take a break"); this produces a high response rate followed by a pause after reinforcement. Variable-ratio schedules involve reinforcement delivery after a variable number of responses with a set mean (i.e., a slot machine that pays out once every 100 pulls, on average); this produces a high and steady response rate. Schedules can also be based on time rather than number of responses. Fixed-interval approaches (i.e., providing a break every 30 minutes, regardless of how much work got done) and variable-interval approaches (i.e., praising a child for playing quietly every 5 minutes on average, with both longer and shorter intervals between praising) produce moderate but steady response rates and are more sustainable to keep up than ratio schedules.

The target response requirements to produce reinforcement can also be adjusted to accelerate learning and behavior change. *Shaping* is the process of delivering reinforcement for a behavior that is already in the individual's repertoire (i.e., providing tablet access for wearing new glasses for 30 seconds without taking them off); once that behavior is strengthened, the behavioral requirement is incrementally increased over time and repeated successful trials (e.g., keeping the glasses on for 60 seconds, then 2 minutes, then 5 minutes, and so on) until the intended target is reached. Another mechanism for accelerating change is the use of *prompting*; this antecedent-focused strategy may involve the establishment of a new, clear discriminative stimulus so that the individual is more aware of the available contingencies. This approach may include coaching parents to deliver a clear "Pick up the block" instruction rather than vague "Can you help mommy clean up?" questions, the addition of a gesture indicating what to do and how to do it, and even physical hand-over-hand guidance to eliminate any ambiguity regarding what behavior is expected. Prompt fading, the gradual removal of artificial antecedent stimuli once the target behavior is established, will ensure that the individual does not become overly reliant on this support (prompt dependent).

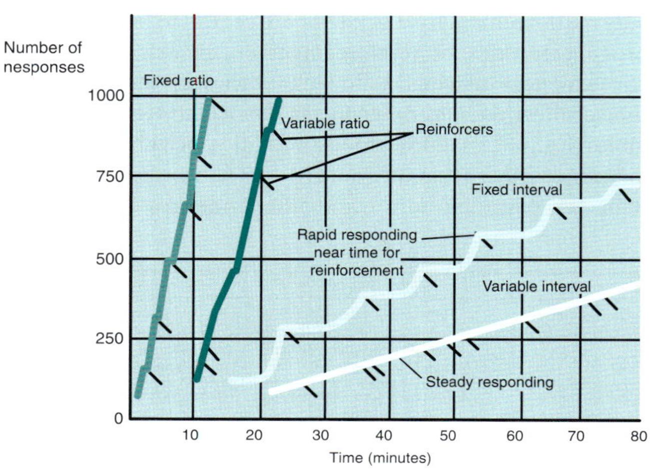

Fig. 4.3 Variations in the rate of behavioral response as a function of the schedule of reinforcement delivery. Adapted from Cooper et al. (2007). *Applied behavior analysis* (2nd ed.). Pearson.

Not infrequently, undesired behaviors are unintentionally prompted, reinforced, and shaped by environmental contingencies (e.g., a child who has inadvertently learned that a certain four-letter word generates continuous high-value attention from surrounding adults, especially under the stimulus control of grandma). Rather than attempting to change this behavior by adding even more attention to the mix (scolding, explanations, arguing, etc.), the family can instead focus on removing or withholding reinforcement following the target behavior. The process of removing or withholding reinforcement from a behavioral contingency is called *extinction* (and also accurately conceptualized as negative punishment, since it is a behavior-reduction technique). Often referred to as planned ignoring in cases when attention is the reinforcer, the speed with which extinction effectively suppresses the behavior depends on the strength of the behavior, the individual's learning history, and the fidelity of application (i.e., mostly ignoring but occasional responding is equivalent to a variable schedule, which is quite reinforcing). Even perfect application of extinction will likely be followed by an extinction burst. As shown in Fig. 4.4, a steady rate of behavioral responding immediately increases when the reinforcement is discontinued, and the response rate only diminishes over time. A known limitation to clinical procedures (e.g., planned ignoring) that rely on an extinction process is the results are often temporary, with the punished behavior likely to reappear once the punishment procedure is withdrawn (spontaneous recovery). To mitigate this, extinction might be augmented with a simultaneous reinforcement-based plan where an alternative behavior is intentionally reinforced at a high rate (i.e., teaching the child to say "I love you!" to grandma instead of using inappropriate words to get her attention).

The entire field of applied behavior analysis (often used in the treatment of children with autism; see Chapter 94) is almost exclusively based on the basic operant processes of learning and behavior change described here, along with complex iterations and extensions of these concepts (including a

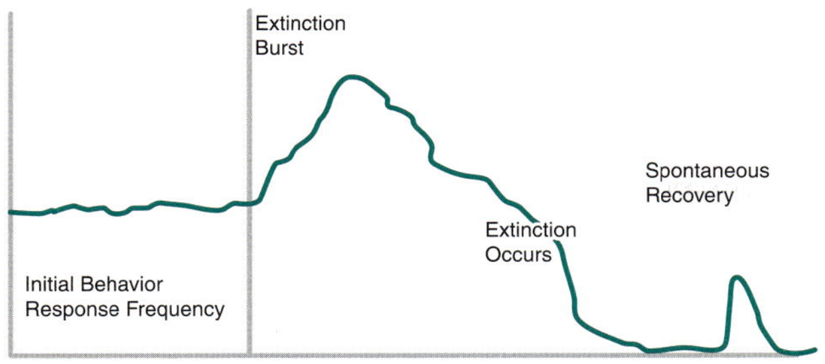

Fig. 4.4 Rate of behavior after reinforcement delivery is discontinued. Adapted from Cooper et al. (2007). *Applied behavior analysis* (2nd ed.). Pearson.

whole branch devoted to applying these ideas to verbal behavior and language development). That said, operant paradigms become more difficult to test (and often less useful in applied settings) when the behaviors of interest are complex, difficult to measure, or impossible to observe directly.

> After trying many discipline approaches, Emma's parents have concluded that she simply does not understand consequences. They most often use verbal scolding and explanations in response to her aggression ("No! That hurts! You hurt daddy! Not nice."). When Emma screams as the parents start to remove the tablet from her hands, they sometimes allow her to continue to have it at least for another minute. Therefore Emma appears quite adept at detecting the operant contingencies; moreover, the intermittent success she experiences has strengthened her repertoire. Even her scream has been shaped to peak effectiveness, as the aversiveness of the high pitch results in her parents relenting almost immediately. With support from the care team, Emma's parents gradually increase their awareness that Emma is in fact learning all of the time from (sometimes unintentional) teaching, and that the current patterns hold clues for how to help her develop new habits. The team can also prepare the parents to anticipate the extinction burst process after they adopt a consistent, function-based approach.

SOCIAL LEARNING THEORIES

As relevant as the classical and operant conditioning paradigms of behaviorism are for contemporary perspectives on learning and behavior change, much of their influence is felt through the lens of *social learning theories* that emerged as behaviorism evolved in response to the cognitive science revolution (and even psychoanalytic perspectives) of the 1960s and 1970s. While there was no doubt that changes in the environment could reinforce and shape behavior, criticism that all learning could not be explained by the immediate external environment challenged researchers and clinicians to consider what processes might mediate behavior change (Grusec, 1992). Concepts from both social learning theory (emphasizing observational learning processes) and the related social cognitive learning theory (integrating covert, cognitive processes) are both discussed here.

Observational learning is an umbrella term that encompasses processes in which an individual's behavior may change (including the development of new skills and a change in the application of an existing repertoire) as a function of observing the behaviors of others and the ensuing environmental consequences. Simply put, we can learn from the example of others without directly experiencing their example (i.e., without contacting the reinforcers or punishers that influence the behavior of the other person). To that end, *modeling* (the demonstration of a behavior) can inspire imitation of that same behavior. This mechanism has obvious implications for how learning and behavior change in children (and adults, for that matter) may be influenced on a moment-to-moment basis simply by being in the presence of others, whether or not the available models intend to be trying to inspire imitation. Bandura's classic "Bobo doll" experiments demonstrated that externally delivered reinforcement was unnecessary for children to imitate adult models, challenging foundations of operant assumptions. Even verbally mediated models (i.e., a verbal description of a behavior) can inspire imitation. While the imitation of a behavior may be subsequently reinforced by external contingencies once it is performed, intrinsic or self-reinforcement (or—to use behavior analytic language—automatic reinforcement; see Chapter 94) can both evoke and sustain behavioral patterns. *Modeling* is most effective at influencing behavior change when the models are highly salient, when the observer can retain the information cognitively and/or practice it through rehearsal, and when environmental contingencies (e.g., reinforcement) are aligned with the behavior. These parameters inform why children are more likely to imitate some behaviors than others and how interventionists can maximize the likelihood that observational learning processes support the advancement of adaptive behaviors. Note that observational learning can also support changes involving the reduction of behaviors (e.g., observing a classmate get reprimanded for leaving the playground during recess may vicariously discourage other children from following suit).

The cognitive processes that support observational learning have broad implications for learning and behavior change. Specifically, social learning perspectives expand on behavioral conceptualizations that we are products of our environments to describe how individuals also actively select and influence their own environments, which in turn influence their behavior. Self-efficacy is the degree to which you believe you can influence your environment, suggesting that having low and high self-efficacy in a situation would mediate the extent to which behaviors intended to change the environment would be pursued or practiced, what goals a person might select, and how much effort or persistence they apply toward their goals. The extent to which individuals are able to monitor their own behavior, evaluate contingencies, and engage in goal-directed behaviors is termed self-regulation, which in and of itself likely supports learning through a variety of pathways.

Social learning theories are perhaps most prominent in the decades of research on the psychosocial etiologies of and treatments for externalizing behavior disorders in children, advanced in large part by researchers at the Oregon Social Learning Center (Patterson, 1982). While parent behaviors unambiguously influence child learning and behavior, strong conceptual models as well as longitudinal analyses confirm that child behavioral patterns also influence the behaviors of their parents (see Chapter 2). Specifically, inconsistent and indiscriminate parental use of discipline increases child irritability; independently, child irritability also increases inconsistent parent discipline (Lengua & Kovacs, 2005). These bidirectional interactions are termed *coercive processes* because both children and parents learn (through direct operant as well as observational learning mechanisms) that hostile strategies can be at least temporarily effective at influencing the other party's behavior (see Chapter 93 for an extended discussion). This cycle has the potential to repeat and expand exponentially, and the cognitive components of social learning theory effectively explain how chronic negative interaction patterns in childhood set the occasion for very specific beliefs about social interaction (e.g., attributing blame to others, feeling justified in engaging in antisocial behaviors, and characteristics of oppositional defiant disorder; see Chapter 55). The final major implication is that learning and behavior are potentially influenced by a child's broader context, including neighborhood (Chapter 19), culture (Chapter 20), and media exposure (Chapter 21). While some social exposures have well-documented psychosocial consequences (e.g., adverse childhood experiences; see Chapter 15), others (like violent videogames) have not been consistently supported by research.

In Emma's case social learning is most relevant when considering the bidirectional influences that she and her parents have on each other's behavior. Her stubbornness and irritability have very likely occasioned her parents to deviate from management strategies they may have preferred to use. Her parents have implicitly discovered that high-salience strategies like yelling or spanking result in brief but highly reinforcing reductions in Emma's problem behaviors, which in turn serve as models for Emma to imitate (yelling and hitting back at them). Evidence-based strategies (see Chapter 93) explicitly seek to interrupt these coercive interaction patterns.

COGNITIVE AND CONSTRUCTIVIST PERSPECTIVES

If learning occurred solely through associations and reinforcement (as early iterations of behavioral theories proposed), simple repetition would be sufficient for teaching skills and changing behavior. While direct instruction approaches are effective for building content knowledge and shaping foundational skills (e.g., discrete trial teaching; see Chapter 94), teaching complex ideas that learners can apply flexibly and creatively becomes difficult to conceptualize using behavioral terms alone. Cognitive mechanisms that describe how humans "construct" meaning and process information extend traditional behavioral approaches. Here we focus on the implications of these perspectives for learning and behavior change.

Cognitive conflict is one of the postulated learning mechanisms offered by Piaget (see Chapter 3) to explain how children acquire new knowledge and behaviors (Palincsar, 1998). This fundamentally social process occurs when an individual's experiences contradict their existing knowledge, forcing a change in understanding and even behavior to resolve the discrepancy. While data are mixed, theory suggests that the relative developmental levels of a child and their interaction partners matter for acquisition, such that children at similar levels might be more likely to engage and coconstruct new knowledge; these ideas underly child-centered learning environments that facilitate creative interaction and exploration among peers. Vygotsky (see Chapter 3) extended these ideas to further describe how a child's *zone of proximal development* (i.e., what a child can accomplish with scaffolding or collaboration with others, rather than just what the child can accomplish alone) is the best indicator of the child's cognitive abilities. These constructs link learning, previously viewed as an externally driven process, with the internal process of development. Teaching, then, is ideally targeted to the outer extensions of a child's zone of proximal development; practically speaking, cognitive approaches might function in the same way as behavioral shaping (reinforcement of gradually more difficult behaviors) and prompting to increase the probability of the desired response.

Cognitive, social, and personality psychology research has also described mechanisms for how acquired information is integrated and influences behavior (Dodge & Crick, 1990). Cognitive heuristics, often described as mental shortcuts or rules that allow individuals to rapidly apply knowledge to situations, can be developed through experience, including observation, teaching, and coconstruction. Relatedly, cognitive schemas are networks built through experience, association, and other cognitive mechanisms to organize information. Extensions of these ideas to applied areas give rise to concepts such as attribution biases, where an individual's learning history produces a tendency to interpret new information in a specific way and to behave accordingly (e.g., chronic social conflict with others giving rise to the assumption that individuals encountered in the future will have those same hostile intentions). The availability of information in memory (as a function of how frequently it is accessed and rehearsed) has implications for what social cues in the environment are most salient and likely to elicit behavioral responses, as well as how an individual predicts the behaviors of others. Such concepts have been integrated frequently into treatments for antisocial behaviors in youth who have developed cognitive justifications for their actions (see Chapter 55), and evidence suggests correlations between changes in information processing and behavioral improvements.

The fundamental ideas that information storage, organization, and retrieval/application mechanisms have implications for learning and behavior continue to be extended. Contemporary artificial intelligence and computer science research use connectionist models of human cognition and learning, including child development and psychopathology (Stein & Ludik, 1998). Reminiscent of classical conditioning models where repeated pairings link unconditioned and conditioned stimuli (not to mention Hebbian learning at the synaptic level), connectionist models use artificial neural networks to study complex information processing. While operant models require an individual to receive performance feedback (reinforcement or punishment) for the experience to impact future behavior, these models use supervised learning where an existing information set and a desired output can train an internal algorithm (i.e., learn how to produce the desired output) based on the degree of error produced through repeated trials. Systematic adjustment of how every available parameter is weighted in the algorithm provides internal (vs. external) feedback. In contrast, unsupervised learning is atheoretical, allowing the relationships within a data set to drive clustering and categorization of information without external influence. While direct links to neuroscience and behavioral processes remain theoretical, these learning paradigms serve as important models for human information processing.

> Emma's special education teacher closely monitors her abilities and how much she can accomplish with varying degrees of scaffolding. Her individualized education plan goals (e.g., sorting colors correctly in the presence of a model with 80% accuracy) specify the degree of support she will be extended, and as Emma meets her goals the expectation as well as the scaffolding itself can be systematically adjusted. Emma's speech therapist has coached the family on using a consistent combination of stimuli (picture schedule, gestures, and verbal repetition) during daily routines to help Emma connect this information with the activity. Over time, modeling and rehearsal of verbal routines ("ready, set, go!") will help Emma anticipate, participate, request, and complete actions independently. These verbal routines also strengthen the connections among the single words she is already using functionally, which will help her gradually increase the complexity of her verbal output.

EXTENSIONS AND CONTEMPORARY APPLICATIONS

The learning theories described earlier are used to support developmental psychopathology research and intervention approaches in the education arena, mental health care, and across the spectrum of developmental and behavioral pediatrics. Selected critical applications are described here and elaborated in other chapters.

Education

Educational contexts (see Chapters 103 and 104) are perhaps the most obvious venue for considering learning and behavior change applications. Early care and education, early intervention, childhood special education programs, preschools, and primary and secondary schools are all tasked with teaching skills and managing behavior. As a whole, public educational programs rely on an eclectic combination of the theoretical frameworks shared here. Virtually all educators employ foundational operant strategies such as differential reinforcement, shaping, and prompting/prompt fading to encourage skill development; many special education programs use peer models and other inclusion models to foster observational learning. However, the extent to which individual educators and programs adopt an entirely behavioral approach is highly variable. There is even tension at times between behavioral and cognitive/constructivist educational frameworks (Steele, 2005). Data-based comparisons evaluating which methods are most effective for specific student populations and learning objectives exist in only a minority of cases (e.g., Poncy, McCallum, & Schmitt, 2010). Schools vary in terms of how they implement evidence-based practices, allocate resources, and monitor academic and behavioral outcomes; at least part of this variability reflects underlying differences in perspective on how students learn (Ball & Trammell, 2011; Noltemeyer, Palmer, James, & Petrasek, 2019).

Cognitive-Behavioral Therapy

Cognitive-behavioral therapy approaches for youth and adults experiencing a variety of mental health conditions incorporate classical, operant, social learning, and constructivist mechanisms to facilitate learning and behavior change (Benjamin et al., 2011). As detailed in Chapter 98, cognitive-behavioral therapy relies on a tripartite model where behavioral, cognitive, and emotional/affective manifestations interact in mental health conditions, and each aspect of the condition can be targeted in therapy. For example, youth with depression may experience cognitive symptoms that include negative beliefs and appraisals about themselves and their ability to improve their situation in life (termed *cognitive distortions*, and conceptually linked to learned helplessness and low self-efficacy described in social learning theories). These cognitive symptoms might be addressed through cognitive restructuring approaches, where the therapist coaches the youth to engage in reappraisal of overly negative perceptions and identify errors in thinking to build self-efficacy. Behavioral manifestations of depression, such as withdrawing from participation in routines, might be addressed through operant approaches that reestablish structure (e.g., go to soccer practice even if you don't think you will enjoy it) via behavioral activation involving prompts and shaping to help individuals recontact naturally occurring sources of positive reinforcement in their daily lives. Emotional and affective symptoms (e.g., depressed mood, loss of enjoyment) might be further targeted by the reintroduction of stimuli previously associated with positive emotions (listening to a favorite song, looking at photos from a treasured experience, etc.).

Health Care Contexts

Health care certainly focuses on biologically oriented aspects of child development and wellbeing; however, learning and behavioral factors have significant implications for health along with several parameters. Particularly when parents serve as the primary care managers for youth with developmental disabilities and/or mental health concerns, consideration of the with social contingencies and the cognitive factors that facilitate and impede proactive participation in health care is critical. Behavioral, cognitive, and social learning foundations led to the development of the health belief model (Fig. 4.5) (Champion & Skinner, 2008), an ABC-based framework for describing why individuals take steps to prevent, identify, and manage chronic conditions. Cognitive-behavioral models have been applied to enhance parent motivation and positive beliefs regarding mental health services (Chacko et al., 2016). Even models for shared decision making that facilitate collaborative problem solving between families and providers draw on integrated learning frameworks (Adams & Levy, 2017). The *transtheoretical model* (TTM; Prochaska, Redding, & Evers, 2008), as the name implies, intentionally integrates broad perspectives on learning to guide intervention for health and behavior problems. Supported by substantial evidence across a range of targets, TTM engages evidence-based behavioral mechanisms (e.g., stimulus control, reinforcement management, counterconditioning) and cognitive approaches (e.g., consciousness raising, self and social liberation) to move individuals through stages of change toward readiness to fully engage in treatment.

> Emma has wide-ranging needs that will require continuous advocacy and engagement. This is a tall order for already-stressed parents who have conveyed a sense of confusion and helplessness regarding how to proceed in their child's care. The team might employ strategies to explore their beliefs about Emma's current needs, what the family perceives as barriers, and their level of confidence that these barriers can be navigated. Clinicians may also engage in a shared decision-making process to identify and prioritize possible next steps. If Emma's parents are reluctant to pursue formal behavioral parent training, understanding the source of this hesitancy (considering time burden, mental health stigma, doubts about efficacy, cultural mismatch, and other factors) would provide an opportunity to collaborate on considering evidence-based alternatives.

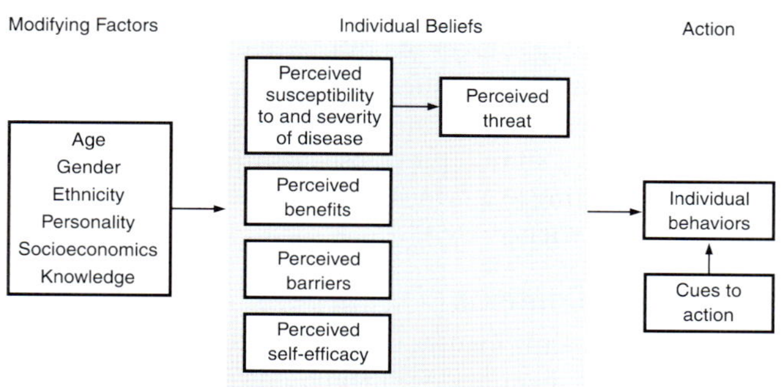

Fig. 4.5 Elements of the health belief model, a framework for describing why individuals take steps to prevent, identify, and manage chronic conditions. (Adapted from Champion, V. L., & Skinner, C. S. [2008]. The health belief model. In K. Glanz, B.K. Rimer, & K. Viswanath [Eds.], ***Health behavior and health education: Theory, research, and practice*** [pp. 45–65]. Wiley & Sons, Inc.)

CONCLUSION

No single perspective has the market cornered when it comes to learning and behavior change, and we hope that following Emma and her family in this chapter underscores how learning paradigms carry important applications in the developmental and behavioral pediatrics arena. Rather than choosing sides, so to speak, we urge you to follow the evidence as it evolves in your areas of practice and to use flexible thinking to identify how different conceptualizations often lead to similar practical applications. Operant mechanisms and parent training grounded in social learning theories will help Emma's parents manage her behavior problems (and reduce their own stress); cognitive and integrative models will help their health care and education professionals engage in shared decision making around how to support her continued growth and development; and cognitive-behavioral models will be available for Emma's parents (and Emma herself, when she is older) to address mental health concerns. Effective providers can "see the forest" in addition to the individual trees, and will convey this guidance clinically without burdening families with excessive theoretical underpinnings. We invite you to apply these same frameworks to your own behavior change as well, as you engage in lifelong learning to support the families you serve and as you educate future generations of pediatric professionals.

REFERENCES

Adams, R. C., & Levy, S. E. (2017). Shared decision-making and children with disabilities: Pathways to consensus. *Pediatrics, 139*(6), e20170956.

Ball, C. R., & Trammell, B. A. (2011). Response-to-intervention in high-risk preschools: Critical issues for implementation. *Psychology in the Schools, 48*(5), 502–512.

Benjamin, C. L., Puleo, C. M., Settipani, C. A., Brodman, D. M., Edmunds, J. M., Cummings, C. M., & Kendall, P. C. (2011). History of cognitive-behavioral therapy in youth. *Child and Adolescent Psychiatric Clinics, 20*(2), 179–189.

Chacko, A., Jensen, S. A., Lowry, L. S., Cornwell, M., Chimklis, A., Chan, E., Lee, D., & Pulgarin, B. (2016). Engagement in behavioral parent training: Review of the literature and implications for practice. *Clinical Child and Family Psychology Review, 19*(3), 204–215.

Champion, V. L., & Skinner, C. S. (2008). The health belief model. In K. Glanz, B. K. Rimer, & K. Viswanath (Eds.), *Health behavior and health education: Theory, research, and practice* (pp. 45–65). Wiley & Sons, Inc.

Cooper, J. O., Heron, T. E., & Heward, W. L. (2007). *Applied behavior analysis* (2nd ed.). Pearson.

Dodge, K. A., & Crick, N. R. (1990). Social information-processing bases of aggressive behavior in children. *Personality and Social Psychology Bulletin, 16*(1), 8–22.

Grusec, J. E. (1992). Social learning theory and developmental psychology: The legacies of Robert Sears and Albert Bandura. *Developmental Psychology, 28*, 776–786.

Lengua, L. J., & Kovacs, E. A. (2005). Bidirectional associations between temperament and parenting and the prediction of adjustment problems in middle childhood. *Journal of Applied Developmental Psychology, 26*(1), 21–38.

Michael, J. L. (2004). *Concepts and principles of behavior analysis*. Association of Behavior Analysis International.

Noltemeyer, A., Palmer, K., James, A. G., & Petrasek, M. (2019). Disciplinary and achievement outcomes associated with school-wide positive behavioral interventions and supports implementation level. *School Psychology Review*, *48*(1), 81–87.

Palincsar, A. S. (1998). Social constructivist perspectives on teaching and learning. *Annual Review of Psychology*, *49*(1), 345–375.

Patterson, G. R. (1982). A social learning approach to family intervention *Coercive family process* (Vol. 3). Castalia.

Poncy, B. C., McCallum, E., & Schmitt, A. J. (2010). A comparison of behavioral and constructivist interventions for increasing math-fact fluency in a second-grade classroom. *Psychology in the Schools*, *47*(9), 917–930.

Prochaska, J. O., Redding, C. A., & Evers, K. E. (2008). The transtheoretical model and stages of change. In K. Glanz, B. K. Rimer, & K. Viswanath (Eds.), *Health behavior and health education: Theory, research, and practice* (pp. 97–121). Wiley & Sons, Inc.

Steele, M. M. (2005). Teaching students with learning disabilities: Constructivism or behaviorism? *Current Issues in Education*, *8*(10). http://cie.asu.edu/volume8/number10/index.html

Stein, D. J., & Ludik, J. (Eds.). (1998). *Neural networks and psychopathology: Connectionist models in practice and research*. Cambridge University Press.

5

The Maternal-Fetal Dyad: Challenges and Adaptations

Amy L. Salisbury, Sara W. Moyer, Shannon Erisman, Patricia A. Kinser, Katheleen Hawes, and Pamela High

For additional material related to the content of this chapter, please see Chapters 2, 6, 49, and 51.

VIGNETTE

Natalie is a partnered, 25-year-old woman, currently at 28 weeks of gestation with her third pregnancy. She brings her 4-year-old son, Jaxon, for an appointment with Dr. Greene, a clinician in a specialty clinic for children with developmental delays. Natalie appears to be sad and irritable, different from her presentation at prior clinic appointments. When Dr. Greene asks how she is doing, she responds, "Not great" and becomes tearful. Dr. Greene recalls that Jaxon was born at 35 weeks of gestational age and has been followed by the clinic since the age of 18 months for mild developmental delays in motor and language skills and sleep difficulties. Natalie had one pregnancy prior to Jaxon, which ended in a spontaneous loss at 12 gestational weeks. Natalie has a history of recurrent major depressive disorder and was treated with venlafaxine, a serotonin-norepinephrine reuptake inhibitor antidepressant, throughout her pregnancy with Jaxon. During his initial clinic visit, she had asked several questions about whether taking medication while pregnant with Jaxon could have contributed to her son's difficulties.

INTRODUCTION

To understand child neurodevelopmental functioning, we must first understand the history of the maternal-child dyadic system from conception. Pregnancy is a dynamic system that comprises the physiologic, anatomic, and psychological components of the woman and her developing fetus within the context of their psychosocial and cultural environment (see Chapter 2). Pregnancy is a time of vast confluence of changes within and among these systems. These changes and the maternal-fetal adaptation to them are influenced by both preconception and current psychological, experiential, and physiologic factors. In this chapter we use the following terms when considering key aspects of maternal-child health: *perinatal* (the time from conception to 12 months postpartum), *prenatal* (conception through infant birth), and *postpartum* (after birth).

In our opening vignette, Natalie's mental health during the current pregnancy may be impacted by her past pregnancy experiences. Inevitably her health status is shared with her fetus. We have yet to learn about Natalie's experiences prior to her first pregnancy or the quality of her current social support; these factors are important to consider in this situation, as mounting evidence suggests that early life and adolescent experiences and current social support may play a significant role in both parental adjustment to pregnancy and parenthood (McDonald, Madigan, Racine, Benzies, Tomfohr, & Tough, 2019). Mental health, stress, and coping have been shown to impact pregnancy outcomes as well as long-term child outcomes (see Chapter 2). Understanding the impact of these adaptations, transactions, and conditions on the pregnant woman and her fetus is critical to health care during pregnancy and throughout the child's development.

This chapter will provide an overview of the inherent adaptations and challenges that may occur in the perinatal period and their potential impact on child development. We focus our information on psychiatric disorders and adverse pregnancy-related events. We will briefly discuss available treatments and what is currently known about their potential impact, compared to the underlying condition, on fetal and child development. We conclude with assessment strategies and recommended actions for each condition in the form of clinical pearls.

PHYSIOLOGIC AND PSYCHOLOGICAL CHALLENGES IN PREGNANCY

Each phase of pregnancy presents ongoing challenges for the maternal-fetal dynamic system that may be met with varying degrees of successful adaptation. A summary of the major adaptations by pregnancy trimester is presented in Table 5.1.

TABLE 5.1 Maternal-Fetal Changes Over Pregnancy and Associated Psychological and Social-Emotional Adaptations

System	First Trimester (0–13 wk)	Second Trimester (14–27 wk)	Third Trimester (28–40+ wk)
Physical/ morphologic	Embryologic development evolves quickly, culminating in the fetal form ~13 wk gestation Primitive embryo movements begin by 7 wk gestation; larger, more frequent movements occur by week 12 No or minimal noticeable physical changes to woman's outward physical form Absence of menses Increasing hCG levels Nausea and fatigue common Vomiting, less common Perception of poor perceived sleep quality with increased daytime sleepiness	Rapid fetal brain development; beginning of myelination Frequent spontaneous movements give way to increasingly stable rest-activity cycles by the end of the second trimester Growth of maternal uterine size, with expansion out of the pelvic cavity Maternal weight gain with altering center of gravity "Quickening"/maternal recognition of fetal movement usually occurs by week 26 Some women may continue to experience nausea and vomiting Blood volume increases, shifting abdominal structures to accommodate uterine size Changes in EEG sleep patterns possible	Accelerated fetal growth, fat stores, and brain development Increasing periods of quiescence as fetal behavioral states emerge Increasing size of the uterus, intermittent contractions of the uterus, and strengthening fetal movements may contribute to maternal physical discomfort Most large fetal movements can be felt by mother More pronounced changes in abdominal structures to accommodate uterine size Sleep becomes more fragmented with additional EEG changes; increased daytime fatigue
Social-emotional	Recognition of pregnancy Reorganization of sense of self, perceptions of others Pregnancy intention, preparation Social support needs increase Prior pregnancy experience, including past pregnancy loss, and psychiatric history and treatment may impact experience of a new pregnancy, increase anxiety, or precipitate changes in treatment due to concerns about taking medication in pregnancy Early mental representation of the fetus may begin	Increased maternal thoughts and images of the fetus; maternal-fetal attachment Most women feel physically well during this time compared to the first trimester Potential for exacerbation of underlying medical conditions or onset of pregnancy-related conditions (e.g., gestational diabetes) There is some evidence of increased onset of depressive mood episodes	Coping with impending delivery Preparation for newborn, transition to parenthood There is some evidence of increased onset of depressive mood episodes and or anxiety

EEG, Electroencephalogram; *hCG*, human chorionic gonadotropin.

This list of adaptations is not exhaustive but is meant to highlight those adaptations that may impact optimal fetal, infant, and child neurobehavioral development.

Women most often suspect a pregnancy after the first missed menstrual period, about 2 weeks after conception, which is considered 4 gestational weeks, calculated as time since the last menstrual period. By the time a woman receives confirmation via a home or laboratory pregnancy test, she may already have begun to experience early physical changes alerting her to the possible pregnancy. Many factors may influence successful adaptation at this time, including an intention to become pregnant, positive social support, ongoing physical and emotional health, and past experiences with adverse pregnancy outcomes, loss, or trauma (Farren, Mitchell-Jones, Verbakel, Timmerman, Jalmbrant, & Bourne, et al., 2018). The recognition of pregnancy may be associated with changes in behavior to protect the fetus. While such changes may represent positive adaptations in the case of decreasing unhealthy habits, such as smoking or drinking alcohol, women may make other decisions, such as to forego needed medication or therapies, without prior consultation with health care providers. Then, changes may precipitate increased medical or psychiatric risk.

The early discomforts associated with the first trimester for some women typically resolve by the week 14 of gestation, which marks the onset of the second gestational trimester. While the second trimester is a time when most women report feeling physically well, it is also a time of vulnerability due to ongoing physiologic changes, including alterations in maternal sleep and circadian rhythms, physical changes in body size and shape, and hormonal and metabolic changes that occur throughout the second and third trimesters. Many women report varying mental representations of their fetus by the second trimester, which is thought to be the foundation for building an attachment to the fetus.

Maternal-fetal attachment is a term used to describe the emotional connection a woman develops with her fetus during pregnancy, expressed in feelings, cognitions, and behaviors. Establishing an emotional connection to the fetus is considered an important part of the process of identification with the maternal role and may lay the groundwork for the mother-infant relationship in the postpartum period. The strength of maternal-fetal attachment increases over the course of pregnancy, particularly after fetal movement can be physically experienced at about 18 weeks of gestation. Several factors may lower the strength of maternal-fetal attachment, including maternal depression and poor social support (McFarland, Salisbury, Battle, Hawes, Halloran, & Lester, 2011). Maternal-fetal adaptation is critical as the early prenatal mother-infant relationship might influence future social, emotional, and cognitive development in the child.

The third trimester presents new challenges to the maternal-fetal dyad. The fetus is growing rapidly and has associated changes in physiology, increased fat distribution, and ongoing brain development. The mother may be experiencing increasing physical discomfort, sleep disturbance, and fatigue while preparing emotionally and otherwise for the impending delivery. Fathers and significant others may also be dealing with preparations and emotional adjustments in anticipation of birth, and this may impact the family's overall relationships. Adapting to these changes successfully contributes to optimal birth outcomes.

While child-focused clinicians may have limited contact with the mother during pregnancy, it is important to understand the impact of maternal mental health on short- and long-term infant and child outcomes. Even in women who have high levels of depressive symptoms during pregnancy, children have better developmental outcomes when their mothers are adequately treated and have decreasing symptoms over time than when their mothers are untreated or undertreated (Park, Brain, Grunau, Diamond, & Oberlander, 2018).

PERINATAL MENTAL HEALTH

A focus on mental health during the perinatal period, from pregnancy through 12 months postdelivery, is essential for all clinicians. A woman may experience psychiatric symptoms at any time in pregnancy, and the likelihood of occurrence is higher if such symptoms were present prior to the pregnancy (Kee et al., 2021). In stark contrast to the prevailing belief that women were protected from mental illness during the perinatal period, recognition that pregnancy and postpartum may be a time of increased risk and vulnerability to mental health disorders is growing; during this time the risk of death by suicide in women is actually heightened (Mangla, Hoffman, Trumpff, O'Grady, & Monk, 2019). Perinatal women may experience mood or anxiety symptoms for the first time, or the symptoms may be recurrences. Evidence of a direct causal pathway between prenatal maternal depression and child and adolescent behavior, emotional functioning, and psychopathology is compelling (Glover, O'Donnell, O'Connor, & Fisher, 2018). The psychological wellbeing of fathers during the pregnancy has also been examined. Men may have different experiences with depression than women and may not seek treatment; however, paternal depression also increases risk for poorer child outcomes after controlling for maternal mental health (Ramchandani, O'Connor, Evans, Heron, Murray, & Stein, 2008). Prevention or treatment of psychiatric conditions remains a priority to promote optimal child development; however, consideration must be given to the potential risks and/or benefits that each treatment may confer.

Perinatal Mood and Anxiety Disorders

In a welcome expansion from a previously narrow focus on postpartum depression, there is growing awareness of the full breadth of mental health difficulties that women encounter throughout the perinatal period. Perinatal mood and anxiety disorder (PMAD) refers to several disorders that may cause distress during pregnancy and up to 12 months after delivery, including bipolar disorder, psychosis, obsessive-compulsive disorder (OCD), posttraumatic stress disorder (PTSD), generalized anxiety disorder (GAD), and panic disorder. A recent, large-scale study reported an increase in PMAD and serious perinatal mental illness from 2006 to 2015 (McKee et al., 2020). Black, Indigenous, and people of color, women of lower socioeconomic status, immigrants and undocumented women, and women with disabilities are at elevated risk for PMAD. However, women from marginalized or disadvantaged communities may be particularly reluctant to disclose mental health concerns, given historical mistreatment and fear of negative consequences, such as involvement of child protective services.

Depressive Disorders

Depression is a leading cause of disability for women and the most common nonobstetric complication of the perinatal period. Perinatal depression can result in negative maternal and infant outcomes, with cognitive, emotional, and behavioral challenges for children of mothers with untreated depression. Prenatal depression occurs at a rate of 10% to 15% overall and appears to be more prevalent as pregnancy progresses. Rates of depression in the first trimester are equivalent to those in nonpregnant women (8%–10%). The prevalence increases in the second and third trimesters, with rates as high as 19% overall (Kinser et al., 2018). In the postpartum period, depression occurs at rates around 20%. However, Latina and Black women report early postpartum symptoms (between 2 and 6 weeks after delivery) at higher rates (47% and 44%, respectively) compared to White women (31%) (Howell, Mora, Horowitz, & Leventhal, 2005). Depression after delivery can be severe; 20% of women with postpartum depression report suicidal ideation (Wisner et al., 2013). Women with postpartum depression often have co-occurring anxiety, which may include anxious attachment or fear of being alone with the baby.

Perinatal depression should be differentiated from the baby blues, a dysphoric 5- to 10-day period that resolves on its own and affects up to 80% of postpartum women (Table 5.2). The baby blues refers to increased tearfulness, anxiety, mood lability, and irritability, and resolves without treatment within a few days. In contrast, depressive disorders are more severe and of longer duration than baby blues, include impairment in functioning, and typically require treatment to resolve.

It may be difficult to differentiate between an unremarkable pregnancy and postpartum symptoms of depression, especially changes in sleep, appetite and weight, and fatigue. Clinicians may minimize or dismiss signs of perinatal depression, assuring mothers their experiences are normal. However,

TABLE 5.2 Comparison of Baby Blues and Postpartum Depression

	Prevalence	Onset	Duration	Treatment
Baby blues	Up to 80%	3–4 days after delivery	<2 weeks	Support
Postpartum depression	20%	Within 12 mo postpartum	Weeks to months	Therapy, medication

the American Academy of Pediatrics (AAP) and other professional organizations recommend incorporating postpartum depression screening into pediatric well-child care. The identification of clinically significant depression may be facilitated using a self-report questionnaire. The Edinburgh Postnatal Depression Scale (EPDS) (Cox, Holden, & Sagovsky, 1987) is widely used and well validated to identify depression and anxiety during pregnancy and postpartum. The EPDS has been translated into numerous languages and has been validated in pregnant and postpartum women across racial, ethnic, and cultural groups in both high- and low-income countries. Scores greater than 7 may indicate mild depression, scores of 13 to 18 suggest moderate depression, and scores above 18 should be considered severe depression (McCabe-Beane, Segre, Perkhounkova, Stuart, & O'Hara, 2016). Clinical judgment should always be used in conjunction with the scores obtained. Another screening option is the Patient Health Questionnaire, a two- or nine-item measure, which has also been validated in an obstetric-gynecologic context but may not be appropriate for all populations.

VIGNETTE

Dr. Greene asks Natalie if she is feeling depressed, and she confirms that she is feeling sad and irritable most of the day, nearly every day, and has been sleeping less than 5 or 6 hours/night. She admits to feeling guilty because she no longer enjoys playing with Jaxon. Dr. Greene asks Natalie to fill out the EPDS survey to learn more about the severity of her symptoms, and her score is 15.

Natalie is endorsing the two main symptoms of depression (depressed mood and anhedonia), and her EPDS score suggests that these symptoms are clinically significant. She is also reporting guilt and distress about her loss of enjoyment of her time with her son. This presentation is clinically significant and requires further assessment for suicidal ideations. It may also require treatment in the form of a referral, such as a "warm hand-off" to mental health care clinicians or trained community-based workers.

Risk and Protective Factors for Perinatal Depression

A history of depression is the most significant risk factor for perinatal depression, conferring a 20-fold increased risk for postpartum depression specifically (Silverman et al., 2017). Risk factors for depression in pregnancy include domestic violence, lack of support, life stress, maternal anxiety, unintended pregnancy, single status, and strained relationship with partner.

Predictors of postpartum depression include symptoms of depression or anxiety during pregnancy, a recent stressful event, perceived lack of support, and traumatic birth. Women with a positive screen for postpartum depression (using an EPDS score of $\geq$10) were more likely to be Black, single, and less educated than White, married, and highly educated (Wisner et al., 2013). Protective factors include perceived social support and resilience, defined as adaptation in the face of adversity.

Risks to Child Outcomes Associated With Perinatal Depression

Prenatal depression is associated with higher risk of obstetric complications, lower gestational age and birthweight, as well as long-term emotional, behavioral, and social problems in the child. Results from preclinical and human studies provide compelling evidence of a direct causal pathway between prenatal maternal depression and child and adolescent behavior, emotional functioning, and psychopathology (Glover et al., 2018). A meta-analysis of 71 studies found that prenatal stress and depression were significant risk factors for child socio-emotional problems independent of other postnatal risk factors, however the effects were greater for those with additional socio-demographic risk (Madigan, 2018).

Postpartum depression is also linked to greater risks for children. Park and colleagues (2018) found that children of mothers with depression were more likely to have behavior problems, including internalizing and externalizing behaviors and attention-deficit/hyperactivity disorder, than children of mothers with low or decreasing depressive symptomatology over time. A high relapse rate of maternal depression can be detrimental to child development, and prompt intervention is essential to avoid impacting the child's pattern of stress responses via hypothalamus-pituitary-adrenal and cortisol reactivity (Lawler, Bocknek, McGinnis, Martinez-Torteya, Rosenblum, & Muzik, 2019). In another recent study, children exposed to maternal depression before age 5 years had 17% greater odds of developmental vulnerability compared to those who were not exposed, with the strongest associations occurring in social-emotional domains (Wall-Wieler, Roos, & Gotlib, 2020). Pediatric clinicians should be aware of maternal mental health and be prepared to refer women for appropriate treatment when possible.

Treatment for Perinatal Depression

VIGNETTE

Natalie reports that she stopped taking her antidepressant medication when she found out she was pregnant, as she feared the same medication was to blame for her son Jaxon's preterm birth and developmental delays. When asked if she has been using alternate treatments for her depression, she reports that she has been using marijuana three to four times per week to relax and sleep better. She says she heard that marijuana is harmless during pregnancy. She recently signed up for prenatal yoga, and her first class is next week.

Natalie's case is not uncommon. Many women fear the impact of medication on their unborn child and prefer nonpharmacologic treatments (Battle, Salisbury, Schofield, & Ortiz-Hernandez, 2013). It is important for women who are contemplating pregnancy or those who are pregnant to have a discussion with their clinicians about benefits and risks associated with treatment and with nontreatment.

Approximately 13% of pregnant women have taken an antidepressant during their pregnancy; serotonin selective reuptake inhibitors (SSRIs) are among the most prescribed drugs in pregnancy. The American College of Obstetrics and Gynecology (ACOG) has published guidelines regarding the use of psychotropic medications in pregnancy as well as treatment recommendations for specific psychiatric conditions based on available data and clinical consensus (Bulletin, 2008). Treatment advice needs to be based on careful consideration of the known risks and benefits of the treatment as well as the severity of the condition, stage of pregnancy, and preferences of the woman. Psychosocial approaches are recommended as a first-line treatment for depression in pregnancy unless the woman experiences suicidality or psychosis; psychotherapy, cognitive behavioral therapy, and interpersonal therapy are effective treatments for prenatal depression (see Chapter 49). For moderate to severe depression, medication may be considered in addition to psychotherapy if the depressive episode occurs after discontinuation of medication or if there is no response or worsening of symptoms to initial evidence-based nonmedication treatment.

Risks to Child Outcomes Associated With Treatment for Perinatal Depression

As indicated, SSRIs are the antidepressants prescribed most often in pregnancy. These inhibitors cross the placenta and affect fetal serotonin signaling, which affects brain development and modulates neurons involved in motor and social behaviors, emotional reactivity, and sleep. Prenatal SSRI exposure contributes to statistically significant adverse obstetric outcomes (Ross et al., 2013). However, the clinical significance of the outcomes is not clear; they were limited to 1.5 times higher risk of preterm birth, half-week earlier gestational age at delivery, and less than 1-g lower birthweight. A meta-analysis of 30 studies showed that antidepressant use in pregnancy was associated with a significantly greater risk of adverse neonatal signs after delivery, specifically respiratory distress and tremors (Grigoriadis et al., 2013). These adverse signs appear to be transient in the first postnatal month but may be more severe and prolonged with concomitant medication exposures such as benzodiazepines (Salisbury et al., 2016). Evidence of the impact of prenatal SSRI exposure on the child after the first postnatal month is inconsistent and complicated by the potential confounding of the underlying maternal condition. However, there is some consistency in the finding of minor motor delays that appear to resolve by 36 months of age. Recent reports that controlled for potential confounding suggested that gastrointestinal complaints may be more common in prenatally SSRI-exposed children than unexposed children (Salisbury, Papandonatos, Stroud, Smith, & Brennan, 2020) and that there may be some impact on specific aspects of social language development (Smearman et al., 2020). The benefits of treating PMAD must be considered for each woman individually.

Scientific evidence of the impact of alternative treatments for depression and anxiety on infant and later outcomes is limited. There is evidence of at least a small to moderate association with better outcomes for children of women who were adequately treated in pregnancy with nonpharmacologic options compared to those whose mothers were not treated (Goodman, Cullum, Dimidjian, River, & Kim, 2018). Several promising nonpharmacologic self-management interventions have received attention for preventing or intervening with perinatal depressive symptoms (e.g., yoga, physical activity), particularly when they are used as adjuncts to usual care (Eustis, Ernst, Sutton, & Battle, 2019).

ACOG guidelines apply to all psychotropic medications used to treat other PMADs. Infants may experience adverse effects from any psychotropic medication; however, the risks of these events may not outweigh the risks of not treating the underlying condition. Prenatal exposure to concomitant psychotropic medications may further increase risk of adverse neonatal signs and events; infants should be monitored closely in the first postnatal month.

Bipolar Spectrum Disorders

Women with a history of bipolar disorder have a recurrence rate of 71% in the perinatal period (Clark & Wisner, 2018). Women with bipolar disorder are more likely to experience a depressive rather than a manic or hypomanic episode during the perinatal period. They are 50% more likely to experience postpartum depression compared to women with a history of unipolar depression (Clark & Wisner, 2018). The Mood Disorder Questionnaire (MDQ) is a useful screening instrument for bipolar disorder and has been validated in postpartum women. A score of 7 or higher indicates a positive screen, in addition to functional impairment.

The decision to maintain or initiate medication for a pregnant or lactating woman requires a careful analysis of the risk of untreated illness compared to risk of medication effects on fetus/baby. Lithium, anticonvulsants, and second-generation antipsychotics are typically used to treat bipolar disorder; valproic acid is discouraged due to negative fetal effects, and carbamazepine is similarly avoided unless it was used prepregnancy and switching medications could prove harmful (Clark & Wisner, 2018). Women with bipolar disorder could utilize bright light therapy, if taking an antimanic agent, and if they are able to follow a specific protocol to avoid activation of mania.

Postpartum Psychosis

Postpartum psychosis occurs in 1 or 2 of 1000 live births and is considered a psychiatric emergency in the early postpartum period, requiring immediate treatment. Symptoms typically emerge over the first 2 weeks after delivery, with highest risk between days 2 and 4. Postpartum psychosis involves disorganization, delirium-like confusion, depersonalization, insomnia, and irritability, with abnormal thoughts (often persecutory in nature) and mood disturbance presenting as depression, mania or agitation, or mixed (Osborne, 2018). Postpartum psychosis is considered a manifestation of bipolar disorder rather than a primary psychotic disorder. However, following an episode of postpartum psychosis, 43.5% of women had an isolated episode of postpartum psychosis, and 56.7% experienced a chronic course of bipolar illness, suggesting that postpartum psychosis may not always precipitate chronic bipolar disorder (Gilden, Kamperman, Munk-Olsen, Hoogendijk, Kushner, & Bergink, 2020).

The strongest risk factor for postpartum psychosis is a history of bipolar disorder; 20% to 30% of women with a bipolar diagnosis experience postpartum psychosis. Other risk factors include a previous psychotic episode and history of postpartum mood disorder. Emerging research shows that additional risk factors are primiparity, preeclampsia, sleep disturbance, immune dysregulation, and hormonal changes (Osborne, 2018). Women with a personal or family history of bipolar disorder or postpartum psychosis should seek prophylactic treatment, including sleep restoration as soon as possible after delivery.

Due to the emergent nature of postpartum psychosis, pharmacologic treatment should be administered as soon as possible. Hospitalization is not uncommon for acute symptom stabilization and to ensure safety of mother and baby given elevated risk of suicide and infanticide (Spinelli, 2009). Bergink and colleagues (2015) suggested a four-phase treatment, starting with benzodiazepine to stabilize sleep and target agitation, followed by an antipsychotic and lithium, with remission occurring at about 40 days (median length of treatment).

Anxiety Disorders

Perinatal anxiety disorders are increasingly becoming the subject of study; however, prevalence and incidence rates vary widely, and meta-analysis and systematic reviews are scarce. Anxiety disorders occur at a rate of 4% to 39% during pregnancy and 15% postpartum (Goodman, Chenausky, & Freeman, 2014). Perinatal anxiety disorders have a prevalence of 13% to 22%, higher than rates of perinatal depression. Anxiety in pregnancy is related to an increased risk of postpartum depression and other maternal-child health sequelae.

GAD is the most commonly diagnosed anxiety disorder, including in the perinatal period. Around 10% of pregnant women and 7% to 8% of postpartum women meet diagnostic criteria for GAD. Pregnant and postpartum women are 1.5 to 2 times more likely to have OCD compared to the general population. Perinatal OCD may be distinct from OCD that occurs outside the perinatal period; for instance, obsessions during pregnancy tend to focus on contamination, while unwanted thoughts during the postpartum period often focus on harm coming to the infant (Abramowitz, Schwartz, Moore, & Luenzmann, 2003).

Posttraumatic Stress Disorder

Between 50% and 80% of women experience a potentially traumatic event in their lifetime. PTSD refers to the persistent constellation of symptoms after a traumatic event, including reexperiencing or intrusive thoughts, avoidance, increased arousal, and functional impairment (American Psychiatric Association, 2013). The traumatic event may have occurred before pregnancy or during the perinatal period, including a traumatic childbirth experience. Women who feel dismissed, humiliated, or invalidated, or whose births included emergency or subjectively frightening medical intervention, are at increased risk for developing PTSD (Beck, Driscoll, & Watson, 2013). Lifetime prevalence for PTSD in women is 12% to 14%, with 8% prevalence during pregnancy (Kessler, Petukhova, Sampson, Zaslavsky, & Wittchen, 2012).

Sociodemographic risk factors include less education, poverty, living in high-crime areas, and teen pregnancy. Childbirth-specific risk factors include an instrumental delivery, cesarean section, general anesthesia, third- or fourth-degree tears, and manual removal of placenta. Protective factors include advanced maternal age (>35 years), multiparity, epidural use, skin-to-skin contact with infant, and having a respected birth plan.

Panic Attacks and Panic Disorder

Panic disorder has a prevalence of 1.3% to 2% in the perinatal period (Ross & McLean, 2006). Panic attacks may occur independently from a panic disorder. Due to the nature of the symptoms, the onset of panic attacks often results in seeking care at an urgent care or an emergency department before an accurate diagnosis is made. Panic disorder is typically considered when the panic attacks are recurrent, unexpected, and associated with significant distress or fear of having another panic attack.

Treatment for Perinatal Anxiety Disorders

Psychotherapy is the first-line treatment for mild to moderate perinatal anxiety disorders in the perinatal period, specifically cognitive behavioral therapy and mindfulness-based behavioral therapies (Thorsness, Watson, & LaRusso, 2018). SSRIs are recommended in addition to psychotherapy for the treatment of moderate to severe anxiety or refractory anxiety disorders. Benzodiazepines may be prescribed in the short term for severe anxiety or insomnia, and lorazepam is preferred for pregnant and lactating women (Thorsness et al., 2018).

Pediatric In-Office Interventions for Perinatal Mood and Anxiety Disorders

Pediatric visits present a unique opportunity for PMAD screening and intervention. Mother-baby cues may signal a PMAD, including lack of attunement between mother and baby or a lack of positive emotion toward baby (either observed or reported by mother, upon prompting). A clinician may also ask the mother about perceived support (e.g., "How much support do you feel like you have? Who is helping you?"), sleep (e.g., "Are you getting enough sleep yourself? When do you catch up on sleep? Are you able to sleep when you get the chance?"), and parenting self-efficacy (e.g., "How confident are you feeling about your role as a mother?") (Umylny, German, & Lantiere, 2017). Screening for depression in pregnant and postpartum women can be a powerful tool for reducing depression symptoms and prevalence, regardless of interventions following screening. The AAP first recommended screening for postpartum depression in pediatric primary care practice in a clinical report in 2010 followed by updated recommendations in 2019 to incorporate both the recognition and management of perinatal and postpartum depression in pediatric practice (Earls, Yogman, Mattson, & Rafferty, 2019). If clinicians suspect or confirm maternal depression via screening, they should provide a referral to a behavioral health provider. Important interventions can be delivered in the exam room. Perhaps most important is to demystify and normalize symptoms, emphasizing three key points to the mother: (1) You are not alone, (2) you are not to blame, and (3) you will get better.

The US Preventive Services Task Force took this recommendation one step further, stating that all adults, including pregnant and postpartum women, should be screened for depression as part of primary care (Siu et al., 2016). These recommendations are supported by the Centers for Medicare and Medicaid Services due to the mounting evidence of detrimental impact of maternal depression on child health and development, with support for financial coverage for this screening for Medicaid-eligible mothers. In addition, states may use the child's Medicaid to cover maternal depression screening for non–Medicaid-eligible mothers during the well-child visit. Provisions were made to allow reimbursement for treatment for the mother when both the child and the mother are present, treatment focuses on the effects of the mother's condition on the child, and services are for the direct benefit of the child (visit https://www.medicaid.gov/federal-policy-guidance/downloads/cib051116.pdf). Box 5.1 provides suggestions regarding the clinical vignette.

BOX 5.1 Brief In-Office Intervention

When Detecting PMAD Symptoms: Demystify and Normalize Symptoms

Praise Natalie's use of yoga to improve mood and her desire to spare her developing fetus harm. Discourage use of marijuana; as there is some evidence of harmful effects on the fetus that may persist into childhood (Nashed, Hardy, & Laviolette, 2021).

Referrals

Discuss with obstetrician and with Natalie's former mental health provider and prescriber of antidepressants about her mental health and treatment recommendations. Consider referral to Maternal Infant Early Childhood Home Visiting (MICHV) for maternal support during and after pregnancy (https://mchb.hrsa.gov/maternal-child-health-initiatives/home-visiting-overview).

Resources

Free online toolkit: https://www.dchealthcheck.net/resources/healthcheck/mental-health-tools.html

AAP.org website with perinatal depression resources: https://www.aap.org/en-us/advocacy-and-policy/aap-health-initiatives/Screening/Pages/Maternal-Depression.aspx

Postpartum Support International: https://www.postpartum.net/

American College of Obstetrics and Gynecology infographic on marijuana in pregnancy: https://www.acog.org/womens-health/infographics/marijuana-and-pregnancy

TRAUMATIC BIRTH EXPERIENCES

Up to 45% of new mothers report experiencing traumatic childbirth (Beck, 2019). A traumatic birth experience is determined by the mother's perception of the birth; it is not a clinical classification. What a woman perceives as a birth trauma may be perceived as routine to obstetric providers, especially when the infant outcome is positive. For example, an unplanned cesarean section is often considered somewhat routine for clinicians, yet this can be perceived by the mother as a traumatic experience. The elements of birth trauma can occur during any phase of childbearing, such as prenatal experiences, but are primarily associated with a woman's labor and delivery experience. Other examples of traumatic birth experiences include stillbirth/infant death, emergency cesarean section/infant distress, cardiac arrest, inadequate medical care, fear of epidural, congenital anomalies, inadequate pain relief, postpartum hemorrhage/manual removal of placenta, forceps/vacuum extraction/skull fracture, severe toxemia, premature birth, separation from infant in neonatal intensive care unit, prolonged painful labor, rapid delivery, and a degrading experience.

Prenatal factors predictive of traumatic birth include previous traumatic birth, prenatal PTSD, child sexual abuse, and previous history of a mood/anxiety disorder necessitating psychotherapy. Predictors also relate to the nature and circumstances of the delivery (e.g., high levels of medical involvement, extremely painful labor, and delivery type). There are subjective factors related to a woman's perception of traumatic birth, such as feelings of powerlessness during labor and perception of lack of caring and support.

Posttraumatic Stress

Traumatic childbirth is an extreme stressor that can lead to mental health problems such as depression, anxiety, and PTSD. It can also have long-term chronic consequences. Posttraumatic stress symptoms can interfere with mother-child interaction, lead to subsequent parenting problems, and impact child development (Cook, 2018). Posttraumatic stress symptoms related to childbirth can flare up on the anniversary of the birth trauma. What is normally a joy-filled time, a child's birthday, can become a day of dread and suffering for women if that child's birth was traumatic. Additionally, subsequent pregnancies after traumatic birth can be anxiety filled if a woman is fearful of history repeating itself (Beck, 2015).

Posttraumatic stress is a common acute response to a traumatic experience. If these symptoms persist, PTSD may develop. Not all women develop PTSD after a traumatic birth. Beck and colleagues (2019) found prevalence rates of elevated posttraumatic stress symptoms ranging from 0.8% to 26% after traumatic childbirth. Posttraumatic stress predictors that occur before childbirth include prior trauma in childhood or adulthood and a history of psychiatric disorders. Predictors that occur after childbirth are poor support during labor and delivery from clinicians, partners and family members, cesarean birth, negative birth experiences, and comorbidity with postpartum depression.

Traumatic Birth and Disenfranchised Grief

When childbirth does not go as planned and is perceived as traumatic, women may experience a significant grief response. If the outcome (e.g., a live birth) is perceived positively by observers, a new mother may not feel that she is able to discuss her emotional response to her perceived loss. This concept is known as disenfranchised grief. Doka (2002) defines disenfranchised grief as grief that is not or cannot be openly acknowledged or socially validated and supported. Women who do not receive support as mourners and are not able to express their grief may develop a prolonged grief response and subsequent depression. Providing resources for grief counseling and support may reduce the development of serious mental health problems after a traumatic birth.

Clinical Implications of Traumatic Birth

Prevention of Traumatic Birth

While not all traumatic births can be prevented, certain strategies can enhance a woman's childbirth experience. Most importantly, it is imperative to treat all women with dignity and respect and to involve them in decision making during the process of labor. Nurses, obstetric providers, doulas, and partners can provide much needed support to women during childbirth (Beck, 2015).

Prevention of PTSD After Traumatic Childbirth

To reduce posttraumatic stress symptoms it is essential to provide women with the opportunity to debrief before discharge from the hospital after childbirth, in essence creating space to discuss their perceptions of the childbirth experience. The postpartum obstetric follow-up visits and the infant's well-baby visits are also important opportunities for clinicians to ask questions and assess for posttraumatic stress symptoms. Suggested posttraumatic screening instruments to be considered include Primary Care PTSD Screen, The Davidson Trauma Scale, the PPQ1, and PPQ2 (Hynan, Mounts, & Vanderbilt, 2013). Validating a woman's childbirth experience, providing caring support, assessing for traumatic stress and other mental health problems, and providing mental/behavioral health resources when necessary are essential to the wellbeing of families after traumatic birth.

FOURTH TRIMESTER AND BEYOND

The postpartum period is typically defined as the first year after delivery, and the early postpartum period, or fourth trimester, is the first 12 weeks after delivery. The entire postpartum period is a time of ongoing and significant change for mothers and families. The time of greatest risk to maternal wellbeing may be 6 to 12 months postdelivery when death by suicide in postpartum women was found to be highest (Grigoriadis et al., 2017). Although the first obstetric visit is traditionally scheduled at 6 weeks postpartum, it is often missed by many women because of the challenges of childcare during that time, making the fourth trimester a sensitive period during which many maternal health needs will be unmet. Due to the relative frequency of recommended routine pediatric visits in the first postnatal year, the pediatric clinician may be the only clinician delivering care during this vulnerable period. Much of the focus is on assessment of the infant; this structure may leave many women feeling unheard and unseen during this time. Given PMAD is one of the most common obstetric complications, and that these symptoms can lead to detrimental consequences, it is essential for the clinician to consider the maternal-infant dyad when providing care to the infant in the early postpartum period (Moyer & Kinser, 2021). By focusing on the maternal-infant dyad together as a unit, the clinician will help prevent women from suffering in silence and therefore enhance the wellbeing of the developing infant.

VIGNETTE

Natalie gives birth to a healthy, full-term infant girl, Maya. However, she had a prolonged labor, failure to progress to fully dilated, and ultimately delivered Maya by emergency cesarean section. Dr. Kim, pediatrician, is scheduled to meet with Natalie and her family prior to discharge from the hospital. When Dr. Kim walks into the room, she finds Natalie alone with the baby and breastfeeding. Although Natalie reports "feeling fine," she becomes tearful when asked about her partner, stating that "he had to go back to work." Dr. Kim examines the infant and finds her to be within normal limits, with a small hemangioma noted on the left shoulder. During the assessment of the newborn, Natalie asks many questions, repeatedly asks if the baby is okay, and if hemangiomas can be caused by medications or marijuana. Dr. Kim observes that Natalie is very anxious and is holding her infant tightly in her arms during their conversation. Dr. Kim recommends a consultation with the psychiatric consultation liaison team.

Clinical Pearls for the Fourth Trimester and Beyond

Following are recommendations for the clinical care of women after delivery.

- Although screening tools, such as the EPDS, can be helpful for detecting maternal depression, do not depend solely upon scores, particularly in cases when maternal behaviors seem divergent from the scores. It is essential to have nuanced conversations with women about your observations, and these conversations can go a long way toward supporting maternal mental health (see Box 5.1 and 5.2).
- PMAD can manifest in many ways. Keep an eye out not only for typical depressive symptoms (crying, difficulty sleeping when having the opportunity), but also for other symptoms such as anxiety, obsessive thoughts and compulsive behaviors, confusion, irritability, and restlessness.
- Clinicians need to be alert near a child's birthday for emotional distress in mothers who have experienced a traumatic birth. Screening for PTSD and providing follow-up may be necessary to avert a crisis.

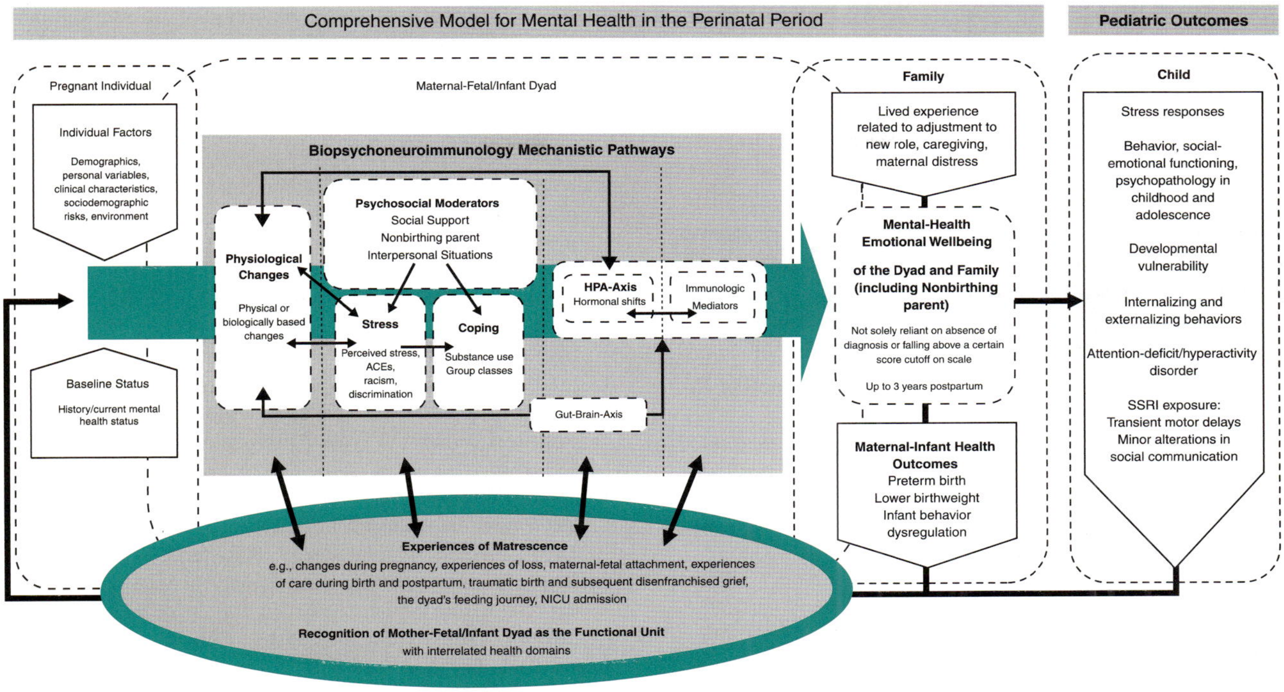

Fig. 5.1 Comprehensive model for maternal-child dyadic mental health during the perinatal period. ***ACEs***, Adverse childhood experiences; ***HPA***, hypothalamic-pituitary-adrenal; ***NICU***, neonatal intensive care unit; ***SSRI***, serotonin selective reuptake inhibitors. Adapted from Moyer, S. W., & Kinser, P. A. [2021]. A comprehensive conceptual framework to guide clinical practice and research about mental health during the perinatal period. *Journal of Perinatal and Neonatal Nursing, 35*[1], 46–56. https://doi.org/10.1097/JPN.0000000000000535.

Framework for Interplay of Maternal-Child Health

Given what is known about the relationship between maternal mental health and the healthy development of children, it is essential for all pediatric clinicians to be aware of maternal mental health throughout the perinatal period, including far into the postpartum period, and to be prepared to refer women for appropriate treatment, if possible (see Chapter 2). Indeed, research on early brain development, toxic stress, epigenetics, and adverse childhood experiences informs our knowledge that maternal mental health forms a critical environment for health, development, and learning during infancy and across the lifespan. Fig. 5.1 provides a framework for clinicians to consider regarding the interplay of biopsychosocial and neuroimmunologic pathways linking maternal, dyadic, family, and child health (Moyer & Kinser, 2021). The pathways linking stress, coping, social support, and other moderators of mental health are critical to understand in the context of child development. The pediatric clinician is a unique position to acknowledge matresence (i.e., the developmental process of becoming a mother) in the care of the maternal-child dyad. Aspects of matrescence may include clinical variables (e.g., physiologic changes), experiences specific to this time of development (e.g., perinatal health care experiences, the dyad's infant feeding journey), and the individual lived experiences of women related to pregnancy and early parenthood (e.g., adjustment to new role, caregiving, returning to work, and maternal distress [relational, environmental, and psychological stress] specific to mothers) (Moyer & Kinser, 2021). Examples from the clinical case vignette presented in this chapter have been included as a visual representation of the aspects relating to this patient.

CONCLUSION

How might a clinician address the family in the continuing case vignette? It would be relevant to provide education based on two key facts: (1) The postpartum period lasts for 1 full year, and perhaps as long as 3 years; and (2) mental wellness is an important focus for both maternal and child health during this time. The clinician could provide the mother with information that maintenance of mental wellness requires full attention to one's biopsychosocial wellbeing, from rest, recovery, and nutrition through awareness of mental health symptoms. The clinician must acknowledge the complexity of experiences of matrescence, reminding the woman that each woman has a unique experience of becoming a mother and affirming the value and complexity of this individual lived experience. After screening with a validated scale, a nuanced conversation should follow that involves demystifying and validating symptoms. The mother should be empowered to recognize her own symptoms and seek assistance from friends, family members, and clinicians whenever she has concerns about her mental wellness. Additionally, the clinician could remind her to recognize social support systems that could surround her during the postpartum period, provide anticipatory guidance about resources (Box 5.2), and provide a warm hand-off if referrals to local mental health clinicians are indicated. By focusing on the maternal-infant dyad together as a unit, the clinician may prevent women from suffering in silence and thereby may enhance the well-being of the developing infant and family.

BOX 5.2 Resources for Discussions About Maternal Mental Health and Referrals for Enhanced Care

Discussion Topics

- What has your experience been of becoming a mother to this child? (matresence)
- What are your priorities today for the health of yourself and your child? (focus on maternal-infant dyad)
- I see that your score was __ on the EPDS. This corresponds to ___ (no, mild, moderate, severe) depression risk. How does that fit with your current experience?

Referrals

- Local mental health professionals
- Postpartum Support International (with perinatal-specific support groups and clinicians)
- Maternal Infant Early Childhood Home Visiting (MIECHV) programs sponsored by the Health Resources and Services Administration (HRSA) Maternal Child Health Bureau (MCHB) and the Administration for Children and Families (ACF) provide evidence-based home visiting for at-risk families during pregnancy and in the early childhood years. Their goal is to identify family needs, including mental health needs, to support young families and to promote healthy parenting practices. Sponsored programs include Nurse Family Partnership and Parents as Teachers, in 30% of American counties in 2021 (https://mchb.hrsa.gov/maternal-child-health-initiatives/home-visiting-overview).

REFERENCES

Abramowitz, J. S., Schwartz, S. A., Moore, K. M., & Luenzmann, K. R. (2003). Obsessive-compulsive symptoms in pregnancy and the puerperium. *Journal of Anxiety Disorders*, *17*(4), 461–478. https://doi.org/10.1016/s0887-6185(02)00206-2

American Psychiatric Association. (2013). Diagnostic and statistical manual of mental disorders (5th ed.). https://doi.org/10.1176/appi.books.9780890425596

Battle, C. L., Salisbury, A. L., Schofield, C. A., & Ortiz-Hernandez, S. (2013). Perinatal antidepressant use: Understanding women's preferences and concerns. *Journal of Psychiatric Practice*, *19*(6), 443–453. https://doi.org/10.1097/01.pra.0000438183.74359.46

Beck. C. T. (2015). Middle range theory of traumatic childbirth: The ever-widening ripple effect. *Global Qualitative Nursing Research*, *2* https://doi.org/10.1177/2333393615575313. 2333393615575313

Beck, C. T., Casavant, S. (2019). "Synthesis of Mixed Research on Posttraumatic Stress Related to Traumatic Birth." *Journal Obstet Gynecol Neonatal Nurs 48*(4): 385–397.

Beck, C. T., Driscoll, J., & Watson, S. (2013). *Traumatic childbirth*. Routledge.

Bergink, V., Burgerhout, K. M., Koorengevel, K. M., Kamperman, A. M., Hoogendijk, W. J., Lambregtse-van den Berg, M. P., & Kushner, S. A. (2015). Treatment of psychosis and mania in the postpartum period. *American Journal of Psychiatry*, *172*(2), 115–123. https://doi.org/10.1176/appi.ajp.2014.13121652

Bulletin, A. P. (2008). Clinical management guidelines for obstetrician-gynecologists number 92: Use of psychiatric medications during pregnancy and lactation (0029-7844 Print).

Clark, C. T., & Wisner, K. L. (2018). Treatment of peripartum bipolar disorder. *Obstetric and Gynecology Clinics of North America*, *45*(3), 403–417. https://doi.org/10.1016/j.ogc.2018.05.002

Cox, J. L., Holden, J. M., & Sagovsky, R. (1987). Detection of postnatal depression: Development of the 10-item Edinburgh Postnatal Depression Scale. *British Journal of Psychiatry*, *150*, 782–786.

Doka, K. (Ed.), (2002). *Disenfranchised grief: New directions, challenges, and strategies for practice*. Research Press.

Earls, M., Yogman, M., Mattson, G., & Rafferty, J. (2019). Incorporating recognition and management of perinatal depression into pediatric practice. *Pediatrics*, *143*(1), e20183259. https://doi.org/10.1542/peds.2018-3259

Eustis, E. H., Ernst, S., Sutton, K., & Battle, C. L. (2019). Innovations in the treatment of perinatal depression: The role of yoga and physical activity interventions during pregnancy and postpartum. *Current Psychiatry Reports*, *21*(12), 133. https://doi.org/10.1007/s11920-019-1121-1

Farren, J., Mitchell-Jones, N., Verbakel, J. Y., Timmerman, D., Jalmbrant, M., & Bourne, T. (2018). The psychological impact of early pregnancy loss. *Human Reproduction Update*, 24(6), 731–749. doi:10.1093/humupd/dmy025

Gilden, J., Kamperman, A. M., Munk-Olsen, T., Hoogendijk, W. J. G., Kushner, S. A., & Bergink, V. (2020). Long-term outcomes of postpartum psychosis: A systematic review and meta-analysis. *Journal of Clinical Psychiatry*, *81*(2). https://doi.org/10.4088/JCP.19r12906

Glover, V., O'Donnell, K. J., O'Connor, T. G., & Fisher, J. (2018). Prenatal maternal stress, fetal programming, and mechanisms underlying later psychopathology—a global perspective. *Development and Psychopathology*, *30*(3), 843–854. https://doi.org/10.1017/S095457941800038X

Goodman, J. H., Chenausky, K. L., & Freeman, M. P. (2014). Anxiety disorders during pregnancy: A systematic review. *Journal of Clinical Psychiatry*, *75*(10), e1153–1184. https://doi.org/10.4088/JCP.14r09035

Goodman, S. H., Cullum, K. A., Dimidjian, S., River, L. M., & Kim, C. Y. (2018). Opening windows of opportunities: Evidence for interventions to prevent or treat depression in pregnant women being associated with changes in offspring's developmental trajectories of psychopathology risk. *Development and Psychopathology*, *30*(3), 1179–1196. https://doi.org/10.1017/S0954579418000536

Grigoriadis, S., VonderPorten, E. H., Mamisashvili, L., Eady, A., Tomlinson, G., Dennis, C. L., … Ross, L. E. (2013). The effect of prenatal antidepressant exposure on neonatal adaptation: A systematic review and meta-analysis. *Journal of Clinical Psychiatry*, *74*(4), e309–320. https://doi.org/10.4088/JCP.12r07967

Grigoriadis, S., Wilton, A. S., Kurdyak, P. A., Rhodes, A. E., VonderPorten, E. H., Levitt, A., … Vigod, S. N. (2017). Perinatal suicide in Ontario, Canada: A 15-year population-based study.

Canadian Medical Association Journal, *189*(34), E1085–E1092. https://doi.org/10.1503/cmaj.170088

Howell, E. A., Mora, P. A., Horowitz, C. R., & Leventhal, H. (2005). Racial and ethnic differences in factors associated with early postpartum depressive symptoms. *Obstetrics & Gynecology*, *105*(6), 1442–1450. https://doi.org/10.1097/01.AOG.0000164050.34126.37

Hynan, M. T., Mounts, K. O., & Vanderbilt, D. L. (2013). Screening parents of high-risk infants for emotional distress: Rationale and recommendations. *Journal of Perinatology: Official Journal of the California Perinatal Association*, *33*(10), 748–753. https://doi.org/10.1038/jp.2013.72

Kee, M. Z. L., Ponmudi, S., Phua, D. Y., Rifkin-Graboi, A., Chong, Y. S., Tan, K. H., ... Meaney, M. J. (2021). Preconception origins of perinatal maternal mental health. *Archives of Women's Mental Health* https://doi.org/10.1007/s00737-020-01096-y

Kessler, R. C., Petukhova, M., Sampson, N. A., Zaslavsky, A. M., & Wittchen, H. U. (2012). Twelve-month and lifetime prevalence and lifetime morbid risk of anxiety and mood disorders in the United States. *International Journal of Methods in Psychiatric Research*, *21*(3), 169–184. https://doi.org/10.1002/mpr.1359

Kinser, P. A., Thacker, L. R., Lapato, D., Wagner, S., Roberson-Nay, R., Jobe-Shields, L., ... York, T. P. (2018). Depressive symptom prevalence and predictors in the first half of pregnancy. *Journal of Womens Health (Larchmt)*, *27*(3), 369–376. https://doi.org/10.1089/jwh.2017.6426

Lawler, J. M., Bocknek, E. L., McGinnis, E. W., Martinez-Torteya, C., Rosenblum, K. L., & Muzik, M. (2019). Maternal postpartum depression increases vulnerability for toddler behavior problems through infant cortisol reactivity. *Infancy*, *24*(2), 249–274. https://doi.org/10.1111/infa.12271

Madigan, S., Oatley, H., Racine, N., Fearon, R. M. P., Schumacher, L., Akbari, E., ... Tarabulsy, G. M. (2018). A meta-analysis of maternal prenatal depression and anxiety on child socioemotional development. *Journal of the American Academy of Child and Adolescent Psychiatry*, *57*(9), 645–657. https://doi.org/10.1016/j.jaac.2018.06.012. e648

Mangla, K., Hoffman, M. C., Trumpff, C., O'Grady, S., & Monk, C. (2019). Maternal self-harm deaths: An unrecognized and preventable outcome. *American Journal of Obstetrics and Gynecology*, *221*(4), 295–303. https://doi.org/10.1016/j.ajog.2019.02.056

McCabe-Beane, J. E., Segre, L. S., Perkhounkova, Y., Stuart, S., & O'Hara, M. W. (2016). The identification of severity ranges for the Edinburgh Postnatal Depression Scale. *Journal of Reproductive and Infant Psychology*, *34*(3), 293–303. https://doi.org/10.1080/02646838.2016.1141346

McDonald, S. W., Madigan, S., Racine, N., Benzies, K., Tomfohr, L., & Tough, S. (2019). Maternal adverse childhood experiences, mental health, and child behaviour at age 3: The all our families community cohort study. *Preventive Medicine*, *118*, 286–294. https://doi.org/10.1016/j.ypmed.2018.11.013

McFarland, J., Salisbury, A. L., Battle, C. L., Hawes, K., Halloran, K., & Lester, B. M. (2011). Major depressive disorder during pregnancy and emotional attachment to the fetus. *Archives of Womens Mental Health*, *14*(5), 425–434. https://doi.org/10.1007/s00737-011-0237-z

McKee, K., Admon, L. K., Winkelman, T. N. A., Muzik, M., Hall, S., Dalton, V. K., & Zivin, K. (2020). Perinatal mood and anxiety disorders, serious mental illness, and delivery-related health outcomes, United States, 2006-2015. *BMC Womens Health*, *20*(1),150. https://doi.org/10.1186/s12905-020-00996-6

Moyer, S. W., & Kinser, P. A. (2021). A comprehensive conceptual framework to guide clinical practice and research about mental health during the perinatal period. *Journal of Perinatal and Neonatal Nursing*, *35*(1), 46–56. https://doi.org/10.1097/JPN.0000000000000535

Nashed, M., Hardy, D., & Laviolette, S. (2021). Prenatal cannabinoid exposure: Emerging evidence of physiological and neuropsychiatric abnormalities. *Frontiers of Psychiatry*, *11*, 624275. https://doi.org/10.3389/fpsyt.2020.624275

Osborne. L. M. (2018). Recognizing and managing postpartum psychosis: A clinical guide for obstetric providers. *Obstetric and Gynecology Clinics of North America*, *45*(3), 455–468. https://doi.org/10.1016/j.ogc.2018.04.005

Park, M., Brain, U., Grunau, R. E., Diamond, A., & Oberlander, T. F. (2018). Maternal depression trajectories from pregnancy to 3 years postpartum are associated with children's behavior and executive functions at 3 and 6 years. *Archives of Women's Mental Health*, *21*(3), 353–363. https://doi.org/10.1007/s00737-017-0803-0

Ramchandani, P. G., O'Connor, T. G., Evans, J., Heron, J., Murray, L., & Stein, A. (2008). The effects of pre- and postnatal depression in fathers: A natural experiment comparing the effects of exposure to depression on offspring. *Journal of Child Psychology and Psychiatry*, *49*(10), 1069–1078. https://doi.org/10.1111/j.1469-7610.2008.02000.x

Ross, L. E., Grigoriadis, S., Mamisashvili, L., Vonderporten, E. H., Roerecke, M., Rehm, J., ... Cheung, A. (2013). Selected pregnancy and delivery outcomes after exposure to antidepressant medication: A systematic review and meta-analysis. *JAMA Psychiatry*, *70*(4), 436–443. https://doi.org/10.1001/jamapsychiatry.2013.684

Ross, L. E., & McLean, L. M. (2006). Anxiety disorders during pregnancy and the postpartum period—a systematic review. *Journal of Clinical Psychiatry*, *67*(8), 14

Salisbury, A., O'Grady, K., Battle, C., Wisner, K. L., Anderson, G. M., Stroud, L. R., ... Lester, B. M. (2016). The roles of maternal depression, serotonin reuptake inhibitor treatment, and concomitant benzodiazepine use on infant neurobehavioral functioning over the first postnatal month. *American Journal of Psychiatry*, *173*(2), 147–157. https://doi.org/10.1176/appi.ajp.2015.14080989

Salisbury, A. L., Papandonatos, G. D., Stroud, L. R., Smith, A. K., & Brennan, P. A. (2020). Prenatal antidepressant exposures and gastrointestinal complaints in childhood: A gut-brain axis connection? *Developmental Psychobiology* https://doi.org/10.1002/dev.21966

Silverman, M. E., Reichenberg, A., Savitz, D. A., Cnattingius, S., Lichtenstein, P., Hultman, C. M., ... Sandin, S. (2017). The risk factors for postpartum depression: A population-based study. *Depression and Anxiety*, *34*(2), 178–187. https://doi.org/10.1002/da.22597

Siu, A. L., Bibbins-Domingo, K., Grossman, D. C., Baumann, L. C., Davidson, K. W., Ebell, M., ... Pignone, M. P. (2016). Screening for depression in adults. *JAMA*, *315*(4), 380. https://doi.org/10.1001/jama.2015.18392

Smearman, E. L., Hendrix, C. L., Winiarski, D. A., Johnson, K. C., Smith, A. K., Ousley, O. Y., ... Brennan, P. A. (2020). School-age social behavior and pragmatic language ability in children with prenatal serotonin reuptake inhibitor exposure. *Development and Psychopathology*, *32*(1), 21–30. https://doi.org/10.1017/S0954579418001372

Spinelli. M. G. (2009). Postpartum psychosis—detection of risk and management. *American Journal of Psychiatry*, *166*(4), 405–408.

Thorsness, K. R., Watson, C., & LaRusso, E. M. (2018). Perinatal anxiety: Approach to diagnosis and management in the obstetric setting. *American Journal of Obstetrics and Gynecology*, *219*(4), 326–345. https://doi.org/10.1016/j.ajog.2018.05.017

Umylny, P., German, M., & Lantiere, A. (2017). Treating postpartum mood and anxiety disorders in primary care pediatrics. *Current Problems in Pediatric and Adolescent Health Care*, *47*(10), 254–266. https://doi.org/10.1016/j.cppeds.2017.08.003

Wall-Wieler, E., Roos, L. L., & Gotlib, I. H. (2020). Maternal depression in early childhood and developmental vulnerability at school entry. *Pediatrics*, *146*(3), e20200794. https://doi.org/10.1542/peds.2020-0794

Wisner, K. L., Sit, D. K., McShea, M. C., Rizzo, D. M., Zoretich, R. A., Hughes, C. L., … Hanusa, B. H. (2013). Onset timing, thoughts of self-harm, and diagnoses in postpartum women with screen-positive depression findings. *JAMA Psychiatry*, *70*(5), 490–498. https://doi.org/10.1001/jamapsychiatry.2013.87

6

Infancy

Marilyn Augustyn, Mei Elansary, and Barry Zuckerman

For additional material related to the content of this chapter, please see Chapters 2, 3, and 6.

VIGNETTE

Rosaria is tightly swaddled as the midwife hands her to her mother. Following a 36-hour labor, her mother is exhausted but grateful to hold her baby for the first time. Rosario instinctively nestles into the crook of her mother's arm and turns her head toward her breast. Awkwardly, she attempts to find her mother's nipple, but when she finds it, she is too tired to suckle. She calmly rests there by her mother. Over the next few hours, she learns to breastfeed, looks toward her mother's adoring face, and turns to her mother's soft voice. In 24 hours her mother takes her home. Rosario joins a household with four older siblings, her grandmother, and another family. She breastfeeds every 2 to 3 hours, and she lets her siblings gawk and poke at her, when she is alert, and cries when she gets drowsy. Her mother returns to work after 2 weeks at home. At that point, Rosario is cared for primarily by her grandmother and siblings. Her parents work long hours to provide the financial resources for their family, limiting their time with Rosario and her siblings. Nonetheless, Rosario continues to thrive in her loving family.

"There is no such thing as a baby, only a baby and an adult." Winnicot

INTRODUCTION

Following birth, infants do not stand alone but continue to be part of an *ex utero* external dyadic regulatory system. Parents provide resources to supplement the infant's capacity to regulate homeostasis. Infant crying, sucking, wriggling, lidded eyes smiling are the external behaviors that signal the need for a caregiver to respond by providing the support the infant needs. These events influence what happens next in the child's life. In many ways the development in the first year of life has the steepest trajectory of developmental changes and brain growth of any other developmental epoch. The rapid changes integrate infants into their social world and simultaneously allow them to begin to function autonomously, if only in limited domains. However, social conditions and governmental policies can influence the earliest stages of infant development. Infants need at least one responsive caregiving adult; nonparental guardians can fit the bill under circumstances, as we have seen in the opening vignette.

This chapter discusses the multiple developmental processes that occur during the first year of life. For each developmental process, possible normal variations and indications for clinical concern are described. The theoretical foundation of the chapter is the transactional model (Sameroff & Chandler, 1974), which asserts that infants, caregivers, and their environment mutually determine the child's developmental and behavioral outcome (see Chapter 2). Seen in these terms, child development is more than a two-way street; it is an intimate and complex interaction. Caregiving, through good times and adversity, impacts the child's neurophysiology and structural changes in the brain; the social environment becomes embedded in biology.

NEUROLOGIC INDICATORS OF NEONATAL MATURITY

State Organization/Sleep

Healthy full-term infants display a regular series of distinct states over time. The study of behavioral states in infants has attracted wide interest as an indicator of the functional integrity of the central nervous system (CNS) during the fetal, neonatal, and infant periods of development (Table 6.1). Maturational changes in neonatal state periodicities have been correlated with later neurodevelopmental outcome; earlier maturation of electrophysiologic and behavioral patterns of quiet sleep in the newborn period predict higher performance on cognitive tests at preschool and school age (Scher, 2005; Shellhaas et al., 2017).

Sleeping and waking states in infancy reflect the competency of the CNS, and they modulate the infant's interactions with the external environment. An infant's behavior differs, depending on whether the infant is in a sleep, drowsy, or alert state, as described in the vignette. A visual stimulus that captures the attention of a quietly awake infant does not elicit a response from an aroused, crying infant. Cyclic activity of the autonomic nervous system mediates the infant's responsivity to the external environment and regulates numerous homeostatic functions. Neonatal behavioral and psychophysiologic measures of state organization highlight maturational differences between preterm and term infants that could affect their responses to caregiving (see Chapter 34). Overall, sleep regulation and consolidation represent critical developmental processes that occur in the first years of life.

TABLE 6.1 Neonatal State Classification Scale

State	Characteristics
Quiet sleep	Regular breathing, eyes closed; spontaneous activity confined to startles and jerky movements at regular intervals. Responses to external stimuli partially inhibited, any response is likely to be delayed. No eye movements, and state changes are unlikely after stimuli or startles than in other states.
Active sleep	Irregular breathing, sucking movements, eyes closed. Rapid eye movements detected underneath the closed lids. Infants also have some low-level and irregular motor activity. Startles occur in response to external stimuli and can produce a change of state.
Drowsiness	Eyes may be open or closed; eyelids often flutter; activity level variable and interspersed with mild startles. Drowsy newborns are responsive to sensory stimuli with delay, and state change frequently follows stimulation.
Alert inactivity	A bright alert look, with attention focused on sources of auditory or visual stimuli; motor activity is inhibited while attending to stimuli.
Active awake	Eyes open, high motor activity, thrusting movements of extremities, and occasional startles set off by activity; reactive to external stimulation with increased startles or motor activity. Discrete responses are difficult to note because of general high activity level.
Crying	Intense irritability in the form of sustained crying, and jerky limb movement. This state is difficult to break through with stimulation.

Adapted from Brazelton, T. B. (1984). *Neonatal Behavioral Assessment Scale* (2nd ed.). Heinemann.

Clinical Implications

The infant's control of state, responsiveness to environmental input, and sleep-wake patterns show wide individual variations. A crying infant who quiets down when picked up and a drowsy one who becomes wide-eyed at the sound of mother's voice delight caregivers. Infants who cannot sustain an alert, receptive state unless assisted by an adult who swaddles them or gently restrains their hands may challenge adult caregivers. Methods to assist such infants in maintaining alertness include swaddling them and minimizing extraneous sounds or images when the infant is trying to focus.

Clinical supervision of sleep disorders requires an understanding of the normal developmental and individual variability in children's sleep patterns. Newborns typically sleep 16.5 hours per day, 6-month-olds sleep approximately 14.25 hours, and 1- to 2-year-olds sleep approximately 13 hours a day including naps (Ferber, 2006). The clinician can help parents devise strategies that gradually mold the infant's innate biologic rhythms into socially convenient patterns (see Chapters 70 and 92, which specifically discuss clinical interventions and sleep). New parents may require help with distinguishing active or rapid eye movement (REM) sleep occurring every 50 to 60 minutes with waking. Infants moan, groan, move around, and may even open their eyes while in REM sleep, which uninformed parents may interpret as a signal to feed or intervene, leading to waking up a sleeping baby and delaying the development of sustained sleep.

Sensory Maturation

Sensory systems undergo rapid changes during the last trimester of pregnancy and the first several months after birth. An orderly sequence characterizes the functional development of the sensory systems of infants *in utero*; the tactile and auditory systems develop early. The visual system is the last sensory system to start functioning during gestation and the least well developed at birth. Sensory abilities in infants mature rapidly during the first year of life. The newborn's vision is optimal at 19 cm, a visual acuity of about 20/120. By 8 months of age, visual acuity improves to 20/30, nearly as good as normal adult acuity.

Clinical Implications

Parents subliminally monitor their infant's responses to sensory input and modulate input to enhance the infant's responsiveness. A mother may move her head slowly back and forth until the infant's expression signals that her face is in focus. Parents slow the tempo of their speech and elongate and amplify words, often called parentese, to maintain infant's attention. Research shows positive brain-related changes in response to parentese versus normal adult speech cadence (Kuhl et al., 2014).

The Brazelton Neonatal Behavioral Assessment Scale (NBAS) was developed by T. Berry Brazelton and colleagues in the early 1970s to measure newborn behavior, to identify and understand normal variability, and to know the impact of prematurity and drug exposure on behavioral functioning (Brazelton, 1995). The NBAS has been shortened to the Newborn Behavioral Observation (NBO) tool to train clinicians to be observers of newborn behavior, respond effectively to newborn needs, and be utilized as a clinical relationship-building tool (Nugent et al., 2007).

Colic is a common condition that is likely related to temperamental characteristics of low sensory threshold to stimulation. Colic typically resolves in a predictable time course by 3 months with or without medical therapy in most cases. The most important role of the health care professional in colic is to educate, reassure, and support families (Fireman, 2006).

Clinicians may need to provide explicit guidance for families whose infants are unusually hypersensitive or unresponsive, which is common among premature or small-for-gestational-age infants. Sounds and sights that are attractive to most infants are aversive to hypersensitive infants. Although most infants prefer to track a moving face that is making sounds, hypersensitive infants may avert their gaze, vomit, or startle when confronted with simultaneous visual and auditory stimulation. With these infants, stimulation can be adaptively offered to one sense at a time. Extraneous stimuli, such as bright lights and loud music, should be decreased. When parents express concern that their infant does not seem to hear or see, the infant should be formally assessed.

SOCIAL-EMOTIONAL DEVELOPMENT

Attachment

Attachment describes the enduring and specific affective bond that children develop with caregivers. The infant's behavior signals, including crying, fussing due to hunger or cold, quiet alert, and sleepy, are learned through trial and error. These behaviors allow caregivers to respond effectively to meet the infant's needs leading to feelings of safety and security. Maternal depression, other mental health problems, alcohol and drug use, and domestic violence can interfere with understanding and responsiveness, which may be experienced by the infant as a stress or adversity (see Chapter 5). As we saw in the opening vignette, the primary caregiver may not be one of the parents. It may be other family members or childcare providers who interact with the child regularly.

The infant also contributes to this dyadic relationship. An alert infant who reacts readily to parents' faces and responds promptly to consoling maneuvers enhances parents' positive feelings and a sense of competence. A drowsy, relatively hypotonic infant who provides less satisfying feedback may diminish parents' emotional satisfaction.

Security of attachment is predicted by (1) caregivers' current representations of their own childhood experiences as expressed by their attachment experiences and (2) caregivers' sensitive responsivity to their infants' cues during the first year of life. Self-understanding of their upbringing enhances the adult's ability to be good parents. Clinicians can support parents' self-understanding by asking key questions (Zuckerman & Zuckerman, 2019).

Most families require several months before they learn to identify and respond effectively to their infant's needs for food, rest, or social interaction. By 3 months of age, the child and caregivers achieve social synchrony manifested by reciprocal vocal and affective exchanges. Adult displays of pleasure are followed by smiling, cooing, and movement in the infant.

The next important step in the attachment process is the development of a clear preference for primary caregivers. By 3 to 5 months of age, an infant stops crying more readily for familiar caregivers than for strangers. Infants usually smile sooner and more brightly for their parents than for other adults, and this clear behavioral preference enhances the parents' formation of positive emotional ties to their infant.

Initially, attachment figures provide a sense of security through their physical presence. Later in the first year, infants internalize their relationship with attachment figures, leading to an internal model of security. By 18 months of age, infants can conjure an image of the attachment figure in their mind (memory), which helps comfort them when the parent is not present.

The creation of a secure relationship of attachment requires consistent availability of adults who are affectionate and responsive to the child's physical and emotional needs. The adults are often the infant's parents, but, as in the vignette, may be other caregivers, based on circumstances. Other factors include mutuality and synchrony, stimulation, positive attitude, and emotional support. Without a secure home base, infants cannot move outward effectively.

Children given the opportunity to develop a secure relationship are better able to build positive relationships with peers and unrelated adults and to cope with stress than children without a home base.

The research method commonly used to describe infant attachment is the strange situation (Ainsworth, 1979). The purpose of this classic paradigm is to assess the quality of an infant's attachment to parents and to evaluate an infant's capacities for coping with stress when a parent leaves the infant's presence and then returns. Attachment theory describes four categories of response at the time of reunion with the caregiver (Table 6.2).

Clinical Implications

The clinician should attempt to identify parental problems, such as depression, excessive drug and alcohol use, and/or past or concurrent adversity (see Chapter 5), which can interfere with sensitive responses that are needed for secure attachment. A two- and three-generation family history often has important implications for the preventing or mitigating intergenerational transmission of mental health conditions.

Clinicians are able to observe and reinforce parent behaviors that promote attachment. When a parent attends to the infant's signals and interest, engages in a shared moment of communication, and shows enjoyment in the infant's face and voice, clinicians should acknowledge the parent's responsiveness. Conversely, if parents exhibit a monotone with their baby, impatience with diaper changes, or emotional disconnection, clinicians should inquire about the parents' feelings and practices in an effort to detect whether the family may require enhanced support. Clinicians can model responsive joyful interactions with the child to coach parents unobtrusively and respectfully to explore the relational capacity of the child. Clinicians may consider using a digital application, such as Small Moments, Big Impact (2021), developed for new parents with weekly segments for the first 6 months to promote parent and infant emotional wellbeing.

When mothers do not respond to their infant's attempts to get their attention, often called a mismatch, the infant responds with distress as indicated by crying, turning away, and jerky movements. This infant response is normal, inevitable, and occurs commonly while parents are driving, cooking, or speaking on the phone. Mismatches are "repaired" when caregivers eventually respond to their infant's distress. After repair, young infants often show joy in the reconnection, likely indicating a sense of trust. This sequence is one of

TABLE 6.2 Categories of Attachment Based on the Strange Situation Classificationa

Category	Description
Secure attachment	1. Reunites with the caregiver and uses the caregiver to become calmed 2. Returns to play quickly Implication: The child's signals have typically be responded to in a respectful, caring manner. This pattern is associated with development of later positive social relationships.
Avoidant attachment	1. No overt response to the return of the caregiver 2. Continues play as though the caregiver did not leave and return Implications: This pattern suggests the child's signals are rarely perceived or responded to in an effective manner. Avoidant attachment predicts later difficulty relating to peers and the emergence of a poorly developed sense of self.
Ambivalent attachment	1. Turns to the mother upon reunion, but become fretful and not easily soothed 2. Does not return to play Implications: This pattern predicts a later level of uncertainty and anxiety in social situations.
Disorganized attachment	1. Chaotic and/or self-destructive behavior upon reunion 2. Does not return to play Implications: This pattern is ascribed to recurring situations when a parent repeatedly causes a state of fear in a child, by expressing excessive anger, withdrawing, or creating a setting in which the child is offered no hope of comfort or safety, or no relief from distress.

[a]The category is defined by the child's behavior on reunion after a brief separation.

the origins of empathy development. Alternatively, when mismatches are not repaired most of the time, the infant's secure attachment may be undermined, and neurophysiology may be disrupted.

Separation

Negotiation of separation, both psychological and physical, poses a continuous challenge to parents and children. In Mahler's theory, separation refers to the internal processes by which the child evolves a satisfying identity as an individual, distinct from the parents (Mahler et al., 1975). Physical separations may enhance or impede the child's ability to develop a comfortable individuality. Responsive caregivers encourage the infant's security and independence. A complementary process of acceptance of the child's internal separation occurs within the parents. Some parents accept an infant's total dependence and have difficulty tolerating a toddler's striving for an independent identity.

Cultural Variations of Parenting Related to Social-Emotional Development

Attachment and separation, discussed earlier, reflect a Western framework. Western cultures emphasize autonomy, individual achievement, self-reliance, and self-assertiveness, which all require parents to offer frequent praise, favor verbal feedback over physical contact, and promote independent behaviors. In contrast, parents in other cultures, particularly in Asian, African, and Latin American countries, tend to value interdependence, collective achievement, sharing, and collaboration. Parenting behaviors that reinforce these traditional concepts originate in agrarian society in which the community survival requires pooling limited resources (food, water, shelter) and distributing them equitably. However, due to economic growth, increased educational opportunity, and skills needed for modern jobs, many of these cultures, with the exception of those living in rural areas, are gradually adopting Western attitudes (Greenfield, 2007).

Feeding is an example of a cross-cultural parenting difference that can have profound impact on the infant. Cultures oriented toward autonomy may emphasize self-feeding, whereas cultures oriented toward interdependence may allow parents to spoon-feed children to older ages. Cultural variations related to sleep are also significant. In an autonomy-oriented approach to sleep parents put children to sleep in their own cribs or rooms. This decision requires the infant to self-regulate. In an interdependence-oriented approach to sleep adults and children share the bed. These traditions should be acknowledged when providing standard pediatric recommendations that may conflict with predominant cultural practices.

Clinical Implications

Infants and toddlers who have experienced chronically inconsistent nurturing may seem uninterested in exploring the surrounding world and may appear clingy without the presence of obvious stress. Other infants may appear actively angry and distrustful of their primary caregivers, ignoring or resisting caregivers' efforts to comfort them after brief separations or stress.

A serious disturbance of the attachment process may be suspected when otherwise typically developing infants between the ages of 9 months and 2 years fail to show a preference for familiar caregivers in response to stress. Such behavior should alert the clinician to search for developmental delay, serious family dysfunction, neglect, or abuse, as described later under Consequences/Biologic Embedding of Early Adversity.

The child's and parents' responses to everyday experiences of physical separation, such as bedtime, childcare, and parental travel, vary widely. Brief, predictable physical separations from the parents may facilitate successful psychological separation for young children. When parents express apparently disproportionate anxiety about their child's wellbeing during routine separations, they are often expressing their ambivalence about the child's evolution of independence. Explicit discussion of the parents' feelings about internal and external separations can be more effective than reassurance about the ostensible concern.

Difficulties with separation become acute when, at 7 to 9 months of age, children begin to show separation distress, crying whenever the caregiver leaves their presence. Clinicians can help parents recognize that the separation distress results from normal object permanence (see Chapter 3 and as described later). Parents can facilitate the formation of these relationships with strangers by their physical availability to the child as the relationship is first formed. Childcare providers or babysitters should be introduced with a parent present and slowly increasing the duration of separation depending on whether it is a strange or home setting. The child's age and temperament should also be considered. Regressive behavior on reunion with the parent should be expected and is normal.

Because the separation process is mutual, clinicians should be alert to parental issues that can unintentionally sabotage the child's establishment of a separate identity. Identity formation may be particularly in jeopardy when the parents perceive the child as unusually "vulnerable" because of past illness or factors that make a child special (e.g., only boy, last child). A recent loss in the parents' lives, such as a death or divorce, also can threaten the normal separation process. Such parents can become overprotective, leading to the vulnerable child syndrome with separation difficulties, insufficient setting of limits, somatic concerns, and overuse of the health care system (Pearson & Boyce, 2004). A clinician who encourages parents to discuss their real or imagined losses can help to liberate the parent and the child.

Social Referencing and Joint Attention

Infants look to their primary caregiver for signals (smile, comfort, fear) about how to deal with new experiences, a phenomenon referred to as social referencing. It emerges from the age of 7 to 10 months and forms a foundation for social learning and social appraisal in adulthood. When approached by a stranger, a 7-month-old infant looks to the parent to see if it is okay to allow this stranger to approach. If the parent smiles comfortably, the infant is more likely to remain calm. If the parent is upset, the child is more likely to cry.

In parallel, joint attention, referring to the capacity to coordinate attention with others regarding objects and events, emerges. Joint attention begins when the infant is about 6 months of age and continues to 18 months. It is associated with future language, cognitive, and social skills. Joint attention then becomes triadic, meaning that the child can direct the attention of one person actively to share in the child's experience of another person or object, often a toy. These two phenomenon are critical milestones of social-emotional development.

Clinical Implications

Encouraging parents to engage their child in conversation, song, and natural eye contact is important from the first days of life. Joint attention provides the opportunity for infants to get the most out of caregivers reading to them; they can look back and forth from book to parent's face with all its emotions with reading and eye contact. Monitoring for the appearance of social referencing and joint attention in the first 2 years of life has become a focus of great attention in efforts for earlier identification of developmental disorders, such as autism spectrum disorders (see Chapter 41).

Autonomy and Mastery

Autonomy refers to the achievement of behavioral independence. Mastery describes the child's quest for competence. These complementary processes require that caregivers and infants continually renegotiate control of the infant's bodily functions and social interactions to prevent struggles over feeding, sleep, toileting, and exploration. Self-consoling behavior marks the beginning of autonomy. A crying infant tries to bring the hand to the mouth, then sucks and stops crying. Sucking facilitates the infant's ability to regulate the level of arousal. Infants who engage in frequent hand sucking cry less than other infants. Sucking on sucrose may reduce further a reaction to a painful stimulus possibly through a neurally mediated pathway. As infants mature, the repertoire for self-consolation expands to include rhythmic behaviors, such as body rocking (20% of all children) and head banging or rolling (6% of all children); these behaviors usually begin between 6 and 10 months of age.

Clinical Implications

The child's struggles for autonomy and mastery produce varying degrees of discord depending on the temperamental style of the child and the characteristics of the caregivers. Clinicians' use of the construct of temperament (i.e., the how of behavior) can facilitate successful negotiation of this developmental stage.

Temperament

Children's behavior can be described as consisting of three components: (1) the *what* of behavior, (2) the *why* of behavior, and (3) the *how* of behavior. The latter can be considered temperament, children's behavioral style, which is different than what they do or why they do it (see Chapter 80). Although not fixed, temperamental characteristics are likely to be consistent over time, especially when the interplay between the individual and the environment remains relatively stable.

Clinical Implications

A poor fit between the child's temperament and the demands and expectations of parents and other caretakers may cause struggles and parental distress, while a good fit makes life easy for everyone (see Chapter 80). A classic example is predictability of biologic functioning. A child with predictable rhythms sleeps, eats, and eliminates at roughly the same time each day. A child with irregular rhythms in these areas can be confusing to many parents. Approach or withdrawal refers to the nature of a child's initial response to new stimuli (e.g., new foods). A child with positive approach likes new foods, enjoys the first bath, approaches strangers regularly, and sleeps well in new surroundings. A child with a negative or withdrawal approach rejects the first taste of infant cereal, will not fall a sleep in strange beds, and keeps a distance from new people. This lack of predictability can confuse parents and thus lead to feeding and sleeping difficulty. When combined with the temperamental characteristic of slow adaptability, negative responses to selected stimuli can continue over a long period of time. High-intensity responding children cry loudly when distressed; low-intensity responsive children whimper or cry softly. In the face of a challenging temperamental characteristic parents of such children tend to blame themselves, believing they must be doing something wrong. When more than one difficult characteristic cooccurs, parental competency and patience are challenged. It is important that clinicians communicate to parents that it is the child's temperament, not their fault nor their child's so-called bad behavior.

Clinical management should focus on reinterpreting the child's behavior from adjectives such as *naughty* or *disobedient* to manifestations of temperament such as *irregular biologic rhythms* or *slowly adaptive*. A better fit between parents' expectations and children's behavior can be created if parents understand their child's temperament and how to avoid unnecessary expectations and subsequent conflict. The clinician may not be able to change a child's inherent temperament but can change the parents' expectations and behavioral responses to them to create a better fit.

Consequences/Biologic Embedding of Early Adversity

A landmark retrospective study demonstrated that adverse childhood experiences (ACEs) predicted poor long-term health and behavioral outcomes, underscoring the importance of the life-course approach for prevention and early intervention (Felitti et al., 1998) (see Chapters 2 and 15). This finding has led to decades of research that has confirmed this finding and elucidated pathways of how social factors occurring in utero and in the first years of a child's life play a role in establishing a lifelong trajectory of physical and mental health problems. The impact of adversity on infants occurs within the context of caregiver-infant relationship. Caregivers with mental health problems such as depression, addiction, and posttraumatic stress disorder are at particular risk of impaired interaction with infants, in turn leading to alterations in the developing brain and immunologic, metabolic, and cardiovascular systems of the infant (Nelson et al., 2020) (see Chapter 5). These alterations may lead to negative developmental outcomes, including subsequent learning and behavior problems, obesity, heart disease, depression, substance abuse, and higher rates of school dropout and unemployment (Berens et al., 2017). Differences in impact are based on intensity, frequency, duration, and timing of adverse events as well as the context of a child's life (e.g., presence of positive supports) (Nelson et al., 2020) and individual neurophysiologic characteristics, especially hypersensitivity to stimuli (Boyce, 2016; Nelson et al., 2020). These findings have generated approaches to clinical screening, identifying protective and resiliency factors, and developing and evaluating interventions (Shonkoff & Garner, 2012). Efforts to mitigate the impact of adversity in early childhood often focus on caregiver-child interactions, as responsive interactions buffer the impact of social adversity (Bick et al., 2015).

Events during early life may be preferentially embedded due to the presence of so-called sensitive periods during infancy and early childhood (i.e., windows of rapid development and heightened responsiveness to both negative and positive experiences). A compelling example of sensitive periods comes from the study of high-quality foster care as an intervention for early institutionalization with its accompanying lack of responsive caregiving in Bucharest, Romania (Nelsonet al., 2014). Children who remained institutionalized suffered lasting effects on brain development and later health, including decreased brain activity, reduced gray and white matter volume, and dysregulation of their stress response systems (Nelson, 2017). Children born in institutionalized care who were placed in high-quality foster care before age 2 years had significantly improved outcomes.

MOTOR DEVELOPMENT

Fine Motor Development

It is in large part through motor acts that infants expand beyond their vision, their experience of the world, and further develop and express perception, emotion, and cognition. Between 2 and 3 months of age, the weakening of the obligatory asymmetric tonic neck reflex and expansion of accommodative abilities permit infants to look at their hands and touch one hand with the other. During the third month of life, as the world of close proximity comes into focus, infants begin swiping at objects with loosely fisted hands. At this stage, infants swipe with one hand only, but by 6 months of age they reach persistently toward objects in the midline, at first with both hands and then with one.

Between 3 and 6 months of age, the coordination of grasping and reaching gradually comes under visual guidance and voluntary control. During early reaching efforts, grasping may occur, but only after the hand has contacted the object. After 6 months of age, infants begin to shape their hands for grasping in the horizontal or vertical plane of the desired object immediately before touching it. By 9 months of age, shaping of the hand occurs before the object is reached. At 1 year old, children orient the hand in the appropriate plane when starting to reach for an object.

When the infant can reliably obtain an object, clumsy whole-hand grasping becomes progressively refined. At 4 months of age, the infant holds an object between fingers and palm; at 5 months of age, the thumb becomes involved. By 7 months of age, thumb and fingers can grasp and retain an object without resting on the palm at all. At this time, the infant uses a raking motion between the thumb and several fingers to scoop up small objects. By 9 months of age, the infant manipulates small objects with a neat pincer grasp, using thumb and forefinger perpendicular to the surface. Every nook and cranny are now accessible to the infant's exploration, which increases the chance for injury or accidental ingestion.

Gross Motor Development

Three processes enable the infant to attain upright posture and the ability to move the limbs across the body's midline: (1) balance of flexor and extensor tone, (2) decline of obligatory primary reflexes, and (3) evolution of protective and equilibrium responses. First, the flexed newborn posture gradually unfolds until 6 months of age; infants can extend their legs so far that they can put their toes in their mouth. Second, the decline and integration into voluntary patterns of initially obligatory primary reflexes (e.g., the Moro or asymmetric tonic neck reflex) permit the infant more flexible movement. A 1-month-old infant cannot look to one side or the other without assuming the fencing posture of the asymmetric tonic neck reflex. Third, to sit and walk, the infant must establish equilibrium and protective responses (e.g., the parachute reflex).

Clinical Implications

The age range for normal development of motor skills is wide. An important tenet is not to focus on a rigid timetable of motor milestones but to appreciate the trajectory of the ongoing process. Generally, infants learn to maintain new positions weeks to months before they can attain them voluntarily. Many infants at 6 months of age sit briefly unsupported if placed in that position but cannot get themselves into a sitting position until 8 months of age. Most children cannot walk independently until 4 to 5 months after they have learned to pull themselves up to a standing position. The developmental route to walking varies with the child's tone and temperament. Temperamentally inactive children or children who adapt slowly may not attempt independent walking until long after they are neurologically able to do so. Conversely, very active infants start taking steps as soon as they can stand. During the second year of life, these active infants rarely walk if they can run.

Parents are often relieved to know that within the wide range of normal variation there is no correlation between intelligence and the age at which gross motor skills are acquired. No single motor skill can be used as an indicator of neurologic integrity or dysfunction. Generally, the clinician should investigate when delayed milestones are associated with global delays, opisthotonic posturing, persistent fisting of the hands, consistent disuse of a limb or side of the body, obligatory and prolonged infantile reflexes, or failure to develop a neat pincer grasp by the first birthday. The diagnosis of cerebral palsy and other motor disabilities is described in Chapter 39.

COGNITIVE DEVELOPMENT

The developmental theories of Jean Piaget provide a useful clinical framework for understanding infant cognitive growth (see Chapter 3). Piaget believed that infants are active initiators, not passive recipients; they begin to modify behavior in response to environmental demands. Infants can take in (assimilate) information and use it to revise (accommodate) existing mental structures, which Piaget called schemas.

Piaget organized cognitive development during the sensorimotor period (birth to 2 years of age) into six stages (Table 6.3). Each stage represents a temporary equilibrium between the infant's skills and the environment's challenges. A toy that is too familiar no longer engages the toddler who prefers the greater challenges posed by the contents of the kitchen cupboard. Conversely, a completely unsolvable problem (e.g., a crayon presented for a 9-month-old infant to use) does not hold the infant's interest. Children are active learners; their cognitive development requires opportunities for exploration and manipulation that are neither too easy nor too hard. Two core concepts of infant cognition, object permanence and causality, develop in the first year of life, and play is important in advancing both.

Object Permanence

Newborns behave as though the world consists of shifting images that cease to exist when they are no longer perceived. "Out of sight, out of mind" is a description of the infant's world during the first stage of sensorimotor development (stage I). By 2 months of age, infants continue to look expectantly at a person's empty hand after an object has been dropped from sight (stage II). Between 4 and 8 months of age, infants locate a partly hidden object and visually track objects through a vertical trajectory. If infants see an object being hidden, however, they do not search for it (stage III). Between 9 and 12 months of age, infants can find an object that they see hidden (stage IV). At this age, however, infants cannot retrieve an object that is moved in plain view from one hiding place to another. By 18 months of age, infants reliably find objects after multiple changes of position as long as those changes are observed, but they cannot deduce the whereabouts of an object if they do not see it being moved (stage V). By age 2 years, toddlers have sufficient symbolic abilities to infer a hidden object's position from other cues without actually observing it being moved to that position (stage VI). People and things now reliably exist for toddlers as stable entities whether or not they are perceptually present—an important achievement that has implications for separation and attachment behaviors.

Causality

Piaget observed an orderly sequence of changes in the child's understanding of causal relationships over the first 2 years of life. First, infants learn to recreate satisfying bodily sensations by maneuvers, such as thumb sucking (primary circular reaction). At about 3 months of age, infants begin to use causal behaviors to recreate accidentally discovered, interesting effects (secondary circular reaction). Infants at this age repeatedly kick the mattress once they have discovered by chance that this behavior sets in motion a mobile above the bed. During the second year of life, toddlers become experimenters, intent on causing novel events such as winding up a toy to make it move instead of just pushing it (tertiary circular reactions).

TABLE 6.3 Piagetian Stages

Piagetian Stage	Age	Object Permanence	Causality	Play	Receptive Language	Expressive Language
I	Birth–1 mo	Shifting images	Generalization of reflexes		Turns to voice	Range of cries (hunger, pain)
II	1–4 mo	Stares at spot from which object disappeared (looks at hand after yarn drops)	Primary circular reactions (thumb sucking)		Searches for a human speaker with eyes	Cooing; vocal contagion
III	4–8 mo	Visually follows dropped object through vertical trajectory (tracks dropped yarn to floor)	Secondary circular reactions (recreates accidentally discovered environmental effects [e.g., kicks mattress to shake mobile])	Same behavioral repertoire for all objects (bangs, shakes, puts in mouth, drops)	Responds to own name and to tones of voice	Babbling; four distinct syllables
IV	9–12 mo	Finds an object after watching it hidden	Coordination of secondary circular reactions	Visual motor inspection of objects; peek-a-boo	Listens selectively to familiar words; responds to "no" and other verbal requests	First real word; "jargoning"; symbolic gestures (shakes head "no")
V	12–18 mo	Recovers hidden object after multiple visible changes of position	Tertiary circular reactions (deliberately varies behavior to create novel effects)	Awareness of social function of objects; symbolic play centered on own body (drinks from toy cup)	Can bring familiar object from another room; points to parts of body	Many single words—uses words to express needs; acquires 10 words by 18 mo
VI	18 mo–2 yr	Recovers hidden object after invisible changes in position	Spontaneously uses nondirect causal mechanisms (uses key to move wind-up toy)	Symbolic play directed toward doll (gives doll a drink)	Follows series of two or three commands; points to picture when named	Telegraphic 2-word sentence

Play

A child's play provides a window through which we come to better understand the child. For example, an infant's handling of objects also reflects a progressive understanding of the world. At 5 to 6 months of age, an infant can reliably reach and grasp attractive objects. At this stage, the infant subjects all toys to the same behavioral repertoire; a toy car, a bell, and a spoon all are mouthed, shaken, banged, and dropped. By 9 months of age, the infant systematically manipulates the object to inspect it with eyes and hands in all orientations, showing the cognitive ability to process information simultaneously instead of sequentially.

By the first birthday, the infant shows understanding of the socially assigned function of objects (e.g., pushing a toy car, ringing a bell). Next, early representational play, which reflects a stable concept of objects, appears. At first, such play centers on the child's own body as the child "drinks" from a toy cup or puts a toy telephone to the ear. Between 17 and 24 months of age, the child's thought and play become less egocentric. Now the child offers the drink to a doll. When the child becomes facile in the use of symbols (24–30 months of age), truly imaginative play begins with the onset of symbolic play.

COMMUNICATION

Communication consists of speech, language, and complex nonverbal and pragmatic skills (see Chapter 44). Infants acquire reciprocal communication through interaction with responsive sources. Screen media have negligible effects on early language learning in infants. To gain the child's attention, parents, talk to their infant is saturated with affect. Children who are sung to throughout the day often learn these "musical words" early because of the strong affect and melody with which they are presented. Parents and infants begin to construct the basis for language before infants can understand or produce a single word.

During the first year, through games and caregiving rituals, children learn to take turns communicating. With vocalization and nonverbal cues, caregivers and infants learn to direct each other's attention to interesting environmental events, to signal needs and feelings. Between 1 and 3 months of age, the infant develops a range of nondistress vocalizations, onomatopoetically described as cooing. The caregiver's contingent responses to these early vocalizations shape the infant's vocalization into back-and-forth conversation-like patterns.

By 4 to 6 months of age, infants can produce vowel sounds and some consonants called babbling. By late in the first year, infants produce repetitive two-syllable combinations, such as *mama* and *dada*, although at this time these combinations have no symbolic reference. Soon thereafter, the first true words usually refer to parents and other family members because the infant's concept of object permanence occurs for people before inanimate objects. Between 10 and 15 months of age, infants speak their first real words or expressive language. During this time, infants also begin to use symbolic gestures, such as shaking the head to indicate "no." Most 1-year-old infants respond to simple commands, such as "bye-bye" or "no-no," and most 15-month-old children can point to one or two body parts indicating receptive language skills.

Clinical Implications

The rate and quality of the infant's progression through linguistic development is sensitive to caregiving practices. Children who hear more language will develop language more quickly than children who have limited input. Clinicians can model talking to infants. Pronunciation is not a focus of concern for children younger than 3 years of age since there is a developmental progression of letter sounds children can make up to age 6 years.

Isolated speech difficulties from either anatomic or neurologic abnormalities may be seen in children with normal language skills. Such children often have difficulty with other oral-motor behaviors, such as eating or blowing kisses, or with other fine motor skills. Through exposure to books, signs, and songs, infants gradually become exposed to more words. Book sharing establishes the enjoyable joint activity of pointing and naming of objects, which is the first step in early literacy (Zuckerman & Needlman, 2020).

PHYSICAL GROWTH

Caregivers must provide infants with nutrients to sustain the rapid growth of body and brain, which is greater during the first 2 years of life than at any other time after birth. Seventy percent of adult brain growth occurs by 2 years. At birth, the infant's small, elongated mouth, combined with forward and backward movements of the tongue, squeeze the nipple creating positive pressure so that milk is suckled. By 3 months infants become progressively efficient at true sucking, which employs negative pressure to obtain milk from the nipple. By 9 to 12 months of age, the development of the pincer grasp permits the child to eat finger foods followed by the ability to use a spoon and hold a cup or bottle. Parental concerns about messiness, decreased appetite, and selective tastes emerge at this time.

Clinical Implications

Newborn boys are larger than newborn girls at birth, and they continue to grow at a faster rate during the first 3 to 6 months of life. After the first 6 months of life there are no sex differences in infant growth rate. A severely decreased rate of weight gain for children under 2 years usually reflects inadequate nutrition or complicating illness, not immutable genetic potential, and should be evaluated. Two-thirds of normal infants cross percentile measurements in length, while their genotype for height is established by 2 years of age. Premature infants should be evaluated according to their corrected age (current postnatal age minus the number of weeks the child was premature).

CONCLUSION

An understanding of infant development and behavior and parental attributions and responses provides a transactional framework to nurture the child's primary attachments involved in the beginnings of internal security, self-control, empathy, and learning. There are vast cultural differences in the approaches caregivers take with children, and there are many different ways to raise a healthy and well-adjusted infant. Moreover, there is wide individual variation in the age at which children reach developmental milestones in infancy. Clinicians can support the range of approaches that families and caregivers use with infants, provided that they are grounded in responsive and respectful practices. Clinicians play a critical role in responding to caregiver concerns to promote a healthy psychosocial environment for the infant. In addition, identification of developmental or behavioral problems through developmental surveillance, screening, assessment, and treatment can often prevent or ameliorate later problems.

REFERENCES

Ainsworth. M. D. S. (1979). Infant-mother attachment. *American Psychologist*, *33*, 932.

Berens, A. E., Jensen, S. K. G., & Nelson, C. A. (2017). Biological embedding of childhood adversity: From physiological mechanisms to clinical implications. *BMC Medicine*, *15*(1), 135.

Bick, J., Zhu, T., Stamoulis, C., Fox, N. A., Zeanah, C., & Nelson, C. A. (2015). Effect of early institutionalization and foster care on long-term white matter development: A randomized clinical trial. *JAMA Pediatrics*, *169*(3), 211–219.

Boyce. W. T. (2016). Differential susceptibility of the developing brain to contextual adversity and stress. *Neuropsychopharmacology*, *41*, 142–162.

Brazelton. T. B. (1995). *Neonatal Behavioral Assessment Scale* (3rd ed.). Mac Keith Press.

Felitti, V. J., Anda, R. F., Nordenberg, D., et al. (1998). Relationship of childhood abuse and household dysfunction to many of the leading causes of death in adults. The Adverse Childhood Experiences (ACE) Study. *American Journal of Preventive Medicine, 14*(4), 245–258.

Ferber. R. (2006). *Solve your child's sleep problems: New, revised, and expanded edition.* Simon & Schuster.

Fireman. L. (2006). Colic. *Pediatric Reviews, 27*, 357–358.

Greenfield. P. (2007). Cultural change and human development. *New Directions for Child & Adolescent Development, 1999*(83), 37–59.

Kuhl, P. K., Ramírez, R. R., Bosseler, A., Lotus Lin, J. F., & Imada, J. (2014). Infants' brain activity in response to speech. *Proceedings of the National Academy of Sciences, 111*(31), 1238–11245.

Mahler, M., Pine, F., & Bergman, A. (1975). *The psychological birth of the human infant.* Basic Books.

Nelson. C. A. (2017). Hazards to early development: The biological embedding of early life adversity. *Neuron, 96*(2), 262–266.

Nelson, C. A., Bhutta, Z. A., Burke Harris, N., Danese, A., & Samara, M. (2020). Adversity in childhood is linked to mental and physical health throughout life. *BMJ*, m3048. https://doi.org/10.1136/bmj.m304.

Nelson, C. A., Fox, N. A., & Zeanah, C. H. (2014). *Romania's abandoned children: Deprivation, brain development and the struggle for recovery.* Harvard University Press.

Nugent, J. K., Keefer, C. H., Minear, S., Johnson, L. C., & Blanchard, Y. (2007). *Understanding newborn behavior and early relationships: The Newborn Behavioral Observations (NBO) system handbook.* Paul H Brookes Publishing.

Pearson, S., & Boyce, W. T. (2004). The vulnerable child syndrome. *Pediatrics in Review, 25*(10), 345–349.

Sameroff, A. J., & Chandler, M. J. (1974). Reproductive risk and the continuum of caretaking causality. *Review of Child Development Research, 4*, 187–244.

Scher. A. (2005). Infant sleep at 10 months of age as a window to cognitive development. *Early Human Development, 81*, 289–292.

Shellhaas, R. A., Burns, J. W., Hassan, F., Carlson, M. D., Barks, J. D. E., & Chervin, R. D. (2017). Neonatal sleep-wake analyses predict 18-month neurodevelopmental outcomes. *Sleep, 40*(11), zsx144. https://doi.org/10.1093/sleep/zsx144.

Shonkoff, J. P., & Garner, A. S. (2012). Committee on Psychosocial Aspects of Child and Family Health; Committee on Early Childhood, Adoption, and Dependent Care; Section on Developmental and Behavioral Pediatrics. The lifelong effects of early childhood adversity and toxic stress. *Pediatrics, 129*(1), e232–e246.

Small Moments, Big Impact. (2021). https://www.smallmomentsbigimpact.com.

Zuckerman, B., & Needlman, R. (2020). 30 years of reach out and read: Need for a developmental perspective. *Pediatrics, 145*(6).

Zuckerman, B., & Zuckerman, P. (2019). Parental self-understanding: Key to preventing problems. In *Zuckerman Parker handbook of developmental and behavioral pediatrics for primary care* (4th ed.). Wolters Kluwer.

7

Toddlerhood and the Preschool Years

Rosmary Ros-DeMarize, Silvia Pereira-Smith, and Michelle M. Macias

For additional material related to the content of this chapter, please see Chapters 41, and 44.

VIGNETTE

Nicky is a handsome, healthy 3-year, 6-month-old boy who was referred for "behavior and developmental concerns" by his primary care clinician. His parents are worried because he is having trouble communicating and becomes easily upset. Nicky began using single words at 12 months of age, phrases shortly before his second birthday, and short sentences by about 36 months of age. He currently has considerable difficulty expressing his thoughts. In addition, he is only about 75% intelligible to his parents and 50% intelligible to strangers. He throws tantrums that last about 30 minutes several times per week, typically triggered when he is unable to communicate effectively, is not getting his way, or experiences unexpected changes in his routine. Nicky sleeps through the night in his own bed, feeds himself with utensils, and helps with dressing. He is toilet trained for urine and stool during the day. He runs smoothly, rides a tricycle, and likes to draw with a crayon. He began preschool about 2 months ago. His teachers note that he is affectionate with the adults and his peers in the classroom, is motivated by praise, and is progressing with early preacademic skills such as counting and letter recognition. However, he does not remain seated during classroom activities, refuses to participate in selected classroom activities, especially answering questions at circle time, and has been aggressive with teachers on occasion, again mostly at circle time.

INTRODUCTION

This chapter describes developmental and behavioral considerations during toddlerhood and the preschool period. For our purposes here, toddlerhood refers to the period between 18 and 36 months of age, and the preschool period refers to the period between 3 and 5 years of age. Hallmarks of both periods include significant increases in receptive and expressive language skills, growth of social-emotional development and play, and increases in adaptive skills. The chapter will:

1. Review developmental domains (e.g., communication, motor, social-emotional, cognitive, adaptive) as they relate to the toddler and preschool periods
2. Review overarching concepts important for development such as self-regulation and school readiness
3. Discuss clinical implications for providers, including screening/assessment and appropriate recommendations for parents

DEVELOPMENTAL DOMAINS

The toddler and preschool years are characterized by remarkable changes in development, with acquisition of a repertoire of skills critical to a child's overall development and functioning. Table 7.1 reviews developmental expectations by domain. Looking broadly, children enter toddlerhood completely dependent on caregivers for almost all aspects of their lives and leave the preschool years with elaborate, well-developed skills. This remarkable acquisition of skills is well characterized in the Erikson stages of development (see Chapter 3). In the toddler years children seek autonomy. If that desire is not well negotiated, then they are left with a sense of shame. In the preschool years children demonstrate increasing initiative. If they cannot succeed with self-directed activities, then the result is a sense of guilt.

Communication

The development of communication involves evolution of both speech and language (see Chapter 44) and supports other important developments. The capacity to understand language and effectively communicate intentions, ideas, and emotions is necessary for virtually all aspects of learning. Receptive language advances result in the toddler learning from what people say in addition to what they do. Toddlers quickly learn that speech is a more efficient means of communication than gestures or facial expressions alone. Between 18 and 24 months of age, astounding changes in communication occur as toddlers experience a "word explosion," rapidly moving from using single words to combining words into phrases and then sentences. They use language to communicate their desires and emotions and to learn what is going on around them. By 3 years of age, children talk about past experiences and use language to pretend. By 4 years of age, children can tell stories and express their thoughts and ideas. Because young children think faster than they can talk, up to about 3.5 years of disfluent speech (known as developmental or typical disfluency) sometimes results in whole word or phrase repetition.

Language acquisition involves complex interactions between biologic, psychosocial, and environmental factors. Wide variation is found in the rate of speech and language development. Yet, children who learn two languages simultaneously generally follow the same pattern of language development as monolingual language learners (Li, 2005). Although,

TABLE 7.1 Developmental Milestones by Domains

Age	Communication	Gross Motor	Fine Motor	Adaptive	Social-Emotional	Cognitive
18 mo	• Uses about 6–10 words (other than names) • Uses giant words (e.g., "thank you"), then two-word phrases (19–24 mo) • Identifies at least two body parts • Points to at least one picture in book	• Walks up stairs with two feet per step with hand held • Sits in small chair • Carries toy while walking • Throws ball a few feet while standing • Runs with toddler gait	• Scribbles • Imitates vertical stroke • Builds three/four-cube tower	• Helps dress and undress self • Begins to scoop with spoon	• Engages with others for play • Points to object of interest to draw attention to it • Turns and looks at adults if something new happens • Gives kisses	• Matches pairs of objects • Copies doing chores
2 yr	• Uses 50 words • Combines two words into sentence • Follows two-step command • Points to ~10 pictures in book • Speech is 50% intelligible to strangers	• Walks down stairs with two feet per step holding rail • Kicks ball • Runs with coordination	• Stacks objects • Turns book pages • Uses hands to turn objects (such as knobs, toys, lids)	• Takes off some clothing • Scoops and feeds self with spoon, spilling little	• Plays alongside other children (parallel) • Plays with more than one toy at the same time	• Uses toys for simple play, like pushing a toy car • Tries to use switches or buttons on a toy • Sorts objects • Matches objects to pictures
2.5 yr	• Uses pronouns correctly • Understands "just one" • Follows two-step directions • Follows two prepositions (*in, on*)	• Begins to walk up stairs with alternating feet • Jumps in place • Walks backward 10 steps • Runs well without falling	• Grasps crayon with thumb and fingers instead of fist	• Urinates in toilet • Spears food with fork	• Engages in pretend or imitative play • Uses objects to pretend, like feeding a block to a doll as if it were food	• Shows simple problem-solving skills, like standing on a small stool to reach something • Names at least one color • Matches colors
3 yr	• Uses three word sentences • Speech is 75% intelligible to strangers • Understands simple prepositions (e.g., *on, under*) • Answers "what" and "where" questions	• Pedals tricycle • Ascends stairs alternating feet • Jumps forward • Balances on one foot for 3 s	• Copies a single circle • Cuts with child scissors • Unbuttons large button • Strings small beads	• Urinates independently • Puts on coat, jacket, or shirt by self • Eats independently	• Plays cooperatively and shares • Early imaginative play	• Does puzzles with 3 or 4 pieces • Picks the bigger of two items when asked • Draws 2–3 part person • Understands big/small • Knows age and gender

TABLE 7.1 **Developmental Milestones by Domains—cont'd**

Age	Communication	Gross Motor	Fine Motor	Adaptive	Social-Emotional	Cognitive
4 yr	• Uses four-word sentences • Speech is 100% intelligible to strangers • Answers "when" questions • Tells stories • Follows three-step command • Points to things that are same vs. different	• Gallops • Balances on one foot for 4–8 s • Hops on one foot two/three times • Standing broad jump 1–2 ft • Throws ball overhead 10 ft	• Draws cross • Copies square • Unbuttons and buttons medium-size buttons • Grasps pencil with thumb and fingers instead of fist	• Independent for bowel habits • Brushes teeth • Dresses and undresses with minimal assistance	• Engages in well-developed imaginative play • Engages in group play • Labels emotions in self (happy, sad, fear, anger)	• Knows full name • Names at least a few colors of items • Understands simple time words (yesterday, tomorrow, morning, night) • Knows what comes next in a well-known story • Draws a person with 4+ body parts
5 yr	• Understands left and right on self • Understands adjectives • Produces rhyming words • Answers "why" questions • Defines simple words • Tells stories with beginning, middle, end	• Balances for 8–10 s on one foot • Jumps backward • Skips	• Writes first name • Copies triangle • Can button 1-in buttons	• Completes simple chores well • Bathes independently • Dresses independently	• Plays games with rules or turn taking with other children • Likes to sing, dance, or act for others • Tries not to hurt others while playing • Apologizes for mistakes	• Counts to 10 • Identifies some single-digit numbers and letters • Uses simple time words (yesterday, tomorrow, morning, night) • Keeps attention for at least 5 to 10 min during activities

Adapted from Accardo & Capute, 2005; Aylward, 1995; Beery et al., 2010; Bly, 2000; Glascoe et al., 2016; Oller et al., 2012; Robins et al., 2014; Squires et al., 2009.
Note. These milestones generally represent the mean or average age of performance of these skills when available.

on average, girls use more words than boys between 12 and 30 months of age, boys are only modestly behind and typically develop words within the accepted time frame (Leaper & Smith, 2004). Delays in speech and language development are rarely due solely to bilingual exposure or to sex.

Toddlers enter the word combination period at around 18 to 24 months of age. Children begin combining two-word phrases once they spontaneously use enough single words to label, request, and comment. Initially, word combinations may be holistic phrases or giant words; these are phrases the child often hears used together such as "thank you" or "let's go." Next, the child combines words into novel phrases such as "more juice" or "bye-bye mama." By 24 months of age, toddlers combine words into two-word sentences with a verb + noun, such as "eat cookie" or "read book" (Oller et al., 2012).

Following the initial word combination period is the sentence formation period. A rough rule of thumb is that 90% of children use two-word sentences at 2 years, three-word sentences by 3 years, and four-word sentences by 4 years of age (Flipsen, 2006). Sentences become more complex as the child's comprehension of grammar and language advances. By 3 to 4 years of age, children comprehend and use prepositions, adjectives, and adverbs and begin to ask and answer questions. Semantics (word meanings) and syntax (grammar) improve over time, and by 5 years of age children completely master grammatical tense marking. As children learn the rules of social communication, pragmatic language skills are refined. By 4 to 5 years of age, most children regularly use language to discuss emotions and feelings (Oller et al., 2012) (see Social-Emotional Development, later).

Receptive language also develops in an orderly fashion during these years. A child's receptive vocabulary is much larger than the number of words used expressively. The rule of thumb is that a child should be able to follow two-step directions by 2 years of age, two prepositional commands by age 2.5 years, and three-step commands by 3 years of age.

Children master sounds at different ages depending on the difficulty of producing the sound. More difficult sounds such as consonants /j/, /r/, /l/, /v/ and blends may not be mastered until the end of the preschool period. A formula for expected intelligibility level of toddlers and preschoolers to unfamiliar listeners is: age in years/4 × 100 = % understood by strangers. Therefore by 4 years of age, a child should be 100% intelligible to strangers even if the child has not yet mastered all consonants and blends (Flipsen, 2006).

Motor Skills

Gross Motor Skills

Progression of gross motor abilities grants toddlers and preschool-aged children the power to explore their environment, which in turn allows them to enhance other skills such as the development of autonomy. By 18 months of age, toddlers are typically walking. With practice, their gait becomes steadier, and their stance narrows, due to improved core tone. At age 2 years, improved balance provides children with the ability to run, climb, kick a ball, and walk up or down stairs (initially 2 feet per step, then alternating by the end of this year). By the third birthday, children's enhanced balance skills allow them to stand on one leg, jump, and ride a tricycle. Over the next 2 years, gross motor skills become more complex; they acquire the ability to hop, skip, jump backward, and ride a bicycle. There is a wide variation in milestone achievement in gross motor skills, especially in the advanced skills (e.g., some children will always struggle with balancing on a bicycle). Regression in gross motor skills is an unusual finding and warrants an evaluation by a physician.

Fine Motor Skills

Fine motor skill progression in this developmental period allows children to begin manipulating their environment. Abilities that are developed in the beginning of toddlerhood include spontaneous scribbling and stacking three cubes to make a tower, followed by imitation of vertical or circular strokes at age 24 months. Hand preference is typically established between 2 and 3 years of age. Children put these fine motor skills into their functional activities. At about age 2, they assist with undressing and dressing. Their feeding skills also improve; they progress from feeding themselves with their fingers to using utensils, such as spearing food with a fork. At 30 months of age, a more mature pencil grasp is developed, which involves holding a pencil between the thumb and forefinger. Children can copy a circle and cut with scissors at age 3 years, copy a cross at 3.5 years, copy a square at 4 years, and copy a triangle at 5 years. It is important to note that writing skills not only include fine motor abilities but are also influenced by language, memory, and attention. In regard to dressing, children can undress themselves (usually socks and pants first, then shirts) at 3 years, button and place shoes on the correct foot at 4 years, and tie shoes by 5 years.

Adaptive Functioning

Autonomy and Fear

The transition from dependence on caregivers to the development of autonomy is often first noted after children begin walking and becomes more pronounced as they improve motor skills in toddlerhood. Temperament plays a prominent role in this process (see Chapter 80); some children are risk averse and stay close to familiar adults, while others are sensation seeking and may wander far from their home base. Other developmental skills, including cognitive abilities and communication, also facilitate this progression. Children become increasingly able to engage with their environment beyond their caregivers.

Though children generally seek autonomous discovery, exploring "the unknown" may trigger fear. That fear causes them to "check in" with their caregiver(s) who can then provide them with feelings of familiarity and safety. The need for reassurance can be confusing for caregivers as they try to balance granting their children freedom to explore while providing them comfort when they become overwhelmed by fear or curiosity. Anticipatory guidance regarding the development of autonomy and accompanying fear is multifaceted. It should include implementation of safety precautions given that children may test boundaries and place themselves in potentially unsafe situations (e.g., climbing on high furniture). It should mention that children may seek reassurance from caregivers, even becoming physically clingy if their exploration triggers fear. Substantial cultural differences characterize expectations of autonomy in toddlers and preschool children. For example, Eurocentric cultures tend to emphasize autonomy while African, Asian, Latin American, and Indigenous cultures often value interdependence.

Toilet Training

Readiness for toilet training often emerges after 18 months of age, and attainment of this important skill is completed by 3 years of age for many children. Readiness is signaled by an interest in sitting on a toilet and is often accompanied by a desire to not be soiled. Developmental skills that support the toilet training process include the ability to communicate regarding the need to use the toilet and motor skills to remove clothing and sit on the toilet. At this age, children's ability to imitate others using the toilet also facilitates their learning.

Training consists of both the child learning internal elimination cues and caregivers educating the child on the expected steps for completing this complicated task. Learning elimination cues tends to occur more quickly for girls than boys. The methods of caregiver education are strongly influenced by cultural factors (e.g., elimination communication).

Caregivers can often feel frustration during this process. Ultimately it is the toddler who must learn to control body movements. Many children respond well to a toileting schedule that is timed with their eating schedule to take advantage of the gastrocolic reflex. A reward system may be used during the toilet training process (see Chapter 4). However, it should reward cooperative tasks, such as sitting on the toilet, and not only successful completions. Some children prefer a child-size toilet, whereas others favor a standard toilet. It is highly recommended that children have a footstool provided if they use the standard toilet to help prop their legs, to allow for natural defecation positioning.

Assessment and intervention may be indicated for children who have had minimal progress with toilet training by age 3 years since it may be an indication of a serious condition. The most common medical cause for delayed toilet training is functional constipation, which can be diagnosed via history and physical examination. Interventions may consist of caregiver education about constipation, disimpaction of stool, subsequent maintenance of regular bowel movements (possibly with medication), and behavior strategies to improve toileting habits and behaviors (e.g. having consistent bowel movements inside the bathroom regardless if the child is on the toilet or in a diaper) (Law et al., 2016) (see Chapter 69). Teaching children with neurodevelopmental conditions to use the toilet should include consideration of their cognitive level; they may not yet possess the fundamental developmental skills needed for toilet training when they reach the appropriate chronologic age. Diagnostic criteria for encopresis include age of at least 4 years and at least 5 years for enuresis (American Psychological Association [APA], 2013) (see Chapter 69).

Feeding and Eating

Early healthy eating patterns can have a long-lasting impact on future health. It is not uncommon for children to become more selective during the toddler period than they were in infancy, as they flex their growing autonomy. They also may eat less during the toddler-preschool years than they did during infancy because of a decreasing rate of growth. Health care providers should share the importance of a varied diet and discuss age-appropriate portions with caregivers. However, socioeconomic status and culture may play roles in many aspects of eating, including food choices, food variety, and expectations for mealtime behavior. Federal grants and programs are available to assist families of young children gain access to healthy food and to avoid food insecurity. Children with neurodevelopmental conditions such as autism spectrum disorder (ASD) may have highly restrictive feeding patterns that require a multidisciplinary approach for treatment. The evaluation of extreme or persistent feeding or eating difficulties, such as highly restricted food choices, may require a team approach: examination by a health care provider for possible contributing medical conditions, assessment of nutritional needs by a dietician, evaluation of oromotor skills by a speech-language pathologist, and assessment of orosensory issues by an occupational therapist.

Sleeping

Though maturation of sleep architecture develops throughout childhood, sleep patterns should become consistent by toddlerhood, including the ability to fall asleep independently and sleep through the night. Night terrors and nightmares may present during toddlerhood and the preschool years. Most of the sleep-related issues that present in this era have a behavioral component (see Chapter 70). They may involve bedtime refusal or resistance and prolonged night awakenings that require caregiver involvement. Consistency, to the extent possible, is key. A child's bedtime and wakeup time should be about the same time every day. Sleep hygiene is also important. A 30-minute bedtime routine that is the same every night should consist of low-stimulation activities such as a warm bath and reading a book in the room where the child sleeps. Screen time should be limited 1 to 2 hours before bed, with all screens (including television, phones, and tablets) out of the child's bedroom (see Chapter 21). Naps should be geared to the child's age and developmental needs; long naps or too many naps can result in sleeplessness at night. Effective behavior modifications at bedtime for behavioral insomnia include issuing a limited number of "bedtime passes," use of written or visual schedules for bedtime routines, and caregiver redirection to return to bed without any reinforcement. The diagnostic workup for children presenting with sleepwalking, night terrors, or nightmares requires a focused history (including inquiry of family history of childhood parasomnias), a good sleep diary to assess for sleep deprivation, plus a physical examination. Cultural differences in regard to sleep practices are common (e.g., bedsharing) and should be explored with families to assist with shared decision making about sleep practices (Owens, 2005). The constellation of frequent nightly snoring, observed apneas, and/or daytime somnolence is concerning for obstructive sleep apnea and may indicate need for a polysomnogram. Restless sleep (including involuntary jerking movements during sleep) may suggest restless leg syndrome or periodic limb movement disorder. Low serum ferritin levels may lead to abnormal sleep movements, and the condition may improve with supplemental iron.

Social-Emotional Development

The toddler to preschool period is marked by significant growth within social-emotional skills. During toddlerhood, children's ability to use nonverbal communication skills and to participate in social reciprocity improves. Toddlers learn to express their likes and dislikes. Their increasing social skills leads to the emergence of peer relationships, especially during the preschool period. These developments change the social world of the child during this developmental period.

Nonverbal Communication and Social Reciprocity

During the toddler period, children increase their use of nonverbal communication strategies, including their range of gestures, to initiate joint attention. Around 18 months of age, children start combining words with gestures when making requests and sharing their interests. Typical progression involves using congruent gestures with words (e.g., pointing to a ball and saying "ball") then using gestures to augment words (e.g., pointing to a ball and saying "red"). In addition, the types of gestures that children use shift. Conventional gestures (e.g., clapping to indicate excitement) and informational or instrumental gestures (e.g., head shaking, nodding, shoulder shrugging) typically emerge in infancy. The development of descriptive or iconic gestures follows in toddlerhood. Descriptive gestures involve acting out or representing objects or events (e.g., demonstrating a kicking motion when explaining that the ball was kicked, making a gesture to indicate "small" when referring to size).

Joint attention refers to the ability to direct another individual's attention to objects, other individuals, or events. By 18 months of age, children can initiate, sustain, and consistently respond to joint attention. This skill relies on their ability to use gestures and coordinated eye contact to direct the attention of others. Clinicians should encourage parents to model and encourage use of gestures in their children. Indeed, greater use of gestures early on has been associated with later greater expressive language skills (Goldin-Meadow, 2015).

The development of social reciprocity within the toddler period is marked by the use of shared enjoyment through an increase in range of facial expressions. During this time, children use complex facial expressions beyond emotional extremes (e.g., happiness, frustration). Complex facial expressions may include guilt, confusion, sneakiness, shyness, and anticipation. Importantly, during this period children direct these expressions at others for the purposes of communicating affective states and are beginning to read emotions in others.

Social Skills and Peer Relationships

Social skills during the preschool period include sharing, turn taking, helping, and engaging in reciprocity during interactions. During the preschool period, social skills become increasingly important as children navigate initial peer relationships in the early childhood education setting. During this period, children expand social reciprocity beyond interactions with caregivers to other individuals across settings (e.g., showing and giving toys to another child on the playground instead of just showing toys to a caregiver at home). Conversational skills also become more advanced during the preschool period. Children are able to initiate and sustain conversations by following another's lead and, importantly, demonstrate interest in others by asking simple questions about the thoughts, feelings, and experiences of others.

During the preschool years children begin to demonstrate preferences and desires to interact with certain peers. They are able to name peers. At this point, children also begin to demonstrate understanding of simple social cues, such as indications that they are accepted or rejected by a peer.

Play Skills

Play is one of the primary forms of learning for young children and serves as the foundation for development across cognitive, motor, and social-emotional domains. By 18 months of age, children's play tends to become less egocentric than it was during infancy and more consistently social; children involve others and objects as agents (e.g., feeding a doll). Symbolic play typically arises between 18 and 24 months and involves using novel objects to represent other objects (e.g., pretending that buttons are food on a toy plate). At this stage, parallel play predominates; children play with similar toys alongside each other without interaction. During the preschool period, play advances to interactive and creative play that is collaborative in nature. Preschoolers use schemas that they learn from their environment to rehearse roles (e.g., pretending to cook, use tools). They play "dress-up" while pretending to take on different characters (e.g., pretending to be a movie character, animal, or adult).

Emotional and Moral Development

Considerable emotional and moral development takes place during the preschool years, which helps preschoolers establish values, conceptualizations of right and wrong, empathy, and altruism. The emergence of these values becomes feasible as theory of mind skills develop in preschoolers. Theory of mind refers to the ability to understand that others have differing beliefs, perspectives, and experiences from one's own. Preschoolers begin to develop a sense of right and wrong based on reinforcement from their environment (e.g., being reprimanded or praised by parents, responses from peers) and progress to understand reasons for rules (e.g., not hitting because it hurts others). Emotional development is underscored by the ability to recognize emotions in the self and others and leads to the development of empathy and altruism. As preschoolers begin to notice emotions in others, they develop responses that are often encouraged by caregivers (e.g., giving a hug or pacifier to a crying infant sibling). Lastly, self-regulatory abilities (described in further detail later) play a large role in emotional development as well.

Cognitive Development

Before the second birthday, cognitive development takes place primarily via sensorimotor exploration of the environment. According to Piaget's (1983) theory of cognitive development (see Chapter 3), during the final stage of the sensorimotor period (18–24 months), toddlers begin to understand causality to achieve new desired outcomes (e.g., using a key to operate a toy). Piaget's (1983) preoperational period characterizes the remainder of toddlerhood and the preschool period. This stage is marked by reduction in the reliance on sensorimotor exploration and the emergence of symbolic thought. Symbolic thought during this period is evidenced by role playing and using novel objects to play pretend. Children develop schemas based on their experiences of the world and begin to accommodate their schemas with ongoing exposure to novel events. Socialized gender roles may also begin to emerge during this period based on schemas children have formed through observational learning. During this period, children's imagination and limited logical reasoning skills lead to difficulties discerning between reality and fantasy (e.g., superheroes, monsters). Lastly, during the preschool period, emerging executive functioning skills (discussed in further detail later) underscore cognition and impact other areas of development.

Let's reflect upon the vignette at the beginning of this chapter regarding the various developmental domains we have discussed. You may have noticed that Nicky exhibits a pattern of relative strengths and weakness. He is overall healthy and demonstrates appropriate gross and fine motor skills. With regard to adaptive skills, he is also on track: sleeping through the night, demonstrating independence with feeding, and having achieved daytime continence. However, Nicky currently presents with possible language delays and poor articulation that compromises his intelligibility, even for his parents. Speech and language delays are likely contributing to frustration at not being understood by others and causing him to engage in disruptive behaviors at home and school.

A comprehensive speech and language assessment could establish the nature and degree of his communication difficulties. While his difficulties with expressive language and speech are apparent, the assessment should include receptive skills as well as expressive language and speech. The results of this assessment will direct interventions designed to capitalize on his strengths and to improve his communication skills (see Chapter 107). He may be able to get speech-language services in the community or, if he is found eligible, he may be enrolled in a special education preschool program (see Chapter 104).

OVERARCHING CONCEPTS IMPORTANT FOR TODDLER-PRESCHOOL DEVELOPMENT

The Developing Brain

The neurologic underpinnings of brain development during the toddler and preschool years are increasingly well understood due to advances in neuroscience techniques. Neural connections formed through interaction of genes and environment/experiences proliferate in the first year of life, followed by reduction of connections through synaptic pruning (Shonkoff & Phillips, 2000). It is in the toddler and preschool years that pruning begins for brain regions involved in language and cognitive function. Brain circuitry becomes more refined and efficient; complex circuits are built on earlier simple circuits. Myelination, which has been ongoing since the prenatal period, proceeds rapidly in these circuits, insulating nerve cells and resulting in increased conduction velocity and efficient communication. Patterns of experience define and stabilize patterns of synaptic connections and optimize the toddler's and preschooler's ability to adapt to the environment.

Development of Self-Regulation

Changes across developmental domains that occur during the toddler and preschool periods may be impacted by global skills that span across domains. Self-regulation represents a multidimensional construct involving the control of emotions, attention, and actions (Vohs & Baumeister, 2004). Components of self-regulation have been divided into two broad categories: (1) Emotion regulation describes behaviors that involve the regulation of emotional expression, and (2) executive functioning skills describe cognitive abilities that typically require conscious effort, such as inhibitory control and working memory, and that facilitate planning and organizing.

Emotion Regulation

Domains of emotion regulation relevant for toddlers and preschoolers include reactivity or emotional lability and self-soothing. Within the toddler years, difficulties with the ability to self-soothe independently, without adult intervention, are common and underscore the tantrums that are typical of the "terrible twos." Tantrums are extremely common during the toddler period; however, their frequency, duration, and intensity are largely based on skills in emotion regulation. Frequent, persistent, or extreme tantrums may be a significant clinical concern, especially when the tantrums are accompanied by aggression and/or self-harm. High emotional lability, accompanied by negativity, may also be clinically concerning when tantrums and behavior problems lead to significant impairment in daily routines. As children progress into the preschool years, ability to regulate negative emotions increases, and emotional lability decreases. These skills become important for following classroom routines, interacting appropriately with peers, and navigating novel demands.

Executive Functioning

Executive functioning skills that emerge during the preschool period include inhibitory control, flexibility, and working memory. Inhibitory control refers to the ability to suppress a typical or well-practiced response to a stimulus. In young children inhibitory control is needed for successfully playing games, such as *Simon Says* or *Red Light Green Light*. Cognitive flexibility involves shifting attention as the demands of the environment or ongoing tasks change. These skills are assessed by tasks that require children to sort cards accurately first by one dimension, such as color, and then, suddenly, by another dimension, such as shape. Working memory involves holding information temporarily in mind while performing tasks. For adults, remembering a telephone number while dialing the number engages working memory. For preschoolers, working memory skills are especially important in the school environment. For example, they must remember their question while they are raising their hand, even if another child gets called on before they do.

School Readiness

Although traditional conceptualizations of school readiness emphasized the importance of emergent academic skills, more recent models have taken a multidimensional approach highlighting the importance of academic, behavioral, and social-emotional readiness (see Chapter 83). According to Rimm-Kaufman and Pianta's (2000) ecological and dynamic model of transition, the transition to kindergarten is marked by increased academic, behavioral, and social demands coupled with decreased supervision and need for autonomy. Not surprisingly, self-regulation skills, including executive functioning and emotion regulation, have been implicated as essential for school readiness (Ursache et al., 2012). Executive functioning skills in the classroom allow students to modulate attention, while emotion regulation skills facilitate the control of emotions and frustration related to novel demands. Both executive functioning and emotion regulation have been associated with emergent academic skills (Clark et al., 2010).

Recalling the opening vignette, Nicky was not only delayed in the development of language and speech, but also had challenges controlling his behavior at home and at school. These symptoms reflect difficulties with self-regulation. His tantrums are more frequent and last longer than would be expected for his developmental level; he has difficulties calming, has difficulty managing negative emotions, and shows unpredictable aggressive behavior. Nicky also has challenges in the classroom in terms of emotion regulation and executive functioning skills. For instance, remaining seated in the classroom requires inhibitory control and the ability to sustain attention to ongoing tasks, even when those tasks are dif-

ficult for him. He must remember classroom expectations to remain seated; he is expected to regulate negative emotions that arise with frustration or challenge. To fully understand and intervene appropriately, further information would be needed from his caregivers on his overall emotional regulation and coping skills. However, it is likely that he will need interventions at home and in his preschool classroom. Implementation of a plan to improve emotion regulation and executive functioning skills is important to prepare him for the even greater demands of a kindergarten classroom when he turns 5 years old.

CLINICAL PERSPECTIVES: CONDITIONS COMMONLY PRESENTING IN THE TODDLER AND PRESCHOOL YEARS

The purpose of early detection of developmental and behavioral problems in the toddler and preschool years, as in any other epoch of childhood and adolescence, is prevention and intervention. Primary prevention involves recognizing warning signs of potential issues, thereby intervening before problems arise. Secondary prevention involves identifying mild disorders and providing interventions to alleviate the problems. Tertiary prevention involves prompt treatment and intervention for more significant disorders, thereby mitigating potential comorbidity or functional limitation. Early detection of developmental and behavioral problems relies on evidence-based methods of screening and assessment (see Chapter 79). Developmental and behavioral screening results in a risk categorization (e.g., low, moderate, high risk) whereas assessment generally confers a diagnosis. Table 7.2 lists developmental screening tools for use in the toddler-preschool period. In this section we discuss conditions that are likely to present during this era. We will consider tools for screening and strategies or tools for assessment.

TABLE 7.2 Commonly Used Developmental Screening Tests for Children in the Toddler-Preschool Age Range

General Developmental Screening

Parent Report

- Ages and Stages Questionnaires-3 (ASQ3), 1–66 mo
- Parents' Evaluation of Developmental Status (PEDS), birth–8 yr
- Parents' Evaluation of Developmental Status: Developmental Milestones (PEDS:DM), birth–11 yr
- Survey of Well-Being of Young Children (SWYC): Developmental Milestones, 2–60 mo

Objective Screeners (direct testing/elicitation screens)

- Capute Scales (Cognitive Adaptive Test/Clinical Linguistic and Auditory Milestone Scale), 1–36 mo
- Brigance Early Childhood Screens-III, 0–35 mo, 3–5 yr
- Battelle Developmental Inventory Screening Test-II (BDIST-2), 6 mo–8 yr
- Kaufman Brief Intelligence Test-2 (K-BIT), 4 yr+

Language Screening

- Communication and Symbolic Behavior Scales: Developmental Profile Infant-Toddler Checklist (CSBS:DP-ITC), 2–24 mo

Autism Spectrum Disorder Screening

Parent Report

- Modified Checklist for Autism in Toddlers, Revised With Follow-Up (M- CHAT-R/F), 16–30 mo
- The Parent's Observations of Social Interactions (POSI), 16–36 mo
- Social Communication Questionnaire (SCQ), 4 yr+

Objective Screeners

- Screening Tool for Autism in Toddlers (STAT), 18–35 mo

Promising Tools

- Early Screening for Autism and Communication Disorders, 12–36 mo
- Rapid Interactive Screening Test for Autism in Toddlers (RITA-T), 12–36 mo

Adapted from Lipkin, P. H., & Macias, M. M. (2020). Promoting optimal development: Identifying infants and young children with developmental disorders through developmental surveillance and screening. *Pediatrics, 145*(1).

Developmental Delay

While motor delays and disorders may present during infancy, delays in cognitive, language, social, and adaptive skills are likely to present later, during the toddler-preschool period. Within well-child care, surveillance regarding a child's development should occur at all visits. The American Academy of Pediatrics recommends formal developmental screening be administered in the medical-home setting at specific intervals (i.e., 9, 18, and 30 months, at minimum) (Lipkin & Macias, 2020). Screening tools include parent report and direct elicitation measures. Diagnostic testing measures are used after a screening test indicates need for detailed assessment. Generally, diagnostic measures are administered by direct testing, though parent report assessment tools are available.

Developmental delay may occur in one or more domains: gross motor, fine motor, language, social-emotional, and cognitive. A formal diagnostic developmental evaluation should include a comprehensive developmental assessment. In addition, familial and psychosocial history and a physical and neurologic examination may identify undetected medical conditions and/or an underlying genetic abnormality. The laboratory workup depends on the findings of this evaluation. It is important to connect families of children with developmental delay to early intervention (see Chapter 103) and/or special education programs (see Chapter 104) in addition to appropriate therapy (see Chapters 106 and 107) aimed at addressing impairment related to the specific delay(s). If a child is impacted by adverse childhood experiences (ACEs), trauma-informed interventions may mitigate negative outcomes since it is known that toxic allostatic stress caused by ACEs disrupts developmental trajectories (Shonkoff et al., 2012) (see Chapter 15).

Autism

Autism spectrum disorder (see Chapter 41) is a neurodevelopmental condition characterized by qualitative impairments in social communication/interaction and restricted/repetitive behaviors. ASD can first be reliably diagnosed in children in the toddler-preschool era. The prevalence rate of ASD is 1 in 44 in US children, and the condition is present in all racial and socioeconomic groups (Maenner et al., 2021). However, many children are not diagnosed until almost school age, missing valuable opportunity for intervention. Racial and ethnic disparities are found in the prevalence of ASD and access to early evaluation and diagnosis (Maenner et al., 2020).

The American Academy of Pediatrics has established policy for autism surveillance and screening, with recommendations for surveillance at all preventive care visits and formal screening at 18 and 24 months of age (Hyman et al., 2020). Screening tools are based on core social communication deficits and to varying degrees on restricted and repetitive behaviors. Level 1 autism screens are almost exclusively parent report measures (e.g., Modified Checklist for Autism in Toddlers [M-CHAT]); at this writing, promising brief observation screens are available or in development. Level 2 screens are intended to detect ASD in referred or high-risk children and require specific training prior to administration (e.g., Screening Tool for Autism in Toddlers [STAT]) (see Table 7.2).

A comprehensive assessment of children with a positive screen should consist of a full history, diagnostic interview, an observational evaluation, and developmental assessment. A clinician with expertise in the various presentations of ASD is most appropriate to conduct the comprehensive assessment. Management includes a referral to early intervention (see Chapter 103) and/or special education programs (see Chapter 104) and behavioral interventions (see Chapter 94) that address core impairment of ASD plus treatments for coexisting conditions, if present.

Behavior and Social-Emotional Problems

Behavioral and social-emotional concerns are common during the toddler and preschool years. Surveillance and screening for these problems are also recommended at preventive care visits (Weitzman & Wegner, 2015).

Caregivers of toddlers and early preschool-aged children often report that the child has difficulty sustaining attention and curbing activity or impulses. However, it is challenging to differentiate normative behavior from clinical conditions at this young age. One consideration is whether the child meets criteria for attention-deficit/hyperactivity disorder (ADHD) (see Chapter 46). Given the high levels of inattention and overactivity in toddlers and preschoolers, it is important to focus on the intensity of behaviors, their impact on daily functioning across settings, and whether they lead to safety concerns. The diagnosis of complex ADHD can be considered in children whose symptoms are severe, functionally impairing, or comprising safety. A formal assessment should include verification of prior diagnoses, evaluation of conditions that may be causing symptoms, and coexisting conditions.

TABLE 7.3 Commonly Used Behavioral Screening Tests for Children in the Toddler-Preschool Age Range

General (Broadband) Behavioral Screening
• Ages and Stages: Social-Emotional-2 (ASQ:SE-2), 1 mo–6 yr
• Brief Infant-Toddler Social and Emotional Assessment (BITSEA), 12–36 mo
• Pediatric Symptom Checklist, 4–16 yr
• Strengths and Difficulties Questionnaire (SDQ), 3–17 yr
• Preschool Pediatric Symptom Checklist (PPSC), 18–60 mo
Condition-Specific (Narrow Band) Behavioral Screening
Disruptive Behavior Problems
• Eyberg Child Behavior Inventory (ECBI), 2–16 yr
Attention-Deficit/Hyperactivity Disorder (ADHD)
• Preschool ADHD-IV Rating Scale, 3–5 yr
• Vanderbilt ADHD Diagnostic Rating Scales, 4–18 yr

Adapted from Weitzman, C., & Wegner, L. (2015). American Academy of Pediatrics Section on Developmental and Behavioral Pediatrics, Committee on the Psychosocial Aspects of Child and Family Health, and Council on Early Childhood, Society for Developmental and Behavioral Pediatrics promoting optimal development: screening for behavioral and emotional problems. *Pediatrics, 135*(2), 384–395.

Management of ADHD in toddlers and preschoolers should prioritize behavioral and educational interventions and treatment plans for coexisting conditions (Barbaresi et al., 2020). Medication is rarely a first-line treatment in this age range unless the impairment is severe or access to interventions is severely limited.

Many toddlers and preschoolers experience fears and worries. Differentiating typical worries from excessive fears and worries that interfere with daily activities is paramount for early targeted treatment. Similarly, young children in this age range may exhibit persistent sadness consistent with depression. Behavior screens and assessment tools can be global/broadband or single condition/domain-specific rating scales (Table 7.3). Although research on screening in younger children is limited, measures with good psychometric properties are available, including some in the public domain.

RECOMMENDATIONS AND EVIDENCE-BASED INTERVENTIONS

Strategies for Increasing Positive Behavior

Parenting toddlers and preschoolers may be difficult for many adults. Tantrums and oppositional behaviors are normative as children exercise autonomy and initiative. When they are aroused, they may also have difficulties with the ability to regulate emotions and self-soothe. This developmental period is often referred to as the "terrible twos." However, the challenging behaviors are likely to begin around 18 months and persist throughout the preschool years.

A critical element of parenting and caregiving for children in this age range is to create a context of warmth and responsiveness. Children misbehave because they do not know the rules or cannot reliably follow the rules. It is important for parents and caregivers to maintain a good relationship with children, even if the children's behavior violates rules or expectations. Clinicians may remind parents not to take their child's misbehavior personally.

For younger toddlers (i.e., 18 months–2 years), anticipatory strategies are paramount. Parents can be encouraged to make simple modifications to the environment or routines to prevent misbehavior (e.g., removing objects from reach that are problematic). When used appropriately, distraction and redirection also work well, especially with toddlers and especially when they are just beginning to engage in the undesirable behavior. It is also important to pair words with gestures and/or signs for younger children so that they understand what is being asked of them. Toddlers may not yet understand the rules or the consequences. Thus it is wise to prevent cycles of escalation. Alternative strategies may be appropriate for preschoolers who are able to understand and follow the rules and who can link their behavior with specific consequences, such as timeouts (described later).

Positive reinforcement, based in operant behavioral principles, is effective for increasing appropriate behaviors (see Chapter 4). Across the toddler-preschool age range, a valuable strategy for parents is to praise positive behaviors, those behaviors that the parents want to see. In that way their children receive attention for appropriate behaviors, which makes those behaviors more likely to occur (see Chapter 4). For younger toddlers (i.e., 18 months–2 years) positive attention includes nonverbal strategies such as smiles, clapping, and excited vocalizations. As children's receptive language skills increase, positive attention may include specific praise statements. Labeled praise (e.g., "Good job staying next to me") is highly effective at increasing those specific behaviors. For preschoolers who may engage in inappropriate behaviors as a form of attention seeking, parents are encouraged to use planned ignoring for the undesirable behaviors paired with positive attention for the "positive opposites" of those behaviors. Scheduling daily "special time" to play with their child can be helpful; during the designated time parents may practice reinforcing positive behaviors. For children between 2 and 7 years old, as receptive language skills increase, parents have many available strategies to promote positive behaviors: praise positive behaviors with highly specific input ("Good job playing so gently with the toys"), describe what the child is doing ("You are building a tower"), reflect on what the child says (child says "I made a house," and parent responds, "Yes, you made a red house"), and avoid criticisms and commands. In addition to verbal praise, tangible reinforcers may be helpful to encourage appropriate behaviors for preschoolers. For instance, daily reward charts using small reinforcers (e.g., stickers, tokens, raffle tickets) can be used to promote the completion of important daily routines, such as brushing teeth without objection or putting away toys without reminders.

To be effective, parents should make their commands and directions extremely simple and clear. As receptive language skills may still be emerging, even in the late toddlerhood and the preschool years, clear instructions give the child the best chance of responding appropriately. Here are tips for effective commands:

- Avoid commands phrased as questions (e.g., say "Please put the blocks away" instead of "Can you please clean up?")
- Present commands one at a time
- Ensure that the child is attending (eye contact) before giving a command
- Make commands specific (e.g., "Sit with your bottom on your chair" instead of "Behave" or "Be good")

Managing Challenging Behavior

Preschoolers may not comply, even with well-constructed commands offered in the context of a warm and nurturing environment. For children who can understand consequences, including most preschoolers, parents should provide warnings and then move to appropriate consequences (e.g., timeout, loss of privilege) for noncompliance.

Timeout is an effective discipline strategy for children ages 2 to 7 years. It can be used as a consequence for noncompliance or for aggressive behaviors. Clinicians often need to coach parents to use timeout wisely. First, parents should plan where the child will spend the timeout. The timeout should be in a location in the home that is free from distractions and where the parent can still monitor the child. An adult-size chair in a common living space is ideal. Second, parents should plan on the duration of the timeout. Approximately 3 minutes has been shown to be an effective length of time for children between 2 and 7 years old (Zisser & Eyberg, 2010). It is important for clinicians to offer parents suggestions as a backup plan when the child refuses to sit on the timeout chair. For instance, backups may include having a timeout room where the child can be placed when refusing to sit in the chair or directly returning the child to the chair repeatedly without providing reinforcement. Importantly, when backups like a timeout room are used, parents should return the child to the timeout chair to ensure that these backups do not become an escape from the timeout chair. Lastly, it is also recommended to suggest that parents get children to comply with the original command, a command that they initially refused, after completion of the timeout.

Many variations and alternatives to timeout may also have a role in behavior management (see Chapter 93). Helping families to establish their approach to misbehavior must consider their values, cultural beliefs, and personal history. Close monitoring of families in which the caregivers struggle with parent behavior management may reduce cycles of escalating parent-child conflict.

Therapeutic Referrals for Clinically Significant Concerns

For children who are experiencing clinically significant behavioral challenges and require further support, a number of evidence-based behavioral therapies are available. Behavioral parent training (also referred to as Parent Training in Behavior Management) is an evidence-based approach for treating behavior problems in children. It empowers parents as agents of change through didactic methods and coaching sessions, based on behavioral principles (Pelham & Fabiano, 2008). Parent–Child Interaction Therapy (PCIT) is among the most well-established behavioral parent training programs (Zisser & Eyberg, 2010) for children 2 to 7 years old. It involves coaching parents on positive parenting techniques, such as differential attention and timeout, to decrease maladaptive behaviors and increase appropriate behavior. PCIT is traditionally delivered within 12 to 20 individual 1-hour sessions, including live coaching of parent-child interactions by a therapist working behind a one-way mirror and providing guidance via an earpiece ("bug-in-the-ear"). Another well-established parent training program that has an expansive research base is Triple P (Positive Parenting Program) (Sanders, 2012). The Triple P system offers a hierarchy of programs depending on a family's level of needs. Standard Triple P (Level 4) constitutes the level of intervention that is appropriate for children with clinically significant levels of behavioral challenges. It includes 10 1-hour sessions of didactic information presented to parents on positive parenting skills to decrease disruptive behaviors. Triple P is available via group format (Group Triple P), and adaptations exist for young children with developmental delays (Stepping Stones).

Avoiding and Managing Elopement and Other Threats to Safety

Children in this age range may wander away from their caregivers or home. This behavior is called elopement. Elopement often occurs in toddlerhood as children seek to further their autonomy and/or become captivated by their expanding environment. Elopement is quite worrisome to caregivers, especially if the child's fear development is not established enough to notice when safety is in danger. Other threats to safety include children climbing on furniture or taking risks on the playground.

To promote autonomy while also keeping the child safe, prevention is the key. Implementing safety measures (e.g., locks at the top of doors, gates, or use of a safety harness) and electronics that alert adults to the child's location (e.g., home alarm system, tracking device) reduce the chances of elopement. For children at high risk for elopement, such as those with developmental disorders, the use of multiple safety strategies allows additional time for adult intervention to occur before a child is successful in an attempt to leave. Clear rules for safety and logical or natural consequences for unsafe behavior are also appropriate. Anticipatory guidance regarding these issues should include discussion about possible barriers to prevention and intervention use since differences in caregiver use of appropriate strategies may depend on familial factors such socioeconomic status or cultural norms.

Promoting Social Engagement and Prosocial Behavior

Parents often ask clinicians for recommendations to promote their child's social engagement. Exposure to positive social situations and appropriate modeling within those settings facilitate the development of prosocial behaviors. Thus clinicians may encourage families to provide opportunities for their child to play with other children routinely. Child care centers and preschools provide opportunities for social engagement among children, ideally under the watchful eye of skilled caregivers. Playdates among children and/or families are an alternative way of increasing social opportunities. When planning a successful playdate, families should arrange developmentally appropriate activities for children to engage with, provide ample toys and activities to prevent challenges, and go over behavioral expectations in a developmentally appropriate manner (e.g., stating rules). Modeling appropriate play and sharing may also promote successful playdates along with scaffolding as needed and frequent positive reinforcement.

Media use is unlikely to promote prosocial behavior (see Chapter 21). Watching television and playing videogames often isolates young children from peers. Interactions via media are not truly interactive and reciprocal. Media has many examples of aggressive and inappropriate behavior, which is easy for young children to imitate.

Prosocial behavior is supported by strong language and speech skills. For children with challenges in initiating and sustaining conversations, speech therapy that focuses on pragmatic language skills may be encouraged. Parents are also encouraged to label emotions they are feeling and that they observe their child feeling to aid with emotion recognition and model appropriate emotion regulation. Playing games with children has many positive features. Most games require turn taking. For older preschoolers, competitive games provide opportunities for managing negative emotions associated with losing and can be used to foster emotion regulation skills.

Early Intervention and Transition to School-Based Services

For children with significant developmental delays and/or clinically significant behavioral challenges, early intervention services and school-based services may be important components of a comprehensive plan. The Individuals with Disabilities Education Act (IDEA) includes provisions important to toddlers and preschoolers with or at risk for developmental disabilities (see Chapters 103, 104, and 113). Part C of IDEA specifies provisions for federal programming to offer early intervention services for children birth to 3 years old (see Chapter 113). Once eligibility is confirmed, an Individualized Family Service Plan (IFSP) is developed to include services such as home-based early intervention/care coordination, speech therapy, occupational therapy, and physical therapy.

As children near their third birthday, typically families are transitioned to Part B services (also discussed in Chapter 113). During the preschool years, these services typically include half-day special education programs and/or mainstream preschool enrollment with additional supports or services pushed into the school setting. As the transition from Part C to Part B services occurs, it is important to suggest to families to initiate outpatient supportive therapies as needed. This ensures that families will continue to receive home- or clinic-based therapies once early intervention ends and services are transferred to school.

How can the clinician support Nicky's parents in managing his aggression? A sensitive clinician may suggest positive parenting strategies such as praise for appropriate behaviors. Given his delays in language and speech, the use of active ignoring for negative behaviors, such as tantrums, may be more effective than explanations of why his behavior is inappropriate. Given his age and appropriate developmental skills in thinking and playing, Nicky's parents may also consider using a timeout system for inappropriate behaviors such as aggression. Labeling his emotions and modeling appropriate coping skills to manage negative emotions may promote his self-regulation.

CONCLUSION

Toddlerhood and the preschool years are an exciting period in a child's life during which they learn many different skills and begin developing their own unique personality. As clinicians, it is crucial to monitor children's development across multiple developmental domains. Primary care should include surveillance and regular screening. Parents and caregivers are likely to be proud of children's achievement of milestones and simultaneously face demanding struggles that are common to these eventful years. Clinicians can provide caregivers with the tools they need to help them support their child and maintain equanimity.

It is important to provide support regarding concerns that may be indicative of serious conditions. For example, in reflecting upon the vignette earlier in this chapter, Nicky's presentation raised concerns about his developmental skills. Early language development was within normal limits, but advanced language skills and intelligibility were below what is expected for his age. He could likely benefit from a formal assessment of speech and language skills, and likely speech therapy would be warranted. Nicky was also struggling with emotional regulation and impulsivity. Counseling to his parents about how to manage his behavior was one approach to giving the child support. If the parents were to have difficulties or his inattention, opposition, or aggression became more pronounced, then professional referrals would be warranted. For children in this dynamic age range, the use of standardized developmental and behavioral screening tools and appropriate assessments can guide anticipatory guidance, counseling, referrals, and treatment.

REFERENCES

Accardo, P. J., & Capute, A. J. (2005). *The Capute Scales: Cognitive Adaptive Test/Clinical Linguistic & Auditory Milestone Scale (CAT/CLAMS)*. Brookes Pub.

American Psychological Association. (2013). *Diagnostic and statistical manual of mental disorders* (5th ed.). APA.

Aylward. G. (1995). *Bayley infant neurodevelopmental screener*. Academic Press.

Barbaresi, W. J., Campbell, L., Diekroger, E. A., Froehlich, T. E., Liu, Y. H., O'Malley, E., … Chan, E. (2020). Society for Developmental and Behavioral Pediatrics clinical practice guideline for the assessment and treatment of children and adolescents with complex attention-deficit/hyperactivity disorder. *Journal of Developmental & Behavioral Pediatrics*, *41*, S35–S57.

Beery, K., Buktenica, N., Beery, N., & Keith, E. (2010). *Developmental test of visual-motor integration* (6th ed.). NSC Pearson.

Bly. L. (2000). *Motor skills acquisition checklist*. Psychological Corporation.

Clark, C. A., Pritchard, V. E., & Woodward, L. J. (2010). Preschool executive functioning abilities predict early mathematics achievement. *Developmental Psychology*, *46*(5), 1176.

Flipsen. P., Jr. (2006). Measuring the intelligibility of conversational speech in children. *Clinical Linguistics & Phonetics*, *20*(4), 303–312.

Glascoe, F. P., Marks, K. P., Poon, J. K., & Macias, M. M. (2016). *Identifying and addressing developmental-behavioral problems*. PEDStest.com.

Goldin-Meadow, S. (2015). Gesture as a window onto communicative abilities: Implications for diagnosis and intervention. *Perspectives on Language Learning and Education*, *22*(2), 50–60.

Hyman, S., Levy, S., & Myers, S. (2020). Council on Children with Disabilities, Section on Developmental and Behavioral Pediatrics. Identification, evaluation, and management of children with autism spectrum disorder. *Pediatrics*, *145*(1), e20193447.

Law, E., Yang, J. H., Coit, M. H., & Chan, E. (2016). Toilet school for children with failure to toilet train: Comparing a group therapy model with individual treatment. *Journal of Developmental & Behavioral Pediatrics*, *37*(3), 223–230.

Leaper, C., & Smith, T. E. (2004). A meta-analytic review of gender variations in children's language use: Talkativeness, affiliative speech, and assertive speech. *Developmental Psychology*, *40*(6), 993.

Li, R. (2005). U.S. Department of Education, U.S. Department of Health and Human Services. Workshop summary. Childhood bilingualism: Current status and future directions.

Lipkin, P. H., & Macias, M. M. (2020). Promoting optimal development: identifying infants and young children with developmental disorders through developmental surveillance and screening. *Pediatrics*, *145*(1).

Maenner, M. J., Shaw, K. A., & Baio, J. (2020). Prevalence of autism spectrum disorder among children aged 8 years—autism and developmental disabilities monitoring network, 11 sites, United States, 2016. *MMWR Surveillance Summaries*, *69*(4), 1.

Maenner, M. J., Shaw, K. A., Bakian, A. V., et al. (2021). Prevalence and characteristics of autism spectrum disorder among children aged 8 years—Autism and Developmental Disabilities Monitoring Network, 11 sites, United States, 2018. *MMWR Surveillance Summaries, 70*(SS-11), 1–16. http://dx.doi.org/10.15585/mmwr.ss7011a1

Oller, J. W., Oller, S. D., & Oller, S. N. (2012). *Milestones: Normal speech and language development across the lifespan*. Plural Publishing.

Owens. J. A. (2005). Introduction: Culture and sleep in children. *Pediatrics*, *115*(1), S201–S203.

Pelham, W. E., & Fabiano, G. A. (2008). Evidence-based psychosocial treatments for attention-deficit/hyperactivity disorder. *Journal of Clinical Child & Adolescent Psychology*, *37*(1), 184–214.

Piaget. J. (1983). Piaget's theory: *Handbook of child psychology (chap 1)*. Wiley.

Rimm-Kaufman, S. E., & Pianta, R. C. (2000). An ecological perspective on the transition to kindergarten: A theoretical framework to guide empirical research. *Journal of Applied Developmental Psychology*, *21*(5), 491–511.

Robins, D. L., Casagrande, K., Barton, M., Chen, C.-M. A., Dumont-Mathieu, T., & Fein, D. (2014). Validation of the

Modified Checklist for Autism in Toddlers, revised with follow-up (M-CHAT-R/F). *Pediatrics, 133*(1), 37–45.

Sanders. M. R. (2012). Development, evaluation, and multinational dissemination of the triple P-positive parenting program. *Annual Review of Clinical Psychology, 8*, 345–379.

Shonkoff, J. P., Garner, A. S., Committee on Psychosocial Aspects of Child and Family Health, Committee on Early Childhood, Adoption, and Dependent Care, Section on Developmental and Behavioral Pediatrics. (2012). The lifelong effects of early childhood adversity and toxic stress. *Pediatrics, 129*(1), e232–e246.

Shonkoff, J. P., & Phillips, D. A. (Eds.). (2000). From neurons to neighborhoods: The science of early childhood development. In *The developing brain* (chap. 8, pp. 182–193). National Academy Press.

Squires, J., Bricker, D. D., & Twombly, E. (2009). *Ages & Stages Questionnaires*. Paul H. Brookes.

Ursache, A., Blair, C., & Raver, C. C. (2012). The promotion of self-regulation as a means of enhancing school readiness and early achievement in children at risk for school failure. *Child Development Perspectives, 6*(2), 122–128.

Vohs, K. D., & Baumeister, R. F. (2004). Understanding self-regulation: An introduction. In *Handbook of self-regulation: Research, theory, and applications* (pp. 1–9). The Guilford Press.

Weitzman, C., & Wegner, L. (2015). American Academy of Pediatrics Section on Developmental and Behavioral Pediatrics, Committee on the Psychosocial Aspects of Child and Family Health, and Council on Early Childhood, Society for Developmental and Behavioral Pediatrics promoting optimal development: screening for behavioral and emotional problems. *Pediatrics, 135*(2), 384–395.

Zisser, A., & Eyberg, S. M. (2010). Parent-child interaction therapy and the treatment of disruptive behavior disorders. In J. R. Weisz & A. E. Kazdin (Eds.), *Evidence-based psychotherapies for children and adolescents* (pp. 179–193). The Guilford Press.

8

Middle Childhood

David Alan Ansel

For additional material related to the content of this chapter, please see Chapters 18, and 104.

VIGNETTE

The PS134 school community readied for its field day finale, a mixed-grade tug-of-war. Noah, age 10 and academically at the top of his class, was feeling down. He'd won no ribbons. His best friend Jaxson had teamed with classmate Aaliyah instead of him and they had won every event. Aaliyah now led some kids in a rap song Noah's mother forbade, so he didn't know the lyrics. He squeezed next to Aaliyah on the rope and tickled her. "Stop it, there's no room, our team's full," she said. Noah yelled, "No fair," prompting his mom's intervention. The 6- and 7-year-old boys watching yelled "Cooties!"

As Noah returned to his team, embarrassed, Coach Delgado blew his whistle for quiet. Behind Noah, 8-year-old Kenji dropped the rope, looking scared. "Buck up! You can do it!" Kenji's father shouted from the sidelines. Coach yelled, "Go!" Teachers chanted, "Teamwork!" while parents cheered "Pull! Pull!" Noah spotted his dad arriving late. "Get up, you baby!" Noah said to Kenji and pulled on the rope as hard as he could. If he could win just one ribbon, his dad might not yell when they get home. The air horn blasted, Noah's entire team was yanked onto the ground, and in victory Aaliyah hugged Jaxson. Her mom passed out "I'm a Winner" t-shirts to everyone, but Noah's dad said, "Losers don't deserve prizes!"

INTRODUCTION

Children approximately 6 to 12 years old are colloquially called school age, a cultural remnant of our educational history. Elementary school became available to most economic classes in America well before high school, kindergarten, or preschool did. Freud called the period "latency," a supposed calm between the storms of early childhood and adolescence. Parenting gets easier for many, but children are not dormant through this time—crucial changes happen while crossing the long bridge from dependence to independence. Erickson cast the main developmental task as resolving industry versus inferiority, but children must also grapple with social, moral, physical, and self-regulatory challenges along the way. Piaget focused on cognition, particularly the disappearance of magical thought and emergence of logical thought, dubbing this "the stage of concrete operations." The word *concrete* does not do justice to the thinking of children during this period, however. While there is much they still cannot fully comprehend, children's powers of reasoning, intuition, problem solving, insight, and creativity are steadily increasing. Indeed, it is during middle childhood that abilities such as multiple perspective taking, inference drawing, and use of metaphor begin to emerge. Freud also referred to this as "the golden age of childhood." Oft repeated, this is perhaps the most apt moniker of all. Children really come into their own during these years. They begin living lives outside the home (i.e., forming relationships, joining teams, pursuing interests, doing work, and accomplishing things). They develop their own opinions and tastes, a moral compass, and a sense of self. They test limits and exercise self-control. Most are fairly well behaved, hewing closely to rules and routine. They hold adults in high esteem (e.g., "I want to be just like you, Dad") even if jealous of their powers. When adults look back on their own childhood, or on their parenting years, this is the time most clearly and fondly recalled. In this chapter we refer to the period as middle childhood.

Human middle childhood corresponds roughly to what primatologists call the juvenile period. Defined biologically as the time between adrenarche and gonadarche, the animal is no longer completely dependent on parents for survival but is not yet sexually mature. In all social mammals this is a period of rapid learning through play, which becomes increasingly social and competitive (i.e., imitating and preparing for adult life). Human culture tends to prolong juvenility by a few years, marking its termination by social, emotional, and cognitive rather than physiologic puberty.

More than anything else, school is what defines middle childhood in modern societies (see Chapter 18). The character of school changes beyond kindergarten. No longer an adjunct to or substitute for the family, it becomes an equally if not more important place where different rules apply and different authority figures matter. For most children school becomes the primary venue for both learning and play. At school children are their own actors; they can try out different roles, personas, behaviors, and peer alliances. School is also a place of little privacy. Children at this age become acutely aware of the ways they and their classmates differ from each other ("I'm fat, she's short"; "I have curly hair, he talks funny"; "She has more toys/nicer clothes/a bigger house than I do"), as seen in the opening vignette. Children this age are very sensitive to how teachers and classmates may judge them. They learn how to hide their feelings. Noah, in the opening vignette, is better at hiding his feelings than Kenji because

TABLE 8.1 Influences on Development in Middle Childhood

Intrinsic	Extrinsic
• Personality/temperament • Genetics and epigenetics • Internalized long-term effects of ACEs • Cognitive strengths, weaknesses • Medical illness/toxins/metabolism • Physical strengths, weaknesses (injury, physical anomaly or disability) • Nutrition	• School quality (goodness of fit) • School programs (resources) • Cultural (political, historical) • Relational (family, community) • Economic (resource availability) • Ongoing stress (toxic or adaptive) • Climate and ecology • Safety (toxins, violence) • Therapeutic services

ACEs, Adverse childhood experiences.

he is older. School-age children discern what is "in" or "out" and choose to conform or not. Hierarchies or pecking orders come to define both social and academic success. Some children start to be ostracized by peers and, unfortunately, sometimes even by teachers. Adjustment to this new school environment is the foremost test of middle childhood. How children navigate this transition and come to see themselves in this new milieu sets the stage for everything that follows.

School provides a setting and primary stimulus for the many developmental changes and challenges of middle childhood. Children must make alliances and find acceptance beyond the family with both adults and peers. They are expected to handle new levels of freedom and responsibility while developing their capacity for restraint, kindness, empathy, emotional self-regulation, and work. They experience an increasing sense of morality, identity, and role in community, while mastering ever more complex knowledge and skills. These tasks are all closely interwoven, with school being the usual integrating force. Interruption or significant deviation from the cultural norm (e.g., homeschooling) in an individual's school experience has the potential to negatively impact not only learning but development and later adaptation. However, developmental progress is also strongly influenced by a variety of factors beyond school. These can be categorized simply as intrinsic or extrinsic (Table 8.1), but they really overlap and interact over time. School is thus one very significant part of a much wider system of risk, protective, and promoting factors with which the child interacts in bidirectional, mutually influential ways (see Chapters 2 and 18).

DEVELOPMENTAL PROGRESSION

Transition From Early Childhood

The expected biologic age of juvenile transition in humans is 5 to 6 years. The shift from the Piagetian preoperational thinking to concrete operations typically happens at 6 to 7 years. Kindergarten was originally conceived to ease the passage from preschooler to student, from early into middle childhood. The topic of school or kindergarten readiness is covered elsewhere (see Chapter 83). Not every child is ready at age 5. Some very precocious youngsters will be at age 4, while some struggle to make the leap even at 6. Clinical judgment about the current life stage of a child is more important than chronologic age alone.

Physical Changes

The biologic markers of the juvenile transition are eruption of the first permanent molars and adrenarche. Adrenal androgens have powerful effects on brain functioning. They promote neurogenesis. They modulate gamma-aminobutyric acid (GABA) and glutamate receptors. They can be converted to estrogen and testosterone, thereby activating sexually differentiated brain pathways for the first time since prenatal development, triggering the many brain and cognitive changes of middle childhood (DelGiudice, 2018).

Between 6 and 12 years the brain grows from approximately 75% to nearly 98% of its adult size. More importantly, it becomes more organized and efficient through progressive processes of myelinization of white matter, new axonal projections, synaptogenesis, and synaptic pruning, all of which have profound effects on structure and function. A notable thickening of the corpus callosum proceeds in a front-to-back wave between 5 and 13 years. Relative gray matter thickening occurs in the frontal cortex and language areas, with relative thinning in areas associated with movement and sensory perception. Numerous studies involving functional magnetic resonance imaging (cortical activation) and diffusion tensor imaging (development of white matter tracts) (see Chapter 89) support increasing specialization of different regions of the brain and efficiency of the communication tracks between them. Feedback loops between the forebrain and midbrain transform. Transmission between subcortical regions and between the two hemispheres improves. Cortical activation during specific tasks becomes more localized and specialized. All this change enables the more flexible regulation of thoughts and actions in the presence of competing stimuli, as well as the more selective responses and cognitive control observed during middle childhood (Mah & Ford-Jones, 2012). Broadly, changes in brain size and structure during middle childhood are subtle, but the changes in function, localization, and differentiation are dramatic.

Middle childhood is also a time of profound physical growth, with increasing accumulation of both muscle and fat, so a nadir in the body mass index also marks the juvenile transition. Children's interest in their own bodies changes at this age as well, becoming less about sensory experience and physical needs, and more about form and capabilities. Between 6 and 12 years, boys grow from ~65% to ~88% and girls from ~70% to ~95% of their final adult height. The physiologic/endocrine onset of puberty brings on the fastest linear growth during the final third of middle childhood, often well before the cognitive/emotional transition into adolescence. The dissonance creates a risky time when individual children may look older than they think or feel. Similarly, many children in this age group participate in competitive team sports, the risks and physical demands of which may outpace the child's neuromotor readiness. It is no wonder therefore that rates of sports injuries peak in the last half of middle childhood.

Expected Achievements

In middle childhood the main trunks of development branch, branch again, then intertwine. Milestones can be listed and categorized (Table 8.2), but they affect one another in a web of interdependency. Variability in the rate and sequence of milestone attainment is greater than at younger ages, so expected age windows are wide and overlapping. In our vignette Noah is adept academically, his friend Jaxson socially, and Aaliyah verbally. Milestones are often spoken about in this age group using educational rather than medical or psychological vernacular. Social and emotional development becomes maturity. Language milestones become verbal skills. Cognitive abilities are reflected in attention, learning, academic performance, and executive functions. Most importantly, early childhood delays, when they do not resolve, manifest in the elementary school classroom as problems or disabilities. Clinicians may need to draw connections for parents and teachers between concerns in the two age ranges, prospectively in early childhood ("We better pay attention to this now, or else …") and retrospectively in middle childhood ("Given the early history of …, the child may now be struggling with …").

Cognition (Thinking)

Around age 6, a metamorphosis occurs in the way children think. Entering the Piagetian stage of concrete operations, magical ideas are replaced by logic, and impulsiveness is replaced by reflection (see Chapter 3). Children become less egocentric and begin to consider other perspectives. They understand cause and effect more clearly and rationally.

TABLE 8.2 Developmental Milestones of Middle Childhood

	6–8 Yr	8–10 Yr	10–12 Yr
Attention/ Executive Functions	• Sustain attention to task • Inhibit unwanted behavior	• Make short- to medium-term plans • Active working memory improves	• Able to plan/execute long-term projects, budget time
Memory/ Sequencing	• Follows three-step directions • Digit span four to five • Can talk about "yesterday" and "tomorrow" • Able to form episodic memories • Able to form paired associations	• Follows four- to five-step directions • Digit span five to six • Meshed associations • Benefits from vicarious memory (through reading or storytelling by adults in family or clan) • Increased use of recall strategies (mnemonics, categorization)	• Follows six- to seven-step directions • Digit span seven • Can plan long-term project • Solve problems with sequential reasoning • Faster retrieval/automaticity
Visual/ Spatial	• R/L discrimination • Transition from local to global visual processing • Ability to understand maps and navigate from place to place	• Crossed laterality understood • Letter/word reversals gone • Understands visual diagrams and instructions	• 3D visualization • Understands complex figures/ diagrams
Motor	• Tripod pencil grip • Emergence of an adult-like gait • Zippers, buttons, shoelaces • Rides two-wheel bicycle	• Synkinesia/overflow movements gone • Manipulates small objects easily • Able to master basic skills of most sports	• Able to master advanced skills of many sports
Language	• Names >5 objects in 30 sec • Vocabulary >5000 words • Mastered basic syntax of language • Able to carry on reciprocal conversation • Words have single, concrete meanings • Can tell stories with consistent topic and sequence • Adverbs absent • Language used to learn about world (questioning)	• Rapid naming >8 • Vocabulary >20,000 words • Increased use/understanding of embedded clauses • Starting to appreciate dual meanings of single words • Emerging use of adverbs • Starting to use simple simile and idiom • Improving ability to tell jokes, distinguish fantasy from reality	• Rapid naming >11 • Vocabulary >50,000 words • Fully appreciates hidden/dual meanings of words/phrases • Starting to understand ambiguity, irony, metaphor, paradox, symbolism • Mastery of adverbs

Continued

TABLE 8.2 Developmental Milestones of Middle Childhood

	6–8 Yr	8–10 Yr	10–12 Yr
Social Skills and Thinking	• Able to initiate and respond to social overtures • Take turns, share, cooperate • Make/maintain friendships based on friendships based on shared activities, proximity, similarity • Cross-cultural differences in prosocial behavior begin to emerge	• Friendships based on common interests, mutual acceptance, admiration, loyalty, shared values/ attitudes • Increasing ability to manage group dynamics, including teams • Starting to juggle multiple relationships and social hierarchy • Able to put self in someone else's shoes and show empathy • Able to see self through someone else's eyes	• Friendships characterized by increasing emotional intimacy, support, self-disclosure • Can manage conflicting allegiances, take multiple perspectives, adopt different persona in different groups • Increasing ability to manipulate truth for own gains
Moral Thinking	• Rule based (law and order) • Goal to gain approval/rewards; maintain friendly relations • Recognizes good/bad intentions as relevant	• Still rule based • Goal to avoid punishment, maintain social order • Starting to consider general principles (fairness, justice)	• Become aware that rules can be arbitrary and therefore subject to question—morally right/legally right not necessarily the same • Ability to consider multiple perspectives and conflicting values/interests • Increased emphasis on individual rights
Emotion Regulation	• Aware their own thoughts and feelings are private and different than others	• Identify feelings • Talk about feelings • Consider alternative attributions	• First romantic/sexual attractions • Able to disguise or feign emotion • Increased mentalizing (i.e., the ability to understand and reason about mental states)
Reading	• Knows that print carries meaning • Knows letters are associated with sounds (phonemic awareness) and words are made up of phonemes • Knows sound-symbol (phoneme-grapheme) relationships • Learning to read: decoding, word attack skills, sight words	• Reading to learn rather than learning to read • Chapter books, expanding comprehension and memory • Asks questions while reading, rereads if confused • Explains characters' personality, motivations • Aware of different genres	• Reads critically, draws conclusions • Summarizes and discusses • Provides supporting details • Able to integrate information from multiple sources • Increasing complexity, fluency, speed
Writing	• Writes name • Copies words and sentences	• Writing to communicate ideas • Creative writing	• Multiple forms/styles of written communication
Math	• Single → multdigit addition, subtraction; regrouping • Understanding simple fractions	• Multiplication, division, • Fractions, percents • Word problems • Understanding of negative numbers	• Roots, powers • Operations with negative numbers • Basic geometry • Prealgebra

Note: The rows above each represent distinct domains of development, but almost everything in middle childhood development depends on many other things. Problems in one domain will reverberate in several others.

Rather than relying on intuition or immediate sensory perception, they reason. Children become able to generalize observations, deriving rules that pertain to other situations. They apply principles such as conservation (constancy of measures) and reversibility to transformations. They understand order, distance, time, and rudimentary probability and are increasingly able to factor multiple variables into their thinking.

Children in middle childhood love rules, whether externally imposed or self-generated, whether about behavior or the physical world. They enjoy discovering, knowing, explaining, imposing, testing, challenging, and breaking rules. The nuance, complexity, and sophistication of their application grows gradually between age 6 and 12. Rules provide security and a sense of control. If they see something confusing, they seek to understand through rules. If they break a rule, they may be testing adult limits or applying different rules to the situation. Often the latter relates to rules about fairness or rules about who should make the rules. By the second half of middle childhood, children become better able to balance multiple competing rules, but rules remain the organizing system of their thoughts.

Learning typically becomes highly pleasurable and quite motivating in middle childhood, thus children accumulate an ever-expanding fund of knowledge. They grow to appreciate spatial or temporal relations and follow sequential operations. They integrate data from multiple sources and apply previous knowledge and experience to current situations. As a result they can interpret, draw inferences, and reach conclusions. Because of their increasing awareness of the outside world, school-age children are particularly interested in knowing about and understanding differences (e.g., between bodies, families, religions, and countries). "How" and "why" questions often predominate.

Among the different types of memory (Table 8.3), familiarity and short-term memory are relatively well formed during early childhood. Active working memory, associative memory, and episodic memory all show marked gains during middle childhood. Kids at this age display faster retrieval and automaticity, they move from paired associations to meshed associations, and they start to use support strategies like mnemonics and categorization. Semantic organization strategies emerge for search and retrieval, as does metacognition (thinking about thinking), which allows children to start, for example, judging the accuracy of their recall. The result is a greatly improved ability to monitor and manipulate information. Episodic memory supports independence in daily activities as well as the development of a sense of self (forming the basis of a "life story"). Deficits in episodic memory have been found in school-age children who have hypoxic or traumatic brain injury, depression, posttraumatic stress disorder, and fragile X syndrome (Ghetti & Bunge, 2012). They have also been implicated as an early (prepsychotic) sign of schizophrenia (Erlenmeyer-Kimling et al., 2000).

The stage of concrete operations also brings with it steadily expanding executive and attentional capacities. At this age, children learn to deliberately direct, sustain, and shift their focus. They may choose to follow adult direction or conform with their peers, or they might decide to pursue their own interests or make their own judgments about salience instead. Either way they should show improving task persistence with a growing ability to preview, predict, plan, set goals, and stave off fatigue. Impulsivity and the need for short-term reward to motivate action should shrink as well. Finally, children in this age group become able to divide their attention. They can build a model and listen to a story simultaneously. This ability (combined with their growing language skills) means that when adults are talking within earshot, children are listening and making some (possibly incomplete or distorted) sense of what they hear (especially if they think the conversation relates to them).

TABLE 8.3 Types of Memory

- Familiarity = recognition that "I've been here/seen this before"
- Short-term memory = immediate recall of recent events
- Active working memory = the ability to hold multiple representations in mind simultaneously while associating, processing, or acting on them
- Associative memory = remembering that this goes with or is caused by that
- Episodic memory = the ability to encode, store, and retrieve specific events along with the context in which they happened

School-age children frequently undergo IQ (cognitive) testing. Both IQ and overall cortical thickness are relatively stable and highly heritable traits, but regional neuroanatomic markers of intelligence vary with age, correlating roughly with the maturational changes going on at those times (Schmitt et al., 2019; Shaw et al., 2006). Intelligence, however, is a fuzzy and controversial construct. What these tests actually measure are expressive/receptive verbal, visual-spatial, graphomotor, memory, sequencing, executive, and problem-solving skills along with processing speed (see Chapter 85). Other aspects of intelligence (emotional, social, musical, artistic) are ignored. Because intelligence develops in the context of experience and culture, cognitive tests always contain an element of inherent bias. Factors that affect how children perform on intelligence tests also change with time. IQ scores at age 5 to 6 are primarily determined by the richness of the home and preschool environment the child has experienced, while by age 11 to 12 genetic inheritance plays a much larger role (Bouchard, 2009). Measured intelligence correlates only loosely with academic and social success. Despite all these limitations IQ test results affect diagnoses, educational placement, and eligibility for services—never more so than during middle childhood.

Social

The nature of both friendship and play changes dramatically as a child enters middle childhood, based on emotional needs and advances in social and moral thinking (see Table 8.2). At younger ages, friendships are determined by proximity and often are adult mediated. Starting around age 6, however, children display a new ability to initiate social interaction, choosing and making their own friends based on mutual interest or attraction. This development is supported by growing capacities to perceive the feelings and motivations of others and provide support, encouragement, or sympathy. Children are now able to modify their behavior in response to the feelings or opinions of others and to balance the ideas of competition versus cooperation. School-age children negotiate with each other about where, when, and what they should play and are able to agree on the rules.

Play is crucial to a child's emotional development. Children rehearse and replay experiences that are confusing, anxiety provoking, or threatening. As children move from preoperational to concrete operational thinking, their play becomes more social and reality based. Middle childhood play emphasizes role playing, problem solving, skill development, and competition. For the first time there are winners and losers, and winning is important. Sports participation begins and becomes a preferred activity for many. Other games are usually learned from peers rather than from parents, reflect the prevailing culture, and carry a strict set of rules that teach cultural norms. It becomes possible to cheat, and playing fair matters. Computer or video games are not fundamentally different than older forms of play in any of these characteristics, although concerningly they may be more violent in their imagery (see Chapter 21).

Children at this age want to grow up. They want to be like adults and have adult powers. They look forward excitedly to landmarks, such as losing their first tooth or going to middle school. Pretend play imitates the adult world and is often repeated, with minor variations, to gain mastery. Children may play at transgressing limits, practicing their ability to tolerate fear or arousal. Children who are exposed to age-inappropriate material in media or elsewhere may try to integrate it into their play. Early middle childhood (age 6–8) often represents the peak of segregation between the sexes (as the younger kids in our vignette enforce by calling "cooties"). At this age, play may also reflect narrowly defined gender norms—with boys chasing, scaring, fighting, hurting, or ruling and girls cooking, decorating, entertaining, or caretaking—although the degree of such differentiation is influenced by prevailing school and community culture. Later in middle childhood (age 9–11) marks the awakening of the first sexual and romantic attractions. These too are initially explored, tested, practiced, and processed in play (as Noah's attraction to Aaliyah in our vignette illustrates).

The desire to grow up and the need to rehearse confusing or emotional experiences are also reflected in the literature children read. Juvenile fiction features strong heroes, villains, and orphans. Heroes are always good; villains are very bad. Stories often involve new rules, secret knowledge, and superpowers. The protagonist is frequently a child with magical powers or a relationship to someone with magical powers. Stories may involve children solving mysteries, being kidnapped, helpless, or lost. Parents are mostly absent. Bad feelings are usually displaced onto others, and most of the time there are happy endings. Book series that feature familiar characters in new situations are particularly appealing. Reading can help school-age children work through many of the challenges of this age and may serve as a substitute for play in those who are, for one reason or another, socially isolated.

Language

Typically, developing 6-year-olds use words as their primary means to reconstruct the past and represent the future. They have begun using language to express ideas, assist in problem solving, and support memory and imagination. They have a receptive vocabulary of 5000 to 10,000 words, and word finding has become easier. They have mastered the basic syntax of their language and should be 95% to 100% intelligible when they speak, even to strangers. Any developmental speech dysfluency (stuttering) they had as a preschooler should be gone. They can tell a story and fluently describe their own actions, thoughts, and feelings. Throughout middle childhood, kids display increasing length and grammatical complexity in their utterances. Adverbs, embedded clauses, and figurative language gradually appear. By age 12 a child's vocabulary surpasses 50,000 words. As they ready themselves for adolescence, late school-age children employ irony, paradox, and double or hidden meanings and become effective at using language to influence others (Merritt, 2012; Nippold, 2016).

During middle childhood, children become adept in the social uses of language (pragmatics). Their ability to listen and take other people's perspectives into account grows. They start talking in groups of more than two people. They learn to adjust what and how they speak for the audience, taking context into account. Humor progresses from memorized jokes to demystification to word play over the course of the age range. They become better at maintaining and smoother at shifting topic appropriately during conversation. The social conventions of speech for their culture become fully internalized.

Emotional Development

Human beings at all ages experience the same range of emotions: happiness to joy, fear to terror, annoyance to anger, sadness to despair. These emotions are experienced on three levels: neurobiologic (brain and autonomic nervous system, leading to somatic symptoms), behavioral (affect, facial expression, crying, hitting, withdrawing), and cognitive (thinking, speaking). The frequency, intensity, and behavioral expressions of emotion vary based on personality, temperament, life circumstances, and preferred coping skills (Table 8.4). Coping skills are cognitive strategies used for emotional regulation. They can be either adaptive or maladaptive, depending on the situation, and when counterproductive are often called defenses.

TABLE 8.4 Emotional Coping Strategies

Strategy	Description
Expression, sharing	"I feel...," "I did..."
Denial/repression	Conscious/unconscious
Avoidance, repression	Don't think about it, bottle it up
Discussion, attribution	Comparing one's own experience to that of others
Rationalization/ intellectualization	Explaining something away, "they were just lucky"
Modesty, humor, face-saving	Turning it into a joke, concealing true feelings/intentions
Displacement, sublimation*	Turning feelings toward a less threatening object
Dissociation, fantasy	Becoming disconnected from real experience
Projection	"They hate me," when really you hate them
Regression	Retreating to younger or more primitive behaviors
Reaction formation*	Expressing opposite emotion (e.g., tenderness for jealousy)
Aim reduction/ compensation	Shooting lower or higher than what one really wants

TABLE 8.4 Emotional Coping Strategies— Cont'd

Strategy	Description
Altruism, undoing	Satisfying needs, making up for wrongs through helping others
Relaxation techniques	Deep breathing, progressive muscle exercises, guided imagery
Internalization	Negative self-talk (may lead to depression, anxiety)
Passive aggression	Indirectly expressing anger or other negative feelings
Externalization, acting out	Anger, blaming others, aggression (often leads to discipline)

*Reaction formation and sublimation are often considered hallmark coping strategies during latency, but school-age children are capable of displaying/utilizing any and all of the above.

The cognitive and language advances of middle childhood enable children to think rationally about their own feelings and coping strategies. Responses to strong emotions become less reflexive and more reflective, planned, and controlled. Children also become able to consciously separate their internal experience from affect and behavior, so they can hide or talk about emotions if they choose. New coping skills can be considered and tried; existing ones can be rejected, modified, or consciously extinguished. The school-age child can be taught to utilize strategies such as deep breathing, progressive muscle relaxation, guided imagery, and even meditation. In middle childhood counseling and psychotherapeutic methods relying on language start to be effective, but children at this age can also disguise their true intentions or attempt to "split" parents (i.e., play one against the other).

Academic Learning

School-age children are oriented toward learning. Their cognitive, language, and social development have brought them to a point of readiness, and thus academically oriented schooling begins at this age in virtually all cultures. Academic expectations (curricula) vary both geographically and over time. A typical sequence of academic milestones is outlined in Table 8.2. Most students can learn what they are taught when they are taught, regardless of the specific timing or teaching methods used. For some, their learning style (determined by an unusual set of neurodevelopmental strengths and weaknesses) demands particular instructional approaches, and a mismatch of learning to teaching style will express as learning difficulty or disability.

Children at this age first learn to read, then read to learn, and finally (hopefully) love to read. The best predictors of reading performance in elementary school, at least for European languages, are being read to frequently as a preschooler, listening comprehension, and phonemic awareness (the understanding that words can be broken down into sequences of sounds, and these phonemes are represented by graphemes consisting of letters or groups of letters).

Writing progresses from copying to communicating to expressing complex ideas, and from single letters to words to sentences to paragraphs and stories or essays. A distinction should be made between the mechanics (handwriting, grammar, spelling, punctuation) and the content (ideas, vocabulary, sequencing) of writing. Difficulties with mechanics are more common, less concerning, and are amenable to bypass strategies (cursive, keyboarding, dictation, voice recognition, automated spelling and grammar checkers). Writing mechanics and content should be judged (and perhaps graded) separately, and mechanical obstacles should never be allowed to hold a child back from progress in learning and practicing writing as a means of expression.

During the early elementary grades, children become proficient using the four basic math operations, first with single digits, then with multiple digits requiring regrouping. They learn zero, negative numbers, and basic fractions (though many have an intuitive sense of these already). Later they learn word problems and how to work with negatives, fractions, decimals, and percents. In late elementary they are introduced to roots, powers, basic geometry, and prealgebraic principles. Math pedagogy in elementary school often leans heavily on memorization of math facts and the expectation that children should be able to explain their work. Assessment of the former emphasizes speed, the later language, both of which can be relative weaknesses for some children who otherwise have a natural aptitude for math. The abilities of such a child may go unrecognized, unappreciated, and unrewarded.

Home, Self-Care, and Community Living

Middle childhood represents a coming-out period for most children, the time when they first leave the family and interact, at least semiautonomously, with the outside world. They start building a life of their own. Social, cognitive, academic, and adaptive milestones together enable this transition. School-age children learn to navigate their world safely and independently, be it the streets of their neighborhood, the public transit system of their city, or the halls of their school. Older children in this stage can be taught to travel long distances by themselves via rail or air. A bicycle becomes not just a toy but a means of transportation. They learn to make phone calls, shop at a store, and surf the web. They know how and when to summon help, and they recognize and respond to danger. They should be able to wash, bathe, dress, make a bed, clean up, and cook a meal. Thus at home, they can mostly take care of themselves. They can also learn to use tools or machinery, tie knots, pitch a tent, tack a horse, plant and harvest a crop, and safely handle knives and fire. Thus they can handle steadily increasing responsibilities to either help with domestic tasks or contribute to the family economy (foraging, farming, family business, household chores). During the latter half of the age range (9–12 years) they can take on increasing responsibility for the care of younger siblings as well. However, just because they can perform these tasks does not mean they should. Parents must strike a balance between nurturing, protecting, and supporting their school-age child on the one hand and fostering a growing sense of independence and responsibility on the other. When children are overscheduled or given too much work, not enough space may be left for the play and social interaction necessary to meet the challenges of this age.

Tasks and Challenges

In the journey from early childhood to adolescence, children form a conscience (moral compass) and develop a self-image (identity). Hopefully they also find both internal (self-esteem) and external (peer group) acceptance. How a child meets and experiences these challenges often sets the stage for later life. Signs of difficulty adjusting or unmet emotional needs at this age may show up as internalizing (depression, anxiety) or externalizing behaviors (tantrums, aggression, lying, stealing, oppositionality, defiance), somatic symptoms (headaches, abdominal pain, sleep disturbance), or academic struggles (focus, learning, completing schoolwork).

Adaptation to School

Adjustment to school is never a trivial or minor event. Most children share common insecurities (e.g., "Maybe I'm stupid," "Nobody will like me," "What if I fail?"). Success requires them to pay attention, persevere, master fears, delay gratification, and forge new alliances in ways that represent a profound reordering of their previous life rhythms and priorities. They must develop the capacity for tolerating frustration and a willingness to try again after failure, which come from earlier experiences in the emotional safety and love from their parents. They must internalize and generalize a new set of rules, with their associated sanctions, personified by a new cast of authority figures. Teachers and administrators soon become the highest power, elevated above parents, but school-aged children are influenced by many adults, including other school staff, coaches, clergy, parents of peers, and even (vicariously) media figures. As they start to compare, children's own images of their parents evolve toward a more nuanced and realistic view. Parents are not always good or right, are no longer seen as omnipotent, but are rather just one of many powerful forces they must reckon with, as each of the children in our vignette does in different ways.

Conscience Formation

Naturally interested in differences and confronted with differing rules in various settings from assorted adults, school-age children start to examine contrasting values, traditions, roles, and expectations. Reconciling these allows them to internalize the values of both family and culture and propels their moral thinking forward. They come to experience feelings of modesty, embarrassment, and disgust. More importantly, they leave behind the purely transactional model of early childhood to develop their own independent sense of right and wrong. Initially rule and conformity (i.e., law and order) driven, ethical principles (e.g., justice) and intent gain influence by the latter half of middle childhood.

Achieving Mastery

Children take great pride in accomplishments during middle childhood. They may also feel shame and embarrassment when they do not live up to expectations, as reflected in Noah's reactions in the vignette. New knowledge and skills can be acquired in many areas aside from school and academics, including sports, clubs, hobbies, and home life. It is important for all children to have areas in which they feel competent, confident, and experience success. School-age children can see through false praise, but they need adult recognition to nurture their strengths and interests; a sense of competency in one realm may provide the resiliency needed to persevere on difficult tasks or areas of relative weakness.

Social Acceptance

Elementary school children pick their own friends. Parents usually are not (and should not be) involved. The mutuality of this process is daunting and delicate (e.g., "Should I approach them, or wait for them to invite me in?"). Although many catch on easily, structured activities (team sports, field days, interest-based clubs) help some children initiate contact with others and learn the "dance." Close friendships provide opportunities for mutual exploration, play, and growth. The number and intensity of close friendships made at this age may set a lifelong pattern. Having at least one or two close friends is very important for all children, however, as it provides protection from rejections and resiliency during psychosocial stress. In the long run children without any close friends are at higher risk of depression, suicide, substance abuse, school failure, and externalizing behaviors.

Friends explore the world and grow together, but they also form groups and exclude others. Bullying emerges at the beginning of middle childhood, and peaks in intensity near the transition to adolescence. Thus the need to balance social integration with social competition to determine one's place in the social hierarchy also appears at this age. Integration calls for prosocial behaviors such as doing favors for others, demonstrating skills, and displaying loyalty; competition demands more aggressive behaviors to earn status, reputation, friends, and allies (e.g., "Should I be an individual or conform?" "Should I lead or follow?" "Should I fight or retreat?" "Should I tell the truth or back this person up?" "Should I support or compete?" "Whose side am I on?"). In the moment, case-by-case decisions must be made many times every school day. How a child strikes these balances depends on many variables (Fig. 8.1). Social demands like these contribute to an early peak in the emergence of both externalizing and internalizing psychopathology at this age. A child's degree of success in this realm can also have lifelong implications for social, economic, and reproductive success.

Self-Regulation

Moving from dependency to autonomy requires a child to exercise new types of self-control. Parents have expectations (e.g., "Buck up," "Use your words," "Don't cry," "Fight back")

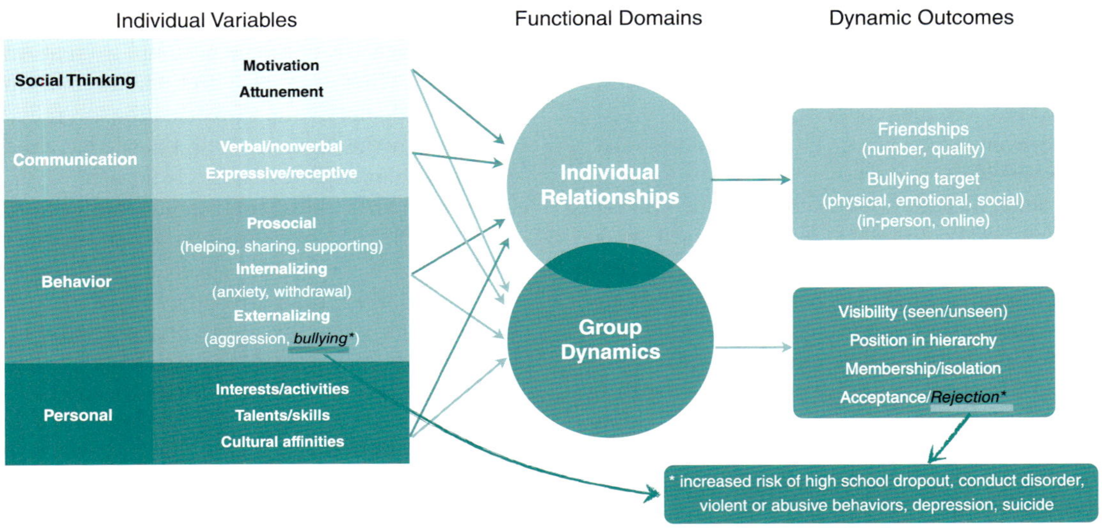

Fig. 8.1 Social adaptation. Social success is dependent on many individual variables mediated through individual relationships and group dynamics. Having no friends, or only superficial friendships, or being socially "unseen" is relatively benign. However, being a bully, being chronically victimized by bullies, or rejected by the entire peer group is associated with poor behavioral, psychosocial, and educational outcomes.

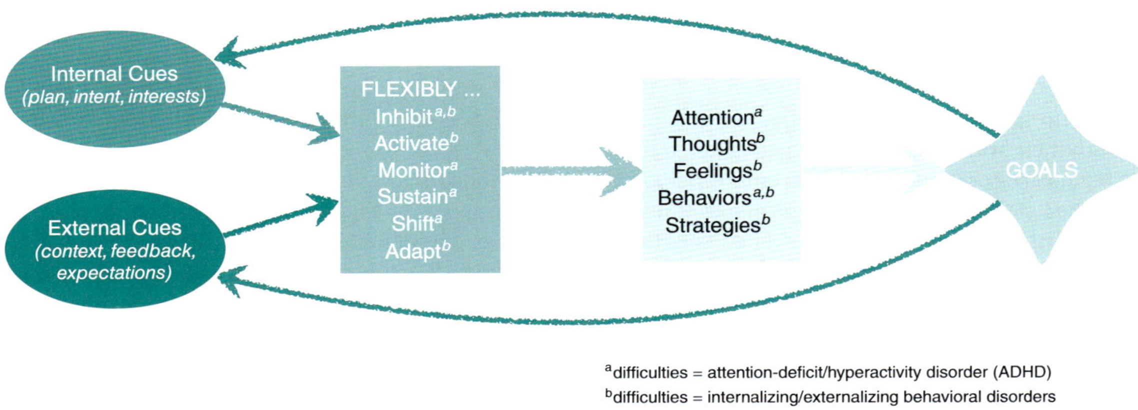

Fig. 8.2 Self-regulation, also known as executive function skills, emotional regulation, or effortful control. Self-regulation is a lot like a thermostat, but one that controls many variables at once. Children must learn to constantly monitor and evaluate their own environment and internal state, comparing to desired "settings." They must then up- or down-regulate ***(left rectangle)*** various systems ***(right rectangle)*** to bring about change in the desired direction.

and so does school (e.g., "Cooperate," "Sit still," "Ask for help," "Raise your hand"). To meet them, children must regulate their own appetites, drives, emotions, and behaviors. They must modulate their levels of excitement, arousal, activity, effort, and focus to match context and demands. They must learn to inhibit impulses and tolerate waiting, worry, frustration, and compromise. Self-regulation calls on a complex set of related abilities and functions (Fig. 8.2), which go by many names (executive skills, emotional regulation, effortful control). The skills involved start out intentionally and typically become internalized and automatic with practice, like riding a bicycle. Self-regulation skills can be taught by parents and teachers through modeling, cueing, and gradual withdrawal of adult support as the child demonstrates increasing competence (Florez, 2011).

Self-regulation is fundamental to successful adaptation at all stages of life. Better regulation measured in childhood predicted adult income, wealth, security, occupational prestige, lack of substance abuse, and lack of criminal convictions. This finding was true even when intelligence and socioeconomic status were controlled for, and even between sibling pairs (Moffitt et al., 2011). How well an individual child develops self-regulatory capacities during middle childhood is impacted by many factors, including heritable personality traits, resiliency factors (or lack thereof), early experiences (either positive or negative in nature), and the timing and structure of environmental influences (parental support, modeling, and teaching). There are ways to quickly assess self-regulation skills in a clinical setting that do not depend solely on parent and teacher report, such as the head-toes-knees-shoulders (HTKS) task (Ponitz, McClellan, Matthews, & Morrison, 2009; Wanless et al., 2011).

Self-Image

Its true roots are even earlier, but middle childhood (not adolescence) is when identity starts to be actively explored, expressed, questioned, and revised. For instance, while gender-type preferences (cis or trans) seen in the play of preschool children remain stable over time (Gülgöz et al., 2019) (see Chapter 76), it is during middle childhood that children start consciously comparing themselves to others and making deliberate choices about how to express their identity. Most adults would recognize their 12-year-old but not their 5-year-old selves. Throughout middle childhood, children undergo a cyclic process of self-questioning and reconstitution (e.g., "Where do I come from?" "Am I valued and by whom?" "Who do I like?" "What do I enjoy?" "What am I good at?" "Will trying harder pay off?" "How do I compare to others?" "What if I fail?" "What do I want to be when I grow up?"). This inquiry leads to an increasingly clear and differentiated set of beliefs about themselves, or self-concept, and a related but more malleable set of feelings, or self-esteem. Noah's self-image is threatened in our vignette as he compares himself to Jaxson, and his family to other families. At this age children show pride (or shame) in family, culture, and community. They get to know themselves and become comfortable (or not) with their body and their personality. They locate themselves in the social pecking order and develop opinions (accurate or not) about their own strengths and weaknesses. Feedback received from both peers and adults strongly influences these developments. The way adults offer praise, criticism, and advice determines whether a child adopts a fixed or a growth mindset (see Chapter 101).

Cultural Influences

What is considered normal child behavior, and what constitutes typical teaching and parenting, is strongly mediated by culture (see Chapter 20). Parental expectations, moral attitudes, and the way families interact with the larger community vary among ethnic groups. Even within relatively monolithic cultures (European, Asian, Latino) there can be great differences in parental expectations across nationalities and other subgroups (Super et al., 2008). It is also at this age that children themselves first become aware of cultural stereotypes, and this awareness occurs earlier among members of stereotyped minorities.

Parents are the first creators and mediators of culture for their children during early childhood. In middle childhood, however, teachers and peers play a larger role. Through media (see Chapter 21) culture exerts direct influence as well. As a result, first-generation immigrant children often begin to deviate from their parents' culture during middle childhood—a phenomenon that can cause conflict and consternation. Many studies show that children develop skills more quickly in areas that carry particular importance within their own culture. When assessing children for developmental and/or behavioral difficulties it is important not to make cultural assumptions. Questions should be designed to ascertain what constitutes children's developmental niche within their own culture, such as:

- Where, with whom, and doing what does the child spend each day?
- What customs, traditions, and assumptions guide parental behaviors?
- What are the parents' expectations for their child (relevant to the problem being discussed)?
- How do the parents view their role versus the role of teachers, peers, professionals, others?

It is important to put this information alongside what you know about a child's personality and temperament and think about the goodness of fit between the child and the cultural expectations.

Readiness for Adolescence

We define the end of middle childhood and transition to adolescence (see Chapter 9) by cognitive, emotional, and social changes rather than biologic markers. The hormonal onset of puberty usually occurs during the last third of middle childhood. Adolescent readiness has not been studied in the same way school or kindergarten readiness has, but one could conceive of it as when a child has met most milestones of middle childhood and overcome most of the challenges facing a school-age child. Key signs may include the following:

- Reads critically, draws conclusions, is able to integrate information from multiple sources
- Shows emerging understanding of irony, paradox, ambiguity, metaphor, and sarcasm
- Is able to complete multistep, long-term assignments independently, with minimal support
- Friendships begin to show more self-disclosure and mutual emotional support
- Manages conflicting allegiances, adopts different persona in different groups
- Considers multiple perspectives and conflicting values/interests
- Knows morally right and legally right are not necessarily the same
- Considers individual rights in addition to rules
- Shows increasing curiosity about world beyond immediate surroundings/experience
- Can handle significant responsibility without supervision
- First explicit, conscious romantic or sexual attractions are starting to emerge

There is considerable individual age variability when the adolescent transition happens. It might be as early as 10 to 11 or as late as 14, but 12 to 13 is the most common age. Recognizing when a juvenile has turned into an adolescent is a shared responsibility of clinicians, teachers, and parents. Whether a particular 12-year-old is still in middle childhood or has entered adolescence has implications for the conduct of the medical visit and the advising of parents.

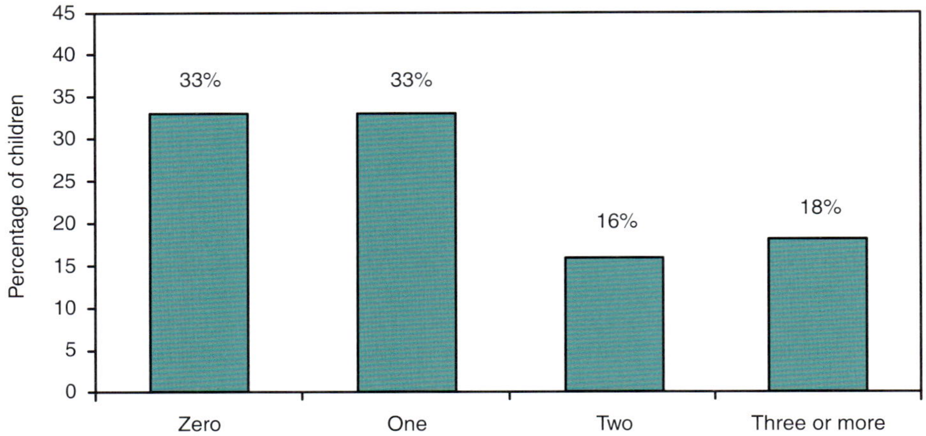

Fig. 8.3 Numbers of comorbid conditions in ADHD. (From Larson, K., Russ, S. A., Kahn, R. S., & Halfon, N. [2011]. Patterns of comorbidity, functioning, and service use for US children with ADHD, 2007. *Pediatrics, 127*[3], 462–470.)

WHEN THINGS GO AWRY—PATTERNS OF DYSFUNCTION

The most common developmental-behavioral diagnoses made during middle childhood are attention-deficit/hyperactivity disorder (ADHD), learning disabilities, oppositional-defiant disorder, and anxiety disorders. The criteria for each are based on symptoms seen at a surface level: learning delay, academic underachievement, distractibility, hyperactivity, tantrums, worry, avoidance, or other problematic behaviors. Symptoms are driven by underlying forces, however, which can be difficult to elucidate and untangle. Emotions, psychosocial stressors, and neurodevelopmental strengths or weaknesses can all contribute. Multifactorial causation is not unusual (see Chapter 2), and similar underlying struggles can express differently at a behavioral level in different children. Comorbidity becomes the rule, not the exception, during middle childhood. Conditions are also not always what they seem to be. Learning differences or emotional problems can create the appearance of ADHD. Oppositional or externalizing behavior may be driven by mood. Social anxiety and obsessive compulsiveness sometimes look a lot like autism. Thus when children qualify for several diagnoses at once, thinking about cause versus effect can help avoid therapeutic misadventures. Conversely, some children fail to meet criteria for any diagnosis despite significant impairment because they straddle boundaries between disorders. Keep an open mind and keep asking questions (e.g., "What else might be going on?" "What if we are wrong?" "How could we approach this differently?") especially when a child is not responding to interventions.

Attention Deficits

Inattention and/or impulsivity are the lens through which many parents and teachers prefer to view middle childhood school and behavior difficulties. ADHD (see Chapter 46) is less stigmatized and more socially accepted than alternative explanations. Treatment is less costly and more accessible. Assessment is simpler as well, with American Academy of Pediatrics (AAP) guidelines (Wolraich et al., 2019) available for diagnosis and management by primary care providers inside the medical home. Two-thirds of children with ADHD suffer from at least one, and one-third have two or more, other disorders, however. (Larson, Russ, Kahn, & Halfon, 2011) (Fig. 8.3).

Learning Differences

When school-age children struggle academically it is important to provide them with help promptly, before they fall too far behind. The AAP has published guidance for the

TABLE 8.5 American Academy of Pediatrics Guidance on School-Aged Children Who Are Not Progressing Academically

- Care coordination should take place in the medical home.
- Pediatricians need to understand special education law and procedures, including right to free appropriate public education, least restrictive environment, how to read an individualized education plan (IEP), and related laws (§504 of the Rehabilitation Act of 1973).
- Pediatricians should take an active role in prevention, identification, diagnosis, and treatment of academic progress problems.
- Pediatricians may take an active role in the initiation, development, and implementation of IEPs and 504 plans.
- Many factors need to be considered when choosing an approach to evaluation.
- Pediatricians should develop relationships with colleagues in other fields serving these children.
- Pediatricians should understand the different goals of evaluation in different settings.
- Payers should consider covering such care.

Adapted from Rey-Casserly, C., McGuinn, L., & Lavin, A. (2019). School-aged children who are not progressing academically: Considerations for pediatricians. *Pediatrics, 144*(4), e20192520.

involvement of primary care physicians in the evaluation and management of these children (Table 8.5) (Rey-Casserly, McGuinn, & Lavin, 2019). Special education law (see Chapters 104 and 113) stipulates every child in the United States between 3 and 22 years old is entitled to a free and appropriate public education in the least restrictive environment capable of meeting each child's needs. Children found eligible under at least 1 of the 13 special needs categories receive an individualized education plan (IEP), which may provide for specialized classroom placement and/or a variety of services, modifications, and accommodations within the mainstream. Specific learning disability (SLD) (see Chapter 47) is the most common reason children qualify for special education services, accounting for 35% to 40% of all IEPs (and an even higher percentage during middle childhood). The next four most frequent eligibility categories are speech-language impairment (see Chapter 44), which often turns into SLD as children move from preschool to school age, other health impairment (not limited to but often used for ADHD), intellectual disability (see Chapter 40), and autism (see Chapter 41).

Peer Problems and Bullying

Peers are any group of similar-age children interacting with each other in one place at one time (typically a school, neighborhood, or village). Friendships are individual relationships formed between peers. Establishing a secure place among peers is crucial to all school-age children (see Chapter 17). Having and keeping at least one close friendship can be a highly protective factor against the adverse emotional consequences of other social difficulties, which are common. Several factors predispose to social struggles (Table 8.6), but any child can experience them, and no one risk factor makes them inevitable.

Bullying is not merely simple conflict, disagreement, or competition. Bullying begins with the inclusion of some and the exclusion of others. It progresses to behavior (by one or more children toward one or more others) intended to establish, maintain, and exploit power. Bullies use intimidation, threats, embarrassment, extortion, manipulation, planned betrayal, and calculated aggression as means to create feelings of fear, shame, or low self-esteem in their victim(s). Bullying first appears in early elementary and peaks during middle school. It occurs most often in unstructured contexts, such as the lunchroom, hallways, bathrooms, recess yard, or cyberspace.

Being either a victim or perpetrator of bullying is a common experience (~20% each) in middle childhood. Some children (~5%) are both in different contexts. Most cases of bullying are isolated, short-term events. Whether bullying becomes a persisting pattern of behavior in the perpetrator depends on temperament, home environment, and the response of authority figures. How traumatizing bullying is to the victim depends on the severity and context of the event, its duration, whether it recurs, the resiliency of the child, and how it is handled by the adults in the child's world. Clinicians, teachers, and school administrators investigating possible bullying should ask about context, patterns, relationships, perceptions, and attributions. If they did not directly witness the bullying, they should hear several versions of the story from different observers. The parties should not be made to confront each other, however. Forced apologies will not help. Mediation or other conflict-resolution approaches assume a false equivalency, which can retraumatize the victim(s) and may inadvertently reward the bully(s). Perpetrators need to learn that bullying behavior is not tolerated and will not work because their teachers "see through them" and thus cannot be fooled. Victims need to know that the bullying is not their fault, their peers support them, and adults will protect them in the future.

Long-term bullying outcomes vary but can be poor for victims, perpetrators, and bystanders. Many bullies become repeat offenders. Habitual bullies do worse in school, have lower educational attainment, display more externalizing psychopathology, and are more likely to engage in substance abuse, domestic violence, and criminal behaviors as adults than nonhabitual bullies. Victims of an isolated bullying event usually recover, but chronic bullying leaves scars in its victims, including social anxiety, depression, and a negative self-image. Sometimes bullying becomes a persistent pattern

TABLE 8.6 Risk Factors for Social Difficulty

Risk Factor	Examples and Issues
Presence of a disability (interfering with participation)	Physical or functional, accommodations required
Differences in appearance (from the group)	Skin color, ethnicity, size/habitus, physical deformity
Differences in cultural practice (from the group)	Dress, grooming, religious observance
Speech, language, communication problems	Expressing self verbally, understanding others
Social thinking (cognition) deficits	Autism, social pragmatic communication disorders
Learning difficulty, difference, delay	The receipt of special education services
Emotional dysregulation	Cries easily, frequent displays of emotion
Internalizing behaviors	Anxiety, withdrawal
Externalizing behaviors	Aggression, hyperactivity, bullying (can cut either way, also being socially rewarded in some cases)

toward a particular child by many perpetrators. Peer rejection is when a child is shunned by most or all of a peer group. Once established, peer rejection is a highly stable characteristic over time and is even likely to relapse in a new venue and peer group. It is a serious social outcome of bullying, causing persistent feelings of isolation and low self-esteem in the victim, which are highly associated with later depression, aggression, conduct disorder, and suicide (see Fig. 8.1) (McDonald & Rubin, 2017).

Unfortunately, bullying and peer rejection are problems that cannot be easily solved on a case-by-case basis. A preventive approach is needed at a school, district, or community-wide level. Antibullying programs with the greatest demonstrated success are those in which students, teachers, and parents are all actively engaged. They combine teacher training (to recognize bullying quickly and unambiguously), a true zero-tolerance policy, and activities aimed at changing school culture to support and celebrate individual differences. The latter teach children problem-solving, empathy, and perspective-taking skills. All these measures together promote helpful bystander responses (intervening to help victims, reporting to the authorities, rather than avoiding involvement by turning away), which is the key to reductions in bullying. Such programs need strong leadership from the top of a school or district, they do not tend to work as grassroots, parent- or teacher-sponsored, bottom-up initiatives. Many manualized programs exist, but they are only likely to be helpful when implemented as intended. When schools select wisely from among the whole-school bullying prevention programs that have strong evidence of effectiveness and are feasible to implement in their setting, they are likely to experience important and sustained beneficial effects for all students (see Chapter 17).

Emotional and Behavioral Difficulties

When parents ask if a behavior is normal, it is best not to dichotomize but see the behavior along a spectrum from highly adaptive/appropriate to extremely maladaptive/disruptive. Maladaptive behavior that is not disruptive is often called internalizing because the harm is directed inward. Externalizing, disruptive behaviors attract greater attention sooner but may actually be adaptive in certain situations. Several variables impact the likelihood a school-age child will experience emotional difficulties:

- Early toxic stress from adverse childhood experiences (ACEs)
- Parenting skills and ongoing parental stress/impairment
- Developmental challenges (motor, language, learning difficulties)
- Social difficulties (bullying, peer rejection)
- Temperament (usually apparent from early infancy)
- Coping skills and resiliency
- Family history of mental illness

Children with developmental delays, autism, or intellectual disability often possess greater awareness of their differences than appreciated by parents and teachers. They may also experience emotion that exceeds their ability to understand, communicate, or cope, resulting in misbehavior that is easily misunderstood by adults. On the other hand, emotional difficulties can hinder social success or learning in otherwise typically developing children. They may masquerade as autism or ADHD, interfere with standardized testing, or create the impression of a learning or intellectual disability.

Externalizing Behavior

Impulsive, hyperactive, attention-seeking, and aggressive behaviors (see Chapters 49 and 55) are disruptive to classroom and family life. Therefore they are likely to prompt stronger discipline and greater concern than internalizing behaviors. Verbal and physical aggression occur most frequently in the context of tantrums. Tantrums occur in four phases:

1. *Prodrome,* during which the child is visibly irritable, tense, bored, or restless. Most parents can learn to recognize this phase and they report knowing something is coming.
2. *Blowup,* during which the child loses all emotional self-control and manifests the most upsetting behaviors.
3. *Letdown,* during which the child may be withdrawn, depressed, remorseful, or still angry but no longer acting out. The child may apologize or make self-deprecating remarks during this phase.
4. *Recovery,* when everything returns to normal, as if nothing ever happened.

It is important for parents to learn to intervene in the prodromal (first) phase of this cycle. Once the blowup happens, it is too late to teach coping skills. Intervening means identifying and talking about feelings. The parent might say, "Something seems to be bothering you." Ultimately, children may learn to do this strategy for themselves (the goal). If the first stage is missed, it is best to wait until it is all over and things are back to normal (stage 4). At that point, parents can revisit the episode when everyone is calm and employ some of the problem-solving techniques discussed in Table 8.7.

Anxiety and Internalizing Behavior

Anxiety in preadolescent children is relatively undifferentiated, often presenting with symptoms that cross boundaries between different subtypes (see Chapter 51). The presentation in an individual child can change dramatically with age. The most common forms of anxiety in middle childhood are social anxiety, somatization (which often progresses to panic disorder as a child approaches adolescence), pathologic perfectionism, and school avoidance. When separation anxiety (more common in preschoolers) persists into middle childhood is often due to a history of trauma and loss. Anxiety can sometimes be predicted by an infant with an inhibited temperament, identifiable at a very young age and moderately heritable. It is also created or exacerbated by a variety of ACEs (Rapee, Schniering, & Hudson 2009), overprotective or negative parenting, as well as cognitive biases to either overrespond to threat or interpret ambiguity in a negative fashion (something that can be taught or discouraged by parents, teachers, and therapists).

Anxiety is the most common psychiatric problem in middle childhood, with an estimated prevalence of 15% to 20%. Anxiety during elementary school strongly predicts later mood disorders, substance use, academic underachievement,

TABLE 8.7 Counseling Parents: How to Promote Emotional Regulation

1. **Give permission to feel/language to talk about feelings:**
   - **Ask** about, acknowledge, accept
     "How you feel?" "I see you're worried" "It's okay to feel mad" "Feelings are never wrong, but we need to …"
   - **Avoid** directives/negation/disapproval
     "Calm down" "Don't be sad" "You shouldn't be …" "Boys don't cry"
   - **Identify**, reflect, and discuss
     "Tell me what happened" "Maybe you feel scared that …"
   - **Sympathize** and share
     "I don't blame you for feeling …" "I remember a time …"

2. **Encourage positive self-talk:**

Encourage positive self-talk:	Discourage negative:
"I did my best"	*"I'm a failure"*
"Next time I'll do better"	*"I might as well give up"*
"I can handle this"	*"I can't handle it"*
"I'm not going to let it get to me"	*"I'm no good"*
"I can do it, it just takes practice"	*"I can't do anything right"*
"She didn't do it on purpose, it was an accident"	*"She doesn't like me"*
"This happens to everyone sometimes"	*"He was out to get me"*

3. **Use typical triggers as an opportunity to teach and practice problem solving (employ this either before the meltdown or when things have returned to normal, not in the midst of a tantrum):**
   - **Define** the trigger and the emotional reaction: ⟷ Discuss, role play when relaxed
   - **Brainstorm** what I could do about it: ⟷ Generate multiple possible solutions (good/bad)
   - **Evaluate** what would happen if …: ⟷ Think through consequences of each solution
   - **Implement** the chosen solution: ⟷ What will it take for me to follow through?
   - **Review** the result: ⟷ How did it turn out?

4. **Practice relaxation and "turtle" skills for physiologic/somatic responses:**
   - **Okay** to take a timeout when feeling strong feelings: ⟷ Go to a safe place or imagine you are a turtle and withdraw inside shell
   - **Deep** breathing exercises: ⟷ Stop, take a deep breath, count to 100
   - **Guided** imagery: ⟷ Close your eyes, imagine you are in your turtle shell, treehouse, beach, etc.
   - **Progressive** muscle relaxation: ⟷ Start with feet and work up
   - **Meditation**: ⟷ Never too young to start, many do-it-yourself apps (HeadSpace, Calm, Breath2Relax, Pacifica)

5. **Use timeouts/token economies for specific behaviors:**
   - **Ignore** what you can: ⟷ Any attention, even negative, can be more reinforcing than none
   - **Have a positive** baseline: ⟷ Consequences lose their impact if everything is always negative
   - **Pick your battles** wisely: ⟷ Focus only on dangerous, disruptive, hurtful behaviors
   - **Timeout**: ⟷ Withdrawal of attention for unwanted behavior
     - 1 min/yr of age; child must be quiet for last half to be released
     - Predetermined (boring) space used only for this purpose
     - Parent should be matter of fact, unemotional when it's over
   - **Token economy**: ⟷ Rewards for desired behaviors
     - Tokens, stars, stickers, or points accumulated, "Cashed in" for specified rewards
     - Privileges, parental time, special activities preferred over material things

6. **Promote open communication, self-awareness, and a growth mindset (see Chapter 101):**
   - **Recognize** and praise efforts (not just results):
     - Progress not perfection, "catch 'em being good"; avoid praising "easy" successes
   - **Use** positive, forward-looking language:
     - *"That was great, you calmed yourself down" "I'm so proud of you for …" "You are becoming a person who can stay cool and control your own anger …"*
   - **Be** on the lookout for use of words (even for negative emotions):
     - Self-restraint, efforts at independent problem solving, use of coping strategies
   - **Use** zones of regulation (blue/green/yellow/red) to monitor and communicate about emotional state:
     - (coordinate with school);
     - Teach child to engage coping strategies/problem-solving skills in yellow and blue zones
   - **Frame** failure/frustration as universal and good:
     - Everybody fails; use as an opportunity to learn and become better

7. Model skills:
   Don't escalate or overreact to child
   Avoid tantrums (verbal or physical) of your own
   Calmly verbalize your own feelings, and the reasons for them
   Never blame others or expect them to fix it for you

   Articulate coping strategies: Talk through your own problem solving in front of the child ("I'm frustrated so I'm making things worse. I think I'll take a break to calm down, then come back later and try again"; "That made me mad, but I understand … maybe things will go better for me next time") and even suicide (see Chapter 50) (Woodward & Fergusson, 2001). It is a great masquerader, frequently mistaken as ADHD, SLD, oppositional defiant disorder, or even high-functioning autism (Allen, Benningfield, & Blackford, 2020). Even when recognized, it tends to be undertreated; 80% of cases fail to receive appropriate evidence-based care even though anxiety has been shown to respond well to a variety of interventions (cognitive behavioral therapy, parent training, psychopharmacology) (Walkup et al., 2008) and can be prevented by school-based programs (Neil & Christensen, 2009). Undertreatment is partially due to a lack of appropriate resources in the community (Merikangas et al., 2010, 2011) and partly due to a misperception among physicians, especially those in primary care, that anxiety is less dangerous and less impairing than mood disorders (Tulisiak et al., 2017). Successful intervention during middle childhood lowers later risk for depression and suicide (Keeton et al., 2019), although relapse rates are high (Ginsburg, 2018).

Depression is less common in middle childhood than during adolescence, and less common than anxiety or mood dysregulation. Although suicidal ideation occurs frequently, serious suicidality (intent, attempts, plans, and completed suicide) is quite rare. Depression at this age also tends to be chronic rather than acute. School-age children are more likely to fit the *Diagnostic and Statistical Manual of Mental Disorders,* fifth edition (*DSM-5*) criteria for persistent depressive disorder than major depression. Therefore instructions commonly found in depression screening instruments to report only symptoms occurring in the last 2 weeks may not be appropriate for this age group. It would be better to ask about symptoms displayed frequently over the last year.

CLINICAL IMPLICATIONS

Concerns about development, learning, or behavior are among the most common reasons children see their pediatrician (20%–30% of all visits). Parents often raise concerns in this area, or a clinician may uncover them with a few insightful questions, even during visits with a different agenda. Clinicians have their biggest impact on preschoolers through their parents, by influencing parenting behavior. During middle childhood interactions with the doctor can become helpful for the child directly, especially when the child feels listened to, seen, respected, and understood.

Approach to the Visit

To work effectively with children in middle childhood, any adult (teacher, coach, therapist, or health care clinician) must gain their trust (see Chapters 75 and 77). Younger children trust based on parental demeanor toward the new/strange adult. Adolescents can bestow trust based either on the role/credentials of the provider or on the relationship they build with them. In middle childhood a child's trust is always built on the relationship and must be earned in that context, whether it is the introductory phase of psychotherapy, the first visit to a doctor, or the first few weeks in a new classroom. Adults gain children's trust by being attentive and showing interest in what the child is saying and expressing through play or behavior. Meet children where they are in terms of interests and affect, but do not put on an act. Children know when you are being genuine. If they are in the room, do not leave them out of conversations with their parents. The skills of motivational interviewing can be highly effective at this age, not only for motivating change but for gaining trust as well. Be nonjudgmental, reflect back to them what you hear, then take it another step. Give them a voice, especially in decisions that affect them. The legal power of consent still lies with parents at this age, but it is best if school-age children assent to care. Obtaining that assent is a shared responsibility of parents and clinicians. Children ought to understand what is going to happen, why, and what the expected benefits, risks, and side effects are to the extent they are cognitively able and emotionally ready. Their questions or worries should be addressed in a manner appropriate to their mental age. School-age children are capable of sabotaging care. Proceeding over their expressed objection should be done with circumspection by parents and physicians, only when felt to be absolutely necessary, and only with respectful and empathetic explanation of the reasons.

Prior to the onset of adolescence, a child's need for (and right to) privacy from their parents is quite limited, and a parent's right to know about and control what happens with their child usually takes precedence. Most verbal children in middle childhood are happy to talk with you (if you gain their trust). Unlike an adolescent, they will not usually withhold information just because their parents are present. Indeed, most children this age will happily say anything in front of their parents or even their friends' parents (as any parent who has ever driven school carpool knows). Many children at this age develop a sense of modesty about their body, which should be respected by parents and physicians. Parents can be asked to turn away while examining private parts, which should otherwise be clothed or covered. Beyond this exam, in most cases there is usually nothing that needs to be done or discussed with the child that parents should not be present for during middle childhood. Exceptions to this general rule include when child abuse is suspected, psychometric testing is being conducted, or situations where significant family discord/conflict exists. If you must examine or interview a latency-age child without the parent present, it is best to do so with a third person in the room.

Conversely, during middle childhood there are many reasons to want to interview parents alone, without the child present. Parents of school-age children are more likely than parents of preschoolers to be angry with or blame children for presenting problems. They may be reasonably reluctant to discuss school, behavior, family financial, or marital issues in front of the child. Children at this age will always be listening if they think the conversation is about them or their family, even when they do not appear to be, but they may only partially understand what they hear. They may be frightened or come away with harmful misperceptions that could have been avoided by having them be out of the room (e.g., "I'm dumb," "I'm in trouble," "Mom and Dad are fighting").

Private feedback to the parents may or may not be necessary, but the child should usually receive some direct feedback as well. Near the transition to adolescence a combined/hybrid approach to the visit may need to be used in which some time is spent alone with both child and parent(s).

School-age children know how to be examined. Aside from modesty and needle phobia, most have no difficulty cooperating with a physical exam (see Chapter 75). They are also now accustomed to talking with adults outside their family. These factors allow reversing the typical preschool encounter workflow: Focus first on the child rather than the parent(s). This design sends positive messages about respect, responsibility, and involvement in their own health care. It telegraphs that you are primarily there for them, not their parents, and it "grabs" them in a way that is more likely to keep them engaged. First, greet and introduce yourself to the child. Acknowledge the adult(s) briefly or invite the child to introduce them to you, then turn right back and launch into the child interview. Most parents will get (and even appreciate) what you are doing, but if necessary nonverbal signals can be sent that "it's not your turn yet." Do not begin with the question, "What brings you in today?" The child may not know, and such questioning can feel threatening; if needed, this information can be gathered ahead of time from parents by a nurse or medical assistant. Instead, say, "Tell me about yourself" or "What's been going on lately?" Kids age 6 to 8 years may struggle to field such an open-ended question, in which case you should move quickly to more closed-ended inquiry. Most 9- to 12-year-olds should have no trouble running with it, however. After interviewing the child, a pediatric clinician may move straight to a physical examination. Comment on what you see and what you are looking for (school-age children are usually fascinated and very glad to hear that they are normal). Some shy or anxious kids do better being examined first because they may need time to warm to the situation, so you can start the interview as the exam proceeds. Once you are done interviewing and examining, dismiss the child and talk to the parent(s) alone (this may present logistical challenges depending on your clinic layout and staffing). Call the child back in to provide feedback at the end.

Sexuality

School-aged children have sexual feelings that are not latent but often are suppressed or sublimated. Nevertheless, sexual thoughts cause excitement in children at this age, and they have a great deal of curiosity about anatomic differences, functions, gender roles, and identity (see Chapters 73 and 76). They are quite sensitive to subtle messages about what is normal and whether these thoughts are okay to talk about. They may feel guilt for having sexual thoughts and feelings, and they may develop shame if they latch on to the idea that they themselves are not normal. It is during middle childhood that many lesbian, gay, bisexual, transgender, questioning (LGBTQ) youth first self-identify, and they are at particular risk for developing self-esteem and adjustment difficulties related to feeling different.

Throughout middle childhood, there is a growing awareness of sexuality and of what constitutes appropriate versus inappropriate, public versus private behavior. At least 90% of boys and 50% to 60% of girls masturbate before they enter adolescence. As they progress through the age range it becomes increasingly prevalent but more hidden. Thus parents of children in the earlier half of middle childhood are more likely to be aware of (and concerned about) the behavior. Professionals should frame this discovery in the context of normal development and help parents to see it as an opportunity for teaching and discussion.

In the face of all this it is unwise for parents or clinicians to be silent about sexuality with school-age children. At best, this leads to ignorance and a feeling that, metaphorically, there is an elephant in the room; at worst, peers media, or even pornography fill the gap. Open discussion about gender and sexuality with parents and professionals during middle childhood prevents misinformation and sets the stage for open discussion with partners later in life, the basis for both consent and the establishment of satisfying intimate relationships. For LGBTQ youth it may be even more important to provide a foundation for self-esteem and acceptance that will support their adjustment throughout the lifespan. Therefore discussion about sexuality should begin as soon as a child starts to ask questions or shows interest in body parts, and certainly no later than the early elementary school years. The topic should be framed in its proper context of feelings and relationships. By the time they are 8 years old, however, children should know about the body changes they can expect when puberty begins. Before entering middle school, all children should have a basic knowledge about how pregnancy happens (and can be prevented), the nature of consent, and sexually transmitted illnesses.

Trauma and Loss

Children regularly experience loss and separation. Parental divorce, losing a friend, moving to a new town, transitioning to a new classroom, or discontinuing psychotherapy are but a few common examples. Sometimes these events are unexpected, but often they can be anticipated. In the latter instance it is best to prepare the child and, if possible, arrange for a way to say goodbye and bring closure to the relationship. Feeling deserted and not allowed a farewell may cause the child to reject both the lost attachment and the replacement (such as a new teacher). Adults should talk honestly but simply about what happened (or is going to happen) in a way that gives the child permission to feel and express emotions.

Death of a loved one is the ultimate loss. In middle childhood children comprehend that death is irreversible and universal. They can understand the dead are no longer here with us and the basic beliefs about death of most religions. It is normal for school-age children to focus on physical processes (such as the means of death or details about burial/cremation) about which adults may be squeamish. Children this age should usually be allowed to attend funerals if they were close to the deceased because it provides closure in the same way as it does for adults and it provides a useful model for how adults share feelings and give/accept emotional support.

Child abuse (see Chapter 15) frequently goes unreported or remains unsubstantiated in middle childhood because of the child's own confused and ambivalent feelings. Abuse may leave no outward physical signs, as is often the case with sexual abuse. School-age children may identify strongly with the perpetrator, especially if the person is also a source of love and protection. The abuse may be scary, painful, or disgusting to them, while at the same time providing attention, power, or serving some other unmet emotional need. Victims often feel guilty and responsible themselves. Furthermore, they have often been told not to tell, with accompanying threats they are old enough to understand but not old enough to be skeptical of.

Children of the 21st century have unprecedented exposure to disasters, war, and terrorism (see Chapter 22), both direct and indirect, through media (see Chapter 21). Children this age have a greater capacity to understand these events than younger children do, but still find them very confusing. They often harbor inaccurate fears and ideas about what is going on. Their view tends to be focused on their own safety and that of their immediate family members. These thoughts can become even more traumatizing if they are separated from their parents and family. When this happens, the sooner family reunification occurs, the better.

School-aged children can react to trauma with acute distress, developmental regression, internalizing and/or externalizing behaviors, reenacting the trauma in play, and in some cases development of posttraumatic stress disorder. Certain types of traumas are more harmful than others: Sustained or repeated trauma is more harmful than brief trauma, trauma that involves permanent loss or disruption of established lifestyle is worse than trauma that involves fear without loss, and intentionally inflicted trauma is more harmful than natural disasters or so-called acts of God. News about a disaster, war, or other atrocity as conveyed through the media can have the effect of repeating the exposure and magnifying the harm. During such events, parents should attempt to limit their children's news consumption (Pine, Costello, & Masten, 2005).

Collaboration—It Takes a Village

Teachers are particularly important in supporting the development of school-age children. Positive relationships with teachers are strongly correlated with a child's academic success and can mitigate other psychosocial and neurodevelopmental risk factors (Liew, 2012). During middle childhood the influence of other adults (coaches, counselors, cops, clergy, therapists, shopkeepers, bus drivers, and neighbors) also grows. Community resources such as childcare, sports leagues, and recreational programs available to children can be vitally important, especially for children with single and/or working parents. Recreational activities can help children with psychopathology maintain physical, academic, and social competencies on a par with other children (Browne, Byrne, Roberts, Gafni, & Whittaker, 2001). More physically active youth been shown to have larger basal ganglia and hippocampi and show better attention, coordination, and memory skills (Bidzan-Bluma & Lipowska, 2018). As trusted expert members of their community, pediatric professionals have the potential to impact middle childhood development and quality of life well beyond the exam room. Clinicians should foster good working relationships with their local schools, with leaders of local sports and recreational programs, and with colleagues in other disciplines working with children in their community. They can provide advice at both a population and an individual level, reaching out and collaborating around specific children or groups of children. Medical and educational privacy laws (e.g., Health Insurance Portability and Accountability Act, Family Education Rights and Privacy Act) do not always serve a child's best interests in this regard. They were never meant to be barriers to collaboration, but in practice often can be. Clinicians caring for school-age children should therefore consider routinely asking parents to sign a release of information for their child's school (and perhaps other key adults) at their yearly health maintenance visit, in advance of a specific need to collaborate.

Advising Parents (and Teachers)

Middle childhood can be a most wonderful, relatively carefree time for families raising children. Parenting styles that focus on supporting autonomy while setting limits result in stronger self-regulation skills than authoritarian styles focused on control and compliance (see Chapter 13). Clinicians can encourage all parents to convey a clear sense of right and wrong in a gentle, noncritical manner. Explain how to be consistent in expectations and responses, both over time and between parents. When two parents disagree about discipline, presenting a united front is more important than which of them is right.

Children need to be given permission to feel, and home should be a safe space to talk about emotions. Children who develop the language of emotions experience benefits beyond emotional regulation later in life, including improved ability to ask for and receive help, a greater tendency to support and express concern for others, and ultimately find it easier to achieve intimacy and stability in their relationships. Parents can also support their child's social development through participation in athletics, clubs, cultural activities, play dates, and sleepovers, but parents should avoid overscheduling. Children also need time for unstructured free play. Parents should encourage independence but stay involved by being a coach, scout leader, or classroom parent.

It is important to set aside a regular study time with minimal distractions after school or in the evening. Parents should be available to assist but avoid doing the homework for the child. Parents should give a child gradually increasing responsibilities around the house commensurate with the child's abilities and, if possible, provide an allowance to teach budgeting and saving skills. In general, rewards and privileges should be earned. Finally, clinicians should reassure parents (and teachers) that there is a lot they can do themselves to promote self-regulation and help the child develop a healthy self-concept (see Table 8.7), and that help is available from many quarters when needed.

CONCLUSION

In our opening vignette three children wrestle with the challenges of middle childhood in different ways. Despite its image of tranquility relative to early childhood and adolescence, this is an age of profound growth and change. Middle childhood is a coming-out period, the time when most children start building a life beyond the family and an identity of their own. Improving powers of reasoning, memory, and self-regulation supports the acquisition of new skills and knowledge at a dizzying pace. Adjusting to the classroom and finding acceptance among peers are the key early challenges. School provides the milieu, peers the medium, and play the means by which the majority of 6- to 12-year-old children explore the world and practice for adult life. In the process they develop and continually refine emotional coping skills, self-concept, and a moral sense. Parents considering home schooling must think carefully about how their children will meet these developmental challenges without such a coming-out period.

The school-age child is capable of cooperating with clinicians, carrying on a conversation, and being included in shared decision making about their own care. Clinicians who focus on them first, respect their voice, understand their world, and who can be authentic gain the child's trust. Trusted adults can speak honestly and simply to children during middle childhood about sexuality, media, societal upheaval, separation, trauma, and loss. By doing so, they help the child process experiences and sort their questions into the proper context. Parents can encourage and model talking about feelings but should take care about what a child this age sees and overhears. Adult conversations, especially about the child or family, may be misconstrued in harmful ways. Direct or indirect exposure to some adult activities can be traumatizing or may reinforce inappropriate ideas and behaviors.

In recent years middle childhood concerns have often taken a backseat to other developmental stages in policy decisions about the commitment of public resources. This situation may be changing, however, as a result of the COVID-19 pandemic. As this book is being written, an entire generation of schoolchildren is experiencing profound, long-lasting disruptions to their schooling and social experiences. Some are suffering more obviously and acutely than others, but society will be dealing with long-term impacts on their development for decades to come. The consequences will shed new light on the importance of school and community, and on the vital role pediatricians and mental health clinicians play in local and national advocacy. Parents face new challenges also, and many are under immense strain. Lucky families who manage to cope successfully may someday look back on this time with gratitude for the precious gift of extra time together during childhood's golden years.

REFERENCES

Allen, K. B., Benningfield, M., & Blackford, J. U. (2020). Childhood anxiety—If we know so much, why are we doing so little? *JAMA Psychiatry*, *77*(9), 887. https://doi.org/10.1001/jamapsychiatry.2020.0585.

Bidzan-Bluma, I., & Lipowska, M. (2018). Physical activity and cognitive functioning of children: A systematic review. *International Journal of Environmental Research and Public Health*, *15*(4), 800. https://doi.org/10.3390/ijerph15040800.

Bouchard, T. J. (2009). Genetic influence on human intelligence (Spearman'sg): How much? *Annals of Human Biology*, *36*(5), 527–544. https://doi.org/10.1080/03014460903103939.

Browne, G., Byrne, C., Roberts, J., Gafni, A., & Whittaker, S. (2001). When the bough breaks: Provider-initiated comprehensive care is more effective and less expensive for sole-support parents on social assistance. *Social Science & Medicine*, *53*(12), 1697–1710. https://doi.org/10.1016/s0277-9536(00)00455-x.

DelGiudice, M. (2018). Middle childhood: An evolutionary-developmental synthesis. In N. Halfon, C. B. Forrest, R. M. Lerner, & E. M. Faustman (Eds.), *Handbook of life course health development* (pp. 95–107). Cham (CH). Springer Open.

Erlenmeyer-Kimling, L., Rock, D., Roberts, S. A., Janal, M., Kestenbaum, C., Cornblatt, B., . . . Gottesman, I. I. (2000). Attention, memory, and motor skills as childhood predictors of schizophrenia-related psychoses: The New York High-Risk Project. *American Journal of Psychiatry*, *157*(9), 1416–1422. https://doi.org/10.1176/appi.ajp.157.9.1416.

Florez, I. R. (2011). Developing young children's self-regulation through everyday experiences. *Young Children; National Association for the Education of Young Children*, *66*(4), 46–51.

Ghetti, S., & Bunge, S. A. (2012). Neural changes underlying the development of episodic memory during middle childhood. *Developmental Cognitive Neuroscience*, *2*(4), 381–395. https://doi.org/10.1016/j.dcn.2012.05.002.

Ginsburg, G. S., Becker-Haimes, E. M., Keeton, C., Kendall, P. C., Iyengar, S., Sakolsky, D., . . . Piacentini, J. (2018). Results from the Child/Adolescent Anxiety Multimodal Extended Long-Term Study (CAMELS): Primary anxiety outcomes. *Journal of the American Academy of Child & Adolescent Psychiatry*, *57*(7), 471–480. https://doi.org/10.1016/j.jaac.2018.03.017.

Gülgöz, S., Glazier, J. J., Enright, E. A., Alonso, D. J., Durwood, L. J., Fast, A. A., . . . Olson, K. R. (2019). Similarity in transgender and cisgender children's gender development. *Proceedings of the National Academy of Sciences*, *116*, 24480–24485. https://doi.org/10.1073/pnas.1909367116.

Keeton, C. P., Caporino, N. E., Kendall, P. C., Iyengar, S., Lee, P., Peris, T., . . . Ginsburg, G. S. (2019). Mood and suicidality outcomes 3–11 years following pediatric anxiety disorder treatment. *Depression and Anxiety*, *36*(10), 930–940. https://doi.org/10.1002/da.22944.

Larson, K., Russ, S. A., Kahn, R. S., & Halfon, N. (2011). Patterns of comorbidity, functioning, and service use for US children with ADHD, 2007. *Pediatrics*, *127*(3), 462–470.

Liew, J. (2012). Effortful control, executive functions, and education: Bringing self-regulatory and social-emotional competencies to the table. *Child Development Perspectives*, *6*(2), 105–111. https://doi.org/10.1111/j.1750-8606.2011.00196.x.

Mah, V. K., & Ford-Jones, E. L. (2012). Spotlight on middle childhood: Rejuvenating the "forgotten years." *Paediatrics & Child Health*, *17*(2), 81–83. https://doi.org/10.1093/pch/17.2.81.

McDonald, K. L., & Rubin, K. H. (2017). Peer relationships and influence in childhood: *Reference Module in Neuroscience and Biobehavioral Psychology*, Elsevier. https://www.sciencedirect.com/science/article/pii/B9780128093245065123.

Merikangas, K. R., He, J. -P., Burstein, M., Swanson, S. A., Avenevoli, S., Cui, L., . . . Swendsen, J. (2010). Lifetime prevalence of mental disorders in U.S. adolescents: Results from the National Comorbidity Survey Replication–Adolescent Supplement (NCS-A). *Journal of the American Academy of Child & Adolescent Psychiatry*, *49*(10), 980–989. https://doi.org/10.1016/j.jaac.2010.05.017.

Merikangas, K. R., He, J. -P., Burstein, M., Swendsen, J., Avenevoli, S., Case, B., . . . Olfson, M. (2011). Service utilization for lifetime mental disorders in U.S. adolescents: Results of the National Comorbidity Survey-Adolescent Supplement (NCS-A). *Journal of the American Academy of Child & Adolescent Psychiatry*, *50*(1), 32–45. https://doi.org/10.1016/j.jaac.2010.10.006.

Merritt, D. (2012). *Typical speech and language development for school-age children: A checklist for school nurses.* http://ctserc.org/component/k2/item/130-typical-speech-and-language-development-for-school-age-children

Moffitt, T. E., Arseneault, L., Belsky, D., Dickson, N., Hancox, R. J., Harrington, H., . . . Caspi, A. (2011). A gradient of childhood self-control predicts health, wealth, and public safety. *Proceedings of the National Academy of Sciences*, *108*(7), 2693–2698. https://doi.org/10.1073/pnas.1010076108.

Neil, A. L., & Christensen, H. (2009). Efficacy and effectiveness of school-based prevention and early intervention programs for anxiety. *Clinical Psychology Review*, *29*(3), 208–215. https://doi.org/10.1016/j.cpr.2009.01.002.

Nippold, M. A. (2016). *Later language development: School-age children, adolescents, and young adults* (4th ed.). PRO-ED.

Pine, D. S., Costello, J., & Masten, A. (2005). Trauma, proximity, and developmental psychopathology: The effects of war and terrorism on children. *Neuropsychopharmacology*, *30*(10), 1781–1792. https://doi.org/10.1038/sj.npp.1300814.

Ponitz, C. E. C., McClellan, M. M., Matthews, J. S., & Morrison, F. J. (2009). A structured observation of behavioral self-regulation and its contribution to kindergarten outcomes. *Developmental Psychology*, *45*(3), 605–619. https://doi.org/10.1037/a0015365.

Rapee, R. M., Schniering, C. A., & Hudson, J. L. (2009). Anxiety disorders during childhood and adolescence: Origins and treatment. *Annual Review of Clinical Psychology*, *5*(1), 311–341. https://doi.org/10.1146/annurev.clinpsy.032408.153628.

Rey-Casserly, C., McGuinn, L., & Lavin, A. (2019). School-aged children who are not progressing academically: Considerations for pediatricians. *Pediatrics*, *144*(4), e20192520. https://doi.org/10.1542/peds.2019-2520.

Schmitt, J. E., Raznahan, A., Clasen, L. S., Wallace, G. L., Pritikin, J. N., Lee, N. R., . . . Neale, M. C. (2019). The dynamic associations between cortical thickness and general intelligence are genetically mediated. *Cerebral Cortex*, *29*(11), 4743–4752. https://doi.org/10.1093/cercor/bhz007.

Shaw, P., Greenstein, D., Lerch, J., Clasen, L., Lenroot, R., Gogtay, N., . . . Giedd, J. (2006). Intellectual ability and cortical development in children and adolescents. *Nature*, *440*(7084), 676–679. https://doi.org/10.1038/nature04513.

Super, C. M., Axia, G., Harkness, S., Welles-Nystrom, B., Zylicz, P. O., Parmar, P., . . . Mcgurk, H. (2008). Culture, temperament, and the "difficult child": A study in seven western cultures. *International Journal of Developmental Science*, *2*(1–2), 136–157. https://doi.org/10.3233/dev-2008-21209.

Tulisiak, A. K., Klein, J. A., Harris, E., Luft, M. J., Schroeder, H. K., Mossman, S. A., . . . Strawn, J. R. (2017). Antidepressant prescribing by pediatricians: A mixed-methods analysis. *Current Problems in Pediatric and Adolescent Health Care*, *47*(1), 15–24. https://doi.org/10.1016/j.cppeds.2016.11.009.

Walkup, J. T., Albano, A. M., Piacentini, J., Birmaher, B., Compton, S. N., Sherrill, J. T., . . . Kendall, P. C. (2008). Cognitive behavioral therapy, sertraline, or a combination in childhood anxiety. *New England Journal of Medicine*, *359*(26), 2753–2766. https://doi.org/10.1056/nejmoa0804633.

Wanless, S. B., McClelland, M. M., Acock, A. C., Ponitz, C. C., Son, S. H., Lan, X., Morrison, F. J., Chen, J.-L., Chen, F.-M., Lee, K., Sung, M., & Li, S. (2011). Measuring behavioral regulation in four societies. *Psychological Assessment*, *23*(2), 364–378. https://doi.org/10.1037/a0021768.

Wolraich, M. L., Hagan, J. F., Allan, C., Chan, E., Davison, D., Earls, M., Evans, S. W., Flinn, S. K., Froehlich, T., Frost, J., Holbrook, J. R., Lehmann, C. U., Lessin, H. R., Okechukwu, K., Pierce, K. L., Winner, J. D., & Zurhellen, W. (2019). Clinical practice guideline for the diagnosis, evaluation, and treatment of attention-deficit/hyperactivity disorder in children and adolescents. *Pediatrics*, *144*(4), e20192528. https://doi.org/10.1542/peds.2019-2528.

Woodward, L. J., & Fergusson, D. M. (2001). Life course outcomes of young people with anxiety disorders in adolescence. *Journal of the American Academy of Child & Adolescent Psychiatry*, *40*(9), 1086–1093. https://doi.org/10.1097/00004583-200109000-00018.

9

Adolescence

Bonnie Halpern-Felsher, Marcia Zorrilla, Adrienne Lazaro, and Arash Anoshiravani

For additional material related to the content of this chapter, please see Chapters 2, 3, 4, 49, 50, 51, 74, and 75.

VIGNETTES

- *Vignette 1: Ally, age 12 years, looks in the mirror and hardly recognizes herself. It feels to her like overnight she grew 4 inches and gained hips and breasts. She isn't sure how she feels about this new body. However, she really likes the clothing she has just bought, identical to her best friend's.*
- *Vignette 2: Like many of her friends, Yasmine, a 16-year-old high school sophomore, is thinking about having sex. She knows about the risks of getting a sexually transmitted infection (STI) but does not know how to talk to her boyfriend about birth control. Despite having been together for 4 months, she is worried that he will be angry with her if she asks him to wear a condom. He may even refuse to be her boyfriend anymore.*
- *Vignette 3: Colin is excited to go to college but is worried about how a decision to go to his first-choice school may negatively impact his family's financial status. He is also reluctant to go as far away as he had originally planned because it would mean putting great distance between himself and his new partner. He is writing lists of pros and cons about each potential school to make a good decision.*
- *Vignette 4: Justin is being persistently pressured by his friends to try vaping. He is curious about it as he has heard about vaping for so long. But he has also heard about the health harms, and he is afraid to get in trouble. He isn't sure what to do. He is looking for help in making his decision.*

INTRODUCTION

Adolescence is the dynamic period between middle childhood and adulthood. Definitions of adolescence vary. The American Academy of Pediatrics (AAP) defines adolescence as the period from ages 11 to 21 (Hagan, Shaw, & Duncan, 2007), whereas the World Health Organization (WHO) defines it as the period from ages 10 to 19 and youth as the period from 15 to 24 years (n.d.). Many consider adolescence to begin with the onset of puberty, typically marked by breast enlargement and the onset of menses, or development of pubic hair and testicular enlargement. Regardless of definition, most experts do not view adolescence as a single age group, but as three distinct but overlapping phases: early adolescence (~10–13 years old), reflected in Vignette 1; middle adolescence (~14–16 years old), reflected in Vignette 2; and late adolescence (~≥17 years old), as reflected in Vignette 3 (Table 9.1).

Adolescence is a period of significant and rapid physical, cognitive, psychosocial, and emotional growth. It is also a time when adolescents make decisions about school, health and healthcare, friends, and whether to engage in a range of behaviors that could have profound implications on their health and wellbeing. While normal and normative, these decisions and the resulting behaviors can be very stressful and can have long-lasting consequences, as reflected in Vignette 4.

In this chapter we discuss the multiple dimensions of adolescent development. We approach adolescent decision making, health, and behavior using two frameworks: the biopsychosocial model and the ecological systems theory of development (see Chapter 2). Both emphasize that multiple factors converge to explain adolescent development. According to the biopsychosocial model (Engel, 1977), development and health are determined by the reciprocal interactions between biology, psychology, and social factors. Similarly, according to the ecological systems model (Bronfenbrenner & Morris, 2007), development takes place through reciprocal interactions between the individual and the persons, objects, and symbols in their immediate environment, and these relationships are impacted by the immediate and remote environment.

DEVELOPMENTAL CHANGES DURING ADOLESCENCE

Adolescents go through rapid physical, cognitive, psychosocial, and emotional changes. The changes vary as a function of stage of development. Table 9.1 describes these changes within early, middle, and late adolescence.

Physical Development

Adolescence is a phase of physical changes and growth spurts. Three dramatic changes occurring during puberty include an increase in height, an increase in weight, and sexual/reproductive development. The timing of onset, rate of change, and ultimate appearance vary widely across individuals. Variability in timing and rate of puberty are based on many factors, including genetics, nutrition, medical conditions, and racial and ethnic background, to name a few.

TABLE 9.1 Developmental Stages During Adolescence

Tasks	Early: 10–13 Yr	Mid: 14–16 Yr	Late: ≥17 Yr
1. Independence	Emotionally breaks from parents and prefers friends to family	Ambivalence about separation	Integration of independence issues
2. Body image	Adjustment to pubescent changes	"Trying on" different images to find real self	Integration of satisfying body image into personality
3. Sexual drives	Sexual curiosity; occasional masturbation	Sexual experimentation; individuals may be viewed as sex objects	Beginning of intimacy and caring
4. Relationships	Unisexual peer group; adult crushes	Begin heterosexual peer group; multiple adult role models	Individual relationships more important than peer group
5. Career plans	Vague and even unrealistic plans	Emerging plans may still be vague	Specific goals and specific steps to implement them
6. Conceptualization	Concrete thinking	Fascinated by new capacity for thinking	Ability to abstract
7. Value system	Decline in superego, testing of moral system of parents	Self-centered	Idealism; rigid concepts of right and wrong; other-oriented; asceticism

From Felice, M. E. (1992). Adolescence. In D. M. Levine, W. B. Carey, & A. C. Crocker (Eds.), *Developmental-behavioral pediatrics* (2nd ed., p. 69). WB Saunders.

While children assigned male at birth (referred to subsequently as "boys") and children assigned female at birth (referred to subsequently as "girls") are similar in height and weight during early childhood, rapid changes occurring during adolescence alter the course for both girls and boys. Increases in height and growth spurts happen at different stages for girls and boys. For girls, the growth spurt begins approximately 2 years earlier than boys, starting, on average, at ages 9 to 10, lasting about 2 years. During this time, girls increase in height by about 3 inches per year. For boys, the growth spurt begins on average at ages 11 to 12 lasting about 2 years. During this time, boys increase in height by about 4 inches per year. During early adolescence, girls are as tall or taller than boys of the same age, but by the end of adolescence, boys are typically taller than are girls (Bordini & Rosenfield, 2011).

Changes in weight, adipose tissue distribution, and muscle mass typically occur at approximately the same time as the gain in height. Weight, in general, almost doubles for all adolescents. Adolescent girls develop a greater amount of body fat than adolescent boys, with changes in adipose tissue distribution varying in adolescent girls and boys. In adolescent girls there is a redistribution of fat to hips and breasts, whereas in adolescent, boys there is less fat overall and increased lean muscle mass and strength.

Skeletal features that undergo changes during adolescence include changes to the face and skull. Adolescent boys acquire thicker and heavier bones in their skull and brow prominence compared to girls. There is increased long bone length (relative to height) and increased bone density. Bone density affects weight and skeletal strength, laying the foundation for bone health through the rest of the individual's life. Discussions with adolescents and their parents regarding bone health, diet, and physical activity are therefore especially important in increasing bone health and ultimately preventing osteoporosis later in life.

Pubertal and Hormonal Development

Physical maturation and the development of secondary sexual characteristics during adolescence results in the individual evolving toward an adult appearance and in adolescents experiencing different culturally determined expectations for cognition, language, social skills, emotional regulation, interests, and activities. Sometime in late childhood, production of adrenal androgens increases before there are any physical signs of puberty. This increased production of adrenal androgens can be approximately contemporaneous with an increasing pulsatile secretion of gonadotropin-releasing hormone during sleep. Gonadotropin-releasing hormone secretion results in increasing levels of luteinizing hormone (LH) and to a lesser extent follicle-stimulating hormone (FSH). In females FSH stimulates follicle growth in the ovary and the production of aromatase. LH stimulates ovarian thecal cells to produce androgens; aromatase converts androgens to estrogens in the FSH-stimulated granulosa cells. Later in puberty, under separate control mechanisms, a mid–menstrual cycle surge of estradiol results in an elevation of LH to trigger ovulation (Joffe & Blythe, 2003). In males LH stimulates the Leydig cells in the testes to produce testosterone; later, FSH stimulates testicular Sertoli cells to support the development of sperm.

Other hormones are also released during puberty. The pituitary secretes human growth hormone, regulated by growth hormone–releasing factor and somatostatin that are also from the hypothalamus. Growth hormone–releasing factor is released in a pulsatile fashion during sleep. Insulin-like growth factor I (IGF-I or somatomedin C) and IGF-II are produced by the liver and influence growth, particularly growth rate, as do thyroxine and the corticosteroids. Parathyroid hormone, 1,25-dihydroxyvitamin D, and calcitonin affect skeletal bone mineralization. The release, surge, and interaction of these hormones result in the physical changes observed during adolescence.

In girls the first sign of puberty is usually the development of breast buds, which occurs between the ages of 8 and 10 years. The growth of pubic hair, further development of breasts, a height spurt, a weight spurt, and menarche then follow in a well-described pattern (Tanner, 1962). Menarche signifies the end of pubertal development in girls. Girls typically experience puberty about 2 years earlier than boys.

In boys the first sign of puberty is usually darkening of the scrotal skin, enlargement of the testes, and lengthening of the penis, all of which occur between the ages of 10 and 12 years. The proliferation of pubic hair, additional enlargement of the genitalia, and a height spurt follow over the next 2 to 6 years (Tanner, 1962). Other pubertal changes, such as acne, axillary hair, deepening of the voice, and the growth of chest hair in boys, also are characteristic, but vary from one individual to another, depending on genetic and cultural factors. Most of the changes of puberty occur in early adolescence (see Table 9.1), but a subset of young men continues to grow taller into their early 20 s.

Motor Skill Development and Coordination

As adolescents grow rapidly, they may become awkward or clumsy as they get used to changing length of limbs and bodies. Strength increases in most children, though generally more so in boys than in girls. Strength and agility are promoted by physical exercise, participation in sports, and ongoing practice. During rapid growth periods, the growth plates (or physes) and large tendon insertion sites of adolescent bones cannot handle as much force and stress as mature adult bones, making adolescents more prone to overuse injuries and fractures, especially in organized sports.

Brain Development

Significant changes occur in brain structure and function during adolescence and into young adulthood. Gray matter areas of the brain, which are involved in motor and sensory functions and in processing emotions and rewards (i.e., the amygdala and limbic systems), have already matured during childhood. However, areas involved in higher level processing, such as organization, planning, self-monitoring, self-control, and working memory, continue to mature during this developmental stage. These higher level skills are collectively called executive functions. The prefrontal cortex is one of the last areas of the brain to develop and generally does not fully mature until early adulthood (approximately age 25) (Casey, Giedd, & Thomas, 2000; Casey, Jones, & Hare, 2008).

During adolescence, gray matter volume decreases, though gray matter density increases. Following the synaptic overproduction and increased neuronal connections of childhood, the adolescent and young adult brain selectively "prunes" itself. The remaining neuronal synapses become more efficient and adept at transmitting information between neurons. The process of pruning occurs in a back-to-front direction with the frontal lobes pruned last (Gogtay et al., 2004).

Along with the maturation of the gray matter regions, white matter, defined as the fiber bundles or tracts that connect brain regions, is also evolving. Advanced magnetic resonance imaging studies show that diffusion in white matter becomes more directional during adolescence, a change indicative in part of increased myelination. Increased myelination increases the efficiency and speed of neuronal connections and communication. The regions in which this white matter changes take place include the prefrontal cortex, again likely leading to greater speed and efficiency in decision making, selective attention, and information processing. The process of myelination also occurs in a back-to-front manner with the frontal lobes becoming myelinated later (Gogtay et al., 2004).

Dopamine receptors, which are connected to the limbic system of the brain responsible for emotions, rewards, and punishment, increase during adolescence. These processes have been shown to continue through age 25, with large individual differences in rate and amount of brain growth over time. This late maturation of dopamine receptors may lead adolescents to act more impulsively, choose more risky behaviors, and make decisions influenced by the emotional and reward centers of the brain compared to emerging adults (Casey et al., 2008). This development would suggest that during early adolescence rational thinking may be overridden by emotions or the desire for rewards.

Cognitive Development

Abstract Thinking

Adolescents become increasingly capable of thinking abstractly as opposed to strictly thinking concretely (see Chapter 3). This development allows adolescents to think logically not only about concrete objects and issues in the present but also about abstract, future, or hypothetical issues. Advances in cognitive skills also allow adolescents to consider multiple aspects of their actions and decisions at one time, assess potential positive and negative consequences of each decision, and plan with consideration of contingencies. Adolescents also become increasingly capable of metacognition, or the ability to "think about thoughts." Metacognition allows adolescents to merge knowledge from past experiences with reflective thinking about current challenges of a new task or problem, review and reflect on possible strategies, and eventually solve or resolve challenges. Metacognitive processes are thought to be largely responsible for helping adolescents successfully counterbalance an array of conflicting thoughts and emotions "new" to their experience, by virtue of rapid biologic growth and dramatically expanding life experiences. Adolescents' abilities to process information rationally and to reason through a decision emerge as young as age 10 and approach adult levels by age 16 (Steinberg, Graham, O'Brien, Woolard, Cauffman, & Banich, 2009). Their ability to apply logical thinking is facilitated by formal education, which in the later grades and ages promotes logical, scientific, and creative thinking.

Language Development

While most adolescents have learned the basics of language before adolescence, the use of both the written and spoken word becomes more sophisticated and refined during adolescence than during middle childhood, corresponding with their emerging cognitive advances. Language during this period involves long sentences, diverse vocabulary, figurative language, sarcasm, and persuasion. Formal education also promotes these developmental changes, whereby adolescents are often required to deliver expository speeches or to debate in school. Social language skills also mature. Adolescents learn and appreciate the communicative needs of individuals and audiences and thereby become increasingly able to adjust their language accordingly.

Emotional Development and Intensity

As adolescents are developing physically, cognitively, and socially, they are also developing emotionally. Indeed, because the human brain develops from the posterior to anterior, the parts of the brain most responsible for generating emotions develop early. During adolescence, individuals make decisions using emotional reasoning, especially the early adolescent years. Further, adolescents tend to have more intense emotions, and unpredictable and extreme mood swings, than children of younger ages. Adolescence is a time known for mood swings and emotionality, and during this time it is especially important for clinicians, parents/caregivers, teachers, and others involved in the life of teens to take the time to calmly listen to the needs and emotions of adolescents.

Self-Regulation

Accompanying other aspects of development is the development of self-regulation, or the ability to regulate one's emotions and behaviors. Adolescents' psychosocial maturity, such as the ability to consider long-term consequences and rewards, to resist impulsivity, and to resist peer pressure, contribute to the development of self-regulation. These abilities are served by the anterior regions of the brain that develop in adolescence and emerging adulthood, with the ultimate milestone of developing increased independence and decision-making abilities.

Psychosocial Development

Personal Identity Development

The development of a sense of self is one of the significant tasks of adolescence. Personal identity development occurs throughout the lifespan. It is during adolescence that important questions predominate an individual's thinking: "Who am I?" "What will I become in life?" "What do I want to be when I grow up?" and "Am I doing a good job?" Many characteristics contribute to the adolescent's self of sense, including gender, race/ethnicity, culture, class, political and religious views. These facets are influenced by family, friends, schools, and society.

Adolescents develop their identity in a social context, following the biopsychosocial model. They try to understand how they fit into their world, comparing themselves to others around them, and deciding to which social group they want to belong. Adolescents are also developing their ethnic, religious, and gender identities at this time, again deciding with which group of people they wish to affiliate.

Adolescents may show multiple facets of their personal identity. A 16-year-old whose parents were born in Mexico and is an American citizen may self-identify as a Mexican American. She may speak only Spanish at home and English in school. Mexican holidays and celebrations may be celebrated with her family while she may participate in American holidays such as the Fourth of July with her friends. Tension may develop for the teen and her family as she tries to navigate both worlds. Adolescents' identity typically solidifies as the individual approaches early adulthood.

Autonomy Development

Adolescents' physical maturity allows them to look like adults. At this stage of their psychosocial and emotional development, society accepts that adolescents can take on increasing responsibility. These trends translate into adolescents' desire to participate in, and eventually dictate, their health and social decisions. Adolescents look for opportunities to make decisions. Indeed, experiences with such decisions-making, serve as practice for making decisions later in life.

Perspective Taking

Perspective taking is the ability to recognize how the thoughts and actions of one person can influence those of another, and to imagine how others might see them. This domain pulls together the advances in cognitive and social development. Social perspective taking also involves the ability to recognize that other people may have different points of view, or a different knowledge set from one's own. The ability to take others' perspectives continues to develop in early adolescence, stabilizing and becoming similar to adults' abilities by about age 16. Susceptibility to peer pressure generally decreases by age 16. Impulsivity, including making quick and reflexive decisions, steadily declines starting at around age 10. Future perspective taking, including the ability to think further into the future and consider possible positive and negative outcomes associated with choices, is generally mature by age 16, though experience and education continue to refine these skills well past age 16 (Steinberg et al., 2009).

Peer Relationships

Developing mutually satisfying peer relationships is an important developmental task in adolescence (see Chapter 17). Friendship formation and survival are about acceptance and trust. Friendships form around groups of youth with similar interests, lifestyles, and cultural backgrounds. Often, friendships are same sex during early adolescence and expand to include all genders by high school. As adolescents seek autonomy from parents, socializing with their peer groups becomes very important. Positive peer relationships contribute to adolescents' wellbeing, as adolescents get to test new roles (e.g., being a good listener, the comedian in the group, the outspoken one) in a safe space with peers.

As adolescents get to test new roles, however, problems may arise. Bullying and other forms of negative behaviors also increase during adolescence. Bullying behavior needs to be addressed by adults immediately to ensure safety for the youth being bullied but also for the youth who is doing the bullying, allowing the adolescent to recognize that this form of behavior is unacceptable and inappropriate.

Family Relationships

Parents are typically important influences in the youth's identity development for promoting and supporting individuation, the process of achieving a sense of individuality distinct from the identity of others. Individuation in adolescents may be displayed through separation from the family and through self-assertion, especially in cultures that value independence over interdependence. These changes lead to adjustments to family relationships during adolescence (see Chapter 12). This period can be stressful between the parent/caregiver and youth, as adolescents enact their need for autonomy and individuation. Youth often test limits with their parents/caregivers, which is a normal part of adolescence as they navigate the world into adulthood. Frequently, youth "push" parents away while simultaneously wanting to stay close to them.

Parents/caregivers do well to set safe boundaries and consistent guidelines so that youth feel a sense of stability and are able to approach the dramatic changes in their lives without becoming overwhelmed. Even though it may not seem like it for many parents, youth need them for love, support, and security. Providing a home environment that fosters connectedness, where there is open, respectful communication among all parties promotes healthy identity development. In health care clinicians may play a critical role assisting both parents and youth to communicate with each other, educating them on what is expected during adolescent development and normalizing these stages of identity development.

Gender

Gender refers to the attitudes, feelings, and behaviors that a culture associates with an individual's biologic sex (see Chapter 75). Gender identity refers to an individual's deeply felt feelings of being a boy, a man, or a male; a girl, a woman, or a female; or an alternative gender (e.g., two-spirit, genderqueer, gender nonconforming, nonbinary). For alternative genders, the external presentation is independent from sexual orientation and sex assigned at birth. As health care clinicians it is important to ask adolescent patients their gender pronouns and then to make sure and use their stated pronouns. Doing so fosters an inclusive environment and affirms, not assumes, their gender identity. It also supports their mental health and wellbeing by raising their self-esteem and lowering their risk for depression or other mental health and behavioral issues.

Sexual Orientation

Sexual orientation develops during the preteen and teenage years and refers to whom an individual is attracted and with whom one wants to have an intimate or sexual relationship (see Chapters 73 and 74). A youth may identify as straight, lesbian, gay, bisexual, pansexual, or asexual. Straight refers to being attracted to members of the other sex; a lesbian is defined as a woman attracted to other women; the word *gay* generally refers to men attracted to men, but also some lesbians use the term. Bisexual people are attracted to both men and women. Pansexuals are attracted toward people regardless of their sex or gender identity. Asexual people have romantic but no sexual attraction to others. Sexuality is fluid during adolescence, and it may be common for adolescents to change their sexual orientation as they explore their identities (Stewart, Spivey, Widman, Choukas-Bradley, & Prinstein, 2019).

Adolescents often worry about how their family members and friends would react if they were to disclose their sexual orientation or gender. Many adolescents feel happier and less stressed after they share their sexual orientation with their family, especially if their family is supportive. Others may not feel safe coming out because of fears of rejection, homophobia, bullying, and other threats. Some adolescents do not disclose their sexuality or gender identity until adulthood. For parents, the news that their child is not straight may be unexpected. Some parents may feel confusion, shame, anger, or sadness, whereas others may feel worry and concern. Other parents immediately are accepting and supportive. Parents in the current era are more accepting of their child's sexual orientation than in the past; nonetheless, they often need time to adjust to the news. Unfortunately for some adolescents, they are rejected by family members who ask them to leave the home. In clinical care it is thus important to provide a safe and confidential space when meeting with adolescent patients to enable a full and honest discussion about gender and sexuality. An adolescent may want to discuss the coming out process, sexual and/or reproductive health, gender-affirming healthcare and/or ask for advice on how to talk to parents. Clinicians often have opportunities to educate parents about sexual orientation and how acceptance promotes an adolescent's health and wellbeing. The clinician may be able to bring family members to a place of understanding.

Race/Ethnic Identity

Race is a social construct and refers to the characteristics and features used to classify a group of people. The meaning of race is not fixed and has changed over time. Ethnicity refers to the membership of a particular cultural, national, or racial group that has a shared culture, language, place of origin, and religion. For example, among two Black people, one may be Dominican and another may be American. Ethnic identity, in particular, is shaped by family socialization. Ethnic identity is also influenced by media, the arts, literature, and global affairs.

Supporting the health and wellbeing of adolescents should include discussion of and understanding about racial and ethnic identity. The demographics of the United States are changing: The US Census Bureau (2018) predicts that less than half of children in the United States are projected to be non-Hispanic White (49.8% of the projected 74 million children age <18 years) by 2020 (updated data not available yet); the percentage of children who are two or more races is projected to more than double, from 5.3% currently to 11.3% in 2060. This demographic shift will bring important opportunities and challenges for health care systems, education systems, and other systems that adolescents and their families encounter. Adolescents from diverse backgrounds are likely to have different behaviors, beliefs, values, and other aspects of culture. Cultural humility that seeks lifelong personal reflection, growth, and learning around issues of culture in relation to service delivery (Tervalon & Murray-Garcia, 1998) will be more important than ever across all these systems in supporting the health and wellbeing of racially/ethnically diverse adolescents.

Social Consciousness

Consciousness can be considered individuals' self-awareness of their thoughts, feelings, and memories, guided by their moral compass and values. Social consciousness is consciousness shared by others (like-minded folks) in a society. Climate change, gun violence in schools, police brutality, animal rights, LGBTQ (lesbian, gay, bisexual, transgender, queer and/or questioning) rights, and others are examples of issues that some youth care deeply about. Social consciousness develops at an early age. Adolescents are influenced by family, peers, religion, schools, the media, community, and world events. These factors raise their awareness about multiple social issues. During mid- and late adolescence, youth may want to "do something" about the injustices they see and/or experience; youth often want to make a change in the larger society.

Youth activism has long been a feature of the adolescent experience, as evidenced by their participation in the civil rights movement in the 1960s to the gun control rallies in 2017–2018, to protests of George Floyd's murder by police in 2020 during the COVID-19 pandemic. What has changed recently is how youth organize and mobilize. Currently, adolescents rely primarily on social media to organize and disseminate information. For example, in 2018 March for Our Lives organized the largest youth gathering to protest gun violence in schools using social media platforms. The availability of the internet facilitates youth connecting to causes and becoming a part of something larger than themselves and doing a world of good. Health care clinicians can help youth identify their passions, interests, and dreams, and support and guide them with their choices.

Awareness of Social Justice

Many adolescents personally experience oppression, ableism, racism, sexism, and other "isms" on a daily basis. The lens of intersectionality suggests that the traits that encourage negative social reactions intersect and overlap (Crenshaw, 1989). For example, in the United States an adolescent Black girl with disabilities may experience both racism and ableism. She is more likely to be economically disadvantaged, further affecting her life experiences. These factors, and the social reactions they trigger, influence physical and mental health outcomes, including quality of life, life expectancy, and access to adequate health care. Stress associated with racism, sexism, ableism, and related social attitudes greatly and negatively impact the mental health of adolescents, placing them at increased risk for anxiety, depression, and suicidality.

Health care clinicians can start tackling these issues by first becoming educated on these "isms" through self-study or continuing education. As clinicians become more comfortable in starting these types of conversations with adolescents, they should address these stressors via either screening for ACEs (adverse childhood experiences) or assessing the mental health impacts of the stressors, counseling adolescents about strategies for mitigating the impact of the stress, and, if appropriate, making referrals to trauma-informed mental health services (Valdez, 2020). Collectively, clinicians who work with adolescents may want to consider advocating for youth by raising awareness of these topics in professional organizations, becoming involved with local organizations that are working against oppression, and acting as a resource for adolescents who are experiencing these "isms" at their schools. With the youth's permission, it may be as simple as making a phone call to a teacher or school counselor to mobilize action.

CONTEXTUAL INFLUENCES

Adolescents are trying to determine who they are in relation to their peers, family, community, culture, and society. As such, they scan their environment for information about external expectations, social norms, their real and perceived value (or lack thereof) to society, acceptance by peers/society, alienation by peers/society, access (or lack thereof) to resources/support, and external validation. This environmental sensitivity can result in a high prioritization of peers' opinions ("but everyone else is doing it"), heightened responses to nonparental authority figures ("I didn't pass that class because Mr. Matthews has it out for me"), desire to redefine familial dynamics ("I'm not a little kid anymore"), and increased attention to social issues ("that's just not fair"). The relative importance of these factors varies as a function of adolescent stage (see Table 9.1). Clinicians may explore with the adolescent patient how different contextual influences impact their psychosocial and personal identity development. The biopsychosocial model of development encourages consideration of multiple environmental influences on adolescent development (see Chapter 2).

Role of Social Media

The role of social media has become increasingly important to adolescents during the past decade (see Chapter 21). Social media is easily accessed through applications on smartphones, which keep adapting to increase appeal to the audience and to respond to consumer trends. A study by the Pew Institute shows that at least 95% of US adolescents have or have access to a smartphone (Anderson & Jiang, 2018). Social media is a platform for the sharing of ideas, mutual interests, and trends, such as music, dance, or fashion. Social media presents a means for youth to socialize and establish new peer friendships and relationships. It offers a way to feel connected and supported online, especially for certain groups such as LGBTQ and disabled youth. During the COVID-19 pandemic, social media became a lifeline for many adolescents who were unable to socialize with friends due to shelter-in-place restrictions. Even as the restrictions based on the COVID-19 pandemic begin to fade, the role of social media remains essential for many adolescents.

There is a dark side to social media. The anonymity in social media allows for victimization, such as cyberbullying (disseminating negative judgments about individuals), sexting (transmitting provocative or frankly sexual messages, videos, or photographs), and forms of child abuse. It is not uncommon for adolescents to see criminal activities taking place on social media, including drug sales. It is also not uncommon for adolescents to open up on social media regarding issues facing them, such as intimate partner violence and self-cutting as a form of self-harm.

Social media and mental health issues may become closely tied. For example, social media may allow an adolescent to meet other (apparently) same-aged peers, relieving them of the social anxiety they might experience with in-person encounters. Yet, relying on social media worsens their verbal communication skills. Poor mental health is associated with high use of social media, especially among young women (Karim, Oyewande, Abdalla, Ehsanullah, & Khan, 2020). Additionally, adolescent social media use is difficult for parents to monitor. Social media applications, such as Snapchat, are ephemeral. Youth may create several social media accounts, each for different audiences, such as parents, friends, and employers, and may use varying levels of privacy settings for each audience. In clinical encounters with adolescents it is important for clinicians to educate both youth and parents about the benefits and harms of using social media.

Schools

Schools are social structures for learning and acquiring knowledge (see Chapter 18). Adolescents are expected to attend regularly, to complete homework assignments, and to pass tests that assess their learning. Schools also provide opportunities for adolescents to develop special skills and talents, such as music, sports, and leadership, through extracurricular activities and sports teams.

Schools vary greatly, even within the same school district, in terms of academics and course options, electives, extracurricular activities, and sports. While some adolescents are exposed to a wide range of academic subject material and educational challenges, from general education to advanced placement (AP) classes, other adolescents, especially in underresourced schools, experience more limited choices in terms of classes and difficulty levels. Students in the latter settings may grapple with outdated textbooks, a rotation of substitute teachers, and crowded classrooms. Students may fall behind age and grade expectations due to poor teaching, limited educational opportunities, learning disabilities, or behavioral challenges leading to suspensions and/or expulsions. These students find it increasingly difficult to catch up and often lose interest in studying or even attending school. Many schools also offer limited extracurricular activities and fail to ignite interest or passion in any facet of the adolescents' lives. Some students conclude that school is irrelevant to what they are experiencing in their personal lives, such as challenging family issues (e.g., parent illness, loss of employment, death), immigration issues, housing problems, and/or their own health issues. These students are at risk for dropping out before high school graduation.

Schools offer a place where adolescents socialize with each other, inside and out of class. They develop and end friendships and romantic relationships; they learn to navigate various cliques and social groups. In class they may work on projects as teams, learning important skills such as negotiation and conflict resolution. Students may participate in school functions such as school dances, sports rallies, and arts performances, refining their sense of self and other. Adolescents may also participate in other activities outside of school with friends such as parties, sleepovers, and other social gatherings.

Schools provide an opportunity for adolescents to connect with caring and trusted adults who are not their parents or caregivers. Adults serve as teachers, coaches, or school clinic staff, such as a health educator, nurse, or school counselor. These caring and trusted adults may serve as mentors for individual students, providing guidance and support. A meaningful adult relationship may make a real difference in the lives of adolescents, especially disconnected youth who lack a supportive network. Having someone who believes in you and cares about you can foster an adolescent's wellbeing and boost confidence throughout the adolescent years (Murphey, Bandy, Schmitz, & Moore, 2013). Of course, schools also vary in the adult-student ratio, the quality of student support services, and the culture regarding the roles adults play for the adolescent students. In well care for adolescents a detailed assessment of the nature of the adolescent's school and school experiences is critical for understanding their lives.

Work

The answer to the question, "What do you want to be when you grow up?" starts to take shape during middle school but may not produce consistent answers until late high school or beyond (see Chapter 10). Career exploration often occurs in schools, with events such as career days or job/internships fairs. Oftentimes schools receive information on jobs and internships from community agencies, such as nonprofits, hospitals, and corporations. Extracurricular activities may sharpen an adolescent's interests in types of work or careers. Early adolescents who cannot work because of age restrictions may accept internships, positions on youth board/councils, and/or volunteer opportunities. Middle and late adolescents may accept employment opportunities. Typically, entry-level jobs for adolescents in the United States are often in the retail and food industries. However, fortunate adolescents may get entry-level jobs as coaches or teachers, particularly if they have experience (e.g., a successful gymnast might land a job coaching gymnastics for young children). Depending on the type of work the adolescent finds, work may lead to future educational or social opportunities and may offer meaningful mentoring.

The world of work prepares adolescents for adulthood. They learn about responsibility, work ethics, and getting along with people who are diverse in age, abilities, gender, socioeconomic status, education levels, and race/ethnicity. Importantly, they learn about money management. For some adolescents, work is a necessity. They may need to work to contribute to household expenses. Immigration status can affect adolescents' ability to attain and maintain employment and/or limit their employment opportunities. Work competes with other activities (such as homework, chores, and extracurricular activities) and can expose a youth to more adultlike behaviors. In health care clinicians should address with adolescents whether they work, how they manage their time, and how work impacts their health (e.g., sleep, nutrition, and stress, as well as academic performance and engagement in health risk behaviors).

Cultural Influences on Adolescents

Culture refers to the beliefs, values, and customs, among other components, that are learned and shared by a group of people and passed on from one generation to the next. Cultural identity frequently overlaps with race and ethnicity. However, in the United States there is also wide diversity within racial and ethnic groups. Again, in the United States there are many different cultures influencing adolescents in distinctive ways. Some cultures emphasize independence, self-reliance, and relative autonomy. Other cultures foster interdependence, group cohesion, and social responsibility. Cultures try to leave their mark on adolescents. Cultural heritage may be supported at home, schools, and within the larger community. Schools contribute through programs that value diversity, such as awareness months (e.g., Black History month, National Asian American and Pacific Islander month, Hispanic Heritage month). In the clinical realm it is important to evaluate adolescents' relationships to their respective culture. Some adolescents readily embrace their cultural heritage. Others may resist these forces. Either way, adolescents may need support.

Religion

Religion and religiosity among adolescents vary greatly. For some adolescents, religion provides structure, lifestyle, and community. Parents are a major influence on whether an adolescent has a religious affiliation. Depending on adolescents' experiences with their religious affiliation, they may decide to stay in their parents' religion, modify their religion or religious practices, change religion, or completely abandon religion. Some adolescents may feel ambivalent if their religion conflicts with their personal or peers' beliefs (e.g., premarital sex, sexual identity, abortion, or suicidal ideation). Other adolescents use the organized structure and rules of their religion to promote a healthy lifestyle (e.g., vegetarianism). Whether in organized religions or not, engaging in prayer, meditation, and chanting may help adolescents reduce stress and maintain their mental health.

Religion and spirituality may be utilized as a coping mechanism for some, but not all, adolescents. In health care it is important for clinicians to ask about religious affiliation, practices, and dedication, recognizing the diversity found in religious expression. Asking adolescents about their religious background may be a conversation starter. The questions allow the clinician to get to know the adolescent, how the adolescent identifies, and the meaning the adolescent assigns to religion.

ASSESSING ADOLESCENTS' HEALTH AND HEALTH BEHAVIORS

Decision Making During Adolescence

As noted in the opening vignettes, adolescents are called on to make many decisions that have direct and significant implications on their long-term health, such as whether to engage in risky sexual behaviors, smoke tobacco or electronic cigarettes (e-cigarettes), drink alcohol, or use illicit drugs. Many theories of health-related behavior, such as the theory of reasoned action, theories of planned behavior, and the health belief model, argue, as their names imply, that behavior-related decisions result from deliberate, rational, and analytic processing. The models conceptualize that competent and rational decision making considers all of the options of engaging and not engaging in the behavior and weighing the risks and benefits of each behavioral option. Both perceived options and consequences are theorized to predict intentions to engage in behavior, which in turn predicts actual behavior. Full execution of decision making expects that individuals will consider the risks and the benefits of each option and decision. These theories, while useful, may not fully take into consideration the influence external factors have on individual decision making.

Adolescents' decision making tends to be more influenced by social and emotional factors than adults' decision making. For the adolescent, the process of decision making is situated within the set of psychosocial, cognitive, emotional, experiential, and contextual changes that define adolescence. For example, the adolescent in Vignette 2 was able to identify and understand the risks of having unprotected sex; however, she might still decide to have unprotected sex if she thinks it will strengthen her relationship with her partner. Thus in health care when discussing decisions regarding behaviors with adolescents, it is important to discuss not only the rational side of decision making but also the emotional costs and benefits.

Risk and Benefit Perceptions

An important component of decision making is the extent to which adolescents can accurately judge risks and benefits associated with health-related behaviors. The popular lure is that adolescents think they are invulnerable to harm. However, this belief does not play out in the scientific literature, which instead shows that adolescents, like adults, overestimate their risk for experiencing negative outcomes (e.g., their risk of becoming pregnant if they have unprotected sex) compared to statistical data. In fact, adolescents generally perceive greater risk than adults. Further, like adults, adolescents have an optimistic bias in their estimation of risk: They judge their personal risk of harm to be lower than risk to others. Such risk perceptions and their influence on behavior are moderated by life experiences. For example, adolescents who see a lot of violence in their neighborhood believe they are more susceptible to crime than adolescents with less experience of violence. Adolescents who see ads promoting e-cigarette use perceive lower risk of vaping than those who miss those ads, and those with lower perceived risk are more likely to use. The perception of low risk is an independent predictor of increased engagement in a variety of health-compromising behaviors.

Adolescents may also have distortions in their perception of benefits. Overestimates of benefits, regardless of perception of risk, are independent predictors of increased engagement in a variety of health-compromising behaviors, including underage drinking, tobacco use, and sexual behavior. Additionally, the order in which adolescents hear information about risks and benefits can significantly influence their health-related decision making. These findings highlight the importance of collaboration and communication between all parties involved in making medical decisions to avoid misperceptions and pitfalls in making decisions.

Comprehensive Assessments of Health: HEADSS

The most common causes of morbidity and mortality in adolescents are behaviorally mediated (e.g., car accidents, suicide, homicide). Thus a comprehensive health assessment must systematically survey the relevant issues and factors that influence adolescents' behaviors. HEADSS is an evolving psychosocial assessment tool that allows clinicians to get a sense of the various domains that can affect an adolescent's life and health. HEADSS is a mnemonic based on the first letters for those domains that should be routinely evaluated in clinical settings: **h**ome, **e**ducation/employment, **a**ctivities, **d**rugs/substances, **s**exuality, and **s**uicide/depression. Other important areas for assessment include: Eating, Sleep, Spirituality, Safety, and Strengths. Safety and Strengths are most often elicited, assessed, and elevated throughout each section for he HEADSS assessment. Table 9.2 includes sample questions to ask within each of the categories. This psychosocial assessment can be an effective screening tool for risk factors and can be used to identify resiliency factors.

In completing the HEADSS assessment it is important to ensure conditional confidentiality upfront to promote patient comfort, trust, and honesty. The clinician should promise that everything discussed between the patient and health care provider is confidential unless the patient is considering self-harm or harm to someone else, or someone is hurting the patient. When administering the HEADSS assessment, the questions should be asked in curious, straightforward, matter of fact, nonjudgmental ways. Clarifying follow-up questions can be useful. Throughout the visit, the clinician should use judiciousness about the adolescent's comfort and willingness to expand on answers. The goal of the HEADSS assessment is not "Gotcha!"; rather, the goal is to understand young people's experiences, behaviors, beliefs, values, and immediate safety concerns related to the various domains of their life. Through use of the evaluation, the clinician seeks to identify opportunities to provide accurate health education, positive reinforcement of healthy behaviors, recommendations for harm reduction regarding unhealthy/dangerous behaviors, behavioral change management, or outside specialty referrals as needed. Next we present a few of the areas on which to concentrate and the data supporting the focus.

Drugs/Substances

According to 2019 Youth Risk Behavior Survey data, in the past 30 days about 6% of adolescents had used cigarettes, 33% had used e-cigarettes, almost 6% had smoked cigars, and 4% used smokeless tobacco. Cannabis use is also common, with 15% of 8th graders, 34% of 10th graders, and 44% of 12th graders reporting ever use (defined as used any amount in their lifetime); almost 7% of 8th graders, 18% of 10th graders, and 22% of 12th graders having used in the month, and 6% of 12th graders reporting daily use. Almost 30% of adolescents reported past 30-day use of alcohol, and almost 15% reported binge drinking (Centers for Disease Control and Prevention [CDC], 2019).

Sexuality

An assessment of sexuality includes discussion of gender identity, sexual orientation, and relationships with others, including intimate partners. Sexual behavior encompasses a range of behaviors, from kissing to petting to masturbation to oral, vaginal, or anal sex. According to the latest national data (CDC, 2019), almost 40% of adolescents have ever had vaginal sex, and almost 30% had sex in the past 30 days. Approximately 45% did not use a condom at their last sexual encounter, putting them at risk for pregnancy and STIs.

Sleep

A hallmark of adolescence involves changes in sleep patterns (see Chapter 70). Related to the biologic changes of puberty, adolescents' typical natural sleep cycle is to want to fall asleep at around 1 a.m. and sleep in until about 10 a.m. However, adolescents still require about 9 hours of sleep, although very few adolescents get that amount of sleep. Unfortunately, typical school days start around 8 a.m. and end around 3 p.m., which conflicts with the normal adolescent biologic schedule. As such, there have been movements to change the school schedule, with varying success. Sleep problems can also be the hallmark of depression. Differentiating normal adolescent sleep from excessive or inadequate sleep is important as a component of evaluating mood disturbances.

Suicide/Depression

Depression among adolescents is unfortunately common, with lifetime prevalence among 13- to 18-year-olds having a major depressive disorder at about 11%, with a 12-month prevalence of almost 8%; these rates are greater among females than males and older than younger adolescents. Predictors of adolescent depression include experience of trauma, family history of depression, family conflict, chronic illness, and identifying as LGBTQ. Adolescents with major depression are at greater risk of suicide. Thus it is imperative that clinicians screen all adolescents for depression. The AAP recommends annual screening using the Patient Health Questionnaire-9 (PHQ-9). Once a patient screens positive for depression, it is then important to help the person obtain treatment (Miller & Campo, 2021). For more information on depression, see Chapters 49 and 50.

TABLE 9.2 **Elements of a HEADDSS Evaluation**

H	Home	Who lives with the young person? Where? Do they have their own room? What are relationships like at home? What do parents and relatives do for a living? Ever institutionalized? Incarcerated? Recent moves? Running away? New people in home environment?
E	Education/employment	School/grade performance—any recent changes? Any dramatic past changes? Favorite subjects—worst subjects? (include grades) Any years repeated/classes failed Suspension, termination, dropping out? Future education/employment plans? Any current or past employment? Relations with teachers, employers—school, work attendance?
A	Activities	On own, with peers (what do you do for fun? where? when?) With family? Sports—regular exercise? Church attendance, clubs, projects? Hobbies—other activities? Reading for fun—what? TV—how much weekly? favorite shows? Favorite music? Does young person have car, use seat belts? History of arrests—acting out, crime?
D	Drugs/substances	Use by peers? Use by young person? (include tobacco, alcohol) Use by family members? (include tobacco, alcohol) Amounts, frequency, patterns of use/abuse, and car use while intoxicated? Source—how paid for?
S	Sexuality	Orientation? Degree and types of sexual experience and acts? Number of partners? Masturbation? (normalize) History of pregnancy/abortion? Sexually transmitted diseases—knowledge and prevention? Contraception? Frequency of use? Comfort with sexual activity, enjoyment/pleasure obtained? History of sexual/physical abuse?
S	Suicide/depression	Sleep disorders (usually induction problems, also early/frequent waking or greatly increased sleep and complaints of increasing fatigue) Appetite/eating behavior changes Feelings of boredom Emotional outbursts and highly impulsive behavior History of withdrawal/isolation Hopeless/helpless feelings History of past suicide attempts, depression, psychological counseling History of suicide attempts in family or peers History of recurrent serious accidents Psychosomatic symptomology Suicidal ideation (including significant current and past losses) Decreased affect on interview, avoidance of eye contact—depression posturing Preoccupation with death (clothing, media, music, art)

Adapted from HEADSS for Adolescents. http://chipts.ucla.edu/assessment/Assessment_Instruments/Assessment_pdf_New/Assess_headss_pdf.pdf.

TREATING ADOLESCENTS

General Considerations

Clinicians should strive to assess adolescents' stage of cognitive development when recommending treatment approaches or options. Clinicians should also include the important adults (e.g., parents, guardians) in the treatment/decision making to the extent possible and safe. Early adolescents and those who are more concrete thinkers may need adult involvement to understand the treatment, participate in decision making, and adhere to the plan. They also need clinicians to provide clear explanations and directions focused on them (sometimes even separately from adults), while the clinicians avoid coming across as sounding paternalistic. It is important to ground any such discussions in what the adolescent cares about (e.g., smoking can make your skin age prematurely and your breath stink; this asthma medicine will make your breathing so much more comfortable and less scary; vaping can affect how fast you can run or how well you can play basketball; using/getting hooked on marijuana or other substances costs a lot of money). Middle adolescents and those who are abstract thinkers may be able to understand the connections between their health, their behaviors, and environmental factors around them. They can be encouraged and allowed to think about issues on their own rather than being told what to do (Box 9.1).

Late adolescents may participate in advanced abstract thinking to see the role much larger forces may be playing on their health and on their broader environment. Seeing those connections can be a motivating factor for health behavior change, treatment plan adherence, and even broader social/political advocacy (e.g., "Yes, it does seem that US drug policy has had many negative social and health impacts. I wonder if you have read about the impacts the drug producing and smuggling cartels have had on the daily lives of regular people in central and south America or in Afghanistan?").

BOX 9.1 How to Engage Teens in Discussion About the Contextual Factors in Their Health Decisions

- Smoking tobacco: "Have you noticed the tobacco companies have most of their advertising in poorer communities? Why do you think they do that?"
- Drinking alcohol: "It sounds like the boys at the parties you go to really encourage you and the other girls to drink as much alcohol as possible. Why do you think they do that?"
- e-cigarette: "Have you noticed all the hip online ads and the cool colors the tobacco/e-cig/vaping corporations use with their products? Who do you think they might be targeting? Why would they do that?"
- Becoming sexually active: "I know it sounds crazy that people recommend condoms during sex even though they don't feel as good as no condoms. Why do you think people keep recommending condoms anyway? How do you think those reasons/concerns might or might not affect you?"

Consent and Confidentiality

In most US states age 18 years is considered the age of majority. Before that age, parents or legal guardians must give consent. However, the strong consensus among clinicians and adolescent development experts is that adolescents can and do have capacity to make certain health decisions for themselves, even when they are under the age of majority. Pragmatically, many adolescents will forego needed care, especially in the sensitive areas of sexual or reproductive health and mental/behavioral health, if they must get their parents' consent to access such care. Studies find that when adolescents are promised confidentiality and have a say in the decisions about their health, they experience improved access and outcomes. For these reasons, most US states allow adolescents under the age of majority to consent for their own care related to the following issues:

- Pregnancy prevention and management
- STI prevention and treatment
- Behavioral health treatment (including therapy and psychoeducation, but not psychoactive medication initiation)

This ability to consent for these sensitive services also implies confidentiality related to care provided for minors, as disclosures to the adults in their lives may cause psychological discomfort (at best) and physical safety concerns (at worst). Clinicians are in a powerful position to encourage and facilitate increased communication between adolescents and the adults in their lives. They should not place themselves in a position of keeping secrets from their patients. However, clinicians must also respect these adolescents' autonomy and preferences to the extent possible, both to build and maintain rapport and trust and to keep their highest risk patients safe (e.g., in situations of violence in the home and child emotional/sexual/physical abuse).

Trauma-Informed Care

Clinicians working with adolescents must keep a high index of suspicion for the presence of past or ongoing ACEs in the lives of their patients (see Chapter 15). Although formal universal screening for children, adolescents, youth, and their caregiving adults has been encouraged as a way of identifying and providing extra support for those impacted by multiple ACEs or trauma, adolescents may not feel comfortable sharing their difficult past or present. Clinicians must be aware that often difficult behaviors in adolescent patients may be the result of trauma. For example, traumatic experiences might be reflected in the angry response to a diagnosis of a STI, or withdrawal when the clinician asks sensitive questions related to their health circumstances, or by a catastrophic reaction out of proportion to the "long wait" they've had to endure before seeing their doctor. The adolescents' response of "just give me my medicine and let me get out of here NOW!" may reflect their past negative experiences around betrayal and breaking of trust more than perceived inefficiency or incompetence of the clinician. A trauma-informed approach incorporates, first and foremost, an understanding that trauma is common and that it may have impacted anyone a clinician is seeing, regardless of age, gender, race/ethnicity, or socioeconomic class. Trauma-informed care aims to promote a sense of safety, empowerment, and healing for all patients, all of which may be more difficult for traumatized teens than for their peers in the medical setting. The power differential between clinician and patient, requests to take off clothing for exams, and physically or emotionally invasive exams and questions can all make for a difficult experience for those who have experienced serious trauma. Thus creating a sense of safety, empowerment, and healing starts with building rapport, demonstrating empathy and compassion, and respecting adolescents' autonomy. Examples of this approach include the following:

- Introducing oneself calmly and kindly
- Asking about their agenda and concerns for the visit
- Listening to the adolescent patient with genuine interest and curiosity
- Explaining upfront issues of confidentiality and what the visit might look like
- Explaining clearly any sensitive parts of a physical exam and their importance
- Following up on their stated agenda
- Asking patients if what has been discussed makes sense and is okay to them
- Asking if they are okay with discussing some concerns on your agenda as a clinician
- Respecting their requests to stop an interview or exam if or when it becomes particularly uncomfortable for them

It is important to recognize that trauma is not addressed or "solved" in one visit. Therefore clinicians should support adolescents through the long journey of healing that may involve eventual referral to experienced mental health clinicians. Clinicians should not get frustrated that a patient cannot "move on."

The Broader Context of Health Management

Health interventions, in both community and clinical settings, commonly intervene with an individual, either their knowledge, attitudes, and behaviors and/or their body. However, research demonstrates that social, cultural, and economic circumstances are often major determinants of health. Effective interventions consider these external layers of influence. This comprehensive view is particularly important in the care of adolescents.

Consider the infamously ineffective program known as the D.A.R.E. "Just Say No" campaign. This campaign aimed to reduce illicit drug use among adolescents. It focused almost exclusively on increasing adolescents' knowledge about drugs. It used what would be considered scare tactics and taught insufficient refusal skills that amounted to, as the name suggests, just saying no. This campaign failed to consider how peer relationships, familial norms, and access to mental health support factored into a young person's decision to use drugs. As such, the campaign was ineffective in preventing drug use (West & O'Neal, 2004). Another example is when clinicians recommend a thorough diet and exercise program to adolescent patients only to see at their next visit that they didn't adhere to the instructions. Perhaps powerful determinants of health at play were not addressed, such as limited access to grocery stores in the patient's community, limited time to prepare fresh meals due to balancing multiple jobs, or limited access to safe outdoor space to exercise. Educating an individual does not factor in the greater social-ecological environment that influences health behavior. Focus on the individual adolescent is often insufficient to create sustained behavior change.

Recent public health efforts related to tobacco control, by most standards, have been largely successful in changing individual- and population-level behavior. Successful tobacco control efforts target multiple layers of the environment. A multipronged approach inspired by the ecological systems model (Bronfenbrenner & Morris, 2007) introduces many interventions, including changing social norms around smoking, funding free quitlines, increasing taxes, thereby decreasing accessibility of tobacco to adolescents, and creating indoor smoke-free policies. The significant and sustained decreases in smoking prevalence, particularly among adolescents and youth, are attributed to the integration of multiple environmental levels on tobacco control interventions (US Department of Health and Human Services [HHS], 2014).

External forces exert powerful influences on adolescents. These forces include factors such as familial economic stability, education access and quality, health care access and quality, neighborhood and built environment, and social and community support access and quality. These factors may be referred to as social determinants of health (HHS, 2020). The environmental factors are bidirectional: Youth receive feedback from their environment, and they also exert their influence onto the environment. These influences can be both negative and positive, known as risk factors and protective factors, respectively. Some influences are conscious, and some are not. Some are changeable by the individual, and some are not. Health care and related interventions should recognize the role of these external factors in health outcomes. Strategic questions may help patients identify potential solutions to improve their own health in a way that fits *their* reality. This approach has the added benefit of empowering adolescent patients to identify and have ownership of their health.

Engagement of Microsystems and Mesosystems

In the ecological systems model (Bronfenbrenner & Morris, 2007) the microsystem is a direct intervention with the adolescent's immediate environment, including family, school, and neighborhood. The recommended treatment may be reducing potentially harmful risk factors and promoting helpful protective factors. For example, a clinician might give an adolescent with diabetes practical advice to take a postdinner walk in the neighborhood to help manage blood sugar levels. However, the clinician must consider additional levels of the system, such as whether the patient lives in a community where it is physically safe to walk or whether the adolescent has family responsibilities that would take priority, such as providing childcare for younger siblings. The mesosystem represents interactions among microsystems. In this case adolescents may be able to take advantage of support groups and in-school programs or community resources and clubs. Adolescents may be able to leverage their own mesosystem, adding to their sense of control. Training in techniques such as motivational interviewing can be a fast way to elicit tailored solutions for patients and their families (Miller & Rollnick, 2012; MINT, 2020).

Exosystems and Macrosystems

Continuing to use the constructs from the ecological systems model (Bronfenbrenner & Morris, 2007), the exosystem includes settings or events that the individual may not actively participate in but that nonetheless have an impact on the adolescent's health or development. The macrosystem is the larger cultural context and includes socioeconomic status and ethnicity. The US Department of Health and Human Services (2020) defines social determinants of health as "the conditions in the environments where people are born, live, learn, work, play, worship, and age that affect a wide range of health, functioning, and quality-of-life outcomes and risks." The influence of these social determinants of adolescent health is complex and may temper the clinician's adoption of clinical guidelines and practice. Clinicians may have limited influence in the exosystem and macrosystem. However, it is important to stay informed of the social determinants of health faced by adolescents. Education and health interventions should be tailored to patient's reality. A recent example is the dramatic changes of the COVID-19 pandemic. This external factor has had a profound impact on adolescent physical and mental health. In addition, the pandemic has exacerbated health disparities, the "preventable differences in the burden of disease, injury, violence, or opportunities to achieve optimal health that are experienced by socially disadvantaged populations" (CDC, 2008). Disparities in technologies of digital health and learning, mental wellbeing, domestic violence, substance use disorders, and access to telehealth are just some of the known effects currently being studied (Lachman, 2020). Clinicians should consider how pandemic shelter-in-place requirements, online education, limited social interactions, disruption of work experiences, and pressures on parents all might play a role in adolescents' ability or inability to adhere to a treatment plan. Addressing social determinants of health may involve joining advocacy efforts in your local area, nationally, or in your clinical specialty in addition to heightened awareness in the clinic.

Chronosystems

The ecological systems model (Bronfenbrenner & Morris, 2007) also considers how changes over time may influence an individual's development. Consider how the 2008 economic recession in the United States affected an early 20-year-old, recent college graduate (e.g., fewer employment opportunities, higher average student debt) compared to a 13-year-old graduating eighth grade and starting high school (e.g., budget cuts in the school can affect quality of education, family stressors due to economic instability). As clinicians it is important to understand and consider these time-related effects when treating adolescents. In the care of adolescents strategies to understand critical factors in the chronosystems are as follows:

- Review publications annually to learn which illicit substance is most prevalent among adolescents in your area
- Learn what social media apps are popular among adolescents to identify how you might leverage them in your practice
- Consider how national or regional events may influence your adolescent patients

SPECIAL POPULATIONS AND DEVELOPMENTAL CONSIDERATIONS

Adolescent populations share attributes and experiences; however, subpopulations may experience distinctive forces that impact their development and behavior. The construct of intersectionality describes how individuals, here adolescents, may experience multiple adverse experiences. For example, teen parents are at higher risk for having grown up in poverty. Moreover, their children are at increased risk of growing up in poverty; those children are then more likely than the general population to land in the foster or juvenile justice system and end up homeless in adolescence or adulthood.

Adolescent Parents

Birth rates for women aged 15 to 19 years in the United States have been dropping over time. The reasons for the declines seem to be a combination of abstention from sexual activity and increased use of birth control compared to previous eras. However, the pregnancy rate among adolescents remains higher in the United States than in other developed countries. Racial, ethnic, and geographic disparities are prominent.

Adolescents who become pregnant require enhanced medical care during the pregnancy. Moreover, the risk factors that lead to early pregnancy often put adolescents at risk for other health problems, including mental health problems and depression, infections and STIs, violence from intimate partners, and poverty. Health risks specifically associated with teen parenting include poor prenatal care, physical and emotional abuse, STIs during pregnancy, poor nutrition, substance use/abuse during pregnancy, preterm labor, and premature births. Teen pregnancy may disrupt social and educational development (changing/dropping out of schools, losing peer networks, losing parent/family supports). These disruptions lead to loneliness, increasing the possibility of mental health disorders, including postpartum depression (see Chapter 5). The disruption of education may lead to limited employment opportunities, poverty, and homelessness. Thus in many situations the outcomes of teen pregnancy are worse than the outcomes of later pregnancy for both teen parents and their children. Health care for adolescents should include strong social service components, regular mental health screenings, nutritional support, and emotional support.

Adolescents in Foster Care

Teens often enter the foster care because either they or their families are experiencing a crisis. Rates vary widely by state.

Adolescents in foster care are likely to experience more instability in placements than younger children.

Adolescents in foster care often exhibit issues due to being traumatized, and often report ACEs that result in challenges achieving trust with others (see Chapter 15). For foster youth, regular health care is often mandated. Though the intentions of this policy are good, a rapid assessment may not be adequate, and delayed general primary care may result in lack of a medical home. The lack of a medical home coupled with foster youth often moving homes results in disjointed and unstable health care. Mental health issues are often stigmatized among foster youth. High caseloads for social workers make it difficult to establish meaningful and clinically effective health care. Foster youth are often medicated with psychoactive medications; continuation of psychiatric medications often makes it more difficult for permanent placement, especially for adolescents and youth.

Youth who do not achieve reunification with their parents, or adoption or guardianship from foster care before a set age (often 18 years but increased to ≥21 years in some states), are said to have "aged out" of the system. Compared to adolescents who find a permanent home, these aged-out youth are likely to have more negative experiences, such as early pregnancy, homelessness, or dropping out of school. Finally, youth in foster care are more likely than others of the same age to end up in the juvenile justice system, unfortunately making health and life outcomes worse than we see in the general population.

Adolescents and Youth in the Justice System

Adolescents in the justice system have typically also experienced past or ongoing ACEs and trauma in childhood. Other risk factors for landing in the juvenile justice system include poor access to health care after childhood; poor connections to positive adult role models; substance abuse at an early age, even as young as 9 to 11 years old, leading to decreased/delayed cognitive and socioemotional development; and poor access to mental health services. The stigma around mental health issues may lead to underutilization of needed mental health resources, especially for adolescent males who are trying to achieve cultural expectations for masculinity. Youth involved in juvenile justice, to mitigate negative feelings, often engage or attempt to engage in risk behaviors, including risky sexual behavior, escalating substance use/dependence/addiction, violence, and early death. Girls in juvenile justice may have experienced early sexual debut as a consequence of disconnection from caring parental/paternal relationships, which is then associated with higher-risk reproductive health behaviors, increased risk for STIs, early pregnancy, sexual coercion, rape, and trafficking. Youth may "self-medicate" by using alcohol, tobacco, cannabis, and other illicit drugs to deal with anger, depression, anxiety, and posttraumatic stress, further contributing to risks to remain in juvenile justice. Youth may seek and find a community and "family" with other disenfranchised and traumatized youth, including gangs.

Youth from marginalized communities are more likely to be seen as "problems," "delinquent," and "criminal" by law enforcement and are more frequently arrested at younger ages than youth from resourced communities. A cycle begins: racial/ethnic disparities in arrests, detention in juvenile facilities, and rearrest/entrenchment in the justice system leads to worse life and health outcomes, including higher mortality rates for youth from marginalized communities. These youth also typically receive less mental health care that they need to rehabilitate, recover, and return to society as contributing members.

Adolescents who have experienced delinquency or have been involved in the justice system may exhibit developmental delays, learning disabilities, and early manifestations of psychiatric disorders. Fragile X, Kleinfelter, fetal alcohol syndrome, brain injuries from childhood abuse, dyslexia, and other learning disabilities are prevalent among youth involved in the juvenile justice system. Further, youth who have been involved in the justice system often have limited capability and capacity to resist pressure, temptation, encouragement; they become involved in risky, criminal, or violent activities (e.g., robberies, carrying weapons) without full understanding of potential consequences to the victims, themselves, or their families. The youth with developmental disorders often "take the fall" for severe charges (rape, attempted murder, murder) either because they cannot comprehend the magnitude of the situation or because their peer group has inculcated a self-serving code of behavior that encourages one member to not "snitch" on others who actually engaged in the criminal activity. Those charged with severe crimes may spend significantly more time in detention as issues of competency are hashed out between lawyers, forensic psychologists, probation officers, and judges.

Adolescents Who Are Immigrants

Adolescents may show up at the US-Mexico border accompanied by a legal guardian, family members, extended family member, or family friend. Unaccompanied youth might have parents, siblings, or other family members who were left behind in their home country. Regardless, youth may or may not have a copy of their health/immunization records and may or may not have any needed medications with them. Many have physical or emotional trauma prior to leaving their home country (e.g., drug gangs, paramilitary groups), as well as trauma experienced during travel to the United States (e.g., sexual assault/rape, physical abuse, weeks/months with food and housing insecurity). Experiences vary once the adolescents arrive at the United States. Immigrant youth at the border may be detained with varying conditions. They may be connected with advocacy and legal groups that may assist them to find health care, housing, educational, and legal resources. Those able to find family members already in the United States or who land in communities with large immigrant populations may find support and security. Those without family or communities of support may not get connected with housing, educational, or legal services and may end up homeless, engaged in survival behaviors, and/or at risk for involvement in the justice system.

The clinical examination of immigrant youth must be multifaceted. It should include evaluation of nutrition and growth; inventory of traumatic experiences in their home country, including loss of family members, physical/emotional/sexual trauma and/or abuse; possible infections such as tuberculosis, parasites, STIs if appropriate; and vaccine history. Importantly, these youth will require connection to a primary care medical home that will have an ongoing, longitudinal relationship with them: catchup immunizations for all youth lacking vaccinations or lacking official documentation from home countries, longitudinal therapeutic relationships with licensed mental health clinicians to address the difficult circumstances they may have experienced migrating to and living in the United States, and routine adolescent health care.

MENTAL HEALTH IN ADOLESCENCE

Almost 15% of children and adolescents experience a mental disorder (Bruha, Spyridou, Forth, & Ougrin, 2018); nearly half of mental disorders present by age 14 and 75% by age 24 (Kessler, Berglund, Demler, Jin, Merikangas, & Walters, 2005). Pediatricians and other primary care clinicians are oftentimes the entry point for adolescents and their families seeking behavioral health services and treatment. Barriers facing primary care clinicians in assessment and referral include limited training, lack of confidence in treating mental health problems, and unfamiliarity with reimbursement codes for treatment of mental health problems (Heneghan, Garner, Storfer-Isser, Kortepeter, Stein, & Horwitz, 2008).

Parents/caregivers, in general, may not follow up on mental health referrals for their adolescent due to the stigma associated with labeling of children and adolescents with mental illness (Heneghan et al., 2008). For parents of children and adolescents with special needs, additional barriers may include time constraints, the burden of "another appointment," and the emotional weight of an added diagnosis. Cultural differences also play a role in accessing mental health services. In a US study of parents of children ages 2 to 17 (N = 85,637) the odds of receiving mental health service varied based on ethnic and racial backgrounds (Lu, 2017). White children had higher odds of receiving mental health services when compared to Latino and Black children. Low mental health literacy, cultural mistrust of mental health clinicians, lack of culturally competent health care clinicians, and underresourced neighborhoods were important barriers to accessing mental health services.

The ecological systems model (Bronfenbrenner & Morris, 2007) encourages us to consider how the time era affects children's development. The outbreak of COVID-19 has profoundly impacted educational and family systems. The reduction or closure of onsite learning in schools severely reduced access to school services, including school-based mental health services. Parents experienced multiple stressors, including deaths of family members, loss of jobs, and the need to assume new roles as teachers for their children. Parents and teachers might have been unable to buffer their children's stress because of their own stressors, which in turn worsened youth mental health (Courtney, Watson, Battaglia, Mulsant, & Szatmari, 2020). These factors may affect the mental health of adolescents for considerable time after the pandemic subsides.

The most prevalent mental disorder among adolescents is anxiety, followed by mood disorders, including depression (Hawes, 2020).

Anxiety

Anxiety is the most common disorder among adolescents aged 13 to 17 years (Kessler et al., 2012) (see Chapter 51). An anxiety disorder differs from everyday worries in that the symptoms are severe, long lasting, and interfere with the adolescent's ability to function in school, at home, and in the community. Teens with anxiety may experience physical symptoms, such as muscle tension, stomachaches, headaches, pain, or fatigue. An anxiety disorder may have begun early in infancy or childhood but may become more obvious and more pronounced during adolescence. Managing anxiety in adolescence requires counseling or therapy to educate the adolescent about new approaches to potentially worrysome situations. Medication may be required to allow the adolescent to resume everyday functions.

Mood Disorders

Mood disorders are a group of depressive disorders that include disruptive mood dysregulation disorder, major depressive disorder, and persistent depressive disorder (dysthymia) (see Chapter 49). Major depressive disorder is the most severe, disabling, and chronic form of depression. Teen depression is usually characterized by persistent sadness and a loss of motivation to participate in activities. Behavioral changes include sleep disturbances, often difficult to distinguish from the typical altered sleep that occurs in adolescence. Other behavioral changes include agitation or restlessness, anger, self-harm such as cutting or burning, and considering suicide. It is associated with negative academic, social, and health outcomes, including recurrence of depression in adulthood, substance use, and increased suicide risk (Lewandowski et al., 2013). As with anxiety, a multimodal approach of therapy and medication may be required for serious cases.

Suicidal Behavior

In 2018 suicide was the second leading cause of death among children ages 10 to 14 and youth ages 15 to 24 (National Institute of Mental Health, n.d.). Research from the CDC's 2019 Youth Risk Behavior Survey indicates that 18.8% of high school students reported suicidal ideation. Additionally, prevalence of suicidal ideation was highest among students who identified as gay, lesbian, or bisexual (46.8%); female (24.1%); and White (19.1%) (Ivey-Stephenson, 2020). Suicidal ideation is not exclusive to middle and high school-aged youth. A research study of children (n = 11,814) aged 9 to 10 years found that children as young as age 9 had suicidal thoughts (DeVille et al., 2020).

Risk factors for suicide include a previous suicide attempt. The CDC's 2019 Youth Risk Behavior Survey indicated that 8.9% reported prior suicide attempt (Ivey-Stephenson, 2020). Also, prevalence of suicide attempts was highest among students who identified as gay, lesbian, or bisexual (23.4%); Black (11.8%); and female (11%). Additionally, data from the National Longitudinal Survey of Adolescent Health (Add

Health) found that youth who have lost a friend to suicide are themselves at increased risk for suicidal ideation and attempts, and higher rates of depression during the first year after the loss (Feigelman & Gorman, 2008). This is significant to note given the importance of peers among adolescents.

Other risk factors for suicide include childhood trauma (e.g., physical, sexual, and emotional abuse), being in the child welfare system, bullying (either as a victim or perpetrator), experiencing a stressful event (e.g., death of peer or parent), access to lethal means of suicide (e.g., guns, medications), and feelings of hopelessness and loss of control (Substance Abuse and Mental Health Services Administration, 2020). Family-level risk factors include family history of depression and suicidal behavior, underresourced households, family breakup, and substance use disorders (Bilsen, 2018). Pediatric and adolescent health care can play a major role in prevention, identification and early treatment for adolescents at risk for suicide (see Chapter 50).

CONCLUSIONS

The Healthy People 2023 (http://www.healthypeople.gov) argued for a four-pronged approach to reducing adolescent and young adult morbidity and mortality, including (1) increasing quality and years of life, (2) eliminating health disparities, (3) creating health-promoting environments, and (4) promoting health across the lifespan. The National Research Council (NRC) and the Institute of Medicine report, Adolescent Health Services: Missing Opportunities (2009), made the point that despite the importance of establishing healthy behaviors during adolescence/young adulthood and the impact that prevention and intervention efforts can have on health, there is a lack of programs and services that target adolescents and young adults. This inadequacy is particularly problematic because individuals missing out on opportunities for intervention during this adolescent period are at high risk for difficulties as they transition to emerging adulthood (see Chapter 10). Healthy People 2023 has as one of its objectives to "increase the proportion of children with mental health problems who get treatment" from 73% to 83% (Healthy People 2030, 2020). This goal may be difficult to achieve. The COVID-19 pandemic has amplified anxiety levels among adolescents (Sahoo & Biswal, 2020). As more research emerges from the mental health impacts of COVID-19, mental health disorders among children and adolescents continue to worsen without concomitant increases in resources and services. Primary care clinicians may have to become supports for families and adolescents while awaiting increased availability of mental health professionals. It has become increasingly important for clinicians to be vigilant when it comes to early identification and referral to treatment of mental disorders for adolescents. Most of the research that currently exists on this age period focuses on factors that lead to risky behavior. We also need to study factors that promote healthy behavior in adolescents so we can be informed about what to recommend in counseling and therapy. Addressing the complex and often life-threatening interactions among biopsychosocial changes of adolescence demands that we break down traditional institutional and academic boundaries within health care to create robust coalitions and collaborations dedicated to the welfare of adolescents and youth.

REFERENCES

Anderson, M., & Jiang, J. (2018). Teens, social media & technology 2018. *Pew Research Center, 31*(2018), 1673–1689.

Bilsen, J. (2018). Suicide and youth: Risk factors. *Frontiers in Psychiatry, 9*. https://doi.org/10.3389/fpsyt.2018.00540

Bordini, B., & Rosenfield, R. L. (2011). Normal pubertal development: Part II: Clinical aspects of puberty. *Pediatrics in Review, 32*(7), 281–292. https://doi.org/10.1542/pir.32-7-281

Bronfenbrenner, U., & Morris, P. A. (2007). The bioecological model of human development. *Handbook of Child Psychology* (Vol. 1).

Bruha, L., Spyridou, V., Forth, G., & Ougrin, D. (2018). Global child and adolescent mental health: Challenges and advances. *London Journal of Primary Care, 10*(4), 108–109. https://doi.org/10.1080/17571472.2018.1484332

Casey, B. J., Giedd, J. N., & Thomas, K. M. (2000). Structural and functional brain development and its relation to cognitive development. *Biological Psychology, 54*(1–3), 241–257.

Casey, B. J., Jones, R. M., & Hare, T. A. (2008). The adolescent brain. *Annals of the New York Academy of Sciences, 1124*(1), 111–126. https://doi.org/10.1196/annals.1440.010

Centers for Disease Control and Prevention. (2008). *Community health and program services (CHAPS): Health disparities among racial/ethnic populations*. US Department of Health and Human Services.

Centers for Disease Control and Prevention. (2019). *Youth risk behavior surveillance system (YRBSS)*. CDC.

Courtney, D., Watson, P., Battaglia, M., Mulsant, B. H., & Szatmari, P. (2020). COVID-19 impacts on child and youth anxiety and depression: Challenges and opportunities. *The Canadian Journal of Psychiatry, 65*(10), 688–691. https://doi.org/10.1177/0706743720935646

Crenshaw, K. (1989). Demarginalizing the intersection of race and sex: A black feminist critique of antidiscrimination doctrine, feminist theory and antiracist politics. *University of Chicago Legal Forum, 1989*(1), 31.

DeVille, D. C., Whalen, D., Breslin, F. J., Morris, A. S., Khalsa, S. S., Paulus, M. P., & Barch, D. M. (2020). Prevalence and family-related factors associated with suicidal ideation, suicide attempts, and self-injury in children aged 9 to 10 years. *JAMA Network Open, 3*(2), e1920956. https://doi.org/10.1001/jamanetworkopen.2019.20956

Engel, G. L. (1977). The need for a new medical model: A challenge for biomedicine. *Science, 196*(4286), 129–136.

Feigelman, W., & Gorman, B. S. (2008). Assessing the effects of peer suicide on youth suicide. *Suicide and Life-Threatening Behavior, 38*(2), 181–194. https://doi.org/10.1521/suli.2008.38.2.181

Gogtay, N., Giedd, J. N., Lusk, L., Hayashi, K. M., Greenstein, D., Vaituzis, A. C., . . . Toga, A. W. (2004). Dynamic mapping of human cortical development during childhood through early adulthood. *Proceedings of the National Academy of Sciences, 101*(21), 8174–8179.

Hagan, J. F., Shaw, J. S., & Duncan, P. M. (2007). *Bright futures: Guidelines for health supervision of infants, children, and adolescents*. American Academy of Pediatrics.

Hawes, D. J. (2020). Diagnosis of adolescent mental health disorders. In *The encyclopedia of child and adolescent development* (pp. 1–11). American Cancer Society. https://doi.org/10.1002/9781119171492.wecad334

Healthy People 2030. (2020). *Increase the proportion of children with mental health problems who get treatment—MHMD-03.* https://health.gov/healthypeople/objectives-and-data/browse-objectives/mental-health-and-mental-disorders/increase-proportion-children-mental-health-problems-who-get-treatment-mhmd-03

Heneghan, A., Garner, A. S., Storfer-Isser, A., Kortepeter, K., Stein, R. E. K., & Horwitz, S. M. (2008). Pediatricians' role in providing mental health care for children and adolescents: Do pediatricians and child and adolescent psychiatrists agree? *Journal of Developmental & Behavioral Pediatrics, 29*(4), 262–269. https://doi.org/10.1097/DBP.0b013e31817dbd97

Ivey-Stephenson, A. Z. (2020). Suicidal ideation and behaviors among high school students—Youth Risk Behavior Survey, United States, 2019. *MMWR Supplements, 69.* https://doi.org/10.15585/mmwr.su6901a6

Joffe, A., & Blythe, M. J. (2003). *Handbook of adolescent medicine: State of the art reviews 14/2.* Hanley & Belfus.

Karim, F., Oyewande, A. A., Abdalla, L. F., Ehsanullah, R. C., & Khan, S. (2020). Social media use and its connection to mental health: A systematic review. *Cureus, 12*(6).

Kessler, R. C., Avenevoli, S., Costello, E. J., Georgiades, K., Green, J. G., Gruber, M. J., . . . Merikangas, K. R. (2012). Prevalence, persistence, and sociodemographic correlates of DSM-IV disorders in the National Comorbidity Survey Replication Adolescent Supplement. *Archives of General Psychiatry, 69*(4), 372–380. https://doi.org/10.1001/archgenpsychiatry.2011.160

Kessler, R. C., Berglund, P., Demler, O., Jin, R., Merikangas, K. R., & Walters, E. E. (2005). Lifetime prevalence and age-of-onset distributions of DSM-IV disorders in the National Comorbidity Survey Replication. *Archives of General Psychiatry, 62*(6), 593–602. https://doi.org/10.1001/archpsyc.62.6.593

Lachman, P. (2020). Where to make a difference: Research and the social determinants in pediatrics and child health in the COVID-19 era. *Pediatric Research*, 1–4.

Lewandowski, R. E., Acri, M. C., Hoagwood, K. E., Olfson, M., Clarke, G., Gardner, W., . . . Horwitz, S. M. (2013). Evidence for the management of adolescent depression. *Pediatrics, 132*(4), e996–e1009. https://doi.org/10.1542/peds.2013-0600

Lu, W. (2017). Child and adolescent mental disorders and health care disparities: Results from the National Survey of Children's Health, 2011–2012. *Journal of Health Care for the Poor and Underserved, 28*(3), 988–1011. https://doi.org/10.1353/hpu.2017.0092

Miller, L., & Campo, J. V. (2021). Depression in adolescents. *New England Journal of Medicine, 385*(5), 445–449.

Miller, W. R., & Rollnick, S. (2012). *Motivational interviewing: Helping people change.* Guilford Press.

MINT. (2020). *Motivational interviewing network of trainers (MINT).* https://motivationalinterviewing.org/

Murphey, D., Bandy, T., Schmitz, H., & Moore, K. A. (2013). Caring adults: Important for positive well-being. *Child Trends, 7.*

National Institute of Mental Health. (n.d.). Suicide. https://www.nimh.nih.gov/health/statistics/suicide#part_154968

Sahoo, H., & Biswal, R. K. (2020). *Impact of Covid 19 on mental health: Whether India is prepared to handle the crisis?* https://mpra.ub.uni-muenchen.de/100765/

Steinberg, L., Graham, S., O'Brien, L., Woolard, J., Cauffman, E., & Banich, M. (2009). Age differences in future orientation and delay discounting. *Child Development, 80*(1), 28–44.

Stewart, J. L., Spivey, L. A., Widman, L., Choukas-Bradley, S., & Prinstein, M. J. (2019). Developmental patterns of sexual identity, romantic attraction, and sexual behavior among adolescents over three years. *Journal of Adolescence, 77*, 90–97.

Substance Abuse and Mental Health Services Administration (SAMHSA). (2020). Treatment for suicidal ideation, self-harm, and suicide attempts among youth (pp. 64). *SAMHSA Publication, PEP20-06-01-002.*

Tanner, J. M. (1962). *Growth at adolescence* (2nd ed.). Thomas.

Tervalon, M., & Murray-Garcia, J. (1998). Cultural humility versus cultural competence: A critical distinction in defining physician training outcomes in multicultural education. *Journal of Health Care for the Poor and Underserved, 9*(2), 117–125.

US Census Bureau. (2018). *Older people projected to outnumber children.* https://www.census.gov/newsroom/press-releases/2018/cb18-41-population-projections.html

US Department of Health and Human Services. (2014). *The health consequences of smoking—50 years of progress: A report of the Surgeon General.* US Department of Health and Human Services, Centers for Disease Control and Prevention.

US Department of Health and Human Services. (2020). *Social determinants of health—Healthy People 2030.* https://health.gov/healthypeople/objectives-and-data/social-determinants-health

Valdez, P. (2020). What can I do? A call for pediatric providers to engage in antiracism and social justice for the health of their patients. *Journal of Developmental and Behavioral Pediatrics: JDBP, 41*(7), 504–505. https://doi.org/10.1097/DBP.0000000000000853

West, S. L., & O'Neal, K. K. (2004). Project DARE outcome effectiveness revisited. *American Journal of Public Health, 94*(6), 1027–1029.

World Health Organization. (n.d.). *Adolescent health.* https://www.who.int/westernpacific/health-topics/adolescent-health

10

Transition to Adulthood

Kimberly Burkhart, Marie A. Clark, Courtney E. Batt, and Nancy J. Roizen

For additional material related to the content of this chapter, please see Chapters 9 and 105.

> **VIGNETTE**
>
> Evelyn is a 17-year-old girl with attention-deficit/hyperactivity disorder (ADHD) who is beginning her senior and final year of high school. She is experiencing a significant amount of stress as she thinks about all the decisions that she must make this year. Her parents would like her to attend college. She has several friends who are applying to college and a few friends who plan to enter the workforce right after high school. Her boyfriend has not yet decided about his plans after high school. She is weighing all this information and is tending to agree that college is a reasonable next step to take. However, she is not sure what she wants to study in college or what career path appeals most to her. She wants to have a purposeful life and meaningful career, though she does not want work to dominate her life in the future. Evelyn recognizes that she remains reliant on her parents in everyday life. She is engaged in several extracurricular activities but has difficulty keeping track of her schedule and all the things she needs for each activity without parental reminders. Evelyn's pediatrician has been treating her ADHD with medication over the past 10 years. Evelyn has not thought about which physician might continue to prescribe her medication as she gets older. She still relies on her parents to arrange for the monthly refills of her prescription.

INTRODUCTION

The developmental stage that spans the years of 16 to 21 has been termed emerging adulthood (Maree & Twigge, 2016). This transition to adulthood, however, especially in the current era, can last well into the late 20 s. The era is marked by exploration, adaptation, increased cognitive control, planning, and decision making. Routes through the transition are highly individual. Pathways of transition to adulthood are characterized by the nature of relationships, especially romantic relationships, including marriage and parenthood; the duration of education; the nature of employment and resulting financial status; and other social engagements. The formation of the young adult is largely influenced by early periods of development; however, social relationships, including family and peer interactions, play a critical role in how young adults develop. Ecological theories also highlight the importance of neighborhood, community, and society for impacting health and development (see Chapter 2).

This chapter focuses on multiple aspects of emerging adulthood. Developmental processes include neurologic, cognitive, and social changes. We describe psychosocial development in terms of several categories of participation from the International Classification of Functioning, Disability and Health (https://www.who.int/standards/classifications/international-classification-of-functioning-disability-and-health): interpersonal or social relationships; major life areas of education and work with their impacts on finances and homeownership; and community, social, and civic life, including religion and political life. Finally, we consider health needs and transition into the adult health care system for physical and mental health.

THE DEVELOPMENTAL PROCESS

Developmental psychological theories vary in their conceptualization of adulthood (see Chapter 3). Psychoanalytic or psychosexual theories, such as Freudian theory, suggest that development occurs through a series of psychosexual stages, ending in the genital stage. The primary developmental task of adulthood is forming a healthy sexual relationship, which is dependent upon the unconscious mind and experiences in childhood. Psychosocial developmental theories, such as Eriksonian stage theory, suggest that success in adulthood is measured to the extent to which intimacy is achieved in comparison to isolation. According to this theory, a strong sense of self must be developed before a successful intimate relationship can be established. If a positive self-concept is not developed, then young adults may experience feelings of loneliness and emotional isolation. Learning theories (see Chapter 4) posit that the environment shapes development to adulthood through conditioning (classical and operant) and social learning. Cognitive developmental theory focuses on the development of mental processes that culminate in abstract logical thinking and are facilitated through biologic changes.

The transition to the adult state in our modern era, regardless of theory, is more complicated and prolonged than ever before. The nuanced approach to studying adulthood is to investigate this transitional phase, known as late adolescence and emerging adulthood, as separate from adulthood. According to Arnett's theory, emerging adulthood consists of identity exploration, changes in romantic partners, and educational and occupational selection. It is defined as a self-focused stage in which there are many opportunities to explore both in terms of education/occupation and in relationships. This exploration can cause the individual stress and anxiety. This new stage in development, the emerging adulthood phase, is associated with delayed entry into the workforce, which often leads to large financial and emotional burden on middle-aged parents (Swanson, 2016).

During this developmental stage in Western cultures, independence is the primary psychosocial task. Family, school, and the job market determine the pathways by which adolescents develop into young adults. The importance of independence varies as a function of cultural and socioeconomic variables. Importantly, social disadvantage and exposure to adverse childhood experiences (ACEs) can negatively affect this transition. Higher levels of wellbeing, satisfaction in life, and self-acceptance are associated with higher levels of autonomy and a more coherent self-structure. Independence for young adults is based on their ability to analyze and adapt to a variety of settings and situations. Research suggests that those who marry, cohabitate, or attend college are more likely to make healthful choices than those who enter the workforce or are single parents (Frech, 2014). Those who are socially disadvantaged, as defined as lack of family support, academic failure, and difficulty holding down a job, display the lowest level of wellbeing (Melendo et al., 2020). Low levels of wellbeing are associated with increased substance use, engagement in risky sexual behavior, and being the victim of gun violence as well as attempted and completed suicide (Centers for Disease Control and Prevention [CDC], 2016). With the opportunity for increased independence comes the challenge of engaging in healthy decision making.

Neurologic Processes

The brain maturation that occurs during the transition from adolescence to young adulthood leads to greater efficiency of neural processing. The limbic system connects to the prefrontal cortex, which coordinates emotional and behavioral regulation. The prefrontal cortex continues to mature. This developmental process allows for greater ability to plan, control impulses, and to be cognitively flexible. Adolescence is a critical period in which the brain is particularly susceptible to stress. When paired with genetic factors and environmental influences, stress can cause disturbance in biologic processes that can create alterations in both mental and physical health functioning. Epidemiologic evidence suggests that adverse early life experiences, such as abuse or neglect, can lead to behavioral changes and psychiatric disturbances in adulthood (Lockart et al., 2018). These changes in functioning are in part due to the constant activation of the hypothalamic-pituitary-adrenal (HPA) axis, which is associated with chronic stress. Positive parenting has been shown to moderate the effect of ACEs, including socioeconomic disadvantage.

Cognitive Processes

Cognitive control and executive function skills continue to develop at this stage and into adulthood. Cognitive control is less influenced by negative emotional influences in young adulthood than at earlier stages, as lateral and ventromedial prefrontal circuits continue to develop. This ongoing development leads to greater cognitive regulation of emotions. Moreover, the cortical regions that support self-representations continue to develop into the third decade of life. Working memory, defined as the ability to hold information in mind for short periods of time in the service of other cognitive tasks, improves in young adulthood as does the temporal foresight, which is critical for planning and decision making. As we see in the opening vignette, Evelyn is having difficulty keeping track of her activities. Improving her skill here would be helpful as she anticipates moving away from her family. Evelyn could use external reminders to help her stay organized and prioritize activities and choices. It is anticipated that as Evelyn's prefrontal cortex continues to develop and executive functioning improves, her brain connectivity and functioning, as well as self-concept (i.e., self-appraisal, independence, and agency), will further develop (Davey et al., 2016).

Social Processes

There is a shift from self-oriented thinking and behavior to prosocial behavior. This shift is needed to be able to control behavior in a context-dependent manner, adapt to new environments, and develop intimate relationships. In addition, social decision-making processes also evolve by the time adulthood is reached when individuals are responsible for their own decisions. However, independence in decision making is highly influenced by environmental factors such as culture.

PSYCHOSOCIAL DEVELOPMENT

Interpersonal and Social Relationships

The transition from late adolescence to adulthood represents a continuation of the developmental tasks launched in adolescence. The main tasks of psychosocial development during adolescence, derived from Erikson's psychosocial stages model, involve changes in a young person's relationships. The changes include achieving independence from parental figures, developing relationships within peer groups, and exploring romantic and sexual relationships. It is during this transition to adulthood that successful individuals form strong friendships and romantic relationships. Erikson's developmental stage characterizes adolescence as the struggle of intimacy versus isolation. The end goal of a successful transition, depending on culture, may include social and financial independence from the family of origin and, possibly, the establishment of one's own family unit.

Family of Origin

The physical transition away from the family home for many used to occur during the period of evolution from adolescence to young adulthood. However, particularly in the current era, this transition may be delayed by social and financial factors. Recent studies have demonstrated that families of older adolescents and young adults are providing increased support for longer periods of time than they had historically. These trends are attributed to increases in the proportion of late adolescents and young adults participating in higher education and the later establishment of full-time employment and marriage. In addition, even when young adults physically move away from the family home, parents or caregiving adults may continue to provide valuable advice and financial support (Wightman et al., 2013).

The varying paths that older adolescents take during the transition to adulthood are largely dependent on their culture, environment, resources, and education. The transition is particularly challenging for young adults who have not experienced a consistently supportive family structure, such as those aging out of foster care; these young adults may be expected to operate totally independent in the world, while many of their peers are still receiving much-needed support from family (Keller et al., 2007). While pregnancy rates among adolescents have been declining, adolescent parents and their children are at higher risk for significant physical and psychosocial complications (Pinzonet al., 2012).

Friends

As adolescents become more comfortable with their own identity, they tend to move away from peer group friendships toward a focus on individual friendships; the peer group values driving individuals in middle adolescence become less important in late adolescence and emerging adulthood. Young adults further the development of individual relationships by establishing intimate relationships, characterized by sharing personal information and emotional closeness, with people they interact with on a regular basis, such as at school, work, or through existing friends. Intimacy increases from high school to college particularly in women's relationships. Men's relationships in late adolescence and early adulthood are more likely to focus on shared activities than are women's relationships; men, as a group, show higher levels of attachment avoidance than emotional closeness. While friendship networks continue to increase throughout the transition from late adolescence to young adulthood, the quality and function of friendships may change, particularly as individuals begin to become partners, cohabitate, and marry. Romantic partners take on supportive roles previously filled by friends (Wrzus et al., 2016).

Romantic/Sexual Relationships

Romantic relationship trajectories are influenced by socioeconomic factors, education, and cultural norms, as well as prior familial and peer group relationships. All these forces contribute to when individuals establish romantic relationships, how long the relationships last, and what are considered acceptable activities within those relationships. One study found that young adults from lower socioeconomic status transition earlier to cohabitating and marriage than young adults from middle- and upper-class groups (Meier & Allen, 2008).

Similar to friendship development, as adolescents transition to adulthood, partners are chosen less often based on the approval of the peer group and more often based on interpersonal characteristics, such as compatibility (Collins, 2003). Increasing amounts of time are spent with romantic partners. Higher levels of wellbeing are seen in individuals within romantic relationships than in individuals without those connections. However, the benefits of romantic relationships are moderated by the quality and satisfaction of the relationship (Gómez-López et al., 2019).

Within health care, as patients become more engaged in romantic and sexual relationships, it is important to address pregnancy planning and prevention, protection from sexually transmitted infections, and issues of consent with all patients in a developmentally appropriate manner (Pinzon et al., 2012). In addition, clinicians should understand the spectrum of sexual orientation (see Chapters 73 and 74) and gender identity (see Chapter 76) to provide appropriate counseling as it pertains to romantic and sexual relationships (Institute of Medicine, 2011).

Marriage and Parenthood

Among all ages, in 2016 half of US adults were married, which is down 9% over the past quarter century, and far below the peak of 72% in 1960 (Parker & Stepler, 2017). In 2016 27.4 years was the median age for a first marriage for women and 29.5 for men, thus most Americans are marrying after the young adult transition period. In 2015 marriage rates were linked to education level; 65% of adults 25 years or older with a 4-year college degree were married compared to 50% of those with no education beyond high school. Marriage rates differed by race and ethnicity; 54% of Whites over age 18 were married compared to 61% of Asians, 46% of Hispanics, and 30% of Blacks. Those of any age who are never married but would like to be married most frequently cite not having found the right person (59%) as the explanation. However, of those ages 18 to 29, 51% cite not being financially stable and 31% cite not being ready to settle down (Parker & Stepler, 2017).

Over the past few decades, births in the United States have been declining, and the vast majority of these births were to women between the ages 20 and 39 years. The percentage of women with children at age 15 to 19 years is 3.1%, at 20 to 24 years is 21.4%, and at 25 to 29 years is 45.8% (Statista Research Department, 2021).

Education

A natural transition point occurs at the end of high school at which the young adult must decide whether to pursue additional education or to join the workforce. Additional educational opportunities may take the form of vocational training or studies at the college or university level. This decision depends on the individual's personal interests, goals, strengths, and abilities of the young adult. It is also influenced by cultural and socioeconomic factors. Peers and family provide important sources of support in this process. In the opening vignette though Evelyn needs to address her plans for education when she completes her senior year, at 18 years of age, she needs to integrate her family's values and preferences, the experiences of her peers, and her romantic partner to make her decision as well.

Emerging adults who have met criteria for special education and have an individualized education plan (IEP) may continue receiving public educational services until the end of the school year in which they turn 22 years old (see Chapter 113). Discussions about transition at age 22 must begin at age 16, as mandated by the Individuals with Disabilities Education Act (IDEA). This discussion should be included as part of the IEP and should be updated each year. During this time, the team, including the individual and family, consider how long the young adult continues public schooling and options for the young adult when schooling is completed.

With changes in US society over the last century, higher education has become key to economic and social success (Baker, 2014). The proportion of students pursuing higher education has increased approximately 25% over the last 2 decades (National Center for Educational Statistics [NCES], 2021). At the same time, the cost of higher education has increased, leading to higher levels of student debt. The average student loan debt, after adjusting for inflation, increased from $15,200 in 1989–1990 to $26,300 in 2011–2012 (Woo & Velez, 2017). A significant racial disparity exists in student debt levels; Black students experience higher levels of debt and more difficulty paying it off compared to White peers (Addo et al., 2016).

Students who begin college coursework may not complete a degree program. The NCES (2021) reports that 62% of students who began studies for a bachelor's degree at a 4-year institution in the fall of 2012 completed a degree at the same institution within 6 years. This rate was higher for females (65%) than for males (59%). Lack of degree completion may hinder job prospects for these students. Those who do not complete their degree are more likely to move back in with their parents (a phenomenon known as boomeranging) than those who complete their degree (Houle & Warner, 2017).

Young adults who have learning differences may request accommodations in higher education. Although IDEA does not extend to colleges and universities, Section 504 of the Rehabilitation Act of 1973 and the Americans with Disabilities Act ensure that young adults with disabilities receive appropriate accommodations. The young adult must register as a student with disabilities to receive accommodations, a barrier for some individuals. Accommodations may include support for notetaking, ability to audio-record lectures, provision of a laptop computer, and the ability to take exams in a separate location (US Department of Education, 2011)

Work and Finances

This generation of emerging adults, like Evelyn in the opening vignette, is committed to finding steady jobs and good careers. The nature of the work is often more important than salary. However, they, like Evelyn, consider work as one component of the variety of roles and activities that contribute to their lives. Thus compared to previous generations, they do not necessarily consider work as their primary focus. Many emerging adults can put off financial independence until they are older. They may mix higher education with full-time work. Similarly, they may return to live in a parental home after a period of residential independence. A study of 25- to 26-year-olds in a longitudinal study of youth development reported the prevalence of the role configurations listed in Table 10.1 (Eliason et al., 2015).

Finances

Major developmental milestones in emerging adulthood for individuals 18 to 28 years old include financial independence. Four patterns of financial attributes and behaviors of emerging adults in the United States are listed in Table 10.2. Individuals who are financially precarious lack financial socialization opportunities, have lower access to banking services, have the poorest actual and perceived financial literacy, and have high usage of alternative financial services, such as payday lending. The majority of those in this category have a low income, are male, and non-White. By contrast, individuals who are financially stable are moderate to high in all the same indicators. Married participants were more likely than unmarried young adults to be in the financially striving or at-risk groups. Participants with a bachelor's or higher degree were more likely to be in the financially stable group (Sinha et al., 2018)

Several societal economic trends have complicated the goal of financial independence. Table 10.3 presents the financial data on consumer units or households. Listed are the two largest consumer units for two young adult age groups: the under 25-year-olds and the 25- to 34-year-olds. Financial data illustrate the issues of poverty in the young adult population who may not have completed their education at less than 25 years of age and the population of 25- to 34-year-olds who are likely to be financially established.

TABLE 10.1 Prevalence of Role Configurations in Individuals Age 25 to 26 Years in the United States

Role	Prevalence
Traditional student	0.24
Stably employed singles	0.22
Working single parent	0.19
Married working parent	0.17
Married working nonparent	0.10

TABLE 10.2 Patterns of Financial Attributes and Behaviors of Emerging Adults in the United States

Financial Status	Prevalence
Precarious	0.32
Financially at risk	0.36
Financially striving	0.10
Financially stable	0.22

TABLE 10.3 Financial Characteristics Comparing Emerging Adults and Adults (Households) Reference Person

Characteristic	<25 Yr	25–34 Yr
Income before taxes	<$15,000	>$100,000
Number consumer units	2,824,401	4,294,191
Income before taxes	$6,261	$148,922
Income after taxes	$6,538	$122,209
Age of reference person	20.6 yr	30.4 yr
Average number in consumer unit	1.3	3.0
Earners in consumer unit	0.8	2.0
Home owner	3%	65%
Renter	97%	35%
College	71%	92%
>1 vehicle owned or leased	42%	94%
Average annual expenditures	$18,018	$90,276
Food	$3,281	$10,921
Housing	$6,000	$30,290
Apparel and services	$947	$3,265
Transportation	$2,304	$14,086
Health care	$515	$5,167
Entertainment	$736	$4,541
Personal care products and services	$267	$1,003
Reading	$33	$95
Education	$3,061	$1,869
Tobacco products and smoking supplies	$115	$250
Miscellaneous	$120	$777
Cash contributions	$107	$1,928
Personal insurance and pensions	$324	$14,979
Sources of Income and Personal Taxes		
Money income before taxes	$6,261	$148,922
Wages and salaries	$3,944	$138,882
Self-employment income	$95	$8,069
Social Security	$63	$481
Interest, dividends, rental income	$36	$701
Public assistance, Supplemental Security Income, SNAP	$550	$33
Unemployment and workers' compensation	$195	$481
Other income	$1,378	$274
Personal taxes (contains some imputed values)	($277)	$26,714

Adapted from US Bureau of Labor Statistics. (2018). *Consumer expenditure survey, 2016–2017.*

Households and Homeownership

Millennials (ages 18–35 in 2016) are the largest living generation but have fewer number of households compared to other generations, including Generation X (ages 36–51). The millennials continue to live under their parents' roof or in a college dorm. Millennial households have a high proportion living in poverty, are racially and ethnically diverse, headed by minorities, and likely to be unmarried. They also dominate the ranks of renters. In addition, about half of cohabiting-couple households are headed by a millennial. They also have surpassed other generations in number of household heads who are single mothers (Fry, 2017).

Community Life

Religious and Spiritual Life

For young adults, involvement in a religious community provides a potential opportunity for identity development. It provides an ideology with a system of beliefs with a social and spiritual context for identity formation. Several trends in religious involvement in the early 21st century are more marked in young adults than in older adults. Reported religious involvement declines from 17-year-olds to 23-year-olds (Hardy et al., 2010). Overall, the proportion of the US population that reports being religious is declining, especially among young adults, and those who do not identify with any organized religion is growing. Of millennials (those ages 18–24), more than one-third are unaffiliated. Within the various religions represented in the United States, those aged 18 to 29 years represent about 17% to 34% (https://www.pewforum.org/religious-landscape-study/age-distribution). Interestingly, interfaith marriages have increased from 19% in 1960 to 39% in 2010.

Political Life and Civic Engagement

Emerging and young adults constitute a larger share of the population than other age cohorts. Table 10.4 describes the proportion of adults in each age group who have taken part in civic or political activities in the past 12 months. Examples of these activities include signing a petition, contributing money to a political cause, attending a rally, and contacting the local government (Smith et al., 2009). Young adults have comparable involvement as older adults.

TABLE 10.4 Proportion of Young Adults Engaged in Civic Engagement and Political Activities in the Last 12 Months

Group	Any Activity	1–2 Activities	3–4 Activities	5+ Activities
Total	63%	34%	16%	13%
Age 18–24	59%	34%	13%	13%
Age 25–34	62%	34%	14%	14%

Data from Smith, A., Schlozman, K.L., Verba, S., & Brady, H. (2009). *The current state of civic engagement in America.* Retrieved from https://www.pewresearch.org/internet/2009/09/01/the-current-state-of-civic-engagement-in.

HEALTH CARE NEEDS AND TRANSITION

Physical Health Care

Health care transition is the process of transition from a pediatric-centered medical practice to an adult-centered medical practice. It is important to note that this transition may not be a one-time event but a long-term process. During the process, patients must become prepared for a new model of care in which they, rather than their parents, are responsible for performing the necessary tasks involved in maintaining health. Many discrete tasks for adolescents and young adults to master within this process include making appointments, learning about medications, refilling prescriptions, and independently providing family and personal medical history. The recommendation is that this process starts at age 12 years and progresses continuously. While the transfer ideally occurs between 18 and 21 years of age, this timing may vary widely based on an individual's health status and on the clinical setting (Lebrun-Harris et al., 2018). In the opening vignette Evelyn's pediatrician should assess her for readiness to transition to adult health care and prepare her by encouraging her incrementally to take on the tasks that are expected of her as an adult managing her own health.

A joint report by the American Academy of Pediatrics, American Academy of Family Physicians, and American College of Physicians supports and describes a process for transitions in health care (American Academy of Pediatrics, American Academy of Family Physicians, and American College of Physicians-American Society of Internal Medicine, 2002). Transfer to adult health care without an appropriate transition process has been associated with negative outcomes such as medication nonadherence and missed medical appointments, both of which may lead to adverse health outcomes and preventable complications (Pai & Ostendorf, 2011). A structured transition results in positive outcomes, including increases in medication adherence and routine screening assessments. Moreover, smooth transitions were associated with improved clinical measures, such as decreases in anxiety scores, hemoglobin A1c levels in patients with diabetes, and in death and graft loss in transplant patients (Gabrielet al., 2017).

Many barriers to medical transition have been identified in various studies, including difficulty leaving familiar providers for new ones, accessing appropriate providers with associated insurance difficulties, and negative perceptions of the adult model of care. The transition process can also be challenging for clinicians. Infrastructure and skills to support transition often do not exist within the pediatric practice. Studies have found that inadequate recognition and addressing of patients' needs on the part of the pediatric clinician is a barrier to successful transition. In addition, while resources may exist to support clinicians through the health care transition, their implementation may seem daunting and time consuming due to lack of specific processes in place to assist clinicians (Gray et al., 2018).

Simplifying the process into six core elements, a process supported through the Got Transition resource center (www.gottransition.org), may make implementation more manageable. These elements include transition and care policy/guide, tracking and monitoring, transition readiness, transition planning, transfer of care, and transfer completion. Providers can access free toolkits to assist them in expanding the availability of resources for adolescents, young adults, and their families in the process of transition from pediatric to adult providers.

Through the transition process, logistical aspects, including insurance coverage and confidentiality, should be addressed as these factors impact the quality of care. Patients and caregivers should be aware of insurance changes and that once a patient turns 18 years old, caregivers may no longer be able to access patient records due to Health Insurance Portability and Accountability Act privacy laws. However, in many states even before a patient turns 18 years old, select topics such as sexual and mental health are confidential (Ford et al., 2004).

Data suggest that the vast majority of adolescents and emerging adults are not receiving appropriate health care transition planning. It is the responsibility of all members of a young adult's care team to ensure that a comprehensive transition plan is in place and discussed with the patient and family.

Mental Health

Mental health needs are high in young adulthood. The four most prevalent mental health disorders in adulthood include ADHD, anxiety disorders, posttraumatic stress disorder, and depressive disorders (Table 10.5). ADHD is more common in males, and internalizing disorders are more common in females. Moreover, based on the National Comorbidity Survey Replication Study, 75% of mental illness present by age 24 (Innocenti & Price, 2005). In this developmental era severe and pervasive mental health disorders, in particular personality disorders and schizophrenia (see Chapter 52), may emerge or be diagnosed.

Studies suggest that those who have experienced poverty in childhood have increased mental health problems in adolescence and adulthood. Higher levels of ACEs are associated with alterations in hormonal balance and immune system functioning. These changes may cause a rewiring of the brain, which in turn may make individuals more susceptible to vulnerabilities and other stressors (Miller et al., 2009). In young adulthood ACEs have been associated with unhealthy behaviors and outcomes, including higher levels of substance use and poor mental health, cigarette use, and obesity (Mersky et al., 2013). Higher levels of ACEs in childhood are associated with higher-risk sexual behaviors in women and an increased risk of sexual victimization during the college years

TABLE 10.5 Prevalence of Mental Health Disorders in Adulthood

Diagnosis	Prevalence		
	Overall	Males	Females
Attention-deficit/hyperactivity disorder	4.4%	5.4%	3.2%
Generalized anxiety disorder	2.7%	1.9%	3.4%
Posttraumatic stress disorder	3.6%	1.8%	5.2%
Major depressive disorder	7.1%	5.3%	8.7%

(Hillis et al., 2001). Exposures to ACEs and trauma, as well as having neurodevelopmental disabilities and mental health disorders, have been associated with increased involvement in the criminal justice system in adulthood. This association is amplified when there has been marginalization and inequality (Hughes et al., 2020).

CONCLUSION

In summary, the period of emerging adulthood is in a state of flux in the modern era. While the developmental processes seem stable, many changes in the nature of education and work have shifted the activities within psychosocial development. Domestic milestones of partnership, marriage, parenthood, education, work, and finances show increasingly diverse pathways and extended timelines. Racial, ethnic, cultural, and socioeconomic demographics contribute to the individual pathways. It is important to remember there are multiple ways to become an adult.

REFERENCES

Addo, F. R., Houle, J. N., & Simon, D. (2016). Young, black, and (still) in the red: Parental wealth, race, and student loan debt. *Race and Social Problems*, *8*(1), 64–76.

American Academy of Pediatrics, American Academy of Family Physicians, & American College of Physicians-American Society of Internal Medicine. (Dec 2002). A consensus statement on health care transitions for young adults with special health care needs. *Pediatrics, 110*(6 Pt 2), 1304–1306. PMID: 12456949.

Baker, D. P. (2014). *The schooled society: The educational transformation of global culture*. Stanford University Press.

Centers for Disease Control and Prevention. (2016). *Fatal and nonfatal injuries reports*. https://www.cdc.gov/injury/wisqars/facts.html.

Collins, W. (2003). More than myth: The developmental significance of romantic relationships during adolescence. *Journal of Research on Adolescence*, *13*(1), 1–24.

Davey, C. G., Pujol, J., & Harrison, B. J. (2016). Mapping the self in the brain's default mode network. *Neuroimage*, *132*, 390–397.

Eliason, S. R., Mortimer, J. T., & Vuolo, M. (2015). The transition to adulthood: Life course structures and subjective perceptions. *Social Psychology Quarterly*, *78*(3), 205–227.

Ford, C., English, A., & Sigman, G. (2004). Confidential health care for adolescents: Position paper of the society for adolescent medicine. *Journal of Adolescent Health*, *35*(2), 160–167.

Frech, A. (2014). Pathways to adulthood and changes in health-promoting behaviors. *Advances in Life Course Research*, *19*, 40–49.

Fry, R. (2017). *5 facts about millennial households*. Pew Research Center. https://www.pewresearch.org/fact-tank/2017/09/06/5-facts-about-millennial-households/.

Gabriel, P., McManus, M., Rogers, K., & White, P. (2017). Outcome evidence for structured pediatric to adult health care transition interventions: A systematic review. *Journal of Pediatrics*, *188*, 263–269. e15. https://doi.org/10.1016/j.jpeds.2017.05.066.

Gómez-López, M., Carmen, V., & Ortega-Ruiz, R. (2019). Well-being and romantic relationships: A systematic review in adolescence and emerging adulthood. *International Journal of Environmental Research and Public Health*, *16*(13), 2415. https://doi.org/10.3390/ijerph16132415.

Gray, W., Megan, N., Schaefer, R., Resmini-Rawlinson, A., & Wagoner, S. T. (2018). Barriers to transition from pediatric to adult care: A systematic review. *Journal of Pediatric Psychology*, *43*(5), 488–502.

Hardy, S. A., Pratt, M. W., Pancer, S. M., Olsen, J. A., & Lawford, H. L. (2010). Community and religious involvement as contests of identity change across late adolescence and emerging adulthood. *International Journal of Behavioral Development*, *35*(2), 125–135.

Hillis, S. D., Anda, R. F., Felitti, V. J., & Marchbanks, P. A. (2001 Sep–Oct). Adverse childhood experiences and sexual risk behaviors in women: A retrospective cohort study. *Family Planning Perspectives, 33*(5), 206–211. PMID: 11589541.

Houle, J. N., & Warner, C. (2017). Into the red and back to the nest? Student debt, college completion, and returning to the parental home among young adults. *Sociology of Education*, *90*(1), 89–108.

Hughes, N., et al. (2020). Health determinants of adolescent criminalisation. *Lancet Child and Adolescent Health*, *4*(2), 151–162. https://doi.org/10.1016/S2352-4642(19)30347-5.

Innocenti, G. M., & Price, D. J. (2005). Exuberance in the development of cortical networks. *Nature Reviews Neuroscience*, *6*(12), 955–965.

Institute of Medicine. (2011). *The health of lesbian, gay, bisexual, and transgender people: Building a foundation for better understanding*. National Academies Press.

Keller, T. E., Cusick, G. R., & Courtney, M. E. (2007). Approaching the transition to adulthood: Distinctive profiles of adolescents aging out of the child welfare system. *Social Service Review*, *81*(3), 453–484.

Lebrun-Harris, L. A., McManus, M. A., Ilango, S. M., Cyr, M., McLellan, S. B., Mann, M. Y., & White, P. H. (2018). Transition planning among US youth with and without special health care needs. *Pediatrics*, *142*(4), e20180194. https://doi.org/10.1542/peds.2018-0194.

Lockart, S., Sawa, A., & Niwa, M. (2018). Developmental trajectories of brain maturation and behavior: Relevance to major mental illnesses. *Journal of Pharmacological Sciences*, *137*, 1–4.

Maree, J. G., & Twigge, A. (2016). Career and self-construction of emerging adults: The value of life designing. *Frontiers in Psychology*, *6*. https://doi.org/10.3389/fpsyg2015.02041.

Meier, A., & Allen, G. (2008). Intimate relationship development during the transition to adulthood: Differences by social class. *New Directions for Child and Adolescent Development*, *119*, 25–39.

Mersky, J. P., Topitzes, J., & Reynolds, A. J. (2013). Impacts of adverse childhood experiences on health, mental health, and substance use in early adulthood: A cohort study of an urban, minority sample in the U.S. *Child Abuse and Neglect*, *37*, 917–925.

Miller, G. E., Chen, E., Fok, A. K., Walker, H., Lim, A., Nicholls, E. F., Cole, S., & Kobor, M. S. (2009). Low early-life social class leaves a biological residue manifested by decreased glucocorticoid and increased proinflammatory signaling. *Proceedings of the National Academy of Sciences*, *106*, 14716–14721.

National Center for Educational Statistics. (2021). *Undergraduate enrollment*. https://nces.ed.gov/programs/coe/indicator_cha.asp.

Pai, A., & Ostendorf, M. (2011). Treatment adherence in adolescents and young adults affected by chronic illness during the health care transition from pediatric to adult health care: A literature review. *Children's Health Care*, *40*(1), 16–33.

Parker, K., & Stepler, R. (2017). *As U.S. marriage rate hovers at 50%, education gap in marital status widens. News in the numbers.* Pew Research Center. https://www.pewresearch.org/fact-tank/2017/09/14/as-us-marriage-rate-hovers-at-50-education-gap-in-marital-status.

Pinzon, J. L., Jones, V. F., Committee on Adolescence, & Committee on Early Childhood. (2012). Care of adolescent parents and their children. *Pediatrics, 130*(6), e1743–1756. https://doi.org/10.1542/peds.2012-2879.

Sinha, G., Tan, K., & Zhan, M. (2018). Patterns of financial attributes and behaviors of emerging adults in the United States. *Children and Youth Services Review, 93*, 178–185.

Smith, A., Schlozman, K. L., Verba, S., & Brady, H. (2009). *The current state of civic engagement in America*. Pew Research Center. https://www.pewresearch.org/internet/2009/09/01/the-current-state-of-civic-engagement-in.

Statista Research Department. (2021). Percentage of childless women in the United States in 2018, by age. https://www.statista.com/statistics/241535/percentage-of-childless-women-in-the-us-by-age/.

Swanson, J. A. (2016). Trends in literature about emerging adulthood: Review of empirical studies. *Emerging Adulthood, 4*(6), 1–12.

US Bureau of Labor Statistics. (2018). *Consumer expenditure survey, 2016–2017*.

US Department of Education. (2011). *Students with disabilities preparing for postsecondary education: Know your rights and responsibilities*. https://www2.ed.gov/about/offices/list/ocr/transition.html.

Wightman, P., Patrick, M., Schoeni, R., & Schulenberg, J. (2013). *Historical trends in parental financial support of young adults*. Population Studies Center Research (Report No. 13-801).

Woo, J., & Velez, E. (2017). *The debt burden of bachelor's degree recipients*. US Department of Education. Stats in Brief. https://nces.ed.gov/pubs2017/2017436.pdf.

Wrzus, C., Zimmermann, J., Mund, M., & Neyer, F. J. (2016). Friendships in young and middle adulthood. In M. Hojjat & A. Moyer (Eds.), *The psychology of friendship* (pp. 21–38). Oxford University Press.

11

End-of-Life, Death, and Bereavement

Michelle R. Brown, Julie Good, and Barbara Sourkes

For additional material related to the content of this chapter, please see Chapters 59 and 63.

VIGNETTE

Emmanuel is a 14-year-old boy born with epidermolysis bullosa (EB), a rare genetic blistering skin disease, who develops acute worsening fatigue, shortness of breath, and severe cachexia with loss of 18% of his body weight. He is diagnosed with heart failure and a large left ventricular thrombus and is admitted to intensive care.

While Emmanuel had attended elementary school every day, when he moved to middle school he developed foot pain that interfered with his ability to ambulate. Three weeks ago, his weight rapidly declined and he "seemed to stop enjoying life." He spent the majority of his time indoors watching movies, whereas previously he liked swimming in the family pool with his siblings and dog.

Emmanuel initially appears bothered by conversations regarding his prognosis. He is vigilant of his parents' reactions to news and often makes comments such as, "I'm okay, mom. Don't worry about me." He apologizes when he is having a tough day. Emmanuel is reticent to express his own feelings; however, he has no history of anxiety and depression nor has he appeared sad during the current admission.

It is unclear if Emmanuel is aware of his prognosis or whether he is downplaying his feelings regarding the disease progression in an attempt to protect his family. He and his parents participate in an online EB listserve, and he has known about other children who have died. The team encourages the parents to engage with Emmanuel about the possibility that he is approaching end of life. His parents share perspectives with Emmanuel about their own mortality and extend the conversation to include him. The team empowers Emmanuel and his parents to express preferences and to listen closely to one another's emotions and concerns. Together, the parents and team offer Emmanuel a choice to relax food and drink restrictions, explaining the potential burdens of this change. They also help him to consider options for life-prolonging interventions and symptom management. The team explores the possibility of returning home, which Emmanuel ultimately declines. He celebrates his 15th birthday in his hospital room. A few days later, his clinical condition rapidly worsens, and he becomes more somnolent. Given diminished quality of life with no pathway to recovery, the parents, supported by the team, decide to discontinue cardiac medications, and Emmanuel dies peacefully in their arms.

APPROACHING END OF LIFE

The process of an individual's death is as unique as the life that precedes it and is influenced by the nature and trajectory of the illness. In this chapter we focus on the death of a child. Approaching end of life may be the result of a predictable worsening of a prolonged illness or a precipitous and unexpected deterioration. Many diseases afford long periods of relative health and life engagement, a recovery to a prior level of functioning, when the threat of death recedes from view (Together for Short Lives, 2018). Physical changes and symptom burden that accompany acute or worsening chronic illness exact a considerable toll on an individual's ability to cope regardless of the life stage.

Children's developmental level shapes both how illness impacts their evolving sense of personal identity and their understanding of death. Infants and toddlers experience death as threatened separation from loved ones. Preschool-aged children generally view death as frightening, although often as temporary and reversible. That being said, children who have experienced or witnessed illness or loss often have a precociously mature understanding of death. Visible markers of illness (e.g., dramatic changes in weight, wheelchair dependence) can lead children to question, "Am I still me?" School-aged children's sense of self is threatened when illness limits their ability to participate in their everyday activities, and fearfulness may accompany their deepening understanding of the finality of death. For adolescents, illness thwarts typical drive toward autonomy as they find themselves increasingly reliant on parents just when they ordinarily would be negotiating their independence. As adolescents become more capable of considering existential issues in a way younger children often cannot, illness also prompts contemplation on the meaning of their life.

As some children and adolescents mourn the loss of attaining future goals, they may also express hope, even when death is imminent. Their hopes may be fairly immediate (e.g., to graduate with their class) or be steeped in the fantasy of an open future (e.g., having children). Families and clinicians can mistake the child's fantasy life for ignorance or denial, sometimes commenting, "Doesn't that child know he is going to die? Someone needs to tell him." While a rigid adherence to magical beliefs for the future may signal fear and avoidance, most children live with ongoing fluctuations in hope, an adaptive process in extraordinary life circumstances.

Sibling relationships are a crucial axis within the family (Muriel et al., 2022). The questions, concerns, and fears of healthy siblings often mirror those of the dying child: All face the threatened losses of a sense of control, identity, and relationships. For siblings who are absent from the hospital setting or shielded from medical updates, lack of information or misinformation may heighten anxiety. A feeling of shame at having a "different" family, anger around diminished attention and nurturance from parents, or being expected to take on responsibilities within the household can further heighten a sibling's distress. Despite such challenges, the bond between the healthy siblings and the ill child is an invaluable reciprocal source of support that is too often overlooked.

For parents facing their child's illness and death, time is not only shortened, but its order is shattered. Typical tasks of parenthood are disrupted and supplanted by the exigencies of medical care. Parents stand on the precipice between what exists in the present and what is yet to come. If parenting other children, they are inevitably torn between the needs of their dying child and those of the siblings who will remain.

Communication

Research has shown that young children often want to know prognostic information, even when the outlook is poor, and parents who share do not regret doing so. Yet, this guideline is not universal. Rather, attention must be paid to the unique characteristics of each child in determining the amount and type of information to disclose (Sisk et al., 2016).

Parents often delay or avoid discussions with their children about the possibility of death. They are unsure of how to initiate such conversations and fear unleashing overwhelming emotion that they feel ill equipped to handle. They may avoid the topic in an attempt to shield their child from the family's grief, or for fear of instilling terrifying thoughts that their child has not yet considered. Some parents worry that discussion of death may impede their child's ability to maintain hope. They may discourage questions from the child (e.g., "You don't need to worry about that") or provide overly optimistic responses (e.g., "You are going to be just fine"). Yet, many children who have lived with the cumulative toll of illness and treatment have acquired an accurate understanding of their impending death long before others discuss it with them. Most basic, parents may be reluctant to discuss death with their child because *they* feel overwhelmed by the reality of the prognosis and are struggling to cope with their own distress. In some instances withholding information may reflect their refusal to accept death as a possible outcome for their child (van der Geest et al., 2015).

Children who sense their parents' discomfort and avoidance often refrain from discussing their illness, prognosis, or emotional response in an effort to shield their parents from additional distress (Sisk et al., 2016). Unfortunately, this mutual pretense can result in increased anxiety for both children and parents as it perpetuates silence and isolation and prevents opportunities to ask questions, express fears, and seek support. Health care providers can help to break down barriers between children and parents by modeling open-ended exploration of goals and values. Box 11.1 presents topics to explore with parents and children.

Culture

How cultural beliefs and values define the roles of children, parents, and extended family in turn shape how death is discussed. The locus of decision making may depend on how collectively family is defined and determine whether the parents defer to one authority figure within the family or to a larger group of extended family (Zahedi, 2011). Collectivist cultures are more likely to support withholding information to protect the child from the perceived harms of disclosure (Rosenberg et al., 2016), such as taking away the child's hope and hastening the dying process (Wiener et al., 2013). Some cultures perceive that open discussions about death deprive children of their sense of security and rob parents of their role

BOX 11.1 Exploring Goals and Values

Understanding illness	What has the medical team told you about your (child's) illness? What is a good or bad day like for you(r child)? How do you prefer to receive medical information? Have you had experience with medical care before or had sick loved ones?
Hopes and fears	What are your biggest hopes and worries? What do you worry the most about happening in the future? What do you think the medical team worries about?
Spiritual context	Do you have spiritual faith or religious beliefs that are important to you? Would you share with me what gives you strength right now?
Cultural context	Are there family rituals or beliefs that are important to you?
Social context	Who do you look to for support? Are there other trusted adults in your child's life who they may confide in—in addition to you? When there are medical decisions to discuss, who do you choose to discuss the options with?

Note: Adapted with permission from Practical Aspects of Palliative Care Communication, by L. Ragdale et al. (Ragdale, October, & Scanlon, 2022). *Interdisciplinary pediatric palliative care.* Oxford University Press.

as protectors. While providers must be attentive to cultural beliefs, presumptions about disclosure of information preferences based on a family's race, ethnicity, or country of origin should be avoided (Cole & Kodish, 2013), as overgeneralizations and misinterpretations can result in families receiving less information than they actually desire (Ilowite et al., 2017).

Religious and spiritual beliefs can be crucial at end of life: from making sense of and ascribing meaning to the experience, to finding and defining hope, to providing guidance in decision making; to giving emotional sustenance at times through the power of rituals (Robinson et al., 2006). Importantly these beliefs may also provide a clear framework for the family's communication with their dying child.

Planning for the End of Life

When the death of a child is anticipated, health care providers can partner with children and their families to understand their immediate concerns, alleviate symptoms, provide clear anticipatory guidance, and explore hope. Hope is multifaceted: Seeming incongruent wishes for a cure or a miracle often coexist with an aspiration to complete a legacy task or to achieve a peaceful death. It can be helpful to explain the dynamic nature of hope, whereby priorities may (or may not) shift from one day to the next. Inviting hope in (e.g., "Tell me what you are worried about now and what you hope for") opens a door to a process whereby children and families can experience an increased sense of control in the direction of their lives. Such conversations also help to eliminate the false dichotomy of a "good" versus "bad" death. This exploration may begin early in the illness trajectory, even when the end of life is not expected for years to come.

Advance care planning enables families to express their goals for the type of care desired at end of life. Although parents have legal decision-making authority, there is increasing belief that children and adolescents should be invited, to the degree they desire, to participate in planning their care (American Academy of Pediatrics, 2000; Hinds et al., 2005). Many adolescents explicitly request the wish to be included (Lyon et al., 2004). Advance care planning tools such as Voicing My Choices (Zadeh et al., 2015) and My Wishes (Aging with Dignity, 2018) use a developmentally appropriate approach to facilitate such conversations. Public initiatives such as The Conversation Project (theconversationproject.org) are also valuable. Even in the absence of a written document, the discussion process fosters collaborative decision making and articulation of a clear treatment plan.

When death is imminent, care shifts toward the optimization of the child's comfort and can be provided in a variety of settings. While the majority of children (~56%) die in the hospital (Carroll et al., 2011), a growing number die in the home (Feudtner et al., 2007). Infrequently, children die in free-standing hospices or long-term care facilities. When the possibility for planning exists, some families choose to remain in (or return to) the hospital for the child's death. Reasons for preferring the hospital include strong relationships with their hospital "family"; inadequate space, resources, and/or limited social supports at home; and specific cultural and/or religious beliefs. Other families want their children to be cared for at home, in familiar surroundings where family and friends can more freely visit. In these instances families are usually supported by home nursing or hospice. Regardless of preference, it is crucial that providers respect the family's choice and reassure them that they can change course at any time. Studies have shown that families' opportunity to plan for the child's death in their preferred location may be a more important variable than the actual location of death; it was associated with parental perceptions of high-quality end-of-life care (Dussel et al., 2009).

As families plan for end of life, many find value in sharing special activities to celebrate the child's life. These may include legacy or memory-making activities (e.g., organizing photographs and videos, creating art or music, handprints). Beyond the shared experience, these activities can facilitate the expression of anticipatory grief that may not otherwise be spoken by children and their families. Psychological and/or spiritual support (e.g., mental health professionals, chaplains, and clergy) can be invaluable during this closing chapter.

DEATH

Death itself may be sudden or gradual, and can be unpredictable in its nature and timing. This uncertainty can be hard for families and practitioners alike and may lead to a sense that "something more" should be done. At this time, the focus is to optimize the child's comfort. Some signs of approaching death can be upsetting to witness, but loved ones should be assured that they are part of a natural process. These may include sleeping more; eating and drinking less or stopping entirely; increasing, slowing, or pauses of respiration (often cyclic); open mouth breathing; wet breath sounds from pooling secretions; loss of bowel and bladder control; cooling and color changes to the child's extremities; and restlessness.

BEREAVEMENT

The impact of the death of a loved one is multilayered. Family identities are challenged, as parents, siblings, and extended family members must redefine their relationship to one another in the absence of the deceased child. If this was an only child, parents are stripped of their role as caregiver and must cope with changes in identity: "Am I still a parent?" Single parents face different stresses as they may feel isolated in their grief. Additional factors invariably affect the grief response, such as history of other losses, birth order of the bereaved child, and the role of extended caregivers. Family members may each respond differently to the death, with no one "right way." While some may grieve openly, others' grief may be less visible. Regardless, bereavement follow-up comprises a crucial part of the continuum of care.

Providers may feel hesitant about contacting a bereaved family, fearing they may remind the family of their loss or incite anger at the outcome. However, families are often comforted by condolence letters from or conversations with practitioners who cared for their child. Providers may consider sharing

BOX 11.2 Loss, Grief, and Bereavement Resources

For Families	
Dougy Center	https://www.dougy.org
Courageous Parents Network	https://courageousparentsnetwork.org
National Alliance for Grieving Children	https://childrengrieve.org
What's Your Grief	https://whatsyourgrief.com
For Schools, Students, and Teachers	
Coalition to Support Grieving Students	https://grievingstudents.org
Supporting Grieving Students: A Handbook for Teachers and Administrators	https://www.stanfordchildrens.org/content-public/pdf/a-handbook-for-teachers-and-administrators.pdf
For Clinical Trainees and Clinicians	
The AAP Resilience in the Face of Grief and Loss Curriculum	https://www.aap.org/en-us/advocacy-and-policy/aap-health-initiatives/hospice-palliative-care/Pages/Resilience-Curriculum.aspx

their sadness, referencing a fond memory, offering that it was a privilege to care for the child, and acknowledging the bereaved person's role in the child's life. Bereavement resources, including online materials and referrals for local support groups or counseling, can be extremely valuable (Box 11.2).

CONCLUSION

The death of a child, as we observed in Emmanuel's case in the opening vignette, is the endpoint of an illness continuum that extends from the child who is seriously ill, to a child who is living under the threat of death, to a child who is dying. Caring for these children and families can result in deeply felt attachment and loss. The importance of self-care in coping with the death of a child, as we observed in Emmanuel's case in the opening vignette, cannot be overestimated. Facets of self-care include seeking the support of colleagues, drawing strength from personal relationships, and finding enjoyment and creativity in interests and activities. Most profoundly, the ability to turn inward and reflect allows for the integration of one's own experience and for the provision of optimal care of children and their families (Sourkes et al., 2022).

REFERENCES

Aging with Dignity. (2018). *My wishes*. www.fivewishes.org.

American Academy of Pediatrics. (2000). Palliative care for children. *Pediatrics*, *106*(2 Pt 1), 351–357.

Carroll, J. M., Wright, J. L., & Frankel, L. R. (2011). Settings of care. In J. Wolfe, P. S. Hinds, & B. M. Sourkes (Eds.), *Textbook of interdisciplinary pediatric palliative care* (pp. 64–73). Elsevier/Saunders.

Cole, C. M., & Kodish, E. (2013). Minors' right to know and therapeutic privilege. *American Medical Association Journal of Ethics*, *15*(8), 638–644. https://doi.org/10.1001/virtualmentor.2013.15.8.ecas1-1308.

Dussel, V., Kreicbergs, U., Hilden, J. M., Watterson, J., Moore, C., Turner, B. G., Weeks, J. C., Wolfe, J. (2009). Looking beyond where children die: Determinants and effects of planning a child's location of death. *Journal of Pain and Symptom Management*, *37*(1), 33–43. https://doi.org/10.1016/j.jpainsymman.2007.12.017.

Feudtner, C., Feinstein, J. A., Satchell, M., Zhao, H., & Kang, T. I. (2007). Shifting place of death among children with complex chronic conditions in the United States, 1989–2003. *JAMA*, *297*(24), 2725–2732. https://doi.org/10.1001/jama.297.24.2725.

Hinds, P. S., Drew, D., Oakes, L. L., Fouladi, M., Spunt, S. L., Church, C., & Furman, W. L. (2005). End-of-life care preferences of pediatric patients with cancer. *Journal of Clinical Oncology*, *23*(36), 9146–9154. https://doi.org/10.1200/JCO.2005.10.538.

Ilowite, M. F., Cronin, A. M., Kang, T. I., & Mack, J. W. (2017). Disparities in prognosis communication among parents of children with. *cancer: The impact of race and ethnicity. Cancer*, *123*(20), 3995–4003. https://doi.org/10.1002/cncr.30960.

Lyon, M. E., McCabe, M. A., Patel, K. M., & D'Angelo, L. J. (2004). What do adolescents want? An exploratory study regarding end-of-life decision-making. *Journal of Adolescent Health*, *35*(6), e521–526. https://doi.org/10.1016/j.jadohealth.2004.02.009. 529.

Muriel, A. C., Rosenberg, A., & Sourkes, B. M. (2022). Children's voices: The experiences of patients and their siblings. In J. Wolfe, P. S. Hinds, & B. M. Sourkes (Eds.), *Interdisciplinary pediatric palliative care*. Oxford University Press.

Ragdale, L., October, T., & Scanlon, C. (2022). Practical aspects of palliative care communication. In J. Wolfe, P. Hinds, & B. Sourkes (Eds.), *Interdisciplinary pediatric palliative care*. Oxford University Press.

Robinson, M. R., Thiel, M. M., Backus, M. M., & Meyer, E. C. (2006). Matters of spirituality at the end of life in the pediatric intensive care unit. *Pediatrics*, *118*(3), e719–729. https://doi.org/10.1542/peds.2005-2298.

Rosenberg, A. R., Wolfe, J., Wiener, L., Lyon, M., & Feudtner, C. (2016). Ethics, emotions, and the skills of talking about progressing disease with terminally ill adolescents: A review. *JAMA Pediatrics*, *170*(12), 1216–1223. https://doi.org/10.1001/jamapediatrics.2016.2142.

Sisk, B. A., Bluebond-Langner, M., Wiener, L., Mack, J., & Wolfe, J. (2016). Prognostic disclosures to children: A historical perspective. *Pediatrics*, *138*(3). https://doi.org/10.1542/peds.2016-1278.

Sourkes, B. M., Liben, S., & Papadatou, D. (2022). Witness to suffering: The clinician experience. In J. Wolfe, P. S. Hinds, & B. M. Sourkes (Eds.), *Interdisciplinary pediatric palliative care*. Oxford University Press.

Together for Short Lives. (2018). *A guide to children's palliative care: Supporting babies, children and young people with life-limiting and life-threatening conditions and their families* (4th ed.). Bristol. www.togetherforshortlives.org.uk.

van der Geest, I. M., van den Heuvel-Eibrink, M. M., van Vliet, L. M., Pluijm, S. M., Streng, I. C., Michiels, E. M., Pieters, R., & Darlington, A. S. (2015). Talking about death with children with incurable cancer: Perspectives from parents. *Journal of Pediatrics*, *167*(6), 1320–1326. https://doi.org/10.1016/j.jpeds.2015.08.066.

Wiener, L., McConnell, D. G., Latella, L., & Ludi, E. (2013). Cultural and religious considerations in pediatric palliative care. *Palliative and Supportive Care*, *11*(1), 47–67. https://doi.org/10.1017/S1478951511001027.

Zadeh, S., Pao, M., & Wiener, L. (2015). Opening end-of-life discussions: How to introduce Voicing My CHOiCES™, an advance care planning guide for adolescents and young adults. *Palliative and Supportive Care*, *13*(3), 591–599. https://doi.org/10.1017/S1478951514000054.

Zahedi, F. (2011). The challenge of truth telling across cultures: A case study. *Journal of Medical Ethics and History of Medicine*, *4*, 11.

12

Understanding Child Development and Behavior in the Context of Family Systems

Jessica Moore, Christina Mulé, and Susan H. McDaniel

For additional material related to the content of this chapter, please see Chapter 10, 13, 81, 97, and 117.

VIGNETTE

The Martin Family

Karen and Scott married in their late 40s, after each ended their first marriages. Both brought biological children to their blended family: Karen's daughters (Emily and Sara) and Scott's sons (Brett and Justin) all were older adolescents when they married. The transition to a blended family was difficult at first. Eventually the family adjusted to the change, settling into roles as stepparents and stepsiblings. Karen and Scott wanted their "own" children and began this journey by foster parenting.

After caring for numerous school-aged children, they were asked to foster a baby boy, Micah, who was born prematurely due to alcohol and substance exposure. Micah arrived at Karen and Scott's home after spending 3 weeks in the neonatal intensive care unit (NICU). He was small, fussy, and had difficulty with feeding and sleeping. Despite these challenges, after months of fostering, Karen and Scott decided to legally adopt Micah.

Micah immediately received early intervention services due to his high risk of developmental delays. Even with these services, Karen and Scott noticed language delays and hyperactive behavior, and developmental testing revealed cognitive delays. Eventually, Micah was diagnosed with fetal alcohol spectrum disorder (FASD), language disorder, attention-deficit/hyperactivity disorder (ADHD), and intellectual disability (ID).

Micah, now 7 years old, continues to experience communication deficits and extreme emotion and behavior regulation challenges. Karen describes Micah as quite volatile when he does not get his way or when requests are made of him. He destroyed property in the home, aggresses toward others (particularly Karen), disrobes, and intentionally urinates/defecates on floors. Karen admits that her limit-setting skills are not strong. Karen frequently relies on Scott when she can no longer manage Micah. Scott tells Karen how better to manage these challenging situations, but she perceives his advice as a criticism of her parenting. Micah's siblings, especially Justin and Sara, often step in to provide respite for Karen and Scott. Recently Emily welcomed her own first child, and has had less involvement in Micah's care. Karen regretfully admits that she wishes that she had never adopted Micah. Karen and Scott began couples therapy to repair their marriage, and a parenting behavioral intervention training program to increase their effectiveness with Micah and decrease the tensions in their family.

INTRODUCTION

The construct of "family" has predictable features. The family itself has a developmental life cycle within which its members grow, it has a structure that defines relationships, it has a culture of its own, as well as the race and ethnicities of its members, and it has a process that organizes the functioning of family relationships. These features exist regardless of whether a family member's development is neurotypical or not and are essential to fully understanding children with developmental and behavioral disabilities. This chapter aims to enhance child health clinicians' understanding of child development and behavior from a family systems perspective with a focus on children with developmental and behavioral disabilities. The first half of the chapter serves as an overview of family systems theory, discusses the role of family in the context of development, and introduces the family life cycle. A case vignette is included to illustrate these family systems concepts. The second half of this chapter describes milestones in a family's life cycle that are unique to developmental and behavioral disabilities. This section includes multiple case vignettes to demonstrate the diversity of families with developmental and behavioral disabilities over time. Each case vignette describes the family with a genogram (Fig. 12.1 provides a key).

Families vary in many other ways, including their biologic connections, cohabitation, legal binds, and demographics. All these features have direct impact on its members, including their children with special needs. Taken broadly, family is a group of people connected and bonded either emotionally, biologically, or legally, usually with long-lasting and meaningful relationships (McDaniel et al., 2005). In the United States today children live in a variety of family situations, including single parent, two-parent, blended, multifamily, and multigenerational family homes. Primary caregivers are parents (adopted or biological), stepparents, grandparents, older siblings, and/or extended family members and close family friends (also known as fictive family). Marital status, cohabitation, racial, gender, and sexual identities vary. Over time, families, have evolved to be more fluid and inclusive in their composition (Brown et al., 2016).

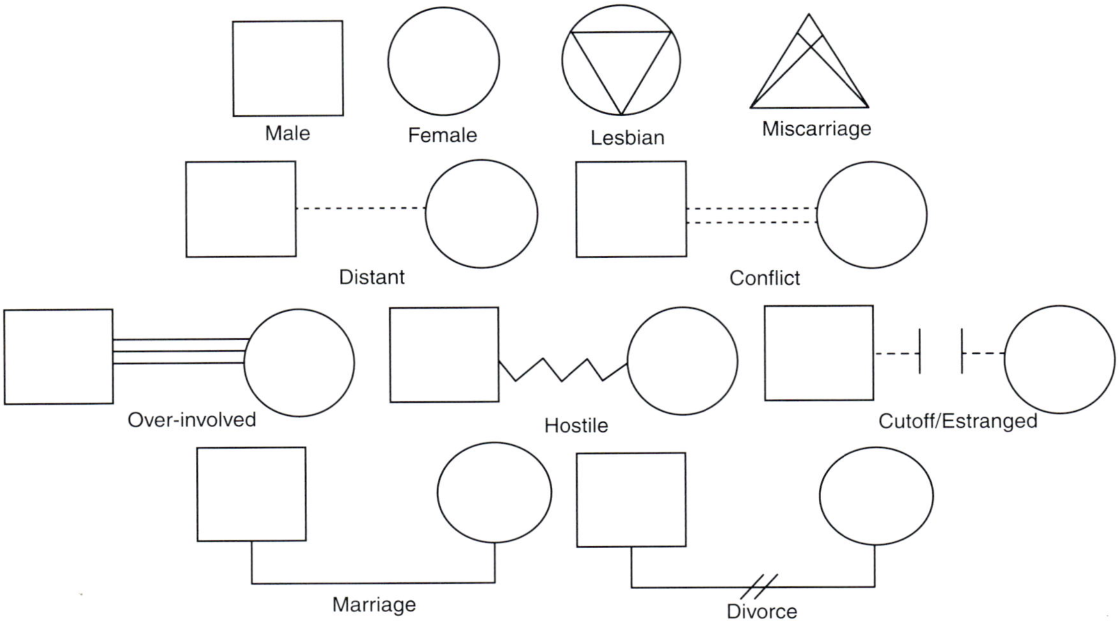

Fig. 12.1 Genogram key. (Adapted from McGoldrick, M., Gerson, R., & Petry, S. [2020]. *Genograms: Assessment and intervention* [4th ed.]. W.W. Norton & Company.)

Family systems theory states that all families are interconnected, intertwined, and dynamic (Goldenberg & Goldenberg, 2012). Instead of viewing a family as individual members who determine their own course, a family systems lens views families as a unit with multiple interacting parts and recursive patterns of behaviors that reinforce functioning (adaptive or not) and create a homeostasis that perpetuates family dynamics until some significant force changes family functioning.

A FAMILY SYSTEMS PERSPECTIVE ON CHILD DEVELOPMENT AND BEHAVIOR

Clinicians who adopt a systemic lens move from thinking of family members as collateral reporters and implementers of treatment recommendations, to partners who understand the child's health as intertwined in family health, behavior, resources, and supports. The Martins (Fig. 12.2) illustrate some of the ways people form a new family. For Emily, Sara, Brett, Justin, and Micah, their sibship evolved as the result of divorce, marriage, and fostering to adoption. At each of these transitions, a family reorganizes to adjust to new roles and responsibilities, and settle into their cohesive family dynamic. When first blending families, Emily and Brett fought over the "oldest sibling" role, exposing Karen and Scott's differences in parenting. With time, tensions settled, and Karen and Scott acclimated to their roles as parent, stepparent, and spouse. When Karen and Scott welcomed Micah as a foster child, Emily, Sara, Brett, and Justin were in high school and beginning the process of "leaving home." Micah's adoption replaced Justin as the "baby" of the family and shifted his role to include childcare responsibilities. Family systems theory recognizes the reality that Micah's development will be influenced by the dynamics that evolved along with his blended family.

ROLE OF THE FAMILY SYSTEM IN DEVELOPMENT

Family systems form a nest from which humans explore their world. According to the US Census Bureau, in 2019 approximately 73,525,000 children lived in family households. Of this group, 70% lived in two-parent homes (biological, stepparent, adoptive parents, and other partners) and 21% with single mothers. Ten percent of children live with at least one grandparent, 80% with siblings, and less than 1% in homes with only nonbiologically related individuals (US Bureau of the Census, 2019). The importance of parents and other primary caregivers in children's development is well documented. Less recognized, however, are the important roles that siblings, grandparents, extended family members, and family of choice also play in health and development (Table 12.1).

Parents/Primary Caregivers

Parental figures (e.g., parents and other primary caregivers) are responsible for providing basic needs to children, including the food, shelter, safety, and protection that are integral for survival and development. Beyond these basic needs, parental figures are the formative base for attachment, emotional support, and emotional wellbeing in a child's life (Bowlby, 1988; Fearon & Belsky, 2016). They model language, social behavior, and emotion regulation in each interaction with their child. The quality and frequency of parent-child interactions stimulate brain development, scaffold new skills, set expectations for behaviors, and shape foundational understandings of social relationships (Byford et al., 2012).

Parental figures are responsible for decisions related to health care and education. They may monitor and promote healthy preschool and school-age peer relationships, and they

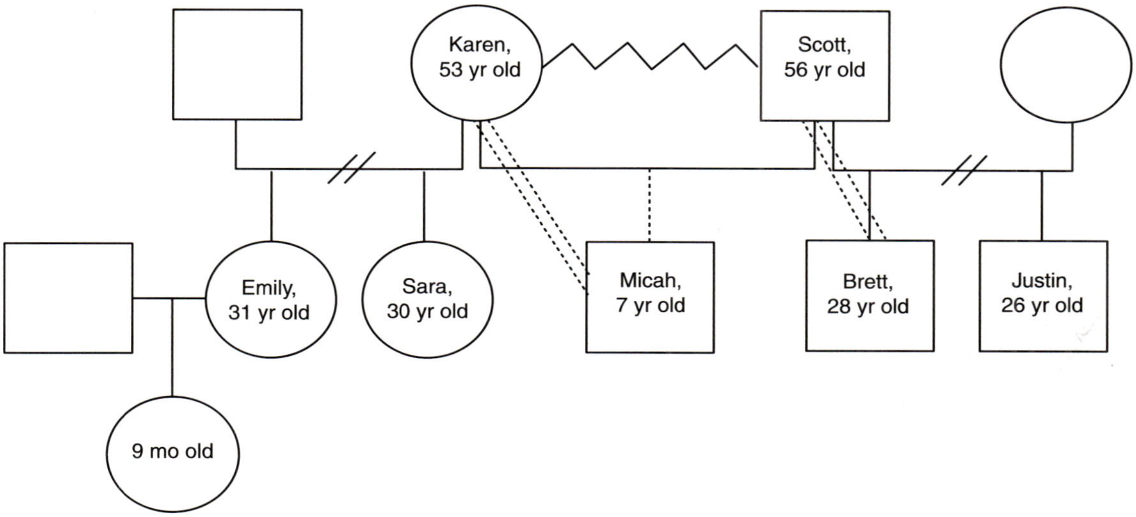

Fig. 12.2 The Martin family genogram.

can provide opportunities for interaction with broader community resources, including connection to religious communities and extracurricular activities. In healthier family systems parent-child relationships create environments that promote the child's successful physical, cognitive, and social/emotional development (Ainsworth et al., 1978; Groh et al., 2014). In less healthy systems parental figures can have lasting maladaptive influences on children's growth (Cyr et al., 2010; Pierce et al., 2020). For Micah, the attention and stimulation, health care access, and enrichment experiences Karen and Scott provided were especially critical when working with his developmental delays.

A parental figure's approach to parenting is determined in part by their own experience as a child (Bailey et al., 2009) and often is delivered in collaboration (or conflict) with another parenting figure (see Chapter 13). The intergenerational transmission of parenting is well documented for both adaptive and harsh parenting practices. When two or more parental figures are involved, their branches of family influence can intertwine, so parenting styles may vary between parents. Parents ideally negotiate these disagreements. When this does not occur, they risk inconsistency, conflict, and confusion for their child. Parental figures receive input, both solicited and unsolicited, from grandparents, extended relatives, and close friends. All approaches are embedded within the context of the family's culture. We return to our first case example to illustrate these points:

Karen and Scott come from different family backgrounds. Scott's parenting borrows from his father's military roots, and he is more controlling and rigid when disciplining his children. Karen's parenting also mirrors her parents' style, leaning toward permissive at times. When they started coparenting, these differences brought moments of conflict and tension and were confusing for their children. Their biggest differences

TABLE 12.1 Family Roles and Child Development, Assuming Healthy Family Relationships

Family Member Role	Contributions to Psychological, Cognitive, Motor, and Social-Emotional Development
Parental figure	• Supplies basic needs and offers a safe environment for exploration and development • Provides emotional support that promotes emotional intelligence, self-confidence, academic development • Plays and provides attention to stimulate physical, language, social, and cognitive growth • Monitoring and behavioral management to ensure safety and shape social behavior
Grandparents	• Offer wisdom, teaching, and family traditions that affect parenting practices and children's socialization • Support (emotional, childcare, and/or financial) can reduce parental stress and create resources for enrichment and opportunity • Relationships with grandchildren can offer emotional support and guidance • Play and attention can similarly simulate physical, language, social and cognitive growth
Siblings	• Play and rivalry stimulates physical development, problem solving, negotiation, emotion regulation, and social skills
Extended relatives and family of choice	• Can offer diverse emotional support, financial, childcare resources

were exposed during sibling conflict. Over time and with communication, Karen and Scott reconciled their parenting differences and established a collaborative approach, even when not seeing eye to eye. This was especially helpful to Justin, as he experimented with risky peers in adolescence and required more monitoring, discipline, and attention.

When parents are under duress, the foundation for their child's development can be compromised, with consequences that can last generations (Deater-Deckard & Panneton, 2017). While parental stress is normative, it can be amplified for parental figures of children with chronic illness or with developmental and behavioral disability. These caregivers can also experience stress related to their own mental or physical illness, problems in romantic relationships, domestic violence, coparenting after divorce, financial strain, discrimination, work stress, or problems in the extended family system. Parental stress can affect epigenetic markers during reproduction, prenatal development, and daily parent-child interactions (Deater-Deckard & Panneton, 2017). Parental figures under considerable stress often have reduced capacity to respond to their child with emotional warmth and can be at higher risk for perpetrating physical or emotional abuse (Chan et al., 2017; Greene et al., 2020). Even without the presence of physical violence, chronic marital discord and/or contentious divorce can create a family dynamic that loses focus on the role/responsibilities of parenting and instead centers on marital conflict and resentment. Children's needs in these situations can become a currency for conflict instead of collaborative parenting. Similar issues arise if other family members have serious, ongoing conflict.

Clinicians who appreciate these family dynamics understand the importance of assessing family functioning as part of their regular care of children. For example, in addition to asking who lives in a child's home, it is important to inquire about the quality of family members' relationships, what stressors and supports a parental figure experiences, and how they approach parenting their child.

Grandparents

Grandparents play dual roles as both grandparent to their grandchild and parent to their adult child in a family. They model and guide parenting; facilitate family connection, traditions, and customs; and, when possible, may offer emotional support, childcare, and financial resources to their children and grandchildren. Extended life span, reduced family size, increased maternal employment, and high costs of childcare have increased the presence and influence of many grandparents on subsequent generations (Dunifin & Bajracharya, 2012; Sadruddin et al., 2019). A grandparent's role differs according to a family's culture, structure, proximity, and socioeconomic needs. In cultures that prioritize extended family, grandparents may be the center for family connection. Grandparents can live within a multigenerational home or be a custodial guardian when the parent is absent. Alternatively, they may live in close proximity or at a long distance. Across the life span, a grandparent's role can evolve from caregiver for young grandchildren to an important confidant or emotional support as grandchildren enter adolescence and adulthood.

Despite these many important roles, only a small body of research is dedicated to grandparenting relative to studies on parenting (Sadruddin et al., 2019). We do know the quality of parent-grandparent relationships often influences grandparent access to and impacts grandchildren and their development. Parental divorce similarly can affect a grandparent's role, depending on custodial relationships and residual family conflict. Sociodemographic factors such as age, race, class, gender, parental education, and socioeconomic status are also strong predictors of grandparents' overall involvement. In particular, grandparent age, gender, and proximity are linked to the quality of the grandparent-child relationship. Broadly, younger, more proximally located, and maternal grandparents tend to have better grandparent- and grandchild-reported relationship quality. Grandparents in Black families more often have a role in discipline and parenting when compared to White families, and Black teens more often identify their grandparent as a significant adult influence. Families with lower income disproportionately depend on grandparents (usually maternal grandmothers) for childcare and/or financial support. Single and divorced mothers more frequently use grandparents for support and informal childcare needs. In addition, grandparents are the most likely surrogates in situations of parental incarceration or incapacity (Dunifin & Bajracharya, 2012).

When parents and grandparents have positive working relationships, consistent parenting practices, and low conflict, together they provide strong parenting practices that promote healthy development for the children (Sadruddin et al., 2019). Grandparents can buffer the negative impact of parental stress by providing emotional support (to their grandchild and/or their adult child), childcare, and (at times) financial assistance. They can also promote cognitive, motor, social, and academic development through their own direct interactions with their grandchildren, or by modeling these skills for their adult children. However, grandparents also can have negative influences on child outcomes if they are frequently critical or harsh. Discord between parents and grandparents can undermine parental authority, add to family stress, and result in conflict and hostility in family life. The variety of factors that influence family dynamics and relationship quality are likely to explain why some studies validate the positive impact of grandparent relationships while others show null or negative results (Dunifin & Bajracharya, 2012; Sadruddin et al., 2019).

The grandparent influence in the Martin family was complicated by the age gap between siblings and the timing of Micah's needs and Emily's child's birth. Although Karen and Emily have a strong positive relationship, Karen and Scott were unable to offer Emily childcare as Micah's needs were too intensive. Emily appreciated Karen's emotional support, although Karen felt guilty witnessing Emily's childcare-related stress because she could not offer the same level of grandparent support as she received from her own mother.

Siblings

Sibling relationships are another family subsystem that is recognized as important yet relatively understudied. Like in the Martin family, modern family structures establish sibling relationships in a myriad of ways. Siblings can be connected genetically, sharing one or both biological parents. Siblings are also bonded through adoption, foster families, parents' new relationships (dating or marriage), and cohabitation. For many, siblings are the most long-standing relationship in a person's life. Navigating sibling interactions offers unique opportunities for social-emotional learning through modeling, play, rivalry, and support. Siblings can be a resource for strength and resilience; however, they can also be a source of stress.

Early sibling literature highlighted the effect of birth order, sibling achievement, temperament, family size, and gender on sibling relationships (McHale et al., 2012). Subsequent work has shifted to understanding the effect of sibling relationships on developmental outcomes. Social learning theory identifies siblings as major contributors to social development and skills (Dunn, 1983). Siblings mimic and shape each other's behavior and gain skills in perspective taking, emotion recognition, and problem solving through everyday play, conflict, rivalry, and negotiation. These social-cognitive skills generalize outside of the family to peer and other social relationships (McHale et al., 2012). Children's identity development and individuation also are affected by their sibling experiences, as each works to find their unique role in the family.

Siblings can alter family dynamics and add significant stress to a family. When a sibling has special needs, family resources can be diluted or unevenly spread, in turn affecting the energy of other family members that is available to the nonimpaired sibling. This phenomenon is part of normal family growth when developmental needs between siblings are in conflict. For example, the birth of a younger sibling inevitably reduces the parents' availability to their older child. Or, an academically gifted older sibling may set an unattainable expectation for younger siblings with average or below-average academic ability. Negative sibling impact can manifest more chronically with significant sibling illness, behavior difficulty, and conflict with parental figures. With stressed parents in dysfunctional situations, siblings can become each other's support and buffer, or they can bully and perpetrate abuse on a vulnerable child in the family. The latter experiences cause distress and, depending on severity, can pose significant safety concerns in the home. Early aggressive dynamics can also generalize outside of family life, promoting subsequent adjustment and behavior disabilities (McHale et al., 2012; Patterson et al., 1984).

In the Martin family the older siblings, Emily and Brett, were close enough in age for their normal rivalry to provide opportunities to practice and learn conflict management skills. Sarah and Justin benefited from navigating their biological parent's shared attention within the blended family. Micah's sibling relationships were different because he was much younger than the other Martin children. As Micah's siblings were involved in his care, they contributed to his cognitive, physical, and social-emotional development. Without siblings close to his age, Micah had less early experience with conflict resolution, sharing, and peerlike play.

Extended Relatives and Family of Choice

In addition to the family relationships described earlier, children also spend time with other extended family members and friends (so-called families of choice). These family members may play a significant role in caregiving and can be a vital resource for emotional or financial support. Having a full understanding of the important people in the family system of a child with developmental and behavioral disabilities will inform and enhance care, regardless of biologic, legal, or traditional bonds. Simply asking children and caregivers, "Who's important in your life?" can unearth important sources of support and information.

FAMILY LIFE CYCLE

The development of a family system does not have an obvious beginning or end; it is simultaneously cyclic and sequential. To pick a starting point, nuclear families in Western cultures often evolve from a romantic union (e.g., marriage). With the birth of children, they become a young family, adjusting to the demands of parenthood. Young families become families with school-aged and then adolescent children, and must navigate the changing developmental needs of their children and the demands of schools, while also dealing with the ongoing redefinition of parental roles, identities, and romantic relationships. As children launch to adulthood, parents may adjust to an "empty nest" for those whose children leave. The family system restarts as these adult children may partner and start another branch in the family. Parents then become grandparents, address questions of retirement, health, and end-of-life concerns. During this time, typical adult children often become involved in parental caretaking to various degrees. The death of a family member, although impactful and sometimes challenging, is an event rather than an ending for a family system.

Considering multiple generations in a family across time, the family system's development includes a combination of individual and family life cycle events occurring at one time (Combrinck-Graham, 1985) (Table 12.2; Fig. 12.3). For example, as an adolescent encounters puberty and tasks of independence and identity formation, the parents may simultaneously experience a midlife period of reevaluating and redefining their identities; at the same time, grandparents may retire, experience illness, and/or reach end-of-life milestones. Layered together, each of these individuals and subgroups interact dynamically within their respective developmental contexts, and the stressors experienced by one developmental task interact with those experienced by others.

The family life spiral model (Combrinck-Graham, 1985) provides a framework for understanding family systems across time. Transitions in family structure, including birth

TABLE 12.2 Family Life Cycle Stages

Life Cycle Stage	Description
Coupling	Courting followed by a commitment to long-term partnership
Childbearing/early childhood years	Transition to parenthood and the birth of a new generation of children
Families with school-age children	Families establish routines and navigate school systems, and children focus on learning and establish peer relationships
Families with adolescents	Children transition through puberty, explore their identities, and families deal with their children's developmental needs for autonomy and independence
Middle adulthood with children "leaving home"	Families reorganize roles and relationships to support independence and the development of new families for their young adult children
Grandparenting and retirement	Parents may become grandparents as they move to retirement from work
Older adulthood and end of life	Families care for and cope with loss of aging adults

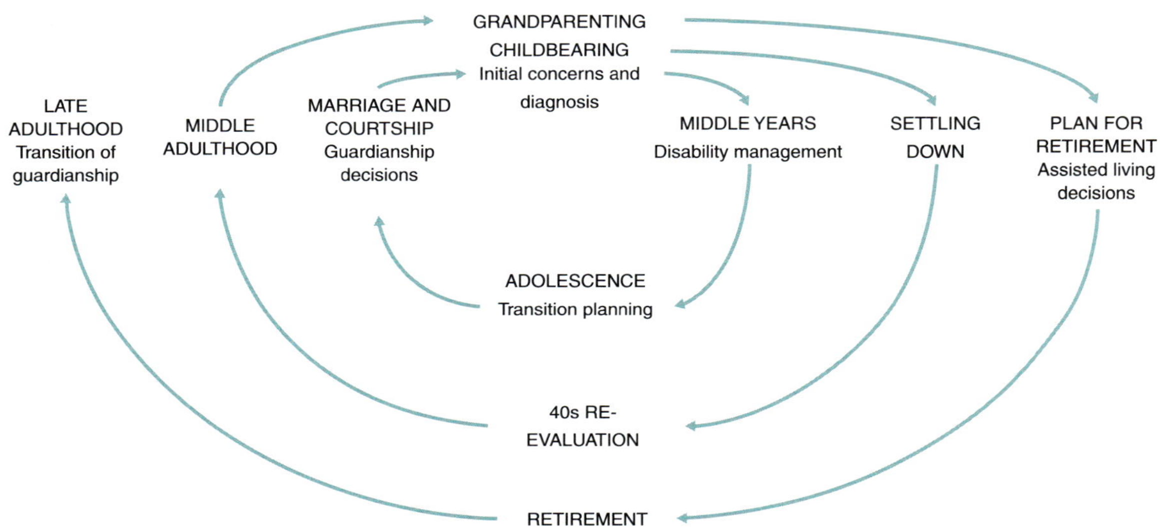

Fig. 12.3 The family life spiral for families with children with developmental and behavioral disabilities. Adapted from Combrinck-Graham, L. (1985). A developmental model for family systems. *Family Practice, 24,* 139–150.

of a new child, weddings, and retirement, are thought of as centripetal periods, when family members come together to redefine, bond, and reorganize around change. This was true for the Martins when Karen and Scott married. Periods when family members distance, reevaluate themselves, or assert independence are described as centrifugal and characterized by more separation between family members. The Martin family experienced a centrifugal phase when the older children launched and left home. Family success during centrifugal times depends on the strength of bonds and organizations made during centripetal times. Families oscillate between centripetal and centrifugal periods throughout their life cycle, and the timing and frequency of these oscillations depend on the developmental spacing and specific needs of family members. With these family concepts in mind, the next section of this chapter applies these concepts to families with children with disabilities. Family systems concepts are applicable to families of all ability statuses.

DEVELOPMENTAL DELAYS AND DISABILITIES IN A FAMILY LIFE CYCLE CONTEXT

Families of children with developmental and behavioral disabilities face transitions and milestones specific to their child's needs within the family's life cycle stage. Fig. 12.3 overlays these milestones onto the family life cycle described earlier. This section reviews these events and offers case examples for illustration. Of note, the model depicted in Fig. 12.3 illustrates the life cycle of a three-generation family spaced about 25 years apart; it can be modified to account for variability in family members' age, marital status, cultural norms, and children.

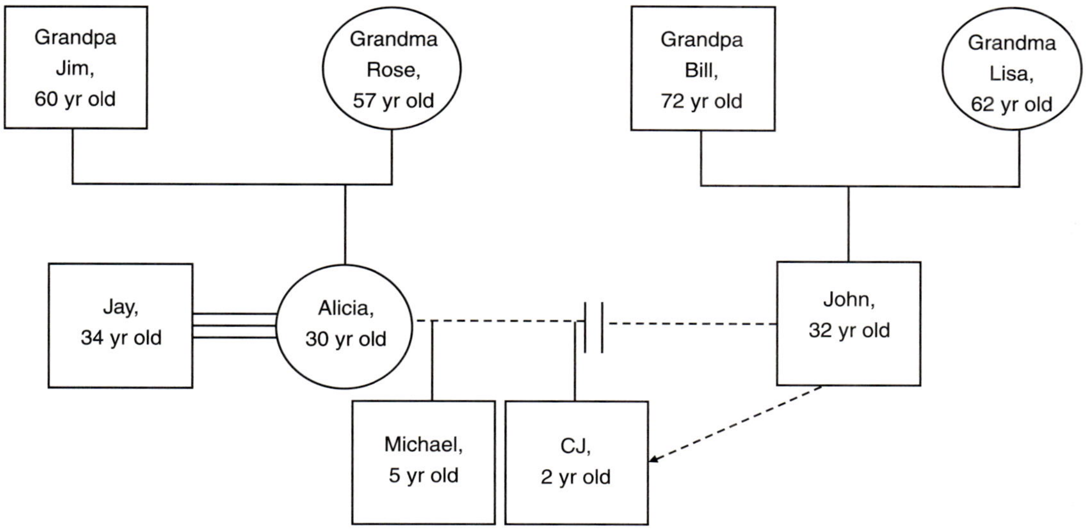

Fig. 12.4 Jackson family genogram.

Initial Concerns and Diagnosis

Identifying initial developmental and/or behavioral concerns and obtaining a diagnosis are a critical starting point for many families who have children with developmental and behavioral disabilities. Often developmental pediatricians or other specialty health care professionals are the first to deliver definitive diagnostic news and education. While parental figures may suspect a developmental disability, the transition from concern to diagnosis can still be challenging. Diagnoses delivered within a systems framework sharpen assessment and can enhance a family's understanding of their child's needs and set the stage for adaptive coping and family organization. Take, for example, the Jackson family (Fig. 12.4):

The Jackson Family

Alicia is a Black single mother to Michael (5 years old) and CJ (2 years old). After separating from the children's father, John, who is estranged, Alicia moved in with her parents, Jim and Rose, who support her in caring for her children while she works as a special educator. Alicia is also close with her older brother, Jay, a surrogate father figure to her boys.

CJ's language development has been slow. Alicia's parents believe that CJ will speak when he is ready. Although they have tried to reassure Alicia, she worries that there is something more significant happening. She also suspects that CJ's paternal grandfather has autism spectrum disorder (ASD). Alicia decided to pursue a developmental evaluation with a specific question of possible ASD.

CJ underwent a full developmental evaluation. While his language development was delayed and he demonstrated attention and behavior difficulties, he demonstrated neither social communication concerns nor the presence of restricted and repetitive behaviors. CJ did not meet diagnostic criteria for ASD; instead, he was diagnosed with a language delay.

Alicia and CJ's developmental-behavioral pediatrician (DBP) worked together to develop a treatment plan that incorporated the family's goals for CJ. CJ was referred to early intervention, which provides in-home and remote speech and language therapy and occupational therapy. Grandpa Jim and Grandma Rose continue to question the diagnoses offered by the developmental evaluation, but have agreed to support Alicia in getting CJ support. While Alicia is at her workplace, Grandma Rose works with the speech-language and occupational therapists in the home.

Early detection and intervention for developmental delay is a widely endorsed goal. During the first 2 years of life, US children see primary care clinicians frequently, with intent to monitor growth and development (Bright Futures/American Academy of Pediatrics, 2020). Still, most developmental screening in primary care relies on caregiver report through clinical interview or screening tools (see Chapter 81); direct observation of developmental milestones is limited to the time and context of well visits. The limited time any child spends with a clinician makes caregivers' information and concerns integral to early detection and connection with services. Family beliefs and cultural practices related to developmental disability, language, health care literacy, and access play a significant role in the initial detection and diagnosis of a disability (Kroening et al., 2016; Marshall et al., 2016). Before bringing a concern to a professional, a caregiver typically consults a family member, close ftriend, or leader in the community. A family's experience and knowledge of disability can equip them to identify divergence from a normative developmental trajectory. However, for families without this experience, or those whose culture or beliefs do not include disability, concerns may be dismissed, minimized through reassurance, and/or stigmatized (Kroening et al., 2016). A family systems approach to disability surveillance includes an assessment of a family's cultural background and baseline understanding of development and disability.

In the case of the Jackson family Alicia has a professional background that helped her understand CJ's language development as delayed and in need of evaluation. Also, Alicia and her children were supported by her parents, and their secure relationship provided emotional support, childcare, and financial resources. With these needs addressed, Alicia had the means and bandwidth to notice, worry about, and act on her concerns for CJ. Alicia's parents hold different views than their daughter on development and, when consulted, provided reassurance that CJ will catch up. Without her background in childhood education, Alicia may have been reassured and less likely to pursue evaluation. Or she may have gone along with her parents' view because of her dependence on them for childcare and financial support.

Following evaluation and initial diagnosis, families typically transition their roles and responsibilities to include disability. There are a range of normative reactions to a new diagnosis, including but not limited to relief, grief, shock, anger, anxiety, and guilt (Seligman & Darling, 2007). It is important to recognize that each family member may experience this transition differently. Asynchrony between family members' responses, if not normalized, can inflate emotions and delay acceptance of a diagnosis.

CJ's grandparents, for example, at first rejected his language delay diagnosis. Worried they might disengage with early intervention and misunderstand CJ's behaviors, the DBP invited CJ's grandparents to a meeting with CJ and his mother to discuss issues about diagnosis and treatment. The clinician listened carefully to the grandparents' concerns and respectfully provided them with education about CJ's strengths and needs. In the end, this family conference resulted in CJ's grandparents accepting his diagnosis and engaging with his support services.

A systemic lens on diagnosis extends beyond symptoms and criteria, considering the impact of family on screening, evaluations, and service engagement. In practice, this requires consistent assessment, monitoring, and follow-up for family knowledge, attitudes, and dynamics toward development, diagnosis, and services. Time invested in family-level assessment can be essential to the efficacy of any intervention to support the child.

Family Management and Organization

Once a diagnosis is established, families must adjust to managing a child's disability across a lifetime. The extent of this adjustment varies widely according to the severity and nature of the disability; however, management of disability typically increases demands on caregiver time and attention. The sequelae of this change can ripple through the family system, with both positive and negative outcomes. Consider the next example (Fig. 12.5):

The Harrington Family

April and Audrey were career-oriented women who wanted to start a family together. They selected a sperm donor, and at age 39, April was able to get pregnant with their first child, Ali, via intrauterine insemination (IUI). When Ali turned 2 years old, April and Audrey were ready to try for a second child. This time, conception was difficult due to further advanced maternal age. IUI resulted in pregnancy and eventual miscarriage. April was told that in vitro fertilization (IVF) might be her only hope of getting pregnant again. Fertility treatment was expensive and emotionally taxing, but they persisted. April eventually became pregnant, and the couple started to share their dreams of who this child would become. They brought a baby boy into the world and named him, Alex.

As Alex grew older, Audrey began to question whether his development was on track. April remarked Audrey was overreacting and that "he just needs time." Eventually, Alex's pediatrician recommended a developmental evaluation. The couple then learned that Alex met criteria for ASD.

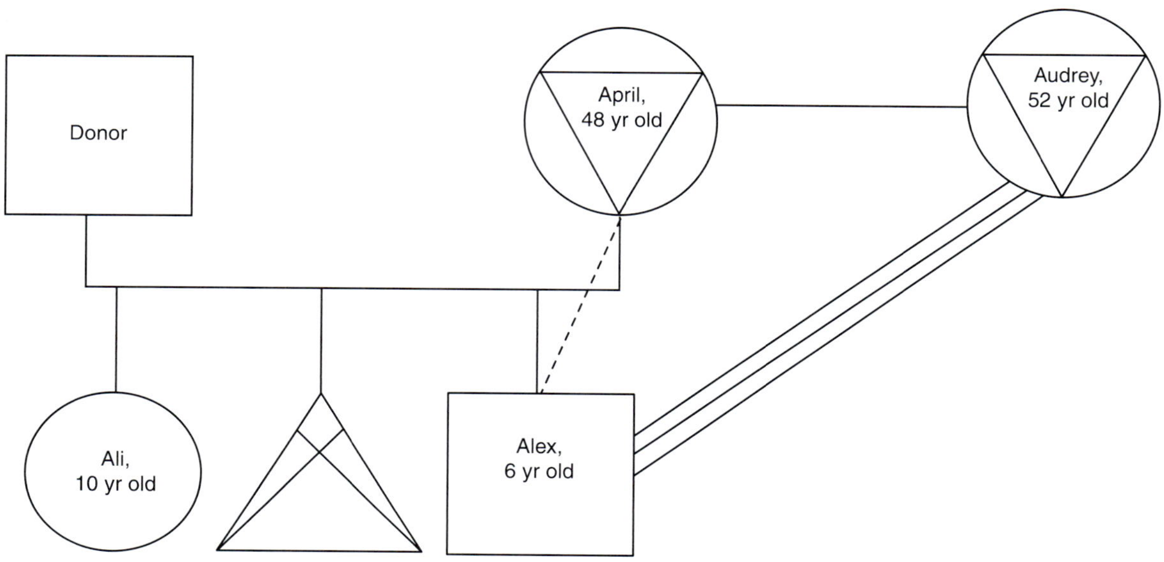

Fig. 12.5 Harrington family genogram.

At 6 years old, Alex was supported by an individualized education plan (IEP), which offered him a separate classroom for children with autism, speech-language therapy, occupational therapy, and physical therapy. Clinically, he worked with a new DBP who focused on psychopharmacologic intervention, as well as a pediatric psychologist who supported the family in multisystemic interventions that focused on Alex, the family, and community systems involved in his care. Finally, at home, Alex received applied behavior analysis for 25 hours/week. Due to the chronicity and severity of his impairment, Alex's family also received respite care, which allowed April and Audrey to spend individual time with Ali. The process of developing a team of professionals was challenging; April and Audrey terminated their relationship with numerous professionals before settling in with people they trust and respect.

Despite the extensive intervention, Alex frequently engaged in vocal and motor stereotypy, which caused April to become dysregulated. Alex's stereotypy and April's dysregulation have resulted in isolation from their extended family and friends. The more her anxiety grew, the more she yelled at Alex to "STOP," which made her feel guilty and wholly ineffective. The more April yelled, the more Audrey felt pulled to intervene. Meanwhile this behavior by her brother made Ali feel that she needs to be a perfect child to make her parents happy. This dynamic resulted in tensions in their marital relationship, with April becoming more distant and Audrey trying to draw her near. Alex's pediatric psychologist referred April and Audrey to a couples therapist who worked with them to strengthen their relationship and diminish the tendency to polarize when under stress.

Like Alex, many children with disabilities need a team-based intervention, including clinicians from multiple areas of medicine and disability services (e.g., pediatricians, medical specialists, psychologists, speech pathologists, occupational therapists, physical therapists, feeding specialists, special educators). Parents must navigate new, complicated systems (social services, special education, and disability services) to establish appropriate care and then regularly and frequently collaborate with a variety of professionals. This task is both daunting and chronic. With each new school year or developmental step, caregivers advocate for services and reorient a new team to their child's needs and goals. Simultaneously, caregivers may encounter more challenging behaviors (much like Alex's vocal stereotypy), adding another layer of stress to the family system (Hayes & Watson, 2013).

For some parents, the caregiving role brings personal growth, purpose, and meaning (Peer & Hillman, 2014). Positive attitudes (e.g., acceptance, viewing disability as a gift), consistent routines, and social support are qualities that can produce resiliency in children and their families (Maul & Singer, 2009). However, as is the case with April and Audrey, these challenges can also result in significant parental stress and burnout. Without intervention and support, caregiver burden can have negative implications for parental mental health, achievement at work, and marital satisfaction (Corcoran et al., 2015).

Parental figures of children with disabilities often experience social isolation resulting from stigma-related friction or distancing from friends and family (Corcoran et al., 2015; Mitter et al., 2019). This is true for April and Audrey, who avoided family gatherings because of Alex's vocal stereotypy. Birthday parties, family events, and larger community functions can be more challenging for children with behavioral and developmental disabilities. Often these events are sensory overloads, disruptive to routine, and require social skill and navigation. Children with more significant behaviors and/or cognitive impairment are more likely to struggle in these scenarios. When family members or friends cannot flex to accommodate disability needs, family tension can increase, and these social functions can become stressors rather than supports. Family and friends who accommodate to disability needs (e.g., hosting a party that offers a quieter space for sensory breaks or taking turns monitoring an impulsive child at a community event) reduce the risk of social isolation for the caregiver and/or the child.

Childcare challenges can also contribute to isolation and parental stress when specialized caregiving is required. For these families, the adolescent next door or an eager relative may not be equipped to safely babysit. Without respite resources, self-care for parental figures can be compromised, increasing the potential of parental stress and burnout. Conflict and tension can ignite when grandparents or extended relatives are unable or unwilling to babysit, especially if the intergenerational family script sets expectations for childcare. Asking parents about their isolation and social support can reveal a need for respite resources that otherwise may not surface. In many communities local agencies and groups sponsor events and activities for families of children with disabilities. These resources connect families who have common lived experience, offering events that are disability friendly.

Siblings are also strongly influenced by how a family manages disability. Often, siblings of youth with developmental disabilities are well adjusted and sometimes demonstrate superior social competence and self-esteem (Mitchell et al., 2016). Ali, for example, is especially empathic to others' needs. These outcomes are variable, however, and depend on temperament of the sibling and the health of the larger family system. In Ali's case her empathy for her parents led her to try to resolve marital conflict between them until they decided to seek couples counseling, taking her out of that unofficial and burdensome role. Difficult behaviors (e.g., aggression, impulsivity, rigidity, stereotypies, intense tantrums) and spillover from unmanaged parental stress can affect sibling behaviors and wellbeing and reduce overall family cohesion (Mitchell et al., 2016).

Transitions, Adulthood, and Family Life Cycle

Transition to adulthood (see Chapter 10) is an especially significant phase in the lifecycle of a family with an older adolescent or young adult with developmental or behavioral disabilities. Between adolescence and adulthood, systems that families worked hard to master, change (sometimes abruptly) and dependable supports dissipate. School services end, medical teams shift, and new challenges emerge related to postsecondary schooling, employment, decision-making support, and independence. Successful connection with adult services requires preparation and time. Although evidence suggests that family and adolescent involvement improve transition outcomes, their input is too often ignored during the planning process (Hetherington et al., 2010; Wong et al., 2020).

Professionals working with transition-age children will find that their families often simultaneously experience other significant life cycle changes: Siblings launch and start new families, parents retire, and families care for aging adults. Family-oriented anticipatory guidance about transition planning benefits from understanding the child and family in the context of their culture and life cycle challenges. Consider the following case illustration (Fig. 12.6):

The Massa Family

Paulina and Vinny came from Italian families and both were health care professionals. The couple felt fortunate to welcome two sets of twins into the world, girls Clara and Beth, and boys Frankie and Tony, each set only 2 years apart. As the twin boys were born, the parents noticed developmental differences between their twin girls who were now 2 years old. Beth did not talk, and she engaged in unusual motor mannerisms. After evaluation, she was diagnosed with ASD. As caregivers in their professional lives, Paulina and Vinny thought "we can handle this" and sought treatment for Beth. Two years went by, and Paulina and Vinny noticed the same developmental characteristics in their boys, and both also were diagnosed with ASD.

Now with three children with ASD, Paulina left her job to care for the children full time. Coming from large Italian families, they felt supported and believed they were equipped to manage their children's care.

As the three children with ASD grew older, the intensity of their needs became more apparent. None of them developed language, and all three were self-injurious and aggressive toward others, even with significant pharmacologic and behavioral interventions. Because Vinny had to work outside of the home, Paulina leaned on Clara to help manage the other children. Paulina felt guilty about this and for neglecting Clara's needs as a teenager. When Clara left for college, her parents wanted her to have time for herself and enjoy being young, but the fatigue of constant caregiving also began to set in.

Although Paulina and Vinny adapted to their children's diagnoses and embraced their roles and responsibilities as caregivers, transitioning the children to adulthood was challenging. They recognized that Beth, Frankie, and Tony would soon age out of school and pediatric services and into adult care systems. At the same time, Clara was launching to adulthood and gaining independence from the family. Vinny and Paulina were reevaluating their lives and looking carefully at their retirement plan. As is true for many families with children with developmental disabilities, the family was entering a centrifugal period of their life cycle at a time when Beth, Frankie, and Tony would need increased attention and care.

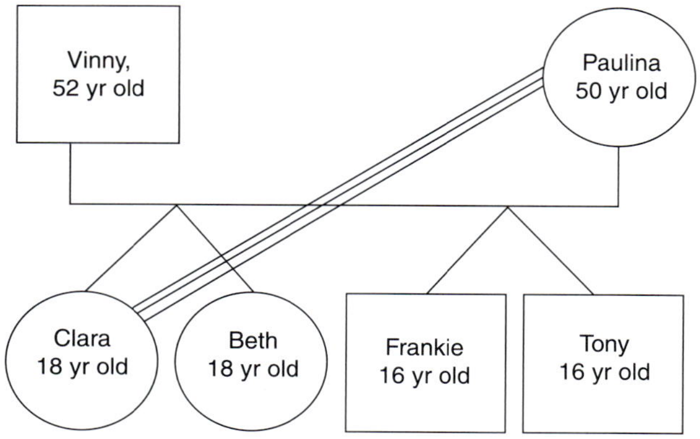

Fig. 12.6 Massa family genogram.

For parental figures, transition planning brings difficult decisions fraught with a myriad of emotions, including excitement, pride, anxiety, guilt, grief, and fear.

Paulina and Vinny, together with their children, had to say goodbye to the school staff who had worked with them for many years and transition from their pediatric specialists to adult primary care. For Paulina, these experiences represented a significant loss, triggering grief and sadness. They were referred to a family therapist to support communication and emotional processing related to their children's transition. Although new to therapy themselves, Vinny and Paulina were receptive to a vetted resource from the trusted professionals who knew their family so well. With this added support, they could more successfully navigate the changes ahead.

Parental figures and adolescents can have different goals for their future and contrasting feelings about their transition. Teens are developmentally primed to prefer separation, autonomy, and independence (Soenens et al., 2017). An adolescent with a developmental disability may plan to move out or attend college away from home, secure a job, or get a license to drive. Parental figures worried about their adolescent may not support these goals and instead set protective and sometimes appropriate limits that inadvertently impede self-determination. Coparents and other family members can disagree about transition choices or have incongruent emotional responses to change. When a parental figure is unsupportive, these emotionally loaded decisions can bring added stress to families, causing marital distress and/or parent-teen conflict (McKenzie et al., 2016). Decisions about long-term care and supportive living are embedded in cultural values, caregiver health, and financial resources.

Supported decision making is a major component of transition planning for families of adults with intellectual, physical, and/or social impairment (see Chapter 117). Posttransition, parental figures, adult children, and siblings are influenced by the quality of transition planning and adult services (Seltzer et al., 2011). Many describe their extended parenting role positively, noting high satisfaction with the opportunity to care for their adult children. However, satisfaction with long-term caregiving can be reduced when adult services are insufficient and leave families to fill service gaps (Samadi et al., 2020).

Long-term parenting also becomes risky for older adults. In comparison to other parents, parent caregivers of adults with disabilities are more likely to have worsening depressive and physical health symptoms starting in their 60s and intensifying through the end of their lives, especially if cohabiting with their adult child with disability (Namkung et al., 2018). If this becomes the case for Vinny and Paulina, Clara may then be asked to take over caregiving for her siblings *and* her aging parents. This may result in a pileup of family life cycle tasks as these caregiving needs could come when Clara is launching her career, having children of her own, and/or a spouse to consider. Successful navigation of these transitions hinges on proactive, frequent, and effective family communication, as well as effective medical, psychological, and social services (Lee et al., 2019). Much like the Massa family, a referral to family therapy may help in this process. One framework well suited for supporting families with developmental disabilities is medical family therapy (McDaniel et al., 2014). Medical family therapy employs a biopsychosocial systems approach to psychotherapy, assuming that health, illness, and relational concerns are all biopsychosocial in nature. Themes of agency (individual efficacy) and communion (meaningful connection between patient and family, and with the medical team) are emphasized, aligning well with the values of self-determination, collaboration, and strength-based care celebrated in the developmental disability community. This framework can provide an opportunity for in-depth communication about difficult topics for the patient, family, and, at times, the health professionals (see Chapter 97 for an overview and examination of family therapy). (For additional reading with this perspective we recommend Allmond et al., 1999; McDaniel et al., 2005, 2014.)

SUPPORTING FAMILIES: A SUMMARY AND CONCLUSION

This chapter encourages clinicians to understand children and their development in the context of their family and the family's developmental lifecycle. Parental figures, grandparents, siblings, extended relatives, and family members of choice play significant roles in development and health. Attention to family context when screening for, evaluating, and tracking development will enhance care. This biopsychosocial systems approach (McDaniel et al., 2005) includes understanding a family's life cycle stage and identifying what transitions and stressors are relevant across generations at a single point in time, and is especially relevant in the assessment and treatment of individuals with developmental and behavioral disabilities.

Family health, which can include remarkable strengths and support as well as stress and conflict, plays a critical role in all children's development. Given this reality, routinely viewing the care of children with developmental and behavioral disabilities through a family systems lens can be very useful. In addition, families often benefit from referral to family therapy, which can be as important to a child's development as speech, occupational, or physical therapy, medication management, and applied behavioral analysis. Effective referrals for all these services start with a systemic understanding of families and their needs.

REFERENCES

Ainsworth, M. D. S., Blehar, M. C., Waters, E., & Wall, S. (1978). *Patterns of attachment*. Lawrence Erlbaum Associates.

Allmond, B. W., Tanner, J. L., & Gofman, H. F. (1999). *The family is the patient: Using family interviews in children's medical care*. Williams & Wilkins.

Bailey, J. A., Hill, K. G., Oesterle, S., & Hawkins, J. D. (2009). Parenting practices and problem behavior across three generations: Monitoring, harsh discipline, and drug use in the intergenerational transmission of externalizing behavior. *Developmental Psychology*, *45*(5), 1214–1226.

Brown, S. L., Stykes, J. B., & Manning, W. D. (2016). Trends in children's family instability, 1995–2010. *Journal of Marriage and Family*, *78*(5), 1173–1183.

Bowlby, J. (1988). *A secure base: Clinical applications of attachment theory*. Brunner-Routledge.

Bright Futures/American Academy of Pediatrics. (2020). *Recommendations for preventative pediatric health care*. American Academy of Pediatrics. https://downloads.aap.org/AAP/PDF/periodicity_schedule.pdf

Byford, M., Kuh, D., & Richards, M. (2012). Parenting practices and intergenerational associations in cognitive ability. *International Journal of Epidemiology*, *41*, 263–272.

Chan, J. C., Nugent, B. M., & Bale, T. L. (2017). Parental advisory: Maternal and paternal stress can impact offspring neurodevelopment. *Biological Psychiatry*, *83*, 886–894.

Combrinck-Graham, L. (1985). A developmental model for family systems. *Family Practice*, *24*, 139–150.

Corcoran, J., Berry, A., & Hill, S. (2015). The lived experience of US parents of children with autism spectrum disorders: A systematic review and meta-synthesis. *Journal of Intellectual Disabilities*, *19*, 356–366.

Cyr, C., Euser, E. M., Bakermans-Kranenburg, M. J., & Van IJzendoorn, M. H. (2010). Attachment security and disorganization in maltreating and high-risk families: A series of meta-analyses. *Development and Psychopathology*, *22*, 87–108.

Deater-Deckard, K., & Panneton, R. (2017). Unearthing the developmental and intergenerational dynamics of stress in parent and child functioning. In K. Deater-Deckard & R. Pannton (Eds.), *Parental stress and early child development*. Springer.

Dunifin, R., & Bajracharya, A. (2012). The role of grandparents in the lives of youth. *Journal on Family Issues*, *33*, 1168–1194.

Dunn, J. (1983). Sibling relationships in early childhood. *Child Development*, *54*(4), 787–811.

Fearon, R. P., & Belsky, J. (2016). Precursors of attachment security. In J. Cassidy & P. R. Shaver (Eds.), *Handbook of attachment: Theory, research, and clinical applications* (pp. 291–313). Guilford Press.

Greene, C. A., Haisley, L., Wallace, C., & Ford, J. D. (2020). Intergenerational effects of childhood maltreatment: A systematic review of the parenting practice of adult survivors of childhood abuse, neglect, and violence. *Clinical Psychology Review*, *80*, 101891.

Groh, A. M., Fearon, R. P., Bakermans-Kranenburg, M. J., Van IJzendoorn, M. H., Steele, R. D., & Roisman, G. I. (2014).

The significance of attachment security for children's social competence with peers: a meta-analytic study. *Attachment and Human Development, 16*, 103–136.

Goldenberg, H., & Goldenberg, I. (2012). *Family therapy: An overview* (8th ed.). Cengage Learning.

Hayes, S. A., & Watson, S. L. (2013). The impact of parenting stress: A meta-analysis of studies comparing the experience of parenting stress in parents of children with and without autism spectrum disorder. *Journal of Autism and Developmental Disorders, 43*(3), 629–642.

Hetherington, S. A., Durant-Jones, L., Johnson, K., Nolan, K., Smith, E., Taylor-Brown, S., & Tuttle, J. (2010). The lived experiences of adolescents with disabilities and their parents in transition planning. *Focus on Autism and Other Developmental Disabilities, 25*(3), 163–172.

Kroening, A., Moore, J., Welch, T., Halterman, J., & Hyman, S. (2016). Developmental screening of refugees: A qualitative study. *Pediatrics, 138*, 1–11.

Lee, C., Burke, M. M., & Stelter, C. R. (2019). Exploring the perspectives of parents and siblings toward future planning for individuals with intellectual and developmental disabilities. *Intellectual and Developmental Disabilities, 57*(3), 198–211.

Marshall, J., Kirby, R. S., & Gorski, P. A. (2016). Parent concern and enrollment in intervention services in young children with developmental delays: 2007 National Survey of Children's Health. *Exceptional Children, 82*(2), 251–268.

Maul, C. A., & Singer, G. H. S. (2009). Just good different things: Specific accommodations families make to positively adapt to their children with developmental disabilities. *Topics in Early Childhood Special Education, 29*(3), 155–170.

McDaniel, S. H., Campbell, T. L., Hepworth, J., & Lorenz, A. (2005). *Family oriented primary care* (2nd ed.). Springer.

McDaniel, S. H., Doherty, W., & Hepworth, J. (2014). *Medical family therapy and integrated care* (2nd ed.). American Psychological Association.

McGoldrick, M., Gerson, R., & Petry, S. (2020). *Genograms: Assessment and intervention* (4th ed.). W. W. Norton & Company.

McHale, S. M., Updegraff, K. A., & Whiteman, S. D. (2012). Sibling relationships and influences in childhood and adolescence. *Journal of Marriage and Family, 74*, 913–930.

McKenzie, K., Oullette-Kuntz, H., Blinkhorn, A., & Demore, A. (2016). Out of school and into distress: Families of young adults with intellectual and developmental disabilities in transition. *Journal of Applied Research in Intellectual Disabilities, 30*(4), 774–781.

Mitchell, D. B., Szczerepa, A., & Hauser-Cram, P. (2016). Spilling over: Partner parenting stress as a predictor of family cohesions in parents of adolescents with developmental disabilities. *Research in Developmental Disabilities, 49-50*, 258–267.

Mitter, N., Ali, A., & Scior, K. (2019). Stigma experienced by families of individuals with intellectual disabilities and autism: A systematic review. *Research in Developmental Disabilities, 89*, 10–21.

Namkung, E. H., Greenberg, J. S., Mailick, M. R., & Floyd, F. J. (2018). Lifelong parenting of adults with developmental disabilities: Growth trends over 20 years in midlife and later life. *American Journal on Intellectual and Developmental Disabilities, 123*(3), 228–240.

Patterson, G. R., Dishion, T. J., & Bank, L. (1984). Family interaction: A process model of deviancy training. *Aggressive Behavior, 10*(3), 253–267.

Peer, J. W., & Hillman, S. B. (2014). Stress and resilience for parents of children with intellectual and developmental disabilities: A review of key factors and recommendations for practitioners. *Journal of Policy and Practice in Intellectual Disabilities, 11*(2), 92–98.

Pierce, M., Hope, H. F., Kolade, A., Gellatly, J., Osam, C. S., Perchard, R., Kosidou, K., Dalman, C., Morgan, V., Prinzio, P. D., & Abel, K. M. (2020). Effects of parental mental illness on children's physical health: Systematic review and meta-analysis. *The British Journal of Psychiatry, 217*, 354–363.

Sadruddin, A. F. A., Ponguta, L. A., Zonderman, A. L., Wiley, K. S., Grimshaw, A., & Panter-Brick, C. (2019). How do grandparents influence child health and development: A systematic review. *Social Science and Medicine, 239*, 112476.

Samadi, S. A., McConkey, R., & Abdollahi Boghrabadi, G. (2020). Parental satisfaction with caregiving across the life span to their children with developmental disabilities: A cross-sectional study in Iran. *International Journal of Environmental Research and Public Health, 17*(5), 1576.

Seligman, M., & Darling, R. B. (2007). *Ordinary families, special children: A systems approach to childhood disability*. The Guilford Press.

Seltzer, M. M., Floyd, F., Song, J., Greenberg, J., & Hong, J. (2011). Midlife and aging parents of adults with intellectual and developmental disabilities: Impacts of lifelong parenting. *American Journal on Intellectual and Developmental Disabilities, 116*(6), 479–499.

Soenens, B., Vansteenkiste, M., & Van Petegem, S. (Eds.). (2017). *Autonomy in adolescent development: Towards conceptual clarity*. Taylor Francis.

US Bureau of the Census. (2019). America's families and living arrangements: 2019. https://www.census.gov/data/tables/2019/demo/families/cps-2019.html

Wong, V., McGrew, J., & Ruble, L. (2020). Predicting the outcomes of parents of transition-age youth or young adults with ASD. *Journal of Autism and Developmental Disorders, 50*, 2723–2739.

13

Parenting and Parenting Behavior

Caitlin F. Canfield, Erin Roby, Kimberly Burkhart, Renée Boynton-Jarrett, and Alan L. Mendelsohn

For additional material related to the content of this chapter, please see Chapters 6, 12, 20, and 21.

VIGNETTE

Parents and their newborns continued to trickle into the community center meeting room for the Parents of Newborns group. As they waited for the meeting to start, Sarah began chatting with Jen, who was sitting next to her. "I'm so looking forward to this group! I thought everything would come naturally, but now I'm really struggling," Sarah said. "I was exactly the opposite," said Jen. "I was so anxious, I read everything I could!" Both women agreed that becoming a parent was stressful, and they realized just how much they needed support from others.

PARENTING AND CHILD DEVELOPMENT

Parenting Styles and Dimensions

As these new parents quickly discovered, becoming a parent is a major life transition that introduces new challenges. Research suggests that having children adds to daily stressors and can have negative impacts on partner and other relationships. At least 20% of new mothers experience postpartum depression, and distress seems to increase for both mothers and fathers across the perinatal period (Nomaguchi & Milkie, 2003). However, there is wide individual variation, and despite the stress, parents report feeling positive and happy about their new role (Lerner & Nightingale, 2016). Regardless of how they weather the transition to parenthood, parents quickly develop a parenting style that impacts everything from feeding to later school involvement.

Classical models of parenting styles, based on the extensive research of Baumrind and colleagues (1966), focused on levels of responsivity and demandingness. These models originally included authoritative, authoritarian, and permissive styles and were later expanded to include a rejecting/neglecting style (Table 13.1). Overall, research has linked authoritative parenting, characterized by high warmth and expectations, with positive child outcomes, but the applicability of these broad parenting styles across cultures and environments is questionable (Smetana, 2017). Some research has indicated that authoritarian parenting styles lead to better child outcomes when families live in high-risk environments and among some ethnic minority immigrant groups. Recent studies of Asian and Middle Eastern parents have indicated that differences occur at the individual rather than the group or societal level, and that, contrary to stereotypes, styles similar to authoritative parenting are predominant across these cultures. Given this variability, recent research has focused on specific domains of parenting, including warmth and demandingness, but also autonomy granting, structure, and others, and how styles and behaviors may change in specific situations. When examined this way, it is clear that parenting styles vary depending on a child's needs or a parent's goals and that children's outcomes show similar variation (Smetana, 2017). Further, focusing on specific domains may provide a better fit across cultures; one study examining parenting domains in Latinx families found that the majority could be classified as protective, similar to the authoritative style in increased sensitivity and expectations, but providing for little autonomy (Rodriguez et al., 2009).

Relational Health

Parents and their practices play a critical role in supporting their child's physical, cognitive, and socioemotional health. Family systems theory recognizes the interconnected, bidirectional relationships between family members and is the basis for the concept of relational health—one's sense of emotional connectedness to important others (see Chapter 12). Early relational health begins in infancy in the parent-child bond and is closely associated with attachment (see Chapter 6). It is associated with a number of developmental outcomes across domains, including mental health through adulthood, and is a key predictor of resilience among children who have experienced adversity (Bethell et al., 2019). Because early relational health is so important for healthy child development, it has become a key focus for both preventive and targeted interventions aimed at improving children's outcomes. Pediatric primary care has been increasingly utilized as a platform for low-cost, population-level implementation (Table 13.2).

The Role of Fathers

The parenting literature, until recently, has focused primarily on mothers, with the role of fathers left largely unexplored (Cabrera et al., 2000). However, recent research has indicated that father-child relational health is equally important as that of mother-child. Early father involvement is related to a more regulated physiologic stress response (i.e., cortisol

TABLE 13.1 Parenting Styles

		Expectations/Demands/Control	
Warmth/Sensitivity/ Responsivity		High	Low
	High	**Authoritative** *Firm but flexible* Clear boundaries, high expectations, nurturing communication	**Permissive** *Nurturing and lenient* Inconsistent boundaries, poor communication, indulgent
	Low	**Authoritarian** *Strict and aloof* High expectations, stringent rules, low warmth	**Neglectful/Rejecting** *Uninvolved and detached* Uninterested, low warmth, few interactions, self-absorbed

Adapted from Baumrind, D. (1966). Effects of authoritative parental control on child behavior. ***Child Development***, 887–907.

TABLE 13.2 Parent-Child Interventions With Impacts on Parenting and Child Development That Have Been Implemented in the Health Care Setting

Intervention	Session Type	Core Component(s)	Delivery Context
General Parenting Support			
Family Foundations	Group	Discussion around improved communication	Prenatal/postnatal maternal care
HealthySteps (HS)	Individual	Developmental support	Primary care
Reach Out and Read (ROR)	Individual, group	Provision of books, modeling, information	Primary care
Smart Beginnings	Individual	Review of parent-child interaction, motivational interviewing	Primary care + Home
Touchpoints	Individual	Video vignettes, modeling	Primary care
Video Interaction Project (VIP)	Individual	Recording and review of parent-child interaction	Primary care
Targeted Behavioral Support			
Incredible Years (IY)	Group	Video vignettes, role play, modeling	Primary care adaptation
Positive Parenting Program (Triple P)	Individual or group	Discussion, role play, information	Primary care adaptation
Parent-Child Interaction Therapy (PCIT)	Individual or group	Live feedback during parent-child interaction	Health care adaptation

Adapted from Peacock-Chambers, E., Ivy, K., & Bair-Merritt, M. (2017). Primary care interventions for early childhood development: A systematic review. ***Pediatrics, 140***(6).

reactivity) and executive function in middle childhood (Roby et al., 2021), and a recent systematic review found overall positive child outcomes linked to high father involvement. Further, when fathers are disengaged during interactions, children are more likely to develop early externalizing behaviors (Sarkadi et al., 2008). These findings highlight the important role fathers play in child health and development, and suggest that consideration should be given to all parents and other caregivers in understanding influences on children's development within the family system.

PARENTING ACROSS THE LIFESPAN

As children grow, parents' expectations and practices change, leading to changes in parenting styles and the role of parents in children's development as they get older.

Parenting in Infancy

Parents of newborns or neonates, those in the first 28 days following birth, face unique challenges that accompany this developmental time period because human infants are not self-sufficient in any capacity and require care in all areas for survival. In fact, parenting responsibilities are arguably the greatest during infancy, from birth into the second year of life, because they involve round-the-clock care, including feeding, diapering, cleaning, and comforting infants who have not yet learned how to self-soothe.

Infants are particularly susceptible to the experiences present in their home and other environments due to rapid changes in early brain development. The large degree of brain plasticity during the 0- to 12-month period means that parents have the capacity to exert a great deal of influence on children's development. These issues are of particular interest because parents spend markedly more time in interactions with their infants than with their children during other developmental periods.

In the following sections we address three key parenting issues during infancy, including breastfeeding, infant sleep, and establishing routines around reading, talking, and play.

Breastfeeding

Breastfeeding is considered the safest and healthiest way to feed infants and is associated with short- and long-term outcomes that span a range of important domains for both infants and mothers. Given these benefits, the American Academy of Pediatrics (AAP) guidelines recommend exclusive breastfeeding for the first 6 months, continued through the first year of life if possible. In the United States, approximately 75% of new mothers breastfeed their infants (AAP Section on Breastfeeding, 2012). Despite high overall adherence to guidelines for breastfeeding, there are disparities across race/ethnicity, socioeconomic status, and maternal age. For instance, while over 80% of Hispanic/Latino mothers initiated breastfeeding, less than 60% of Black mothers did so. There are a variety of factors that contribute to mothers' decisions to initiate and maintain breastfeeding, including breastfeeding knowledge, familial/social/cultural norms and support, work and childcare environment, differences in hospital practices (e.g., providing samples of formulas at discharge, adherence to AAP guidelines for feeding after birth), and problems with lactation. Black mothers, mothers with low income, and young mothers may be disproportionally impacted by these issues and face greater barriers to breastfeeding (AAP Section on Breastfeeding, 2012). For instance, one study found that the largest percentage of mothers who decided to stop breastfeeding at any point between birth and 12 months did so because they worried their infant was not being satisfied by breast milk alone (Li et al., 2008). This perception was highest among Hispanic mothers with very low income. Incorporating breastfeeding curriculum into education for clinicians and advocacy by current clinicians can help to improve mothers' breastfeeding knowledge and confidence, and in turn promote breastfeeding rates (AAP Section on Breastfeeding, 2012).

Infant Sleep

Infant sleep is incredibly important as it is posited to facilitate neural processes such as synapse formation and pruning. Sleep states also allow for the development of the neurosensory and motor systems and for dreaming and memory consolidation to occur (Tarullo et al., 2011). In addition to promoting healthy brain functioning, infant sleep has been linked to numerous positive developmental outcomes, including cognition, language, executive functioning, and more general learning (Tarullo et al., 2011).

Most parents of newborns would agree that their baby spends a great deal of time sleeping. Infants' sleeping and waking cycles tend to shift over the first year of life with sleep episodes initially distributed across the 24-hour period in 3- to 4-hour increments changing to a longer single episode during the night over time that is similar in length (Burnham et al., 2002). It may come as a surprise to new parents that infants do not initially sleep through the night and do not begin to consolidate their sleep until around 6 months. Some infants take longer to make this transition than others, with nearly 60% of 6-month-olds and over 40% of 12-month-olds not sleeping through an 8-hour increment during the night (Burnham et al., 2002).

This transition can pose significant challenges for parents who may be awakened multiple times per night as infants adjust to longer durations of sleep. The ways that parents respond to their infant during this process is based on a variety of factors, including beliefs, expectations, culture, personality, personal history, and infant temperament. Parental distress and parenting style may also affect parents' response and have been linked to sleep and sleep problems from infancy through early childhood (Tyler et al., 2019). However, accumulating evidence suggests that infants who fall asleep with limited assistance from their caregivers wake up fewer times per night and in episodes that last less time than infants who receive high levels of assistance in getting to sleep (e.g., being held, nursed, rocked). These differences are posited to emerge from variation in how different bedtime routines support infants' ability to develop self-regulatory skills (Morrell & Cortina-Borja, 2002). Parents can help their child sleep by learning the signs of sleep readiness, including fussiness, rubbing eyes, and yawning. Setting a daily routine for bedtime that is calming and includes safe sleep practices can help to facilitate sleep through the night. This may include reading, singing, and allowing the infant to become tired before placement into the crib while still awake.

Establishing Routines for Language-Rich Interactions

Research shows that children's exposure to language-rich home environments plays a large role in their development across domains that are important for school readiness and academic achievement, including language, cognition, and social-emotional development. Some infants are exposed to more language in their homes and early learning environments than others, and this difference in both number of words spoken and experience with reciprocal parent-child interactions translates into disparities in child outcomes that have been called "the word gap" (Brooks-Gunn & Markman, 2005). Researchers, practitioners, and policymakers suggest that establishing early routines for reading, talking, and playing can reduce these disparities by supporting parent-child interactions that enhance cognitive, language, and social-emotional development (Weisleder et al., 2019). Reading aloud and play have been shown to support verbal and social parent-child interactions, thereby enhancing child cognition. Starting these routines in infancy can create habits around these behaviors and ensure that children will be exposed to a language-rich environment over the course of childhood.

Parenting in the Toddler and Preschool Years

The toddler period coincides with children (1) beginning to walk on their own and (2) increasing dramatically in their ability to communicate through language, generally between

18 and 24 months of age. The preschool period begins at 36 months and spans through age 5 years, or until children enter kindergarten. Many milestones are met during the toddler and preschool years that give way to new autonomy on the part of the child but also new challenges from the perspective of parents, who must begin to set limits, outline rules and routines, and keep their now mobile and active child safe. In the following sections we address several key issues that are relevant to the preschool and toddler years, including promoting autonomy and discipline.

Supporting Autonomy

During this period parents play two important roles. One is providing opportunities for developing autonomy, exploration, and learning. The other is providing sufficient boundaries and teaching social norms and rules. Parents can help children to develop autonomy and self-esteem by providing them with opportunities to make their own decisions when feasible, following and taking interest in children's interests and activities, and ensuring children have the opportunity to take part in successfully completing tasks (Grolnick et al., 2002). In addition, providing scaffolding (i.e., help that is just beyond a child's abilities without solving a problem for the child) can help children to tackle challenges that are beyond their ability without creating frustration. Engaging in these kinds of strategies not only improves children's ability to problem solve but also supports the development of children's self-regulatory capacities both concurrently and longitudinally.

Discipline

Discipline refers to a system of teaching and nurturing that is used in the context of raising children (Howard, 1996). Toddlers and preschool children need outside support from caregivers and teachers in learning to conform to rules and social standards. Creating clear rules and delivering consistent consequences help children learn which behaviors are acceptable and unacceptable, to internalize these rules, and over time develop a sense of responsibility and self-control. Discipline techniques will be most effective in the context of a parent-child relationship characterized by positive relational health, in which the parent is viewed as a positive role model that the child feels loved by and seeks to emulate. Discipline and teaching techniques should vary across time and be paired to children's developmental level.

During the toddler and preschool years, rules are often established around safety concerns and routines. Parents can reduce the likelihood of conflict during this period by proactively setting up the child's environment to be free from dangerous or "off limits" items, setting predictable daily routines, and by having consistent reactions to behavior. The most effective technique for managing behavior is the promotion of positive behavior by providing positive reinforcement (praising positive behavior), modeling behavior and conflict management, and ignoring misbehavior (Solnick et al., 1977). This latter technique is particularly important in the context of temper tantrums, as trying to reason with or reprimand a child during a tantrum provides attention (even if negative in nature), which can reinforce the behavior (Wilder & Hodges, 2020). Parents can also use redirection (identifying the expected behavior without calling attention to the unwanted behavior), offering choices (giving choices when a child feels powerless) and encouraging communication (asking and helping the child to communicate wants and needs) (Committee on Psychosocial Aspects of Child and Family Health, 1998). Approaches such as timeout (i.e., removing the child from a stressful or emotional situation and allowing time to calm down alone) or, for some older preschool children, removal of privileges (e.g., access to a desired activity) may work if parents provide appropriate, immediate, and clear consequences and explain the reason for the consequence in a calm and empathetic manner (Committee on Psychosocial Aspects of Child and Family Health, 1998). Other forms of punishment such as verbal reprimands are discouraged except when used infrequently and in important (i.e., dangerous) circumstances where a behavior needs to be extinguished immediately. Lastly, corporal or physical punishment should not be used. Research has shown that physical punishment as a primary discipline strategy is not effective, is a risk factor for child maltreatment, and is associated with numerous negative outcomes (Bauman & Friedman, 1998; Choe et al., 2013).

Parenting in Middle Childhood

Middle childhood spans the ages 6 through 12, years that correspond with early elementary school through the transition to adolescence. During this period, children expand their environments and personal roles and begin to take on more responsibility. They reduce the amount of time they spend directly with family and caregivers, and increase their engagement in school and extracurricular activities. Children in the middle childhood period also make changes in their sense of self and begin to engage in social comparison. In the following sections we address two key issues that apply to the middle childhood period, academic achievement and screen time.

Academic Achievement

Academic achievement, including children's performance in elementary school and their scores on standardized tests, has become a key focus for parents during middle childhood, as these abilities set the stage for later success in high school and beyond (Casillas et al., 2012). Over the last several decades parent involvement in children's school (e.g., attending meetings, volunteering) has steadily increased. Research overwhelmingly demonstrates that parent involvement in children's learning is positively related to achievement, and this association is consistent across ages and is maintained even after controlling for child intelligence (Topor et al., 2010).

Children's academic achievement can be explained in part by how they respond to challenges and whether they view their intelligence and abilities as fixed (i.e., innate) or as the result of hard work. Importantly, parents can support children's responses to challenges by praising their efforts rather than their intelligence. Doing so is thought to result in what Dweck and colleagues (2008) have referred to as "a growth mindset," in which children view ability as something that can be increased by trying harder (i.e., not fixed). Children with this perception are more likely to set mastery goals for themselves (aimed to improve skills and intrinsically motivated) rather than performance goals (aimed to show intelligence and extrinsically motivated) and to display mastery responses (persistence and positive emotions) to both high and low challenges rather than giving up (Fig. 13.1).

There are well-documented racial and ethnic disparities in academic achievement that have persisted for decades. However, more recently, socioeconomic disparities have become even more pronounced. Research shows that the income gap in achievement is wide upon entry to kindergarten and does not change over the elementary school years (Reardon, 2011). However, as described earlier, the growth mindset is predictive of academic achievement across all socioeconomic strata (Claro et al., 2016). One study showed that children from low-income homes were less likely to hold this kind of mindset than their higher-income peers, but that among those who did have this mindset, it acted as a buffering effect against the effect of low income on achievement, suggesting that children from all income backgrounds can benefit from viewing achievement as a direct result of effort (Claro et al., 2016).

Screen Time

One of the most challenging issues facing parents today is how to navigate their child's use of technology and exposure to screen time. Children now have more access to media and screens than ever before, and research suggests exposure has both benefits and risks (see Chapter 21). Key benefits include exposure to a vast range of ideas and information that may promote creativity or new skills, and increased capacity to connect socially. Risks include increased likelihood of obesity, problems with sleep, and exposure to dangerous interactions (e.g., bullying, explicit messages) (AAP Council on Communications and Media, 2016).

Children's use of media is strongly correlated with parents' use of media across a number of different platforms (e.g., television, computer, smartphone), and studies show that parents' media use influences parent-child interactions (Radesky et al., 2015). In one study, nearly 25% of mothers with school-age children spontaneously used their mobile device during a parent-child activity, which resulted in those mothers talking less and initiating fewer nonverbal interactions (Radesky et al., 2015). Parents also report that mobile devices, which are widely accessible, are difficult to monitor in terms of the content being accessed or downloaded. The AAP (2016) recommends developing a family media plan that is tailored to children's age, health, temperament, and developmental stage and takes into account the importance of children's need for physical activity, plenty of sleep, and time spent away from media.

Parenting Adolescents

Parent-child relationships begin to change in adolescence. Although parental warmth and discipline continue to remain important, a key developmental task for adolescents is to establish autonomy. As adolescents strive for greater independence, parents need to adapt their approach from a vertical to a horizontal parenting style, which results in a more egalitarian relationship.

Parenting Styles in Adolescence

Based on the self-determination theory, there are three needs that must be met for individual growth (Ryan & Deci, 2017): autonomy, competence, and relatedness. Adolescents experience autonomy when they feel that they have chosen their own behavior, have control over the behavior, and have chosen behavior that is consistent with their principles. Competence refers to a feeling of effectiveness in handling day-to-day challenges and interpersonal relationships (Ryan & Deci, 2017). Relatedness is a sense of feeling loved and cared for, and in return being able to establish closeness with others by reciprocating feelings of love and kindness. Parents can support or thwart meeting these psychological needs. Parents' ability to support an adolescent's autonomy, competence, and relatedness is associated with the degree to which an adolescent

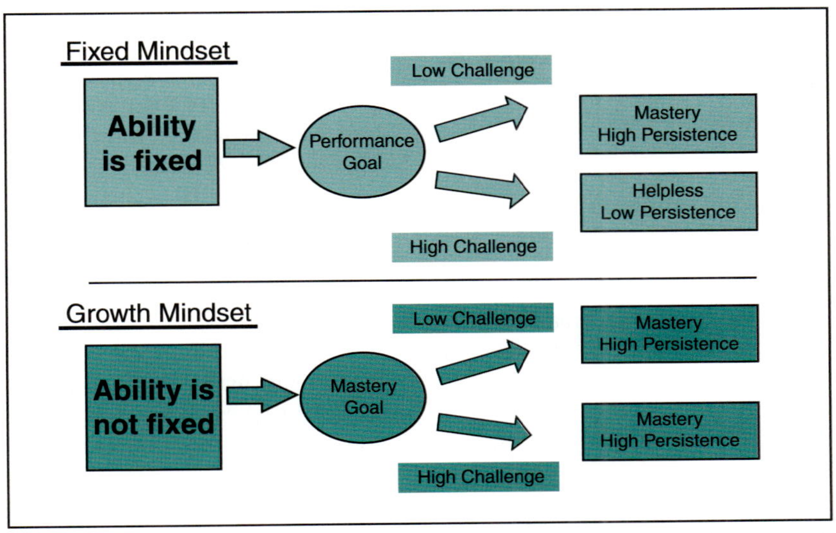

Fig. 13.1 Academic achievement. Fixed versus growth mindsets: impacts on goals and responses to challenges.

displays adaptive psychological and social functioning and academic success (Costa et al., 2019).

Furthermore, the six dimensions of parenting mentioned earlier are consistent with the self-determination theory: autonomy support versus psychological control, structure versus chaos, and warmth versus rejection. Autonomy is associated with a greater ability to cope, whereas the use of parent psychological control has been associated with worse adolescent adjustment, including externalizing and internalizing symptoms, increased delinquency and depression, and poorer academic performance (Lansford et al., 2014). However, parent knowledge of their adolescent child's peers, emotions, and routines, when not used to control adolescents' behavior, is associated with positive adolescent outcomes, including decreases in externalizing behavior problems. Structure involves developing clear expectations and age-appropriate limit setting. Consistent parenting is associated with higher academic achievement and self-regulation, and inconsistent parenting is associated with lower levels of cognitive functioning and increased behavioral problems. Warmth refers to a parent's positive regard and emotional availability and is associated with improved social functioning. Rejection, however, includes hostility and explosive discipline and is associated with depression and suicidality. Findings have shown that autonomy, structure, and warmth mediate the relationship between parenting and adolescents' adjustment (Costa et al., 2019).

Adjustment and Peer Relationships

Parental warmth in adolescence is associated with greater adolescent adjustment. Adolescents who reported higher parental support exhibit improved adjustment. While there are gender differences in parenting (Box 13.1), adolescents whose parent-child relationship is marked with warmth show greater attachment to parents and peers, lower peer victimization and involvement in bullying, and better school success. Parental warmth serves as a protective factor against school failure, delinquency, and substance use. In other words, parents set the tone for their adolescent's emotional and social adjustment, with socialization practices of the same-sex parent having a greater effect (Bully et al., 2019).

Adolescents of both sexes who have supportive parents are more likely to be in satisfying friendships. That is, adolescent friendships tend to mirror their relationship with parents. For example, adolescents whose fathers are cooperative and engage in collaborative problem solving imitate this approach with their friends (Flynn et al., 2018). Parents and peers impact positive development in adolescence. Adolescents who perceive their parents as authoritative or permissive, rather than authoritarian, show increased wellbeing. Although some studies have indicated benefits of authoritative parenting over permissive styles for younger children, it may be that the responsiveness and autonomy-granting that are characteristic of both authoritative and permissive parenting styles are especially important for wellbeing during adolescence, such that both styles lead to increased self-esteem and life satisfaction. Additionally, those with higher quality friendships report increased happiness and self-esteem (Raboteg-Saric & Sakic, 2014).

BOX 13.1 Gender Differences in Parenting

Gender differences have been found in parenting adolescents. Historically, fathers play a more critical role in gender socializing, whereas mothers are more consistent and socially scripted in their approach. It is thought that gender identification increases during adolescence and same-gender parent-adolescent dyads form. Adolescent females tend to report higher parental support. Studies are inconsistent, however, in terms of the degree of control between adolescent females and males. Regardless of adolescent gender there is greater divergence when comparing parent and adolescent perception of parental support and control in early adolescence with greater convergence reported with an increase in adolescent age.

Adapted from Mastrotheodoros, S., Van der Graaff, J., Deković, M., Meeus, W. H., & Branje, S. J. (2019). Coming closer in adolescence: Convergence in mother, father, and adolescent reports of parenting. *Journal of Research on Adolescence, 29*(4), 846–862.

PARENTING IN CONTEXT

Throughout the lifespan, parents approach the task of parenting in the context of the greater environment and contexts in which they live. The stressors of poverty and racism impact the resources, both material and emotional, that parents can devote to their children. Further, the additional complexities of raising a child with developmental disabilities change both parenting practices and the potential impacts of those practices. We talk about each of these in more detail, using autism spectrum disorder (ASD) as an exemplar developmental disability.

Poverty

When faced with the additional stressors related to poverty, parents may feel they do not have the bandwidth for positive interactions with their child. In fact, in low-socioeconomic status environments, parents have been observed as harsher, with more punitive discipline strategies. Although there is evidence that impacts of poverty on child development increase the longer they live below the poverty line, acute declines in income lead to greater family conflict and, in turn, more hostile parenting (Roubinov & Boyce, 2017). Further, the impacts of poverty on children's mental health and later adult health outcomes are mediated, at least in part, by negative relationships with parents and other family members early in life (Grant et al., 2003).

Poverty may impact parenting through two distinct but not mutually exclusive pathways. The first pathway, called the family stress path, indicates that poverty leads to more distress in parents—increased mental health symptoms and partner conflict—which negatively impact parenting practices. The second pathway, the family investment path, posits that families living in poverty do not have the capital to provide for their child's development, either through material goods (e.g., books, toys), parental involvement, or opportunities for later education and employment. There has been limited research on the family investment pathway, but a large body of literature provides evidence for the family stress model across family structure, child age, environment, and with a few exceptions race and ethnicity (Roubinov & Boyce, 2017).

Racism

Racism, a system of advantage where opportunity and value are assigned based on socially constructed categories, is entrenched in American society and culture, and is an established social determinant of mental and physical health (Pachter & Garcia-Coll, 2009).

Children are attuned to race from an early age, and racial identity formation is a complex and relational process that develops through stages (Fig. 13.2). Many caregivers, though, delay discussions of racial identity and racism due to discomfort and misestimating the timing of children's processing of race and racial injustice (Sullivan et al., 2021). White parents are also more likely to have conversations that deemphasize racial differences (color blindness) and fail to describe racist policies, overlooking systemic racism that connects privilege and power to those socially constructed differences (Vittrup, 2018).

Parents can help children recognize and understand historical and contemporary processes that marginalize and mistreat people of color and advantage White people by engaging in conversations about race and racism with their children from an early age, increasing exposure to diversity through books with racially and ethnically diverse characters, and expanding social connections beyond immediate social circles. Parents and caregivers can also discuss incidents of racial injustice with their children, share stories of resilience and strength to promote healing, and role model their own growth toward antiracism by validating efforts to promote social change and justice and addressing their own biases.

Racial Socialization

Racial socialization is actively communicating with children and youth about experiences informed by race and racism. This may buffer racial trauma, which stems from direct or indirect (vicarious) social forces and interpersonal dynamics that are associated with racism and threaten wellbeing, and may lead to anxiety, poor immune functioning and sleep, and impaired daily activity (Pachter & Garcia-Coll, 2009).

Racial socialization incorporating experiences and relationships, as well as language that positively affirms a child's identity, can help children develop a sense of connection and pride within a racial-ethnic or cultural community. Strategies to incorporate racial socialization that include opportunities to explore cultural pride in combination with preparation for addressing bias have been shown to be successful (Anderson & Stevenson, 2019).

It is important for providers to recognize that the act of talking with children about race and racism may be stressful for parents. Actively supporting caregivers with resources and through multidisciplinary teams may (1) increase their competency to engage with children to appraise a situation as one that involves racism, (2) build self-efficacy in coping through strategies to understand and manage threat, and (3) ultimately resolve the situation (see Chapter 20).

Colorism

Colorism is prejudicial or preferential treatment associated with skin tone. Colorism can impact family processes, experiences of discrimination, and ways that parents racially socialize their children. Similar to racism, social hierarchies associated with skin tone that elevate lighter skin to browner-skinned individuals can lead to microaggressions and traumatic stress (Landor et al., 2011). Parenting behaviors may be impacted by colorism, and parents may value their child's racial phenotype (skin, hair, facial features) to different degrees, based on historical trauma and internalized oppression, including both personal experiences and intergenerational trauma (Tharps, 2016). To counteract colorism, caregivers can use daily interactions intentionally as opportunities to affirm and celebrate beauty, can welcome questions and invite conversations about skin color, and can embrace opportunities for exposure to diverse skin colors and representations in books, media, and community (Tharps, 2016).

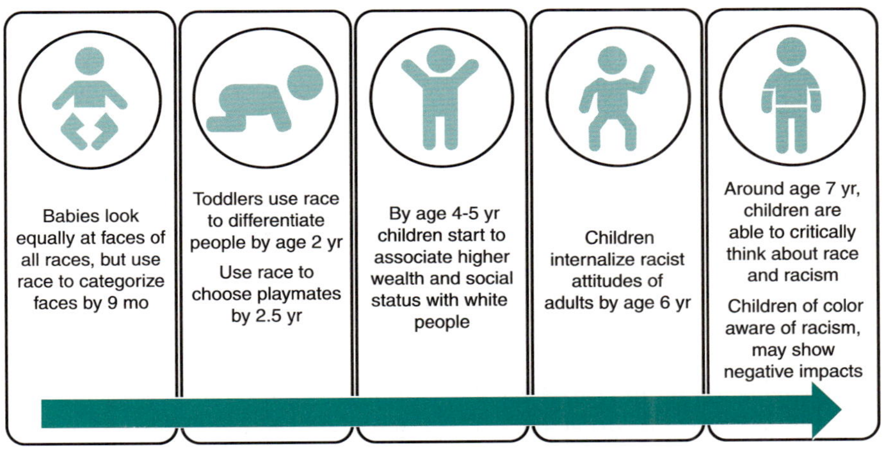

Fig. 13.2 How infants and young children understand race and racism.

Black children are more likely to be perceived as older than their age or as adults. Clinicians can support parents in navigating the implications of these perceptions, particularly in encounters with police, educators, and health care providers. "The talk" has been popularized as a strategy for caregivers, educators, and clinicians to help teach children protective strategies for police encounters, but we presently do not have data on the effectiveness of these strategies. "The talk" may also signal an expectation that Black children can prematurely assume adult roles and responsibilities in the face of institutional racism (Burton, 2007).

Parenting that is attuned to the context of racism applies to all families. Antiracism is an active practice that involves action and learning. Caregivers can proactively embrace racial socialization, help children explore their racial identities, and teach, role model, and reinforce antiracist practices. Finally, caregivers can use clear language to describe racism and racial justice and role model their own efforts to reduce bias.

Parenting Children With Developmental Disabilities

Studies of parenting children with developmental disabilities are far less common than those of parenting with typically developing children. The studies that do exist consistently indicate that parenting children with special health care needs results in more parenting stress, and parents of children with developmental disabilities report higher stress than parents of children with chronic medical illnesses (Gupta, 2007). A qualitative study of the experience of parenting a child with developmental disabilities indicated that these parents face both challenges—including mental and physical exhaustion, blame and stereotypes from others, and negative impacts on other family relationships—and rewards, with coping strategies allowing hope for their children's development (Nurullah, 2013). In this context, authoritative parenting may actually increase stress for parents, as it is difficult to implement (Woolfson & Grant, 2005). However, there is an overall positive impact of positive parenting practices on the functional outcomes of young children with developmental disabilities (Dyches et al., 2012).

The literature on parenting in the context of developmental disabilities most often examines developmental disabilities in general terms, grouping together children with a variety of disorders. However, studies specifically examining parenting of children with ASD have been emerging, and thus we turn to this research now.

Autism Spectrum Disorder

Parents of youth with ASD tend to be less confident in their parenting and may experience increased parental stress. This has been associated with depression and hopelessness. Moreover, research has shown that both children with ASD and their parents have increased psychopathology, which may have a negative bidirectional effect on the parent-child relationship. In fact, some studies suggest that the emotional and behavioral problems that are often comorbid with ASD may be more closely associated with family wellbeing than with core ASD symptomatology (Yorke et al., 2018). Keen and colleagues (2010) found that by providing parenting support at the time of an ASD diagnosis, there was reduced parent stress and a positive influence on children's adaptive behavioral functioning and social communication, highlighting the important role parents play on child outcomes.

Studies have looked at the parent-child relationship among children with ASD through their response to the "strange situation" procedure. These studies indicate that approximately 50% of these children exhibited secure attachment to their mothers, and mothers of secure children were found to be more sensitive and responsive than others (Rutgers et al., 2004). Children with ASD were more likely than neurotypical children to have a delayed response to their mothers' return, and increased autism severity was associated with fewer prosocial behaviors at reunion.

Play, children's natural medium for communication, serves an important role in the parent-child relationship, but differences in play among children with ASD may have negative effects on both the child and parents' sense of self-efficacy. Studies have shown that mother-child interactions with ASD youth had more mismatched emotion-engagement states. Additionally, children spent more time attending to objects (Naber et al., 2008). A parent's coping style can also impact parent-child interactions; those who solve problems more flexibly tend to have fewer negative emotions and improved functioning (Crowell et al., 2019). In a study conducted by Roman-Oyola and colleagues (2018), both mothers and fathers identified intrinsic motivation and internal control as facilitating improved engagement of the child.

Compared to mothers of typically developing youth, mothers of children with ASD use simpler strategies to provide comfort when the child is emotionally dysregulated, such as physical comfort and a holding gaze. In a longitudinal study, mothers' warmth, relationship quality, and praise were associated with decreases in problem behaviors and repetitive behaviors (Ostfeld-Etzion et al., 2015). Parents with ASD youth often use the strategy of accommodation (i.e., making adaptations to regulate their child's affect), including by modifying demands, limiting exposure to stressors, and/or by avoiding conflict in an attempt to prevent aggressive outbursts (O'Nions, 2018). In general, parents of children with ASD are more lenient, using fewer rules and discipline (Maljaars et al., 2014). On the other hand, in the context of a frustrating event, authoritarian parenting was associated with an increase in a child's attempts to self-regulate (Crowell et al., 2019).

CLINICAL IMPLICATIONS

Parenting has large impacts across all aspects of child development and behavior, from early childhood through adolescence, and with implications for outcomes across the life course. Parenting and parent-child relationships therefore represent a central consideration in developmental-behavioral pediatrics, as well as in all areas of general and subspecialty pediatric clinical practice. Substantial heterogeneity in parenting practices across developmental periods, populations/cultures, and other family/child characteristics represents further consideration. Both theoretical frameworks and empirical data can be utilized to inform efforts to enhance developmental outcomes and prevent disparities through support for parenting.

REFERENCES

American Academy of Pediatrics Council on Communications and Media. (2016). Media and young minds. *Pediatrics*, *138*(5), e20162591.

American Academy of Pediatrics Section on Breastfeeding. (2012). Breastfeeding and the use of human milk. *Pediatrics*, *129*(3), e827–e841.

Anderson, R., & Stevenson, H. (2019). RECASTing racial stress and trauma: Theorizing the healing potential of racial socialization in families. *American Psychologist*, *74*(1), 63.

Bauman, L. J., & Friedman, S. B. (1998). Corporal punishment. *Pediatric Clinics of North America*, *45*(2), 403–414.

Baumrind, D. (1966). Effects of authoritative parental control on child behavior. *Child Development*, 887–907.

Bethell, C., Jones, J., Gombojav, N., Linkenbach, J., & Sege, R. (2019). Positive childhood experiences and adult mental and relational health in a statewide sample: Associations across adverse childhood experiences levels. *JAMA Pediatrics*, *173*(11), e193007.

Brooks-Gunn, J., & Markman, L. B. (2005). The contribution of parenting to ethnic and racial gaps in school readiness. *The Future of Children*, 139–168.

Bully, P., Jaureguizar, J., Bernaras, E., & Redondo, I. (2019). Relationship between parental socialization, emotional symptoms, and academic performance during adolescence: The influence of parents' and teenagers' gender. *International Journal of Environmental Research and Public Health*, *16*(12), 2231.

Burnham, M. M., Goodlin-Jones, B. L., Gaylor, E. E., & Anders, T. F. (2002). Nighttime sleep-wake patterns and self-soothing from birth to one year of age: A longitudinal intervention study. *Journal of Child Psychology and Psychiatry*, *43*(6), 713–725.

Burton, L. (2007). Childhood adultification in economically disadvantaged families: A conceptual model. *Family Relations*, *56*(4), 329–345.

Cabrera, N., Tamis-LeMonda, C. S., Bradley, R. H., Hofferth, S., & Lamb, M. E. (2000). Fatherhood in the twenty-first century. *Child Development*, *71*(1), 127–136.

Casillas, A., Robbins, S., Allen, J., Kuo, Y. L., Hanson, M. A., & Schmeiser, C. (2012). Predicting early academic failure in high school from prior academic achievement, psychosocial characteristics, and behavior. *Journal of Educational Psychology*, *104*(2), 407.

Choe, D. E., Olson, S. L., & Sameroff, A. J. (2013). The interplay of externalizing problems and physical and inductive discipline during childhood. *Developmental Psychology*, *49*(11), 2029.

Claro, S., Paunesku, D., & Dweck, C. (2016). Growth mindset tempers the effects of poverty on academic achievement. *Proceedings of the National Academy of Sciences*, *113*(31), 8664.

Committee on Psychosocial Aspects of Child and Family Health. (1998). Guidance for effective discipline. *Pediatrics*, *101*(4), 723–728.

Costa, S., Sireno, S., Larcan, R., & Cuzzocrea, F. (2019). The six dimensions of parenting and adolescent psychological adjustment: The mediating role of psychological needs. *Scandinavian Journal of Psychology*, *60*(2), 128–137.

Crowell, J. A., Keluskar, J., & Gorecki, A. (2019). Parenting behavior and the development of children with autism spectrum disorder. *Comprehensive Psychiatry*, *90*, 21–29.

Dweck, C. S. (2008). *Mindset: The new psychology of success*. Random House Digital, Inc.

Dyches, T. T., Smith, T. B., Korth, B. B., Roper, S. O., & Mandleco, B. (2012). Positive parenting of children with developmental disabilities: A meta-analysis. *Research in Developmental Disabilities*, *33*(6), 2213–2220.

Flynn, H. K., Felmlee, D. H., Shu, X., & Conger, R. (2018). Mothers and fathers matter: The influence of parental support, hostility, and problem solving on adolescent friendships. *Journal of Family Issues*, *39*(8), 2389–2412.

Grant, K. E., Compas, B. E., Stuhlmacher, A. F., Thurm, A. E., McMahon, S. D., & Halpert, J. A. (2003). Stressors and child and adolescent psychopathology: Moving from markers to mechanisms of risk. *Psychological Bulletin*, *129*(3), 447.

Grolnick, W. S., Gurland, S. T., DeCourcey, W., & Jacob, K. (2002). Antecedents and consequences of mothers' autonomy support: An experimental investigation. *Developmental Psychology*, *38*(1), 143.

Gupta, V. B. (2007). Comparison of parenting stress in different developmental disabilities. *Journal of Developmental and Physical Disabilities*, *19*(4), 417–425.

Howard, B. J. (1996). Advising parents on discipline: What works. *Pediatrics*, *98*(4), 809–815.

Keen, D., Couzens, D., Muspratt, S., & Rodger, S. (2010). The effects of a parent-focused intervention for children with a recent diagnosis of autism spectrum disorder on parenting stress and competence. *Research in Autism Spectrum Disorders*, *4*(2), 229–241.

Landor, A., Simons, L. G., Simons, R. L., Brody, G. H., & Gibbons, F. X. (2011). The role of religiosity in the relationship between parents, peers, and adolescent risky sexual behavior. *Journal of Youth and Adolescence*, *40*(3), 296–309.

Lansford, J. E., Laird, R. D., Pettit, G. S., Bates, J. E., & Dodge, K. A. (2014). Mothers' and fathers' autonomy-relevant parenting: Longitudinal links with adolescents' externalizing and internalizing behavior. *Journal of Youth and Adolescence*, *43*(11), 1877–1889.

Lerner, C., & Nightingale, M. O. (2016). Tuning in: Parents of young children speak up about what they think, know, and need. *Zero to Three*, *37*(1), 44–49.

Li, R., Fein, S. B., Chen, J., & Grummer-Strawn, L. M. (2008). Why mothers stop breastfeeding: Mothers' self-reported reasons for stopping during the first year. *Pediatrics*, *122*(2), S69–S76.

Maljaars, J., Boonen, H., Lambrechts, G., Van Leeuwen, K., & Noens, I. (2014). Maternal parenting behavior and child behavior problems in families of children and adolescents with autism spectrum disorder. *Journal of Autism and Developmental Disorders*, *44*(3), 501–512.

Mastrotheodoros, S., Van der Graaff, J., Deković, M., Meeus, W. H., & Branje, S. J. (2019). Coming closer in adolescence: Convergence in mother, father, and adolescent reports of parenting. *Journal of Research on Adolescence*, *29*(4), 846–862.

Morrell, J., & Cortina-Borja, M. (2002). The developmental change in strategies parents employ to settle young children to sleep, and their relationship to infant sleeping problems, as assessed by a new questionnaire: The Parental Interactive Bedtime Behaviour Scale. *Infant and Child Development*, *11*(1), 17–41.

Naber, F. B., Bakermans-Kranenburg, M. J., Van Ijzendoorn, M. H., Swinkels, S. H., Buitelaar, J. K., Dietz, C., van Daalen, E., &

Van Engeland, H. (2008). Play behavior and attachment in toddlers with autism. *Journal of Autism and Developmental Disorders, 38*(5), 857–866.

Nomaguchi, K. M., & Milkie, M. A. (2003). Costs and rewards of children: The effects of becoming a parent on adults' lives. *Journal of Marriage and Family, 65*(2), 356–374.

Nurullah, A. S. (2013). "It's really a roller coaster": Experience of parenting children with developmental disabilities. *Marriage & Family Review, 49*(5), 412–445.

O'Nions, E., Happé, F., Evers, K., Boonen, H., & Noens, I. (2018). How do parents manage irritability, challenging behaviour, non-compliance and anxiety in children with autism spectrum disorders? A meta-synthesis. *Journal of Autism and Developmental Disorders, 48*(4), 1272–1286.

Ostfeld-Etzion, S., Golan, O., Hirschler-Guttenberg, Y., Zagoory-Sharon, O., & Feldman, R. (2015). Neuroendocrine and behavioral response to social rupture and repair in preschoolers with autism spectrum disorders interacting with mother and father. *Molecular Autism, 6*(1), 1–13.

Pachter, L., & Garcia-Coll, C. (2009). Racism and child health: A review of the literature and future directions. *Journal of Developmental Behavioral Pediatrics, 30*(3), 255–263.

Peacock-Chambers, E., Ivy, K., & Bair-Merritt, M. (2017). Primary care interventions for early childhood development: A systematic review. *Pediatrics, 140*(6).

Raboteg-Saric, Z., & Sakic, M. (2014). Relations of parenting styles and friendship quality to self-esteem, life satisfaction and happiness in adolescents. *Applied Research in Quality of Life, 9*(3), 749–765.

Radesky, J. S., Schumacher, J., & Zuckerman, B. (2015). Mobile and interactive media use by young children: The good, the bad, and the unknown. *Pediatrics, 135*(1), 1–3.

Reardon, S. F. (2011). The widening academic achievement gap between the rich and the poor: New evidence and possible explanations. *Whither Opportunity, 1*(1), 91–116.

Roby, E., Piccolo, L. R., Gutierrez, J., Kesoglides, N., Raak, C., Mendelsohn, A. L., & Canfield, C. (2021). Father involvement in infancy predicts behavior and response to chronic stress in middle childhood in a low-income Latinx sample. *Developmental Psychobiology*

Rodriguez, M. M. D., Donovick, M. R., & Crowley, S. L. (2009). Parenting styles in a cultural context: Observations of "protective parenting" in first-generation Latinos. *Family Process, 48*(2), 195–210.

Román-Oyola, R., Figueroa-Feliciano, V., Torres-Martínez, Y., Torres-Vélez, J., Encarnación-Pizarro, K., Fragoso-Pagán, S., & Torres-Colón, L. (2018). Play, playfulness, and self-efficacy: Parental experiences with children on the autism spectrum. *Occupational Therapy International, 2018.*

Roubinov, D. S., & Boyce, W. T. (2017). Parenting and SES: Relative values or enduring principles? *Current Opinion in Psychology, 15*, 162–167.

Rutgers, A. H., Bakermans-Kranenburg, M. J., van Ijzendoorn, M. H., & van Berckelaer-Onnes, I. A. (2004). Autism and attachment: A meta-analytic review. *Journal of Child Psychology and Psychiatry, 45*(6), 1123–1134.

Ryan, R. M., & Deci, E. L. (2017). *Self-determination theory: Basic psychological needs in motivation, development, and wellness.* Guilford Publications.

Sarkadi, A., Kristiansson, R., Oberklaid, F., & Bremberg, S. (2008). Fathers' involvement and children's developmental outcomes: A systematic review of longitudinal studies. *Acta Paediatrica, 97*(2), 153–158.

Smetana, J. G. (2017). Current research on parenting styles, dimensions, and beliefs. *Current Opinion in Psychology, 15*, 19–25.

Solnick, J. V., Rincover, A., & Peterson, C. R. (1977). Some determinants of the reinforcing and punishing effects of time out. *Journal of Applied Behavior Analysis, 10*(3), 415–424.

Sullivan, J., Wilton, L., & Apfelbaum, E. P. (2021). Adults delay conversations about race because they underestimate children's processing of race. *Journal of Experimental Psychology: General*

Tarullo, A. R., Balsam, P. D., & Fifer, W. P. (2011). Sleep and infant learning. *Infant and Child Cevelopment, 20*(1), 35–46.

Tharps, L. L. (2016). *Same family, different colors: Confronting colorism in America's diverse families.* Beacon Press.

Topor, D. R., Keane, S. P., Shelton, T. L., & Calkins, S. D. (2010). Parent involvement and student academic performance: A multiple mediational analysis. *Journal of Prevention & Intervention in the Community, 38*(3), 183–197.

Tyler, D., Donovan, C. L., Scupham, S., Shiels, A. L., & Weaver, S. A. (2019). Young children's sleep problems: The impact of parental distress and parenting style. *Journal of Child and Family Studies, 28*(8), 2098–2106.

Vittrup, B. (2018). Color blind or color conscious? White American mothers' approaches to racial socialization. *Journal of Family Issues, 39*(3), 668–692.

Weisleder, A., Cates, C. B., Harding, J. F., Johnson, S. B., Canfield, C. F., Seery, A. M., Raak, C. D., Alonso, A., Dreyer, B. P., & Mendelsohn, A. L. (2019). Links between shared reading and play, parent psychosocial functioning, and child behavior: Evidence from a randomized controlled trial. *The Journal of Pediatrics, 213*, 187–195.

Wilder, D. A., & Hodges, A. C. (2020). *Tantrums. The encyclopedia of child and adolescent development* (pp. 1–11). John Wiley & Sons.

Woolfson, L., & Grant, E. (2005). A comparison of parenting of developmentally disabled and typically developing children. *Proceedings of the British Psychological Society, 13*(1), 42.

Yorke, I., White, P., Weston, A., Rafla, M., Charman, T., & Simonoff, E. (2018). The association between emotional and behavioral problems in children with autism spectrum disorder and psychological distress in their parents: A systematic review and meta-analysis. *Journal of Autism and Developmental Disorders, 48*, 3393–3415.

14

Foster Care and Adoption: Implications for Developmental and Behavioral Pediatrics

*Kida Ingram and Lisa Prock**

For additional material related to the content of this chapter, please see Chapters 15, 37, and 56.

> **VIGNETTE**
>
> *James is a 10-year-old young man in grade 4 with a history of prenatal exposure to at least tobacco, marijuana, and opiates (reported to be both heroin and suboxone use during pregnancy). He resided with his birth mother and siblings until 18 months of age and then transitioned to foster care. He resided in three different foster homes with several brief periods of returning to his birth mother's care and ultimately transitioned to an adoptive family at 4 years of age. James currently presents with the challenges of attending and learning in school. His parents appreciate that reading is hard for him, and they are working with his school system to provide him with specialized support for reading. James appears inattentive and impulsive at times, but there are no concerns about hyperactivity. His parents wonder how much of his current challenges are related to his prenatal substance exposure and experiences during his first 4 years of life before joining their family. His teachers and his pediatrician suspect that he may have attention-deficit/hyperactivity disorder (ADHD).*

INTRODUCTION

The story of James in our case vignette highlights some complexities inherent in foster care and adoption—namely, transition is not always a single event, and experiences prior to a transition can be extremely variable. We begin with defining terms used to describe the experiences of children and their families during transitions associated with foster care and/or adoption and beyond.

Key Terms and Definitions

Although children with a history of foster care and adoption often have similar experiences prior to placement and may have overlapping risk and resilience factors at the time of their placement into nonparental care, the goals of the foster care and adoption systems are quite different. This chapter focuses on the experiences of children impacted by US foster care and adoption systems. Policies and procedures vary across states and countries, thus we encourage readers to become familiar with policies and procedures in their specific localities. For the purposes of this chapter, we summarize the goals of these systems as follows:

- The foster care system provides direct and ideally transient support for a child who has experienced presumed abuse or neglect. The aims generally include child protection and family reunification, which involves returning a child to reside with the birth parents.
- In contrast, adoption provides a permanent transition of a child to a family not including the birth parents, which may be voluntary or court mandated.

There are three primary paths through which children are adopted in the United States, each of which support different groups of children joining adoptive families: domestic private adoption, domestic public adoption, and international adoption (Table 14.1).

In this chapter we examine the implications for children experiencing foster care and/or adoption. We note similarities and differences between these groups, with a focus on the best available evidence regarding child outcomes. We also highlight important gaps in current knowledge.

Epidemiology

Many children transition either temporarily or permanently into nonparental care each year in the United States. Approximately 2% of children permanently transition to join their families via adoption each year, with the majority joining their family either as infants via domestic adoption or following foster care with a much smaller number joining their families via international adoption. In addition, more than 1% of children in the United States experience significant neglect and/or abuse who transition into foster care every year. Importantly, 5% to 6% of US children will be placed in foster care from 0 to 18 years of age (Wildeman & Emanuel, 2014; Turney & Wildeman, 2016). Children living in foster care, compared with other children, disproportionately come from low-income families and are ethnic and racial minorities (roughly 10% of Black children and 15% of Indigenous children). At any point in time, more than 400,000 children in the United States are in foster care, with approximately one-third in relative homes and approximately one-fourth with a goal of adoption (Child Welfare Information Gateway, 2020).

*Address correspondence to Lisa Prock MD, MPH at lisa.prock@childrens.harvard.edu or at Boston Children's Hospital, 300 Longwood Avenue, Boston, MA 02115

TABLE 14.1 Types of Adoption in the United States in 2021

Adoption Type	Demographics	Comments
Domestic private adoption	Child typically joins family at birth	Voluntary placement of a child for adoption; unplanned pregnancy and risk of substance use (~80% of birth mothers); open adoption highly preferred by birth families
Domestic public adoption	Child may join family as infant or older child	Typically high-risk placement (e.g., parental rights not yet terminated; placement due to substance exposure)
International adoption	Child rarely joins family before 1 yr of age	Increasingly special needs (e.g., severe cardiac concerns, cleft lip/palate, severe epilepsy) are identified prior to adoption, in contrast to international adoption population decades ago

FAMILY AND CHILD PREPARATION

In our opening case vignette James was transitioning to an adoptive family after multiple foster care placements, including one where he resided with extended family members (kinship placement). As a result it is expected that his transition to an adoptive family may raise questions about the permanency of his placement as well as his role in leading to this transition.

Children and families receive variable information when transitioning to a new family. When children transition to foster care, rarely is there an opportunity for advanced planning and discussion with older children. For infants, preparation of a child about a family transition is challenging. However, for children who have had many placements like James in our case above, it is important to explain in a developmentally appropriate manner why the transition has occurred and that the child is not responsible for the transition. Many older children will ask about ongoing contact with their foster care parents and communication should be supported when possible.

Prospective families receive a range of preparation to support children. With respect to foster care, most US states require prospective foster parents to participate in didactic sessions where they are introduced to a number of potential risk factors that may impact the health and wellbeing of their future foster or adoptive child (Table 14.2). Foster families are not given a great deal of choice about a child transitioning to their home, and they are routinely provided with little information about a foster child's previous experiences and needs. Prospective adoptive parents are also increasingly expected to participate in educational seminars prior to adopting a child. Some agencies require prospective parents to consult with "a physician experienced with adoption," but many do not. However, like parenting a birth child, each child and each family situation is unique. As a result, "preadoption consultations" often review limited information and attempt to describe the range of potential postadoptive outcomes (Mason et al., 2014).

TRANSITION CONSIDERATIONS

With any child transitioning to a new foster or adoptive family, many factors impact a child's transition, including but not limited to each child's age and previous experiences as well as

TABLE 14.2 Risk and Protective Factors That May Impact Developmental and Behavioral Outcomes for Adopted Children

Preadoptive Factors
Genetic factors (e.g., cognitive abilities, learning disabilities, mental health concerns)
Prenatal health (e.g., maternal nutrition, prenatal exposure to substances of abuse, prescription medications)
Preadoptive living situation (e.g., orphanage, foster care, birth family, presence or absence of at least one nurturing caretaker/role model/protector)
Preadoptive medical concerns (e.g., unremediated hearing loss or vision loss, malnutrition)
Postadoptive Factors
Family factors (e.g., parental emotional attunement capacity, fiscal and time capacity, number of caretakers/children in the home)
Developmental supports (e.g., access to typical play, speech and language supports such as early invention programs, special education system [individualized education plan, 504], and remedial supports such as speech-language, occupational therapy, physical therapy)
Mental health supports (e.g., trauma-based cognitive behavioral therapy, behavioral supports for symptoms of autism, psychoeducation for child/family regarding postadoptive grief/loss and identity development)
Relationship support for family (e.g., adoption competent therapists understanding and supporting families by suggesting "when to worry and when to not")
Community supports (e.g., routine family/friends for family, especially friends/families who look like adoptee/adoptive family; friends with a history of adoption)

the capacity of each receiving family to support any given child. For example, if a child is transitioning to a family whom the child knows, the immediate transition may be a bit smoother as the caretaker(s) and the child know each other. On the other hand, if a child is transitioning to a completely unknown setting and/or the child speaks a different language than the caretakers or educators, there may be more challenges.

Several behaviors are quite common for foster or adoptive children transitioning from neglectful and/or abusive situations to a new setting.

Feeding Challenges

Children with a history of nutritional neglect and/or rigid feeding schedules with limited flexibility regarding their eating time and food variety may present as voracious eaters in a setting with ample food security. Some children may not sense hunger or satiety, but rather react to seeing food preparation with panic. Families can support children by at least initially encouraging them to eat when requested (unless a child is overeating to the point of vomiting, which suggests a need for portion control by caretakers) and offering healthy snacks whenever desired. For older children, this may also include providing portable packages of snacks to take on trips, to school, and whenever away from a ready food supply.

Sleep Problems

Children experiencing neglect in their home settings may either be left in cribs or expected to regulate their sleep independently while their environment is unpredictable. Self-soothing habits may include rocking at bedtime or seeking another person with whom to sleep. For children exposed to yelling, domestic violence, sirens, or alarms during the night, hypervigilance to sounds is common. Families can support children by developing healthy sleep hygiene strategies (e.g., consistent sleep schedule, limitation of screens/distractions prior to bedtime and in sleeping quarters, and allowing children to check in as needed with parents while staying in their room [even if it means having parents sleep in their room]).

Need for Control

Children who have lived with parents who are not able to adequately care for themselves, for example, due to impairment from mental health concerns or substance abuse, may present as expert caretakers of siblings or even of foster or adoptive parents (referred to as parentification). Parents can be encouraged to overtly explain the parent-child dynamic, emphasizing that going forward in a foster or adoptive home caring for other siblings is the role of a parent.

DEVELOPMENTAL AND BEHAVIORAL OUTCOMES WITHIN THE CONTEXT OF ADOPTION

For children with a history of adoption, preadoptive and postadoptive risk factors (see Table 14.2) and a child's trajectory in the adoption process may impact a child's outcomes (Table 14.3). As a result, each adoptive child's circumstances are unique. We recommend the following guiding principles when interpreting the literature on outcomes of children with a history of foster care or adoption. First, while foster care and/or adoption may be a fact of a child's history, the individual

TABLE 14.3 Examples of Postadoptive Developmental/Behavioral Trajectory Contextual Considerations

Factor	Examples of Implications
Age at adoption	Younger children have fewer challenging experiences prior to joining families while older children have more preadoptive life experiences which may be positive or negative.
Number of placements prior to joining permanent family	Transitioning immediately to an adoptive family (norm with private domestic infant adoption) is optimal for children's outcomes when compared with time spent with birth family and/or multiple foster placements or residing in an orphanage.
Time since joining a family	Time transitioning to a new family must be considered within the context of age at transition to a foster or adoptive family. For example, children's growth and development 1 yr after joining a family as a newborn as opposed to 1 yr after joining a family as a 6-yr-old has different implications for a child's likelihood of continued developmental/behavioral change.
Trajectory since joining a family	Honeymoon periods (weeks or month where a child seems to be doing relatively well, without behavioral challenges) for older children may be followed by increased behavioral concerns. But 10 yr after adoption of a toddler, development and behavioral trajectory more likely reflect child's potential.
Current or previous relationship with birth and/or foster families	Intermittent interactions with birth family members may be positive or may contribute to behavioral exacerbations. The loss of meaningful birth/foster family members may have different meaning for children based on their developmental age and experiences.
Stage of adoptive identity development	Transracial/transethnic adoption may trigger identity concerns as early as preschool. Identity development includes integration and making sense of one's history, which may be in opposition to the expectations and desires of joining a family for older adoptees and must consider potential transracial/transethnic placement.

factors related to one's preadoptive and postadoptive experiences are more relevant to predicting long-term outcomes than purely a history of adoption alone. Second, positive and negative preadoptive and postadoptive factors as well as the timing of exposures and transitions dynamically influence developmental trajectories for children with a history of adoption. Therefore the theory of risk and protective mechanisms, which suggests that an accumulation of risk factors contributes to less optimal developmental outcomes while protective factors may buffer negative effects of the risks (Rutter, 2012), provides a useful framework for interpreting this literature. With respect to adoption, transitioning to an adoptive family may reflect a significant protective mechanism and often changes a child's trajectory by decreasing exposure to some risk factors over time. Third, resilience may be a useful concept for understanding variations in outcomes among children with a history of foster care placement or adoption. Resilience can be defined as reduced vulnerability to environmental risk experiences, the overcoming of a stress or adversity, or a relatively good outcome despite risk experiences (Rutter, 2012) and appreciating variations in outcome among individuals who have experienced significant stress or adversity. Despite the challenges in examining long-term developmental and behavioral outcomes for children and young adults with a history of foster care placement and/or adoption, we describe evidence from the literature regarding implications of specific risk factors while emphasizing the unique aspects of each child's experience. We then review the limitations of the current literature and identify opportunities for future research.

Cognitive and Educational Outcomes Following Adoption

Cognitive abilities are influenced by genetic and environmental factors throughout childhood and adolescence. Largely positive outcomes have been described for domestically adopted infants with respect to both development and attachment security. Research also suggests that the majority of children adopted at older ages with special needs have positive outcomes with their adoptive families. Joining a caring and nurturing family, whether via birth or adoption, is a protective factor; but for some children, even the most optimal family environment will not completely ameliorate preadoptive experiences.

Studies examining the heritability of cognitive abilities often use "adoption status" as a predictor variable. However, one metaanalysis reviewing 62 studies and including 77,767 adopted children (van Ijzendoorn et al., 2005) considered the potential positive or negative impact of adoption at various ages on cognitive (intelligence quotient [IQ]) and academic outcomes for children and adults. Their study suggested that adoption alone was not a predictor of IQ. Specifically, they found that overall IQ of adopted children did not vary significantly from their nonadopted environmental siblings or peers.

Risk for learning disabilities has been widely described in the adoptive population. The same metanalysis described earlier (van IJzendoorn et al., 2005) found that despite no statistically significant difference in mean IQ score between those who had been adopted and the general population, adoptive status doubled a child's chance of having learning disabilities requiring special education or other services (12.8% for children with a history of adoption vs. 5.5% for nonadopted children). Statistics from the United Kingdom describe that children with a history of adoption do worse academically than their peers when controlled for possible confounders such as IQ (Teyhan et al., 2018). In addition, adoption after the age of 1 year predicted less optimal school achievement when compared with nonadopted peers. Other factors associated with learning disabilities such as family history were not examined. Importantly, for older children with a history of international adoption, it may take 4 to 6 years or more before children have achieved a communicative language level in their new primary language. The experience for an older adopted child of losing a primary language and acquiring a new primary language in the adopted home and educational setting is far more challenging than for a child who is becoming bilingual while adding a second language but continuing to learn and communicate in a primary language with strong skills. This primary language transition can also impact a child's academic outcomes until the child is fluent in a new language.

Mental Health Issues and Support Seeking Following Adoption

Children with a history of adoption have historically been overrepresented in both inpatient and outpatient mental health facilities. Of adopted children, 5% to 12% are seen in outpatient mental health settings, representing 2.5 to 6 times the population rate for children in general (Haugaard, 1998). It is most likely that this disparity reflects a complex combination of genetic and environmental risk factors (gene-environment correlation) (Lehto et al., 2020). Also, on average, adoptive families have increased financial capacity to access support (Hellerstedt et al., 2008) and may have a lower threshold for engaging with mental health professionals to access services. In some cases access to mental health services may be transient and/or required to address urgent transition issues. For example, for children with a history of domestic public adoption, ongoing counseling after they join a new family may be an expected part of the transition process. Children with known significant trauma history or anxiety/mood issues often benefit from long-term therapy, but accessing support at the time of transition may not represent a long-term mental health need.

Although questions are frequently asked about mental health outcomes given a child's history of adoption in childhood, other factors may also predict behavioral outcomes than a child's adoptive status. For example, certain risk factors (e.g., prenatal substance exposure, preplacement deprivation, older age at adoptive placement) increase a child's likelihood of social and emotional concerns in childhood and beyond. Increasing age (especially adoption >24 months of age) and history of multiple adversities at the time of adoption have been associated with an increased risk of both internalizing and externalizing symptoms (Fisher, 2015). Analysis of data provided for the National Longitudinal Study of Adolescent Health suggests that early maltreatment and peer-family relations were associated with antisocial behavior, but adoption status alone contributed little or no additional predictive power (Grotevant et al., 2006). Although, overall, epidemiologic studies suggest that adoptees are at increased risk of behavioral and mental health concerns, type of adoption may also impact the relative degree of risk.

One metaanalysis (Juffer & van IJzendoorn, 2005) considered behavior problems and mental health referrals for children with a history of international adoption or domestic adoption in contrast to nonadopted controls in a range of developed countries (Europe, North America, Asia) and reviewed 64 articles regarding behavioral problems and 34 articles about mental health referrals published between 1961 and 2004. The authors drew four main conclusions. First, adoptees (n = 25,281 cases; 80,260 controls) were more likely to present with behavioral problems than nonadoptees, although effect sizes were small (d, 0.16–0.24). Second, adoptees were overrepresented in mental health settings. Third, international adoptees demonstrated more behavioral concerns than nonadopted controls, but effect sizes were small (d, 0.07–0.11). Fourth, international adoptees showed fewer total externalizing and internalizing behavior problems than domestic adoptees and were less often referred to mental health services (international adoptees d, 0.37; domestic adoptees d, 0.81).

One systematic review suggested that at least a subpopulation of children with a history of international adoption are at greater risk of long-term developmental, behavioral, and emotional concerns when compared to the general population (Cederblad et al., 1999). This comprehensive review, commissioned by the Swedish government, suggested that children with a history of international adoption have a two to three times greater chance of later psychiatric problems and relationship difficulties when compared with their nonadopted peers. In general, the older a child was at the time of adoption, the greater the risk of later being identified as having psychiatric or social adjustment concerns. Although several studies do not support a significantly greater risk for major developmental and psychiatric concerns after international adoption, sampling bias and validity of outcome measurements may have influenced the conclusions reached in some studies. Cederblad concluded that a small proportion of the adoptees may show severe symptoms and may be overrepresented in clinical samples, whereas many children who are healthy and develop well are only documented in larger cohort studies.

Perception of mental health concerns can vary depending on the reporter. For example, one study examining the mental health of US adolescents adopted both domestically and internationally under 2 years of age (Keyes et al., 2008) looked at parent, teacher, and child self-reports and used a structured diagnostic interview (Diagnostic Interview for Children and Adolescents [DICA]) to compare adolescents' profiles with *Diagnostic and Statisical Manual of Mental Disorders*, fourth edition (*DSM-IV*) diagnostic criteria for behavioral and emotional concerns. Despite some limitations in their approach, the researchers found that most individuals adopted as infants did not meet diagnostic criteria for any disorder, but a subset of adoptees appeared to be at risk for externalizing disorders (effect size 0.18–0.46.) For example, the odds of meeting criteria for oppositional defiant disorder (ODD) or ADHD were approximately twice as high in this study's adoptees compared with nonadoptees. In contrast, the prevalence of conduct disorder, major depressive disorder, and separation anxiety disorder were not associated with adoption status. Interestingly, even though children adopted internationally joined their families at significantly later ages than domestic adoptees, they were at statistically less risk of externalizing concerns compared to domestic adoptees after controlling for other variables, including family socioeconomic status and gender. It is also noteworthy that teachers rated international adoptees as more anxious than nonadoptees, although parents and children did not report anxiety symptoms. Overall, adolescents with a history of adoption (whether domestic or international) in this study were significantly more likely to have had contact with a mental health professional (approximately twice as likely) compared with nonadopted peers.

As a typical part of the identity development process, adolescents naturally are expected to consider who they are in the world, including how they came to be part of an adoptive family and making sense of their adoptive history, which may impact the degree of testing and acting out behaviors in adolescence. Some investigators have described that children who have been residing with their family for more than 12 years demonstrated fewer externalizing behaviors. For transracial adoptees, it has been hypothesized that given obvious differences in physical appearance when compared with their adoptive parent(s), greater awareness of their adoptive status may contribute to increased behavioral concerns prior to adolescence (Juffer, 2006). In addition to a greater awareness of their adoptive status, transracially adopted youth face different hurdles in their processes of identity development. Successfully navigating these hurdles, or struggling to cope with them, may play an important role in their need for more mental health support. Furthermore, transracially adopted youth are much more likely to be exposed to racism and discrimination within and outside of multiracial families. Santana et al. (2007) found that after adjusting for age, sex, and socioeconomic status, adolescents who reported *ever* perceiving discrimination in their lives were 97% more likely to also report symptoms of major depression and 69% more likely to report feeling unhappy, as compared to individuals who did not report discrimination. Again, it is critical to note that the nature of international adoption and the acceptability of transracial adoption have changed dramatically over the past several decades and therefore the generalizability of existing studies is limited.

Fewer studies have examined the complex relationship between birth family history, adoptive family history, and substance abuse. One study suggests that a birth parent history of substance use approximately doubles the odds of an adopted person's history of substance use compared to baseline population risk. Interestingly, birth sibling history of drug use and adoptive sibling history of drug use were nearly identical in impacting an adoptee's risk of substance use (odds ratio [OR] 1.84 for birth siblings; OR 1.95 for adoptive siblings) (Kendler et al., 2012). In other words both birth and adoptive family factors significantly impact one's use of substances.

Impact of Preadoptive Deprivations: Lessons Learned From Studies of Previously Institutionalized Children

Studies of previously institutionalized children provide unique insight into resilience and vulnerability among children. Both resilience and vulnerability to severe deprivation have been described by researchers examining the postadoptive trajectory of internationally adopted children with a history of institutionalization.

Deprivation may occur on a range of levels and to various degrees and may have an impact on a child's health and wellbeing on three different planes: (1) basic nutritional, hygiene, and medical needs; (2) stimulation and opportunity to engage with the environment in a way that supports motor, cognitive, language, and social development; and (3) stable interpersonal relationships allowing children to develop an attachment relationship with a consistent caregiver (Nelson et al., 2011). Importantly, although these levels of deprivation may be theoretically described and separated, they are not independent factors in a child's real-life experience. However, an appreciation of these different planes of support or deprivation informs our understanding of factors that may impact children residing with either families or in institutions. Some aspects of a child's preadoptive history are easier to ascertain than others. For example, while access to nutrition can be crudely observed by examining a child's growth chart, access to a stable interpersonal relationship is much harder to quantify. Although it is likely that access to adequate nutrition increases the likelihood of having interpersonal relationships with those providing the nutrition, the degree of deprivation suffered before adoption is essentially impossible to determine for any child and may be significant.

Although all families and child welfare institutions are unique, the overwhelmingly negative long-term impact of institutional life on a child's growth and development has been well described for more than a century in many different countries. Fortunately, children transitioning from living in orphanages to living with foster or adoptive families have demonstrated an immense human capacity for developmental plasticity and recovery of many functions. Three well-designed longitudinal epidemiologic studies examining children adopted from Romania to the United Kingdom and to Canada (Canadian-Romanian study) or transitioning from institutional care to foster care in Romania shed insight on preadoptive experiences and postplacement resiliency.

Taken together, these studies demonstrate significant cognitive, behavioral, and emotional improvement for previously institutionalized children throughout childhood and adolescence—albeit recovery is not always complete. In general, previously institutionalized children have been reported to have relatively higher rates of inattention, hyperactivity, difficulty with emotional regulation, and elevated levels of anxiety as well as difficulties later in life with intimate social attachments, emotional regulation, and interpretation of facial expression (Zeanah et al., 2011). In general, most children are expected to demonstrate healthy attachments with their adoptive parents, although the classification of their attachment relationship with their adoptive parent is more likely to be insecure (Fox et al., 2017). Indiscriminate friendliness is common (more than two-thirds of previously institutionalized preschool children) and may persist for years following adoption (Fox et al., 2017). Despite an increased risk of long-term concerns on a population level, cognitive and emotional improvement following transition to adoptive families is still expected for the majority of children transitioning to a foster or adoptive family. Similarly, it is expected that children without a history of institutionalization, but with some degree of deprivation, may also experience some degree of postadoptive recovery of functioning. Delays in or variations from the normal progression of a child's development prior to adoption have been attributed to multiple factors common for children residing in institutions or depriving environments, including but not limited to malnutrition, emotional neglect via lack of a consistent emotional connection with caretakers, and lack of developmentally stimulating opportunities or experiences. Additional factors such as prenatal exposure to alcohol, environmental exposures (including lead), and genetic or neurologic disorders may also cause or contribute to children's developmental outcomes, although these factors may not be identified prior to adoption. In general, postadoptive improvements of children's developmental skills and behaviors are routinely expected when children join their families even following a history of institutionalization. However, persistent developmental or behavioral concerns after years of residing with adoptive parents may represent innate disorders, irreversible consequences of early life experiences, or a combination.

Certain factors, such as quality of care and length of institutionalization, are especially predictive of outcomes. Both historical and contemporary studies confirm a relationship between length of time and quality of care received while a child resides in an institution and that child's long-term health and development following adoption. Length of time residing in an institution is positively correlated with a child's risk of presenting with developmental, behavioral, and emotional concerns after international adoption (Bos et al., 2011; Rutter, 2012; Zeanah et al., 2011). In one study examining children with a history of residing in Romanian orphanages timing of placement with foster families correlated with improvements in cognitive, language, behavioral, emotional, and attachment outcomes and were most significant for children with the least time in an orphanage (Smyke et al., 2010; Zeanah & Humphreys, 2018). Longitudinal studies of children adopted from Romanian orphanages into adoptive families in the United Kingdom suggested no measurable differences between children adopted prior to 6 months of age and age-matched peers without a history of institutionalization. Other investigators have found that with less depriving environments, outcomes for children adopted at less than 12 or 24 months were indistinguishable from noninstitutionalized peers. Quality of care provided in an institution is also correlated with children's postadoptive outcomes, as orphanages associated with improved child health and development outcomes typically provide children with adequate nutrition and health care, a lower child-to-caregiver ratio, a lower total number of caregivers over the life of the child, and caregivers who recognize and respond to the distress and vocalizations of children (Bos et al., 2011). Unfortunately, despite this well-documented fact, most children residing in an institution do not experience preferred institutional conditions or high-quality foster care (McCall et al., 2012).

Although concerns with self-regulation have been widely described for previously institutionalized children (Juffer & van Ijzendoorn, 2005), there is a fair amount of variability with respect to outcomes described in different populations. Zeanah et al. (2011) have estimated that approximately 20% of previously institutionalized children (compared with ~6% of US children) will reach a clinical threshold for an anxiety disorder, while 19% of previously institutionalized children (compared with ~9% of US children) meet criteria for ADHD (Roskam et al., 2014). Internalizing concerns (such as anxiety or depression) have been described in some samples of previously institutionalized children (Casey et al., 2009), while others have not described an increase in such concerns for previously institutionalized children (Johnson et al., 2010). Some studies have suggested that internalizing symptoms (vs. externalizing symptoms) are much more likely to improve after joining a stable family (Bos et al., 2011; Zeanah et al., 2011), but follow-up into adolescence has not yet been described.

Relative to children remaining in orphanage care, previously institutionalized children demonstrated dramatic improvements in developmental domains over time despite well-described growth and developmental delays at the time of joining families (Groark & McCall, 2011). Long-lasting developmental concerns for previously institutionalized children have specifically been described for children adopted after 6 months of age. Despite overall cognitive competence, specific vulnerabilities have been described for previously institutionalized children, including relative weaknesses with executive functioning, language, and memory (Fox et al., 2017).

Mental health concerns remained for children transitioning out of foster care despite developmental and cognitive improvements. Even in preschool years, a substantial number of children with a history of institutionalization presented with diagnosable psychiatric disorders (53% of children ever institutionalized vs. 22% of children never institutionalized). However, relatively shortly after transitioning to foster care homes, children demonstrated greater attention to tasks and greater positive affect in comparison to their still institutionalized peers (Bos et al., 2011). Children transitioned to caring and committed foster families from institutions (at a mean age of 22 months) were comparable to never institutionalized peers with resolution of internalizing symptoms (anxiety, mood symptoms). The impact on improvement of internalizing symptoms was especially notable for girls. Unfortunately, a similar impact of foster care was not noted for externalizing behavioral symptoms for children of either gender, suggesting that these symptoms are less amenable to recovery by transitioning to new living circumstances (Bos et al., 2011).

Limitations and Current Knowledge Gaps

Predicting future developmental, behavioral, and mental health outcomes for children with a history of foster care and/or adoption is challenging for a variety of reasons. Importantly, children may experience a wide range of life circumstances, including risk and resilience factors before joining their foster or adoptive families that may have an impact on their later health, development, and long-term potential and outcomes, including prenatal substance exposure and trauma (see Chapters 15, 37, and 56). As a result, outcomes for children with a history of foster care and/or adoption vary.

Importantly, when considering possible long-term outcomes for children with a history of foster care and/or adoption, it is critical to acknowledge that the penultimate long-term outcomes relevant for any child are in fact how they function in adulthood, not the behaviors noted shortly or even several years after transition to a family. However, adult outcome studies considering experiences of foster care or adoption in childhood are limited. Published reports primarily reflect the experiences of populations of children who joined their families decades earlier than children currently being adopted, whose experiences are different. The landscape of foster care as well as that of domestic and international adoption, including preadoptive and postadoptive experiences and preparation of both children and families, has changed dramatically over the past several generations, most notably with an increase in open adoptions and changes in international adoption. As a result, even post–foster care and postadoption outcomes currently available and described for individuals in adulthood may not be entirely reflective of current preadoptive experiences and post-adoptive experiences of children and adolescents with a contemporary history of foster care and/or adoption. Additionally, evidence about the outcomes of children with a history of foster care and/or adoption is typically based on population level outcomes, whereas individual outcomes are harder to predict for any given child.

Ideally, studies of long-term outcomes following foster care or adoption of a child would consider child, family, and geographic specific variables as they may impact developmental, behavioral, and emotional outcomes for children from infancy through adulthood (see Tables 14.2 and 14.3). Relevant postadoptive outcomes may include those measurable in childhood (e.g., cognitive and learning abilities) and later functional outcomes (e.g., employment status, emotional health in adulthood) as well as considering issues that may impact identity development (e.g., impact of adoption and transracial adoption on identity development) well into adulthood. Unfortunately, to date no study has carefully examined preadoptive genetics and experiences, postadoptive experiences, and individual, family, or community variables impacting long-term developmental, academic, or emotional outcome in adults with a history of adoption.

IDENTITY DEVELOPMENT CONSIDERATIONS POSTADOPTION

Ethnic/Racial Identity

Ethnic/racial identity (ERI) is important when considering transracial and transethnic foster care and adoption. ERI refers to the personal attitudes toward and feelings of belonging to a particular racial and/or ethnic group and affects development across the life span, including social-emotional wellbeing. Stronger ERI predicts higher levels of self-esteem and overall wellbeing into adulthood (Ghavami et al., 2011). Importantly, positive ERI development can provide a buffer to the well-documented, widespread deleterious effects of perceived discrimination (see Marks et al., 2015 for a systematic review).

The development of one's ethnic identity is a dynamic process that occurs through exploration and commitment. Parental support (Radina & Cooney, 2000) and family ethnic socialization (Umaña-Taylor & Fine, 2004) can facilitate ERI and are important roles for adoptive families. ERI can promote adjustment and buffer the negative social-emotional, physical health, academic, and wellbeing effects of discrimination (Castle et al., 2011; Marks et al., 2015).

When considering other ways in which foster and adoptive parents can support ERI development, it is important to consider *socialization*, which is the main factor by which children and adolescents are exposed to, taught about, and internalize the skills, behavioral patterns, and values needed to function in the culture in which they are growing up (Maccoby, 2007). For adopted children, particularly with relation to ERI development, this includes socialization to their home culture. When interviewed as adults about their experiences in developing their identities in White adoptive families (Zhou et al., 2011), common themes arose among Korean adult adoptees regarding their adoptive families' attempts at socialization. These themes may transfer to other groups and can inform guidance for families.

- **Limited exposure:** Although their adoptive parents attempted to increase ethnic socialization to their home culture by taking them to Korean restaurants, enrolling them in cultural camps, and occasionally celebrating Korean holidays at home, adoptees reported that their exposure to Korean culture was infrequent and insufficient. In considering these findings, adoptive transracial and transethnic adoptive parents should seek out cultural socialization experiences for their children with regular frequency and across a wide range of modalities. Prospective adoptive parents should learn about their child's culture of birth and examine socialization experiences for their children that may include more in-depth exposures to a child's racial and ethnic background.
- **Language:** Limited proficiency in the language of the participants' home culture created a barrier to accessing cultural experiences, led to feelings of inauthenticity, and inhibited socialization experiences and ERI development. While individual family factors may differ, specifically, with a child's desire to learn the language of the home culture, exposure to and opportunities to learn that language are important for families to consider.
- **Colorblindness and racism:** Adult adoptees in the sample reported that their families either adopted a colorblindness mentality (e.g., not acknowledging their adopted children as people of color and thus avoiding necessary conversations about race and discrimination) or one of open racism and biased attitudes toward other racial/ethnic groups and people of color, in an attempt to erase racial and ethnic differences in their adoptive families. Transracial/ethnic families should have regular open conversations about race, racism, and stereotypes that are relevant to their children of color. Such factors can promote family socialization and ERI.

The phenotypical differences between transracially or transethnically adopted youth and their families may make adoption status more salient, much sooner than children who are not transracially or transethnically adopted. However, parents can use these differences, most likely to be noticed by younger children asking, "Why do I look different from mommy/daddy?", to start early conversations about adoption, race, and identity, openly and honestly.

Much of the research to date has focused on transethnic adoptions, with a strong focus on culture (e.g., Asian children adopted into White families), despite the growing number of transracially adopted children. Researchers have highlighted the complexity of racial socialization and ERI development faced by adopted children of color and their White families. While these factors share some overlap with transethnically adopted youth, racial socialization varies in unique ways from cultural and ethnic socialization and should be treated as a distinct process. Future research should examine different factors faced by adoptees who are of a different race than their adoptive families.

Adoption Identity Discussions

Children with a history of adoption will incorporate this fact into their life story. For some children, this is just a fact of their history. But for others, especially if they have previously resided with their birth family or if they have ongoing contact with their birth parents and/or extended birth family members, questions may arise more frequently. One important consideration for families is to realize that children's own adoption story is theirs to share, not the family's. Understanding the difference between secrecy (where a child is not aware of the history) and privacy (sharing information as needed, such as in medical settings and in response to a child's questions) can be helpful. For example, multiethnic families may be asked questions about adoption by strangers and can choose to respond that they are not interested in discussing the topic. Caring family members, friends, and strangers may ask questions out of curiosity, but that does not mean each question needs to be answered.

Many events in the life of a child, adolescent, or adult may trigger questions about the adoptive history. School assignments discussing a family tree and genetics discussions (e.g., eye color) may highlight one's differences from the adoptive family. Life events such as considering marriage and having a child may also raise questions about one's own birth history. Siblings joining the family (whether by birth or adoption) and adoption of a pet may also raise new questions. Adoptive parents can support their children by being open to answering questions and preparing for some routinely expected questions. Given the particular importance of identity development in multiethnic youth, these questions may happen earlier, or with more frequency, in response to life events, questions from outside observers, or in response to incidents of racism or discrimination.

Some individuals with a history of adoption who do not have an open adoption are interested in searching to learn as much as possible about their birth family, which has become ever easier with the evolution of technology and social media. Some people also reach out to meet their birth family, which may be declined or accepted, and they may even meet with their birth family. Many adopted people find it helpful to work with a therapist experienced with search and reunification processes to support them along the way.

PRACTICE AND POLICY IMPLICATIONS

Clinical research provides guidance regarding practice and policy for children raised without permanent parents, including those with a history of institutionalization and/or foster care. Infants and young children reared in most child welfare institutions experience delays in their physical, neurobiologic, cognitive, and social-emotional development (McCall et al., 2012). For children who transition to family environments (i.e., adoptive or foster families), immediate and substantial catchup is observed in all domains. However, delays in all developmental domains can persist at higher-than-expected rates even after transitioning to families. As a result, children should be referred for early intervention, school-based supports, and mental health services if questions arise.

A range of longitudinal studies suggest that transition to a caring and supportive family, whether adoptive or foster, promotes improved developmental progress for children who have experienced abuse and neglect. Increased time in a challenging environment and age at placement with a foster or adoptive family are important predictors of outcomes. As a result, child welfare policies need to reduce the amount of time any child spends in a neglectful and/or abusive environment.

CONCLUSION

Foster care placement and/or adoption is an important albeit single aspect of an individual's story. Children presenting with developmental and behavioral challenges who also have a history of foster care and/or adoption like James in the opening vignette, are expected to make progress after transitioning to a new family. However, early trauma, prenatal substance exposure, and other experiences prior to transitioning to a family may contribute to potential developmental and behavioral challenges that must be addressed in the broader context of the individual's unique traits, family, community, and society. Clinicians can play an important role in promoting optimal outcomes for children and their families through preadoption planning and postadoption support. Ultimately, practitioners and policies must work to ensure all children have access to supportive and nurturing caregivers, but professionals should appreciate that even the most healthy environment and developmental supports may not be able to remediate some children's challenges prior to transitioning to a foster or adoptive setting. Early identification and treatment of potential learning and regulatory difficulties as well as supporting healthy adoptive and racial/ethnic identity are important in supporting all children with a history of foster care and/or adoption.

REFERENCES

Bos, K., Zeanah, C., Fox, N., Drury, S., McLaughlin, K., & Nelson, C. (2011, Jan/Feb). Psychiatric outcomes in young children with a history of institutionalization. *Harvard Review of Psychiatry*, 15–24.

Casey, B. J., Glatt, C. E., Tottenham, N., Soliman, F., Bath, K., Amso, D., Altemus, M., Pattwell, S., Jones, R., Levita, L., McEwen, B., Magariños, A. M., Gunnar, M., Thomas, K. M., Mezey, J., Clark, A. G., Hempsted, B. L., & Lee, F. S. (2009). Brain-derived neurotrophic factor as a model system for examining gene by environment interactions across development. *Neuroscience, 164*, 108–120. https://doi.org/10.1016/j.neuroscience.2009.03.081.

Castle, H., Knight, E., & Watters, C. (2011). Ethnic identity as a protective factor for looked after and adopted children from ethnic minority groups: A critical review of the literature. *Adoption Quarterly*, *14*(4), 305–325.

Cerderblad, M., Höök, B., Irhammar, M, & Mercke, A. (1999). Mental health in international adoptees as teenagers and young adults. An epidemiological study. *Journal of Child Psychology and Psychiatry,* 1239–1248.

Child Welfare Information Gateway. (2020). *Foster care statistics 2018*. US Department of Health and Human Services, Administration for Children and Families, Children's Bureau. https://www.childwelfare.gov/pubPDFs/foster.pdf.

Fisher. P. A. (2015). Review: Adoption, fostering, and the needs of looked-after and adopted children. *Child and Adolescent Mental Health*, *20*(1), 5012. https://doi.org/10.1111/camh.12084.

Fox, N. A., Nelson, C. A., & Zeanah, C. H. (2017). The effects of psychosocial deprivation on attachment: Lessons from the Bucharest Early Intervention Project. *Psychodynamic Psychiatry*, *45*(4), 441–450. https://doi.org/10.1521/pdps.2017.45.4.441.

Ghavami, N., Fingerhut, A., Peplau, L. A., Grant, S. K., & Wittig, M. A. (2011). Testing a model of minority identity achievement, identity affirmation, and psychological well-being among ethnic minority and sexual minority individuals. *Cultural Diversity & Ethnic Minority Psychology, 17,* 79–88. https://doi.org/10.1037/a0022532.

Groark, C. J., & McCall, R. B. (2011). Implementing changes in institutions to improve young children's development. *Infant Mental Health Journal, 32*(5), 509–525. https://doi.org/10.1002/imhj.20310.

Grotevant, H., van Dulmen, M., Dunbar, N., Nelson-Christinedaugter J., Christensen, M., Fan, X., & Miller, B. C. (2006). Antisocial behavior of adoptees and nonadoptees: Prediction from early history and adolescent relationships. *Journal of Research on Adolescence*, *16*, 105–131.

Haugaard. J. J. (1998). Is adoption a risk factor for the development of adjustment problems? *Clinical Psychology Review*, *18*(1), 47–69.

Hellerstedt, W. L., Madsen, N. J., Gunnar, M. R., Grotevant, H. D., Lee, R. M., & Johnson, D. E. (2008). The International Adoption Project: Population-based surveillance of Minnesota parents who adopted children internationally. *Maternal and Child Health Journal, 12*, 162–171.

Johnson, D. E., Guthrie, D., & Smyke, A. T., (2010). Growth and associations between auxology, caregiving environment, and cognition in socially deprived Romanian children randomized to foster vs ongoing institutional care. *Archives of Pediatrics & Adolescent Medicine, 164*, 507–516.

Juffer, F. (2006). Children's awareness of adoption and their problem behavior in families with 7-year old internationally *adopted children. Adoption Quarterly, 9*(2–3), 1–22. https://doi.org/10.1300/J145v09n02_01.

Juffer, F., & van Ijzendoorn, M. H. (2005). Behavior problems and mental health referrals of international adoptees: A meta-analysis. *JAMA, 293*(20), 2501–2515.

Kendler, K. S., Sundquist, K., Ohlsson, H., Palmér, K., Maes, H., Winkleby, M. A., & Sundquist, J. (2012). Genetic and familial environmental influences on the risk for drug abuse: A national Swedish adoption study. *Archives of General Psychiatry, 69(7),* 690–697. https://doi.org/10.1001/archgenpsychiatry.2011.2112.

Keyes, M., Sharma, A., Elkins, I. J., Iacono, W. G., & McGue, M. (2008). The mental health of US adolescents adopted in infancy. *Archive of Pediatrics & Adolescent Medicine, 162*(5), 419–425.

Lehto, K., Hägg, S., Lu, D., Karlsson, R., Pedersen, N., & Mosing, M. (2020). Childhood adoption and mental health in adulthood: The role of gene-environment correlations and interactions in the UK biobank. *Biological Psychiatry, 87*(8), 708–716.

Maccoby, E. E. (2007). Historical overview of socialization research and theory. In J. E. Grusec & P. D. Hastings (Eds.), *Handbook of socialization: Theory and research*. Guliford Press.

Marks, A. K., Ejesi, K., McCullough, M. B., & Garcia Coll, C. (2015). The development and implications of racism and discrimination. In R. M. Lerner & M. E. Lamb (Eds.), *Handbook of child psychology and developmental science, socioemotional processes* (7th ed.). John Wiley & Sons.

Mason, P. W., Johnson, D. E., & Prock, L. A. (2014). *Adoption medicine: Caring for children and families. American Academy of Pediatrics Council on Foster Care. Adoption and kinship care.* American Academy of Pediatrics.

McCall, R., van IJzendoorn, M., Juffer, F., Groark, C., & Groza, V. (2012). *Children without permanent parents: Research, practice and policy*. Wiley-Blackwell.

Nelson, C. A., III, Bos, K., Gunnar, M. R., & Sonuga-Barke, E. J. (2011). The neurobiological toll of early human deprivation. *Monographs of the Society for Research in Child Development, 76*(4), 127–146. https://doi.org/10.1111/j.1540-5834.2011.00630.

Radina, E., & Cooney, T. (2000). Relationship quality between multiracial adolescents and their biological parents. *American Journal of Orthopsychiatry, 70*, 445–454.

Roskam, I., Stievenart, M., Tessier, R., Muntean, A., Escobar, M. J., Santelices, M. P., Juffer, F., Van Ijzendoorn, M. H., & Pierrehumbert, B. (2014). Another way of thinking about ADHD: The predictive role of early attachment deprivation in adolescents' level of symptoms. *Social Psychiatry and Psychiatric Epidemiology, 49*(1), 133–144. https://doi.org/10.1007/s00127-013-0685-z.

Rutter. M. (2012). Resilience as a dynamic concept. *Development and Psychopathology, 24*, 335–344. https://doi.org/10.1017/S0954579412000028.

Santana, V., Almeida-Filho, N., Roberts, R., & Cooper, S. P. (2007). Skin color, perception of racism, and depression among adolescents in Brazil. *Child and Adolescent Mental Health, 12,* 125–131. https://doi.org/10.1111/j.1475-3588.2007.00447.x.

Smyke, A. T., Zeanah, C. H., Fox, N. A., Nelson, C. A., & Guthrie, D. (2010). Placement in foster care enhances quality of attachment among young institutionalized children. *Child Development, 81,* 212–223. https://doi.org/10.1111/j.1467-8624.2009.01390.x.

Teyhan, A., Wijedasa, D., & Macleaod, J. (2018). Adult psychosocial outcomes of men and women who were looked-after or adopted as children: Prospective observational study. *BMJ Open, 8*, 3019095. https://doi.org/10.1136/bmjopen-2017-019095.

Turney, K., & Wildeman, C. (2016). Mental and physical health of children in foster care. *Pediatrics, 138*(5), e20161118.

Umaña-Taylor, A. J., & Fine, M. A. (2004). Examining ethnic identity among Mexican-origin adolescents living in the United States. *Hispanic Journal of Behavioral Sciences, 26*, 36–59. https://doi.org/10.1177/0739986303262143.

van Ijzendoorn, M. H., Juffer, F., & Klein Poelhuis, C. W. (2005). Adoption and cognitive development: A meta-analytic comparison of adopted and non-adopted children's IQ and school performance. *Psychological Bulletin, 131*, 301–316.

Wildeman, C., & Emanuel, N. (2014). Cumulative risks of foster care placement by age 18 for US children, 2000–2011. *PLoS One, 9*(3), e92785. https://doi.org/10.1371/journal.pone.0092785. eCollection 2014.

Zeanah, C. H., & Humphreys, K. L. (2018). Child abuse and neglect. *Journal of the American Academy of Child and Adolescent Psychiatry, 57*(9), 637–644. https://doi.org/10.1016/j.jaac.2018.06.007.

Zeanah, C. H., Gunnar, M. R., McCall, R. B., Kreppner, J. M., & Fox, N. A. (2011). Sensitive periods (VI). *Monographs of the Society for Research in Child Development, 76*, 147–162.

Zhou, X., Kim, J., Lee, H., & Lee, R. M. (2011). Korean adoptees as parents: Intergenerationality of ethnic, racial, and adoption socialization. *Family Relations, 70*(2), 637–632. https://doi.org/10.1111/fare.12439.

15

Trauma, Resilience, and Child Development

Marsheena Murray and Robert D. Keder

For additional material related to the content of this chapter, please see Chapters 22 and 115.

VIGNETTE 1

Krystal is an 8-year-old girl with an extensive trauma history. Local Child Protective Services (CPS) first removed her from her mother's home at the age of 2 years for neglect and parental substance abuse. After 8 months she was reunified with her mother, who was engaged to her current boyfriend. Krystal remained in the care of her mother from age 3 to 8 years and then was removed again due to reports of sexual abuse by her stepbrother and witnessing domestic violence between her mother and stepfather. Once again in CPS custody, Krystal also reported a history of continued parental substance abuse and neglect.

Krystal presents to your outpatient clinic at age 8 years, during this second placement in foster care. Krystal was referred for an assessment due to academic problems, severe inattention, poor focus, hyperactivity, and at times aggressive behaviors. She dislikes school and has past diagnoses of oppositional defiant disorder and bipolar disorder. Her treatments have focused on these diagnoses but have been relatively unsuccessful. Her CPS worker asks for an assessment and treatment recommendations.

VIGNETTE 2

Miguel is an 8-year-old boy with an extensive trauma history. He arrived in the southwestern United States at age 2 years as a refugee from a country in Central America. He and his older sister were separated from their mother at the border and later placed in the care of their maternal aunt, who lives in a New England state and holds a green card. He endured years of food insecurity and was noted to have several developmental delays when he arrived at his aunt's care. Early Intervention (IDEA Part C) services were started. Miguel qualified for special education services on his third birthday, but services were rescinded on his sixth birthday due to his progress. His mother and father were later able to join him at age 6 years and live with him, his aunt, and his aunt's partner. A year later, his mother died of complications of late diagnosed ovarian cancer, and his father was incarcerated and deported for involvement in drug trafficking. He has been working with a school social worker for support since then.

Now at age 8, Miguel is an honor roll student and loves his teachers and friends at school and is very close with his aunt. He was always an easygoing child but started experiencing anxiety since his mother passed away and he was separated from his father. He has maintained his grades, but his weight has increased and he is now overweight for his age. Additionally, his uncle developed problematic drinking behaviors, and his aunt (continued legal guardian) is experiencing domestic violence. They arrive for his routine pediatric well-care visit, and his anxiety and the domestic violence are flagged on clinical screening tools. You are considering your next steps in management as you page your clinic social worker to join you during the visit.

FRAMEWORKS: TRAUMA, TOXIC STRESS, AND RESILIENCE

Trauma

As Krystal's story illustrates, trauma can have a large impact on developing children. Likewise, Miguel's story illustrates several experiences of trauma but different outcomes. In this chapter we examine child development in the context of trauma, adversity, and resilience.

Definition of Trauma

The American Psychological Association defines trauma as "an emotional response to a terrible event like an accident, rape or natural disaster." The Substance Abuse and Mental Health Services Administration (SAMHSA) focuses on three *E*s of trauma: events, experiences of events, and effect. Specifically, the idea is that individual trauma is the result of an event that is experienced as physically or emotionally harmful or life threatening and that has lasting adverse effects on the person's functioning (i.e., mental, physical, social, or emotional). While we recognize other groups may use different definitions of trauma, in this chapter we use this inclusive and comprehensive definition.

Prevalence

In the United States 70% of adults have experienced some form of trauma during their lifetimes (i.e., an estimated 223 million people). In samples taken from individuals receiving behavioral health services the estimates of trauma increase to over 90%. For children, one epidemiologic study found that almost 60% of the youth surveyed experienced one potentially traumatic event in the past year (Finkelhor et al. 2013); 48% had experienced more than one traumatic event.

Types of Trauma

Table 15.1 outlines different types of trauma with definitions and examples. Trauma can be further grouped into one of three categories: acute, chronic, or complex traumas. Acute traumas are events that occur at a specific time and place and are usually short lived (e.g., a car accident, or physical assault that occurs one time). In contrast, chronic traumas are ongoing and occur repeatedly over long periods (e.g., ongoing childhood sexual abuse, witnessing domestic violence). Complex trauma refers to multiple traumatic events, often of an invasive, interpersonal nature. These events are severe and pervasive, such as profound neglect. They may occur early in life and disrupt many aspects of the child's development and the formation of a sense of self. Since these events often occur with a caregiver, they interfere with the child's ability to form a secure attachment. Many aspects of a child's healthy physical and mental development rely on this primary source of safety and stability.

Implications of Trauma

The timing of traumatic experiences may affect outcomes. Early childhood trauma refers to trauma that occurs before the age of 6 years. Experiencing trauma during such a critical developmental period can have a substantial impact. Young children's brains are still rapidly developing, making them more vulnerable to the impact of trauma. Early trauma has been associated with reduced size of the brain cortex, which functions in memory, attention, thinking, language, consciousness, and perceptual awareness.

Trauma has substantial impacts across different domains for developing children. Experiencing trauma can bring forth a wide range of emotional responses, including intense feelings of fear, loss of trust in others, decreased sense of personal safety, guilt, and shame. Table 15.2 delineates the impact of trauma. These presentations may differ based on chronologic age and developmental level or other factors (Box 15.1).

Adverse Childhood Experiences, Toxic Stress, and Adversity

Both Krystal and Miguel, at age 8 years, have experienced multiple ACEs. As you read in this section, you will learn the significant impact that ACEs can play throughout both Krystal's and Miguel's development into adulthood.

TABLE 15.1 Types of Trauma With Definitions and Examples

Trauma Type	Definition	Examples
Abuse	Infliction of injury	Physical abuse: an act that results in physical injury to a child or adolescent Sexual abuse: any interaction between a child and an adult (or another child) in which the child is used for the sexual stimulation of the perpetrator or an observer Emotional abuse: abuse that is emotional in nature Bullying: a deliberate and unsolicited action with the intent of inflicting social, emotional, physical, and/or psychological harm to someone who often is perceived as being less powerful
Neglect	Failure to care for properly	Physical neglect: failure to provide the basic necessities that a child needs to survive and thrive Educational neglect: failure to meet needs with regard to schooling and education Medical neglect: failure to provide necessary medical or mental health treatment
Loss	Death or separation from a loved one	Death of loved one Incarceration of a caregiver
Medical	Medical traumatic stress: trauma responses of children and their families to single or multiple medical events	Admission to an intensive care unit for anaphylaxis Diagnosis of cancer and subsequent treatments
Natural disaster	Weather events that pose life-threatening risks	Hurricanes, earthquakes, tornadoes, wildfires, tsunamis, and floods, as well as extreme weather events such as blizzards, droughts, extreme heat, and wind storms
Violence	The use of physical force to inflict harm	Domestic violence: witnessing violence between mother and a partner Neighborhood violence: witnessing someone being shot at a park or outside of one's home Acts of terrorism: shootings, bombings, or other types of attacks

TABLE 15.2 Examples of the Impact of Trauma on Domains of Wellbeing

Domain	Examples of Impact
Development	Difficulties focusing or learning in school Memory problems
Physical health	Experience stomachaches or headaches Poor appetite, poor growth, or digestive problems
Mental health	Difficulties managing emotions Difficulties navigating and adjusting to life's changes
Relationships and attachment	Inability to trust others Difficulty making/keeping friends

BOX 15.1 Children's Reactions to Trauma

Reactions to trauma will vary depending on multiple factors, including:

- Age and developmental stage
- Temperament
- Perception of danger faced
- Trauma history (cumulative effects)
- Adversities faced following the trauma
- Availability of adults who can offer help, reassurance, and protections

The Origin of ACEs

The Centers for Disease Control and Prevention (CDC) and Kaiser Permanente adverse childhood experiences (ACEs) study is one of the largest and most impactful investigations into childhood abuse and neglect and the subsequent impact on adult health and wellbeing. The original study was conducted at Kaiser Permanente over the course of 2 years (1995–1997). The sample included over 17,000 participants who participated in both physical exams and surveys regarding their childhood experiences and current health status and behaviors (Table 15.3). This study divided trauma into three groups: abuse, neglect, and household challenges. The results indicated that ACEs are common. Specifically, almost two-thirds of participants reported at least one ACE, and more than 20% reported experiencing three or more ACEs. The study findings support a dose-response relationship between ACEs and negative health and wellbeing outcomes (i.e., the more ACEs, the higher the risk for negative outcomes). This study demonstrated a powerful relationship between childhood experiences and adult emotional health, physical health, and major causes of mortality in the United States (Fig. 15.1).

TABLE 15.3 Adverse Childhood Experiences (ACEs)

Abuse	Neglect	Household Dysfunction
Physical	Physical	Divorce/parental separation
Emotional	Emotional	Domestic/partner violence
Sexual		Caregiver with mental health needs
		Caregiver with substance abuse
		Incarcerated caregiver

Role of Race in ACEs

The role of race in ACEs was not specifically addressed in the original CDC/Kaiser study. Race impacts the likelihood of ACEs (Sacks & Murphey, 2018). Specifically, in the United States 61% of Black children and 51% of Hispanic children experienced at least one ACE, compared to 40% of White children and 23% of Asian children. Clearly there is an adverse impact of being a person of color in a society where both systemic and institutional racism are rampant. Racism and discrimination are the foundations of many ACEs, including parental incarceration, neighborhood violence, and poverty.

Neurobiology of Toxic Stress

Advances in the field of genetics over the 20th century inform our understanding of the interplay between nature and nurture. The science of epigenetics demonstrates the interaction between environment and DNA. Gene-environment studies offer insight into why children respond differently to their environments. Two models serve as organizing frameworks. The diathesis-stress model suggests that certain genetic differences

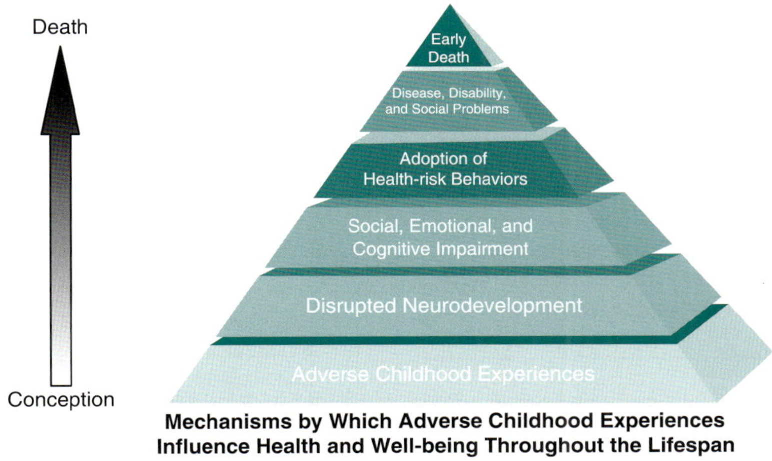

Fig. 15.1 The adverse childhood experiences (ACEs) pyramid. (From http://www.acestudy.org/.)

place individuals at risk for poor outcomes in harsh environments (Caspi et al., 2002). More recently, the differential susceptibility model posits that individuals with certain genetic variations do worse in harsh environments but may have even better outcomes compared to peers without these variations in positive environments (Belsky & Pluess, 2009). While more work is needed, this field enhances our understanding of the interplay of nature, nurture, and health.

Stress physiology offers important insight into the consequences of toxic stress. The physiologic response of the body to stressful situations involves the hypothalamic-pituitary-adrenocortical axis and the sympathetic-adrenomedullary system. These regulate the production of stress hormones: corticotropin-releasing hormone (CRH), cortisol, norepinephrine, and adrenaline in response to activation of the parasympathetic nervous system resulting in elevation of inflammatory cytokines and other mediators. The effects depend on the intensity and duration of stressors presented in relationship to protective factors. They range from brief but adaptive physiologic responses (e.g., increased heart rate, alertness) to long-term maladaptive responses (e.g., wear and tear across organ systems). In regard to the effect of stress and stress responses on young children, the National Scientific Council on the Developing Child developed a framework consisting of three different types of stress responses: positive, tolerable, and toxic. A positive stress response is a normal and healthy response to brief and mild stressors (e.g., first day of school). Positive stress responses when supported by protective, stable, and nurturing relationships offer opportunities for growth and can foster resilience. A tolerable stress response is associated with experiences that are more severe in intensity and/or duration and are often considered nonnormative experiences in children's development. Examples include ACEs as defined in the original CDC/Kaiser study (e.g., parental incarceration) but also include other situations such as natural disasters (e.g., a global pandemic) (see Chapter 22), problems with social-political systems (e.g., racism), and death in a family. Supportive and protective adult relationships can make such experiences tolerable by reducing the cascade of harm caused by stress response systems. A toxic stress response is the result of intense and prolonged or frequent activation of these stress response systems in the absence of protective and supportive adult relationships. Examples include all of those noted for tolerable stress responses. Toxic stress responses during critical periods of development result in changes in brain architecture and derail healthy development (Garner et al., 2012).

Resilience

While both Krystal and Miguel have each experienced complex traumatic events, their outcomes are different. These cases highlight that adversity and trauma alone do not determine developmental outcomes and help introduce resilience.

Defining Resilience

Here we define resilience as the ability to maintain positive outcomes in the face of adversity. Resilience is the result of an interplay of intrinsic and extrinsic factors as well as sets of skills that can be modeled, nurtured, learned, and practiced. However, among all resilience factors the single most common and critical protective factor is the provision of safe, stable, and nurturing relationships (Garner & Saul, 2018). Understanding the roles of risk, adversity, and resilience are fundamental to the field of developmental and behavioral pediatrics. It is through this framework that positive developmental trajectories can be promoted on the individual (clinical) level as well as on a population (public health) level.

Resilience Factors

Resilience factors help explain the different outcomes experienced by Krystal and Miguel. We see that Krystal has experienced several disruptions in her opportunity to maintain and develop a relationship with a protective and nurturing adult. Meanwhile, although Miguel experienced significant disruption in accessing this type of relationship at age 2 years, he has had access to the stability and support of his aunt as well as the positive and supportive climate of his school community.

Resilience represents a complex interaction between intrinsic and extrinsic factors (Boxes 15.2 and 15.3). Understanding these factors allows for promoting resilience on both the individual and the population level. The American Academy of Pediatrics (AAP) emphasizes that safe, stable, and nurturing relationships are the single most important factor in buffering adversity and building resilience (Garner et al., 2021).

Ongoing research has increasingly focused on the vital role of external and ecological factors that promote positive outcomes (Table 15.4). In one study investigators examined the effects of positive childhood experiences, which included children's ability to talk to family about their feelings, knowing that family stands with them during difficult times, participating in and enjoying community traditions, having a sense of belonging in high school, feeling supported by friends, having at least two nonparent adults who take genuine interest in them, and feeling safe and protected by an adult at home (Bethell et al., 2019). This study found that positive

BOX 15.2 Internal/Individual Traits Associated With Resilience

- High self-esteem
- Strong self-efficacy
- Internal locus of control
- External attributions of blame
- Optimism
- Grit (determination in the face of obstacles)
- Cognitive and emotional flexibility
- Reappraisal ability
- Social skills
- Flight inhibition/ability to face fears
- Easygoing temperament
- Sense of belonging

TABLE 15.4 Modifiable Resilience Factors Relevant to Pediatric Clinical Practice

Level	Resilience Factor	Description
Individual	Cognitive traits: positive appraisal style and executive function skills	Positive appraisal styles, defined by optimism and confidence about one's ability to manage adversity, are associated with resilience to adversity. Improved executive function, especially cognitive flexibility and inhibitory control, is also associated with resilience to adverse childhood experiences (ACEs)
Family	Parenting	Responsive parenting and good parental relationships foster resilience. The HPA axis normalizes in traumatized children when parenting improves.
	Maternal mental health	Maternal mental health problems are associated with risk for trauma as well as less sensitive parenting (a resilience factor); identifying and treating maternal psychopathology could foster resilience in children and prevent ACEs.
Individual/family	Self-care skills and household routines	ACEs are associated with poor sleep, nutrition, and exercise habits. Teaching children self-care skills and using consistent routines at home are associated with healthy resilient development.
	Trauma understanding	Educating children and families about trauma in pediatric settings and through trauma-focused interventions builds resilience.

Traub, F., & Boynton-Jarrett, R. (2017). Modifiable resilience factors to childhood adversity for clinical pediatric practice. *Pediatrics, 139*(5).
HPA, Hypothalamic-pituitary-adrenocortical.

childhood experiences were associated with reduced odds of behavioral health problems and increased odds of reporting social support even after adjusting for ACEs.

Recently, Malhi and colleagues (2019) proposed a useful framework that integrates the neurobiologic and psychosocial underpinnings of resilience. The model uses a floodwall as an analogy and consists of four components. First, intrinsic factors from birth (e.g., temperament) form a foundation for resilience. The height of this foundation provides a baseline tolerance for stress that varies among individuals. Second, interconnected neurobiologic and psychosocial constructs (e.g., healthy neurodevelopment and learned behaviors) support resilience. These interconnected constructs form a floodwall or barrier that prevents the stress from overflowing and harming the individual. Third, a supportive environment supports active processing and regulation of neurobiologic and psychosocial factors to build and promote adaptive resilience. Such environments allow individuals to continue to build and support the flood wall of resilience as it experiences adversity. Fourth, the presence of adversity in a magnitude allows for safe testing and implementation of the neurobiologic and psychosocial constructs being built. When the magnitude of adversity (flood waters) exceeds the capacity of the first three components (the foundation, the floodwall, and the adaptive real-time supports) to withstand it, negative outcomes can occur (Malhi et al., 2019).

CLINICAL INTERVENTIONS

Screening, Assessment, and Diagnosis of Trauma

The clinician must properly assess trauma history to ensure accurate diagnoses for Krystal and Miguel. Clinicians can mistake or misinterpret trauma symptoms, which can often result in misdiagnosis.

Screening

Screening can help identify children who have experienced trauma by eliciting trauma-related symptoms. Policymakers, advocates, and clinicians have increasingly called for universal screening for trauma in systems such as pediatric clinics. When conducting universal screening, clinicians must be prepared to link families to further mental health assessment and ensure safety throughout this process by reporting trauma if it has not been reported (i.e., contact CPS), ensuring child safety (e.g., assess risk of suicide among children), and creating a treatment approach (e.g., refer and ensure linkage to services as needed).

Assessment

Ideally the assessment should involve a multidisciplinary team. An ideal team would include medical, behavioral health, and educational expertise with additional support as needed. Box 15.4 includes key steps for conducting a comprehensive assessment of trauma.

Treatment and Trauma-Informed Care

Krystal would likely benefit from receiving a trauma-specific treatment such as trauma-focused cognitive behavioral therapy (TF-CBT). As you read about trauma-informed care, consider how much your clinic/institution implements these principles. Likewise, Miguel and his aunt are experiencing acute trauma, and their safety must be assessed. His anxiety is likely related to a long-term accumulation of trauma.

Definition and Principles of Trauma-Informed Care

It is important to distinguish trauma-focused services from the concept of trauma-informed care. Trauma-focused services or trauma-specific treatments refer to evidence-based and best practice treatment models that facilitate recovery from problems resulting from the experience of trauma. These treatments

BOX 15.3 External/Ecological Supports Associated With Resilience

- Supportive/nurturing attachment to caregivers
- Opportunities for skill building using scaffolding-based approaches
- Opportunities to experience and cope with manageable stressors
- Building healthy emotional self-regulation skills
- Use of faith, cultural, and other traditions to build stability
- Access to family and parenting supports especially for at-risk infant-caregiver dyads
- Access to high-quality early childhood education
- Addressing physiologic needs by addressing food, financial, and housing insecurity
- Access to social-emotional learning curricula
- Engagement at school
- Positive school climate

BOX 15.4 Key Steps for Conducting a Comprehensive Assessment of Trauma

- Assess for a wide range of traumatic events. Determine when traumatic events occurred so that they can be linked to developmental stages.
- Assess for a wide range of symptoms (beyond posttraumatic stress disorder), risk behaviors, functional impairments, and developmental changes.
- Gather information using a variety of methods (clinical interviews, standardized measures, and behavioral observations).
- Gather information from multiple informants (e.g., child, caregivers, teachers, other providers).

directly address the emotional, behavioral, and physiologic impact of trauma on an individual's life and facilitate improvement in related symptoms and functioning: they are designed to treat the consequences of trauma. Given the range of possible responses to trauma, not all patients with trauma histories need to or choose to access trauma-focused services.

In contrast, trauma-informed care is a global, universal precautions approach to providing quality care. Trauma-informed care can be applied to all aspects of health care and to all patients. Trauma-informed care is a strengths-based service delivery framework that is grounded in an understanding of, and responsiveness to, the disempowering impact of experiencing trauma. It seeks to maximize physical, psychological, and emotional safety in all health care encounters, not just those that are specifically trauma focused, and creates opportunities to rebuild a sense of control and empowerment while fostering healing through safe and collaborative patient-clinician relationships. See Box 15.5 for specific applications of trauma-informed care.

The SAMHSA outlines six key principles of trauma-informed care:

1. *Safety:* Safety is the first and most important principle. The staff and the people they serve should feel physically and psychologically safe throughout the system. The physical setting is safe, and interpersonal interactions promote a sense of safety. Patients determine if they feel safe or not. The institution or clinicians cannot decide when patients should feel safe.
2. *Trustworthiness and transparency:* The system operations and decisions are conducted with transparency and the goal of building and maintaining trust among clients and their family members, as well as staff. Clinicians are able to provide patients with transparency in treatment.
3. *Peer support and mutual self-help:* Peers are defined as individuals with shared lived experiences of trauma. With the prevalence of trauma, many individuals can offer some form of peer support and mutual self-help. These are key vehicles for establishing safety and hope, building trust, empowerment, enhancing collaboration, and using the stories and lived experiences to promote recovery and healing.
4. *Collaboration and mutuality:* With this principle, importance is placed on partnering between staff and clients. This includes all staff from clerical and housekeeping to professional staff and administrators. Through this principle, they are able to show and demonstrate that healing happens in relationships and in the meaningful sharing of power and decision making. The system recognizes that everyone has a role to play in a trauma-informed approach.
5. *Empowerment, voice, and choice:* Each individual's strengths and experiences are recognized and built upon. There is a belief about resilience, ability to heal, and promote recovery from trauma. Clinicians must understand that historic

BOX 15.5 Applications of Trauma Informed Care

Outpatient Setting

- Involving patients in the treatment process
- Screening for trauma
- Training staff in trauma-specific treatment approaches
- Engaging referral sources and partnering organizations
- Pay attention to staff's own trauma and self-care
- Understand maladaptive behaviors we see in patients from a trauma perspective
  - Think "What happened to you?" not "What is wrong with you?"
  - Understand maladaptive behavior from a faulty coping style (sick) perspective rather than from a volitional (bad) perspective.
- Model healthy/adaptive interactions, emotional stability, good coping skills, problem-solving skills

Inpatient Setting

- Meet the patient's needs
- Good staff/team communication to minimize splitting
- Set limits in a firm but kind manner; be consistent
- Work with team/unit staff to develop a unified safety plan for high-risk situations
- Allow the opportunity for the patient to regain control without coercive measures
- Debriefings are important; debrief staff and the patient after a code
- Do not take verbalizations/actions personally; keep a professional empathic boundary

power differentials have led to diminished voice and choice and even coercive treatments in the past. In trauma-informed care patients are supported in shared decision making, choice and goal setting to determine the plan of action they need to heal and move forward. Through this, self-advocacy skills are taught and strengthened.

6. *Cultural, historical, and gender issues:* The system actively moves past cultural stereotypes and biases, offers culturally responsive services, leverages the healing value of traditional cultural connections, and recognizes and addresses historical trauma. It offers policies, protocols, and processes that are responsive to the racial, ethnic, and cultural needs of individuals served; and it recognizes and addresses historical trauma.

Promoting Resilience

Understanding the science underlying the progression in Krystal's and Miguel's development allows clinicians to promote and build positive outcomes. All children and their families can benefit from developing healthy, strong, and supportive relationships and adaptive coping skills. Here we present a framework of opportunities that can be implemented in clinical settings.

Using a Resilience-Building Framework

Clinicians can apply their understanding of trauma, adversity, and resilience to promote positive health care outcomes and trajectories. The Health Outcomes from Positive Experiences (HOPE) framework builds on our understanding of ACEs. This framework is a holistic model that approaches the complex interplay of ecological, biologic, and developmental factors that result in positive health trajectories. It recognizes the need to identify and mitigate ACEs while also supporting positive childhood experiences (Burstein et al., 2021).

HOPE focuses on outcomes in four domains of development: physical development (e.g., adequate growth and nutrition, disease prevention, healthy physical activity), cognitive development (e.g., language, executive functioning skills), social development (e.g., secure attachments with trusting adults, self-advocacy skills), and emotional development (e.g., development emotional self-regulation skills, positive identity formation) (Sege & Browne, 2017). HOPE uses the four building blocks of relationships, environments, engagement, and emotional growth.

Building Resilience in Clinical Settings

Regular visits and established relationships with families offer clinicians a unique opportunity to promote resilience during visits. Experts have recommended using a tiered approach (Garner & Saul, 2018). Tier 1 includes anticipatory guidance, trauma screening, and resilience promotion. Several tools can help clinicians identify traumatic stress in children (Table 15.5). Clinicians can also offer concrete guidance on positive discipline strategies, encourage healthy routines (e.g., shared reading), and screen for caregiver behavioral health conditions. Once children and families are at risk, tier 2 supports such as referrals and closer monitoring are needed. Clinicians should build strong partnerships with community-based organizations and leverage existing system-based models (e.g., Help Me Grow) to ensure they can connect families to additional support seamlessly when needed. Tier 2 should also include close surveillance of children at risk such as those in foster care, children of parents with complex health/mental health needs, and all children experiencing ACEs. We also encourage communication with school and community providers such as teachers, coaches, and counselors. Finally, once children demonstrate red flags or symptoms of stress (e.g., anxiety, depressions, disruptive behaviors, substance use, school failure) tier 3 supports should be implemented. Clinicians can refer to specialists as indicated by need (e.g., psychologists, developmental-behavioral pediatricians, child and adolescent psychiatrists) for evidence-based treatment and intervention. Interdisciplinary care models (see Chapter 115) are well suited for tiered approaches.

TABLE 15.5 Instruments for Assessing Traumatic Stress in Young Children

Name	Author	Age
Child Behavior Checklist (CBCL)	Achenbach and Rescorla (2001)	1.5–5 yr
Posttraumatic Stress Disorder Semi-Structured Interview and Observation Record	Scheeringa and Zeanah (1994)	0–4 yr
Posttraumatic Symptom Inventory for Children (PT-SIC)	Eisen (1997)	4–8 yr
Preschool Age Psychiatric Assessment (PAPA)	Egger and Angold (2004)	2–5 yr
PTSD Symptoms in Preschool Aged Children (PTSD-PAC)	Levendosky et al. (2002)	3–5 yr
Traumatic Events Screening Inventory-Parent Report Revised (TESI-PRR)	Ghosh et al. (2002)	0–6 yr
Trauma Symptom Checklist for Young Children (TSCYC)	Briere et al. (2001)	3–12 yr
Violence Exposure Scale for Children-Preschool Version (VEX-PV)	Shahinfar et al. (2000)	4–10 yr
Violence Exposure Scale for Children-Revised Parent Report (VEX-RPR)	Shahinfar et al. (2000)	For parents of preschool-aged children aged 4–10 yr

Secondary Trauma, Resilience, and Self-Care for Clinicians

In helping children like Krystal and Miguel who have experienced trauma, clinicians themselves can experience significant emotional reaction. Such secondary trauma is common, and the next section offers strategies to manage it.

Secondary trauma, also known as vicarious trauma, is emotional stress that results when an individual hears about the firsthand trauma experiences of another. For clinicians, care of traumatized children may take an emotional toll that can impact their functioning and quality of life. Clinicians need to be aware of the potential effects of this indirect trauma exposure. Awareness allows clinicians to take care of themselves, and helps them to provide the best care possible for the children they serve. To decrease the impact of secondary trauma it is important that providers engage in self-care (Boxes 15.6 and 15.7).

BOX 15.6 Ways to Improve Self-Care

- Pay attention to personal emotional wellbeing and coping
- Create personal plan for self-care
- Address four key areas: emotional, physical, psychological, and spiritual health
- Learn to process with supervisor/colleagues; debrief

BOX 15.7 Seven Ways to Engage in Self-Care

1. Maintain friendships. Be sure to connect regularly with friends and loved ones. Do things together that bring you joy.
2. Set a bedtime. Get into the routine of getting quality sleep. Putting down electronics 1 hr before bed will improve sleep. Try relaxation or meditation if you have trouble.
3. Accept help when you need it. You do not have to deal with things alone. If you are worried or stressed, talk to someone (e.g., friend, loved one, therapist, doctor).
4. Exercise regularly. This reduces stress levels and improves your health.
5. Eat a balanced diet.
6. Be kind to yourself. Encourage and reward yourself, for achievements, big or small. Allow yourself grace to make mistakes.
7. Plan something to look forward to, whether that be a weekend hike, vacation, or even a happy hour with friends.

SYSTEMIC INTERVENTIONS

Addressing Trauma in Schools

Systemic interventions help address the wide reach of trauma. For children, schools are an ideal setting for such interventions. Cognitive Behavioral Intervention for Trauma in Schools (CBITS) is a program that was developed to reduce the negative effects of trauma (e.g., symptoms of posttraumatic stress disorder, depression, and other behavioral issues) and improve children's functioning (e.g., grades and attendance, peer and parent support, and coping skills) (Jaycox et al., 2018). School-based mental health professionals (e.g., social workers, counselors, psychologists) implement the program. Schools that have implemented CBITS have had significantly higher retention rates, with 98% of patients completing treatment, compared to only 37% with traditional outpatient treatment (Jaycox et al., 2010). CBITS is effective among diverse populations, including students who recently immigrated, urban youth, and youth of color (Jaycox et al., 2002, 2010; Stein et al., 2003).

Building Resilience in Schools

Dray and colleagues (2017) conducted a metaanalysis to examine the effect of universal, school-based, resilience-focused interventions on the mental and emotional wellbeing in children and adolescents. The study found that resilience-focused interventions were effective relative to a control in reducing depression symptoms, internalizing problems, externalizing problems, and general psychological distress. These findings suggest that universal resilience-focused interventions are promising in both children and adolescents especially when a cognitive-behavioral therapy–based approach is used. Additional studies are needed as there was a limited number of trials providing data sufficient for metaanalysis, and this remains an area for further research.

Building Resilience Through Policy

Policies at the clinical and systemic level can help promote resilience. The AAP recognizes the interdisciplinary need for clinicians to partner with schools, community organizations, and other stakeholders to support optimal developmental trajectories for all children (Garner et al., 2021). Clinicians, parents, teachers, and coaches to legislators and other civic leaders can all play an important role. Clinicians have a unique opportunity to serve as a voice for children at the local, state, and federal levels. The AAP also highlights the importance of working with key stakeholders to translate advances in understanding developmental science for policymakers to promote positive outcomes on the population health level (Garner et al., 2012).

On the clinical level, we encourage readers to implement trauma-informed care, use trauma and resilience screening tools, and regularly collaborate with school and other community-based professionals to address trauma and promote resilience in their practices and health systems. On the systemic level, we encourage readers to advocate at the local, state, and federal levels to continue to address and mitigate complex social determinants of health (e.g., food security, housing, parent mental health, school funding for evidence-based interventions). Additionally, we advocate for continued funding to further research that can enhance our understanding of successful individual and public health level interventions to mitigate trauma and promote resilience. We also advocate for continued development of educational models to promote best practices to be disseminated to all stakeholders involved in the health and wellbeing of children.

FURTHER CONSIDERATIONS

An understanding of trauma, adversity, toxic stress, and resilience provides us with a comprehensive model by which to promote healthy outcomes on the individual and population levels. This requires reassessing current models and reimbursement structures in health care and other sectors. This science calls for further investigation of the benefits of transitioning from an illness model of health care to a wellness and outcomes-focused model.

CONCLUSION

Krystal and Miguel represent many but not all of the children encountered in developmental-behavioral pediatric settings. Krystal has experienced significant trauma and toxic stressors with a dearth of resilience-promoting factors. Meanwhile, Miguel with a similar experience of trauma and adversity had a very different developmental trajectory due to the strong, stable, and supportive relationships he experiences with his aunt, school team, and care professionals.

Each of these cases has themes and problems that offer several opportunities of contact. Care in these cases calls for clinicians to do more than just assess for immediate safety, especially in Miguel's case with concern for active domestic violence at home, but also how to ensure safe, positive, and equitable outcomes. Taken together, these cases illustrate the importance of care that helps build skills and supports resilience among all children.

REFERENCES

Achenbach, T. M., & Rescorla, L. A. (2001). *Manual for the ASEBA school-age forms & profiles*. University of Vermont, Research Center for Children, Youth, & Families.

Belsky, J., & Pluess, M. (2009). Beyond diathesis stress: Differential susceptibility to environmental influences. *Psychological Bulletin, 135*(6), 885–908.

Bethell, C., Jones, J., Gombojav, N., Linkenbach, J., & Sege, R. (2019). Positive childhood experiences and adult mental and relational health in a statewide sample: Associations across adverse childhood experiences levels. *JAMA Pediatrics, 173*(11), e193007.

Briere, J., Johnson, K., Bissada, A., Damon, L., Crouch, J., Gil, E., Hanson, R., & Ernst, V. (2001). The Trauma Symptom Checklist for Young Children (TSCYC): Reliability and association with abuse exposure in a multi-site study. *Child Abuse & Neglect, 25*(8), 1001–1014.

Burstein, D., Yang, C., Johnson, K., Linkenbach, J., & Sege, R. (2021). Transforming practice with HOPE (healthy outcomes from positive experiences). *Maternal and Child Health Journal*, 1–6.

Caspi, A., McClay, J., Moffitt, T. E., Mill, J., Martin, J., Craig, I., Taylor, A., & Poulton, R. (2002). Role of genotype in the cycle of violence in maltreated children. *Science, 297*(5582), 851–854.

Dray, J., Bowman, J., Campbell, E., Freund, M., Wolfenden, L., Hodder, R. K., McElwaine, K., Tremain, D., Bartlem, K., Bailey, J., Small, T., Palazzi, K., Oldmeadow, C., & Wiggers, J. (2017). Systematic review of universal resilience-focused interventions targeting child and adolescent mental health in the school setting. *Journal of the American Academy of Child & Adolescent Psychiatry, 56*(10), 813–824.

Egger, H. L., & Angold, A. (2004). The Preschool Age Psychiatric Assessment (PAPA): A structured parent interview for diagnosing psychiatric disorders in preschool children. In R. DelCarmen-Wiggins & A. Carter (Eds.), *Handbook of infant, toddler, and preschool mental health assessment* (pp. 223–243). Oxford University Press.

Eisen, M. (1997). The Development and Validation of a New Measure of PTSD for Young Children. Unpublished Manuscript.

Finkelhor, D., Turner, H. A., Shattuck, A., & Hamby, S. L. (2013). Violence, crime, and abuse exposure in a national sample of children and youth: An update. *JAMA Pediatrics, 167*(7), 614–621.

Garner, A. S., & Saul, R. A. (2018). *Thinking developmentally: Nurturing wellness in childhood to promote lifelong health*. American Academy of Pediatrics.

Garner, A. S., Shonkoff, J. P., & Committee on Psychosocial Aspects of Child and Family Health, Committee on Early Childhood, Adoption, and Dependent Care, Section on Developmental and Behavioral Pediatrics. (2012). Early childhood adversity, toxic stress, and the role of the pediatrician: Translating developmental science into lifelong health. *Pediatrics, 129*(1), e224–e231.

Garner, A., Yogman, M., & Committee on Psychosocial Aspects of Child and Family Health, Section on Developmental and Behavioral Pediatrics, Council on Early Childhood, (2021). Preventing childhood toxic stress: Partnering with families and communities to promote relational health. *Pediatrics, 148*(2). e2021052582.

Ghosh, C., Ford, J., Racusin, R., Acker, M., Bosquet, K., Rogers, C., & Edwards, J. (2002). *Trauma events screening inventory-parent report revised*. San Francisco: The Child Trauma Research Project of the Early Trauma Network and The National Center for PTSD Dartmouth Child Trauma Research Group.

Jaycox, L. H., Cohen, J. A., Mannarino, A. P., Walker, D. W., Langley, A. K., Gegenheimer, K., Scott, M., & Schonlau, M. (2010). Children's mental health care following Hurricane Katrina: A field trial of trauma-focused psychotherapies. *Journal of Traumatic Stress: Official Publication of The International Society for Traumatic Stress Studies, 23*(2), 223–231.

Jaycox, L., Langley, A., & Hoover, S. (2018). *Cognitive Behavioral Intervention for Trauma in Schools (CBITS)* (2nd ed.). RAND Corporation.

Jaycox, L. H., Stein, B. D., Kataoka, S. H., Wong, M., Fink, A., Escudero, P. I. A., & Zaragoza, C. (2002). Violence exposure, posttraumatic stress disorder, and depressive symptoms among recent immigrant schoolchildren. *Journal of the American Academy of Child & Adolescent Psychiatry, 41*(9), 1104–1110.

Levendosky, A. A., Huth-Bocks, A. C., Semel, M. A., & Shapiro, D. L. (2002). Trauma symptoms in preschool-age children exposed to violence. *Journal of Interpersonal Violence, 17*, 150–164.

Liu, D., Diorio, J., Day, J. C., Francis, D. D., & Meaney, M. J. (2000). Maternal care, hippocampal synaptogenesis and cognitive development in rats. *Nature Neuroscience, 3*(8), 799–806.

Malhi, G. S., Das, P., Bell, E., Mattingly, G., & Mannie, Z. (2019). Modelling resilience in adolescence and adversity: A novel framework to inform research and practice. *Translational Psychiatry, 9*(1), 1–16.

Sacks, V., & Murphey, D. (2018). *The prevalence of adverse childhood experiences, nationally, by state, and by race or ethnicity. Child Trends*. Retrieved from: https://www.childtrends.org/publications/

prevalence-adverse-childhood-experiences-nationally-state-race-ethnicity.

Sege, R. D., & Browne, C. H. (2017). Responding to ACEs with HOPE: Health Outcomes from Positive Experiences. *Academic Pediatrics*, *17*(7), S79–S85.

Shahinfar, A., Fox, N. A., & Leavitt, L. A. (2000). Preschool children's exposure to violence: Relation of behavior problems to parent and child reports. *American Journal of Orthopsychiatry*, *70*(1), 115–125.

Sheeringa, M. S., & Zeanah, C. H. (1994). *PTSD semi-structured interview and observation record for infants and young children*. Department of Psychiatry and Neurology, Tulane University Health Sciences Center, New Orleans, LA.

Stein, B. D., Jaycox, L. H., Kataoka, S. H., Wong, M., Tu, W., Elliott, M. N., & Fink, A. (2003). A mental health intervention for schoolchildren exposed to violence: A randomized controlled trial. *JAMA*, *290*(5), 603–611.

Traub, F., & Boynton-Jarrett, R. (2017). Modifiable resilience factors to childhood adversity for clinical pediatric practice. *Pediatrics*, *139*(5):e20162569.

16

Childcare

W. Steven Barnett and Anna Malia Beckwith

For additional material related to the content of this chapter, please see Chapters 6 and 19.

> **VIGNETTE**
>
> *Avery's parents raised several concerns about childcare during their 1-month well child visit. Avery's mother has 6 weeks paid leave; the father is self-employed with no leave options. Concerns include potential developmental effects of parental separation, starting at different ages, long hours, and different types of care, and health risks from group care. One option is for Avery's grandmother to provide care part time while Avery's father or mother reduce their work time. However, this would reduce the family's income and harm their career progress, and they have difficulty meeting expenses as it is. It seems that whatever choice they make will be stressful.*
>
> *Planning for childcare and work after the birth of a child poses difficult challenges for parents. Avery's family benefitted from paid leave, an option not available to everyone. Parents may choose not to use nonparental childcare before age 1 year, but many cannot afford to make this choice, and most will use regular childcare by age 1 year. The challenges parents face are not just financial, but involve complex child development issues. Lost income from forgone employment can negatively impact child health and development, while childcare can have positive or negative impacts depending on the child and family, quality of care, and context.*
>
> *Clinicians can provide information that helps parents make these difficult decisions. Fortunately for Avery and her parents, their clinician talked with them about the importance of responsive adult-child interactions and rich language environments in parental and nonparental care as well as minimizing screen time. Their clinician also has at hand information on the local Early Head Start and childcare resource and referral agency.*

TYPES OF CHILDCARE

Childcare encompasses a wide range of different arrangements for young children (Gable, 2014). For school-age children, the public schools are the largest provider of childcare supplemented by before- and after-school care and a variety of summer programs. Several types of nonparental care serve children prior to kindergarten: relative, nonrelative, and center. Relative and nonrelative care are provided in the child's own home or another home. All childcare potentially supports learning and development, and parental employment. However, arrangements vary considerably in their support for learning and development and their hours and convenience as a work support.

The terms parents and caregivers use for childcare are as varied and unstandardized as the arrangements themselves: babysitting, nannies, daycare, family home daycare or childcare, preschool, pre-K or prekindergarten, child development or early learning center, Head Start, and Educare (Gable, 2014). These names more clearly identify differences in where the arrangements are located and in hours than in the quality of care provided and its support for learning and development.

Children experience multiple types of childcare arrangements sometimes in combination and typically changing as they grow older (Chaudry et al., 2021). For example, a child might attend a childcare center part-time in the morning followed by grandparent care in the afternoon. In the first 3 years of life home care is more common; from age 3 years on, children are more likely to attend centers as their primary childcare arrangement.

CHILDCARE ARRANGEMENTS

Most children begin regular childcare by age 1 year, and the vast majority attend a center-based program prior to kindergarten (Chaudry et al., 2021). Public funding has greatly expanded to support these services in recent years, yet there remain large inequalities in childcare arrangements with the lowest use of care, especially higher-quality center care, by parents with less education and income. In 2020 the COVID-19 pandemic greatly disrupted childcare arrangements (Barnett & Jung, 2021). Many parents withdrew children from care, especially centers, and many center-based programs, especially public programs, shifted to remote learning and no longer provided in-person care.

In 2019 about 60% of children not yet in kindergarten participated in at least one regular nonparental care arrangement (Barnett & Li, 2021). Participation varied from 42% prior to age 1 year to more than 80% at age 5 years before kindergarten (Fig. 16.1). Relative and nonrelative care decline with age, while weekly center care increases from less than 15% before age 1 year to more than 70% at ages 4 and 5 years. This pattern reflects both parents' beliefs and attitudes about what is best for the child and the realities of access and affordability (Chaudry et al., 2021). Infant and toddler child care is much more expensive than care for older preschoolers who can be provided with quality care in larger groups with fewer staff (Chaudry et al., 2021). In addition, the availability of free public programs is greater for children ages 3 and, especially, 4 years.

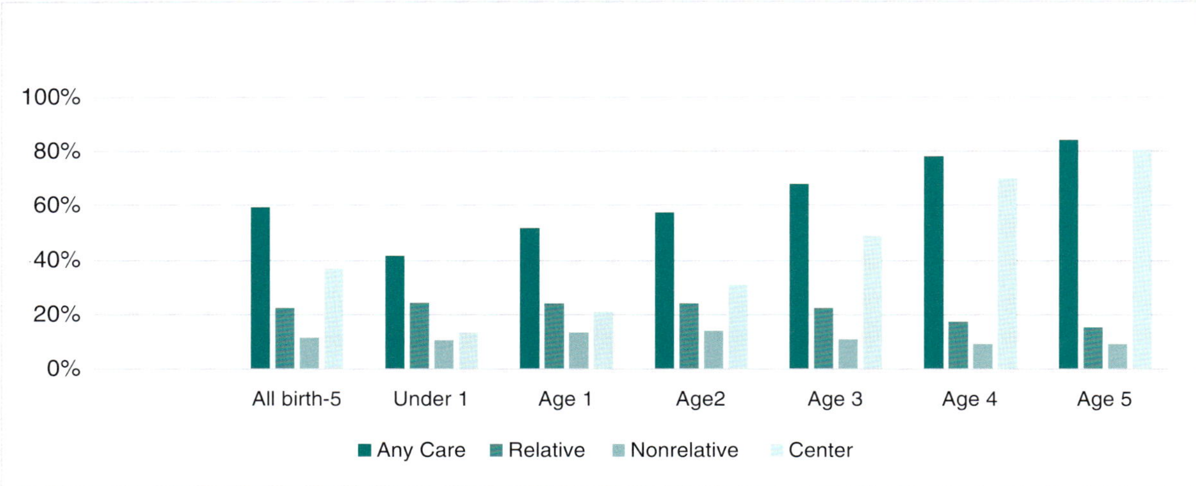

Fig. 16.1 Childcare arrangements by age, 2019 (Barnett & Li, 2021).

Government support for early childhood care and education services has expanded access to child care with the greatest benefits to low-income families as many public programs limit eligibility based on income (Chaudry et al., 2021). State childcare subsidies limit eligibility to low-income families. Federally funded Head Start and Early Head Start primarily serve children in poverty. Most state- and local-funded preschool programs limit eligibility by income, though a growing number are universal. One constraint is that public programs often lack adequate funding to serve all eligible families, and this characterizes childcare subsidy programs, Head Start and Early Head Start, and even some "universal" preschool programs. The bottom line is that childcare participation rates rise steadily with family income, many low- and moderate-income families cannot access quality childcare, and access to quality center-based care is U-shaped with young children in middle-income families having the lowest participation rates (Barnett & Li, 2021).

DEFINING QUALITY IN THE CHILDCARE SETTING

Recognition of factors associated with a high-quality childcare experience is crucial to parents and pediatric clinicians, as research has shown positive impacts across multiple domains with provision of high-quality early childhood education (Barnett, 2021). Improved cognition and academic achievement scores have been observed in recipients of this care. More recently, physical health benefits, including significantly lower prevalence of risk factors for cardiovascular and metabolic diseases in adulthood, were found to be associated with high-quality care (Campbell et al., 2014). Therefore benefits of a high-quality early childcare experience may last a lifetime (Barnett, 2021). However, childcare often is not of high quality—and has no developmental benefits—while poor-quality care has been found to have (modest) negative impacts on development (Barnett, 2021).

Traditionally quality has been defined by process quality (a child's experiences) and structural quality (program features). Particularly important for process quality are strong, sustained relationships with caregivers who are highly responsive to children (Chaudry & Sandstrom, 2020). Structural quality that supports good interactions is more readily regulated by state licensing standards, which may fall below expert recommendations (Gable, 2014). Greater than 75% of states currently utilize a quality rating and improvement system (QRIS) (Donoghue, 2017). A QRIS sets specific quality levels, which are defined by evidence-based, measurable levels, often represented as a star rating. These ratings tend to be weakly related, at best, to process quality (Chaudry et al., 2021). Much of the childcare parents use is neither rated by a QRIS nor licensed by states (Chaudry et al., 2021). The American Academy of Pediatrics (AAP) is one of many national organizations that has created standards and a system for voluntary accreditation (Donoghue, 2017). Indicators of quality in childcare are summarized in Table 16.1.

Staffing factors play key roles in determining the quality of a childcare setting. Dedicated, nurturing, attentive adults are paramount to a successful experience. The clinician should be aware of guidelines regarding adult-to-child ratios and group size (Table 16.2). When responsible for fewer children, a caregiver is better able to ensure each child's safety and provide sufficient attention to emotional and learning needs. Provision of a small-group setting also ensures peer exposure to support social learning.

Childcare settings vary considerably regarding standards for staff education or training (Donoghue, 2017), which may impact the opportunity for educational and emotional enrichment of attendees. Compensation may not be adequate to retain staff with bachelor's or associate's credentials in early childhood education (Whitebook et al., 2018), and provision of career development opportunities may be limited. Without formal training in early childhood development and behavior, it may be difficult for staff to implement a developmentally appropriate curriculum or address behavior concerns. Annually 5000 children are expelled from childcare settings; this rate far exceeds that of school-aged peers, and the rate is higher for boys and Black children (Donoghue, 2017; Meek & Gilliam,

TABLE 16.1 Quality Indicators in the Childcare Setting

1. Staffing	2. Environment	3. Health Preparedness	4. Education and Emotional Enrichment
• Ratio for sufficient supervision • Relationship: family member vs. center based • Qualifications, education • Sufficient criminal history background check • Provider turnover	• Cleanliness • Injury prevention: equipment/toy safety • Food storage, preparation • Toxic product storage	• Safe sleep practices • Medication administration • Infection control, immunization status • Nutrition • Physical activity • Emergency procedures: first-aid training, disaster preparation	• Curriculum focused on child development, with clear schedule of activities • Behavior management strategies that focus on positive guidance and avoid negative punishment techniques, such as yelling, harsh criticism, or physical punishment • Access to age-appropriate learning materials (books, blocks, puzzles, art materials) • Focus on language exposure: staff understanding of the value of speaking to infants/toddlers, reading to the young child

Adapted from American Academy of Pediatrics; American Public Health Association; National Resource Center for Health and Safely in Child Care and Early Education. (2013). *Stepping stones to caring for our children* (3rd ed.). https://reader.aappublications.org/stepping-stones-to-caring-for-our-children/.

TABLE 16.2 Recommended Childcare Staffing

	Center Based		Family Childcare	
Child Age	**Ratio**	**Group Size**	**Child Number by Age**	**Ratio**
Birth–12 mo	1:3	≤6	None <2 yr	1:6
13–30 mo	1:4	≤8	One <2 yr	1:4
31–35 mo	1:5	≤10	Two <2 yr	No others recommended
36 mo	1:8	≤16		

Adapted from American Academy of Pediatrics; American Public Health Association; National Resource Center for Health and Safely in Child Care and Early Education. (2013). *Stepping stones to caring for our children* (3rd ed.). https://reader.aappublications.org/stepping-stones-to-caring-for-our-children/.

2016). When preschool teachers were provided with behavioral health consultation, however, a significant decrease in rate of expulsion (Meek & Gilliam, 2016) was observed. Thus with provision of staff education and support, the ability of a child with behavior concerns to remain in a childcare setting was improved.

Retention of childcare staff may also be challenging. This is very problematic as the development of strong, secure relationships with care providers allows an infant or toddler the confidence to explore the world and learn (Ahnert et al., 2006). Furthermore, a secure relationship with a care provider is associated with improved emotional regulation, attention, memory, planning skills, and self-control (Tarullo et al., 2009).

Children with disabilities can benefit from inclusion in childcare, though finding high-quality childcare suitable for inclusion can be challenging. Early Head Start and Head Start exempt children with disabilities from income-eligibility requirements and offer opportunities for higher-quality care and coordination of special services (see Chapter 103) in inclusive settings (Chaudry et al., 2021).

Finally, health preparedness, including infection control and vaccination monitoring, is an important quality and safety indicator. Childcare attendance is a potential risk factor for upper respiratory tract infection and acute otitis media (Silverstein et al., 2003), though risks may be decreased through infection control measures. The onset of the COVID-19 pandemic resulted in increased scrutiny of infection control in childcare settings. The measures introduced successfully decreased childcare's contribution to COVID-19 transmission to adults (Gilliam et al., 2020), showing the potential of strong infection control in childcare settings.

CLINICIANS' ROLES

There are many ways a clinician may serve to improve the quality of childcare for individual patients, via participation in community programs, or through support of state and federal regulations or funding opportunities (Donoghue, 2017).

At the individual patient level, the clinician should include an assessment of childcare quality indicators during well-child visits. Though parents may not be aware of all environmental or health policy considerations at their child's childcare center, this process will serve to educate parents on potential areas of concern or strength within their childcare arrangement. The clinician may also direct parents to a simple checklist for use when visiting childcare programs (Donoghue, 2017).

Serving as an educator to childcare staff regarding a patient's medical or behavioral health diagnoses and potential impacts on classroom function is another key role for the clinician (Alkon et al., 2003). When a child is expelled from daycare, a visit to the clinician's office is often not far behind. However, it is possible that expulsion could be prevented through proactive communication regarding a child's accommodation needs and successful behavior management strategies (Meek & Gilliam, 2016).

Communication between the clinician and childcare provider is even more important for children with special healthcare needs. Clinicians may be asked to provide written care or action plans to support staff in the management of a healthcare concern.

At the community level, clinicians may serve as childcare health consultants, conducting safety and health assessments for local programs (Donoghue, 2017). Clinicians may volunteer to provide educational sessions for childcare staff regarding common health topics such as medication administration, safe sleep practices, or encouragement of nutrition and physical activity. Additionally, clinicians may consult on the development of health and safety policies for the center.

At the state or national level, the clinician may provide input to QRIS implementers, assisting with translation of research to measurable quality outcomes. Participation in legislative groups, available via the AAP, provides the opportunity to influence policymakers through testimony and letter-writing campaigns.

CONCLUSION

Most children experience nonparental childcare before school entry, with most entering such care before age 2 years. Nevertheless, childcare access is highly unequal and children of parents with less education and income may struggle to obtain quality care. Public subsidies and programs such as Head Start target children from lower-income families but are far from adequate to serve all eligible families. High-quality childcare, especially when sustained over time, can benefit children's learning, development, and health over a lifetime. However, childcare often is not of high quality, and poor quality care may negatively impact development. Clinicians can help to improve the quality of childcare for individual patients by offering guidance to parents on assessment of quality and choosing care, as demonstrated in our vignette. Avery's clinician educated her parents to components of a quality childcare setting: responsive adult-child interactions, language-rich environment, and minimization of screen time. The clinician also provided information on Early Head Start and childcare resources.

Beyond the individual patient, the clinician is able to provide guidance via participation in community programs and by supporting improvements in public policy. Expulsion or exclusion of children who might benefit most from care is all too common, particularly for boys and Black children. Clinicians can help programs to better support children rather than exclude them. Other important roles clinicians can play include educating childcare staff and policymakers regarding health issues, quality, and the value of improvements in infection control, a much-heightened concern since the COVID-19 pandemic that began in 2020.

REFERENCES

Ahnert, L., Pinquart, M., & Lamb, M. E. (2006). Security of children's relationships with nonparental care providers: A meta-analysis. *Child Development*, *77*(3), 664–679.

Alkon, A., Ramler, M., & MacLennan, K. (2003). Evaluation of mental health consultation in child care centers. *Early Childhood Education Journal*, *31*(2), 91–99.

American Academy of Pediatrics; American Public Health Association; National Resource Center for Health and Safely in Child Care and Early Education. (2013). *Stepping stones to caring for our children* (3rd ed.). https://reader.aappublications.org/stepping-stones-to-caring-for-our-children/.

Barnett, W. S. (2021). *NEPC Review: The drawbacks of universal pre-k: A review of the evidence*. National Education Policy Center. http://nepc.colorado.edu/thinktank/universal-pre-k.

Barnett, W. S., & Jung, K. (2021). *Eight ways the pandemic continues to harm early learning and development*. NIEER.

Barnett, W. S., & Li, Z. (2021). *Original analyses of data from the National Household Education Survey 2019 Early Childhood Program Participation Public Use Data File*. NIEER.

Campbell, F., Conti, G., Heckman, J. J., Moon, S. H., Pinto, R., Pungello, E., & Pan, Y. (2014). Early childhood investments substantially boost adult health. *Science*, *343*(6178), 1478–1485.

Chaudry, A., Morrissey, T., Weiland, C., & Yoshikawa, H. (2021). *Cradle to kindergarten: A new plan to combat inequality* (2nd ed.). Russell Sage Foundation.

Chaudry, A., & Sandstrom, H. (2020). Child care and early education for infants and toddlers. *Future of Children*, *30*(2), 165–190.

Donoghue, E. A. (2017). Quality early education and child care from birth to kindergarten. *Pediatrics*, *140*(2), e20171488. https://doi.org/10.1542/peds.2017-1488.

Gable, S. (2014). *The states of child care: Building a better system*. Teachers College Press.

Gilliam, W. S., Malik, A. A., Shafiq, M., Klotz, M., Reyes, C., Humphries, J. E., Murray, T., Elharake, J. A., Wilkinson, D., & Omer, S. B. (2020). COVID-19 transmission in US child care programs. *Pediatrics*, *147*(1), e2020031971.

Meek, S. E., & Gilliam, W. A. (2016). Expulsion and suspension as matters of social justice and health equity. *Discussion Paper*. National Academy of Medicine.

Silverstein, M., Sales, A. E., & Koepsell, T. D. (2003). Health care utilization and expenditures associated with child care attendance: A nationally representative sample. *Pediatrics*, *111*(4), e371–e375. https://doi.org/10.1542/peds.111.4.e371.

Tarullo, A., Obradović, J., & Gunnar, M. (2009). Self-control and the developing brain. *Zero to Three*, *29*, 31–37.

Whitebook, M., McLean, C., Austin, L. J. E., & Edwards, B. (2018). *Early Childhood Workforce Index—2018*. Center for the Study of Child Care Employment, University of California. http://cscce.berkeley.edu/topic/early-childhood-workforce-index/2018/17.

17

Peers

*Gary Kwok and Katie A. Devine**

For additional material related to the content of this chapter, please see Chapters 21, 41, and 110.

VIGNETTE

Twelve-year-old Ana recalls feeling nervous about returning to school after losing her hair during cancer treatment. When a friend posted a picture of them together online, another girl made mean comments. "It really hurt. But my friend stood up for me, and that was the last mean thing said."

Peer relationships make critical contributions to healthy social-emotional development. Children benefit from the social and emotional support that friends offer, and they learn important social skills by interacting with peers. Healthy relationships, like Ana's, can buffer children from negative effects of poor interactions with peers. Yet successfully navigating the social world of peers can be challenging, particularly for youth with special health care needs, and persistent problems with peers can have detrimental consequences. This chapter provides an overview of the importance of peer relationships, reviews potential problems children experience, and gives practical recommendations for clinicians when screening for these issues.

SOCIAL DEVELOPMENT AND THE IMPORTANCE OF PEER RELATIONSHIPS

Establishing relationships with other children is a major developmental task of childhood. Understanding how social development typically progresses through different developmental stages helps identify problems in relating to others that may more broadly impact a child's development (Parker et al., 2006). The foundations for building future social relationships start in infancy, as babies learn to interact with and mimic others. From the preschool years and beyond, children spend increasingly more time with peers and social play and interactions become more complex. Friendships, defined as reciprocal relationships with mutual liking and affection (Howes et al., 1988), begin to form and become more stable, mature, and complex with age. Children's normative preference for same-sex friendships begins in preschool and intensifies during the school-age years. Adolescents tend to have fewer friendships than during late childhood, but these friendships are typically more intimate and influential, corresponding to adolescents' growing autonomy.

It is widely recognized that developing and sustaining healthy peer relationships affects many social and emotional outcomes for children. Peer acceptance, the degree to which a child is liked by peers, is linked to social competence, or one's ability and skills to initiate, manage, and sustain positive social and emotional experiences. Social competence at a young age has been linked to a number of positive adult social-emotional outcomes, including educational achievement, stable employment, crime, substance use, and mental health (Joneset et al., 2015).

PROBLEMS IN PEER RELATIONSHIPS

Problems in peer relationships can be characterized along several domains: peer rejection, social isolation/withdrawal, peer victimization or bullying, and a lack of any reciprocal friendships. Peer rejection is defined as social exclusion due to perceived individual deficits or bias due to group membership (Mulvey et al., 2017). Peer rejection can occur in many forms, such as excluding a child completely, preventing a child access to other group members or resources, or verbal or physical aggression toward the rejected child (Asher et al., 2012). Social isolation/withdrawal occurs when a child removes oneself or avoids peers, which may be due to shyness, anxiety, poor social skills, or preference to spend time alone. Data suggest that aggressive, disruptive, or withdrawn behavior can lead to peer rejection and/or social withdrawal, leading to a perpetuating cycle that puts these children at increased risk of continuous rejection and social withdrawal (Rubin et al., 2015). These behaviors may or may not meet the definition of peer victimization. Peer victimization, or bullying, is defined as being repeatedly and intentionally harassed, assaulted, or aggressed upon by one or more peers with a power differential between the victim and perpetrator(s) (Espelage & Colbert, 2016; Turner et al., 2011). Peer victimization can take a number of forms, including physical assault, physical intimidation, verbal, social or relational, and electronic (Turner et al., 2011). Metaanalytic review of 80 studies found prevalence rates of 35% for traditional bullying and 14% for cyberbullying among adolescents (Modecki et al., 2014). Longitudinal data suggest that different subgroups

*Address correspondence regarding this chapter to Katie A. Devine, PhD, MPH, Rutgers Cancer Institute of New Jersey, 195 Little Albany Street, New Brunswick, NJ 08903. Email: katie.devine@rutgers.edu; Telephone: 732-235-7549

of children experience different victimization trajectories across the formal schooling years, with about 24% experiencing chronic and stable bullying across time (Ladd et al., 2017). Boys are more likely to be both perpetrators and victims of bullying, especially physical bullying, but girls tend to begin using social forms of bullying at earlier ages than boys (Williams & Guerra, 2007). While physical bullying declines with age, verbal, social, and cyberbullying tend to increase between the ages of 11 and 15 and peak around the transition from middle school to high school.

In today's society the ubiquity of mobile devices (see Chapter 21) has brought increased attention to electronic or cyberbullying, which tends to occur less frequently than traditional bullying but with similar detrimental effects (Modecki et al., 2014). Examples of cyberbullying include sending harassing or threatening messages via text message, email, or social media; posting derogatory comments about someone on a website or social networking platform; or spreading rumors about someone in an online setting (Hinduja & Patchin, 2009). These types of behaviors may be difficult to identify, as they frequently occur outside the direct observation of adults and therefore may require children to report these behaviors to trusted adults. A recent metaanalysis found that perpetrators of cyberbullying were more likely to be male, of older age, engage in frequent online activities, show aggressive cognitions, be offline victims and bullies, have internalizing and externalizing problems, have antisocial personality traits, experience negative family environment and school climate, and have negative peer influences (Guo, 2016). The same metaanalysis found that victims of cyberbullying shared similar risk factors, but were more likely to be female and have poor self-esteem. In addition, there is high overlap between cyberbullying and traditional bullying, with children who experience cyberbullying also reporting experiencing other forms of bullying, particularly relational and verbal bullying (Waasdorp & Bradshaw, 2015).

Peer victimization is concurrently and longitudinally predictive of a number of physical, emotional, and academic consequences, including internalizing (e.g., school-related fear, poor academic adjustment, anxiety, depression, loneliness, self-blame, low self-esteem, poor self-concept, suicidal ideation and attempts) and externalizing problems (e.g., disruptiveness, argumentativeness, aggression, truancy, delinquency, substance use, and subsequent bullying/peer victimization) (Zych et al., 2015). Some data suggest that cyberbullying is more strongly related to suicidal ideation than traditional bullying (van Geel et al., 2014). Together, evidence strongly suggests that it is critical to identify children experiencing victimization through routine screening (e.g., asking about peer relationships using open-ended questions) and to intervene to prevent long-term negative consequences.

CHILDREN WITH SPECIAL HEALTH CARE NEEDS AS A POTENTIALLY VULNERABLE POPULATION

Children with Special Health Care Needs (CSHCN) are a potentially vulnerable group due to the characteristics of their health or developmental conditions or the impact of the condition on emotional and social functioning. For example, certain conditions, such as autism spectrum disorder, are characterized by impairment in social interactions (see Chapter 41). Children diagnosed with other health conditions such as asthma, diabetes, or cancer may experience significant disruption to school participation and daily activities that interfere with social functioning. In 2017–2018 approximately 13.6 million US children (18.5%) had at least one special health care need, and almost two-thirds (65.9%) of those children were either moderately or significantly impacted by their conditions (Maternal and Child Health Bureau, 2020). CSHCN are also at greater risk for mental health and behavioral problems compared with children without special health care needs (Maternal and Child Health Bureau, 2020).

Chronic illness can disrupt participation in daily activities and hinder a child's social development such as making and keeping friends (Sisk et al., 2018). Metaanalyses have shown children with chronic illnesses have worse social functioning on average, though there is significant variability across conditions, and children with neurologic conditions such as spina bifida or seizure disorders tend to have the poorest social competence (Pinquart & Pfeiffer, 2015; Pinquart & Teubert, 2012). Evidence suggests, that problems in forming friendships and peer group membership are worse for adolescents with more highly externally visible conditions (Pinquart & Pfeiffer, 2015).

CSHCN are more likely to be victims of physical, relational, verbal, and cyberbullying, as well as illness-specific teasing (Pinquart, 2016). They are also more likely to be perpetrators themselves (Pinquart, 2016), suggesting a need for routine assessment of victimization experiences among CSHCN.

IMPLICATIONS FOR CLINICIANS

The American Academy of Pediatrics (AAP) encourages pediatric clinicians to regularly monitor children's development during well-child visits; screen for behavioral, developmental, and social-emotional concerns using validated tools at recommended ages; and ensure that comprehensive developmental evaluations are completed if risks are identified (Weitzman & Wegner, 2015). Identifying and addressing problems in peer relationships is an important aspect of these routine screenings.

Given negative consequences for both victims and perpetrators of bullying, clinicians should focus on prevention, screening, identifying, and supporting patients who are affected by bullying and their families. Prevention efforts include promoting child and family strengths during well-visits by helping families identify their own strengths, teaching families strategies for promoting optimal development, encouraging positive social relationships, and providing feedback to families based on observations or their reports. Clinicians can model open communication about bullying and encourage parents to regularly communicate with their children about these issues. Clinicians may also advocate for antibullying campaigns in their communities and schools. General screening recommendations include asking about

BOX 17.1 Sample Resources for Clinicians and Families About Bullying

Resource	Description
Centers for Disease Control and Prevention (CDC) https://www.cdc.gov/violenceprevention/youthviolence/bullyingresearch/fastfact.html	A fact sheet about bullying and how to prevent it
American Academy of Family Physicians (AAFP) https://www.aafp.org/about/policies/all/violence-harassment-school-bullying.html	AAFP's policy against violence, harassment, and school bullying
Cyberbullying Research Center https://cyberbullying.org/	Best practices in bullying and cyberbullying prevention and response, statistics, presentations, state laws, activities, tip sheets, handouts, current news, and more
US Department of Health and Human Services https://www.stopbullying.gov/	A federal government website with information on bullying, cyberbullying, prevention, and response
STOMP Out Bullying https://www.stompoutbullying.org/	STOMP Out Bullying is the leading national antibullying and cyberbullying organization for kids and teens in the United States

peer relationships as well as bullying-related issues using indirect, open-ended questions (e.g., "Do you feel safe at school?" "How do you get along with other kids?"); asking about online and social media use; asking about bullying if children present with multiple somatic problems, school avoidance, or self-harm; and screening for mental health problems among patients who report being bullied or bullying (Stephens et al., 2018). Parents should also be asked about any notable changes in behavior or mood. While these questions can be asked as part of a routine health history interview, clinicians can also screen using validated paper or electronic measures (e.g., Pediatric Symptom Checklist, the HEEADSSS [*h*ome environment, *e*ducation/employment, *e*ating, peer-related *a*ctivities, *d*rugs, *s*exuality, *s*uicide/depression, *s*afety] interview, myAssessment mobile app [Bradford & Rickwood, 2015], and the Rapid Assessment for Adolescent Preventive Services [Salerno et al., 2012]). Among adolescents, electronic tools may even increase disclosure about sensitive topics. Providing the adolescent with a confidential opportunity to disclose to the clinician without the parent present may also enhance reporting.

Once bullying has been identified, clinicians should screen for mental health problems and arrange for quality behavioral health interventions if needed. Models of behavioral health care range from coordinated care to fully integrated care (Ramirez et al., 2020), and it is critical for clinicians to establish a system to help children and families obtain this care. Recent data suggest that integrative care models increase access to quality behavioral health services without substantial additional costs (Walter et al., 2019). Clinicians should also become familiar with school-based professionals and assist parents in working productively with schools to address bullying that occurs there (see Chapter 110). Box 17.1 provides practical resources for clinicians and families.

CONCLUSION

Peer relationships are a critical part of social and emotional development for children and adolescents. Pediatric clinicians offer essential preventive, screening, and intervention resources to help families promote positive peer relationships and foster optimal social-emotional development for their children. As a trusted resource for families, clinicians can give patients like Ana and their families the opportunity to discuss peer relationships and get help for peer problems.

REFERENCES

Asher, S. R., Rose, A. J., & Gabriel, S. W. (2012). Peer rejection in everyday life: *Interpersonal rejection*. Oxford University Press. https://doi.org/10.1093/acprof:oso/9780195130157.003.0005

Bradford, S., & Rickwood, D. (2015). Acceptability and utility of an electronic psychosocial assessment (myAssessment) to increase self-disclosure in youth mental healthcare: A quasi-experimental study. *BMC Psychiatry*, *15*(305), 1–13. https://doi.org/10.1186/s12888-015-0694-4

Espelage, D. L., & Colbert, C. L. (2016). School-based bullying: Definition, prevalence, etiology, outcomes, and preventive strategies. In M. K. Holt & A. E. Grills (Eds.) , *Critical issues in school-based mental health: Evidence-based research, practice, and interventions* (pp. 132–144). Routledge/Taylor & Francis Group.

Guo. S. (2016). A meta-analysis of the predictors of cyberbullying perpetration and victimization. *Psychology in the Schools*, *53*(4), 432–453. https://doi.org/10.1002/pits.21914

Hinduja, S., & Patchin, J. W. (2009). *Bullying beyond the schoolyard: Preventing and responding to cyberbullying*. Sage Publications (Corwin Press).

Howes, C., Rubin, K. H., Ross, H. S., & French, D. C. (1988). Peer interaction of young children. *Monographs of the Society for Research in Child Development*, *53*(1), 1–92. https://doi.org/10.2307/1166062

Jones, D. E., Greenberg, M., & Crowley, M. (2015). Early social-emotional functioning and public health: The relationship between kindergarten social competence and future wellness. *American Journal of Public Health*, *105*(11), 2283–2290. https://doi.org/10.2105/AJPH.2015.302630

Ladd, G. W., Ettekal, I., & Kochenderfer-Ladd, B. (2017). Peer victimization trajectories from kindergarten through high school: Differential pathways for children's school engagement and achievement? *Journal of Educational Psychology*, *109*(6), 826–841. https://doi.org/10.1037/edu0000177

Maternal and Child Health Bureau. (2020). *Children with special health care needs NSCH data brief.* Health Resources and Services Adminstration.

Modecki, K. L., Minchin, J., Harbaugh, A. G., Guerra, N. G., & Runions, K. C. (2014). Bullying prevalence across contexts: A meta-analysis measuring cyber and traditional bullying. *Journal of Adolescent Health*, *55*(5), 602–611. https://doi.org/10.1016/j.jadohealth.2014.06.007

Mulvey, K. L., Boswell, C., & Zheng, J. (2017). Causes and consequences of social exclusion and peer rejection among children and adolescents. *Report on Emotional & Behavioral Disorders in Youth*, *17*(3), 71–75. http://www.ncbi.nlm.nih.gov/pubmed/30100820

Parker, J. G., Rubin, K. H., Erath, S. A., Wojsklawowicz, J. C., & Buskirk, A. A. (2006). Peer relationships, child development, and adjustment: A developmental psychopathology perspective. In D. Cicchetti & D. J. Cohen (Eds.), *Developmental psychopathology: Theory and method* (pp. 419–493). John Wiley & Sons, Inc.

Pinquart. M. (2016). Systematic review: Bullying involvement of children with and without chronic physical illness and/or physical/sensory disability—a meta-analytic comparison with healthy/nondisabled peers. *Journal of Pediatric Psychology*, *42*(3), 245–259. https://doi.org/10.1093/jpepsy/jsw081

Pinquart, M., & Pfeiffer, J. P. (2015). Solving developmental tasks in adolescents with a chronic physical illness or physical/sensory disability: A meta-analysis. *International Journal of Disability, Development and Education*, *62*(3), 249–264. https://doi.org/10.1080/1034912X.2015.1020922

Pinquart, M., & Teubert, D. (2012). Academic, physical, and social functioning of children and adolescents with chronic physical illness: A meta-analysis. *Journal of Pediatric Psychology*, *37*(4), 376–389. https://doi.org/10.1093/jpepsy/jsr106

Ramirez, L. Y., Myers, B. R., & Stancin, T. (2020). Models of consultation in primary care settings. In B. Carter. & K. Kullgren. (Eds.), *Clinical handbook of psychological consultation in pediatric medical settings. Issues in clinical child psychology* (pp. 63–74). Springer. https://doi.org/10.1007/978-3-030-35598-2_6

Rubin, K. H., Bukowski, W. M., & Bowker, J. C. (2015). Children in peer groups. In R. M. Lerner, M. Bornsteint, & T. Leventhal (Eds.), *Handbook of child psychology and developmental science* (pp. 175–222). John Wiley & Sons, Inc.

Salerno, J., Marshall, V. D., & Picken, E. B. (2012). Validity and reliability of the rapid assessment for adolescent preventive services adolescent health risk assessment. *Journal of Adolescent Health*, *50*(6), 595–599. https://doi.org/10.1016/j.jadohealth.2011.10.015

Sisk, C., Chitiyo, G., & Akenson, A. (2018). Predictors of social relationships for children with special health care needs. *Journal of Pediatric Nursing*, *42*, 92–99. https://doi.org/10.1016/j.pedn.2018.03.009

Stephens, M. M., Cook-Fasano, H. T., & Sibbaluca, K. (2018). Childhood bullying: Implications for physicians. *American Family Physician*, *97*(3), 187–192. http://www.ncbi.nlm.nih.gov/pubmed/29431974

Turner, H. A., Finkelhor, D., Hamby, S. L., Shattuck, A., & Ormrod, R. K. (2011). Specifying type and location of peer victimization in a national sample of children and youth. *Journal of Youth and Adolescence*, *40*(8), 1052–1067. https://doi.org/10.1007/s10964-011-9639-5

van Geel, M., Vedder, P., & Tanilon, J. (2014). Relationship between peer victimization, cyberbullying, and suicide in children and adolescents. *JAMA Pediatrics*, *168*(5), 435–442. https://doi.org/10.1001/jamapediatrics.2013.4143

Waasdorp, T. E., & Bradshaw, C. P. (2015). The overlap between cyberbullying and traditional bullying. *Journal of Adolescent Health*, *56*(5), 483–488. https://doi.org/10.1016/j.jadohealth.2014.12.002

Walter, H. J., Vernacchio, L., Trudell, E. K., Bromberg, J., Goodman, E., Barton, J., Young, G. J., DeMaso, D. R., & Focht, G. (2019). Five-year outcomes of behavioral health integration in pediatric primary care. *Pediatrics*, *144*(1), e20183243. https://doi.org/10.1542/peds.2018-3243

Weitzman, C., & Wegner, L. (2015). Promoting optimal development: Screening for behavioral and emotional problems. *Pediatrics*, *135*(2), 384–395. https://doi.org/10.1542/peds.2014-3716

Williams, K. R., & Guerra, N. G. (2007). Prevalence and predictors of internet bullying. *Journal of Adolescent Health*, *41*(6), S14–S21. https://doi.org/10.1016/j.jadohealth.2007.08.018

Zych, I., Ortega-Ruiz, R., & Del Rey, R. (2015). Systematic review of theoretical studies on bullying and cyberbullying: Facts, knowledge, prevention, and intervention. *Aggression and Violent Behavior*, *23*, 1–21. https://doi.org/10.1016/j.avb.2015.10.001

18

Schools as a Milieu

Anson J. Koshy and Mary Yarus

For additional material related to the content of this chapter, please see Chapters 19,104 and 113.

VIGNETTE

Angela Ramirez is an 11-year-old girl who is fluent in both English and Spanish. Angela's parents emigrated from Mexico to the United States when she was 2 years old. Her father speaks little English, and her mother speaks only Spanish. Angela qualified for English as a Second Language (ESL) supports in preschool, which continued through first grade. In first grade she qualified for special education supports, specifically speech and language therapy under a classification of speech or language impairment. In the third grade updated psychoeducational testing noted a full-scale IQ of 90 and poor performance in reading, spelling, and writing. By fourth grade, she was diagnosed with attention-deficit/hyperactivity disorder, predominantly inattentive presentation by her pediatrician and prescribed a long-acting stimulant medication.

Since starting middle school 12 months ago, Angela has been struggling with peer interactions and has not been as engaged in classroom learning. She is regularly handing in assignments late or not at all and has few explanations for her missing homework. The middle school is much further away from her inner-city apartment where she lives with her three younger siblings, mother, father, and maternal grandfather. Her grandfather has recently taken ill, and Angela has taken on additional responsibilities at home to care for him. Angela previously met with a school counselor regularly in elementary school and had a close relationship with her teacher. However, now in a much larger middle school, staff turnover is high, and resources for students are limited. Her classes are overcrowded, and the accommodations she previously received have not carried over to middle school. The condition of her middle school is in disrepair, and there are concerns about poor supervision of students before and after school.

Angela's teachers report that she seems more isolated and withdrawn. Her grades have declined. Her teachers have requested Angela's parents seek out guidance from her pediatrician for further medical workup and intervention.

INTRODUCTION

Angela's story illustrates the complex interaction between child, family, school, community, and societal factors that influence academic performance. In Angela's case her declining academic performance and disengaged behavior in the classroom are signs of underlying developmental-behavioral health and social concerns that are affecting her wellbeing. Schools can play a vital role in identifying developmental-behavioral concerns and supporting child wellbeing. However, Angela's case highlights how school-level factors such as limited resources, high staff turnover, and classroom overcrowding can inhibit a school's ability to support children and can negatively affect outcomes. Unfortunately, like Angela, children from historically marginalized communities, who face intense social needs, often attend underresourced schools that must deal with such challenges.

Like Angela's parents, many caregivers seek guidance from developmental-behavioral clinicians when academic and behavioral concerns arise in the classroom. To address these concerns effectively, clinicians must consider child-level factors such as innate potential, strengths, and needs in the broader context of the child's family, neighborhood, and school. While many clinicians consider psychosocial factors in the evaluation of a child's school functioning, characteristics of the school and classroom may receive less attention. This chapter reviews characteristics of the school environment and physical features that can affect child outcomes. We also review the vital role of the school environment in promoting physical health and wellbeing, particularly for children from low-income backgrounds and children with special health-care needs and disabilities. We close the chapter by highlighting implications for clinician practice and advocacy.

SCHOOL ENVIRONMENT

Schools are complex organizations made up of diverse stakeholders (e.g., administrators, teachers, staff, students, parents, and others). Dynamic forces, including interactions between these stakeholders; policies and politics at the local, state, and federal level; and shifts in societal and cultural norms, all shape the priorities and day-to-day activities that compose the school environment for a student. Factors such as emphasis on academics; commitment to diversity, equity, and inclusion; support for teachers and staff; strategies to address behavioral concerns; and availability of extracurricular activities shape the students' experiences and in turn influence outcomes.

Academic Emphasis

In 1983 the report, *A Nation at Risk: The Imperative for Educational Reform*, by the National Commission on

Excellence in Education, called for a shift in emphasis of US educational systems toward improved academic achievement. In calling for higher standards to prepare US students for the demands of the 21st century and the challenges of a global economy, the report triggered numerous reform initiatives with a focus on assessment, academic standards, and accountability. This focus culminated in the passage of the No Child Left Behind Act of 2001 and its successor, the Every Student Succeeds Act of 2015, which were both reauthorizations of the Elementary and Secondary School Act first passed in 1965. These laws codified expectations for educational excellence and school accountability, while triggering an impassioned, national debate on such issues as charter schools, vouchers and parental choice, teacher qualifications and training, school finance, and valid indicators of academic achievement (see Chapter 113 for more information).

While many of the same debates are ongoing, it is clear that children benefit when there is an appropriate emphasis on academics in schools. Such an emphasis may be reflected in the frequent assignment of homework, high teacher expectations for students' academic achievement, the display of children's work on classroom walls, total teaching time per week, a high rate of students' use of the school library, and group (as opposed to individual teacher) planning of courses and lessons with monitoring and advice provided by department heads.

Diversity, Equity, and Inclusion

The mid-20th century was marked by legislative achievements, court decisions, and social movements that have influenced efforts to promote diversity, equity, and inclusion in US public schools. In a 1954 unanimous decision in the landmark case *Brown v. Board of Education of Topeka* the US Supreme Court ruled that US state laws enforcing racial segregation in public schools were unconstitutional. A second decision in *Brown II* (1955) ordered states to desegregate schools. In the civil rights era of the 1960s and 1970s concerns with schools in the United States focused on issues of equality and community inclusion, as expectations for racial integration and the mainstreaming of children with disabilities in the least restrictive educational environments influenced school planning and design. Around this time, President Lyndon B. Johnson signed the Elementary and Secondary Education Act of 1965 into law. This law provides federal funding to primary and secondary education, including for instructional materials, professional development, and supporting parental involvement, with a primary goal of addressing racial/ethnic and income-based achievement gaps. Along these lines, the Bilingual Education Act was the first federal legislation that recognized the needs of students with limited English proficiency. Passed in the wake of the civil rights movement, this act signaled that the federal government recognized that US public schools needed bilingual education programs to address the needs of children learning more than one language.

Another landmark decision by the US Supreme Court in 1982 directly impacted the right to a public education for immigrant children. The case *Plyer v. Doe* struck down legislation in Texas denying school district funding for the education of undocumented children from kindergarten to the grade 12. The court ruled that the undocumented status of children could not be a basis for depriving them of an education, and the ruling further supported the tenant for a free appropriate public education for all children in the United States.

Despite this progress, the COVID-19 pandemic has illustrated how the struggle for diversity, equity, and inclusion in schools continues. Lockdowns in response to the pandemic forced many supports to suddenly stop, and students of color suffered disproportionately, including students who are immigrants and English language learners (ELLs) like Angela in the opening vignette. In the early days of the pandemic certain states, including parts of Virginia, California, and Maryland, began seeing ELL students fall behind more significantly than their peers academically. The *New York Times* (Kim, 2020) reported that the increase in Connecticut absentee rates for ELL students was second only to homeless students when accounting for either in-person or remote learning attendance. These findings illustrate the need for continued vigilance and advocacy among clinicians and other professionals to support diversity, equity, and inclusion in schools.

Teacher Training and Support

Low-income and at-risk students are often served in urban schools, and teachers in these settings often demonstrate lower credentials or qualifications when compared to teachers placed in more affluent schools in suburban areas. Urban schools are inherently at greater risk to provide lower-quality instruction for students who are often most in need. However, some studies have shown that teacher qualifications, whether it be duration of teaching or licensure scores, do not directly impact student achievement (Buddin, 2010). Research in the last 2 decades shows how teachers differ from one another in ways that go beyond their qualifications and how these differences impact student achievement and long-term outcomes. For example, (Chetty, Friedman & Rockoff, 2014) found that students who are assigned to high-value-added teachers (value-added refers to teachers' impact on student performance) are more likely to graduate from high school, attend college, and gain successful employment.

Teacher and school assessment professionals require a clear understanding of the wide range of developmental, behavioral, and learning differences impacting all learners. Understanding early signs of learning differences such as dyslexia is critical to ensure young students are identified and evidence-based interventions are provided as early as possible to promote optimal outcomes. It is critical to ensure that teachers and assessment personnel are aware of early signs of learning disabilities and have the training to recognize and intervene with evidence-based supports when indicated (see Chapter 104).

Teachers and Peers

The most powerful school models for promoting resilience among disadvantaged children are those that foster strong and supportive teacher-student relationships and actively buffer the effects of adversity on children. However, research has shown that high teacher turnover negatively impacts achievement for all students, and the highest rates of turnover impact low-income students and students of color disproportionately (U.S. Department of Education, Office for Civil Rights, 2014). Schools experiencing staffing shortages have increased need for substitute teachers, higher rates of canceled classes, and underprepared instruction. The financial costs of teacher turnover are well established and include the additional expenses related to recruitment, hiring, and training, which could be allocated to other resources. Of note, teacher attrition rates in the United States have not always been an issue and were lower when salaries were more competitive and working conditions were more supportive. Returning to the opening vignette, Angela had strong relationships with her teacher and counselor in elementary school, but was unable to develop similar relationships in the larger middle school where there was high teacher and staff turnover. Such relationships with caring professionals can be critical to uncovering the stress Angela is experiencing at home and providing appropriate supports in a timely manner.

Student interactions with teachers and peers in the classroom make major contributions to the school environment and influence student social, behavioral, and academic development. Students rely on their observations of how a teacher interacts with their classmates when forming perceptions of a classmate's likability (Hughes & Kwok, 2007). Students observe how a teacher interacts with a classmate in the classroom, which can contribute to a classroom consensus about that child's reputation and influence how classmates interpret the child's behavior. Supportive relationships with teachers may reduce the risk of peer rejection (Hughes & Kwok, 2007). Returning to Angela's case, it would be important to inquire about her perceptions of her teachers as well as how she perceives she is doing socially with peers at school to better understand additional factors that may be impacting her academic performance.

Peer interactions within and outside of the classroom foster a climate characterized as nonacademic, and the amount of time spent with peers has a significant impact on a learner's achievement. Regardless of their own ability level, students who affiliate with low-achieving peers have significantly lower achievement scores than students who affiliate with high-achieving peers. Despite the importance of peer group membership for educational outcomes, it is often overlooked during the assessment process. Assessments conducted in school should consider peer group membership during the monitoring of student academic and behavioral performance.

Positive Behavior Supports

Academic and behavioral outcomes can be improved when general standards for classroom discipline are set by the school, as opposed to being left to individual teachers. School-wide positive behavior supports are an approach conducive to optimizing a learning environment in school and can be seen as an alternative for traditional reactive or punitive consequences to minimize problem behaviors. The underpinnings of school-wide behavioral supports are based on evidence-based practices in the fields of education and behavior, including applied behavior analysis. This type of support is often organized into tiers, including instruction provided to all students, and behavioral expectations are relayed to students in a concise, clear, and positive way. Systems are in place to monitor and promote appropriate behavior. Students who are not responsive to this universal level of instruction are provided with more intensive interventions. Students who continue to struggle to respond to the aforementioned interventions receive even more intensive and individualized behavior supports, which correspond with the highest tier. Positive behavior supports that are implemented school-wide are designed to improve learning by increasing total time students are in school and engaged with instruction. Some studies have shown that use of school-wide positive behavior supports can decrease ineffective disciplinary practices producing gains in student behavior and overall school climate (Nocera, Whitbread, & Nocera, 2014).

Extracurricular Activities

Participation in extracurricular activities or activities led by an adult during the school day but outside of the typical classroom has been championed as a strategy to further support cognitive and social emotional learning among students. Research has found that adolescents involved in extracurricular activities learn skills that can be applied both in and out of the classroom (Feldman & Matjasko, 2005). Rates of participation for low-income students are lower than peers from higher-income backgrounds. The Pew Research Center (2015) found children from families making less than US $30,000/year were 10% to 20% less likely to participate in extracurricular activities. The Individuals with Disabilities Education Act has helped to provide a more inclusive school environment for children with disabilities, but this is less consistent for extracurricular programs. One study found that over 60% of parents of children with disabilities reported that their child never participated in clubs, teams, or similar organizations in the school or community setting (Coster et al., 2012). However, opportunities for children to be involved in structured activities outside of the classroom have been found to serve as a protective factor that has been associated with positive social and academic outcomes (Spencer, McDermott, Burton, & Kochman, 1997). For children with various disabilities, participation in extracurricular activities has been shown to establish better social outcomes and indirectly decrease bullying incidents (Bills, 2020).

PHYSICAL FEATURES

In this section we review how physical aspects of the school environment such as size and space, neighborhood factors, and structural and technology features of schools can affect student outcomes.

Size and Space

The mid to late 20th century in the United States featured a rapid shift toward the consolidation of schools, which resulted in larger student populations and construction of larger school buildings (Bindler et al., 2002). This trend was largely motivated by the idea that larger schools could offer more academic opportunities while minimizing the cost per student (Bindler et al., 2002). More recent evidence challenges this idea by suggesting that smaller schools may be better equipped to promote academic success especially for children from disadvantaged backgrounds (Leithwood & Jantzi, 2009). More specifically, smaller school sizes are associated with enhanced student achievement, improved attendance, and higher graduation rates (Leithwood & Jantzi, 2009). One potential mechanism is that smaller schools can offer opportunities for community building among teachers, students, and parents, which can facilitate effective governance and learning environments (Bindler et al., 2002). However, school size alone does not guarantee such processes or outcomes, and other factors such as funding, staffing, and leadership likely play an important role.

Studies on the effects of class size also offer differing results. Class size appears to have modest but statistically significant effects on mathematics and reading achievement growth, but these effects decline as students progress through school (Rivkin, Hanushek, & Kain, 2005). Importantly, smaller class sizes would require more teachers and more classrooms, greatly increasing already-stretched public school budgets. This could lead to a tradeoff between teacher quality and class size, particularly in schools serving disadvantaged populations that are already difficult to staff.

In summary, while school and class sizes are often among the most debated issues in school reform, definitive answers remain elusive and require additional research. When interpreting this literature, we remind readers that although important, school and class size do not determine student outcomes alone and should be considered in the context of other factors.

Neighborhood Factors

The primary community group a child belongs to outside of the immediate family often lies within the school community. Public education has traditionally been tied directly to housing through the assignment of residences to specified school zones. Across the United States it is difficult for families from low or moderate incomes to afford suitable housing in a transit-rich community with access to high-performing public schools. Research has shown that housing characteristics vary across school zones, with larger houses and single-family homes more commonly seen inside of higher-performing zones (Kane, Staiger, & Cellini, 2005).

Few states extend transportation services to students attending schools of choice that lie outside of a residentially assigned school zone. Families that choose a school outside of the zoned public school must often arrange their own transportation. As a result, families with accessible transportation options have more options for school enrollment.

Neighborhood violence negatively impacts academic performance, particularly for children residing in neighborhoods with high crime rates (Burdick-Will et al., 2011; Schwartz, Laurito, Lacoe, Sharkey, & Gould, 2016; Sharkey, 2010; Sharkey et al., 2014). The climate within each school can play a critical role in helping students cope with external stressors experienced outside of the school setting. Many schools are viewed as safe havens for children in high-crime neighborhoods (Laurito, Lacoe, Schwartz, Sharkey, & Ellen, 2019). Schools can support community engagement by allowing access to physical facilities and extending the learner's educational environment into the broader community. Schools often have large gathering spaces and recreational grounds for sports or play that may otherwise not be readily available in the community (see Chapter 19).

Structure and Technology

Several factors have been shown to positively impact academic outcomes for learners in school-based settings. Access to abundant natural light while also limiting the effects of glares or overheating is important alongside high-quality electric lighting (Barkmann et al., 2012). Similarly, maintaining comfortable temperatures can impact both teacher's wellbeing and academic performance of learners (Goodman et al., 2018; Haverinen-Shaughnessy & Shaughnessy, 2015; Sadick & Issa, 2017). Students in underresourced neighborhoods typically contend with aging schools with uncomfortable temperatures, dust, mold, poor ventilation, and poor lighting (Filardo, Vincent, Sullivan, 2019). There may also be aging water infrastructures that can lead to harmful environmental exposures from as lead, copper, and other materials contaminating drinking water (American Society of Civil Engineers, 2017). Poor environmental factors can lead to increased asthma and respiratory cases as well as other health concerns. Illnesses lead to absenteeism, which can greatly reduce student performance.

Schools are increasingly using technology to support learning in and outside of the classroom. Technology use can allow students to learn at their own pace and provide students with more diverse learning opportunities and experiences. However, an international study into the impacts of heavy financial investments in school technologies from 2015 noted mixed outcomes. There was some evidence that moderate use of computers in the classroom tended to assist learning outcomes, but technology could also distract from intensive teacher-student interaction that supports conceptual understanding and higher-order thinking (Organisation for Economic Co-operation and Development, 2015).

THE SCHOOL'S ROLE IN PROMOTING PHYSICAL HEALTH AND WELLBEING

Schools have long served a critical role in identifying and intervening on behalf of learners who present with a range of socioeconomic, medical, and developmental-behavioral concerns. In this section we highlight specific areas in which school environments can affect physical health and wellbeing: mitigating food insecurity, identifying children at risk for maltreatment, and administering medications and conducting health screenings.

Food Insecurity

Food insecurity is lacking consistent access to enough food for every member in a household to live a healthy and active life.

The US Department of Agriculture (USDA) Household Food Insecurity report from 2020 noted that more than 35 million people in the United States experience hunger. Households with children are more likely to experience food insecurity, and schools play an important role in supporting these children. The National School Lunch Program (NSLP) is one of the earliest examples of federal school-based programs and remains in place to this day serving millions of children. Signed into law by President Harry Truman in 1946, this program provides low- or no-cost meals to children on school days. The program plays an important role in mitigating the harmful effects of food insecurity and illustrates how schools support health and wellbeing beyond academic performance. Children in households with incomes below 130% of the poverty level or those whose families receive Supplemental Nutrition Assistance Program (SNAP) or Temporary Assistance of Needy Families (TANF) qualify for free meals. Families whose incomes are between 130% and 185% of the poverty level qualify for reduced-price meals.

During summer months, millions of children in the United States suffer from hunger and food insecurity due to a lack of access to school lunch programs. The USDA funds summer food service programs to establish summer meal delivery across the country for eligible children; however, many families are not aware of these programs or how to access them. Clinicians can help raise awareness about these programs. The COVID-19 pandemic highlighted inequities, including food insecurity, which disproportionately impacted students from lower-income families who depend on a reduced or free school lunch for regular meals during the week. News coverage during the height of the 2020 pandemic often included scenes of long lines for food distribution and schools providing meals that parents could pick up and take home to ensure their children were accessing regular meals during the week.

Child Maltreatment/Abuse

In most states school employees (teachers, counselors, and other school staff) are mandated reporters of child abuse and are legally obligated to report signs of abuse or neglect to appropriate authorities in a timely manner. During a typical school week, students spend much of their time with their teachers. According to the Children's Bureau (2020), the Child Maltreatment Report 2018 noted that nearly 67% of reports to Child Protective Services (CPS) of suspected child abuse were from professionals, with educational professionals making up the largest cohort of reporters. As such, education professionals must be prepared to identify early signs of abuse and neglect, and professional development in this area is critical to help ensure child safety.

Medication Administration and Health Screening

With increasing numbers of children with special health care needs that require medication administration daily, the need for school nursing staff can be in direct competition with other resources when school funding supports are limited. The American Academy of Pediatrics (AAP, 2009) supports medication administration in schools by a full-time licensed registered nurse on campus to administer routine and emergency medications. This preferred option is followed by having a licensed practical nurse on campus and then as a last resort the delegation of nursing duties to unlicensed assistive personnel as long as this is consistent with state regulations (AAP, 2009). Although schools that receive federal funds are required to provide reasonable accommodations based on Section 504 of the Rehabilitation Act, there is wide variability in the implementation of accommodations when it comes to medication administration. Clinicians can advocate for optimal school-based health care by supporting the role of nursing in schools.

Screening for vision and hearing concerns in public schools provides critical opportunities to identify sensory impairments for low-income students. Children from low-income families are less likely to see an eye care provider compared to families with incomes greater than 200% of the federal poverty level (Centers for Disease Control and Prevention, 2018). As of 2016, 40 states have required screening for vision for students in public schools; however, the means of doing so vary across states. One study that examined rates of chronic health conditions by race and ethnicity in children found that Hispanic students were more likely to report visual impairment compared to Black or White peers (Kitsantas, Kornides, Cantiello, & Wu, 2013). Full-time nurses in schools can help ensure that children have access to necessary vision and hearing screens to help children better meet their full potential in the learning environment.

ROLE OF CLINICIAN AS AN ADVOCATE

The powerful influence of school environments on student performance and wellbeing has important implications for clinician practice and advocacy. For children experiencing school difficulties, clinicians should consider children's strengths and needs within the context of their environment at home and at school. Clinicians should also ensure that psychological, educational, and developmental assessments are not considered in isolation. Instead, clinicians should interpret findings from careful history taking, observations, and assessments within the broader context of these environments when considering medical diagnoses, educational classifications, interventions, and treatment plans.

As influential members of the community, clinicians can bring familiarity of local resources and scientific credibility to advocate for school environments that promote optimal child wellbeing. Clinicians can offer support and guidance to schools, boards of education, and parent groups. Clinicians can also advocate for school policies such as funding for school nurses to provide reliable care for children with special health care needs. Familiarity with the organization of schools, including the administrative, financial, and communication structures, can enable the clinician to advocate more effectively for developmentally appropriate policies that enhance the school environment such as positive behavior supports.

Returning to the opening vignette, Angela's clinician could gain critical insight into her declining academic performance and diminishing engagement in the classroom by asking questions about Angela's school environment. For example, upon learning about conditions such as high staff turnover, overcrowded classrooms, and inconsistent implementation of her individualized education plan (IEP) supports, the clinician can help Angela's parents request an IEP team meeting to reassess her supports, ensure access to counseling services, and consider updated psychoeducational testing if indicated. The clinician might also link the family to an educational advocate who can offer support in making these requests. Angela's clinician can also link her and her family to community-based behavioral health supports, which could offer additional support.

CONCLUSION

The school environment has major impacts on child well-being, and schools play a key role in promoting physical health and safety for children. Developmental-behavioral clinicians must be aware of these important contributions to inform their practice and use their knowledge to advocate for school environments that promote optimal outcomes for all children.

REFERENCES

American Society of Civil Engineers. (2017). *2017 Infrastructure Report Card. A comprehensive assessment of America's infrastructure.* https://www.infrastructurereportcard.org/wp-content/uploads/2016/10/2017-Infrastructure-Report-Card.pdf

Bills, K. L. (2020). Helping children with disabilities combat negative socio-emotional outcomes caused by bullying through extracurricular activities. *Journal of Human Behavior in the Social Environment, 30*(5), 573–585.

Bindler, S., Diamond, B. M., Hill, B., Hoffman, J. L., Howley, C. B., Kent Lawrence, B., ... Washor, E. (2002). *Dollars and sense: The cost effectiveness of small schools.* Concordia and Knowledge Works Foundations.

Buddin, R., & Gema, Z. (2010). *What teacher characteristics affect student achievement? Findings from Los Angeles public schools.* RAND Corporation. https://www.rand.org/pubs/research_briefs/RB9526.html

Burdick-Will, J., Jens, L., Raudenbush, S. W., Sampson, R. J., Sanbonmatsu, L., & Sharkey, P. (2011). Converging evidence for neighborhood effects on children's test scores: An experimental, quasi-experimental, and observational comparison. In G. J. Duncan & R. J. Murnane (Eds.), *Whither opportunity? Rising inequality, schools, and children's life chances.* Russell Sage Foundation.

Centers for Disease Control and Prevention (CDC). (2018). *Visual impairment and use of eye-care services and protective eyewear among children, United States 2002.* http://www.cdc.gov/mmwr/preview/mmwrhtml/mm5417a2.htm

Chetty, R., Friedman J. N., & Rockoff J. (2014). Measuring the impacts of teachers I: Evaluating bias in teacher value-added estimates. American Economic Review, 104(9), 2593–2632.

Coleman-Jenson, A., Rabbitt, M., Gregory C. A., & Singh. A. (2021). Household food security in the United States in 2020 (p. 298). U.S. Department of Agriculture, Economic Research Service.

Council on School Health. (2009). Policy statement—Guidance for the administration of medication in school. Pediatrics, 124(4), 1244–1251.

Coster, W., Law, M., Bedell, G., Liljenquist, K., Kao, Y. C., Khetani, M., & Teplicky, R. (2012). School participation, supports and barriers of students with and without disabilities. *Child: Care, Health and Development, 39*, 535–543.

Feldman, A. F., & Matjasko, J. L. (2005). The role of school-based extracurricular activities in adolescent development: A comprehensive review and future directions. *Review of Educational Research, 75*, 159–210.

Filardo, M., Vincent, J. M., Sullivan, K. (2019). How crumbling school facilities perpetuate inequality. *Phi Delta Kappan, 100*(8), 27–31.

Goodman, J., Hurwitz, J. P., & Smith, J. (2018). *Heat and learning [working paper].* National Bureau of Economic Research.

Haverinen-Shaughnessy, U., & Shaughnessy, R. J. (2015). Effects of classroom ventilation rate and temperature on students' test scores. *PLoS One, 10*(8), e0136165. https://doi.org/10.1371/journal.pone.0136165

Hughes, J., & Kwok, O. (2007). Influence of student-teacher and parent-teacher relationships on lower achieving readers' engagement and achievement in the primary grades. *Journal of Educational Psychology, 99*, 39–51.

Kane, T. J., Staiger, D. O., & Cellini, S. (2005). *School quality, neighborhoods and housing prices: The impacts of school desegregation.* National Bureau of Economic Research.

Kim, J. (2020 December 29). *With remote learning, a 12-year-old knows her English is slipping away. The New York Times.* https://www.nytimes.com/2020/12/29/nyregion/coronavirus-english-language-students.html

Kitsantas, P., Kornides, M. L., Cantiello, J., & Wu, H. (2013). Chronic physical health conditions among children of different racial/ethnic backgrounds. *Public Health, 127*(6), 546–553.

Laurito, A., Lacoe, J., Schwartz, A. E., Sharkey, P., & Ellen, I. G. (2019). School climate and the impact of neighborhood crime on test scores. *The Russell Sage Foundation Journal of the Social Sciences: RSF, 5*(2), 141–166.

Leithwood, K., & Jantzi, D. (2009). A review of empirical evidence about school size effects: A policy perspective. *Review of Educational Research, 79*(1), 464–490.

Nocera, E., Whitbread, K., & Nocera, G. P. (2014). Impact of school-wide positive behavior supports on student behavior in the middle grades. *Research in Middle Level Education, 37*(8).

Organisation for Economic Co-operation and Development (OECD). (2015). *Students, computers and learning: Making the connection.* OECD Publishing.

Pew Research Center. (2015). *Children's extracurricular activities. Social and demographic trends project.* http://www.pewsocialtrends.org/2015/12/17/5-childrens-extracurricular-activities/

Rivkin, S., Hanushek, E. A., & Kain, J. F. (2005). Teachers, schools, and academic achievement. *Econometrica, 73*, 417–458.

Sadick, A.-M., & Issa, M. H. (2017). Occupant's indoor environmental quality satisfaction factors as measures of teachers' well-being. *Building and Environment, 119*, 99–109.

Schwartz, A. E., Laurito, A., Lacoe, J., Sharkey, P., & Gould, E. I. (2016). *The academic effects of chronic exposure to neighborhood violence. Maxwell School [working paper 195].* Syracuse University, Center for Policy Research.

Sharkey, P. (2010). The acute effect of local homicides on children's cognitive performance. *Proceedings of the National Academy of Sciences*, *107*(26), 11733–11738.
Sharkey, P., Schwartz, A. E., Gould, E. I., & Lacoe, J. (2014). High stakes in the classroom, high stakes on the street: The effects of community violence on students' standardized test performance. *Sociological Science*, *1*(14), 199–220.
Spencer, M. B., McDermott, P. A., Burton, L. M., & Kochman, T. J. (1997). An alternative approach to assessing neighborhood effects on early adolescent achievement and problem behavior. In J. Brooks-Gunn, G. J. Duncan, & J. L. Aber (Eds.), *Neighborhood poverty: Policy implications in studying neighborhoods* (vol. 2, pp. 145–162). Sage.
U.S. Department of Education, Office for Civil Rights. (2014). Dear Colleague Letter: Resource comparability. Washington, DC.
U.S. Department of Health & Human Services, Administration for Children and Families, Administration on Children, Youth and Famlies, Children's Bureau. (2020). *Child Maltreatment 2018.* https://www.acf.hhs.gov/cb/data-research/child-maltreatment

19

Neighborhoods and Personal Networks

Sarah E. Dubner and Lynne C. Huffman

For additional material related to the content of this chapter, please see Chapters 2, 18, 27 and 110.

VIGNETTE

Luciana is a 24-month-old girl, born after an uncomplicated pregnancy to Gloria, a 22-year-old Latina first-time mother. Luciana was a healthy baby; at her 2-year well-child visit, the pediatrician noted that she uses "mama" to call her mother, but she does not yet have any single words. They live in a low-resource high-density neighborhood with one small park that is poorly maintained. Gloria has a highly developed and extensive social network that includes multiple generations living in the same house and growing professional relationships through her job as a health care advocate. In the neighborhood there are other parents of young children who Gloria considers friends. How might knowing her neighborhood inform the pediatrician's assessment and recommendations? How might Gloria's networks help Luciana flourish?

DEFINING THE NEIGHBORHOOD AND THE PERSONAL NETWORK

Neighborhood

For children, the neighborhood is the relatively small environmental range and inherent relationships of home, school, and community that, together, determine the fabric of daily life. Although this sphere widens as children grow older and become more independent, this definition is intended to recognize the central importance of a child's functional environment in determining the material resources and human interaction so necessary to a child's health and social wellbeing. In defining the neighborhood unit of analysis for research purposes options have expanded over the past decade. These include census information and local knowledge of boundaries in cities, health districts, police districts, and school districts. Administrative data sources rely on bureaucratically defined units that vary across systems (health, education, law enforcement, social services) but tend to overlap to some extent. Such definitions of neighborhoods have primarily been limited to city or regional studies and often are used in conjunction with census data. More ethnographic accounts of neighborhoods emphasize the fact that individuals perceive boundaries differently. Some studies rely on participants' ratings of neighborhoods, including perceptions of the contexts encountered during daily activities. The predominance of research investigating neighborhood effects on child health has used census tract data. Tract boundaries are delineated with the advice of local communities working under Census Bureau guidelines and typically reflect prominent physical features that define neighborhoods (e.g., major streets, railroads) as well as important social and ethnic divisions.

Personal Network

The personal network of the child overlaps with and is distinct from the neighborhood, encompassing sources and pathways of social support. The personal network is characterized by the absence of common social boundaries, differentiating it from the concept of social groups. Network members may be defined generally as people outside of the parent or child's immediate household with whom they share affective or material activities and exchanges. Networks may also be defined by a particular type of relationship or exchange (e.g., networks of preschool children within a classroom and social emotional development) or health outcome (e.g., networks of adolescents who use nicotine products). Qualitative and quantitative approaches complement each other in the study of networks and health. The field of social network analysis as applied to health focuses on relationships between individuals or entities, rather than traditional methodologies that assess relationships between attributes of individuals. Such methods can be applied to analyze disease transmission or information dissemination among individuals, or it can be used to assess how social structures, relationships, social support, and social capital influence health and behaviors. The network paradigm can further be applied to systems-level health. Social network analysis can take a sociocentric or egocentric approach. The sociocentric approach seeks to understand entire networks of communities, while the egocentric approach seeks to model the networks related to an individual. Measurements of network structure and function seek to quantify the quantity, quality, and type of social ties, as well as emotional, instrumental, and information support, social norms and attitudes, and availability of community-based resources that may impact development, health attitudes and behaviors, and outcomes. Anthropologic and ethnographic approaches deepen investigation of the network relationship to health from the individual to societal level.

NEIGHBORHOOD

Mechanisms of Effect

Neighborhood factors explain 5% to 10% of the variation in children's development, wellbeing, and health (Leventhal, Dupéré, & Shuey, 2015). The means by which neighborhood influences child health can take many forms; several models have been proposed, with significant shifts since 2000.

In Bronfenbrenner's ecological systems model child development is influenced by multiple nested levels of the surrounding environment, starting with the microsystem (the immediate family), followed by the mesosystem, exosystem, macrosystem, and chronosystem (see Chapter 2). The five systems are interrelated. In this theoretical model (Fig. 19.1) (Scott, 2016) the neighborhood occupies the exosystem level labeled "local environment, formal networks and services." Recently, Minh, Muhajarine, Janus, Brownell, & Guhn, (2017) utilized this ecological systems theory and postulated diverse mechanisms by which neighborhood characteristics affect early child development (Table 19.1).

This theoretical framework also emphasizes place-based characteristics (i.e., where neighborhood effects occur) and child characteristics (i.e., for whom development and health are most affected). To examine the utility of this framework longitudinal data are important, and analytic approaches that consider mediators and moderators are essential for understanding the causal pathways of neighborhood effects. A mediator explains the process by which two variables are related, while a moderator variable affects the strength and direction of that relation.

Tung, Cagney, Peek, and Chin (2017) have recognized the importance of neighborhood in their three-axis model of health inequity. Race and poverty represent two axes of the model. Place is a third axis comprising built environment and social environment. Place is regarded as a local phenomenon, predominantly captured in neighborhoods and street-level units (not county, state, or national level units).

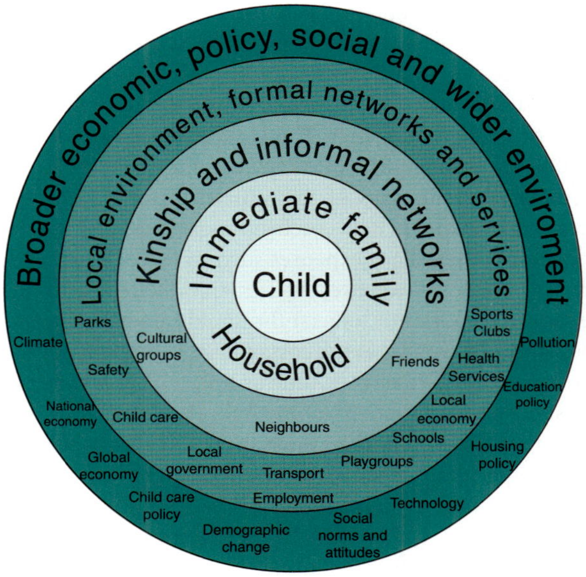

Fig. 19.1 Bronfenbrenner's ecological model. Diagram by Joel Gibbs based on Bronfenbrenner's (1979) ecological model. Adapted from Scott, K. [2016]. *Housing children: South Auckland. The Housing Pathways Longitudinal Study*. https://doi.org/10.13140/RG.2.2.24769.76645

Recent Trends in Neighborhood Research

Economic Disadvantage

Components of economic disadvantage: Income poverty, material hardship, family health. Despite being a common focus of discussion and research, economic disadvantage has defied a single

TABLE 19.1 Theoretical Links Between Neighborhoods and Child Development Outcomes

Mechanism of Effect	Conceptual Linkage	Examples of Metrics
Structural	Neighborhood disadvantage/advantage	• Income/wealth, employment • Education (e.g., school, childcare) • Immigrant concentration • Family structure • Social disconnection • Housing (e.g., housing quality) • Living environment (e.g., crowding) • Population density
Structural	Social stratification	• Gender • Race/ethnicity • Class
Social-interactive	Collective efficacy/social disorganization Norms Social networks [see this chapter] Family level	• Parents' perceived social or physical disorder • Fear of victimization • Safety • Parental depression • Adverse life events (e.g., family financial crisis, family death)
Institutional	Institutional resources	• Classroom instructional quality • Childcare quality • Neighborhood services
Geographical	Isolation, remoteness	• Distance to services
Environmental	Toxins, pollutants, noise	• Air pollution levels

definition. In large measure economic disadvantage is treated as synonymous with income poverty. Most often, for purposes of policy formulation and research, poverty is defined as a measure of subsistence: the income level that permits the maintenance of physical efficiency. The United States has been using the Official Poverty Measure (OPM) since the 1960s. There are major shortcomings of this official measure. It does not account for in-kind benefits such as food stamps and tax credits or for nondiscretionary expenses such as out-of-pocket health care and childcare expenses. It uses an outdated definition of the family. Importantly, official thresholds are not adjusted for geographic differences in the cost of living, which have become increasingly important over time as housing costs have grown to assume a larger share of family budgets. The OPM's statistical shortcomings compelled the National Academy of Sciences to converge upon a set of recommendations for improving the measure of poverty, resulting in the Supplemental Poverty Measure (SPM) (Short, 2016). The SPM improves on the official measure by more fully accounting for resources, expenses, and resource sharing, comparing household resources against poverty thresholds that are adjusted for modern standards of living as well as differences in costs of living across the United States, and applying a broader definition of the household.

More recently and less frequently, other components of economic disadvantage, including material hardship and adult health, have been considered in research that addresses the health and development of poor children. Material hardship is informally described as the inability to make ends meet and comprises inadequate housing, food insecurity, and unmet medical need. Adult health, specifically the health problems of adults in families with children, is another component of economic disadvantage. Parental illness can make it harder for parents to provide for their children, result in work limitations, and increase risk of joblessness.

Dynamics of disadvantage according to individual and family characteristics. Conceptualization of disadvantage also has shifted with regard to measurement over time of individual and family characteristics (i.e., age and race/ethnicity). The timing, duration, and community context of income poverty also have demonstrated to matter for child outcomes. Early experience of poverty, long periods of poverty, and high neighborhood concentration of poverty lead to worse child outcomes. Despite the common belief that childhood poverty has been a relatively stable phenomenon in American history, rates of childhood poverty are sensitive to economic and social trends. As a group, larger proportions of children are in poverty (using an SPM measure) compared to adults (e.g., in 2014, 17.5% of children in poverty and 15.9% of adults in poverty). Trends in income poverty among children differ greatly by race/ethnicity. Between 1970 and 2014, non-Hispanic Black and Latino children had higher poverty rates than non-Hispanic White children. During this period, poverty rates for non-Hispanic Black, Latino, and non-Hispanic White children declined (55.3% to 28.2%, 48.9% to 28.2%, and 18% to 9.6%, respectively) (Pac, Nam, Waldfogel, & Wimer, 2017). Use of the SPM measure highlighted an important antipoverty role of government safety net programs, especially for non-Hispanic Black and Latino children. Safety net programs include three types: cash benefits (e.g., Temporary Assistance for Needy Families [TANF]), in-kind benefits (e.g., Supplemental Nutrition Assistance Program [SNAP], housing subsidies, Special Supplemental Nutrition Program for Women, Infants, and Children [WIC]), and tax credits (e.g., earned income tax credit [EITC], child tax credit [CTC]). Trends over the past decade show a shift from cash benefit programs to in-kind and tax credit programs (Pac et al., 2017).

Restricted Physical Environment (Increased Density, Diminished Green Space)

Questions about how population exposure to natural environments may benefit health outcomes now are being addressed by the emerging field of environmental epidemiology. Reviews that have considered these questions in the context of neighborhoods conclude that various measures of exposure to residential greenness (i.e., vegetation level) or green spaces such as parks, gardens, and forests are beneficial for multiple measures of health. Most reviews focus largely on adult experience.

For children, in particular, there are fewer studies. Recent research trends in the child population include (1) inclusion of multiple, possibly related physical and social predictors (e.g., greenspace, air pollution, socioeconomic deprivation); (2) consideration of both positive and negative effects; (3) the use of normalized difference vegetation index (NDVI) to quantify greenness (the NDVI is based on satellite data and represents land surface reflectance of visible and near-infrared portions of the electromagnetic spectrum with higher numbers indicating more greenness); and (4) deliberate analysis of the implications of research results for policymakers who seek to translate evidence into feasible and achievable targeted interventions.

For example, one study showed that higher "greenness" surrounding residences was associated with lower prevalence of child overweight and excessive screen time and was not associated with asthma or allergic rhinoconjunctivitis (Dadvand et al., 2014). Exposure to outdoor surrounding greenness, especially greenness surrounding schools, has been shown to be associated with increases in working memory and reduction of inattentiveness. These associations were partly mediated by reduced air pollution.

In September 2016 a workshop entitled "Exploring Potential Pathways Linking Greenness and Green Spaces to Health" took place in Munich-Herrsching, Germany (Markevych et al., 2017). Participants concluded that the pathways by which greenspace can benefit health include reducing harm (e.g., decreased exposure to environmental stressors such as noise and heat), restoring capacities (e.g., stress recovery), and building capacities (e.g., encouragement of physical activity). Workshop recommendations related to future research included enhancement/expansion of study designs, exposure assessment, analytic methods, and study areas (most research has been conducted in high-income countries in Europe, North America, and Australia).

Geographic Mobility and Residential Instability

A child's ability to thrive can be greatly enhanced by stable and familiar surroundings. Stability and familiarity breed opportunities to master developmental tasks and to develop secure relationships. Changing neighborhoods, especially frequent changes, may place the child at risk for academic, behavioral, emotional, and potentially health problems. An analysis of data from the 2011/2012 National Survey of Children's Health showed that the number of moves in a child's life is inversely associated with flourishing (as measured by items addressing child self-regulation/curiosity and school engagement) (Gjelsvik, Rogers, Song, Field, & Vivier, 2019). Having three or more moves in childhood was associated with less flourishing for both poor boys and nonpoor girls, with no associations found for nonpoor boys or poor girls. Of note, because this study was correlational in design and the timing of the moves was not reported, investigators could not assess for sensitive time periods and could not determine if decreased flourishing was an immediate or delayed response. In a large, multisite, clinical sample of predominantly urban, low-income families of young children, Sandel and colleagues (2018) found that compared with caregivers in stable housing, caregivers with multiple moves had increased likelihood of fair and/or poor health and maternal depressive symptoms. Among children in households with multiple moves compared with those in stable housing, there was increased likelihood of developmental risk. Households with multiple moves also experienced increased likelihood of household hardships, including child food insecurity, inability to afford child health care, and paying for health care while sacrificing other essentials.

Research on the complex experience of residential mobility highlights the need for evolving theoretical and methodologic approaches. Results of the systematic review by Cotton (2016) highlight the importance of neighborhood context. Neighborhood-level variables increase risk of unwanted adolescent outcomes, including teen pregnancy, violent behaviors, and smoking. When families move, the destination neighborhood is an important indicator of risk. Adolescents moving from one disadvantaged neighborhood into another are at increased likelihood for violent offending, yet the risk decreases when relocating to a less disadvantaged neighborhood. However, for adolescents involved in the juvenile justice system recidivism increases, no matter the direction of the move (Wolff, Baglivio, Intravia, Greenwald, & Epps, 2017). Moving upward has the most negative effect for adjudicated male adolescents, while moving downward has the most negative effect for female youth.

In the positive direction higher neighborhood concentration of immigrants is associated with decreased school victimization (Foster & Brooks-Gunn, 2013). The US experience is different from other nations. Flouri, Mavroveli, & Midouhas, (2013) explored the impact of residential mobility within disadvantaged UK neighborhoods. Researchers observed that neighborhood and socioeconomic deprivation explained the association between mobility and children's emotional problems. Specifically, findings concluded that there were no significant differences between movers and nonmovers within this British sample. It is possible that this variation in findings reflects the economic, political, cultural, and geographic variation between the United Kingdom and the United States. Research investigating the influence of culture on residential mobility and associated outcomes is warranted.

Neighborhood Effects on Infants

Neonatal and Infant Mortality

Neonatal and infant mortality rates have long been recognized as sensitive indicators of social conditions. In the United States infant mortality rates have declined markedly during the past 8 decades. However, infant and child mortality rates are substantially higher in rural areas than in urban areas. Within rural areas, Black and American Indian/Alaska Native infants have higher infant mortality rates than White infants. Infant and child mortality rates are also higher in communities with higher poverty rates, regardless of rural-urban residence or race/ethnicity. In 2010–2014 the infant mortality rate for Black infants in rural counties with a poverty rate of ≥20% (9.4/1000 live births) was almost three times as high as in counties with a poverty rate of <5% (*Health Resources and Services Administration & Office of Health Equity, 2018*).

The influence of poverty on birthweight distribution is modulated primarily by the health of the mother before and during pregnancy; maternal health reflects the adequacy of nutrition, age, parity, health-related behaviors (e.g., smoking, alcohol use, illicit drug use), and a range of social stresses. In addition to elevating the chance that an infant will be born at low birthweight, poverty can also increase the risk that an infant will die, even among neonates of comparable birthweights. This occurs primarily when poverty, often accompanied by inadequate health insurance coverage, affects access to tertiary care facilities. Causes of the health disparities reported here are multifactorial in nature. Differences in social and built environments, socioeconomic and living conditions, health-risk behaviors such as tobacco use, obesity, lack of access to healthy foods, and access to and use of quality health care services are important social determinants contributing to persistent health disparities between population groups and geographic areas.

In 2014 a systematic review and metaanalysis examined evidence on the relation between neighborhood deprivation and the risks for preterm birth, small-for-gestational age, and stillbirth (Vos, Posthumus, Bonsel, Steegers, & Denktaş, 2014). The metaanalysis ($n = 7$ studies, including 2,579,032 pregnancies) assessed the risk of adverse perinatal outcomes by comparing the most deprived neighborhood quintile with the least deprived quintile. Deprivation did not have a standard definition; however, studies described neighborhood characteristics that included local unemployment, housing deprivation, domestic overcrowding, low neighborhood income, and high crime. Compared to the least deprived quintile, odds ratios for adverse perinatal outcomes in the most deprived neighborhood quintile were significantly and similarly increased for preterm delivery, small-for-gestational age, and stillbirth (odds ratios of 1.23, 1.31, and 1.33, respectively) (Fig. 19.2). The authors concluded that living in a deprived neighborhood is associated with these adverse perinatal outcomes. They were unable to draw specific conclusions about the extent to which the effect of neighborhood deprivation goes beyond the effect of poor individual level of socioeconomic status.

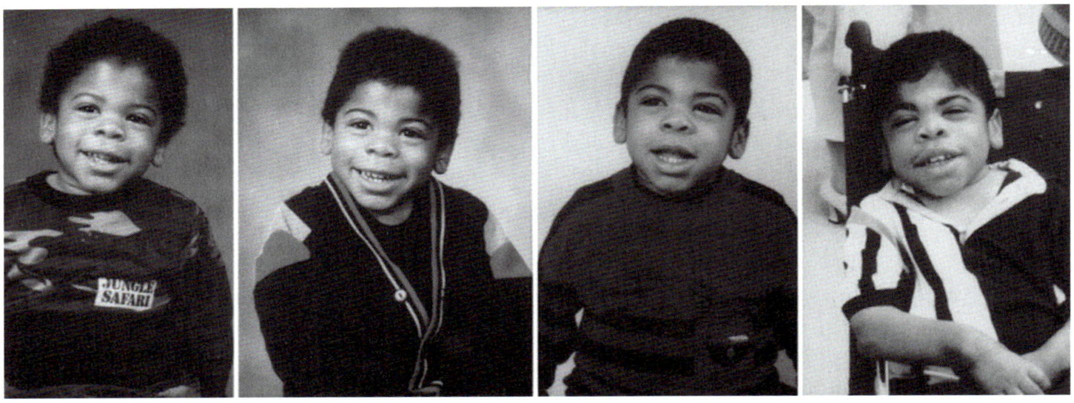

Fig. 19.2 Mild progression of classic features of Hunter syndrome (MPS II). The patient had minimal evidence of MPS II at initial evaluation for developmental delay. Photographs at ages 3 to 6 years demonstrate progression to classic coarse facial features, accompanied by organomegaly and dysostosis multiplex, observed at 10 years of age *(right)*.

Nutrition and Growth

One example of research addressing neighborhood characteristics and infant nutrition is the Yourkavitch, Kane, & Miles, (2018) study of breastfeeding practices. In this study the authors constructed indices of neighborhood disadvantage and neighborhood affluence and examined their associations with breastfeeding in multilevel models, controlling for individual-level characteristics. The associations of neighborhood disadvantage and affluence with breastfeeding practices differed by race/ethnicity. The likelihood of any breastfeeding decreased with worsening neighborhood disadvantage only for Hispanic women and increased for White women. The likelihood of any breastfeeding increased with improving neighborhood affluence for all except Hispanic women. Authors concluded that there were race/ethnic differences in associations between neighborhood disadvantage or affluence and breastfeeding practices at the time of hospital discharge. It is possible that specialized support improving access to services would be beneficial.

Neighborhood Effects on Children

Intellectual Development

We have known for decades that poor children are at increased risk for problems of cognitive and behavioral development. Any experience of poverty is associated with less favorable family situations and child outcomes than never being poor. Being poor later in childhood tends to be more detrimental than early poverty; children in chronically poor families show lower cognitive performance than do other children.

More recent studies reinforce and extend this understanding by including assessment of brain growth as well as cognitive skills. In a cross-sectional study Taylor, Cooper, Jackson, & Barch, (2020) assessed whether neighborhood poverty (beyond household income) accounts for differences in brain and cognitive skill development in a large sample of school-aged children. The authors reported that after accounting for household income, greater neighborhood poverty was associated with lower scores across all cognitive domains measured by the National Institutes of Health Toolbox Cognition Battery (e.g., verbal ability, attention, executive functioning, working memory, reading ability, processing speed) and with decreased brain volume in prefrontal and right hippocampal brain areas.

School Readiness and Achievement

Other research has attempted to separate the effects of neighborhood poverty and family poverty on children's academic skills and classroom behavior (see Chapter 18). As noted previously, the concentration of economic disadvantage in residential neighborhoods is increasingly recognized as a potentially important context that creates burdens on families beyond their own individual economic circumstances. Living in severely disadvantaged communities appears to be an exacerbating factor that contributes to worse child outcomes than family poverty alone. After reviewing studies of children and adolescents, Leventhal et al. (2015) concluded that high neighborhood socioeconomic status (SES) predicts better school readiness, academic achievement, and educational attainment among children, whereas lower neighborhood SES predicts worse behavior and mental health outcomes among children. However, they found that neighborhood SES (high or low) generally explains only 5% to 10% of the variance in developmental outcomes—a small effect—after accounting for child and family characteristics.

Psychological Wellbeing and Ethnic Density

Ethnic density or immigrant concentration is a concept that has emerged in the literature examining neighborhood effects on behavioral, emotional, and mental health concerns. There is a longer history of study for adults; in these projects the classic ethnic density effect is described as better health for individuals from minority ethnic groups if they live in neighborhoods with a larger concentration of people from their own group. Explanations for this include the hypothesis that own-group concentration helps to reduce exposure to the direct prejudice of the majority group and increase levels of mutual support.

Only a few studies have considered the effect of ethnic density on psychological wellbeing in childhood and adolescence. Xue, Leventhal, Brooks-Gunn, & Earls, (2005) investigated a group of 5- to 11-year-old children to determine whether children's anxiety and depression were associated with neighborhood structural characteristics (concentrated disadvantage, immigrant concentration, and residential stability) and whether neighborhood social processes (collective efficacy and organizational participation) underlie such effects. In this work the variable concentrated disadvantage represented characteristics, including poverty rate, receipt of public assistance, and unemployment. The authors found that, in general, children living in low-SES neighborhoods had more internalizing mental health problems than those in high-SES neighborhoods. Within each SES level, children living in neighborhoods with more minority residents had more problems than children living in neighborhoods with fewer minority residents. After accounting for individual and family characteristics, children living in neighborhoods marked by concentrated disadvantage were more likely than their peers in more advantaged neighborhoods to have internalizing problems. Of note, living in neighborhoods with high immigrant concentration or residential instability had no significant effects on children's mental health in this study (after controlling for concentrated disadvantage). In the Zhang, Beauregard, Kramer, & Bécares. (2017) study data were used from two nationally representative birth cohort studies, the US Early Childhood Longitudinal Study-Birth Cohort and the UK Millennium Cohort Study, to estimate the association between own ethnic density and behavioral and cognitive development at 5 years of age. Findings showed differences in ethnic density associations with child outcomes within and between the United States and United Kingdom, suggesting that neighborhood ethnic density effects also may reflect larger social and economic contexts. Authors argue that researchers should take area deprivation into account when estimating ethnic density effects and when developing policy initiatives targeted at strengthening and improving the health and development of racial and ethnic minority children. Overall, the results of studies to date indicate substantial heterogeneity in ethnic density effects on child outcomes. Future research addressing limitations related to sample size, inadequate adjustment for area deprivation, and poorly specified theoretical frameworks will improve our understanding of ethnic density effects.

Neighborhood Effects on Adolescents

Violence-Related Mortality

Homicide, the most extreme consequence of interpersonal violence, led to more than 2000 deaths among adolescents ages 10 to 19 years in 2019, with the highest incidence concentrated in urban settings and among Black youth. Culyba et al. (2016) assessed associations between environmental neighborhood features and adolescent homicide to identify targets for future place-based interventions. Using a population-based case control study design, 13- to 20-year-old adolescents who died by homicide between 2010 and 2012 were compared to control 13- to 20-year-old participants matched on sex and indoor-outdoor location at the time of each index case participant's homicide. Standardized techniques were used to photograph case and control participant outdoor locations. In adjusted analyses multiple features of city streets, buildings, and natural surroundings were associated with adolescent homicide. The presence of street lighting, illuminated walk/don't walk signs, painted marked crosswalks, public transportation, parks, and maintained vacant lots were associated with decreased likelihood of homicide. These results suggest multiple modifiable environmental features that might be targeted in future randomized intervention trials designed to reduce youth violence by improving neighborhood context.

Involvement in the Criminal Justice System

Neighborhood disadvantage has an effect on a known gender gap in violent crime—that is, males, more than females, engage in violent crime. Specifically, as the level of neighborhood disadvantage increases, the gender gap for adolescents engaged in violent crime decreases. It is believed that this is explained by gender differences in peer influence. Neighborhood disadvantage increases exposure to peer violence for both sexes, but peer violence has a larger effect on violent offending for females than for males. Zimmerman and Messner (2010) noted that females have more intimate friendships than males, and peer intimacy moderates the association between peer violence and self-reported violent behavior.

With regard to community disadvantage there are supported reasons to believe it may be beneficial to crime-reduction efforts to improve adolescents' contexts (increased resources, better schools, employment opportunities for youth and their families) as well as implications for increasing crime (relative deprivation, increased scrutiny and surveillance by neighbors and police, especially of males).

High School Completion

Higher neighborhood SES decreases the chances of failing to graduate from high school. Rural, compared to urban, setting also is a protective factor for high school graduation (Wall-Wieler, Roos, Chateau, & Rosella, 2016). Sustained exposure to disadvantaged neighborhoods has a detrimental effect on high school graduation. Growing up in the most (compared to the least) disadvantaged quintile of neighborhoods is estimated to reduce the probability of graduation from 96% to 76% for Black children, and from 95% to 87% for non-Black children (Wodtke & Parbst, 2017).

Wickrama, Simons, & Baltimore, (2012) used longitudinal, prospective data from waves 1 and 4 of the National Longitudinal Study of Adolescent Health ($n = 13,450$; 53% females) to assess the effect of educational level attainment on economic stability in early adulthood. Results indicated that youth who were Black, from disadvantaged communities, and from lower-SES families achieved significantly lower levels of earnings, assets, and job quality during young adulthood. Young adults' educational level partially mediated the influences of family and race/ethnicity influences on young adults' socioeconomic attainment. These findings underline the importance of social context as well as educational opportunities during adolescence for economic stability in early adulthood.

PERSONAL NETWORKS

Mechanisms of Effect

Multiple theoretical frameworks define child and parent personal networks in relation to child development. In Bronfenbrenner's ecological systems theory (see Fig. 19.1) children's social roles and interpersonal relations are part of the microsystem within which development occurs. Family social networks are among the exosystems that indirectly influence the child's lived experience. Personal networks are also central to the life-course theory of development in which "lives are lived interdependently, social and historical influences are expressed through this network of shared relationships" (Elder, 1998. p. 1).

Social integration and belonging relate to health and wellbeing (Smith & Christakis, 2008). Personal networks exert their effects on health through social support (whether perceived or actual), social norms and attitudes, availability of community-based resources, social engagement, and direct contact between individuals (Smith & Christakis, 2008). The value of networks may be as ecological or group-level social capital (e.g., civic participation, trust, expectations of reciprocity, social organizations), as conceptualized by Putnam (Hunter, Neiger, & West, 2011). Alternatively, the value of networks may be considered as resources that accrue to individuals as participants in a network, as described by Bourdieu (Hunter et al., 2011). This model postulates that the network and network ties, namely characteristics such as social structure, power, and disparities in access to resources, are the mechanisms by which social determinants exert their effect on health (Hunter et al., 2011). The focus of this chapter is primarily on this second definition of personal networks and on individual-level social capital on health. Aspects of personal networks have been identified as the underlying reason for relations between socioeconomic standing and health outcomes (e.g., network size and composition) and associated with parent education. Individuals with higher SES are more likely to consult expert professionals as well as to have family or friends who are experts.

Personal networks influence child health and development directly via their effect on the child and indirectly through their effects on parents. Variables directly affecting child cognitive and social development include social stimulation, new experiences, and provision of observational models and opportunities for active participation. Indirect support through the parents include (1) access to direct assistance, (2) provision of child-rearing controls, and (3) availability of role models. Berkman, Glass, Brissette, and Seeman (2000) synthesized social network theories, Durkheim's work on social integration and suicide, and attachment theory, generalized beyond child development to postulate that networks influence health through provision of influence and support.

Diffusion describes the way a contagion, whether a disease, belief, action, or information, spreads through networks. Mechanisms of diffusion of simple (e.g., virus) and complex (e.g., health behaviors such as smoking) contagions differ. A number of variables can be defined and generated to understand the formation and evolution of network structure in general and as it relates to health. Homophily describes the similarity of network members or ties on particular characteristics (e.g., "birds of a feather"). Centrality measures assess individual or group influence or leadership. Structural metrics include degree (number of ties a network member has to other members), density (how connected network members are to each other), small worlds (low-density, highly clustered networks with short overall path lengths), ties (connections between network members from which community is formed), among others.

Recent Trends in Personal Networks Research

The concept of social capital, though variably defined, has existed for over 100 years. Personal networks and social capital have been studied in depth in fields such as sociology. More recently, the fields of sociology and public health have come together to leverage the expertise and methods of social network analysis to understand how networks affect health and to develop network interventions to affect change.

A large body of work exists to describe the relationships between social support and health. Individual measures of trust in others have been found to be more highly correlated than income with lower levels of psychological distress and better self-rated health (Kawachi & Kennedy, 1999). Similarly, individual measures of social isolation are associated with poorer health, illness, and even death (Smith & Christakis, 2008).

As computing power has increased, the field of network research has grown to include more complex analyses of social networks themselves as they relate to health. Smith and Christakis (2008) argue that characterizing social relations and the ways in which individuals are connected elucidate relevant aspects of the whole that are not explained by or present in individual measures. Collaborations between public health researchers and sociologists over the past 20 to 30 years have expanded the methods and depth of investigations. Sociologists have brought expertise in influence and information diffusion and network function, and the interaction between race, gender, and class, and networks. The interaction of sociology and health has allowed classic sociologic principles to bring new perspectives to health. For instance, while one may focus on close relationships or densely connected networks, "weak ties" can bridge disparate and otherwise unrelated groups and are critical to diffusion of information or disease. Concepts such as weak ties and small worlds are now being utilized to design network interventions that focus not only on an individual but also on those to whom they are connected. This is a potential powerful tool for behavior change and disease prevention.

The rise of online communities and networks has raised new questions and potential opportunities in the understanding of networks and health. Online communities may be important sources of informational support. Online communities may have features unavailable in offline communities that can be beneficial to health. For instance, anonymity in online communities may allow discussion of topics taboo in an individual's community (Zhang & Centola, 2019). On the other hand, adolescents' offline risk-taking behavior has been found to be influenced by online peer behavior. Advances in mobile and wearable technology are allowing new and innovative approaches to research the influence of online and offline networks on behavior (Zhang & Centola, 2019).

Networks Across the Life Span

Personal networks evolve over the lifespan. In social convoy theory the core relationships among network members are relatively stable, and the peripheral relationships change and differ in closeness depending on a person's circumstances (Wrzus, Hänel, Wagner, & Neyer, 2013). Normative and non-normative life events change social networks. Changes such as puberty are a time of expanding networks as individuals build ties outside the family and have first romantic relationships, necessary to the development of autonomy and information acquisition. Parenthood is often accompanied by a constricting network, both for practical reasons such as changes in free time and for psychological reasons such as increased focus on the child and partner. Parents may also selectively maintain relationships with others with similar attitudes toward children. Events such as death of a close family member, divorce, and geographic relocation generally serve to decrease the size of networks.

Neonatal and Infant Health

Parents mediate their infant's interaction with the world. Aspects of social capital, including social mistrust, perceived unfairness, and perceived lack of helpfulness, have been associated with infant mortality in multiple studies, some showing that they account for up to 43% of the variance in infant mortality (Hunter et al., 2011). In the simplest child network, the parent-child dyad, the mental and physical health of the parent or child affects the other. Maternal depression is associated with multiple markers of poorer health and adjustment, including more behavior problems, mood disorders, hospitalizations, respiratory illness, and more (Smith & Christakis, 2008). The role of genetics versus environment in these relations is not yet elucidated.

Greater heterogeneity in parent personal networks is generally associated with better child health. The composition of parent networks influences resources available to parents and children. Research has primarily focused on mothers. In poorer households extended kin and coresident network members are important sources of support. This has been demonstrated across cultures, though is sensitive to cultural context. Kana'iIaupuni, Donato, Thompson-Colón, and Stainback (2005) framed the Mexican concepts of *confianza* and *compadrazgo* (godparenting) as important mechanisms of reciprocal exchange that promote child health. Mothers without social support were associated with rating their child's health as poor, whereas networks with more face-to-face contact were associated with more favorable ratings of child health.

On an individual level, people in parents' social networks influence common and important basic health decisions such as vaccination (Brunson, 2013) and sleep practices (Moon et al., 2019), with different network compositions associating with different decisions. For instance, in a study of network influence on infant safe sleep practices networks primarily exclusively composed of kin had greater influence on sleep practices than did more diverse networks. Diverse networks are associated with a variety of more positive outcomes than more restricted or homogenous networks. The reasons are likely multifactorial. People with diverse networks may have more sources of social resources and may be exposed to a greater diversity of viewpoints. Weak ties are important sources of new information, and the authors hypothesize that this may be a reason that attitudes toward recommended safe sleep practices were more positive in expansive networks.

Children

Parent network resources relate to child thriving beyond infancy. A recent and ongoing longitudinal study of 1082 mother-child dyads in Tennessee (Conditions Affecting Neurocognitive Development and Learning in Early Childhood [CANDLE]) has investigated the connections between networks and aspects of cognitive development. They have reported that large maternal social networks were positively associated with Bayley Scales of Infant Development–III cognitive domain scores at age 2 years and that children of mothers with many neighborhood members in their networks had better cognitive development (Shin et al., 2019).

Young children's early life relationships influence development and skills across domains. Play networks in preschool are an important area of study as children learn language, social, and cognitive skills through play with other children. Interactive play provides experiences for building shared meaning, developing emotional regulation, and reciprocity.

Personal networks of children are especially relevant to children with developmental disabilities. Chen, Lin, Justice, & Sawyer, (2019) studied 465 preschoolers across 64 inclusive classrooms in two states. Compared to children without disabilities, children with disabilities had lower centrality in play networks and were more likely to be marginalized or isolated. Homophily played an important role. Not only were they less likely to form play networks, but they were 1.5 times more likely to play with peers with a similar level of disability. While language ability similarly correlated with play network formation, the influence of the child's disability status uniquely influenced their play networks.

As children enter the school years, both their and their parents' relationships within the school are important to developmental outcomes. A diverse network with strong family support promotes wellbeing and may protect against problems such as depressive symptoms (Manalel & Antonucci, 2020). Bussing et al. (2003) showed that high levels of instrumental support in parent networks of elementary school students lowered the odds of attention-deficit/hyperactivity disorder (ADHD) mental health treatment, while caregiver strain increased likelihood of ADHD treatment.

Adolescents

The transition from childhood to adolescence marks an inflection point for personal network development. Peer networks become larger and peer relationships intensify. As with adults, adolescent networks with diverse sources of support are generally associated with better wellbeing and health. Youth health and characteristics themselves are related to their social network composition and structure. Adolescents with poor health have smaller networks and have lower centrality in their global networks than those in good health (Haas, Schaefer, & Kornienko, 2010). In one study of adolescents with high functioning autism those students were more frequently isolated or peripheral compared with their typically developing peers in classroom networks, despite being in inclusive settings (Locke, Ishijima, Kasari, & London, 2010). In addition, their connections were more likely to be to each other rather than to typically developing peers.

Mood, both positive and negative, diffuses through networks. A recent systematic review of offline and online networks and adolescent wellbeing found that healthy moods within offline networks can improve the probability of recovering from depression, while having more friends with worse moods can make individual moods worse. In addition to mood, self-esteem was positively associated with network size, and loneliness was negatively associated with the number of reciprocated friendships (Webster, Dunne, & Hunter, 2021). The National Longitudinal Study of Adolescent to Adult Health (Add Health) has been used to examine many features of adolescent networks, including the diffusion of mood and suicide. Suicidal ideation in girls, in particular, was related to social network position (Bearman & Moody, 2004). Schools with densely connected social networks had lower suicidal ideation in girls, but not boys, and lower likelihood of suicide attempts among boys. Social isolation and having friends who themselves were not friends were associated with increased suicidal ideation in girls. Further highlighting the salience of social networks, suicide attempts in friends affected suicidal ideation and attempts more than suicide attempts in family members.

Several investigations have connected academic achievement to network variables. Calvó-Armengol, Patacchini, & Zenou. (2009) found positive associations between centrality within larger social networks and educational outcomes. Based on a large natural experimental design study of students in Tel Aviv who nominated friends with whom to be placed for middle school, Lavy and Sand (2012) modeled that having more reciprocated friendships predicted significantly improved scores on standardized tests and that nonreciprocal friends offset the effects of reciprocal friends.

Peer and social relations have been linked in various ways to both positive and negative health behaviors in adolescents, including smoking, alcohol use, eating and dieting, sleep, and illicit substance use beyond biologic or genetic associations. Since behaviors diffuse through a network (peer contagion), it is important to consider how adolescents are grouped in settings such as school and the juvenile justice system. Studies point to development of interventions that incorporate the adolescent's social network, either by providing peer support or altering the network in some way to effect behavior change (Smith & Christakis, 2008). Indeed, because peer social influence wanes as individuals leave adolescence and enter adulthood, network interventions are a potentially powerful tool to affect health particularly in adolescents.

Network Effects on Health Care

The entities connected in a network need not be individuals. A network lens is also applied to relations between groups or organizations. A recent systematic review assessed the networks of health care professionals as they relate to effectiveness and sustainability in quality of care and patient safety (Cunningham et al., 2012). They reported that nursing directors were more central in their networks than medical directors and "hence better adapted to gathering and disseminating information" (p. 243). Meanwhile, medical directors were "embedded in more densely connected networks (cliques)" (p. 243), making them better instruments of change, while less densely connected nursing director networks were better for accessing information. Nonclinical managers were important to brokerage, forming bridges to disseminate information, and influence between groups. Network stability and decreased fragmentation over time related to network effectiveness. They concluded that network analysis can improve information flow and interaction in networks and that understanding local and global network characteristics such as bridges, brokers, and centrality may be useful in improving coordinated care.

NEIGHBORHOODS AND PERSONAL NETWORKS: STRATEGIC ACTIVITIES

Applying Knowledge to Interventions

Engaging Clinicians

Many things clinicians do can be reexamined through a neighborhood or social network lens. Think back to the opening vignette and the challenges and opportunities presented by the child's neighborhood and her family's social networks. Clinicians can identify opportunities for involvement by identifying their personal communities, whether geographic or disease focused. Clinicians can bring their professional expertise and resources to activities intended to strengthen neighborhood communities and networks. As noted by Hyde-Peters and Simkiss (2016):

> *Paediatricians in hospital practice may struggle to see how they can be involved with communities to develop social capital, though all hospitals are in a place and have neighbourhoods. Also, not all communities are geographical; as well as online communities, some communities are created by medical illness, so there are online communities and support organisations for almost all diseases and medical conditions. Hospital paediatricians can start with engaging with the community of patients with the diseases they treat, such as cystic fibrosis, diabetes or sickle cell anaemia. They can support these communities by signposting, legitimizing the support network and contributing to the social capital." (p. 208)*

Engaging Communities

Clinicians can only do so much by providing information or serving in a consultative role. It is essential for clinicians to reach beyond professional boundaries. Enthusiasm for transdisciplinary work can result in the creation of colocated biopsychosocial teams that can support complete neighborhood-based care for children. It also is important to engage communities by increasing community participation, empowerment, and control/ownership. These levels of engagement are associated with health improvement. With increasing community coproduction and ownership, there can be greater impact.

Engaging Public Health Professionals and Federal Programs

Public health professionals can broaden our conceptualizations of how neighborhoods and social networks affect child outcomes. As one example, in an attempt to move beyond the unidimensional concept of neighborhood poverty the Child Opportunity Index has been constructed by public health policymakers to describe relative child neighborhood opportunity (Acevedo-Garcia et al., 2014). Through a web-based mapping system, the Child Opportunity Index offers a valuable new tool to the housing and community development

BOX 19.1 Emerging Topics in Neighborhood and Network Research

- Identification of meaningful units of analysis at neighborhood level
- Enrichment of the study of neighborhood racial health disparities to include examination of racism and racial hierarchies
- Consideration of community effects when studying individual-level interventions
- Examination of network characteristics that are associated with improved individual infant, child, and adolescent outcomes
- Design of network-based interventions to impact child and adolescent behavior and health

fields that focuses on children and facilitates analyses of racial/ethnic inequities.

Advancing Research

A number of emerging research areas need pursuit. Exemplar topics include accurate measurement of neighborhood characteristics, interrogating and dismantling systemic bases of health disparities, understanding population-level effects on individuals, and developing neighborhood- and network-sensitive interventions to promote child development (Box 19.1).

CONCLUSION

For children, the neighborhood and network are the relatively small environmental range and inherent relationships of home, school, and community that, together, determine the fabric of daily life. The neighborhood appears to influence child health through institutional resources and collective efficacy as well as through human relationships and home environment. How these mechanisms interact depends on neighborhood structural characteristics, family income, socioeconomic status, child characteristics such as age, and the health outcome in question. Children living in poor neighborhoods or with limited network resources experience elevated rates of developmental and medical problems and a greater likelihood that these problems will produce deleterious outcomes. However, rich social networks may mitigate the effects of limited resource neighborhoods, as in the opening vignette. A variety of clinical and community-level interventions, both private and public in nature, may enhance a network's or a neighborhood's capacity to provide a stable and safe environment for optimal child health outcomes.

REFERENCES

Acevedo-Garcia, D., McArdle, N., Hardy, E. F., Crisan, U. I., Romano, B., Norris, D., Baek, M., & Reece, J. (2014). The child opportunity index: Improving collaboration between community development and public health. *Health Affairs (Millwood)*, *33*, 1948–1957. https://doi.org/10.1377/hlthaff.2014.0679

Bearman, P. S., & Moody, J. (2004). Suicide and friendships among American adolescents. *American Journal of Public Health*, *94*, 89–95.

Berkman, L. F., Glass, T., Brissette, I., & Seeman, T. E. (2000). From social integration to health: Durkheim in the new millennium. *Social Science & Medicine*, *51*, 843–857. https://doi.org/10.1016/S0277-9536(00)00065-4

Brunson, E. K. (2013). The impact of social networks on parents' vaccination decisions. *Pediatrics*, *131*, e1397–e1404. https://doi.org/10.1542/peds.2012-2452

Bussing, R., Zima, B. T., Gary, F. A., Mason, D. M., Leon, C. E., Sinha, K., & Garvan, C. W. (2003). Social networks, caregiver strain, and utilization of mental health services among elementary school students at high risk for ADHD. *Journal of the American Academy of Child & Adolescent Psychiatry*, *42*, 842–850. https://doi.org/10.1097/01.CHI.0000046876.27264.BF

Calvó-Armengol, A., Patacchini, E., & Zenou, Y. (2009). Peer effects and social networks in education. *The Review of Economic Studies*, *76*, 1239–1267. https://doi.org/10.1111/j.1467-937X.2009.00550.x

Chen, J., Lin, T. -J., Justice, L., & Sawyer, B. (2019). The social networks of children with and without disabilities in early childhood special education classrooms. *Journal of Autism and Developmental Disorders*, *49*, 2779–2794. https://doi.org/10.1007/s10803-017-3272-4

Cotton, B. P. (2016). Residential mobility and social behaviors of adolescents: A systematic review of the literature. *Journal of Child and Adolescent Psychiatric Nursing*, *29*, 177–187. https://doi.org/10.1111/jcap.12161

Culyba, A. J., Jacoby, S. F., Richmond, T. S., Fein, J. A., Hohl, B. C., & Branas, C. C. (2016). Modifiable neighborhood features associated with adolescent homicide. *JAMA Pediatrics*, *170*, 473–480. https://doi.org/10.1001/jamapediatrics.2015.4697

Cunningham, F. C., Ranmuthugala, G., Plumb, J., Georgiou, A., Westbrook, J. I., & Braithwaite, J. (2012). Health professional networks as a vector for improving healthcare quality and safety: A systematic review. *BMJ Quality & Safety*, *21*, 239–249. https://doi.org/10.1136/bmjqs-2011-000187

Dadvand, P., Villanueva, C. M., Font-Ribera, L., Martinez, D., Basagaña, X., Belmonte, J., … Nieuwenhuijsen, M. J. (2014). Risks and benefits of green spaces for children: A cross-sectional study of associations with sedentary behavior, obesity, asthma, and allergy. *Environmental Health Perspectives*, *122*, 1329–1335. https://doi.org/10.1289/ehp.1308038

Elder, G. H. (1998). The life course as developmental theory. *Child Development*, *69*, 1. https://doi.org/10.2307/1132065

Flouri, E., Mavroveli, S., & Midouhas, E. (2013). Residential mobility, neighbourhood deprivation and children's behaviour in the UK. *Health & Place*, *20*, 25–31. https://doi.org/10.1016/j.healthplace.2012.12.002

Foster, H., & Brooks-Gunn, J. (2013). Neighborhood, family and individual influences on school physical victimization. *Journal of Youth and Adolescence*, *42*, 1596–1610. https://doi.org/10.1007/s10964-012-9890-4

Gjelsvik, A., Rogers, M. L., Song, L., Field, A. E., & Vivier, P. M. (2019). Residential mobility and flourishing among United States school-age children, 2011/2012 National Survey of Children's Health. *Maternal and Child Health Journal*, *23*, 522–529. https://doi.org/10.1007/s10995-018-2664-1

Haas, S. A., Schaefer, D. R., & Kornienko, O. (2010). Health and the structure of adolescent social networks. *Journal of Health and Social Behavior*, *51*, 424–439. https://doi.org/10.1177/0022146510386791

Health Resources and Services Administration, & Office of Health Equity. (2018). *Health Equity Report 2017*. U.S. Department of Health and Human Services.

Hunter, B. D., Neiger, B., & West, J. (2011). The importance of addressing social determinants of health at the local level: The case for social capital. *Health & Social Care in the Community, 19*, 522–530. https://doi.org/10.1111/j.1365-2524.2011.00999.x

Hyde-Peters, Z., & Simkiss, D. (2016). Social capital and community development in child health. *Paediatrics and Child Health, 26*, 205–211. https://doi.org/10.1016/j.paed.2016.02.004

Kana'iIaupuni, S. M., Donato, K. M., Thompson-Colón, T., & Stainback, M. (2005). Counting on kin: Social networks, social support, and child health status. *Social Forces, 83*, 1137–1164.

Kawachi, I., & Kennedy, B. P. (1999). Income inequality and health: Pathways and mechanisms. *Health Services Research, 34*, 215–227.

Lavy, V., & Sand, E. (2012). *The friends factor: How students' social networks affect their academic achievement and well-being? (No. w18430)*. National Bureau of Economic Research. https://doi.org/10.3386/w18430

Leventhal, T., Dupéré, V., & Shuey, E. A. (2015). Children in neighborhoods (vol. 4) *Handbook of child psychology and developmental science: Ecological settings and processes* (7th ed., pp. 493–533). John Wiley & Sons, Inc.

Locke, J., Ishijima, E. H., Kasari, C., & London, N. (2010). Loneliness, friendship quality and the social networks of adolescents with high-functioning autism in an inclusive school setting. *Journal of Research in Special Educational Needs, 10*, 74–81. https://doi.org/10.1111/j.1471-3802.2010.01148.x

Manalel, J. A., & Antonucci, T. C. (2020). Beyond the nuclear family: Children's social networks and depressive symptomology. *Child Development, 91*, 1302–1316. https://doi.org/10.1111/cdev.13307

Markevych, I., Schoierer, J., Hartig, T., Chudnovsky, A., Hystad, P., Dzhambov, A. M., … Fuertes, E. (2017). Exploring pathways linking greenspace to health: Theoretical and methodological guidance. *Environmental Research, 158*, 301–317. https://doi.org/10.1016/j.envres.2017.06.028

Minh, A., Muhajarine, N., Janus, M., Brownell, M., & Guhn, M. (2017). A review of neighborhood effects and early child development: How, where, and for whom, do neighborhoods matter? *Health & Place, 46*, 155–174. https://doi.org/10.1016/j.healthplace.2017.04.012

Moon, R. Y., Carlin, R. F., Cornwell, B., Mathews, A., Oden, R. P., Cheng, Y. I., … Wang, J. (2019). Implications of mothers' social networks for risky infant sleep practices. *The Journal of Pediatrics, 212*, 151–158.e2. https://doi.org/10.1016/j.jpeds.2019.05.027

Pac, J., Nam, J., Waldfogel, J., & Wimer, C. (2017). Young child poverty in the United States: Analyzing trends in poverty and the role of anti-poverty programs using the Supplemental Poverty Measure. *Child and Youth Services Review, 74*, 35–49. https://doi.org/10.1016/j.childyouth.2017.01.022

Sandel, M., Sheward, R., Cuba, S. E., de Coleman, S. M., Frank, D. A., Chilton, M., … Cutts, D. (2018). Unstable housing and caregiver and child health in renter families. *Pediatrics, 141*. https://doi.org/10.1542/peds.2017-2199

Scott, K. (2016). *Housing children: South Auckland. The Housing Pathways Longitudinal Study*. https://doi.org/10.13140/RG.2.2.24769.76645

Shin, E. K., LeWinn, K., Bush, N., Tylavsky, F. A., Davis, R. L., & Shaban-Nejad, A. (2019). Association of maternal social relationships with cognitive development in early childhood. *JAMA Network Open*, e186963. https://doi.org/10.1001/jamanetworkopen.2018.6963

Short, K. S. (2016). Child poverty: Definition and measurement. *Academic Pediatrics, Child Poverty in the United States, 16*, S46–S51. https://doi.org/10.1016/j.acap.2015.11.005

Smith, K. P., & Christakis, N. A. (2008). Social networks and health. *Annual Review of Sociology, 34*, 405–429. https://doi.org/10.1146/annurev.soc.34.040507.134601

Taylor, R. L., Cooper, S. R., Jackson, J. J., & Barch, D. M. (2020). Assessment of neighborhood poverty, cognitive function, and prefrontal and hippocampal volumes in children. *JAMA Network Open, 3*, e2023774. https://doi.org/10.1001/jamanetworkopen.2020.23774

Tung, E. L., Cagney, K. A., Peek, M. E., & Chin, M. H. (2017). Spatial context and health inequity: Reconfiguring race, place, and poverty. *Journal of Urban Health, 94*, 757–763. https://doi.org/10.1007/s11524-017-0210-x

Vos, A. A., Posthumus, A. G., Bonsel, G. J., Steegers, E. A. P., & Denktaş, S. (2014). Deprived neighborhoods and adverse perinatal outcome: A systematic review and meta-analysis. *Acta Obstetricia et Gynecologica Scandinavica, 93*, 727–740. https://doi.org/10.1111/aogs.12430

Wall-Wieler, E., Roos, L. L., Chateau, D. G., & Rosella, L. C. (2016). What predictors matter: Risk factors for late adolescent outcomes. *Canadian Journal of Public Health, 107*, e16–e22. https://doi.org/10.17269/cjph.107.5156

Webster, D., Dunne, L., & Hunter, R. (2021). Association between social networks and subjective well-being in adolescents: A systematic review. *Youth & Society, 53*, 175–210. https://doi.org/10.1177/0044118X20919589

Wickrama, K. A. S., Simons, L. G., & Baltimore, D. (2012). The influence of ethnicity and adverse life experiences during adolescence on young adult socioeconomic attainment: The moderating role of education. *Journal of Youth and Adolescence, 41*, 1472–1487. https://doi.org/10.1007/s10964-012-9764-9

Wodtke, G. T., & Parbst, M. (2017). Neighborhoods, schools, and academic achievement: A formal mediation analysis of contextual effects on reading and mathematics abilities. *Demography, 54*, 1653–1676. https://doi.org/10.1007/s13524-017-0603-1

Wolff, K. T., Baglivio, M. T., Intravia, J., Greenwald, M. A., & Epps, N. (2017). The mobility of youth in the justice system: Implications for recidivism. *Journal of Youth and Adolescence, 46*, 1371–1393. https://doi.org/10.1007/s10964-016-0498-y

Wrzus, C., Hänel, M., Wagner, J., & Neyer, F. J. (2013). Social network changes and life events across the life span: A meta-analysis. *Psychological Bulletin, 139*, 53–80. https://doi.org/10.1037/a0028601

Xue, Y., Leventhal, T., Brooks-Gunn, J., & Earls, F. J. (2005). Neighborhood residence and mental health problems of 5- to 11-year-olds. *Archives of General Psychiatry, 62*, 554–563. https://doi.org/10.1001/archpsyc.62.5.554

Yourkavitch, J., Kane, J. B., & Miles, G. (2018). Neighborhood disadvantage and neighborhood affluence: Associations with breastfeeding practices in urban areas. *Maternal and Child Health Journal, 22*, 546–555. https://doi.org/10.1007/s10995-017-2423-8

Zhang, N., Beauregard, J. L., Kramer, M. R., & Bécares, L. (2017). Neighbourhood ethnic density effects on behavioural and cognitive problems among young racial/ethnic minority children in the US and England: A cross-national comparison. *Population Research and Policy Review, 36*, 761–804. https://doi.org/10.1007/s11113-017-9445-1

Zhang, J., & Centola, D. (2019). Social networks and health: New developments in diffusion, online and offline. *Annual Review of Sociology, 45*, 91–109. https://doi.org/10.1146/annurev-soc-073117-041421

Zimmerman, G. M., & Messner, S. F. (2010). Neighborhood context and the gender gap in adolescent violent crime. *American Sociological Review, 75*, 958–980. https://doi.org/10.1177/0003122410386688

20

Celebrating Sociocultural Diversity in the Exam Room and Addressing Racism and Bias

Irene M. Loe, Adiaha Spinks-Franklin, and Kate E. Wallis

For additional material related to the content of this chapter, please see Chapter 2.

VIGNETTE

Omari presented to developmental-behavioral pediatrics at 67 months for concerns about his communication and behavior. He recently had been expelled from a private school because of behavioral issues, so this appointment was urgently needed to help his family find appropriate educational and therapeutic supports.

Omari's parents had emigrated from Ethiopia before his birth and identify as Black. They speak English and Amharic. Between 20 and 25 months, Omari's health insurance lapsed, but otherwise he was continuously followed in the same primary care pediatric practice since birth.

Omari's parents reported that they had early concerns about his development. He screened at-risk on a general developmental screen at 9 months, but no action was taken. Later, when Omari was 16 months old and was not using any words, he began early intervention (EI). His parents thought that he was making progress because he began using single words to communicate, so they did not continue services when he aged out of EI at age 3 years. They later reported uncertainty about when a child is expected to reach each developmental milestone.

At 48 months, Omari's pediatrician referred him for a speech-language evaluation, as he was still only using single words to communicate. That evaluation led to referral for this assessment for concerns for autism spectrum disorder (ASD).

Omari demonstrated behaviors consistent with ASD, including difficulties with personal space, limited eye contact and gestures, and hand-flapping. His speech was very delayed. After they heard the diagnosis, Omari's parents wondered how the diagnosis had been missed for so long.

Adapted from Wallis, K. E., Buttenheim, A. M., & Mandell, D. S. (2021). Insights from behavioral economics: A case of delayed diagnosis of autism spectrum disorder. *Journal of Developmental & Behavioral Pediatrics, 42*(2), 109–113.

INTRODUCTION

This case highlights the myriad ways that a patient and family's sociocultural characteristics may impact how a child's developmental trajectory is perceived by caregivers and clinicians, when and how a child may present for care when concerns are identified, and how that care is delivered. Previous considerations of a child's sociocultural context focused on the experiential factors that may impact development and the debate between the relative importance of nature and nurture. Many developmental theories acknowledge the role of culture in shaping a child's development. Lev Vygotsky, a Russian psychologist, developed the sociocultural theory, which recognizes the role that social interactions and cultural experiences play in a child's cognitive development (Rosa & Tudge, 2013). Building on this, Urie Brofenbrenner's ecological systems theory examines the interactions of a child within the child's broader environment, including with family, school, religion, and culture (Rosa & Tudge, 2013). Various theories of child development acknowledge what psychologist Barbara Rogoff (2003, pp. 3–4) summarizes as: "people develop as participants in cultural communities. Their development can be understood only in light of the cultural practices and circumstances of their communities—which also change."

For a child with special health care needs, recent explorations of a child's cultural influences have become more introspective, examining the ways that a child's and family's sociodemographic characteristics may impact how they interact with the health care system to produce differential experiences and results. At least since the landmark report, "Unequal Treatment: Confronting Racial and Ethnic Disparities in Health Care," was published by the Institute of Medicine in 2003, the social determinants of health (SDOH) have been recognized to impact developmental and other health outcomes in a differential manner, depending on the racial or ethnic identities of patients and families. The SDOH are defined as the "conditions in the environments in which people are born, live, learn, work, play, worship, and age that affect a wide range of health, functioning, and quality-of-life outcomes and risks" (US Department of Health and Human Services, 2020). Such conditions include the social, economic, and physical characteristics of the place in which an individual finds oneself. Housing security, having access to quality education and health care, and experiences of racism and other forms of discrimination are all independent but related examples of SDOH (Paradies et al., 2015). An individual's sociodemographic characteristics, including race, ethnicity, preferred language(s), immigration status, sexual orientation, gender identity, income, wealth, religion, and educational attainment, are undeniably linked to many of these determinants and may result in disparities in care and outcomes.

In the field of developmental-behavioral pediatrics there are numerous examples of ways that a child's sociodemographic characteristics and the SDOH impact their experiences. For example, decades of research indicate disparities in the likelihood that a child, like Omari, from a minoritized racial or ethnic group is identified with ASD, and at what age (Mandell, Listerud, Levy, & Pinto-Martin, 2002). The term *minoritized* reflects that minority racial/ethnic status is not inherent but reflects a history of systematic oppression. Use of the term *BIPOC* (which references Black, Indigenous, and People of Color) also acknowledges the legacy of discrimination against individuals from these groups. Historically, BIPOC children with ASD have been identified at lower rates and later ages than White children, although those gaps appear to be shrinking (Baio et al., 2018). After adjusting for important factors such as family income and student academic achievement, Black and Hispanic children are less likely to be identified with a disability and receive special education (Morgan et al., 2019). Race and racism are apparent in many facets of developmental-behavioral pediatric practice, but much remains to be learned.

In this chapter we explore the ways that children's sociocultural environment and experiences of racism may impact their developmental trajectory and ethnic/racial identity development, as well as the ways that sociocultural factors should be considered and celebrated in developmental-behavioral pediatric care.

DEFINING RACIAL TERMINOLOGY

The story of Omari and his family highlights the complexities of how race, culture, racism, clinician implicit biases, and SDOH influence child development, behavior, and health, and families' experiences with health care systems. Children are reared within the context of their families, communities, and environments. Within the United States, race, culture, and racism play very prominent roles in how parents teach, guide, protect, and support their children. Studies have found that clinicians are less likely to provide anticipatory guidance, appropriate developmental surveillance, and family-centered care to Black, Latinx, and Asian American children and families, and to families with limited English proficiency (Zuckerman, Mattox, Sinche, Blaschke, & Bethell, 2014). Although we recognize that in other countries terms such as *race* and *ethnicity* have very different meanings and usages, we will focus on the US historical context for this chapter.

Pediatrics has begun to examine the roles that race, racism, other forms of discrimination, and social justice play in the lives of children (Trent, Dooley, & Dougé, 2019), but has not systematically addressed these concerns for children who have developmental disabilities and behavior disorders. Unfortunately, clinician behaviors play an important role in contributing to health disparities of children of color who have developmental and behavioral concerns. Primary care pediatricians are less likely to provide family-centered care or ask Black parents and Spanish-speaking Latinx parents about concerns they have about their child's development, even when the child is at high risk for developmental delays (Zuckerman et al., 2014). Black and Latinx children with special health care needs have higher unmet mental health needs compared to White children with special health care needs, even when adjusting for several sociodemographic factors (Ngui & Flores, 2007). Pediatricians are less likely to refer US Black, Latinx, and Asian children and children with foreign-born parents for EI services (Wallis et al., 2020). Clinicians are less likely to treat Black and Latinx children with attention-deficit/hyperactivity disorder and to treat them for shorter periods of time (Coker et al., 2016). In total, clinicians are not giving equitable care to BIPOC children who have developmental disabilities and behavior disorders, which contributes to health disparities.

In light of all of these findings, the field of developmental-behavioral pediatrics has not trained fellows or practicing clinicians to understand, address, or negotiate the roles that race, racism, social justice, and physician implicit racial bias play in the lives of children who have developmental disabilities and behavior disorders. This section will provide developmental-behavioral pediatric clinicians with foundational vocabulary, concepts, and terminology to help them develop basic racial literacy skills. The concepts reviewed may shed light on how the clinician can provide improved family-centered, culturally respectful care to Omari and his family.

Race

Race is a recent human invention, a social construct designed to divide members of a society into a hierarchy of social, economic, and political advantage or disadvantage based on a set of randomly selected normal human variations in phenotype. Race was invented in the late 1600s by the landowning European colonists in what is now the United States as a means of maintaining their economic, political, and social dominance over other groups deemed to be inferior. Race categories were used to create a caste system in the United States into which people were thrust from birth for the remainder of their lives, into which their offspring were born. Racial categories are fluid and have changed over the course of centuries to include some and exclude others from the dominant White racial caste classification (e.g., individuals of Irish, Polish, and Italian backgrounds have been accepted into White racial categories over time). Race is not biologic. People do not inherit race. People inherit ancestry; race is placed upon them by society at birth. Race is not a risk factor for disease because race is not biologic. People who are put into subordinate racial caste status have been historically and systematically targeted for and denied access to economic, political, educational, and social power and resources. Therefore experiences with racism in all its forms and other SDOH are risk factors for disease and poor health outcomes.

Ethnicity

Ethnicity is another societal category used in the United States to further divide people into subgroups based on certain shared traditions, values, history, language, ancestry, region of origin, or other common experiences. Larger "racial" groups can be broken into smaller "ethnic" groups. For example, the Asian race could be further divided into multiple ethnicities, including Chinese or Indian; Latinx race into the ethnicities of Mexican or Puerto Rican; White race into the ethnicities of French or Irish; and Black race into the ethnic groups Haitian or African American. Within these "ethnic groups" are even more cultural groups. For example, in India, Nigeria, and China, hundreds of different languages, cultures, and traditions exist within the geographic boundaries of those countries. In the United States a person classified as Nigerian American could be Igbo, Yuroba, Fulani, Hausa, or any of the numerous other ethnic groups within Nigeria. In some instances the terms *race* and *ethnicity* are used interchangeably; however, for clarification in this section, we differentiate between the category of "race" and the subcategory of "ethnicity."

Racism

Racism refers to the system of oppression based on the superiority of people considered White and the inferiority of people considered non-White. Racism has many levels, including institutionalized, interpersonal, and internalized (Table 20.1) (Jones, 2000).

Racism also has multiple forms, including colorblind racism, cultural racism, environmental racism, gendered racism, and medical racism (Table 20.2).

Microaggressions

Microaggressions are casual, ordinary, daily actions that communicate a derogatory message to members of historically oppressed and marginalized groups. In the domain of racism microaggressions are acts of interpersonal racism committed toward a member of a historically targeted racial group. Examples of microaggressions include commenting on how well a person speaks English.

Implicit Racial Bias

Implicit bias refers to an unconscious preference for or against a person, idea, or thing. Implicit racial bias refers to the unconscious preference for one racial group and distaste for other racial groups. The majority of people in the United States espouse pro-White and anti-Black, anti-Latinx, anti-American Indian implicit racial bias and pro-light skin and anti-dark skin implicit bias against adults and children. The majority of physicians (including pediatricians) and other clinicians in the United States have the same implicit racial biases as those found in the larger society and endorse pro-White/anti-Black, pro-White/anti-Hispanic, pro-White/anti-American Indian, and pro-light skin/anti-dark skin implicit racial biases in adults and children as measured by the Implicit Association Test (IAT) (Maina, Belton, Ginzberg, Singh, & Johnson, 2018). Pro-White implicit racial biases influence the way in which clinicians deliver health care. These clinicians give worse care to their patients of color than they do to White patients, contributing to medical racism. Physicians with pro-White implicit racial bias demonstrate paternalistic communication styles with non-White patients and receive lower ratings on patient satisfaction surveys from BIPOC patients (Maina et al., 2018).

Racial/Ethnic Socialization

Racial/ethnic socialization refers to the process of preparing children for living within a racially hostile society by transferring information about race and ethnicity from adult to child (Hughes et al., 2006). Racial socialization includes both verbal and nonverbal racial and ethnic communication between families and youth about racialized experiences (Table 20.3).

TABLE 20.1 Levels of Racism

Level of Racism	Description	Examples
Institutionalized racism (also called structural or systemic racism)	Differential access to the goods, services, and opportunities of society by race category, including: • Material conditions: education, health care, economic stability, housing, clean environment (e.g., the social determinants of health) • Access to power: information, resources, political voice Can be legalized, normative, and codified throughout the structure of society through policies, practices, traditions, and laws	Housing segregation policies Inequities in public education funding Pay inequities by race and sex Differences in sentencing practices in the criminal legal system
Interpersonal racism (also called personally mediated racism)	Acts of discrimination and prejudice based on race category by members of a dominant racial caste against a member of a subordinated racial caste Microaggressions are everyday acts of interpersonal racism	Denying someone service based upon race Assuming a Black, Indigenous, and People of Color (BIPOC) person is not in a leadership position but is in a service position Harsher punishment of BIPOC boys in public schools
Internalized racism	An individual believes in and accepts the system of White supremacy and racial oppression of BIPOC	BIPOC person believes in own inferiority and seeks to change oneself to become more like the dominant caste by rejecting own cultural heritage and practices

TABLE 20.2 **Forms of Racism**

Form of Racism	Definition	Example
Colorblind racism	Denying the ongoing impact of racism in society Belief that historic racism should not be considered in any way to account for current racial disparities	Minimizing experiences of racism described by a colleague Blaming BIPOCs for the racial oppression they experience
Cultural racism (i.e., Whiteness)	The assumption that being White is the norm, regular, or baseline measure by which all others should be compared and measured	Using the term "American" as synonymous with being White Superheroes portrayed as White people
Environmental racism	Policies that are designed to place marginalized racial groups into living environments that increase their risk of poor health outcomes	The practice of redlining, where neighborhoods with large populations of Black, Latinx, and immigrant populations were deemed "hazardous" and were systematically disinvested The placement of highways with resultant pollution in neighborhoods with higher numbers of BIPOC residents
Gendered racism	Intersection of racism and sexism that Black, Indigenous, and People of Color (BIPOC) women experience	Gendered racial pay gap: BIPOC women make less money than White women doing the same job Gendered racial unemployment rates: BIPOC women have higher unemployment rates than White women even when controlling for educational level and parity
Medical racism	The ways in which racism influences the practice of medicine historically and currently that leave traditionally marginalized groups with poor health care access and poor health outcomes	Physicians with pro-White/anti-Black, anti-Latinx, anti-American Indian implicit racial bias give worse health care to BIPOC patients

TABLE 20.3 **Racial-Ethnic Socialization Practices**

Racial-Ethnic Socialization Practice	Definition	Examples
Cultural socialization	Building a healthy cultural identity by teaching children about their heritage and ancestry; emphasizing cultural values, norms, and traditions; and exposing children to cultural symbols and representations in the home	Displaying ethnocentric art in the home, speaking native languages at home, reading children's literature that reflects the home culture positively, listening to cultural music, selecting dolls and toys that reflect the home culture
Preparation for bias	Training children to recognize and respond to all forms of racism, including both overt and covert forms, institutional and interpersonal racist experiences	Teaching teens how to interact with police officers, coaching children on how to deal with peer-on-peer interpersonal racism, modeling ways to address microaggressions in public places
Promotion of mistrust	Emphasizing the need for wariness and distrust in interracial interactions	Talking to children and teens about racially stressful encounters, such as police shootings of unarmed Black people
Egalitarianism and silence about race	Explicitly encouraging children to value individual qualities over racial group membership or avoiding any mention of race in discussions with their children	Deciding not to address acts of interpersonal or institutional racism that is displayed in the media, such as antiimmigrant rhetoric

Racial Literacy

Racial literacy refers to the explicit practice of building knowledge and skills about race as a social construct and how to identify and respond to racialized experiences (Twine, 2004). Racial literacy refers to the skills parents teach their children to deal with discriminatory racial encounters in the moment. Racial literacy encompasses the ability to read, recast, and resolve the language of racially

BOX 20.1 Strategies for RECASTing Racial Stress

Strategy	Definition	Example
Read	Decoding, interpreting, and appraising discriminatory racial encounters (DRE) as being a threat or not. Appraising one's coping tools and strategies for managing the racial stress	Observing the participants' behaviors and emotional state in the DRE
Recast	If the DRE is perceived to be a threat, then calculate, locate, and communicate one's own racial stress response in order to deescalate the threat	Perform a "body check" to observe one's own physiologic and psychological reaction to the DRE, including one's thoughts, feelings, and bodily sensations in the moment
Resolve	Deciding how to respond to the DRE in the moment, so as not to under- or overreact to the situation	Employing problem-solving choices that will be healthy and productive in resolving the DRE Avoiding emotionally laden reactions

stressful encounters (Anderson & Stevenson, 2019). Just as literacy refers to the ability to decode, encode, and comprehend written words, racial literacy includes the ability to decipher the underlying racialized messages in a discriminatory racial encounter, determine whether the encounter is a threat to one's safety or life, and then employ effective strategies for deescalating the racially stressful encounter (Box 20.1).

Social Determinants of Health

Negative SDOH are risk factors for poor physical and mental health outcomes. Racism (in all levels and forms) negatively influences all of the domains of SDOH and contributes to poor mental and physical health outcomes, and shorter life expectancies (Table 20.4) (Paradies et al., 2015).

RACIAL AWARENESS AND RACIAL IDENTITY DEVELOPMENT IN CHILDHOOD

In this section we review how children demonstrate racial awareness across different periods of childhood using a developmental framework based on the Piagetian theory of cognitive development (see Chapter 3).

Newborn to Toddler (Birth–2 Years)

In this earliest phase Piaget's sensorimotor stage is characterized by learning through grasping, looking, and listening. Newborns show no preexisting preferences based on differences in normal human variation as measured by visual preference or recognition bias (Anzures et al., 2013). Infants do recognize major differences in normal human

TABLE 20.4 The Impact of Racism on the Social Determinants of Health

Social Determinant of Health	Definition	Racism's Impact
Economic stability	The opportunity to earn a steady income that allows people to meet their health needs	Unemployment inequities: when controlling for educational attainment and other factors, US Black, Latinx, and Asian people have significantly higher unemployment rates than White people. Job applicants with Black-sounding names are less likely to be called for an interview compared to job applicants with White-sounding names
Education access and quality	Access to educational opportunities that help children and adolescents do well in school	Public school funding inequities: school districts serving the largest populations of Black, Latinx, or American Indian students receive less per student in state and local funding than those serving the fewest students of color, an estimated $23 billion nationally
Health care access and quality	Access to comprehensive, high-quality health care services	Black and Latinx parents are less likely to report having a medical home and have higher rates of being uninsured
Neighborhood and built environment	Create neighborhoods and environments that promote health and safety	Residential housing segregation Lack of green space Food deserts Communities with concentrated poverty
Social and community context	Social and community support, including relationships and interactions with family, friends, coworkers, and community members	Overpolicing of Black, Indigenous, and People of Color communities Experiences of community violence

variation (e.g., pigmentation, shape of face/eyes/nose/lips, facial hair). By 3 months of age, infants primarily exposed to those with similar human variations to their own prefer to look at those faces rather than faces with other variations, a phenomenon called the other race effect (ORE) that has been identified from childhood to adulthood (Anzures et al., 2013). Generally, from 3 to 6 months of age, infants show preferences for groups that they have been exposed to most, typically the infant's own group. It appears that infant reactions to group status may serve to assist in attachment during infancy by differentiating caregivers from strangers (Williams et al., 2020). There is no evidence suggesting that infants discriminate against social partners on the basis of race. Studies show that 10-month-olds accept toys equally from own- and other-race individuals, and that 2-year-olds give toys equally to own- and other-race individuals (Kinzler & Spelke, 2011).

Preschool and Early Childhood (3–5 Years)

In Piaget's framework children move into the preoperational stage from age 2 to 7 years. This stage is characterized by egocentrism and difficulty seeing things from the perspective of others, the development of symbolic thinking, and expanded pretend play but continued thinking in very concrete terms. The age-related developmental progression of race as a concept in children starts first with showing knowledge of color categories prior to conceptual awareness of racial categories (Phillips Swanson, Cunningham, Youngblood, & Beale Spencer, 2009). Preschoolers demonstrate a lot of interest in physical characteristics of themselves and others, as well as interest in observable cultural characteristics such as language and dress (Derman-Sparks, Tanaka Higa, & Sparks, 1980; Van Ausdale & Feagin, 2001). By age 3 to 4 years, children categorize by racial group based on skin color, may comment on different skin colors or tones, and ask questions that help them make classifications. While figuring out racial identity, preschoolers are also learning colors and begin to distinguish the meaning of colors applied to objects and the social meaning of colors when applied to race (Derman-Sparks et al., 1980). Children may ask why people with different skin tones are all considered Black, even when they belong to the same family. By age 5 to 6 years, children can accurately identify racial labels based on socially constructed skin color identities, such as Black or White (Phillips Swanson et al., 2009). Clinicians can encourage parents to speak openly when children observe differences in skin color; by doing so, they normalize discussions about race (Anderson & Douge, 2019; Derman-Sparks et al., 1980).

Early in this stage racial prejudice has not developed, although older children in this age group may begin to absorb cultural stereotypes from social learning experiences (Phillips Swanson et al., 2009). Children age 3 to 4 years show no preference for own- or other-race peers when choosing playmates, unlike 5-year-olds, who tend to choose own-race over other-race children (Kinzler & Spelke, 2011). As young as age 5 years, children will also share more toys with unknown individuals that match their own race than with those of different races (Kinzler & Spelke, 2011). By age 5 to 7 years, children show more positive evaluations (e.g., clean, good, friendly) of own-race children and more negative evaluations (e.g., dirty, naughty, unfriendly) of other-race children compared to younger children (Box 20.2) (Aboud, 2003). During this period parents should be conscious of themselves as role models in their interactions with others, embrace a diverse social network, and increase children's exposure to people of other races and cultures, through diverse books, travel, events, or settings, such as daycare, preschool, and school (Anderson & Douge, 2019; Winkler & Hagerman, 2021).

BOX 20.2 Historical Insights

Early measurement of racial bias in childhood was exemplified by the famous doll studies of Kenneth and Mamie Clark, in which 3- to 7-year-old children were asked to assign positive or negative attributes to White or Black dolls. Replication of the Clark studies conducted from the 1940s to 1980s found Black children reporting White (Eurocentric) preferences when assigning positive attributes to Black and White pictures or dolls. The Clarks' findings were instrumental in the *Brown v. Board of Education* 1954 decision to integrate schools and paved the way for increased interest in children's development of racial identity (Phillips Swanson et al., 2009). William Cross, a social psychologist, is credited with first proposing the concept of racial identity development through what is now known as the Cross model on the psychology of nigrescence (1978). Nigrescence refers to the process of becoming Black. Cross developed a five-stage model of racial identity for Black Americans: Preencounter, encounter, immersion/emersion, internalization, and internalization-commitment.

Middle Childhood (6–11 Years)

Children are moving into Piaget's concrete operational stage (age 7–11 years), which is characterized by more logical, but still concrete, thinking and by reasoning from specific information to a general principle. Children are less egocentric and more sociocentric (i.e., thinking about how others might think and feel) and have awareness that others might not share their feelings or opinions. Piaget also identified reciprocity, the understanding of interaction between individuality and group membership, and that we are all humans and members of specific subgroups with both similar and different needs. Early in middle childhood, children's sense of self-identity evolves to include group identity (i.e., they are part of a group that is different from other groups). Distinct groupings can apply to social groups, recognized as "ingroup" versus "outgroup" (Burkholder, D'Esterre, & Killen, 2019). Five- to 8-year-olds become more peer oriented and have a greater sense of fairness in group games that is foundational in developing moral sense and understanding of the unfairness of racism (Derman-Sparks et al., 1980). Indeed, children at this stage become more aware of racism against their group and can internalize racist experiences. At this stage, clinicians can encourage parents to point out racial stereotypes and emphasize fairness when discussing experiences of racial bias and discrimination (Anderson & Douge, 2019; Winkler & Hagerman, 2021).

Older children show greater ability to differentiate others on the basis of race or ethnicity than preschoolers. By age 8 years, children understand racial classification beyond simple physical features and characteristics. By age 10 years, children recognize social stereotypes associated with racial groups (Phillips Swanson et al., 2009). Between ages 9 and 12 years, preadolescents deepen their understanding of racial and cultural identity, including historical and geographic aspects, as well as ancestry. With age, children are also better able to understand the interaction between personal and group identity and that their identity includes multiple facets such as race/ethnicity, gender, and socioeconomic class. An increase in name-calling based on various identities can be seen, but children also have greater empathy about name-calling. They also have deepening awareness of racism in terms of historical and institutional dimensions. Piaget's concept of reciprocity aids preadolescents in their understanding of differentiating majority and minority perspectives (Derman-Sparks et al., 1980).

There is greater variability in middle to late childhood with regard to the dissonance reported between social stereotypes and the impact this understanding has on a child's personal identity (Phillips Swanson et al., 2009). Differences relate to the child's social cognitive abilities and socialization experiences at home and school. The expanding social world provides societal perceptions that may contribute to the variability in self-esteem and racial attitudes in older children. Studies find that parents' racial socialization of children is associated with more positive self-concept compared to children who are not provided this support against racial stereotypes (Hughes et al., 2006; Phillips Swanson et al., 2009).

Given children's increased understanding of racial stereotypes and racism, middle childhood is considered an ideal time to discuss racial biases and prejudice, although developmentally appropriate discussions can begin even earlier to combat implicit biases and internalized racist messages. Parents should actively engage in open talks with children about race and racism so that children see them as trusted sources of information (Anderson & Douge, 2019; Van Ausdale & Feagin, 2001). When children make comments about race based on events at school or in the media, it is important to ask them how they feel and why they think the way they do in order to understand their perspective. When parents don't know the answer to children's questions, they can invite the child to join them in seeking out answers (Winkler & Hagerman, 2021).

Adolescence (≥12 Years)

Adolescents are moving into Piaget's formal operational stage, in which operations are carried out on ideas rather than objects. Thinking is increasingly logical and systematic, and includes abstract ideas, the ability to follow an argument, and hypothetical problem solving with multiple solutions. At this stage, moral development is typically complete. Values are solidified, including racial attitudes and stereotypes, but may undergo change or questioning when faced with a major or life-changing event that challenges existing beliefs (Williams et al., 2020). BIPOC adolescents may be faced with the reality of unfair encounters with law enforcement; this is a specific area of pediatric counseling—"the talk," which includes pediatrician and parent discussions on how youth can stay safe during such encounters (Maroney & Zuckerman, 2018). Adolescents often have a strong sense of fairness and justice and may be able to act on social and racial justice issues.

Identity formation is often recognized as a primary psychosocial goal of adolescence. Ethnic racial identity (ERI), or the manner in which one draws meaning from experiences as a member of a racial group, is an important facet of identity and can promote positive adjustment in the face of risk or adversity (Williams et al., 2020). Several models of ERI have been developed for various groups (Daniel Tatum, 2017). In Jean Phinney's three-stage progression model the process begins in adolescence: (1) unexamined ethnic identity—individuals have not explored their identity and may absorb the values or attitudes of the majority culture; (2) ethnic identity search—individuals actively explore their ethnic identity; and (3) ethnic identity achievement—characterized by acceptance, internalization, and clear understanding of one's ethnic identity, individuals come to terms with cultural differences between their ethnic group and the majority culture (Daniel Tatum, 2017).

Although many individuals begin to examine their ethnic/racial identity in adolescence, the process is not necessarily linear and is heavily contextual (i.e., driven by major events in an individual's social environment) (Williams et al., 2020). Evaluation of personal and group identity in adolescence can move in both positive and negative directions. For adolescents of color, this can manifest as positive self and group identification, acting out internalized racism against themselves or others, or some combination of both. For White adolescents, a continuum also occurs, in that they may demonstrate active racism in speech and behavior, take a colorblind or passive stance without examining privilege of the majority race, or reject colorblindness and take an active antiracism stance. Such categorizations of individuals are overly simplistic; studies on prejudice in childhood and adolescence highlight the complexity of intergroup relationships between racial ingroups and outgroups and the context in which situations occur (Burkholder et al., 2019). Children may demonstrate prejudice through intergroup peer inclusion and exclusion, stereotypes about outgroup members, and bias or assumptions about similarity of ingroup members. Some studies have shown that group knowledge and the awareness of social hierarchies can lead to rejection of prejudice and promotion of fairness for those involved. Intergroup friendships and the ability to view outgroup members as individuals, not just as products of group membership, can also combat prejudice in childhood (Burkholder et al., 2019).

Clinicians can encourage parents to combat stereotypes by confronting their own biases, discussing stereotypes with children, and encouraging children to view members of other groups as individuals. Perhaps one of the best ways to have children view other children as individuals is through intergroup friendships. Encouraging diversity in multiple aspects of families' daily lives, including through conversation about other groups' histories and customs, can help cultivate shared curiosity and understanding. Parents can also support adolescents' ERI through racial literacy and racial socialization strategies (Anderson & Stevenson, 2019; Hughes et al., 2006), including sharing positive messages about ethnic racial pride and preparing children for encounters of discrimination.

CULTURAL HUMILITY

Cultural humility requires clinicians to engage in self-reflection of their own beliefs and traditions, while engaging with and learning about those of the people around them (Yeager & Bauer-Wu, 2013). Cultural humility acknowledges that group-level characteristics do not adequately describe an individual's lived experiences. Clinicians instead humbly recognize their own limited knowledge of another's cultural beliefs and experiences. Experiences can also be viewed through a historical lens, recognizing the ways that groups have faced discrimination over time. Additionally, cultural humility acknowledges that even for clinicians who belong to dominant cultural groups (e.g., those of White race), a reflection on one's own cultural norms, values, and traditions is required to fully engage with members of other groups. A prior iteration of this concept, cultural competence, was criticized for its impossibly lofty goal of asking clinicians to attain knowledge of all the cultural factors associated with each particular cultural group to which patients may belong. Cultural humility should not hinder explorations and knowledge-seeking about other cultural experiences. But acknowledging the limits of one's ability to attain knowledge about another's cultural experiences is important.

Children and families, especially those with an individual with a disability, may have intersectional identities that place them at increased risk for experiencing various forms of discrimination (Crenshaw, 2017). It is important to recognize how those experiences intersect to produce injustices that might exceed what members of any single identity group experience. For example, engagement with the criminal justice system differs for Black and White children, and for children with and without identified disabilities. Black children with intellectual disability are more likely to be involved with the juvenile justice system than their White nondisabled counterparts, a risk that likely comes from the intersection of race and disability (Mendoza, Blake, Marchbanks, & Ragan, 2019). Cultural humility offers clinicians the ability to explore with patients their intersectional identities.

In every clinical encounter it is incumbent upon clinicians to pause and reflect on their own identity and cultural beliefs before engaging with others. Even when clinicians and families share membership in racial, ethnic, religious, socioeconomic, or other groups, each person's experience is unique. Reflecting on their own beliefs and potential biases can open clinicians up to learning more about the lived experience of their patients and families they encounter. This requires asking open-ended questions about how a family perceives and describes various components of their identity, experiences with various SDOH, and how a family's beliefs may impact perceptions of the child and disability. The term *structural competency* describes this focus on the broader forces that may impact patient health (Metzl & Hansen, 2014).

An extension of this concept asks clinicians to actively identify their own implicit biases and to then develop strategies to mitigate the negative effects of those biases. All humans have biases and are more likely to rely on those biases when making decisions in ambiguous situations, moments of stress or fatigue, or when they must make a decision based on incomplete information (scenarios that are common in clinical medicine). Thus identification of one's implicit biases, which can be measured through tools such as the IAT (available through Project Implicit: https://implicit.harvard.edu), can help to uncover automatic preferences that may impact decision making on the individual level. Techniques such as mindfulness and reflection can reduce activation of stereotypes (Marcelin, Siraj, Victor, Kotadia, & Maldonado, 2019). Increasing contact across groups can serve to reduce reliance on stereotypes in decision making.

Mitigating the effects of one's implicit biases and engaging in culturally respectful, family-centered care are critical in developmental-behavioral pediatrics. Inquiring about the unique experiences that families face in an open and honest manner can demonstrate one's commitment to practicing cultural humility. For example, clinicians may be tasked with weighing conflicting and ambiguous information, such as when rating scales completed by teachers indicate behavioral concerns but family rating scales do not. Clinicians may consider whether a child's behavior is being accurately represented in each environment or whether discrimination may be contributing to this discrepancy in scores. When safety planning, families may fear using publicly available mental health or crisis services, or contacting law enforcement. Discussing these situations honestly with families can allow clinicians to adjust diagnostic, treatment, and crisis plans for children to address these concerns.

Beyond relying on individual clinicians to practice cultural humility, national standards were developed to ameliorate disparities faced by racial and ethnic minorities, individuals with limited English proficiency and low health literacy, and other minoritized groups. The national Culturally and Linguistically Appropriate Services (CLAS) standards, enhanced and released in 2013, guide health care organizations to deliver services that are responsive to individuals' beliefs, preferences, and communication needs.

In the field of developmental-behavioral pediatrics a particular challenge exists with respect to provision of multicultural care: the validation of screening and diagnostic tools for diverse patient populations. For example, a systematic review found that while several screening instruments to identify developmental concerns among Hispanic populations in the United States have been translated into Spanish, none had undergone rigorous evaluation of cultural validity and reliability (Bevan, Liu, Wallis, & Pinto-Martin, 2020). A popular tool that screens for ASD was found to have lower accuracy (specificity and positive predictive value) among children of color and those from lower-income households (Guthrie et al., 2019). Thus screening and diagnostic tools must be used and interpreted with caution, as their accuracy may differ based on a child's or family's sociodemographic characteristics or cultural backgrounds.

PUTTING CULTURAL HUMILITY INTO PRACTICE: A RETURN TO OMARI'S CASE

When Omari presented to developmental-behavioral pediatrics for his evaluation, his parents reflected on their prior experiences. They felt that at times, Omari's pediatrician had reassured them and advised them to watch and wait before seeking developmental assessment and therapies, even when they shared their concerns. Because they were unsure of the age that a child would be expected to reach certain milestones, they did not feel that they were able to push for additional evaluations or support. And later, when they began to see some progress and Omari began using single words to communicate at around 36 months, they felt reassured that perhaps their earlier worries had been unfounded. Now that Omari had been asked to leave his private school and teachers in his public school were continuing to report concerns about his behaviors, his parents were again very worried. They wondered if their child's race and the family's status as immigrants and speakers of English as a second language impacted the care they had received or Omari's treatment in school. They reported feeling unsure of how to navigate the various educational and medical systems to get Omari additional support.

In Omari's case practicing cultural humility would have required clinicians to avoid assumptions about parents' linguistic abilities or preferences, to have inquired about their expectations for Omari's developmental milestones, to have explored parents' beliefs about Omari's behaviors, and to have asked about perceptions of experiences with racism and discrimination. Omari's parents perceived that their pediatrician took an approach of watchful waiting and minimized their concerns, an experience reported by other Black families, who report needing to engage in aggressive advocacy to have concerns adequately heard and addressed (Pearson & Meadan, 2018). When his parents offered their beliefs that Omari's progress in meeting early speech milestones was sufficient, which led to their discontinuation of intervention services at 36 months, clinicians could have probed more about the parents' goals for Omari's communication skills and could have offered support about next steps to continue services if this was desired by parents.

Open communication between caregivers and clinicians lends itself to shared decision making when developing diagnostic and treatment plans. Additionally, research corroborates the parents' concerns that Omari, as a Black boy, may have suffered from lower expectations (Rowley et al., 2014) or from misperceptions of his behaviors as more aggressive (Neitzel, 2018), which may have resulted in the failure to act upon his early developmental concerns and in kindergarten expulsion, respectively. Explicitly inquiring about experiences of discrimination or racism is important. The Perceptions of Racism in Children and Youth (PRaCY) is a validated tool to measure such experiences (Pachter, Szalacha, Bernstein, & Coll, 2010). This information can give clinicians an opportunity to discuss ways that discrimination may be impacting how a child is perceived by others. Additionally, experiences of discrimination may have impacted Omari's parents' interactions with educational and public systems, which may have led to their decision to discontinue EI therapies. An honest discussion with families like Omari's about their experiences may also serve to validate their perceptions, to allow them to prepare to respond to any situations that may arise in the future, and to help Omari develop his own racial identity.

CONSIDERATIONS FOR CARE OF CHILDREN IN IMMIGRANT FAMILIES

Children in immigrant families, defined as children who are foreign born or who are born in the United States and have at least one parent who is foreign born, are a large and growing population (Linton & Green, 2019). Immigrant children and families face particular challenges, but they also have unique sources of resilience that may result in better health outcomes than their risk factors would suggest, a phenomenon referred to as the immigrant paradox (Teruya & Bazargan-Hejazi, 2013). Practicing cultural humility when caring for children in immigrant families is particularly important, given the diversity of immigrant children and families in terms of native country, experience with Western medicine practices, education levels, English proficiency, and levels of acculturation in the United States (Linton & Green, 2019). For children who have limited English proficiency, school-based services for English-language learners can be incorporated into educational plans under federal law. Families are also entitled to services and translation of materials and should be encouraged to request that these services be implemented to allow parental participation in their child's educational programming.

An additional consideration for caring for children in immigrant families is recognition of the discrimination and trauma that they may have experienced. Fear regarding family's immigration status and risk of deportation can impact children's behaviors, learning, and development (Yoshikawa & Kholoptseva, 2013). Building trust with patients and families over time may allow them to feel comfortable disclosing information about their experiences and immigration status. The American Academy of Pediatrics immigrant health toolkit suggests that instead of directly asking about household members' immigration status, clinicians may consider asking if a family member has left or is potentially going to leave the family for any reason, which may shed light on this information but be more acceptable. If families share this information, it is important to confirm that the information is confidential, will not impact a child's care, and that the information will not be shared with immigration enforcement agencies. Documenting this information in the patient's health record must be carefully considered, but accounting for the impact of these stressors on patients and families is important for providing holistic care.

CONCLUSION: PROMOTING RESILIENCE BY CELEBRATING DIVERSITY

While much of developmental-behavioral pediatric care by its nature focuses on a child's challenges or needs, clinicians can also incorporate a strengths-based approach, which encourages reflections on an individual's or family's strengths and can promote resilience (Brito & Boller, 2020). Broadly, a strengths-based approach consists of identifying family and individual strengths, providing feedback on those strengths, and using these identified strengths to engage families in shared decision making. This can include asking families about their favorite qualities in their child, about where they go when they need additional support or strength, and about what they as a family do really well. Delivering patient-centered care, which is tailored to their beliefs and preferences, is key to promoting resilience among patients.

In particular, a family's cultural beliefs, traditions, and supports should be considered strengths that clinicians and caregivers alike can draw upon. Clinicians can show genuine curiosity and openness to learning about different beliefs and practices and may learn about new ways of celebrating children and families. Practicing cultural humility and celebrating this diversity in the exam room is one step toward breaking down barriers and ensuring families feel welcome to share and fully participate in their children's care. Box 20.3 provides additional sources of reading on the important topics discussed in this chapter.

BOX 20.3 For Additional Reading

- American Academy of Pediatrics' Immigrant Health Toolkit: https://www.aap.org/en-us/advocacy-and-policy/aap-health-initiatives/Immigrant-Child-Health-Toolkit/Pages/Immigrant-Child-Health-Toolkit.aspx
- American Academy of Pediatrics' Strengths-Based Approach: https://www.aap.org/en-us/advocacy-and-policy/aap-health-initiatives/HALF-Implementation-Guide/communicating-with-families/Pages/Strength-Based-Approach.aspx
- American Anthropological Association Statement on Race: https://www.americananthro.org/ConnectWithAAA/Content.aspx?ItemNumber=2583
- Bonilla-Silva, E. (2015). The structure of racism in color-blind, "post-racial" America. *American Behavioral Scientist, 59*(11), 1358–1376.
- Goodman, A. H., Moses, Y. T., & Jones, J. L. (2019). *Race: Are we so different?* John Wiley & Sons.
- Johnson, T. J. (2020). Intersection of bias, structural racism, and social determinants with health care inequities. *Pediatrics, 146*(2), e2020003657.
- Maina, I. W., Belton, T. D., Ginzberg, S., Singh, A., & Johnson, T. J. (2018). A decade of studying implicit racial/ethnic bias in healthcare providers using the implicit association test. *Social Science & Medicine, 199*, 219–229. https://doi.org/10.1016/j.socscimed.2017.05.009.
- Powell, R. (2000). Overcoming cultural racism: The promise of multicultural education. *Multicultural Perspectives, 2*(3), 8–14.
- Project Implicit: https://implicit.harvard.edu
- Schnierle, J., Christian-Brathwaite, N., & Louisias, M. (2019). Implicit bias: What every pediatrician should know about the effect of bias on health and future directions. *Current Problems in Pediatric and Adolescent Health Care, 49*(2), 34–44.
- Understanding Race: www.understandingrace.org
- US Department of Health and Human Services National Standards for Culturally and Linguistically Appropriate Services (CLAS) in Health and Health Care: https://thinkculturalhealth.hhs.gov/clas
- Wilkerson, I. (2020). *Caste: The origins of our discontents.* Random House.

REFERENCES

Aboud, F. E. (2003). The formation of in-group favoritism and out-group prejudice in young children: Are they distinct attitudes? *Developmental Psychology*, 39(1), 48–60.

Anderson, A., & Douge, J. (2019). Talking to children about racial bias. Healthy Living: Emotional wellness—Building resilience. *American Academy of Pediatrics.* https://www.healthychildren.org/English/healthy-living/emotional-wellness/Building-Resilience/Pages/Talking-to-Children-About-Racial-Bias.aspx

Anderson, R. E., & Stevenson, H. C. (2019). RECASTing racial stress and trauma: Theorizing the healing potential of racial socialization in families. *American Psychologist*, *74*(1), 63–75.

Anzures, G., Quinn, P. C., Pascalis, O., Slater, A. M., Tanaka, J. W., & Lee, K. (2013). Developmental origins of the other-race effect. *Current Directions in Psychological Science*, *22*(3), 173–178.

Baio, J., Wiggins, L., Christensen, D. L., Maenner, M. J., Daniels, J., Warren, Z., … Dowling, N. F. (2018). Prevalence of autism spectrum disorder among children aged 8 years—Autism and Developmental Disabilities Monitoring Network, 11 Sites, United States, 2014. *MMWR Surveillance Summaries*, *67*(6), 1–23. https://doi.org/10.15585/mmwr.ss6706a1

Bevan, S. L., Liu, J., Wallis, K. E., & Pinto-Martin, J. A. (2020). Screening instruments for developmental and behavioral concerns in pediatric Hispanic populations in the United States: A systematic literature review. *Journal of Developmental & Behavioral Pediatrics*, *41*(1), 71–80.

Brito, A., & Boller, K. (2020). Changing the pediatric paradigm: Focusing on strengths. *Pediatric Clinics of North America*, *67*(2), 247–258. https://doi.org/10.1016/j.pcl.2019.12.010

Burkholder, A. R., D'Esterre, A. P., & Killen, M. (2019). Intergroup relationships, context, and prejudice in childhood. In H. E. Fitzgerald, D. J. Johnson, D. Baolian Qin, F. A. Villarruel, & J. Norder (Eds.), *Handbook of children and prejudice: Integrating research, practice, and policy*. Springer.

Coker, T. R., Elliott, M. N., Toomey, S. L., Schwebel, D. C., Cuccaro, P., Tortolero Emery, S., … Schuster, M. A. (2016). Racial and ethnic disparities in ADHD diagnosis and treatment. *Pediatrics*, *138*(3) e20160407.

Crenshaw, K. (2017). *On intersectionality: Essential writings*. The New Press.

Cross, W. E. (1978). The Thomas and Cross models of psychological nigrescence: A review. *Journal of Black Psychology*, *5*(1), 13–31. https://doi.org/10.1177/009579847800500102

Daniel Tatum, B. (2017). *Why are all the Black kids sitting together in the cafeteria? And other conversations about race*. Basic Books, Perseus Books, LLC.

Derman-Sparks, L., Tanaka Higa, C., & Sparks, B. (1980). Children, race and racism: How race awareness develops. *Interracial Books for Children Bulletin*, *11*(3/4), 3–9.

Guthrie, W., Wallis, K., Bennett, A., Brooks, E., Dudley, J., Gerdes, M., … Miller, J. S. (2019). Accuracy of autism screening in a large pediatric network. *Pediatrics*, *144*(4).

Hughes, D., Rodriguez, J., Smith, E. P., Johnson, D. J., Stevenson, H. C., & Spicer, P. (2006). Parents' ethnic-racial socialization practices: A review of research and directions for future study. *Developmental Psychology*, *42*(5), 747–770. https://doi.org/10.1037/0012-1649.42.5.747

Jones, C. P. (2000). Levels of racism: A theoretic framework and a gardener's tale. *American Journal of Public Health*, *90*(8), 1212–1215. https://doi.org/10.2105/ajph.90.8.1212

Kinzler, K. D., & Spelke, E. S. (2011). Do infants show social preferences for people differing in race? *Cognition*, *119*(1), 1–9. https://doi.org/10.1016/j.cognition.2010.10.019

Linton, J. M., & Green, A. (2019). Providing care for children in immigrant families. *Pediatrics*, *144*(3), e20192077. https://doi.org/10.1542/peds.2019-2077

Maina, I. W., Belton, T. D., Ginzberg, S., Singh, A., & Johnson, T. J. (2018). A decade of studying implicit racial/ethnic bias in healthcare providers using the Implicit Association Test. *Social Science & Medicine*, *199*, 219–229. https://doi.org/10.1016/j.socscimed.2017.05.009

Mandell, D. S., Listerud, J., Levy, S. E., & Pinto-Martin, J. A. (2002). Race differences in the age at diagnosis among medicaid-eligible children with autism. *Journal of the American Academy of Child and Adolescent Psychiatry*, *41*(12), 1447–1453. https://doi.org/10.1097/00004583-200212000-00016

Marcelin, J. R., Siraj, D. S., Victor, R., Kotadia, S., & Maldonado, Y. A. (2019). The impact of unconscious bias in healthcare: How to recognize and mitigate it. *The Journal of Infectious Diseases*, *220*(2), S62–S73. https://doi.org/10.1093/infdis/jiz214

Maroney, T., & Zuckerman, B. (2018). "The talk," physician version: Special considerations for African American, male adolescents. *Pediatrics*, *141*(2), e20171462.

Mendoza, M., Blake, J. J., Marchbanks, M. P., & Ragan, K. (2019). Race, gender, and disability and the risk for juvenile justice contact. *The Journal of Special Education*, *53*(4), 226–235.

Metzl, J. M., & Hansen, H. (2014). Structural competency: Theorizing a new medical engagement with stigma and inequality. *Social Science & Medicine*, *103*, 126–133. https://doi.org/10.1016/j.socscimed.2013.06.032

Morgan, P. L., Woods, A. D., Wang, Y., Hillemeier, M. M., Farkas, G., & Mitchell, C. (2019). Are schools in the U.S. south using special education to segregate students by race? *Exceptional Children*, *86*(3), 255–275. https://doi.org/10.1177/0014402919868486

Neitzel, J. (2018). Research to practice: Understanding the role of implicit bias in early childhood disciplinary practices. *Journal of Early Childhood Teacher Education*, *39*(3), 232–242.

Ngui, E. M., & Flores, G. (2007). Unmet needs for specialty, dental, mental, and allied health care among children with special health care needs: Are there racial/ethnic disparities? *Journal of Health Care for the Poor and Underserved*, *18*(4), 931–949. https://doi.org/10.1353/hpu.2007.0102

Pachter, L. M., Szalacha, L. A., Bernstein, B. A., & Coll, C. G. (2010). Perceptions of Racism in Children and Youth (PRaCY): Properties of a self-report instrument for research on children's health and development. *Ethnicity & Health*, *15*(1), 33–46. https://doi.org/10.1080/13557850903383196

Paradies, Y., Ben, J., Denson, N., Elias, A., Priest, N., Pieterse, A., … Gee, G. (2015). Racism as a determinant of health: A systematic review and meta-analysis. *PLoS ONE*, *10*(9), e0138511.

Pearson, J., & Meadan, H. (2018). African American parents' perceptions of diagnosis and services for children with autism. *Education and Training in Autism and Developmental Disabilities*, *53*, 17–32.

Phillips Swanson, D., Cunningham, M., Youngblood, J., & Beale Spencer, M. (2009). Racial identity development during childhood. In H. A. Neville, B. M. Tynes, & S. O. Utsey (Eds.), *Handbook of African American psychology* (pp. 269–281). Sage Publications.

Rogoff, B. (2003). *The cultural nature of human development*. Oxford University Press.

Rosa, E. M., & Tudge, J. (2013). Urie Bronfenbrenner's theory of human development: Its evolution from ecology to bioecology. *Journal of Family Theory & Review*, *5*(4), 243–258.

Rowley, S. J., Ross, L., Lozada, F. T., Williams, A., Gale, A., & Kurtz-Costes, B. (2014). Framing Black boys: Parent, teacher, and student narratives of the academic lives of Black boys. In L. S. Liben & R. S. Bigler (Eds.), *Advances in child development and behavior* (pp. 301–332, Vol. 47). JAI.

Teruya, S. A., & Bazargan-Hejazi, S. (2013). The immigrant and Hispanic paradoxes: A systematic review of their predictions and effects. *Hispanic Journal of Behavioral Sciences, 35*(4), 486–509.

Trent, M., Dooley, D. G., & Dougé, J. (2019). The impact of racism on child and adolescent health. *Pediatrics, 144*(2), e20191765. https://doi.org/10.1542/peds.2019-1765

Twine, F. W. (2004). A white side of black Britain: The concept of racial literacy. *Ethnic and Racial Studies, 27*(6), 878–907. https://doi.org/10.1080/0141987042000268512.

US Department of Health and Human Services. (2020). *Social determinants of health.* https://www.healthypeople.gov/2020/topics-objectives/topic/social-determinants-of-health

Van Ausdale, D., & Feagin, J. R. (2001). *The first R: How children learn race and racism.* Rowman and Littlefield Publishers, Inc.

Wallis, K. E., Buttenheim, A. M., & Mandell, D. S. (2021). Insights from behavioral economics: A case of delayed diagnosis of autism spectrum disorder. *Journal of Developmental & Behavioral Pediatrics, 42*(2), 109–113.

Wallis, K. E., Guthrie, W., Bennett, A. E., Gerdes, M., Levy, S. E., Mandell, D. S., & Miller, J. S. (2020). Adherence to screening and referral guidelines for autism spectrum disorder in toddlers in pediatric primary care. *PLoS ONE, 15*(5), e0232335. https://doi.org/10.1371/journal.pone.0232335

Williams, C. D., Byrd, C. M., Quintana, S. M., Anicama, C., Kiang, L., Umaña-Taylor, A. J., … Whitesell, N. (2020). A lifespan model of ethnic-racial identity. *Research in Human Development,* 1–31. https://doi.org/10.1080/15427609.2020.1831882

Winkler, E. N., & Hagerman, M. A. (2021). *How kids learn about race: Embrace Race.* https://www.embracerace.org/resources/how-children-learn-about-race.

Yeager, K. A., & Bauer-Wu, S. (2013). Cultural humility: Essential foundation for clinical researchers. *Applied Nursing Research, 26*(4), 251–256. https://doi.org/10.1016/j.apnr.2013.06.008

Yoshikawa, H., & Kholoptseva, J. (2013). *Unauthorized immigrant parents and their children's development: A summary of the evidence.* Migration Policy Institute.

Zuckerman, K. E., Mattox, K. M., Sinche, B. K., Blaschke, G. S., & Bethell, C. (2014). Racial, ethnic, and language disparities in early childhood developmental/behavioral evaluations: A narrative review. *Clinical Pediatrics (Philadelphia), 53*(7), 619–631.

21

The Influence of Digital Media on Children and Families

Tiffany Munzer

For additional material related to the content of this chapter, please see Chapters 13, 67, and 70.

> **VIGNETTE**
>
> *Matthew, a 7–year old boy with attention-deficit/hyperactivity disorder (ADHD), presents for a routine well-child visit, and you are the clinician. While you and his mother catch up on how Matthew has been doing, he uses his mother's smartphone to watch videos on YouTube. His mother notes that she is worried about his school performance but reports he is otherwise healthy. He lives at home with his mother, father, and 4-year-old sister, and he is currently in second grade in the local public school district. He has difficulty remembering to turn in his homework, seems distracted during independent work times, and frequently refuses to complete schoolwork at home. Therefore his mother would like to consider an increase in his ADHD psychostimulant medication. His mother also notes, "He is on a screen almost all day." She asks for recommendations on screen media. Specifically, Matthew's mother would like to know to what extent his screen use is causing him to have a harder time focusing in school and whether it is harmful for his development. She is looking for resources to help curb his screen media use.*

PREVALENCE OF DIGITAL MEDIA

Digital media use, which includes use of mobile devices such as smartphones, traditional television, and computers, is increasingly a fixture in children's lives. The overall duration of use has increased over the last decades. Smartphones and tablet devices have made it easier to access digital content from anywhere, at any time. In 2020 97% of households owned a smartphone, and 75% of households owned a tablet device. In 2020 a survey of parents conducted by Common Sense Media found that young children (0–8 years of age) spend approximately 2.5 hours per day using digital media (Rideout & Robb, 2020). Objective measures of tablet play have found that preschoolers spend about 2 hours per day on mobile devices, and their parents spend approximately 3 hours per day on their devices (Radesky et al., 2020). In 2019 preteens (8–12 years of age) spent just under 5 hours per day using digital media, and teens (13–18 years of age) spent about 7 hours per day using digital media—not including screen use for school or homework (Rideout & Robb, 2019). During the COVID-19 pandemic, when many US schools turned to remote learning to curb the spread of the virus, digital media became a more integral family fixture, providing opportunities for education, connection with peers, entertainment, and parents' work.

EVOLUTION OF DIGITAL MEDIA

The rapid pace of technological development in the last century has surpassed the pace of research and therefore the ability to understand digital media's effects on children in an evidence-based manner. The television was invented in 1927 with wide adoption in the 1950s after World War II when black-and-white televisions became more popular in the United States. Home personal computers entered the market in 1977, with wide adoption in the 1980s. More recently, the modern smartphone was invented in 2007 with the Apple iPhone, and tablet devices were invented in 2011, with wide and rapid adoption in the 2010s. These personal devices are highly portable and have a seamless and intuitive interface that is easily accessible by young children and families. As a result, they have revolutionized how children consume screen media. Whereas prior forms of digital content were accessible in the form of television—which could be turned on and off, and would not accompany children to stores, restaurants, or other activities of daily living—these portable forms of digital media increase the importance of understanding not just duration of use but frequency and quality of content as well.

CONTENT

Though quantity of viewing time is associated with wellbeing and physical risk factors (e.g., overweight, obesity, hypercholesterolemia), the quality of content is also associated with sleep, language development, emotion regulation, aggression, and social-emotional competence in both positive and suboptimal ways. Therefore the term *screen time*, which was traditionally used to describe the duration of media use, has been replaced with *screen media* to capture the nuances of content, duration, and format. One challenge with characterizing what children watch is the expansive variety of videos and content now available through platforms such as YouTube. Individuals may develop such content with sponsorships or advertisements embedded in these videos, which are highly unregulated.

As of 2020, parents reported that young children (0–8 years) spent the majority (73%) of their daily screen media use watching videos—either through television, streamed content, or online videos—and these platforms have changed rapidly. In 2020 most young children received their content from online apps/websites such as YouTube or Netflix.

PARENT ROLE IN MEDIA

The amount of content to navigate makes it more important and challenging for already-busy parents to be involved in their young children's media consumption. The task of media supervision is often at odds with the multitude of demands and stressors that families are facing in their daily lives. Anecdotally, children's engagement with digital media might be an opportunity for parents to work on getting dinner on the table, attend other tasks, or just take a breather for themselves. In such ways digital media can alleviate stressors or play a role in helping families get work done, as long as it does not create greater conflict in the family system.

Parents serve an important role in helping children understand content in digital media and in learning to use it safely. Prior work in children's television viewing has identified three ways in which parents might scaffold their children's screen media consumption: (1) coviewing (e.g., watching a show together), (2) instructive mediation (e.g., teaching/talking about what children are viewing), and (3) restrictive mediation (e.g., setting limits and choosing what children view) (Valkenburg, Krcmar, Peeters, & Marseille, 1999). With the advent of tablet and smartphone devices, parental guidance and support around digital media have evolved. More work is needed to understand how parents can best scaffold their children's technology use over a tablet or smartphone device, teach their children about digital citizenship (i.e., teaching about the responsible use of technology), and set ground rules with online safety.

Parents not only have the daunting task of managing their children's screen media use but also their own digital media use habits. Digital media can be used as a tool to connect with others, access work remotely, or provide entertainment. One major challenge is that digital media is designed to have compelling and enticing content. This content sustains the user's attention, which may decrease parents' ability to notice and respond to others in their environment. Yet, responsive caregiving facilitates children's development of emotion regulation and language skills (see Chapter 13). Indeed, prior work has found associations between greater "technoference" (i.e., parent distraction with technology) and child behavior problems (McDaniel & Radesky, 2020). When parents seek advice around digital media use with children, consider helping the parents reflect on when and how they are using digital media, proactively plan their media use when possible, and set aside times of the day to take breaks from a digital device as a family. This approach to screen media use may create a positive example for young children. However, a recent randomized trial of adolescents participating in a family digital media plan did not find significant changes in media rule engagement compared to controls (Moreno, Binger, Zhao, & Eickhoff, 2021). Additional work is needed to understand how a family digital media plan might provide role modeling for young children and whether it can create boundaries around digital media use for all in a household.

> *You ask Matthew what he likes to watch and play on his tablet. He replies, "I like playing Fortnite, watching YouTubers play Minecraft, and when Ryan unboxes toys from Ryan's World." When Matthew recalls what he enjoys playing on his tablet, his mother replies, "Oh, I didn't know you played Fortnite."*

It is very challenging to supervise all of the screen media content that children consume. As illustrated in the chapter-opening vignette, clinicians may have opportunities to acknowledge the difficulties with keeping up with children's digital media consumption; engage in an open, nonjudgmental conversation with parents; assess parents' and children's possible motivation for change; and consider next steps with feasible but actionable recommendations. For example, resources such as CommonSenseMedia.org can offer parents ideas for replacements with age-appropriate content such as apps, movies, or videogames.

ASSOCIATIONS WITH HEALTH OUTCOMES AND CHILDREN'S WELLBEING

Overview

Screen media use is associated with child health and wellbeing outcomes. This section will focus on four outcomes (sleep, obesity, language development, executive functioning), address hypothesized mechanisms, review important considerations when interpreting the literature, and offer practical recommendations. A large body of work has examined screen media in the form of television and videos. Less is known about tablet and mobile devices, therefore some of this evidence may be extrapolated from the literature on television and videos.

Sleep

Insufficient sleep affects 30% of children (from toddlers through adolescents), with shorter sleep duration and lower sleep quality being associated with greater challenges in emotional regulation, greater behavioral difficulties, and less optimal academic performance across childhood (LeBourgeois et al., 2017; see Chapter 70). Screen media use is a modifiable environmental factor related to sleep. Excessive duration of screen media use is strongly associated with insufficient sleep, possibly due to arousing effects of the content and effects of light-emitting screens on suppression of endogenous melatonin production (Arora, Broglia, Thomas, & Taheri, 2014). The American Academy of Pediatrics (AAP) and American Academy of Sleep Medicine recommend limiting screen-based activities 30 minutes before bedtime and avoiding screen-based devices in children's bedrooms (Radesky & Christakis, 2016). On the other hand, educational content may reduce the risk of future sleep problems. In one study greater viewing of prosocial and educational content by preschoolers improved sleep problems in follow-up 6 to 18 months later (Garrison & Christakis, 2012).

During your visit with Matthew, his mother also brings up that he is having difficulties with sleep onset. She notes that he does not have a television in his room, but he will charge the tablet on his nightstand and play with the tablet to fall asleep at night. There are times when she hears him awakening in the middle of the night but is unsure if he is using the device.

The presence of tablet devices in the bedroom makes it easier to have access to content that may be arousing for children. The clinician can guide parents on ways to limit access to such a device immediately before sleep. For example, consider creating a "bed" for the tablet in another room, even tucking it in while it is charging may help eliminate the temptation of reaching over to play with a device right before bed or in the middle of the night.

Obesity

Epidemiologic studies have revealed associations between higher screen media use, generally television, during childhood and greater risk of overweight/obesity across the life span (Robinson et al., 2017; see Chapter 67). Preschoolers who watched 2 or more hours of television per day experienced an increased risk of overweight at 36 months and 54 months of age (Lumeng, Rahnama, Appugliese, Kaciroti, & Bradley, 2006). Greater childhood TV exposure is associated with greater prevalence of overweight into adulthood. For every 1 hour of television viewed during the weekend at 5 years, the odds ratio for adult obesity increased by 7% (Viner & Cole, 2005). Greater quantity of screen media (primarily television) is also associated with hypertension, hypercholesteremia, insulin resistance, and metabolic syndrome (Hancox, Milne, & Poulton, 2004). There are a few hypothesized mechanisms, which may help explain these associations. Exposure to advertisements that promote calorically dense foods during screen media use may lead to greater consumption of such foods. During YouTube videos, for instance, advertisements often occur in the form of a child social media influencer consuming calorically dense foods, with 90% of influencers in one YouTube content analysis consuming unhealthy branded items (Alruwaily et al., 2020). Consumption of snacks and meals during screen media use may reduce satiety cues and therefore increase the risk of overeating. Lastly, excessive use of screen media may displace opportunities for physical activity. Recommendations to reduce the risk of obesity around screen media are to reduce exposures to advertisements and reduce snacking/eating behaviors while viewing screens.

Language Development

Screen media exposure is negatively associated with language development in the early childhood years. Infants and young toddlers have more difficulty translating information from a screen into the real world, known as the video deficit effect (Krcmar, 2010). In a 2020 metaanalysis of 42 studies of children 12 years and younger, greater quantity of screen hours and background television was associated with lower language skills. Meanwhile, higher-quality educational programming and coviewing with an adult were independently associated with stronger child language skills. Educational television programming such as *Sesame Street, Dora the Explorer, Blue's Clues, Arthur, Clifford*, and *Dragon Tales* were associated with greater preschooler vocabularies and expressive language scores (Linebarger & Walker, 2005). Aspects of these TV shows, which are associated with better language outcomes, include narrative, storylike content, and elements that elicit child engagement (Linebarger & Walker, 2005). Clinicians can encourage families to seek out media content with these characteristics and help them apply developmental principles (see later) that can guide when to introduce children to media.

Executive Functioning

Children's executive functioning skills, such as the ability to sustain attention with tasks, carry out plans, delay gratification, and regulate their emotions, have strong associations with future educational achievement and job attainment. There are cross-sectional and longitudinal associations between greater screen media use (primarily television) and challenges with executive functioning in young children (Radesky & Christakis, 2016). It is also possible that these associations are bidirectional (i.e., children with greater social-emotional difficulties may gravitate toward screen media or receive greater exposure to screen media at a younger age, as a soothing technique). For instance, fussy babies were more likely to have received greater screen media exposure during infancy and during toddlerhood (Radesky, Silverstein, Zuckerman, & Christakis, 2014). Certain characteristics may make children more or less susceptible to certain types of content. In a randomized trial a media diet consisting of fast-paced television was associated with greater externalizing symptoms in preschoolers who were boys but not in other children (Christakis et al., 2013). However, digital media can also be used as a tool to promote social-emotional regulation and development. Indeed, one study from 2016 found associations between exposure to *Daniel Tiger's Neighborhood* while parents were also watching and preschoolers' positive social-emotional development (Rasmussen et al., 2016). Another study of preschool children found greater ability to delay gratification after playing with an educational application compared with viewing a cartoon (Huber, Yeates, Meyer, Fleckhammer, & Kaufman, 2018).

Matthew may gravitate toward digital media because of the intense reinforcing design features. Videogames in particular have strong visual features and immediate rewards (tokens, points) for accomplishing certain levels that are highly reinforcing for children with ADHD. Such games are designed to hold one's attention for long periods of time, and for children who struggle with executive functioning skills it makes it harder to resist such design features. Matthew may be predisposed toward enjoying such digital content, and such highly reinforcing digital content may make it harder for him to sustain attention for other less-compelling activities, which may be less immediately rewarding (e.g., homework, chores). Because of these characteristics, children with ADHD may be more likely to develop problematic digital media habits and therefore need more comprehensive behavior plans to identify positive replacement content and set limits around technology use.

CHILDREN'S DEVELOPMENTAL STAGES AND ASSOCIATIONS WITH DIGITAL MEDIA

Associations between children's media and children's development depend largely on how children optimally learn during each life stage. This section reviews associations between media use and children's development from infancy through adolescence, and how parents and clinicians can promote development in concert with an increasingly digital environment. Table 21.1 summarizes general recommendations from the 2016 AAP screen media guidelines (Radesky & Christakis, 2016; Reid Chassiakos, Radesky, Christakis, Moreno, & Cross, 2016).

Infancy

Infant Development and Screen Media

The body of work on infant screen media has often used experimental paradigms to understand how infants transfer information from a screen to the real world, how infants behave in the presence of a screen, and how parents respond to their infants in the presence of screens. There are also studies focused on cross-sectional and longitudinal associations between infant screen media exposures and developmental outcomes.

Infant development occurs in the context of a trusted caregiver. Infants learn more readily from in-person interactions compared to videos of similar interactions. This concept is known as the video deficit effect, as described earlier (Barr, 2010). One study found pronounced video deficit effects at 13 to 20 months of age—such children learned best from their mother's live demonstrations, followed by mother's video demonstration, then a stranger's video demonstration. With touchscreen tablets, infants were less able to transfer information from a three-dimensional (3D) to two-dimensional (2D) world (and vice versa), compared with transferring information from a 2D to 3D world (Zack, Barr, Gerhardstein, Dickerson, & Meltzoff, 2009).

There are small to moderate associations between greater duration of infant screen media exposure per day and greater parent depression symptoms, and greater infant regulation challenges, possibly due to displacement of other developmental activities. When infants were exposed to background television, they engaged in less sustained toy play, and the conversation from their parents was less robust (Kirkorian, Pempek, Murphy, Schmidt, & Anderson, 2009). Other work has found challenges in parents' responsivity to infant cues when parents themselves are engaged with a

TABLE 21.1 Recommendations for Parents by Child Age

Age Group	Developmental Principles	Ideas for Parents
Infants	• Have difficulties translating information from a screen to real life • Caregivers take the biggest role in promoting infant development through attachment	• Limit screen media to video chatting • Provide ample time for other developmentally enriching activities
Toddlers/preschoolers	• Receptive language skills and visuospatial skills have matured, making it easier for toddlers to learn from digital media • Children still rely on caregivers to translate information and get the "most" out of digital media	• Choose high-quality educational content • Watch together when possible • Limit screens to <1 hr/d
School-age children	• Mature problem-solving abilities help school-age children take a greater role in more independent digital media and in reflecting on experiences • Identifying privacy issues and advertisements is challenging for school-age children, therefore they require adult support	• Choose high-quality educational content • Watch together when possible • Reflect with your child on digital media and promote digital citizenship • Provide ample time for other developmentally enriching activities
Adolescents	• Peer relationships and connecting with others become a more prominent aspect of online engagement	• School-age tips are applicable • Limit digital distractions when completing school work • Consider supervising teenager's social media accounts on a regular basis

screen device, with possible implications on infant development in this context (Haughton, Aiken, & Cheevers, 2015).

Relevance for Parents/Clinicians Caring for Infants

Infant development is tightly nested within the caregiving environment, with responsive, sensitive caregivers being an essential driving force of development. A tablet or digital device is unable to replicate contingent, in-person caregiving interactions that are critical for building these foundations. Cognitively, infants have trouble transferring information from a digital device to the real world. Therefore the AAP recommends limiting infant screen media exposure, with the exception of video chat services such as FaceTime or Skype. Video chat has the advantage of contingent input from a responsive caregiver (though not in-person), which serves as an opportunity to connect with distant friends or relatives.

Toddlers and Preschoolers

Toddler/Preschooler Development and Screen Media

By the toddler and preschool years, preschoolers start to spend approximately 2 hours per day on a tablet device, with the majority of this time viewing videos such as YouTube (Radesky et al., 2020). The AAP and World Health Organization recommend limiting daily duration of screen media use to less than 1 hour per day, but most children at ages 2 and 3 years exceed such screen media guidelines (Madigan, Racine, & Tough, 2020).

As toddlers and preschoolers develop greater receptive language skills, they develop improved capacity for learning and transferring information from a screen. Therefore content of digital media becomes more important during this developmental period. Apps should encourage active participation, be meaningful for the child, facilitate social interaction, and have a clear learning goal (Hirsh-Pasek et al., 2015). High-quality shows such as *Sesame Street, Daniel Tiger's Neighborhood, Blue's Clues*, and *Dora the Explorer* are associated with enhanced language/literacy, social-emotional competence, and academic skills (Rasmussen et al., 2016). However, many children are not viewing such educational content. Indeed, a 2020 content analysis of young children's (0–8 years of age) YouTube browsing histories found that one in five videos contained ads that were not age appropriate, almost half of the videos featured promoted products for children to buy, one in four videos were intended for older target audiences, and three in ten videos contained physical violence. When the content that is widely available to children is at odds with expert recommendations for high-quality digital play and content, it becomes all the more challenging for parents to extensively vet the content their children are viewing. Coviewing is one potential albeit time-intensive solution to understanding what children are viewing. Coviewing can also help toddlers/preschoolers who still have more limited cognitive flexibility and therefore continue to have some difficulties with gleaning information from a screen. Coviewing may help in translating information from a 2D surface to their daily life. However, one caveat with coviewing is that sometimes the personal nature of a tablet or mobile device may interfere with the parent's and child's ability to engage with each other (e.g., toddlers may be at risk for preferring to play or view a tablet independently, and may engage in behaviors that do not promote social reciprocity) (Munzer, Miller, Weeks, Kaciroti, & Radesky, 2019).

Relevance for Parents/Clinicians Caring for Toddlers/Preschoolers

Language and social-emotional outcomes in the toddler and preschool years account for a high degree of variance across the life span. High-quality content, providing plenty of opportunities for other developmentally enriching activities, and coviewing are strategies for families with children this age. For parents looking for high-quality educational content there are several resources that can serve as a guide for choosing content. The website commonsensemedia.org contains several rating systems and identifies educational apps, TV shows, and movies, which are sorted by age range (from the toddler years to the adolescent years). PBS kids includes funding from the Corporation for Public Broadcasting, whose mission is to ensure access to noncommercial high-quality content. Though there are often times when coviewing is not possible, given the many competing demands and pressures faced by families, coviewing does confer some advantages to children. Specifically for toddlers and preschoolers, parents can help promote active participation, make the content more engaging, and relate it back to their daily life making it more meaningful. Lastly, though high-quality content has associations with better child language and social-emotional development during the preschool years, ample time to engage in play, physical activity, and reading is also important for toddler/preschooler development. Therefore limiting the duration of total screen media consumed per day to less than 1 hour, as advised by the AAP, may help ensure families engage in these other enriching activities.

School Age

School-Age Children's Development and Screen Media

School-age children are building key problem-solving skills, learning how to negotiate and engage with their peers, and developing more varied interests. School-age children are also gaining more critical-thinking skills and can take a more active role as a consumer of digital media. Schools may also introduce and/or integrate the use of tablets or computers as a learning tool. The same principles of high-quality educational content and setting limits on the duration of time spent each day using screen media apply to school-age children to provide optimal time for other developmental activities that support problem solving, social competence, and emotion regulation.

Apps can be a good learning tool when there is a specific educational goal; however, most are not reviewed by a developmental psychologist or educational specialist despite claiming educational benefits. Most target rote skills such as ABCs or memorization and do not challenge children to flexibly problem solve, which tends to occur in the context of peer and adult relationships (Hirsh-Pasek et al., 2015). There is evidence to support some improvements with language development when using high-quality language apps. Among children 5 to 7 years old, carefully designed apps have demonstrated promise in improving vocabulary and literacy skills (Chiong & Shuler, 2010). When electronic books are developed with limited distractions there is evidence they support literacy in kindergarteners (Korat & Shamir, 2008). There is also similar evidence suggesting that targeted mathematics practice on apps may support development of these concepts. One content analysis of mathematics apps found that many focused on number place and value (including addition and subtraction), units of measurement, and fractions and decimals (Larkin, 2013). In one study using an app that promoted learning about physical science kindergarteners performed better manipulating physical science concepts on the app when they had a greater understanding of the same physical science concepts in real life, compared to children who did not have an understanding of these physical science concepts (Zacharia, Loizou, & Papaevripidou, 2012). Therefore for young school-age children, apps may be best used when children have a baseline idea of these concepts in the real world, and again when learning goals are clearly defined.

Because children have a greater level of autonomy during the school-age years compared with the preschool years, they are more able to deftly access different types of content and engage with screens in ways that a preschooler would not be able to, and operate a mobile device in a more independent way. Though they may be able to search YouTube on their own, find and download apps on their own, their understanding of privacy and online safety may still be quite limited (Zhao et al., 2019). Additionally, managing online privacy is increasingly challenging given how much information and data are collected on each individual, and children in particular do not understand the risks of having their data collected. In one focus group study with children, average age 8.5 years, most were unaware of the implicit data collection but did care about who might access this sensitive information (Zhao et al., 2019). However, talking about online privacy together with a parent may help children understand the risks and challenges with online safety. One study tested an electronic book app, which provided tips and tricks for children aged 7 to 9 years to optimize privacy and safety online, which was met with favorable feedback from both children and parents (Zhang-Kennedy & Chiasson, 2016).

Relevance for Parents/Clinicians During School Age

Because children at this age are naturally curious, logical, and rules based, parents and clinicians can leverage these skills developmentally to introduce them to more reflective, critical thinking around digital media. The same guidelines for school-age children apply when choosing high-quality educational content and coviewing; however, now children have greater reflective capacities that parents and teachers can leverage to promote digital citizenship and online safety. Similarly, in the office visit, it can help to ask children what their favorite games or shows to watch are, asking them what they like about that particular programming, asking them who created the particular content, why they think the content was created, and what enables them to create such content (e.g., discussing consumerism and identifying ads together) (Reid Chassiakos et al., 2016). Duration and time limits around digital media continue to be important at this age so that children can engage in developmentally enriching activities outside of digital media, including ensuring children have time for 1 hour per day of physical activity, adequate sleep, and avoiding screen media at least 1 hour before bed.

In asking Matthew about the toy reviews in Ryan's World he reveals he did not realize they were often hidden advertisements promoting certain toys or foods. In asking about other online safety behaviors he denies ever having contacted an individual online that he has not met in-person. He has used apps from PBS Kids in the past, and he liked them. You also ask him about other hobbies and interests, and he reveals that he loves playing soccer, reading books such as Wayside School, and learning about animals.

A clinician might use this as an opportunity to positively reinforce Matthew's reading habits and interest in animals and sports. A clinician can also positively reinforce family's support of these positive and screen-free developmental activities. This may also provide an opportunity to search commonsensemedia.org for shows about animals—and mention that the website has several ideas, tools, and information about digital citizenship.

Adolescence

Teenagers are developing their sense of independence and self apart from their parents, with robust peer interactions; they may also engage in risk-taking behaviors, which translate to the online environment. The online environment includes social media, peer influences, and more ways to interact and engage with others. Parents continue to play an important role in helping their adolescents navigate digital media. Social media use patterns and rates have grown substantially over the last decade, and in 2018 a Pew Research Center survey found that 97% of 13- to 17-year-olds use a social media platform such as Facebook, Instagram, Snapchat, or YouTube, and 45% report being online "almost constantly."

Social media has both benefits and drawbacks for teenagers—with more complicated associations with their wellbeing. Social media might allow for connection to peers and may enable adolescents who identify with a certain group (e.g., LGBTQ, adolescents experiencing a chronic illness) to find support with others who are going through similar circumstances. However, there are downsides to excessive use of social media, with a possible dose-response effect with the quantity of social media consumed. For instance, in 2017 a survey-based study of about 120,000 15-year-olds in the United Kingdom who completed a media diary found a U-shaped relationship, or Goldilocks effect, between the quantity of social media consumed and mental health. Those who had no to very limited social media use or excessive social media use showed worse mental health outcomes than those who had a "sweet spot" of screen media use for watching television, playing videogames, using the computer, and using smartphones. For each of these categories, the sweet spot varied as did the weekday versus weekend use. For instance, they found that for smartphone use, 1 hour and 57 minutes of use per day was the inflection point before wellbeing started to decline; on weekends, smartphone use increased to 4 hours and 17 minutes before adolescent wellbeing started to decline (Przybylski & Weinstein, 2017). The authors also surmised that how adolescents are using digital media and content is likely associated with psychological wellbeing, though this was not captured in their study. Another study elucidated adolescents' affective states and wellbeing in a survey and additional qualitative interviews with teenagers. Researchers found, in general, a majority of participants report feeling happy and amused; however, when engaging in the qualitative interview, they found affective responses to be more complicated. For instance, teenagers noted they used digital media for the opportunity of self-expression and found both affirmation and concern regarding the judgment of others. When teens were browsing content, they reported feelings of admiration, envy, entertainment, and boredom. Regarding peer connections online, teens identified sentiments of closeness and connection in addition to isolation and disconnection. Such work points to the complex nature of digital media, and individual responses and affective states can vary even widely between and within individuals (Weinstein, 2018).

Relevance for Parents/Clinicians During the Adolescent Years

Screen media often provides an opportunity to connect and relate to peers in the teenage years, and some engagement with social and screen media confer benefits to mental health. However, after a certain inflection point, such benefits may decline. Recommendations for parents of teenagers might include placing consistent limits on hours per day of digital media (including locations and type of media used). Parental involvement in monitoring social media accounts may be helpful. Clinicians may also wish to recommend ongoing conversations about online citizenship (including cyberbullying), and avoiding use of screen media that is unrelated to schoolwork, during homework, to minimize distractions (Reid Chassiakos et al., 2016). Lastly, promotion of other positive developmental activities such as in-person social activities, physical activity through organized sports, and clubs/groups, which promote each adolescent's unique interests and offer a sense of belonging, are important.

DISPARITIES AND ACCESS

Digital media use occurs in the context of other psychosocial factors and structures. There are disparities and discrepancies in how children are able to access digital content, which were highlighted during the COVID-19 pandemic. Black, Latinx, and rural communities are among those at greatest risk of having limited or no Internet access (Katz, Gonzalez, & Clark, 2017). In 2017 over half of parents reported that their Internet connectivity was insufficient to access information or complete work (Katz et al., 2017). A survey from May 2020 found that 12% to 34% of students in the country did not have any access to the Internet. When families lack the access to the technology they need, they are also lacking access to opportunities that can support their children's learning and wellbeing. Understanding these barriers and addressing the structural forces that contribute are critical to promoting children's development equitably.

PRACTICAL APPLICATIONS

Digital media has the potential to confer many developmental benefits when used in concert with supportive caregivers and when choosing high-quality content. However, excessive digital media use may pose challenges with physical health and wellbeing. Basic principles to optimize children's engagement with digital media include (1) choose high-quality educational content (two resources might include the commonsensemeda.org website and PBS Kids); (2) use digital media to connect with others (e.g., FaceTime, social media in the adolescent years), engaging together (coviewing); (3) make sure there are opportunities to engage in other important unplugged, in-person developmental activities (e.g., physical activity); (4) help children reflect on what they are viewing, who might be creating the content and why, and what data or information might be collected from the user; and (5) discuss online safety. Additionally, digital media should be designed to consider children's cognitive needs and development. Partnering with individuals with expertise in children's development may facilitate design choices that support development. Furthermore, regulations, which promote children's privacy standards online and appropriate enforcement of such regulations, are important in protecting young children from unknowingly having their data collected.

Resources

For those interested in reading and learning more about digital media and children's development, other notable resources include the AAP guidelines on digital media in young children (Radesky & Christakis, 2016) and the AAP Family Media plan (https://www.healthychildren.org/English/media/Pages/default.aspx).

REFERENCES

Alruwaily, A., Mangold, C., Greene, T., Arshonsky, J., Cassidy, O., Pomeranz, J. L., & Bragg, M. (2020). Child social media influencers and unhealthy food product placement. *Journal of Pediatrics*, *146*(5), e20194057. https://doi.org/10.1542/peds.2019-4057%

Arora, T., Broglia, E., Thomas, G. N., & Taheri, S. (2014). Associations between specific technologies and adolescent sleep quantity, sleep quality, and parasomnias. *Sleep Medicine*, *15*(2), 240–247. https://doi.org/10.1016/j.sleep.2013.08.799

Barr, R. (2010). Transfer of learning between 2D and 3D sources during infancy: Informing theory and practice. *Developmental Review*, *30*(2), 128–154.

Chiong, C., & Shuler, C. (2010). *Learning: Is there an app for that. Paper presented at the Investigations of young children's usage and learning with mobile devices and apps*. The Joan Ganz Cooney Center at Sesame Workshop.

Christakis, D. A., Garrison, M. M., Herrenkohl, T., Haggerty, K., Rivara, F. P., Zhou, C., & Liekweg, K. (2013). Modifying media content for preschool children: A randomized controlled trial. *Pediatrics*, *131*(3), 431–438.

Garrison, M. M., & Christakis, D. A. (2012). The impact of a healthy media use intervention on sleep in preschool children. *Pediatrics*, *130*(3), 492–499. https://doi.org/10.1542/peds.2011-3153

Hancox, R. J., Milne, B. J., & Poulton, R. (2004). Association between child and adolescent television viewing and adult health: A longitudinal birth cohort study. *Lancet*, *364*(9430), 257–262. https://doi.org/10.1016/s0140-6736(04)16675-0

Haughton, C., Aiken, M., & Cheevers, C. (2015). Cyber babies: The impact of emerging technology on the developing infant. *Psychology Research*, *5*(9), 504–518.

Hirsh-Pasek, K., Zosh, J. M., Golinkoff, R. M., Gray, J. H., Robb, M. B., & Kaufman, J. (2015). Putting education in "educational" apps: Lessons from the science of learning. *Psychological Science in the Public Interest*, *16*(1), 3–34.

Huber, B., Yeates, M., Meyer, D., Fleckhammer, L., & Kaufman, J. (2018). The effects of screen media content on young children's executive functioning. *Journal of Experimental Child Psychology*, *170*, 72–85. https://doi.org/10.1016/j.jecp.2018.01.006

Katz, V. S., Gonzalez, C., & Clark, K. (2017). Digital inequality and developmental trajectories of low-income, immigrant, and minority children. *Pediatrics*, *140*(2), S132–S136.

Kirkorian, H. L., Pempek, T. A., Murphy, L. A., Schmidt, M. E., & Anderson, D. R. (2009). The impact of background television on parent–child interaction. *Child Development*, *80*(5), 1350–1359.

Korat, O., & Shamir, A. (2008). The educational electronic book as a tool for supporting children's emergent literacy in low versus middle SES groups. *Computers Education and Information Technologies*, *50*(1), 110–124.

Krcmar, M. (2010). Can social meaningfulness and repeat exposure help infants and toddlers overcome the video deficit? *Media Psychology*, *13*(1), 31–53. https://doi.org/10.1080/15213260903562917

Larkin, K. (2013). Mathematics education: Is there an app for that? Paper presented at the Annual Meeting of the *Mathematics Education Research Group of Australasia* (MERGA).

LeBourgeois, M. K., Hale, L., Chang, A. -M., Akacem, L. D., Montgomery-Downs, H. E., & Buxton, O. M. (2017). Digital media and sleep in childhood and adolescence. *Pediatrics*, *140*(2), S92–S96.

Linebarger, D. L., & Walker, D. (2005). Infants' and toddlers' television viewing and language outcomes. *American Behavioral Scientist*, *48*(5), 624–645.

Lumeng, J. C., Rahnama, S., Appugliese, D., Kaciroti, N., & Bradley, R. H. (2006). Television exposure and overweight risk in preschoolers. *Archives of Pediatrics Adolescent Medicine*, *160*(4), 417–422.

Madigan, S., Racine, N., & Tough, S. (2020). Prevalence of preschoolers meeting vs exceeding screen time guidelines. *JAMA Pediatrics*, *174*(1), 93–95. https://doi.org/10.1001/jamapediatrics.2019.4495%

McDaniel, B. T., & Radesky, J. S. (2020). Longitudinal associations between early childhood externalizing behavior, parenting stress, and child media use. *Cyberpsychology, Behavior, Social Networking*, *23*(6), 384–391. doi:10.1089/cyber.2019.0478. Epub 2020 Feb 25.

Moreno, M. A., Binger, K. S., Zhao, Q., & Eickhoff, J. C. (2021). Effect of a family media use plan on media rule engagement among adolescents: A randomized clinical trial. *JAMA Pediatrics*. https://doi.org/10.1001/jamapediatrics.2020.5629%

Munzer, T. G., Miller, A. L., Weeks, H. M., Kaciroti, N., & Radesky, J. (2019). Parent-toddler social reciprocity during reading from electronic tablets vs print books. *JAMA Pediatrics*, *173*(11), 1076–1083.

Przybylski, A. K., & Weinstein, N. (2017). A large-scale test of the goldilocks hypothesis: Quantifying the relations between digital-screen use and the mental well-being of adolescents. *Psychological Science*, *28*(2), 204–215.

Radesky, J., & Christakis, D. (2016). Media and young minds. *Pediatrics*. https://doi.org/10.1542/peds.2016-2591

Radesky, J. S., Silverstein, M., Zuckerman, B., & Christakis, D. A. (2014). Infant self-regulation and early childhood media exposure. *Pediatrics*, *133*(5), e1172–e1178.

Radesky, J. S., Weeks, H. M., Ball, R., Schaller, A., Yeo, S., Durnez, J., ... Barr, R. (2020). Young children's use of smartphones and tablets. *Pediatrics*, *146*(1), e20193518. https://doi.org/10.1542/peds.2019-3518

Rasmussen, E. E., Shafer, A., Colwell, M. J., White, S., Punyanunt-Carter, N., Densley, R. L., & Wright, H. (2016). Relation between active mediation, exposure to Daniel Tiger's Neighborhood, and US preschoolers' social and emotional development. *Journal of Children and Media Psychology*, *10*(4), 443–461.

Reid Chassiakos, Y., Radesky, J., Christakis, D., Moreno, M. A., & Cross, C. (2016). Children and adolescents and digital media. *Journal of Pediatrics*, *138*(5), e20162593. https://doi.org/10.1542/peds.2016-2593%

Rideout, V., & Robb, M. B. (2019). *The Common Sense Census: Media use by tweens and teens*. Common Sense Media.

Rideout, V., & Robb, M. B. (2020). *The Common Sense Census: Media use by kids age zero to eight*. Common Sense Media.

Robinson, T. N., Banda, J. A., Hale, L., Lu, A. S., Fleming-Milici, F., Calvert, S. L., & Wartella, E. (2017). Screen media exposure and obesity in children and adolescents. *Pediatrics*, *140*(2), S97–S101. https://doi.org/10.1542/peds.2016-1758K

Valkenburg, P. M., Krcmar, M., Peeters, A. L., & Marseille, N. M. (1999). Developing a scale to assess three styles of television mediation: "Instructive mediation," "restrictive mediation," and "social coviewing". *Journal of Broadcasting Electronic Media*, *43*(1), 52–66.

Viner, R., & Cole, T. (2005). Television viewing in early childhood predicts adult body mass index. *Journal of Pediatrics*, *147*(4), 429–435. https://doi.org/10.1016/j.jpeds.2005.05.005

Weinstein, E. (2018). The social media see-saw: Positive and negative influences on adolescents' affective well-being. *New Media Society*, *20*(10), 3597–3623.

Zacharia, Z. C., Loizou, E., & Papaevripidou, M. (2012). Is physicality an important aspect of learning through science experimentation among kindergarten students? *Early Childhood Research Quarterly*, *27*(3), 447–457.

Zack, E., Barr, R., Gerhardstein, P., Dickerson, K., & Meltzoff, A. N. (2009). Infant imitation from television using novel touch screen technology. *The British Journal of Developmental Psychology*, *27*(Pt 1), 13–26. https://doi.org/10.1348/026151008x334700

Zhang-Kennedy, L., & Chiasson, S. (2016). *Teaching with an interactive e-book to improve children's online privacy knowledge.* Paper presented at the Proceedings of the the 15th International Conference on Interaction Design and Children.

Zhao, J., Wang, G., Dally, C., Slovak, P., Edbrooke-Childs, J., Van Kleek, M., & Shadbolt, N. (2019). *'I make up a silly name' Understanding Children's Perception of Privacy Risks Online.* Paper presented at the Proceedings of the 2019 CHI Conference on Human Factors in Computing Systems.

22

Natural and Human Disasters

David J. Schonfeld and Thomas P. Demaria

For additional material related to the content of this chapter, please see Chapters 15.

VIGNETTE

Bridgett, a 9-year-old girl with high-functioning autism spectrum disorder, presents with sleep difficulties and separation protests upon returning home after a 5-day evacuation caused by a wildfire. On the first night of evacuation, she stayed at a relative's home about 30 minutes away while her parents tried to protect the home from the approaching wildfire; during that time, she was very anxious about the safety of her parents and cried and asked to be with them. Her parents rejoined her the next day, and they shared a bedroom in the relative's home. Since returning home Bridgett has refused to sleep alone in her bedroom, crawls into her parents' bed when she awakens in the middle of the night alone, and gets upset if a parent leaves during the day without her. The parents reported that Bridgett watched news coverage about homes in their community being destroyed by the fire while at the relative's home; they did not allow her to watch any media coverage once they were in their own home, and they avoided any discussion about the fire so as not to upset her. When talking alone with the child, the pediatrician learned that the girl was having dreams about the fire and remained worried that the fire would return; she was not aware that the fire had been fully contained. She felt guilty that the school was damaged as were homes of her classmates, while her home was not damaged. The pediatrician provided advice to the parents about how to talk to and support the girl and manage her sleep problems; the parents gradually increased expectations for independence until her problems resolved within a couple weeks.

THE IMPACT OF DISASTERS ON CHILDREN

Children may experience both short- and long-term effects of disasters on their developmental trajectory, behavior, emotional adjustment, academic learning, psychosocial functioning, and physical health (Chrisman & Dougherty, 2014; Maclean et al., 2016). Children with intellectual, neurodevelopmental, physical, and socioemotional disabilities, such as Bridgett in the opening vignette, are often uniquely vulnerable to these impacts and require additional support and accommodations to promote adaptation and recovery.

Natural Versus Manmade Disasters

A disaster is a natural or manmade catastrophe that may result in temporary or ongoing disruptions in community services; exposure to life-threatening events and deaths of family members and friends; insecurity about basic human needs such as food, water, and housing; and disruptions in families and communities that may be too overwhelming for children and their families to cope with in the absence of external support (Becker-Blease et al., 2010). Natural disasters include severe weather or other environmental events (e.g., hurricanes causing flooding, wildfires, or pandemics); manmade disasters (e.g., terrorism or chemical spills) result from intentional or unintentional human actions. Distinguishing between natural and manmade disasters may be complex, as natural disasters often involve an element of human error, malfeasance, or neglect, which contributes to the occurrence and/or impact of the environmental hazard. In general, disasters that are felt to be intentional or otherwise avoidable may result in more emotional reactions. This chapter will not include discussion of terrorism or school/community shootings or violence, although many of the same considerations may apply in those contexts as well.

In a representative sample of US children aged 2 to 17 years 13.9% reported lifetime exposure to disaster, and 4.1% reported experiencing a disaster in the past year (Becker-Blease et al., 2010). The number of children affected by natural disasters is only expected to rise as climate change continues. Large-scale disasters, such as the recent COVID-19 pandemic, have the potential to impact virtually all children.

Major disasters typically generate extensive media coverage. Indirect exposure to disasters through content from television, radio, print, and online or social media may create additional exposures to frightening images and news that worsen adjustment difficulties for those with direct involvement. This, too, causes distress and adjustment difficulties even for those children with no direct exposure (Bernstein & Pfefferbaum, 2018).

The Vulnerability of Children, Especially Those With Disabilities

Children are especially vulnerable to disasters because of their limited coping skills and dependence on social supports, which place them at a greater risk for a range of adjustment difficulties, including bereavement, transitory symptoms of distress and posttraumatic stress (PTS), and symptoms of anxiety and depression (Grolnick et al., 2018). Especially at risk are children who have disabilities, are dependent on others for their functioning, rely on medical technology, and/or live in poverty (Dziuban et al., 2017). Disasters can also undermine the systems of safety that are in place to protect children, leaving them more vulnerable to interpersonal violence, physical and sexual abuse, and opportunistic crimes, and place children with a wide range of disabilities at even greater risk (Boon et al., 2011; Pfefferbaum et al., 2013).

ADJUSTMENT REACTIONS OF CHILDREN FOLLOWING DISASTERS

Children may demonstrate a wide range of adjustment reactions after a disaster, as outlined in Tables 22.1 and 22.2, which include both internalizing and externalizing problems as well as somatic reactions (Pfefferbaum et al., 2013). Caregiver and/or teacher feedback is helpful for identifying externalizing symptoms, whereas asking children directly about their feelings appears to be the best way to assess internalizing symptoms following a disaster (Self-Brown et al., 2017). Many children, though, may actively hide or fail to show their distress, leading parents and other adults to underestimate the negative impacts on children.

Most children who are exposed to a traumatic event will experience transitory posttraumatic stress (PTS) or an acute stress disorder without necessarily developing posttraumatic stress disorder (PTSD). PTS typically decreases substantially within the first year, with symptoms no longer of concern in most situations within 2 years after a disaster (Terasaka et al., 2015).

TABLE 22.1 Common Symptoms of Adjustment Reactions in Children After a Disaster

- Sleep problems: difficulty falling or staying asleep, frequent night awakenings or difficulty awakening in the morning, nightmares, or other sleep disruptions
- Eating problems: loss of appetite or increased eating
- Sadness or depression: may result in a reluctance to engage in previously enjoyed activities or a withdrawal from peers and adults
- Anxiety, worries, or fears: children may be concerned about a repetition of the traumatic event (e.g., become afraid during storms after surviving a tornado) or show an increase in unrelated fears (e.g., become more fearful of the dark even if the disaster occurred during daylight); this may present as separation anxiety or school avoidance
- Difficulties in concentration: disruption in the ability to learn and retain new information or to otherwise progress academically
- Substance abuse: the new onset or exacerbation of alcohol, tobacco, or other substance use may be seen in children, adolescents, and adults after a disaster
- Risk-taking behavior: increased sexual behavior or other reactive risk-taking can occur, especially among older children and adolescents
- Somatization: children with adjustment difficulties may present instead with physical symptoms suggesting a physical condition
- Developmental or social regression: children (and adults) may become less patient or tolerant of change, revert to bedwetting, or become irritable and disruptive
- Posttraumatic reactions and disorders: see Table 22.2

From Schonfeld, D. J., & Gurwitch, R. H. (2012). Children in disasters. In A. Y. Elzouki, F. B. Stapleton, R. J. Whitley, W. Oh, H. A. Harfi, & H. Nazer (Eds.), *Textbook of clinical pediatrics* (2nd ed., pp. 687–698). Springer-Verlag.

TABLE 22.2 Symptoms of Posttraumatic Stress Disorder

Exposure: The child is exposed to actual or threatened death, serious injury, or sexual violence. This may be through the child's direct experience; by witnessing the traumatic event, especially when involving a caretaker; or by the child learning that the traumatic event occurred involving a close family member or friend without any direct experience or witnessing of the event by the child. The following symptoms must occur for >1 mo:

Intrusion
- The child has repeated distressing memories and/or dreams (nightmares) about the traumatic event; it is not required for children to remember the content of these distressing dreams. For some children, repetitive play activities may involve themes or aspects of the traumatic event.
- The child may display a loss of awareness of present surroundings (dissociation) and act as if the traumatic event is reoccurring (flashbacks).
- The child may experience intense or prolonged psychological distress and/or physiologic reactions at exposure to internal or external cues that symbolize or resemble the traumatic event.

Avoidance
- The child attempts to avoid distressing memories, thoughts, feelings, activities, and/or places that are reminders of the traumatic event.

Negative Alterations in Cognitions and Mood
- The child has problems remembering important aspects of the traumatic event.
- The child maintains negative beliefs or expectations about oneself, others, or the world.
- The child has thoughts about the cause or consequences of the traumatic event that lead to blame of self/others.
- The child experiences negative emotional states, such as depression, and has trouble experiencing and expressing positive emotions.
- The child shows a markedly diminished interest or participation in significant activities, including play.
- The child feels distant from others, which may lead the child to become socially withdrawn and avoid people, conversations, or interpersonal situations.

Increased Arousal and Reactivity Associated With the Traumatic Event
- Irritable and angry outbursts (extreme temper tantrums)
- Reckless or self-destructive behavior
- Hypervigilance
- Exaggerated startle response
- Problems with concentration

From Schonfeld, D. J., & Gurwitch, R. H. (2012). Children in disasters. In A. Y. Elzouki, F. B. Stapleton, R. J. Whitley, W. Oh, H. A. Harfi, & H. Nazer (Eds.), *Textbook of clinical pediatrics* (2nd ed., pp. 687–698). Springer-Verlag.

An understanding of these adjustment reactions can help identify children most in need of additional support and/or mental health services, both in the short term and over time. Mental health triage in the immediate aftermath of the disaster should focus on reactions most likely to indicate an urgent need for mental health services, as outlined in Table 22.3.

Knowledge of common adjustment reactions can also inform anticipatory guidance and guide supportive interventions provided to caregivers, educators, and other caring adults in the aftermath of a disaster. For example, sleep difficulties are very common in the aftermath of a disaster and can lead to problems with attention, concentration, academic functioning, and emotional adjustment. Advice to caregivers on how to promote sleep hygiene may be challenging in the immediate aftermath of a disaster, especially when families are living in shelters or other temporary locations, but is important to promoting adjustment (Schonfeld et al., 2015).

Risk Factors for Adjustment Difficulties

Preexisting factors, the nature of the disaster experience, and subsequent factors, as outlined in Table 22.4, determine in part how children adjust to the additional stressors resulting from a disaster. A prior history of mental health (e.g., depression or anxiety) and/or substance abuse problems, history of prior or concurrent losses or traumatic experiences, and limited coping skills render children more vulnerable. In addition, contextual factors increase children's vulnerability, including whether their family lives in a hazardous location, has limited financial resources, and/or endures discrimination because of their minority group status (Ronoh et al., 2015). Social support, especially that provided by the child's family, has been consistently identified as the main protective factor (Lai et al., 2017). A rapid return to a safe, predictable, and comfortable routine within the child's daily environment and overall community lessons the stress on children and accelerates the recovery process.

TABLE 22.4 Factors Associated With an Increased Risk of Adjustment Problems After a Disaster

- Previous psychopathology, significant losses, attachment disturbances, limited coping skills, or other traumatic events
- Socioeconomic differences that result in lower levels of postdisaster resources and support

Nature of Disaster Experience

- Injury of the child or death or injury of those close to the child
- Nature and extent of exposure, including number of deaths, physical proximity to disaster, and extent of personal loss. Humanmade disasters, especially terrorist attacks that have a high degree of intentionality, generally create reactions that are more prevalent and long-lasting
- Extent of exposure to horrific scenes (including indirectly through the media)
- Child's perception (at the time of the event) that one's life was in jeopardy

Subsequent Factors

- Personal identification with the disaster or victims
- Separation of child from parents or other important caregivers as result of event
- Loss of property or belongings; need to relocate or other disruption in daily routine or environment
- Parental difficulty in coping, substance abuse, mental illness
- Lack of supportive family communication style
- Lack of community resources and support

From Schonfeld, D. J., & Gurwitch, R. H. (2012). Children in disasters. In A. Y. Elzouki, F. B. Stapleton, R. J. Whitley, W. Oh, H. A. Harfi, & H. Nazer (Eds.), *Textbook of clinical pediatrics* (2nd ed., pp. 687–698). Springer-Verlag.

TABLE 22.3 Adjustment Reactions Indicating the Need for Urgent Mental Health Services in Immediate Aftermath of a Disaster

- Dissociative symptoms, such as detachment, derealization, or depersonalization, which may present in children as appearing confused, distant, daydreaming, or distant. Dissociation at the time of exposure has been found to be the most significant predictor of later posttraumatic stress disorder
- Extreme confusion or inability to concentrate or make even simple decisions
- Evidence of extreme cognitive impairment or intrusive thoughts
- Intense fear, anxiety, panic, helplessness, or horror
- Depression at the time of the event (Lai et al., 2013)
- Uncontrollable and intense grief
- Suicidal ideation or intent
- Marked physical complaints resulting from somatization

Adapted from Schonfeld, D., & Demaria, T. (2020). Supporting children and families in the aftermath of disasters. In C. J. Goodhue & N. Blake (Eds.), *Nursing management of pediatric disaster* (pp. 289–300). Springer Nature.

Children with intellectual, neurodevelopmental, or language disabilities who cannot readily communicate their distress verbally may instead express their feelings in nonverbal ways. They may show a range of behaviors, including a reappearance of challenging and disruptive behaviors that they demonstrated in the past or greater intensity in current behaviors. They may have more difficulty regulating their emotions, demonstrate regressive behaviors, or begin or increase self-stimulating behaviors.

BEREAVEMENT IN CHILDREN

Children who experience the death of a close family member or friend as a result of a disaster are more likely to have prolonged PTS symptoms (King et al., 2015) and to develop later emotional difficulties (Pfefferbaum et al., 2013). Even outside the context of a disaster, bereavement can have both immediate and long-lasting impacts on children's emotional adjustment, psychological functioning, academic achievement, developmental trajectory, and social and behavioral adaptation.

Children's Conceptual Understanding of Death

For children to cope with the death of someone close, they first need to understand what it means when someone dies. Research has shown that there are four major concepts about death: irreversibility, finality (nonfunctionality), causality, and universality (inevitability) (Speece & Brent, 1984). These concepts, and the implications of an incomplete understanding of each one, are outlined in Table 22.5. On average, children acquire an understanding of these concepts at a developmental age between 5 and 7 years. Children who have experienced a personal loss may develop a substantial understanding of these concepts at a much younger age; education has also been shown to advance conceptual understanding (Schonfeld & Kappelman, 1990).

TABLE 22.5 Concepts of Death and Implications of Incomplete Understanding for Adjustment to Loss

Irreversibility: death is a permanent phenomenon from which there is no recovery or return

- Example of incomplete understanding: the child expects the deceased to return, as if from a trip
- Implication of incomplete understanding: failure to comprehend this concept prevents the child from detaching personal ties to the deceased, a necessary first step in successful mourning

Finality (nonfunctionality): death is a state in which all life functions cease completely

- Example of incomplete understanding: the child worries about a buried relative being cold or in pain; the child wishes to bury food with the deceased
- Implication of incomplete understanding: may lead to preoccupation with physical suffering of the deceased and impair readjustment

Inevitability (universality): death is a natural phenomenon that no living being can escape indefinitely

- Example of incomplete understanding: the child views significant individuals (i.e., self, parents) as immortal
- Implication of incomplete understanding: if not viewing death as inevitable, the child is likely to view death as punishment (either for actions or thoughts of the deceased or the child), leading to excessive guilt and shame

Causality: the child develops a realistic understanding of the causes of death

- Example of incomplete understanding: the child who relies on magical thinking is apt to assume responsibility for the death of a loved one by assuming that bad thoughts or unrelated actions were causative
- Implication of incomplete understanding: tends to lead to excessive guilt that is difficult for the child to resolve

Reprinted from Schonfeld, D. (1989). Crisis intervention for bereavement support: A model of intervention in the children's school. *Clinical Pediatrics (Philadelphia), 28*(1), 29.

Conceptual understanding of death should be viewed as a necessary precondition for coping, but not sufficient in and of itself. Older children, and even adults, may comprehend these concepts but find it difficult to accept the reality after a personal loss. They may imagine that they see later someone who has died in a crowd even though they understand irreversibility; they may find themselves at times talking to someone who has died even when they know that all life functions cease upon death. They likely will question the cause of death, although they understand the real cause. They may voice surprise that someone close to them has died despite understanding the universality of death (Schonfeld & Demaria, 2020a).

Literal misinterpretations and misconceptions about death may limit children's understanding of death and complicate children's grief. Children who are invited to draw a picture to be placed in the casket of a deceased family member may assume that the person who has died still can see the picture and is conscious of being buried. Magical thinking may cause grieving children to feel more personal responsibility for a death, assuming that their unrelated actions or negative thoughts and feelings were responsible for the death (Schonfeld & Demaria, 2020a). It is therefore helpful to inquire about children's understanding of the concepts of death, as well as their personal worries or fears, after the death of someone close to them, especially for children with intellectual or neurodevelopmental disabilities.

Practical guidance on how to approach death notification in the context of a disaster is available through the American Academy of Pediatrics (Chung et al., 2019). Free online video-based and print resources addressing a wide range of topics on how to support grieving children can be found at the Coalition to Support Grieving Students (www.grievingstudents.org) (see Chapter 11).

GUILT

Guilt is commonly experienced after the death of someone close and can be seen after disasters unassociated with deaths. Children may wonder what they did or failed to do that caused or contributed to a disaster, even when there is no objective reason for such feelings. At some level, children (and indeed adults) may find that feeling in some way responsible for a disaster provides some initial relief because it may provide the illusion of control. If the child believes there is something the child did to cause or contribute to a death or disaster, then it follows there is something the child can do to decrease the risk or recurrence. Appreciating instead that they may have no responsibility and therefore likely have little control over future disasters or death may at some level be harder to accept. But the illusion of control does not provide any real protection, and the resulting guilt complicates adjustment. It is important to inquire about guilt and to provide reassurance to children of lack of responsibility even when guilt has not been identified and there is no logical reason to be present.

SECONDARY AND CUMULATIVE LOSSES AND STRESSORS

Ongoing stress, multiple losses, and frequent reminders of the disaster can lead to thoughts of helplessness and hopelessness (Bonanno et al., 2010), which can intensify endorsement of beliefs about personal blame and foster depression. How children view their world and their future often changes following a disaster; disasters may increase children's sense of personal vulnerability.

Disasters often exacerbate preexisting stressors such as financial pressure faced by the family, parental depression, or parenting challenges (Scaramella et al., 2008). The secondary stressors and losses experienced by children in the aftermath of a disaster not only prolong posttraumatic reactions but may become the primary cause of ongoing adjustment reactions. For example, if a caregiver becomes unemployed or underemployed because of damage from a wildfire, which results in financial stress among adults in the family and in turn contributes to marital discord or worsening of substance use or mental illness of the caregiver, the adjustment difficulties may be due to these parental reactions or a concern that a caregiver may leave. It should not be assumed that all ongoing reactions to a disaster are due to the trauma of the disaster itself (e.g., in this case the wildfire), nor that trauma treatment will be effective for these issues. Because of the many stressors and losses faced by children and families in the aftermath of a disaster, the need to adopt a more holistic approach to assessing adjustment and promoting coping and resiliency among children and families after a disaster is recommended. This requires an assessment of current life circumstances and functioning and not focusing solely on potential reactions to the cause of the disaster itself (Schonfeld & Demaria, 2015).

In the context of large-scale disasters resulting in displacement of populations migrant and refugee children often must contend with extensive secondary and cumulative losses and stressors after the death of a caregiver which, by themselves, can be overwhelming and threaten the safety, health, and overall wellbeing of children. Family and community members may be missing and presumed dead; families may not have been able to bury the deceased or follow other cultural practices and traditions associated with mourning. These secondary losses and stressors can complicate or prolong the grieving process. Initial efforts should focus on meeting the basic needs of families such as for food, shelter, and safety; reunification with family and establishing communication with extended family or community members; and ensuring all children have a trusted, consistent, and nurturing caregiver. It is critical that children are kept safe from additional harm and not placed in settings that may increase the risk of physical or sexual abuse and neglect (Schonfeld, 2021).

TRAUMA AND GRIEF TRIGGERS AND ANNIVERSARY REACTIONS

In the aftermath of a disaster distressing memories and feelings may resurface from prior crises and losses, whether they be related to the current disaster or even completely unrelated. For example, memories of a wildfire 3 years ago may heighten anxiety in children as they evacuate their home again amid concerns of flooding from an approaching hurricane. Children may acutely miss a parent who died of cancer 5 years prior as they struggle to adjust to destruction of their home by a tornado.

After a disaster, children may see a temporary increase in posttraumatic reactions from subsequent reminders of the disaster. An impending storm, or even very windy weather, may serve as a trauma trigger and resurface or worsen anxiety in children who once experienced a tornado or hurricane. Grief triggers involve reminders of the person who died that cause an unanticipated but generally brief resurgence of some of the feelings associated with the loss. Virtually anything that reminds children of the person that died may serve as a grief trigger: the smell of perfume worn by their mother, the sound of someone's voice like their brother's, the mention of a town where they vacationed with their grandmother, the favorite cookies of their brother, or simply a teacher asking students to have their parents sign a permission slip. As such, grief triggers are difficult to anticipate and hard to prevent. It is helpful to explain triggers to children and let them know they commonly occur and develop a safety plan for management when they occur in public settings such as a classroom. For example, educators can provide permission for students to temporarily leave a classroom to go sit in the library for a few minutes or talk with a school professional (e.g., school counselor, nurse, psychologist, or social worker) and identify a discreet way to communicate the need that doesn't draw attention to the student at a time of distress (e.g., the child may take a tissue from a box near the door to signal to the teacher he is experiencing a grief trigger before stepping out of the classroom). Children who know they can leave the room if they feel overwhelmed and avoid embarrassing themselves in front of peers by crying in public often find that the feelings of distress pass quickly. They are likely to have less of a need to leave knowing that they can and remain instead in the classroom and engaged with the classroom lesson (Schonfeld & Quackenbush, 2021).

Anniversaries of the disaster are often associated with media coverage, including video or sound clips and commentary that may serve as a trauma trigger. Schools and communities should incorporate the input of children and youth in commemorative and memorialization events and activities, which may be held shortly after the disaster and on anniversaries, and can help promote adjustment and recovery and counter feelings of helplessness (Schonfeld & Quackenbush, 2021).

EFFECTIVE COMMUNICATION WITH CHILDREN FOLLOWING DISASTERS

Children should be notified about a disaster that has, or may, impact them as information becomes available. Attempts to protect them from such information often result in confusion and additional distress, increase the chance children

TABLE 22.6 Practical Suggestions for How Clinicians Can Facilitate Communication and Provide Support to Children After a Disaster

For children undergoing medical evaluation or treatment:

- Minimize exposure to potentially traumatic content by drawing curtains or closing doors in sites delivering emergency medical care to shield children from suffering and distress of others; turn off televisions and radios in sites where care is being provided to children. Remind clinicians that children often overhear conversations among the health care team.
- Use alternatives to invasive or painful procedures and treatments; when required, provide adequate sedation or analgesia.
- Allow caregivers and other family members to remain with children. This may be particularly important for children with disabilities and other special needs as these caregivers may be uniquely aware of their children's medical needs and strategies that have, in the past, helped their children to cope with distress. Encourage caregivers to use calming techniques that have been helpful in the past when their children were distressed (e.g., attention refocusing techniques such as a calming touch or distraction).
- Time spent on understanding the child's psychological distress and implementing effective brief interventions may shorten the overall time for the encounter and expedite the delivery of appropriate emergency medical care. Psychological distress may present as signs and symptoms, such as tachycardia, tachypnea, confusion, or pain that mimic physical conditions or worsen symptoms caused by physical etiologies and complicate both evaluation and medical management.
- Provide information about testing and treatment procedures in simple and direct terms, avoiding jargon and unnecessary detail. Frame interventions in positive terms (e.g., "I am asking you to swallow this medicine, which will help you stay healthy" rather than "If you don't take this medicine right away, you may become very ill").

For all children:

- Ensure that children's (and families') basic needs are being met; refer to appropriate resources as indicated.
- Ask children what they already know about or have heard about the disaster. Look for misinformation, misunderstandings, and misconceptions, especially those that may cause or add to fears or concerns.
- Ask what questions, concerns, or worries they may have. Remember that children often have very different concerns than adults, sometimes based on their limited, incomplete, or incorrect information or understanding.
- While providing honest reassurance, do not attempt to minimize concerns expressed by children. Listen actively and empathically. Avoid telling children how they ought to feel (e.g., "Many children have told me that they are upset and scared. How are you feeling?" rather than stating, "You must be scared").
- Provide basic information in simple and direct terms. Avoid jargons and unnecessary details. There are two basic reasons for communication during disasters: to provide reassurance and to provide practical information about steps people can take to protect themselves and those they care about during the disaster. Aim to communicate information that falls into these two categories, both in discussions with children and families or when communicating to the general public. Advise families and children to limit their media exposure.
- Inquire about the personal experiences of children and their families, to identify risk factors for adjustment difficulties, and about how they are coping. If children are reluctant to share their concerns, explore with them who they might feel comfortable talking with and invite them to speak when they feel ready to do so.
- Suggest coping techniques that children may wish to use.
- Refer for behavioral health support as indicated.

will receive incomplete or inaccurate information that contributes to worries or concerns based on misunderstandings, and make it likely that they will ultimately find out from overhearing conversations or from less reliable and appropriate sources of information. Such withholding of information may undermine the trusting relationship children hold with key adults in their lives, such as parents/caregivers and educators, thereby impacting their sense of security during a crisis. If children sense that adults are unwilling or uncomfortable talking about such matters, or are not being honest and genuine in their discussion, they are less likely to share their concerns or seek support.

Table 22.6 offers are some practical suggestions for how clinicians, including those delivering medical care in the immediate aftermath of a disaster, can facilitate communication and provide support to children after a disaster (Schonfeld & Demaria, 2020b; Schonfeld et al., 2015).

SOCIAL SUPPORT FROM CAREGIVERS AND OTHER CARING ADULTS

Research has consistently demonstrated that social support is the main protective factor for children in the aftermath of disasters (Lai et al., 2017). Parents and other important caregivers and family members should remain with children to the extent possible as separation can heighten a child's distress (Pfefferbaum et al., 2017). This is especially important for children with disabilities and other special needs because of the unique role caregivers often play in supporting these children even outside the context of a disaster. Parental reactions, parenting styles, and family interactions can influence children's postdisaster functioning (Cobham et al., 2016). Parental and child mental health following a disaster are interrelated, with each family member influencing the emergence and continuance of symptoms in other family members, possibly due to the strain posed on communication pathways and conflict resolution skills (Bountress et al., 2020).

PSYCHOSOCIAL SUPPORT IN THE AFTERMATH OF A DISASTER

Promoting Effective Coping Strategies

Initially, children generally should be encouraged to naturally process their experiences and utilize their personal resources to cope with their feelings. Intervening clinically too soon after a disaster might be ineffective or even damaging, disrupting naturally occurring recovery processes by undermining self-efficacy or available community support (Wolmer et al., 2017). In addition, a primary focus on PTS reactions may not address the complexity and full breadth of emotional and behavioral responses that may emerge because of secondary stressors (Pfefferbaum et al., 2014a).

Children's culture and engagement with that culture should be considered. Families can be asked to share protective aspects of their culture following a disaster and can help inform the clinician about how best to support children (Hunt et al., 2018). This cultural sensitivity is important as a culture can shape a child's appraisal of what is stressful as well as the coping strategies that are used (Bernstein & Pfefferbaum, 2018). Children's unique personal, social, cultural, and religious backgrounds may also influence the way grief is expressed and how mourning rituals are conducted (Holte Kofod, 2017).

A range of interventions are appropriate for implementation in the weeks and months after a disaster. These include psychological first aid (PFA), family outreach, psychoeducation, social support, and anxiety-reduction techniques (Pfefferbaum et al., 2013).

Early Interventions—Psychological First Aid

Critical incident stress debriefing or management (CISD or CISM) strategies were initially developed for professional first responders (e.g., police and fire) but have at times been used with children after major crisis events. Psychological debriefing of this nature is usually administered soon after disaster exposure and involves telling people their reactions are "normal" and encouraging them to share details of the upsetting event and their feelings even if they are reluctant to do so, with the intention of helping them better understand the upsetting experience. CISD/CISM has not been shown to be effective and, in some studies, has been shown to be harmful. Compulsory debriefing of victims of trauma is discouraged (Chung et al., 2019); the American Academy of Child and Adolescent Psychiatry (AACAP) recommends it be used only with "caution" (Pfefferbaum et al., 2013).

An intervention called psychological first aid appears to be more promising and is currently considered best practice, although there is, to date, limited research demonstrating that PFA contributes more to adjustment than the passage of time and natural recovery (Grolnick et al., 2018). PFA involves offering psychoeducation and supportive services to foster effective and normative coping strategies and adjustment as well as to accelerate the natural healing process, and identifying family and community supports and resources as well as how to access them.

Psychoeducation for both children and their parents can be helpful in the management of reactions and guide parents on how to provide effective support and to monitor the need for mental health services. Helping parents address their own distress may increase their perceptiveness and responsiveness to their children's needs.

Long-Term Interventions

Problem-focused or active coping includes activities such as seeking information or attempting to change the circumstances or thoughts about the event in some way. Cognitive restructuring is one type of active coping, which includes thought stopping, self-talk, and positive imagery to address children's intrusive thoughts, cognitive distortions, misattributions, and harmful thought patterns. The use of "coping" puppets and collages, role plays using coping skills, and construction of a book on coping to share with a caring adult are examples of some techniques that are used (Pfefferbaum et al., 2014c). Research has confirmed the effectiveness of cognitive-behavioral therapy (CBT) in multiple forms, delivered both to individual children (e.g., trauma-focused CBT [TFCBT]) and groups (e.g., cognitive-behavioral intervention for trauma in schools [CBITS]) (Grolnick et al., 2018; Wolmer et al., 2017).

Far less research has explored interventions for bereavement and loss that are often experienced by children after a disaster (Grolnick et al., 2018). This may be because many professionals view grief as a normative reaction and best managed with supportive services rather than formal treatment (Pfefferbaum et al., 2013). Similarly, it has been difficult to accumulate research evidence of efficacy of interventions when applied to children impacted by disasters but who demonstrate adjustment reactions that are either insufficient in number or degree to qualify for a mental health diagnosis (Grolnick et al., 2018).

USE OF PSYCHOTROPIC MEDICATIONS

Stress reactions following a disaster are very common and generally resolve without active treatment. Psychotropic medications should not be used immediately after the disaster to blunt children's awareness or to reduce typical emotional reactions such as crying. This may undermine children's understanding of the event and their ability to acknowledge and express their distressing feelings, which ultimately is important for recovery (Schonfeld & Demaria, 2015). When used, medications should be considered part of a comprehensive treatment plan, which includes psychotherapy, case management support, and active family involvement. Pharmacologic treatments should be directed by a mental health clinician with expertise in the treatment of posttraumatic disorders. In this context psychopharmacologic interventions should focus on target symptoms, such as acute onset of anxiety, depression, agitation, or aggressive behavior, that significantly limit a child's psychosocial functioning (Pfefferbaum et al., 2013).

RESILIENCY AND POSTTRAUMATIC GROWTH

Early support for children should focus on reinforcing natural resilience by enhancing children's and families' strengths and resources. Psychotherapeutic interventions should be reserved for children showing significant distress and impairment in functioning (Pfefferbaum et al., 2017).

Resilience is the positive coping ability demonstrated following serious threats to adaptation and development using ordinary rather than extraordinary processes (Masten, 2001). Individuals who are resilient can cope with a crisis without much external support but may still experience similar amounts of distress. Resiliency, however, is different from recovery, which may require an extended period of time. Resilience reflects the ability to maintain stability during the recovery process (Bonanno et al., 2010) which, however, may falsely lead caregivers to conclude that their children are no longer experiencing distress.

Resilience can be understood as the interplay among personal characteristics, protective contextual factors, and the severity of the stressors faced by the child. Personal resiliency capacity has been found to include beliefs about personal mastery, a sense of being connected to others, and the capacity for emotional regulation (Prince-Embury, 2011). After a disaster, resiliency and positive adaptation can be fostered by promoting problem solving and ingenuity, enhancing motivation to overcome challenges, fostering a sense of purpose and hope, encouraging supportive relationships, addressing attachment needs, and providing security through the demonstration of leadership by role models (Masten, 2020). Parents can be encouraged to also provide age-appropriate opportunities for their children to gain a sense of control and engage in decision making so that children can restore meaning in their lives and achieve confidence that they can master challenges they may face and contribute to their own recovery (Masten, 2020).

Following a disaster, some children will display significant transformation or growth. Posttraumatic growth (PTG) refers to a positive change experienced as a result of undergoing a traumatic event, which includes feelings of strength, closer relationships, an appreciation of life, a recognition of new possibilities, and spiritual development (Self-Brown et al., 2017). PTG appears related to the parent's own PTG, wherein parents provide their child with positive reframing coping advice and modeling (Kilmer & Gil-Rivas, 2010).

CONSULTATION TO SCHOOLS

The Value of Universal Supports

In the aftermath of major disasters adjustment difficulties are likely to be widespread, and large numbers of children may be impacted. In such a context support should be offered at the population level. Schools often serve as a critical means to reach such large numbers of children and are well positioned to provide universal supports to all children and to monitor adjustment over time. It is therefore important that educators and other school professionals become familiar with strategies to provide support to children in distress, such as those encompassed in PFA; these same techniques can be used as well for children dealing with personal or family crises.

After a major disaster, adjustment difficulties will be pervasive and persistent, and most children will not seek or receive traditional mental health services. The primary strategy for providing support after a disaster should be based on offering universal support to all children to promote coping and resiliency, rather than exclusively relying on a clinical approach involving screening, evaluation, diagnosis, referral, and treatment for children perceived to be at risk of having a mental illness. This should be coupled with resources for additional mental health services for those needing more than universal support.

Advice for Educators

Childhood is a time of rapid intellectual development, so children are uniquely vulnerable to difficulty in attention and learning that may be seen in the aftermath of disasters and contribute to problems with academic performance (Peek, 2008). Effective schools support resiliency, including strong leadership, caring relationships, collective pride, a sense of belonging for students, positive routines, good communication, and opportunities to learn new skills (Masten, 2020). Schools also provide a natural venue for conducting public health activities such as delivering psychoeducation and social support, assessing and monitoring affected children, and identifying and triaging children with problems that warrant more professional attention (Pfefferbaum et al., 2014b). Schools and teachers are therefore very important in the recovery of children, especially those with special needs, following a disaster (Stough et al., 2017). When relocation of children or closure of schools results from the disaster, children may be separated from educators and support professionals who are familiar with them, which may be particularly problematic for children with disabilities and other special needs. Even when children remain with familiar staff, the staff may be preoccupied with their own losses and impact from the disaster.

While children benefit from a return to routine and predictability after a disaster that may be provided by resumption of school and learning, it is critical that schools modify expectations and student workloads to align with students' current learning abilities as they recover their cognitive, emotional, and social functioning. If academic expectations even temporarily exceed children's learning capacity, school may emerge as a source of additional distress for children rather than as a source of support to promote recovery (Schonfeld & Quackenbush, 2021).

PERSONAL IMPACT OF DISASTERS ON CLINICIANS AND PROFESSIONAL SELF-CARE

Clinicians who live within the community impacted by a large-scale disaster will often be dealing with the personal impact of the disaster on themselves as well as their friends and family. They often must work in austere settings with limited resources and supports to practice medicine at a time when patient care needs are greatly increased. The psychological strains inherent in continuing to provide medical service during disasters may place clinicians at risk for emotional difficulties, substance abuse, and maladaptive coping responses, including the tendency to work beyond one's limits and neglect self-care. These risks may be intensified by medical training and culture, which emphasize emotional control and suppressing personal feelings, unrealistic expectations of personal invulnerability, and a commitment to taking care of others before taking care of oneself (Mull et al., 2019).

The psychological impact of working with those who have suffered trauma and loss has been variously referred to as vicarious traumatization, compassion fatigue, or, more simply, burnout. Vicarious traumatization is described as the emotional and psychological reactions that are triggered by the experience of empathic engagement with patients who are survivors of traumatic events such as those experienced by children in disasters. Burnout is commonly found in those exposed to a high level of stress as part of their work and includes emotional exhaustion, depersonalization, and a reduced belief in personal and professional competency (Romani & Ashkar, 2014).

The importance of routinely maintaining self-care strategies becomes even more critical following a disaster because of the increased emotional and social burdens clinicians may experience in this context. Clinicians should create realistic professional expectations and recognize and celebrate small successes within their team. Practicing daily personal stress management and healthy practices (e.g., sleep, diet, exercise.) should be followed in addition to drawing on social supports and professional support as indicated.

CONCLUSION

Natural and human disasters may perturb children's developmental trajectory, behavior, emotional adjustment, academic learning, psychosocial functioning, and physical health. Children with disabilities, such as Bridgett in the opening vignette, may be particularly vulnerable. In the assessment of children after disasters, adjustment reactions should be differentiated from PTSD and reactions related to grief distinguished from those due to trauma. Coping and resiliency are promoted by providing the child and family with open, honest communication and advice and with instrumental and social support. Clinicians should also appreciate the personal impact of working with children and families after disasters and practice professional self-care.

REFERENCES

Becker-Blease, K. A., Turner, H. A., & Finkelhor, D. (2010). Disasters, victimization, and children's mental health. *Child Development*, *81*(4), 1040–1052. https://doi.org/10.1111/j.1467-8624.2010.01453.x.

Bernstein, M., & Pfefferbaum, B. (2018). Posttraumatic growth as a response to natural disasters in children and adolescents. *Current Psychiatry Reports*, *20*(5), 37. https://doi.org/10.1007/s11920-018-0900-4.

Bonanno, G. A., Brewin, C. R., Kaniasty, K., & Greca, A. M. (2010). Weighing the costs of disaster: Consequences, risks, and resilience in individuals, families, and communities. *Psychological Science in the Public Interest*, *11*(1), 1–49. https://doi.org/10.1177/1529100610387086.

Boon, H., Brown, L., Tsey, K., Speare, R., Pagliano, P., Usher, K., & Clark, B. (2011). School disaster planning for children with disabilities: A critical review of the literature. *Journal of Special Education*, *26*(3), 223–237.

Bountress, K. E., Gilmore, A. K., Metzger, I. W., Aggen, S. H., Tomko, R. L., Danielson, C. K., Williamson, V., Vladmirov, V., Ruggiero, K., & Amstadter, A. B. (2020). Impact of disaster exposure severity: Cascading effects across parental distress, adolescent PTSD symptoms, as well as parent-child conflict and communication. *Social Science & Medicine*, *264*, 113293. https://doi.org/10.1016/j.socscimed.2020.113293. Epub ahead of print.

Chrisman, A. K., & Dougherty, J. G. (2014). Mass trauma: Disasters, terrorism, and war. *Child and Adolescent Psychiatric Clinics of North America*, *23*(2), 257–279. https://doi.org/10.1016/j.chc.2013.12.004. viii.

Chung, S., Foltin, G., & Schonfeld, D. J. (Eds.). (2019). *Pediatric disaster preparedness and response topical collection.* American Academy of Pediatrics. https://www.aap.org/en-us/advocacy-and-policy/aap-health-initiatives/Children-and-Disasters/Pages/Pediatric-Terrorism-And-Disaster-Preparedness-Resource.aspx#:~:text=The%20American%20Academy%20of%20Pediatrics%20Pediatric%20Disaster%20Preparedness,health%20professionals%20in%20hospital%20and%20other%20care%20settings.

Cobham, V. E., McDermott, B., Haslam, D., & Sanders, M. R. (2016). The role of parents, parenting and the family environment in children's post-disaster mental health. *Current Psychiatry Reports*, *18*, 53. https://doi.org/10.1007/s11920-016-0691-4.

Dziuban, E. J., Peacock, G., & Frogel, M. (2017). A child's health is the public's health: Progress and gaps in addressing pediatric needs in public health emergencies. *American Journal of Public Health*, *107*(2), S134–S137. https://doi.org/10.2105/AJPH.2017.303950.

Grolnick, W. S., Schonfeld, D. J., Schreiber, M., Cohen, J., Cole, V., Jaycox, L., & Zatzick, D. (2018). Improving adjustment and resilience in children following a disaster: Addressing research challenges. *American Psychologist*, *73*(3), 215–229. https://doi.org/10.1037/amp0000181.

Holte Kofod, E. (2017). A brief historization of contemporary Western grief practices and understandings. *Nordic Psychology*, *69*(1), 47–60. https://doi.org/10.1080/19012276.2016.1267914.

Hunt, M., Pal, N. E., Schwartz, L., & O'Mathúna, D. (2018). Ethical challenges in the provision of mental health services for children and families during disasters. *Current psychiatry reports*, *20*(8), 60. https://doi.org/10.1007/s11920-018-0917-8.

Kilmer, R. P., & Gil-Rivas, V. (2010). Exploring posttraumatic growth in children impacted by Hurricane Katrina: Correlates of the phenomenon and developmental considerations. *Child Development*, *81*(4), 1211–1227. https://doi.org/10.1111/j.1467-8624.2010.01463.x.

King, L. S., Osofsky, J. D., Osofsky, H. J., Weems, C. F., Hansel, T. C., & Fassnacht, G. M. (2015). Perceptions of trauma and loss among children and adolescents exposed to disasters—A mixed-methods study. *Current Psychology*, *34*, 524–536. https://doi.org/10.1007/s12144-015-9348-4.

Lai, B. S., La Greca, A. M., Auslander, B. A., & Short, M. B. (2013). Children's symptoms of posttraumatic stress and depression after a natural disaster: Comorbidity and risk factors. *Journal of Affect Disorders*, *146*(1), 71–78.

Lai, B. S., Lewis, R., Livings, M. S., Greca, A. M., & Esnard, A. (2017). Posttraumatic stress symptom trajectories among children after disaster exposure: A review. *Journal of Traumatic Stress*, *30*(6), 571–582. https://doi.org/10.1002/jts.22242.

Maclean, J. C., Popovici, I., & French, M. T. (2016). Are natural disasters in early childhood associated with mental health and substance use disorders as an adult? *Social Science & Medicine*, *151*, 78–91. https://doi.org/10.1016/j.socscimed.2016.01.006.

Masten. A. S. (2001). Ordinary magic: Resilience processes in development. *The American Psychologist*, *56*, 227–238.

Masten. A. S. (2020). Resilience of children in disasters: A multisystem perspective. *International Journal of Psychology* https://doi.org/10.1002/ijop.12737. Epub ahead of print.

Mull, C. C., Thompson, A. D., Selbst, S. M., Miller, E. G., Rappaport, D. I., Gartner, J. C., Jr., & Bowman, W. R. (2019). A call to restore your calling: Self-care of the emergency physician in the face of life-changing stress—Part 1 of 6. *Pediatric Emergency Care*, *35*(4), 319–322. https://doi.org/10.1097/PEC.0000000000001807.

Peek. L. (2008). Children and disasters: Understanding vulnerability, developing capacities, and promoting resilience. *Children, Youth and Environments*, *18*(1), 1–29.

Pfefferbaum, B., Jacobs, A. K., Jones, R. T., Reyes, G., & Wyche, K. F. (2017). A skill set for supporting displaced children in psychological recovery after disasters. *Current Psychiatry Reports*, *19*(9), 60. https://doi.org/10.1007/s11920-017-0814-6.

Pfefferbaum, B., Shaw, J., & American Academy of Child and Adolescent Psychiatry (AACAP) Committee on Quality Issues (CQI). (2013). Practice parameter on disaster preparedness. *Journal of the Academy of Child and Adolescent Psychiatry*, *52*, 1224–1238. https://doi.org/10.1016/j.jaac.2013.08.014.

Pfefferbaum, B., Sweeton, J. L., Newman, E., Varma, V., Nitiéma, P., Shaw, J. A., Chrisman, A. K., & Noffsinger, M. A. (2014a). Child disaster mental health interventions, part I: Techniques, outcomes, and methodological considerations. *Disaster Health*, *2*(1), 46–57. https://doi.org/10.4161/dish.27534.

Pfefferbaum, B., Sweeton, J. L., Newman, E., Varma, V., Noffsinger, M. A., Shaw, J. A., Chrisman, A. K., & Nitiéma, P. (2014b). Child disaster mental health interventions, part II: Timing of implementation, delivery settings and providers, and therapeutic approaches. *Disaster Health*, *2*(1), 58–67. https://doi.org/10.4161/dish.27535.

Pfefferbaum, B., Sweeton, J. L., Nitiéma, P., Noffsinger, M. A., Varma, V., Nelson, S. D., & Newman, E. (2014c). Child disaster mental health interventions: Therapy components. *Prehospital & Disaster Medicine*, *29*(5), 494–502. https://doi.org/10.1017/S1049023X14000910.

Prince-Embury, S. (2011). Assessing personal resiliency in the context of school settings: Using the resiliency scales for children and adolescents. *Psychology in the Schools*, *48*(7), 672–685.

Romani, M., & Ashkar, K. (2014). Burnout among physicians. *Libyan Journal of Medicine*, *9*, 23556. https://doi.org/10.3402/ljm.v9.23556.

Ronoh, S., Gaillard, J. C., & Marlowe, J. (2015). Children with disabilities and disaster preparedness: A case study of Christchurch, Kōtuitui. *New Zealand Journal of Social Sciences Online*, *10*(2), 91–102. https://doi.org/10.1080/1177083X.2015.1068185.

Scaramella, L. V., Sohr-Preston, S. L., Callahan, K. L., & Mirabile, S. P. (2008). A test of the family stress model on toddler-aged children's adjustment among Hurricane Katrina impacted and nonimpacted low-income families. *Journal of Clinical Child & Adolescent Psychology*, *37*(3), 530–541.

Schonfeld. D. J. (1989). Crisis intervention for bereavement support: A model of intervention in the children's school. *Clinical Pediatrics (Philadelphia)*, *28*(1), 29.

Schonfeld, D. J. (2021). Children's understanding of and adjustment to death in the aftermath of a crisis. In C. Harkensee, K. Olness, & B. E. Esmaili (Eds.), *Child Refugee and migrant Health: A manual for health professionals*. Springer Nature, 57–66.

Schonfeld, D. J., & Demaria, T. (2020a). Supporting grieving students. In E. Rossen (Ed.), *Supporting and educating traumatized students: A guide for school-based professionals* (2nd ed.). Oxford University Press.

Schonfeld, D. J., & Demaria, T. (2020b). Supporting children and families in the aftermath of disasters. In C. Goodhue & N. Blake (Eds.), *Nursing management of pediatric disaster*. Springer. https://doi.org/10.1007/978-3-030-43428-1-12.

Schonfeld, D. J., Demaria, T., Disaster Preparedness Advisory Council, & Committee on Psychosocial Aspects of Child and Family Health. (2015). Providing psychosocial support to children and families in the aftermath of disaster and crisis: A guide for pediatricians. *Pediatrics*, *136*(4), e1120–e1130.

Schonfeld, D. J., & Gurwitch, R. H. (2012). Children in disasters. In A. Y. Elzouki, F. B. Stapleton, R. J. Whitley, W. Oh, H. A. Harfi, & H. Nazer (Eds.), *Textbook of clinical pediatrics* (2nd ed., pp. 687–698). Springer-Verlag.

Schonfeld, D. J., & Kappelman, M. (1990). The impact of school-based education on the young child's understanding of death. *Journal of Developmental and Behavioral Pediatrics*, *11*(5), 247–252.

Schonfeld, D. J., & Quackenbush, M. (2021). *The grieving student: A guide for schools* (2nd ed.). Brookes Publishing.

Self-Brown, S., Lai, B., Patterson, A., & Glasheen, T. (2017). The impact of natural disasters on youth: A focus on emerging research beyond internalizing disorders. *Current psychiatry reports*, *19*(8), 53. https://doi.org/10.1007/s11920-017-0798-2.

Speece, M. W., & Brent, S. B. (1984). Children's understanding of death: A review of three components of a death concept. *Child Development*, *55*(5), 1671–1686.

Stough, L. M., Ducy, E. M., & Kang, D. (2017). Addressing the needs of children with disabilities experiencing disaster or terrorism. *Current Psychiatry Reports*, *19*(4), 24. https://doi.org/10.1007/s11920-017-0776-8.

Terasaka, A., Tachibana, Y., Okuyama, M., & Igarashi, T. (2015). Post-traumatic stress disorder in children following natural disasters: A systematic review of the long-term follow-up studies. *International Journal of Child, Youth and Family Studies*, *6*(1), 111–133. https://doi.org/10.18357/ijcyfs.6120151348.

Wolmer, L., Hamiel, D., Pardo-Aviv, L., & Laor, N. (2017). Addressing the needs of preschool children in the context of disasters and terrorism: Assessment, prevention, and intervention. *Current Psychiatry Reports*, *19*(7), 40. https://doi.org/10.1007/s11920-017-0792-8. PMID: 28536808

23

Biological Mechanisms of Human Development and Behavior

Ellen Roy Elias

VIGNETTE

A 5-year-old boy was born at 28 weeks of gestation following a pregnancy notable for conception via in vitro fertilization (IVF), maternal hypertension, and polyhydramnios. The diagnosis of Beckwith-Wiedemann syndrome (BWS) was made after birth due to the presence of macrosomia, macroglossia, and a large omphalocele. The diagnosis of BWS was confirmed by molecular testing, demonstrating changes in the imprinted region on chromosome 11. He was hospitalized for 10 months after birth in the neonatal intensive care unit (NICU). He required a tracheostomy with ventilatory support and gastrostomy feedings during early infancy. He experienced hypoglycemia during the first few months of life, which resolved with tolerance of feeds. His omphalocele was repaired at age 2 years. Now at the age of 5 years, he continues to have a tracheostomy, but only requires oxygen when ill and is no longer on a ventilator. He is nourished both orally with solids and via his gastrostomy tube for fluids. Developmentally, he is ambulatory and is learning to ride a bike. He can feed and dress himself, but he speaks in sentences with some articulation issues due to his large tongue. He knows colors and shapes and is starting to learn letters. He is potty trained. He has an individualized education plan and receives physical and occupational therapy and speech therapy supports.

INTRODUCTION

In the decade or so that has passed since the publication of the previous edition of this textbook truly extraordinary advances in science and medical care have occurred. There is now an infinitely greater understanding of normal embryologic, physiologic, and genetic mechanisms involved not only in human reproduction but in the normal process of being a healthy and functioning person. The identification of thousands of molecular mutations that can affect these processes and result in a person with medical and developmental challenges is much better understood. This has resulted in scientific advances that allow testing of molecular and metabolic derangements and tests that have moved from research techniques to standards of medical care and evaluation. Our knowledge about normal human reproduction and embryology has also exploded. The field of advanced reproductive technology currently allows couples to have children who previously would have not been able to raise families. This chapter explores some of these advances and how they are important for the developmental pediatrician. This chapter will also be a roadmap to where to find more detailed information regarding these exciting issues elsewhere in this textbook.

WHERE DOES ONE START WHEN ASSESSING CHILDREN WITH DEVELOPMENTAL DISABILITIES FOR UNDERLYING BIOLOGIC DIAGNOSES?

Although trying to navigate scientific and genetic advances can be daunting, pediatricians have many important skills to help them determine if there might be an underlying biological/genetic diagnosis in play. These essential medical skills are discussed in this section.

History

Obtaining a past medical history is critically important, especially information regarding the pregnancy and delivery (Box 23.1). Difficulty with conception and a need for advanced reproductive technology to conceive can be important clues to underlying genetic factors. A history of prior miscarriage, especially more than two fetal losses, can also be important to discern. This raises the suspicion of a possible genetic issue such as a balanced translocation in a parent. Complications during the pregnancy, such as bleeding or hypertension, can also indicate an underlying medical or genetic problem in the fetus.

Prenatal screening is quite routine. This includes bloodwork from the pregnant woman and scans, including ultrasound and magnetic resonance imaging (MRI). It is important to determine if there were any prenatal studies obtained, such as maternal bloodwork for a quad screen or cell-free DNA.

BOX 23.1 Important Information to Obtain Regarding the Pregnancy

Age, gravida and para status of mother at delivery
Mode of conception: vaginal vs. cesarean section
Gestational length
Bleeding or spotting
Illness
Teratogenic exposure
Medications
Quickening
Maternal hypertension
History of infertility or fetal loss

Subtle abnormalities on the quad screen (e.g., a low fetal estriol) can be a clue to metabolic diagnoses in the fetus, such as the cholesterol metabolic defect in Smith-Lemli-Opitz syndrome. Elevated alpha-fetoprotein suggests open skin defects such as myelomeningocele or omphalocele. Ultrasounds or other radiologic imaging done during the pregnancy can raise the suspicion of an underlying birth defect or genetic disorder. More invasive procedures obtained, such as chorionic villus sampling or amniocentesis, can give additional molecular, chromosomal, and metabolic clues to underlying diagnosis. A maternal history of problems such as HELLP syndrome can be associated with disorders of fatty acid metabolism.

Findings on prenatal imaging, including ultrasound and MRI, can be extremely helpful not only in raising the suspicion of an underlying genetic problem in the fetus prior to delivery but may also lead to important decisions as to timing of delivery, mode of delivery, and what kind of supports and resuscitation might be required at delivery. This information may even dictate where the baby should be delivered, to be close to appropriate interventions that might be required emergently. Prenatal genetic testing is now becoming more routine, and even highly sophisticated genetic testing such as next-generation sequencing, whole exome sequencing, and even whole genome sequencing have been utilized to make correct diagnoses prior to delivery and to help guide appropriateness of interventions following birth. For example, it is now possible to prenatally diagnose skeletal dysplasia, which can help prepare the family for a possible lethal outcome or need for intense NICU support before the baby is delivered.

While obtaining a history about a patient being evaluated for a developmental disability, it is essential to inquire regarding the mode of delivery (Box 23.2) and to document any perinatal complications. Gestational age at delivery as well as complications of delivery are important to ascertain. Knowing the Apgar score and whether any resuscitation or interventions after delivery were required can help explain subsequent neurologic issues such as seizures or abnormal tone. Presence of unusual facial features or limb abnormalities, as well as any birth defects diagnosed after birth, can provide clues to making an underlying syndromic diagnosis.

Information about the postnatal course (Box 23.3) is also important to obtain. Inquiring about feeding and respiratory issues is important, especially if they arise soon after birth. The presence of any metabolic concerns such as hypoglycemia or electrolyte abnormalities can lead to the diagnosis of an inborn error of metabolism.

BOX 23.2 Important Information to Obtain Regarding the Delivery

Mode of delivery
Anesthesia
Hemorrhage or abnormal bleeding
Length of labor
Birth order if multiples
Medications given to mother
Fetal monitoring
Natural, induced, or emergency delivery
Post natal Events
Apgars
Resuscitation required
Birth weight/length and OFC
Breathing problems
Feeding problems
Hypoglycemia
Hyperbilirubinemia
Stay in nursery vs. NICU
Age at discharge
Any surgical events
Oxygen at discharge
Medications at discharge

BOX 23.3 Important Information to Obtain Regarding the Perinatal Course

Apgars and any resuscitation required
Birthweight/length and occipitofrontal circumference
Breathing problems
Feeding problems
Metabolic issues, including hypoglycemia and hyperbilirubinemia
Stay in the neonatal intensive care unit vs nursery
Age and weight at discharge
Neonatal surgical events
Oxygen at discharge
Medications at discharge

The medical course during infancy and early childhood can help provide important information. Reviewing growth curves can help show that the child has thrived nutritionally or has demonstrated malnutrition. The history of any significant illnesses such as meningitis or hospitalizations for severe illness or injury may impact developmental progress. Neurologic issues such as seizures that require medication or markedly abnormal tone are important clues to underlying genetic problems. If a brain MRI has been performed, it can demonstrate brain malformations or other problems (e.g., worsening hydrocephalus) that may impact health, nutrition, and development.

One of the most important components to a good history is the family history (Box 23.4). Obtaining a three-generation pedigree (Box 23.5) is sometimes the clue that leads to a diagnosis and is an essential part of the pediatric history in the evaluation of a child presenting with developmental disabilities. It is important to inquire if there are any other individuals in the

BOX 23.4 Important Questions to Ask About Family History

History of infertility or fetal loss in mother, her siblings and parents
Consanguinity
Any individuals with developmental disabilities or behavioral problems such as autism, especially in the patient's siblings and parent's siblings
Any individuals with birth defects
Any deaths during early infancy or childhood
Any individual with epilepsy
History of multiple miscarriages; should ask further about a possible clotting disorder with questions that include a history of early stroke, deep vein thrombosis, or pulmonary emboli
Ethnic background in parents; if they are both from the same country, it is good to ask if they are from the same small village or isolated area, which can unmask consanguinity

BOX 23.5 Three-Generation Pedigree

A three-generation pedigree is important to document, and contains information about the child, the child's parents, siblings, grandparents, aunts, uncles, and cousins. Drawing a pedigree is not that difficult and can provide very useful information. See the references provided for details.

Resources can be found here:

National Society of Genetic Counselors: http://www.nsgc.org/About/FamilyHistoryTool/tabid/226/Default.aspx

Bennett, R. L., French, K. S., Resta, R. G., & Doyle, D. L. (2008). Standardized human pedigree nomenclature: Update and assessment of the recommendations of the National Society of Genetic Counselors. *Journal of Genetic Counselors, 17*, 424–433.

family who have developmental disabilities. For example, if the mother has a brother with intellectual disabilities or autism, an X-linked disorder such as fragile X syndrome might be suspected (Neri, Schwartz, Lubs, & Stevenson, 2018). The presence of parental consanguinity is associated with an increased risk for an autosomal recessive disorder. As mentioned, a history of infertility or multiple fetal losses can increase the possibility of a parental chromosomal abnormality (see Box 23.4 with important questions to ask in the family history).

Physical Examination

After the history, the physical exam is the next critical part of the evaluation of the patient with developmental disabilities. Assessment of growth parameters is the first critical step. Is the child too large or too small, and is the head normal or macro- or microcephalic? The facial features and appearance of the pinnae can provide critical clues; pediatricians may not have formal training in dysmorphology but can clearly have a sense of whether features appear normal or not. Chapter 77 provides further details about the physical exam in the evaluation of children with developmental disabilities.

Evaluation of the skin can provide important clues, including pigmentary abnormalities and pattern of hair growth. The genitalia should always be inspected as even subtle abnormalities can give important clues to an underlying genetic diagnosis. For example, hypospadias is often seen in males with a 22q11 deletion, which is a common chromosome abnormality seen in patients with both developmental and behavioral issues. Lastly, a close examination of the extremities can be revealing. Even subtle 2-3 toe syndactyly can be the only outside sign of the common genetic disorder Smith-Lemli-Opitz syndrome resulting in intellectual disabilities and autism.

ADVANCES IN MEDICAL CARE

The child described in the opening vignette exemplifies many of the issues involved in the evaluation and care of a child with complex medical and developmental issues. He was conceived using advanced reproductive technology. Although these techniques, including IVF, result in thousands of healthy infants born per year, disorders resulting from errors in imprinting may be seen with increased frequency in children conceived with this technology. Chapter 24 describes genetic disorders and associated mechanisms leading to further discussion of disorders arising from imprinting errors, an epigenetic mechanism that can cause significant medical and developmental consequences.

The child in the vignette was born prematurely and required many services provided in a tertiary level NICU. The ability to care for such tiny and complex infants has shown great progress over the years. Chapter 34 provides a comprehensive discussion of the developmental consequences of preterm delivery.

In addition to the superb medical services offered in NICUs, other medical concerns can lead to the need for intense inpatient hospitalization and management. Injuries to the brain resulting from motor vehicle accidents, falls, infections, malignancies, and vascular events can also necessitate inpatient care and management as well as have developmental consequences. Medical and surgical advances and increasingly sophisticated radiologic techniques have led to improved survival and outcome following these kinds of events. For further discussion on these topics, see Chapters 32, 33, and 60.

Once a child has survived a complex hospitalization, whether from issues surrounding birth and underlying genetic defects to injuries sustained at any age, and is discharged home, the care of that child by home caregivers and pediatricians can be a complex and daunting task. Care of the child at home may entail nursing supports and durable medical equipment. Chapter 59 shows a comprehensive approach to the care of the child with medical complexity.

Home developmental services are essential for young children from ages birth to 3 years and may include the support of therapists from early intervention, which can be either home or center based. These services have become more available and accessible. For children ages 3 to 21 years, educational and therapeutic services are often obtained at school. Planning for this is important, including educating parents to advocate for their child's emotional and behavioral needs as well as academic needs, while supporting medical issues in a safe way.

Nutritional concerns are extremely common and can significantly impact developmental outcome. Nutritional deficiencies can have developmental consequences, with iron deficiency being one of the most common and well-described concerns. Nutritional advances have been made that can lead to better growth and health, allowing children to have a better potential for developmental advancement. The development of new formulas and a better understanding of nutritional deficiencies and how to correct them has led to significant improvements in medical and developmental outcome for children. Chapter 35 provides a detailed look at nutrition.

Inborn errors of metabolism are rare genetic diseases that can present with developmental delays, abnormal muscle tone, medical complications, and characteristic abnormalities on laboratory testing. Most of these disorders are inherited in an autosomal recessive pattern. Symptoms include hypoglycemia, abnormal liver function with cholestasis, and hyperammonemia; these can be clues to devastating inborn errors of metabolism. The improvements in newborn screening have allowed detection of many of these disorders soon after birth, which can prevent developmental consequences and allow the provision of lifesaving treatments and interventions. Understanding when to suspect these rare disorders and when to request the help of a genetic specialist is important for the developmental pediatrician to know. Chapter 36 details a comprehensive approach toward the diagnosis of inborn errors of metabolism.

Better and more sophisticated imaging techniques have evolved that allow an improved understanding of underlying central nervous system developmental disorders. These include disorders of brain dysgenesis (see Chapter 29), epilepsy (see Chapter 31), brain injury (see Chapter 32), neuromuscular disorders (see Chapter 30), and progressive disorders of neurodegeneration (see Chapter 36). The types of imaging that would give the best help in making a clear diagnosis and more in-depth discussion of the different types of imaging are discussed in Chapter 89.

Advances outside of medical care and knowledge can impact understanding of underlying biologic and genetic mechanisms. Broadened availability of Internet-based communication has allowed the more rapid spread of knowledge between scientists, researchers, and physicians, and between physicians and their patients. Although many families seek the information available from "Dr. Google" or have access to specialists via telehealth, being able to interpret and guide families to a better understanding of the child's underlying issues remains in the realm of an in-person and knowledgeable physician. The popularity of and ease in using Zoom conferencing has blossomed during the COVID-19 pandemic and has allowed continued sharing of knowledge despite the inability to have large scientific meetings or family support group sessions.

ADVANCES IN GENETICS

The field of genetics has changed significantly since the last version of this text was published. This has led to major improvements in the ability to diagnose underlying genetic and metabolic disorders that can cause developmental disabilities. Advances have been extraordinary and include marked improvements in the sensitivity of genetic testing and the ability to detect subtle chromosome abnormalities using microarray and subtle gene defects using next-generation sequencing panels. Chapters 24 and 25 provide details about these advancements and technologies.

The evolution of new genetic testing technologies includes whole exome and whole genome sequencing (Anazi et al., 2017; Bowling et al., 2017; Fitzgerald et al., 2015; Freed et al., 2020). Publications in 2016 and 2020 (Huang, Zhu, Qu, & Mu, 2016; Ilyas 2020) have advocated using these technologies to make diagnoses in critically ill infants and children in the ICU setting, and even have proposed doing this testing prenatally (Sparks et al., 2020). Confirming a diagnosis can lead to improved medical care, more appropriate conversations about prognosis, and better recurrence risks for families (Vissers, Gilissen, & Veltman, 2016; Waggoner et al., 2018; Wang, Wang, Wang, Chen, & Sheng, 2020). See Chapters 24 and 36 for more details.

Our understanding of embryology, mechanisms of teratogenic effects, and molecular mechanisms causing interruptions in normal organ development have advanced significantly in the past decade. Even birth defects as common as spina bifida have been studied with advances made as to genetic etiologies, as well as medical and surgical interventions that improve health and quality of life. Recent publications have described the benefits of folate supplementation to women both preconception and during early pregnancy in reducing the rate of neural tube defects. However, the more than 25 years of folate supplementation in normal foods such as grains and bread has not eradicated the incidence of spina bifida. Furthermore, despite intensive research in this area, all the genes causing neural tube defects are still not known (Lemay et al., 2019; Lupo, 2017; Murdoch et al., 2014; Wolujewicz & Ross, 2019).

The advent of techniques that fall under the umbrella of personalized medicine can provide a variety of information from genealogy to testing to determine dose of medications and which medication might be most effective to help patients. This is now frequently done by psychiatrists and some developmental pediatricians to help determine which medications might be most effective to help patients with behavioral disorders. The advent of in-home personalized genetic testing has increased significantly, and patients often come to their physicians for help with interpretation regarding their underlying risks for developing certain conditions. The reported results of these kinds of tests can be quite confusing, leading to error and misinterpretation of findings. These for-profit genetic testing companies frequently offer the support of a genetic counselor to help with interpretation, which is often advisable for both patients and their physicians.

Knowledge about the underlying molecular cause of a disease helps lead to the development of disease-specific interventions and potential cures (Monroe et al., 2016; Oegema et al., 2020; Pivalizza & Lalani, 2020). Advances in treatment cross a wide range of interventions, including medical and surgical interventions, and more complex and sophisticated interventions, including bone marrow transplant and gene therapy (Waldrop et al., 2020). Use of pleuripotent stem cell technology may allow future cures of rare and severe diseases. See Chapter 36 for a more detailed discussion about the future of therapeutic interventions for patients with developmental disabilities and rare metabolic disorders.

In summary, there is an underlying biologic/genetic etiology for many patients with developmental disabilities and genetic disorders. The tools available to diagnose underlying conditions have made significant advances (Oegema et al., 2020; Vissers et al., 2016; Wang et al., 2020). This new knowledge can bring better treatment, better prediction of recurrence risks, and more hope for families who have children with developmental and behavioral challenges.

REFERENCES

Anazi, S., Maddirevula, S., Faqeih, E., Alsedairy, H., Alzahrani, F., et al. (2017). Clinical genomics expands the morbid genome of intellectual disability and offers a high diagnostic yield. *Molecular Psychiatry*, *22*, 615–624.

Bowling, K. M., Thompson, M. L., Amaral, M. D., Finnila, C. R., Hiatt, S. M., et al. (2017). Genomic diagnosis for children with intellectual disability and/or developmental delay. *Genome Medicine*, *9*, 43. https://doi.org/10.1186/s13073-017-0433-1

Fitzgerald, T. W., et al. (2015). Deciphering developmental disorders study: Large-scale discovery of novel genetic causes of developmental disorders. *Nature*, *519*(7542), 223–228.

Freed, A. S., et al. (2020). Rapid exome sequencing leads to changes in management. *Journal of Pediatrics*, *226*, 202–212.

Huang, J., Zhu, T., Qu, Y., & Mu, D. (2016). Prenatal, perinatal and neonatal risk factors for intellectual disability: A systemic review and meta-analysis. *PLoS One*, *11*, e0153655.

Ilyas, M., Mir, A., Efthymiou, S., & Houlden, H. (2020). The genetics of intellectual disability: Advancing technology and gene editing. *F1000Research*.

Lemay, P. (2019). Whole exome sequencing identifies novel predisposing genes in NTD. *Molecular Genetics and Genomic Medicine*, *7*(1), e00467.

Lupo, P. J. (2017). Genetic epidemiology of neural tube defects. *Journal of Pediatric Rehabilitation Medicine*, *10*(3–4), 189–194.

Monroe, G. R., Frederix, G. W., Savelberg, S. M. C., de Vries, T. I., Duran, K. J., van der Smagt, J. J., Terhal, P. A., van Hasselt, P. M., Kroes, H. Y., Verhoeven-Duif, N. M., Nijman, I. J., Carbo, E. C., van Gassen, K. L., Knoers, N. V., Hövels, A. M., van Haelst, M. M., Visser, G., & van Haaften, G. (2016). Effectiveness of whole-exome sequencing and costs of the traditional diagnostic trajectory in children with intellectual disability. *Genetics in Medicine*, *18*, 949.

Murdoch, J. N., Damrau, C., Paudyal, A., Bogani, D., Wells, S., Greene, N. D. E., Stanier, P., & Copp, A. J. (2014). Genetic interactions between planar cell polarity genes cause diverse NTD's in mice. *Disease Mechanisms*, *10*, 1154.

Neri, G., Schwartz, C. E., Lubs, H. A., & Stevenson, R. E (2018). X-linked intellectual disability update 2017. *American Journal of Human Genetics*, *176*(6), 1375–1388.

Oegema, R., Barakat, T. S., Wilke, M., Stouffs, K., Amrom, D., Aronica, E., Bahi-Buisson, N., Conti, V., Fry, A. E., Geis, T., Andres, D. G., Parrini, E., Pogledic, I., Said, E., Soler, D., Valor, L. M., Zaki, M. S., Mirzaa, G., ... Donato, N. D. (2020). International consensus recommendations on the diagnostic work-up for malformations of cortical development. *Nature Reviews Neurology*, *16*(11), 618–635.

Pivalizza, P., & Lalani, S. R. (2020). Intellectual disability in children: Evaluation for a cause. *UpToDate*.

Sparks, T. N., Lianoglou, B. R., Adami, R. R., Pluym, I. D., Holliman, K., Duffy, J., Downum, S. L., Patel, S., Faubel, A., Boe, N. M., Field, N. T., Murphy, A., Laurent, L. C., Jolley, J., Uy, C., Slavotinek, A. M., Devine, P., Hodoglugil, U., Van Ziffle, J., ... Norton, M. E. (2020). Exome sequencing for prenatal diagnosis in nonimmune hydrops fetalis. *NEJM*, *383*(18), 1746.

Vissers, L. E., Gilissen, C., & Veltman, J. A. (2016). Genetic studies in intellectual disability and related disorders. *Nature Reviews Genetics*, *17*, 9.

Waggoner, D., Wain, K. E., Dubuc, A. M., Conlin, L., Hickey, S. E., Lamb, A. N., Martin, C. L., Morton, C. C., Rasmussen, K., Schuette, J. L., Schwartz, S., & Miller, D. T. (2018). Yield of additional genetic testing after chromosomal microarray for diagnosis of neurodevelopmental disability and congenital anomalies: A clinical practice resource of the American College of Medical Genetics and Genomics (ACMG) on behalf of the ACMG Professional Practice and Guidelines Committee. *Genetics in Medicine*, *20*(10), 1105–1113.

Waldrop, M. A., Karingada, C., Storey, M. A., Powers, B., Iammarino, M. A., Miller, N. F., Alfano, L. N., Noritz, G., Rossman, I., Ginsberg, M., Mosher, K. A., Broomall, E., Goldstein, J., Bass, N., Lowes, L. P., Tsao, C. Y., Mendell, J. R., & Connolly, A. M. (2020). Gene therapy for spinal muscular atrophy. *Pediatrics*, *146*(3), e20200729.

Wang, J., Wang, Y., Wang, L., Chen, W. Y., & Sheng, M. (2020). The diagnostic yield of intellectual disability: Combined whole genome low coverage sequencing and medical exome sequencing. *BMC Medical Genomics*, *13*, 70. https://doi.org/10.1186/s12920-020-0726-x

Wolujewicz, P., & Ross, M. E. (2019). The search for genetic determinants of human neural tube defects. *Current Opinions in Pediatrics*, *31*(6), 739–746.

24

Genetic Disorders and Their Associated Mechanisms

Jessica Duis and Ellen Roy Elias

For additional material related to the content of this chapter, please see Chapters 25, 28, 31, 40, and 41.

VIGNETTE

Amanda, a 14-month-old female with a developmental delay and hypotonia, has been referred by her pediatrician. Her parents have noted persistent "jumps" and "tremor" when falling asleep. She is described as a happy baby with an infectious laugh. Amanda's mother states she loves her bath time. The parents report exhaustion because it seems like their daughter does not need to sleep, and she goes to bed well but is up multiple times overnight. They have to bring her in their bed to get any sleep.

INTRODUCTION

Concerns regarding development are often associated with the presenting feature of genetic conditions and syndromes. The approach to genetic testing to identify a genetic cause for neurodevelopmental disabilities is changing, and a wide breadth of knowledge of these disorders offers the opportunity to support suspected diagnoses such as autism spectrum disorder (ASD) and to consider the patient's care holistically. This chapter will focus on unique patterns of inheritance that require specialized genetic testing and Mendelian disorders of neurodevelopment for which broad next-generation sequencing panels are currently available. Chromosomal anomalies are outside the scope of this chapter and are covered elsewhere.

Molecular studies offer high diagnostic accuracy to confirm many of these disorders; however, consideration of the differential diagnosis is essential. In many cases it is possible to predict the phenotype on the basis of specific DNA changes, known as genotype-phenotype correlation. We focus on epigenetic mediated disorders, including imprinting disorders and Mendelian disorders of the epigenetic machinery, which significantly impact neurodevelopment (Fahrner & Bjornsson, 2019). Specific Mendelian disorders will be considered in particular with respect to a changing landscape of personalized therapies. Somatic mosaicism and particular considerations in testing are also covered. Multifactorial conditions include those caused by multiple genes and environmental factors. Many types of developmental disabilities are due to this form of inheritance.

Knowledge about an underlying genetic condition can facilitate prevention, such as preconception treatment with diet or vitamins in future pregnancies of mothers who have phenylketonuria. Finally, teratogenic mechanisms play a role in causing a significant number of developmental disabilities. Clearly, environmental factors and underlying genetic tendencies combine to affect brain formation and function from early in embryonic life throughout childhood. The natural history of these many conditions reflects a changing phenotype with age. Management of most disorders is multidisciplinary, including medical genetics, pediatrics, and developmental services. A greater understanding of genetic and molecular mechanisms is beginning to allow us to better understand the etiology and management of many developmental disorders.

EPIGENETIC MECHANISMS OF DISEASE

Epigenetics

The Human Genome Project greatly contributed to our current comprehension of molecular biology and disease processes. In revealing that we have approximately 23,000 genes we learned that there are additional factors that influence the timing and expression of genes critical to development. Specifically, critical regulatory elements exist for genes, and depending on the unique interplay of these regions with transcription factors, a gene may have distinct roles depending on timing or tissue location. Epigenetics refers to changes in the expression of genes based on determinants of gene function such as chromatin confirmation, as opposed to changes in the genome sequence itself. These changes are transmitted from cell to cell and maintained by several mechanisms, including modifications to the DNA such as DNA methylation, histone modifications that alter chromatin packaging or access, and substitution of specialized histone variants that mark chromatin associated with particular sequences or regions of the genome. Chromatin changes respond quickly to the environment and are more transient, exerting an ability to respond quickly to the changes of the cell, or can be long term. Growing evidence suggests that there is an important role of epigenetics in neurodevelopmental disorders and therefore some knowledge of this field is essential to developmental medicine (Nussbaum et al., 2007).

Genomic Imprinting

Allelic imbalances play a role in gene expression for both autosomes and the X chromosome. Genomic imprinting is a mechanism by which an allele from a specific parent of origin is expressed. In this case the choice of the chromosome expressed is nonrandom. It requires the introduction of epigenetic marks at the level of the germline of a particular parent. This leads to monoallelic expression of a gene or chromosomal region. The process of imprinting occurs during gametogenesis as a means of marking the contribution of chromosomes from the mother or father. After conception, the specific imprint silences expression of the allele within the imprinted region. Imprinting may be tissue specific, in which some tissues have monoallelic expression from a parent of origin, which other tissues show biallelic expression. Imprinting is maintained in the tissues through the duration of the individual's life. However, the process is reversible in a manner that allows for a paternally derived allele in female offspring to be remarked with a maternal imprint in her gametes. Similarly, a maternally derived allele in male offspring is remarked with a paternal imprint in his gametes. Control of this process is mediated by imprinting centers located within imprinted regions throughout the genome. More than 100 genes are imprinted across the genome primarily on chromosomes 7, 11, 14, 15, 16, and 20.

Disorders Associated With Genomic Imprinting

Angelman Syndrome

Angelman syndrome (Fig. 24.1) was initially described as "happy puppet" syndrome in 1965 in individuals with happy demeanor and awkward movements with truncal ataxia (Angelman, 1965). Children with Angelman syndrome present with hypotonia and developmental delay with severe expressive language delays and motor impairment. They may have feeding difficulties and gastroesophageal reflux disease (see Fig. 26.1). Neurologic problems include tremor, abnormal electroencephalographic patterns, seizures, and ataxia. Characteristic features include a happy demeanor, excitability, hypermotoric behavior, anxiety, sleep concerns, and sensory seeking. Angelman syndrome is a contiguous gene syndrome localized at 15q11.2-q13 due to absent maternal expression of the gene *UBE3A* in the central nervous system. The incidence is between 1 in 12,000 and 1 in 20,000 live births. Specific DNA methylation testing may detect 70% to 80%, including those with a deletion of chromosome 15q11.2q13, paternal uniparental disomy of chromosome 15, or an imprinting center defect. A mutation in the maternally inherited copy of the gene *UBE3A* is detected in approximately 10% of cases (Dagli et al., 1998/2017; Driscoll et al., 1998/2017).

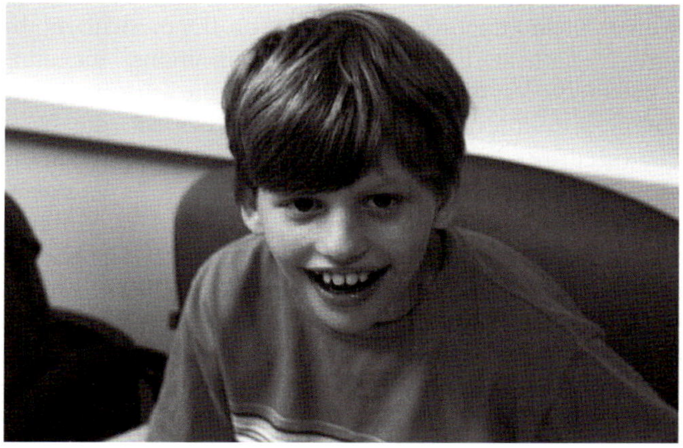

Fig. 24.1 Angelman syndrome in a 10-year-old boy.

Developmental issues include neonatal hypotonia, movement disorders with ataxia, seizures, gross motor and fine motor delay, and speech delay. Gait changes may occur over time in a maladaptive pattern. Frequently, the developmental quotient is less than 50. There is often tremor, awkward gait, excessive laughter, and absent speech. Features of ASDs are described in Angelman syndrome. It is now known that mutations in the *MECP2* gene at Xq28 (the gene for Rett syndrome) can modify imprinting of the gene *UBE3A* at 15q11 and cause clinical autism in some individuals with Angelman syndrome. This may be one of the first descriptions of two genetic syndromes in which a mutation in one gene, such as in *MECP2*, which normally would result in a different disorder called Rett syndrome, modifies the expression of another gene, namely *UBE3A*, such that children with Angelman syndrome present with autism because of the interaction between these two genes. Individuals with mosaic Angelman syndrome often have developmental delay and autistic features.

Management guidelines include a multidisciplinary approach with specialists in genetics, neurology, child development, physical medicine and rehabilitation, gastroenterology, orthopedics, physical therapy, occupational therapy, and speech and language pathology, including a specialist in augmentative and assistive communication devices. Personalized therapies are in development for Angelman syndrome. Support groups include https://www.angelman.org and https://cureangelman.org.

Prader-Willi Syndrome

In 1956 Prader, Labhart, and Willi characterized the unique clinical natural history of neonatal hypotonia, failure to thrive, onset of hyperphagia, developmental delay, short stature, characteristic facies with tall forehead and bitemporal narrowing, almond-shaped eyes, scoliosis, small hands and feet with tapered fingers, hypothalamic hypogonadism, delayed puberty, and often morbid obesity by midchildhood (Fig. 24.2). Prader-Willi syndrome (PWS) is localized to 15q11.2, the Prader-Willi critical region, which is an imprinted region (Cassidy & Schwartz, 2006). The incidence of PWS is between 1 in 10,000 and 1 in 25,000 births. There are a number of genetic mechanisms that can explain imbalance at the 15q11.2 region. Deletion of a paternal chromosome at 15q11.2q13 occurs in 70% of patients. With either the chromosomal or molecular FISH deletion, the recurrence rate in a sibling is less than 1%. An additional 25% of individuals will present with PWS due to maternal disomy at 15q11.2, frequently due to meiotic nondisjunction followed by trisomic rescue. Again, recurrence risk is less than 1% but may be related to a parental Robertsonian translocation. Finally, a few individuals with PWS have an imprinting mutation that

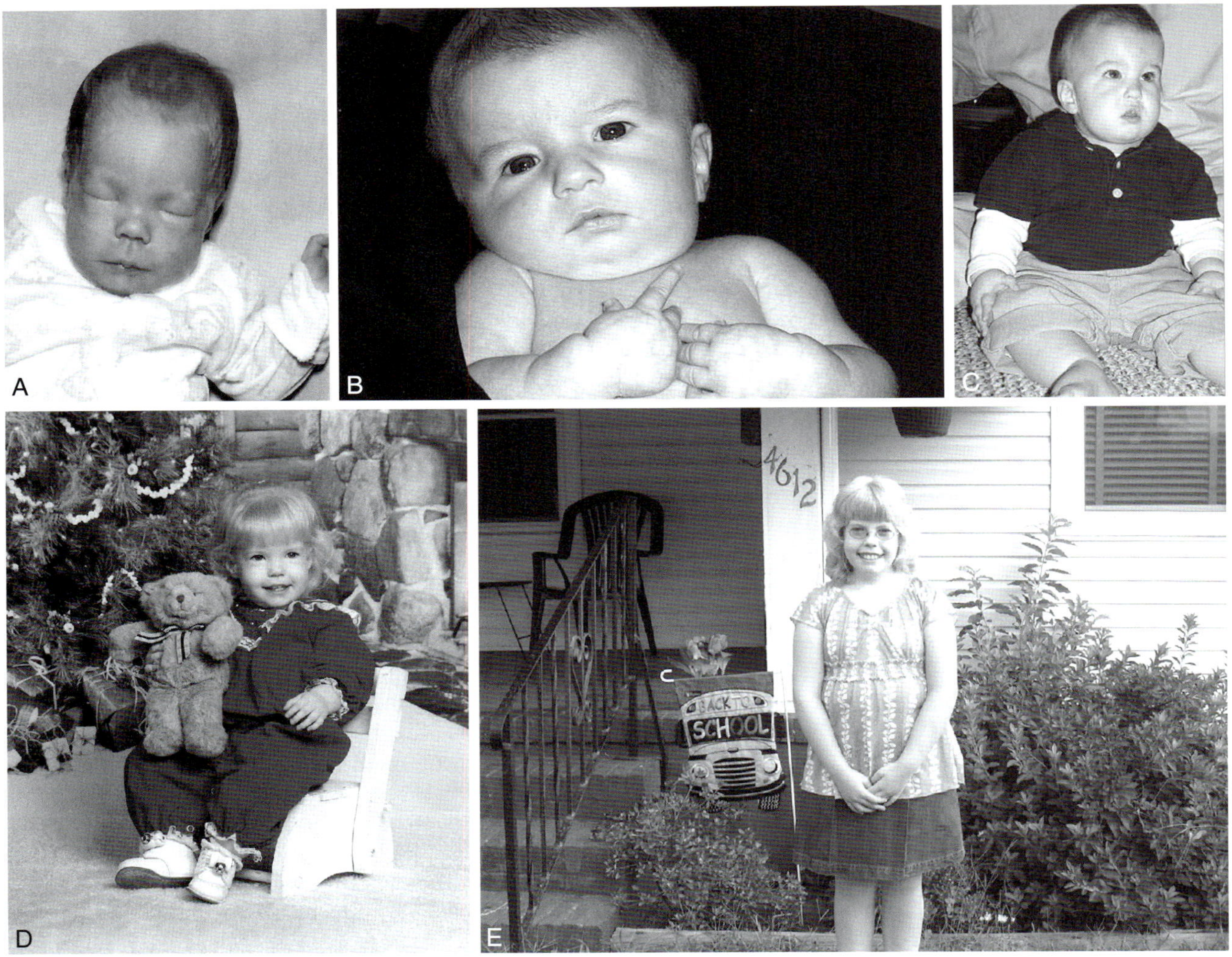

Fig. 24.2 Prader-Willi through the years: (a) 8-week-old boy, (b) 5-month-old, (c) 1-year-old boy, (d) 2-year-old girl, (e) 11-year-old girl.

modifies the expression of the entire region. Those individuals with an imprinting gene mutation may have a recurrence risk as high as 50% if there is a deletion that is detected in the imprinting control region located in the *SNRPN* gene; however, most cases are due to an epimutation, which does not have a recurrence risk.

Developmental issues in children with PWS focus primarily on profound hypotonia at birth, with gross motor, fine motor, and speech delays often related to apraxia of speech. Individuals progress through nutritional phases with onset of hyperphagia reported to occur in the age range of 6 to 8 years old. The behavioral phenotype of PWS is unique and includes behavioral rigidity, insistence on sameness, perseveration, self-injurious behaviors such as skin picking, generalized anxiety, behavioral outbursts, and obsessive-compulsive behaviors. Individuals with PWS are prone to psychosis, particularly if they have the maternal uniparental disomy subtype. Features of ASDs, including repetitive behaviors, social-emotional difficulties, and communication deficits, are common, and a referral to behavioral therapies to assist in environmental modifications is often helpful.

Individuals with PWS require management by a multidisciplinary team, including geneticists, endocrinologists, sleep specialists, psychiatrists, orthopedists, gastroenterologists, behavioral therapists, physical therapists, and occupational and speech therapists. Management guidelines include use of human growth hormone from the time of diagnosis throughout adulthood, which may provide additional benefits beyond growth, including a reported impact on IQ, particularly the verbal quotient. Environmental modifications, including restricting access to food often by locking the refrigerator and pantry, impact level of anxiety in the individual with PWS. Food security is key and includes routine mealtimes, planning ahead, and use of visual schedules in addition to environmental controls. Other important medical issues include monitoring for osteoporosis with bone densitometry and clinical monitoring for scoliosis. Endocrine follow-up and treatment of growth, osteoporosis, and hypogonadism can significantly improve quality of life for these children. Sleep-disordered breathing is common in PWS and requires management by a sleep specialist. Increasingly it is recognized that excessive daytime sleepiness and features of narcolepsy contribute to irritability and behavioral outbursts. Consideration of stimulants often used in narcolepsy may be helpful. In addition, psychiatric management requires strict environmental control. Use of medications such as selective serotonin reuptake inhibitors, which can be activating, requires care due to propensity to develop aggression and psychotic features. Diabetes can occur in the setting of obesity. Support groups include Foundation for Prader-Willi Research (https://www.fpwr.org) and Prader-Willi Syndrome Association USA (https://www.pwsausa.org).

Beckwith-Wiedemann syndrome

Beckwith-Wiedemann syndrome (BWS; or exomphalos, macroglossia, gigantism syndrome) was initially described by Wiedemann in 1964 and Beckwith in 1969 (Beckwith, 1969). Major findings in BWS include macrosomia, macroglossia, lateralized overgrowth, omphalocele or umbilic hernia, embryonal tumor in childhood, visceromegaly involving intraabdominal organs, cytomegaly of the fetal adrenal cortex, renal anomalies (including structural differences), nephromegaly, nephrocalcinosis, and/or later development of medullary sponge kidney, anterior linear ear lobe creases, and/or posterior helic ear pits. Minor criteria include pregnancy-related findings (including polyhydramnios and prematurity), neonatal hypoglycemia, vascular lesions (including nevus simplex or hemangiomas), characteristic facies (including midface retrusion and infraorbital creases), structural cardiac anomalies, diastasis recti, and advanced bone age. Diagnosis prompts implementation of screening for embryonal tumors. Tumors occur in 4% to 7% and include Wilms tumor, adrenal carcinoma, gonadoblastoma, and hepatoblastoma. Even with a classic presentation in the newborn period there is spontaneous resolution of many of the problems, the omphalocele after surgical correction, and macroglossia with time. The chromosomal localization involves an imprinted region of critical genes located on chromosome 11p15.5. BWS is heterogeneous; 85% of cases are sporadic, but in some there is an apparent autosomal dominant inheritance with variable expressivity. In other cases contiguous gene duplication at 11p15 results from a defect of maternal gene expression or specific mutations in the p57 *(CDKNIC)* or in the *NSD1* gene. Microdeletions, including methylation of *H19*, can also cause BWS by loss of *IGF2* imprinting, as can microdeletion of the entire *LIT1* gene. Increased risk of BWS is associated with assistive reproductive technology. Diagnostic testing by methylation studies of the 11p15.5 region can identify approximately 75% of affected individuals. Reflex testing to include sequencing of the *CDKN1C* gene should be performed if methylation studies are normal (Shuman et al., 2000/2016).

Development may be compromised by hypoxemia or profound hypoglycemia in the newborn period. In most individuals with BWS development is normal. There may be an increased risk of neurodevelopmental concerns, including attention-deficit/hyperactivity disorder (ADHD).

Management needs to address the airway, feeding, and speech problems if there is significant macroglossia. Scoliosis may be manifested in adolescence. It is important to screen for hepatoblastoma by serum alpha-fetoprotein determinations every 3 months in the first 3 years and to screen for other embryonal tumors with a complete abdominal ultrasound examination quarterly until 7 years of age. Specific genetic subtypes, in particular, uniparental disomy of 11p15 or gain of methylation at IC1 are at highest risk of Wilms tumor and hepatoblastoma. Loss of methylation at IC2 is associated with a lower risk for tumor development. Identification of intragenic variants on the maternally inherited copy of *CDKN1C* is associated with neuroblastoma, ganglioneuroblastoma, and acute lymphocytic leukemia.

Support groups include Beckwith-Wiedemann Children's Foundation (www.beckwith-wiedemannsyndrome.org) and Beckwith-Wiedemann Syndrome Family Forum (www.beckwith-wiedemann.info).

Silver-Russell Syndrome

Silver-Russell syndrome (SRS) was first described by Silver in 1953 and Russell in 1954 and originally thought to be unique disorders. Suggestive findings include small size for gestational age, postnatal growth failure, relative macrocephaly at birth, frontal bossing with a prominent forehead, body asymmetry (limb length discrepancy), and feeding difficulties. Features suggestive of the condition include triangular facies, fifth-finger clinodactyly, and micrognathia with narrow chin. Hypoglycemia may require aggressive management. Other features include gastroesophageal reflux disease, oral motor challenges, feeding aversion, and poor appetite. Genitourinary abnormalities may require management by a multidisciplinary team specializing in disorders of sexual development. Growth failure is proportionate, and head growth is normal. The Netchine-Harbison Clinical Scoring System (NH-CSS) is utilized as a diagnostic scoring system. Clinical diagnosis is established in an individual who meets at least four of the NH-CSS clinical criteria—prominent forehead/frontal bossing and relative macrocephaly at birth plus two additional findings—and in whom other disorders have been ruled out (Saal et al., 2002/2019).

The chromosomal localization involves an imprinted region of critical genes located on chromosome 11p15.5. Genetic testing is consistent with hypomethylation on chromosome 11p15.5 or maternal uniparental disomy of chromosome 7. Recently, maternal uniparental disomy of chromosome 16 was reported in association with an RSS phenotype. If initial testing is unrevealing, consideration of a multigene panel with *IGF1, CDKN1C, PLAG1*, and *HMGA2* should be considered. An underlying molecular cause is only identified in 60% of cases.

Developmental concerns include motor and cognitive delays and learning disabilities. Speech delays appear to be the most common. A multidisciplinary team includes genetics, endocrinology, feeding specialists, otolaryngology, urology, dental, and developmental pediatricians. Treatment includes growth hormone therapy, management of hypoglycemia, comprehensive feeding management (including nutritional supplements), treatment of gastroesophageal reflux disease, appetite stimulants, and monitoring/management of limb length discrepancy. Referral for early interventional therapies and an individualized education plan are required to manage delays. Psychological counseling is needed to address psychosocial concerns.

Support groups include Silver-Russell Syndrome Global Alliance (https://silverrussellsyndrome.org) and The Magic Foundation (https://www.magicfoundation.org/Growth-Disorders/Russell-Silver-Syndrome/).

MENDELIAN DISORDERS OF THE EPIGENETIC MACHINERY

The Mendelian disorders of the epigenetic machinery are most often characterized by intellectual disability. They result from mutations in genes encoding components of the epigenetic machinery. These include DNA methylation and histone machinery. Genes are classified as writers, erasers, or readers of epigenetic marks and chromatin remodelers (Table 24.1).

Somatic Mosaicism

Mosaicism occurs when there is a postzygotic change in which a mutation in a single cell gives rise to unique clonal descendants. This can impact any cell or tissue within a developing embryo and occur at any point making it challenging to assess the extent of involved tissue. It can be purely isolated to the tissues of the embryo (somatic) or restricted to the germline (germline mosaicism), or present in both. These delineations are very challenging, as failure to isolate the mutation in a subset of cells from a readily accessible tissue such as blood or buccal cells does not rule out its presence, especially in the germline. Perhaps the best example of a syndrome associated with somatic mutations that manifests often with developmental concerns includes PIK3CA-associated segmental overgrowth disorders of the brain, namely megalencephaly-capillary malformation (MCAP) syndrome. Characteristic features of MCAP include megalencephaly associated with neurologic findings of hypotonia, seizures, and mild to severe intellectual disability and cutaneous capillary malformations with focal or generalized overgrowth. Additional findings can include digital anomalies (syndactyly, polydactyly) and cortical malformations such as polymicrogyria (Fig. 24.3). The appearance of segmental or patchy abnormalities of the skin may alert the provider to consider mosaicism and obtaining more clearly affected tissue such as the skin for genetic testing.

Mendelian Genetic Syndromes and Conditions

Rasopathies

Approximately, 1 in 1000 newborns are impacted by germline or somatic gain-of-function mutations in the components of the RAS-mitogen-activated protein kinase (RAS/MAPK) pathway, which result in developmental disorders categorized as the rasopathies. This is due to the essential role of this pathway in proliferation, differentiation, and migration in the central nervous system. Neurodevelopmental disabilities associated with these disorders include developmental delay, seizures, neurocognitive deficits, and structural malformations.

Neurofibromatosis Type I

Neurofibromatosis (von Recklinghausen neurofibromatosis or NF1) was described by Crowe and associates (1956) in individuals who had at least six café au lait spots of more than 1.5 cm in diameter. National Institutes of Health clinical guidelines for diagnosis of NF1 include at least two of the following: (1) six café au lait spots of more than 5 mm in diameter, (2) axillary or inguinal freckling, (3) Lisch nodules (hamartomatous tufts of pigment on the iris) in individuals older than 10 years, (4) optic glioma, (5) bony pseudarthrosis (particularly the tibia), (6) skin neurofibromas or a plexiform neurofibroma of the subcutaneous tissues, and (7) first-degree relative with neurofibromatosis.

Infants may have a few café au lait spots, but by 3 years of age, axillary and inguinal freckling becomes more common. Median age at onset of optic gliomas is 4 years, and Lisch nodules and neurofibromas may not appear until after adolescence. Scoliosis may require surgery in adolescence, and pain and paresthesias from neurofibromas become a primary problem in early adulthood. There are no current standard treatments of neurofibromatosis, but many clinical studies are under way to evaluate treatment protocols. Neurofibromatosis occurs in all populations at an incidence of approximately 1 in 3500 live births. Fifty percent of cases appear to be new mutations, but that may be difficult to determine without mutation analysis of the gene *NF1* at 17q11.2 that codes for neurofibrin,

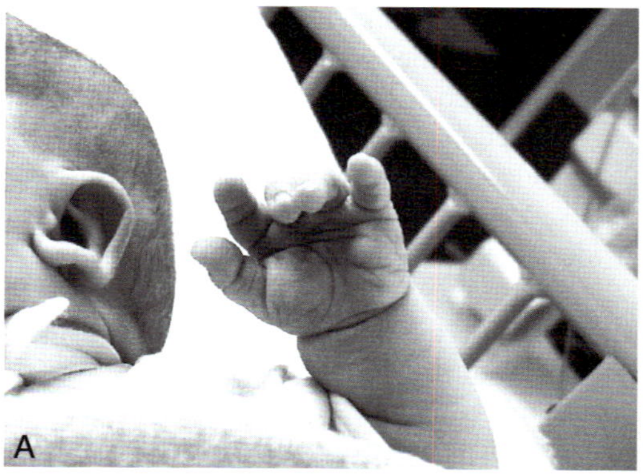
A

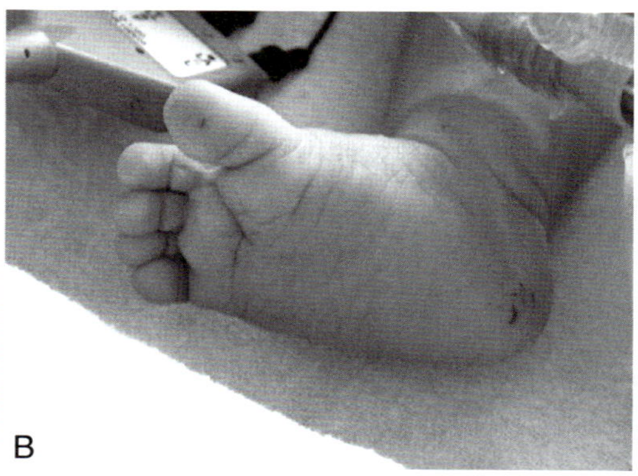
B

Fig. 24.3 Costello syndrome, 4-month-old girl.

TABLE 24.1 Mendelian Disorders of the Epigenetic Machinery

Disorder	Gene	Clinical Features	Developmental Features	Prevalence	Inheritance	References
Writers: Introduce Various Chemical Modifications on DNA and Histones						
Kabuki syndrome 1	*KMTD2* *KDM6A**	Postnatal growth deficiency; congenital heart defects; genitourinary anomalies; gastrointestinal anomalies, including anal atresia, ptosis, and strabismus; typical facial features (long palpebral fissures with eversion of the lateral third of the lower eyelid, arched and broad eyebrows, short columella, large and prominent or cupped ears), persistent of fetal finger pads	Intellectual disability commonly mild to moderate; deficits in comprehension and expressive language, deficits in adaptive skills, audio-verbal learning is a strength; ADHD, reports of autism	1:32,000–1:86,000	AD X-linked*	Adam, M. P., Hudgins, L., & Hannibal, M. (2011/2019). Kabuki syndrome. In M. P. Adam, H. H. Ardinger, R. A. Pagon, et al. (Eds.), ***GeneReviews***. University of Washington. https://www.ncbi.nlm.nih.gov/sites/books/NBK62111/
Kleefstra syndrome	*EHMT1* ~50% are due to a heterozygous deletion of 9q34.3	Childhood hypotonia, distinctive facial features, hypermetropia, congenital heart defects, GU anomalies, severe respiratory infections, epilepsy/febrile seizures, psychiatric disorders, extreme apathy or catatonic-like features after puberty	Intellectual disability moderate to severe; severe expressive language delay, autistic-like features; mood and psychotic disorders	1:120,000 with neurodevelopmental disorder	AD	Kleefstra, T., & de Leeuw, N. (2010/2019). Kleefstra syndrome. In M. P. Adam, H. H. Ardinger, R. A. Pagon, et al. (Eds.), ***GeneReviews***. University of Washington. https://www.ncbi.nlm.nih.gov/books/NBK47079/
Sotos syndrome	*NSD1*	Distinctive facial appearance, overgrowth (height and/or head circumference >2 SD above the mean), advanced bone age, cardiac anomalies, cranial MRI/CT abnormalities, hypermobile joints, renal anomalies, scoliosis, seizures	Developmental delay, mild to severe intellectual disability; autism spectrum disorder	1:14,000 live births	AD	Tatton-Brown, K., Cole, T. R. P., & Rahman, N. (2004/2019). Sotos syndrome. In M. P. Adam, H. H. Ardinger, R. A. Pagon, et al. (Eds.), ***GeneReviews***. University of Washington. https://www.ncbi.nlm.nih.gov/books/NBK1479/
Rubinstein-Taybi syndrome	*CREBBP* *EP300*	Distinctive facial features, broad and often angulated thumbs and halluces, failure to thrive in first few months of life, short stature, ocular anomalies, hearing loss, respiratory difficulties, congenital heart defects, GU anomalies, recurrent infection and severe constipation, obesity	Moderate-to-severe intellectual disability; behavioral features include impulsivity, distractibility, instability of mood and stereotypies, autistic-like behavior (62%) and anxiety	1:100,000–1:125,000 in the Netherlands	AD	Stevens, C. A. (2002/2019). Rubinstein-Taybi syndrome. In M. P. Adam, H. H. Ardinger, R. A. Pagon, et al. (Eds.), ***GeneReviews***. University of Washington. https://www.ncbi.nlm.nih.gov/books/NBK1526/

(continued)

TABLE 24.1 Mendelian Disorders of the Epigenetic Machinery

Disorder	Gene	Clinical Features	Developmental Features	Prevalence	Inheritance	References
Koolen-De Vries syndrome	*KANSL1*	Psychomotor developmental delay, neonatal/childhood hypotonia, dysmorphic features, hypermobility, hypermetropia, deformities of the spine and/or feet, epilepsy, GU anomalies, congenital heart defects	Mild to moderate intellectual disability, speech delay, behavior is friendly and cooperative	1:55,000	AD	Koolen, D. A., Morgan, A., & de Vries, B. B. A. (2010/2019). Koolen-de Vries syndrome. In M. P. Adam, H. H. Ardinger, R. A. Pagon, et al. (Eds.), *GeneReviews*. University of Washington. https://www.ncbi.nlm.nih.gov/books/NBK24676/
Erasers: The Specialized Domain Containing Proteins That Identify and Interpret Those Modifications						
Townes-Brocks syndrome	*SALL1*	Imperforate anus, dysplastic ears, sensorineural or conductive hearing loss, thumb malformations, renal disease with or without malformations, congenital heart disease, foot malformations, GU anomalies	Intellectual disability in 10%	1:250,000	AD	Kohlhase, J. (2007/2016). Townes-Brocks syndrome. (2007/2016). In M. P. Adam, H. H. Ardinger, R. A. Pagon, et al. (Eds.), *GeneReviews*. University of Washington. https://www.ncbi.nlm.nih.gov/books/NBK1445/
Readers: Dedicated Group of Enzymes Proficient in Removing These Chemical Tags						
Smith-Magenis syndrome	*RAI1* ~majority have a heterozygous 17p11.2 deletion that includes *RAI1*	Distinctive physical features, feeding difficulties, failure to thrive, hypotonia, hyporeflexia, prolonged napping, generalized low level of activity, developmental delay, intellectual disability, childhood-onset abdominal obesity	Mild to moderative intellectual disability, behavioral abnormalities, including stereotypies, maladaptive and self-injurious behaviors, sensory issues, anxiety, ADHD, frequent outbursts, sleep disturbance	1:15,000	Autosomal dominant	Smith, A. C. M., Boyd, K. E., Brennan, C., et al. (2001/2019). Smith-Magenis syndrome. In M. P. Adam, H. H. Ardinger, R. A. Pagon, et al. (Eds.), *GeneReviews*. University of Washington. https://www.ncbi.nlm.nih.gov/books/NBK1310/
Rett syndrome	*MECP2*	Developmental stagnation starting at 6–18 mo, regression in language and motor skills, repetitive, stereotypic hand movements replace purposeful hand use, fits of screaming and inconsolable crying, episodic apnea and/or hyperpnea, gait ataxia and apraxia, tremors, seizures, acquired microcephaly, abnormal tone, involuntary movements	Severe intellectual disability, autistic features, panic-like attacks, bruxism, developmental regression	1:10,000–1:23,000 female births	X linked	Kaur, S., & Christodoulou, J. (2001/2019). *MECP2* disorders. In M. P. Adam, H. H. Ardinger, R. A. Pagon, et al. (Eds.), *GeneReviews*. University of Washington. https://www.ncbi.nlm.nih.gov/books/NBK1497/

(continued)

TABLE 24.1 Mendelian Disorders of the Epigenetic Machinery

Disorder	Gene	Clinical Features	Developmental Features	Prevalence	Inheritance	References
Remoderlers: Nucleosome Maintenance						
CHD2-related neurodevelopmental disorders	*CHD2*	Early-onset epileptic encephalopathy (6 mo–4 yr), associated regression	Cognitive slowing or regression with onset of seizures, autism spectrum disorders common	1:91,862 Danish births	AD	Khaikin, Y., & Mercimek-Andrews, S. (2016). *STXBP1* encephalopathy with epilepsy. In M. P. Adam, H. H. Ardinger, R. A. Pagon, et al. (Eds.), ***GeneReviews***. University of Washington. https://www.ncbi.nlm.nih.gov/books/NBK396561/
CHARGE syndrome	*CHD7*	Coloboma, heart defect, choanal atresia, retarded growth and development, genital hypoplasia, ear anomalies (hearing loss common), cranial nerve anomalies, seizures, GU anomalies, cleft lip and/or palate, hypothyroidism, tracheoesophageal anomalies	Developmental delay, intellectual disability, delayed motor milestones may be secondary to sensory and balance deficits	1:8500–1:15,000	AD	van Ravenswaaij-Arts, C. M., Hefner, M., & Blake, K., et al. (2006/2020). CHD7 disorder. In M. P. Adam, H. H. Ardinger, R. A. Pagon, et al. (Eds.), ***GeneReviews***. University of Washington. https://www.ncbi.nlm.nih.gov/books/NBK1117/
Alpha-thalassemia X-linked intellectual disability syndrome	*ATRX*	Distinctive craniofacial features, genital abnormalities, hypotonia, developmental delay, intellectual disability, mild alpha-thalassemia in 75%, osteosarcoma, growth impairment including microcephaly and short stature, GU anomalies	Mild to profound developmental delay/intellectual disability	>200 worldwide	X linked	Stevenson, R. E. (2000/2020). Alpha-thalassemia X-linked intellectual disability syndrome. In M. P. Adam, H. H. Ardinger, R. A. Pagon, et al. (Eds.), ***GeneReviews***. University of Washington. https://www.ncbi.nlm.nih.gov/books/NBK1449/
Floating-harbor syndrome	*SRCAP*	Typical craniofacial features, low birthweight, short stature, bone age delay, skeletal abnormalities, hyperopia and/or strabismus, conductive hearing loss, seizures, gastroesophageal reflux, GU anomalies	Severe receptive and expressive language impairment; hypernasality and high-pitched voice, mild to moderate intellectual disabilities; difficulties with temperament and behavior	Unknown	AD	Nowaczyk, M. J. M., Nikkel, S. M., & White, S. M. (2012/2019). Floating-harbor syndrome. In M. P. Adam, H. H. Ardinger, R. A. Pagon, et al. (Eds.), ***GeneReviews***. University of Washington. https://www.ncbi.nlm.nih.gov/books/NBK114458/

AD, Autosomal dominant; ***ADHD***, attention-deficit/hyperactivity disorder; ***GU***, genitourinary; ***MRI/CT***, magnetic resonance imaging/computed tomography; ***SD***, standard deviation.
*KDM6A is often called Kabuki syndrome type 2. It is X linked. It would more appropriately be placed in the category of the eraser.

a tumor suppressor protein. Most disease is thought to be due to a constitutional mutation resulting in truncation of the neurofibrin protein. This protein is a critical substrate in many important signaling pathways, and deficient protein results in insufficient tumor suppressors. At this time, there is limited genotype-phenotype correlation; however, DNA testing to identify a mutation or large deletion in an affected family member can be beneficial in prenatal diagnosis when there is a 50% recurrence risk.

Developmental manifestations show a wide variability of phenotypic expression. Of patients with NF1, 25% to 50% may have learning disabilities, and 5% to 10% have intellectual disabilities. Some neurologic and developmental problems are specifically related to the degree of central nervous system involvement with tumors; but even in individuals with no identifiable central nervous system abnormalities there is an increased likelihood of learning problems. Social communication ability is a challenge in this disorder. Reports vary, but individuals with NF1 have as high as a four- to fivefold increased risk of ASDs when studied in large population databases. These individuals were significantly less likely to receive a community-based ASD diagnosis and understand nonverbal communication. In addition, individuals with NF1 are more likely to have attention-deficit disorder of the inattentive type that may be underrecognized.

The National Institutes of Health consensus management guidelines include monitoring for tumors, especially optic glioma in a young child, by ophthalmologic examination and diagnostic imaging studies. Monitoring of children for hypertension due to renal arterial dysplasia can be critical. Multidisciplinary follow-up of children by specialists in pediatrics, neurology, and orthopedics and developmental specialists is recommended. When to perform brain magnetic resonance imaging needs to depend on the neurologic examination findings and reported symptoms. Teachers, therapists, and early infant evaluation and therapy are indicated on an individual basis. Support groups include Children's Tumor Foundation (www.ctf.org) and Neurofibromatosis, Inc. (www.nfinc.org).

Noonan Syndrome

Noonan syndrome (NS) was first described by Jacqueline Noonan, a cardiologist who had noted that children with valvular pulmonic stenosis shared the characteristic physical appearance with short stature, webbed neck, hypertelorism, and low-set ears. In 1968 Noonan published "Hypertelorism With Turner Phenotype." Characteristic features of NS include short stature, congenital heart disease (pulmonary valve stenosis often with dysplasia; atrial and ventricular septal defects, branch pulmonary artery stenosis, and tetralogy of Fallot), hypertrophic cardiomyopathy (20%–30%), developmental delay, webbed neck, pectus deformities of the chest, cryptorchidism, coagulation defects, lymphatic dysplasias, and ocular abnormalities.

Developmental features include mild intellectual disability and, in particular, language impairments. Joint hyperextensibility and hypotonia contribute to a delay in developmental milestones. The average age of sitting unsupported is 10 months and for walking is 21 months. Fifty percent of individuals meet the diagnostic criteria for a developmental coordination disorder, and impaired manual dexterity is significantly correlated with verbal and nonverbal intellectual functioning. Twenty-five percent have learning disabilities, and 10% to 15% require special education. Intellectual disabilities are generally mild. Articulation difficulties are common. Language delay can be related to hearing loss, perceptual motor disabilities, or articulation difficulties. The average age of first words is around 15 months, and two-word phrases on average emerge at 31 to 32 months.

NS is an autosomal dominant disorder. There are many genes associated with this diagnosis, including *PTPN11* (50%), *SOS1* (13%), *RAF1* (5%), *RITI* (5%), *BRAF, LZTR1, MAP2K1, NRAS*, and *RRAS2*. Management requires a multidisciplinary team, including genetics, developmental medicine, cardiology, urology, endocrinology, occupational, physical, and speech therapies. Growth hormone is of benefit for short stature. Guidelines for management are available at Dyscerne—Noonan Syndrome Guideline Development Group (https://rasopathiesnet.org/wp-content/uploads/2014/01/265_Noonan_Guidelines.pdf).

Costello Syndrome

Costello syndrome (fasciocutaneous skeletal syndrome) is due to a germline mutation in an *HRAS* gene that normally causes cancer when it is affected by somatic mutations. Costello syndrome was initially described by Costello (1977) with "mental subnormality and nasal papillomata." Clinical features include dysmorphic facies with epicanthal folds, depressed nasal bridge, broad mouth and coarse features, normal head circumference but short stature, developmental delay, and intellectual disability with cutis laxa and deep soft creases in the palms and soles (Fig. 24.4). Cardiac malformations are often complicated by dysrhythmias and hypertrophic cardiomyopathy. Benign tumors such as nasolabial, perioral, and anal papillomas are common, and malignant tumors (ganglioneuroblastoma, bladder cancer, embryonal rhabdomyosarcoma, and other malignant neoplasms) occur in up to 17% of mutation-positive cases. Individuals may present *in utero* with polyhydramnios,

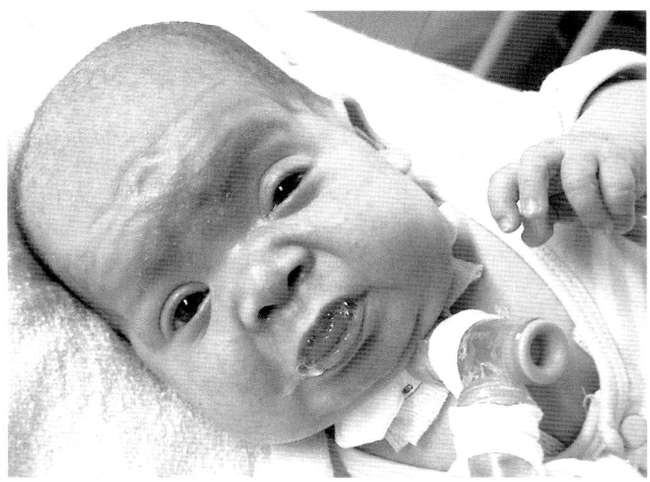

Fig. 24.4 Costello syndrome at age 4 months.

macrosomia, and occasionally cardiac arrhythmias. Infantile hypotonia and failure to thrive require gastrostomy tube placement in half of cases. Features are suggestive of ASD in early infancy, and this improves by age 4 years. In childhood developmental delay with coarsening facial features and papillomas develop; by adolescence, short stature, intellectual disability, characteristic facies with nasolabial papillomas, and thick, coarse, darkened skin on the hands and feet are apparent. Diagnosis is established by molecular testing of the *HRAS* gene, which localizes to 11p15.5. Almost all cases at this time have been sporadic. Rare sibling reports are most likely due to germline mosaicism (Gripp& Rauen, 2006/2019).

Developmental problems in the neonatal period include oral motor incoordination and hypotonia that frequently lead to failure to thrive. Global delay in gross and fine motor skills becomes apparent with median age of walking at 2 years and talking at 4 years. Final IQs generally are in the mild to moderate range of intellectual disability. It is notable that many infants and children with this disorder have a unique interpersonally interactive, pleasant, and engaging personality. Management includes cardiac monitoring throughout life as well as a low threshold for evaluation for malignant neoplasms. There are no clear cancer screening guidelines, but abdominal and pelvic ultrasounds are recommended to screen for rhabdomyosarcoma and neuroblastoma every 3 to 6 months until age 8, in addition to annual urinalysis for evidence of hematuria to screen for bladder cancer starting at age 10. Assistance is available with the Costello Syndrome Support Group (www.costellokids.com).

Cardiofaciocutaneous Syndrome

Cardiofaciocutaneous (CFC) syndrome is caused by mutation in four known genes, including *BRAF* (75%), *MAP2K1* and *MAP2K2* (25%), and *KRAS* (<2%). Clinical features include congenital heart disease (pulmonic stenosis, septal defects, hypertrophic cardiomyopathy, rhythm disturbances); dysmorphic features; cutaneous anomalies (xerosis, hyperkeratosis, ichthyosis, keratosis pilaris, eczema, pigmented moles, hemangiomas, palmoplantar hyperkeratosis); sparse, curly, fine, or thick woolly or brittle hair; eyelashes or eyebrows that are absent or sparse; dystrophic or fast-growing nails; cognitive disabilities from mild to severe; and an increased risk of malignancy (acute lymphoblastic leukemia) (Rauen, 2007/2016).

Intellectual disability varies from mild to severe. Hypotonia and developmental delays are common. Additional neurologic findings include seizures, abnormal electroencephalogram, cortical tract findings, hydrocephalus, frontal lobe hypoplasia, agenesis of the corpus callosum, abnormal myelination, Chiari malformation, and pachygyria.

Management requires care by a multidisciplinary team, including cardiology, genetics, dermatology, gastroenterology and nutrition, endocrinology, orthopedics, ophthalmology, developmental medicine, neurology, occupational, physical, and speech therapies. Treatments include consideration of growth hormone, regular echocardiograms and electrocardiograms, and monitoring for scoliosis. Support can be found at CFC International (https://www.cfcsyndrome.org).

Connective Tissue Disorders

Connective tissue disorders typically affect the cardiovascular system, eyes, skeleton, lungs, skin, and dura mater. Cognitively individuals are most often typical; however, developmental disabilities may be associated with some disorders such as Shprintzen-Goldberg syndrome and homocystinuria. Some may have neuropsychiatric manifestations at rates greater than predicted in the general population such as Marfan syndrome, which appears to be associated with an increased risk of schizophrenia (Lemberg & Thompson, 2010; Van Den Bossche et al., 2012).

Marfan Syndrome

Marfan syndrome (type 1) includes a group of connective tissue disorders predominantly due to fibrillin 1 abnormalities. Marfan (1896) described the first classic patients; Boerger (1914) first noted ectopia lentis; and McKusick (1956) delineated cardiovascular complications. Fibrillin 1 is a protein found in almost every tissue. Mutations in the gene *FBN1* include cardiovascular, skeletal, and eye manifestations. Other tissues frequently involved are the skin, lungs, and dura of the central nervous system. Classic features of Marfan syndrome type 1 include dilation or dissection in the aorta at the level of the sinus of Valsalva, myopia with ectopia lentis, scoliosis with pectus excavatum or carinatum, arachnodactyly of the fingers and toes, spontaneous pneumothorax, dural ectasia, and striae or stretch marks of the skin. Other typical skeletal manifestations include disproportionate stature with an upper/lower segment ratio of less than 0.86 and a facial gestalt with a long narrow face, high arched palate, and crowded teeth. The phenotype evolves with age so that infants may have only skeletal or cardiac findings; toddlers may have a characteristic facial gestalt, myopia, and stretchy skin; and a 5-year-old may have mitral valve prolapse and lax joints. In contrast, a 14-year-old first diagnosed with a fibrillinopathy may present with only mildly disproportionate but not necessarily tall stature, spontaneous pneumothorax, pectus excavatum, mildly dilated aortic outlet, and high myopia. In adults who have not been previously recognized fibrillinopathy may present as spontaneous ruptured thoracic aorta, dislocated lens, glaucoma, cataracts, arthritis, varicosities, and life-threatening complications in pregnancy, including uterine rupture. The incidence of type 1 fibrillinopathies is approximately 1 in 5000 to 10,000 with no ethnic, geographic, or gender preference. The gene *FBN1* is located at 15q11.2 and codes for the elastin protein fibrillin 1. A mutation in *FBN1* is found by sequencing in approximately 93% of individuals who have clinical findings of Marfan syndrome type 1. Marfan syndrome type 2, also called Loeys-Dietz syndrome (LDS), is due to mutations in transforming growth factor-beta receptor 2. Often these patients have additional manifestations, such as craniosynostosis, hypertelorism, bifid uvula/cleft palate, cutaneous findings, and congenital heart malformations. Congenital Marfan syndrome presents in the first 6 months of life. Loss of the central coding region for the protein appears to result in this more severe and potentially life-threatening form of the disorder, whereas errors in C-terminal processing primarily cause only skeletal manifestations.

Intellectual disability, hypotonia, and epilepsy may be more prevalent in hypochondroplasia and may present prior to disproportionate short state. Frequently, achondroplasia is sporadic and may be associated with advanced paternal age. Homozygous mutations are lethal *in utero* or in early infancy. Although most children with achondroplasia are cognitively normal, developmental issues may be seen. Lax joints and low muscle tone contribute to early apparent gross motor developmental delay. In addition, hydrocephalus due to narrowing at the foramen magnum may lead to more generalized delays. Short broad hands and lax joints often contribute to initial fine motor delays, and recurrent otitis media due to eustachian tube dysfunction leads to chronic hearing loss and can affect speech development. Psychological problems stemming from body image issues complicated by neurologic and musculoskeletal problems need to be addressed.

Management guidelines include prenatal genetic counseling, with chorionic villus sampling, amniocentesis, or cord blood sampling for mutation analysis if identification is made by ultrasound examination early or if one of the parents has achondroplasia. A genetic skeletal survey in the newborn period often can confirm a clinical diagnosis. Because up to 4% of individuals with achondroplasia may die in the first year of a combination of obstructive and central apnea, early measurement of the foramen magnum with magnetic resonance imaging and sleep study are recommended by 6 months of age or earlier, regardless of clinical symptoms such as snoring, nighttime apnea, and extensor posturing that may increase the urgency of diagnostic studies. Audiologic evaluation is repeated by 6 months, and aggressive treatment of recurrent otitis media and neurosurgical, orthopedic, and pulmonary problems is performed as needed. Recently, guidance to management was updated by the American Academy of Pediatrics. Support groups include the Human Growth Foundation (www.hgfound.org), Little People of America (www.lpaonline.org), and The Magic Foundation (www.magicfoundation.org).

Multifactorial Conditions

Multifactorial disorders are those that can be differentiated from conditions that follow Mendelian inheritance patterns. Characteristics of these disorders include interaction with environmental factors that may modify the risk of the disease and concordance rates among monozygotic and dizygotic twins that contradict rates predicted when Mendelian inheritance is present. The disease may have a gender predilection, and first-degree relatives of the individual more rarely impacted have a risk of being affected and impact a specific ethnic group. Examples of disordered multifactorial etiologies include ASDs in some cases, coronary artery disease, obesity cleft lip and palate, and congenital heart disease.

Cleft Lip and Palate

Cleft lip with or without cleft palate is usually due to multiple genes and often unknown environmental factors. Incidence of cleft lip with or without cleft palate is 1 in 1000 live births. There are more than 500 different syndromes that may be associated with clefting. Cleft lip is more common among Asian (1.7 per 1000) and American Indian (3.6 per 1000) live births. It is less common than average in Blacks at 1 in 2500. Males are more frequently affected than are females. Cleft palate with or without cleft lip occurs in approximately 1 in 2000 births and is more common in females. Cleft palate is more likely than cleft lip to have a strongly inherited basis. Multiple genes are associated with both simple and syndromic cleft lip or cleft palate. Embryologically, the lip closes between 5 and 6 weeks and the palate by 10 weeks of gestation. Women with seizure disorders who take anticonvulsant medications have an increased risk of facial clefting, as do individuals with alcohol exposure or maternal glucose intolerance. Multifactorial recurrence for a couple with no family history and one child with cleft lip or palate is approximately 3% to 5%. This is the same as the occurrence for offspring of individuals with simple clefting. If the clefting is associated with a specific syndrome, however, the recurrence is much more difficult to predict and depends on the specific underlying diagnosis. For example, with autosomal dominant van der Woude syndrome, although the gene is inherited by 50% of the offspring, the specific occurrence of clefting depends on the penetrance of that gene in the family. Penetrance is calculated by comparing the number of individuals who have the gene with the members who actually have cleft lip or palate. For most multifactorial clefts in which neither parent has a cleft, the recurrence risk actually varies between 2% and 8%. Genetic testing is often unrevealing unless there is an association with a specific condition, such as deletion 22q11.2 syndrome; Di George syndrome needs to be considered if there appears to be a familial pattern for velopharyngeal insufficiency, especially with cardiac problems observed by history, family history, or physical examination. Testing of most children with cleft palate for deletion 22 is reasonable, and as array comparative genomic hybridization (CGH) becomes more refined and cost effective, panels to look at syndromic or nonsyndromic clefting genes will also become more readily available.

For simple nonsyndromic clefting, developmental issues are related to speech and language complicated by palatal insufficiency and articulation. There may be additional structural malformations of the oropharynx, tongue, and lip compounded by conductive hearing loss due to eustachian tube dysfunction and chronic ear infections that compromise speech and language development.

Management is optimized by a multidisciplinary team, including specialists in plastic surgery, oral surgery, dentistry, speech pathology, occupational therapy (particularly for feeding issues), genetics, and education. Support groups for children with facial clefts include Operation Smile, an international program for children with craniofacial anomalies (www.operationsmile.org), the Cleft Palate Foundation (www.cleftline.org), and the March of Dimes Birth Defects Resources (www.marchofdimes.com).

Congenital Heart Disease

Multiple genes have been identified for both syndromic and nonsyndromic congenital heart disease. One common gene *(VEGF)* is localized at chromosome 22q11.2/DiGeorge syndrome/deletion 22/velocardiofacial critical region. Mutations in *TBX1* in this region are also found in individuals with "conotruncal facial" syndrome with cardiac malformations. Teratogens causing congenital heart defects include maternal diabetes and alcohol. The incidence of congenital heart disease is approximately 1 in 125 live-born infants. Some children have heart defects on the basis of heart-face or heart-hand syndromes. The majority of children, however, do not have associated dysmorphic features. Genes, including variations in *HRAS* or *VEGF* or *TBX1*, contribute to a number of cardiac defects, including hypertrophic cardiomyopathy. All children with congenital heart defects should have chromosome analysis and array CGH. Because additional loci, such as the velocardiofacial locus at chromosome 10p, are being identified, there is potential for specific array CGH for nonsyndromic or syndromic congenital heart defects.

Developmental progress is compromised by early persistent cyanosis, failure to thrive, or chronic illness. Aggressive medical and surgical management and optimization of nutrition to minimize failure to thrive will also have an impact on development. All children with congenital heart defects need to have the benefit of multidisciplinary management, including specialists in pediatrics, cardiology, cardiac surgery, development, genetics, and therapies. Support groups include the March of Dimes Birth Defects Resources (www.marchofdimes.com) and the National Organization for Rare Disorders (www.rarediseases.org).

CHARGE Syndrome

CHARGE syndrome (CHARGE association or Hall-Hittner syndrome) is an acronym for the combination of *c*oloboma, *h*eart anomaly, choanal *a*tresia, *r*etardation, and *g*enital and *e*ar anomalies. Clinical features include ocular coloboma that can be peripupillary, iris, retinal, macular, or nerve; choanal atresia or stenosis; cranial nerve dysfunction; and characteristic small, posteriorly rotated, cupped simple ears. It is uncommon for a child to have all manifestations of this association. The term CHARGE should be restricted to infants with at least three major malformations, including choanal atresia or coloboma combined with cardinal malformations, heart, ear, and genital. Growth retardation, especially low birthweight, should not be used in the definition. The incidence of CHARGE syndrome is approximately 1 in 10,000, and gene localizations include chromosomes 8q12.1 and 7q21.1. The gene *CHD7*, chromodomain helicase DNA binding protein, at 8q21.1 is known to be associated with CHARGE syndrome, but other genes are no doubt also involved. The basic genetic mechanism, however, continues to be described as multifactorial because although the gene may be inherited in a dominant fashion, there are many other genes as well as known and unknown environmental factors that affect the expression of those genes. Diagnostic testing should include at least CGH array with high-resolution banded chromosomes, although most individuals will have normal results with these tests. Sequence analysis of *CHD7* coding region detects mutations in 60% to 65% of individuals. Large *CHD7* deletions, however, are uncommon. *CHD7* sequencing is possible and can be valuable for preconception counseling and prenatal diagnosis when the result is positive.

Most children with CHARGE association have delayed milestones and hypotonia. Development is complicated by dual sensory vision and hearing impairment as well as by vestibular dysfunction. Management in neonates requires immediate evaluation of airway, feeding, heart, and hearing. Tracheostomy or surgical correction of choanal atresia may often be necessary. Speech and language, occupational, nutrition, and physical therapies are important, and with failure to thrive, gastrostomy tube and nutrition services are critical. It is important to monitor hearing closely because children with CHARGE association can have normal IQ and be compromised by hearing and visual deficits. School and psychological services need to be provided by specialists in management of the deaf and blind. Special attention is often required for airway problems (even as older children) with anesthesia, and regular ophthalmologic and audiologic evaluations are important. Pubertal evaluation for hypogonadal hypogonadism is indicated in some children.

The support group is CHARGE Syndrome Foundation (www.chargesyndrome.org).

Neural Tube Defects

See Chapter 59 in which particularly folic acid prevention of neural tube defects is described.

Teratogens

Fetal Alcohol Syndrome

Refer to Chapter 37 for information on fetal alcohol syndrome.

Maternal Diabetes

There are specific effects of maternal glucose concentration and glucose intolerance that correlate with the three stages of alcohol embryopathy, depending on the timing of exposure: alcohol-related birth defects, fetal alcohol exposure, and fetal alcohol syndrome. First-trimester glucose intolerance can result in malformations, especially congenital heart defects. Maternal glucose intolerance in the second trimester can result in central nervous system, brain development, developmental, and learning issues. Third-trimester maternal glucose intolerance results in the classic infant of a gestational diabetic mother. Maternal glucose intolerance is becoming identified as a teratogen regardless of whether the mother has diabetes mellitus or is identified at 28 weeks to have gestational diabetes during gestation. Some birth defects may be due to first-trimester hypoglycemia in women with only a familial history of diabetic tendency. This can be evidently severe in infants with malformations when there is maternal obesity or genetic predisposition in a family, such as deletion 22q11.2. The website for the American Diabetes Association is www.diabetes.org.

VIGNETTE

Amanda's chromosomal microarray showed a 15q11.2q13 deletion. Follow-up methylation studies were consistent with Angelman syndrome.

REFERENCES

American Heart Association Rheumatic Fever, Endocarditis, and Kawasaki Disease Committee, American Heart Association Council on Cardiovascular Disease in the Young, American Heart Association Council on Clinical Cardiology, American Heart Association Council on Cardiovascular Surgery and Anesthesia, Quality of Care and Outcomes Research Interdisciplinary Working Group. (2007). Prevention of infective endocarditis: Guidelines from the American Heart Association: A guideline from the American Heart Association Rheumatic Fever, Endocarditis, and Kawasaki Disease Committee, Council on Cardiovascular Disease in the Young, and the Council on Clinical Cardiology, Council on Cardiovascular Surgery and Anesthesia, and the Quality of Care and Outcomes Research Interdisciplinary Working Group. *Circulation*, *116*, 1736–1754. (Erratum in 2007;116, e376–e377).

Angelman, H. (1965). Ueber zwei Falle von Arachnodaktylie. *Monatsschr Kinderheilk*, *13*, 335–

Beckwith, J. B. (1969). Macroglossia, omphalocele, adrenal cytomegaly, gigantism, and hyperplastic visceromegaly. *Birth Defects Original Article Series*, *5*(2), 188.

Boerger, F. (1914). Ueber zwei Falle von Arachnodaktylie. *Monatsschr Kinderheilk*, *13*, 335.

Cassidy, S., & Schwartz, S. (2006). *Prader-Willi syndrome: Gene tests/gene reviews*. University of Washington.

Crowe, F. W., Schull, W. J., & Neel, J. V. (1956). *A clinical, pathological, and genetic study of multiple neurofibromatosis*. Charles C Thomas Publishers.

Dagli, A. I., Mueller, J., & Williams, C. A. (1998/2017). Angelman syndrome. In M. P. Adam, H. H. Ardinger, & R. A. Pagon, et al. (Eds.), *GeneReviews*. University of Washington.

Driscoll, D. J., Miller, J. L., Schwartz, S., & Cassidy, S. B. (1998/2017). Prader-Willi syndrome. In M. P. Adam, H. H. Ardinger, & R. A. Pagon, et al. (Eds.), *GeneReviews*. University of Washington.

Fahrner, J. A., & Bjornsson, H. T. (2019). Mendelian disorders of the epigenetic machinery: Postnatal malleability and therapeutic prospects. *Human Molecular Genetics*, *28*(2), R254–R264.

Glorieux, F. H., Bishop, N. J., Plotkin, H., Chabot, G., Lanoue, G., & Travers, R. (1998). Cyclic administration of pamidronate in children with severe osteogenesis imperfecta. *New England Journal of Medicine*, *339*(14), 947–952.

Gripp, K. W., & Rauen, K. A. (2006/2019). Costello syndrome. In M. P. Adam, H. H. Ardinger, & R. A. Pagon, et al. (Eds.), *GeneReviews*. University of Washington.

Lemberg, M., & Thompson, A. W. (2010). Marfan syndrome and schizophrenia: A case report and literature review. *General Hospital Psychiatry*, *32*(2), 228. e9–228.e10.

Marfan, A., (1896). Un cas de déformation congénitgale des quatres membres, plus prononcée aux extremités, caractérisée par l'allongement des os avec un certain degré d'amincissiment. *Bulletins et memoires de la Société medicale des hôpitaux de Paris*, *13*, 220–228.

McKusick, V. A., (1956). *Heritable disorders of connective tissue* (1st ed.). Mosby.

Noonan, J. A., (1968). Hypertelorism with Turner phenotype. A new syndrome with associated congenital heart disease. *American Journal of Diseases of Children* (1960), *116*(4), 373–380.

Nussbaum, R. L., McInnes, R. R., Willard, H. F., Hamosh, A., & Thompson, M. W. (2007). *Thompson & Thompson genetics in medicine*. Saunders/Elsevier.

Rauen, K. A. (2007/2016). Cardiofaciocutaneous syndrome. In M. P. Adam, H. H. Ardinger, & R. A. Pagon, et al. (Eds.), *GeneReviews*. University of Washington.

Rossi, V., Lee, B., & Marom, R. (2019). Osteogenesis imperfecta—Advancements in genetics and treatment. *Current Opinion in Pediatrics*, *31*(6), 708–715.

Rousseau, F., Bonaventure, J., Legeai-Mallet, L., Pelet, A., Rozet, J., Maroteaux, P., Le Merrer, M., & Munnich, A. (1994). Mutations in the gene encoding fibroblast growth factor receptor-3 in achondroplasia. *Nature*, *371*, 252–254.

Saal, H. M., Harbison, M. D., & Netchine, I. (2002/2019). Silver-Russell syndrome. In M. P. Adam, H. H. Ardinger, & R. A. Pagon (Eds.), *GeneReviews*. University of Washington.

Shuman, C., Beckwith, J. B., & Weksberg, R. (2000/2016). Beckwith-Wiedemann syndrome. In M. P. Adam, H. H. Ardinger, & R. A. Pagon, et al. (Eds.), *GeneReviews*. University of Washington.

Sirota, P., Frydman, M., & Sirota, L. (1990). Schizophrenia and Marfan syndrome. *The British Journal of Psychiatry*, *157*, 433–436.

Van Den Bossche, M. J., Van Wallendael, K. L., Strazisar, M., Sabbe, B., & Del-Favero, J. (2012). Co-occurrence of Marfan syndrome and schizophrenia: What can be learned? *European Journal of Medical Genetics*, *55*(4), 252–255.

25

Chromosome Disorders and Inheritance Patterns

Aaina Kochhar and Naomi J.L. Meeks

For additional material related to the content of this chapter, please see Chapters 24, 26, and 27.

VIGNETTES

1. *A 32-year-old G1P0 is seen for a routine 20-week ultrasound. There is a history of multiple miscarriages in her own mother as well as her grandmother. She also has a maternal uncle with Down syndrome (trisomy 21). The ultrasound demonstrates fetal intrauterine growth retardation (IUGR), cystic hygroma, and likely double outlet right ventricle. The patient was then referred to a maternal fetal medicine center where follow-up fetal magnetic resonance imaging (MRI) confirmed the congenital heart defect and identified holoprosencephaly and a cleft lip. Amniocentesis was offered, and fluorescence in situ hybridization (FISH) studies confirmed trisomy 13. Follow-up karyotype demonstrated a fetal karyotype of 46,XY,t(13;21),+13. Maternal karyotype was performed identifying a balanced 13:21 Robertsonian translocation.*
2. *A 6-year-old boy comes to your developmental pediatrics clinic for management of attention-deficit/hyperactivity disorder (ADHD). Pregnancy and birth history are unremarkable. He met his motor milestones on time but has had speech delays first identified by around 18 months of age. He has delays in development and is not meeting grade-level expectations in his first-grade class; he still struggles with speech and is working on learning his letters and numbers. His parents and teachers report he is easily distracted. He is nondysmorphic and normally grown. His father reports that he also struggled with speech and ADHD as a child. As part of your management, you offer genetic testing with a chromosomal microarray based on his developmental delays. The result returns and identifies a 16p11.2 deletion.*

INTRODUCTION

Chromosomal disorders are an important cause of miscarriage in pregnancies and multiple congenital anomalies and developmental delays in the pediatric population. Understanding the genetics of chromosomal conditions and how to test for them is essential for providing comprehensive care in these patients. Though many are referred to genetic specialists for evaluation, other specialists such as developmental pediatricians may encounter these patients first and can play an important role in identifying diagnoses that have additional developmental, medical, and reproductive implications. In this chapter we address the different numeric and structural chromosomal abnormalities, patterns of inheritance, and cytogenetic techniques used to diagnose chromosomal disorders.

KARYOTYPE

Our genomic material (DNA) is organized into structures called chromosomes. There are 23 pairs with one-half of each pair from each parent. These can be visualized during mitosis under a microscope. To perform a karyotype, blood or other biologic sample (e.g., buccal cells, saliva, skin, products of conception, bone marrow, chorionic villi, or amniocyte) is treated in a cytogenetics laboratory with a mitogen to stimulate mitosis in preparation for cell division. Cells processed for routine (low-resolution) chromosome analysis are stained on glass slides to yield a light-and-dark band pattern across the arms of the chromosomes. This band pattern is characteristic and reproducible for each chromosome. With the use of different staining techniques, different banding patterns result: G, Q, and R banding. The most commonly used is G banding. The layout of chromosomes in a predetermined order is called a karyotype. The chromosomes are organized in pairs from largest to smallest in size. The largest chromosome pair is labeled "1" with the smallest chromosome pair labeled "22." Pair 23 is the sex chromosomes with two X chromosomes in a typical female and an X and a Y chromosome in a typical male (Fig. 25.1). The typical structure of a chromosome includes a short upper segment or arm (the p arm), a narrowed region in the middle (the centromere), and a longer lower segment (the q arm). The banding pattern is labeled from lowest number to highest starting from the centromere and moving distally to the ends of the chromosome. This allows a description of a location on a chromosome with accuracy and consistency. For example, 16p11.2 refers to the first band next to the centromere of the p arm on chromosome 16 (Fig. 25.2).

High-resolution chromosome analysis is the study of more elongated chromosomes in prometaphase of mitosis, which allows visualization of the banding pattern in greater detection of smaller, more subtle chromosome rearrangements. This technology is useful for determining abnormalities in structure and arrangement, including detection of extra or missing chromosomes, unbalanced rearrangements (deletions, duplications, translocations), and some balanced rearrangements (inversions, translocations). It can also detect

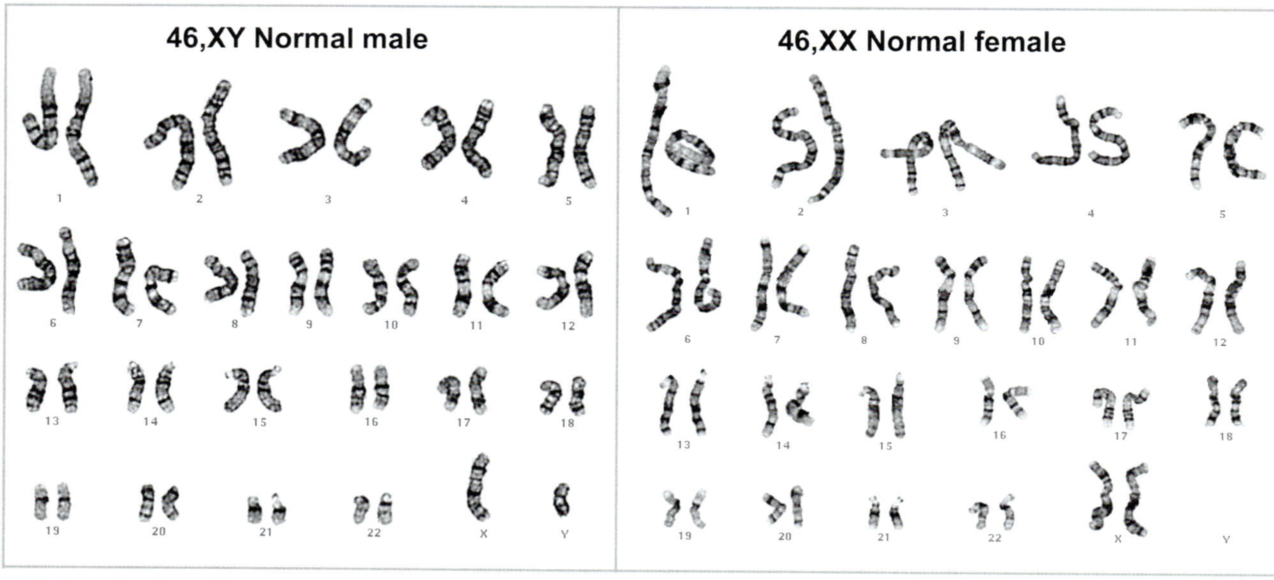

Fig. 25.1 Normal male and female karyotypes.

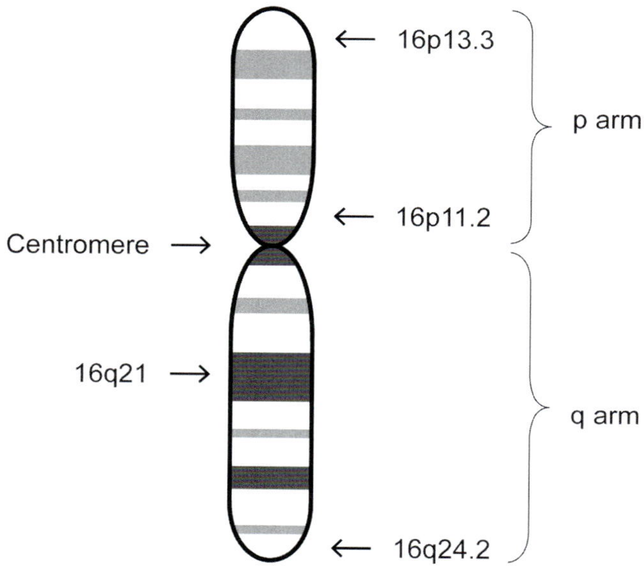

Fig. 25.2 Example of chromosome structure.

atypical structures such as a ring or marker chromosome, which is, respectively, a circular or extra structure that can include genetic material from any other chromosome. These are denoted with common symbols, including del (deletion), dup (duplication), inv (inversion), ish (*in situ* hybridization), i (isochromosome), pat (paternal origin), mat (maternal origin), and r (ring chromosome). A karyotype has limited utility, however, for detecting copy number variation for rearrangements of less than 5 Mb (million base pairs) in size.

FLUORESCENCE *IN SITU* HYBRIDIZATION

Karyotypes often take a week or more to result, and in some cases identification of abnormal overall chromosome number (aneuploidy) is important for clinical care particularly in the neonatal period. FISH is a powerful technique that labels a known chromosome sequence with DNA probes attached to fluorescent dyes, thus enabling visualization of specific regions of chromosomes by fluorescent microscopy. There are many kinds of probes, including paint probes (a mixture of sequences throughout one chromosome), sequence-specific probes, centromere probes, and telomere probes. Sequence-specific probes are primarily used currently, though many others were used in the past. FISH can detect submicroscopic structural rearrangements undetectable by classic cytogenetic techniques and can identify marker chromosomes. Marker chromosomes are chromosome material identified on karyotype that does not have the typical appearance of well-characterized chromosomes, so its genomic content is unknown. FISH also allows interphase cells (lymphocytes, amniocytes) to be screened for numeric abnormalities such as trisomy 13, 18, or 21 and sex chromosome aneuploidy. However, because of the possible background or contamination of the signal, the abnormality must be confirmed by conventional chromosome analysis.

COMPARATIVE GENOMIC HYBRIDIZATION AND MICROARRAY

Comparative genomic hybridization (CGH), also known as a chromosomal microarray, is a molecular cytogenetic method of screening for genetic copy number variation. This test is beneficial for finding smaller copy number imbalances that cannot be found by high-resolution karyotype. Genomic DNA from a patient and a control is labeled by fluorescent dyes and competitively hybridized to chromosomal targets. The copy number balance between the two samples is reflected by their signal intensity ratio. The alterations are classified as DNA gains and losses and reveal a characteristic pattern that includes changes at chromosomal and subchromosomal levels. Depending on the platform, copy number changes, including as little as one or two exons, may be detectable. Individual laboratories establish thresholds for detection and reporting of clinically relevant changes, so understanding of the limitations of the test ordered is important. Typically a result is reported as cytogenetic description of the involved chromosomal band (i.e., 16p11.2 deletion) as well as the exact chromosomal coordinates and copy number (i.e., 29,567,295-30,177,916 x1). A notation such as "Hg19" is included to denote which genomic reference sequence (genome build) was used for that test. Periodically, new genome builds become the standard, and the numbering in specific genomic regions may change. This is relevant when comparing testing from year to year or between patients.

Also included in the laboratory report for a chromosomal microarray is a classification of any identified copy number variant. The current classification scheme includes "Pathogenic," "Likely Pathogenic," "Uncertain Significance," "Likely Benign," and "Benign." By convention, copy number variants that fall into the categories "Likely benign" and "Benign" are not included on laboratory reports as they are not thought to be clinically significant. The classification of the copy number variants is made based on knowledge of common clinically significant copy number variants, review of the genes included in the altered region, incidence of the copy number variant in healthy populations, and whether the variant is de novo (meaning it is brand new in the affected individual) or inherited from a parent. Variants classified as of uncertain significance are reviewed for clinical and medical actionability at the time of testing and then should be revisited periodically to evaluate for updated interpretations or reclassification.

Another type of result that may be seen on a chromosomal laboratory report can include runs of homozygosity. These occur in cases of consanguinity or uniparental disomy. Uniparental disomy and clinically associated conditions are discussed in Chapter 24. Multiple runs of homozygosity most often indicate that the parents of the patient share a common ancestor, and this is evidence for consanguinity. On their own, most runs of homozygosity do not have clinical significance; it does, however, raise the risk that the patient may have an underlying autosomal recessive disorder. Further evaluation by a clinical geneticist is recommended in those circumstances.

Genetic testing has the potential to yield complex and unexpected results. It is important before ordering genetic testing, particularly in the case of ordering a chromosomal microarray, that the patient and family receive genetic counseling about the testing and types of possible results. Counseling topics include discussion of the variant classification scheme, including variants of uncertain significance. It should also include the risk to identify clinically unrelated findings, consanguinity, or nonpaternity/maternity if parental testing is involved. Chromosomal microarrays have become the first line in genetic testing in children with developmental delays, autism spectrum disorder (ASD), and multiple congenital anomalies. It is also used in the prenatal setting as well as to characterize tumors in oncology. Testing should be considered in patients with any of the abovementioned symptoms, and referral to a genetics specialist in the case of either positive or nondiagnostic results is recommended.

BALANCED AND UNBALANCED TRANSLOCATIONS

Balanced translocations occur when genetic material is transferred to a location other than its typical position. The total genomic content is normal, but the genetic information resides in a different place on the chromosomes. This can occur in several types of arrangements, including inversions on one chromosome, transfer of material to a different chromosome, and rearrangements where two genomic regions switch places (reciprocal translocation) (Fig. 25.3). In most cases these rearrangements do not cause clinical symptoms, but the possibility that the rearrangement will disrupt a gene or alter a regulatory element is a concern. Determining when balanced rearrangements cause clinical symptoms is challenging because there are no reliable clinical assays to determine when that is the case. In some cases breakpoints of rearrangements can be sequenced, which may support the disruption of a gene or a regulatory element, but these cases are rare.

An example of a common balanced translocation is the presence of a balanced Robertsonian translocation (see Fig. 25.3). Robertsonian translocations occur when two chromosomes are fused, such as two copies of chromosome 13 being fused together. A balanced carrier of a Robertsonian translocation will have 45 total chromosomes instead of 46 because the two fused chromosome 13s are counted as one chromosome. This does not have any clinical consequences for the carrier personally because the total genomic content is normal.

Clinical consequences of being a balanced translocation carrier become apparent at reproduction The balanced carrier is now predisposed to chromosome mis segregation in the gametes, which can result in an unbalanced translocation in the offspring. This can result in increased incidence of miscarriage or chromosomal copy number variants. In the previous example there would be an increased risk to have a miscarriage in fetuses with monosomy 13 and to have a child with trisomy 13. In families that have multiple miscarriages through multiple generations it is advisable to consider the possibility of a balanced translocation in the family and perform testing with high-resolution chromosomes to look for this.

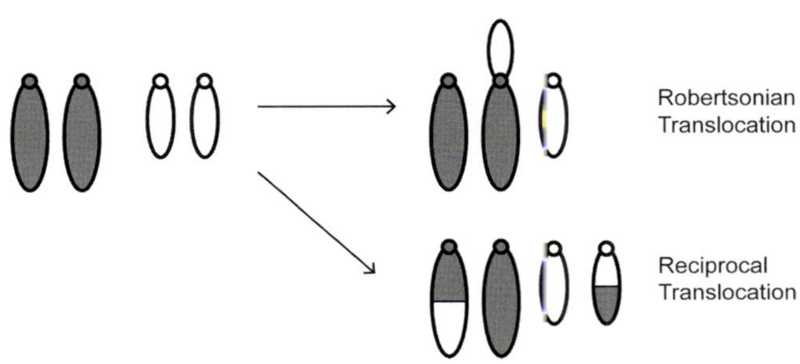

Fig. 25.3 Robertsonian translocation.

COPY NUMBER VARIANTS

Copy number variants encompass a broad category of conditions and can range in size from very small (on the order of thousands of bases) to very large (on the order millions of bases). The severity of the conditions is dictated by the gene content of the copy number variants in the setting of the patient's genetic and environmental baseline. There are many well-described copy number variants with significant clinical implications to the patients. The topic is too large to cover in detail here, but a description of several common conditions is included.

22q11.2 Deletion Syndrome

22q11.2 deletion syndrome (also known as DiGeorge syndrome, Shprintzen syndrome, velocardiofacial syndrome) is a deletion of 1.5 to 3 Mb that occurs in 1 of 4000 to 5000 live births. Diagnosis can be made through FISH studies or chromosomal microarray. Individuals with this condition can have a wide spectrum of symptoms, including developmental delays, intellectual disability, congenital cardiac anomalies (primarily conotruncal defects), velopharyngeal insufficiency, feeding and speech difficulties, immunodeficiency, short stature, and increased risk for behavioral and mental health concerns. Inheritance for the condition is autosomal dominant; it is inherited about 7% of the time. Dysmorphic features can include prominent ears, epicanthal folds, hypoplastic nares, and a triangular-shaped upper lip. Confirmation of this diagnosis is important to screen for known medical complications. Ideally, patients should be followed in a multidisciplinary setting to assist with coordination of complex care. Practice guidelines have been developed to guide the care of these patients (Bassett et al., 2011). Referral to a multidisciplinary setting is ideal for ongoing management.

Williams Syndrome (7q11.23 Deletion)

Williams syndrome is a contiguous gene deletion at 7q11.23 that occurs in 1 of approximately 7500 live births. Diagnosis can be made through FISH studies or chromosomal microarray. Individuals with Williams syndrome have symptoms that include short stature, developmental delays, hypercalcemia, hypothyroidism, kidney anomalies, cardiac defects (including supravalvular aortic stenosis), and distinctive facial features (malar flattening, wide full lips, long philtrum, stellate iris pattern, and small jaw). Patients benefit from screening for the hormone abnormalities, kidney ultrasounds, referral for interventional therapies and support, and management by cardiology specialists. This condition has variable expressivity though is fully penetrant. It is unlikely to be inherited from a parent if neither is asymptomatic. However, a balanced chromosome 7 inversion has been reported in unaffected parents; this can be detected by karyotype. This increases the risk to have a child with Williams syndrome.

16p11.2 Deletion

16p11.2 deletion can cause developmental delays, ASD, ADHD, other neuropsychiatric disorders, and seizures. Physically, some individuals have macrocephaly, cerebellar tonsillar ectopia, and obesity in adolescence and adulthood. However, there are individuals with none, some, or all of these features demonstrating that this finding has incomplete penetrance and is likely influenced by other genetic or environmental factors. Most (80%) of the time the deletion is de novo.

ANEUPLOIDY

Aneuploidy is a numeric chromosome abnormality caused by the gain or loss of one or more chromosomes. Aneuploidy can affect the autosomes (most commonly in trisomy 21, 18, or 13) and/or sex chromosomes (45X, 47XXY). The most common chromosomal mechanism for aneuploidy is nondisjunction, which is the failure of a pair of chromosomes to disjoin or separate properly during meiosis, usually during meiosis 1. Nondisjunction can also occur in a mitotic division after formation of the zygote and result in mosaicism. In partial aneuploidy there is gain or loss of part of a chromosome. Polyploidy is the addition of a complete haploid set of chromosomes, as in 69,XXX or 69,XYY.

TRISOMY

Trisomy is the presence of three copies of a chromosome rather than the normal two copies. Most trisomic embryos are lost in early pregnancy. The most common type of trisomy in liveborn infants is trisomy 21 or Down syndrome (47,XX+21 or 47,XY+21). With rare exceptions, other trisomies seen in liveborns include trisomy 18 and 13. It is notable that these autosomes (13, 18, 21) are the three with the lowest number of genes located on them; presumably, trisomy for autosomes with a greater number of genes is lethal in most instances. Trisomy for sex chromosomes, such as XXX or XXY, has fewer deleterious effects on development, and most of these trisomies result in term live births.

Trisomy 21

See Chapter 27 for a full discussion of trisomy 21 (Down syndrome).

Trisomy 13

Trisomy 13 is a chromosomal disorder caused by the presence of an extra chromosome 13. The newborn incidence of trisomy 13 is approximately 1 in 5000. Most trisomy 13 fetuses spontaneously abort in the first trimester. Ongoing pregnancy is complicated by IUGR and abnormal ultrasound findings that include congenital heart defects and midline brain lesions (e.g., holoprosencephaly). Newborns with trisomy 13 have dysmorphic facial features, scalp cutis aplasia, microcephaly, microphthalmia, brain malformations, congenital heart defects (most commonly ventricular septal defect and patent ductus arteriosus), cleft lip and/or palate, omphalocele, and postaxial polydactyly. Mortality is high in neonates and infants with trisomy 13 due to complex and multiple congenital anomalies. Those who survive usually have feeding difficulties, failure to thrive, and profound intellectual disability.

Trisomy 18

Trisomy 18 is caused due to the presence of an extra chromosome 18 (Fig. 25.4). The newborn incidence is approximately 1 in 3500; however, the incidence at conception is much higher with most trisomy 18 pregnancies resulting in spontaneous abortion. Abnormalities such as severe IUGR, congenital heart lesions, and diaphragmatic hernia are frequently detected by ultrasound examination. The newborn with trisomy 18 has distinctive features with microcephaly, prominent occiput, small malformed ears, overlapping clenched fingers, and rocker-bottom heels. Hypertonia is a typical finding. Most newborns have congenital heart disease and other congenital anomalies such as undescended testes in males. There is high mortality in newborns and infants with trisomy 18. Those who survive are affected by profound intellectual disability, feeding difficulties, and failure to thrive.

The combined total prevalence of trisomy 13 and 18, which includes elective termination of pregnancies, stillbirths, and live births, is approximately 1 in 1800, making the occurrence of a fetus or baby with either of these chromosomal disorders a relatively common event. Each of these chromosomal disorders consists of a recognizable pattern of multiple congenital anomalies, an increased neonatal and infant mortality, and marked cognitive and motor disability in older children.

Due to the medically serious nature of the outcomes, the traditional approach to management in the newborn and early infancy periods has been to withhold technological support and surgery. In the last decade, however, a rich dialogue has emerged in the literature; one view makes the case for pure comfort care for the benefit of the child, while the other view supports full intervention in appropriate situations. There is a growing consensus for using a model of providing care in patients with trisomy 13 and 18 that uses shared decision making between the family and the health care providers as a foundational principle.

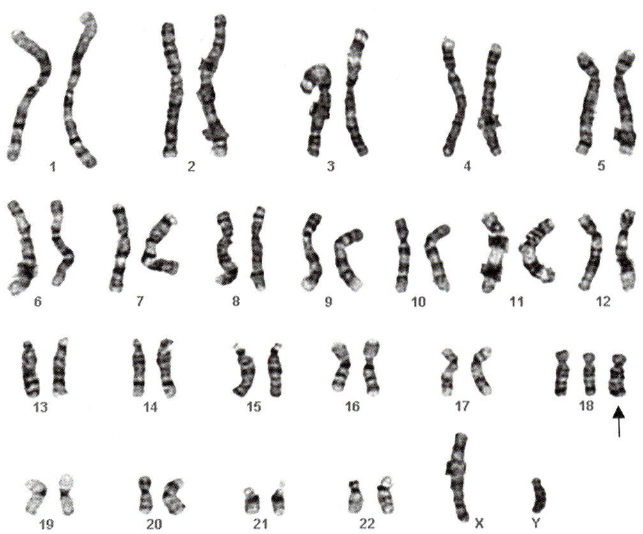

Fig. 25.4 Trisomy 18 karyotype.

MONOSOMY

See Chapter 26 for a discussion on monosomy.

MOSAICISM

Mosaicism is the presence of at least two different cell lines in an individual or tissue, with a common origin from a single zygote. When an individual has a chromosomal abnormality, that abnormality is typically present in all the body's cells. However, sometimes two or more chromosome complements can be present in an individual, and this phenomenon is referred to as mosaicism. It is usually caused by nondisjunction in early postzygotic mitotic division. Mosaicism can be numeric or structural and is typically detected by conventional karyotype methods. It can also be suspected based on interphase FISH analysis or array CGH.

The presence of mosaicism for chromosomal abnormalities can influence the severity of the clinical phenotype, with mosaic individuals potentially exhibiting clinical features at the milder end of the spectrum. The overall impact of mosaicism depends on the nature of the chromosomal abnormality, the proportion of different chromosome complements, and the different tissues affected by mosaicism. Routine genetic testing on a blood sample identifies mosaicism in the blood or germline but is not an accurate reflection of the presence or absence of mosaicism in other tissues such as brain, heart, and bone marrow.

ATYPICAL CHROMOSOME STRUCTURE

Isochromosome

An isochromosome is a chromosome in which one arm is missing and the other is duplicated in a mirror-image fashion. A person with 46 chromosomes carrying an isochromosome therefore has a single copy of the genetic material of one arm (partial monosomy) and three copies of the genetic material of the other arm (partial trisomy). The most common isochromosome is that of the long arm of the X chromosome, i(Xq), in some individuals with Turner syndrome. Refer to Chapter 26 for discussion on Turner syndrome, which is caused by numeric abnormalities involving the X chromosome in females.

Ring Chromosomes

A ring chromosome is formed when a chromosome undergoes two breaks, and the broken ends of the chromosome reunite in a ring structure. They are usually in addition to normal chromosome complement and are referred to as supernumerary ring chromosomes. When the centromere is within the ring, a ring chromosome is expected to be mitotically stable.

Inversions

An inversion is a structural chromosome abnormality whereby a single chromosome undergoes two breaks and is reconstituted, with the segment between the chromosomes inverted. There are two different types of inversion patterns: pericentric inversions (include the centromere) with a break in each arm of

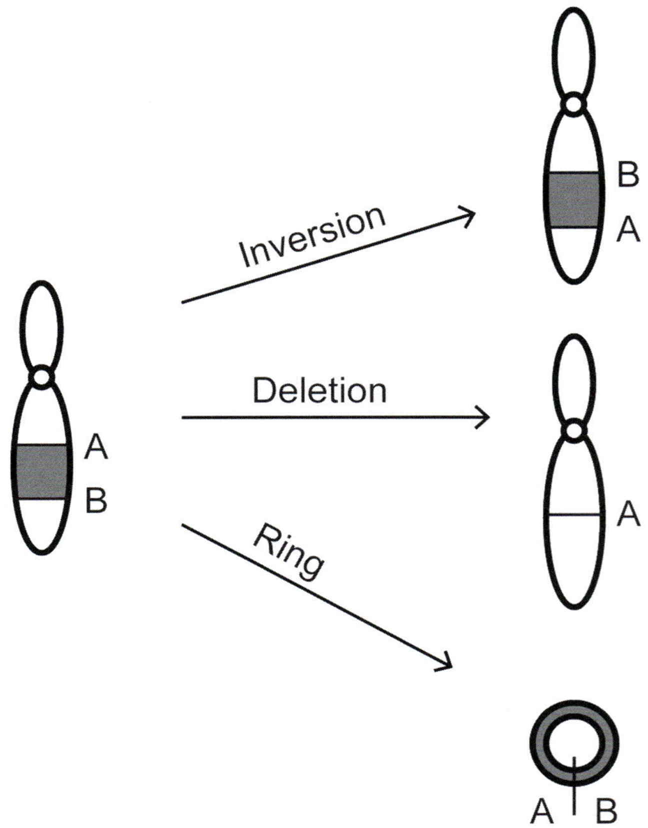

Fig. 25.5 Examples of a chromosome inversion, deletion, and ring chromosome.

the chromosome and paracentric inversions (not including the centromere) with the two breaks occurring on the same arm of the chromosome.

Inversions are associated with an overall balanced chromosome complement for the carrier—that is, there is no net gain or loss of chromosome material, and therefore the carrier of an inversion is not clinically affected. However, there are reproductive clinical consequences, with carriers of inversions at risk for producing abnormal gametes, which in turn can lead to progeny with an unbalanced chromosome complement leading to increased risk for spontaneous miscarriage, infertility, and/or birth of baby with multiple congenital anomalies.

Examples of these atypical chromosome formations can be seen in Fig. 25.5.

INHERITANCE PATTERNS

VIGNETTES

1. *A 6-month-old girl presents with recurrent lower respiratory tract infections, loose stools, and failure to thrive. She has normal developmental milestones. Exam is notable for height and weight below 3rd percentile, with no dysmorphic features and a normal neurologic exam. A three-generation pedigree is obtained, and family history is negative for any similar health concerns. Both parents are of Northern European descent. Extensive testing identifies her to be affected by cystic fibrosis, an autosomal recessive condition.*
2. *An 8-year-old boy with previously normal growth and development presents with a 6-month history of change in behavior, decline in school performance, and 1-week history of decline of vision. On exam he is noted to have a slightly more "tan" appearance than the rest of his family members with no other dysmorphic facial features. Family history is negative except for maternal grandfather with history of unexplained leg weakness and Addison disease in his 50s. MRI brain shows areas of white matter abnormality in the parietal and occipital regions of the brain, raising suspicion for X-linked adrenoleukodystrophy, an X-linked recessive condition.*
3. *An 18-month-old girl presents with a 6-month history of gross motor and speech delay and recent onset of repetitive hand movements. Exam is notable for microcephaly but no dysmorphic features. Also noted are repetitive hand wringing movements and unsteady broad-based gait. Family history is negative for any developmental delay, ASD, or microcephaly. Genetic testing identifies a single pathogenic mutation in the MECP2 gene confirming a diagnosis of Rett syndrome, an X-inked dominant condition.*

Autosomal Dominant Inheritance

Autosomal dominant inheritance refers to the situation where the genetic cause for a condition maps to an autosome, may be equally likely to occur in males or females and can be inherited from either parent. Autosomal dominant conditions occur when one of the two copies of the associated gene is not functioning normally. The second copy of the gene is not sufficient to make up for the impairment of the first.

A pedigree is a visual depiction of a genetic condition and how it exists in a family. By convention, squares represent males, circles represent females, each horizontal line of individuals represents a generation with the oldest generation at the top and the youngest generation at the bottom. Children and parents are connected by vertical lines and affected individuals are denoted with a shaded square or circle. Fig. 25.6 shows an example of an autosomal dominant pedigree.

There are many factors that impact how an autosomal dominant condition is manifested, so these must all be taken into account when assessing an individual or a family for an autosomal dominant condition.

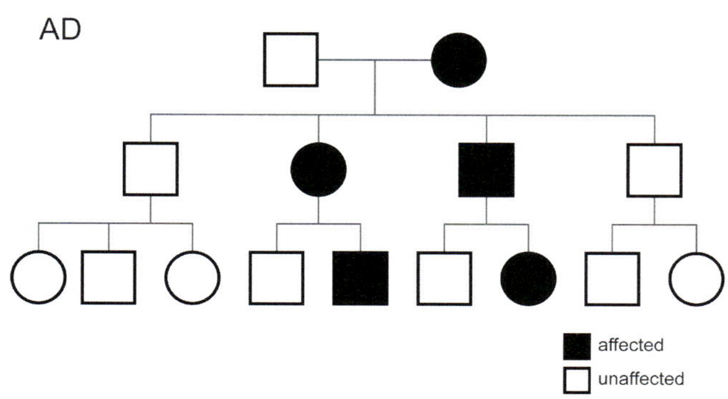

Fig. 25.6 Autosomal dominant pedigree.

Penetrance

Penetrance refers to whether an individual with a genetic condition manifests symptoms. In conditions with full penetrance every individual in a family who carries the genetic mutation for the condition will have symptoms. In conditions with reduced penetrance some individuals will not show symptoms, and thus it may appear that the condition skips generations.

Expressivity

Expressivity refers to the symptoms an individual may show. In syndromic conditions there are often symptoms that may impact different organ systems, but with variable expressivity one affected individual may demonstrate one symptom while another individual in the same family may demonstrate a different symptom. An example of a condition with variable expressivity is neurofibromatosis type 1, which is a condition that causes abnormal cell growth and is often associated with multiple café au lait macules and neurofibromas. One individual with neurofibromatosis type 1 may have optic gliomas, while another has bone deformities.

Age of Onset

Age of onset is an important factor to consider in autosomal dominant conditions. Some disorders do not manifest symptoms until adulthood or later. For instance, an individual may carry a genetic change that causes an increased risk for breast cancer, but breast cancer does not typically occur until adulthood even though a pediatric patient may carry the genetic predisposition. In some autosomal dominant conditions, particularly those associated with trinucleotide repeat disorders (discussed in Chapter 30) such as Huntington disease, anticipation can be seen. Anticipation is where the severity of the disease increases and/or the age of onset decreases in subsequent generations.

Allelic Heterogeneity and Locus Heterogeneity

Each copy of a chromosome, gene, or marker is referred to as an allele. In many autosomal dominant conditions genetic changes in a particular gene may cause different symptoms or conditions. This is seen in genes such as *LMNA* in which some individuals manifest dilated cardiomyopathy and some individuals manifest a congenital muscular dystrophy with variants in the same gene. This is called allelic heterogeneity. Locus (also called genetic) heterogeneity, by contrast, is where similar conditions may be caused by genetic changes in many different genes. This is seen in the case of nonsyndromic hearing loss where genetic variants in dozens of different genes are associated with bilateral sensorineural hearing loss.

Sex Limited Conditions

Finally, though a disease may have autosomal dominant inheritance, there are some conditions in which the disease is sex limited, meaning it does not necessarily impact both sexes equally. This can include genetic predispositions to ovarian or prostate cancer in which the organ does not exist in both sexes.

Autosomal Recessive Inheritance

Autosomal recessive disorders occur due to mutations in genes encoded on the autosomes. Affected individuals have a mutation at both alleles at a given locus—that is, both copies of the specific gene have a mutation, and there is no normal copy of the gene. Carriers for autosomal recessive disorders carry a mutation on one of the alleles at the locus, while the other allele is wild type or normal. Carriers for autosomal recessive diseases, also referred to as heterozygotes, are clinically unaffected and do not manifest any phenotypic features of the disease, as one normal copy of the gene is able to compensate and prevent the disease from occurring. Because an individual inherits only one of the two alleles at each locus from one parent, homozygotes must have inherited a mutant allele from each parent (barring new mutation or uniparental disomy, which is rare in autosomal recessive disorders). Fig. 25.7 shows a pedigree demonstrating autosomal recessive inheritance.

In clinical vignette 1 the child is affected with cystic fibrosis, which is an autosomal recessive disorder. Both parents are carriers for cystic fibrosis but are clinically unaffected. Unless couples pursue prenatal genetic carrier screening they are usually unaware of their carrier status. Of note, prenatal genetic carrier screens only offer testing for common genetic conditions.

Aspects of Autosomal Recessive Inheritance

Consanguinity. A consanguineous relationship is one between individuals who are related (second cousins or closer). The incidence of autosomal recessive disorders is higher in consanguineous unions due to common ancestors and a shared gene pool. Consanguinity of the parents of a patient with a genetic disorder is strong evidence but not proof for the autosomal recessive inheritance of that condition. Consanguinity, however, is not the most common explanation for an autosomal recessive trait. The mating of unrelated individuals, who by chance happen to be carriers for the same disease, is by far the most common reason for autosomal recessive disease, particularly if the carrier frequency for that condition is high in the general population.

Inbreeding. Individuals from a small population tend to choose their partners from the same geographic area for geographic, cultural, or religious reasons. While parents do not consider

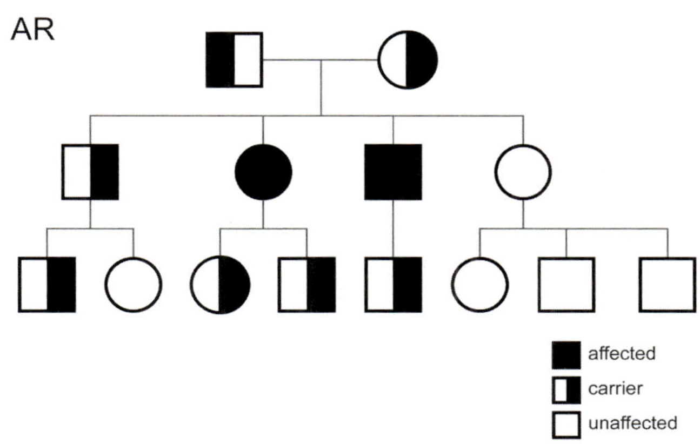

Fig. 25.7 Autosomal recessive pedigree.

themselves related in this situation, they may have common ancestry within the past few generations.

Founder effect. Founder effect is the high prevalence of a genetic disorder in an isolated or inbred population, as many members of the population are derived from a common ancestor who harbored a disease-causing mutation. The affected individuals in the population are all homozygous for the same mutation (founder mutation).

Carrier frequency. The risk for two unrelated individuals to have a child affected with an autosomal recessive disorder depends on the carrier frequency for that disorder in the general population. An autosomal recessive disorder is inherited through both parents, which means that both must carry one normal and one mutant copy of the allele. Therefore the chance that a person who is a carrier for a mutant allele has a child with disease is based partly on the chance that the partner is also a carrier of a mutant allele for that condition. Knowledge of the carrier frequency of a disease is clinically important for risk assessment and genetic counseling.

There are certain small groups in which the carrier frequency for rare disease gene mutations is much higher than the general population. Such groups, also known as genetic isolates, become separated from the general population by religious, cultural, language, or geographic barriers. Although these individuals are not consanguineous, the chance of mating with another individual who is carrier for the same condition is quite high. For example, the incidence of Tay-Sachs disease, which is a rare neurodegenerative condition, is much higher among Ashkenazi Jews in North America than the general population, about 1:3600. This number has fallen by 90% with the advent of population-based carrier frequency screening.

X-Linked Inheritance

X-linked diseases are caused by mutations in genes on the X chromosome. Disorders with X-linked inheritance patterns affect males and females differently based on the fact that males have one and females have two X chromosomes. X-linked dominant and recessive patterns of inheritance are distinguished based on the expression of disease phenotype in heterozygous females.

X-Linked Recessive Disease

X-linked recessive diseases are expressed in all males who carry the mutation (hemizygous) and only in those females who are homozygous (both alleles of the gene carry the mutation). An example would be X-linked adrenoleukodystrophy (XALD), in which affected males have a mutation in the *ABCD1* gene on the X chromosome and present with childhood onset of adrenal dysfunction and leukodystrophy associated with progressive neurologic decline. Affected males who do not develop the cerebral form remain at high risk for developing adrenomyeloneuropathy (AMN) as adults. Carrier females do not typically manifest the cerebral form of the disease.

Manifesting heterozygotes. Women who are heterozygous for X-linked recessive conditions but are symptomatic are referred to as manifesting heterozygotes. This is thought to be the results of skewed X inactivation pattern, where the mutation found on one of the X alleles is being read more than the 50/50 chance, which is expected. Skewed X inactivation can cause carrier females to manifest a phenotype, which is generally more mild than is seen in a male with the same mutation.

X-Linked Dominant Disease

In diseases with X-linked dominant pattern of inheritance heterozygous females are affected. X-linked hypophosphatemia rickets is a common example of X-linked dominant inheritance pattern, where females are mildly affected and have a variable expression of disease. Some X-linked dominant disorders such as Rett syndrome have a severe presentation in affected females and can be perinatal lethal in males.

X-linked dominant inheritance can be distinguished from autosomal dominant inheritance by the lack of male-to-male transmission (as males transmit their Y chromosomes to their sons and not the X). Affected males have no affected sons and no normal daughters.

REFERENCES

Bassett, A. S., McDonald-McGinn, D. M., Devriendt, K., Digilio, M. C., Goldenberg, P., Habel, A., Marino, B., Oskarsdottir, S., Philip, N., Sullivan, K., Swillen, A., Vorstman, J., & International 22q11.2 Deletion Syndrome Consortium. (2011). Practical guidelines for managing patients with 22q11.2 deletion syndrome. *The Journal of Pediatrics*, *159*(2), 332–339. e1. https://doi.org/10.1016/j.jpeds.2011.02.039

Carey, J. C., & Kosho, T. (2016). Perspectives on the care and advances in the management of children with trisomy 13 and 18. *American Journal of Medical Genetics Part C Seminars in Medical Genetics*, *172C*, 249–250. https://doi.org/10.1002/ajmg.c.31527

Kaur, S., & Christodoulou, J. (2001/2019). *MECP2* disorders. In M. P. Adam, et al. (Eds.), *GeneReviews*. University of Washington. https://www.ncbi.nlm.nih.gov/books/NBK1497/

Lockwood, W., Chari, R., Chi, B., & Lam, W. L. (2006). Recent advances in array comparative genomic hybridization technologies and their applications in human genetics. *European Journal of Human Genetics*, *14*, 139–148. https://doi.org/10.1038/sj.ejhg.5201531

Morris, C. A. (1999/2017). Williams syndrome. In M. P. Adam, et al. (Eds.), *GeneReviews*. University of Washington. https://www.ncbi.nlm.nih.gov/books/NBK1249/

Nussbaum, R., McInnes, R. R., & Willard, H. F. (2016). *Thompson and Thompson genetics and medicine* (8th ed). Elsevier.

Perovanovic, J., & Hoffman, E. P. (2018). Mechanisms of allelic and clinical heterogeneity of lamin A/C phenotypes. *Physiological Genomics*, *50*(9), 694–704. https://doi.10.1152/physiolgenomics.00128.2017

Raymond, G. V., & Moser, A. F. (1999/2018). X linked adrenoleukodystrophy. In M. P. Adam, et al. (Eds.), *GeneReviews*. University of Washington. https://www.ncbi.nlm.nih.gov/books/NBK1315/

Riggs, E. R., et al. (2020). Technical standards for the interpretation and reporting of constitutional copy-number variants: A joint consensus recommendation of the American College of Medical Genetics and Genomics (ACMG) and the Clinical Genome Resource (ClinGen). *Genetics in Medicine*, *22*(2), 245–257. https://doi.10.1038/s41436-019-0686-8

26

Sex Chromosome Aneuploidy

Kristen Wigby, Talia Thompson, Mariah Brown, Nicole Tartaglia, and Shanlee Davis

For additional material related to the content of this chapter, please see Chapter 24.

VIGNETTE

Gregory is an 8-year-old boy presenting to developmental pediatrics for learning and behavioral difficulties. Milestones included walking independently at 15 months, first words at 16 months, and lack of two-word phrases at 28 months, prompting initiation of speech-language therapy. Academically, he receives reading group intervention but still struggles to complete grade-level work. His parents describe challenges establishing peer relationships, anxiety, and low frustration tolerance leading to episodes of crying, withdrawal, and escape behaviors. Examination revealed stature at the 90th percentile and mild diffuse hypotonia with no dysmorphic features.

Psychological assessment revealed overall cognitive abilities at the 40th percentile, with strengths in nonverbal skills relative to verbal domains. Neuropsychology testing led to diagnoses of specific learning disability in reading, inattentive attention-deficit/hyperactivity disorder (ADHD), and moderate deficits in executive functioning. Speech-language results showed higher-order expressive language skills, including pragmatic language below the 10th percentile. Social-emotional evaluation revealed symptoms of anxiety and emotional immaturity. Gregory also had challenges with social communication, including conversational reciprocity and reading social cues; however, he did not meet criteria for autism spectrum disorder (ASD).

Due to the history of developmental delays and the current presentation of neurodevelopmental diagnoses across multiple domains, genetic testing was performed revealing a diagnosis of 47,XXY/Klinefelter syndrome. This diagnosis was helpful in explaining his history of developmental and behavioral challenges, provided additional support for implementation of an individualized education plan (IEP), and led to referrals for genetic counseling and endocrinology. Medication treatment for ADHD was initiated with positive results, and Gregory began therapy for anxiety and emotional regulation.

INTRODUCTION

Humans have 23 pairs of chromosomes. The first 22 pairs (chromosomes 1–22) are the autosomes and are the same for males and females. The 23rd pair are the sex chromosomes, or the X and Y chromosomes, and these determine the biologic sex of an individual. Typically females have two X chromosomes (46,XX) and males have one X and one Y chromosome (46,XY). Aneuploidy is the genetic term describing a difference from the typical chromosome number, and thus sex chromosome aneuploidy (SCA) conditions are defined as genetic conditions with an atypical number of X and/or Y chromosomes.

As a group, SCA conditions have many names and may be called sex chromosome abnormalities, sex chromosome disorders, sex chromosome variations, or X&Y chromosome variations. There are many different forms of SCA, including monosomies, trisomies, tetrasomies, and pentasomies (Table 26.1; Fig. 26.1), with an estimated overall prevalence rate of 1 in 400 births. Trisomy conditions are the most common, followed by monosomy X, and tetrasomy and pentasomy conditions become increasingly rare. SCA conditions are generally not inherited and result from one or more nondisjunction errors in meiosis I and/or meiosis II during formation of the sperm or oocyte, or by postzygotic nondisjunction. SCA conditions with X chromosome aneuploidy have been associated with advanced maternal age due to increased nondisjunction events in aging oocytes. In conditions with Y chromosome aneuploidy (i.e., XYY, XXYY), the extra chromosome(s) is(are) usually paternal in origin. A comparison of the general medical and neurodevelopmental features across the different SCA conditions is shown in Table 26.2, and each feature is described in more detail in the syndrome-specific sections that follows.

The estimated prevalence of 1 in 400 is based on results of newborn screening studies; however, SCA conditions are not currently included in the newborn screening panels used in clinical practice. Thus diagnosis of SCA relies on genetic testing ordered by medical providers. SCA conditions can be diagnosed either in the prenatal period or postnatally, usually by standard karyotype or microarray. Studies that compare actual diagnosis rates to the 1:400 birth prevalence show that there is currently marked underascertainment of SCA cases, with the majority of cases not identified during the lifetime. Currently it is estimated that only ~50% of Turner syndrome (TS), ~40% of males with XXY, and ~10% of individuals with trisomy X or XYY are diagnosed during the lifetime. For the tetrasomy and pentasomy conditions is not known due to their rarity; however, due to the presence of multiple extra chromosomes these conditions are associated with increased rates of congenital malformations, dysmorphic features, and more significant neurodevelopmental involvement, and thus are more likely to come to medical attention and receive genetic testing.

TABLE 26.1 Sex Chromosome Aneuploidy Subtypes

		SCA Condition	Other Names	Prevalence
Males	Trisomies	47,XXY	Klinefelter syndrome	1:650
		47,XYY	Jacobs syndrome	1:1000
	Tetrasomies	48,XXYY		1:18,000
		48,XXXY		1:30,000
		48,XYYY		<20 cases reported
	Pentasomies	49,XXXXY		1:85,000
		49,XXXYY		<20 reported cases
		49,XXYYY		<20 reported cases
		49,XYYYY		<20 reported cases
Females	Monosomy	45,X	Turner syndrome	1:2500[a]
	Trisomy	47,XXX	Trisomy X, triple X	1:1000
	Tetrasomy	48,XXXX	Tetrasomy X	1:100,000
	Pentasomy	49,XXXXX	Pentasomy X	1:150,000
All sex chromosome aneuploidies:				1:400 births

[a]Includes other genetic causes of Turner syndrome, including X chromosome mosaicism, Xq isochromosome, Xp deletion, and ring X chromosome.

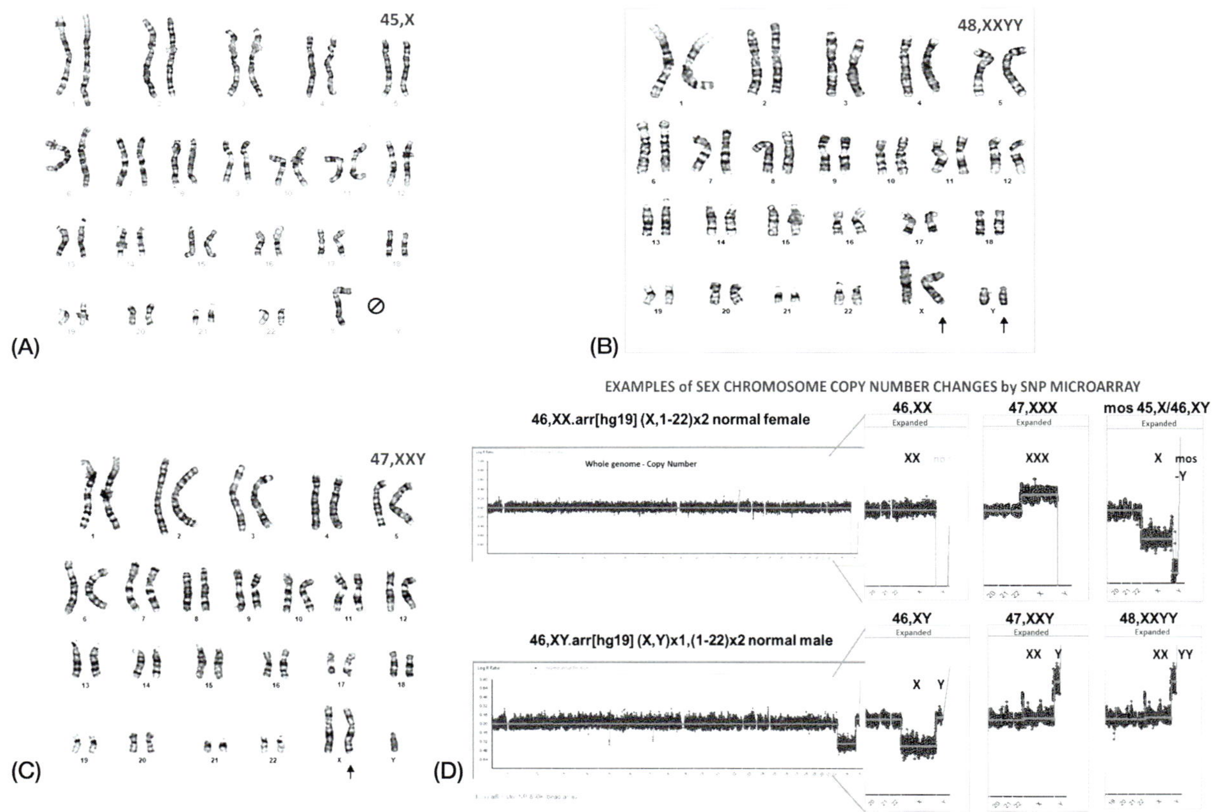

Fig. 26.1 Sex chromosome aneuploidy conditions as seen on karyotype/chromosome analysis (a) 45,X Turner syndrome, (b) 47,XXY Klinefelter syndrome, (c) 48,XXYY syndrome or by (d) SNP microarray. Note typical chromosome copy number in 46,XX and 46,XY expanded figure, followed by examples of sex chromosome aneuploidy SNP microarray readings in females (Trisomy X and mosaic 45,X/46,XY Turner syndrome) and males (47,XXY Klinefelter synddrome and 48,XXYY). Figures provided by Colorado Genetics Laboratory, University of Colorado, Anschutz Medical Campus and Billie Carstens of the Colorado Genetics Laboratory.

TABLE 26.2 Comparison of Neurodevelopmental, Psychological and Clinical Features of Sex Chromosome Aneupolidy (SCA) Conditions

	XXY/KS	XYY	Trisomy X	Tetrasomy/Pentasomy	Turner X
Early development	Delayed milestones 50–70% (mild) Expressive < receptive language delays Gross motor/motor planning			Delayed milestones >80% (mild–severe) Expressive < receptive language	20–30% delayed milestones Motor celays more common than language
Mean full-scale IQ	90–95		80–85	More severely affected	95–100
Intellectual disability	~5%		~10%	>50% tetrasomy >90% pentasomy	~5–10%
Cognitive profile	Nonverbal (NV) and visual-spatial (VS) domains > verbal domains				Verbal > NV and VS domains
Learning/ academics	Language-based learning disabilities (LD) Language disorders				Math LD
Executive function deficits	Increased risk in all SCA conditions				
Adaptive functioning delays	Increased risk in all SCA conditions				
Attention-deficit/ hyperactivity disorder (ADHD)	~15–30% ADHD-inattentive subtype most common	~30–75% ADHD-combined subtype most common	~15–30% ADHD-inattentive subtype most common	~75% XXYY ADHD-combined subtype most common Other conditions: Increased risk	~25% ADHD-combined subtype most common (hyperactivity prominent)
Social/autism spectrum disorder (ASD)	~10–15% ASD	~30% ASD	~20% ASD	>50% XXYY Limited research but increased risk in other conditions	Social difficulties common, minimal ASD research
Anxiety/ depression	Increased risk in all SCA conditions				
Stature	Tall	Tall	Tall	Tetrasomies: Tall Pentasomies: Tall or short	Short stature
Hormone/ reproductive	Microorchidism (95% at puberty) Testicular failure: hypogonadism/ testosterone deficiency Fertility problems	Normal puberty and testosterone Mild risk of fertility problems	Increased risk Premature ovarian failure	Males with extra Xs: same as XXY Females: increased risk of premature ovarian failure	~90% gonadal dysgenesis/ovarian failure Spontaneous puberty 5–10% Spontaneous pregnancy 2–5%
Congenital malformations	Rare[a]	Rare[a]	Rare[a]	More common[b]	More common[c]

[a]Congenital malformations in all trisomies may include cardiac septal defects. Trisomy X is also associated with renal abnormalities and hip dysplasia.
[b]Congenital malformations in tetrasomy/pentasomy SCA conditions may include cardiac septal defects, renal malformations, radioulnar synostosis, cleft palate/velopharyngeal insufficiency, clubfoot.
[c]Congenital malformations in Turner syndrome may include congenital health disease (coarctation of aorta/bicuspid aortic valve most common), renal malformations, lymphedema/neck webbing, ear malformations.

The reasons behind the low ascertainment rate of the sex chromosome trisomies and TS are multiple. First, as described later in the sections on each SCA condition, there is wide variability in both the physical and the neurodevelopmental phenotypic presentation within each phenotype. The majority do not have intellectual disability, and there is considerable overlap with the general population resulting in testing of only the most affected. Second, for the SCA trisomies, characteristic facial features and physical findings are often subtle and variable between individuals (Fig. 26.2), associated medical problems are common in the general population, and the presence of tall stature does not typically raise concern unless extreme. An exception to this is the almost universal finding of microorchidism in males with XXY starting in adolescence; however, this finding is often either not examined or not recognized. For TS, facial and physical features are somewhat more recognizable, and medical conditions such as congenital heart malformations, short stature, and amenorrhea usually prompt genetic workup. However, not all TS cases show these features, and a large percentage remain undiagnosed. Third, many of the neurodevelopmental and psychological diagnoses associated with SCA trisomies and TS such as learning disabilities, ADHD, motor skills deficits, language disorders, and anxiety disorders alone do not meet the threshold of current genetic testing guidelines. As a result, medical providers do not often consider genetic testing for these diagnoses, despite many patients having a constellation of physical findings, developmental history, and current symptoms to justify genetic testing. Genetic testing is more likely, however, in those who present with symptoms of autism or more severe developmental delay. Finally, there is a general lack of knowledge by many medical providers about the features and constellation of symptoms seen in SCA conditions and subsequently decreased diagnosis.

The landscape of genetic testing is changing rapidly, however, and genetic testing in clinical practice is increasing overall as research has advanced, testing costs have decreased, and there has been more public interest in genetic causes of medical and neurodevelopmental conditions. The most significant change for the SCA field has been the introduction of noninvasive prenatal screening (NIPS, also called noninvasive prenatal testing [NIPT]) in prenatal care, which allows for fetal DNA to be identified from peripheral blood of pregnant women starting at 10 weeks of gestation. This technology identifies many cases of SCA, and prenatal care guidelines now support use of NIPS in all pregnancies. While most women undergo NIPS to identify Down syndrome or for fetal sex determination, findings of SCA are very common. Prior to NIPS it was estimated that only 5% to 10% of all SCA cases were identified during the prenatal period; however, the rate of prenatal SCA diagnosis is markedly increasing with more widespread use of NIPS and is estimated that 6 to 10 times more infants will be diagnosed with SCA in the prenatal period. Prenatal NIPS results are not diagnostic and should always be confirmed by postnatal genetic testing, and by amniocentesis if diagnostic confirmation is desired in the prenatal period. The growing number of infants with a known SCA diagnosis at birth has many implications for primary care providers and developmental pediatricians, as an increasing number will be presenting to practices for medical care, developmental screening, and seeking care for associated neurodevelopmental problems. Thus it is important for providers to have knowledge of care guidelines for the medical, developmental, and psychological features of SCA conditions.

TURNER SYNDROME

Genetics and Diagnosis of Turner Syndrome

Definition and Prevalence of Turner Syndrome

TS was named after the endocrinologist Henry Turner who in 1938 originally described a series of seven females ages 15 to 23 years with a constellation of features, including short stature, webbed neck, low posterior hairline, primary amenorrhea and underdeveloped secondary sex characteristics, cubitis valgus, and average cognitive abilities. These early reports preceded the identification of the chromosomal basis of TS in 1959, when it was discovered that TS was caused by the loss of a second intact X chromosome in a female. Today TS is defined as a SCA condition that results from complete

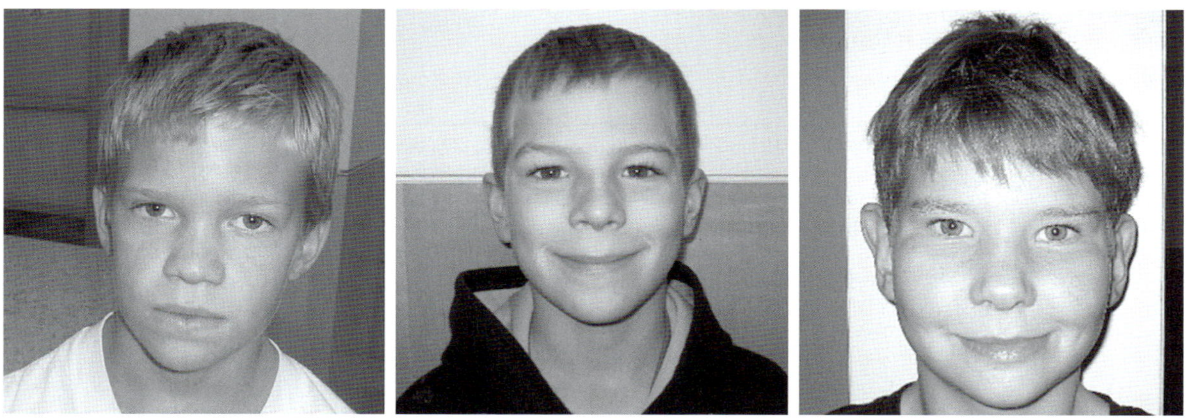

Fig. 26.2 Minimal dysmorphic facial features in males with XXY, XYY and XXYY syndromes highlight need for clinicians to be aware of developmental-behavioral presentation and common medical findings in individuals with sex chromosome disorders, as well as low testicular volume in males with an extra X chromosome after pubertal onset. Also note mild hypertelorism and facial asymmetry in XXYY.

(monosomy) or partial loss of one of the two X chromosomes in a phenotypic female with at least one of the recognized manifestations of TS.

TS occurs in 1 in 2500 liveborn females but is more common in fetuses that are spontaneously miscarried or born stillborn. The majority of 45,X fetuses present as growth disorganized embryos that spontaneously abort during the first trimester of pregnancy 99% of the time. These monosomies represent about 10% of early spontaneous abortions. Some 45,X fetuses are detected on ultrasound examination in the second trimester, typically as a fetus with a cystic hygroma or a more generalized fluid collection (e.g., hydrops fetalis). Additional prenatal findings can include congenital heart and renal malformations, most frequently preductal coarctation and horseshoe kidney. The majority of these fetuses are stillborn.

Of those that survive to term, clinical features vary, and a diagnosis of TS can be made at different timepoints from the prenatal period to adulthood. The diagnosis is made by cytogenetic testing, most commonly karyotype or chromosomal microarray. In infancy and early childhood, many cases are identified due to congenital malformations or characteristic physical features. Later cases are primarily identified due to short stature or delayed puberty and in adulthood due to ovarian failure and infertility.

Genetic Variations and Mechanisms in Turner Syndrome

Increasing use of cytogenetic testing, both in the prenatal and postnatal clinical settings, has expanded on the variability of genetic findings in females with TS. Nearly half of females with TS have a complete loss of one X chromosome (45,X or monosomy X). Monosomy may result from nondisjunction error or chromosome lag, where a chromosome may lag at anaphase and be excluded from the new nucleus. The remaining females with TS have a partial loss of one X chromosome or mosaic loss of part or all of one X chromosome, including X chromosome mosaicism, Xq isochromosome, Xp deletion, or a ring X. Mosaicism is defined as two or more genetically distinct cell populations within the same individual. There are multiple mosaic forms of TS, which can include 45,X/46,XX, 45,X/46,XX/47,XXX, 45,X/47,XXX, 45,X/46,XY, or other variants. Mosaic forms of TS arise due to a postzygotic nondisjunction error or chromosome lag in the developing fetus. The level of mosaicism may vary between tissues and by the age of the individual. A ring X chromosome usually results from a terminal break in both chromosome arms followed by fusion of the broken ends. Monosomy X and mosaic TS karyotypes are both sporadic events that do not tend to recur within families. The important exception is that females with TS due to a partial Xp deletion can be inherited, and parental karyotypes to evaluate for inheritance are recommended.

45,X/46,XY mosaicism can present as phenotypic females, with genital ambiguity, or as phenotypic males. It is important to note that phenotypic males (e.g., 45,X/46,XY or other karyotype variations) are not included in the diagnostic definition of TS and are recognized as a separate clinical entity. In addition, as it is now recognized that women may lose an X chromosome in a portion of their cells as part of the aging process, a woman over 50 years with low-level mosaicism (<5% of cells contain 45,X) would not meet the definition of TS. Finally, females with X chromosome deletions distal to Xq24 typically have primary or secondary amenorrhea without other features of TS and therefore are also not considered to have TS.

Genotype-Phenotype Correlations in Turner Syndrome

The spectrum of manifestations of TS result from the lack of a second intact X chromosome. Studies of females with various TS karyotypes have made several observations of karyotype-phenotype correlations, although these findings are variable and may not always apply to all females with a particular TS karyotype. These include observations in mosaic TS females, with the caveat that mosaicism in the blood may not reflect mosaicism in other tissues, and those with a ring X chromosome. Congenital heart anomalies and lymphatic defects occur less frequently in females with mosaic 45,X/46,XX karyotypes, and when these manifestations are present they tend to be less severe in comparison to nonmosaic TS (45,X) females. Furthermore 45,X/46,XX females are more likely to have spontaneous pregnancies, although they are at increased risk for spontaneous miscarriage. Females with 45,X/46,XX/47,XXX or 45,X/47,XXX karyotypes are also considered to have a milder phenotype. Finally, variable degrees of intellectual disability have been reported in females with ring X chromosome; however, the degree of intellectual disability does not appear to correlate with the size of the ring X chromosome or absence of *XIST* in the ring X. While these karyotype-phenotype correlations can be helpful for refining genetic counseling it is recommended that all females with a TS karyotype or 45,X cell line receive surveillance and care based on current TS clinical practice guidelines.

Clinical Features of Turner Syndrome

Physical and Medical Features of Turner Syndrome

Infants with TS may present in the newborn period with dysmorphic physical features, including low hairline, webbing of the neck, low-set ears, high arched palate, wide-spaced nipples, and lymphedema. These features should prompt genetic testing. However, many girls with TS will not have any of these features, particularly if there is mosaicism for a typical 46,XX cell line. Therefore many girls with TS are not diagnosed in the newborn period.

Short stature is nearly universal in girls with TS and is the most common feature leading to TS diagnosis in the school-age years. Often girls are born small for gestational age and fail to have catchup growth, have a low-normal growth velocity in the childhood years, and lack a pubertal growth spurt. Without intervention the average height of adult women with nonmosaic 45,X is 4 ft 8 inches tall. Growth hormone treatment is approved for use in girls with TS and short stature, resulting in about 0.4 inch extra per year of treatment. If growth hormone treatment is started late or there is a poor response, the low-potency oral androgen oxandrolone has shown to have synergistic effects on growth but does have potential unwanted side effects, including virilization. These growth-promoting treatments should be managed by a pediatric endocrinologist.

Most girls with TS will have primary ovarian insufficiency resulting in hypogonadism and infertility. Often this occurs well before pubertal age, but a minority of girls will have enough ovarian function for spontaneous thelarche (~30%) or menarche (~20%). For girls with primary ovarian insufficiency, low-dose transdermal estradiol starting at age 11 to 12 years is advised to induce secondary sexual characteristics, contribute to pubertal growth, and improve long-term bone and cardiovascular health. Reproductive medicine advances may improve fertility options for girls with some remaining oocytes.

Congenital and acquired heart disease affect more than half of all girls with TS and require lifelong cardiology monitoring. Left-sided structural defects, including bicuspid aortic valve (15%–30%), coarctation of the aorta (~15%), and aortic dilation are the most common and should prompt genetic evaluation for TS if diagnosed in a female. Cardiac imaging is required at least every 5 years even in the absence of physical exam findings or previously identified abnormalities. Arterial hypertension is also common, and due to the risk of aortic dilation and dissection this should be treated promptly. Additional comorbidities include structural renal disease (horseshoe kidney), orthopedic conditions (hip dysplasia, scoliosis, osteoporosis), autoimmune diseases (thyroid, celiac, vitiligo, type 1 diabetes), recurrent otitis media, sensorineural or conductive hearing loss, ophthalmologic concerns (strabismus, refractory errors), and cardiometabolic conditions (obesity, type 2 diabetes, dyslipidemia, liver dysfunction).

Developmental and Psychological Features of Turner Syndrome

Infants and toddlers with TS have an increased risk for developmental delays across all domains, although many present with typical early development. Infants born with congenital heart malformations or other medical problems that require medical or surgical intervention(s) in the first years of life are at increased risk for delays, as are young children with hearing loss.

The neuropsychological and social-emotional risks in TS have been well characterized, although like all SCA conditions they vary widely in their presentation between individuals (Hutaff-Lee, Bennett, Howell, & Tartaglia, 2019). Studies of cognitive abilities in TS show that mean full-scale IQ is only slightly lower than the population mean, and individual scores generally follow a normal distribution such that a percentage also have above-average cognitive abilities. Cognitive profiles most often show higher scores in the verbal compared to nonverbal domains, highlighting important challenges with visual-spatial skills that can affect daily life. A subgroup of individuals with TS present with more significant cognitive involvement, and it is estimated that about 5% to 10% have intellectual disability.

Despite average cognitive abilities, individuals with TS may present with academic challenges due to a combination of learning disabilities and other neuropsychological features such as executive function deficits, attentional problems, and slow processing speed. Research has suggested that up to 75% of females with TS will experience some level of math difficulties, and up to 50% meet criteria for a specific learning disability in math. There is also an increased risk for attention deficits, and up to 25% meet criteria for ADHD. While all ADHD subtypes can be present, hyperactive/impulsive symptoms are often higher in TS compared to typical females. Executive function difficulties in TS can include challenges with working memory and difficulties with inhibition, flexibility, organization, and planning. Fine motor and motor coordination difficulties are also common and can affect handwriting, daily living skills, and physical activities.

There is also an increased risk for social-emotional difficulties, including challenges with developing and maintaining peer relationships and reading social cues. Generally, social challenges do not meet criteria for ASD; however, in some cases social communication difficulties can be more significant and include other behavioral features leading to a diagnosis of ASD. The lifetime prevalence of anxiety or depression in TS is as high as 50%, and it is common for anxiety symptoms to emerge in early childhood. Overall, many subtypes of anxiety have been reported, including generalized anxiety, social anxiety, specific phobias, and obsessive-compulsive behaviors. Further, as some children and adolescents may require frequent medical procedures, blood draws for hormone levels, or growth hormone injections, anxiety related to medical procedures may occur.

Screening and Treatment Recommendations for Turner Syndrome

The International Clinical Practice Guidelines for the care of girls and women with Turner syndrome were published in 2017 and include evidence-based recommendations for screening and management (Gravholt et al., 2017). These detailed guidelines emphasize a multidisciplinary approach to caring for TS and should be referenced whenever providing care. In brief, medical recommendations include endocrinology for growth hormone treatment, pubertal monitoring and estrogen/progesterone treatment, and ongoing screening for thyroid and other cardiometabolic risks. Further, cardiology management and routine surveillance for hearing and vision deficits and autoimmune diseases are among the universal screening recommendations. Genetic counseling is encouraged for all families with a child with TS, and preconception counseling is recommended for any female with TS who has spontaneous menarche or has a karyotype that may be associated with preserved fertility (e.g., 45,X/46,XX, partial Xp deletions, or other X chromosome structural anomalies).

For the developmental-behavioral pediatrician, care for TS requires knowledge of the medical, neurodevelopmental, and social-emotional features, with important consideration of how medical features can impact development and behavior. Treatment guidelines specify that neuropsychology or other behavioral health specialists are integrated into the care team and that developmental and behavioral screenings are conducted annually until adulthood. These screenings should target the specific challenges associated with TS as described earlier, including early development, learning/academic problems, ADHD, social development, and emotional difficulties such as anxiety. Other important recommendations include referral for neuropsychological assessments at key transitional stages in schooling and implementation of academic supports and accommodations. Educational recommendations can include special education and evidence-based interventions for learning disabilities and supports for executive functioning deficits, ADHD, slow processing speed, and social-emotional difficulties. If needed, IEP recommendations can also include considerations for short stature such as desk/chair size and locker location. It is important to consider medical conditions associated with TS when evaluating behavioral symptoms, such as considering new-onset hearing loss when evaluating symptoms of inattention or the potential of thyroid or other hormonal abnormalities contributing to symptoms of depression or anxiety.

Treatment for neurodevelopmental disorders such as ADHD should follow ADHD treatment guidelines that include a combination of educational and behavioral supports as well as medication treatment, with special consideration of medical features that may be present in TS. Stimulant medications can be effective; however, consultation with cardiology prior to beginning stimulant medications is important for those with a history of heart malformations, arrythmias, or hypertension. Stimulants can also decrease appetite, and thus weight and growth should be monitored closely to ensure that caloric intake is sufficient to support ongoing growth especially in those also treated with growth hormone. Nonstimulant medications for ADHD can also be effective in TS. As with other neurodevelopmental disorders, medication treatment should begin at conservative doses and be increased slowly to obtain symptom control while monitoring side effects.

Symptoms of anxiety and/or depression should be addressed with psychotherapy strategies and consideration of medication treatments. Psychological techniques based in cognitive behavioral therapy (CBT) are often effective for anxiety and depression symptoms. Other features of TS should be considered when evaluating for triggers of anxiety (e.g., math or learning difficulties contributing to anxiety in the school setting or social communication difficulties leading to social anxiety). Medications are also often included in the treatment plan for symptoms of anxiety and depression, most commonly selective serotonin reuptake inhibitor (SSRI) medications; however, other classes such as alpha agonists or propranolol may be helpful. Again, medical history and current cardiac status should be considered when selecting medications, as some can prolong cardiac QT interval, which may be contraindicated for some patients. Benzodiazepines can be effective for situational or medical procedure–related anxiety.

XXY/KLINEFELTER SYNDROME

Genetics and Diagnosis of XXY/Klinefelter Syndrome

XXY (also known as Klinefelter syndrome [KS]) is an SCA condition characterized by the presence of an additional X chromosome in a male. The clinical features of XXY were first described by Dr. Harry Klinefelter in 1942, and it was later discovered to be due to an extra X chromosome by Dr. Patricia Jacobs in 1959. The diagnosis is made by various chromosome analysis techniques, usually karyotype or microarray. The supernumerary X chromosome in XXY arises due to a nondisjunction event in meiosis I or II. In nearly one-half of cases the supernumerary X chromosome is due to a paternal nondisjunction event, while it is maternal in origin in the other 50%. The second X chromosome undergoes X inactivation as in females; however, 15% to 20% of X chromosome genes escape X inactivation, and overexpression of these genes and their downstream effects lead to the clinical features of KS. The quest to identify the specific genes and pathways is underway (see Genetic Research in SCA, later). About 10% of cases show mosaicism with 46,XY cell lines, which typically results in a milder phenotype and improved fertility. Conversely, mosaicism with the different tetrasomy and pentasomy SCA conditions can also occur often leading to a more complex presentation (see Tetrasomy and Pentasomy Conditions, later).

The prevalence of KS is approximately 1 in 650 male births. Diagnoses may be made at different times throughout the life span when various clinical features present for care, although it is estimated that ~60% remain undiagnosed during their lifetime. Currently, ~10% are identified in the prenatal period, although this rate is increasing due to increased noninvasive prenatal testing. Only another 5% are diagnosed in infancy or childhood because of speech delays, hypotonia, motor delays, learning disabilities, autism, or behavioral problems, despite almost 70% presenting with these clinical findings. With increased awareness of clinical features of KS, there is opportunity for developmental pediatricians to decrease this discrepancy by increasing genetic testing in this age group. An additional 10% of cases of KS are diagnosed in adolescence due to physical features (i.e., tall stature, microorchidism, gynecomastia) and/or incomplete puberty caused by hypogonadism (testosterone deficiency), and 15% are identified in adulthood during evaluation for infertility or hypogonadism.

Clinical Features of XXY/Klinefelter Syndrome

Medical and Physical Features of XXY/Klinefelter Syndrome

There is significant phenotypic variability in KS with some individuals significantly affected by the developmental and medical features, while others have milder features (Davis et al., 2016). Facial dysmorphic features are not universal and are usually subtle when present, including epicanthal folds or hypertelorism. Tall stature, or stature taller than expected for the family history, is noted in many males with KS and usually becomes more evident during the second decade of life.

Primary testicular insufficiency resulting in hypogonadism (testosterone deficiency) is a hallmark feature of KS and is nearly universal (Fig. 26.3). Testicular development appears to be abnormal from early in life. Hypogonadism may start as early as fetal life or early infancy. Infants with KS have a higher prevalence of underdeveloped genitalia and cryptorchidism, reduced germ cell number in testicular

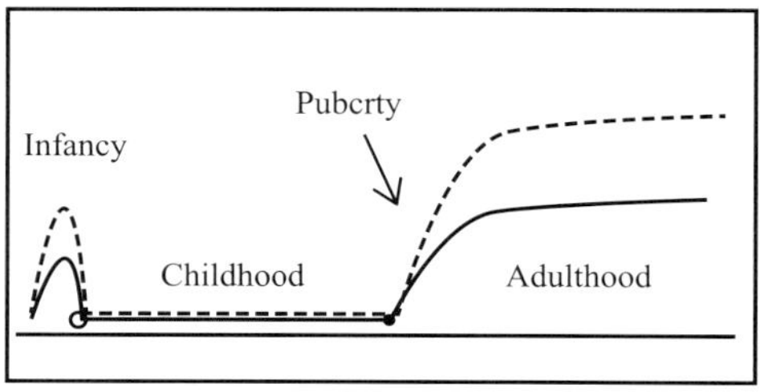

Fig. 26.3 Testosterone levels over the lifespan in Klinefelter syndrome *(solid)* compared to typical male *(dashed)*. (From Davis, S., Howell, S., Wilson, R., Tanda, T., Ross, J., Zeitler, P., & Tartaglia, N. [2016]. Advances in the interdisciplinary care of children with Klinefelter syndrome. *Advances in Pediatrics, 63*[1], 15–46. https://doi.org/10.1016/j.yapd.2016.04.020.)

biopsies, and smaller testicular size. A systematic review summarizing testosterone levels during the minipuberty of infancy found ~20% of infants had testosterone below the normal range, and all were below the median (Aksglaede et al., 2020). Studies investigating the potential benefits of testosterone supplementation in infancy are being conducted (Davis, Reynolds, Dabelea, Zeitler, & Tartaglia, 2019). Androgen supplementation during childhood prior to puberty has shown modest benefits in body composition, visual-motor integration, and anxiety symptoms; however, it also led to precocious puberty and therefore is not recommended as standard of care at this time.

In adolescence, boys with KS typically have a normal age of onset of puberty, but progression often stalls in mid-to-late puberty due to testicular failure and lack of sufficient testosterone production (Pizzocaro et al., 2020). Testicular size is universally small in postpubertal males with KS due to a reduction in the germ cells that make up the bulk of the testis volume and is a clinical finding often overlooked during adolescent primary care. Gynecomastia likely occurs in similar rates in pubertal boys without KS (~50%) but may be more likely to persist in KS, especially if initiation of testosterone treatment is delayed. It is recommended that boys with KS see an endocrinologist for pubertal monitoring starting around 10 years of age or at the first sign of puberty, whichever comes first. Testosterone replacement therapy is considered standard of care when there is evidence of testicular insufficiency to support normal pubertal development. Sperm production is impaired, leading to impaired fertility and azoospermia in most cases. Advances in reproductive technology are promising, however, and with current microsurgical techniques sperm can be found in the testes for in vitro fertilization in up to 50% of men with KS who wish to have biological children.

Children and adolescents with KS are at risk of other medical conditions, including musculoskeletal concerns (elbow abnormalities, pes planus, joint laxity), atopic conditions (asthma, allergies, eosinophilic esophagitis), neurologic differences (hypotonia, tremor, white matter magnetic resonance imaging [MRI] abnormalities, seizures), cardiac septal defects, velopharyngeal insufficiency, autoimmunity, certain malignancies, and dental problems. Rates of these findings vary widely depending on the samples studied; however, clinicians should recognize the increased risk for these conditions in males with KS and pursue appropriate screening and management. Adults with KS are known to have a high prevalence of disorders related to insulin resistance, including metabolic syndrome, type 2 diabetes mellitus, dyslipidemia, fatty liver disease, osteoporosis, and a higher prevalence of cardiovascular disease, peripheral vascular disease, and thromboembolic events. Thus screening and lifestyle counseling for these adult conditions should begin in adolescence.

Developmental-Behavioral Features of XXY/Klinefelter Syndrome

Although developmental outcomes are highly variable in XXY there is a clear pattern of increased risk for developmental delay (Tartaglia et al., 2020). Approximately 70% of young boys with XXY show mild speech delays, with relative strengths in receptive language and more impairment in expressive communication. Developmental dyspraxia of speech can be a component of the early expressive language delays. Problems with motor coordination, motor planning, and low tone can also contribute to delayed gross motor milestones (e.g., average age of first steps is 14–15 months). Treatment recommendations include close developmental monitoring starting in infancy, with standardized developmental assessments at 9- to 12-month intervals starting in the first year of life through 5 years of age. Implementation of early intervention for speech, physical, and occupational therapy is indicated if delays are identified.

Overall, cognitive abilities are generally in the average range, although mean full-scale IQ scores are approximately 10 to 15 points less than those of sibling controls, often with a profile of stronger nonverbal skills compared to verbal domains. Processing speed and working memory are also often affected. Despite average cognition, high rates of language-based learning disabilities (e.g., dyslexia/reading disabilities), language disorders, and executive function deficits cause many children with XXY to struggle in school and require supports through a 504 plan or IEP. Neuropsychological and speech-language evaluations are recommended in school-age children with XXY to evaluate for learning disabilities, executive function deficits, and language disorders, including childhood apraxia of speech and higher-level pragmatic communication deficits (Bishop et al., 2019). Fine and gross motor deficits and graphomotor problems are also common, and children may benefit from occupational therapy interventions and assistive technology in the classroom. Low physical endurance, daytime fatigue, and overall strength challenges also sometimes occur and may benefit from physical therapy and increased physical activity.

Children with XXY are at increased risk for a variety of neurodevelopmental, behavioral, and social-emotional disorders. Attention deficits are common, with ~35% meeting criteria for ADHD (primarily inattentive type). In addition, shy and withdrawn temperaments combined with language delays and social immaturity can interfere with social development. Children with XXY have increased risk for ASD, and those who do not meet full criteria for a diagnosis may still demonstrate deficits in social communication skills or sensory processing difficulties. Anxiety and mood disorders (e.g., depression, dysthymia) are also common and often underlie or contribute to behavioral challenges presenting in this population. ADHD, anxiety, mood, and social skills should be assessed and treated with therapy and psychopharmacologic interventions as indicated, with therapy approaches adapted as necessary for language deficits. Neuroimaging studies show that brain maturation lags 1 to 2 years compared to typical males, and this is evident in a subset where social-emotional maturity may lag behind same-age peers but improves in their 20 s. For some, the combination of learning, executive functioning, and emotional features contribute to lower overall adaptive functioning in adulthood than expected for their cognitive abilities. However, adult outcomes for males with XXY are as broad as in the general population, and many successfully achieve occupational success and higher education.

XYY SYNDROME

Genetics and Diagnosis of XYY

XYY syndrome is a SCA condition characterized by the presence of an additional Y chromosome in a male. The additional Y chromosome arises from a sporadic nondisjunction event in meiosis I or II during sperm production in the father. The prevalence of XYY is estimated to be 1 in 1000 male births, although studies estimate that up to 90% of XYY males are undiagnosed. As with the other SCAs, prenatal ascertainment is increasing due to rising use of NIPS, and NIPS results should always be confirmed by postnatal genetic testing and by amniocentesis if diagnostic confirmation is desired in the prenatal period. Although initially publicized as such, the diagnosis of XYY is not associated with increased aggressive or criminal behaviors. Males with XYY syndrome may be diagnosed by prenatal screening for other fetal aneuploidies or they may be identified postnatally when genetic testing is ordered for developmental delays, ASD, or medical features such as tall stature, joint laxity, or seizures. Given the lack of other distinctive associated medical problems to prompt genetic testing, if not identified in the prenatal period the majority of males with XYY remain undiagnosed.

Clinical Features of XYY

Physical and Medical Features of XYY

As with other SCAs there is variability in the features exhibited in XYY (Bardsley et al., 2013). Birthweight, length, and head circumference are normal in infants with XYY. Tall stature is the most prominent physical feature in XYY, with most at or above the 75th percentile for height and stature taller than expected for the family history. Tall stature usually becomes more evident during the adolescent years. Facial dysmorphic features are not universal and are usually subtle when present, including epicanthal folds or hypertelorism.

Testes and penile size are within the normal range in men with XYY. Males with XYY generally have normal male hormone production with a slight increase in fertility problems. Some males with XYY have reported cryptorchidism and hypospadias; however, overt hypogonadism or testosterone deficiency is not commonly associated with XYY. Further, the extra Y chromosome does not lead to elevated testosterone levels compared to typical males, despite some false reports of this on the internet.

There is an increased prevalence of type 2 diabetes and cardiovascular diseases, with both conditions yielding a standardized mortality ratio of 2.2 in men with XYY. Studies of cardiometabolic features in younger cohorts with XYY are lacking; however, a recent study in youth with XYY showed higher prevalence of cardiometabolic features (dyslipidemia, abdominal adiposity), along with a potential relationship with testicular hormones. Similar to KS, males with XYY are at risk of other health conditions, including congenital anomalies, musculoskeletal concerns (elbow abnormalities, pes planus, joint laxity), atopic conditions (asthma, allergies, eosinophilic esophagitis), neurologic differences (hypotonia, white matter MRI abnormalities, seizures, tremor), autoimmunity, velopharyngeal insufficiency, and dental problems. Seizures are reported in about 10%, often in association with more significant neurocognitive involvement; however, this relationship contains ascertainment bias as those with neurocognitive involvement are more likely to undergo genetic testing. Rates of these different medical problems within the XYY population vary depending on the population studied; however, clinicians should have familiarity with the risks present in XYY diagnosis and pursue appropriate screening and clinical management.

Developmental-Behavioral Features of XYY

Although developmental outcomes in XYY vary considerably, a majority of young boys with XYY present with mild speech delays, with relative strengths in receptive language and more significant impairment in expressive communication (Tartaglia et al., 2020). Developmental dyspraxia of speech can be a component of the early expressive language delays. Problems with motor coordination, balance, motor planning, and low tone can also contribute to delayed gross motor milestones. Close developmental monitoring starting in infancy is recommended, with standardized developmental assessments at 9- to 12-month intervals starting in the first year of life through 5 years of age. Implementation of early intervention for speech, physical, and occupational therapy is indicated if delays are identified. If features of apraxia of speech are apparent, additional speech therapy techniques supporting motor planning of speech are important, in addition to strategies for language stimulation.

Overall, cognitive abilities for boys with XYY are generally in the average range, with mean full-scale IQ approximately 5 to 10 points less than normative means. Despite average cognition, high rates of learning disabilities, language disorders, and executive function deficits cause many children with XYY to struggle in school and require supports through a 504 plan or IEP. Psychoeducational assessment, including speech-language evaluation, should be obtained in school-age children with XYY to evaluate for learning disabilities as well as language impairment, including childhood dyspraxia of speech and higher-level pragmatic communication deficits.

Gross motor coordination and balance deficits as well as graphomotor problems are also common, and children may benefit from physical and occupational therapy interventions and assistive technology in the classroom.

Children with XYY are at increased risk for a variety of neurodevelopmental, behavioral, and social-emotional disorders. Given the high risk, screening for challenges across all affected domains should be completed on a yearly basis. Attention deficits and hyperactivity/impulsivity are common, with up to 75% of a clinical sample meeting criteria for ADHD. Children with XYY also have increased risk for social skills deficits and social communication difficulties, and studies show that 15% to 30% meet criteria for a diagnosis of ASD (Tartaglia et al., 2017). Anxiety, low frustration tolerance, and mood dysregulation can also be common, and may underlie many behavioral challenges from a young age through adolescence. ADHD, anxiety, and mood symptoms should be assessed and treated with behavioral and psychopharmacologic interventions as indicated, with therapy approaches adapted as necessary for language deficits. Social skills groups and other interventions for social development, as well as occupational therapy strategies to improve self-care, sensory symptoms, and self-regulation, may be indicated. For some, the combination of learning, executive functioning, and emotional features contributes to lower overall adaptive functioning in adulthood than expected for their cognitive abilities. However, adult outcomes for males with XYY are as broad as in the general population, and many successfully achieve occupational success and higher education.

TRISOMY X/47,XXX

Genetics and Diagnosis of Trisomy X

X47,XXX (also known as triple X, and herein referred to as trisomy X) is a SCA characterized by the presence of an additional X chromosome in a phenotypic female. Trisomy X arises due to a nondisjunction error in meiosis I or II during the formation of gametes. Cytogenetic studies have revealed that the supernumerary X chromosome in females with trisomy X can be either maternal or paternal in origin; however, of those studied, the supernumerary X chromosome was maternal in origin in ~80% and associated with advanced maternal age. In females with mosaic trisomy X (46, XX/47, XXX) the supernumerary X arises due to a postzygotic nondisjunction error in the developing fetus.

The prevalence is 1 in 1000 liveborn females. As with XYY syndrome, it is estimated that only 10% of females with trisomy X are identified during their lifetime. Low clinical ascertainment can be partially attributed to the lack of a distinct recognizable physical phenotype, and to many being asymptomatic or showing only mild physical or neurodevelopmental concerns. Therefore, similar to XYY, descriptions in the medical literature of females with trisomy X apply to females currently aware of their diagnosis and likely underrepresent more mildly affected and asymptomatic females.

Females with trisomy X are diagnosed by cytogenetic testing obtained in either the prenatal or postnatal setting. Historically, a small percentage of females were identified prenatally due to screening for fetal aneuploidies in mothers with advanced maternal age. However, rates of prenatal ascertainment of females with trisomy X are rising with increased use of NIPS. The positive predictive value of NIPS for the SCA conditions is lower compared with autosomal aneuploidies, and a positive NIPS screen should be confirmed with a diagnostic test (e.g., karyotype of fetal cells from amniocentesis or postnatal peripheral blood sample). NIPS has also led to identification of many adult women with previously unrecognized trisomy X (after ruling out trisomy X in the fetus). Postnatally, ascertained cases of trisomy X are most commonly identified as part of a diagnostic evaluation for hypotonia or developmental delays in early childhood, ASD, or medical features such as tall stature, joint laxity, seizures, or ovarian failure/infertility.

Clinical Features of Trisomy X

Medical and Physical Features of Trisomy X

Many females with trisomy X have no obvious physical features, although subtle and variable physical differences such as hypertelorism, epicanthal folds, fifth finger clinodactyly, pes planus, joint laxity, tall stature, and hypotonia can be present (Wigby et al., 2016). Echocardiogram and renal ultrasound are recommended due to congenital cardiac and genitourinary anomalies in an estimated 10% to 15% with trisomy X, though surgical interventions are not usually needed. Seizures, in particular focal onset impaired awareness seizures, are present in 5% to 10% and tend to be well controlled with anticonvulsant medications. Other potential neurologic features include tremor, white matter MRI abnormalities, and motor coordination deficits. Low physical endurance often impacts physical activities and quality of life. Other associated medical conditions may include atopic conditions (asthma, allergies, eosinophilic esophagitis), hip dysplasia, velopharyngeal insufficiency, autoimmunity, hypothyroidism, sleep disorders, and dental problems. Rates of these findings vary widely depending on the study; however, clinicians should recognize the increased risk for these conditions in females with trisomy X and pursue appropriate screening and management.

Puberty and fertility have traditionally been considered to be normal. A small proportion of females with trisomy X may be identified as adults as part of diagnostic evaluation for premature ovarian failure (POF), although the prevalence of POF remains unknown. Recent studies have reported adolescents with trisomy X with smaller ovarian volumes and lower anti-Müllerian hormone levels compared with age-matched controls, suggesting diminished ovarian reserve. Further dedicated study of the natural history of fertility and hormonal variability in trisomy X is an important area that will help inform medical care.

Developmental-Behavioral Features of Trisomy X

Developmental outcomes in trisomy X vary considerably; however, there is a clear pattern of increased risk for early developmental delays (Tartaglia et al., 2020). Prospective studies have shown that over half of young girls with trisomy X present with mild speech delays, with relative strengths in receptive language compared to expressive communication and some showing features of developmental dyspraxia of speech. Problems with motor coordination and low tone can also contribute to delayed gross motor milestones, and motor deficits may persist through adolescence. Close developmental monitoring starting in infancy is recommended, with standardized developmental assessments at 9- to 12-month intervals starting in the first year of life through 5 years of age. Early intervention therapies, including speech, physical, and occupational therapy, are recommended when delays are identified.

Overall, cognitive abilities in girls with trisomy X are more impaired than in the other sex chromosome trisomies, with higher frequencies of mild intellectual disability (~15%) and average full-scale IQ scores approximately 10 to 15 points lower than normative means (Urbanus, van Rijn, & Swaab, 2020). The characteristic profile includes higher nonverbal IQ than verbal IQ. Working memory and processing speed can also be affected. Higher rates of learning disabilities, language impairment, and executive function deficits cause many girls with trisomy X to struggle in school and require supports through a 504 plan or IEP. Psychoeducational assessment, including speech-language evaluation, should be obtained in school-age children every 3 years to evaluate for learning disabilities and language impairment (or more frequently if needed), including evaluation for higher-level language, comprehension, and pragmatic communication skills (Bishop et al., 2019). Gross motor coordination deficits, low strength and endurance, and graphomotor problems are also common into adolescence, and these often benefit from physical and occupational therapy interventions as well as assistive technology in the classroom.

Girls with trisomy X are at increased risk for psychological distress across the life span, primarily with internalizing behaviors such as anxiety, depression, social withdrawal, and low self-esteem. In early childhood, anxiety can present as selective mutism. Attention deficits are also common, with up to 35% meeting criteria for ADHD inattentive type. There is also increased risk for social-emotional immaturity and social communication difficulties, with an estimated 10% meeting criteria for a diagnosis of ASD. Anxiety, mood, ADHD, and social skills should be assessed and treated with behavioral and psychopharmacologic interventions as indicated. Social skills groups and other interventions for social development, as well as occupational therapy strategies to improve sensory processing problems and self-regulation, are recommended as indicated. The combination of cognitive deficits with social-emotional features contributes to adaptive functioning levels that are often lower than expected for cognitive abilities. Research supports that females with prenatally ascertained trisomy X have higher IQ scores and adaptive functioning levels compared to those with a postnatal diagnosis, although they remain at risk for learning disabilities, ADHD, and anxiety. Those with mosaicism (46,XX/47,XXX) tend to have milder symptoms compared to nonmosaic females. Research on adult outcomes of females with trisomy X shows more psychological symptoms and lower quality of life compared to the general population; however, outcomes are very broad, and many achieve occupational success and higher education.

TETRASOMY AND PENTASOMY CONDITIONS (XXYY, XXXY, XYYY, XXXXY, XXYYY, TETRASOMY X, PENTASOMY X)

Genetics of Sex Chromosome Tetrasomy and Pentasomy

Tetrasomy and pentasomy SCA conditions can occur in all different combinations of X and Y chromosomes up to a total of five sex chromosomes; however, they are much less common compared to the trisomies (see Table 26.1). Tetrasomy and pentasomy SCAs occur by mechanisms of double nondisjunction events during formation of oocytes or spermatids, or by very early postzygotic nondisjunction of typical XX or XY embryos. Mosaicism with other trisomy or typical cell lines is also often seen.

Clinical Features of Tetrasomy and Pentasomy Conditions

Overall, the features of the tetrasomy and pentasomy conditions overlap with the trisomy conditions; however, there are higher rates of physical dysmorphic features and congenital malformations, and more significant neurodevelopmental involvement (Tartaglia, Ayari, Howell, D'Epagnier, & Zeitler, 2011) (see Table 26.2). Congenital heart malformations (usually septal defects), torticollis, renal malformations, talipes equinovarus, cleft palate, velopharyngeal insufficiency, radioulnar synostosis, thromboembolic events, MRI white matter and corpus callosum abnormalities, hypotonia, joint laxity, tremor, and seizure disorders are more common compared to the general population across both sexes. Tall stature is also often associated, although some with pentasomy conditions have short stature. Echocardiogram and renal ultrasound are recommended at diagnosis.

Males may also present with cryptorchidism or small genitalia. Any male with one or more extra X chromosomes will manifest the same features of hypogonadism (testosterone deficiency) and impaired fertility as seen in XXY, and management by endocrinology for testosterone treatment is important. Further medical risks occur in adulthood as described in the trisomy conditions earlier. Females are also more likely to have other genitourinary malformations and hip dysplasia. Females are at increased risk for delayed menarche or early ovarian failure, although in some puberty is normal, and larger studies are needed to understand sex hormones and reproductive function. The trisomy X section earlier describes additional medical features and treatment recommendations also appropriate for tetrasomy and pentasomy X.

As the number of X and/or Y chromosomes increases, there are more significant impacts on brain development. Delayed milestones are almost universal across all conditions, with both speech and motor milestones affected. Speech-language delays can be significant and typically include expressive delays with features of apraxia of speech, with some having minimal verbal speech until 6 to 7 years of age, and a small percentage remain mostly nonverbal. Mild intellectual disability occurs in approximately 50% to 60% of tetrasomy conditions and 75% to 85% of pentasomy conditions. Verbal cognitive skills are typically lower compared to nonverbal/visual-spatial abilities, which may fall in the low-average to average range; however, overall adaptive outcomes tend to correlate more with verbal scores. Language disorders and academic challenges (especially in reading and writing) are almost universal. Fine and gross motor coordination and planning are typically often impacted.

Other neurodevelopmental and psychological diagnoses, including ADHD, ASD, and anxiety disorders, are frequent. In XXYY syndrome, ~80% meet criteria for ADHD and 50% meet criteria for ASD. Both occur at high rates in the other conditions, although large studies are lacking. Behavioral dysregulation, including tantrums, meltdowns, avoidant behaviors, low frustration tolerance, and aggression, may occur in some patients, more commonly in the male tetrasomy/pentasomy conditions compared to females. These are often exacerbated by language challenges, anxiety, poor executive functioning, and sensory sensitivities. In females with tetrasomy and pentasomy X, externalizing behaviors are less common, although meltdowns and sensory sensitivities can occur, and features of anxiety such as selective mutism are also common.

Treatment recommendations for all conditions include comprehensive assessment at diagnosis and at key timepoints thereafter that includes evaluation of cognitive, language, academic, motor, social, emotional, executive functioning, sensory, and adaptive functioning, Treatment for behavioral challenges should include adaptations of psychological or behavioral therapy approaches targeting appropriate developmental and language levels. Traditional psychological therapies may have decreased effectiveness due to frequent expressive language challenges and tendency to become withdrawn or frustrated with high-language environments. Antecedents for behavioral challenges often include anxiety, challenges with self-expression, or feeling overwhelmed. Psychopharmacologic treatments are frequently an important component of the treatment plan as indicated for anxiety, depression, ADHD, or mood regulation. Selective mutism in females often responds well to SSRI treatment. In those males with an extra X chromosome who typically develop hypogonadism, testosterone therapy started conservatively when deficiency emerges does not typically exacerbate underlying behavioral challenges; however, it also does not markedly improve them except in some cases of late diagnoses where hypogonadism is longstanding and more severe. It is recommended that testosterone therapy is started separately from other psychological or psychopharmacologic treatments and that other conditions such as ADHD or anxiety are treated per recommendations for those conditions rather than expecting testosterone to improve emotional or behavioral concerns.

GENETIC RESEARCH IN SEX CHROMOSOME ANEUPLOIDIES

The clinical features associated with SCAs result from the missing or extra sex chromosomes in general; however, the genetic mechanisms or specific genes explaining the phenotypic variability are mostly unknown. Studies have explored whether the parent-of-origin of the extra X chromosomes in X chromosome aneuploidy conditions (or the single X in TS) are related to the phenotype; however, results have been variable and not consistently duplicated. In X aneuploidy conditions in both males and females, the additional X chromosome(s) undergo(es) the epigenetic mechanism of X inactivation, and incomplete or skewed X inactivation ratios have also been evaluated in small studies with inconsistent results. In addition, an estimated 20% to 30% of genes on the inactivated X chromosome "escape" inactivation and remain actively expressed. Thus increased dosage of these genes is postulated as a mechanism of phenotypic differences, but specific genes have not yet been identified.

When examining phenotypic variability, some studies show risk factors for poorer outcomes also known to be risks in the general population. For example, multiple SCA studies have supported that background familial factors such as the presence of learning disabilities, mental health conditions, language disorders, ADHD, or autism also confer additional risk for presence and severity of these features in SCA conditions. Environmental factors such as adverse childhood events are also associated with more complex clinical presentations.

Only a few specific genes have been identified that are associated with clinical features of the SCA conditions. The *SHOX* gene is located in one of the two segments of the sex chromosomes called the pseudoautosomal regions, which are short regions of homologous genes on the X and Y chromosomes. Genes in this region escape X inactivation and are thus expressed from all the sex chromosomes that are present. The *SHOX* gene is involved in bone growth, and the copy number of *SHOX* is associated with the stature differences in the SCA conditions: One copy in monosomy X leads to the short stature in TS, while three or more copies lead to tall stature associated with XXY/KS and other sex chromosome trisomies and tetrasomies. Other potential genes involved in SCA phenotypes include polymorphisms in the X chromosome androgen receptor gene associated with some physical manifestations in XXY, and *NLGN4Y* expression differences are associated with autism. Researchers looking for genotype-phenotype correlations have traditionally focused efforts on sex chromosome genes. However, recent studies show that patterns of gene expression in SCA are much more complex than would be expected from traditional X and Y gene dosage theories and that SCA conditions are associated with dysregulation of hundreds to thousands of autosomal genes as well (Raznahan et al., 2018). These findings add a great deal of complexity to the quest to understand the pathophysiology of the phenotypic findings in SCA conditions, and newer complex -omic approaches such as epigenomics, transcriptomics, and metabolomics are being pursued to identify genes and downstream pathways responsible for SCA phenotypes.

PATIENT AND PROFESSIONAL RESOURCES

Patients, parents/caretakers, and professionals should be directed to national advocacy organizations, including the Association for X&Y Chromosome Variations (AXYS) (www.genetic.org), Turner Syndrome Global Alliance (www.tsgalliance.org), Turner Syndrome Society of the United States (www.turnersyndrome.org), or XXYY Project (www.genetic.org) for support, care guidelines, updated research findings, and research opportunities. A family-friendly version of the 2017 clinical practice guidelines for TS is available in English and Spanish at http://schererclin.com/tspatiented2017/.

CONCLUSION

In conclusion, SCA conditions are common in the general population and often present with nonspecific manifestations. Mild developmental delays, learning challenges, and social deficits may be the first symptoms of these conditions, as illustrated in the case vignette. Developmental and Behavioral Pediatricians should therefore be aware of these subtle signs and symptoms that may lead to the diagnosis, as well as be able to guide individualized evaluation and management after a diagnosis has been made.

REFERENCES

Aksglaede, L., Davis, SM., Ross, JL., Juul, A. (2020). Minipuberty in Klinefelter syndrome: Current status and furture directions. *American Journal of Medical Genetics Part C, 184*(2), 320–326.

Bardsley, M., Kowal, K., Levy, C., Gosek, A., Ayari, N., Tartaglia, N., . . . Ross, J. L. (2013). 47,XYY syndrome: Clinical phenotype and timing of ascertainment. *Journal of Pediatrics, 163*(4), 1085–1094.

Bishop, D. V. M., Brookman-Byrne, A., Gratton, N., Gray, E., Holt, G., Morgan, L., . . . Thompson, P. A. (2019). Language phenotypes in children with sex chromosome trisomies. *Wellcome Open Research, 3*, 143.

Davis, S., Howell, S., Wilson, R., Tanda, T., Ross, J., Zeitler, P., & Tartaglia, N. (2016). Advances in the interdisciplinary care of children with Klinefelter syndrome. *Advan ces in Pediatrics, 63*(1), 15–46.

Davis, S. M., Reynolds, R. M., Dabelea, D. M., Zeitler, P. S., & Tartaglia, N. R. (2019). Testosterone treatment in infants with 47,XXY: Effects on body composition. *Journal of the Endocrine Society, 3*(12), 2276–2285.

Gravholt, C. H., Andersen, N. H., Conway, G. S., Dekkers, O. M., Geffner, M. E., Klein, K. O., . . . International Turner Syndrome Consensus Group, (2017). Clinical practice guidelines for the care of girls and women with Turner syndrome: Proceedings from the 2016 Cincinnati International Turner Syndrome Meeting. *European Journal of Endocrinology, 177*(3), G1–G70.

Hutaff-Lee, C., Bennett, E., Howell, S., & Tartaglia, N. (2019). Clinical developmental, neuropsychological, and social-emotional features of Turner syndrome. *American Journal of Medical Genetics Part C: Seminars in Medical Genetics, 181*(1), 126–134.

Pizzocaro, A., Vena, W., Condorelli, R., Radicioni, A., Rastrelli, G., Pasquali, D., . . . King, Klinefelter ItaliaN Group, (2020). Testosterone treatment in male patients with Klinefelter syndrome: A systematic review and meta-analysis. *Journal of Endocrinological Investigation, 43*(12), 1675–1687.

Raznahan, A., Parikshak, N. N., Chandran, V., Blumenthal, J. D., Clasen, L. S., Alexander-Bloch, A. F., . . . Geschwind, D. H. (2018). Sex-chromosome dosage effects on gene expression in humans. *Proceedings of the National Academy of Sciences of the United States of America, 115*(28), 7398–7403.

Tartaglia, N., Ayari, N., Howell, S., D'Epagnier, C., & Zeitler, P. (2011). 48,XXYY, 48,XXXY and 49,XXXXY syndromes: Not just variants of Klinefelter syndrome. *Acta Paediatrica, 100*(6), 851–860.

Tartaglia, N., Howell, S., Davis, S., Kowal, K., Tanda, T., Brown, M., . . . & Ross, J. (2020). Early neurodevelopmental and medical profile in children with sex chromosome trisomies: Background for the prospective eXtraordinarY Babies Study to identify early risk factors and targets for intervention. *American Journal of Medical Genetics Part C: Seminars in Medical Genetics, 184*(2), 428–443. https//:doi.org/10.1002/ajmg.c.31807.

Tartaglia, N. R., Wilson, R., Miller, J. S., Rafalko, J., Cordeiro, L., Davis, S., . . . Ross, J. (2017). Autism spectrum disorder in males with sex chromosome aneuploidy: XXY/Klinefelter syndrome, XYY, and XXYY. *Journal of Developmental and Behavioral Pediatrics, 38*(3), 197–207.

Urbanus, E., van Rijn, S., & Swaab, H. (2020). A review of neurocognitive functioning of children with sex chromosome trisomies: Identifying targets for early intervention. *Clinical Genetics, 97*(1), 156–167.

Wigby, K., D'Epagnier, C., Howell, S., Reicks, A., Wilson, R., Cordeiro, L., & Tartaglia, N. Expanding the phenotype of triple X syndrome: A comparison of prenatal versus postnatal diagnosis. *American Journal of Medical Genetics Part A, 170*(11), 2870–2881.

Down Syndrome

Francis Hickey and Karen Kelminson

In memory of Dr. William I. Cohen (1947–2009).

For additional material related to the content of this chapter, please see Chapters 23 and 25.

> **VIGNETTE**
>
> *Paula is a 15-year-old girl with Down syndrome (DS). DS was diagnosed in the prenatal period after having abnormal first-trimester screening and confirmed with amniocentesis in the second trimester. A small ventricular septal defect was detected on an echocardiogram performed at birth and spontaneously closed in the first few years of life. Paula had oral feeding difficulties in infancy and early childhood. She was found to have pharyngeal dysphagia and aspiration and required thickening of thin liquids until age 5 years. She started developmental therapies through early intervention programs in early infancy and transitioned to public preschool at age 3 years where she continued therapies and started special education. At age 3 she had a polysomnogram, which demonstrated obstructive sleep apnea. She underwent adenotonsillectomy, which resulted in improvement in sleep apnea. Paula thrived in school where she participated in mainstream classes and her special education program. At age 8 years she was diagnosed with Hashimoto hypothyroidism and started therapy with levothyroxine. In the preteen years Paula started to gain weight quickly, out of proportion to linear growth. She has been followed in a multidisciplinary nutrition and weight management clinic. With encouragement from this clinic to begin a structured exercise program, Paula started to take part in Special Olympics and participates in track and basketball. She is in her first year of high school and is involved in extracurricular basketball and dance teams. After high school, Paula will attend a transition program through the school district and will focus on learning vocational skills.*

DOWN SYNDROME

DS is the most common genetic disorder causing intellectual disability. This discussion of its diagnosis and management serves the dual purpose of reminding the clinician of the important features of this condition and providing a model for the management of other developmental disabilities, combining a comprehensive understanding of the biologic disorder and an appreciation of how the parents, extended family, and community respond to the child and the child's unique needs.

Life for a family with a child with DS has improved in recent decades. Life expectancy has increased in individuals with DS, from the 20s in the 1980s to the 60s currently. Parents have been very involved in improving community and educational access and its quality, along with being the drivers in medical access and compliance with the medical guidelines. Other community changes started in the 1970s with deinstitutionalization of individuals with disabilities, including closing of institutions and federal legislation to guarantee education. There still are challenges in equity of access to services such as community, educational, and medical services.

HISTORY OF DOWN SYNDROME

Recent evidence indicates individuals with DS have existed since ancient times. Earliest depictions were from statues in 1500 BC in Mesoamerica. The oldest archeologic evidence of an individual with DS is a 9-year-old in England between AD 700 and 900. In the Middle Ages infants with DS are depicted as the infant Christ with the Madonna.

John Langdon Down, the lead physician at a hospital for individuals with intellectual disabilities in Surrey, England, chronicled the physical phenotype and intellectual disability in this identifiable syndrome. Down published his report in 1885 and noted common findings, including hearing/vision deficit, increased seizures, shortened lifespan, and poor circulation in this population.

Jérôme Lejeune discovered the presence of an extra chromosome 21 (trisomy 21) in individuals who fit Down's description in 1959. DS occurs in 1/691 live births or 1/150 conceptions. The higher rate for conceptions reflects the fact that one of four spontaneous abortions is a fetus with trisomy of any kind.

GENETICS

Three different chromosomal abnormalities are associated with individuals who have the phenotypic appearance of DS: trisomy 21, translocations, and mosaicism. Of individuals with the physical appearance of DS, 95% have trisomy 21, which is the presence of an extra chromosome 21 as a result of nondisjunction. In nondisjunction the chromosomes fail to pair or fail to exchange genetic material. This usually occurs at the first meiotic division, although it can occur at the second meiotic division as well. The extra chromosome is most often of maternal origin, but paternal origin occurs as well; in one study 7% of the infants received the extra chromosomal material from their fathers. Nondisjunction occurs sporadically in individuals of all ages; however, the association of increasing maternal age and trisomy reflects a well-known age-related increase in meiosis I nondisjunction. Although trisomy 21 occurs sporadically, empirically the rate of recurrence of trisomy 21, irrespective of age, is 1%. Nevertheless, for most women, the age-related risk predominates. At age 35 years, the risk is approximately 1 in 250. Although there are more parents who delay childbearing into their 30s and beyond, most of the infants with DS are born to mothers younger than 35 years. Women 35 years and older account for only about 7% of births each year (and approximately 20% of infants with DS). Consequently, the other 80% are born to women younger than 35 years.

Of individuals with DS, 3% to 4% have a translocation with the extra chromosomal material "stuck" to another chromosome. The extra chromosome 21 may be commonly attached to either chromosome 14 or chromosome 15. Fifty percent of translocations occur *de novo* and have a low risk of recurrence in subsequent pregnancies; however, 50% are inherited from a normal parent with a balanced translocation. These families have a high risk of recurrence in subsequent pregnancies. Therefore parents of children with translocations are encouraged to obtain a karyotype to determine whether they are balanced carriers and therefore at risk of having a subsequent child with DS. In this case siblings of the child with DS need testing to determine if they are also carriers of a balanced translocation.

Lastly, 1% to 2% of children have mosaicism, in which only some cells have the extra chromosome. This usually represents nondisjunction in an early postzygotic mitosis. The extent of affected tissues with an extra chromosome 21 varies with the timing of the event. Mosaicism can also occur by loss of the extra chromosome in early cell lines, so-called trisomy rescue. The greater the proportion of tissues with an extra chromosome 21, the greater likelihood that the individual will have the characteristic DS phenotype. On the other hand, individuals with only a small proportion of cells affected may never be detected because they would be unlikely to be karyotyped.

Mosaic forms of DS tend to cause confusion for both the families and physicians, who often assume that children with mosaicism have a milder form of DS. This statement is partially correct; depending on the tissues involved, an individual who has some cell lines with an extra chromosome 21 may be indistinguishable from the typical child. However, most children with mosaicism and the full phenotypic expression of DS will show typical characteristics.

PRENATAL SCREENING AND DIAGNOSIS

In January 2007 the American College of Obstetricians and Gynecologists (ACOG) issued a practice bulletin recommending that all pregnant women be screened for DS, starting with a first-trimester blood test for free beta-human chorionic gonadotropin and pregnancy-associated plasma protein A together with an ultrasound examination for nuchal translucency. Those at risk would be offered genetic counseling and the option of chorionic villus sampling or second trimester amniocentesis. In addition, neural tube screening with maternal serum alpha-fetoprotein determinations would be offered to women who undergo the first-trimester screening. The ACOG further recommends that those women who are not screened in the first-trimester obtain serum screening with alpha-fetoprotein, estriol, human chorionic gonadotropin, and inhibin A (ACOG, 2007). These recommendations elicited a strong negative reaction from the various national DS organizations, including the National Down Syndrome Congress and the National Down Syndrome Society. These groups expressed consternation that these guidelines promoted early identification for the purpose of termination of the pregnancy and offered to collaborate with ACOG to provide accurate information about the lives of people with DS to families faced with these decisions.

Cell-free DNA prenatal screening started in 2012 at the recommendation of ACOG at gestational age 10 to 16 weeks. An abnormal cell-free DNA test indicates an increased risk of the birth of an infant with a trisomy, including DS. It is important nondirective information from a counselor or provider enables parents to balance risks, limitations, and benefits of prenatal screening and diagnosis with issues involved in raising a child with DS or planning termination. This discussion infrequently occurs.

MAKING THE DIAGNOSIS IN THE NEWBORN PERIOD

The diagnosis of DS is first suggested by a variety of phenotypic characteristics that together indicate the consideration of this diagnosis (Table 27.1). The facial appearance of the child is often the first clue: flat profile, up-slanted palpebral fissures, epicanthal folds, flat nasal bridge, small auricles (external ears), nuchal fat pad, and short head (brachycephaly). Infants born vaginally often have edema of the face and eyelids, making it more difficult to detect the eye findings. On the other hand, central hypotonia, manifested as low muscle

TABLE 27.1 **Phenotypic Characteristics in Down Syndrome**
Hypotonia
Small brachycephalic head
Epicanthal folds
Flat nasal bridge
Upward slanting palpebral fissures
Brushfield spots
Macroglossia
Small ears
Excess skin at the nape of the neck
Single transverse palmar crease
Wide space between the first and second toes
Short fifth fingers with clinodactyly

tone, may make the diagnosis easier, whereas relatively normal tone will confound the picture.

The definitive diagnostic procedure is the chromosomal karyotype. Ordinarily, karyotype results may take up to 1 week, even longer if they are sent to a commercial laboratory. Interphase fluorescent *in situ* hybridization for trisomy 21 can be done to expedite the diagnosis but should always be followed by a karyotype to detect translocations or mosaicism.

INFORMING THE FAMILY

We recommend informing parents of suspicion of a DS diagnosis as soon as feasible. It is important to allow the newborn's mother to recover from immediate delivery and to wait until her husband, partner, or support person and infant are present together in a private setting. In this case offering the family a private hospital room is ideal. We recommend that the delivering medical provider and the primary care provider for the infant be present to discuss the diagnosis of DS. It is important to offer a balanced approach to information, and always offer congratulations for the birth of the new baby. Up-to-date printed information on DS given to the family can help serve as a first reference for questions about the diagnosis. We also recommend offering access to other families with children with DS and/or DS support organizations. Clinicians should be aware of realities and possibilities for healthy, productive lives of individuals with DS in society.

HEALTH CONCERNS IN INDIVIDUALS WITH DOWN SYNDROME

Gastrointestinal Disorders

Congenital gastrointestinal tract malformations, such as duodenal atresia and imperforate anus, occur in approximately 12% (Hickey et al., 2017) of children with DS. Vomiting and the inability to tolerate feedings in the first 12 hours of life warrant immediate investigation. The diagnosis of intestinal obstruction may be the first clue to the diagnosis of DS. Prenatal ultrasound findings of a "double bubble" or polyhydramnios may suggest the diagnosis *in utero*. These conditions are rarely occult, and the obvious need for intervention makes it impossible to overlook them. Hirschsprung disease is 25 times more likely to occur in individuals with DS than in the typical child. Failure to pass meconium in the first 24 hours of life may be the first clue to this condition. Severe constipation in infancy is an indication for evaluation for Hirschsprung disease by a pediatric gastroenterologist or a pediatric surgeon because of the high mortality associated with enterocolitis in the untreated child. Chronic constipation is reported in 30% of individuals with DS. It is often successfully treated with dietary interventions or stool softeners. Failure to respond should suggest further evaluation for Hirschsprung disease or hypothyroidism.

Gastroesophageal reflux occurs commonly and needs to be treated to prevent the consequences of acid reflux. Children with DS may have oral-motor dysfunction with swallowing difficulties and aspiration. A swallow study should be considered to evaluate dysphasia for signs of aspiration or recurrent respiratory infections, although often silent aspiration. An aerodigestive team (otolaryngologist, pulmonologist, and gastroenterologist) can be particularly helpful in this regard. Celiac disease (gluten enteropathy) is reported to occur in 7% to 14% of individuals with DS. In addition to the usual symptoms of bloating, diarrhea, and failure to thrive, children with DS may have no symptoms of malabsorption. If screening with tissue transglutaminase (TTG) is positive, refer to a gastroenterologist to confirm the diagnosis. A biopsy is necessary before treatment with a gluten-free diet.

Ophthalmologic Difficulties

Ophthalmologic difficulties are common in children with DS, and it is important to ensure optimal visual function. Dense congenital cataracts occur more frequently in DS than in the general population. The absence of a red reflex on funduscopic examination is an indication of emergent ophthalmologic referral. Cataract extraction is critical because amblyopia can occur rapidly, within 7 days in children younger than 1 year. Overall, cataracts are estimated to occur in 15% of individuals with DS, and fortunately, most of them are visually insignificant. Children with DS have an increased incidence of strabismus, nasolacrimal duct stenosis, and nystagmus. The detection of these conditions warrants timely referral. Because refractive errors occur in 50% of children with DS, they should be referred for routine ophthalmologic evaluation by 6 months of age in the absence of obvious ocular disease and yearly exams are recommended. Keratoconus is noted with increased frequency in DS. It is a cause of progressive loss of vision due to severe astigmatism and abnormal corneal anatomy. Early identification and intervention is important (Imbornoni et al., 2020).

Audiologic and Ear, Nose, and Throat Problems

Ear, nose, and throat problems are common in children with DS. Because of the characteristic midfacial hypoplasia, manifested as narrow airways, eustachian tubes, sinus ostia, and external auditory canals, children with DS are at increased risk for recurrent otitis media, nasopharyngitis or sinusitis, and the consequences of chronic serous otitis media. This is of significance, given the well-known difficulties in expressive language development in children with DS. At 6 years old 25% of children with DS have permanent hearing loss (Nightengale et al., 2017). The DS guidelines recommend hearing test every 6 months until 3 years of age, then annual testing (American Academy of Pediatrics [AAP], 2011). The team of physicians caring for the child must ensure optimal hearing to avoid the undesirable consequence of suboptimal language development. Common upper airway abnormalities include laryngomalacia, tracheomalacia, and subglottic stenosis. Such children need an ear, nose, and throat evaluation, often including laryngobronchoscopy. Children with DS have frequent episodes of croup, and this may reflect silent reflux causing laryngeal irritation.

Sleep Difficulties

Children and adults with DS frequently have a variety of sleep abnormalities. The anatomic features noted earlier, together with hypotonia, contribute to an increased incidence of obstructive sleep apnea. Even normally sized tonsils and adenoids may lead to relative obstruction, and adenoidectomy or tonsillectomy may be indicated in the presence of obvious symptoms. Some youngsters sleep sitting up and leaning forward. However, children with DS often are restless sleepers, awakening or arousing several times during the night. It is unclear whether this represents undetected airway obstruction without apnea (related to the collapse of the airway and the arousal of the child in response) or a separate, central phenomenon. In addition to the negative consequences of hypoxemia and disordered sleep on daytime wakefulness, untreated obstructive sleep apnea has been associated with significant cardiac morbidity, such as pulmonary hypertension. One study of children with DS showed that 80% had abnormal sleep evaluations when abnormal arousals were included. Because parental reports of abnormal sleep do not correlate well with the results of sleep studies, clinicians should strongly consider an evaluation by a pediatric sleep center in the face of these symptoms, including full polysomnography. Although adenotonsillectomy is the first procedure performed, 50% of patients may still have obstruction after this procedure, and therefore a postoperative sleep study is needed to define the nature of the residual obstruction, which might include glossoptosis, hypopharyngeal collapse, lingual tonsillar hypertrophy, or adenoidal regrowth in the case of previous adenoidectomy. The growing awareness of sleep disorders in children with DS and the increase in sleep studies have led to the use of positive-pressure airway devices, such as continuous positive airway pressure and bilevel positive airway pressure. Although these devices are challenging to use, the efforts of pediatric sleep specialists are often able to successfully desensitize children to them.

Cardiovascular Disease

Congenital heart anomalies are the most common birth defects in children with DS. A recent large population-based cohort study demonstrated that just over 65% of children with DS had cardiovascular abnormalities (Heinke et al., 2020). This analysis demonstrates that simple cardiac septal defects, atrial septal defect (32.5%) and ventricular septal defect (20.6%), are more common than atrioventricular septal defect (14%–17%). More complicated structural heart defects, including coarctation (1.7%) and tetralogy of Fallot (2.7%), are seen less commonly. Pulmonary hypertension is also common in children with DS, with an incidence of up to 28% (Bush et al., 2018). Pulmonary hypertension is most commonly transient (70%) with a median duration of 8 months, less commonly persistent (15%) and recurrent (15%). Obstructive sleep apnea, dysphagia, and respiratory infection are associated with recurrent pulmonary hypertension (Bush et al., 2018).

Endocrinology

Thyroid disorders are common in childhood and adolescence. Hypothyroidism occurs frequently, in 17.5% to 35% of infants and children. Hyperthyroidism is less common, occurring in approximately 2% of children with DS. Many show persistent mild elevations of thyroid-stimulating hormone with low normal thyroxine levels. It is debated if these differences represent compensated hypothyroidism or if normal levels of thyroid hormones are different in children with DS.

Type 1 diabetes mellitus is also three to eight times more common in children with DS compared to the general population. DS is associated with an increased incidence of autoimmune disorders, including thyroid abnormalities, celiac disease, juvenile-onset diabetes mellitus, juvenile rheumatoid arthritis, and alopecia areata.

Hematology

Hematologic abnormalities are common in infancy and childhood. Infants with DS often present with polycythemia, which quickly resolves. Erythrocytes show a persistent macrocytosis in two-thirds of individuals with DS. One-third of children with DS have white blood cells in the 5th percentile or below (Roizen & Amaraose, 1993). Thrombocytopenia occurs commonly in newborns with DS, and it is usually transient although it may be part of a transient myeloproliferative disorder, which is found in 10% of infants. This condition is manifested by pancytopenia, hepatosplenomegaly, and circulating blasts. The majority of neonates fully recover within the first 3 months of life. Death occurs rarely and is associated with higher white blood cell levels at diagnosis, higher bilirubin levels, and failure of blood count to normalize. Children with DS are at much higher risk for developing leukemia than the general population; approximately 1% of children with DS develop leukemia (Massey et al., 2006). Of infants with transient myeloproliferative disorder, 20% to 30% develop acute megakaryocytic leukemia in the first 5 years of life. Both transient myeloproliferative disorder and acute megakaryocytic leukemia are associated with somatic mutations of the *GATA1* gene, which encodes hematopoietic transcription factor (Hitzer et al., 2003). Acute myeloid leukemias have extremely high rates of remission and very low rates of relapse in children with DS compared with typically developing children. Historically mortality of acute lymphoblastic leukemia was higher in DS compared with other children. More recently, these outcomes are comparable with risk-adapted therapies (Whitlock, 2006).

Infectious Disease and Immunology

Children with DS are more likely to suffer infectious and autoimmune disease. Children have many nonimmunologic abnormalities that increase susceptibility to infection, including craniofacial abnormalities, lower airway abnormalities, hypotonia, dysphagia, and aspiration of food contents that contribute to higher susceptibility to infection. Several abnormalities of the immune system are associated with DS, including decreased T- and B-cell counts, decreased naive lymphocytes, impaired mitogen-induced T-cell proliferation, reduced specific antibody responses to immunizations, and defects of neutrophil chemotaxis (Ram & Chinen, 2011). Although it is rare, children with DS have been reported to have a deficiency of immunoglobulin G subclasses 2 and 4 in the face of normal total immunoglobulin G. Children with repeated serious infections, such as pneumonia and empyema, need to have quantitative immunoglobulins measured. Furthermore, children with recurrent pneumonia should be evaluated for gastroesophageal reflux and aspiration. Children with DS who meet standard cardiac and pulmonary criteria for respiratory syncytial virus prophylaxis are urged to receive palivizumab to prevent infection during the winter months because their narrow airways put them at increased risk for serious morbidity.

Musculoskeletal Disease

Ligamentous laxity is a common finding in children with DS. Together with hypotonia, children present as floppy and flexible. It is rare to see congenitally dislocated hips in children with DS, although hip problems do occur in adolescence. Adolescents also are prone to patellar dislocation. The most potentially serious problems caused by ligamentous laxity are related to the occiput and cervical spine. Screening of the cervical spine has not been recommended by AAP since 2011 DS guidelines. Approximately 13% of individuals with DS have more than 4.5 mm of distance between the atlas and the dens on lateral cervical spine radiographs on comparison of the neutral view with full flexion and full extension. These individuals have been described as having atlantoaxial instability and have been, in the past, considered at risk for the development of spinal cord compression. A small percentage of individuals with DS (estimated at 1%–2%) will develop spinal cord compression from this excess movement. The belief that atlantoaxial instability is an asymptomatic precursor of cord compression as well as the desire to prevent any possible injury led to the recommendation that all individuals participating in Special Olympics have such studies performed. However, recent reviews of the literature have suggested that such screening may not be necessary and that individuals who are at risk for such spinal cord catastrophes either have symptoms or signs (neck pain, weakness in the upper extremities, gait disturbance, bladder or bowel problems, or hyperreflexia and presence of Babinski sign) or have been subjected to manipulation of the neck. All children with DS should have their deep tendon reflexes examined at visits so any marked change can be evaluated. Symptomatic individuals must be referred for neurosurgical evaluation and treatment, which consists of fusion of C1 and C2 (Caird et al., 2006).

Neuropsychiatric Concerns

Intellectual Disability

Individuals with DS have a large range of cognitive impairment. IQ in DS ranges from mild (50–70), to moderate (35–50), to occasionally severe (20–35) (AAP, 2011).

Autism Spectrum Disorder

Autism spectrum disorder is more common in children and adults with DS. Whereas the incidence of autism spectrum disorder in the general population is reported at 1.7%, current evidence suggests that the prevalence in DS is approximately 16% (Richards et al., 2015). Children with DS and autism spectrum disorder are found to have more profound intellectual disability and increased aberrant behavior, particularly stereotypy, anxiety, and social withdrawal (Carter et al., 2007). Children with DS seem to be more likely to develop the so-called disintegrative form of autism, in which a child with adequate development of cognitive, language, and adaptive skills undergoes a dramatic regression with the emergence of typical autistic features.

Down Syndrome Disintegrative Disorder

DS disintegrative disorder has been documented in adolescents and young adults with DS found to have regression of previously attained language, communication, and social skills, with some patients progressing to mutism. Mood symptoms are often present, including depression, anxiety, and social withdrawal. Symptoms appear acutely over 6 months and then stabilize in most patients. About 58% of patients have partial or full recovery, 7.5% have worsening of symptoms, and 35% have stabilization of symptoms (Rosso et al., 2020).

Attention-Deficit/Hyperactivity Disorder

This common neuropsychiatric disorder occurs more frequently in children with DS than in typically developing children. It is important to control for the child's developmental age in using standardized ratings. Be mindful of underlying undiagnosed medical problems, such as hyperthyroidism, hearing loss, and sleep disturbances, that may be responsible for the inattention or overactivity. In general, children with DS respond well to current medical management with stimulant therapy, although it is wise to start with smaller than usual doses because of heightened sensitivity to psychoactive medications.

Epilepsy

The frequency of seizures in individuals with DS ranges from 1% to 13% (Goldberg-Stern et al., 2001). Half of these seizures can be attributed to an underlying medical problem (such as cardiovascular disease, infection, trauma, perinatal problems, or, more rarely, moyamoya disease), and the other 50% are idiopathic. Of note, infantile spasms occur more frequently in children with DS. Although they are usually associated with poor neurodevelopmental outcome, timely recognition of this disorder along with rapid institution of treatment correlates with better outcomes. Children who had a delay in beginning treatment and who had a long time until the spasms stopped had a lower developmental quotient and a higher incidence of autistic features (Eisermann et al., 2003).

Dementia

Alzheimer dementia is common in individuals with DS over age 40 years. By 50 years of age, individuals have a 20% risk of Alzheimer dementia, and by 65 years of age, they have an 80% risk. Individuals with epilepsy have been shown to have an increased propensity for developing Alzheimer dementia (McCarron et al., 2014).

HEALTH CARE GUIDELINES FOR CHILDREN AND ADULTS

A variety of screening protocols have been developed to ensure optimal health and well-being for children and adults with DS. The most recent version is the Health Supervision for Children with Down Syndrome, developed jointly by the Committee on Genetics of the AAP and the Down Syndrome Medical Interest Group and published in *Pediatrics* (AAP, 2011). This protocol was designed to supplement, not replace, the standard well-child care protocols of the AAP and the American Academy of Family Physicians. Table 27.2 gives a brief summary of the recommended screenings and evaluations for children with DS. The Global Down Syndrome Foundation published health guidelines for adults with DS in 2020. These guidelines address screening for mental health and dementia, screening or treatment of diabetes, cardiovascular disease, obesity, osteoporosis, atlantoaxial instability, thyroid disease, and celiac disease (Tsou et al., 2020).

TABLE 27.2 Down Syndrome Health Care Guidelines

Guideline	Age	Additional Information
Genetic counseling, genetic testing	Prenatal Birth	
Complete blood count (CBC) to r/o transient myeloproliferative disorder, polycythemia	Birth	
Echocardiogram	Birth Adolescence	Repeat in adolescence to screen for acquired mitral or aortic disease
Swallowing assessment if feeding problems or signs of aspiration	Any age	
Family support/parent group	Every age	Parent to parent contact, support groups, current books and pamphlets
Hemoglobin	Annually beginning at age 1 yr	If hemoglobin <11, screen for iron deficiency with ferritin, reticulocyte hemoglobin content
Audiology evaluation	Birth: newborn screen 6 mo–3 yr: every 6 mo 3–18 yr: annually	
Ophthalmologic exam	Start at 6 mo Age 1–5 yr: annually Age 5–13 yr: every 2 yr Age 13–18 yr: every 3 yr	
Celiac disease screening	Beginning at age 3 yr, repeat every 3 yr	Test more frequently with concerning symptoms
Thyroid screening	Birth: state newborn screen 6–18 mo: every 6 mo 2–18 yr: annually	
Cervical spine imaging	After age 3 yr	X-rays only with myopathic signs or symptoms
Sleep study	Prior to age 4 yr	
Developmental support	Birth–3 yr: early intervention program 3 yr–school age: public school system	Discuss self-help, attention-deficit/hyperactivity disorder, obsessive-compulsive disorder, wandering, transition to middle school
Sexual development and behaviors	Start at age 13 yr	Discuss contraception, sexually transmitted disease prevention, recurrence risk for offspring
Facilitate transition	Start at age 13 yr	Discuss guardianship, financial planning, vocational training, group home, work settings
Preventative care	Annually	Monitor for constipation, obstructive sleep apnea, aspiration

Adapted from Sie Center for Down Syndrome. (2013 update). Down Syndrome Healthcare Guidelines (2011 revision) Record Sheet. *Pediatrics, 128*, 393–406.

GROWTH AND DEVELOPMENT

Children with DS grow in length and height at a slower rate than typically developing children. The mechanism is multifactorial, including metabolic and endocrine abnormalities related to the presence of extra genetic material. This growth retardation begins prenatally. Children with DS should be plotted on DS-specific growth charts, which exist for both boys and girls from birth to 18 years of age. Growth charts for head circumference are available up to age 36 months. New DS-specific growth charts have been published, created from a sample of children with DS in the United States. These new charts show marked improvement in growth in children age 0 to 36 months. School-age and adolescent children with DS continued to show a tendency to become overweight or obese. Body mass index charts were also developed, demonstrating that average body mass index values were nearly 1 SD above the median of the standard Centers for Disease Control and Prevention growth charts (Zemel et al., 2015).

Children with DS have delays in all areas of development: gross and fine motor, cognitive, language, and personal-social. Expressive (verbal) language abilities tend to be more delayed than cognitive and receptive language skills. Children with DS from 0 to 3 years of age are eligible for early intervention services. This federally funded program provides a range of developmental services, rendered by child development specialists, occupational therapists, physical therapists, and speech-language pathologists. The services are provided in the home. After 3 years of age, local school districts are responsible for providing educational services. Individuals with disabilities are eligible for educational programming through the age of 21 years.

EDUCATION

In general, families and advocates support inclusive education opportunities for students with DS, including the least restrictive environment provisions in the Individuals with Disabilities Education Act. In more recent years there has been steady development of inclusive education for children with DS. Research indicates that appropriate education provided in inclusive settings offers the best opportunities for children with DS, who need to learn with their nondisabled peers with the necessary individual support to make this successful. Research indicates that it is difficult to provide a maximally effective learning environment in a special education classroom. Children learn from their peers, so watching and participating alongside their typically developing peer group will provide learning opportunities throughout the day. Expectations in the classroom are higher in mainstream schools. Inclusion helps parents and teachers to do more to ensure that friendships with nondisabled peers carry on outside of school. Although children with DS have additional educational needs, they also have many of the same needs as other nondisabled pupils of their age. They will make the most rapid progress if they are fully socially included and accepted, benefiting from age-appropriate role models and from the benefits of feeling that they are part of the ordinary community. This social acceptance will have a profound effect on self-confidence, self-identity, and self-esteem. "If we wish to make a difference to the life experiences of children and adults with disabilities, all children need to grow and learn together. We need to realize that individuals with DS have strengths and weaknesses and that everyone has a contribution to make to a caring society" (Hughes, 2006).

TRANSITION

The transition process involves taking steps toward building independence, planning for the future, and transitioning to adult health care. Medical care needs to be transferred to adult physicians for primary and specialty care if appropriate. Starting this process in early adolescence is ideal so that transition can happen as an individual with DS approaches age 18 years. The following legal support can be helpful in approaching transition:

- Power of attorney allows individuals with trisomy 21 to appoint someone to make decisions on their behalf.
- Guardianship provides a designated person legal authority to make decisions for an individual that the court decides is "incapacitated." The court also determines the scope of the guardian's authority. Limited guardianship may be appropriate for individuals who are able to make some decisions on their own. General guardianship may be more appropriate for individuals with more severe intellectual disability.
- Representative payee is a person or organization appointed by the Social Security Administration to receive Social Security funds for individuals who cannot manage their own benefits.
- Waivers are state-provided services and benefits that may allow the individual to live more independently and promote community living. Benefits may include support for recreation, educational/vocational opportunities, home assistance with daily living, and transportation.
- Achieving a Better Life Experience (ABLE) Act of 2014 allows individuals with disabilities and their families to set up a tax-advantaged savings account for expenses pertaining to their disability.
- Special needs trust, as part of estate planning, is an instrument customized to address the unique circumstances of each family. It allows the beneficiary to remain eligible for need-based government benefits, such as Medicaid and Supplemental Security Income.
- Vocational training provides individuals the ability to maximize success and enjoyment of employment.

CONCLUSION

Children with DS provide a multifaceted opportunity to integrate our expertise in the medical, developmental, and emotional issues surrounding the diagnosis and management of this common condition. Our efforts to use current knowledge to minimize the impact of the medical and developmental challenges in the service of promoting maximal functional adaptation of the individual with minimal personal burden to the family make this endeavor both challenging and satisfying. Despite many medical complications, our patient Paula has gone on to have a healthy and happy childhood and adolescence. Due to continued research and medical advances, Paula has a bright future ahead.

REFERENCES

American Academy of Pediatrics Committee on Genetics. (2011). Health supervision for children with Down syndrome. *Pediatrics*, *128*(2), 393–406.

American College of Obstetrics and Gynecology. (2007). Screening for fetal chromosomal abnormalities. Practice Bulletin No. 77. *Obstetrics and Gynecology*, *109*(1), 217–228.

Bush, D., Galambos, C., Ivy, D. D., Abman, S., Wolter-Warmerdan, K., & Hickey, F. (2018). Clinical characteristics and risk factors for developing pulmonary hypertension in children with Down syndrome. *Journal of Pediatrics*, *202*, 212.

Caird, C. M. S., Wills, B. P., & Dormans, J. P. (2006). Down syndrome in children: The role of the orthopaedic surgeon. *Journal of the American Academy of Orthopaedic Surgeons*, *14*, 610–619.

Carter, J. C., Capone, G. T., Gray, R. M., et al. (2007). Autistic-spectrum disorders in Down syndrome: Further delineation and distinction from other behavioral abnormalities. *American Journal of Medical Genetics Part B*, *144*, 87–94.

Eisermann, M. M., DeLaRaillère, A., Dellatola, G., et al. (2003). Infantile spasms in Down syndrome—Effects of delayed anticonvulsive treatment. *Epilepsy Research*, *559*(12), 21–27.

Goldberg-Stern, H., Strawsburg, R. H., Patterson, B., et al. (2001). Seizure frequency and characteristics in children with Down syndrome. *Brain & Development*, *23*, 375–378.

Heinke, D., Isenburg, J. L., Stallings, E. B., et al. (2020). Prevalence of structural birth defects among infants with Down syndrome, 2013-2017: A US population-based study. *Birth Defects Research*, 1–14. https://doi.org/10.1002/bdr2.1854.

Hickey, F., Wolter-Warmerdam, K., Hickey, E., Yoon, J., & Daniels, D. (2017). Pediatric comorbidities and medical complications identified in children with Down syndrome. *Journal of Down Syndrome Chromosomal Abnormalities*, *3*(124), 2472–1115.

Hitzer, J. K., Cheung, J., Li, Y., et al. (2003). GATA1 mutations in transient leukemia and acute megakaryoblastic leukemia of Down syndrome. *Blood*, *101*, 4301.

Hughes, J. (2006). Inclusive education for individuals with Down syndrome. *Down Syndrome News and Update*, *6*(1), 1–3. https://doi.org/10.3104/practice.370.

Imbornoni, L., Wise, R., Taravella, M., et al. (2020). Keratoconus and corneal morphology in patients with Down syndrome at a pediatric hospital. *Journal of American Association of Pediatric Ophthalmology and Strabismus*, *24*, 140.e1–5.

Massey, G. V., Zipursky, A., Chang, M. N., et al. (2006). A prospective study of the natural history of transient leukemia in neonates with Down syndrome. Children's Oncology Group study POG-9481. *Blood*, *107*, 4606.

McCarron, M., McCallion, P., Reilly, E., & Mulryan, N. (2014). A prospective 14-year longitudinal follow-up of dementia in persons with Down syndrome. *Journal of Intellectual Disability Research*, *58*(1), 61–70. https://doi.org/10.1111/jir.12074.

Nightengale, E., Yoon, P., Wolter-Warmerdam, K., Daniels, D., & Hickey, F. (2017). Understanding hearing and hearing loss in children with Down syndrome. *American Journal of Audiology*, *26*(3), 301–308. https://doi.org/10.1044/2017_AJA-17-0010. PMID: 28854301.

Ram, G., & Chinen, J. (2011). Infections and immunodeficiency in Down syndrome. *Clinical & Experimental Immunology*, *164*, 9.

Richards, C., Jones, C., Groves, L., & Moss, J. (2015). Prevalence of autism spectrum disorder phenomenology in genetic disorders: A systematic review and metaanalysis. *Lancet Psychiatry*, *2*, 909–916.

Roizen, N., & Amaraose, A. (1993). Hematologic abnormalities in children with Down syndrome. *American Journal of Medical Genetics*, *46*, 510.

Rosso, M., Fremion, E., Santoro, S., Oreskovic, N. M., Chitnis, T., Skotko, B. G., & Santoro, J. D. (2020). Down syndrome disintegrative disorder: A clinical regression syndrome of increasing importance. *Pediatrics*, *145*(6), e20192939. https://doi.org/10.1542/peds.2019-2939.

Tsou, A. Y., Bulova, P., Capone, G., et al. (2020). Medical care of adults with Down syndrome: A clinical guideline. *JAMA*, *324*(15), 1543–1556. https://doi.org/10.1001/jama.2020.17024.

Whitlock, J. A. (2006). Down syndrome and acute lymphoblastic leukemia. *British Journal of Haematology*, *135*, 595.

Zemel, B. S., Pipan, M., Stallings, V. A., et al. (2015). Growth charts for children with Down syndrome in the United States. *Pediatrics*, *136*(5), e1204–e1211. https://doi.org/10.1542/peds.2015-1652.

28

Fragile X Syndrome and *FMR1* Variants

Susan Howell, Elizabeth Coan, Kristen Slaymaker, Randi Hagerman, and Nicole Tartaglia

For additional material related to the content of this chapter, please see Chapters 40 and 41.

VIGNETTE

Sam is a 2.5-year-old boy who presents with delayed milestones, including walking at 18 months and first words at 28 months of age. He also has gaze avoidance, auditory sensitivities, and repetitive body-rocking and hand-flapping. History includes term pregnancy conceived via assisted reproduction in 35-year-old parents. He had surgical placement of ear tubes at 24 months due to recurrent otitis media. He has sleep challenges, hypotonia, poor motor coordination, and pes planus. Family history is significant for a typical 5-year-old brother and 7-year-old sister diagnosed with a math learning disability and inattentive attention-deficit/hyperactivity disorder (ADHD). His mother endorsed a family history of anxiety disorder in herself and her sister, and cessation of menses at age 34 years. Sam's maternal first cousin has autism and intellectual disability. His father is healthy. His maternal grandfather is 70 years with 3 years of progressive tremors and loss of balance diagnosed as ataxia and Parkinsonism.

Sam was diagnosed with global developmental delay and autism spectrum disorder (ASD). Microarray results showed 46,XY karyotype, and fragile X DNA test showed a full mutation with over 200 CGG repeats in the FMR1 gene with full methylation. Genetic counseling, including family history, led to cascade testing identifying a fragile X syndrome (FXS) full mutation in his sister and his cousin, a premutation in his mother leading to a diagnosis of fragile X primary ovarian insufficiency (FXPOI) and anxiety symptoms consistent with fragile X–associated neuropsychiatric disorder (FXAND). Genetic testing of his grandfather identified a premutation and revealed his neurologic symptoms to be due to fragile X–associated tremor ataxia syndrome (FXTAS) (see pedigree of this family in Fig. 28.2, *p. 3).*

INTRODUCTION

Fragile X syndrome is the most common inherited cause of intellectual disability and the most common single-gene mutation associated with ASD. Clinical features of the syndrome were first described in 1943 by Drs. Martin and Bell, primarily describing a family in which intellectual disability was inherited and linked to the X chromosome. In 1991 Dr. Stephen Warren and colleagues identified the *FMR1* gene as the specific gene affected and subsequently further described the complex genetics of inheritance, including the concept of female carriers of a "premutation" having high risk for having children with FXS. The study of families with children with FXS over subsequent decades led to discovery that having a premutation confers more than just risk of FXS in offspring, but also risk for separate medical and psychiatric conditions associated with the premutation state across the lifespan, including premature ovarian insufficiency (FXPOI), a progressive neurodegenerative disease of aging with predominant symptoms of tremor and ataxia (FXTAS) first described by Dr. Randi Hagerman, and other neuropsychiatric disorders such as anxiety and attentional disorders (FXAND) (Hagerman et al., 2018). While the role of the developmental pediatrician is primarily to care for children and adolescents with FXS, mutations in the *FMR1* gene can affect multiple generations, and it is often the developmental pediatrician who is the first to find the mutation in a family. Thus, understanding the inheritance and clinical features of all *FMR1*-associated conditions is important to identify others with FXS, those at risk for having children with FXS, and to identify premutation carriers who may have or carry risk for premutation-associated conditions.

FXS is estimated to occur in approximately 1 in 4000 males and 1 in 6000 females, and it has been reported in all races and ethnicities with studies suggesting a slightly lower rate in the Asian population. FXS and *FMR1*-associated conditions are diagnosed by specific fragile X DNA test, and current guidelines by the American Academy of Pediatrics and American College of Medical Genetics recommend fragile X DNA testing as part of the first-tier genetic testing for children presenting with global developmental delays, ASD, or intellectual disability. Recent studies show the average age of FXS diagnosis is 3 to 3.5 years, which is delayed compared to the average age of first parental concern (12 months of age) and also frequently after younger siblings are born. Thus it is common to have multiple cases of FXS in a family. Following diagnosis, care guidelines include a combination of medical, neurodevelopmental and behavior evaluations, and treatments as described in this chapter, along with genetic counseling to solicit a detailed family history for pedigree analysis and recommendations for cascade testing of at-risk family members in the nuclear and extended family.

GENETICS OF FRAGILE X

The name fragile X initially originated from the fragile site observed on the X chromosome of affected individuals when cells were grown in folate-deficient media for cytogenetic analysis. The 1991 discovery of the fragile X mental retardation 1 gene (*FMR1*) located at Xq27.3 transformed current diagnostics to utilize DNA analysis to measure the number of trinucleotide repeats of the DNA bases cytosine-guanine-guanine (CGG) in the 5′ untranslated portion (promoter region) of the gene. At the time of description of the gene, mental retardation was the accepted medical diagnosis for the current definition of intellectual disability. However, the *FMR1* gene name was changed in 2022 to be called the fragile X messenger ribonucleoprotein 1 gene to replace the outdated nomenclature with a term more descriptive of the gene product's function.

Typical unaffected individuals are found to have 5 to 44 CGG repeats in the *FMR1* gene, whereas carriers of the *FMR1* premutation are classified based on larger CGG repeats identified, with full mutations over 200 CGG repeats resulting in FXS due to methylation and subsequent *FMR1* silencing (Fig. 28.1). In extremely rare cases the underlying genetic defect has been attributed to a deletion or point mutation, resulting in a loss of function of *FMR1*. The protein produced from the *FMR1* gene, fragile X messenger ribonucleoprotein (FMRP), is a regulator of posttranscriptional RNA metabolism and translation for many other messages important for synaptic maturation and plasticity, dendrite and axon development, and clinically associated with learning and memory.

FMR1 transgenerational mutation expansion occurs by genetic anticipation, in which the CGG repeats become larger (and clinically more severe in cases with >200 repeats) when transmitted from one generation to the next. *FMR1* mutations are classified in ranking size as grey zone (45–54 CGG repeats), premutation (55–200 CGG repeats), and full mutation (>200 CGG repeats).

The grey zone, also described as the intermediate mutation (44–54 CGG repeats), is commonly found in the general population, with an estimated prevalence of approximately 1:66 females and 1:112 males. These smaller expansions in *FMR1* have been termed grey zone alleles based on the lower likelihood of the CGG repeat increasing and causing FXS in later generations. Grey zone alleles have been reported to expand over two generations to a full mutation, but typically it takes at least three generations. While most grey zone/intermediate mutations occur in unaffected individuals, associated risks for FXTAS-like or Parkinsonian manifestations in carriers have been reported.

The premutation (55–200 CGG repeats) is commonly found in the general population, with an estimated prevalence of approximately 1 in 200 females and 1 in 500 males. Premutation alleles are unstable in maternal transmission and may significantly expand in CGG repeat length, often transforming from a premutation to a full mutation (>200 CGG repeats) in the next generation. Male premutation carriers transmit the premutation to all daughters (not sons, as sons inherit the Y chromosome from their father); however, the premutation is typically stable in paternal transmission, and the repeat length is unlikely to significantly expand when paternally inherited. Premutation carriers are at risk for developing fragile X premutation–associated disorders, including FXPOI, FXTAS, and FXAND, described in more detail later. See Fig 28.2 for an example pedigree demonstrating inheritance and clinical features.

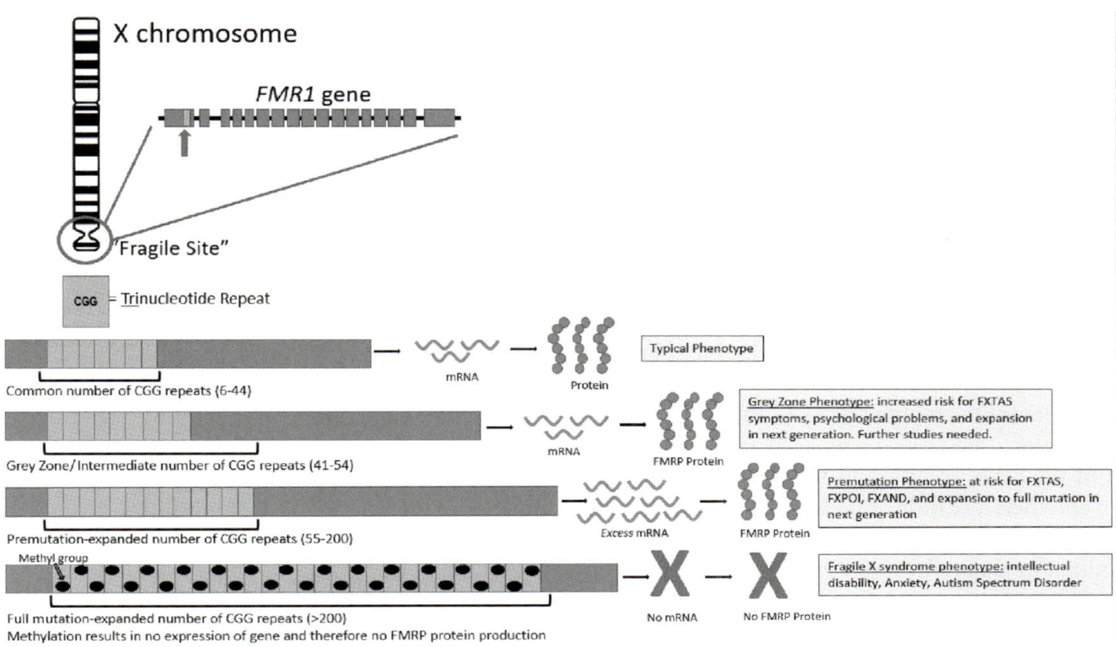

Fig. 28.1 The *FMR1* gene promoter region classified by CGG repeat number with transcription and translation effects.

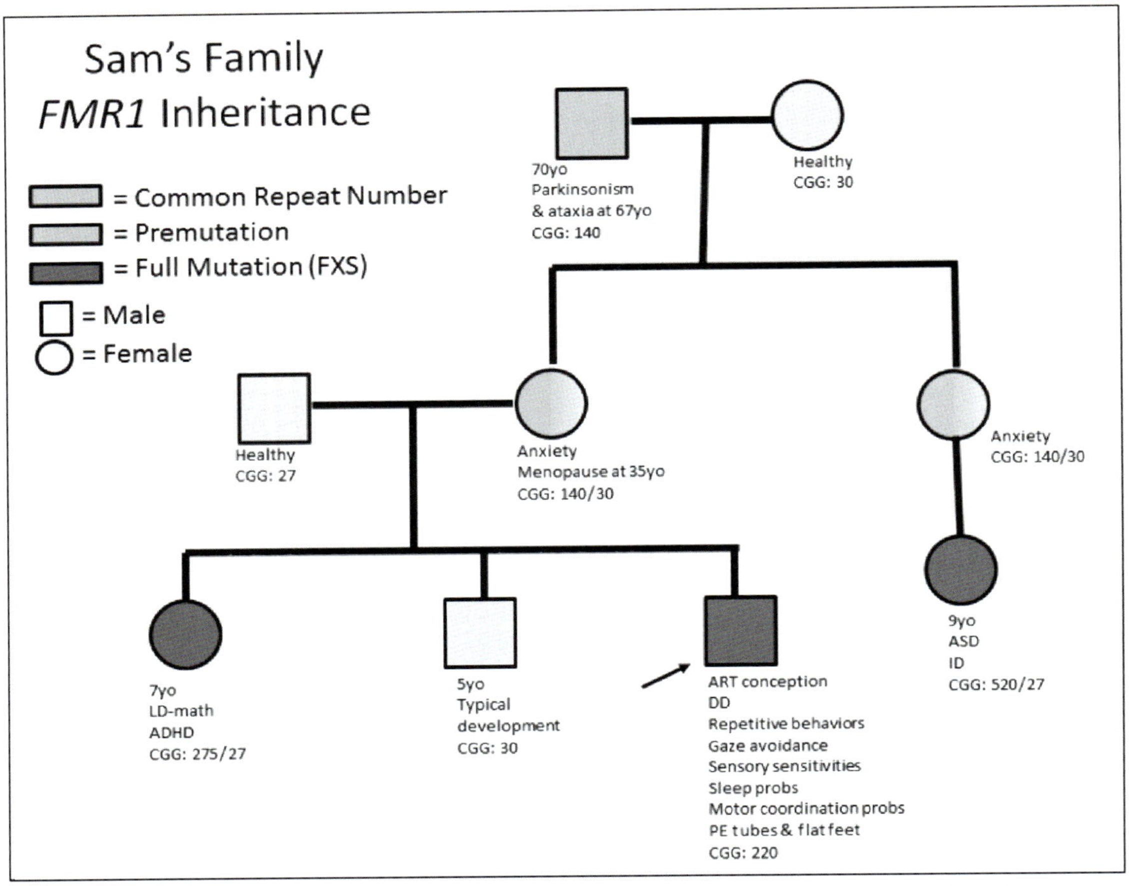

Fig. 28.2 Example pedigree of familial *FMR1* inheritance and clinical presentations among family members (see chapter-opening vignette). *ADHD*, Attention-deficit/hyperactivity disorder; *ART*, advanced reproductive technology; *ASD*, autism spectrum disorder; *CGG*, number of cytosine-guanine-guanine repeats on the X chromosome(s); *DD*, developmental delay; *ID*, intellectual disability; *LD*, learning disability; *PE tubes*, pressure equalization tubes.

Factors that influence the risk for expansion from a premutation to a full mutation when inherited include the sex of the carrier parent, the carrier parent's CGG repeat number, and the presence and count of AGG (adenine-guanine-guanine) interruptions embedded within the carrier parent's *FMR1* CGG expansion, sometimes called AGG anchors. The presence of AGG interruptions serves to stabilize CGG repeats during transmission to the next generation, with the greatest stabilizing impact occurring when the mother's premutation is 60 to 100 CGG repeats and multiple AGG interruptions are embedded. Maternal premutation transmissions lacking AGG interruptions within this 60 to 100 CGG repeat range pose the risk for CGG repeat expansion into a full mutation in the next generation. Maternal premutation expansions with over 100 CGG repeats almost universally expand to a full mutation in the next generation regardless of the number of AGG anchors.

The full mutation (>200 CGG repeats) leads to hypermethylation of the gene, resulting in suppression of mRNA transcription and therefore little or no FMRP production. It is the absence or deficiency of FMRP that causes FXS. Females with a full mutation generally have a milder clinical presentation compared to males due to the presence of the second X chromosome, which expresses *FMR1* and produces FMRP, although this can be dependent on X inactivation ratios (the percentage of cells with the normal *FMR1* allele on the inactive X chromosome).

Phenotypic variability is commonly observed in males and females with FXS, with a common source attributed to mosaicism. Both repeat size mosaicism (mosaicism among various mutation size categories: full mutation/premutation/intermediate) and methylation mosaicism (a lower methylation fraction despite >200 CGG repeats) may contribute to various levels of FMRP production. While it remains difficult to extrapolate the effects of mosaicism identified in peripheral blood to all tissues throughout the body, partial FMRP expression may be sufficient to positively impact clinical outcomes.

FRAGILE X SYNDROME

Physical, Medical, and Motor Features of FXS

Physical features commonly associated with FXS include large head circumference, long face, large or prominent ears (often with cupping and smoothness of the pinnae), high-arched palate, hyperextensible joints especially evident in the hands (including double-jointed thumbs), smooth velvety skin, hypotonia, and pes planus (Fig. 28.3). In males, macroorchidism (large testicles) can emerge beginning in puberty, and there is increased risk for inguinal hernias.

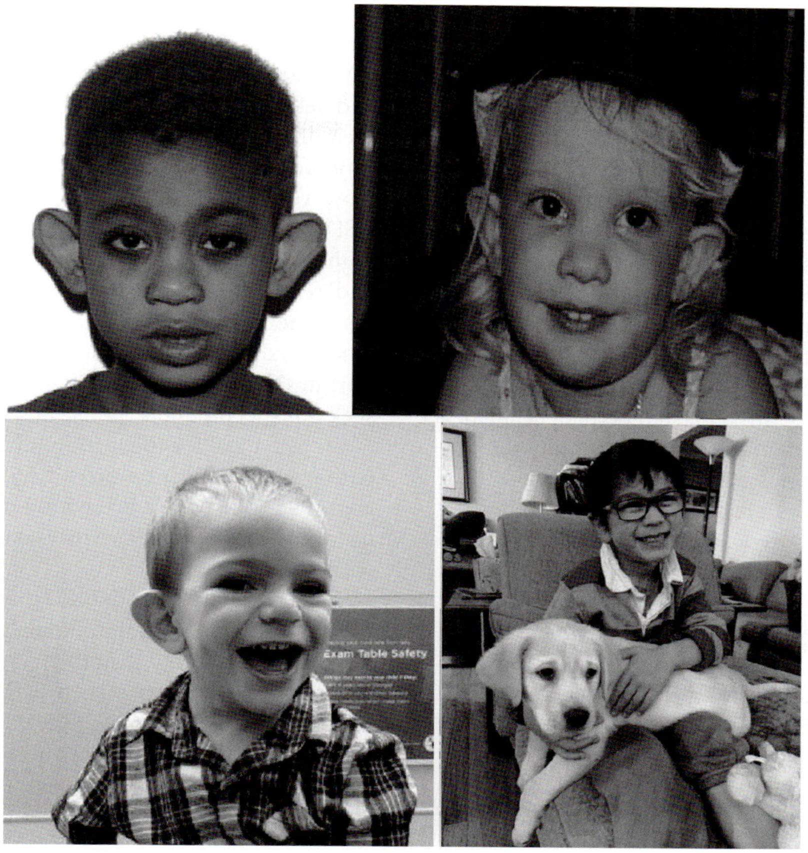

Fig. 28.3 Facial features of fragile X syndrome.

However, approximately 30% of children with FXS do not have obvious physical features, thus DNA testing should not be dependent on these features and is indicated in any child with developmental delay of unknown etiology, intellectual disability, or ASD.

Medical problems associated with FXS include increased risk for strabismus (~15%), recurrent otitis media often requiring tympanostomy tubes (~40%–50%), gastrointestinal symptoms such as gastroesophageal reflux, chronic constipation or loose stools, and sleep disorders (~50%–70%), including challenges with falling asleep, staying asleep, and increased risk for obstructive sleep apnea. Feeding difficulties are common in infancy. Approximately 10% to 15% of males and 5% of females have a cooccurring seizure disorder, typically presenting around 6 years of age. Connective tissue laxity is common and underlies the increased risk for hernias, joint dislocations, pes planus/ankle pronation, and mitral valve prolapse. Males and females with FXS are fertile. While research on aging in FXS is minimal, age span is estimated to be normal or just slightly reduced compared to the general population.

A subpopulation of full mutation FXS includes those with the Prader-Willi phenotype (FXPWP). This phenotype includes clinical features of obesity, hyperphagia, and small genitalia or delayed puberty, but without cytogenetic or methylation abnormalities at 15q11-13 as in typical Prader-Willi syndrome (PWS). Many cases also present with marked hypotonia and feeding difficulties in infancy similar to PWS. The similarities between this subset of patients with FXS and those with typical PWS have been attributed to lower mRNA expression of CYFIP1, a protein in the 15q deleted region of PWS that is regulated by FMRP.

Individuals with FXS also commonly have hypotonia and motor skill delays. Early motor milestones are often delayed, with average age of sitting at 8 to 9 months and walking independently at 18 months in males with FXS. Other neuromotor deficits often include challenges with balance and motor coordination. Fine motor deficits coupled with joint laxity in the hands can affect handwriting and self-care skills.

Developmental-Behavioral and Cognitive Features of FXS

The behavioral phenotype of FXS is characterized by symptoms across many different domains of functioning, and like most genetic disorders there is broad phenotypic variability between affected individuals. Further, symptoms within the FXS phenotype present differently in males compared to females, where males almost universally show moderate intellectual disability while only approximately one-third of females have intellectual disability. In infancy and early childhood delayed milestones in motor and speech-language domains are common and the most typical reason for genetic testing leading to the FXS diagnosis. Typical age for walking independently is around 18 months, and first words around 24 to 26 months, although there is a wide range as seen in typical children. Speech-language disorders, stereotyped language, and perseverative speech are very common in children with FXS, although approximately 10% are nonverbal or minimally verbal into adulthood.

Behavioral challenges in childhood in both males and females can include inattentive behaviors with or without hyperactivity/impulsivity, leading to a diagnosis of ADHD in up to 80% of males and 35% of females. Anxiety, sensory sensitivities, and hyperarousal are also often frequently seen, with anxiety symptoms sometimes presenting as extreme shyness or selective mutism, more commonly in females. Other prominent symptoms of anxiety include social anxiety, specific phobias, irritability or emotional lability, and obsessive or perseverative behaviors. Individuals with FXS also often demonstrate repetitive or stereotyped behaviors, including physical motor mannerisms such as body rocking or hand flapping, stereotypic speech patterns, ritualized or repetitive activities, and/or restricted interests. Gaze avoidance and poor eye contact are also common. The combination of anxiety and sensory sensitivities, as well as challenges with communication, can lead to behavioral escalations and low frustration tolerance, which can subsequently be associated with the possibility of self-injury (often hand or arm self-biting) and aggressive or destructive behaviors (Hagerman & Hagerman, 2020).

The combination of behavioral symptoms described and higher rates of social communication deficits often leads to consideration of the cooccurrence of ASD. Approximately 50% of boys and 20% of females with FXS meet *Diagnostic and Statistical Manual of Mental Disorders*, fifth edition (*DSM-5*) criteria for ASD. The profile of ASD symptoms and behaviors overlaps with those seen in idiopathic autism, including language deficits, decreased eye contact/gaze avoidance, and stereotyped speech and motor behaviors. However, compared to idiopathic autism, individuals with ASD and FXS often show more prominent social withdrawal, higher levels of anxiety, and less intense complex repetitive and restricted behaviors as measured by ASD diagnostic instruments. However, individuals with FXS and ASD also tend to exhibit a more pronounced degree of social motivation in that they often initiate simple social exchanges and seek out specific social praise and approval in a manner that is not as typical for those individuals who present with idiopathic autism. The presence of ASD is associated with lower cognitive skills, more behavioral challenges and medication use, and higher rates of seizures compared to those with FXS without ASD.

While most males with FXS fall in the moderate intellectual disability range, only approximately one-third of females have intellectual disability. Another one-third of females instead show milder symptoms such as learning disabilities (most commonly in math), borderline cognitive functioning, attention deficits/ADHD, executive functioning deficits, motor coordination deficits, and anxiety symptoms. The remaining females with a full mutation can have very few cognitive or

TABLE 28.1 Evaluate Checklist for Evaluation and Treatment of Children and Adolescents With Fragile X Syndrome (FXS)

FXS: Evaluation Checklist	
Referrals for evaluations and treatments	Developmental skills (birth–3 yr) or cognitive assessment (≥4 yr) for ID or learning disabilities, adaptive functioning Speech-language/communication evaluation OT/PT evaluation of fine and gross motor skills Sensory sensitivities/sensory processing Evaluation for autism and/or ADHD if not previously completed Psychological/behavioral therapies (as indicated for anxiety, outbursts, irritability, aggressive behavior, self-injury) Special education/IEP supports
Genetic counseling	Family history (≥3-generation pedigree) with targeted inquiry for relatives at risk for having FXS, fragile X premutation, or with symptoms of premutation-associated conditions Coordinate fragile X testing for siblings or other family members as indicated
Medical evaluations	Audiology evaluation Vision/strabismus examination Examination related to connective tissue laxity (pes planus, hernias, scoliosis) GI disorders, including feeding, reflux, constipation, loose stools Consideration of increased risk for seizures Cardiac examination Management of sleep disorders
Psychopharmacologic treatment	Consideration of medication treatments for anxiety, attention/ADHD, irritability, aggression, self-injury, hyperarousal, sleep disorders
Family support	Refer to advocacy and support groups for family, siblings Provide educational materials or resources Connect with social work, community services for disabilities

ADHD, Attention-deficit/hyperactivity disorder; *GI*, gastrointestinal; *ID*, intellectual disability; *IEP*, individualized education plan; *OT*, occupational therapy; *PT*, physical therapy.

behavioral/emotional symptoms, many not being identified until motherhood following FXS diagnosis in their child. Cognitive profiles of individuals with FXS often show relative weaknesses in sequential processing of information, auditory and visual attention, working memory, response inhibition, cognitive flexibility, and arithmetic reasoning.

Evaluation and Treatment Approaches for FXS

Management of the child with FXS requires an interdisciplinary team approach that includes community and school-based therapies and educational supports, medical screenings and treatments, and consideration of medication treatments. Upon a new diagnosis, it is common that the individual is already receiving treatment for developmental or behavioral challenges; however, the combination of therapies, behavioral supports, and special education should be reconsidered in the context of the new FXS diagnosis. Evaluations for new diagnoses should include assessment of developmental or cognitive skills, academic testing, speech-language, motor, social-emotional evaluation including anxiety disorders and assessment for ASD, sensory processing, behavioral concerns, attention/ADHD, executive functioning, and self-care/adaptive skills (Martin et al., 2013). Genetic counseling is also important for family counseling and cascade genetic testing recommendations, as well as connecting families with resources including advocacy organizations and community supports. The pediatrician plays many important roles, including educating families, therapists, and school settings about FXS; making referrals for appropriate evaluations and therapies; providing guidance for best practices in assessment of children with FXS; and helping to provide coordination of medical screenings and medication management for behavioral and psychological symptoms of FXS. Table 28.1 includes guidance for the child's medical provider following a new diagnosis.

FXS specialists have made considerable efforts to identify and describe optimal methods of psychological and behavioral assessment, including validation of many standardized psychological tests and behavioral measures in FXS and alternative FXS-specific scoring methods for some measures of cognition and behavior such as the Stanford-Binet 5 and Aberrant Behavior Checklist. Detailed strategies to help therapists and other professionals obtain optimal results when evaluating individuals with FXS have been developed. Examples include preparation due to heightened anxiety such as practice visits to a testing setting and social stories, demonstration of the requested task to completion due to strengths in simultaneous processing, and visual supports such as task completion sticker charts or checklists due to visual strengths. Environmental adaptations due to sensory sensitivities and monitoring for physical and behavioral signs of increasing hyperarousal are important so evaluators can respond with breaks or positive supports. Detailed recommendations for assessment of all domains (cognition, behavior, language, motor, adaptive) have been developed for professionals, including research on specific standardized measures in FXS and considerations for behavioral supports for testing. These can be found in the NFXF Consensus document "Assessment of Fragile X Syndrome" that should be shared with all therapists and psychologists evaluating children with FXS at https://fragilex.org/understanding-fragile-x/fragile-x-syndrome/assessment-fxs.

Speech-Language Therapy

Most individuals with FXS show delays in language development, many of which are clearly recognizable by the age of 2 years. Challenges often span many aspects of speech-language development targeted by speech-language therapists, including difficulties with receptive and expressive language, vocal production challenges, atypical patterns of speech (i.e., repetitive or perseverative speech, atypical intonation, and/or stereotyped phrases), and social communication difficulties. Speech-language therapy is typically a critical component of therapy programming from early intervention into adolescence, and given the strong visual memory skills in FXS should include consideration of additional approaches such as picture exchange or other forms of augmentative communication. Recent research studies have shown improved speech-language outcomes in FXS with therapy approaches such as parent-initiated language intervention that can be delivered by telehealth.

Occupational Therapy

Occupational therapy is typically a critical component in care of children with FXS both in the school setting and in private therapy targeting many other aspects of fine motor, self-care, self-regulation, and sensory processing challenges. Difficulty with sensory-based hyperarousal is often one of the largest challenges for individuals with FXS, often causing significant interruption in their ability to learn and manage their behavior across settings. As a result, occupational therapy is almost always part of the treatment plan to help families/caregivers and individuals with FXS to understand their unique sensory needs and sensitivities. Occupational therapists can help develop sensory diets (to provide sensory environments and activities optimal to each individual) so that hyperarousal, anxiety, and overall self-regulation can be maintained. Beyond sensory needs of FXS, occupational therapists also support development of self-care skills, social and play skills, fine motor skills and coordination, and adaptive community/work skills.

Physical Therapy

Motor coordination and delayed motor milestones are common in FXS, and physical therapists should be considered as a component of the treatment plan to target these areas. Many physical therapists also manage fitting and monitoring of orthotics if needed for pes planus that is affecting motor coordination or gross motor development.

Special Education

Special education services are almost always part of the treatment protocol given the typical cognitive profile in FXS that includes intellectual disability in almost all males and high rates of intellectual and learning disabilities in females. In US public schools special education services are provided based on legal guidelines set by individual states as they are for other disabilities, which can sometimes be difficult to navigate for families as they work with different systems of care and support. Similarly, different state and school districts will often have different approaches to how educational support is provided. This includes programs such as response to intervention, multitiered systems of support, inclusion programs, and the provision of individualized education plans. Sometimes additional advocacy for special education supports is needed for females with FXS who do not meet criteria for intellectual disability but instead have learning disabilities, ADHD, executive function deficits, autism, or social anxiety that will still benefit from supports and therapies in the school setting. More information on the specifics of approaches specific to educational supports in FXS can be found in the consensus documents entitled "Educational Guidelines for Fragile X Syndrome" for early childhood, elementary and middle/ high school students at https://fragilex.org/our-research/treatment-recommendations/.

Behavioral Therapies

Behavioral symptoms associated with FXS can interfere with daily life and limit opportunities in the community, causing challenges for the individual with FXS, as well as for their families, peers, and teachers. As a result, behavioral treatments in FXS are largely focused on the encouragement and teaching of appropriate prosocial behaviors and the reduction of maladaptive or inappropriate ones. Good behavioral intervention relies on consistent patterns of responding to specific behaviors across people and environments so coordination of the plan between parents and the full treatment team is needed to elicit the best outcomes.

Applied behavior analysis (ABA) therapy is based on the science of learning and behavior, with overall goals of increasing behaviors that are helpful and decreasing behaviors that are harmful or interfere with learning or other important activities of an individual's daily life. ABA is recognized as a first-line treatment for young children with autism, but the principles that inform ABA can be applicable for all individuals. Like all therapeutic interventions, ABA therapy is most effective when personally tailored to the individual. ABA is sometimes criticized because of the lack of flexibility in its application, and it is important to adapt the ABA approach for individuals with FXS.

The most commonly overlooked factor is the crucial role anxiety and hyperarousal play in the behavioral challenges seen in many individuals with FXS. When this aspect is not taken into consideration when applying ABA-based principles, ABA interventions may lead to greater behavioral upset and increased anxiety. Good behavioral intervention for children with FXS needs to prioritize their unique learning style and approach teaching with these differences in mind. Some prominent considerations for successfully adapting ABA for FXS include:

- Adjusting or softening the mass trial approach, especially when requiring a specific face-to-face response
- Honoring the tendency for individuals with FXS to learn simultaneously rather than sequentially for academic as well as self-care tasks and other community skills
- Relinquishing the need to force eye contact to start social interactions
- Allowing for substantial rapport building or social warm-up time to encourage anxiety and hyperarousal to become more regulated prior to systemic instruction or intervention

Research into ABA adaptations for individuals with FXS is currently underway, though general treatment guidelines are accessible on the National Fragile X Foundation website.

Psychological and Social Skills Therapies

Psychological therapies can target symptoms of anxiety, behavior, and development of social skills. Strategies such as cognitive-behavioral therapy (adapted to cognitive levels as needed) can be very helpful, especially in females with FXS who are often higher functioning and more verbal compared to males. Careful and slow desensitization approaches for fears/phobias, anxiety in new settings, and medical procedures can be helpful. Social skills groups should be considered for children with social challenges. While psychologists specializing in FXS are rare, identifying those experienced in disabilities and/or autism often have the skill set necessary to learn and adapt strategies for FXS.

Medical Evaluations and Treatments in FXS

Medical evaluations. Medical evaluations in infancy should include close evaluation for connective tissue abnormalities such as congenital hip dislocation, as well as addressing any feeding problems or reflux. In childhood tympanostomy tubes are often needed for recurrent otitis media, thus timely referral to otolaryngology and audiology assessments when ear infections begin is important. Ongoing evaluation for strabismus and vision is important. Evaluation for possible orthotics may be needed if pes planus and ankle pronation impact motor development or cause pain with activity. Neurology care should occur in the event of clear seizures, and electroencephalography should be considered for other atypical spells or movements. Seizures typically respond to standard anticonvulsant therapies. Physical examination should include close evaluation for related connective tissue abnormalities, including joint laxity, flat feet, hernias, scoliosis, and cardiac abnormalities. There is increased mitral valve prolapse, and cardiology should be consulted for any cardiac symptoms or arrythmias (Lozano, Azarang, Wilaisakditipakorn, & Hagerman, 2016). Macroorchidism can occur starting in puberty in males and typically does not require treatment, although examination is important as hydroceles, hernias, and other testicular abnormalities can still occur, and supportive underwear is a helpful recommendation for some males. Females often have typical menarche and menses. Hormonal treatments to lessen or inhibit menstruation should be considered for some who have challenges with managing hygiene or who have marked emotional symptoms with menses, and for pregnancy prevention.

Psychopharmacologic medications. Psychopharmacologic medications are a common component of the treatment plan for individuals with FXS from early childhood through adulthood, targeting associated concerns such as anxiety, ADHD, irritability/aggression, self-injury, and sleep. A national survey of over 1000 FXS families showed that 61% of males and 38% of females were being treated with at least one medication for behavioral symptoms. Generally, psychopharmacologic treatments follow the recommendations for other children with autism or developmental disabilities, including optimizing behavioral therapies and supports, considering medical symptoms that may contribute to behavioral symptoms, and conservative dosing when initiating treatment. Many children with FXS do well with alpha-agonists or stimulant medication for ADHD, selective serotonin reuptake inhibitors (SSRIs) for anxiety, melatonin or clonidine for sleep, and atypical antipsychotics for autism, mood instability, or aggression. Recent research shows safety in use of the SSRI sertraline at an earlier age than typically started in children with developmental disabilities, with placebo-controlled studies showing some benefit to motor, visual perceptual, and language outcomes in children 2 to 6 years of age (Hagerman & Hagerman, 2020).

Targeted treatment medications. Neuroscience research on the effects of low FMRP has led to identification of specific neurobiologic abnormalities underlying the thin, immature dendritic spines and weakened connections of fragile X synapses. FMRP acts as a repressor of translation for many other proteins involved in synaptic development and function, and lack of FMRP leads to dysregulation of many proteins subsequently affecting neurotransmitter systems, including overactivity of glutamate pathways and underactivation of inhibitory GABA-mediated pathways. Medications targeting these pathways with a hope of improving synaptic functioning, cognitive outcomes, and behavioral symptoms are called targeted treatments (Erickson et al., 2017). These studies began in animal models in 2004, and many agents such as mGluR5 antagonists, GABA agonists, phosphodiesterase inhibitors, among others have been shown to improve synaptic morphology, seizures, memory, and anxiety in fragile X knockout mice. Human trials of targeted treatments began in 2005, and many compounds have been studied with variable results, although none yet with convincing results needed for US Food and Drug Administration (FDA) approval. Clinical trials of new agents with improved study designs are ongoing (Budimirovic et al., 2017). Many FDA-approved medications also target pathways impaired by the lack of FMRP, and research studies and off-label clinical use of these medications are ongoing in fragile X clinics. These include medications such as minocycline, metformin, trazodone, cannabidiol (CBD), and acamprosate. Parents of children with FXS will often inquire about off-label use of these and other targeted treatment medications, and it is important for the medical provider caring for patients with FXS to be aware of the current research on safety and efficacy of these agents (Hagerman & Hagerman, 2020).

FMR1 PREMUTATION–ASSOCIATED DISORDERS

Premutation expansions (55–200 CGG repeats) are associated with elevated levels of *FMR1* mRNA, which is the opposite of what occurs in FXS (>200 CGG repeats) where the gene is methylated and little or no mRNA is produced (see Fig. 28.1). Most individuals with the premutation are intellectually normal with normal FMRP production; however, the elevated mRNA can lead to clinical diagnoses called fragile X premutation–associated disorders (see later). Additional medical problems more common in premutation carriers than the general population include hypertension, seizures, fibromyalgia, migraines, hypothyroidism, and other autoimmune problems. At the upper end of the premutation range (>175 CGG repeats), the level of FMRP can be 30% to 50% lower, and features of FXS such as prominent ears or hyperextensible joints are common (Hagerman & Hagerman, 2020).

The mechanisms of pathology in these conditions are currently being studied; however, known mechanisms include RNA toxicity where the elevated mRNA sequester proteins important for neuronal and mitochondrial function lead to enhanced oxidative stress. In some reports an abnormal protein FMRpolyG may be produced because of translation of the mRNA that does not begin at the AUG normal start site (RAN translation), so a repetitive polyglutamine tail is on the FMRP protein that is toxic to neurons. Premutation-associated conditions are important for the medical provider to recognize as they can play an important role in the understanding and management of a family with a child with FXS or with a premutation childhood disorder.

Fragile X–Associated Tremor Ataxia Syndrome

FXTAS is a neurodegenerative disorder that occurs in approximately 40% of males and 15% of females with the premutation. FXTAS usually begins with tremor in the early 60s, and higher CGG repeat numbers are associated with earlier onset of symptoms (Hagerman & Hagerman, 2020). Balance problems or ataxia begin 1 or 2 years after tremor followed by memory and executive function deficits. Emotional problems such as frontal disinhibition, anxiety, or depression are common, and further cognitive decline into dementia is seen in 50% of males with FXTAS. Females develop FXTAS less frequently and less severely than males. The central nervous system develops white matter disease that involves the middle cerebellar peduncles (MCP sign) in 60% of males but only 10% of females. FXTAS is also associated with lower extremity neuropathy, autonomic problems, Parkinsonian features, mood lability, and chronic pain symptoms. FXTAS is caused by the elevated mRNA so those with a full mutation and no mRNA do not develop FXTAS. However, rare cases of FXTAS have been reported in those with the full mutation with methylation mosaicism and elevated mRNA levels. Premutation carriers with symptoms of FXTAS need to be evaluated by a movement disorder neurologist and should have magnetic resonance imaging (MRI). The finding of the MCP sign is diagnostic of FXTAS when tremor or ataxia occur. Other MRI features include white matter disease in the splenium of the corpus callosum and the periventricular area along with brain atrophy. The neuropathology of FXTAS includes eosinophilic intranuclear inclusions in neurons and astrocytes throughout the brain but also in peripheral neurologic and organ tissues (Hall et al., 2016).

Fragile X–Associated Primary Ovarian Insufficiency

The premutation is the most common genetic mutation leading to early ovarian failure or menopause before age 40, a condition termed FXPOI. FXPOI occurs in 15% to 20% of women with the premutation, and an additional 20% experience menopause between 40 and 45 years of age (Noto, Harrity, Walsh, & Marron, 2016). Ovarian insufficiency is associated with fertility problems, and fragile X in a family is sometimes identified from infertility evaluations. Women with FXPOI should be referred for consultation with an obstetrician/gynecologist related to potential hormonal evaluation and treatment. Women of all ages with the premutation desiring future pregnancies should be aware of the risk for FXPOI, and be referred to reproductive medicine for evaluation of ovarian reserve and discussion related to reproductive options.

Fragile X–Associated Neuropsychiatric Disorders

FXAND is the most common set of disorders associated with the premutation, and the neuropsychiatric problems include depression, anxiety, obsessive-compulsive disorder, ASD, ADHD, insomnia, chronic pain, and chronic fatigue (Hagerman et al., 2018). Approximately 50% of those with the premutation can experience FXAND, and symptoms often start in childhood. Children with the premutation can present with ADHD, shyness, social anxiety, and sometimes ASD. Usually, however, children with the premutation do not have intellectual disability unless an additional genetic abnormality is found. In boys found to have the premutation through cascade testing of a family, only 8% have ASD and 38% have ADHD. In adults FXAND is a common problem, and approximately 50% of carriers experience significant anxiety and/or depression. This is important to recognize and refer for treatment in the mothers of fragile X children seen in developmental clinics as this can affect their ability to care for their child and family. Psychotic thinking with delusions and/or hallucinations is less common but require prompt treatment if present. Problems of chronic pain are more common in female carriers who have fibromyalgia and in those who experience migraines or neuropathy associated with FXTAS. Usually FXAND symptoms of anxiety or depression respond well to SSRIs in childhood or adulthood, although treatment with a therapist is typically very helpful in addition to daily exercise (Hagerman & Hagerman, 2020).

GENETIC COUNSELING AND CASCADE TESTING

Genetic counseling for FXS and associated disorders is commonly multifaceted due to the multigenerational and inherited nature of *FMR1* mutations. Families are frequently faced with variable implications for both nuclear and extended family members at risk for both full mutation and premutation-associated disorders and problems, while simultaneously processing a new diagnosis for the proband identified and implications for the individual's and family's future. It is also increasingly common that some female carriers are being incidentally identified during routine prenatal carrier screening in the absence of family history.

Once an *FMR1* mutation (pre or full) is identified in an individual, genetic counseling for the individual and family should ensue (McConkie-Rosell et al., 2005). Counseling should include solicitation of a detailed family history (3+ generation pedigree) to identify those at risk of carrying a premutation or full mutation, with targeted inquiry for male or female relatives with diagnoses or symptoms of:

- Developmental delays, intellectual disability, learning disabilities, and/or special education supports
- ASD and ADHD
- Anxiety disorders or other mental health diagnoses
- Females with primary ovarian insufficiency, infertility, irregular menses
- Adults with Parkinson disease, tremors, ataxia, cognitive decline, psychiatric changes, dementia

Genetic counseling should occur soon after a new diagnosis as there are often other females of childbearing age in the extended family, and the family itself may be interested in having additional children. Counseling should provide a detailed discussion about the diagnosis and management, as well as *FMR1* inheritance, clinical presentation of all fragile X–associated disorders, reproductive options (as appropriate), guidance for sharing information with identified at-risk family members, family and community support resources, research opportunities, and referrals to medical and psychological providers as indicated.

RESOURCES FOR PROVIDERS AND FAMILIES

A new diagnosis of FXS or associated disorder and its implications can be extremely difficult and emotional for individuals and families. It is common for parents to experience feelings of grief and guilt, as well as newly diagnosed adult patients to feel despair. Individual or family counseling can be helpful in processing these complex emotions and monitor for extreme grief. Parents of children with FXS often find significant support in connecting with other parents. Siblings of children with FXS also often need support. While there is currently no cure for FXS or associated disorders, families often find participation in advocacy efforts and/or research studies empowering. Various organizations are available to patients, families, and professionals:

- The National Fragile X Foundation (NFXF; www.fragilex.org) serves patients, their families, and professionals by focusing on advocacy, community support, awareness, education, and research.
- The NFXF Community Support Network (https://fragilex.org/community/) is a network of parent/family groups connecting families more locally to provide support throughout the country.

- Social networking sites, such as Facebook and Twitter, have dedicated fragile X groups.
- The Fragile X Clinical & Research Consortium (FXCRC; https://fragilex.org/fxcrc-and-clinics/) is a national collaboration of dedicated fragile X clinics providing comprehensive consensus-based treatment recommendations (consensus documents) (https://fragilex.org/our-research/treatment-guidelines/).
- The FRAXA Research Foundation (www.fraxa.org) serves a primary goal of funding research to find a cure for FXS.

REFERENCES

Budimirovic, D. B., Berry-Kravis, E., Erickson, C. A., Hall, S. S., Hessl, D., Reiss, A. L., … Kaufmann, W. E. (2017). Updated report on tools to measure outcomes of clinical trials in fragile X syndrome. *Journal of Neurodevelopmental Disorders*, *9*, 14. https://doi.org/10.1186/s11689-017-9193-x

Erickson, C. A., Davenport, M. H., Schaefer, T. L., Wink, L. K., Pedapati, E. V., Sweeney, J. A., … Berry-Kravis, E. (2017). Fragile X targeted pharmacotherapy: Lessons learned and future directions. *Journal of Neurodevelopmental Disorders*, *9*, 7. https://doi.org/10.1186/s11689-017-9186-9

Hagerman, R. J., & Hagerman, P. (Eds.). (2020). *Fragile X syndrome and premutation disorders: New developments and treatment.* MacKeith Press. https://doi.org/10.1111/dmcn.14726

Hagerman, R. J., Protic, D., Rajaratnam, A., Salcedo-Arellano, M. J., Aydin, E. Y., & Schneider, A. (2018). Fragile X-associated neuropsychiatric disorders (FXAND). *Frontiers in Psychiatry*, *9*, 564. https://doi.org/10.3389/fpsyt.2018.00564

Hall, D. A., Robertson, E., Shelton, A. L., Losh, M. C., Mila, M., Moreno, E. G., … O'Keefe, J. A. (2016). Update on the clinical, radiographic, and neurobehavioral manifestations in FXTAS and *FMR1* premutation carriers. *Cerebellum*, *15*(5), 578–586. https://doi.org/10.1007/s12311-016-0799-4

Lozano, R., Azarang, A., Wilaisakditipakorn, T., & Hagerman, R. J. (2016). Fragile X syndrome: A review of clinical managemen. *Intractable & Rare Diseases Research*, *5*(3), 145–157. https://doi.org/10.5582/irdr.2016.01048

Martin, G. E., Ausderau, K. K., Raspa, M., Bishop, E., Mallya, E., & Bailey, D. B. (2013). Therapy service use among individuals with fragile X syndrome: Findings from a US parent survey. *Journal of Intellectual Disability Research*, *57*(9), 837–849. https://doi.org/10.1111/j.1365-2788.2012.01608.x

McConkie-Rosell, A., Finucane, B., Cronister, A., Abrams, L., Bennett, R. L., & Pettersen, B. J. (2005). Genetic counseling for fragile X syndrome: Updated recommendations of the National Society of Genetic Counselors. *Journal of Genetic Counseling*, *14*(4), 249–270. https://doi.org/10.1007/s10897-005-4802-x

Noto, V., Harrity, C., Walsh, D., & Marron, K. (2016). The impact of *FMR1* gene mutations on human reproduction and development: A systematic review. *Journal of Assisted Reproduction and Genetics*, *33*, 1135–1147. https://doi.org/10.1007/s10815-016-0765-6

29

Nervous System

Elizabeth Troy and Padmini Palat

For additional material related to the content of this chapter, please see Chapters 25, 36, 39, 40, and 59.

VIGNETTE

A 7-week-old term infant presented with signs of increased intracranial pressure, including fussiness, persistent downgaze, and rapidly increasing head circumference. Urgent brain magnetic resonance imaging (MRI) (Fig. 29.1A, B) revealed obstructive hydrocephalus secondary to webbing at the cerebral aqueduct. An endoscopic third ventriculostomy was performed but complicated by a hemorrhagic stroke (see Fig. 29.1C). A ventriculoperitoneal shunt was ultimately placed. The infant developed acute symptomatic seizures, which were treated with levetiracetam that was subsequently weaned at 3 months of age. Two months later the patient developed subtle seizures, described as facial grimace with gaze deviation up and to the right. An electroencephalogram confirmed infantile spasms with a background of hypsarrhythmia. The spasms were refractory to vigabatrin but resolved with adrenocorticotropic hormone. Repeat MRI (see Fig. 29.1D) demonstrated a well-functioning ventriculoperitoneal shunt as well as volume loss of the left-sided structures. At 2 years of age, the toddler remained seizure-free off medications. Right spastic hemiparesis delayed the child's motor development, but the child was able to make consistent gains and ambulate with a gait trainer. The patient's language was advanced for age, and social and language development was typical for age. The progress was attributed to timely diagnosis of congenital hydrocephalus, rapid recognition of seizures, and early initiation of medical treatment and intensive therapy.

This chapter reviews congenital malformations and childhood vascular diseases of the brain in the context of typical neurodevelopmental anatomy. The clinical vignette illustrated how a thorough history and physical examination led to the appropriate diagnosis and treatment.

PRENATAL BRAIN DEVELOPMENT

The adult human brain consists of more than 100 billion neurons with 60 trillion synapses, as well as a rich network of nonneuronal glial cells that have a supportive function. Brain development begins in the third week of gestation, extending at least through late adolescence. This process encompasses a complex series of events operating within a genetically determined framework adapting to a constantly changing milieu. Disruption of either gene expression or environmental input can adversely affect brain development.

The first major step in human embryonic brain development involves the formation of the neural plate, which occurs by day 20 of conception. The neural plate subsequently folds over to form the neural plate.

The anterior end of the neural tube forms brain vesicles that forms brain vesicles that represents the primary organization of the central nervous system (CNS). Discernible patterns of organization of the sensorimotor neocortex, diencephalon, midbrain, hindbrain, and spinal cord are present by the end of the embryonic period at 8 completed weeks. The primitive ventricular system is lined by neural progenitor cells in a transient ventricular zone. Neuron production in this zone begins at day 42. Different populations of neurons migrate away from the proliferative regions of the ventricular zone to form gray matter in many regions of the brain.

Much of the fetal period from the ninth week to term is characterized by ongoing neuronal production, migration, and differentiation. Neuronal axons and dendrites form pathways that ultimately make up the white matter of the brain. Major nerve fiber pathways are established by the end of the prenatal period. The proliferation and migration of glial progenitors continue for an extended period after birth. Myelination of the brain is mostly a postnatal process that continues well into the second and third years of life.

NEUROANATOMY

The brain is the most complex human organ. Historically the study of brain disease by clinicians and neuropathologists contributed to mapping of different brain functions to specific anatomic regions. Recent advances in genetics and the advent of sophisticated functional brain imaging have added to this evolving process. Clinical medical practice continues to rely on discerning normal from abnormal brain function by means of a neurologic examination.

Supratentorial Anatomy

It is useful to think of the brain as contained in two compartments separated by a layer of dura mater known as the tentorium. The supratentorial brain consists of the cerebral hemispheres, thalami, basal ganglia, and hypothalamus. Each cerebral hemisphere has an outer cortex of neuronal gray matter folded to form sulci and gyri, with an inner white matter of connecting fibers transmitting information between the cortex and deeper brain structures. Each cerebral hemisphere controls the function of the contralateral half of the body. There are four

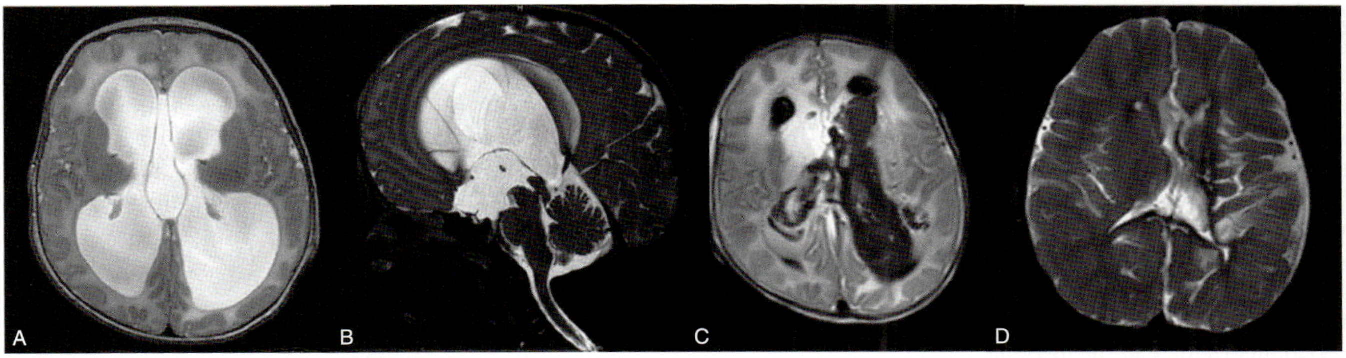

Fig. 29.1 Congenital hydrocephalus *(A, B)*; hemorrhagic stroke *(C)*; volume loss following hemorrhagic stroke *(D)*.

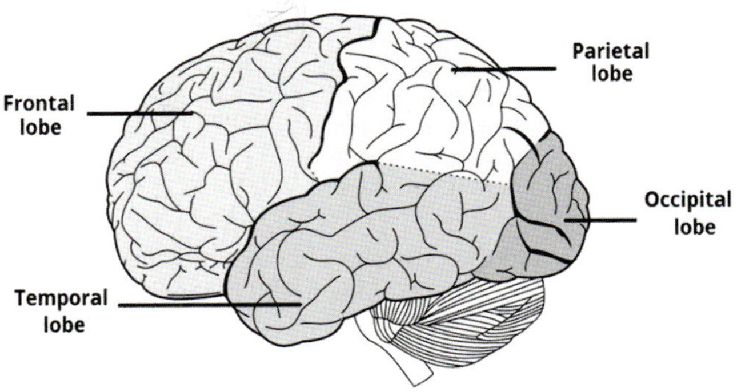

Fig. 29.2 Lateral view of cerebral cortex. (From https://teachmeanatomy.info/neuroanatomy/structures/cerebrum)

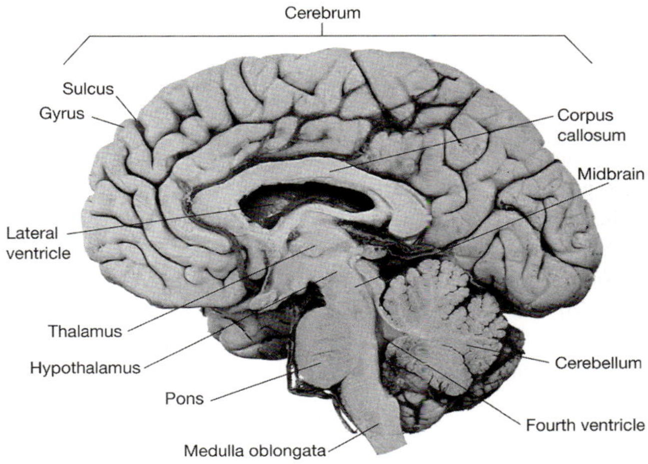

Fig. 29.3 Ventricular system Neuroanatomy. An Illustrated Colour Text. Crossman, Alan R, PhD DSc; Neary, David, MD FRCP. Published January 1, 2020. Pages 55–50. 2020. Fig. 6.2 Median sagittal section of the brain showing the ventricular system.

lobes of the cerebral cortex (Fig. 29.2). The frontal lobe controls voluntary movements, language, and cognitive and executive function. The speech area is located in the left frontal lobe in most individuals, hence the left hemisphere is considered dominant. The parietal lobe is the sensory receptive area and transmits spatial information to the motor cortex. The temporal lobe controls memory, language comprehension, emotional processing, and auditory function. The occipital lobe is responsible for visual functions, including object and face recognition, visuospatial processing, depth perception, and color determination. The two sides of the cerebrum communicate through the corpus callosum, which is a broad midline tract of white matter between hemispheres.

The thalami function as relay stations for sensory and motor signals and regulate consciousness and alertness. The hypothalamus controls the autonomic nervous system and works in conjunction with the pituitary gland to mediate endocrine functions. The basal ganglia initiate and integrate movements. The pineal gland regulates circadian rhythm and influences pituitary sex hormone secretion.

Infratentorial Anatomy

The infratentorial brain consists of the cerebellum and brainstem that occupy the posterior fossa. The cerebellum is composed of two cerebellar hemispheres and the midline vermis. The brainstem continues downward into the spinal cord through the foramen magnum and includes the midbrain, pons, and medulla (Fig. 29.3). The cerebellum functions in coordination and motor planning, with the laterally placed cerebellar hemispheres controlling ipsilateral limbs and the midline vermis the neck and trunk. In addition, the role of the cerebellum in cognitive function is being increasingly recognized. The midbrain controls eye movements and processes auditory and visual signals. The pons has nuclei that regulate respiration and sleep in addition to mediating the functions of several cranial nerves. The medulla oblongata controls vital functions such as respiration and heart rate.

The cranial nerves (CN) have been named for their functions and are designated by Roman numerals. CNI (olfactory nerve) and CNII (optic nerve) mediate smell and vision, respectively, and are located above the tentorium. CNIII, CNIV, and CNVI (oculomotor, trochlear, and abducens nerves) control eye movements with CNIII also responsible for accommodation and pupillary constriction. CNIII and CNIV emerge from the midbrain; CNV, CNV1, CNVII, and CNVIII from the pons. CNV (trigeminal nerve) is responsible for facial sensation and motor control of masticatory muscles. Other facial muscles are controlled by CNVII (facial nerve), which also carries taste fibers from the anterior two-thirds of the tongue and supplies salivary and tear glands. CNVIII (vestibulocochlear nerve) has auditory and vestibular functions. CNIX (glossopharyngeal nerve) controls palatal sensation and taste in the posterior one-third of the tongue. CNX (vagus nerve) has a long course with a wide range of function, including motor control of the pharynx, palate, and larynx; sensory innervation of larynx, pharynx, heart, and abdominal viscera; parasympathetic supply to smooth muscles of the trachea and bronchi; and control of heart rate. CNXI (accessory nerve) controls neck and shoulder musculature, and CNXII (hypoglossal nerve) is the motor nerve of the tongue muscles. CNIX, CNX, CNXI, and CNXII all originate in the medulla.

Spinal Cord and Peripheral Nervous System

The spinal cord extends from the foramen magnum to the first lumbar vertebra. It contains central gray matter consisting of spinal neurons surrounded by white matter made of ascending sensory and descending motor tracts. The peripheral nervous system includes the spinal nerves and the autonomic nervous system. There are 31 pairs of spinal nerves that are segmentally organized and named in relation to vertebral bodies. C1 to C7 cervical spinal nerves emerge from the spinal cord above their corresponding vertebrae, C8 and the remaining spinal nerves exit below their vertebral levels. The spinal nerves divide into branches and then organize into peripheral nerves with motor and sensory functions.

The sympathetic and parasympathetic pathways of the autonomic nervous system control involuntary functions. The sympathetic pathways originating in the hypothalamus descend to the spinal cord for distribution to the effector organs via the peripheral nervous system. The parasympathetic pathways are mediated by cells in the brainstem and sacral spinal cord and also reach their destination via peripheral nerves.

Meninges

The meninges are composed of three membranes, organized from superficial to deep layers as dura mater, arachnoid mater, and pia mater. These membranes are present intracranially and travel the length of the spinal canal. The dura mater is a thick fibrous structure composed of two layers—periosteal and meningeal. Dural venous sinuses are present between these two layers. The arachnoid membrane is a thin membrane deep to the dura mater. Invaginations of the arachnoid membrane, known as arachnoid granulations, traverse the dura mater and facilitate absorption of cerebrospinal fluid (CSF). The subarachnoid space lies between the arachnoid and pia mater, and CSF and bridging veins are present here. The pia is a thin delicate membrane that adheres to the surface of the brain and spinal cord. The pia and arachnoid layers are collectively referred to as the leptomeninges. The meninges receive sensory innervation predominantly via terminal branches of the trigeminal nerve.

Cerebrovascular Circulation

The intracranial arterial system is divided into an anterior and a posterior circulation with a Circle of Willis anastomosis (Fig. 29.4). The anterior circulation is supplied by the internal carotid arteries, and the posterior circulation by the vertebral arteries. The intracranial venous system is composed of dural venous sinuses as well as a collection of smaller veins (Fig. 29.5).

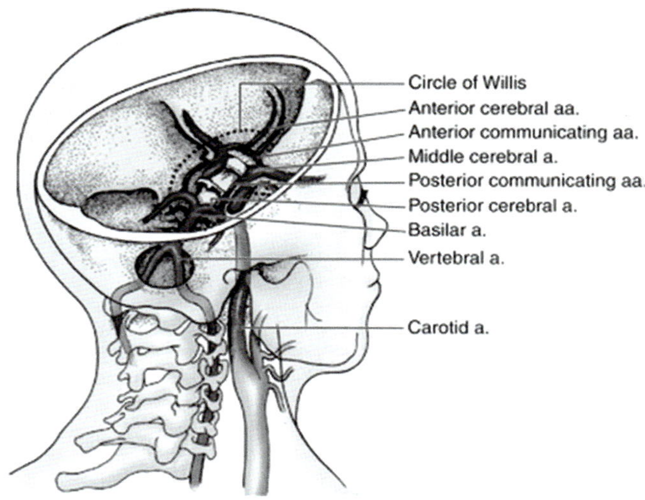

Fig. 29.4 Intracranial arterial circulation. From Introdution to vascular ultrasonography expert consult. 2012.

Cerebrospinal Fluid Circulation

CSF is produced by the choroid plexus and circulates within the ventricular system composed of four ventricles–lateral (right and left), third, and fourth ventricles. The lateral ventricles form the frontal, occipital, and temporal horns. They drain via the foramen of Monro into the third ventricle, which is located between the thalami. CSF then traverses the cerebral aqueduct into the fourth ventricle, which lies between the dorsal brainstem and cerebellum. The fourth ventricle drains via the foramina of Luschka and Magendi into the subarachnoid space around the spinal cord. CSF then recirculates to ultimately be reabsorbed into the venous system via arachnoid granulations.

NEUROLOGIC HISTORY AND PHYSICAL EXAMINATION

History

In child neurology, the history and physical examination are vital to reaching the proper diagnosis. It is essential to include the child in the interview while simultaneously engaging the parents or caregivers to provide supportive information.

The initial portion of the history is driven by the chief complaint. Chronology is important, as distinguishing between acute, chronic, or progressive conditions directs the acuity of the workup. In contrast, many neurologic conditions are paroxysmal, such as spells, headaches, or abnormal movements. The description of these episodes, including details before and after, leads toward a diagnosis. For instance, tunnel vision and head rush prior to an event are suggestive of vasovagal syncope, and an unusual smell or sense of déjà vu

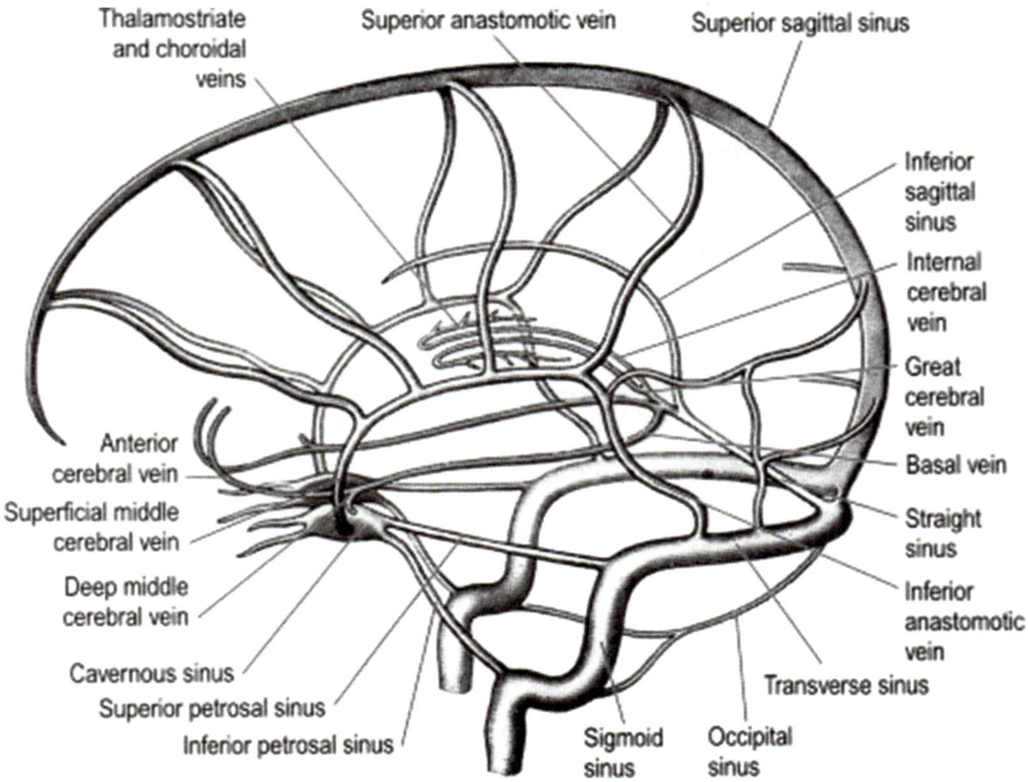

Fig. 29.5 Intracranial venous circulation. (From Greenlee, J. E. [2010]. Suppurative intracranial thrombophlebitis. In *Handbook of Clinical Neurology* [vol. 96, pp. 101–123]. Elsevier. https://doi.org/10.1016/S0072-9752(09)96008-0)

can be indicative of temporal lobe seizures. For abnormal movements, an urge to move followed by release of tension is supportive of a motor tic, but an early-morning jerk resulting in dropping an object is suggestive of a myoclonic seizure. Presence of symptoms during sleep is also helpful. Seizures and dystonia persist during sleep while tics, stereotypies, and chorea abate. Triggers, worsening or alleviating factors, and degree of functional impairment or injury are other valuable features.

A birth and developmental history should be obtained for every pediatric patient. Inquire about the course of the pregnancy, including the presence of fever, sick symptoms, or vaginal bleeding; medication or substance use; and gestational age at time of delivery. Assess whether a neonatal intensive care unit stay was necessary and, if so, the interventions that were required. Breech presentation, decreased movements, or failure to progress are suggestive of a neuromuscular disorder. Fetal hiccups could indicate seizures in utero. A complete medical history should also be obtained. Congenital heart disease can raise suspicion of other malformations. Risk factors for brain injury, such as intracranial infection, head injury, or stroke, should be elicited.

All domains of development, including gross and fine motor, language, cognitive, and social, should be evaluated. For younger children, obtain a course of developmental milestones, including age at sitting, walking, first word, and establishment of hand preference. Discuss whether they have been getting physical, occupational, speech, behavioral, and other therapies. For older children it is important to inquire on school performance. A variety of academic or psychiatric conditions such as learning disability, intellectual disability, anxiety and/or depression, and attentional problems are comorbidities of neurologic diagnoses. A social history can provide context to the family and home structure.

A thorough review of systems to investigate for other system involvement is useful. Discuss the child's growth as well as safety of chewing and swallowing. Choking or coughing following liquids or solids is worrisome for a neuromuscular process. Evaluate for hearing or vision concerns. Discuss whether the child needs breathing assistance with special apparatus or supplemental oxygen. Bowel or bladder difficulties could be suggestive of spinal cord pathology. All patients with neurologic conditions are at risk for sleep problems, so difficulty with sleep onset, nighttime awakenings, sleepwalking, or other movements during sleep should be elicited.

Lastly, it is important to discuss family history. Many neurologic diseases are genetic in etiology, and it is helpful to distinguish between inherited and non-inherited conditions. Drawing a pedigree can identify possible patterns of inheritance.

General Examination

A complete examination always begins with a quality general physical examination. Review vital signs and growth parameters with attention to the head circumference. If macrocephaly or microcephaly is identified, measurement of parents' heads can indicate a familial component. Observe the head shape. Plagiocephaly is suggestive of torticollis. Scaphocephaly or brachycephaly could indicate craniosynostosis. Atypical facial features, such as frontal bossing, eye or ear position, or midface hypoplasia raise suspicion for an underlying genetic condition. A skin examination looks for neurocutaneous stigmata, such as café au lait spots. On cardiac examination, auscultate the heart rhythm and for presence of a murmur. On the abdominal examination, palpate for hepatosplenomegaly, which can be seen with a storage disorder. Pectus excavatum is a sign of hypotonia. Decreased range of motion of major joints is suggestive of increased tone. Other atypical features such as clinodactyly or single palmar crease indicate an underlying genetic syndrome.

Neurologic Examination

The neurologic examination begins from the instant the provider enters the clinic room. Many details are gleaned from observation of children and adolescents, but this is most true in infants and toddlers or children with autism spectrum disorder or other neurodevelopmental conditions. The details of the neurologic examination are provided in Table 29.1.

TABLE 29.1 Neurologic Examination

	Examination Maneuvers	Pathology
Mental status	Level of alertness, orientation, attention, follow commands	Global brain for cognitive abilities, frontal lobe for executive function
Speech	Content, quality, cadence of speech, conversation, naming objects, repetition	Cerebellar function Aphasia: frontal or temporal lobes
Cranial Nerves **Optic nerve (II)**	Visual fields by bringing toys/fingers into periphery, visual acuity, fundoscopy, afferent of pupillary light reflex	Visual pathway is from retina > optic nerve > optic tracts > occipital lobe
Oculomotor (III), Trochlear (IV), Abducens (VI)	Fixation and tracking in an infant Ability to follow an object in all directions Efferent of pupillary light reflex (CNIII)	Midbrain function Lateral gaze palsy is suggestive of increased intracranial pressure
Trigeminal (V)	Sensation in the upper, middle, and lower face: muscles of mastication	Pontine function
Facial (VII)	Upper face: eyebrow raise, eye closure Lower face: smile, puff of cheeks Taste to anterior 2/3 of tongue	Upper motor neuron: lower face only; lower motor neuron: upper and lower face Pontine function
Vestibulocochlear (VIII)	Hear finger rub or clap Balance	Pontine function
Glossopharyngeal (IX)	Afferent for gag reflex; taste posterior 1/3 of tongue	Medullary function
Vagus (X)	Efferent for gag reflex; parasympathetic to heart and gastrointestinal tract	Medullary function
Accessory (XI)	Shoulder shrug (trapezius); turn of head to the left and right (sternocleidomastoid)	Medullary function
Hypoglossal (XII)	Protrude tongue and move side to side	Upper motor neuron: deviates contralaterally; lower motor neuron: deviates ipsilaterally
Motor	Bulk: overall size of muscles Tone: passive range of motion of all limbs Strength: confrontational testing or observation of functional movements	Upper motor neuron: increased tone and weakness; lower motor neuron: decreased tone and weakness
Sensation	Light touch, pinprick, temperature, vibration, and proprioception	Large fiber/posterior column of cord: ↓ proprioception/vibration Small fiber: ↓light touch
Reflexes	Biceps, brachioradialis, triceps, pateller, and Achilles Pathologic: Hoffman, suprapubic, crossed adductor	Upper motor neuron: hyperreflexia and pathologic reflexes Lower motor neuron: hyporeflexia
Coordination	Finger taps, finger to nose, heel to shin	Cerebellar function
Gait	Stance; casual gait; toe, heel, and tandem walk	Assessment of cerebellar function, vestibular system, strength, and large fiber nerves

TABLE 29.2 Primitive Reflexes Based on Description and Timing

Reflex	Description	Appears	Disappears
Moro	Infant's arms abduct with startle	28 wk gestation	3–6 mo
Palmar	Infant's fist closes into grasp with touch of palm	28 wk gestation	3–4 mo
Stepping	Infant appears to walk when held upright	32 wk gestation	2 mo
Tonic neck	With infant's head turned to one side, ipsilateral arm extends and contralateral arm flexes	Birth	4–6 mo
Parachute	When lowered to ground, infant will extend arms forward to prop	6–7 mo	Persists

Techniques in Infants

Most of the neurologic examination in an infant is observational, but there are a host of examination features that are unique to the infant period. Neonates naturally have a flexed posture. A frog-leg position, slip through with vertical suspension, or inability to maintain head at neutral with horizontal suspension are signs of hypotonia. Opisthotonos or early rolling from back to belly are signs of hypertonia. Primitive reflexes can also be assessed (Table 29.2). Asymmetry in these reflexes can be a subtle sign of weakness.

Telehealth

The COVID-19 pandemic has ushered in an expansion of telemedicine. This opportunity for patient care can be immensely valuable for the clinician. A history can be obtained as easily via telehealth as in person, and it is valuable to observe the patient at home as social stressors can be more apparent. Children with autism spectrum disorder or other neurodevelopmental conditions typically are more comfortable in their home rather than in a new clinic environment. Challenges include difficulty for a young child to interact with a screen or patients in whom a fundoscopic or neuromuscular examination is required.

Indications for Imaging

Chief complaint, history, and physical examination guide the decision to obtain head imaging, and acuity of symptoms influences the modality of computed tomography (CT) or MRI. In head trauma, CT head should be obtained for any patient who has altered mental status or signs of skull fracture and should be considered for patients with a severe mechanism of injury, loss of consciousness, severe headache, or vomiting (Kuppermann et al., 2009). For developmental delay, imaging is included in first-tier testing if the patient has neurocutaneous stigmata or a focal neurologic deficit such as spastic hemiparesis. MRI brain is considered standard of care in epilepsy unless patient has a typical presentation for a well-described pediatric epilepsy syndrome such as childhood absence epilepsy. If red flags are observed with headache, then head imaging is required.

CENTRAL NERVOUS SYSTEM MALFORMATIONS

Malformations of the CNS, comprising the brain and spinal cord, account for a significant proportion of congenital anomalies. A 2019 multicenter population-based European study identified 9.8 cases of cerebral malformations per 10,000 births (Morris et al., 2019). Spina bifida has a marked geographic variation in incidence ranging from 0.77 to 6.1 per 1000 live births in South Africa to an estimated 3.5 per 1000 live births in the United States (Ntimbani, Kelly, & Lekgwara, 2020).

Brain malformations are an important cause of developmental delay, intellectual disability, motor impairment, and intractable childhood epilepsy. Spinal dysraphism can impact bladder and bowel function as well as mobility.

Genetic factors as well as the intrauterine environment influence CNS development. Chromosome abnormalities and single gene disorders have been identified in many CNS malformations. Prenatal exposure to certain toxins such as alcohol, drugs such as retinoic acid and valproate, virus infections such as cytomegalovirus, hyperthermia, ionizing radiation, trauma, maternal metabolic dysfunction, and nutritional factors have been linked to a variety of prenatal brain and spinal cord disorders. The timing of exposure of the fetal brain and spinal cord to an external agent appears critical (e.g., spina bifida results from exposure to an adverse agent between day 21 and day 28 of gestation).

A single agent can cause a spectrum of brain abnormalities, as in the case of prenatal Zika virus infection leading to microcephaly, parenchymal calcifications, defective neuronal migration, corpus callosum abnormalities, ventriculomegaly, and posterior fossa abnormalities (VHP et al., 2020). Conversely, there can be an overlap of causes for the same malformation, such as agenesis of corpus callosum that can be due to fetal alcohol exposure or a variety of genetic or neurometabolic disorders. The 2019 European population study of congenital brain malformations showed that 48% of all cases had an isolated cerebral anomaly, 25% had associated noncerebral anomalies, and 27% were identified with a chromosomal abnormality or a known genetic or teratogenic syndrome (Morris et al., 2019).

Major advances in clinical genetics and improved imaging with MRI brain, including fetal MRI imaging, are leading to earlier and more accurate diagnoses of CNS malformations.

Precise pathologic mechanisms may not be identified in an individual patient due to the complex interplay of genes with metabolic and environmental factors, but genetic counseling should be offered once an anatomic abnormality is identified on brain imaging. A search for an identifiable genetic cause can include karyotype, chromosome microarray, targeted gene panels, and whole exome or genome sequencing. Details about genetic testing are discussed in Chapter 25.

An exact diagnosis can help to determine the recurrence risk in subsequent pregnancies, and this allows appropriate reproductive counseling. Early detection of a malformation can lead to intervention such as prenatal closure of spina bifida and shunt surgery for congenital hydrocephalus. Brain and spinal cord malformations caused by adverse intrauterine conditions may be preventable.

Neuroimaging with brain MRI is the most common diagnostic tool used to identify CNS malformations in clinical practice, and this section uses MRI to illustrate many of these conditions. It is important to recognize the broad range of neurodevelopmental effects in many of these disorders, keeping in mind that a clinically insignificant finding may be discovered when a patient undergoes neuroimaging for head trauma or other reasons.

CNS malformations have been classified in various ways. Commonly used systems divide malformations according to the anatomic area of involvement as well as embryologic underpinnings, often incorporating genotype correlations.

Forebrain and Cerebral Cortex

Holoprosencephaly

Holoprosencephaly is a severe defect that refers to incomplete division of the forebrain. The most severe form is alobar holoprosencephaly where there is no separation of the cerebral hemispheres, the thalami are fused, and there is a single large ventricular cavity (Fig. 29.6). The cerebellum and brainstem are normally formed. This malformation is typically associated with severe facial and ocular abnormalities. Congenital heart disease and polydactyly may also be noted. Severe intellectual disability, rigidity, intractable seizures, apnea, growth hormone deficiency, diabetes insipidus, and temperature instability are common neurologic manifestations. Severe cases are generally identified early, though incomplete subtypes may be detected only at a later age.

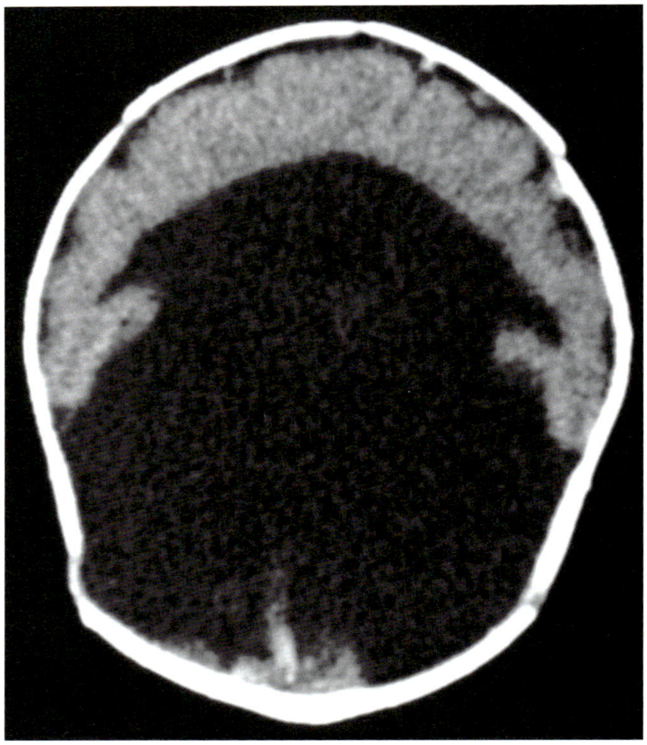

Fig. 29.6 Alobar holoprosencephaly.

Genetic disorders are identified in 25% to 50% cases (Tekendo-Ngongang, Muenke, & Kruszka, 2020). These include trisomy 13 (the most common genetic cause), trisomy 18, other chromosome deletions or duplications, monogenic disorders such as Smith-Lemli-Opitz syndrome, and several nonsyndromic single-gene abnormalities such as sonic hedgehog gene mutations (Dubourg, Kim, Watrin, , Tayrac, de, Odent, David, & Dupé, 2018). Maternal diabetes mellitus is another prenatal risk factor. Any child with holoprosencephaly deserves a full genetic evaluation so that appropriate counseling may be offered.

Agenesis of Corpus Callosum

The corpus callosum is the largest interhemispheric white matter tract in the brain and is formed between gestational weeks 13 and 19. Agenesis of the corpus callosum (ACC) can occur as an isolated finding on MRI (Fig. 29.7) but is more commonly

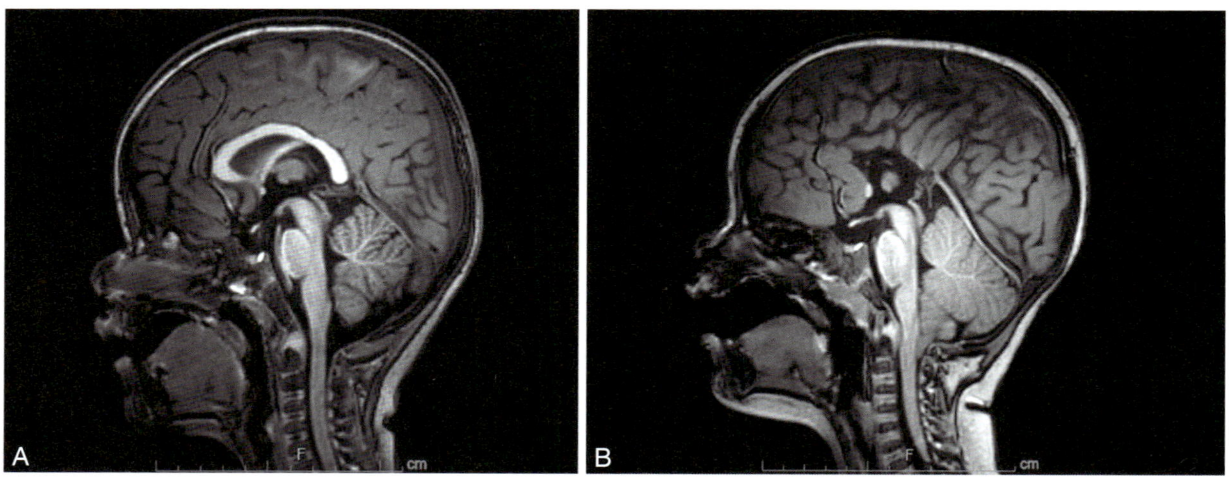

Fig. 29.7 A, typically formed corpus callosum; B, agenesis of corpus callosum.

associated with other disorders of brain development. Partial ACC or hypoplasia of corpus callosum is more commonly seen than complete agenesis. Neurologic findings and developmental disabilities are understandably diverse, ranging from minimum neurologic abnormalities in isolated ACC to more severe problems such as seizures, intellectual disabilities, and motor dysfunction. Deficits in problem solving and social skills as well as autism spectrum disorder can occur.

A large number of genetic causes have been described, including chromosomal syndromes, copy number variations, and pathogenic variants of single genes (Edwards, Sherr, Barkovich, & Richards, 2014). Abnormal development of the corpus callosum has been noted in several enzyme deficiencies affecting cellular metabolism, including pyruvate dehydrogenase deficiency and fumarase deficiency. Disorders of cholesterol synthesis such as Smith-Lemli-Opitz syndrome and desmosterolosis particularly affect corpus callosum formation. A higher rate of ACC has been reported in individuals with fetal alcohol syndrome, a finding of significant public health importance. Interestingly a cause has not been identified in Aicardi syndrome, the clinically well-characterized triad of ACC, chorioretinal lacunae, and infantile spasms occurring in girls.

Septo-Optic Dysplasia

Septo-optic dysplasia encompasses a the classical triad of agenesis of the septum pellucidum and/or corpus callosum, hypoplasia of the hypothalamic-pituitary axis, and optic nerve hypoplasia. At least two of the three criteria are required for diagnosis. It is one of the top causes of congenital vision loss in developed countries. Neuroendocrine disturbance including growth hormone deficiency and diabetes insipidus may result, and a full endocrinology evaluation is warranted. The presence of additional brain malformations is often referred to as septo-optic dysplasia spectrum disorder, which increases the severity of neurologic manifestations such as epilepsy, spasticity, and intellectual disability.

Septo-optic dysplasia is usually a sporadic disorder, but familial cases have been described. A combination of prenatal environmental factors and genetic predisposition appears to play a causative role (Ganau, Huet, Syrmos, Meloni, & Jayamohan, 2019).

Lissencephaly

Lissencephaly, meaning "smooth brain," is caused by failure of neuronal migration. Only four of the six layers of cerebral cortex are present. Imaging studies reveal a thickened cortex and paucity of sulci (Fig. 29.8). Enlarged lateral ventricles are noted. Subcortical band heterotropia is a related condition where abnormal bands of neurons are seen beneath a normal cortex. Hypotonia, profound global developmental delays, microcephaly, and intractable seizures are characteristic of lissencephaly. Infantile spasms develop in 35% to 85% of children with classic lissencephaly (Di Donato et al., 2017). Seizures are often intractable, and many patients have Lennox-Gastaut syndrome. Life expectancy is lowered by feeding difficulties that include gastroesophageal reflux and aspiration, epilepsy, and pneumonia.

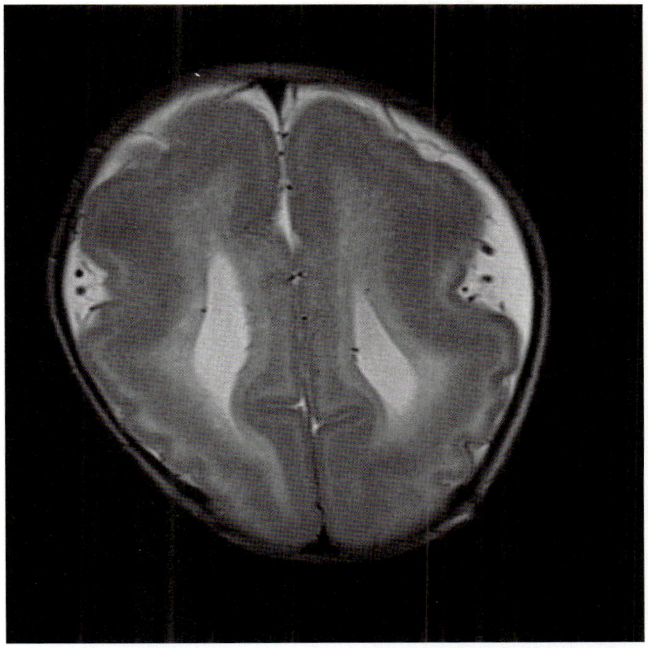

Fig. 29.8 Lissencephaly.

Lissencephaly is a genetically heterogenous disorder. Classical lissencephaly is due to pathogenic changes in the *LIS1* gene. *DCX* pathogenic variant is X-linked and causes lissencephaly in hemizygous males and subcortical band heterotropia in heterozygous females. Multiple congenital anomaly syndromes with lissencephaly include Miller-Dieker syndrome, Baraitser-Winter syndrome, and X-linked lissencephaly with abnormal genitalia.

Polymicrogyria

Polymicrogyria (PMG) is one of the most common brain malformations, accounting for 20% of all disorders of cortical development (Stutterd, Dobyns, Jansen, Mirzaa, & Leventer, 2018). In PMG, cortical gyri are small, crowded, and too numerous (Fig. 29.9). The Sylvian fissures are frequently affected. Clinical findings in PMG are variable, with developmental issues ranging from learning problems to intellectual disabilities. A variety of uni- or bilateral motor deficits and tone abnormalities ranging from spasticity to hypertonia with hyperreflexia may be seen. Epilepsy is common. Bilateral perisylvian PMG results in pseudobulbar palsy with dysphagia along with failure to develop expressive speech, referred to as congenital bilateral perisylvian syndrome.

PMG can result from intrauterine infection, vascular disruption, and toxic, metabolic, and genetic causes. More than 40 contiguous-gene or single-gene disorders have been associated with PMG. Recognizable syndromes with other clinical features include DiGeorge syndrome, 1p36 deletion, megalencephaly-capillary malformation (MCM), or megalencephaly- polymicrogyria-polydactyly-hydrocephalus (MPPH). Metabolic diseases such as Zellweger spectrum disorder and mitochondrial disorders can cause PMG. PMG has also been described in monochorionic twin pregnancies, usually associated with intrauterine co-twin death and twin-to-twin

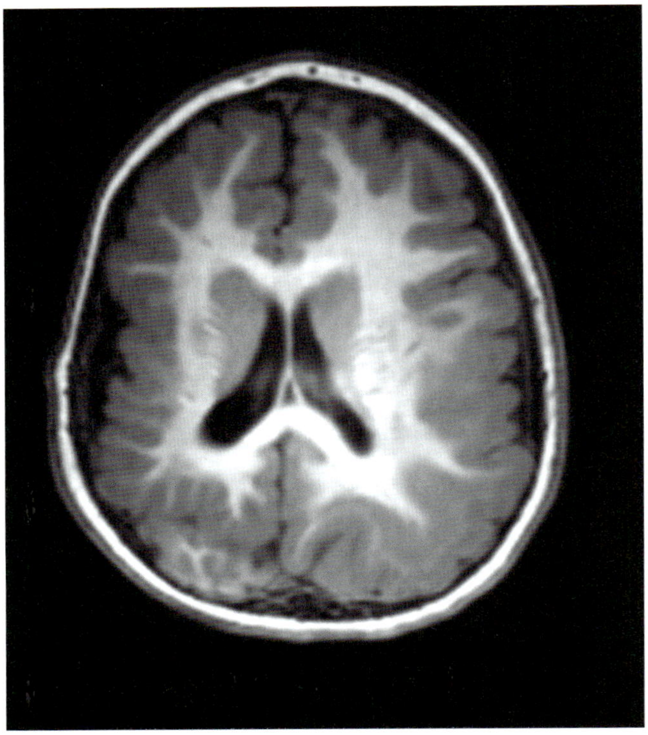

Fig. 29.9 Polymicrogyria: excessive folding of right cerebral cortex.

transfusion syndrome. Congenital cytomegalovirus infection is a well-known etiology, and additional features such as microcephaly, chorioretinitis, and intracranial calcifications can occur. More recently, congenital Zika syndrome virus has been implicated as a cause.

Schizencephaly

Schizencephaly is a specific pattern of PMG characterized by uni- or bilateral clefts on the cortical surface associated with gray matter extending from the cortical surfaces to the ventricular cavity (Fig. 29.10). In closed-lipped schizencephaly the cleft walls are opposed. Open-lipped schizencephaly is associated with a prominent CSF cleft and may be difficult to differentiate from a porencephalic cyst, the latter implying cortical destruction from vascular or infectious insults.

Neuronal Heterotopia

Neuronal heterotropia is caused by abnormal neuronal migration with failure of neurons to reach their destination in the cerebral cortex and can result in epilepsy. It can be recognized on brain MRI as single or multiple nodules lining the lateral ventricles of the brain, or subcortical bandlike or discrete rests of gray matter within otherwise normal white matter (Fig. 29.11).

Focal Cortical Dysplasia

Focal cortical dysplasia consists of areas of abnormal brain anatomy with neuronal dyslamination and abnormal cell types. Focal cortical dysplasia may be asymptomatic or can result in focal onset epilepsy sometimes manifesting only in later life. Not all focal cortical dysplasias are detectable on

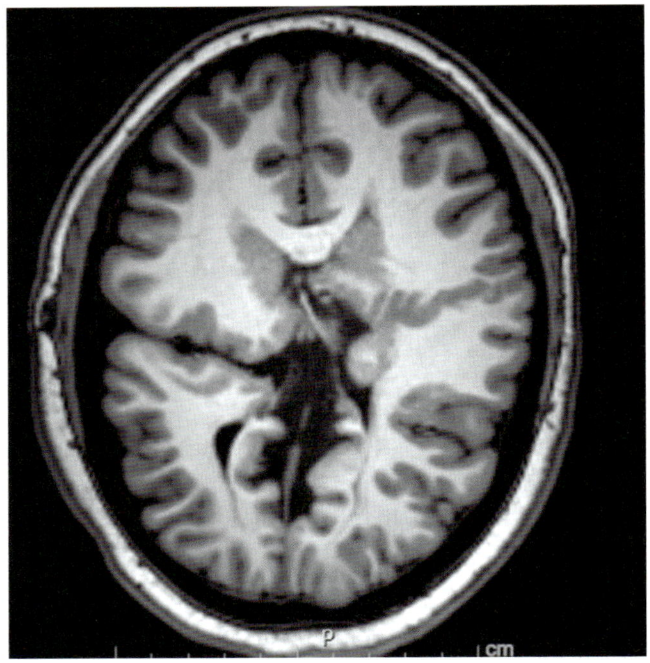

Fig. 29.10 Schizencephaly: cleft in right cerebral hemisphere extending to midline.

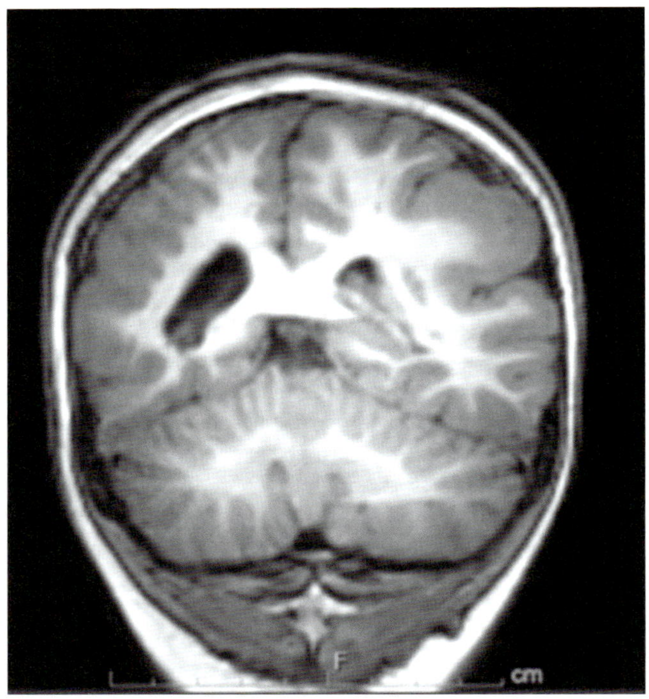

Fig. 29.11 Neuronal heterotopia: areas of gray matter left periventricular white matter *(right)*.

brain MRI and are sometimes diagnosed only by microscopic examination after epilepsy surgery.

Posterior Fossa

Dandy-Walker Malformation

Dandy-Walker malformation refers to hypoplasia and anticlockwise rotation of the cerebellar vermis with cystic dilation of the fourth ventricle (Fig. 29.12). Hydrocephalus is

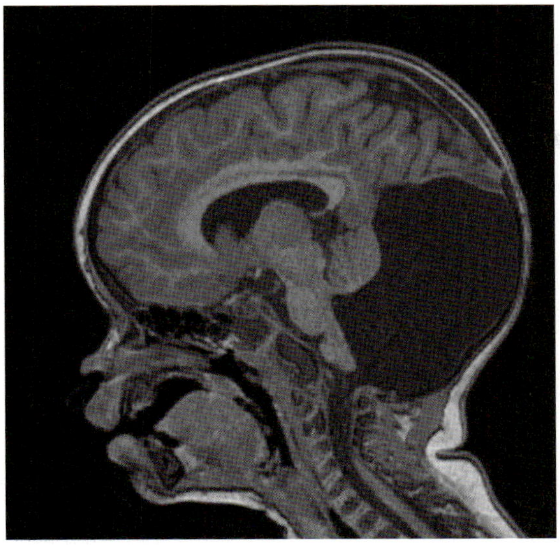

Fig. 29.12 Dandy-Walker malformation.

frequently associated and is often the presenting feature. Other brain malformations occur in more than half the cases. Extracranial abnormalities are often seen, including congenital heart disease, syndactyly, and polycystic kidneys. Involvement of the cerebellum and brainstem typically cause motor delays, hypotonia, and abnormal eye movements. Cognitive delays or epilepsy are seen if there are associated cortical malformations. Patients with Dandy-Walker syndrome often require shunting of hydrocephalus or of the posterior fossa cyst. Prognosis is variable and is worse if there are associated intracranial or extracranial manifestations.

Chromosomal abnormalities occur in approximately 50%, most frequently trisomy 18, trisomy 13, and triploidy. Other causes include teratogens, alcohol, maternal viral infection and diabetes, and a few single-gene disorders (Haddadi, Zare, & Asadian, 2018).

Pontocerebellar Hypoplasia

Pontocerebellar hypoplasia refers to reduced volume of the cerebellum and pons (Fig. 29.13) and is typically associated with severe neurologic symptoms. Many genetic causes have been identified, including tubulinopathies (van Dijk, Baas, Barth, & Poll-The, 2018). Most cases are inherited in an autosomal recessive manner. Some pontocerebellar hypoplasia subtypes cause progressive atrophy, particularly of the pons, and could be subsumed under the category of neurodegenerative brain disease of prenatal onset. Structural brainstem abnormalities can occur in congenital genetic muscle dystrophies such as Fukuyama disease. Joubert syndrome is a genetic disorder with a distinctive cerebellar and brainstem malformation on brain imaging referred to as the molar tooth sign, with associated episodic breathing irregularity and hypotonia. Prematurity with gestational age less than 32 weeks has also been associated with varying degrees of cerebellar hypoplasia.

Chiari I to IV

Chiari I the most common Chiari malformation, seen in 0.6% of pediatric brain MRI studies (McClugage & Oakes, 2019). It refers to downward displacement of cerebellum and tonsils

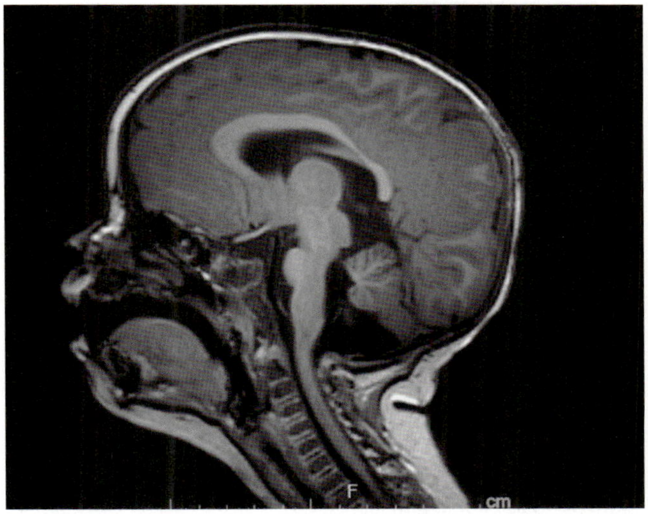

Fig. 29.13 Pontocerebellar hypoplasia.

5 mm or more below the foramen magnum (Fig. 29.14). It can be associated with syringomyelia (central spinal canal dilatation) or bony abnormalities of the skull base.

Symptomatic Chiari I usually presents in adolescents and adults, less commonly in children. The most common features are occipital headache and cervical pain. Infants and young children can have excessive crying and irritability due to pain, but are more likely to be diagnosed when they develop signs of brainstem dysfunction such as central sleep apnea or feeding difficulties. Other symptoms of Chiari I include hydrocephalus or features of spinal cord dysfunction. Surgical management is undertaken in symptomatic cases, but over 93% of Chiari I cases are benign and do not need intervention. Chiari I is generally congenital but can be acquired in a variety of disorders.

Chiari II refers to a combination of abnormalities including a small posterior fossa with low-lying fourth ventricle beaking of the tectal plate, aqueductal stenosis resulting in hydrocephalus, and low-lying cerebellum and vermis (Fig. 29.15). There is almost always an associated meningomyelocele, though some babies may have a tethered or even normal spinal cord.

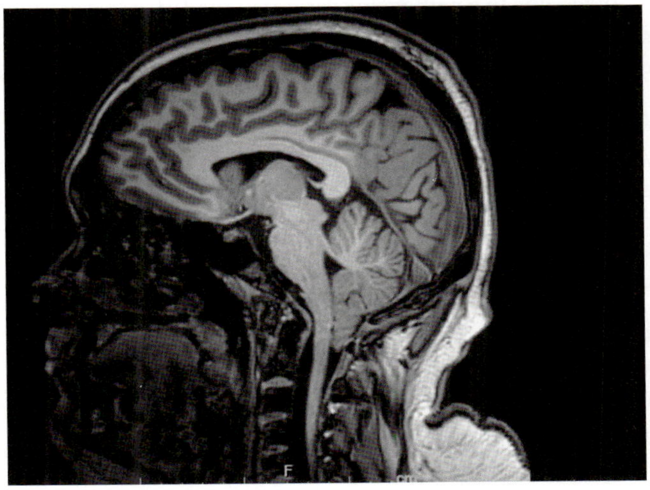

Fig. 29.14 Chiari I malformation.

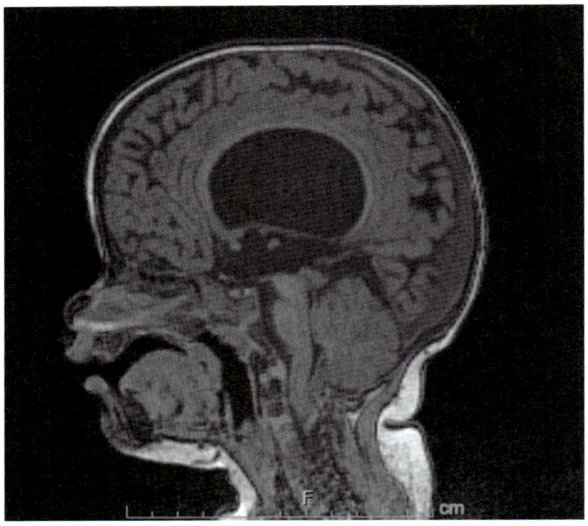

Fig. 29.15 Chiari II malformation.

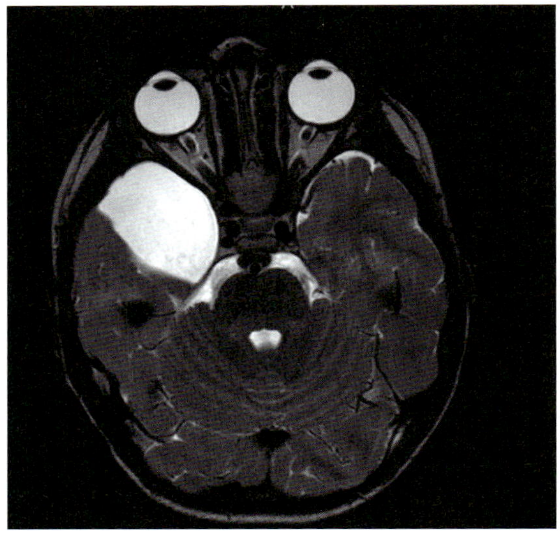

Fig. 29.16 Arachnoid cyst in right middle cranial fossa.

Chiari III refers to an occipital encephalocele with associated herniation of the cerebellum and brainstem through an unfused upper cervical spinal canal, and it results in severe neurologic deficits.

Chiari IV refers to cerebellar hypoplasia.

Cerebrospinal Fluid Pathways

Hydrocephalus

Hydrocephalus has an estimated prevalence of 1.1 per 1000 infants (Tully & Dobyns, 2014) and can be congenital or acquired. Congenital hydrocephalus (Fig. 29.1) is a frequent feature of spina bifida. Dandy-Walker malformation can occur as well as several other brain malformations, including holoprosencephaly, Aicardi syndrome, ACC, lissencephaly, and periventricular heterotropia. The large ventricular size can be detected on prenatal ultrasound or MRI. These babies are often born with large heads, and examination may reveal bulging anterior fontanelle and separated cranial sutures. Surgical interventions such as placement of a ventriculoperitoneal shunt are often necessary.

Congenital hydrocephalus can be due to prenatal infections or a variety of other causes such as an unrecognized intrauterine microhemorrhage. Aqueductal stenosis can be X-linked due to a pathogenic variant in the *L1CAM* gene, but most of the underlying genes resulting in congenital hydrocephalus are still unknown.

Arachnoid Cyst

Arachnoid cyst is a developmental condition characterized by entrapped CSF (Fig. 29.16). It is a common finding on incidental brain imaging and is usually asymptomatic, though seizures or signs of raised intracranial pressure can occur in some children.

Brain Size

Megalencephaly

Megalencephaly refers to brain size and volume greater than 2 SD for age and is usually reflected by a large head size (macrocephaly). In anatomic megalencephaly, the increase in the

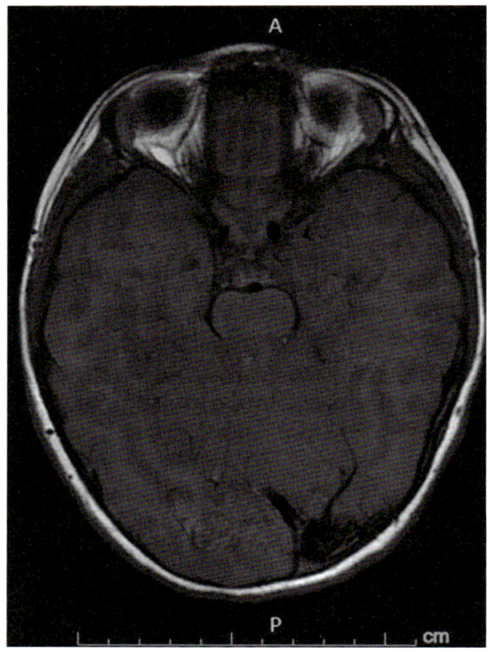

Fig. 29.17 Right hemimegalencephaly.

size or number of brain cells is due to abnormal neuronal development. This can be associated with a range of developmental disabilities.

Hemimegalencephaly refers to increased size of one side of the brain (Fig. 29.17). It generally results in intractable seizures and severe neurologic disabilities.

Megalencephaly can be the result of pathogenic changes in the mTOR pathways such as the PTEN hamartoma tumor syndrome, tuberous sclerosis, and neurofibromatosis type 1. Other recognizable syndromes include MCM, MPPH, epidermal nevus syndrome, and congenital lipomatous asymmetric overgrowth of the trunk with vascular malformations, epidermal nevi, scoliosis/skeletal/spinal anomalies (CLOVES) syndrome. These conditions are frequently associated with body overgrowth and cutaneous hallmarks (Severino et al., 2020).

Microcephaly

Congenital or primary microcephaly is present at birth and is a common feature in several neurodevelopmental disorders. Microcephaly is defined as an occipitofrontal circumference (OFC) below 2 SD for sex, age, and ethnicity. Severe microcephaly is defined as an OFC below 3 SD. Comprehensive clinical evaluation should include serial head circumference measurements. Microcephaly implies reduced cerebral volume, and most children with severe microcephaly present with neurologic symptoms in infancy, including seizures and developmental delays.

Primary microcephaly is considered syndromic when associated with extracranial malformations. Abnormal brain anatomy such as simplified cortical gyral pattern, lissencephaly, gray matter heterotopia, PMG, or abnormalities of deep grey matter or posterior fossa structures occur in more than three-quarter of cases (von der Hagen et al., 2014).

The pathogenesis of primary microcephaly is heterogeneous, ranging from genetic disorders to adverse prenatal factors. Nongenetic causes include infections such cytomegalovirus or Zika virus, early intrauterine stroke, and exposure to alcohol, radiation, or certain drugs. Several hundred genetic syndromes have been associated with microcephaly. It is important to differentiate congenital microcephaly from acquired microcephaly due to postnatal injury to the developing brain from a variety of causes, including severe birth asphyxia or abusive head trauma. In a study of 680 patients with microcephaly, the etiology was ascertained in 59% of all patients, leaving 41% without a definite diagnosis. Genetic causes were identified in about half the patients with a known cause, perinatal brain damage accounted for 45%, and postnatal brain injury for 3% of cases (von der Hagen et al., 2014).

Neural Tube Defects

Abnormal closure of the neural tube can result in a range of disorders, including anencephaly, encephalocele, and spina bifida.

Anencephaly

Anencephaly refers to absence of forebrain development because the anterior end of the neuropore fails to close. It is incompatible with life, and early prenatal detection invariably leads to termination of pregnancy.

Encephalocele

Encephalocele is the presence of a midline cystic mass of meningeal tissue protruding through unfused skull bones. The cavity may also contain brain tissue. It can be anterior or posterior, and the former can be mistaken for a nasal polyp.

Spina Bifida and Myelomeningocele

Please refer to Chapter 59 for detailed discussion.

VASCULAR DISEASE

Perinatal/Neonatal Stroke

Perinatal Arterial Ischemic Stroke

Perinatal arterial ischemic stroke (PAIS) is defined as an embolic or thrombotic event that occurs between 20 weeks of gestation and 28 days of life. The incidence is 10.2 to 29 per 100,000 live births (Armstrong-Wells, Johnston, Wu, Sidney, & Fullerton, 2009; deVeber et al., 2017), and it accounts for approximately 80% of perinatal strokes. The most common presentation is focal seizures in the first week of life, but PAIS can also present with encephalopathy or focal neurologic deficits. A subset of children with presumed perinatal arterial ischemic infarct (PPAIS) are asymptomatic in the neonatal period but present with asymmetry of motor development at about 6 months of age. Diagnosis of PPAIS is confirmed with brain MRI demonstrating cystic encephalomalacia in an arterial distribution (Fig. 29.18). Porencephalic cyst, which is a cystic structure with abutting white matter, can be the result of PAIS or PPAIS in addition to other infectious, traumatic, or genetic etiologies. For both PAIS and PPAIS, the most common arterial distribution is the left middle cerebral artery. There are numerous risk factors for ischemic strokes in neonates. Maternal factors include infection or fever during pregnancy or the perinatal period, chronic medical conditions such as autoimmune disease or coagulation disorders, preeclampsia, and placental insufficiency or abruption. Fetal or neonatal factors include congenital heart disease, intracranial or systemic infection, coagulation disorder, or fetal intolerance of labor. Although fetal distress is a common risk factor, most of these neonates need only minimal if any resuscitation. Acute treatment is focused on treatment of provoking factors, neuroprotective measures, and control of seizures. Neonates rarely require antiplatelet or anticoagulation therapy.

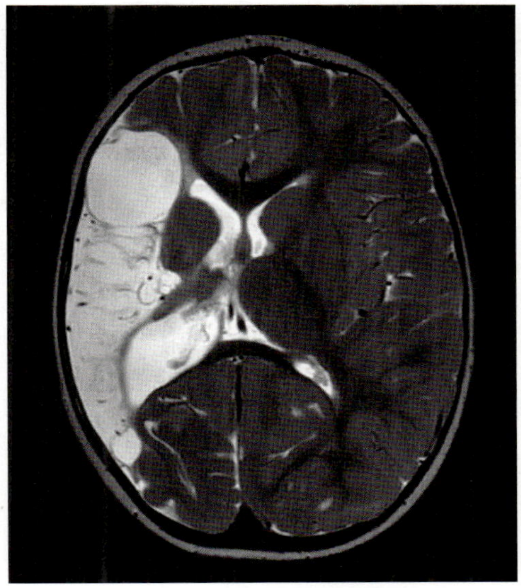

Fig. 29.18 Presumed perinatal arterial ischemic stroke, right MCA.

Neonatal Hemorrhagic Stroke

Neonatal hemorrhagic stroke (NHS) occurs in 6.2 to 15.9 per 100,000 live births (Armstrong-Wells et al., 2009; Cole et al., 2017). It is defined as a hemorrhage within the brain parenchyma (Fig. 29.19), although subarachnoid or intraventricular hemorrhage can be a complication of NHS. Seizures are common at presentation, and neonates are more likely to be encephalopathic with NHS than with PAIS. Risk factors for

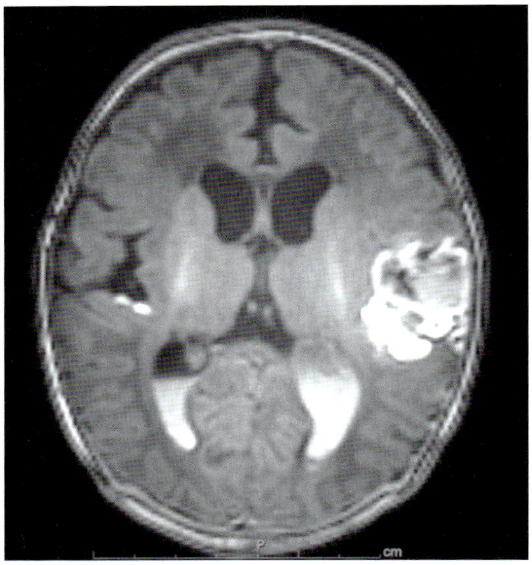

Fig. 29.19 Neonatal hemorrhagic stroke, left.

NHS include primiparity, young maternal age, postmaturity, and fetal distress during delivery. In a minority of patients, NHS is symptomatic of thrombocytopenia, coagulopathy, vitamin K deficiency, or vascular malformation, but the majority of cases are idiopathic. It is uncommon for neonates to need neurosurgical intervention in the acute period as the open fontanelle assists with regulation of intracranial pressure, but they are at risk for developing hydrocephalus in the long term.

Cerebral Sinovenous Thrombosis

Cerebral sinovenous thrombosis (CSVT) is seen in 0.67 per 100,000 children, of which 43% are neonates (deVeber et al, 2001). Presenting symptoms are the same as for PAIS and NHS and are typically due to complications of CSVT, including ischemic or hemorrhagic stroke. Risk factors include systemic or intracranial infection, dehydration, hypercoagulability, congenital heart disease, and delivery complications. Consensus for the use of anticoagulation for neonatal CVST is lacking, so treatment is variable.

Periventricular Venous Infarct

Periventricular venous infarct (PVI) is associated with germinal matrix hemorrhage, but there is a lack of data regarding epidemiology. The germinal matrix is a highly vascular structure adjacent to the lateral ventricles, and injury results in intraventricular hemorrhage leading to infarction of surrounding periventricular white matter. Risk factors include intrapartum complications such as maternal fever or infection, vaginal bleeding, or abdominal trauma. Comparable to PPAIS, delay in motor development is apparent by about 6 months of age. Diagnosis is confirmed with a brain MRI, which classically reveals periventricular white matter loss in an irregular or scalloped fashion.

Hypoxic Ischemic Encephalopathy

Hypoxic ischemic encephalopathy is a common cause of acquired brain injury in the neonatal period. Additional details can be found in Chapter 32.

Childhood/Adolescence Stroke

Childhood Arterial Ischemic Stroke

Childhood arterial ischemic stroke (CAIS) is defined as an ischemic stroke, whether embolic, thrombotic, or due to watershed injury, that occurs in a child aged 28 days to 18 years (Fig. 29.20). The incidence of CAIS is 1.72 per 100,000 (deVeber et al., 2017). Risk factors include congenital heart disease, sickle cell anemia, intracranial or systemic infection, thrombophilia, and autoimmune disorders. Vasculopathies likely account for half of CAIS (deVeber et al., 2017; Wintermark et al., 2014). In contrast to neonates, children are more likely to present with focal neurologic deficits such as hemiparesis, hemisensory loss, aphasia, visual field cuts, cranial nerve dysfunction, or hemiataxia. Seizures are less common than in neonates but more common than in adults. Although the use of intravascular tissue-type plasminogen activator is controversial, endovascular thrombectomy is performed with increasing frequency (Ferriero et al., 2019).

Focal cerebral arteriopathy. Focal cerebral arteriopathy (FCA) is defined as a focal narrowing or irregularity of the distal internal carotid or proximal middle cerebral artery (Fig. 29.21). FCA subtypes are traumatic or inflammatory, specifically following varicella or an upper respiratory infection. Children present with stuttering focal neurologic deficits. Treatment with steroids can be considered.

Moyamoya disease. Moyamoya disease, which is Japanese for "puff of smoke," is a progressive stenoocclusive arteriopathy that typically occurs in the distal internal carotid arteries and can include proximal anterior and middle cerebral arteries. It represents 8% of arterial ischemic strokes in children (Lee, Rivkin, Kirton, deVeber, & Elbers, 2017). Similar to FCA, presenting symptoms can also have a stuttering pattern. Injury can be transient ischemic attack, hemorrhagic stroke, or ischemic stroke. Risk factors include neurofibromatosis 1, Down syndrome, and sickle cell disease. Antiplatelet medication is the most common therapy in the acute period. Surgical revascularization is the treatment of choice to prevent recurrence.

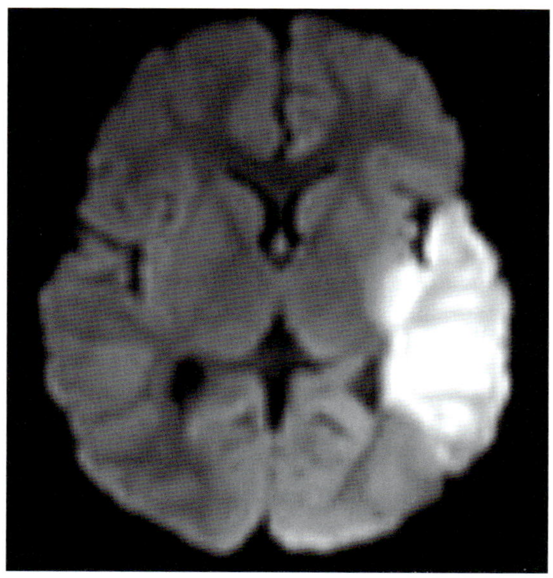

Fig. 29.20 Childhood arterial ischemic stroke, left MCA.

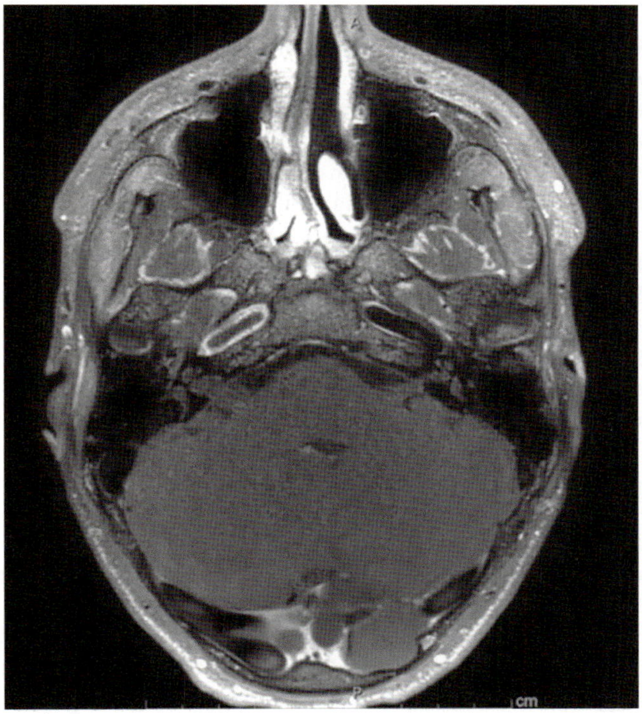

Fig. 29.21 Focal cerebral arteriopathy—inflammation/wall thickening of proximal right middle cerebral artery.

Vasculitis. Vasculitis is inflammation in the arterial wall. Although CNS vasculitides are rare, secondary processes are more common than primary etiologies. CNS vasculitis typically presents with seizures and cognitive decline but can also present with focal neurologic deficits. Patients are at risk for either hemorrhagic or ischemic stroke. Treatment is aimed at the underlying process and commonly includes immunotherapy.

Arterial dissection. Arterial dissection is a tear in the intimal wall of an artery. This leads to clot formation that can embolize. It is most common in an extracranial carotid or vertebral artery. It accounts for approximately 7% of childhood AIS (Rafay, Armstrong, deVeber, Domi, Chan, & MacGregor, 2006). Risk factors are head and/or neck trauma or connective tissue disorders. Treatment is typically with antiplatelet medications.

Cerebral Sinovenous Thrombosis

CSVT has an incidence of 0.67 per 100,000 children of which 57% are nonneonates (deVeber et al., 2001). The most common presenting symptom is headache with features of increased intracranial pressure, such as positional headache, early-morning emesis, or diplopia. It can also present with strokelike symptoms due to complications of CSVT, such as ischemic or hemorrhagic stroke (Fig. 29.22). Risk factors include dehydration, trauma, iron deficiency anemia, malignancy, thrombophilia, autoimmune conditions such as ulcerative colitis, nephrotic syndrome, estrogen-containing contraceptives, otitis, sinusitis, systemic infection, or intracranial infection. Anticoagulation is the mainstay of treatment (Ferriero et al., 2019).

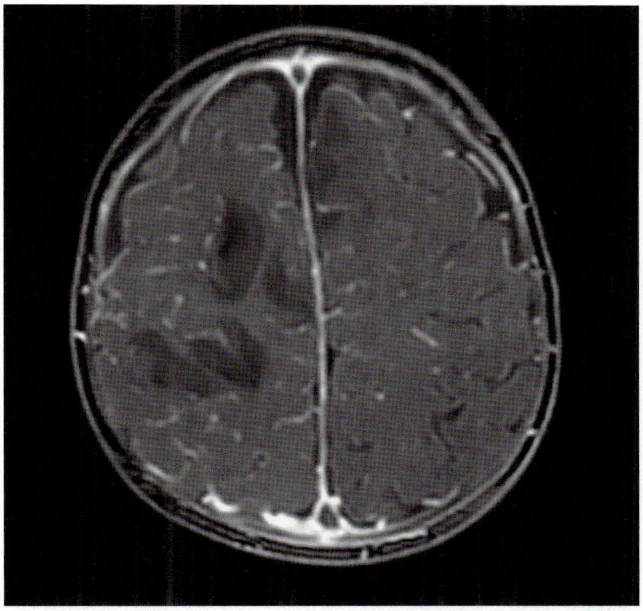

Fig. 29.22 Cerebral sinovenous thrombosis—filling defect in anterior/posterior aspect of superior sagittal sinus.

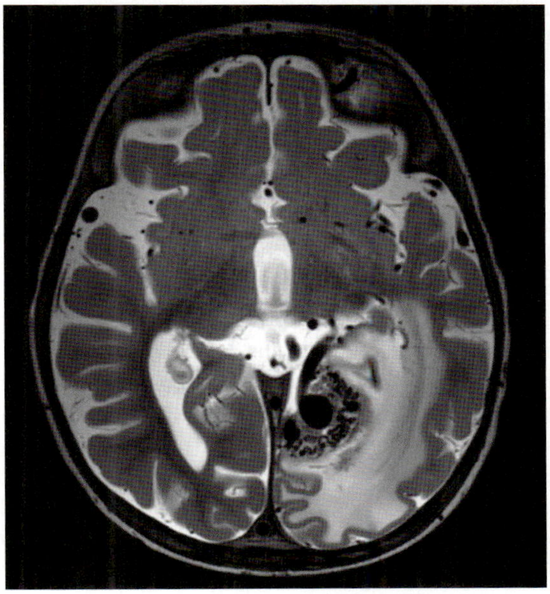

Fig. 29.23 Arteriovenous malformation, left occipital.

Vascular Malformations

Arteriovenous malformation (AVM) and cerebral cavernous malformation (CCM) are the most common types of intracranial vascular malformations. An AVM is a collection of twisted blood vessels with direct arterial-to-venous connection and intervening brain parenchyma (Fig. 29.23). A CCM is a collection of dilated capillaries without intervening brain parenchyma (Fig. 29.24). Both entities can present with headache, focal seizure, or hemorrhagic stroke. A stroke as a complication of AVM tends to be catastrophic. The inheritance pattern for AVM is typically sporadic, whereas CCM is more likely to be familial.

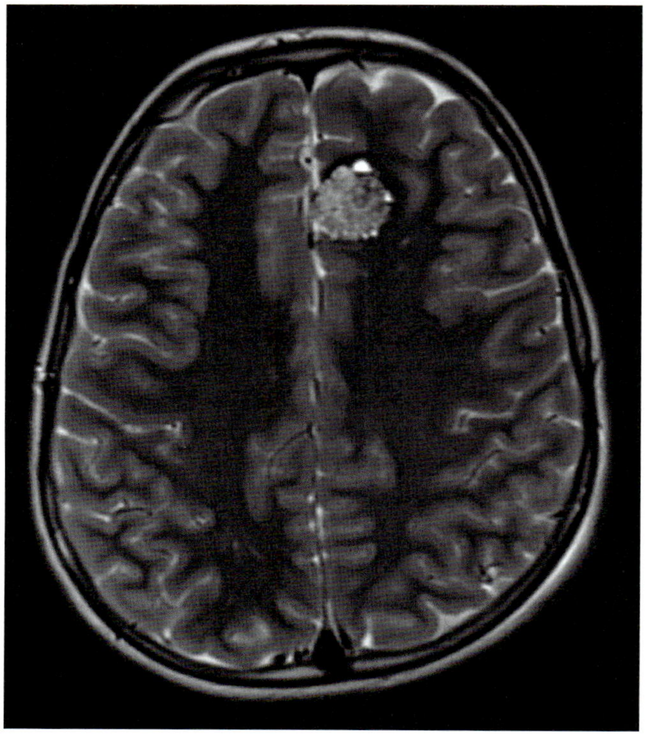

Fig. 29.24 Cavernous malformation, left frontal.

Prognosis

Although the mortality associated with neonatal or childhood stroke is low, the morbidity is high. Children are at risk for sensorimotor deficits, epilepsy, and cognitive or behavioral problems. Children with minimal evidence of parenchymal injury may not have any deficits, whereas children with multifocal parenchymal injury are at highest risk for a severe neurodevelopmental outcome.

The risk of motor impairment with stroke is dependent on location of injury. The risk increases with involvement of the corticospinal tracts, including motor cortex, posterior limb of the internal capsule, or pyramids. PAIS is the most common cause of hemiplegic cerebral palsy. Children with PAIS or CAIS typically have greater impairment in the upper limbs as opposed to venous infarcts with subcortical involvement that predominantly affects lower limbs.

Epilepsy is another common morbidity for children with stroke. Acute symptomatic seizures are more common in neonatal injury than in older children, and the same is true for epilepsy. It is most common in children with PPAIS with an incidence of 36% and is less common in PAIS and CAIS with an incidence of 15% and 7%, respectively (Billinghurst et al., 2017). Cortical injury implicates the highest risk for epilepsy while isolated subcortical injury, as in PVI, has a minimal increased risk. Although first-line treatment is antiseizure medications, children with medically refractory epilepsy should be considered for epilepsy surgery.

Children with prior stroke are at risk for cognitive sequelae. Following perinatal or childhood stroke, most children will have a normal IQ. They are at increased risk for learning disabilities, attentional difficulties, and executive functioning impairment. Neuropsychological testing can identify these challenges and provide tools to the family and school to optimize the child's success.

HEADACHE

Headache is the most common neurological complaint evaluated by a pediatrician or child neurologist. It is important to distinguish between primary and secondary headache, and history is key. Headache characteristics are comprised of location, frequency, quality, severity, and duration of pain. Associated symptoms such as nausea, vomiting, photophobia, phonophobia, pericranial or muscle tenderness, rhinorrhea, and lacrimation are also valuable. Presence of red flags (Box 29.1) should prompt evaluation for secondary headache with neuroimaging. Transient visual obscurations are suggestive of brief periods of increased intracranial pressure. Diagnostic criteria for primary headache syndromes are detailed in the *International Classification of Headache Disorders*, Third Edition (Headache Classification Committee of the International Headache Society, 2013) (Table 29.3).

Migraine

Migraine is seen in 20% of children (Oskoui et al., 2019) with a male predominance until 10 years of age when the prevalence shifts to a twofold increased female risk through adulthood (Victor, Hu, Campbell, Buse, & Lipton, 2010). A family history is present in almost all children. The most common type is migraine without aura, but as many as 20% of children will have migraine with aura. Visual auras may manifest as blind spots or zigzag lines that float across vision. The most common sensory aura is paresthesia of a limb, which will have a marching or spreading quality. It should be differentiated from stroke, which is marked by acute onset numbness in a full vascular territory. Less common presentations of

BOX 29.1 Headache Red Flags

Age <8 yr	Fever	Nocturnal wakening and/or vomiting
Abrupt in onset	Papilledema	Early-morning wakening and/or vomiting
Progressive since onset	Neurocutaneous stigmata	Onset with Valsalva
Whooshing in ear(s)	Focal weakness, numbness, or other deficit	Postural headache
Transient visual obscurations		

TABLE 29.3 **Classification of Migraine, Tension-Type Headache, Trigeminal Autonomic Cephalgias (TACs)**

	Migraine	Tension Type	TACs[a]
Frequency	At least 5 episodes	At least 10 episodes	Variable from >5 or >20 attacks or constant
Duration	Last 4–72 hr	Last 30 min–7 days	2–180 min or continuous
Features	At least 2 of: Unilateral Pulsating Moderate to severe intensity Aggravation with activity At least 1 of: Nausea and/or vomiting Photophobia and phonophobia	At least 2 of: Bilateral Pressing or tightening Mild to moderate intensity Not aggravated by activity Both of: No nausea or vomiting No more than 1 of photophobia or phonophobia	Unilateral—tends to be orbital, supraorbital, or temporal Either or both of: At least 1 of: conjunctival injection, lacrimation, nasal congestion, rhinorrhea, eyelid edema, forehead or facial sweating, miosis, ptosis Restlessness or agitation

[a]Including cluster, paroxysmal hemicrania, and hemicrania continua.

migraine include migraine with brainstem aura (previously known at basilar migraine), hemiplegic migraine, and retinal migraine. Other migraine phenotypes are benign paroxysmal torticollis, benign paroxysmal vertigo of childhood, and cyclic vomiting syndrome.

Treatments for migraine are categorized as abortive or preventative. Nonsteroidal antiinflammatory drugs such as ibuprofen or naproxen are first-line treatments. Acetaminophen can also be considered. Zofran is a common outpatient treatment for nausea. Triptans are now FDA-approved in the pediatric population, beginning at 6 years of age. Triptans are contraindicated in patients with cardiac, cerebrovascular, or peripheral vascular disease; uncontrolled hypertension; hemiplegic migraine; or migraine with brainstem aura. If oral medications are not helpful, patients should present to the emergency department for a migraine cocktail, which is traditionally composed of intravenous fluids, ketorolac, diphenhydramine, and a dopamine receptor antagonist, of which prochlorperazine has the highest efficacy (Sheridan et al., 2018). Other considerations include valproic acid infusion, dihydroergotamine infusion, and occipital nerve block.

Preventative treatment is important for any child with migraine. Headache hygiene is the first step. This focuses on adequate sleep, exercise, nutrition, and hydration; stress reduction; and limited electronic use. A daily medication is indicated for patients with more than one headache per week. For prepubertal children, the initial choice of medication is cyproheptadine. Common side effects are weight gain and sedation. For older children, first-line medications are topiramate or amitriptyline. Common side effects for topiramate are paresthesias, appetite suppression, and cognitive dulling. Common side effects for amitriptyline are sedation, constipation, and dry mouth. Other considerations for preventative therapy are propranolol, onabotulinum toxin A injections, or calcitonin gene-related peptide inhibitors.

Tension-Type Headache

Tension-type headache is the most common headache type seen in children and frequently co-occurs with anxiety and depression. The exact frequency is likely underrepresented as children do not typically present for care. Posture while sitting, and sleeping should be examined to reduce undue stress on musculature of the neck and back. Treatments include relaxation, biofeedback, and physical therapy. Alternative treatments, such as heat therapy, massage, and acupuncture, can also be considered. Only a small proportion of children will require preventative pharmacotherapy.

Trigeminal Autonomic Cephalgias

Trigeminal autonomic cephalgias (TACs) are exceedingly rare in the pediatric population. TACs include cluster headache, paroxysmal hemicrania, short-lasting unilateral neuralgiform headaches, and hemicrania continua. Diagnosis is crucial as there are treatment implications. Supplemental oxygen is used for cluster headache, and indomethacin is prescribed for paroxysmal hemicrania and hemicrania continua.

REFERENCES

Armstrong-Wells, J., Johnston, S. C., Wu, Y. W., Sidney, S., & Fullerton, H. J. (2009). Prevalence and predictors of perinatal hemorrhagic stroke: Results from the Kaiser Pediatric Stroke Study. *Pediatrics*, *123*(3), 823–828. https://doi.org/10.1542/peds.2008-0874

Billinghurst, L. L., Beslow, L. A., Abend, N. S., Uohara, M., Jastrzab, L., Licht, D. J., & Ichord, R. N. (2017). Incidence and predictors of epilepsy after pediatric arterial ischemic stroke. *Neurology*, *88*(7), 630–637. https://doi.org/10.1212/WNL.0000000000003603

Cole, L., Dewey, D., Letourneau, N., Kaplan, B. J., Chaput, K., Gallagher, C., … Kirton, A. (2017). Clinical characteristics, risk factors, and outcomes associated with neonatal hemorrhagic stroke: A population-based case-control study. *JAMA Pediatrics*, *171*(3), 230. https://doi.org/10.1001/jamapediatrics.2016.4151

deVeber, G. A., Kirton, A., Booth, F. A., Yager, J. Y., Wirrell, E. C., Wood, E., … Bjornson, B. H. (2017). Epidemiology and outcomes of arterial ischemic stroke in children: The Canadian Pediatric Ischemic Stroke Registry. *Pediatric Neurology*, *69*, 58–70. https://doi.org/10.1016/j.pediatrneurol.2017.01.016

deVeber, G., Andrew, M., Adams, C., Bjornson, B., Booth, F., Buckley, D. J., … Gillett, J. (2001). Cerebral sinovenous thrombosis in children. *New England Journal of Medicine*, *345*(6), 417–423. https://doi.org/10.1056/NEJM200108093450604

Di Donato, N., Chiari, S., Mirzaa, G. M., Aldinger, K., Parrini, E., Olds, C., … Dobyns, W. B. (2017). Lissencephaly: Expanded imaging and clinical classification. *American Journal of Medical Genetics. Part A*, *173*(6), 1473–1488. https://doi.org/10.1002/ajmg.a.38245

Dubourg, C., Kim, A., Watrin, E., Tayrac, M., de, Odent, S., David, V., & Dupé, V. (2018). Recent advances in understanding inheritance of holoprosencephaly. *American Journal of Medical Genetics Part C: Seminars in Medical Genetics*, *178*(2), 258–269. https://doi.org/10.1002/ajmg.c.31619

Edwards, T. J., Sherr, E. H., Barkovich, A. J., & Richards, L. J. (2014). Clinical, genetic and imaging findings identify new causes for corpus callosum development syndromes. *Brain*, *137*(6), 1579–1613. https://doi.org/10.1093/brain/awt358

Ferriero, D. M., Fullerton, H. J., Bernard, T. J., Billinghurst, L., Daniels, S. R., DeBaun, M. R., … on behalf of the American Heart Association Stroke Council and Council on Cardiovascular and Stroke Nursing, (2019). Management of stroke in neonates and children: A scientific statement from the American Heart Association/American Stroke Association. *Stroke*, *50*(3). https://doi.org/10.1161/STR.0000000000000183

Ganau, M., Huet, S., Syrmos, N., Meloni, M., & Jayamohan, J. (2019). Neuro-ophthalmological manifestations of septo-optic dysplasia: Current perspectives. *Eye and Brain*, *11*, 37–47. https://doi.org/10.2147/EB.S186307

Haddadi, K., Zare, A., & Asadian, L. (2018). Dandy-Walker syndrome: A review of new diagnosis and management in children. *Journal of Pediatrics Review*, *6*(2), 47–52. http://jpr.mazums.ac.ir/article-1-193-en.html

Headache Classification Committee of the International Headache Society (IHS). (2013). The International Classification of Headache Disorders, 3rd edition (beta version). *Cephalalgia*, *33*(9), 629–808. https://doi.org/10.1177/0333102413485658

Kuppermann, N., Holmes, J. F., Dayan, P. S., Hoyle, J. D., Atabaki, S. M., Holubkov, R., … Wootton-Gorges, S. L. (2009). Identification of children at very low risk of clinically-important brain injuries after head trauma: A prospective cohort study. *The Lancet*, *374*(9696), 1160–1170. https://doi.org/10.1016/S0140-6736(09)61558-0

Lee, S., Rivkin, M. J., Kirton, A., deVeber, G., & Elbers, J. (2017). Moyamoya disease in children: Results from the International Pediatric Stroke Study. *Journal of Child Neurology*, *32*(11), 924–929. https://doi.org/10.1177/0883073817718730

McClugage, S. G., & Oakes, W. J. (2019). The Chiari I malformation. *Journal of Neurosurgery. Pediatrics*, *24*(3), 217–226. https://doi.org/10.3171/2019.5.PEDS18382

Morris, J. K., Wellesley, D. G., Barisic, I., Addor, M. -C., Bergman, J. E. H., Braz, P., … Garne, E. (2019). Epidemiology of congenital cerebral anomalies in Europe: a multicentre, population-based EUROCAT study. *Archives of Disease in Childhood*, *104*(12), 1181–1187. https://doi.org/10.1136/archdischild-2018-316733

Ntimbani, J., Kelly, A., & Lekgwara, P. (2020). Myelomeningocele—a literature review. *Interdisciplinary Neurosurgery*, *19*, 100502. https://doi.org/10.1016/j.inat.2019.100502

Oskoui, M., Pringsheim, T., Billinghurst, L., Potrebic, S., Gersz, E. M., Gloss, D., … Hershey, A. D. (2019). Practice guideline update summary: Pharmacologic treatment for pediatric migraine prevention: Report of the Guideline Development, Dissemination, and Implementation Subcommittee of the American Academy of Neurology and the American Headache Society. *Neurology*, *93*(11), 500–509. https://doi.org/10.1212/WNL.0000000000008105

Rafay, M. F., Armstrong, D., deVeber, G., Domi, T., Chan, A., & MacGregor, D. L. (2006). Craniocervical arterial dissection in children: Clinical and radiographic presentation and outcome. *Journal of Child Neurology*, *21*(1), 8–16. https://doi.org/10.1177/08830738060210010101

Severino, M., Geraldo, A. F., Utz, N., Tortora, D., Pogledic, I., Klonowski, W., … on behalf of the European Network on Brain Malformations (Neuro-MIG), (2020). Definitions and classification of malformations of cortical development: Practical guidelines. *Brain*, *143*(10), 2874–2894. https://doi.org/10.1093/brain/awaa174

Sheridan, D. C., Laurie, A., Pacheco, S., Fu, R., Hansen, M. L., Ma, O. J., & Meckler, G. D. (2018). Relative effectiveness of dopamine antagonists for pediatric migraine in the emergency department. *Pediatric Emergency Care*, *34*(3), 165–168. https://doi.org/10.1097/PEC.0000000000000718

Stutterd, C. A., Dobyns, W. B., Jansen, A., Mirzaa, G., & Leventer, R. J. (2018). Polymicrogyria Overview. In M. P. Adam, H. H. Ardinger, R. A. Pagon, S. E. Wallace, L. J. Bean, K. Stephens, & A. Amemiya (Eds.), GeneReviews. University of Washington–Seattle. http://www.ncbi.nlm.nih.gov/books/NBK1329/

Tekendo-Ngongang, C., Muenke, M., & Kruszka, P. (2020). Holoprosencephaly overview. In M. P. Adam, H. H. Ardinger, R. A. Pagon, S. E. Wallace, L. J. Bean, K. Stephens, & A. Amemiya (Eds.), GeneReviews. University of Washington–Seattle. http://www.ncbi.nlm.nih.gov/books/NBK1530/

Tully, H. M., & Dobyns, W. B. (2014). Infantile hydrocephalus: A review of epidemiology, classification and causes. *European Journal of Medical Genetics*, *57*(8), 359–368. https://doi.org/10.1016/j.ejmg.2014.06.002

van Dijk, T., Baas, F., Barth, P. G., & Poll-The, B. T. (2018). What's new in pontocerebellar hypoplasia? An update on genes and subtypes. *Orphanet Journal of Rare Diseases*, *13*(1), 92. https://doi.org/10.1186/s13023-018-0826-2

VHP, L., Aragão, M., Pinho, R., Hazin, A., Paciorkowski, A., Penalva de Oliveira, A., & Masruha, M. R. (2020). Congenital Zika virus infection: A review with emphasis on the spectrum of brain abnormalities. *Current Neurology and Neuroscience Reports*, *20*(11), 49. https://doi.org/10.1007/s11910-020-01072-0

Victor, T., Hu, X., Campbell, J., Buse, D., & Lipton, R. (2010). Migraine prevalence by age and sex in the United States: A life-span study. *Cephalalgia*, *30*(9), 1065–1072. https://doi.org/10.1177/0333102409355601

von der Hagen, M., Pivarcsi, M., Liebe, J., von Bernuth, H., Didonato, N., Hennermann, J. B., … Kaindl, A. M. (2014). Diagnostic approach to microcephaly in childhood: A two-center study and review of the literature. *Developmental Medicine and Child Neurology*, *56*(8), 732–741. https://doi.org/10.1111/dmcn.12425

Wintermark, M., Hills, N. K., deVeber, G. A., Barkovich, A. J., Elkind, M. S. V., Sear, K., … Forsyth, R. (2014). Arteriopathy diagnosis in childhood arterial ischemic stroke: Results of the vascular effects of infection in pediatric stroke study. *Stroke*, *45*(12), 3597–3605. https://doi.org/10.1161/STROKEAHA.114.007404

30

Neuromuscular Disorders

Michele Yang

For additional material related to the content of this chapter, please see Chapters 25, 36, 39, 40, and 59.

VIGNETTE

A 3-year-old boy presents to you for evaluation of global developmental delay. His parents report that his gross motor milestones were delayed, with rolling at 8 months of age and walking at 24 months of age. They felt that from birth he was "floppy" and had poor latch and suck. He has limited language with 20 words. His examination is marked by a long facies, open mouth with a tented upper lip, and a dull appearance of his face. When he walks, he seems to drag his feet. He arises from supine with a Gower maneuver. His family history is notable for a mother with a history of learning delays. She appears to have limited facial expression with a long face. When you shake her hand she seems to have a hard time letting go of your hand.

OVERVIEW OF NEUROMUSCULAR DISORDERS

What Are the Neuromuscular Disorders?

This overview will discuss the group of genetically based neuromuscular disorders, the initial diagnostic workup, and management. This is a genotypically and phenotypically heterogeneous group of disorders of the peripheral nervous system involving the anterior horn cell, nerve, neuromuscular junction, and muscle. Infant and children present with hypotonia, gross and/or fine motor delays, and weakness. While classically the neuromuscular disorders are thought to involve only the peripheral nervous system, central nervous system involvement is increasingly being recognized. Cognitive delays, autism, behavioral problems, and seizures can be seen as the initial presentation. Therefore in any patient presenting with delays this group of disorders should be considered.

Diagnostic Workup of Neuromuscular Disorders

The workup of any patient with developmental delay should begin with a history and an outline of the evolution of the delays, its character, and similar features in family members. It is helpful to establish the course as progressive, static, or saltatory. A progressive disorder may suggest a dystrophy, whereas myopathies are typically static. Saltatory disorders, characterized by exacerbation and partial recovery, can be seen with disorders such as congenital myasthenic syndromes. The quality of fetal movements, breech presentation, and polyhydramnios may suggest *in utero* weakness. Early respiratory or bulbar weakness from birth may also suggest a neuromuscular disorder. A careful neurologic examination is required to verify the localization to the peripheral nervous system but may be daunting in a young infant or uncooperative child. As a rule, the direct approach of examination from head to toe is doomed to failure, particularly with an autistic or shy child. A more successful approach is observation, which often yields more information than attempting a strength examination. Invasive aspects of the examination, such as obtaining reflexes, should be performed last. It is, however, important to establish the pattern of weakness and to check reflexes when considering a neuromuscular disorder (Table 30.1). Therefore the examiner should observe the child throwing a ball, arising from supine (Gower maneuver), climbing stairs, walking/running, jumping, picking up snacks with fingers, and kicking a ball. An infant's spontaneous movements should be observed on the examination table (e.g., presence of a frog-legged position), spontaneous movements against gravity, and grip strength. Formal muscle strength testing of the older child can be graded on the Medical Research Council (MRC) scale of 0 to 5, with a grade of 0 indicating no movement and a grade of 5 indicating full power.

A distinction between hypotonia and weakness needs to be made here, a distinction that can be difficult to make but crucial to the workup. While weak patients are always hypotonic, hypotonic patients may not always be weak. For instance, patients with Down syndrome have hypotonia but do not have muscle involvement or weakness. However, infants with spinal muscular atrophy (SMA) will have both weakness and hypotonia. This distinction is critical when determining the next steps in the workup. Next, the pattern of weakness should be established. Distal weakness, suggested by foot drop or difficulty manipulating objects with the fingers, can suggest a neuropathy. Proximal weakness, with difficulty arising from the floor or climbing stairs, pelvic instability with walking/running, or neck flexion weakness can suggest a myopathy. Other localizing signs include the presence of tremor, which can suggest a neuropathy, and the presence of fasciculations, which can suggest a motor neuron disorder. Pattern recognition of these constellations of signs therefore is the first critical step in the diagnostic workup (Barohn et al., 2014).

TABLE 30.1 Summary of Examination Findings by Localization

Examination Findings	Central	Anterior Horn Cell	Peripheral Nerve	Neuromuscular Junction	Muscle
Strength	Normal or slightly decreased	Decreased	Decreased, distal > proximal	Variable, typically most prominently of face, eye movements, bulbar	Decreased, proximal > distal
Muscle mass	Normal or disuse atrophy	Decreased	Decreased, distal > proximal	Normal or decreased	Can be decreased Can be pseudohypertrophy in dystrophies
Tone	Decreased to evolving increased tone	Decreased	Decreased	Decreased	Decreased
Deep tendon reflexes	Normal to increased	Decreased	Decreased, in distal to proximal fashion, typically out of proportion to weakness	Decreased	Decreased, though preserved until significant weakness
Fasciculations	None	Present	None	None	None
Sensation	Normal	Normal	Decreased, in distal to proximal fashion	Normal	Normal

For any patient with delays, and particularly if one suspects a primary neuromuscular disorder, a serum creatine kinase (CK) should be the first test performed. This is a simple, inexpensive laboratory study that can quickly screen for a primary neuromuscular disorder and shorten the diagnostic odyssey. If the CK is elevated, then an algorithm may be a useful framework in which to start the workup and make appropriate referrals (Fig. 30.1). It is not a comprehensive algorithm but meant as a guide through the initial workup. If the CK is elevated, muscle dystrophies, congenital muscular dystrophies, and limb girdle muscular dystrophies should be considered. However, it should be noted that CKs can be mildly elevated in neuropathies, motor neuron disorders, and myopathies, and the normal range may be related to gender and race (Barohn et al., 2014). The CKs will typically be in the range of the 1000 s for limb girdle muscular dystrophies and as high as 10 times normal in patients with dystrophinopathies. If intellectual disability or autistic-like features are present, then a magnetic resonance image (MRI) of the brain should be performed. An abnormal MRI of the brain may suggest a congenital muscular dystrophy such as due to *LAMA2* or *FKRP* mutations, as these genes are expressed in the central nervous system. If the CK is normal, then other neuromuscular disorders are a possibility if weakness is present. These can include neuropathies, motor neuron disorders, and congenital myopathies and myasthenic syndromes. Of note, the levels of alanine aminotransferase (ALT) and aspartate aminotransferase (AST), traditionally thought of as liver function tests, may also be elevated as these enzymes are also found within myofibers. Therefore in any patient with elevated AST and ALT levels without gastrointestinal signs or symptoms a serum CK should be obtained. Further workup to distinguish between these possibilities can include the following studies:

1. Electrodiagnostic (EDX) testing: Nerve conduction studies (NCSs) and electromyography (EMG) are electrophysiologic tests that assess the function of the the nerve and muscle, respectively. With NCSs, the patient has electrodes placed over the limbs, and a small electrical current is passed transcutaneously to the nerve. The nerve conducts this signal to the recording electrodes, and the response latency, response amplitude, and conduction velocity are calculated. The response amplitude reflects the number of underlying axons, and the latency and conduction velocity reflect the myelination of the nerve. The EMG can determine the chronicity and severity of a neuropathy, the presence of denervating features, and the presence of a myopathy. These are minimally invasive tests, but they can be frightening to a child initially. However, in the hands of an experienced electromyographer, this can be a helpful diagnostic test. The major aim of the EDX examination is localization, and therefore it is important to remember that the EDX examination is an extension of the clinical examination. While nearly every muscle in the body can be studied by needle examination, this is neither desirable nor feasible in the pediatric patient. Therefore approaching the EDX study with a specific question about localization and diagnosis can help both the electromyographer and the patient. The exact etiology cannot be made with EDX studies alone, but localization and the presence of specific findings, such as electrical myotonia, can help guide the diagnostic workup.
2. Muscle biopsy: Traditionally, in the diagnosis of a primary neuromuscular disorder a muscle and/or nerve biopsy had been performed. Analysis of histology, histochemistry, immunohistochemistry, and ultrastructure by light and electron microscopy had been the mainstay of diagnosis

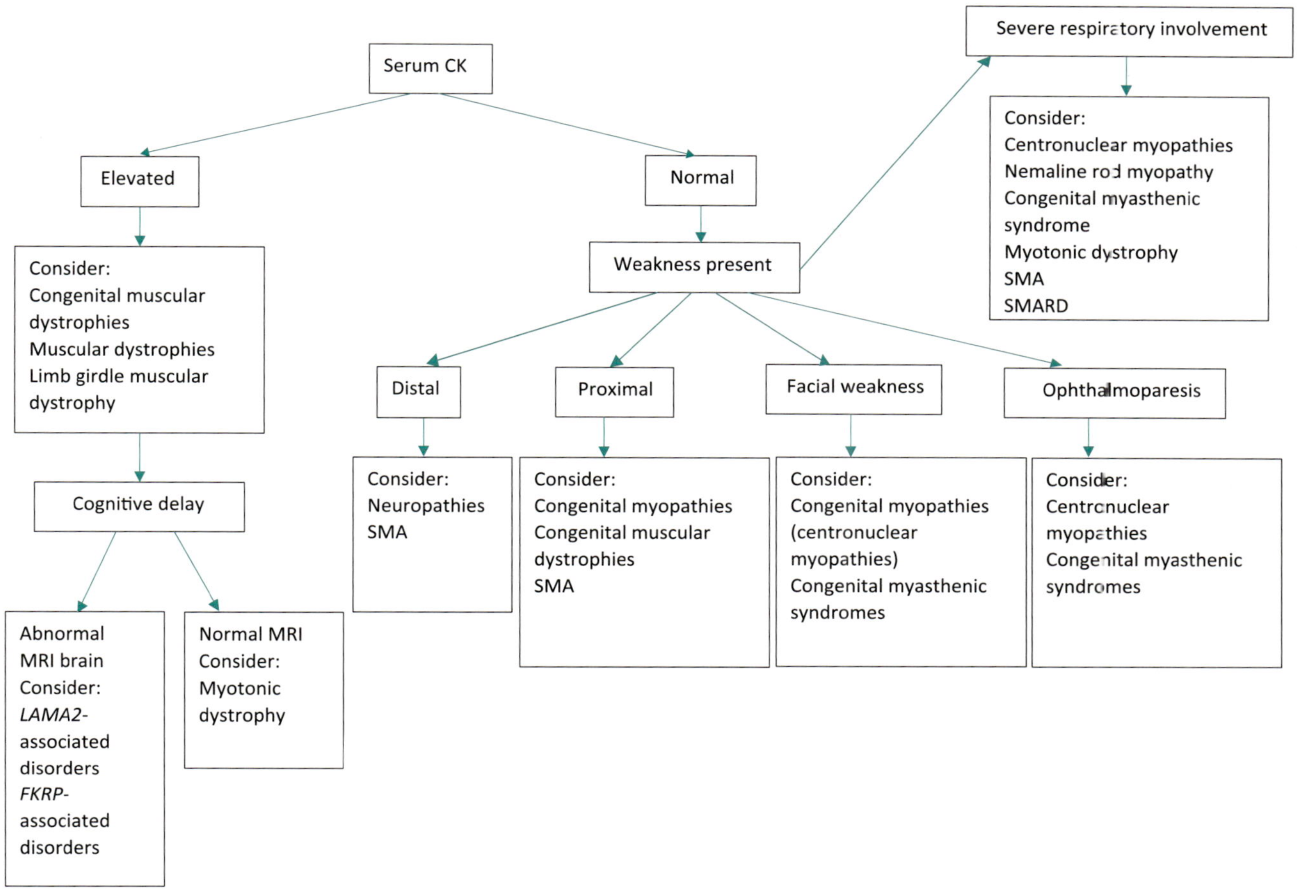

Fig. 30.1 Algorithm for diagnosis of neuromuscular disorders. *CK*, Creatine kinase; *MRI*, magnetic resonance imaging; *SMA*, spinal muscular atrophy; *SMARD*, spinal muscular atrophy with respiratory distress.

particularly for the congenital myopathies and muscular dystrophies. The presence of dystrophic changes, with necrotic muscle fibers, regenerating fibers, and fibrosis, may suggest a muscular dystrophy. Intact muscle fibers with centralized nuclei may suggest a congenital myopathy. Fiber type grouping, with atrophic fibers of the same fiber type, may suggest a neuropathy. Specific antibody stains against specific proteins of the sacrolemmal membrane can identify deficiencies of specific proteins. However, in this era of technological advances in genetic testing, genetic testing is often performed prior to obtaining a biopsy, as genetic testing is often less invasive than a biopsy. In many cases because a specific diagnosis cannot be made by muscle biopsy alone and requires follow-up genetic testing, genetic testing has been performed as a first step to expedite a diagnosis.

3. Imaging: Similarly, muscle imaging with MRI or ultrasound is often performed in favor of a muscle biopsy. The differential involvement of specific muscles by imaging and the appearance of the muscle can be helpful to diagnose specific neuromuscular disorders and suggest a specific gene.
4. Genetic testing: Genetic testing is often performed as the first diagnostic test, after a serum CK, if neuromuscular disorders are suspected. Next-generation sequencing panels, comprised of genes common in the neuromuscular disorders, are commercially available and of relatively low cost compared with single-gene sequencing (Winder et al., 2020). Therefore next-generation sequencing panels are often performed preferentially to single-gene sequencing.
5. Newborn screening: Newborn screening is available for some of the neuromuscular disorders, depending on the state. For instance, SMA testing is available in most states and allows for earlier detection and therefore treatment of a disorder in which, in the past, 90% of infants died in the first 2 years of life (CureSMA, n.d.; Mercuri et al., 2018).

SPECIFIC NEUROMUSCULAR DISORDERS

Neuromuscular disorders can be overwhelming to consider as a group, given the wide range of presentations and increasing number of genes associated with them. For the purposes of this review, we will simplify neuromuscular disorders into a few categories based on localization in the nervous system. We will also discuss the more common specific disorders within each group.

Motor Neuron Disorders

In this group of disorders there is progressive degeneration of the anterior horn cells in the spinal cord, resulting in weakness. The classic disorder is SMA due to biallelic mutations in the *SMN1* gene, resulting in deficiency of the SMN protein. SMA has been traditionally subcategorized further into types based on the highest motor milestone achieved (Montes et al., 2018). Type 1 is the most common type, accounting for 60% of all cases (Mercuri et al., 2018). Without treatment, patients typically develop symptoms before 6 months of age and never develop the ability to sit independently; survival is limited, and most infants die within the first 2 years of life (Finkel et al., 2018). They experience progressive weakness in bulbar, respiratory, and limb muscles. Patients with SMA type 2 typically achieve the ability to sit independently, but they never achieve the ability to stand or walk on their own. Symptoms present between 6 and 18 months of age (Mercuri et al., 2016). Patients with SMA type 3 achieve the ability to walk independently, though they may lose this ability. Symptoms present after 12 months of age, and they live to adulthood. SMA type 4 patients usually present in adulthood and have a normal lifespan. The classifications have shifted, however, in the last decade with improvements in and standardization in the care of patients with SMA (Mercuri et al., 2020; Tizzano & Finkel, 2017). Additionally, earlier recognition of these diagnoses has allowed early intervention with improved care. Advancements in therapies have been particularly exciting for this group of patients. Therapies aimed at increasing the function of the *SMN2* backup gene have included altering *SMN2* mRNA splicing to produce more full-length SMN protein. Antisense oligonucleotides are now commercially available to administer intrathecally, and oral small molecules are in clinical trials. Current intrathecal treatments for viral vector-mediated replacement of *SMN1* genes are also available. Treatments may not address all symptoms but have increased motor function and improved mortality. Nusinersen, a US Food and Drug Administration (FDA)–approved intrathecal treatment, is given in four loading doses over 2 months and then every 4 months for life. Onasemnogene abeparvovce-xioi is approved for patients up to 2 years of age as a gene replacement therapy in a one-time intravenous infusion (Waldrop & Kolb, 2019). Those patients treated earlier appear to have improvement over those treated at later ages (Lowes et al., 2019). The inclusion of SMA on the newborn screen has helped with the early detection of this diagnosis. However, 5% of infants with SMA will not be identified by newborn screening due to an *SMN1* gene point mutation on one allele and a deletion of exon 7 on the other (Mercuri et al., 2018). Therefore a high index of suspicion is required even if the newborn screening does not detect an *SMN1* deletion, so that appropriate follow-up genetic testing may be pursued and that this treatable diagnosis is not overlooked.

Nerve

Inherited neuropathies are one of the most common neuromuscular disorders, occurring with a prevalence of 1 in 2500. This is a genotypically and phenotypically heterogeneous group of disorders, which includes pure motor, pure sensory, sensory-autonomic, and sensorimotor neuropathies. The typical presentation of the inherited sensorimotor neuropathies (also known as Charcot-Marie-Tooth disease [CMT]) is with slowly progressive sensory and motor impairments. Toe walking may be the first presentation, with progression to a high steppage gait. Foot deformities such as pes cavus and hammertoe deformities are common. Muscular atrophy and weakness progress in a distal-to-proximal fashion. Patients report sensory changes, including difficulty with balance, with particular difficulty on uneven surfaces, and with walking in the dark. The subtypes have been classically subdivided into three forms as defined by electrophysiologic findings: demyelinating, axonal, and intermediate types; and by inheritance pattern. EDX studies have an important role in identifying the subtypes. In demyelinating forms the motor NCSs in the upper limbs are below 38 m/sec, and usually <25 m/sec. In axonal forms NCVs are greater than 38 m/sec, and in intermediate forms between 24 and 35 m/sec. About 60% of patients with CMT and a known genetic diagnosis have CMT1A due to a duplication in the *PMP22* gene. A broad range of clinical presentations can be seen, and they can present at any age, from infancy to adulthood. Family history and examination of the parents can be helpful, as the most common forms for CMT are autosomal dominantly inherited. The clinical presentation with slowly progressive distal atrophy, loss of reflexes, and sensory changes in childhood should prompt consideration of an inherited neuropathy. EMG/NCS can help with the localization to the nerve and distinguishing between demyelinating and axonal forms of CMT. Next-generation sequencing panels may help to identify the genetic etiology of some but not all patients (Winder et al., 2020). There are no current treatments for the CMTs other than supportive treatments. However, identification of other associated neurologic and nonneurologic features can be helpful in the management of these patients, including the presence of autonomic involvement, cold-induced hand cramping, and pupillary abnormalities (Werheid et al., 2016). White matter changes can occur in patients with CMTX1 with a presentation of strokelike symptoms, and therefore appropriate counseling of the patients should be made (Niu et al., 2019).

Neuromuscular Junction

Congenital myasthenic syndromes are a group of disorders caused by mutations in genes that regulate or form the neuromuscular junction (Engel et al., 2015). Typically, patients have some degree of baseline weakness, especially of the face and limb muscles, and episodes of increased, fatigable weakness. They typically present in infancy but can present at any stage (Garg et al., 2016). The diagnosis can be made by EDX testing, with an abnormal increment or decrement in compound motor action potential (CMAP) in response to repetitive nerve stimulation. However, this response in the CMAP may not always be seen, given the fluctuating nature of this disorder and the technical challenges of this study in infants and young children. Therefore a high index of suspicion for these disorders is warranted for any patient presenting with fluctuating weakness with prominent involvement of the face, extraocular, and bulbar muscles. The congenital myasthenic syndromes are further subdivided based on the part of the neuromuscular junction involved (i.e., presynaptic, synaptic, or postsynaptic). At this time, there are 32 known genes associated with the congenital myasthenic syndromes (Finsterer, 2019). The role of these genes is complex and is likely prominent in development, as patients with congenital myasthenic syndromes may have other systemic involvement such as cognitive impairment (e.g., due to *COL13A1, MUNC13-1,* and *SNAP25* genes), cerebellar ataxia *(SNAP25)*, microcephaly *(MUNC13-1)*, and neuropathies (*SYT2* and *SLC25A7*) (Finsterer, 2019; Nicole et al., 2017).

Muscle

Disorders of the muscle are typically subdivided by their pathologic features. The muscle biopsies of muscular dystrophies typically show evidence of degeneration and regeneration, with subsequent replacement of the muscle tissue by fibrotic tissue. As a result, clinically, there is progressive weakness, such as seen in boys with Duchenne muscular dystrophy (DMD), and elevated CKs due to the release of the enzyme from the degenerating muscle fibers. In the congenital myopathies histologic and ultrastructural changes in the muscle without significant degeneration are hallmarks of the disorders. CKs are generally normal. Patients can have a static or slowly progressive course, such as seen in patients with *RYR1*-associated congenital myopathy. However, the phenotypic and genotypic spectrum of the muscle disorders is broad: A single gene may cause multiple phenotypes, and a phenotype may be the result of many different gene mutations.

The most common muscular dystrophy in childhood is a dystrophinopathy (i.e., DMD and Becker muscular dystrophy [BMD]). This affects 1 in 3600 to 6000 live male births (Mah et al., 2014; Mendell & Lloyd-Puryear, 2013). Mutations in the *DMD* gene can cause the functional absence of dystrophin at the sarcolemmal membrane, resulting in a DMD phenotype, or a relative deficiency of dystrophy, resulting in the BMD phenotype. The deficiency or absence of dystrophin causes force-contraction injury of the muscle fibers. The chronic and repeated cycles of degeneration and regeneration result in inflammation, which in turn inhibits muscle fiber regeneration. Symptoms first present at 2 to 3 years of age, with delayed gross motor milestones or toe walking. Early signs of weakness include neck flexion weakness and difficulty arising from the floor (Gower maneuver). Patients can present with pseudohypertrophy of the calves, with well-defined, rubbery-textured gastrocnemius muscles. The pseudohypertrophy can also be noted in the brachioradialis muscles. Boys may also have intellectual disability, speech delay, and cognitive impairment; the dystrophin isoform expressed in brain may play a role in this (Banihani et al., 2015; Doorenweerd, 2020). The gradual loss of muscle strength and function occurs over years. Without treatment, patients become wheelchair bound by 13 years of age and require ventilatory assistance by 20 years of age. Corticosteroids are considered standard of care in the treatment of boys with DMD either with prednisone at a dose of 0.75 mg/kg/day or deflazacort at a dose of 0.9 mg/kg/day (Matthews et al., 2016). Treatment with corticosteroids improves muscle function and delays the loss of ambulation by 1.5 years. However, attendant side effects accompany use of steroids and need to be monitored closely. Consensus guidelines for the treatment of boys with DMD were recently updated and include noninvasive ventilation and cough assist, nutritional management, and monitoring for and treatment of cardiomyopathy (Birnkrant et al., 2018a, 2018b). Because boys with DMD are surviving into adulthood, discussion about transition into adulthood and adult care has increasing importance (Birnkrant et al., 2018c). At this time there are two gene-based therapies targeting the loss of dystrophin. Ataluren, granted orphan drug status by the FDA, is a compound that suppresses nonsense mutations, allowing for expression of a truncated dystrophin protein. Eteplirsen, an FDA-approved antisense-oligonucleotide, is designed to induce exon 51 skipping to produce a modified dystrophin protein (FDA, 2016). However, these gene-based therapies only target a specific population, which highlights the need for genetic confirmation so that eligible patients may be identified early and start treatments.

Myotonic dystrophy type 1 (DM1) is a multisystem disorder that can present in the pediatric population, though it is generally thought of as being an adult-onset disorder. DM1 results from a CTG triplet repeat expansion in the *DMPK* gene, which results in accumulation of toxic mRNA in the nucleus of cells (Kamsteeg et al., 2012). This toxic mRNA in turn impacts proteins important in the splicing of multiple proteins, causing multisystem problems. Patients without DM1 have 5 to 34 repeats. In classic DM1 patients have 100 to 1000 repeats and present with distal weakness in the hands, foot drop, and fatigue. The myotonia, which gives this disorder its name, can be elicited by shaking the patient's hand: Delayed release after shaking the hand or the delayed relaxation after voluntary contraction is a demonstration of the myotonia. Other maneuvers to elicit this include percussing the thenar eminence (percussion myotonia), forced eyelid closure with delayed eye opening, and grip myotonia (forced grip with delayed opening of the hand). EDX studies can uncover electrical myotonia, a spontaneous discharge of the muscle membrane with waxing and waning frequency and amplitude. The myotonia may worsen with cold, and improve with repeated contractions (warm-up phenomenon). Adults with DM1 can also have mild facial weakness, cataracts, smooth muscle dysfunction with dysmotility, cardiac conduction defects, endocrine abnormalities, a higher risk for cancers, and hypersomnolence (Ashizawa et al., 2018). Mild intellectual disability may be present as well, though the degree of disability may be overestimated by the dull appearance of the facies due to the weakness in the facial levator palpebrae muscles. The progression typically is slow and correlated with disease duration and size of the repeat expansion (Bouchard et al., 2015). However, infants born to mothers with DM1 may manifest more severe manifestations due to genetic anticipation with expansion of the maternal repeat. Infants with congenital DM1, as presented in the opening case of the chapter, can have severe generalized weakness with hypotonia, and bulbar and respiratory weakness requiring support. They may have an inverted V-shaped or "fish-shaped" upper lip, a sign of the significant facial weakness. Patients who survive the neonatal period gradually attain motor milestones, though they are delayed. About 50% to 60% of patients with congenital DM1 have intellectual disability. Therefore in any neonate who presents with hypotonia pronounced facial weakness, generalized weakness, and respiratory and bulbar weakness this diagnosis should be considered. The parents should be examined in the event that they have mild manifestations of DM1; this is an inexpensive and quick evaluation that can quickly lead to a diagnosis in a patient.

CLINICAL IMPLICATIONS OF A NEUROMUSCULAR DIAGNOSIS

The examples of neuromuscular disorders that were discussed in this chapter highlight the importance of the need for multidisciplinary care in patients with neuromuscular disorders. While the name neuromuscular disorder implies that the primary presenting problem may be weakness, they may initially present to the developmental-behavioral pediatrician for concerns about autism or intellectual disability, and therefore a high degree of suspicion for these disorders is needed. In this new era in which gene-modifying treatments are available it is particularly important to rapidly identify patients who are candidates for these potentially curative therapies.

REFERENCES

Ashizawa, T., Gagnon, C., Groh, W. J., Gutmann, L., Johnson, N. E., Meola, G., ... Winblad, S. (2018). Consensus-based care recommendations for adults with myotonic dystrophy type 1. *Neurology Clinical Practice*, *8*(6), 507–520. https://doi.org/10.1212/CPJ.0000000000000531

Banihani, R., Smile, S., Yoon, G., Dupuis, A., Mosleh, M., Snider, A., & McAdam, L. (2015). Cognitive and neurobehavioral profile in boys with Duchenne muscular dystrophy. *Journal of Child Neurology*, *30*(11), 1472–1482. https://doi.org/10.1177/0883073815570154

Barohn, R. J., Dimachkie, M. M., & Jackson, C. E. (2014). A pattern recognition approach to patients with a suspected myopathy. *Neurology Clinics*, *32*(3), 569–593. https://doi.org/10.1016/j.ncl.2014.04.008. vii.

Birnkrant, D. J., Bushby, K., Bann, C. M., Alman, B. A., Apkon, S. D., Blackwell, A., ... Group, D. M. D. C. C. W. (2018a). Diagnosis and management of Duchenne muscular dystrophy, part 2: Respiratory, cardiac, bone health, and orthopaedic management. *Lancet Neurology*, *17*(4), 347–361. https://doi.org/10.1016/S1474-4422(18)30025-5

Birnkrant, D. J., Bushby, K., Bann, C. M., Apkon, S. D., Blackwell, A., Brumbaugh, D., ... Group, D. M. D. C. C. W. (2018b). Diagnosis and management of Duchenne muscular dystrophy, part 1: Diagnosis, and neuromuscular, rehabilitation, endocrine, and gastrointestinal and nutritional management. *Lancet Neurology*, *17*(3), 251–267. https://doi.org/10.1016/S1474-4422(18)30024-3

Birnkrant, D. J., Bushby, K., Bann, C. M., Apkon, S. D., Blackwell, A., Colvin, M. K., ... Group, D. M. D. C. C. W. (2018c). Diagnosis and management of Duchenne muscular dystrophy, part 3: Primary care, emergency management, psychosocial care, and transitions of care across the lifespan. *Lancet Neurology*, *17*(5), 445–455. https://doi.org/10.1016/S1474-4422(18)30026-7

Bouchard, J. P., Cossette, L., Bassez, G., & Puymirat, J. (2015). Natural history of skeletal muscle involvement in myotonic dystrophy type 1: A retrospective study in 204 cases. *Journal of Neurology*, *262*(2), 285–293. https://doi.org/10.1007/s00415-014-7570-x.

CureSMA. (n.d.). https://www.curesma.org/wp-content/uploads/2020/11/Cure-SMA-State-of-Newborn-Screening-Report-111120.pdf

Doorenweerd, N. (2020). Combining genetics, neuropsychology and neuroimaging to improve understanding of brain involvement in Duchenne muscular dystrophy—A narrative review. *Neuromuscular Disorders*, *30*(6), 437–442. https://doi.org/10.1016/j.nmd.2020.05.001

Engel, A. G., Shen, X. M., Selcen, D., & Sine, S. M. (2015). Congenital myasthenic syndromes: Pathogenesis, diagnosis, and treatment. *Lancet Neurology*, *14*(4), 420–434. https://doi.org/10.1016/S1474-4422(14)70201-7

Finkel, R. S., Mercuri, E., Meyer, O. H., Simonds, A. K., Schroth, M. K., Graham, R. J., ... group, S. M. A. C. (2018). Diagnosis and management of spinal muscular atrophy: Part 2: Pulmonary and acute care; medications, supplements and immunizations; other organ systems; and ethics. *Neuromuscular Disorders*, *28*(3), 197–207. https://doi.org/10.1016/j.nmd.2017.11.004

Finsterer, J. (2019). Congenital myasthenic syndromes. *Orphanet Journal of Rare Diseases*, *14*(1), 57. https://doi.org/10.1186/s13023-019-1025-5

Garg, N., Yiannikas, C., Hardy, T. A., Belaya, K., Cheung, J., Beeson, D., & Reddel, S. W. (2016). Late presentations of congenital myasthenic syndromes: How many do we miss? *Muscle & Nerve*, *54*(4), 721–727. https://doi.org/10.1002/mus.25085

Kamsteeg, E. J., Kress, W., Catalli, C., Hertz, J. M., Witsch-Baumgartner, M., Buckley, M. F., ... Scheffer, H. (2012). Best practice guidelines and recommendations on the molecular diagnosis of myotonic dystrophy types 1 and 2. *European Journal of Human Genetics*, *20*(12), 1203–1208. https://doi.org/10.1038/ejhg.2012.108

Lowes, L. P., Alfano, L. N., Arnold, W. D., Shell, R., Prior, T. W., McColly, M., ... Mendell, J. (2019). Impact of age and motor function in a phase 1/2A study of infants with SMA type 1 receiving single-dose gene replacement therapy. *Pediatric Neurology*, *98*, 39–45. https://doi.org/10.1016/j.pediatrneurol.2019.05.005

Mah, J. K., Korngut, L., Dykeman, J., Day, L., Pringsheim, T., & Jette, N. (2014). A systematic review and meta-analysis on the epidemiology of Duchenne and Becker muscular dystrophy. *Neuromuscular Disorders*, *24*(6), 482–491. https://doi.org/10.1016/j.nmd.2014.03.008

Matthews, E., Brassington, R., Kuntzer, T., Jichi, F., & Manzur, A. Y. (2016). Corticosteroids for the treatment of Duchenne muscular dystrophy. *Cochrane Database of Systematic Reviews*, *5*, CD003725. https://doi.org/10.1002/14651858.CD003725.pub4

Mendell, J. R., & Lloyd-Puryear, M. (2013). Report of MDA muscle disease symposium on newborn screening for Duchenne muscular dystrophy. *Muscle & Nerve*, *48*(1), 21–26. https://doi.org/10.1002/mus.23810

Mercuri, E., Finkel, R., Montes, J., Mazzone, E. S., Sormani, M. P., Main, M., … De Vivo, D. C. (2016). Patterns of disease progression in type 2 and 3 SMA: Implications for clinical trials. *Neuromuscular Disorders*, *26*(2), 126–131. https://doi.org/10.1016/j.nmd.2015.10.006

Mercuri, E., Finkel, R. S., Muntoni, F., Wirth, B., Montes, J., Main, M., … Group, S. M. A. C. (2018). Diagnosis and management of spinal muscular atrophy: Part 1: Recommendations for diagnosis, rehabilitation, orthopedic and nutritional care. *Neuromuscular Disorders*, *28*(2), 103–115. https://doi.org/10.1016/j.nmd.2017.11.005

Mercuri, E., Pera, M. C., Scoto, M., Finkel, R., & Muntoni, F. (2020). Spinal muscular atrophy—Insights and challenges in the treatment era. *Nature Reviews Neurology*, *16*(12), 706–715. https://doi.org/10.1038/s41582-020-00413-4

Montes, J., McDermott, M. P., Mirek, E., Mazzone, E. S., Main, M., Glanzman, A. M., … Mercuri, E. (2018). Ambulatory function in spinal muscular atrophy: Age-related patterns of progression. *PLoS One*, *13*(6), e0199657. https://doi.org/10.1371/journal.pone.0199657

Nicole, S., Azuma, Y., Bauche, S., Eymard, B., Lochmuller, H., & Slater, C. (2017). Congenital myasthenic syndromes or inherited disorders of neuromuscular transmission: Recent discoveries and open questions. *Journal of Neuromuscular Diseases*, *4*(4), 269–284. https://doi.org/10.3233/JND-170257

Niu, J., Dai, Y., Liu, M., Li, Y., Ding, Q., Guan, Y., … Jin, L. (2019). *GJB1* mutation—A disease spectrum: Report of case series. *Frontiers in Neurology*, *10*, 1406. https://doi.org/10.3389/fneur.2019.01406

Tizzano, E. F., & Finkel, R. S. (2017). Spinal muscular atrophy: A changing phenotype beyond the clinical trials. *Neuromuscular Disorders*, *27*(10), 883–889. https://doi.org/10.1016/j.nmd.2017.05.011

US Food and Drug Administration. (2016). https://www.fda.gov/NewsEvents/Newsroom/PressAnnouncements/ucm521263.htm

Waldrop, M. A., & Kolb, S. J. (2019). Current treatment options in neurology—SMA therapeutics. *Current Treatment Options in Neurology*, *21*(6), 25. https://doi.org/10.1007/s11940-019-0568-z

Werheid, F., Azzedine, H., Zwerenz, E., Bozkurt, A., Moeller, M. J., Lin, L., … Claeys, K. G. (2016). Underestimated associated features in CMT neuropathies: Clinical indicators for the causative gene? *Brain & Behavior*, *6*(4), e00451. https://doi.org/10.1002/brb3.451

Winder, T. L., Tan, C. A., Klemm, S., White, H., Westbrook, J. M., Wang, J. Z., … Aradhya, S. (2020). Clinical utility of multigene analysis in over 25,000 patients with neuromuscular disorders. *Neurology Genetics*, *6*(2), e412. https://doi.org/10.1212/NXG.0000000000000412

31

Seizures and Epilepsy

Elizabeth Dubow and Krista Eschbach

For additional material related to the content of this chapter, please see Chapters 24, 25, 29, 36, and 89.

> **VIGNETTE**
>
> *A 9-year-old boy presents to his pediatrician office due to concern for staring spells. His teachers notice that he will briefly daze off and miss pieces of information. This has been present for the last few months. There has been no clear decline in his school performance. These same concerns are also noted at home, and parents occasionally notice mouth and hand movements or eye blinking when it occurs. He is very active with reduced attention, making it hard for parents to know if he is just daydreaming or if there is something else concerning.*

BACKGROUND

Epilepsy affects approximately 50 million people worldwide, and on average, 7.6 per 1000 people have epilepsy during their lifetime (World Health Organization [WHO], 2019). It is estimated that in the United States 1.2% of the population has active epilepsy, which results in 470,000 children with epilepsy (Zack & Kobau, 2017). Epilepsy is associated with many neurocognitive comorbidities. Depression, anxiety, and intellectual disability are seen in approximately 23%, 20%, and 30% to 40% of patients with epilepsy, respectively (WHO, 2019). A 2019 metaanalysis calculated an epilepsy prevalence of 12.1% in individuals with autism and a prevalence of autism in individuals with epilepsy of 9% (Lukmanji et al., 2019). This is much higher than rates of epilepsy or autism in the general population (Christensen et al., 2018; Zack & Kobau, 2017).

Epilepsy is associated with an increased risk of premature morbidity and mortality, including preventable injuries related to seizures (such as falls, drowning, burns, and head injuries) and sudden unexpected death in epilepsy patients (SUDEP) (Talati et al., 2011; WHO, 2019). Approximately, 65% of people living with epilepsy have the potential to be seizure free if appropriately treated and diagnosed (Chen et al., 2018; WHO, 2019). Given this, along with the potential consequences of untreated epilepsy, it is of utmost importance to accurately recognize and diagnose epilepsy.

FIRST-TIME SEIZURE EVALUATION AND MANAGEMENT

It is estimated that approximately 10% of the population will have a seizure at some point in their lifetime (Hauser & Beghi, 2008). Population-based data demonstrate an incidence of unprovoked seizures of 50 to 70 per 100,000 with the highest rates in those under 1 year old and the elderly (Wiebe et al., 2008). The evaluation after a first-time seizure aims to identify etiologies that may acutely alter management, as well as the risk of recurrent seizures.

In the acute setting, after stabilization of the child, it is important to determine if the event was a seizure and if there is any history of similar events (Hirtz et al., 2000). There are events that can easily be mistaken for and misdiagnosed as seizures, and these need to be considered in the differential diagnosis (Box 31.1) (EpilepsyDiagnosis.org, 2020). The evaluation starts with a detailed history of the event and assessment for risk factors for seizures, including both individual specific risk factors and relevant family history. It is also necessary to perform a complete neurologic exam evaluating for subtle focal neurologic symptoms and neurocutaneous findings. It is important to determine if the child has returned to baseline, as failure to return to baseline during the observation period influences evaluation and treatment recommendations.

The American Academy of Neurology (AAN) practice parameter states laboratory tests may be considered as part of the evaluation of a first-time seizure, although they should not be routinely ordered and instead based on individual clinical characteristics (Hirtz et al., 2000). The clinical features that suggest a need for laboratory evaluation include a history of vomiting, diarrhea, or dehydration, as well as failure to return to baseline. Children with a first-time seizure are rarely found to have an unsuspected abnormality in routine laboratory testing. However, children less than 6 months old have a higher likelihood of identifying abnormalities on routine laboratory screening, and thus this testing should more strongly be considered in this age group. Abnormalities in this testing, if present, can help identify a provoked seizure. Toxicology screening should be completed if there is any history of possible toxic ingestions or exposures. A lumbar puncture is also not routinely recommended in the evaluation of a child with a first-time seizure unless there are signs of meningitis or encephalitis (Hirtz et al., 2000). However, in children under 6 months old there is again a stronger consideration for a lumbar puncture as part of the diagnostic evaluation of a first-time seizure. If there is any concern for increased intracranial pressure, then neuroimaging should be performed prior to the lumbar puncture.

The next diagnostic test to consider in the acute evaluation of a first-time seizure is neuroimaging. Features suggestive of

BOX 31.1 Seizure Mimics

Syncope: vasovagal syncope, breathholding spells, hyperventilation syncope, cardiac syncope
Behavioral/psychiatric: inattention, self-gratification, tantrums, panic attacks, hallucinations, psychogenic nonepileptic seizures
Sleep related: parasomnias, sleep myoclonus, restless leg syndrome, narcolepsy-cataplexy
Movement disorders: tics, stereotypies, paroxysmal dyskinesias, episodic ataxias, hyperekplexia, opsoclonus myoclonus ataxia syndrome
Migraine-associated disorders: migraine with aura, benign paroxysmal torticollis/vertigo/tonic upgaze, cyclic vomiting syndrome
Other: shuddering attacks, jitteriness, Sandifer syndrome, spasmus nutans, increased intracranial pressure

Adapted from EpilepsyDiagnosis.org. (2020). *Diagnostic manual*. International League Against Epilepsy. https://www.epilepsydiagnosis.org/

intracranial pathology include a focal onset seizure, abnormal neurologic exam, and persistent altered mental status. The yield of clinically urgent neuroimaging in a focal first-time seizure is 2% to 4% and can often be found on computed tomography (CT) scan (Maytal et al., 2000). Emergent neuroimaging should be performed in children with a postictal focal deficit that is not improving or failure to return to baseline within several hours after the seizure. Additionally, there is a higher yield of emergent neuroimaging in children less than 6 months old and those with predisposing conditions (i.e., sickle cell disease, known malignancy, recent cerebral spinal fluid shunt revision, closed head injury, and neurocutaneous stigmata), and the AAN recommends that imaging in the emergency department should be considered in these scenarios (Harden et al., 2007; Warden et al., 1997). If neuroimaging is obtained, magnetic resonance imaging (MRI) is recommended over a CT scan due to the higher yield of this testing when clinically practical, noting that it is not always possible to obtain MRI in the acute setting (Hirtz et al., 2000).

For patients in which neuroimaging is not obtained acutely, it may be considered in the outpatient setting but is not indicated for all patients with a first-time seizure. In fact, in the absence of high-risk features by history or examination there is a low yield of neuroimaging after a first-time seizure with less than 1% of patients having any type of structural abnormality (Sharma et al., 2003). Features of the history and evaluation associated with a higher yield of nonemergent neuroimaging include significant motor or cognitive impairment or regression, an abnormal neurologic exam, neurocutaneous stigmata, focal seizure in a child younger than 33 months or seizure in any child younger than 24 months, or an electroencephalogram (EEG) that is not consistent with a generalized epilepsy or a self-limited focal epilepsy of childhood (Gaillard et al., 2009; Hirtz et al., 2000; Sharma et al., 2003). These features of the clinical presentation help determine the need for neuroimaging.

An EEG is a key component of the evaluation after a first-time seizure. This is agreed upon as a standard by the AAN in the evaluation of a first-time unprovoked seizure in a child of any age. EEG is not used to alter acute evaluation, but instead is essential to understand the future risk of seizures and provide prognostic information. Furthermore, after a single seizure a diagnosis of epilepsy can be supported if the EEG is sufficiently abnormal. The EEG will also help determine if additional evaluation with neuroimaging is warranted. An EEG is typically not obtained acutely due to postictal effects, but the yield of a routine outpatient EEG is increased (51% vs. 34%) if done early after the first seizure (King et al., 1998; Schreiner & Pohlmann-Eden, 2003). The EEG should aim to capture both wakefulness and sleep and include activation procedures (photic stimulation, hyperventilation, and sleep deprivation). Sleep deprivation further increases the yield of routine EEG studies (King et al., 1998).

Family counseling is also essential after a first-time seizure—this includes seizure safety and first aid—and will be discussed later in this chapter.

RISK OF RECURRENT SEIZURES AND FUTURE EPILEPSY

The risk of recurrent seizures after a single unprovoked seizure is highest in the first 6 to 12 months (Mizorogi et al., 2015; Sartori et al., 2019). This recurrence risk of additional seizures and epilepsy can be further estimated based on the clinical history and associated diagnostic evaluation. In a child with a normal neurologic exam and normal EEG the risk of further seizures in the next 5 years is 32% (Shinnar et al., 1996). However, in children with a known remote symptomatic etiology (hypoxic ischemic encephalopathy, perinatal stroke, etc.) or with an abnormal EEG with focal slowing or epileptiform discharges the risk doubles (66% and 60% at 5 years, respectively) (Shinnar et al., 1996). It is important to note that some individuals without seizures can incidentally have abnormalities on their EEG, including focal epileptiform discharges or slowing, and this is more common in children with autism than the general population. Interictal EEG abnormalities are reported in up to 60% of children with autism independent of any history of seizures (Kim et al., 2006). This highlights the importance of correlation between the EEG results and event of concern to determine the significance of the findings. Additional risk factors for recurrent seizures include history of febrile seizures, seizures arising out of sleep, and family history of febrile seizures or epilepsy (Sartori et al., 2019; Shinnar et al., 1996, 2000).

EPILEPSY DIAGNOSIS AND CLASSIFICATION

The diagnosis of epilepsy was updated by the International League Against Epilepsy (ILAE) in 2014. There are three ways in which diagnostic criteria for epilepsy can be met as outlined in Box 31.2. Note that provoked seizures, where there is a temporary factor that lowers the seizure threshold (such

BOX 31.2 Diagnosis of Epilepsy

2014 ILAE Diagnosis of Epilepsy

1. Two unprovoked seizures at least 24 hr apart
2. Single unprovoked seizure with a probability of seizure recurrence >60%
   a. Structural abnormality on imaging
   b. EEG abnormality, including focal epileptiform discharges or focal slowing
   c. Remote symptomatic etiology
3. Diagnosis of an epilepsy syndrome (see Table 31.1)

EEG, Electroencephalogram; *ILAE*, International League Against Epilepsy.

Adapted from Fisher, R. S., Acevedo, C., Arzimanoglou, A., Bogacz, A., Cross, J. H., Elger, C. E., Engel, J., Forsgren, L., French, J. A., Glynn, M., Hesdorffer, D. C., Lee, B. I., Mathern, G. W., Moshé, S. L., Perucca, E., Scheffer, I. E., Tomson, T., Watanabe, M., & Wiebe, S. (2014). ILAE official report: A practical clinical definition of epilepsy. *Epilepsia, 55*(4), 475–482. https://doi.org/10.1111/epi.12550

as a febrile seizure or acute symptomatic seizures), does not contribute to a diagnosis of epilepsy.

Types of Seizures

Classification of seizure and epilepsy types has changed throughout the years with the most recent definitions published by ILAE in 2017 (Figs. 31.1 and 31.2). Classification of seizure types starts with type of seizure onset: focal, with origin limited to a network within one hemisphere; generalized, originating in bilaterally or widespread distributed networks; or unknown. Focal onset seizures are classified as aware or with impaired awareness. The next differentiation refers to the first prominent symptom at seizure onset, classified as either motor or nonmotor, followed by further descriptions of these motor and nonmotor symptoms. Focal to bilateral tonic-clonic refers to a seizure spreading to involve both hemispheres, formerly referred to as secondary generalization. Generalized onset seizures, in addition to those of unknown onset, are classified according to their first prominent symptom, motor versus nonmotor. Unclassified seizures are reserved only for when the clinician is confident that the event is a seizure but cannot further classify (Fisher et al., 2017a, 2017b).

Types of Epilepsy

In addition to application of the standardized classification of seizure types, it is possible to identify the epilepsy type (focal, generalized, combination, or unknown) (see Fig. 31.2) (Scheffer et al., 2017).

Epilepsy Syndromes

Classification into specific epilepsy syndromes provides prognostic information, including the risk of additional seizure types, potential seizure triggers, likelihood of seizure freedom and epilepsy resolution, and the risks of comorbidities (Scheffer et al., 2017). Identification of the specific epilepsy syndrome can also guide antiseizure medication selection

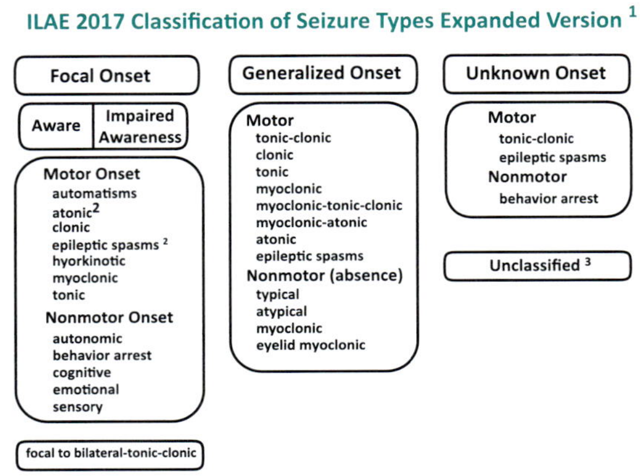

Fig. 31.1 International League Against Epilepsy *(ILAE)* 2017 classification of seizure types. *1*, Definitions, other seizure types, and descriptors are listed in the accompanying paper and glossary of terms. *2*, Degree of awareness usually is not specified. *3*, Due to inadequate information or inability to place in other categories. (From Fisher, R. S., Cross, J. H., French, J. A., Higurashi, N., Hirsch, E., Jansen, F. E., Lagae, L., Moshé, S. L., Peltola, J., Roulet Perez, E., Scheffer, I. E., & Zuberi, S. M. (2017). Operational classification of seizure types by the International League Against Epilepsy: Position paper of the ILAE Commission for Classification and Terminology. *Epilepsia, 58*(4), 522–530. https://doi.org/10.1111/epi.13670)

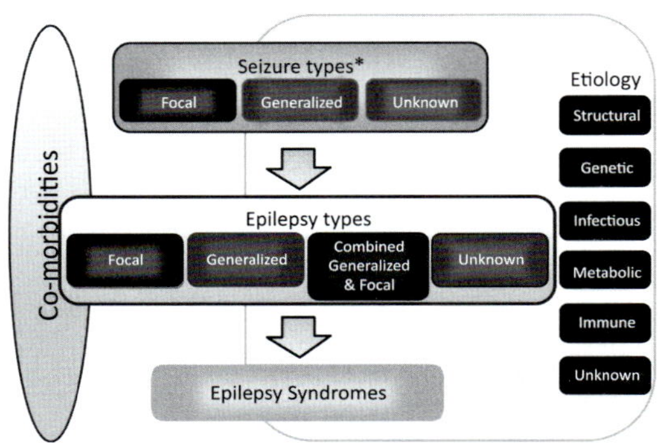

Fig. 31.2 International League Against Epilepsy 2017 classification of epilepsies. *, Onset of seizure. (From Scheffer, I. E., Berkovic, S., Capovilla, G., Connolly, M. B., French, J., Guilhoto, L., Hirsch, E., Jain, S., Mathern, G. W., Moshé, S. L., Nordli, D. R., Perucca, E., Tomson, T., Wiebe, S., Zhang, Y. H., & Zuberi, S. M. (2017). ILAE classification of the epilepsies: Position paper of the ILAE Commission for Classification and Terminology. *Epilepsia, 58*(4), 512–521. https://doi.org/10.1111/epi.13709)

and subsequent evaluation for the epilepsy etiology (i.e., genetic testing). Epilepsy syndromes encompass several combined features and include age of onset, seizure types, seizure triggers, and electrographic and imaging findings (Scheffer et al., 2017). Three main categories of epilepsy syndromes are idiopathic generalized epilepsies (also referred to as genetic generalized epilepsies due to a presumed genetic risk), self-limited focal epilepsies, and epileptic encephalopathies. The term *developmental and epileptic encephalopathy* is used when both the underlying disorder and the epileptic activity additively contribute to neurocognitive and neurobehavioral impairments (Scheffer et al, 2017). Table 31.1 reviews features of some of the more common epilepsy syndromes.

TABLE 31.1 Common Epilepsy Syndromes

Syndrome Name	Age of Onset	Seizure Types	Medications and Treatments	Other
Idiopathic Generalized Epilepsies				
Childhood absence epilepsy (CAE)	2–12 yo (peak 5–7 yo) (EpilepsyDiagnosis.org, 2020; Wirrell, 2016)	Absence seizures • Frequent (multiple per day) • Brief (~10 sec) • Provoked by hyperventilation Can have generalized tonic-clonic seizures, typically in adolescence (EpilepsyDiagnosis.org, 2020; Matricardi et al., 2014; Wirrell, 2016)	Ethosuximide Valproic acid Lamotrigine (Glauser et al., 2010)	Associated with neurocognitive deficits, including ADHD. Seizures are typically self-limited but may evolve to JAE (EpilepsyDiagnosis.org, 2020; Wirrell, 2016). With onset of absence seizures <4 yo, *SLC2A1* mutation (GLUT1 deficiency) should be considered (EpilepsyDiagnosis.org, 2020)
Juvenile absence epilepsy (JAE)	8–20 yo (peak 9–13 yo) (EpilepsyDiagnosis.org, 2020; Wirrell, 2016)	Absence seizures Generalized tonic-clonic seizures (EpilepsyDiagnosis.org, 2020; Wirrell, 2016)	Valproic acid Lamotrigine Ethosuximide (for absences only) (Glauser et al., 2010; Wirrell, 2016)	May have ADHD, learning difficulties (EpilepsyDiagnosis.org, 2020) Remission is rare (Wirrell, 2016)
Juvenile myoclonic epilepsy (JME)	8–25 yo (peak 10–18 yo) (EpilepsyDiagnosis.org, 2020; Wirrell, 2016)	Myoclonic seizures (often early morning) Generalized tonic-clonic seizures Absence seizures can be seen (Wirrell, 2016; Zhang et al., 2019)	Valproic acid Levetiracetam Topiramate (Glauser et al., 2013; Wirrell, 2016; Zhang et al., 2019)	Developmental cognition typically normal (EpilepsyDiagnosis.org, 2020) Remission is rare (Wirrell, 2016)
Self-Limited Focal Epilepsies				
Self-limited childhood epilepsy with centrotemporal spikes	3–14 yo (peak 5–9 yo) (EpilepsyDiagnosis.org, 2020; Weir et al., 2018)	Brief focal motor hemifacial clonic seizures, may include speech arrest, hypersalivation, swallowing/chewing movements. May progress to bilateral tonic-clonic seizures. Seizures are typically brief (<5 min) and 20%–50% of patients have <5 lifetime seizures (EpilepsyDiagnosis.org, 2020; Ross et al., 2020; Weir et al., 2018; Wirrell, 2016)	Medications not always used if seizures are rare (Wirrell, 2016) Oxcarbazepine Carbamazepine Levetiracetam Valproic acid (Glauser et al., 2013; Ross et al., 2020)	Seizures resolve by 12–18 yo. May have behavioral and neuropsychiatric deficits especially during period of active epilepsy. Can be associated with CSWS and LKS (Wirrell, 2016)
Panayiotopoulos syndrome	1–14 yo (peak 4–6 yo) (EpilepsyDiagnosis.org, 2020; Weir et al., 2018; Wirrell, 2016)	Focal autonomic seizures (often with gastrointestinal predominance), typically with eye deviation Seizures are often prolonged (can last hours with autonomic status epilepticus) but infrequent (25% only have a single seizure, 50% have six seizures or fewer) (EpilepsyDiagnosis.org, 2020; Weir et al., 2018; Wirrell, 2016)	Medications not always used if seizures are rare (Wirrell, 2016) Oxcarbazepine Carbamazepine Levetiracetam (Wirrell, 2016)	Seizures resolve by 11–13 yo. Diffuse neuropsychiatric deficits are common especially during the period of active epilepsy (Fonseca Wald et al., 2020)

(Continued)

TABLE 31.1 Common Epilepsy Syndromes—Cont'd

Syndrome Name	Age of Onset	Seizure Types	Medications and Treatments	Other
Epileptic Encephalopathies				
West syndrome	3–24 mo (EpilepsyDiagnosis.org, 2020; Knupp et al., 2016)	Epileptic spasms (EpilepsyDiagnosis.org, 2020; Knupp et al., 2016)	ACTH Vigabatrin Oral corticosteroids (prednisolone) (Knupp et al., 2016; Wirrell, 2016)	Often associated with developmental delay or regression (EpilepsyDiagnosis.org, 2020; Knupp et al., 2016; Wirrell, 2016). Can be associated with structural brain abnormalities, genetic or metabolic etiologies and can be associated with TSC (EpilepsyDiagnosis.org, 2020) May progress to LGS (Wirrell, 2016)
Epilepsy with myoclonic atonic seizures (Doose syndrome)	6 mo–6 yo (peak 2–5 yo) (EpilepsyDiagnosis.org, 2020; Wirrell, 2016)	Myoclonic-atonic seizures May also have absence seizures, generalized tonic-clonic seizures, rarely tonic seizures Can progress to myoclonic status epilepticus or NCSE (EpilepsyDiagnosis.org, 2020; Wirrell, 2016)	Valproic acid Levetiracetam Topiramate Zonisamide Ketogenic diet (Nickels et al., 2018, 2020)	Exclude glucose transporter disorders. Variable prognosis, can have cognitive impairment after seizure onset (EpilepsyDiagnosis.org, 2020; Wirrell, 2016)
Dravet syndrome (severe myoclonic epilepsy of infancy)	6–15 mo (EpilepsyDiagnosis.org, 2020)	Focal and generalized seizures, including: Hemiclonic seizures Atypical absence seizures Myoclonic seizures Atonic seizures (EpilepsyDiagnosis.org, 2020; Wirrell, 2016)	Clobazam Valproic acid Topiramate Levetiracetam Stiripentol Fenfluramine Cannabidiol Ketogenic diet VNS (Eschbach & Knupp, 2019; Knupp & Wirrell, 2018; Wirrell & Nabbout, 2019) Avoid agents that inhibit sodium channels (Wirrell, 2016)	Typical onset is with febrile seizures. Often heat sensitive. Typically have developmental plateau and regression (EpilepsyDiagnosis.org, 2020; Wirrell, 2016)
Lennox-Gastaut syndrome (LGS)	1–7 yo (peak 3–5 yo) (Cross et al., 2017; EpilepsyDiagnosis.org, 2020)	Multiple seizure types, including: Tonic seizures, often from sleep Atonic seizures Atypical absence seizures Generalized tonic-clonic seizures Myoclonic seizures Focal seizures Epileptic spasms (Cross et al., 2017; EpilepsyDiagnosis.org, 2020; Wirrell, 2016)	Valproic acid Lamotrigine Rufinamide Topiramate Clobazam Felbamate Cannabidiol Ketogenic diet VNS Corpus callosotomy Resective surgery (Cross et al., 2017; Wirrell, 2016) Limited evidence: Levetiracetam Zonisamide Perampanel (Cross et al., 2017; Verrotti et al., 2018)	Can have developmental delays preceding epilepsy onset in addition to stagnation and regression after epilepsy onset (EpilepsyDiagnosis.org, 2020; Wirrell, 2016)

TABLE 31.1 Common Epilepsy Syndromes—Cont'd

Syndrome Name	Age of Onset	Seizure Types	Medications and Treatments	Other
Continuous spike-and-wave during sleep (CSWS)	2–12 yo (peak 4–8 yo) CSWS often presents 1–2 yr after seizure onset (EpilepsyDiagnosis.org, 2020; Van Den Munckhof et al., 2015)	May or may not have seizures. If seizures are present, they can be focal or generalized (EpilepsyDiagnosis.org, 2020; Van Den Munckhof et al., 2015).	Benzodiazepines (diazepam) Antiseizure medications (valproic acid, levetiracetam) Oral corticosteroids (prednisolone) Epilepsy surgery (focal resections, hemispherotomy, multiple subpial transection, corpus callosotomy) (Moresco Moresco et al., 2018; Van Den Munckhof et al., 2015; Wirrell, 2016)	Associated with global decline in cognitive, behavioral, and psychiatric skills (EpilepsyDiagnosis.org, 2020; Scheltens-De Boer, 2009; Van Den Munckhof et al., 2015)
Landau-Kleffner syndrome (LKS)	3–8 yo (peak 5–7 yo) (EpilepsyDiagnosis.org, 2020; Moresco et al., 2018)	May or may not have clinical seizures (EpilepsyDiagnosis.org, 2020)	Similar to CSWS	Development of progressive aphasia with previously normal language development (EpilepsyDiagnosis.org, 2020; Moresco et al., 2018; Scheltens-De Boer, 2009)

ACTH, Adrenocorticotropic hormone; *ADHD*, attention-deficit/hyperactivity disorder; *GLUT1*, glucose-1 transporter deficiency syndrome; *NCSE*, nonconvulsive status epilepticus; *TSC*, tuberous sclerosis complex; *VNS*, vagus nerve stimulator; *yo*, years old.

CAUSES OF EPILEPSY

There are many causes of epilepsy. ILAE has proposed broad etiologic categories (see Fig. 31.2). This includes structural, genetic, infectious, metabolic, and immune-mediated etiologies (Scheffer et al., 2017). However, in 43% of children with epilepsy the exact cause remains unknown (Aaberg et al., 2017). Please refer to Chapters 24, 25, 29, 36, and 89 for more detailed information.

EPILEPSY EVALUATION

The evaluation after a diagnosis of epilepsy is based on the age of epilepsy onset, type of epilepsy and epilepsy syndrome, and the presence of comorbid conditions. In children less than 2 years of age with epilepsy it is recommended to obtain neuroimaging with preferably MRI (Gaillard et al., 2009; Wilmshurst et al., 2015). In older children the recommendation for MRI is based on clinical features suggestive of a potential structural cause of seizures (e.g., abnormal neurologic exam, focal seizure with EEG not consistent with a self-limited focal epilepsy, and motor or cognitive impairment) as previously discussed. Neuroimaging is not indicated for children with childhood and adolescent onset idiopathic generalized epilepsy syndromes or childhood epilepsy with centrotemporal spikes that follow a typical course with normal development and response to antiseizure medication (Gaillard et al., 2009).

Additional testing with metabolic and genetic investigations is also considered in the evaluation of epilepsy. The yield of genetic testing is often highest in children with early onset epilepsy and more severe neurodevelopmental impairments (Sands & Choi, 2017). For children with seizure onset less than 2 years of age with absence of a structural lesion on neuroimaging or with drug-resistant seizures, further metabolic and/or genetic testing is recommended (Wilmshurst et al., 2015). The specific testing can be narrowed based on the epilepsy syndrome classification and presentation (e.g., evaluation for glucose transporter deficiency in infants with early onset absence epilepsy). In children with early-life epilepsy (<3 years old) genetic testing can identify the cause of epilepsy in approximately 25% of children who would have previously been classified as having an unknown etiology (Berg et al., 2017). The yield is highest with epilepsy gene panels and whole exome sequencing studies, although abnormalities can also be detected with chromosomal microarray (Berg et al., 2017). The growing potential for precision therapy based on specific genetic diagnoses and the increased availability of testing has altered the role of genetic testing in the evaluation of epilepsy. Additional information about genetic disorders is available in Chapter 24.

TREATMENT OF EPILEPSY

Status Epilepticus and Acute Treatment Options

Status epilepticus refers to an abnormally prolonged seizure and was historically classified as either a seizure lasting 30 minutes or longer or two or more sequential seizures without full recovery in between (Glauser et al., 2016; Trinka et al., 2015). This definition is based on the amount of time for which a continuous seizure is expected to cause irreversible cerebral injury. The current operational definition defines status epilepticus as a single seizure lasting longer than 5 minutes (Trinka et al., 2015). This is based on the knowledge that seizures lasting longer than 5 minutes are likely to continue without intervention, and treatment at this time interval is more likely to prevent ongoing seizures that may cause neuronal injury (Trinka et al., 2015). In the United States between 50,000 and 150,000 people have status epilepticus each year (Glauser et al., 2016). The highest incidence is in children under 5 years of age and the elderly (Wu et al., 2002). There is an increased mortality associated with status epilepticus that, in part, may be related to the underlying cause of status epilepticus or a progressive neurologic condition (Maytal et al., 1989). The neurocognitive outcome after status epilepticus varies based on etiology, duration of seizure activity, and age of patient (Glauser et al., 2016; Jafarpour et al., 2019). The rate of neurologic impairment reported after status epilepticus is widely variable with 6% to 30% of children having new neurologic deficits (Jafarpour et al., 2019). These concerns can arise after a single episode of status epilepticus and highlight the importance of prompt identification and treatment.

The American Epilepsy Society published a guideline for management of status epilepticus in 2016. The first 5 minutes follows standard emergency care with management of airway, breathing, circulation, and disability, as well as identification and correction of treatable causes and obtaining intravenous (IV) access. If the seizure persists for 5 minutes, medications are initiated. The first treatment is with a benzodiazepine (intramuscular midazolam, IV lorazepam, or IV diazepam). If the seizure continues despite these medications, a second-line medication should be given with options including IV fosphenytoin, valproic acid, or levetiracetam, with phenobarbital an alternative option if these medications are not available. After this, if a seizure continues for a total of 40 minutes, options include repeating a second-line medication or starting an infusion of anesthetic medications (midazolam, pentobarbital, propofol, or thiopental) with continuous EEG monitoring (Glauser et al., 2016). These guidelines outline care in the acute prehospital and hospital setting. However, it is also beneficial for caregivers to have access to emergency medications if their child has a prolonged seizure outside of the hospital. Such prehospital medication options include rectal or intranasal diazepam and intranasal or buccal midazolam (Glauser et al., 2016).

Antiseizure Medications

Once a patient is diagnosed with epilepsy, management typically begins with initiating antiseizure medications. Antiseizure medication is not recommended after a first-time seizure unless the diagnosis of epilepsy is established (Hirtz et al., 2000), as studies have not demonstrated improved long-term epilepsy remission rates when antiseizure medication is started after the first seizure (Leone et al., 2016). Approximately, 50% of patients have their seizures controlled with their first appropriately chosen antiseizure medication, with an additional 15% becoming seizure free with their second or third medication (Chen et al., 2018). Choice of antiseizure medication depends on seizure and epilepsy type, side effects of medications, comorbidities, and cost/availability of medications.

Patients who continue to have seizures despite an adequate trial of two appropriately selected and dosed antiseizure medications are considered to have drug-resistant epilepsy. In these patients the likelihood of seizure freedom with their next medication trial is less than 5% (Chen et al., 2018). For these children additional nonmedication options are considered, and referral to an epileptologist is recommended. The nonmedication treatment options that may be considered include dietary therapies and epilepsy surgery. Dietary treatment options include most commonly ketogenic diet, medium-chain triglyceride ketogenic diet, and modified Atkins diet. Surgical treatment options include palliative interventions that typically are not associated with complete seizure freedom (vagus nerve stimulation, responsive neurostimulation, and corpus callosotomy) and surgical resection of an epileptogenic focus, which is associated with higher rates of seizure freedom (i.e., lesionectomy, lobectomy, multilobar resections, and hemispherotomy). Referral to an epileptologist within an epilepsy surgery center is recommended for all patients with drug-resistant epilepsy.

OTHER CONSEQUENCES OF EPILEPSY

Neurocognitive Effects of Epilepsy

Epilepsy is frequently associated with neurocognitive and neuropsychiatric deficits. This can be attributed to the underlying cause, interictal epileptiform activity and seizures themselves, or the effect of therapies. We can see neurocognitive effects even in epilepsy syndromes that often resolve in childhood, such as childhood absence epilepsy and self-limited childhood epilepsy with centro-temporal spikes.

Childhood absence epilepsy is primarily associated with deficits in frontal lobe function, but can include difficulties with visual spatial skills, attention, verbal memory, verbal comprehension, processing speed, executive function, working memory, motor control, and behavioral skills. Although some of these deficits are favored to be caused at least in part by seizures themselves, these deficits can persist in patients whose seizures are well controlled with medications (Cheng et al., 2017; Yildiz-Coksan et al., 2019). Children with childhood absence epilepsy are also commonly diagnosed with attention-deficit/hyperactivity disorder (ADHD), although at times it can be difficult to differentiate inattention from absence seizures themselves (Auvin et al., 2018).

Self-limited childhood epilepsy with centrotemporal spikes is associated with neurocognitive and neuropsychiatric deficits during the period of active epilepsy, but these comorbidities can be present both prior to the onset of seizures and after seizures resolve (Ross et al., 2020). Common comorbidities include ADHD, learning difficulties (Ross et al., 2020), oral language difficulties (Teixeira et al., 2020), developmental coordination disorders (Teixeira et al., 2020), and behavioral concerns (Ross et al., 2020). This syndrome occurs along a spectrum with continuous spike-and-wave during sleep and Landau-Kleffner syndrome, given the activation of electrographic discharges during sleep, which are associated with neurocognitive deficits themselves (Ross et al., 2020).

Sudden Unexpected Death in Epilepsy Patients

It is important to make special note of the concept of SUDEP. Families wish to be informed about this devastating possibility (Harden et al., 2017). SUDEP is defined as "sudden, unexpected, witnessed or unwitnessed, non-traumatic and non-drowning death, occurring in benign circumstances, in an individual with epilepsy, with or without evidence for a seizure and excluding documented status epilepticus, in which postmortem examination does not reveal a cause of death" (Nashef et al., 2012). While the incidence of SUDEP is variable with different epilepsy syndromes (e.g., higher in Dravet syndrome) (Harden et al., 2017), the overall incidence in children is approximately 1 in 4500 (Harden et al., 2017; Scorza et al., 2019). The cause of SUDEP is not clearly known and is favored to reflect a combination of factors, including cardiac arrhythmias, respiratory dysfunction, circulation dysregulation, and seizure-induced hormonal and metabolic changes (Martz et al., 2019; Scorza et al., 2019). The primary risk factors for SUDEP include the presence of generalized tonic-clonic seizures, seizures during sleep, frequent seizures (>3/year), and the absence of seizure freedom (Harden et al., 2017). The most effective way to decrease the risk of SUDEP is to attain seizure freedom, especially from generalized tonic-clonic seizures (Martz et al., 2019). Therefore knowledge of epilepsy management and counseling families about medication adherence is of utmost importance.

Seizure Safety

Seizure safety and first aid is important to review with families after the first seizure. Caregivers should receive education regarding what to do if their child has another seizure and prehospital emergency medication use. A seizure action plan is also often recommended for the school, which outlines what to do if the child were to have a seizure at school.

Specific recommendations regarding safety measures are also commonly reviewed after a first-time seizure. This is important to discuss with patients and families with consideration of activities that pose an added risk if the person were to have a seizure during the activity. The risk of injury from seizures in people with epilepsy is highest in those with uncontrolled seizures (Tomson et al., 2004). The most frequent injuries for people with seizures are head injuries, although notable additional injuries include dental injury, bone fractures, and burns (Salas-Puig et al., 2019; Tomson et al., 2004). The following safety measures are proposed (Noe, 2019): extra supervision while swimming/bathing or taking a shower rather than a bath, avoidance of locking bathroom or bedroom doors, safety around cooking (avoidance of open flames, microwave use vs. a stove top, and decreased temperature on the water heater to reduce scalding), household environment with soft or padded furniture, and epilepsy safety pillows for sleep. Standard recommendations for wearing a helmet when bike riding or horseback riding should also be followed. Overall, the goal is to maximize the quality of life for people living with epilepsy and to not routinely restrict activities, although extra precautions may be needed (Institute of Medicine et al., 2012). Engaging in physical exercise or sports can have a positive impact on children with epilepsy and can typically be done safely depending on the sport and degree of risk (Capovilla et al., 2016). The ILAE Task Force on Sports and Epilepsy has proposed guidelines to help with the decision about when to return to sports and activities based on the level of risk (Capovilla et al., 2016). This guideline follows similar seizure-free intervals as driving regulations for return to high-risk activities (e.g., climbing, wind-surfing, rodeo, diving).

Each state has driving regulations after a first-time seizure and for individuals with epilepsy. Patients should be counseled to stop driving after a first-time seizure. The specific duration of driving restriction varies by state and country, often requiring 3 to 12 months of seizure freedom. It is important that patients and physicians review local laws and regulations, as some states require that physicians report to the state if their patients with epilepsy are driving against medical recommendations. It is essential that both physicians and patients are aware of the medical-legal ramifications around driving for individuals with epilepsy.

EPILEPSY SUPPORT AND RESOURCES

Epilepsy Foundation: epilepsy.com
Cure Epilepsy: cureepilepsy.org (promotes and funds patient-centered research)
American Epilepsy Society: aesnet.org

REFERENCES

Aaberg, K. M., Surén, P., Søraas, C. L., Bakken, I. J., Lossius, M. I., Stoltenberg, C., & Chin, R. (2017). Seizures, syndromes, and etiologies in childhood epilepsy: The International League Against Epilepsy 1981, 1989, and 2017 classifications used in a population-based cohort. *Epilepsia*, *58*(11), 1880–1891. https://doi.org/10.1111/epi.13913

Auvin, S., Wirrell, E., Donald, K. A., Berl, M., Hartmann, H., Valente, K. D., ... Wilmshurst, J. M. (2018). Systematic review of the screening, diagnosis, and management of ADHD in children with epilepsy. Consensus paper of the Task Force on Comorbidities of the ILAE Pediatric Commission. *Epilepsia*, *59*(10), 1867–1880. https://doi.org/10.1111/epi.14549

Berg, A. T., Coryell, J., Saneto, R. P., Grinspan, Z. M., Alexander, J. J., Kekis, M., ... Koh, S. (2017). Early-life epilepsies and the emerging role of genetic testing. *JAMA Pediatrics*, *171*(9), 863–871. https://doi.org/10.1001/jamapediatrics.2017.1743

Capovilla, G., Kaufman, K. R., Perucca, E., Moshé, S. L., & Arida, R. M. (2016). Epilepsy, seizures, physical exercise, and sports: A report from the ILAE Task Force on Sports and Epilepsy. *Epilepsia*, *57*(1), 6–12. https://doi.org/10.1111/epi.13261

Chen, Z., Brodie, M. J., Liew, D., & Kwan, P. (2018). Treatment outcomes in patients with newly diagnosed epilepsy treated with established and new antiepileptic drugs a 30-year longitudinal cohort study. *JAMA Neurology*, *75*(3), 279–286. https://doi.org/10.1001/jamaneurol.2017.3949

Cheng, D., Yan, X., Gao, Z., Xu, K., Zhou, X., & Chen, Q. (2017). Neurocognitive profiles in childhood absence epilepsy: A focus on cognitive dysfunction associated with the frontal lobe. *Journal of Child Neurology*, *32*(1), 46–52. https://doi.org/10.1177/0883073816668465

Christensen, D. L., Braun, K. V. N., Baio, J., Bilder, D., Charles, J., Constantino, J. N., … Yeargin-Allsop, M. (2018). Correction and republication: Prevalence and characteristics of autism spectrum disorder among children aged 8 years—Autism and Developmental Disabilities Monitoring Network, 11 sites, United States, 2012. *MMWR*, *65*(No. SS-13), 1–23. https://doi.org/10.15585/mmwr.mm6745a7

Cross, J. H., Auvin, S., Falip, M., Striano, P., & Arzimanoglou, A. (2017). Expert opinion on the management of Lennox-Gastaut syndrome: Treatment algorithms and practical considerations. *Frontiers in Neurology*, *8*(SEP), 505. https://doi.org/10.3389/fneur.2017.00505

EpilepsyDiagnosis.org. (2020). *Diagnostic manual*. International League Against Epilepsy. https://www.epilepsydiagnosis.org/.

Eschbach, K., & Knupp, K. G. (2019). Stiripentol for the treatment of seizures in Dravet syndrome. *Expert Review of Clinical Pharmacology*, *12*(5), 379–388. https://doi.org/10.1080/17512433.2019.1605904

Fisher, R. S., Acevedo, C., Arzimanoglou, A., Bogacz, A., Cross, J. H., Elger, C. E., … Wiebe, S. (2014). ILAE official report: A practical clinical definition of epilepsy. *Epilepsia*, *55*(4), 475–482. https://doi.org/10.1111/epi.12550

Fisher, R. S., Cross, J. H., D'Souza, C., French, J. A., Haut, S. R., Higurashi, N., … Zuberi, S. M. (2017a). Instruction manual for the ILAE 2017 operational classification of seizure types. *Epilepsia*, *58*(4), 531–542. https://doi.org/10.1111/epi.13671

Fisher, R. S., Cross, J. H., French, J. A., Higurashi, N., Hirsch, E., Jansen, F. E., … Zuberi, S. M. (2017b). Operational classification of seizure types by the International League Against Epilepsy: Position paper of the ILAE Commission for Classification and Terminology. *Epilepsia*, *58*(4), 522–530. https://doi.org/10.1111/epi.13670

Fonseca Wald, E. L. A., Debeij-Van Hall, M. H. J. A., De Jong, E., Aldenkamp, A. P., Vermeulen, R. J., Vles, J. S. H., … Hendriksen, J. G. M. (2020). Neurocognitive and behavioural profile in Panayiotopoulos syndrome. *Developmental Medicine and Child Neurology*, *62*(8), 985–992. https://doi.org/10.1111/dmcn.14417

Gaillard, W. D., Chiron, C., Helen Cross, J., Simon Harvey, A., Kuzniecky, R., Hertz-Pannier, L., & Gilbert Vezina, L. (2009). Guidelines for imaging infants and children with recent-onset epilepsy. *Epilepsia*, *50*(9), 2147–2153. https://doi.org/10.1111/j.1528-1167.2009.02075.x

Glauser, T., Ben-Menachem, E., Bourgeois, B., Cnaan, A., Guerreiro, C., Kälviäinen, R., … Tomson, T. (2013). Updated ILAE evidence review of antiepileptic drug efficacy and effectiveness as initial monotherapy for epileptic seizures and syndromes. *Epilepsia*, *54*(3), 551–563. https://doi.org/10.1111/epi.12074

Glauser, T., Shinnar, S., Gloss, D., Alldredge, B., Arya, R., Bainbridge, J., … Treiman, D. M. (2016). Evidence-based guideline: Treatment of convulsive status epilepticus in children and adults: Report of the guideline committee of the American Epilepsy Society. *Epilepsy Currents*, *16*(1), 48–61. https://doi.org/10.5698/1535-7597-16.1.48

Glauser, T. A., Cnaan, A., Shinnar, S., Hirtz, D. G., Dlugos, D., Masur, D. M., … Adamson, P. C. (2010). Ethosuximide, valproic acid, and lamotrigine in childhood absence epilepsy. *Pediatric Neurology Briefs*, *362*(9), 790–799. https://doi.org/10.1056/nejmoa0902014

Harden, C. L., Huff, J. S., Schwartz, T. H., Dubinsky, R. M., Zimmerman, R. D., Weinstein, S., Foltin, J. C., Theodore, W. H., & Therapeutics and Technology Assessment Subcommittee of the American Academy of Neurology. (2007). Reassessment: Neuroimaging in the emergency patient presenting with seizure (an evidence-based review): Report of the Therapeutics and Technology Assessment Subcommittee of the American Academy of Neurology. *Neurology. 30;69*(18), 1772–1780. https://doi. 10.1212/01.wnl.0000285083.25882.0e

Harden, C., Tomson, T., Gloss, D., Buchhalter, J., Cross, J. H., Donner, E., … Ryvlin, P. (2017). Practice guideline summary: Sudden unexpected death in epilepsy incidence rates and risk factors. *Neurology*, *88*(17), 1674–1680. https://doi.org/10.1212/wnl.0000000000003685

Hauser, W. A., & Beghi, E. (2008). First seizure definitions and worldwide incidence and mortality. *Epilepsia*, *49*(1), S8–S12. https://doi.org/10.1111/j.1528-1167.2008.01443.x

Hirtz, D., Ashwal, S., Berg, A. T., Bettis, D., Camfield, C., Camfield, P., … Shinnar, S. (2000). Practice parameter: Evaluating a first nonfebrile seizure in children: Report of the quality standards subcommittee of the American Academy of Neurology, the Child Neurology Society, and the American Epilepsy Society. *Neurology*, *56*(55), 616–623. https://doi.org/10.1212/WNL.56.4.574

Institute of Medicine (US) Committee on the Public Health Dimensions of the Epilepsies; England, M. J., Liverman, C. T., Schultz, A. M., & Strawbridge, L. M. (Eds.). (2012). *Epilepsy across the spectrum: Promoting health and understanding*. National Academies Press. PMID: 22993876.

Jafarpour, S., Stredny, C. M., Piantino, J., & Chapman, K. E. (2019). Baseline and outcome assessment in pediatric status epilepticus. *Seizure*, *68*, 52–61. https://doi.org/10.1016/j.seizure.2018.04.019

Kim, H. L., Donnelly, J. H., Tournay, A. E., Book, T. M., & Filipek, P. (2006). Absence of seizures despite high prevalence of epileptiform EEG abnormalities in children with autism monitored in a tertiary care center. *Epilepsia*, *47*(2), 394–398. https://doi.org/10.1111/j.1528-1167.2006.00434.x

King, M. A., Newton, M. R., Jackson, G. D., Fitt, G. J., Mitchell, L. A., Silvapulle, M. J., & Berkovic, S. F. (1998). Epileptology of the first-seizure presentation: A clinical, electroencephalographic, and magnetic resonance imaging study of 300 consecutive patients. *Lancet*, *352*(9133), 1007–1011. https://doi.org/10.1016/S0140-6736(98)03543-0

Knupp, K. G., Coryell, J., Nickels, K. C., Ryan, N., Leister, E., Loddenkemper, T., … Consortium, P. E. R. (2016). Respose to treatment in a prospective national infantile spasms cohort. *Annals of Neurology*, *79*(3), 475–585. https://doi.org/10.1002/ana.24594

Knupp, K. G., & Wirrell, E. C. (2018). Treatment strategies for Dravet syndrome. *CNS Drugs*, *32*(4), 335–350. https://doi.org/10.1007/s40263-018-0511-y

Leone, M. A., Giussani, G., Nolan, S. J., Marson, A. G., & Beghi, E. (2016). Immediate antiepileptic drug treatment, versus placebo, deferred, or no treatment for first unprovoked seizure. *Cochrane Database of Systematic Reviews*, 5. John Wiley and Sons Ltd. https://doi.org/10.1002/14651858.CD007144.pub2

Lukmanji, S., Manji, S. A., Kadhim, S., Sauro, K. M., Wirrell, E. C., Kwon, C. S., & Jetté, N. (2019). The co-occurrence of epilepsy and autism: A systematic review. *Epilepsy and Behavior*, *98*, 238–248. https://doi.org/10.1016/j.yebeh.2019.07.037

Martz, G., Duberstein, S., Hill, C., Spanaki-Veralas, M., & Stanton, T. (2019). *AES position statement on SUDEP counseling*. https://www.aesnet.org/about/position-statements/position-statement-on-sudep-counseling

Matricardi, S., Verrotti, A., Chiarelli, F., Cerminara, C., & Curatolo, P. (2014). Current advances in childhood absence epilepsy. *Pediatric Neurology, 50*(3), 205–212. https://doi.org/10.1016/j.pediatrneurol.2013.10.009

Maytal, J., Krauss, J. M., Novak, G., Nagelberg, J., & Patel, M. (2000). The role of brain computed tomography in evaluating children with new onset of seizures in the emergency department. *Epilepsia, 41*(8), 950–954. https://doi.org/10.1111/j.1528-1157.2000.tb00277.x

Maytal, J., Shinnar, S., Moshe, S. L., & Alvarez, L. A. (1989). Low morbidity and mortality of status epilepticus in children. *Pediatrics, 83*(3), 323–331.

Mizorogi, S., Kanemura, H., Sano, F., Sugita, K., & Aihara, M. (2015). Risk factors for seizure recurrence in children after first unprovoked seizure. *Pediatrics International, 57*(4), 665–669. https://doi.org/10.1111/ped.12600

Moresco, L., Bruschettini, M., Calevo, M. G., & Siri, L. (2018). Pharmacological treatment for continuous spike-wave during slow wave sleep and Landau-Kleffner syndrome. *Cochrane Database of Systematic Reviews*, 9. https://doi.org/10.1002/14651858.CD013132

Nashef, L., So, E. L., Ryvlin, P., & Tomson, T. (2012). Unifying the definitions of sudden unexpected death in epilepsy. *Epilepsia, 53*(2), 227–233. https://doi.org/10.1111/j.1528-1167.2011.03358.x

Nickels, K., Kossoff, E. H., Eschbach, K., & Joshi, C. (2020). Epilepsy with myoclonic-atonic seizures (Doose syndrome): Clarification of diagnosis and treatment options through a large retrospective multicenter cohort. *Epilepsia, 62*(1), 120–127. https://doi.org/10.1111/epi.16752

Nickels, K., Thibert, R., Rau, S., Demarest, S., Wirrell, E., Kossoff, E., ... Shellhaas, R. (2018). How do we diagnose and treat epilepsy with myoclonic-atonic seizures (Doose syndrome)? Results of the Pediatric Epilepsy Research Consortium survey. *Epilepsy Research, 144*, 14–19. https://doi.org/10.1016/j.eplepsyres.2018.04.010

Noe, K. (2019). Counseling and management of the risks of living with epilepsy. *CONTINUUM Lifelong Learning in Neurology, 25*(2), 477–491. https://doi.org/10.1212/CON.0000000000000708

Ross, E. E., Stoyell, S. M., Kramer, M. A., Berg, A. T., & Chu, C. J. (2020). The natural history of seizures and neuropsychiatric symptoms in childhood epilepsy with centrotemporal spikes (CECTS). *Epilepsy and Behavior, 103*(Pt A), 106437. https://doi.org/10.1016/j.yebeh.2019.07.038

Salas-Puig, X., Iniesta, M., Abraira, L., & Puig, J. (2019). Accidental injuries in patients with generalized tonic–clonic seizures. A multicenter, observational, cross-sectional study (QUIN-GTC study). *Epilepsy and Behavior, 92*, 135–139. https://doi.org/10.1016/j.yebeh.2018.10.043

Sands, T. T., & Choi, H. (2017). Genetic testing in pediatric epilepsy. *Current Neurology and Neuroscience Reports, 17*(5), 1–11. https://doi.org/10.1007/s11910-017-0753-y

Sartori, S., Nosadini, M., Tessarin, G., Boniver, C., Frigo, A. C., Toldo, I., ... Da Dalt, L. (2019). First-ever convulsive seizures in children presenting to the emergency department: Risk factors for seizure recurrence and diagnosis of epilepsy. *Developmental Medicine and Child Neurology, 61*(1), 82–90. https://doi.org/10.1111/dmcn.14015

Scheffer, I. E., Berkovic, S., Capovilla, G., Connolly, M. B., French, J., Guilhoto, L., ... Zuberi, S. M. (2017). ILAE classification of the epilepsies: Position paper of the ILAE Commission for Classification and Terminology. *Epilepsia, 58*(4), 512–521. https://doi.org/10.1111/epi.13709

Scheltens-De Boer, M. (2009). Guidelines for EEG in encephalopathy related to ESES/CSWS in children. *Epilepsia, 50*(7), S13–S17. https://doi.org/10.1111/j.1528-1167.2009.02211.x

Schreiner, A., & Pohlmann-Eden, B. (2003). Value of the early electroencephalogram after a first unprovoked seizure. *Clinical EEG and Neuroscience, 34*(3), 140–144. https://doi.org/10.1177/155005940303400307

Scorza, F. A., Olszewer, E., Fiorini, A., Scorza, C., & Finsterer, J. (2019). Sudden unexpected death in epilepsy: Rethinking the unthinkable. *Epilepsy and Behavior, 93*, 148–149. https://doi.org/10.1016/j.yebeh.2019.01.002

Sharma, S., Riviello, J. J., Harper, M. B., & Baskin, M. N. (2003). The role of emergent neuroimaging in children with new-onset afebrile seizures. *Pediatrics, 111*(1), 1–5. https://doi.org/10.1542/peds.111.1.1

Shinnar, S., Berg, A. T., Moshe, S. L., O'dell, C., Alemanyy, M., Newstein, D., ... Hauser, W. A. (1996). The risk of seizure recurrence after a first unprovoked afebrile seizure in childhood: An extended follow-up. *Pediatrics, 98*(2), 216–225. www.aappublications.org/news

Shinnar, S., Berg, A. T., O'Dell, C., Newstein, D., Moshe, S. L., & Hauser, W. A. (2000). Predictors of multiple seizures in a cohort of children prospectively followed from the time of their first unprovoked seizure. *Annals of Neurology, 48*(2), 140–147. https://doi.org/10.1002/1531-8249(200008)48:2<140::AID-ANA2>3.0.CO;2-Y

Talati, R., Scholle, J. M., Phung, O. J., Baker, W. L., Baker, E. L., Ashaye, A., ... White, C. M. (2011). Effectiveness and safety of antiepileptic medications in patients with epilepsy. *Agency for Healthcare Research and Quality (US), 12*. https://doi.org/10.1097/00006250-200301000-00014

Teixeira, J. M., Santos, M. E., & Oom, P. (2020). Oral language in children with benign childhood epilepsy with centrotemporal spikes. *Epilepsy and Behavior, 111*, 107328. https://doi.org/10.1016/j.yebeh.2020.107328

Tomson, T., Beghi, E., Sundqvist, A., & Johannessen, S. I. (2004). Medical risks in epilepsy: A review with focus on physical injuries, mortality, traffic accidents and their prevention. *Epilepsy Research, 60*(1), 1–16. https://doi.org/10.1016/j.eplepsyres.2004.05.004

Trinka, E., Cock, H., Hesdorffer, D., Rossetti, A. O., Scheffer, I. E., Shinnar, S., ... Lowenstein, D. H. (2015). A definition and classification of status epilepticus—Report of the ILAE Task Force on Classification of Status Epilepticus. *Epilepsia, 56*(10), 1515–1523. https://doi.org/10.1111/epi.13121

Van Den Munckhof, B., Van Dee, V., Sagi, L., Caraballo, R. H., Veggiotti, P., Liukkonen, E., ... Jansen, F. E. (2015). Treatment of electrical status epilepticus in sleep: A pooled analysis of 575 cases. *Epilepsia, 56*(11), 1738–1746. https://doi.org/10.1111/epi.13128

Verrotti, A., Striano, P., Iapadre, G., Zagaroli, L., Bonanni, P., Coppola, G., ... Curatolo, P. (2018). The pharmacological management of Lennox-Gastaut syndrome and critical literature review. *Seizure, 63*(December), 17–25. https://doi.org/10.1016/j.seizure.2018.10.016

Warden, C. R., Brownstein, D. R., & Del Beccaro, M. A. (1997). Predictors of abnormal findings of computed tomography of the head in pediatric patients presenting with seizures. *Annals of Emergency Medicine*, *29*(4), 518–523. https://doi.org/10.1016/S0196-0644(97)70226-9

Weir, E., Gibbs, J., & Appleton, R. (2018). Panayiotopoulos syndrome and benign partial epilepsy with centro-temporal spikes: A comparative incidence study. *Seizure*, *57*, 66–69. https://doi.org/10.1016/j.seizure.2018.03.002

Wiebe, S., Téllez-Zenteno, J. F., & Shapiro, M. (2008). An evidence-based approach to the first seizure. *Epilepsia*, *49*(1), S50–S57. https://doi.org/10.1111/j.1528-1167.2008.01451.x

Wilmshurst, J. M., Gaillard, W. D., Vinayan, K. P., Tsuchida, T. N., Plouin, P., Van Bogaert, P., … Cross, J. H. (2015). Summary of recommendations for the management of infantile seizures: Task force report for the ILAE Commission of Pediatrics. *Epilepsia*, *56*(8), 1185–1197. https://doi.org/10.1111/epi.13057

Wirrell, E. (2016). Infantile, childhood, and adolescent epilepsies. *CONTINUUM Lifelong Learning in Neurology*, *22*(February), 60–93. https://doi.org/10.1212/CON.0000000000000269

Wirrell, E. C., & Nabbout, R. (2019). Recent advances in the drug treatment of Dravet syndrome. *CNS Drugs*, *33*(9), 867–881. https://doi.org/10.1007/s40263-019-00666-8

World Health Organization. (2019). *Epilepsy: A public health imperative*. WHO.

Wu, Y. W., Shek, D. w, Garcia, P. A., Zhao, S., & Johnson, C. (2002). Incidence and mortality of generalized convulsive status epilepticus in California. *Neurology*, *58*(7), 1070–1076. https://doi.org/10.1212/wnl.58.7.1070

Yildiz-Coksan, S., Aslan, A., Coksan, S., & Okuyaz, C. (2019). Cognitive profile and academic achievement of children with absence epilepsy. *Epilepsy and Behavior*, *95*, 95–99. https://doi.org/10.1016/j.yebeh.2019.04.001

Zack, M. M., & Kobau, R. (2017). National and state estimates of the numbers of adults and children with active epilepsy. *MMWR*, *66*(31), 821–825.

Zhang, Y., Chen, J., Ren, J., Liu, W., Yang, T., & Zhou, D. (2019). Clinical features and treatment outcomes of Juvenile myoclonic epilepsy patients. *Epilepsia Open*, *4*(2), 302–308. https://doi.org/10.1002/epi4.12321

32

Diffuse Acquired Brain Injury

Sarah J. Tlustos, Aaron Powell, and Michael W. Kirkwood

For additional materials related to this chapter, please see Chapters 5, 29, 31, 33, 34, and 39.

VIGNETTE

Jacob is a 15-year-old male, who at 3 years of age sustained a severe traumatic brain injury (TBI) that included left-sided subdural hematoma and diffuse axonal injury. Despite some regression in language and mild right hemiparesis soon after the injury, he seemed largely back to his typical, active self within a few months. As he became older, his teachers noticed problems with reading, math, concentration, and behavior. He received some extra help for academics via an individualized education plan (IEP), but this was discontinued in middle school despite poor classroom achievement because his academic testing was within grade expectations. At home, his parents described behavioral problems such as aggression and frequently changing moods. Now, his mother is worried he may be depressed and is struggling to keep friends. His primary care provider is wondering about the role of the early TBI in his problems.

INTRODUCTION TO DIFFUSE ACQUIRED BRAIN INJURY

Acquired brain injury (ABI) is an umbrella term that refers to a noncongenital brain insult. Pediatric ABI can include TBI, central hypoxic/anoxic insults related to cardiac and pulmonary arrests, stroke, central nervous system neoplasms and infections, and metabolic crises and autoimmune conditions affecting the central nervous system.

ABI can be classified into diffuse versus focal and traumatic versus nontraumatic injuries. Diffuse injuries affect multiple brain regions, whereas focal injuries are largely localized to a contiguous region of the brain. Traumatic brain injuries result from an external biomechanical force (e.g., motor vehicle crash, fall). The current chapter will focus on moderate-severe TBI, which is the most common diffuse brain injury in children that results in significant long-term problems. The chapter will also briefly review pediatric mild TBI and the special case of abusive head trauma (AHT), as well as one of the more common nontraumatic diffuse injuries in children, anoxic/hypoxic brain injury. Focal ABI will be considered in other chapters of this text, as will brain injuries resulting from infectious or autoimmune processes and those occurring during pregnancy or around the time of birth.

Epidemiology

Table 32.1 illustrates the most common types and mechanisms of ABI in children. ABI is a leading cause of morbidity and mortality in children with extremely high costs to patients, families, and society (Schneier, Shields, Hostetler, Xiang, & Smith, 2006). TBI alone had an estimated cost of $1 billion for acute hospitalizations in 2014 (Centers for Disease Control and Prevention, 2019). The estimated lifetime health care costs are exponentially higher for children, as their needs are compounded throughout a lifespan (Slomine et al., 2006). Of course, costs to families and communities are not purely financial, with families of children with brain injury citing higher stress, poorer mental health, and worse family functioning.

Pathophysiology

Diffuse ABI is often broken down into two major stages of injury: primary and secondary. Primary injuries are those that occur at the time of the original insult. Typically these include mechanical disruptions of the brain parenchyma, such as contusions and axonal shearing or neuronal death from cellular energy crises (Tasker, 2006). When compared to adults, children have increased vulnerabilities to traumatic forces for many reasons, including a larger head relative to body size, weaker neck musculature, decreased myelination, and increased brain water content. The main protection against primary brain injuries is prevention, such as seatbelts and child restraints, helmets, modification of playground equipment with lower heights and rubber or wood chips, and gates around pools (Cassidy et al., 2004).

Secondary brain injuries occur in the days or weeks following the initial insult. The major risk factors for continued neuronal injury are inadequate cerebral perfusion resulting from increased intracranial pressure and metabolic crises (Box 32.1). Biochemical cascades play an important role in postinjury inflammation, edema, and apoptosis and are under investigation as potential targets to help in secondary brain injury prevention (Popernack, Gray, & Reuter-Rice, 2015). Management of secondary brain injury is largely the role of neurointensivists. Care of acute brain injury in children should differ from adult care given the multiple differences in

TABLE 32.1 Common Conditions and Mechanisms Resulting in Diffuse and Focal Brain Injury

Diffuse Brain Injury	Common Mechanisms
Traumatic brain injury	Auto crashes, unhelmeted recreation related, falls, abuse
Anoxic/hypoxic-ischemic brain injury	Cardiopulmonary arrest, drowning
Metabolic derangement	Congenital metabolic and genetic disorders
Autoimmune conditions affecting the central nervous system (CNS)	Multiple sclerosis, acute disseminated encephalomyelitis, autoimmune encephalitis
Infectious meningitis and encephalitis	CNS viral/bacterial infections
Toxic exposure	Secondary exposure (e.g., direct inhalation such as carbon monoxide)
Focal Brain Injury	**Common Mechanisms**
Stroke (ischemic or hemorrhagic)	Embolic, blood vessel abnormalities, sickle cell disease, central venous thrombosis
Brain neoplasms	Primary cancers
Empyema/intracranial abscess	Sinusitis

BOX 32.1 Contributors to Secondary Brain Injury

- Hypotension
- Hypoxia
- Hypoglycemia
- Vasospasm
- Edema
- Uncontrolled seizures
- Underlying medical comorbidities
- Posttraumatic hydrocephalus

developmental physiologies, though there is a paucity of evidence-based age-specific protocols at this time (Figaji, 2017).

Injury Grading/Severity

Diffuse brain injuries can be broadly characterized into levels of severity: mild, moderate, and severe (Table 32.2). These categories have demonstrated utility in predicting outcomes. The Glasgow Coma Scale (GCS), adapted for pediatrics (Holmes, Palchak, MacFarlane, & Kuppermann, 2005), at initial point of contact with a medical provider has shown to be an important predictor of outcome. In addition to GCS, a number of severity markers have consistently been linked to pediatric outcomes after TBI, including length and depth of coma, duration of posttraumatic amnesia, duration to follow commands, and neuroimaging abnormalities (Bruns, 2003).

TABLE 32.2 Injury Severity Classification for Traumatic Brain Injury

	Mild	Moderate	Severe
Length of coma/ duration of loss of consciousness	<30 min	30 min–6 hr	>6 hr
Initial Glasgow Coma Scale score	13–15	9–12	3–8
Duration of posttraumatic amnesia	<24 hr	24 hr–1 wk	>1 wk

Taken together, these factors have been associated in dose-response fashion with multiple outcomes, though data are not sufficient to make precise outcome predictions based on any single injury-related variable. While some research has suggested that severity of TBI may become less important over time in predicting longer-term outcome, studies in adults do continue to note a role of injury severity.

Less guidance exists regarding classifying injury severity for etiologies other than TBI. For example, with anoxic/hypoxic-ischemic brain injuries, the initial neurologic exam and GCS, responsivity after withdrawal of sedating medications, and initial neuroimaging findings are generally used to prognosticate in broad terms ("good" vs. "bad" outcomes, such as risk for mortality or severe global impairment). The extent of injury identified on brain magnetic resonance imaging (MRI), classified as cortical, subcortical, or mixed, has also been associated with global outcomes, with mixed findings indicating poorer outcomes (Ramiro, 2015).

Neuroimaging/Electroencephalography

The initial imaging modality of choice in severe brain injury is computed tomography (CT) because it is rapid and can reveal actionable neuropathology such as parenchymal edema and/or herniation, intracranial bleeding, foreign bodies, and fractures. Head CT can also quickly identify unexplained subdural hematoma or hemispheric hypodensity that could alert providers to the potential of AHT (Shaahinfar, Whitelaw, & Mansour, 2015). MRI is better at revealing the soft tissue structures of the brain; however, it is a relatively slow examination and requires sedation for younger children and those who are in an agitated state secondary to their brain injury. The primary goal of MRI in TBI is the identification of diffuse axonal injury, with both diffusion weighted and susceptibility weighted imaging being helpful (Ferrazzano et al., 2019). Total volume of injury (i.e., "lesion burden") demonstrated via susceptibility weighted imaging has been found to relate to neurobehavioral outcomes (Beauchamp et al., 2013).

Electroencephalography (EEG) is commonly utilized in children with more severe brain injuries to identify seizures, a common side effect of brain injury in children. EEG can also help in establishing whether a sleep/wake cycle exists for patients with disorders of consciousness. While there is likely some prognostic utility to EEG, its fidelity increases when viewed in the context of additional prognostic data (Brenner, Freier, Holshouser, Burley, & Ashwal, 2003).

BOX 32.2 Risk Factors for Poorer Outcomes After Diffuse Acquired Brain Injury, Above and Beyond Injury Severity

Individual Risk Factors	Contextual Risk Factors
• Preexisting developmental delays and neurodevelopmental conditions (e.g., learning disabilities, attention-deficit/hyperactivity disorder) • Preexisting mood disorder, anxiety, or other psychiatric conditions • Preexisting adaptive functioning impairments • Genetic risk factors (e.g., APOE4)	• Family distress, family functioning, family burden • Permissive parenting styles • Socioeconomic status (including parental education level)

Plasticity Versus Development and the Role of Age at Injury

While neuroplasticity might seem to be an advantageous quality for brain injury recovery, growing evidence indicates that younger age at diffuse injury portends poorer functional outcomes (Anderson et al., 2010). This is due to several factors, including the hijacking of existing apoptotic cascades, interruption of white matter connectivity, and the vulnerability that a baseline lack of development mastery poses.

Individual and Contextual Predictors of Outcomes

While injury severity is an important predictor of outcome after diffuse ABI, individual and contextual factors are now well established as playing a role, particularly for certain neurobehavioral outcomes such as psychosocial and academic functioning. Individual factors that have shown to be important for prediction of longer-term outcomes include preinjury cognitive/developmental and social-emotional functioning. Contextual factors, including socioeconomic status, family resources, and both preinjury and postinjury family functioning, have also been shown to be important moderators of long-term outcomes, and many of these relationships appear to be bidirectional (Box 32.2). These will be discussed in greater detail within other sections as they pertain to moderate-severe TBI, mild TBI, AHT, and anoxic/hypoxic brain injury.

TABLE 32.3 Common Brain Injury–Associated Impairments and Comorbidities

Sensory	• Olfactory dysfunction • Hearing impairment • Cortical visual impairment • Touch or position sense impairment • Cranial nerve (CN) palsy (most common is CNIII) • Neuropathic pain/allodynia
Central nervous system	• Posttraumatic hydrocephalus • Cerebral atrophy • Posttraumatic headaches • Seizures • Paroxysmal sympathetic hyperactivity • Insomnia/sleep cycle dysregulation
Endocrine	• Cerebral salt wasting • Anterior pituitary dysfunction (SIADH, diabetes insipidus) • Precocious puberty
Nutrition	• Dysphagia • Tube feed dependence • Constipation
Skeletal	• Growing skull fracture • Long bone fractures • Heterotopic ossification
Motor	• Weakness • Motor control impairment (apraxia) • Hypertonicity (dystonia, spasticity, rigidity) • Ataxia

SIADH, Syndrome of inappropriate antidiuretic hormone.

MODERATE AND SEVERE TRAUMATIC BRAIN INJURY

Outcomes

Medically, moderate-severe TBI can result in a wide array of medical comorbidities and impairments affecting multiple different systems (summarized in Table 32.3). Interest in genetic influences on biologic responses to injury and recovery has also increased in recent years. The apolipoprotein e4 (APOE) gene, which is associated with neuron protection and synaptic repair, has been studied the most extensively. Presence of the APOE e4 allele seems to be associated with risk for poorer outcomes for both adults and children (Kassam, Ganon, & Cusimano; McFadyen et al., 2019). However, this relationship appears to have complex interactions with environmental factors, such as parenting style (Trebel-Barna et al., 2016). Similar relationships have recently been described for genes that are associated with dopamine (e.g., catechol-O-methyltransferase enzyme and presence of the T allele of the gene ANKK1 rs1800497), which is associated with cognitive functions, including executive functioning, that are affected by TBI (Kurowski et al., 2016; Smith-Payne et al., 2018).

Cognitively, recovery from moderate-severe TBI, most rapid within the first 3 to 6 months, tends to plateau after approximately 1 to 2 years, and a significant proportion of children have persistent deficits. Research has demonstrated a dose-response relationship between IQ and injury severity; however, age is also an important factor. For children who sustain injuries during the infancy or preschool years, the impact on IQ is fairly global, and they tend to show a slowed rate of cognitive growth over time (Anderson, Godfrey, Rosenfelt, & Catroppa, 2012). As age at injury increases, however, the effects on IQ become more varied. Vocabulary and other basic linguistic skills may be relatively spared, while abilities that rely on more distributed neural networks (e.g., attention, processing speed, learning and memory, problem solving, abstract reasoning) are more vulnerable to insult (Babikian, 2009). Weaknesses in various aspects of executive functioning likely contribute to significant challenges with academic achievement, adaptive functioning, social and emotional-behavioral functioning (Beauchamp et al., 2011), and may increase over the course of childhood as environmental expectations naturally grow more demanding with age (Petranovich et al., 2020). Children injured during infancy or the preschool years are also at risk for difficulties in the acquisition of a broad range of academic skills. Cognitive functioning is strongly related to academic performance, with better verbal story memory and inhibitory control being particularly associated with kindergarten readiness and early reading, spelling, and math. In contrast, TBI in later childhood or adolescence is generally associated with age-appropriate basic academic achievement, likely reflecting the fact that certain core academic skills such as those underpinning reading (decoding, phonologic processing) are fairly well established earlier in childhood and rely on less widely distributed neural networks (Catroppa et al., 2008). When specific skill-based deficits do occur, reduced mathematics and reading comprehension are most common. Despite adequate performance on most standardized academic tests, children injured at any age often display remarkably poor everyday classroom functioning, and sadly many have unmet academic needs (Petranovich et al., 2020; Wade et al., 2020).

Pediatric moderate-severe TBI increases the risk for a variety of psychosocial problems as well, including depressive and anxious symptoms, disruptive behavior disorders such as oppositional defiant disorder, and secondary attention-deficit/hyperactivity disorder (S-ADHD), which has been found to develop in approximately 15% to 20% of children with TBI who did not display premorbid ADHD (Petranovich et al., 2020; Wade et al., 2020). In general, more severe injury and younger age at injury are related to higher levels of postinjury ADHD and behavior problems, with evidence for latent or emerging behavior problems over time for those injured at younger ages. Older age at injury, by contrast, appears to place individuals at higher risk for internalizing problems, including depression and anxiety. A history of preinjury emotional or behavioral difficulties increases this risk. Personality changes such as increased lability, aggression, and disinhibition are relatively common, whereas mania and psychosis are not (Max et al., 2015). Children with TBI tend to also have worse social cognition and social competence, which places them at risk for peer rejection and victimization (Yeates et al., 2013), educational underachievement, antisocial behavior, drug abuse, mood problems, and even suicide (DeRosier & Lloyd, 2010). Persistent functional deficits (Fay et al., 2009) and reduced health-related quality of life are also common after severe TBI; injury during early childhood may lead to increasing adaptive functioning problems over time.

Compared with cognitive outcomes, research suggests psychosocial difficulties are more likely to be multidetermined and less related to injury-specific factors, more likely to show a stable or even worsening pattern over time (Fay et al., 2009), and often cause greater distress for patients and families than cognitive deficits (Petranovich et al., 2020).

Clinical Management

Rehabilitation

The overarching goal of rehabilitation of children after ABI is to maximize recovery and functioning physically, psychologically, cognitively, and socially. This is done by directing therapeutic intervention at functional impairments and engaging and educating the child, family, school, and community (Gordon & di Maggio, 2012). In the case of more severe TBI an interdisciplinary intensive rehabilitation model, typically through an inpatient program, is recommended to maximize early functional return in brain injury recovery and to best prepare the patient and family system for success upon reintegration into the home and community given the child's new functional level. Continued outpatient follow-up with therapies (Table 32.4), rehabilitation physicians, psychologists, neuropsychologists, and educational specialists is also recommended given the frequent continued needs across development (Keenan, Clark, Holubkov, Cox, & Ewing-Cobbs, 2018).

TABLE 32.4 Commonly Recommended Therapy Disciplines and Roles

Discipline	Clinical Focus
Physical Therapy	Big body motor movements such as sitting, standing, transfers, balance, and walking. Help establish home exercise and cardiopulmonary conditioning programs.
Occupational Therapy	Upper body movements, feeding and swallowing, vision and activities of daily living such as bathing, toileting, dressing, and higher-level thinking skills.
Speech Therapy	Speaking and understanding of language, feeding and swallowing, and cognitive skills such as memory and executive functioning.
Behavioral/ Psychological Therapy	Maladaptive behaviors, mood, coping and adjustment using a range of psychological interventions and techniques.

TABLE 32.5 **Commonly Utilized Medications After Traumatic Brain Injury**

Symptom Targets	Example Medications	Mechanism of Action
Alertness and attention	Amantadine	Indirect dopaminergic agonist
	Methylphenidate	Dopaminergic and noradrenergic agonist
	Carbadopa/levodopa	Dopaminergic agonist
	Bromocriptine	Indirect dopaminergic agonist
Paroxysmal sympathetic Hyperactivity (tachycardia, hyperthermia, hypertension, tachypnea, dystonia)	Propranolol	Central beta blocker
	Clonidine	Alpha agonist
	Opiates	Mu agonist
	Dantrolene	Depresses the intrinsic mechanisms of excitation-contraction coupling in skeletal muscle
	Bromocriptine	Indirect dopaminergic agonist, sympatholytic
Hypertonicity	Baclofen	GABA B receptor agonist
	Benzodiazepine	GABA A receptor agonist
	Tizanidine	Alpha 2 adrenergic receptor agonist
	Dantrolene	Skeletal muscle contraction coupling depressant
	Botulinum toxin	Intramuscular snare protein antagonist
Sleep	Melatonin	Melatonin receptor type 1 A agonist
	Trazodone	Serotonin transporter and serotonin type 2 receptor antagonist
	Clonidine	Alpha agonist
	Quetiapine	Serotonin, dopamine, histamine, and adrenergic antagonist
Mood	SSRIs	Serotonin antagonist
	SNRIs	Serotonin and norepinephrine antagonists
	Atypical antipsychotics	Antidopaminergic (D2), mixed noradrenergic, cholinergic, and histaminergic antagonists

SNRI, Serotonin and norepinephrine reuptake inhibitor; *SSRI*, selective serotonin reuptake inhibitor.

Medication Management

Pharmacologic interventions in children with moderate to severe TBI are generally aimed at the following objectives after the acute intensive care phase: controlling sympathetic surges, increasing alertness and attention, restoring sleep/wake cycles, reducing hypertonicity, and stabilizing mood and behavior (Table 32.5).

Neuropsychological Monitoring

Pediatric neuropsychologists evaluate cognition and social-emotional functioning within the context of typical and atypical brain development to inform interventions. Due to the complex and multifaceted influence of developmental, familial-genetic, and social-contextual factors on outcomes after moderate-severe pediatric TBI, regular neuropsychological monitoring is an important component of long-term care. This is particularly true for young children given risks for late-emerging deficits or slowed rates of development over time. Neuropsychological assessments conducted earlier in recovery can be useful for supporting the child and family's community reintegration and securing necessary educational, behavioral, and community-based services. Typically assessments are then recommended regularly over the course of development to continue to monitor for ongoing recovery and/or the emergence of cognitive, emotional-behavioral, and functional problems. This proactive approach can serve to identify problems and risk factors to help support those families who may be least likely (e.g., due to financial or social factors) to seek out or secure services.

Psychological and Behavioral Interventions

Relatively few randomized, controlled studies have investigated psychosocial interventions after pediatric TBI. The limited pediatric TBI-specific research does suggest that interventions derived from traditional applied behavioral analysis methodologies as well as those grounded in the provision of proactive, antecedent-focused support (such as with proactive behavioral intervention supports) are considered evidence-based interventions for TBI (Ylvisaker et al., 2007). Additionally, family-based problem-solving interventions (Wade et al., 2019) using a combination of problem solving, family communication training, and antecedent behavior management have shown utility via multiple randomized controlled clinical trials for improving externalizing and internalizing behavior problems, social competence, and behavior ratings of executive functions, as well as reducing family distress and caregiver depression.

Family-based interventions seem to be more effective than a problem-solving intervention provided to adolescents individually, without the family component (Laatsch et al., 2020).

Cognitive Rehabilitation

While quality data on the results of cognitive rehabilitation interventions in pediatrics remain limited, there has been a significant increase in studies in recent years. A recent systematic review by Laatsch et al. (2020) identified evidence for several practice standards and guidelines. Specifically, attention process training and process-specific attention and memory training paired with metacognitive strategy training were recommended as a practice standard. Family-based interventions for improving executive functioning were recommended as a practice standard, while metacognitive training was put forth as a practice guideline. While there is emerging evidence for specific technology-based interventions without clinician support, such as Cog-Med and Neuropage for improving working memory and memory, it is less clear whether they will be effective for individuals with more severe memory and executive functioning impairments, and to what degree they generalize to daily functioning.

Educational Supports

In the United States the average length of a hospital stay after pediatric TBI has been decreasing in recent decades, and comprehensive outpatient rehabilitation programs have become less available. Thus much postinjury rehabilitation and support is now expected to occur within the educational system. Unfortunately, quality research examining specific educational interventions after pediatric TBI is strikingly absent, perhaps in part because of the significant variability in the needs and settings of each child. A recent systematic review and metaanalysis identified only three qualifying studies published between 1980 and 2017; no statistically significant effects of educational interventions were identified (Linden, Glang, & McKinlay, 2018). Given the lack of direct empirical support, at this point, school intervention following TBI must rely on indirect studies conducted with populations who may display similar manifest problems (e.g., ADHD).

Jacob was referred for a neuropsychological evaluation by his primary care provider given concerns for academic underachievement, mood and behavior problems, and poor social functioning. The evaluation revealed solid intellectual and basic academic skills but weaknesses with fine motor skills, processing speed, attention, memory, and executive functioning. These problems were thought to be contributing to his difficulties keeping up with schoolwork and earning good grades. Further, problems with self-regulation were thought to be contributing to behavioral problems and new symptoms of depression. An increase in educational support was recommended, and he was referred to a pediatric rehabilitation medicine physician for medical management of attention and mood concerns, as well as a family-based problem-solving intervention to further manage his brain injury–related impairments in executive functioning, mood, and behavior.

MILD TRAUMATIC BRAIN INJURY

In the last several decades considerable progress has been made in characterizing outcomes after pediatric mild TBI (aka concussion). Two domains that have received much of the empirical attention are cognitive outcomes measured objectively by performance-based tests and symptom outcomes measured subjectively by parent and/or child report.

When measuring cognitive functioning objectively in the first hours to days after mild TBI, large effects can be seen (Williams, Puetz, Giza, & Broglio, 2015). Most methodologically rigorous studies indicate cognitive deficits resolve rapidly, rarely persisting for more than 1 month (Hung et al., 2014; Williams et al., 2015). When measuring outcome using subjective report, a constellation of symptoms are commonly seen, including headache, dizziness, fatigue, inattention, and forgetfulness. Sport-related concussion studies indicate that pronounced symptomatology is reported in the first hours to days postinjury, with resolution similar to cognitive outcomes in a matter of days to weeks (Chrisman, Rivara, Schiff, Zhou, & Comstock, 2013). More variability is apparent in samples recruited from hospital settings, with a minority of pediatric patients displaying symptoms for some months (Ledoux et al., 2019). By 1 year postinjury, however, persistent symptoms are rare (Hung et al., 2014).

In clinical settings persistent symptoms attributed to a history of mild TBI are common. Such symptoms are influenced by both injury and noninjury factors. One injury-related factor is mild TBI severity. As severity worsens (but still within the mild range) the risk for persistent problems increases. The presence of intracranial abnormalities on conventional neuroimaging is the clearest marker of severity that influences outcome, so these injuries are now known as complicated mild TBI (Hung et al., 2014). The amount of outcome variance explained by injury-related factors diminishes over time, with many persistent postconcussive symptoms driven by nonconcussion factors. For example, persistent symptoms have been found to be associated with demographic factors, premorbid symptomatology, premorbid learning and psychosocial problems, postinjury symptom exaggeration and/or feigning, maladaptive coping, comorbid bodily injury and pain, parental attributional biases, and parental anxiety and family stress (Kirkwood, 2019).

Clinical management early after mild TBI should always include medical providers as minor head trauma can be associated with other pathology, including cervical injury, skull fracture, and intracranial lesions. Another clinical focus soon after injury should be psychoeducation, focused on ensuring the family understands that most youth display initial problems but recover relatively quickly. At some point within the first weeks, transitioning youth back to their usual activities (in which they are unlikely to sustain a repeat concussion) is apt to be helpful, even if they remain symptomatic. For those with persistent symptoms, an active rehabilitation approach that includes physical therapy targeted at cervical, vestibular, visual, and autonomic dysfunction is also likely to be more effective than a rest-based approach (Gauvin-Lepage et al., 2020).

In cases with persistent problems disentangling the multiple factors that can influence symptoms is key to identifying effective specific management approaches. One method to help in this endeavor is neuropsychological assessment, which can be used to not only evaluate cognitive and psychosocial status after TBI but has shown promise in actually reducing persistent postconcussive symptoms (Kirkwood, Peterson, Connery, Baker, & Forster, 2016).

Educationally based management of mild TBI typically involves an initial period of missed school (e.g., 1–3 days) to allow for brief rest before transitioning back with some temporary academic adjustments. Too slow a return to school can serve to protract a child's recovery (e.g., by causing undue stress secondary to feelings of falling behind, being away from friends). Because outcomes after uncomplicated mild TBI are favorable, very few concussed students should need longer-term educational supports.

Sport-based management of pediatric mild TBI is most often focused on whether an athlete is safe to return to play. Experts agree that pediatric athletes should always be removed from competition after a suspected concussion and not be allowed to return until they have undergone a proper evaluation by a provider familiar with mild TBI. Once an athlete is free of all concussion-related problems, consensus guidelines encourage a graduated return to play, with the athlete needing to remain free of new symptoms without medication before progressing in the protocol and being cleared for game play (McCrory et al., 2017).

ABUSIVE HEAD TRAUMA

Research suggests that approximately half of severe TBI in infants can be attributed to AHT and that these children are at higher risk for worse outcomes than nonabusive injuries (Keenan, Presson, Clark, Cox, & Ewing-Cobbs, 2019). As has been noted for children who have sustained accidental injuries, factors such as earlier age at injury (particularly those injured <6 months of age), preinjury developmental delays, and those from lower-income or single-parent homes are at particularly high risk for poorer outcomes. In addition to these well-described general factors, some specific factors seen after AHT are also associated with poorer outcomes such as presence or extent of retinal and vitreous hemorrhages, seizures, and cranial growth deceleration. However, extremely limited research on long-term outcomes after AHT is available; due to the limited repertoire of skills expected for very young children, those injured very young may have a sign-free interval where they have appeared to recover, only to develop emerging deficits years later as they fail to meet expected developmental milestones (Lind et al., 2016). While impairments in motor, visual, and language functioning are common after AHT (up to 50%–60% of children), attention problems are particularly common (nearly 80%).

Alarmingly, Keenan et al. (2019) noted that, although 60% of children with severe TBI sustained in the infancy or toddler period scored in the "assess" range on the Ages and Stages Questionnaire (ASQ-3) 12-months after injury, less than one-third were receiving early childhood intervention services. Thus a substantial proportion of patients with AHT have unmet needs, which may contribute to further gaps in subsequent educational service provision. Children with AHT require close monitoring and should be referred early for services versus taking a wait and see approach.

ANOXIC BRAIN INJURIES

Anoxic brain injury occurs due to a transient restriction of oxygen to the brain and can be caused by any number of events that affect cardiopulmonary function. In the literature a distinction is sometimes made between ischemic injuries, which result from a reduction in cerebral blood flow such as with cardiac arrest, and hypoxemic injuries, which are related to a drop in blood oxygen saturation (where glucose and other necessary metabolic substances may remain available), from obstructed breathing such as drowning or suffocation. Some research suggests that ischemic, compared with hypoxemic, injuries may result in more severe and global impairment (Thaler et al., 2012). Other studies have suggested that injuries associated with near-drowning events are associated with poorest outcomes, though this may vary depending on water temperature as colder water temperature may be protective (Johnson, DeMatt, & Salorio, 2009). GCS, need for extended cardiopulmonary resuscitation, and early seizure activity have been associated with poorer outcomes, though the most robust predictor appears to be duration of unconsciousness. Depending on the duration and intensity of the event, anoxic injuries result in neuronal damage with varying degrees of related impairment. Due to the selective vulnerability of neurons in different brain regions, the cortex, hippocampus, cerebellum, and basal ganglia tend to be most susceptible to interruptions in cerebral blood flow, with more severe injuries potentially affecting deeper regions of the brain.

Compared to moderate-severe TBI, research suggests poorer outcomes overall for children with anoxic brain injury; however, this population has received less attention in the empirical literature and therefore less is known regarding typical outcomes (Johnson et al., 2009). A long-term study comparing anoxic brain injury with TBI (Shaklai, Fish, Simantov, & Groswasser, 2018) noted reduced functional independence, including need for personal assistance, higher rates of special education and/or problems with reintegrating into educational settings, and reduced independence with mobility. As with TBI, younger age at injury was associated with poorer outcomes. In terms of neuropsychological outcomes, memory impairment is most ubiquitous, presumably due to the susceptibility of the hippocampus to anoxic episodes. However, diffuse impairment affecting other neurocognitive domains (motor and sensory functions, aspects of higher-level language, visuoperceptual ability, attention, and executive functions) as well as emotional-behavioral challenges also appear to be quite common. Further, some case examples have demonstrated that long-term memory and neurocognitive impairments can be present in children after anoxic injury even in the absence of findings on brain imaging (Thaler et al., 2012). This highlights the importance of neuropsychological assessment in monitoring developmental outcomes over time, as this modality may offer improved sensitivity to injury-related impairments and provide opportunity to inform and recommend appropriate interventions.

CONCLUSIONS AND FUTURE DIRECTIONS

Diffuse ABI is one of the most prevalent and impactful pediatric diagnoses with implications in long-term medical, physical, cognitive, social-emotional, and functional deficits, particularly for those with more severe injuries and those injured at younger ages. Given these wide-reaching implications, access to specialized interdisciplinary interventions to identify challenges early and improve outcomes is an essential component for the care of children with ABI. Continued research is needed to improve pediatric ABI care in domains of primary and secondary injury prevention, improved prognostic modeling, and more effective and efficient therapeutic interventions at the individual, family system, and societal levels.

REFERENCES

Anderson, V. A., Godfrey, C., Rosenfelt, J. V., & Catroppa, C. (2012). Predictors of cognitive function and recovery 10 years after traumatic brain injury in young children. *Pediatrics, 129*.

Anderson, V., Jacobs, R., Spencer-Smith, M., Coleman, L., Anderson, P., Williams, J., … Leventer, R. (2010). Does early age at brain insult predict worse outcome? Neuropsychological implications. *Journal of Pediatric Psychology, 35*(7), 716–727.

Babikian, T., & Asarnow, R. (2009). Neurocognitive outcomes and recovery after pediatric TBI: Meta-analytic review of the literature. *Neuropsychology, 23*(3), 283–296.

Beauchamp, M. H., Beare, R., Ditchfield, M., Coleman, L., Babl, F. E., Kean, M., … Anderson, V. (2013). Susceptibility weighted imaging and its relationship to outcome after pediatric traumatic brain injury. *Cortex, 49*(2), 591–598.

Beauchamp, M., Catroppa, C., Godfrey, C., Morse, S., Rosenfeld, J. V., & Anderson, V. (2011). Selective changes in executive functioning ten years after severe childhood traumatic brain injury. *Developmental Neuropsychology, 36*(5), 578–595.

Brenner, T., Freier, M. C., Holshouser, B. A., Burley, T., & Ashwal, S. (2003). Predicting neuropsychologic outcome after traumatic brain injury in children. *Pediatric Neurology, 28*(2), 104–114.

Bruns Jr., J. H., (2003). The epidemiology of traumatic brain injury: A review. *Epilepsia, 44*, 2–10.

Cassidy, J. D., Carroll, L. J., Peloso, P. M., Borg, J., von Holst, H., Holm, L., … World Health Organization. (2004). Incidence, risk factors and prevention of mild traumatic brain injury: Results of the WHO Collaborating Centre Task Force on Mild Traumatic Brain Injury. *Journal of Rehabilitation Medicine, 43*, S28–S60.

Catroppa, C., Anderson, V. A., Morse, S. A., Haritou, F., & Rosenfeld, J. V. (2008). Outcome and predictors of fuctional recovery 5 years following pediatric traumatic brain injury (TBI). *Journal of Pediatric Psychology, 33*(7), 707–718.

Centers for Disease Control and Prevention, US Department of Health and Human Services. (2019). *Surveillance report of traumatic brain injury-related emergency department visits, hospitalizations, and deaths—United States 2014*. https://stacks.cdc.gov/view/cdc/78062

Chrisman, S. P., Rivara, F. P., Schiff, M. A., Zhou, C., & Comstock, R. D. (2013). Risk factors for concussive symptoms 1 week or longer in high school athletes. *Brain Injury, 27*(1), 1–9.

Fay, T. B., Yeates, K. O., Wade, S. L., Drotar, D., Stancin, T., & Taylor, H. G. (2009). Predicting longitudinal patterns of functional deficits in children with traumatic brain injury. *Neuropsychology, 23*, 271–282.

Ferrazzano, P. A., Rosario, B. L., Wisniewski, S. R., Shafi, N. I., Siefkes, H. M., Miles, D. K., … Bell, M. J. (2019). Use of magnetic resonance imaging in severe pediatric traumatic brain injury: Assessment of current practice. *Journal of Neurosurgery: Pediatrics, 23*(4), 471–479.

Figaji, A. A. (2017). Anatomical and physiological differences between children and adults relevant to traumatic brain injury and the implications for clinical assessment and care. *Frontiers in Neurology, 8*, 685.

Gauvin-Lepage, J., Friedman, D., Grilli, L., Sufrategui, M., De Matteo, C., Iverson, G. L., & Gagnon, I. (2020). Effectiveness of an exercise-based active rehabilitation intervention for youth who are slow to recover after concussion. *Clinical Journal of Sport Medicine, 30*(5), 423–432.

Gordon, A. L., & di Maggio, A. (2012). Rehabilitation for children after acquired brain injury: Current and emerging approaches. *Pediatric Neurology, 46*(6), 339–344.

Holmes, J. F., Palchak, M. J., MacFarlane, T., & Kuppermann, N. (2005). Performance of the pediatric Glasgow Coma Scale in children with blunt head trauma. *Academy of Emergency Medicine, 12*(9), 814–819.

Hung, R., Carroll, L. J., Cancelliere, C., Cote, P., Rumney, P., Keightley, M., … Cassidy, J. D. (2014). Systematic review of the clinical course, natural history, and prognosis for pediatric mild traumatic brain injury: Results of the International Collaboration on Mild Traumatic Brain Injury Prognosis. *Archives of Physical Medicine and Rehabilitation, 95*(3), S174–S191.

Johnson, A. R., DeMatt, E., & Salorio, C. F. (2009). Predictors of outcome following acquired brain injury in children. *Developmental Disabilities, 15*, 124–132.

Kassam, I., Ganon, F., & Cusimano, M. D. (2016). Association of the APOE-e4 allele with outcome of traumatic brain injury in children and youth: A meta-analysis and meta-regression. *Journal of Neurology, Neurosurgery, and Psychiatry, 87*, 433–440.

Keenan, H. T., Clark, A. E., Holubkov, R., Cox, C. S., & Ewing-Cobbs, L. (2018). Psychosocial and executive function recovery trajectories one year after pediatric traumatic brain injury: The influence of age and injury severity. *Journal of Neurotrauma, 35*(2), 286–296.

Keenan, H. T., Presson, A. P., Clark, A. E., Cox, C. S., & Ewing-Cobbs, L. (2019). Longitudinal developmental outcomes after traumatic brain injury in young children: Are infants more vulnerable than toddlers? *Journal of Neurotrauma, 36*, 282–292.

Kirkwood, M. W. (2019). Mild TBI in children and adolescents. In T. W. Silver & D. B. Arciniegas (Eds.), *Textbook of traumatic brain injury* (3rd ed.). American Psychiatric Publishing.

Kirkwood, M. W., Peterson, R. L., Connery, A. K., Baker, D. A., & Forster, J. (2016). A pilot study investigating neuropsychological consultation as an intervention for persistent postconcussive symptoms in a pediatric sample. *Journal of Pediatrics, 169*, 244–249.e241.

Kurowski, B. G., Backelijauw, B., Zang, H., Martin, L. J., Pilipenko, V., Yeates, K., ... Wade, S. (2016). Influence of catechol-o-methyltransferase (COMT) on executive functioning longitudinally after early childhood traumatic brain injury (TBI): Preliminary findings. *Journal of Neurotrauma*, *34*, 2280–2290.

Laatsch, L., Dodd, J., Brown, T., Ciccia, A., Connor, F., Davis, K., ... Yaeger, L. (2020). Evidence-based systematic review of cognitive rehabilitation, emotional, and family treatment studies for children with acquired brain injury literature: 2006 to 2017. *Neuropsychological Rehabilitation*, *30*(1), 130–161.

Ledoux, A. A., Tang, K., Yeates, K. O., Pusic, M. V., Boutis, K., Craig, W. R., ... Pediatric Emergency Research Canada Concussion. (2019). Natural progression of symptom change and recovery from concussion in a pediatric population. *JAMA Pediatrics*, *173*(1), e183820.

Lind, K., Toure, H., Brugel, D., Meyer, P., Laurent-Vannier, A., & Chevignard, M. (2016). Extended follow-up of neurological, cognitive, behavioral, and academic outcomes after severe abusive head trauma. *Child Abuse and Neglect*, *51*, 358–367.

Linden, M. A., Glang, A. E., & McKinlay, A. (2018). A systematic review and meta-analysis of educational interventions for children and adolescents with acquired brain injury. *NeuroRehabilitation*, *42*, 311–323.

Max, J. E., Wilde, E. A., Bigler, E. D., Hanten, G., Dennis, M., Schachar, R. J., ... Levin, H. S. (2015). Personality change due to traumatic brain injury in children and adolescents: Neurocognitive correlates. *Journal of Neuropsychiatry and Clinical Neurosciences*, *27*(4), 272–279.

McCrory, P., Meeuwisse, W., Dvorak, J., Aubry, M., Bailes, J., Broglio, S., ... Vos, P. E. (2017). Consensus statement on concussion in sport—The 5th International Conference on Concussion in Sport. Berlin, October 2016. *British Journal of Sports Medicine*, *51*(11), 838–847.

McFadyen, C. A., Zeiler, F. A., Newcombe, V., Synnot, A., Steyerberg, E., Gruen, R. L., ... Menon, D. K. (2019). Apolipoprotein E4 polymorphism and outcomes from traumatic brain injury: A living systematic review and meta-analysis. *Journal of Neurotrauma*, 1–13. https://doi.org/10.1089/neu.2018.6052.

Petranovich, C. L., Smith-Payne, J., Wade, S. L., Yeates, K. O., Taylor, G., Stancin, T., & Kurowski, B. G. (2020). From early childhood to adolescence: Lessons about traumatic brain injury from the Ohio Head Injury Outcomes study. *Journal of Head Trauma Rehabilitation*, *35*(3), 226–239.

Popernack, M. L., Gray, N., & Reuter-Rice, K. (2015). Moderate-to-severe traumatic brain injury in children: Complications and rehabilitation strategies. *Journal of Pediatric Health Care*, *29*(3), e1–e7.

Ramiro, J. I. K. (2015). Updates on management of anoxic brain injury after cardiac arrest. *Missouri Medicine*, *112*, 136–141.

Schneier, A. J., Shields, B. J., Hostetler, S. G., Xiang, H., & Smith, G. A. (2006). Incidence of pediatric traumatic brain injury and associated hospital resource utilization in the United States. *Pediatrics*, *118*(2), 483–492.

Shaahinfar, A., Whitelaw, K. D., & Mansour, K. M. (2015). Update on abusive head trauma. *Current Opinions in Pediatrics*, *27*(3), 308–314.

Shaklai, S., Fish, R. P., Simantov, M., & Groswasser, Z. (2018). Prognostic factors in childhood-acquired brain injury. *Brain Injury*, *32*, 533–539.

Slomine, B. S., McCarthy, M. L., Ding, R., MacKenzie, E. J., Jaffe, K. M., Aitken, M. E., ... Grovup, C. S. (2006). Health care utilization and needs after pediatric traumatic brain injury. *Pediatrics*, *117*(4), e663–e674.

Smith-Payne, J. M., Trebel-Barna, A., Zhang, N., Zhang, H., Martin, L. J., Yeates, K. O., ... Kurowski, B. G. (2018). The moderating effect of ANKK1 on the association of family environment with longitudinal executive function following traumatic brain injury in early childhood: A preliminary study. *Journal of Neurotrauma*, *35*, 2796–2802.

Tasker, R. C. (2006). Changes in white matter late after severe traumatic brain injury in childhood. *Developmental Neuroscience*, *28*(4-5), 302–308.

Thaler, N. S., Reger, S. L., Ringdahl, E. N., Mayfield, J. W., Goldstein, G., & Allen, D. N. (2012). Neuropsychological profiles of six children with anoxic brain injury. *Child Neuropsychology*, *19*(5), 479–494.

Trebel-Barna, A., Zang, H., Zhang, N., Martin, L. J., Yeates, K. O., Taylor, H. G., ... Kurowski, B. G. (2016). Does apolipoprotein e4 status moderate the association of family environment with long-term child functioning following moderate to severe traumatic brain injury? A preliminary study. *Journal of the International Neuropsychological Society*, *22*, 859–864.

Wade, S. L., Fisher, A. P., Kaizar, E. E., Yeates, K. O., Taylor, H. G., & Zhang, N. (2019). Recovery trajectories of child and family outcomes following online family problem-solving therapy for children and adolescents after traumatic brain injury. *Journal of the International Neuropsychological Society*, *25*(9), 941–949.

Wade, S. L., Kaizar, E. E., Narad, M. E., Zang, H., Kurowski, B. G., Miley, A. E., ... Zhang, N. (2020). Behavior problems following childhood TBI: The role of sex, age, and time since injury. *Journal of Head Trauma Rehabilitation*, *35*(5), 93–404.

Williams, R. M., Puetz, T. W., Giza, C. C., & Broglio, S. P. (2015). Concussion recovery time among high school and collegiate athletes: A systematic review and meta-analysis. *Sports Medicine*, *45*(6), 893–903.

Yeates, K. O., Gerhardt, C. A., Bigler, E. D., Abildskov, T., Dennis, M., Rubin, K. H., ... Vannatta, K. (2013). Peer relationships of children with traumatic brain injury. *Journal of the International Neuropsychological Society*, *19*(5), 518–527.

Ylvisaker, M., Turkstra, L., Coehlo, C., Yorkston, K., Kennedy, M., Sohlberg, M. M., & Avery, J. (2007). Behavioral interventions for children and adults with behaviour disorders after TBI: A systematic review of the evidence. *Brain Injury*, *21*(8), 769–805.

33

Congenital Infections

Megan Honor Pesch and Terri Stillwell

For additional material related to the content of this chapter, please see Chapter 23.

VIGNETTE

A 4-year-old boy is referred to developmental and behavioral pediatrics for disruptive behavior in the setting of a recently diagnosed speech-language delay and left unilateral profound hearing loss. Through your evaluation you additionally diagnose developmental coordination disorder and autism spectrum disorder. Brain imaging done as part of a cochlear implant evaluation reveals trace calcifications and small cysts. As such, you request his banked dried blood spot card from the neonatal metabolic screen and order cytomegalovirus polymerase chain reaction testing. The test results are positive, confirming the diagnosis of congenital cytomegalovirus infection. You refer to ophthalmology and infectious disease specialists and recommend a vestibular evaluation, applied behavioral analysis, as well as speech and physical therapy. Over the next 2 years you guide the family through a special education evaluation, placement in a classroom with appropriate supports, and closely follow his behavior and development.

INTRODUCTION

Some consider congenital infections more broadly, including those that are acquired intrauterine, transplacentally, and those that are acquired intrapartum or soon after birth, oftentimes referred to as perinatally acquired. For the purposes of this chapter, the term congenital infections refer to intrauterine infections, those that are transplacentally transmitted. Additionally, while bacterial entities such as chorioamnionitis can lead to intrauterine infection, the focus of this chapter will be on TORCH (toxoplasma, other, rubella, cytomegalovirus [CMV], and herpes simplex virus [HSV]) infections and emerging viral infections that are more classically associated with congenital infections and potential for adverse outcomes. Due to lack of standard national or international registries and lack of reporting mechanisms, the true global burden of congenital infections is not known.

Congenital infections may result in significant long-term neurodevelopmental sequelae in some children; however, the spectrum of possible outcomes is wide. Concerns for congenital infections can arise *in utero* due to worrying imaging or maternal symptoms and in the neonatal period as a result of physical signs and symptoms. This concern may also arise later on in infancy and childhood as neurodevelopmental sequelae emerge. The majority of infants born with congenital infections present as asymptomatic and therefore go undiagnosed. The lack of universal screening for these infections has contributed to the difficulty in fully characterizing neurodevelopmental outcomes and delays that may be attributed to silent congenital infections. Presentations can vary from seemingly unaffected to severe neuromuscular and cognitive impairments; it should be noted that congenital infections are thought to be a significant contributor to miscarriage and stillbirth in the United States.

Developmental and behavioral pediatricians can play an important role in the care of children with congenital infections. While infectious disease specialists primarily oversee the acute phase treatment of a congenital infection, developmental and behavioral pediatricians are well positioned to monitor, diagnose, treat, and support children experiencing long-term sequelae. Symptoms may impact behavior and development all within the context of a child's social and family environment. Later in this chapter we will discuss the important role of the developmental and behavioral pediatrician in the care of children with congenital infections.

Overview of the Pathophysiology of Congenital Infections

As noted, this chapter will focus on those infections that are intrauterine, transplacentally transmitted. Perinatally acquired infections will not be discussed and should be considered separately, as their presentations and outcomes differ from congenitally acquired infections. Congenital infections are most often hematogenously spread via the placenta where there are breakdowns or defects in the maternal-to-fetus interface, leading to disseminated infection within the fetus. Once in the fetal circulation, the pathogen proceeds to target organs as it does in routine infection. Placental insufficiency itself can lead to miscarriages, stillbirths, and significant fetal morbidity. Additionally, fetal morbidity is caused by both the pathogen itself and the inflammatory response to the pathogen (Frenkel et al., 2018).

There are multiple maternal factors that influence the degree of fetal infection, including whether it is a primary maternal infection and the degree of maternal viremia, parasitemia, or spirochetemia. Primary infection often results in increased risk for intrauterine transmission. Nonetheless, reinfection with a different strain, serotype, or reactivation of previous infection can also cause congenital infection in the right setting (Frenkel et al.,

2018). If maternal infection burden is high, that increases the amount of pathogen at that maternal-fetal interface, increasing likelihood of transmission. Studies of CMV, toxoplasma, and Zika virus seem to indicate certain strains or serotypes are associated with increased risk for maternal reinfection and increased severity of congenital infection (Frenkel et al., 2018).

The gestational age at which maternal infection occurs is also associated with disease severity. Fetuses infected in the first trimester are more likely to have severe disease as opposed to those infected in the third trimester. Given that central nervous system (CNS) development occurs early in embryogenesis, the CNS is particularly vulnerable during early fetal infection. In fact, many early fetal infections result in fetal demise or significant morbidity (Del Pizzo, 2011; Ericson & Benjamin, 2018; Frenkel et al., 2018). Additionally, for those pathogens that are neurotropic, infection can interfere with replication and migration of neuronal cells leading to tissue damage (Frenkel et al., 2018).

CONGENITAL INFECTIONS AND NEURODEVELOPMENTAL OUTCOMES

Types of Congenital Infections

A growing fetus can be affected by viral, bacterial, fungal, or parasitic pathogens. Incidence of these congenital infections vary based on risk of vertical transmission, community levels of maternal seropositivity, and endemic nature of the pathogen in different countries and regions. Specific fetal pathogens and subsequent congenital sequelae are presented in Table 33.1. This list is not comprehensive and provides an overview of the epidemiology, neonatal presentation, and possible neurodevelopmental sequelae of more commonly seen congenital infections.

TORCH INFECTIONS

TORCH, as mentioned, is an acronym that refers to a group of congenital infections: toxoplasmosis, other, rubella, CMV, and HSV. The "other" category is somewhat ambiguous and may include other less common congenital infections such as those listed in Table 33.1. Although the TORCH infections are all mentioned in Table 33.1, in this section closer attention is devoted to the most common congenital infections, which also have the potential for poorer neurodevelopmental outcomes. These congenital infections are consequently of more importance to developmental and behavioral pediatricians.

Congenital Cytomegalovirus

Congenital CMV (cCMV) is the most common congenital infection in the United States, the leading nongenetic cause of neonatal sensorineural hearing loss (SNHL), and can lead to poorer neurodevelopmental outcomes (Fowler & Boppana, 2018). As such, we have devoted more text to discussing cCMV than other less common infections.

Epidemiology

In the United States 1 in 150 to 200 infants is born with cCMV. Infants born to women from marginalized communities, those with African and/or Hispanic race/ethnicity, as well as those who live in poverty are thought to have a fivefold risk increase (Fowler et al., 2018). The exact US incidence is unknown due to lack of universal neonatal screening and that cCMV is not a reportable disease.

Presentation and Classification of Disease

The classically taught "blueberry muffin" presentation of an infant with cCMV is rare. In reality 85% to 90% of infants are born without visible signs, with most of the remaining 10% to 15% presenting with one or more often subtle signs (e.g., petechiae, late preterm birth, symmetric small for gestational age) (Fowler & Boppana, 2018). As such, it is estimated that only 1% of cases are diagnosed. Other silent symptoms at birth include SNHL, intracranial abnormalities, chorioretinitis, and seizures (Manicklal et al., 2013). cCMV is often classified as "symptomatic" versus "asymptomatic" based on visible signs at birth alone; however, infants with both presentations can have SNHL and may be at risk of later sequelae (Korndewal et al., 2017). This binary classification of a wide spectrum of disease, including the term *asymptomatic*, provides false reassurance to parents and medical providers and has contributed to inconclusive research on neurodevelopmental outcomes.

Neurodevelopmental Outcomes

Based on the limited existing literature, it is thought that 80% of infants born with cCMV will have no long-term sequelae, although this remains an area of active research. The literature to date generally shows that infants born with microcephaly or significant intracranial findings (e.g., neuronal migration disorders) have poorer neurodevelopmental outcomes than those with milder presentations. However, severely symptomatic infants represent 1% to 5% of cCMV cases and contribute to a wide variety of potential outcomes. In general children with cCMV have increased risk of cerebral palsy with a medium correlation to intracranial lesions. Spastic quadriplegia is thought to be more common among children with cerebral palsy and cCMV versus cerebral palsy attributed to other causes. Children with cCMV can also exhibit hypotonia, thought to be due to lenticulostriate vasculopathy adjacent to the basal ganglia (Frankovich et al., 2017). Vestibular disturbances may affect up to 80% of children with cCMV (Pinninti et al., 2021). As such, gross motor delay is common.

Speech and language outcomes have been largely studied in relation to hearing outcomes. SNHL affects 40% of infants born with visible signs at birth and 10% to 15% of infants born without signs at birth. Unique to cCMV is the variable nature of associated hearing loss, which can fluctuate from unilateral or bilateral, sudden onset or progressive over childhood, especially prior to age 5 years (Rawlinson et al., 2017). It is recommended that children with cCMV, regardless of their presentation, have long-term monitoring of their hearing

TABLE 33.1 **Congenital Infections, Pathogens, and Outcomes**

Pathogen	Incidence and Epidemiology Notes	Neonatal Presentation	Childhood Neurodevelopmental Sequelae	Comments
Trypanosoma cruzi (Chagas)	5% of liveborn infants to chronically infected women, endemic in areas of Latin America	Most often no visible signs at birth; fetal growth restriction, encephalitis, hepatosplenomegaly, sepsis, myocarditis, hepatitis	Most congenitally infected infants have no long-term sequelae	
Plasmodium falciparum and *Plasmodium vivax* (malaria)	Varied incidence across endemic areas (5% in Africa, but up to 42% in endemic areas with unstable transmission patterns)	Often asymptomatic, although fetal growth restriction and preterm birth can result from placental compromise. Neonatal symptoms occur at 3–12 wk of age and include fever, irritability, jaundice, hepatosplenomegaly	At present, specific neurodevelopmental sequelae associated with congenital malaria have not been firmly established	Hypothesized mechanism of poorer neurodevelopmental outcomes due to perinatal insult, elevated serum cytokines, and placental infection
Cytomegalovirus	Industrialized nations: 1%–2% live births; > in low SES and marginalized groups. Developing nations: 6%–14% live births; > in areas of higher HIV prevalence	80% have no physical signs +/– SNHL, 10% have one or more subtle signs: SGA, microcephaly, petechiae, hepatosplenomegaly, conjugated hyperbilirubinemia, chorioretinitis +/– SNHL "Blueberry muffin" presentation with multiple signs is rare	SNHL common, which can be progressive over childhood even in infants born without signs at birth. Increased risk of cerebral palsy, vestibular dysfunction, developmental delays, and autism. Those with intracranial findings > risk of intellectual disability, spastic quadriplegia, visual impairment, and global developmental delay	All infants require hearing monitoring throughout childhood. Close monitoring for delays/autism, especially in the setting of vision/hearing loss
Herpes simplex virus	True congenital infection in a liveborn infant rare, neonatal/perinatal infection more common, <0.001% of live births	Cutaneous (vesicular bullous rashes), ophthalmologic, and central nervous system findings (hydrocephalus, white matter lesions, seizures, lethargy, hypotonia, encephalitis, etc.)	Vision loss, severe gross motor, and neurologic impairment in surviving infants. Due to the rarity of congenital disease, the literature describes single cases or small case series who have not presented with a singular phenotype at birth or later in childhood	95% of cases in newborns are acquired in the postpartum and peripartum periods, but not congenitally
Parvovirus B19	Incidence peaks in spring and summer in United States; 3.5% of pregnancies exposed, incidence of congenital infection unclear ~0.03% of live births	Parvovirus does not seem to cause fetal malformations but can cause severe fetal anemia, which may lead to nonimmune fetal hydrops, ventriculomegaly, heart failure, and fetal demise	Most children (99%) have no known adverse neurodevelopmental sequelae. Infants born with hydrops have increased with "abnormal neurodevelopmental outcomes" (10%, e.g., mild ID, fine motor delay). Severe complications (e.g., polymicrogyria, profound ID) are rare	Intrauterine transfusions for parvovirus related increases risk of cerebral palsy and severe developmental disability (~10%)

TABLE 33.1 Congenital Infections, Pathogens, and Outcomes—cont'd

Pathogen	Incidence and Epidemiology Notes	Neonatal Presentation	Childhood Neurodevelopmental Sequelae	Comments
Human immunodeficiency virus (HIV)	Widespread testing and intrapartum antiretroviral treatment have lowered incidence of congenital infections	Most infants are born asymptomatic. Two categories of infants born to HIV+ mothers: HIV exposed but uninfected and HIV+	Children born either HIV exposed but uninfected or HIV+ at risk of lower cognitive and motor abilities (vs. unexposed controls)	
Listeria monocytogenes	Congenital disease is rare. Neonatal listeriosis occurs in 0.09 per 1000 live births, including early onset (congenital) and late onset (perinatal) cases	Increased risk of fetal demise and preterm birth. Early onset disease (~36 hr after birth): sepsis, respiratory distress or pneumonia, meningitis. Late onset disease (5 days–2 wk postpartum): sepsis and meningitis	Long-term outcomes are largely manifestations of neonatal meningitis, including global developmental delay, intellectual disability, cerebral palsy, hearing or vision loss, epilepsy	
Rubivirus (rubella)	Extremely rare in United States, <1000 cases per year	High perinatal mortality rate and preterm birth. Cataracts, congenital heart defects, SNHL, retinopathy, glaucoma, microcephaly	Relatively low incidence of developmental delays and learning difficulties (6%) as compared to other congenital infections. Hearing loss occurs in ~80%, vision loss in ~25%	
Treponema pallidum (syphilis)	Increasing US incidence ~0.1 per 1000 live births, disproportionately affects Black and Hispanic populations; 25% of pregnancies result in intrauterine fetal demise or miscarriage	Early congenital syphilis (symptomatic onset in the first 2 yr of life): hepatomegaly, jaundice, hemolytic anemia, thrombocytopenia, maculopapular rash, osteochondritis	Late congenital syphilis (manifestations after 2 yr of age), occurs in ~40% untreated infants, occurs as a result of scarring from early infection, including osteocutaneous abnormalities (frontal bossing, anterior bowing of shins, widely spaced upper incisors, etc.), as well as vision loss due to glaucoma, SNHL, hydrocephalus, and ID	
Toxoplasma gondii	Global incidence of 1.5 per 1000 live births; highest seroprevalence in Latin America	Most infants present as asymptomatic (80%–90%). Symptomatic infants may have fever, maculopapular rash and classic triad of chorioretinitis, intracranial calcifications, and hydrocephalus	At risk of recurrent chorioretinitis and vision loss	Included in universal newborn screening programs in several developed nations, but not in the United States, Canada, or the United Kingdom
Varicella zoster virus	Congenital varicella zoster is rare, 0.1 per 1000 live births	Clinical features present in ~1% of cases. Skin lesions, neurologic and eye defects, limb hypoplasia, fetal growth restriction, cortical atrophy	Symptoms and organs affected at birth associated with later outcomes. Children born asymptomatic are not at increased risk of poorer neurodevelopmental or behavioral outcomes	

Continued

TABLE 33.1 Congenital Infections, Pathogens, and Outcomes—cont'd

Pathogen	Incidence and Epidemiology Notes	Neonatal Presentation	Childhood Neurodevelopmental Sequelae	Comments
Zika virus	Congenital Zika syndrome refers to the most severely affected infants	Severe microcephaly, brain anomalies, ocular findings, congenital contractures, and neurologic impairment	5%–40% of congenitally exposed infants will have associated long-term sequelae, including severe mobility impairment and gross motor delays due to spasticity, hyperreflexia, posturing, contractures, hip and knee dislocations, club foot. Neuro-irritability (85%), intellectual disability, dysphagia, and SNHL. Ocular findings and vision loss in ~50% of those with persistent microcephaly	Neuroimaging not reliable predictor of developmental outcomes. Long-term outcomes have not yet been studied, particularly in areas of academic achievement, learning, and cognition

ID, Intellectual disability; *SES*, socioeconomic status; *SGA*, small for gestational age; *SNHL*, sensorineural hearing loss.

through age 5, although some recommend monitoring into adolescence (Rawlinson et al., 2017). Children with cCMV may have increased risk of attention-deficit/hyperactivity disorder and executive functioning deficits, although the literature on this is mixed (Korndewal et al., 2017). Autism spectrum disorder (ASD) may also be more common among children with cCMV, which is discussed in more detail later. Of note, early treatment with valganciclovir has been associated with improved hearing and development outcomes at 24 months in infants born with visible symptoms. Use of antiviral medication in infants born without visible signs or with isolated hearing loss has not yet been supported in the literature (Rawlinson et al., 2017).

Congenital Toxoplasmosis

Epidemiology

Toxoplasma gondii is a protozoan parasite that is often related to foodborne and zoonotic infections but can also lead to intrauterine infections. Given toxoplasmosis is not a reportable infection, it is difficult to know the true prevalence of infection in the United States. A recent national survey found 10.42% seropositivity in individuals 6 years and older, with a seroprevalence in childbearing-age women of 7.5%; most of these infections are asymptomatic (Jones et al., 2018). Seroprevalence is much higher in other nations. Roughly 400 to 4000 infants are born with congenital toxoplasmosis in the United States each year. Risk of vertical transmission is higher, while severity of disease is less later in the pregnancy (Contopoulos-Ioannidis & Montoya, 2018).

Presentation and Classification of Disease

At birth, 80% to 90% of infants with congenital toxoplasmosis present as subclinical, without apparent signs. When affected, intracranial calcifications, hydrocephalus, and chorioretinitis are the classic triad of presenting signs in infancy, sometimes presenting months after birth (Frankovich et al., 2017). Chorioretinitis affects 23% of infants born to mothers who received antibiotic treatment during pregnancy, and 73% of those whose mothers did not receive antibiotics (Maldonado et al., 2017). Reduction of visual acuity can occur through the third decade of life. Other presenting symptoms at birth can include hepatosplenomegaly, petechial rash, jaundice, lymphadenopathy, and a spectrum of neurologic findings (Contopoulos-Ioannidis & Montoya, 2018; Maldonado et al., 2017).

Neurodevelopmental Outcomes

Long-term neurodevelopmental outcomes for those with treated and untreated congenital toxoplasmosis are not well researched outside of ocular outcomes. Most work to date has found little to no evidence of increased risk of developmental or cognitive delays in children born with congenital toxoplasmosis who receive treatment as infants, especially those with mild presentations (Maldonado et al., 2017). However, there have been no recent studies examining neurodevelopmental outcomes in children with congenital toxoplasmosis in the last decade. One large study in a European cohort found no difference in risk of motor, speech and language, or cognitive delays at 3 years of age compared to unaffected controls, even when controlling for treatment status (Freeman et al., 2005). Unsurprisingly, children who present with severe neurologic manifestations such as microcephaly, seizures, hydrocephaly, or encephalopathy, who represent a minority of cases, have poorer long-term neurodevelopmental outcomes than those born without neurologic manifestations.

Congenital Syphilis

Epidemiology

Syphilitic disease has been present for centuries. However, the causative agent, *Treponema pallidum*, was not discovered until 1905 (Dobson & Sanchez, 2019). In 2018 the Centers for Disease Control and Prevention (CDC) reported 115,045 new diagnoses of syphilis with 1306 new cases of congenital syphilis (CDC, 2017; Kimball et al., 2020). The number of cases of congenital syphilis was a 261% increase from the number reported in 2013, mirroring the rise in new cases of primary and secondary syphilis diagnoses, primarily impacting minority communities (CDC, 2017; Kimball et al., 2020). Six percent of neonates were stillborn and 33% were symptomatic at birth (Kimball et al., 2020). Neonates born to mothers with earlier stages of syphilitic disease have higher risk of transmission compared to those born to mothers with late-stage disease, correlating to the degree of maternal spirochetemia (Dobson & Sanchez, 2019).

Presentation and Classification of Disease

Signs and symptoms of untreated congenital syphilis may be present at birth or may emerge in the weeks to years after birth. While most neonates born to untreated mothers are asymptomatic (<10% symptomatic at birth), early congenital syphilis (birth–2 years of age, most occur at <3 months of age) may present with fever, rash, hepatosplenomegaly, snuffles, skeletal changes, CNS abnormalities, ocular findings, and low birthweight (Bowen et al., 2015; Dobson & Sanchez, 2019). Late congenital syphilis (defined as presenting after 2 years of age) may not present with signs until several years of age or in rare cases may remain dormant until adulthood. Clinical findings are thought to be related to scarring from early infection and persistent inflammation due to lack of treatment and therefore are often not reversible (Dobson & Sanchez, 2019). Signs and symptoms may include vision loss, bone pain, abnormal sensitivity to light, SNHL, and other CNS symptoms similar to those found in tertiary syphilis as well as cutaneous signs (e.g., saddle nose, peg-shaped incisors, frontal bossing, anal and mouth fissures) (Dobson & Sanchez, 2019; Rawstron & Hawkes, 2017).

Neurodevelopmental Outcomes

Infants exposed to syphilis during pregnancy, regardless of whether they are congenitally infected, are at risk for poorer neurodevelopmental outcomes (Verghese et al., 2018). However, studies of long-term outcomes have been limited by sample size (high perinatal mortality rate) and have included infants born to mothers with known prior syphilis infection who received treatment. In these small studies children with intrauterine syphilis exposure had a high rate of neurodevelopmental impairment (defined as having cerebral palsy, vision or hearing loss, seizure disorder, or cognitive delays) (27%) and speech-language delay (40%) as toddlers (Verghese et al., 2018). Ocular inflammatory processes may also impact vision development, and skeletal abnormalities may also cause extreme pain and decreased mobility.

EMERGING CONGENITAL INFECTIONS

Over the past decade, emerging infections such as Ebola virus, Zika virus, and COVID-19 have been noted to have potential for intrauterine transmission and have raised increasing concerns for congenital infections. In the following sections we focus on Zika virus and SARS-CoV-2, given their role in recent public health emergencies.

Zika Virus

Epidemiology

In 2015 an outbreak of Zika virus in Brazil revealed a causal relationship between the virus and severe congenital anomalies, most notably microcephaly. As of 2019, 87 countries and territories have reported Zika virus transmission (World Health Organization, 2019).

Presentation and Classification of Disease

Zika virus primarily presents as a febrile illness, associated with rash, conjunctivitis, and arthritis or arthralgias in the mother. Vertical transmission of Zika virus can result in intrauterine fetal demise, miscarriage, or severe birth defects, most prominent of which is severe microcephaly (Honein et al., 2017). Zika virus most notably impacts the developing fetal CNS, with 84% to 91% of infants born with brain anomalies (Smoots et al., 2020). Zika-associated microcephaly is distinct from proportional microcephaly and is felt due to disruption in the fetal brain sequence, leading to a collapsed skull with overlapping sutures, a prominent occipital bone, and presence of redundant skin (Moore et al., 2017). The virus may continue replicating in infants' brains after birth, with some infants developing microcephaly between 5 and 11 months of age. Other sequelae include subluxation of large joint, conductive hearing loss, vision loss, abnormal posturing, and exaggerated primitive reflexes, epilepsy, reflux, and severe irritability (Moore et al., 2017).

Neurodevelopmental Outcomes

In general, cognitive outcomes are associated with head circumference at birth, with smaller head circumferences inferring a poorer prognosis. Two-thirds of infants with congenital Zika syndrome are born with severe microcephaly and are therefore expected to have intellectual disability in the severe-profound range. Additional high rates of severe language and motor impairment are also found. It is estimated that most children with congenital Zika syndrome will not attain mastery of developmental milestones beyond the toddler age. Behavioral sequelae may include severe irritability, inconsolability, abnormal sleep patterns, and self-injurious behaviors. Current guidance recommends ongoing developmental, visual, and auditory monitoring for patients with congenital Zika syndrome (Hendrixson & Newland, 2018).

Novel Coronavirus Disease 2019 (COVID-19)

This section was written using the most up-to-date evidence available at the time of the writing of this chapter. Especially in newer emerging infections such as COVID-19, large or longitudinal studies have not been conducted and, as such, preliminary assumptions need to be made with regard to the pathophysiology, presentation, and long-term outcomes of affected neonates. Here we summarize the known data to date and acknowledge that this will continue to be a rapidly changing area.

Epidemiology

In early 2020 the World Health Organization announced the presence of a novel coronavirus, subsequently referred to as COVID-19, which rapidly spread to pandemic levels. Based on the available literature, COVID-19 does not seem to have a high rate of vertical transmission, ranging from 0% to 9%, with most studies finding transmission to be less than 3% (Yang & Liu, 2020). Case reports provide evidence of possible intrauterine transmission. The overwhelming majority of infants born to COVID-19–positive mothers are reported to have favorable outcomes (Yang & Liu, 2020). There is a possible increased risk of preterm birth in neonates born to COVID-19–positive mothers, although these rates may be confounded by iatrogenic premature delivery in mothers with severe disease (Flaherman et al., 2020; Woodworth et al., 2020).

Neurodevelopmental Outcomes

At present, increased risk of neurodevelopmental delays in COVID-19–exposed infants has not been reported; however, the majority of mothers developed symptoms in their third trimester. Three case reports hint at the potential for neurologic involvement; long-term follow-up was not reported (Correia et al., 2020; Lorenz et al., 2020; Vivanti et al., 2020). The impact of COVID-19 on early pregnancy and long-term neurodevelopmental outcomes is unknown but will be an area of particular importance to developmental and behavioral pediatricians.

CONGENITAL INFECTIONS AND HYPOTHETICAL RISK OF AUTISM SPECTRUM DISORDER

In utero infections have been hypothesized to increase risk of ASD by promoting aberrant synaptic pruning by fetal microglia (see Chapter 41 for additional discussion of risk factors for ASD) (Meltzer & Van De Water, 2017). Retrospective analyses using newborn dried blood spot testing have reported cCMV prevalence as high as 5% in children with ASD (Gentile et al., 2017). This remains an area of investigation, with inconclusive evidence, largely due to lack of universal neonatal screening for congenital infections at birth making large prospective observational studies challenging. If congenital infections were found to be a proximal risk factor for ASD, public health interventions around infection prevention could, in theory, lower ASD incidence.

THE ROLE OF THE DEVELOPMENTAL AND BEHAVIORAL PEDIATRICIAN

Developmental and behavioral pediatricians are uniquely positioned to evaluate, monitor, and support children with congenital infections and their families. Depending on the type and severity of a congenital infection, developmental evaluation and ongoing surveillance may be needed, yet may also be outside the comfort of general practitioners. The developmental and behavioral pediatrician may follow children closely in early childhood, while development is rapidly changing, trajectories are being established, and the opportunity for early intervention is available. Developmental and behavioral pediatricians may also oversee the coordination of follow-up with other subspecialists, for instance ensuring that a child with congenital toxoplasmosis receives routine follow-up with a pediatric ophthalmologist. Due to their subspecialty training, developmental and behavioral pediatricians may have a higher index of suspicion for later onset developmental or behavioral sequelae of congenital infections than general practitioners (e.g., suspecting hearing loss in a 4-year-old with asymptomatic cCMV and speech delay, as in the case vignette).

Alternatively, developmental and behavioral pediatricians may also consider silent congenital infections as contributors to current behavioral or developmental challenges. Later diagnosis may aid in obtaining treatment when available, help better understand the possible prognosis, and avoid costly additional workup for genetic contributors. As experts in child development and behavior, developmental and behavioral pediatricians can help disentangle concerns for neurodevelopmental differences and sensory impairments. Neurodevelopmental differences can, at times, mask underlying vision or hearing loss, which in turn can impact neurodevelopment. Other times, developmental delays or behavioral difficulties can be falsely attributed to sensory impairments rather than identified as a separate diagnosis (e.g., a child with cCMV, cerebral palsy, bilateral SNHL, and decreased visual acuity who presents with rigid, repetitive behaviors and social pragmatic delays).

REFERENCES

Bowen, V., Su, J., Torrone, E., Kidd, S., & Weinstock, H. (2015). Increase in incidence of congenital syphilis—United States, 2012–2014. *MMWR*. https://doi.org/10.15585/mmwr.mm6444a3

Centers for Disease Control and Prevention. (2017). *Syphilis—CDC fact sheet (detailed)*. https://www.cdc.gov/std/syphilis/stdfact-syphilis-detailed.htm

Contopoulos-Ioannidis, D., & Montoya, J. G. (2018). Toxoplasma gondii (toxoplasmosis). In *Principles and practice of pediatric infectious diseases*. https://doi.org/10.1016/B978-0-323-40181-4.00273-5

Correia, C. R., Marçal, M., Vieira, F., Santos, E., Novais, C., Maria, A. T., … Tuna, M. L. (2020). Congenital SARS-CoV-2 infection in a neonate with severe acute respiratory syndrome. *Pediatric Infectious Disease Journal*. https://doi.org/10.1097/INF.0000000000002941

Del Pizzo. J. (2011). Focus on diagnosis: Congenital infections (TORCH). *Pediatrics in Review*. https://doi.org/10.1542/pir.32-12-537

Dobson, S., & Sanchez, P. (2019). Syphilis. In Cherry, Harrison, Kaplan, Steinbach, & Hotez (Eds.), *Feigin and Cherry's textbook of pediatric infectious diseases*. Elsevier.

Ericson, J. E., & Benjamin, D. K. (2018). Clinical approach to the infected neonate. In *Principles and practice of pediatric infectious diseases*. https://doi.org/10.1016/B978-0-323-40181-4.00091-8

Flaherman, V. J., Afshar, Y., Boscardin, J., Keller, R. L., Mardy, A., Prahl, M. K., … Gaw, S. L. (2020). Infant outcomes following maternal infection with SARS-CoV-2: First report from the PRIORITY study. *Clinical Infectious Diseases: An Official Publication of the Infectious Diseases Society of America*. https://doi.org/10.1093/cid/ciaa1411

Fowler, K. B., & Boppana, S. B. (2018). Congenital cytomegalovirus infection. *Seminars in Perinatology*. https://doi.org/10.1053/j.semperi.2018.02.002

Fowler, K. B., Ross, S. A., Shimamura, M., Ahmed, A., Palmer, A. L., Michaels, M. G., … Boppana, S. (2018). Racial and ethnic differences in the prevalence of congenital cytomegalovirus infection. *Journal of Pediatrics*. https://doi.org/10.1016/j.jpeds.2018.04.043

Frankovich, J., Egan, M., Mahony, T., Benitz, W., & Shaw, G. (2017). An electronic health record investigation of lenticulostriate vasculopathy features. *American Journal of Perinatology*. https://doi.org/10.1055/s-0036-1585417

Freeman, K., Salt, A., Prusa, A., Malm, G., Ferret, N., Buffolano, W., … Valenti, L. (2005). Association between congenital toxoplasmosis and parent-reported developmental outcomes, concerns, and impairments, in 3 year old children. *BMC Pediatrics*. https://doi.org/10.1186/1471-2431-5-23

Frenkel, L. D., Gomez, F., & Sabahi, F. (2018). The pathogenesis of microcephaly resulting from congenital infections: Why is my baby's head so small? *European Journal of Clinical Microbiology and Infectious Diseases*. https://doi.org/10.1007/s10096-017-3111-8

Gentile, I., Zappulo, E., Pia Riccio, M., Binda, S., Bubba, L., Pellegrinelli, L., … Bravaccio, C. (2017). Prevalence of congenital cytomegalovirus infection assessed through viral genome detection in dried blood spots in children with autism spectrum disorders. *In Vivo*. https://doi.org/10.21873/invivo.11085

Hendrixson, D. T., & Newland, J. G. (2018). Zika virus infection in children. *Infectious Disease Clinics of North America*. https://doi.org/10.1016/j.idc.2017.10.003

Honein, M. A., Dawson, A. L., Petersen, E. E., Jones, A. M., Lee, E. H., Yazdy, M. M., … Jamieson, D. J. (2017). Birth defects among fetuses and infants of US women with evidence of possible Zika virus infection during pregnancy. *JAMA*. https://doi.org/10.1001/jama.2016.19006

Jones, J. L., Kruszon-Moran, D., Elder, S., Rivera, H. N., Press, C., Montoya, J. G., & McQuillan, G. M. (2018). *Toxoplasma gondii* infection in the United States, 2011–2014. *American Journal of Tropical Medicine and Hygiene*. https://doi.org/10.4269/ajtmh.17-0677

Kimball, A., Torrone, E., Miele, K., Bachmann, L., Thorpe, P., Weinstock, H., & Bowen, V. (2020). Missed opportunities for prevention of congenital syphilis—United States, 2018. *MMWR*. https://doi.org/10.15585/mmwr.mm6922a1

Korndewal, M. J., Oudesluys-Murphy, A. M., Kroes, A. C. M., van der Sande, M. A. B., de Melker, H. E., & Vossen, A. C. T. M. (2017). Long-term impairment attributable to congenital cytomegalovirus infection: A retrospective cohort study. *Developmental Medicine and Child Neurology*. https://doi.org/10.1111/dmcn.13556

Lorenz, N., Treptow, A., Schmidt, S., Hofmann, R., Raumer-Engler, M., Heubner, G., & Gröber, K. (2020) Neonatal early-onset infection with SARS-CoV-2 in a newborn presenting with encephalitic symptoms. *Pediatric Infectious Disease Journal*. https://doi.org/10.1097/INF.0000000000002735

Maldonado, Y. A., Read, J. S., Byington, C. L., Barnett, E. D., Davies, H. D., Edwards, K. M., … Zaoutis, T. E. (2017). Diagnosis, treatment, and prevention of congenital toxoplasmosis in the United States. *Pediatrics*. https://doi.org/10.1542/peds.2016-3860

Manicklal, S., Emery, V. C., Lazzarotto, T., Boppana, S. B., & Gupta, R. K. (2013). The "silent" global burden of congenital cytomegalovirus. *Clinical Microbiology Reviews*. https://doi.org/10.1128/CMR.00062-12

Meltzer, A., & Van De Water, J. (2017). The role of the immune system in autism spectrum disorder. *Neuropsychopharmacology*. https://doi.org/10.1038/npp.2016.158

Moore, C. A., Staples, J. E., Dobyns, W. B., Pessoa, A., Ventura, C. V., Da Fonseca, E. B., … Rasmussen, S. A. (2017). Characterizing the pattern of anomalies in congenital zika syndrome for pediatric clinicians. *JAMA Pediatrics*. https://doi.org/10.1001/jamapediatrics.2016.3982

Pinninti, S., Christy, J., Almutairi, A., Cochrane, G., Fowler, K. B., & Boppana, S. (2021). Vestibular, gaze, and balance disorders in asymptomatic congenital cytomegalovirus infection. *Pediatrics*. https://doi.org/10.1542/peds.2019-3945

Rawlinson, W. D., Boppana, S. B., Fowler, K. B., Kimberlin, D. W., Lazzarotto, T., Alain, S., … van Zuylen, W. J. (2017). Congenital cytomegalovirus infection in pregnancy and the neonate: Consensus recommendations for prevention, diagnosis, and therapy. *The Lancet Infectious Diseases*. https://doi.org/10.1016/S1473-3099(17)30143-3

Rawstron, S. A., & Hawkes, S. J. (2017). *Treponema pallidum* (Syphilis). In *Principles and practice of pediatric infectious diseases*. https://doi.org/10.1016/B978-0-323-40181-4.00182-1

Smoots, A. N., Olson, S. M., Cragan, J., Delaney, A., Roth, N. M., Godfred-Cato, S., … Honein, M. A. (2020). Population-based surveillance for birth defects potentially related to Zika virus infection—22 states and territories, January 2016–June 2017. *MMWR*. https://doi.org/10.15585/mmwr.mm6903a3

Verghese, V. P., Hendson, L., Singh, A., Guenette, T., Gratrix, J., & Robinson, J. L. (2018). Early childhood neurodevelopmental outcomes in infants exposed to infectious syphilis in utero. *The Pediatric Infectious Disease Journal*. https://doi.org/10.1097/INF.0000000000001842

Vivanti, A. J., Vauloup-Fellous, C., Prevot, S., Zupan, V., Suffee, C., Do Cao, J., … De Luca, D. (2020). Transplacental transmission of SARS-CoV-2 infection. *Nature Communications*. https://doi.org/10.1038/s41467-020-17436-6

Woodworth, K. R., Olsen, E. O., Neelam, V., Lewis, E. L., Galang, R. R., Oduyebo, T., … Whitehill, F. (2020). Birth and infant outcomes following laboratory-confirmed SARS-CoV-2 infection in pregnancy—SET-NET, 16 jurisdictions, March 29–October 14, 2020. *MMWR*. https://doi.org/10.15585/mmwr.mm6944e2

World Health Organization. (2019). *Zika epidemiology update—July 2019*. https://www.who.int/publications/m/item/zika-epidemiology-update

Yang, Z., & Liu, Y. (2020). Vertical transmission of severe acute respiratory syndrome coronavirus 2: A systematic review. *American Journal of Perinatology*, *37*(10), 1055.

34

Consequences of Preterm Birth

Brittany L. Schwarz and Mary L. O'Connor Leppert

For additional material related to the content of this chapter, please see Chapters 39, 40, and 43.

VIGNETTE

A 3.5-month-old girl presents for an initial primary care visit. She was born at 26 weeks of gestation, with a birthweight of 844g. She was discharged 2 days ago from the neonatal intensive care unit (NICU), and her discharge summary lists diagnoses of extreme preterm birth, grade II intraventricular hemorrhage, bronchopulmonary dysplasia, and medical necrotizing enterocolitis. She had retinopathy of prematurity, but her evaluation just prior to discharge raised no concerns, and she passed her audiology assessment. She is comfortable on room air and mother reports that she is nursing well. Parents would like to know what risks their daughter has for developmental problems in the future.

INTRODUCTION

The 20th century brought tremendous advancement in medical care, but few more spectacular than the management of infants born preterm. At the start of the last century, mortality of preterm infants was high and largely attributable to hypothermia, hypoxia, inadequate nutrition, and infection, but the evolution of care has secured improved healthy survival of the vast majority of the youngest and smallest infants.

Interest in preterm infants began in the mid-19th century with European obstetricians such as Budin and Tarnier in France and von Reuss in Germany, who built prototypes of incubators for controlling temperature and used rudimentary gavage tubes to feed human milk to infants too young to nurse. At the turn of the 20th century, the contributions of great physicians such as Julius Hess formalized care of preterm infants. Hess published the first text on preterm care and opened the first Infant Station in Chicago in 1922, a unit focused on temperature control, feeding techniques, infection prevention, and oxygen delivery for infants born of low or very low birthweight (Dunn, 2001).

The rest of the 20th century brought rapid improvements in neonatal care. Incubators, which had been warm but poorly controlled, became more refined, keeping infants warm to finely tuned temperatures and visible to examiners. Gavage feeds, introduced in the late 19th century with rubber tubing and a solution of milk and corn syrup, evolved to sophisticated calculation of essential nutrients delivered in oral gavage or enteral forms. Oxygen therapy was initially delivered liberally into incubators, and infants suffered high rates of retrolental fibroplasia and blindness; yet without oxygen, mortality and morbidity rates were unacceptably high. The balance between optimal oxygen delivery and improved outcomes has been the study for several decades, continually refined and improved by technology advancements of oxygen delivery modalities. Similar to the iatrogenic consequences of 100% oxygen use, enthusiasm for the use of new antibiotics proved to be an early misadventure in neonatology as toxicities from antibiotics such as chloramphenicol, sulfonamides, and streptomycin became evident in newborns.

At the same time that interventions for the major causes of preterm mortality were evolving, so too was the training of professionals, the organization of NICUs, and the technology for assessing infants. Maternal-fetal medicine and neonatal-perinatal medicine became boarded subspecialties and provided expert training on complex obstetric, fetal, and high-risk infant care. The sum total of advances, including surfactant and antenatal steroid use, has reduced the limit of viability to 23 weeks of gestation and improved survival of a new cohort of incredibly preterm infants.

The consequences of preterm birth and the neonatal complications therein reflect the immaturity of the organ systems of preterm infants and result in higher rates of morbidity. Compared to children born full term, populations of children born preterm have higher prevalence rates for cerebral palsy, cognitive impairment, visual impairment, strabismus, hearing loss, specific learning disabilities, attention-deficit disorder, speech and language delay, executive dysfunction, working memory deficit, visual-perceptual impairment, minor neuromotor dysfunction, and fine motor difficulties (Behrman et al., 2007). NICU follow-up clinics formed to monitor preterm infants for health and neurodevelopmental sequelae after discharge and to determine childhood outcomes of preterm birth and its complications. Guidelines were established for optimal NICU follow-up to assess preterm outcomes, and the American Academy of Pediatrics (AAP, 2008) recommends high-risk clinic follow-up for most preterm infants (Vohr et al., 2004).

EPIDEMIOLOGY OF PRETERM BIRTHS

Incidence of Preterm Birth

The World Health Organization defines preterm birth as a neonate born prior to 37 completed weeks of gestation. For the purposes of nomenclature and risk assessment, preterm births are further divided into extremely preterm (<28 weeks), very preterm (28–31 weeks), moderate preterm (32–34 weeks), and late preterm (34–36 weeks). Infants born preterm are at increased risk for mortality and morbidity compared to infants born full term. In 2018 low birthweight, a surrogate of preterm birth, was the second leading cause of infant mortality in the United States, second only to congenital malformations (Xu et al., 2020). Surviving preterm infants are at increased risk for neurologic and developmental morbidities, which will be discussed throughout the chapter.

Roughly 1 in 10 neonates is born preterm in the United States. The rate of preterm birth increased by 2% in 2019 from 10.02% to 10.23% compared to 2018 data (Martin et al., 2019). Despite this recent increase, the overall rate remains below the peak of 12.8% in 2006 (Martin et al., 2007). The overall decrease is thought to be due to fewer spontaneous preterm births and a decrease in medically indicated preterm deliveries (Frey & Klebanoff, 2016).

Racial Disparities

Racial disparities in preterm birth persist, with a preterm birth rate for non-Hispanic Black women that is 50% higher than Hispanic women and non-Hispanic White women (14.39% compared to 9.97% and 9.26%) (Martin et al., 2019). The etiology of these differences is not well understood and is likely multifactorial, given that the disparity remains after accounting for other preterm birth risk factors, including socioeconomic background and maternal education (Manuck, 2017). Disparities in long-term outcomes between races are compounded by the fact that black preterm infants are more likely to experience a number of neonatal conditions that are associated with morbidity later in life, such as sepsis, intraventricular hemorrhage (IVH), and retinopathy of prematurity (ROP) (Wallace et al., 2017).

Obstetric Dating Practices

One of the difficulties in using gestational age to assess risk in this population is the inherent inaccuracy in establishing a due date, and thereby gestational age. Traditionally, a woman's estimated due date (EDD) is calculated to be 280 days after the first day of her last menstrual period. However, this does not account for differences between women with respect to irregular menstrual cycle length, timing of ovulation, and inaccurate recall of the last menstrual period (Committee Opinion, 2017). Based on these potential discrepancies, the American College of Obstetricians and Gynecologists recommends a first trimester ultrasound to establish or confirm the gestational age of the embryo or fetus (Committee Opinion, 2017). Assessment of gestational age based on first trimester ultrasound is accurate within 5 to 7 days (Committee Opinion, 2017).

For women who do not establish prenatal care during the first trimester, the earliest available ultrasound is used for dating purposes; however, ultrasound accuracy in establishing EDD decreases throughout pregnancy due to increasing individual variation in fetal growth and size later in pregnancy. A late second trimester ultrasound has an accuracy of +/− 10 to 14 days, and this increases to +/− 21 to 30 days in the third trimester (Committee Opinion, 2017). Unfortunately, access to early prenatal care is a major limitation for many women already at increased risk for preterm birth (e.g., minority or lower socioeconomic status [SES] women) and contributes to health disparities surrounding preterm birth. In 2019 83% of non-Hispanic White women initiated prenatal care in the first trimester, compared with only 68% of non-Hispanic Black and 72% of Hispanic women (Martin et al., 2019).

Etiology of Preterm Birth

The etiology of preterm birth is poorly understood. While we often discuss preterm birth as one outcome, there are a number of complex physiologic pathways that are presumed to contribute to preterm birth (Behrman et al., 2007; Frey & Klebanoff, 2016). Risk factors for preterm birth include a number of environmental or social factors (e.g., neighborhood characteristics, low SES, stress, and low educational attainment), maternal medical conditions (e.g., genitourinary infections, low body mass index, periodontal disease), and pregnancy conditions (multiple gestation, use of assisted reproductive technology, polyhydramnios, cervical insufficiency) (Behrman et al., 2007; Frey & Klebanoff, 2016).

Preterm births are frequently referred to as either spontaneous or indicated. Spontaneous preterm birth represents women who present to obstetric care either in preterm labor (defined as regular contractions and cervical dilation at <37 weeks of gestation) or with preterm rupture of membranes. Indicated preterm births, whether via induction of labor or by cesarean section without preceding labor, are initiated by a medical provider in the setting of maternal or fetal indications such as preeclampsia or fetal distress. This oversimplified classification fails to acknowledge the underlying mechanisms leading to preterm labor or indicated delivery, which vary among women and populations. For example, spontaneous preterm births may result from premature activation of the normal labor cascade, stimulation of an inflammatory pathway due to underlying infection, uteroplacental ischemia, uterine overdistension, or other ill-defined immunologic processes (Goldenberg et al., 2008). Despite extensive and ongoing research in this area, a more thorough understanding of these underlying mechanisms is needed to make significant advancements in the prevention of preterm births.

NEONATAL CONDITIONS AND ASSESSMENT OF RISK

Preterm Perinatal Brain Injury

Premature infants, especially those born prior to 32 weeks of gestation, are at risk for intracranial lesions such as IVH and periventricular leukomalacia (PVL), which can lead to adverse neurodevelopmental outcomes. The susceptibility to IVH in preterm infants relates to the impaired autoregulation of cerebral blood flow seen with prematurity, combined with the fragility of capillaries in the germinal matrix (Ballabh, 2010). The germinal matrix is a highly vascularized area within the preterm brain that gives rise to neuronal and glial cell precursors (Bolisetty et al., 2014). PVL, on the other hand, refers to an ischemic injury within the periventricular white matter (Bolisetty et al., 2014). Both types of injury increase the risk for long-term motor abnormalities and cerebral palsy.

Cranial ultrasounds are routinely used to screen preterm infants for intracranial lesions at various time points during their initial hospitalization. Despite recent suggestions to report ultrasound findings with more descriptive language, the severity of IVH is most commonly reported by radiologists as grade I through IV, using a modified Papile classification system (Mukerji et al., 2015). Much of the outcomes literature on perinatal brain injury in preterm infants divides this entity into mild (grade I or II) or severe (grade III or IV), with increasing severity of IVH being associated with higher rates of cerebral palsy and gross motor impairment, even after adjustment for other neonatal morbidities (Mukerji et al., 2015). A recent metaanalysis reported that IVH itself, regardless of severity, is not associated with cognitive delays at 18 to 24 months after adjusting for other neonatal morbidities (Mukerji et al, 2015). The authors do acknowledge, though, that previous school-age outcomes studies assessing academic performance and IQ demonstrated lower cognitive scores for all degrees of IVH (Mukerji et al., 2015).

Cognitive delays are, however, associated with PVL, a type of cerebral white matter injury seen in preterm infants. This type of injury may be focal or diffuse in nature, and can ultimately lead to ventriculomegaly and white matter volume loss (Novak et al., 2018). Often, PVL is not evident on initial cranial ultrasounds obtained shortly after birth, but identified on follow-up exams weeks after birth or on brain magnetic resonance imaging (Novak et al., 2018). These infants are at high risk for cognitive and motor impairment. The rate of Bayley Scales Infant and Toddler Development (Bayley-III) cognitive scores below 70 increases with increasing severity of white matter injury, as does the rate of moderate-severe cerebral palsy (Hintz et al., 2015).

It is important to note that imaging findings do not provide the whole story and do not replace developmental surveillance. In a large multicenter study of infants born less than 28 weeks of gestation roughly half of infants with severe range imaging findings did not demonstrate severe adverse outcomes as toddlers (Hintz et al., 2015). On the other end of the spectrum are reports that up to 30% of infants with birthweight less than 1000 g and normal cranial ultrasounds are subsequently diagnosed with cerebral palsy or have Bayley-II scores below 70 (Laptook et al., 2005).

Bronchopulmonary Dysplasia

The definition and diagnosis of bronchopulmonary dysplasia (BPD) continues to evolve with emerging research and changes in care practices. The term is used to describe the lung injury and abnormal lung development that is commonly seen in preterm infants (Bancalari & Jain, 2018). Many neonatologists look at the need for oxygen supplementation at 28 days of life, in combination with the amount of respiratory support required at 36 weeks corrected gestational age to arrive at a diagnosis of BPD. However, varying definitions of BPD used in clinical trials make it difficult to draw consistent conclusions with respect to outcomes (Bancalari & Jain, 2018; Hines et al., 2017).

A surrogate marker of respiratory disease severity that correlates with neurodevelopmental outcomes is the duration of ventilator dependence (Walsh et al., 2005). The incidence of Mental Developmental Index scores below 70, moderate-severe cerebral palsy, blindness, and deafness all increase for infants that require ongoing mechanical ventilation past 28 days of life, with continued risk increases for each week of ventilator dependence (Walsh et al., 2005). Infants whose lung disease is so severe that they require tracheostomy have the even greater risk for neurodevelopmental impairment when compared to preterm infants without tracheostomy, even after adjusting for confounding variables known to affect developmental outcomes (e.g., birthweight, antenatal steroid exposure, necrotizing enterocolitis [NEC], severe ROP, brain injury) (DeMauro et al., 2014).

Antenatal corticosteroids are administered to women who present in preterm labor to promote fetal lung maturation and have been shown to decrease rates of respiratory distress syndrome and the need for mechanical ventilation in preterm infants (Roberts et al., 2017). They have the additional benefit of decreasing the rates of IVH and NEC (Roberts et al., 2017) and have been associated with improved neurodevelopmental outcomes (Walsh et al., 2005). Postnatal corticosteroids, on the other hand, have a more complicated and controversial relationship within the field of neonatology. When used in the newborn period, corticosteroids facilitate extubation and are associated with a shorter duration of mechanical ventilation (Doyle et al., 2006). These benefits are weighed against a decades-old concern for adverse effects on brain development and neurodevelopmental outcomes (Halliday, 2017). The timing and duration of postnatal corticosteroid use has evolved over time and remains an active area of research in the field. Interestingly, in a study of over 5000 preterm infants postnatal corticosteroids were not associated with neurologic impairment after adjustment for other known risk factors such as antenatal corticosteroids, PVL, and NEC (Walsh et al., 2005).

Retinopathy of Prematurity

ROP is the result of abnormal retinal blood vessel development in preterm infants, placing them at increased risk for visual impairment and blindness. In the United States this abnormal vascularization of the retina occurs in up to 16% of premature infants who require hospitalization for 28 days or longer (Sharma & VanderVeen, 2017). ROP is a progressive disease, and routine screening guidelines are in place to identify severe disease prior to the development of retinal detachment. A description of the disease is reported in stages (1–5) corresponding with the severity of disease and zones (1–3) representing the location on the retina. The higher the stage of ROP and the lower the zone, the more severe the disease (Sharma & VanderVeen, 2017). Standard therapy for infants with vision-threatening ROP consists of laser ablation surgery or intravitreal antivascular endothelial growth factor (anti-VEGF) injections to stop the progression of abnormal vascularization and ultimately prevent blindness. Not all ROP progresses to a severe form. In mild forms spontaneous regression may occur as the retina matures and the infant's clinical status improves. Compared to preterm infants without ROP, infants with any stage of disease are at increased risk for ocular problems, including strabismus, amblyopia, and myopia (Molloy et al., 2016).

Traditionally severe ROP was thought to have a negative effect on cognitive and visual outcomes of preterm infants, specifically in such areas as visual motor integration, visual planning, and visual processing (Molloy et al., 2016). However, previous studies did not control for other neonatal morbidities that influence cognitive outcomes. Molloy et al. (2016) demonstrated that when controlling for morbidities such as abnormal cranial ultrasounds and postnatal corticosteroids, only impairments in visual acuity remained independently attributable to ROP. Severe ROP is most common in infants born at the youngest gestational ages, with IVH, and with a prolonged duration of mechanical ventilation and supplemental oxygen use. Therefore the cognitive outcomes previously attributed to ROP are most likely to be a reflection of ROP occurring in the sickest of babies that are already at risk for adverse neurodevelopmental outcomes (Molloy et al., 2016). Regardless of the mechanism, though, infants with severe ROP are more likely to experience cognitive and visual processing difficulties and hence require close developmental surveillance and early intervention (Molloy et al., 2016).

Necrotizing Enterocolitis

NEC is a known complication of preterm birth, occurring in up to 9% of preterm infants, with an incidence that is inversely proportional to gestational age (Adams-Chapman, 2018; Stoll et al., 2015). The exact etiology of NEC is unclear and thought to be multifactorial. This devastating complication of prematurity presents as a spectrum of disease ranging from feeding intolerance to profound bowel ischemia and necrosis requiring surgical intervention, or even death. The systemic inflammatory response that occurs due to bowel necrosis, in addition to hemodynamic instability, places these infants at risk for central nervous system injury and adverse neurologic outcomes. Unfortunately, the timing of NEC presentation occurs during a vulnerable period in preterm brain development, and the body's cytokine response can lead to white matter injury within the brain.

The literature often divides the diagnosis of NEC into medical NEC or surgical NEC. Medical NEC is treated with bowel rest, parenteral nutrition, and antibiotics. Surgical NEC requires similar treatments; however, the degree of clinical instability also prompts a surgical intervention with either drain placement or laparotomy to remove necrotic bowel. The designation of medical versus surgical NEC has major implications for assessing the risk of future neurodevelopmental outcomes. Infants with a history of medical NEC have neurodevelopmental outcomes that are similar to age-matched infants without NEC. This is in contrast to infants with a history of surgical NEC, which is associated with a 2.3-fold increased risk for neurodevelopmental impairment (Adams-Chapman, 2018).

Surgical NEC is associated with higher rates of a number of neonatal morbidities such as chronic lung disease, late-onset sepsis, and cystic PVL compared to the general preterm population (Adams-Chapman, 2018). These additional morbidities compound the risk for adverse neurodevelopmental outcomes, as discussed earlier in this chapter. Infants with surgical NEC are at high risk for motor and cognitive impairment and are more likely to be diagnosed with cerebral palsy compared to infants with medical NEC or without any NEC diagnosis (Adams-Chapman, 2018).

NEURODEVELOPMENTAL OUTCOMES

Overview

Major neurodevelopmental sequelae of preterm birth include cerebral palsy, sensory impairment, and cognitive delays. These developmental morbidities are commonly identified in the first two years of life. Preterm infants acquire developmental milestones in an orderly, sequential fashion similar to term infants, but at an age corrected to account for the degree of preterm birth. The AAP recommends using corrected age up to 3 years of age, and investigators generally agree that full correction is required to appropriately interpret developmental testing (Engle & AAP Committee on Fetus and Newborn, 2004). There is less agreement, however, on the length of time that corrected age should be applied. For very low birthweight infants, at least 2.5 years is suggested (Vohr, 2007). Lesser neurodevelopmental sequelae such as neuromotor abnormality, language, learning, and behavioral disorders though often functionally impairing are often identified after NICU follow-up visits cease.

The degree of preterm birth along with the nature, severity, and number of neonatal complications associated with preterm birth are strong predictors of neurodevelopmental sequelae. The dichotomous distinction of major and minor sequelae has been used to describe the types of neurodevelopmental outcomes. Those conditions that are identified early and carry with them a lifelong need for intervention and services such as sensory impairment, cerebral palsy, and intellectual disability are considered major sequelae. Minor neurodevelopmental impairments are those typically identified later and are of lower severity but higher prevalence. These conditions include developmental coordination disorder (DCD), language impairments, learning disabilities, behavioral disorders, and mental health disorders. Caution is advised in assuming that minor impairments are less consequential because the frequency of cooccurring disorders is high, and the constellation of these comorbidities is often quite functionally impairing.

The prevalence of all neurodevelopmental sequelae increases with decreasing gestational age. The complications of neurologic insults, IVH, white matter injury, BPD, ROP, and NEC are both markers of the degree of preterm birth and additive contributors to neurologic injury, and ultimately to neurodevelopmental sequelae. The increase in neurodevelopmental sequelae with decreasing gestational age is consistent across broad categories of mild, moderate, severe, and no disability outcomes, and is generally reflective of the same dose effect of preterm birth observed in specific outcome conditions. Across broader outcomes, approximately 95% of moderate to late preterm infants (32–36 weeks) have no disability, 3.4% have mild disability, and 1.8% have moderate-severe disability (Blencowe et al., 2013). Very preterm infants (28–31 weeks of gestational age) escape disability in 66% to 71% of cases and have moderate-severe disability in 12% to 34% of cases, whereas infants born younger than 27 or 28 weeks escape disability in only 34% to 42% of cases and have moderate-severe disability outcomes in 11% to 29% of cases (Blencowe et al., 2013; Marret et al., 2013; Moore et al., 2012; Serenius et al., 2013).

Cerebral Palsy

The prevalence of cerebral palsy in US children ages 3 to 17 years is 0.31%, but in preterm infants the prevalence increases substantially with decreasing gestational age (Zablotsky et al., 2019). In preterm infants cerebral palsy occurs in 0.7% of infants born at 32 to 36 weeks of gestation, in 6.2% to 6.6% born at 28 to 31 weeks, and in 7% to 20% of children born younger than 27 weeks of gestation, with higher rates in lower gestational ages under 27 weeks (Hafström et al., 2018; Himpens et al., 2008; Marret et al., 2013; Moore et al., 2012; Serenius 2013). Extreme prematurity and the presence of abnormal neuroimaging findings pose the greatest risks for cerebral palsy, although half to two-thirds of children with grade IV IVH or PVL on head ultrasound do not have cerebral palsy, and 9% to 10% of children with normal head ultrasounds are diagnosed with cerebral palsy (Broitman et al., 2007; Laptook et al., 2005).

The nature and severity of cerebral palsy seems to be consistent across studies, with 91% to 96% of cerebral palsy classified as spastic in nature. Within the group of children with spasticity, the majority have bilateral involvement (71%–73%) and are more often diplegic (61%) rather than quadriplegic (17%) (Hafström et al., 2018; Himpens et al., 2008). The interpretation of severity of cerebral palsy varies across studies. Some refer to severe cerebral palsy as those children with motor developmental quotient (DQ) less than 50, those unable to sit or unlikely to ever walk, or in more recent reporting those who require physical assistance or powered mobility in most or all settings: a gross motor functional classification system (GMFCS) of IV or V (Oeffinger et al., 2004). Moderate cerebral palsy is often GMFCS III, where walking is expected indoors with the assistance of a device. Moderate-severe cerebral palsy (GMFCS III) occurs in 24% to 39% of preterm children (Oeffinger et al., 2004).

Associated deficits in preterm infants mirror those of the general population of individuals with cerebral palsy. In extreme preterm infants with cerebral palsy over 50% have intellectual disability, 33% have attention-deficit/hyperactivity disorder (ADHD), 22% visual impairment, 18% epilepsy, and 10% hearing impairment (Hafström et al., 2018). In a large systematic review of all individuals with cerebral palsy nearly half had intellectual disability, 24% had epilepsy, 11% were blind, and 4% were deaf (Novak et al., 2012). In both groups, associated deficits were greater in children with higher GMFCS scores, and in the extreme preterm group all children with GMFCS scores of IV or V had intellectual disability (Hafström et al., 2018; Novak et al., 2012).

Intellectual Disability

Intellectual disability is the most frequent major neurodevelopmental impairment of preterm infants. It is a lifelong diagnosis of varying degrees of severity with cognitive measures below 2 SD and commensurate impairments in adaptive function. Preterm outcomes reporting on intellectual disability range broadly in definition of intellectual or cognitive impairment, as well as the measures used and ages at which cognition is assessed. A recent metaanalysis and systematic review of outcomes found that the standardized mean differences (SMD) in IQ measures was lower across all preterm groups (Allotey et al., 2018). The differences in SMD corresponded to the degree of premature birth and were greatest in preterm infants born before 28 weeks of gestation, and still significant in children born at 34 to 37 weeks. SMD deficits were largest in performance IQ measures (PIQ) and full-scale IQ (FSIQ) and least in verbal IQ (VIQ) measures. The deficits in IQ measurements were consistent across preschool and all school-age assessments (Allotey et al., 2018).

Intellectual disability prevalence in preterm infants increases with decreasing gestational age, as does borderline intelligence. Borderline cognition, with IQ measures greater than −1 and less than −2 SD from the mean, does not carry with it the same expectation of lifelong functional impairment, but it certainly puts individuals at a cognitive disadvantage, at least during their educational years. Further, because of the frequency of cooccurring neurodevelopmental or behavioral impairments in preterm children, those with borderline IQ and comorbid conditions may be more functionally impaired than their IQ alone may suggest.

In extreme preterm infants intellectual disability occurs in 8.8% to 16% of survivors, and borderline IQ in 24% to 39% (Adams-Chapman et al., 2018; Cheong et al., 2017; Marret et al., 2013; Moore et al., 2012; Serenius et al., 2013). Collectively it appears that approximately one-third to one-half of preterm infants born before 27 weeks of gestation have IQ scores below the average range (Marret et al., 2013; Pascal et al., 2018; Serenius et al., 2013). In infants born between 28 and 32 weeks of gestation rates of intellectual disability range from 4.9% to 10.7%, and borderline IQ rates range from 18% to 28%, reflecting one-quarter to one-third with IQ scores below average range (Marret et al., 2013). Even children born between 33 and 37 weeks of gestation have intellectual disability rates as high as 5% to 8% and borderline IQ rates of 14% to 19% (Johnson et al., 2015; Marret et al., 2007).

The impact of low or borderline cognition on the academic success of children must neither be underestimated nor viewed in isolation. In addition to their cognitive potential, as estimated by IQ, children born preterm also carry high risk for learning and language difficulties, attention deficits, neuromotor disorders, and mental health disorders. Each additional cooccurring disorder must be viewed in the context of underlying IQ and as a constellation that may impact academic success. Eligibility criteria for services under the Individuals with Disabilities Education Act (IDEA) does not include borderline intelligence, and school individualized education plans (IEPs) often use a single diagnosis for eligibility, which may not represent the entire educational support that an individual child requires.

Neurosensory Impairments

The prevalence of significant vision and hearing impairment in preterm infants is far less than that of cerebral palsy or intellectual disability, but considerably greater than children born at term. As with all major neurodevelopmental impairments, the prevalence of neurosensory impairment increases with decreasing gestational age. Outcome studies vary slightly in reporting of visual impairments, as some separate moderate (low vision) from severe (blindness) impairment, while others combine them. Similarly, hearing impairments are considered severe if the outcome is deafness and moderate if the hearing impairment requires the use of hearing aids.

Extremely preterm infants have a prevalence of moderate-severe vision impairment of 1% to 2.7%, with blindness reported in roughly 1% and low vision reported in 2.9% to 6% (Adams-Chapman et al., 2018; Hirvonen et al., 2018; Marret et al., 2007, 2013; Serenius et al., 2013). Moderate-severe visual impairments occur in 0.4% to 0.9% of infants 27 to 32 weeks of gestation and in 0.8% to 1.47% of infants 33 to 37 weeks of gestation (Hirvonen et al., 2018; Marret et al., 2007). The greatest risk of visual impairment in preterm infants is the presence of ROP, and in particular severe ROP, which requires surgical intervention or more recent use of anti-VEGF therapy (Wallace et al., 2017). Retinal findings direct subsequent follow-up visits, treatment, and the cessation of ROP examinations, including continued follow-up after NICU discharge. Ophthalmologic follow-up is recommended for preterm infants at 4 to 6 months of age, regardless of ROP status, because they are at higher risk for visual acuity differences, strabismus, amblyopia, and other ophthalmologic findings (Fierson, 2018).

Moderate-severe hearing impairments occur in 2.7% to 3% of extreme preterm infants, in 0.4% to 1.1% of infants born 27 to 32 weeks, and in 0.3% to 0.5% of infants born 33 to 37 weeks of gestation (Adams-Chapman et al., 2018; Hirvonen et al., 2018; Marret et al., 2007, 2013). The risk for hearing impairment is correlated to the number of days of mechanical ventilation required in the NICU and prolonged oxygen use (Adams-Chapman et al., 2018; Robertson et al., 2009). The use of ototoxic medications, the presence of hyperbilirubinemia, along with neonatal infection, though not specific to prematurity, do occur more often in premature infants and add to the risk of hearing impairment. The AAP (2007) recommends that all children who spend more than 5 days in the NICU should have an auditory brainstem response performed before discharge and a follow-up audiology evaluation before 24 months of age. In keeping with the Early Hearing Detection and Intervention (EDHI) program recommendations, children should have hearing impairment diagnosis confirmed by 3 months and intervention in place by 6 months of age. Close follow-up and a low threshold for reassessment of hearing is particularly germane to preterm infants as delayed onset and progressive hearing loss occur more frequently in extremely preterm infants (Robertson et al., 2009; van Noort-van der Spek et al., 2017).

Neurosensory impairments in preterm infants often do not occur in isolation. The Neonatal Research Network recently reported that nearly three-quarters of extremely preterm infants with visual impairment and more than one-quarter with hearing impairment also had cerebral palsy (Adams-Chapman et al., 2018). In children born of extreme prematurity who have cerebral palsy about one-half have intellectual disability and 11% to 14% also have significant neurosensory impairment (Adams-Chapman et al., 2018; Moore et al., 2012). The recommendations for hearing assessment and for vision follow-up should bring neurosensory impairment diagnoses to light early, irrespective of whether they occur alone or with other neurodevelopmental impairments. Hearing and vision impairments are generally detected before motor or cognitive disability are diagnosed, and they most certainly affect the approach to therapeutic intervention for subsequent diagnoses.

Neuromotor Abnormality

Cerebral palsy is certainly the most significant motor outcome of preterm birth, but minor neuromotor abnormality or developmental motor coordination disorder are also motor outcomes that occur in 37% of extremely preterm infants evaluated in early childhood and may cause functional limitations (Bolk et al., 2018). DCD is characterized by suboptimal motor function in the absence of neurologic findings. Children with DCD are often less coordinated than same-age peers and may appear clumsy in gross and fine motor activity. Athletic activities that require finesse in coordinating gross motor and eye-hand coordination, such as lacrosse, may be particularly challenging for children with DCD, whereas greater success may be found in sports requiring repetitive movement such as running, swimming, and bicycling. Difficulty with manual dexterity is the most common finding in DCD and may have significant impact on functional adaptive skills such as buttoning, snapping, using scissors, and handwriting (Bolk et al., 2018). Accompanying the diagnosis of DCD are higher rates of both internalizing and externalizing behavioral problems, ADHD, executive dysfunction, social skills, and similar difficulties (Acharya et al., 2016; Bolk et al., 2018).

Language Disorders

The acquisition of language is perhaps one of the most remarkable feats of human development. Preterm infants maintain a language disadvantage with average language performance 0.5 to 1 SD below peers and is both observed early and persists into at least middle childhood or early adolescence (Nguyen et al., 2018). Approximately 11% to 16% of children born very or extremely preterm have moderate to severe language delays in early childhood, with about 6% severely delayed (<-2 SD), and 5% to 9% moderately delayed (<-1 SD) (Moore et al., 2012; Serenius et al., 2013). Moderate to late preterm infants also have persistent deficits in language skills that also average scores of −0.5 to 1 SD, but a greater proportion of children are in the moderate range of delay (Cheong et al., 2017).

Language delays may be expressive, receptive, or a mix of receptive and expressive delay, and they carry different degrees of established risks and comorbidities. Expressive language delays in early childhood are often accompanied by behavioral difficulties arising from the frustration of ineffective communication. Mixed receptive and expressive language impairments, particularly if severe or persistent in early childhood, carry a high risk for language-based learning disabilities, including reading and written language difficulties, and have less desirable educational outcomes (Catts et al., 2008; Connelly et al., 2012; Johnson et al., 2010). Behavioral difficulties, including ADHD, and emotional disorders are more frequent cooccurring disorders in children with specific language impairments as compared with nonlanguage-impaired peers (Yew & O'Kearney, 2013).

Learning

Reports of academic outcomes in preterm infants require consideration of several variables. For example, the age of assessment, the inclusion or exclusion of children with intellectual disability, the definition of learning disability, and age versus grade-level comparisons of academic achievement may all influence the outcomes of such reports. In recent studies, where children with intellectual disabilities are not included in learning outcomes, and variables such as maternal education and SES are considered, there appears to be a substantial learning impact of extreme preterm birth on learning. An estimated 23.5% to 30.9% of children with a history of extremely preterm birth have learning disabilities (Akshoomoff et al., 2017; Squarza et al., 2016). Reading disability occurs in 1% to 6.4% of extremely preterm infants, whereas learning disability in mathematics occurs in 5% to 16%, and 8.3% to 13.7% have more than one disability (Akshoomoff et al., 2017; Squarza et al., 2016). The burden of learning disability in moderate preterm infants is substantially lower than that of extreme preterms, and by late preterm learning disability prevalence is similar to term peers (Chan & Quigley, 2014; Harris & Graham, 2013).

Learning disability diagnoses, however, may not represent the true educational burden of premature birth, as grade retention is more common in preterm infants, and educational services may be provided in the absence of a learning disability diagnosis. At 7 years of age, academic underachievement in reading was noted in 30% of preterms born before 32 weeks, 22% of moderate preterms, 19% of late preterms, and 12% of term infants (Chan & Quigley, 2014). At 11 years of age, 10% of former extremely preterm infants without intellectual disability had reading impairments, 16.8% had math disability, and 42.7% required special education services, while term born classmates had disability rates of 2% in reading, 1.3% in math, and only 10.7% required special education services (Johnson et al., 2011). In addition to the increased need for special education services, school-age children with a history of extremely preterm birth are far more likely than term-age peers to be below grade level or to have been retained in school (Akshoomoff, et al., 2017; Litt et al., 2005). Given all of these considerations, the educational impact of preterm birth is not well represented by the frequency of learning disability alone but on a broader view of the evidence of educational difficulty.

Behavioral Outcomes

ADHD occurs in 16% to 19% of children born very or extremely preterm and appears to be most pervasive in the youngest and smallest of infants (Johnson et al., 2011). It has become clear, however, that ADHD in preterm infants differs from children born at term. Preterm ADHD is more likely to be inattentive type and does not demonstrate the male preponderance, associated conduct disorders, or socioeconomic or family risk seen in classic ADHD (Johnson et al., 2011; Korzeniewski et al., 2017). Additionally, children born before 28 weeks were four times more likely to have social impairment on standardized rating scales and more likely to have symptoms of emotional disorders, particularly social anxiety or generalized anxiety, than were their term-age peers (Johnson et al., 2011; Korzeniewski et al., 2017). Emotional disorders, including anxiety and depression, are nearly four times more common in extremely preterm infants, but the greatest preponderance of emotional disorder reported is anxiety. The constellation of findings of inattentive type ADHD, emotional difficulties, social impairment, and internalizing behavior has been dubbed "the preterm behavioral phenotype" and has grown in evidence and acceptance in the last decade. The prevalence of the preterm behavioral phenotype is as high as 20% in children born extremely preterm (Burnett et al., 2019).

The evaluation of autism in preterm infants is complicated by the frequency of cooccurring diagnoses. Early reports of suspicions of autism in preterm populations were very high based on the results of autism screening measures. Careful evaluations for the diagnosis of autism in preterms must consider mitigators of the autism spectrum disorder, including the higher prevalence of neurosensory, cognitive, communication, and behavioral disorders associated with preterm birth, which may influence the interpretation of screening or evaluation results. Recent evidence suggests that with long-term follow-up, approximately 7% of extremely preterm infants are diagnosed with autism spectrum disorder (Agrawal et al., 2018; Kim et al., 2016).

FOLLOW-UP OF THE PRETERM INFANT

The AAP recommends routine screening of all children for development and motor disorders at 9-, 18-, and 30-month well-child visits, and the principles of screening are perhaps most germane to children born preterm (Lipkin & Macias, 2020; Noritz & Murphy, 2013). The AAP recommends developmental follow-up for preterm infants for periodic assessments to identify delayed or atypical development and ensure timely initiation of early intervention services. Developmental assessments may be provided by a primary care physician with appropriate skills or by specialized multidisciplinary follow-up programs for children who are identified at NICU discharge as having substantial risk (AAP, 2008). It behooves primary care physicians caring for preterm infants to consider the neurodevelopmental risks for individual infants and the ages at which they are most likely diagnosed. Neurosensory deficits are often apparent in the first months of life, motor impairment in the latter part of the first year, and cognitive or language deficits at 2 to 3 years of age. Developmental coordination and behavioral and learning disorders present later, often between preschool and middle childhood.

Neonatal follow-up clinics monitor high-risk infants to provide comprehensive evaluation, identify early signs of neurodevelopmental disability, and facilitate referral infants to appropriate community services. Ideally, the comprehensive assessments utilize a multidisciplinary model, with participation by developmental pediatrics, physical and occupational therapy, nursing, social work, and clinical neuropsychology. The majority of multidisciplinary NICU follow-up programs are associated with academic centers, follow high-risk infants until 24 to 36 months of age, and monitor growth, development, and neurologic status (Kuppala et al., 2012).

CONCLUSION

Premature birth occurs in 1 in 10 live births and is an important, complex public health problem. The etiology of preterm birth is multifactorial, resulting from interrelated biologic, psychosocial, and environmental risk factors that vary in frequency among different populations. Despite medical and technological advancements that have led to dramatic improvements in preterm survival, a significant burden of neurodevelopmental sequelae associated with preterm birth remains. All types of neurodevelopmental outcomes are more common in the youngest and smallest of this vulnerable population. Most preterm survivors do not have major disabilities, and despite the likelihood of minor neurodevelopmental outcomes they are functional as adults who report good quality of life (Saigal, 2013). In the wisdom of Dr. Julius Hess, "I give you these statistics to support our original belief that any effort expended in the care of these smallest prematurely born infants is of inestimable value. Nature has been kind to many…" (Dunn, 2001).

REFERENCES

Acharya, K., Pellerite, M., Lagatta, J., Andrews, B., & Msall, M. E. (2016). Cerebral palsy, developmental coordination disorder, visual and hearing impairments in infants born preterm. *NeoReviews*, *17*(6), e325. https://doi.org/10.1542/neo.17-6-e325.

Adams-Chapman, I. (2018). Necrotizing enterocolitis and neurodevelopmental outcome. *Clinics in Perinatology*, *45*(3), 453–466. https://doi.org/10.1016/j.clp.2018.05.014.

Adams-Chapman, I., Heyne, R. J., DeMauro, S. B., Duncan, A. F., Hintz, S. R., Pappas, A., ... Follow-Up Study of the Eunice Kennedy Shriver National Institute of Child Health and Human Development Neonatal Research Network. (2018). Neurodevelopmental impairment among extremely preterm infants in the Neonatal Research Network. *Pediatrics*, *141*(5). https://doi.org/10.1542/peds.2017-3091.

Agrawal, S., Rao, S. C., Bulsara, M. K., & Patole, S. K. (2018). Prevalence of autism spectrum disorder in preterm infants: A meta-analysis. *Pediatrics*, *142*(3). https://doi.org/10.1542/peds.2018-0134.

Akshoomoff, N., Joseph, R. M., Taylor, H. G., Allred, E. N., Heeren, T., O'Shea, T. M., & Kuban, K. C. K. (2017). Academic achievement deficits and their neuropsychological correlates in children born extremely preterm. *Journal of Developmental and Behavioral Pediatrics*, *38*(8), 627–637. https://doi.org/10.1097/dbp.0000000000000479.

Allotey, J., Zamora, J., Cheong-See, F., Kalidindi, M., Arroyo-Manzano, D., Asztalos, E., ... Thangaratinam, S. (2018). Cognitive, motor, behavioural and academic performances of children born preterm: A meta-analysis and systematic review involving 64 061 children. *BJOG*, *125*(1), 16–25. https://doi.org/10.1111/1471-0528.14832.

American Academy of Pediatrics Committee on Fetus and Newborn. (2008). Hospital discharge of the high-risk neonate. *Pediatrics*, *122*(5), 1119–1126. https://doi.org.proxy1.library.jhu.edu/10.1542/peds.2008-2174.

American Academy of Pediatrics, Joint Committee on Infant Hearing. (2007). Year 2007 position statement: Principles and guidelines for Early Hearing Detection and Intervention programs. *Pediatrics*, *120*(4), 898–921. https://doi.org.proxy1.library.jhu.edu/10.1542/peds.2007-2333.

Ballabh, P. (2010). Intraventricular hemorrhage in premature infants: Mechanism of disease. *Pediatric Research*, *67*(1), 1–8. https://doi.org/10.1203/PDR.0b013e3181c1b176.

Bancalari, E., & Jain, D. (2018). Bronchopulmonary dysplasia: Can we agree on a definition? *American Journal of Perinatology*, *35*(6), 537–540. https://doi.org/10.1055/s-0038-1637761.

Behrman, R. E., Butler, A. S., & Institute of Medicine (US) Committee on Understanding Premature Birth and Assuring Healthy Outcomes. *Preterm birth: Causes, consequences, and prevention*. National Academies Press.

Blencowe, H., Lee, A. C., Cousens, S., Bahalim, A., Narwal, R., Zhong, N., ... Lawn, J. E. (2013). Preterm birth-associated neurodevelopmental impairment estimates at regional and global levels for 2010. *Pediatric Research*, *74*(1), S17–S34. https://doi.org/10.1038/pr.2013.204.

Bolisetty, S., Dhawan, A., Abdel-Latif, M., Bajuk, B., Stack, J., Oei, J.-L., & Lui, K. (2014). Intraventricular hemorrhage and neurodevelopmental outcomes in extreme preterm infants. *Pediatrics*, *133*(1), 55. https://doi.org/10.1542/peds.2013-0372.

Bolk, J., Farooqi, A., Hafström, M., Åden, U., & Serenius, F. (2018). Developmental coordination disorder and its association with developmental comorbidities at 6.5 years in apparently healthy children born extremely preterm. *JAMA Pediatrics*, *172*(8), 765–774. https://doi.org/10.1001/jamapediatrics.2018.1394.

Broitman, E., Ambalavanan, N., Higgins, R. D., Vohr, B. R., Das, A., Bhaskar, B., ... National Institute of Child Health and Human Development Neonatal Research Network. (2007). Clinical data predict neurodevelopmental outcome better than head ultrasound in extremely low birth weight infants. *Journal of Pediatrics*, *151*(5), 500–505, e501–e502. https://doi.org/10.1016/j.jpeds.2007.04.013.

Burnett, A. C., Youssef, G., Anderson, P. J., Duff, J., Doyle, L. W., & Cheong, J. L. Y. (2019). Exploring the "preterm behavioral phenotype" in children born extremely preterm. *Journal of Developmental and Behavioral Pediatrics*, *40*(3), 200–207. https://doi.org/10.1097/dbp.0000000000000646.

Catts, H. W., Bridges, M. S., Little, T. D., & Tomblin, J. B. (2008). Reading achievement growth in children with language impairments. *Journal of Speech, Language, and Hearing Research*, *51*(6), 1569–1579. https://doi.org/10.1044/1092-4388(2008/07-0259).

Chan, E., & Quigley, M. A. (2014). School performance at age 7 years in late preterm and early term birth: A cohort study. *Archive of Disease in Childhood Fetal and Neonatal Edition*, *99*(6), F451–F457. https://doi.org/10.1136/archdischild-2014-306124.

Cheong, J. L. Y., Anderson, P. J., Burnett, A. C., Roberts, G., Davis, N., Hickey, L., ... Victorian Infant Collaborative Study Group. (2017). Changing neurodevelopment at 8 years in children born extremely preterm since the 1990s. *Pediatrics*, *139*(6). https://doi.org/10.1542/peds.2016-4086.

Committee Opinion No. 700: Methods for Estimating the Due Date. (2017). *Obstetrics and Gynecology*, *129*(5), e150–e154. https://doi.org.proxy1.library.jhu.edu/10.1097/AOG.0000000/000002046.

Connelly, V., Dockrell, J. E., Walter, K., & Critten, S. (2012). Predicting the quality of composition and written language bursts from oral language, spelling, and handwriting skills in children with and without specific language impairment. *Written Communication*, *29*(3), 278–302. https://doi.org/10.1177/0741088312451109.

DeMauro, S. B., D'Agostino, J. A., Bann, C., Bernbaum, J., Gerdes, M., Bell, E. F., ... Eunice Kennedy Shriver National Institute of Child Health and Human Development Neonatal Research Network. (2014). Developmental outcomes of very preterm infants with tracheostomies. *Journal of Pediatrics*, *164*(6), 1303–1310. https://doi.org/10.1016/j.jpeds.2013.12.014.e1302.

Doyle, L. W., Davis, P. G., Morley, C. J., McPhee, A., & Carlin, J. B. (2006). Low-dose dexamethasone facilitates extubation among chronically ventilator-dependent infants: A multicenter, international, randomized, controlled trial. *Pediatrics*, *117*(1), 75–83. https://doi.org/10.1542/peds.2004-2843.

Dunn, P. M. (2001). Perinatal lessons from the past. Julius Hess, MD (1876–1955) and the premature infant. *Archives of Disease in Childhood Fetal and Neonatal Edition*, *85*(2), F141–144. https://doi.org/10.1136/fn.85.2.f141.

Engle, W. A., & American Academy of Pediatrics Committee on Fetus and Newborn, (2004). Age terminology during the perinatal period. *Pediatrics*, *114*(5), 1362–1364. https://doi.org.proxy1.library.jhu.edu/10.1542/peds.2004-1915.

Fierson, W. M. (2018). Screening examination of premature infants for retinopathy of prematurity. *Pediatrics*, *142*(6). https://doi.org/10.1542/peds.2018-3061.

Frey, H. A., & Klebanoff, M. A. (2016). The epidemiology, etiology, and costs of preterm birth. *Seminars in Fetal and Neonatal Medicine*, *21*(2), 68–73. https://doi.org/10.1016/j.siny.2015.12.011.

Goldenberg, R. L., Culhane, J. F., Iams, J. D., & Romero, R. (2008). Epidemiology and causes of preterm birth. *The Lancet*, *371*(9606), 75–84. https://doi.org/10.1016/s0140-6736(08)60074-4.

Hafström, M., Källén, K., Serenius, F., Maršál, K., Rehn, E., Drake, H., ... Strömberg, B. (2018). Cerebral palsy in extremely preterm infants. *Pediatrics*, *141*(1). https://doi.org/10.1542/peds.2017-1433.

Halliday, H. L. (2017). Update on postnatal steroids. *Neonatology*, *111*(4), 415–422. https://doi.org/10.1159/000458460.

Hamilton, B. E., Martin, J. A., Ventura, S. J., & Division of Vital Statistics, (2007). *Births: Preliminary data for 2006*. National Center for Health Statistics.

Harris, K. R., & Graham, S. (2013). "An adjective is a word hanging down from a noun": Learning to write and students with learning disabilities. *Annals of Dyslexia*, *63*(1), 65–79. https://doi.org/10.1007/s11881-011-0057-x.

Himpens, E., Van den Broeck, C., Oostra, A., Calders, P., & Vanhaesebrouck, P. (2008). Prevalence, type, distribution, and severity of cerebral palsy in relation to gestational age: A meta-analytic review. *Developmental Medicine and Child Neurology*, *50*(5), 334–340. https://doi.org/10.1111/j.1469-8749.2008.02047.x.

Hines, D., Modi, N., Lee, S. K., Isayama, T., Sjörs, G., Gagliardi, L., ... International Network for Evaluating Outcomes (iNeo) of Neonates. (2017). Scoping review shows wide variation in the definitions of bronchopulmonary dysplasia in preterm infants and calls for a consensus. *Acta Paediatrica*, *106*(3), 366–374. https://doi.org/10.1111/apa.13672.

Hintz, S. R., Barnes, P. D., Bulas, D., Slovis, T. L., Finer, N. N., Wrage, L. A., ... SUPPORT Study Group of the Eunice Kennedy Shriver National Institute of Child Health and Human Development Neonatal Research Network. (2015). Neuroimaging and neurodevelopmental outcome in extremely preterm infants. *Pediatrics*, *135*(1), e32–e42. https://doi.org.proxy1.library.jhu.edu/10.1542/peds.2014-0898.

Hirvonen, M., Ojala, R., Korhonen, P., Haataja, P., Eriksson, K., Gissler, M., … Tammela, O. (2018). Visual and hearing impairments after preterm birth. *Pediatrics*, *142*(2). https://doi.org/10.1542/peds.2017-3888.

Johnson, C. J., Beitchman, J. H., & Brownlie, E. B. (2010). Twenty-year follow-up of children with and without speech-language impairments: family, educational, occupational, and quality of life outcomes. *American Journal of Speech and Language Pathology*, *19*(1), 51–65. https://doi.org/10.1044/1058-0360(2009/08-0083).

Johnson, S., Evans, T. A., Draper, E. S., Field, D. J., Manktelow, B. N., Marlow, N., ... Boyle, E. M. (2015). Neurodevelopmental outcomes following late and moderate prematurity: A population-based cohort study. *Archives of Disease in Childhood. Fetal and Neonatal Edition*, *100*(4), F301–F308. https://doi.org/10.1136/archdischild.-2014-307684.

Johnson, S., Wolke, D., Hennessy, E., & Marlow, N. (2011). Educational outcomes in extremely preterm children: Neuropsychological correlates and predictors of attainment. *Developmental Neuropsychology*, *36*(1), 74–95. https://doi.org/10.1080/87565641.2011.540541.

Kim, S. H., Joseph, R. M., Frazier, J. A., O'Shea, T. M., Chawarska, K., Allred, E. N., … Kuban, K. K. (2016). Predictive validity of the modified checklist for autism in toddlers (M-CHAT) born very preterm. *Journal of Pediatrics*, *178*, 101–107.e102. https://doi.org/10.1016/j.jpeds.2016.07.052.

Korzeniewski, S. J., Joseph, R. M., Kim, S. H., Allred, E. N., O'Shea, T. M., Leviton, A., & Kuban, K. C. K. (2017). Social responsiveness scale assessment of the preterm behavioral phenotype in 10-year-olds born extremely preterm. *Journal of Developmental and Behavioral Pediatrics*, *38*(9), 697–705. https://doi.org/10.1097/dbp.0000000000000485.

Kuppala, V. S., Tabangin, M., Haberman, B., Steichen, J., & Yolton, K. (2012). Current state of high-risk infant follow-up care in the United States: Results of a national survey of academic follow-up programs. *Journal of Perinatology*, *32*(4), 293–298. https://doi.org/10.1038/jp.2011.97.

Laptook, A. R., O'Shea, T. M., Shankaran, S., & Bhaskar, B. (2005). Adverse neurodevelopmental outcomes among extremely low birth weight infants with a normal head ultrasound: Prevalence and antecedents. *Pediatrics*, *115*(3), 673–680. https://doi.org/10.1542/peds.2004-0667.

Lipkin, P. H., & Macias, M. M. (2020). Promoting optimal development: Identifying infants and young children with developmental disorders through developmental surveillance and screening. *Pediatrics*, *145*(1). https://doi.org/10.1542/peds.2019-3449.

Litt, J., Taylor, H. G., Klein, N., & Hack, M. (2005). Learning disabilities in children with very low birthweight: Prevalence, neuropsychological correlates, and educational interventions. *Journal of Learning Disabilities*, *38*(2), 130–141. https://doi.org/10.1177/00222194050380020301.

Manuck. T. A. (2017). Racial and ethnic differences in preterm birth: A complex, multifactorial problem. *Seminars in Perinatology*, *41*(8), 511–518. https://doi.org/10.1053/j.semperi.2017.08.010.

Marret, S., Ancel, P. Y., Marpeau, L., Marchand, L., Pierrat, V., Larroque, B., ... Epipage Study Group. (2007). Neonatal and 5-year outcomes after birth at 30-34 weeks of gestation. *Obstetrics and Gynecology*, *110*(1), 72–80. https://doi.org/10.1097/01.AOG.0000267498.95402.bd.

Marret, S., Marchand-Martin, L., Picaud, J. C., Hascoët, J. M., Arnaud, C., Rozé, J. C., ... EPIPAGE Study Group. (2013). Brain injury in very preterm children and neurosensory and cognitive disabilities during childhood: The EPIPAGE cohort study. *PLoS One*, *8*(5), e62683. https://doi.org/10.1371/journal.pone.0062683.

Martin, J. A., Hamilton, B. E., Osterman, M. J. K., Driscoll, A. K., & Division of Vital Statistics. (2019). *Births: Final data for 2018*. National Center for Health Statistics.

Molloy, C. S., Anderson, P. J., Anderson, V. A., & Doyle, L. W. (2016). The long-term outcome of extremely preterm (<28 weeks' gestational age) infants with and without severe retinopathy of prematurity. *Journal of Neuropsychology*, *10*(2), 276–294. https://doi.org/10.1111/jnp.12069.

Moore, T., Hennessy, E. M., Myles, J., Johnson, S. J., Draper, E. S., Costeloe, K. L., & Marlow, N. (2012). Neurological and developmental outcome in extremely preterm children born in England in 1995 and 2006: The EPICure studies. *BMJ*, *345*, e7961. https://doi.org/10.1136/bmj.e7961.

Mukerji, A., Shah, V., & Shah, P. S. (2015). Periventricular/intraventricular hemorrhage and neurodevelopmental outcomes: A meta-analysis. *Pediatrics*, *136*(6), 1132–1143. https://doi.org/10.1542/peds.2015-0944.

Nguyen, T. N., Spencer-Smith, M., Zannino, D., Burnett, A., Scratch, S. E., Pascoe, L., ... Anderson, P. J. (2018). Developmental trajectory of language from 2 to 13 years in children born very preterm. *Pediatrics*, *141*(5). https://doi.org/10.1542/peds.2017–2831.

Noritz, G. H., & Murphy, N. A. (2013). Motor delays: Early identification and evaluation. *Pediatrics*, *131*(6), e2016–e2027. https://doi.org/10.1542/peds.2013-1056.

Novak, I., Hines, M., Goldsmith, S., & Barclay, R. (2012). Clinical prognostic messages from a systematic review on cerebral palsy. *Pediatrics*, *130*(5), e1285–e1312. https://doi.org/10.1542/peds.2012-0924.

Novak, C. M., Ozen, M., & Burd, I. (2018). Perinatal brain injury: Mechanisms, prevention, and outcomes. *Clinics in Perinatology*, *45*(2), 357–375. https://doi.org/10.1016/j.clp.2018.01.015.

Oeffinger, D. J., Tylkowski, C. M., Rayens, M. K., Davis, R. F., Gorton III, G. E., D'Astous, J., ... Luan, J. (2004). Gross motor function classification system and outcome tools for assessing ambulatory cerebral palsy: A multicenter study. *Developmental Medicine and Child Neurology*, *46*(5), 311–319. https://doi.org/10.1017/s0012162204000519.

Pascal, A., Govaert, P., Oostra, A., Naulaers, G., Ortibus, E., & Van den Broeck, C. (2018). Neurodevelopmental outcome in very preterm and very-low-birthweight infants born over the past decade: A meta-analytic review. *Developmental Medicine and Child Neurology*, *60*(4), 342–355. https://doi.org/10.1111/dmcn.13675.

Roberts, D., Brown, J., Medley, N., & Dalziel, S. R. (2017). Antenatal corticosteroids for accelerating fetal lung maturation for women at risk of preterm birth. *Cochrane Database of Systematic Reviews*, *3*(3), Cd004454. https://doi.org/10.1002/14651858.CD004454.pub3.

Robertson, C. M., Howarth, T. M., Bork, D. L., & Dinu, I. A. (2009). Permanent bilateral sensory and neural hearing loss of children after neonatal intensive care because of extreme prematurity: A thirty-year study. *Pediatrics*, *123*(5), e797–e807. https://doi.org/10.1542/peds.2008-2531.

Saigal, S. (2013). Quality of life of former premature infants during adolescence and beyond. *Early Human Development*, *89*(4), 209–213. https://doi.org/10.1016/j.earlhumdev.2013.01.012.

Serenius, F., Källén, K., Blennow, M., Ewald, U., Fellman, V., Holmström, G., ... EXPRESS Group. (2013). Neurodevelopmental outcome in extremely preterm infants at 2.5 years after active perinatal care in Sweden. *JAMA*, *309*(17), 1810–1820. https://doi.org/10.1001/jama.2013.3786.

Sharma, M., & VanderVeen, D. K. (2017). Identification and treatment of retinopathy of prematurity: Update 2017. *NeoReviews*, *18*(2), e84. https://doi.org/10.1542/neo.18-2-e84.

Squarza, C., Picciolini, O., Gardon, L., Giannì, M. L., Murru, A., Gangi, S., ... Mosca, F. (2016). Learning disabilities in extremely low birth weight children and neurodevelopmental profiles at preschool age. *Frontiers in Psychology*, *7*, 998. https://doi.org/10.3389/fpsyg.2016.00998.

Stoll, B. J., Hansen, N. I., Bell, E. F., Walsh, M. C., Carlo, W. A., Shankaran, S., ... Eunice Kennedy Shriver National Institute of Child Health and Human Development Neonatal Research Network. (2015). Trends in care practices, morbidity, and mortality of extremely preterm neonates, 1993–2012. *JAMA*, *314*(10), 1039–1051. https://doi.org/10.1001/jama.2015.10244.

van Noort-van der Spek, I. L., Goedegebure, A., Hartwig, N. G., Kornelisse, R. F., Franken, M. J. P., & Weisglas-Kuperus, N. (2017). Normal neonatal hearing screening did not preclude sensorineural hearing loss in two-year-old very preterm infants. *Acta Paediatrica*, *106*(10), 1569–1575. https://doi.org/10.1111/apa.13960.

Vohr, B. R. (2007). How should we report early childhood outcomes of very low birth weight infants? *Seminares in Fetal and Neonatal Medicine*, *12*(5), 355–362. https://doi.org/10.1016/j.siny.2007.05.003.

Vohr, B., Wright, L. L., Hack, M., Aylward, G., & Hirtz, D. (2004). Follow-up care of high-risk infants. *Pediatrics*, *114*, 1377–1397. https://doi.org/10.1542/peds.2004-0866.

Wallace, M. E., Mendola, P., Kim, S. S., Epps, N., Chen, Z., Smarr, M., ... Grantz, K. L. (2017). Racial/ethnic differences in preterm perinatal outcomes. *American Journal of Obstetrics and Gynecology*, *216*(3), 306. e301–e312. https://doi.org/10.1016/j.ajog.2016.11.1026.

Walsh, M. C., Morris, B. H., Wrage, L. A., Vohr, B. R., Poole, W. K., Tyson, J. E., ... National Institutes of Child Health and Human Development Neonatal Research Network. (2005). Extremely low birthweight neonates with protracted ventilation: Mortality and 18-month neurodevelopmental outcomes. *Journal of Pediatrics*, *146*(6), 798–804. https://doi.org/10.1016/j.jpeds.2005.01.047.

Xu, J., Murphy, S. L., Kockanek, K. D., & Arias, E. (2020). Mortality in the United States, 2018. *NCHS Data Brief*, *355*, 1–8.

Yew, S. G., & O'Kearney, R. (2013). Emotional and behavioural outcomes later in childhood and adolescence for children with specific language impairments: Meta-analyses of controlled prospective studies. *Journal of Child Psychology and Psychiatry*, *54*(5), 516–524. https://doi.org/10.1111/jcpp.12009.

Zablotsky, B., Black, L. I., Maenner, M. J., Schieve, L. A., Danielson, M. L., Bitsko, R. H., ... Boyle, C. A. (2019). Prevalence and trends of developmental disabilities among children in the United States: 2009–2017. *Pediatrics*, *144*(4). https://doi.org/10.1542/peds.2019-081.

35

Nutritional Disorders

Liliane Diab and Nancy F. Krebs

For additional material related to the content of this chapter, please see Chapter 23.

VIGNETTE

F.G. is a 17-month-old Hispanic female former full-term infant who was admitted for global developmental delay, poor linear growth, hypotonia, and worsening anemia in the setting of exclusive direct breastfeeding. Her weight gain is at approximately the 15th percentile; her linear growth has been at a plateau from 12 months of age and is currently below the 5th percentile; her weight for length is at the 50th percentile; and her head circumference is growing at approximately the 10th percentile. The family is exclusively Spanish speaking. They established care with a primary care physician 4 months prior to admission and discussed concerns about her significant feeding difficulties and the family history of autism and developmental delay (brother). The mother reported F.G. having difficulty starting complementary food and inability to swallow puree except for broth with a spoon. Mother reported that she continues to have good breast milk supply and no difficulty or choking with nursing. She eats a well-varied diet, takes her prenatal vitamins, and reports being in good health except for fatigue that she attributed to taking care of both F.G. and her 3-year-old brother who has special needs. Labs were drawn and they showed hemoglobin (Hgb) of 10.5, hematocrit (Hct) of 31.1, mean corpuscular volume (MCV) of 92.6, and platelet count of 207. F.G. was started on iron and referred for therapies (speech, physical, and occupational), and genetic testing was briefly discussed.

On admission, F.G. had worsening weakness and further regression in her milestones. Physical exam revealed pallor, significant developmental delay, and hypotonia. She was very weak and unable to sit without support. Labs repeated on admission showed Hgb of 5.6, Hct of 16.9, MCV of 90.4, and a platelet count of 28. She was admitted for blood transfusion. Additional detailed history and laboratory testing revealed a diagnosis that required urgent treatment, and an improved outcome could have resulted if the diagnosis had been made earlier.

OVERVIEW OF THE BRAIN-NUTRIENT INTERACTION

The human brain undergoes remarkable changes beginning at approximately 23 to 24 weeks postconceptional age through the first 2 years of life (the critical 1000-day window encompasses the time from conception to one's second birthday). Recent epidemiologic and neurodevelopmental outcomes studies suggest this sensitive period is broader and extends into the third year of life.

Some primary systems and structures that are rapidly developing during this time period are key to executive brain functions that develop later in life. These systems include anatomic regions (e.g., the hippocampus and the striatum, which are both essential for learning and memory) and processes (e.g., myelination and the monoamine neurotransmitter system that is essential for mediating rewards) that are involved in many developmental trajectories.

Some brain functions that are supported by these key circuits may not have clear manifestations at birth. Certain complex processing behaviors, such as attention and multitasking, that develop later in life have their origins in the growth spurt of the prefrontal cortex during the first 6 postnatal months (Cusick & Georgieff, 2016; Georgieff et al., 2018).

Three main factors that have profound effects on the growth of these circuits and connectivity are exposures and inflammation, the presence of social emotional support, and nutritional sufficiency. This chapter will focus on the role of nutrients. Toxic exposures are covered in Chapter 38, and the interaction of failure to thrive and social determinants of health are covered in Chapter 66. We begin with the discussion of some principles of brain-nutrient interactions.

High Metabolic Demands

The rapid development of the brain during the 1000-day critical window accounts for 60% of the body's energy consumption, in contrast with the adult value of ~20%. Many macronutrients and micronutrients are needed to support this rapid growth (Krebs, Lozoff, & Georgieff, 2017). Nutrients that are essential for neurodevelopment during critical and sensitive windows are summarized in Table 35.1.

Timing and Dose of the Nutritional Deficiency

Critical periods and *sensitive periods* are terms used by neuroscientists to describe time epochs of brain vulnerability to environmental factors (e.g., nutrition). These periods coincide with the specific times of rapid development of specific brain regions (e.g., the cortex, the hippocampus, the striatum) and the peak of certain processes (e.g., myelination) that have higher nutrient requirements. Because the brain is not a homogeneous organ, the growth trajectories of its different structures and processes peak at different times and have specific requirements. As a result there are different sensitive periods during which the deficiency of a specific nutrient is most deterministic. Table 35.1 provides a list of critical macro- and micronutrients

TABLE 35.1 Critical Nutrients That Particularly Affect Brain Development in the First 1000 Days

Nutrient	Critical Time	Biomarkers	Suggested Preventive Strategy
Protein	Gestation 4–12 mo of age	Length at birth Z score (LAZ) and linear growth in the first year of life Weight gain from birth–4 mo of age	Optimizing maternal health and nutrition to prevent intrauterine growth restriction Improving protein intake in early life
LC-PUFA	Last trimester of gestation, 2–3 mo postnatal	DHA levels are not routinely checked	Supplementation during pregnancy, lactation, and infancy has yielded mixed results
Iron	Last trimester of pregnancy and 6 mo–3 yr of age	Hemoglobin, red cell indices, ferritin, transferrin saturation, and TIBC	Optimizing iron status starting in the preconception stage and during pregnancy For infants: no need to supplement if consuming iron-fortified formula, but the AAP recommends breastfed infants be supplemented with iron at 1 mg/kg/day starting at 4 mo of age and started on iron-rich food by 6 mo of age Special attention to providing complementary food that is rich in iron and low in phytate for all infants starting at 6 mo of age
Iodine	First trimester of gestation is most critical, last trimester, and infancy–12 yr of age	Urine iodine (median population level <20 indicates endemic deficiency) Goiter	Iodine supplementation before 10 wk gestation is most effective, especially in areas where iodine deficiency is endemic
Zinc	Last 4 mo gestation 6 mo–10 yr	Dietary zinc intake, plasma zinc concentration, and height-for-age of growing infants and children	Optimizing maternal health, timely introduction of complimentary food that is a good source of zinc and low in phytate (fortified cereal, animal products)
Copper	Last trimester of gestation	Copper level and ceruloplasmin	More studies needed
B12	Birth–6 mo of age	Newborn screen detects methylmalonic acidemia and homocysteine	Supplementation is critically important for mothers who follow a vegetarian or vegan diet. Identifying maternal risk factors. Supplementing infants of vegan mothers
Folate	More studies needed	Serum folate, red blood cell folate, and homocysteine level	The US Public Health Service recommends that all women of childbearing age take 400 μg folic acid daily
Choline	More studies needed	More studies needed	Potential benefit of supplementation in the 1000-day window

AAP, American Academy of Pediatrics; *DHA*, docosahexaenoic acid; *LC-PUFA*, long-chain polyunsaturated acids; *TIBC*, total iron-binding capacity.
Adapted from Georgieff, M. K., Ramel, S. E., & Cusick, S. E. (2018). Nutritional influences on brain development. *Acta Paediatrica, 107*(8), 1310–1321; Wachs, T. D., et al. (2014). Issues in the timing of integrated early interventions: Contributions from nutrition, neuroscience, and psychological research. *Annals of the New York Academy of Sciences, 1308*, 89–106; King, J. C., et al. (2015). Biomarkers of nutrition for development (BOND)—Zinc review. *Journal of Nutrition, 146*(4), S858–S885; Bailey, L. B., et al. (2015). Biomarkers of nutrition for development—Folate review. *Journal of Nutrition, 145*(7), S1636–S1680; Derbyshire, E., & Obeid, R. (2020). Choline, neurological development and brain function: A systematic review focusing on the first 1000 days. *Nutrients, 12*(6).

aligned with the time of developmental window when the brain is most vulnerable to their deficiency.

In addition to the timing of a nutritional deficiency, the region or process requirements of the nutrient at the time of deficiency play a major role in determining the phenotype of the deficiency. Iron is a good example where the behavior phenotype of a deficiency varies greatly with the severity of deficiency and the age of the child (Georgieff et al., 2018).

Vulnerability and Plasticity

The increased vulnerability of the brain during the critical epoch of development is counterbalanced by a higher degree of plasticity (repairability). However, as different regions of the brain become highly specialized in serving certain behaviors and learning processes, this plasticity decreases. Recent research using animal models has focused on understanding the developmental plasticity of the brain and using the critical periods as windows of opportunity for early therapeutic interventions to change the time course of a neurodevelopmental condition (e.g., intellectual disability, autism spectrum disorder) into a normal or asymptomatic neurodevelopmental trajectory (Dehorter & Del Pino, 2020).

The Role of the Microbiome

Much of the earlier work regarding the gut-brain axis has focused on obesity, satiety, and digestive health. However, recent research has led to the appreciation of higher-order cognitive and psychological effects of gut-brain reciprocal communication (Cryan et al., 2019). Factors that alter microbiota composition in early life can affect this communication. These include mode of delivery, infections, use of antibiotics, diet and nutritional provision, stressors, and genetics. Breastfeeding is a good example of the emerging evidence about the interaction of diet and gut-brain axis. Results from Project Viva (a US longitudinal prebirth cohort of 1300 pregnant women and their infants) indicate that even after controlling for socioeconomic status, home environment, and maternal IQ, longer breastfeeding duration up to 12 months of age is associated with higher IQ at 7 years of age. Actually the effects of breastfeeding on neurodevelopment were already measurable at 1 year of age. In addition, the beneficial effect of breastfeeding on visual motor abilities at age 3 years seemed greater for women who consumed two or more servings of fish per week (Blomkvist et al., 2019). In the Donor Milk for Improved Neurodevelopmental Outcomes study 840 infants born less than 1500 g were randomized to receive pasteurized nutrient-fortified donor milk or preterm formula as a supplement to their mother's own milk. Cognitive, language, and motor scores (Bayley-III) at 18 months corrected age were not statistically different among the two groups (O'Connor et al., 2016). This supports the hypothesis that the beneficial effects of breastfeeding on neurodevelopment may be due to both nutrients and bioactive nonnutrient factors.

Epigenetics

Epigenetics is an emerging field of science that studies the change in phenotype, based on change in gene expression, due to environmental factors. Intrauterine growth restriction (IUGR) is an example of the interaction of nutritional status and cognitive development via gene modification. Small-for-gestational age (SGA), a form of IUGR, is defined as birth weight less than the 10th percentile for gestational age, so it is a state of fetal malnutrition. IUGR has been associated with disruption of DNA methylation leading to disruptions in gene expression in animal models. These neurobiologic changes are potentially implicated with increased rates of attention deficit disorder, autism, depression, and anxiety among patients with history of IUGR (Georgieff et al., 2018).

CRITICAL MACRONUTRIENTS

Protein

Anthropometrics are a good reflection of the adequacy of macronutrients provision. Linear growth (vs. weight gain) in the first year of life may be especially critical for cognitive development. Linear growth velocity, especially before 12 months of age, significantly impacts the child's IQ later in life. No anthropometric measures after 12 months were associated with the child future IQ (Horta et al., 2017).

Long-Chain Polyunsaturated Fatty Acid

The evidence is mounting on the role of *n*-3 long-chain polyunsaturated fatty acid (LC-PUFA), particularly docosahexaenoic acid (DHA), in brain and retinal development.

LC-PUFA accumulates in the phospholipids of all brain regions and in the retinal photoreceptors. This accumulation occurs primarily during the fetal period through the first 2 years of life. Thus LC-PUFA and especially DHA are critical macronutrients for optimal visual and neurologic development during early life. The developing fetus and the young infant in the 1000-day critical window have limited ability to synthesize *n*-3 LC-PUFA de novo and must acquire it from the placenta, breast milk, or other external sources (formula). Deprivation of *n*-3 LC-PUFA during the 1000-day window has negative effects on memory, learning abilities, and visual acuity (Chmielewska et al., 2019).

The effect of supplementing with LC-PUFA, particularly DHA and arachidonic acid, during gestation, lactation, and early childhood on childhood cognition has been extensively studied. Although systemic reviews and metaanalyses report no significant benefit in cognitive and behavioral development and in visual acuity (Gould, Roberts, & Makrides, 2021), these analyses are possibly limited by the short age window under consideration. Some studies with longer timeframes showed improvement on standardized developmental tests with maternal supplementation with DHA during pregnancy and through the first few months of life (Basak, Mallick, & Duttaroy, 2020). This emphasizes the fact that the effect of nutrition on key brain systems may not be clear until later in life when more complex behavior can be tested (Georgieff et al., 2018).

CRITICAL MICRONUTRIENTS

Iron

Iron deficiency is the most common micronutrient deficiency in the world. The risk of iron deficiency is highest during pregnancy and infancy, which coincides with the 1000-day critical window. Iron deficiency in pregnancy can affect newborn brain structure and lead to compromised recognition memory and slower processing speed. Both effects are proven to continue despite postnatal iron supplementation. Low maternal iron intake has also been associated with autism spectrum disorder and schizophrenia (Georgieff, 2020). The combined exposure to low iron intake and advanced maternal age with metabolic conditions was associated with a fivefold increased autism spectrum disorder risk (Adams et al., 2021).

In 1983 Dr. Frank Oski published the results of his research on iron deficiency without anemia and concluded that even in the absence of anemia, iron deficiency resulted in biochemical alteration of the brain that impaired cognitive behavior. Many more studies followed confirming the importance of iron sufficiency for neurodevelopmental outcomes. Of great concern is the consistent finding among all these studies that prompt treatment of early iron deficiency does not lead to complete brain recovery and that early-life iron deficiency can lead to loss of human potential. Timing of iron supplementation is critical. Studies in areas where iron deficiency is prevalent suggest that iron supplementation during pregnancy was associated with improved neurodevelopmental outcomes, but supplementation of children between 12 and 35 months of age conferred no added benefit (Lynch et al., 2018).

However, mistimed iron supplementation may negatively impact neurodevelopmental outcomes. A 16-year follow-up study of an infant iron supplementation randomized controlled trial in Chile showed that 6-month-old infants with high hemoglobin who consumed iron-fortified formula performed significantly worse on a battery of neurodevelopmental tasks, but infants with low hemoglobin who received the same formula performed significantly better (Gahagan et al., 2019). These results underscore the importance of dose, timing, and host nutritional status for certain critical micronutrients.

The risks and benefits of dietary iron delivery should be carefully considered, especially in less common circumstances of iron overload in infants where it can lead to neurodevelopmental comorbidities. Formula iron fortification significantly improved neurodevelopmental outcomes in both iron-depleted and iron-sufficient children. Iron supplementation can carry more risk than benefit in two cases: (1) the presence of high hemoglobin regardless of the status of ferritin (even if low, this represents a case of polycythemia by volume contraction or for non–iron-related conditions) and (2) in the presence of normal or elevated ferritin even with low hemoglobin (anemia of inflammation) (Georgieff et al., 2019).

Iron deficiency remains one of the top four causes for lost human potential among children worldwide. Optimizing maternal, fetal, and infant iron status is an important strategy for improving neurobehavioral outcomes. However, especially in well-resourced countries, this effort should be guided with appropriate screening and monitoring (Box 35.1).

Iodine

Iodine is critical for thyroid hormone synthesis. Severe iodine deficiency in the first trimester can result in cretinism, which is marked by an IQ of 30, and deficits in hearing, speech, and gait. The impact of mild and moderate iodine deficiency is less studied, but recent research has shown significant improvement in neurodevelopmental outcomes at 18 months of age, when mothers were supplemented with iodine before 10 weeks of gestation (Georgieff et al., 2018). Despite global efforts to achieve universal iodine fortification of staple foods (e.g., salt), maternal iodine deficiency has not been eliminated, including in the critical periconceptional period (Young et al., 2021).

BOX 35.1 Clinical Pearl: Targeted Screening and Treatment for Iron Deficiency

- High-risk infants may need screening earlier than 1 year of age. These include preterm infants and especially late preterm who may not have had supplementation/fortified human milk in nursery, small-for-gestational age infants, infants/young children who have been reliant on prolonged breastfeeding without adequate iron intake from foods or supplements, and infants with rapid postnatal weight gain.
- Infants/children who have received a large percentage of calories from fortified formulas may benefit from screening a few months after they transition to whole milk.
- Screen for iron deficiency with ferritin and an inflammatory marker. Hemoglobin only screens for anemia, which is a late manifestation of iron deficiency.
- Best food sources for iron are infant-fortified cereals and red meat. Iron from vegetables and beans is not well absorbed due to the presence of phytate, polyphenols, or other compounds.
- Treatment dose for iron deficiency without anemia is 3 mg/kg/day and for iron deficiency anemia is 6 mg/kg/day for 2–3 months, then repeat labs.

Vitamin B12 (Cobalamin)

Vitamin B12 is essential for myelination and neuronal development. Newborn infants have limited endogenous stores and are at risk of vitamin B12 deficiency when maternal vitamin B12 status is poor and they are predominantly breastfed. The most common reasons for maternal B12 deficiency are unrecognized pernicious anemia, strict vegetarian diet, and history of gastric bypass. Vitamin B12 deficiency is marked by brain atrophy and nerve demyelination. Symptoms usually start between 4 and 10 months of age and include failure to thrive, developmental regression, tremors, hypotonia, lethargy, irritability, and feeding difficulties. It is very important to note that hematologic findings are not always present.

Vitamin B12 replacement leads to rapid improvement with documented reversal of apathy, hypotonia, anorexia, and tremors, sometimes within days of initiating treatment. Brain atrophy and feeding difficulties may take several months to improve. Unfortunately, despite the dramatic rapid improvement, many infants with vitamin B12 deficiency suffer from long-term cognitive and developmental delay (Green et al., 2017).

The infant in the vignette had vitamin B12 deficiency secondary to undiagnosed maternal pernicious anemia. Detailed history after admission revealed that F.G. was developing normally until 5 months of age. Mother provided pictures of F.G. as an infant smiling and lifting her chest up supported on her arms in a prone position. Unfortunately, the developmental regression was missed and, due to the brother's diagnosis of autism, it was erroneously assumed that there was a genetic etiology. It was further assumed that F.G. was only iron deficient due to her dependence on breast milk, and the high MCV on the initial complete blood count was not noted. This patient was treated with daily, then weekly vitamin B12 injection, but sadly she remains with global developmental delay. Timing can clearly be critical when a micronutrient deficiency coincides with a sensitive period of brain development.

Zinc

Zinc is a structural component in 2500 transcription factors (zinc fingers), a catalyst to more than 300 enzymes, and a regulator for thousands of genes (8% of the human genome). There are 24 zinc transporters that coordinate these cellular functions. Zinc deficiency affects many body functions, most importantly physical growth, the immune and reproductive systems, and neurobehavioral development. To prevent zinc deficiency, a regular adequate dietary intake is needed because, similar to protein, there is no functional reserve for zinc. Conditions associated with zinc deficiency include dietary inadequacies (plant-based/low-meat diet, high phytate, prolonged [>6 months] exclusive breastfeeding), higher zinc requirements (prematurity, IUGR, growth, pregnancy, and lactation), and conditions leading to zinc malabsorption (inflammatory bowel disease, chronic liver disease, diarrhea, cystic fibrosis, etc.) (Lassi et al., 2020).

Vitamin D

Although not considered a critical micronutrient for brain development, we added this small section about vitamin D due to the high prevalence of its deficiency among adults and children worldwide. Various cells and tissues express the vitamin D receptor, which highlights the nonskeletal functions of vitamin D. In addition to rickets and osteopenia, vitamin D deficiency has been associated in epidemiologic studies with increased risk of infections, types 1 and 2 diabetes, multiple sclerosis, cardiovascular disease, dementia, and cancer; however, causality has not been established for any of these observations (Charoenngam, Shirvani, & Holick, 2019).

There continues to be much debate regarding definition of vitamin D deficiency. At present the Institute of Medicine, the American Academy of Pediatrics, and European Society of Paediatric Gastroenterology, Hepatology and Nutrition all suggest 20 ng/mL as the cutoff for deficiency, but the controversy continues with respect to the level of serum 25(OH)D that defines sufficiency.

Circulating 25(OH)D level measured by a reliable assay is the best indicator of vitamin D status. However, universal screening of all patients for vitamin D deficiency is not recommended and should be reserved for high-risk patients such as patients with limited sun exposure (dark or covered skin), exclusively breastfed older infants, patients with malabsorption or who use certain medications that interfere with vitamin D homeostasis, patients with liver and kidney disease, and patients with obesity. The therapeutic and preventive doses of vitamin D are summarized in Table 35.2 (Diab & Krebs, 2018).

BOX 35.2 Clinical Pearl: Over-the-Counter Vitamins Are NOT All the Same

- Poly-Vi-Sol does not contain zinc, iron, or folic acid but does contain 400 IU (10 mcg) vitamin D3.
- Poly-Vi-Sol with Iron (10 mg elemental iron/mL) is intended for prevention NOT treatment of iron deficiency. It contains 400 IU (10 mcg) vitamin D3. It does not contain vitamin B12, folate, or zinc.
- Gummy multivitamins do NOT contain iron or zinc in meaningful quantities.
- Flintstones Complete Hard Chewable Tablet (or its generic equivalent) is a good reference by which to compare other children's multivitamins for completeness.
- Calcium supplementation with TUMS (or its generic equivalent) offers an economic/widely accessible option for calcium carbonate (500–1000 mg/tab).

TABLE 35.2 Therapeutic and Preventive Doses of Vitamin D

Age	Therapeutic Dose	Preventive Dose
Infants 0–1 yr old	2000 IU (50 mcg) per day or 50,000 IU (1250 mcg) once weekly for 6 wk until blood level is >30 ng/mL	400–1000 IU/day (10–25 mcg/day)
Children 1–18 yr old	2000 IU (50 mcg) per day or 50,000 IU (1250 mcg) once weekly for 6 wk until blood level is >30 ng/mL	600–1000 IU/day (15–25 mcg/day)

- Experts estimate that 100 IU (2.5 mcg) of vitamin D2 or D3 daily will raise the blood level of 25(OH)D by 1 ng/mL.
- The higher maintenance dose is for children with risk factors for deficiency (children with obesity, on anticonvulsants or glucocorticoids).

Adapted from Holick, M. F., et al. (2011). Evaluation, treatment, and prevention of vitamin D deficiency: An Endocrine Society clinical practice guideline. *Journal of Clinical Endocrinology and Metabolism, 96*(7), 1911–1930. https://doi.org/10.1210/jc.2011-0385

NUTRITION STATUS ASSESSMENT IN CHILDREN WITH DEVELOPMENTAL DISABILITY

Children with developmental disabilities are at increased risk for under- and overnutrition. Altered body composition and physical activity imply different growth expectations and different recommendations for nutrient intake. Taking this into consideration is essential for accurate assessment of nutritional status and needs. The purpose of this brief review is to provide the reader with resources and practical tips to perform such an assessment.

A nutrition status assessment should include a detailed medical and dietary history (with focus on feeding difficulties and signs of dysphagia), anthropometrics, estimated energy needs, and bone density (ambulatory status, use of anticonvulsant medication, etc.). Table 35.3 summarizes some of the history and physical exam findings that can be associated with micronutrient deficiencies. Laboratory workup must align with risk factors revealed in the history and physical exam.

Anthropometrics, Body Composition, and Bone Density

Standard Growth Charts

Growth assessment typically and most readily includes weight, length (or standing height for children age >2 years), and head circumference measurements. For normative standard, the Centers for Disease Control and Prevention (CDC) recommends the use of the World Health Organization (WHO) standard growth charts for children from birth to 2 years of age, and the CDC reference charts for children ages 2 to 20 years. These charts are available at www.cdc.gov/growthcharts. On both charts, anthropometric measures are expressed as

TABLE 35.3 **Quick Reference for Findings Associated With Micronutrient Deficiencies**

Nutrient	Rash/Skin Findings	Mouth Lesions	Neurologic Symptoms	Anemia	Other
Vitamin A	X				Eye findings, blindness
Thiamine B1			X		Beriberi, congestive heart failure
Riboflavin B2		X			
Niacin B3	X		X		Pellagra
Pyridoxine B6		X	X	X	
Vitamin B12		X	X	X	
Folate		X		X	
Vitamin C	X	X			Bone pain, refusal to walk
Vitamin D					Bone pain, fractures
Vitamin E			X	X	Loss of reflexes
Vitamin K	X	X			
Copper			X	X	Osteopenia, neutropenia
Iron			X	X	
Zinc	X				

percentiles, but more recently Z scores (standard deviation) are recommended for expressing deviations from norms. The use of electronic medical records has facilitated the calculation of Z scores. Normal growth is considered to be Z scores between ±1 for any given measure (Price et al., 2020).

Head circumference is considered a proxy indicator of overall brain growth and should be included in all anthropometrics. However, head circumference is of limited use in cases of micro- or macrocephaly, except to monitor for stagnation of growth or rapid increase, respectively.

Special Growth Charts

Many disease-specific or genetic condition–specific growth charts are published. However, it is important to take into consideration that these charts are mostly descriptive of growth in populations with high risk for nutritional disorders such as growth faltering or sometimes obesity. Many experts recommend using the WHO/CDC infant charts (0–24 months) or the CDC growth chart (2–20 years), and use depends on the child's age and adjusting growth goals based on the clinical scenario. For example, it is not reasonable to aim for over 90% of ideal body weight for patients with Russell-Silver syndrome, and 75% to 85% of ideal body weight is considered acceptable (Wakeling et al., 2017).

Debate exists in regard to the use of specific growth charts for patients with cerebral palsy (CP). In 2011 Brooks, Day, Shavelle, & Strauss, developed CP-specific growth charts stratified by functional ability as defined by the Gross Motor Function Classification System (GMFCS). The complete set of CP-specific growth charts is available at www.lifeexpectancy.org/articles/newgrowthcharts.shtml. The GMFCS level V charts are different for an orally or tube-fed child. In addition, Brooks et al. identified the low-weight threshold associated with increased morbidity and mortality (Scarpato et al., 2017).

Despite this stratification many experts recommend caution when using these growth charts and to consider them only to gain perspective on the broad growth expectations for patients with CP.

In our practice, we use the WHO or the CDC growth chart, but we adjust our goals based on body composition assessment aiming for weight for length or body mass index (BMI) at the 5th or 10th percentile.

Midupper Arm Circumference

Midupper arm circumference (MUAC) can be used as an independent anthropometric tool to screen for and diagnose malnutrition in children 6 to 59 months of age based on WHO standards. Reference ranges and Z scores are available from the WHO for ages 3 months to 5 years at https://www.who.int/tools/child-growth-standards/standards/arm-circumference-for-age and for older children and adults from Frisancho (1981) for ages 1 to 79 years. MUAC correlates to BMI in children and adults and can be used in combination with the triceps skinfold (TSF) thickness to estimate UA muscle area.

Table 35.4 lists classification of nutrition status based on standard anthropometric measures and MUAC. If used, for children with complex medical conditions such as those mentioned earlier, these classifications should be interpreted with particular attention to body composition, growth potential, among other factors.

Triceps Skinfold Thickness

TSF is a measure of the subcutaneous fat in that specific site. It is a sensitive indicator of total body fat and reflects changes in nutritional status. The sensitivity of the TSF makes it a reliable method for measuring progress on short-term goals. When combined with the MUAC, TSF can be used to calculate

TABLE 35.4 Nutritional Status Assessment

Method	No Malnutrition	Mild Malnutrition	Moderate Malnutrition	Severe Malnutrition
Weight for height percent of median	90%	80–89%	70–79%	<70%
Weight for height Z score	>−1	−1−−1.9	−2−−2.9	<−3
BMI Z score	>−1	−1−−1.9	−2−−2.9	<−3
Length/height Z score	Not applicable	No data but Z score <−2 suggests stunting	No data but Z score <−2 suggests stunting	<−3
MUAC for children age 6–59 mo			11.5–12.4 cm	<11.5 cm

BMI, Body mass index; MUAC, midupper arm circumference.

midarm muscle area, which makes it a useful tool for nutrition status assessment in children with altered body compositions and low muscle mass. TSF charts are available at https://www.who.int/childgrowth/standards/tsf_for_age/en/.

Subscapular Skinfold Thickness

The subscapular skinfold thickness is a measure of subcutaneous fat on the trunk. It is helpful in the assessment of body composition. Reference data are available from the WHO at https://www.who.int/tools/child-growth-standards/standards/subscapular-skinfold-for-age.

Body Composition

Taking body composition into consideration is essential in the nutrition status assessment of children with disabilities. Understanding a specific patient's fat and lean body stores is important for preventing under- and overfeeding. A very simple, low-cost, and accurate estimation can be done in an office visit with anthropometric equations that utilize the TSF and MUAC to calculate the UA muscle area and UA fat area. The equations are listed later in Table 35.6 for reference values as provided by Addo et al., (2017).

Bioelectrical impedance analysis and dual-energy X-ray absorptiometry (DXA) can also be used for the assessment of body composition.

Weight Gain Velocity

Table 35.5 presents ranges of normal weight gain velocity. This table was based on the WHO multicenter study. Gaining 50% or less of the normal weight gain per age is considered an indicator of pediatric malnutrition.

TABLE 35.5 Approximate Average Rates of Weight Gain

Age	Weight Gain
Newborn–3 mo	25–30 g/day
3–6 mo	15–20 g/day
6–12 mo	10 g/day
1–3 yr	6 g/day

Arm and Leg Length Measures

Length and height measurements are not always possible in children with developmental disabilities. Segmental measurements of the arm and leg can be used, and specific height predictive equations based on ulnar length and knee height can be applied.

Assessment of Bone Mineral Density

Nonambulatory children are at increased risk of osteopenia and fractures. The International Society for Clinical Densitometry defines osteoporosis in children on the basis of both fracture history and low bone density compared to age and gender reference data. The current recommendations are to measure bone mineral density (BMD) via DXA to identify children and adolescents who will benefit from an intervention to decrease the risk of fractures. A Z score of less than or equal to −2 is considered low BMD; however, a history of fracture is essential to make a diagnosis of osteoporosis (Ward, 2021).

Basic Principles for Assessment of Nutritional Requirements in Children With Disabilities

The best starting point to accurately recommend a nutritional therapy plan is an accurate assessment of nutrition status (i.e., malnutrition, obesity, risk for micronutrient deficiencies) with history, physical exam, and anthropometrics in addition to laboratory workup as needed.

Recommended Dietary Allowance

The recommended dietary allowance (RDA; https://www.nal.usda.gov/fnic/dietary-reference-intakes) is a good starting point for estimating nutritional needs for patients with normal body composition and normal nutrition status. The RDA will require adjustments for children with malnutrition, obesity, acute illness, or chronic conditions. This calculator for health care professionals provides an estimated caloric need, macronutrient requirements, recommended intake, and tolerable upper-level intake for micronutrients (https://www.nal.usda.gov/fnic/dri-calculator/).

Resting Energy Expenditure and Total Energy Expenditure

The resting energy expenditure (REE) accounts for 65% to 70% of total energy expenditure (TEE). The thermic effect of food (TEF) and physical activity (PA) account for the remaining 10% to 15% and 20% to 30%, respectively. The TEF and PA are difficult to quantify and can vary from day to day, especially for PA, so REE is most often used as the best predictor of TEE. REE is multiplied by a PA coefficient based on the estimated physical activity level.

In medically complex children, it is best to measure REE with indirect calorimetry; however, when this is not available REE can be estimated using prediction equations such as the WHO and the Schofield (1985). These estimates are then adjusted using a physical activity level based on the disease state, physical activity, and growth needs. The RDA Estimated Energy Requirement can replace these estimates but may not be as reliable in patients with special needs. Tables 35.6, 35.7, and 35.8 provide resources for applying these calculations in clinical practice. We will end this chapter with two case studies that demonstrate the application of the above mentioned principles when taking care of patients with special needs (Figs. 35.1 and 35.2).

TABLE 35.6 Estimated Energy and Protein Needs for Pediatric Patients

	Age	Energy Needs[a,b,c] (kcal/kg/day)	Resting Energy Expenditure[d] (kcal/kg/day)	Protein: RDA[f] (g/kg/day)	Protein: Hospitalized Patients[g] (g/kg/day)
Infants	0–2 mo	110–130[e]	45–60[e]	1.52*	1.5–2.5
	2–3 mo	102	55	1.52*	1.5–2.5
	4–6 mo	82	55	1.52*	1.5–2.5
	7–12 mo	80	55	1.2–1.5	1.5–2.5
	13–35 mo	82	55	1.05	1.5–2.5
Males	3 yr	85	55	1.05	1.5–2.5
	4–5 yr	70	45	0.95	1.5–2
	6–7 yr	64	40–45	0.95	1.5–2
	8 yr	59	40	0.95	1.5
Females	3 yr	82	55	1.05	1.5–2.5
	4–5 yr	65	45	0.95	1.5–2
	6–7 yr	61	40–45	0.95	1.5–2
	8 yr	59	55	0.95	1.5
Males	9–11 yr	49	30–40	0.95	1.5
	12–13 yr	44	30	0.95	1.5
	14–16 yr	39	30	0.85	1.5
	17–18 yr	37	30	0.85	1.5
	>18 yr	36	30	0.8	1.2–1.5
Females	9–11 yr	42	30–40	0.95	1.5
	12–13 yr	40	30	0.95	1.5
	14–16 yr	33	25	0.85	1.5
	17–18 yr	31	25	0.85	1.5
	>18 yr	34	25	0.8	1.2–1.5

RDA, Recommended daily allowance; *, adequate intake.

Table adapted from 2019 Pediatric Nutrition Handbook, an internal guide at Children Hospital Colorado.

[a]Adapted from Institute of Medicine. (2006). *Dietary reference intakes: The essential guide to nutrient requirements.* The National Academies Press. https://doi.org/10.17226/11537

[b]Adapted from ASPEN Pediatric Nutrition Support Handbook 2nd Edition, 2015

[c]Adapted from Mark R. Corkins (Ed.). (2015). *Pediatric nutrition support core curriculum* (2nd ed.). American Society for Parenteral and Enteral Nutrition (ASPEN).

[d]Adapted from FAO/WHO/UNU. (1985). *Energy and protein requirements.* World Health Organization Technical Report Series 724, 1–206.

[e]Adapted from Tsang, R. C. (2005). *Nutrition of the preterm infant* (2nd ed.). Digital Education Pub.

[f]Adapted from Dietary Reference Intakes: Recommended Dietary Allowance (RDA)

[g]Guidelines for the Provision and Assessment of Nutrition Support Therapy in the Pediatric Critically Ill Patient: Society for Critical Care Medicine and ASPEN, 2017

TABLE 35.7 Using Resting Energy Exposure to Estimate Total Energy Exposure

Patient Population	Factor for Desired Energy Provision	Comments
Obesity	REE × PA– (reasonable amount of calories to create a daily deficit)	500 kcal deficit per day can lead to 1 lb weight loss per week
Underweight	REE × PA + 5 kcal/g/day weight gain desired	For catch-up growth typical goal for weight gain is 150% of normal daily weight gain per age

PA, Physical activity; *REE*, resting energy exposure.

TABLE 35.8 Physical Activity Adjustment Based on Physical Activity Level

Physical Activity Coefficient	Physical Activity Level	Comment
1.0	1.0–<1.4	Sedentary
1.12	1.4–<1.6	Low active
1.24	1.6–<1.9	Active
1.45	1.9–<125	Very active

Adapted from World Health Organization. (1985). Energy and protein requirements. *WHO Technical Report Series 724*, 1–206; Seagle, H. M., et al. (2009). Position of the American Dietetic Association: Weight management. *Journal of the American Dietetic Association, 109*, 330–346.

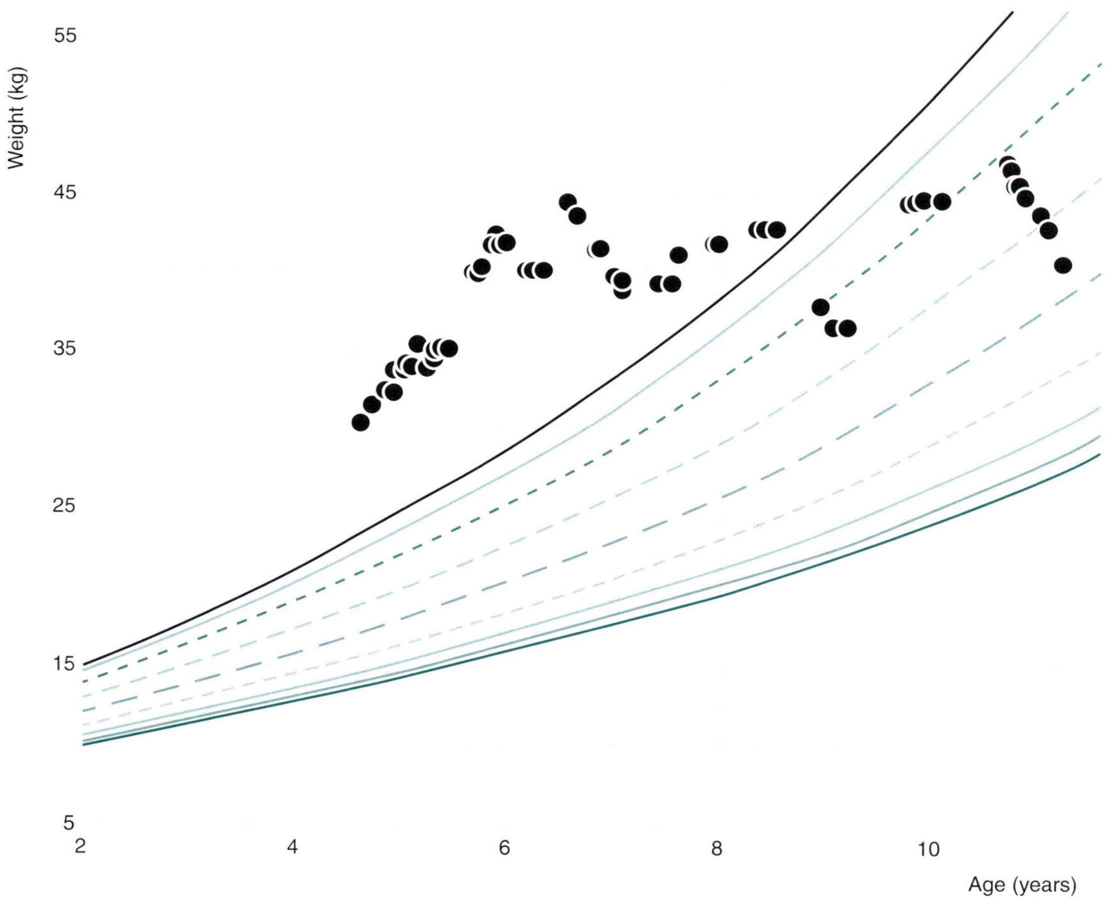

Fig. 35.1 *Case Study 1* A 10-year-old presents with global developmental delay secondary to meningitis in infancy. Using the WHO equation to predict her REE (30 kcal/kg/day) the estimated need was 1200 kcal per day. Indirect calorimetry shows measured REE of 580 kcal. PA estimated to be 1 (patient is sedentary), so she was started on 600 kcal diet per day under the supervision of registered dietitian to ensure complete provision of protein, micronutrients, and essential fatty acids. Patient is successfully losing weight with improvement in her BMI and mobility.

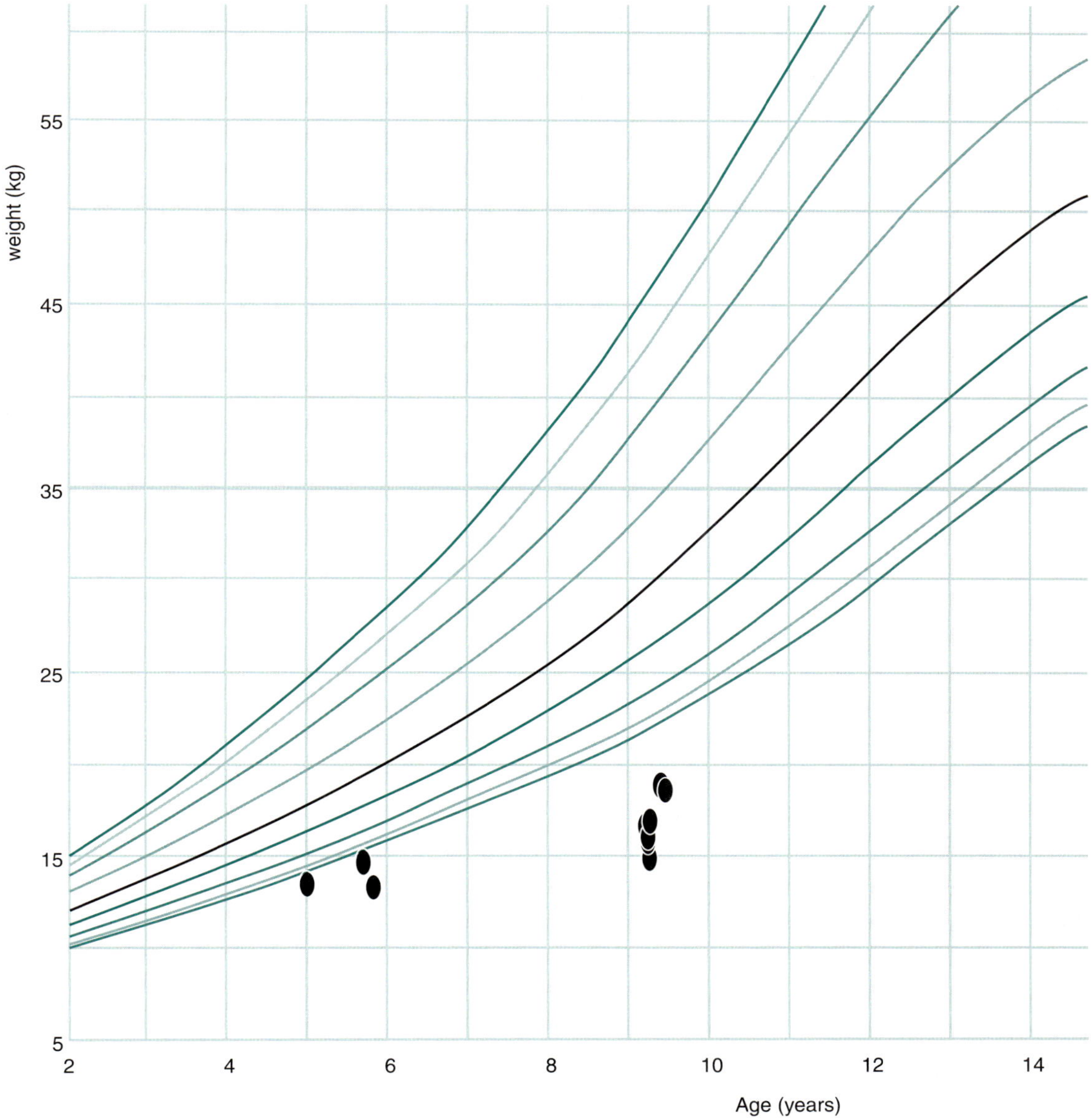

Fig. 35.2 Case Study 2 A 9-year-old presents with CP and poor weight gain that was secondary to medical neglect. Patient is fed via G tube; she was started on 80 kcal/kg/day for catchup growth. Patient gained 8 lb in 2 months and presents for follow-up. Length measurements were not consistent due to contractures. Weight Z score was −3.4. Skinfold Measurements MUAC 170 mm (Z score: −2.04); TSF 11 mm (Z score: −0.66); MAMA 1461 mm^2 (Z score: −2.5) Discussion TSF Z score indicates adequate subcutaneous fat. Low MUAC Z score is due to low muscle mass. Caloric provision was adjusted based on the results to provide adequate intake for growth as patient is considered to be well nourished at this point.

REFERENCES

Adams, J. B. B., et al. (2021). Evidence-based recommendations for an optimal prenatal supplement for women in the U.S., part two: Minerals. *Nutrients*, *13*(6).

Addo, O. Y., Himes, J. H., & Zemel, B. S. (2017). Reference ranges for midupper arm circumference, upper arm muscle area, and upper arm fat area in US children and adolescents aged 1-20 y. *American Journal of Clinical Nutrition*, *105*(1), 111–120.

Basak, S., Mallick, R., & Duttaroy, A. K. (2020). Maternal docosahexaenoic acid status during pregnancy and its impact on infant neurodevelopment. *Nutrients*, *12*(12).

Blomkvist, E. A. M., et al. (2019). Diet and neurodevelopmental score in a sample of one-year-old children—A cross-sectional study. *Nutrients*, *11*(7).

Brooks, J., Day, S., Shavelle, R., & Strauss, D. (2011). Low weight, morbidity, and mortality in children with cerebral palsy: New clinical growth charts. *Pediatrics*, *182*(2), e299–e307.

Charoenngam, N., Shirvani, A., & Holick, M. F. (2019). Vitamin D for skeletal and non-skeletal health: What we should know. *Journal of Clinical Orthopaedics & Trauma*, *10*(6), 1082–1093.

Chmielewska, A., et al. (2019). Effects of prenatal and/or postnatal supplementation with iron, PUFA or folic acid on

neurodevelopment: Update. *British Journal of Nutrition*, *122*(1), S10–S15.
Cryan, J. F., et al. (2019). The microbiota-gut-brain axis. *Physiological Reviews*, *99*(4), 1877–2013.
Cusick, S. E., & Georgieff, M. K. (2016). The role of nutrition in brain development: The golden opportunity of the "first 1000 days". *Journal of Pediatrics*, *175*, 16–21.
Dehorter, N., & Del Pino, I. (2020). Shifting developmental trajectories during critical periods of brain formation. *Frontiers in Cellular Neuroscience*, *14*, 283.
Diab, L., & Krebs, N. F. (2018). Vitamin excess and deficiency. *Pediatric Reviews*, *39*(4), 161–179.
FAO/WHO/UNU, (1985). Energy and protein requirements. *World Health Organization Technical Report Series*, *724*, 1–206.
Frisancho, A. R., (1981). New norms of upper limb fat and muscle areas for assessment of nutritional status. *The American Journal of Clinical Nutrition, 34*(11), 2540–2545. https://doi.org/10.1093/ajcn/34.11.2540
Gahagan, S., et al. (2019). Randomized controlled trial of iron-fortified versus low-iron infant formula: Developmental outcomes at 16 years. *Journal of Pediatrics*, *212*, 124–130.e1.
Georgieff, M. K. (2020). Iron deficiency in pregnancy. *American Journal of Obstetrics and Gynecology*, *223*(4), 516–524.
Georgieff, M. K., Krebs, N. F., & Cusick, S. E. (2019). The benefits and risks of iron supplementation in pregnancy and childhood. *Annual Review of Nutrition*, *39*, 121–146.
Georgieff, M. K., Ramel, S. E., & Cusick, S. E. (2018). Nutritional influences on brain development. *Acta Paediatrica*, *107*(8), 1310–1321.
Gould, J. F., Roberts, R. M., & Makrides, M. (2021). The influence of omega-3 long-chain polyunsaturated fatty acid, docosahexaenoic acid, on child behavioral functioning: A review of randomized controlled trials of DHA supplementation in pregnancy, the neonatal period and infancy. *Nutrients*, *13*(2).
Green, R., et al. (2017). Vitamin B. *Nature Reviews Disease Primers*, *3*, 17040.
Horta, B. L., et al. (2017). Associations of linear growth and relative weight gain in early life with human capital at 30 years of age. *Journal of Pediatrics*, *182*, 85–91.e3.
Institute of Medicine. (2006). *Dietary reference intakes: The essential guide to nutrient requirements*. The National Academies Press. https://doi.org/10.17226/11537
Krebs, N. F., Lozoff, B., & Georgieff, M. K. (2017). Neurodevelopment: The impact of nutrition and inflammation during infancy in low-resource settings. *Pediatrics*, *139*(1), S50–S58.
Lassi, Z. S., et al. (2020). Zinc supplementation for the promotion of growth and prevention of infections in infants less than six months of age. *Cochrane Database of Systematic Reviews*, *4*, CD010205.
Lynch, S., et al. (2018). Biomarkers of nutrition for development (BOND)—Iron review. *Journal of Nutrition*, *148*(1), S1001–S1067.
Mark R. Corkins (Ed.). (2015). *Pediatric nutrition support core curriculum* (2nd ed.). American Society for Parenteral and Enteral Nutrition (ASPEN).
O'Connor, D. L., et al. (2016). Effect of supplemental donor human milk compared with preterm formula on neurodevelopment of very low-birth-weight infants at 18 months: A randomized clinical trial. *JAMA*, *316*(18), 1897–1905.
Oski, F. A., Honig, A. S., Helu, B., Howanitz P. Pediatrics. (1983). Effect of iron therapy on behavior performance in nonanemic, iron-deficient infants. *Pediatrics*, *71*(6), 877–880.
Price, A. A., et al. (2020). Utilization of current diagnostic indicators to characterize pediatric undernutrition among US children. *Nutrients*, *12*(5)., 1409.
Scarpato, E., et al. (2017). Nutritional assessment and intervention in children with cerebral palsy: A practical approach. *International Journal of Food Sciences and Nutrition*, *68*(6), 763–770.
Schofield, W. N., et al. (1985). Predicting basal metabolic rate, new standards and review of previous work. *Human Nutrition. Clinical Nutrition*, *39*(Suppl 1), 5–41.
Tsang, R. C. (2005). *Nutrition of the preterm infant* (2nd ed.). Digital Education Pub.
Wakeling, E. L., et al. (2017). Diagnosis and management of Silver-Russell syndrome: First international consensus statement. *Nature Reviews Endocrinology*, *13*(2), 105–124.
Ward, L. M. (2021). Part I: Which child with a chronic disease needs bone health monitoring? *Current Osteoporosis Reports*.
Young, A. E., Kemp, J. F., Uhlson, C., Westcott, J. L., Ali, S. A., Saleem, S., ... Women First Preconception Maternal Nutrition Trial Group (2021). Improved first trimester maternal iodine status with preconception supplementation: The Women First Trial. *Maternal & Child Nutrition*, *17*(4), e13204.

PEDIATRIC FORMULAS

INFANT FORMULAS

Category	Brands	Features and Comments
Cow-Milk Protein	Similac Advance ***(48:52 whey:casein ratio)*** Similac 24 with Iron Enfamil NeuroPro Enfamil Enspire	With lactose
Partially Hydrolyzed Cow-Milk and Whey Protein	Good Start Gentle ***(100% whey)*** Similac Total Comfort ***(Hydrolyzed protein)*** Enfamil NeuroPro Gentlease Good Start Soothe	Reduced lactose; not hypoallergenic but may prevent atopic disease

INFANT FORMULAS—Cont'd

Category	Brands	Features and Comments
Cow-Milk Protein Without Lactose	Similac Sensitive ***(18:82 whey:casein ratio)***	Lactose free
Soy Protein	Similac Soy Isomil Isomil Prosobee	Lactose free; not for premature infants
Premature	Similac Special Care ***(60:40 20&24 kcal; 50:50 30 kcal whey:casein ratio)*** Enfamil Premature	Cow-milk protein, reduced lactose, 40–50% fat as MCT
Premature Transitional	NeoSure ***(50:50 whey:casein ratio)*** EnfaCare	Standard at 22 kcal/oz; cow-milk protein, reduced lactose, 25% fat as MCT
Semielemental/ Hydrolyzed	Alimentum ***(hydrolyzed protein)*** Pregestimil ***(hydrolyzed protein)*** Nutramigen ***(hydrolyzed protein)*** Gerber Extensive HA	Extensively hydrolyzed formula contains MCT: (Alimentum 33%, Pregestimil 55%, Nutramigen 0%) Hydrolyzed casein, lactose free Used for protein allergy (all) and malabsorption (Alimentum and Pregestimil)
Elemental	EleCare Infant Neocate Infant Puramino Alfamino Infant	Free amino acids and with MCT (EleCare 33%) Used in severe protein allergy or malabsorption
Fat Modified (High Medium-Chain Triglyceride [MCT])	Enfaport ***(60:40 whey:casein ratio)***	30 kcal/oz concentrate; cow-milk protein, lactose free, 83% fat as MCT Typically used for chylous effusions, lymphatic anomalies, or FA oxidation defects
Electrolyte and Mineral Modified	Similac PM 60/40 ***(60:40 whey:casein ratio)***	Cow-milk protein, lactose; reduced electrolytes, minerals, iron

Adapted from 2019 Pediatric Nutrition Handbook, an internal guide at Children Hospital Colorado.

PEDIATRIC FORMULAS

Category	Brands	Features and Comments
Oral Supplements		
Standard, Cow-Milk Protein	Boost Kid Essentials 1.0 Boost Kid Essentials 1.5 with or w/o fiber Scandishake Carnation Breakfast Essentials Nutren 1.0 PediaSure 1.0 without fiber PediaSure 1.0 w/fiber PediaSure 1.5 with or w/o fiber	May or may not contain lactose May or may not provide complete nutrition
Semielemental	Kate Farms Pediatric Peptide 1.5 Pediasure Peptide 1.0 PediaSure Peptide 1.5	Used for malabsorption, contain medium-chain triglyceride (MCT)
Elemental	EleCare Junior Neocate Splash Neocate Jr Puramino	Used for malabsorption or severe protein allergy; contains MCT
Soy Protein	Bright Beginnings Soy Pediasmart Soy	Cow-milk protein free
Clear Liquid	Boost Breeze Ensure Clear	Clear liquid, fruit flavored, fat free; cow-milk protein source For supplemental nutrition only

(Continued)

PEDIATRIC FORMULAS—Cont'd

Category	Brands	Features and Comments
Wound Healing Supplement	Juven Arginaid n/a	Arginaid: L-arginine only Juven: arginine glutamine, and beta-hydroxy-beta-methylbutyrate
Tube Feeding		
Standard, Cow-Milk Protein	Boost Kid Essentials 1.0 Nutren Junior with or w/o fiber *(1.0 kcal/ml)* PediaSure (w/ or w/o fiber) Boost Kid Essentials (w/fiber)	Isotonic, available with fiber or without fiber
High Calorie, Cow-Milk Protein	Boost Kid Essentials 1.5 with or w/o fiber *(1.5 kcal/ml)* PediaSure 1.5 w/ or w/o fiber	For increased caloric needs or fluid restriction
Food-Based Formulas	Compleat Pediatric *(1.0 kcal/ml)* Compleat Pediatric Reduced Calorie *(0.6 kcal/ml)* Kate Farms Pediatric Standard 1.2 *(1.2kcal/ml)* Nourish Compleat Pediatric Organic Blends (*1.0 kcal/ml)* (chicken, plant based) PediaSure Harvest	Consult registered dietitian for details on differences between these formula options
Semielemental	Peptamen Junior *(1.0 kcal/ml)* PediaSure Peptide 1.0 Cal Peptamen Junior with Prebio	Isotonic, contains MCT, some available with fiber
High Calorie, Semielemental	Peptamen Junior 1.5 Kate Farms Pediatric Peptide 1.5 *(both 1.5 kcal/ml)* Peptamen Junior 1.5 with Prebio PediaSure Peptide 1.5	Used for malabsorption, contains MCT
Soy Protein, Cow-Milk Protein Free	Bright Beginnings Soy *(1.0 kcal/ml)* –	Soy-based tube feeding
Elemental	Elecare Junior *(1.0 kcal/ml)* Neocate Splash *(1.0 kcal/ml)* Vivonex Pediatric *(0.8 kcal/ml)* NeoCate Junior Vivonex Pediatric Puramino Toddler Alfamino Junior	For severe protein allergy or malabsorption contains MCT Vivonex Pediatric is low in total fat
Fat Modified (High MCT)	Tolerex *(1.0 kcal/ml)* Portagen Lipistart Monogen	Cow-milk protein, may need essential fat supplement in long-term use
Low Carbohydrate	KetoCal 4:1 Liquid or Powder	1.5 kcal/mL liquid base, or powder to make specific recipe; cow-milk protein, high fat

Table adapted from 2019 Pediatric Nutrition Handbook, an internal guide at Children Hospital Colorado.

36

Inborn Errors of Metabolism

Emily Shelkowitz, Austin Larson, and Peter Baker II

For additional material related to the content of this chapter, please see Chapters 23, and 30.

VIGNETTE

A previously healthy, cognitively above-average 7-year-old male presented to his pediatrician's office for evaluation of attention-deficit/hyperactivity disorder (ADHD). There was concern of inattention and distractibility raised by his new second-grade teacher, a concern not present in the prior school year. His parents had noticed forgetfulness over the past few months, which they attributed to normal "summer vacation silliness." He was noted to have a tan appearance, which was felt to be a result of increased outdoor activities. Finally, a neurologic evaluation had been recommended by his ophthalmologist due to abnormal gaze convergence.

The boy was seen by neurology, and an urgent magnetic resonance imaging (MRI) brain was ordered due to hyperreflexia and mild ataxia on exam. The MRI brain revealed hyperintense signal abnormality of the posterior and cerebral white matter and optic tracts with a Loes score of 18 (see Fig. 36.3). The metabolic specialist on call was notified, very long-chain fatty acid (VLCFA) levels were ordered, and the boy was seen emergently for a presumed diagnosis of X-linked adrenoleukodystrophy (XALD). Molecular genetic testing eventually returned revealing a maternally inherited ABCD1 variant, confirming the diagnosis. Subsequent supportive biochemical testing included an elevation of VLCFAs and an elevated adrenocorticotropic hormone (ACTH) level confirming the complication of adrenal insufficiency.

Following a discussion of the diagnosis and natural history of the disease, the patient was evaluated for bone marrow transplant by multiple transplant teams, locally and at several other centers nationally. The unanimous assessment was that disease progression was so severe that he was not a transplant candidate. All agreed that the transplant process itself would likely accelerate the neuroinflammatory progression of disease before the full efficacy of stem cell engraftment could be seen and disease remission occurred. He was unlikely to survive the transplant without experiencing significant additional morbidity and a high risk of mortality. A referral to a palliative care specialist was made in anticipation of future needs for pain, tone management, nutritional needs, and in-home nursing support. In the ensuing months the boy began to demonstrate more significant motor decline. The disease ultimately progressed, resulting in death only 1 year following the initial diagnosis.

This case illustrates the insidious onset and rapid progression that is typical in males with cerebral XALD. Screening for the disorder in newborns, via detection of elevated VLCFA, was recently added to the national Recommended Uniform Screening Panel. As newborn screening for the condition is adopted by more states, in the future such catastrophic outcomes will hopefully be mitigated. In the interim a level of suspicion should be maintained in school-aged males with new onset behavioral and neurologic changes.

BACKGROUND

Inborn errors of metabolism (IEMs) are a group of heterogeneous inherited disorders that typically arise from enzyme or transporter deficiencies and resultant metabolic perturbations. Until recently, IEMs were almost exclusively diagnosed based on either the accumulation of metabolic pathway intermediates or the deficiency of downstream products. This approach is still valid and often used to screen for IEMs if a patient has suggestive symptoms. Increasingly though, due to improved ease, affordability, and test performance, molecular genetic testing is often used as a primary means of diagnosis. Direct enzymatic testing can also be performed in some cases. As patients with nonspecific symptoms, such as developmental delay, are offered broad genetic testing through next-generation sequencing panels, patients with milder phenotypes or at earlier stages of the disease process are being diagnosed. This shift has ushered in a change in our understanding of the natural history of many metabolic diseases. The advent of broader newborn screening (NBS) in the last 2 decades has also changed the understood natural history of many metabolic diseases, sometimes significantly.

The goal of this chapter is to provide a broad overview of IEMs, highlighting information that is most pertinent to the diagnostic evaluation of a new patient for developmental concerns. We will review aspects of the clinical and family history and physical examination that should raise suspicion for an IEM and discuss the appropriate diagnostic evaluation. Rather than providing a comprehensive review of all IEMs, we will cover specific disorders that are most relevant to the field of developmental-behavioral pediatrics. We will focus on categories of disorders that commonly have neurodevelopmental phenotypes (often in the absence of other signs of systemic disease). Though this is changing, most of these disorders are not NBS targets, and patients may present solely for developmental evaluation. Examples of disease categories that will be discussed in depth are urea cycle disorders, congenital disorders of glycosylation (CDGs), peroxisomal diseases, mitochondrial diseases, lysosomal storage disorders, neurotransmitter metabolism disorders, disorders of amino acid metabolism, and some vitamin-responsive conditions. Common disorders that typically present with metabolic crises or are identified on NBS, such as organic acidemias, are mentioned briefly but are not a focus of this chapter. Similarly, conditions with neurodevelopmental features that are significantly less prominent compared to other features, such as hepatomegaly or hypoglycemia (in the case of glycogen storage disorders) or exercise intolerance or rhabdomyolysis (in the case of disorders of fatty acid oxidation), are not discussed. We will briefly review a few common disorders, galactosemia and phenylketonuria (PKU) in particular, in which patients still exhibit subtle neurodevelopmental deficits for which they might seek the care of a developmental-behavioral pediatrician, despite identification on NBS and early initiation of treatment.

As with all genetic diseases, the field of metabolics is constantly changing as our knowledge of the full spectrum of diseases grows and treatments such as gene therapy and gene editing advance. Thus if in-depth knowledge of any specific condition is required, we would encourage this text to be used as a starting point. Valuable resources such as primary literature sources, GeneReviews, and clinicaltrials.gov can be utilized to obtain the most accurate information about prognosis and up-to-date treatment options.

GENERAL APPROACH

As with all consultations, the initial approach in the evaluation for an IEM in a patient presenting with developmental delay, intellectual disability, behavioral concerns, or developmental regression should focus on a comprehensive history (including birth history), family history, and physical examination.

Pertinent features to consider on perinatal history include growth concerns, anatomic anomalies noted on prenatal scans, decreased fetal movement or abnormal movements, oligo- or polyhydramnios, and fetal hydrops, which has been associated with multiple IEMs including lysosomal storage disorders and congenital defects of glycosylation. Birth history features such as neonatal resuscitation, respiratory insufficiency, prolonged hyperbilirubinemia, or feeding intolerance are important to note. It is also helpful to note the geographic location of birth as the breadth of NBS varies by state and country of birth. For those born outside of a hospital it is important to inquire if the patient has had NBS as part of routine prenatal care.

In reviewing the patient's own medical history it is important to catalog all medical and surgical problems, emergency room visits, and hospitalizations. Historical items that are routine pediatric problems such as recurrent ear infections, evaluation for a brief resolved unexplained event (BRUE, formerly referred to as ALTE), or a febrile seizure may be clues to an underlying IEM. A dietary history should be obtained. Some patients with IEMs may have food aversions, such as to protein or fructose, or intolerance to fasting. Some patients may have a correlation between onset of symptoms and dietary changes (e.g., transition from breast milk to formula or solids, adoption of vegan or vegetarian diet). A developmental history should be obtained with careful attention paid to periods of developmental regression triggered by severe illnesses or fasting.

Family history may offer helpful information. Most IEMs are autosomal recessive, so a history of parental relatedness (such as cousin marriages or parents hailing from the same small town/village) increases the probability of an IEM. The death of male infants in the family may indicate the presence of an X-linked condition (such as ornithine transcarbamylase [OTC] deficiency). If there are multiple generations of affected individuals with matrilineal inheritance, then disorders caused by mutations in mitochondrial DNA should be considered. It is also helpful to inquire about ethnic, national, or religious background as some IEMs have increased prevalence in specific populations due to founder effects and the prevalence of endogamy. Examples include Tay-Sachs disease in the Ashkenazi Jewish population or maple syrup urine disease in the Amish (Table 36.1).

Some findings suggestive of IEMs can be gained from a thorough physical examination (Table 36.2). Other objective findings that are important to note include unusual odors (e.g., maple syrup, sweaty feet, and mustiness) and patterns such as progressive macrocephaly on growth charts (Table 36.3). Results of imaging studies and other clinical investigations (Table 36.4) as well as laboratory studies (Table 36.5) are also important to incorporate into the formulation of a differential diagnosis.

Laboratory Evaluation

Diagnostic patterns of metabolites are often much more informative than isolated concentrations of individual substances. For this reason an initial set of screening tests is performed routinely as a first-tier biochemical assessment. This initial set of screening tests typically consists of analysis of serum amino acids, urine organic acids, serum acylcarnitines, and measurement of serum free and total carnitine levels. These tests, in combination, offer an overview of multiple pathways of lipid, protein, and small intermediary metabolism. For example, elevations or deficiencies in particular amino acids may point to a urea cycle disorder or other disorder of protein metabolism; elevations of organic acids in the urine may point to an organic acidemia or mitochondrial disease; and the presence of specific patterns of elevated acylcarnitines or abnormal ratios may point to a fatty acid oxidation disorder. There are often complementary findings on multiple biochemical tests that aid interpretation. Other first-tier studies include a comprehensive metabolic profile to assess for hypoglycemia, elevations in

TABLE 36.1 **Disorders With Increased Prevalence Depending on Ancestry**

Disorder	Ethnic Groups With Increased Prevalence
Glutaric acidemia type 1	Ojibway-Cree First Nation Canadians of Manitoba and Ontario, South African Xhosa peoples, Pennsylvania Amish, Lumbee Native Americans of North Carolina, and Irish Traveler communities in the Republic of Ireland
Maple syrup urine disease	Mennonite populations of Pennsylvania, Kentucky, New York, Indiana, Wisconsin, Michigan, Iowa, and Missouri
Pyruvate carboxylase deficiency	Type 1: North American Ojibwa, Cree, and Micmac tribes of the Algonquin-speaking peoples Type 2: French, German, and English Europeans
Propionic acidemia	Saudia Arabia, Greenland Inuits, Japanese
Tay Sachs	Ashkenazi Jewish French Canadian Northern Portugal (B1 variant) South Europe (B1 variant)
Canavan disease	Ashkenazi Jewish
Niemann-Pick A	Ashkenazi Jewish
Gaucher I (nonneuropathic)	Ashkenazi Jewish
Sialolipidosis (mucolipidosis type 4)	Ashkenazi Jewish
MPS III	Cayman Islands, Italian, Turkish and Southern European populations
Neuronal ceroid lipofuscinosis	CLN1: Finnish CLN6: Southern Europe, Indian subcontinent, and South America
Glycogen storage disease	I: Ashkenazi Jews III: Inuit population in Nunavik (Canada), North African Jews, Faroese
PMM2-CDG	Swedish, Belgian, and Dutch populations
Carnitine palmitoyl transferase deficiency type 1	Hutterites
Carnitine uptake deficiency	Faroe Islands
Lysinuric protein intolerance	Finnish, Japanese
HHH syndrome	Northern Saskatchewan population of mixed French-Canadian and Aboriginal descent
Citrullinemia type 2	Japanese, Chinese, Taiwanese, Korean
Arginase deficiency	French-Canadian and Portuguese
Cobalamin C	Possibly increased in Hispanic American Populations
Tyrosinemia I	Saguenay-Lac Saint-Jean region of Canada

CLN1, Neuronal ceroid lipofuscinosis type 1; ***CLN6***, neuronal ceroid lipofuscinosis type 6; ***HHH***, hyperornithinemia, hyperammonemia, homocitrullinuria syndrome; ***MPS III***, mucopolysaccharidosis type III; ***PMM2-CDG***, phosphomannomutase 2 (PMM2)-congenital disorder of glycosylation.

aminotransferases, and acid-base status; serum ammonia; serum homocysteine; serum creatine kinase; and serum lactate. Other more specific metabolic analyses are rarely obtained in a child who has not yet been evaluated by a metabolic specialist, but these tests (including such things as urine mucopolysaccharides, serum pipecolic acid) could point to very specific diagnoses and may be valuable in conjunction with molecular genetic test results as a confirmatory test. When an IEM that primarily affects the central nervous system is suspected, a lumbar puncture to analyze metabolites in the cerebral spinal fluid may be indicated; however, this is becoming less common as molecular genetic testing panels become more accessible. Refer to Table 36.5 for a review of laboratory studies helpful in the diagnosis of IEMs.

NEWBORN SCREENING

Any review of IEMs would be incomplete without a discussion of NBS. NBS is a public health project that aims to identify patients with treatable IEMs in a presymptomatic state so that disease-related morbidity and mortality is decreased. The NBS program began in the mid-1960s with the development of the bacterial inhibition assay for diagnosis of PKU. Since that time, with the development of new technologies, NBS has massively expanded. In the late 1990s US states began to adopt tandem mass spectroscopy (MS/MS). For a time, the numbers of conditions screened for varied significantly from state to state. To address this disparity the National Advisory Committee on Heritable Disorders in Newborns and Children was established in 2007 as part of the Health Resources and

TABLE 36.2 Historical Findings Concerning for an Inborn Error of Metabolism

Historical Findings	Diagnoses to Consider
Avoidance of protein	Urea cycle disorders
Episodic regression with illness	Mitochondrial disease
Episodic encephalopathy	Urea cycle disorders
Developmental regression in previously neurotypical preschool/school-aged child	X-linked adrenoleukodystrophy, neuronal ceroid lipofuscinosis, metachromatic leukodystrophy
Self-harming behaviors	Lesch-Nyhan disease
Diurnal symptoms or fluctuating with time of day	GLUT-1, neurotransmitter disorders
Severe hyperactivity	MPS III
Irritability in newborn period	Krabbe, serine synthesis deficiency
Neonatal seizures	Nonketotic hyperglycinemia, sulfite oxidase deficiency, molybdenum cofactor deficiency, pyridoxine disorders
Autism/isolated speech delays	Creatine biosynthesis defects, cerebral folate deficiency, alpha-mannosidosis
Adolescent/adult-onset psychiatric symptoms	Niemann-Pick C, Wilson disease, cerebrotendinous xanthomatosis, mucolipidosis I
Hearing loss	Peroxisomal disorders, mitochondrial disease, mucopolysaccharidoses, mucolipidoses
Vision loss	See Table 36.3 for specific ocular findings
Frequent upper respiratory infections	Mucopolysaccharidoses, alpha-mannosidosis, mucolipidoses

GLUT-1, Glucose transporter type 1 deficiency; *MPS III*, mucopolysaccharidosis type III.

TABLE 36.3 Findings on Physical Examination Concerning for Inborn Errors of Metabolism

General Exam Findings	Diagnoses to Consider
Macrocephaly	Mucopolysaccharidoses, Canavan, Alexander disease, glutaric acidemia, Tay-Sachs, mannosidosis
Progressive microcephaly	Sulfite oxidase deficiency, molybdenum cofactor deficiency
Large fontanelle	Peroxisomal biogenesis disorders
Short stature	Mucopolysaccharidoses, mucolipidoses, oligosaccharidoses
Marfanoid appearance	Homocystinuria
Coarse features	Mucopolysaccharidoses, mucolipidoses, oligosaccharidoses
Upward gaze palsy	Niemann-Pick C
Horizontal gaze palsy	Gaucher III
Ophthalmoplegia	Mitochondrial disease
Inverted nipples	Congenital disorders of glycosylation (CDGs), Menkes, biopterin synthesis disorders, molybdenum cofactor deficiency
Organomegaly	Mucopolysaccharidoses, mucolipidoses, oligosaccharidoses, Niemann-Pick, peroxisomal biosynthesis disorders
Genitourinary anomalies (cryptorchidism, microphallus)	Smith-Lemli-Opitz (SLO), cholesterol biosynthesis disorders, congenital disorders of glycosylation
Extremity anomalies (syndactyly, polydactyly)	SLO and other disorders of cholesterol biosynthesis
Endocrinopathies (hypo-/hyperthyroidism, hyper-/hypoinsulinism adrenal insufficiency)	CDGs, X-linked adrenal leukodystrophy, mitochondrial disorders
Spastic diplegia (scissoring/tip-toe gait) with our corresponding brain MRI findings	Arginase deficiency, cobalamin C, HHH syndrome, dopamine synthesis defects

TABLE 36.3 Findings on Physical Examination Concerning for Inborn Errors of Metabolism—cont'd

General Exam Findings	Diagnoses to Consider
Dyskinesias	Neurotransmitter disorders, Lesch-Nyhan syndrome, creatine synthesis disorders, cerebral folate deficiency, GLUT-1 deficiency, homocystinuria
Ataxia	Pyruvate dehydrogenase deficiency, late-onset Tay-Sachs, late-onset GM1 gangliosidosis, cobalamin disorders, mucolipidosis type 1
Lipodystrophy	CDGs, glycogen storage disorders
Angiokeratomas	Fucosidosis, GM1 gangliosidosis, sialidosis, fucosidosis, mannosidosis
Trichorrhexis nodosa	Argininosuccinic aciduria, argininemia, LPI
Dermatitis/ichthyosis	Cholesterol biosynthesis disorders, steroid sulfatase deficiency, multiple sulfatase deficiency
Cutis laxa	
Distinct odors • Maple syrup • Sweaty feed • Musty/mousy • Cat urine	CDG, Menkes, TALDO • MSUD • IVA, GAII • PKU • Beta-methylcrotonylglycinuria

CDGs, Congenital disorders of glycosylations; *GAII*, glutaric acidemia type II; *GLUT-1*, glucose transporter type 1 deficiency; *HHH syndrome*, hyperornithinemia, hyperammonemia, homocitrullinuria syndrome; *IVA*, isovaleric acidemia; *LPI*, lysinuric protein intolerance; *MSUD*, maple syrup urine disease; *PKU*, phenylketonuria; *TALDO*, transaldolase deficiency.

TABLE 36.4 Clinical Findings Concerning for an Inborn Error of Metabolism

Findings on Specialized Exam or Clinical Studies	Diagnoses to Consider
Dislocated lens	Homocystinuria, sulfite oxidase deficiency, molybdenum cofactor deficiency
Cherry-red spot	Niemann-Pick A, Tay-Sachs, Krabbe, gangliosidoses, galactosidosis, sialidosis, mucolipidosis, Farber disease
Retinitis pigmentosa	Neuronal ceroid lipofuscinosis, peroxisomal disorders, congenital disorders of glycosylation, mitochondrial disorders, MPS II, mevalonic aciduria
Corneal opacities	Mucopolysaccharidoses, Fabry, mucolipidoses, oligosaccharidosis, sphingolipidoses
Lenticular opacities (cataracts)	Peroxisomal disorders, homocystinuria, Smith-Lemli-Opitz, mitochondrial disorders, mevalonic aciduria, cerebrotendinous xanthomatosis
Dysostosis multiplex, gibbus, scoliosis	Mucopolysaccharidoses, mucolipidoses, gangliosides, galactosidosis
Subdural hemorrhage	Glutaric acidemia, Menkes
Punctate calcifications on skeletal imaging	Chondrodysplasia punctata (peroxisomal or cholesterol biosynthesis disorders)
Leukodystrophies	Krabbe, metachromatic leukodystrophy, adrenoleukodystrophy, Canavan disease
Basal ganglia abnormalities	Mitochondrial disease, organic acidemias, Krabbe, GM1 gangliosidosis, molybdenum cofactor deficiency, tetrahydrobiopterin defects
Cerebral calcifications	Adrenoleukodystrophy, GM2 gangliosidosis, Krabbe, mitochondrial disorders, folate disorders, biopterin disorders

MPII, Mucopolysaccharidosis type II.

Services Administration (HRSA). The advisory committee developed the Recommend Uniform Screening Panel (RUSP), which is a list of primary and secondary disorders (often detected using the same metabolites) that states should strongly consider including in their NBS programs. As of July 2018, the RUSP includes 35 primary targets (25 of which are IEMs) and 26 secondary targets (24 of which are IEMs). Refer to the HRSA website for updated recommendations. Currently all 50 US states screen for at least 35 conditions (McCandless & Wright, 2020). The newest metabolic conditions to be added to the RUSP are XALD and mucopolysaccharidosis type 1. Both conditions present with insidious neurodevelopmental decline and have disease-stabilizing therapies that are most efficacious when they are started early in the course of the disease. When evaluating a patient with concerns for these conditions one should consider when these conditions were added to the birth-state's NBS panel. A good reference is the NBS

TABLE 36.5 Laboratory Concerning for an Inborn Error of Metabolism

Laboratory Findings	Diagnoses to Consider
Metabolic acidosis (less significant hyperammonemia)	Organic acidemias
Hyperammonemia with normal pH or metabolic alkalosis	Urea cycle disorders
Absent ketones	Fatty acid oxidation defect
Hypoglycemia	Fatty acid oxidation defects, organic acidemias, congenital disorders of glycosylation, defects of ketogenesis, and ketone body utilization
Hematologic disturbances	Cobalamin defects, Pearson syndrome, disorders of pyrimidine metabolism
High uric acid	Lesch-Nyhan
Low uric acid	Sulfite oxidase deficiency, molybdenum cofactor deficiency
High homocysteine	Homocystinuria, disorders of remethylation, cobalamin disorders
Low homocysteine	Transmethylation defects, sulfite oxidase deficiency, molybdenum cofactor deficiency
Low cholesterol/cholesterol precursors	Smith-Lemli-Opitz and disorders of cholesterol biosynthesis
Elevated creatine kinase	Fatty acid oxidation disorders, mitochondrial disease
Low serum copper	Menkes, Wilsons (also with elevated urine and liver copper)
Elevated succinylacetone	Tyrosinemia type 1
Elevated very long-chain fatty acids	Peroxisomal disorders, specifically X-linked adrenoleukodystrophy in the right clinical context
Low creatine and/or guanidinoacetate in blood or urine	Creatine deficiency syndromes
Elevations of alpha-aminoadipic semialdehyde (AASA), pipecolic acid and 1-piperidine-6-carboxylase (P6C) in cerebrospinal fluid	Disorders of B6 metabolism, specifically pyridoxine-dependent epilepsy
Elevated lactate in the presence of other consistent lab abnormalities (e.g., metabolic acidosis)	Mitochondrial disease, secondary inhibition of mitochondrial function due to another inborn error of metabolism
Pyruvate elevated out of proportion to lactate	Defects of pyruvate metabolism such as pyruvate dehydrogenase deficiency, pyruvate carboxylase deficiency
Elevated 3-methylglutaconic acid	Mitochondrial membrane defects, specifically Barth syndrome
Elevated oxysterols	Niemann-Pick C
Elevated urine ceramide trihexosides, mucopolysaccharides, oligosaccharide, and/or sulfatides	Lysosomal storage disease

CLN1, Neuronal ceroid lipofuscinosis type 1; CLN6, neuronal ceroid lipofuscinosis type 6; HHH, hyperornithinemia, hyperammonemia, homocitrullinuria syndrome; MPS III, mucopolysaccharidosis type III; PMM2-CDG, phosphomannomutase 2 (PMM2)-congenital disorder of glycosylation.

resource center (www.newsteps.org). It should also be noted that most of the conditions reviewed in the text that follows are not currently included in NBS; thus the reported history of a normal NBS does not decrease the likelihood of many of these diagnoses.

DISORDERS PRESENTING WITH HYPERAMMONEMIA

Overview

Ammonia is produced as a byproduct of amino acid catabolism and is excreted as urea as a result of the enzymatic steps of the urea cycle. A deficiency in any of the enzymes or transporters in the pathway is termed a urea cycle disorder. Cumulatively, this category of disease is estimated to have an incidence of 1/35,000 live births. All urea cycle disorders are inherited in an autosomal recessive fashion except for OTC deficiency, which is X linked. The clinical manifestations of hyperammonemia may include vomiting, poor feeding, irritability, tachypnea, and hyperpnea (resulting in respiratory alkalosis) and may lead rapidly to lethargy, coma, seizures, and respiratory arrest. Many urea cycle disorders can have a severe neonatal presentation characterized by vomiting, poor feeding, irritability, tachypnea and hyperpnea, seizures, encephalopathy, and respiratory arrest. Milder conditions or individuals with partially retained enzymatic activity may present later in life with largely neurodevelopmental symptoms or nonspecific manifestations such as changes in appetite, psychiatric symptoms, or sleep disturbance (Häberle et al., 2019; Matsumoto et al., 2019).

A urea cycle disorder should be considered as a diagnosis in the setting of developmental delay, particularly with episodic changes in behavior or psychiatric manifestations. Other episodic symptoms such as headaches/migraines, inattentiveness, abdominal migraines, or cyclical vomiting should raise the index of suspicion for urea cycle disorders, particularly if these symptoms are triggered by dietary intake of protein or intercurrent illnesses. Diagnostic evaluations include baseline biochemical screening labs (quantitative serum amino acids, urine organic acids, a serum acylcarnitine profile, and quantitative urine orotic acid) as well as a serum ammonia level, and a blood gas or set of electrolytes (to assess acid-base status) during an acute episode.

Laboratory interpretation, acute management, and molecular testing should be performed in conjunction with a subspecialist in biochemical genetics. Chronic treatment for many urea cycle disorders includes a protein-restricted diet as well as supplementation of urea cycle intermediates such as citrulline and arginine, and administration of ammonia scavengers such as sodium phenylacetate and sodium benzoate to help promote excretion of ammonia via alternative routes (other than the urea cycle). Liver transplantation is pursued in severe cases, and gene therapy is under investigation for certain urea cycle disorders.

Refer to the following text for a more in-depth discussion of OTC deficiency as well as abbreviated discussions of arginosuccinate lyase deficiency, arginase deficiency, and hyperammonemia, hyperornithinemia, homocitrullinuria (HHH) syndrome. It is important to recognize that the urea cycle disorders discussed here may have later onset chronic presentations that include neurocognitive features.

Ornithine Transcarbamylase Deficiency

OTC is required to convert carbamoyl phosphate and ornithine into citrulline in the mitochondria. OTC deficiency is the most common urea cycle disorder with an estimated incidence of 1/56,000 live births (Lichter-Konecki et al., 2016). Males with severe OTC deficiency present in the neonatal period with progressive encephalopathy, hyperventilation, seizures, and severe respiratory alkalosis. However, recent longitudinal studies suggest that these cases account for only 20% of individuals with OTC deficiency, with the other 80% presenting outside of the neonatal period, even into old age. Males with residual enzyme activity and female heterozygotes, with variable X-inactivation patterns, may present later in life in a decompensation akin to that of the severe neonatal presentation or with less acute symptoms, such as episodic nausea, vomiting, inattention, irritability, headaches, and mood/behavioral changes. Triggering events may include fasting with acute or chronic illness; the use of valproate, haloperidol, systemic corticosteroids, and some chemotherapy drugs; dietary changes such as high-protein diet; and childbirth. Clues to the diagnosis in the clinical history may include lifelong avoidance of protein-containing foods or a history of a neonatal death in a male sibling or relative. Chronic treatment as outlined earlier consists of dietary restriction of protein, supplementation with arginine or citrulline, and the use of ammonia scavengers. Even with chronic treatment, the mortality rate remains high with 24% mortality in neonatal-onset cases and 11% in late-onset cases. Neurocognitive outcomes correlate with the number, severity, and duration of hyperammonemic episodes. Females who have remained asymptomatic or mildly symptomatic have average intellectual ability overall; however, they often have impairments in fine motor skills, attention and executive skills, and nonverbal intelligence. Liver transplant may be pursued for patients in whom metabolic control is not satisfactory with medical management. The long-term effects of liver transplantation on neurodevelopment in these patients remain a subject of study. Gene therapy is currently under investigation.

Argininosuccinic Aciduria

Argininosuccinic aciduria is an autosomal recessive urea cycle disorder that arises from a deficiency in the enzyme argininosuccinic lyase (ASL). It is the second most common urea cycle disorder after OTC deficiency (Erez, Nagamani, & Lee, 2011). It can present in the neonatal period or later in life with symptoms due to hyperammonemic crisis, or later in life with a chronic neurocognitive phenotype associated with gastrointestinal and liver symptoms (most commonly hepatomegaly and elevated transaminases) without hyperammonemia. Cognitive outcomes range from severe intellectual disability to borderline cognitive abilities, and epilepsy is seen in about 40% of patients. The neurobehavioral phenotype varies and includes muscular weakness, cerebellar ataxia, tremor, dysphagia, dystonia, hyperactivity, self-harming behaviors, autism, psychosis, and schizophrenia. Unique features observed in patients with argininosuccinic aciduria include trichorrhexis nodosa, dermatitis, and hypertension. Argininosuccinic aciduria differs from other urea cycle disorders in that a high percentage of patients, even those with the chronic phenotype, have significant long-term neurocognitive deficits even in the absence of any hyperammonemic events.

Arginase Deficiency

Arginase deficiency arises from a deficiency in arginase, the last step in the urea cycle that catalyzes the conversion of arginine to urea and ornithine. It typically does not present with an acute hyperammonemic phenotype but instead is characterized by liver disease (cholestasis, acute liver failure or liver fibrosis) and progressive neurologic disease that includes seizures as well as spastic paraplegia, usually manifesting in the first years of life. Children with arginase deficiency may be misdiagnosed as having cerebral palsy. Cognitive development may plateau, and developmental regression may be observed without treatment. With treatment, normal cognitive outcomes may be achieved in some cases (Sun, Crombez, & Wong, 2020).

Hyperornithinemia, Hyperammonemia, Homocitrullinuria Syndrome

HHH syndrome arises from a deficiency in the ornithine carrier, which causes diminished urea cycle function. HHH syndrome can have a variable age of onset with a minority (<10%) of patients presenting in the neonatal period with a hyperammonemic crisis. Most patients present later in life (roughly 10% in infancy, 50% between 1 and 10 years, and the remainder in adolescence/adulthood) with more chronic symptoms such as developmental delay, hypotonia, hyperactivity, episodic inattention, learning difficulties, cognitive deficits, ataxia, spasticity, and seizures. Approximately 70% of patients have intellectual disability, ranging from mild to severe (Martinelli et al., 2015).

AMINO ACID DISORDERS

Several IEMs have historically been categorized as aminoacidopathies or disorders of amino acid metabolism, many of which are associated with neurocognitive impairments that are preventable or ameliorated by dietary restriction of the offending amino acid.

Phenylketonuria

PKU was the first disorder to be included in NBS. It is an autosomal recessive condition that arises from a deficiency in phenylalanine hydroxylase, the enzyme that converts phenylalanine to tyrosine. Diagnostic findings are high phenylalanine and low tyrosine on NBS or quantitative serum amino acid studies. Phenylalanine hydroxylase requires the cofactor tetrahydrobiopterin (BH4), and phenylalanine may be elevated if the synthesis of BH4 is impaired (refer to Neurometabolic Disorders for more details). PKU was historically associated with severe intellectual disability, a musty (mousy) odor, eczematous rashes, acquired microcephaly, and a hypopigmented complexion (Fig. 36.1). With the advent of NBS, individuals with PKU are now diagnosed as neonates and treated with a low-protein diet. Some patients (depending on genotype) will respond to sapropterin, a synthetic analog of BH4. Pegvaliase enzyme substitution therapy is also approved to treat PKU and allows phenylalanine to be metabolized via an alternative route. Both therapies may allow for liberalization of dietary treatment and discontinuation of protein restriction in some patients. Gene therapy trials are ongoing, as are natural history studies in treated patients (Regier & Greene, 2017).

Adults with PKU may have neurocognitive deficits such as reduced attention span, slowed motor reaction times and slow information-processing abilities, and higher rates of depression and anxiety, particularly at times when their phenylalanine levels are high. Appropriately treated individuals are otherwise healthy and lead fulfilling and productive lives without experiencing significant disease-related morbidity in adulthood. Women with PKU require close follow-up during pregnancy due to the teratogenic effects of high phenylalanine levels on the developing fetus.

Disorders of Hyperhomocystinemia and Hypermethioninemia

Homocysteine and methionine are both sulfur-containing amino acids that are interconverted via a complex set of reactions involved in the methionine demethylation and remethylation pathways. Deficiencies in any of the involved enzymes can cause abnormal elevations in these amino acids. Hyperhomocystinemia and hypermethioninemia are seen in multiple IEMs, some of which are detectable via NBS.

Classic homocystinuria, which is an autosomal recessive condition that arises from cystathionine beta-synthase (CBS) deficiency, is the most common disease in this group. It is characterized by ocular (ectopia lentis, severe myopia), skeletal (marfanoid body habitus), cardiovascular

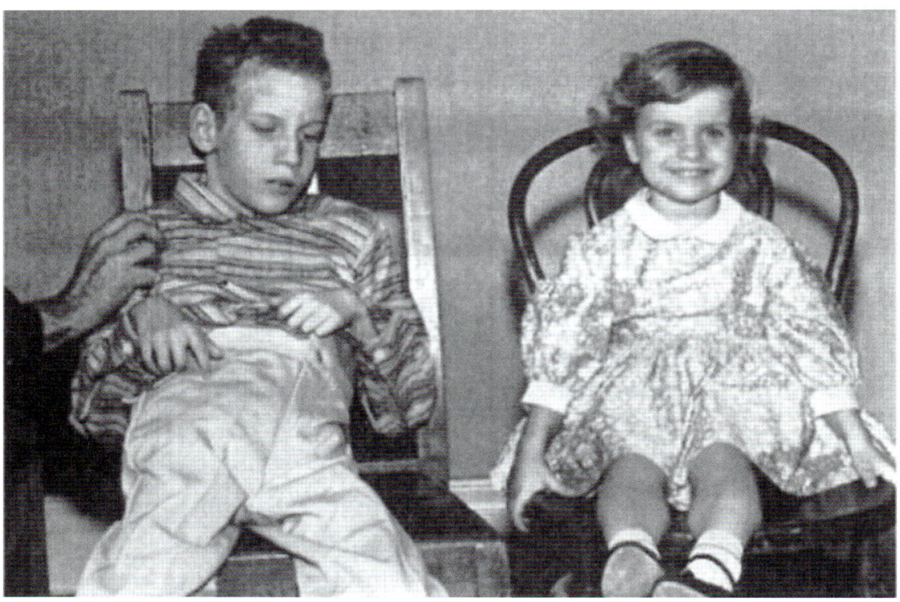

Fig. 36.1 Diet-treated *(right)* patient with phenylketonuria compared to older brother *(left)* who was not treated. (From Centerwall, S. A., & Centerwall, W. R. [2000]. The discovery of phenylketonuria: The story of a young couple, two retarded children, and a scientist. *Pediatrics, 105*[1], 102.)

(thromboembolism), and central nervous system (developmental delays, intellectual disability, seizures, dystonia) manifestations. Some individuals with homocystinuria are diagnosed based on the occurrence of an early thromboembolic event and may have no other manifestations. It can be screened for via detection of elevated homocysteine and methionine and diagnosed based on molecular genetic testing (Morris et al., 2017).

In childhood developmental delays are a common presenting feature of homocystinuria and are typically apparent by 6 years. Ocular manifestations are an even more common presenting feature at the time of diagnosis and are typically apparent by 7.5 years. Cognitive outcomes are highly variable, though it appears that individuals who respond to vitamin B6 supplementation (a cofactor for CBS) may have better outcomes than those who are nonresponsive. Patients identified on NBS and who started treatment earlier have better outcomes compared to those diagnosed later. Anxiety, depression, and obsessive-compulsive behaviors may be present in adolescence and adulthood. All patients are offered a pyridoxine (vitamin B6) supplementation, and approximately 50% respond with reduced homocysteine. A protein-restricted diet along with vitamin B12 and folate supplementation is recommended. The medication betaine is prescribed for most patients and provides an alternative remethylation pathway from homocysteine to methionine.

Nonketotic Hyperglycinemia

Nonketotic hyperglycinemia (NKH) is an autosomal recessive condition that arises from a deficiency of any of the proteins of the glycine cleavage system. As a result of this deficiency glycine accumulates in all tissues in the body, including the central nervous system, and has both neuroinhibitory and neuroexcitatory effects. Biochemical diagnosis is based on detection of elevated glycine concentrations in the plasma and cerebrospinal fluid (CSF). The disease is not included in NBS (Van Hove et al., 2019).

Individuals with severe NKH come to medical attention during the early neonatal period after a birth history of intrauterine hiccups followed by progressive postnatal hypotonia, poor feeding, and apnea. Seizures are often present. Later in infancy (by about 6 months) spasticity and cortical visual blindness develop. Cognitive outcomes vary based on disease severity, which can be predicted based on biochemical, genetic, and neuroimaging findings as well as age and severity of the clinical presentation. Children with the most severe form of the disease make minimal developmental progress. Those with an attenuated form of the disease may not be diagnosed until later infancy or childhood. Those with attenuated disease will have some degree of cognitive impairment and often have severe attentional deficits. Unlike the above-mentioned aminoacidopathies, NKH cannot be treated with dietary protein restriction. Instead, most patients are treated with dextromethorphan, which blocks the N-methyl-D-aspartate receptors in the brain that are impacted by elevated glycine, and with sodium benzoate, which conjugates and facilitates excretion of glycine.

The Tyrosinemias

The tyrosinemias are a group of related IEMs caused by enzymatic deficiencies in the tyrosine catabolic pathway. All three are detected via NBS. Tyrosinemia type I arises from a deficiency of fumarylacetoacetate hydrolase (the fourth enzymatic step in the tyrosine degradation pathway), which results in the accumulation of succinylacetone and fumarylacetoacetate. Biochemical diagnosis is made based on detection of succinylacetone in blood or urine. Untreated, tyrosinemia type I is associated with variable but progressive liver disease, often leading to cirrhosis and hepatocellular carcinoma, renal tubular dysfunction (and vitamin D–resistant rickets due to hypophosphatemia), and intermittent neurologic crises resembling acute intermittent porphyria that may include seizures, posturing, hypertension, and mental status changes. Prior to the advent of effective pharmaceutical therapy death often occurred in the first decade of life. Fortunately, tyrosinemia type I can be treated with 2-(2-nitro-4-trifluoromethylbenzoyl)-1,3-cyclohexanedione (known as NTBC or nitisinone), which blocks a more proximal step in the tyrosine degradation pathway (that of 4-hydroxypyruvate dioxygenase), and prevents the accumulation of fumarylacetoacetate and succinylacetone. With NTBC therapy patients are required to remain on a protein-restricted diet as the tyrosine catabolic pathway remains impaired. Tyrosinemia type I patients treated with NTBC may have borderline or mildly decreased cognitive functioning, which is thought to correlate with elevated blood tyrosine levels. Long-term outcomes of treated patients remain a topic of study (Demirbas, Brucker, & Berry, 2018).

Tyrosinemias type II and III are rare. Both are treated with a protein-restricted diet to reduce tyrosine concentrations in the body. Hypertyrosinemia likely impacts developmental outcomes and can cause formation of painful corneal crystals and hyperkeratosis of the skin of the palms and soles.

ORGANIC ACIDEMIAS

The organic acidemias are a large group of metabolic disorders that arise from deficiencies in the enzymes or enzyme cofactors involved in catalyzing the breakdown of amino acids. The prototypical organic acidemias are propionic acidemia, methylmalonic acidemia, isovaleric acidemia, and maple syrup urine disease. All of the diagnoses discussed in this section are targets for NBS (Schillaci, DeBrosse, & McCandless, 2018).

Except for maple syrup urine disease, these disorders classically present with vomiting, lethargy, and hypotonia due to a high anion-gap metabolic acidosis that is often associated with hypoglycemia and hyperammonemia. Maple syrup urine disease presents with elevations in the branched-chain amino acids, hypertonia, and abnormal movements. These acute episodes are often triggered by the physiologic catabolic state of the first few days of the newborn period while feeding is being established. Adolescent and adult patients with maple syrup urine disease have a very high burden of mental health diagnoses.

Glutaric acidemia type 1 is termed a cerebral organic acidemia because of the lack of systemic biochemical perturbations and lack of nonneurologic symptoms. The enzyme deficiency causes the accumulation of glutaryl-CoA intermediates, which are neurotoxic, and usually presents with acute basal ganglia injury during periods of catabolism. Patients may have severe motor impairment as a result of the basal ganglia injury but do not typically have cognitive impairment.

The cobalamin metabolism disorders are a group of conditions arising from a defect in any of the steps involved in the intracellular transport and conversion of dietary cobalamin (vitamin B12) to its active forms, methylcobalamin (MeCbl) and adenosylcobalamin (AdoCbl), which are cofactors for methionine synthase and methylmalonyl-coenzyme A mutase, respectively. Depending on where the defect occurs, individuals may have symptoms typical of methylmalonic acidemia or clinical features consistent with remethylation disorders (discussed in more depth in the aminoacidopathies section earlier).

Most organic acidemias are managed with dietary restriction of protein to reduce the accumulation of toxic metabolites and with vitamins and supplements, such as carnitine, to boost residual enzyme activity and promote excretion of metabolites, respectively. Liver transplant is recommended to improve neurocognitive outcomes and stabilize disease in some of the organic acidemias, and gene therapy is under investigation for certain disorders. These conditions can be screened for with biochemical analysis of serum amino acids, urine organic acids, and serum acylcarnitines, and diagnoses are typically confirmed with molecular genetic testing. Late-onset presentations of these conditions, which include neurocognitive symptoms, are possible.

NEUROMETABOLIC DISORDERS

Glucose Transporter Type-1 Deficiency

Glucose transporter type-1 (GLUT-1) deficiency is a disorder of glucose transport across the blood-brain barrier that arises from the deficiency of the protein transporter that facilitates the entry of glucose into the brain. It is diagnosed based on the detection of a low CSF glucose level (compared to serum glucose levels). The classic phenotype associated with GLUT-1 deficiency, which accounts for about 90% of cases, includes seizures with onset before 2 years of life with associated microcephaly, developmental delays, and ataxia. Milder cases can have a range of phenotypes, which include early-onset absence epilepsy and paroxysmal symptoms (often exercise induced) such as dyskinesia, epilepsy, choreoathetosis, spasticity, ataxia, dystonia, and alternating hemiplegia. Symptoms may be triggered by fasting or stress. Not all GLUT-1 deficiency patients have epilepsy. Early diagnosis is important because the cerebral energy deficit created by defective glucose transport can be mitigated with initiation of the ketogenic diet, which provides ketone bodies as energetic substrate for the brain. Earlier initiation of ketogenic diet is associated with better neurodevelopmental outcomes. Cognitive outcomes and communication skills are varied and range from mildly to significantly impacted depending on the severity of the patient's disease (Wang, Pascual, & De Vivo, 2018).

Neurotransmitter Disorders

Neurotransmitter disorders are a group of conditions caused by genetic defects in the enzymes involved in the synthesis, degradation, or transport of neurotransmitters or by defects in the cofactors important in the function of these enzymes, such as tetrahydrobiopterin. Examples of neurotransmitter systems include inhibitory (gamma-aminobutyric acid [GABA]), excitatory (aspartate and glutamate), cholinergic (acetylcholine), monoaminergic (adrenaline, noradrenaline, dopamine, and serotonin), and purinergic (adenosine and adenosine mono-, di-, and triphosphate [ATP]) (Mastrangelo, 2020). The diagnosis of a neurotransmitter disorder may be made based on assessment of neurotransmitter metabolites in the CSF or noninvasively with molecular genetic testing. A discussion of specific diseases is beyond the scope of this text; however, this disease category as a whole is important to be aware of as certain disorders are treatable with supplementation of the deficient neurotransmitter(s) or downstream products.

Creatine Deficiency Syndromes

Creatine deficiency syndromes arise from defects in either the synthesis or transport of creatine into the brain. Creatine is a critical component of ATP (and hence cellular energy) metabolism in the brain; thus these conditions present with a predominant neurodevelopmental phenotype. The diagnosis can be made with molecular genetic testing or biochemically, based on characteristic deficiencies of guanidinoacetate, creatine, or creatinine in the blood, urine, and brain (via magnetic resonance spectroscopy), the pattern of which depends on the specific condition. The clinical hallmark of the creatine deficiency syndromes is intellectual disability, with speech impacted more than other developmental domains. The degree of intellectual disability ranges from mild to severe and can be associated with hyperactivity and autism. Creatine transporter deficiency and arginine:glycine aminotransferase (AGAT) deficiency can present with purely developmental concerns and may be treated with oral monohydrate creatine supplementation. Creatine transporter deficiency presents with intellectual disability, and speech delays are universal features. Many patients have behavioral concerns, ADHD, and autism. Additionally, anxiety, aggression, obsessive-compulsive behaviors, and impulsive and self-injurious behaviors have been reported; 60% of patients have seizures, and a minority of patients have hypotonia, ataxia, and dystonia. Unlike AGAT, supplementation with oral monohydrate creatine alone is not sufficient to restore cerebral creatine stores, nor does it improve developmental outcomes (Clark & Cecil, 2015).

Vitamin-Responsive Disorders: Disorders of B6 Metabolism

Pyridoxal 5′-phosphate, the activated form of vitamin B6, plays many important roles in cellular function, including acting as a cofactor for a variety of enzymatic pathways. One such pathway is the synthesis of GABA, one of the main inhibitory neurotransmitters in the brain (Wilson, Plecko, Mills, & Clayton,). Disorders of B6 metabolism give rise to B6-responsive epilepsy syndromes. Pyridoxine-dependent epilepsy (PDE) and pyridox(am)ine-phosphate oxidase (PNPO) deficiency are two examples of disorders that fall into this classification. Both of these conditions present classically, with neonatal seizures that show variable response to pyridoxine supplementation (in the case of PNPO deficiency) and associated with residual development delays despite achievement of seizure control. Atypical forms, presenting outside of the neonatal period, but before age 3 years are also described.

Disorders of Sulfur Amino Acid Metabolism

Isolated Sulfite Oxidase Deficiency

The deficiency of sulfite oxidase results in an accumulation of sulfites that are neurotoxic (Claerhout et al., 2018). The classic presentation is apparent in the first 24 to 72 hours of life with seizures, feeding difficulties, rapidly progressive neonatal encephalopathy, spastic quadriplegia, and opisthotonos with subsequent development of microcephaly and profound developmental impairments. Lens subluxation can be seen in the newborn period. Late-onset sulfite oxidase deficiency presents with developmental delays and regression, a movement disorder characterized by dystonia and choreoathetosis, and ataxia. Symptoms may be progressive or episodic. Initial neuroimaging studies of patients with classic sulfite oxidase deficiency resemble hypoxic ischemic encephalopathy with a loss of gray-white matter differentiation and edema in the cerebral cortex and basal ganglia.

Molybdenum Cofactor Deficiency

Molybdenum cofactor deficiency is an autosomal recessive condition that arises from biallelic defects in any of four genes (*MOCS1, MOCS2, MOCS3*, and *GEPH*) involved in the biosynthesis of molybdenum cofactor. As a result of molybdenum cofactor deficiency the activity of the enzymes that are dependent on molybdenum (i.e., sulfite oxidase, xanthine dehydrogenase/oxidase, and aldehyde oxidase) are impaired. The neurologic symptoms of the disease are due to a deficiency in sulfite oxidase, and thus the presentation and phenotypic features of the disease are like sulfite oxidase deficiency. Molybdenum cofactor deficiency type A (MOSC1) has been treated by supplementation with cyclic pyranopterin monophosphate (cPMP), which is deficient in this form of the condition (Atwal & Scaglia, 2016).

PURINE AND PYRIMIDINE DISORDERS

Inborn errors of purine and pyrimidine metabolism are a broad category of disorders that have symptoms that include disorders of neurodevelopment, renal disease, arthrosis, anemia, cancer predisposition, and immunodeficiency. They are not detected by NBS. Purine and pyrimidines play multiple vital roles in cellular metabolism, including energy transport and conservation, signal transduction and translation, formation of coenzymes, and as substrate for DNA and RNA synthesis.

Disorders of hypoxanthine-guanine phosphoribosyltransferase (HPRT1) deficiency are the most common of the purine and pyrimidine disorders. HPRT1 is an X-linked recessive condition that arises from a deficiency in the conversion of hypoxanthine and guanine to their respective nucleotides IMP and GMP. That conversion is part of the purine salvage pathway for recycling nucleotides. Deficiency of the salvage pathway results in overactive de novo synthesis of purines but impaired recycling of the purines as they get catabolized to uric acid. The diagnosis should be suspected in the setting of uric acid levels. Functional assays of residual enzyme activity are helpful in determining where on the HPRT1 deficiency spectrum a patient may fall.

Patients with Lesch-Nyhan syndrome (LNS) have less than 2% residual enzyme activity. Boys with LNS typically have normal perinatal and neonatal histories. Hypotonia and gross motor delays become evident during late infancy. Parents may notice the appearance of "brick dust" in the diaper caused by uric acid crystals. Over the first few years of life abnormal movements such as opisthotonos, choreoathetosis, ballismus, and dystonia develop. Many boys also develop spasticity, hyperreflexia, and clonus. Most individuals with LNS do not learn to walk. The hallmark of the disease, self-injurious behavior, typically develops between 2 and 4 years of age, but it may arise as early as the first year of life or be delayed until the teenage years. Expressive language skills are varied; however, most patients have typical language comprehension. Cognition is mildly impaired. LNS is not a neurodegenerative condition. The expected lifespan is into midadulthood and is limited by renal disease or respiratory infections from aspiration as well as the sequelae of immobility.

Variants of LNS include HPRT1-related neurologic disease, which is distinguished from LNS by the amount of residual enzyme activity (typically 2%–8%) along with milder motor impairments and lack of self-injurious behavior, and HPRT1-related hyperuricemia (>8% residual enzyme activity), which does not have neurologic involvement (Jinnah et al., 2000; Jinnah, De Gregorio, Harris, Nyhan, & O'Neill, 2020).

Care for boys with LNS is largely supportive. Treatment with allopurinol is effective at lowering uric acid levels, but it does not modify the neurologic or behavioral phenotype of the disease. SAMe (s-adenosyl-L-methionine), which provides purine precursors to the brain, is under investigation as a treatment for self-injurious behaviors and aggression.

DISORDERS OF CARBOHYDRATE METABOLISM

Galactosemia

Galactosemia is an autosomal recessive disorder due to deficiency of galactose-1-phosphate uridylyltransferase. As a result, galactose-1-phosphate and galactitol accumulate and have toxic effects. Neonates and infants can present with failure to thrive, poor feeding, vomiting, hypotonia, liver failure, and *Escherichia coli* sepsis (Demirbas et al., 2018). In the United States, galactosemia is nearly always diagnosed on NBS, and the acute manifestations are reversed with removal of galactose from the diet. Breast milk and cow milk-based formulas are replaced with a nongalactose-containing soy-based formula. Treated patients have generally good health; however, they still have a unique neuropsychiatric profile that includes mild intellectual deficits, delayed speech development (especially verbal dyspraxias), and some difficulties in visual perception, spatial orientation, and performance of visual-motor tasks. The long-term neurocognitive manifestations of galactosemia do not correlate with compliance with diet. Premature ovarian failure is also common despite dietary adherence. The mechanisms of these persistent manifestations in treated patients are currently a subject of research and will hopefully be further elucidated with future investigations.

Congenital Disorders of Glycosylation

CDGs are a large and growing group of disorders that arise from defects in any of the steps along the glycan synthesis or modification pathway (Chang et al., 2018). Glycans are sugar moieties that are attached to proteins or lipids to modify the properties of those molecules. CDGs often present with multisystemic involvement, including failure to thrive, developmental delay, hypotonia, hepatopathy, neurologic disease, ocular abnormalities, endocrine disease (hypoglycemia or hypothyroidism), coagulopathy, enteropathy, and renal disease. Isolated neurologic disease is also common. Biochemical studies such as transferrin isoelectric focusing and N-glycan profiling by mass spectrometry can be used to diagnose some types of CDG, though many CDGs can only be identified with genetic testing. Aside from a few notable exceptions, such as mannose therapy for MPI-CDG, treatment for most CDGs remains supportive; however, targeted therapies are an active area of research.

PMM2-CDG (formerly called CDG-1a) is the most common congenital disorder of glycosylation with an estimated prevalence of 1/20,000 (Schiff et al., 2017). It can present in infancy with severe neurologic and multisystemic disease, in childhood with developmental delays, or in adulthood with mild intellectual disability. Children with PMM2-CDG have a variety of mild facial dysmorphisms, including large dysplastic ears, a long philtrum, a prominent chin, and upslanting palpebral fissures (Fig. 36.2). More recognizable features include inverted nipples and abnormal distribution of adipose tissue, seen in about one-third of PMM2-CDG patients (see Fig. 36.2). Strabismus is seen in about 70% of patients. Children may have speech and motor delays, retinopathy, elevations in hepatic transaminases, seizures, stroke-like episodes, peripheral neuropathy, and thyroid abnormalities. Though intellectual disability is nearly universal, approximately one-half to two-thirds of patients learn to walk independently, and a higher percentage can walk with assistance. Slightly less than half of patients can speak in sentences. Adults may live into their seventh or eighth decade of life and typically have stable, mild neurocognitive deficits but may have progressive musculoskeletal disease (scoliosis/kyphosis, osteopenia, osteoporosis), multiple endocrinopathies (hyperinsulinism, insulin resistance, hyperprolactinemia, and hypogonadotropic hypogonadism), and hypercoagulability. Treatment remains supportive and centers around surveillance for known complications and management of disease manifestations.

PEROXISOMAL DISORDERS

Overview

Peroxisomes are small organelles that contain about 50 different enzymes that enact various anabolic or catabolic functions. Peroxisomal disease is divided into two main categories: (1) disorders that result in a generalized defect in the assembly and function of the peroxisome, called peroxisome biogenesis disorders and (2) disease due to single enzyme deficiencies. As a group they have a combined incidence of 1/5000 (Waterham, Ferdinandusse, & Wanders, 2016). Depending on the specific enzyme that is deficient, different patterns of abnormalities are found in corresponding peroxisomal metabolites. These findings can offer important diagnostic clues that help narrow the diagnostic possibilities when considering genes of interest. Ultimately the specific diagnosis is usually confirmed with genetic testing.

Given that peroxisomes are ubiquitous and found in cells throughout the body, clinical manifestations are usually multisystemic. Symptoms include developmental delay, regression, hypotonia, seizures, cataracts, retinal degeneration, sensorineural hearing loss, and in some cases leukodystrophy, liver dysfunction, or skeletal dysplasia. Peroxisomal disease should be considered in any child with progressive vision and

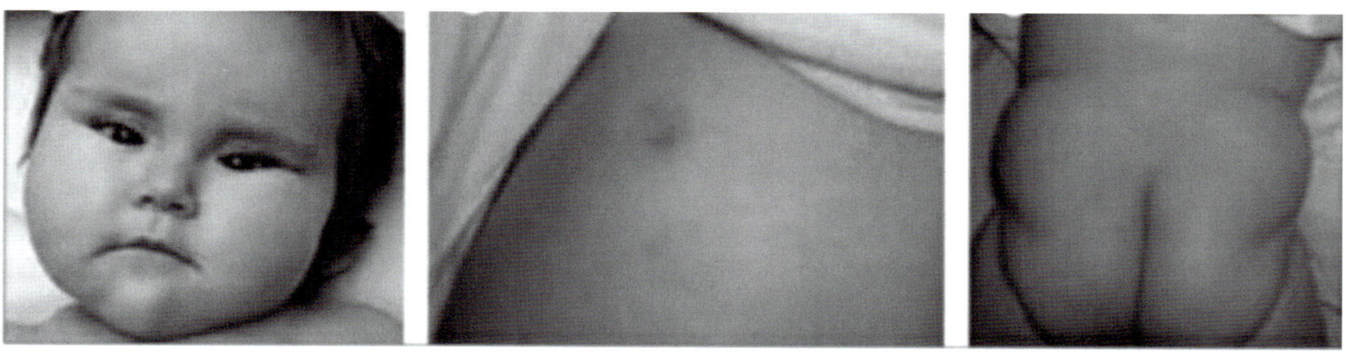

Fig. 36.2 PMM2-congenital disorder of glycosylation. ***(Left)*** Long philtrum, prominent chin, upslanting palpebral fissures and strabismus; ***(middle)*** inverted nipples; ***(right)*** abnormal fat distribution. (From Freeze, H. H., et al. [2012]. Neurology of congenital disorders of glycosylation. *Lancet Neurology, 11*[5], 453–466.)

hearing loss. Unfortunately, for most peroxisomal disorders, treatment largely consists of supportive care, though there are dietary interventions for some disorders as well as medication for some specific manifestations. XALD is a notable exception, and disease-modifying therapy for that disorder will be discussed.

X-Linked Adrenoleukodystrophy

XALD is the most common peroxisomal disorder with an estimated incidence of 1/17,000. It is caused by deficiency of *ABCD1*, which transports very long-chain fatty acids (VLCFAs) into the peroxisome to be catabolized via beta-oxidation. As a result, VLCFAs accumulate in cells throughout the body and have toxic effects. NBS for XALD is variable among states, but the disease is on the recommended uniform screening panel (Turk, Theda, Fatemi, & Moser, 2020).

It is an X-linked partially dominant condition and can affect males and females, though females typically have less severe symptoms with later onset. There are different forms of the disease, and importantly family members with the same genetic change can present with different types of XALD. Most relevant to the field of developmental pediatrics is the childhood cerebral form of ALD (CCALD), which occurs for about 35% of males with XALD.

Onset of CCALD, discussed in the case vignette, usually occurs between 3 and 10 years of age. Boys with XALD have typical neurodevelopment early in life and then present with subtle behavioral, cognitive, and neurologic changes such as changes in the ability to follow directions, diminished clarity of handwriting, incoordination, and seizures. The disease is rapidly progressive and ultimately, if untreated, results in death in a matter of a few years from the time of diagnosis due to rapid demyelination of the cerebral white matter (Fig. 36.3). Adrenomyeloneuropathy, which accounts for 45% of XALD cases, is a more slowly progressing disease characterized by paraplegia and spasticity. It typically manifests by the third decade of life in males and by the fifth to sixth decade in females. Individuals may also present with a history of isolated adrenal insufficiency. CCALD should be considered for a boy with new neurodevelopmental symptoms especially if review of family history elicits such features in maternal relatives.

The timing and nonspecific neurologic findings in CCALD make early diagnosis difficult. The prompt recognition and diagnosis of CCALD is of the utmost importance as it is one of the only peroxisomal diseases that has a disease-modifying treatment: bone marrow transplant, which is only effective if performed in the early stages of disease (after onset of MRI changes but before clinical symptoms worsen). The disease can be screened for with measurement of serum VLCFAs; the diagnosis is usually confirmed with molecular sequencing of the *ABCD1* gene. Adrenal function is abnormal in 90% of symptomatic boys, so assessment of adrenal function should be pursued if the diagnosis of XALD is being considered.

Peroxisomal Biogenesis Disorders: The Zellweger Spectrum

Neonatal adrenoleukodystrophy (NALD), infantile Refsum disease (IRD), and Zellweger syndrome are now typically referred to as peroxisomal biogenesis disorders or Zellweger spectrum disorders. They are autosomal recessive conditions caused by mutations in one of the 14 different *PEX* genes (Braverman et al., 2016). Patients can present with hypotonia, developmental delay, liver dysfunction, progressive sensorineural hearing loss, retinal dystrophy, visual impairment, and enamel defects of the teeth. Patients may also have renal calcium oxalate stones and adrenal insufficiency. NALD is distinguished from IRD by the presence of a leukodystrophy that typically begins in the deep

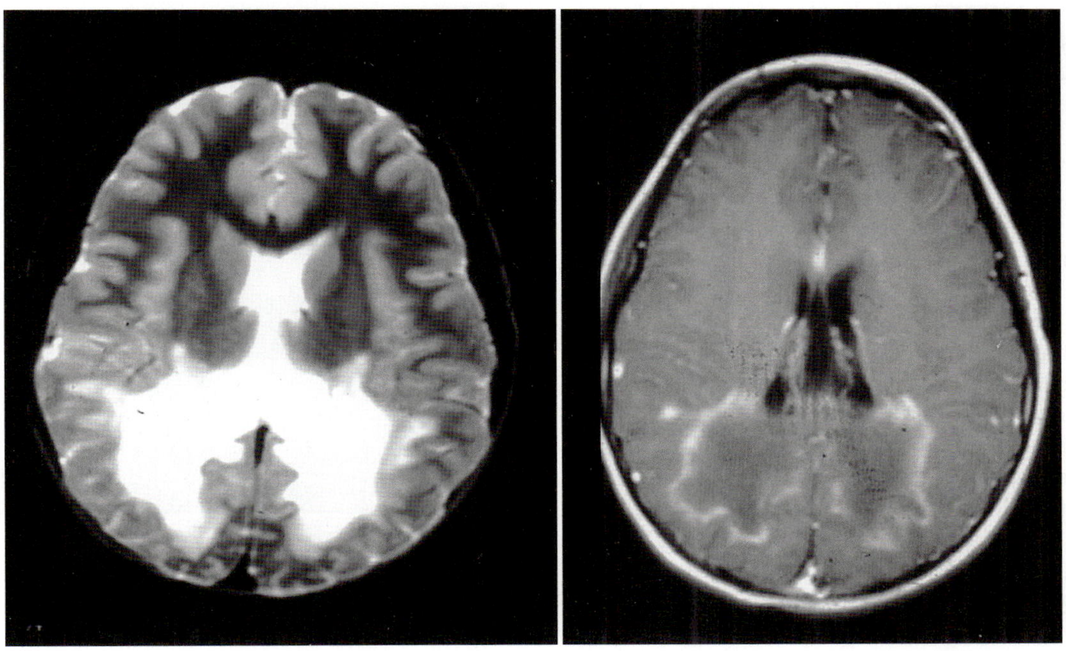

Fig. 36.3 Magnetic resonance imaging of cerebral X-linked adrenaleukodystrophy. *(Left)*T1-weighted image shows extensive parietooccipitcal white matter involvement and right enhancement with gadolinium contrast indicating the lesion is active.

white matter tracks of the cerebellum and progresses, much like in CCALD, to include the remainder of the cerebellar white matter, brain stem, parietooccipital lobes, corpus callosum, and finally the cerebral white matter.

The diagnosis, as in other peroxisomal diseases, is made based on abnormal values of peroxisomal metabolites and genetic analysis of the *PEX* genes. Children who survive the first year of life and have a nonprogressive course have a 77% probability of surviving to school age. For those who do survive, those with milder genotypes may achieve major milestones such as sitting and walking, albeit delayed. A minority of patients are able to speak in sentences and read. Treatment is largely symptomatic.

MITOCHONDRIAL DISEASES

Overview

Mitochondria are complex organelles present in nearly every cell in the body and are involved in many metabolic pathways (most notably oxidative phosphorylation). They are double membrane–bound organelles that are organized into distinct compartments based on the folding of the inner mitochondrial membrane into specialized structures called cristae. The proper functioning of the mitochondria is dependent, in part, on its dynamic three-dimensional structure. Due to their evolutionary origin as a separate bacterial organism, mitochondria uniquely depend on dual genetic codes: (1) the mitochondrial genome (mtDNA), which undergoes the entirety of replication, transcription, translation, and repair within the mitochondrial matrix; and (2) the nuclear mitochondrial genes that encode for proteins, which are transported from the cytosol into the mitochondria. The dual genetic code allows for multiple mechanisms of mitochondrial disease inheritance, which includes autosomal dominant, autosomal recessive, X-linked, and mitochondrial inheritance. Inheritance of disorders caused by mutations in mtDNA occurs in an exclusively matrilineal fashion because the developing embryo derives all of its mitochondria from the oocyte (Gorman et al., 2016).

Mitochondrial disease is defined as any genetic change in the nuclear or mitochondrial genomes that compromises the process of oxidative phosphorylation and consequently results in an impairment of mitochondrial energy generation. Mitochondrial diseases can be classified based on the specific mechanism by which oxidative phosphorylation is defective or by which of the mechanisms necessary for sustaining mitochondrial function (mtDNA maintenance, mitochondrial dynamics, transcription, or translation) is affected.

The prevalence of all forms of mitochondrial disease in children less than 16 years is estimated to be between 5 and 15/100,000 individuals, and mitochondrial disorders are collectively the most common form of inherited neurologic diseases (Rahman, 2020). They can present at any age and can involve just one organ system or be multisystemic. Typically the organs that rely most heavily on aerobic metabolism are most impacted. There is a bimodal distribution of presentations in those less than 3 years and then a wide distribution in the late teenage years into adulthood.

Common, and nonspecific, symptoms of mitochondrial disease in childhood include developmental delay or regression, weakness, failure to thrive, and feeding intolerance. More specific features include ptosis, ophthalmoplegia, cardiomyopathy, sensorineural deafness, optic atrophy, pigmentary retinopathy, and diabetes mellitus. Common central nervous system findings are fluctuating encephalopathy, seizures, dementia, migraine, strokelike episodes, ataxia, spasticity, and dystonia. Some mitochondrial diseases, such as MELAS (mitochondrial myopathy, encephalopathy, lactic acidosis, and stroke-like episodes) or MERFF (myoclonic epilepsy with ragged-red fibers) have a more well-defined and easily recognized phenotype; however, most do not. Due to similar clinical, biochemical, or imaging findings some mitochondrial diseases despite having different genotypic origins have historically been assigned a phenotypic label for descriptive purposes, such as Leigh syndrome, which is defined by the following criteria: the presence of bilateral brainstem or basal ganglia injury (Fig. 36.4), intellectual or motor impairments, and evidence of dysfunction of the mitochondrial respiratory chain or pyruvate dehydrogenase (PDH) complex.

Screening tests for mitochondrial disease include the measurement serum lactate (and pyruvate if lactate is elevated), serum acylcarnitine profile, urine organic acids, serum amino acids, general studies such as assessments of liver function, creatine kinase levels, and a complete blood count, and if available the measurement of the lactate, pyruvate, and amino acids in the CSF. The measurement of serum lactate is prone to error and is nonspecific. Lactate can be elevated due to

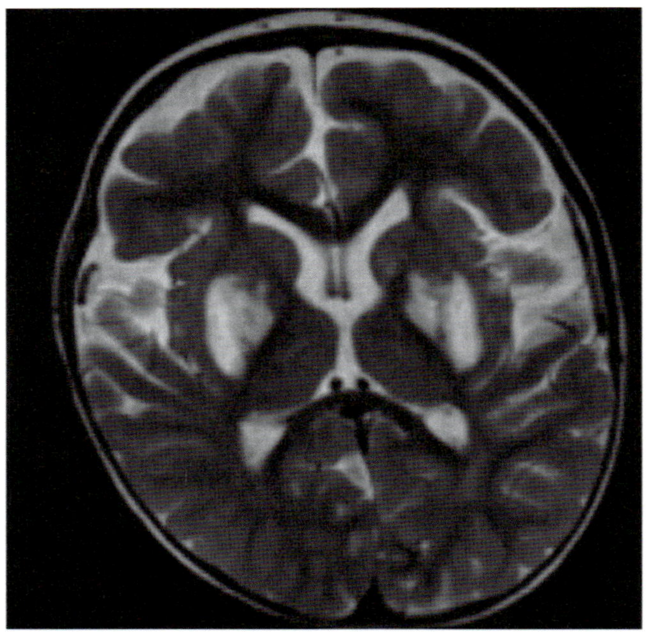

Fig. 36.4 Magnetic resonance imaging of patient with Leigh syndrome due to biallelic *SURF1* mutations. Axial T2-weighted image shows hyperintense lesions in caudate nuclei, putamina, and globus pallidus. (From Sofou, K., et al. [2013]. MRI of the brain in childhood-onset mitochondrial disorders with central nervous system involvement. ***Mitochondrion, 13***, 364–371.)

secondary dysfunction of the mitochondria resulting from impaired tissue perfusion, toxins, or other disease processes and therefore is most helpful when elevated in conjunction with other more specific laboratory findings (see Table 36.4).

With improving technologies and the ability to detect levels of heteroplasmy (variation in the genotype of mitochondrial DNA in an individual) as low as 1% to 2% in the blood, next-generation sequencing is the preferred method for testing for mutations in both the nuclear and mitochondrial genome (Parikh et al., 2015). In many cases genetic testing of the nuclear genome and mtDNA is the preferred first-line diagnostic test for mitochondrial disease. If a diagnosis is not made from genetic testing and clinical suspicion for mitochondrial disease remains high, then more invasive testing of tissue obtained from a muscle or liver biopsy may be employed.

Unfortunately, except for a few specific diagnoses, most mitochondrial diseases are not treatable. Most management is focused on disease surveillance and providing symptomatic care. There is limited evidence to suggest that any specific vitamins, supplements, or combinations thereof are efficacious; however, CoQ10 (ubiquinol), riboflavin, alpha-lipoic acid, creatine, carnitine, vitamin E, and other supplements are often used by patients with mitochondrial disease.

Pyruvate Dehydrogenase Deficiency

PDH complex deficiency is the second most common individual mitochondrial disorder reported in the North American Mitochondrial Disease Consortium (NAMDC) Registry (Barca et al., 2020) with an estimated birth prevalence of 1/50,000 to 1/75,000 live births per year. It is caused by a defect in the enzymatic machinery that catalyzes the oxidative decarboxylation of pyruvate to acetyl Co-A, the starting substrate for the citric acid cycle and the rate-limiting step of aerobic respiration. Due to an energy deficit, patients may present with developmental delays, hypotonia, intermittent ataxia, and episodic developmental regression when energy demands are increased during times of stress, such as febrile illnesses. Other more severe phenotypes include neonatal encephalopathy or Leigh syndrome. Depending on the genetic etiology of PDH deficiency, patients may have characteristic dysmorphic features (narrow head with frontal bossing, wide nasal bridge, upturned nose, long philtrum, and flared nostrils) and congenital brain malformations (such as cerebellar dysgenesis and abnormalities in neuronal migration) (Patel, O'Brien, Subramony, Shuster, & Stacpoole, 2012).

Due to elevated lactate, patients may present with a metabolic acidosis. The primary diagnostic metabolites that raise suspicion for PDH deficiency are pyruvate, lactate, and alanine though it is important to recognize that females with mutations in the X-linked gene *PDHA1* often do not have elevated lactate. Ultimately the diagnosis is made based on molecular genetic identification of pathogenic variants in any of the genes that encode for proteins in the PDH complex.

PDH deficiency can be treated with use of the ketogenic diet. The initiation of the ketogenic diet provides an alternative energy source (ketones) that allows the defective step in energy generation to be bypassed. For PDH deficiency patients initiated on the ketogenic diet, some improvement has been noted in seizure control, gait and balance, quality of sleep, speech and language development, social functioning, frequency of hospitalizations, and survival. Depending on the underlying genetic defect, patients may be treated with thiamine or lipoate, both cofactors for the PDH complex. Dichloroacetate (DCA) is also being studied to help augment enzyme activity.

LYSOSOMAL STORAGE DISORDERS

Overview

Lysosomal storage diseases (LSDs) are a large group of over 50 conditions characterized by lysosomal dysfunction, the majority of which are inherited in an autosomal recessive fashion. Each individual condition is rare, but collectively their incidence is estimated to be about 1/5000 births annually. There are over 80 enzymes present in the lysosome, and most of the LSD arise from defects that interfere with the ability of these enzymes to degrade complex molecules and allow for them to be excreted or recycled. The clinical features of LSD depend on the specific substrates that are stored and their sites of accumulation. Accordingly, most LSDs are categorized by the substrate that accumulates. Examples of stored substrate include mucopolysaccharides, oligosaccharides, sphingolipids, and neuronal ceroid lipofuscin. Examples from each of these categories will be discussed further in this section. A few lysosomal storage disorders are targets for NBS, but the specific disorders tested vary by state.

About 75% of patients with LSDs have central nervous system involvement that can manifest as developmental delays, regression in milestones, or behavioral changes. Many patients will also have systemic involvement, including coarsening of facial features (Fig. 36.5), hearing loss, ophthalmologic abnormalities, skeletal anomalies (see figure), organomegaly, cardiac valvular disease, dermatologic changes, and bone marrow involvement. The presence of these findings on physical examination and laboratory or imaging studies can be clues to the underlying diagnosis (Table 36.6). The age of onset varies from the neonatal period (in those that are severely affected) to adulthood (in milder conditions or in those who have more residual enzyme activity). Most LSDs are progressive, and it is important to recognize and diagnose them promptly, especially those that have specific therapies available (Table 36.7).

LSDs can be diagnosed using urine studies (e.g., glycosaminoglycans, oligosaccharides, sulfatides, and sialic acid) that assess the abundance of accumulated substrate. The specific diagnosis is generally made based on leukocyte enzyme analysis and genetic testing. As of 2020 several LSDs have approved disease-specific treatments. These include substrate reduction therapy, enzyme replacement therapy (ERT), and chaperone therapy to help stabilize the defective enzyme. Hematopoietic stem cell transplant (HSCT) may be considered for some LSDs. As research progresses and our understanding of the pathophysiology of these diseases improves

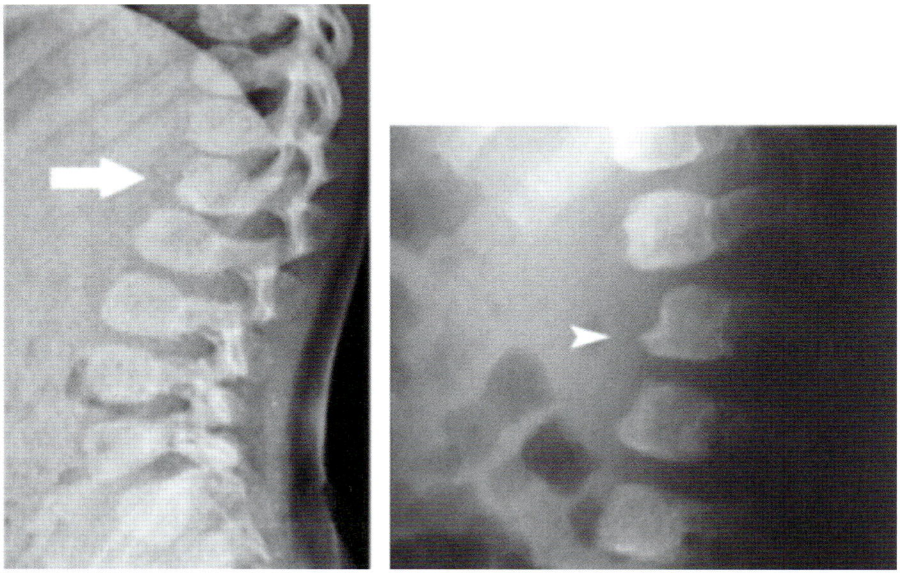

Fig. 36.5 Findings in MPS II. Top series of images shows minimal evidence of MPS II at initial evaluation for developmental delay. Photographs at ages 3 to 6 years demonstrate progression to classic coarse features, accompanied by organomegaly and dystosis multiplex, observed at age 10 years. Bottom shows dystosis dultiplex in a 4-year-old with MPS II. Left image shows rounding of vertebral bodies and right images shows "anterior beaking" with "posterior scalloping" of the vertebral bodies. (From Palmucci, S. et al. [2013]. Imaging findings of mucopolysaccharidoses: A pictorial review. *Insights into Imaging, 4*, 447.)

there is hope that other disease-modifying therapies will become available in the future (Platt, d'Azzo, Davidson, Neufeld, 2018).

Mucopolysaccharidoses

The mucopolysaccharidoses (MPSs) are collectively a group of LSDs that result from the impaired degradation of glycosaminoglycans. Seven different MPSs have been identified with varying degrees of severity, though in general they are all progressive diseases with symptoms such as organomegaly, dysostosis multiplex (see Fig. 36.5), coarse facial features, hearing and vision impairments, and cardiovascular compromise resulting from accumulated storage material. MPS II (Hunter syndrome) and MPS III (Sanfilippo syndrome) are the two most common to occur with neurodevelopmental symptoms as the presenting findings.

Hunter syndrome is an X-linked disorder that arises due to a deficiency in iduronate sulfatase (encoded for by iduronate-2-sulfatase [IDS]), which results in impaired degradation of heparan and dermatan sulfate (Mohamed, He, Singh, & Ferro, 2019). In general, MPS II patients' milestones of early infancy are met on time, with delays not becoming evident until 18 to 24 months of age. Patients tend to plateau developmentally and show signs of hyperactivity, aggression, and obstinacy by 3 to 5 years of age. Hearing loss is a nearly universal feature that is present by age 2 years. MPS II can be viewed as a phenotypic spectrum with the descriptive terms "early progressive" and "slowly progressive" used to describe where within the spectrum a patient falls. Patients with early progressive MPS II have early-onset developmental delays and have onset of systemic symptoms between 2 and 4 years of age, with death typically occurring in the second decade of life, between 10 and 15 years. Patients with slowly progressive MPS II may not have baseline cognitive impairments. They typically show onset of symptoms by around 4 years of age. Patients may survive into adulthood with some surviving into their 50s. MPS II patients have a normal appearance at birth but begin to exhibit somatic manifestations, particularly umbilical hernias, hepatosplenomegaly, recurrent otitis, and coarsening of facial features between 2 and 4 years of age. Changes in facial features are progressive, manifesting as macrocephaly, broad nasal bridge with wide and flattened nasal alae, prominent supraorbital ridges, large jowls, thickened ear lobules and lips, and an enlarged protruding tongue. Short stature with dysostosis multiplex, cardiac vascular abnormalities, hepatomegaly, and upper airway obstruction develop with time as well. ERT with idursulfase was approved in the United States in July 2006 with reductions in urinary metabolites and improvements in visceral symptoms observed; however, it has shown limited clinical benefit in the treatment of neurologic disease. The benefits of other therapies, such as bone marrow transplantation, are unclear at this time. Gene therapy remains under active investigation.

Sanfilippo syndrome is an autosomal recessive disorder that arises due to impaired degradation of dermatan sulfate. It has four subtypes depending on the specific step in dermatan sulfate degradation that is impaired (Andrade, Aldámiz-Echevarría, Llarena, & Couce, 2015). MPS IIIA is generally the most severe and rapidly progressive form. The other forms may have more attenuated phenotypes, and in some rare instances they may not present until adulthood. Symptom onset generally occurs between 2 and 6 years of age, with neurodegeneration worsening between 6 and 10 years. Speech delays are often the first symptom observed by parents. In MPS IIIA gains in fine motor development are generally made through ages 2 to 3 years, and adaptive skills are generally gained through age 4 years. Given the

TABLE 36.6 **Review of Storage Diseases by Clinical Presentation**

Condition	US Prevalence	Usual Age of Onset	Distinguishing Feature(s)	Coarse Facies	Organomegaly	Abnormalities on Neuroimaging	Neurodegeneration	Neurodevelopmental Phenotype
Hurler (MPS1)	1/100,000	By 1 yr with coarsening of features; signs may be present in the first months of life	Dysostosis multiplex and short stature (less apparent or absent in attenuated forms of MPS1)	Y	Y	Focal or diffuse, periventricular, bilateral, T2-hyperintense signal abnormality in the white matter Signal abnormalities most confluent in MPSIII Enlarged perivascular spaces involving white matter, corpus callosum, brainstem and basal ganglia (most pronounced in MPS I/II) Brain atrophy Hydrocephalus (MPS I/II) Enlargement of subarachnoid spaces	Y; initial plateau followed by gradual decline	Normal early on; however, delays apparent by 18 mo
Hurler Scheie (attenuated MPS1)	1/150,000	3–10 yr		Y	Y		N	Normal or mild intellectual disability
Hunter (MPS2) *X linked	1/100,000–1/170,000	2–4 yr		Y	Y		Y; prominent by 6–8 yr	Normal development initially followed by plateau at 2–3 yr (speech > motor) and then decline Poor sleep, hyperactivity, behavioral problems, perseverative chewing, inability to toilet train (note these features may not be present in those with mild forms of disease)
Sanfillipo (MPS3) *Most Common MPS	1/70,000	2–8 yr	Severe sleep disturbances (milder skeletal findings)	Y, but mild	Y, but mild		Y; usually severe after first decade of life Loss of ambulation, spasticity, swallowing difficulties develop in teenage years Process slowed in attenuated form and more challenging to diagnose	Period of normal development followed by decline Speech delays noticeable first Development of severe ADHD, sleep disturbances and behavioral difficulties by 3–4 yr

(Continued)

TABLE 36.6 **Review of Storage Diseases by Clinical Presentation—cont'd**

Condition	US Prevalence	Usual Age of Onset	Distinguishing Feature(s)	Coarse Facies	Organomegaly	Abnormalities on Neuroimaging	Neurodegeneration	Neurodevelopmental Phenotype
Sly syndrome (MPS7)	1/250,000	Variable, prenatal: 10 yr	History of nonimmune fetal hydrops; dysostosis multiplex and short stature	Y	Y		Y, in some	Varying degree of intellectual disability, speech deficits common (MPS1 like)
Multiple sulfatase deficiency	1/1,400,000	Variable, but generally between 2 and 6 yr	Ichthyosis	Y	Y	White matter (periventricular) abnormalities with U fiber sparing, radiating stripes, and severe white matter atrophy	Y, rate varies, those with mild disease may retain limited speech into late childhood and remain ambulatory into teenage years	May have normal development until disease onset
Sialidosis (ML1) type 1	Unknown	Childhood–adolescence	Cherry-red spot myoclonus syndrome	Y/N	Y		Y, develop gait abnormalities and visual deficits	Normal
Sialisodis (ML1) type 2	Unknown	<1 yr		Y	Y		Y	Global delays
I-cell disease (ML2)	1/100,000–1/40,000	Prenatal–early childhood	Microcephaly, skeletal features and organomegaly	Y	Y		Y	Developmental delays (motor > speech/cognitive)
Pseudo-Hurler polydystrophy (ML3)	1/100,000–1/2,500,000	3–5 yr		Y	Y/N		Y	Mild cognitive deficits, speech generally attained at normal age
Sialolipidosis (ML4)	1/40,000	First year of life	Anemia/gastrointestinal issues	Y	N	Dysgenic corpus callosum, white matter dysmyelination, decreased signal intensity in the basal ganglia, and cerebellar atrophy	Y in ~15%	Global DD, most nonambulatory and have limited/absent speech
Galactosialidosis	Unknown	Infantile (birth–7 mo)		Y	Y		Y	
		Adult (>3 yr)		Y	N		Y	Ataxia, seizures, myoclonus

Alpha-mannosidosis	1/500,000	Mild (>10 yr)	Recurrent infections (especially in the first decade of life), dystosis multiplex	Y, mild	Y, mild	Brain MRI including sagittal T_1 and axial T_2 sections reveals a partially empty sella turcica, cerebellar atrophy, and white matter signal modifications	Y, slow	Speech and motor delays, mild-moderate intellectual disability though those with mild disease have normal motor functioning (ski, learn to ride a bike, etc.)
		Moderate (<10 yr)					Y, slow	
		Severe (<10 yr)					Y, rapid	
Beta-mannosidosis	Unknown	Adolescence/adulthood	Angiokeratomas	Y, mild	Y, mild		Y, slow	DD, moderate-severe ID, introversion, hyperactivity/impulsivity/aggression
Fucosidosis	Unknown	Infancy 2 yr	Angiokeratomas, telangiectasias, neuroimaging findings	Y	Y	Low signal in globus pallidus on T2	Y	DD, but do learn to walk
Aspartylglucosaminuria	1/18,500	2–3 yrs	Macrocephaly	N, characteristic facies: hypertelorism, short bulbous nose, small ears, and square-shaped face	N	Decreased signal intensity in susceptibility weighted imaging of the thalamic nuclei	Y, slowly progressing	Developmental delays and severe ADHD early on Continue to make gains until ~13–16 yr Stable period until ~25–28 yr, followed by rapid decline after 30 yr
Schindler disease	Rare	8–15 mo		N	N		Y, develop seizures, loss vision	
Gaucher	1/100,000	Type 2 (<2 yr) 2–4 mo on average		N	Y		Y, rapid, survival beyond 2 yr rare	Severe cognitive impairment, brainstem dysfunction, and pyramidal signs
		Type 3 (childhood/early adolescence) average age 5 yr	Horizontal gaze palsy, thrombocytopenia, anemia, and bone pain	N	Y		Y, slower progression	+/– DD, develop encephalopathy and seizures

(Continued)

TABLE 36.6 Review of Storage Diseases by Clinical Presentation—cont'd

Condition	US Prevalence	Usual Age of Onset	Distinguishing Feature(s)	Coarse Facies	Organomegaly	Abnormalities on Neuroimaging	Neurodegeneration	Neurodevelopmental Phenotype
Krabbe	1/100,000	Infantile (<6 mo; average 3–4 mo)	Extreme irritability and episodic unexplained fever	N	N	Abnormal brain MRI, consistent with demyelination T2-weighted images show involvement of periventricular white matter, deep gray matter, and centrum semiovale as well as enhancement of cranial nerves Subcortical U-fibers may be spared until late in the disease course	Y, first stage hypertonic episodes, followed by permanent posturing and seizures, followed by vision loss and loss of bulbar functions	Developmental plateau followed by regression/neurodegeneration
		Late infantile (7–12 mo)					Y, slower progression compared to early infantile form	Loss of milestones, poor feeding, crying/irritability
		Juvenile (13 mo–10 yr, commonly after 5 yr)				Paresthesias, weakness, ataxia	Y, variable rate of progression	Normal IQ or DD/slow development at disease onset, first sign usually ataxia
Metachromatic Leukodystrophy	1/40,000–160,000	Late-infantile (<30 mo; average age 18 mo)		N	N	+Leukodystrophy	Y, gradual progression, loss of motor milestones, speech, and vision	Gross motor delays (many never walk independently)
		Juvenile (30 mo–16 yr)					Y, progressive gait abnormalities	Decline in school performance may proceed motor changes
		Adult (>16 yr)						Emotional liability, psychosis, seizures
Neiman-Pick A	1/250,000	Infantile–first few months	Massive hepatosplenomegaly	N	Y (presenting sign)	S	Y	Plateau 10–12 mo followed by loss of skills and lack of interest in surroundings
		Intermediate (2–7 yr)						Normal development until 2–7 yr at which point learning problems, hypotonia, and hyporeflexia develop followed by ataxia, cognitive impairment and loss of motor function

Niemann-Pick C	1/100,000	Early infantile (9 mo–2 yr)	Often have a history of cholestatic jaundice	N	+/– when present precedes onset of neurologic disease	Often normal until late stages of disease At that time shows cerebellar and cerebral atrophy and thinning of the corpus callosum	Y, typically do not survive past middle childhood	Hypotonia and gross motor delays, typically nonambulatory
		Late infantile/ juvenile onset (60%–70% of cases)	Vertical gaze palsy and gelastic cataplexy				Y, develop spasticity and pyramidal signs, seizures, impaired swallowing	Delayed language, ataxia, and increasing problems in school
		Adolescent/ adult onset	Vertical gaze palsy, psychiatric symptoms, and dementia					Ataxia, dystonia, dysarthria, movement disorders, and variable cognitive dysfunction
GM1 gangliosidosis	1/100,000–1/200,000	Early infantile–<6 mo		Dysmorphisms–puffy face, moderate macroglossia, hypertrophic gums, depressed nasal bridge	Y		Y, usually rapid after first year of life	Developmental arrest at 3–6 mo
		Late infantile–<3 yr (on average 12–18 mo)		Y/N	Y/N		Y, rapid and severe Develop spastic quadriparesis	
		Adult/ chronic late onset-late childhood–adulthood		Y/N	Y/N		Y, slowly progressive Develop dysarthria, dystonia, and pyramidal signs	Mild cognitive impairment
Tay-Sachs/Sandhoff	1/320,000	Infantile (average 4–6 mo)	Exaggerated startle in infantile form Macrocephaly (by 18 mo)	N	N		Y, rapid, develop blindness, spasticity, and seizures	Initially normal, hypotonia noted at 3–6 mo with regression by 6–10 mo
		Juvenile (2–10 yr)	Ataxia, dysarthria				Y, slower progression, develop seizures and spasticity	Initially normal, ataxia, incoordination and dysarthria are presenting signs

(Continued)

TABLE 36.6 Review of Storage Diseases by Clinical Presentation—cont'd

Condition	US Prevalence	Usual Age of Onset	Distinguishing Feature(s)	Coarse Facies	Organomegaly	Abnormalities on Neuroimaging	Neurodegeneration	Neurodevelopmental Phenotype
		Late onset	Ataxia, dysarthria					Delayed onset of ataxia, dystonia, dysarthria, hypotonia 40% with psychiatric involvement (paranoia or schizophrenia)
Farber	Rare	Varied, can present in adulthood but usually presents in infancy	"JIA-like" Painful joint swelling, contractions, and periarticular subcutaneous nodules	N	Y		Variable	Variable
Neuronal ceroid lipofusinosis (includes 13 different genes)	Reported by gene	Infantile (6–24 mo)	Deceleration of head growth	N	N		Y, visual impairments, seizures, stereotypic hand movements	DD
		Late infantile (2–4 yr)	Speech delay and vision loss				Y, more gradual loss of vision, gait disturbance, seizures, and developmental regression	Presenting feature speech delay
		Juvenile (4–10 yrs)	Vision loss, behavioral changes				Y, blindness presenting feature, develop seizures, dysarthria, behavioral issues/ aggression	Develop echolalic speech
Pompe disease	1/40,000	Infantile	Hypotonia, hypertrophic cardiomyopathy and macroglossia	N	+/- (not seen in adult)		N, symptoms are progressive but cognitive decline not typical	Hypotonia
		Juvenile	Skeletal muscle involvement and progressive respiratory insufficiency (minimal cardiac involvement)					Hypotonia and myopathy Mimics "Duchenne muscular dystrophy"

		Adult (third to fourth decade)	Mimics limb girdle muscular dystrophy Respiratory disease > muscle disease (minimal cardiac involvement)					Weakness of trunk and proximal limbs
Canavan disease		2–4 mo	Head lag, hypotonia, and macrocephaly	N	N	Diffuse white matter abnormalities Classically shows symmetric diffuse low signal intensity on T1W and high signal intensity on T2W	Y, develop spasticity, opisthotonic posturing, optic nerve atrophy, and impaired swallowing	Hypotonia leads to global developmental delays leads to progressive neurodegeneration
Alexander disease	Rare	Neonatal	Megalencephaly	N	N	Leukoencephalopathy with following features: • White matter abnormalities with frontal predominance • Periventricular signal abnormalities • Basal ganglia, thalamic and brainstem abnormalities	Y	Poor feeding and global delays leads to neurodegeneration
		Infantile	Megalencephaly					Variable acquisition of milestone, followed by onset of seizures and regression
		Juvenile	Bulbar symptoms					Language delay, hypophonia or nasal speech, bulbar symptoms may manifest as vomiting and anorexia
		Adult	Bulbar symptoms					Bulbar symptoms (palatal myoclonus), motor/gait abnormalities and cerebellar ataxia

Color coding: red = mucopolysacharridoses, green = mucolipidoses, blue = oligosaccharides, purple = sphingolipidoses, pink = NCL; other = orange.
DD, Developmental delay; *ID*, intellectual disability; *N*, no; *Y*, yes; *yr*, year.

TABLE 36.7 Summary of Treatment Status for Inborn Errors of Metabolism Presenting With Developmental Concerns

Treatable/Significantly Improved Outcomes	Supportive Care/Treatment Minimally Efficacious	Active Clinical Trial/Area of Research
PDE/PNPO	NKH (severe)	CLN3, CLN2
GLUT-1	Most CLNs	UCD
NKH (attenuated)	Most mitochondrial disease/ETC defects	CRTR
UCD	TH (infantile form)	LNS
PDH	CRTR	MPS2
CTX	ISOD, other MoCD	MPS3
TH (dopa-responsive dystonia)	Alexander	Krabbe
AGAT	Gaucher (2/3)	Tay-Sachs
GAMT	NPA	Canavan
CFD	GM1	MLD (infantile)
MoCD due to ***MOSC1***	MSD	AADC
XALD	ML1	Alpha-mannosidosis
NPC	AGU	MLIV
MPS1		
MLD (juvenile/adult)		
GTPCH-1		
Wilson		
Hcy		
Cobalamin disorders		
Ser		
Pompe		

AADC, Aromatic L-amino acid decarboxylase deficiency; *AGAT*, arginine:glycine amidinotransferase deficiency; *AGU*, aspartylglucosaminuria; *CDG*, congenital disorders of glycosylation; *CFD*, cerebral folate deficiency; *CLN*, neuronal ceroid lipofuscinosis 10; *CRTR*, creatine transporter deficiency; *CTX*, cerebrotendinous xanthomatosis; *ETC*, electron transport chain deficiencies; *GAMT*, guanidinoacetate methyltransferase deficiency; *GABA/Gln*, disorders of GABA and glutamine metabolism; *GLUT1*, glucose transporter type 1 deficiency; *GM1*, GM1 gangliosidosis; *GM3*, GM3 synthase deficiency; *hcy*, homocystinuria; *GTPCH-1*, GTP cyclohydrolase 1 deficiency; *ISOD*, isolated sulfite oxidase deficiency; *LNS*, Lesch-Nyhan syndrome; *MLI*, mucolipidosis type I; *MLIV*, mucolipidosis type IV; *MLD*, metachromatic leukodystrophy; *MoCD*, molybdenum cofactor deficiency; *MOSC1*, molybdenum cofactor deficiency type A; *MPS*, mucopolysacharridosis; *MSD*, multiple sulfatase deficiency; *NKH*, nonketotic hyperglycinemia; *NPA*, Niemann-Pick A; *NPC*, Niemann-Pick C; *PBD*, peroxisome biogenesis disorders; *PDE*, pyridoxine-dependent epilepsy; *PNPO*, pyridoxamine-phosphate oxidase deficiency; *Ser*, serine deficiency; *TH*, tyrosine hydroxylase deficiency; *UCD*, urea cycle disorder; *XALD*, X-linked adrenoleukodystrophy.

minimal involvement of the musculoskeletal system, gross motor impairments may not be observed until 5 to 6 years. The neurocognitive profile of MPS III is characterized by cognitive regression, severe hyperactivity, anxiety, aggression, and sleep disturbances. Sleep disorders (which occur in 80%–90% of patients) consist of difficulties falling asleep and frequent nocturnal awakenings, with complete reversal of the day-night rhythm in some patients. Epilepsy has been observed in about 30% of patients. Unlike the other MPS disorders, patients with MPS III may have only mild systemic features such as recurrent otitis, femoral head necrosis, mild hepatomegaly, subclinical cardiac abnormalities, and subtle facial coarsening with a protruding philtrum, synophrys, and hypertrichosis (Fig. 36.6). To date, there are no effective therapies for MPS III; however, research exploring the possibilities of ERT, substrate reduction therapy, chaperone therapy, and gene therapy is ongoing.

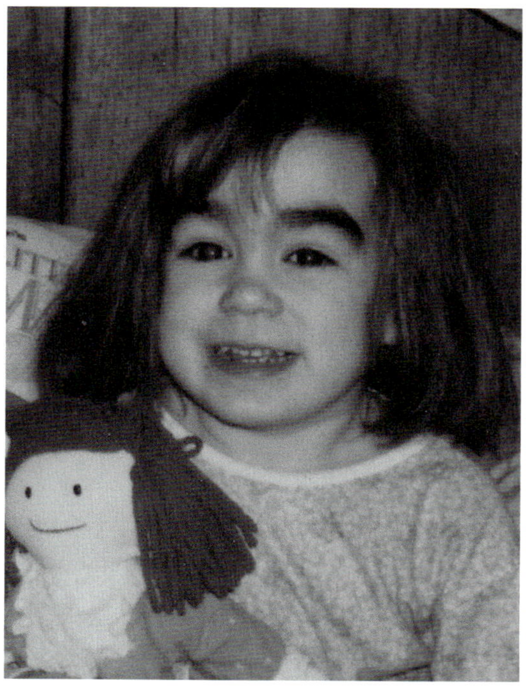

Fig. 36.6 Subtle facial coarseness and hypertrichosis in a patient with MPS III, age 3 years.

Niemann-Pick C

Niemann-Pick C is an autosomal recessive lipid storage disease that arises from abnormalities in the trafficking of endocytosed cholesterol. It can be identified by abnormalities in serum oxysterols and urinary bile acids (Geberhiwot et al., 2018). The typical presentation occurs in childhood with the insidious onset of clumsiness, eventually progressing to ataxia, vertical supranuclear gaze palsy (VSGP), and dementia. Dystonia and seizures are common. Gelastic cataplexy may develop in about 20% of patients. Dysarthria and dysphagia eventually become disabling. The life expectancy is variable, but death usually occurs in the late second or third decade of life. Adolescents and adults are more likely to present with dementia or psychiatric symptoms such as hallucinations and delusional thoughts mimicking depression and schizophrenia. This form of the disease progresses more slowly compared to the classic childhood form. A neonatal form of the disease presenting with fetal hydrops or cholestatic liver disease can occur with severe enzyme deficiency. Miglustat, a substrate reduction therapy originally implemented in Gaucher disease, has been used with some success in slowing disease course.

Neuronal Lipofuscinosis

The neuronal ceroid lipofuscinoses (NCLs) are a group of LSDs characterized by neurodegeneration and intracellular accumulation of ceroid lipofuscin due to defects in any of the 13 genes that have been associated with NCL (Mole et al., 2019). Together they represent the most prevalent class of childhood neurodegenerative diseases. Visual loss is a common feature among many of the NCLs, which vary by the age of symptom onset, presenting feature, and rate of neurodegeneration. The diagnosis is made using genetic testing. In some cases characteristic pathology findings in the skin or ocular mucosa may be helpful in confirming the diagnosis.

DISORDERS OF CHOLESTEROL METABOLISM

Disorders of Cholesterol Synthesis: Smith-Lemli-Opitz Syndrome

Cholesterol has numerous functions in normal cellular physiology: it is a component of the cell membrane and myelin sheath in the central nervous system, a precursor to steroid hormones that influence prenatal and postnatal development, and a precursor to the synthesis of bile acids. It is also important to highlight that cholesterol is impenetrable to the blood-brain barrier, which forms between 12 and 18 weeks of gestation, and that after this point in fetal development the brain becomes entirely dependent on endogenous sources of cholesterol (Kanungo, Soares, He, & Steiner, 2013). Thus it is not surprising that defects in cholesterol synthesis can have widespread impact on body morphology, neurodevelopment, and other systems. The cholesterol biochemical synthetic pathway is highly complex, and human diseases have been associated with defects in many of the enzymatic steps (Table 36.8).

Smith-Lemli-Opitz syndrome (SLOS) is an autosomal recessive disorder with an estimated prevalence of 1/20,000 to 1/40,000 (Kanungo et al., 2013) that arises from a deficiency in 7-dehydrocholesterol reductase (7DHCR), which catalyzes the final step of cholesterol synthesis. The condition is identified by measuring levels of 7- and 8-dehydrocholesterol, which are elevated in the serum of affected individuals. Serum cholesterol levels will be normal in ~90% of SLOS patients, and it is therefore not a sensitive diagnostic test. The phenotypic spectrum of SLOS is varied and may range from a milder disorder, characterized by isolated learning and behavioral

TABLE 36.8 Phenotypes of Disorders of Cholesterol Synthesis

Condition	Inheritance	Cognitive Profile	Distinguishing Feature	Dysmorphic Features
Sterol C4 methyl oxidase deficiency (SC4MOL)	AR	Variable ID	Dermatologic phenotype: severe dermatitis/ichthyosis	Y
Congenital hemidysplasia with ichthyosiform nevus and limb defects (CHILD)	X-linked dominant (lethal in males in the hemizygous state)	Normal in females	Dermatologic phenotype: inflammatory nevus with waxlike scaling and a marked affinity for skinfolds, unique lateralization, and strict midline demarcation	Y
CK syndrome	X-linked dominant (females typically unaffected)	Mild to severe ID, speech delay, self-mutilating tendencies	Tall stature, kyphosis, arachnodactyly, and hyperextensible joints	Y, long, narrow face, almond-shaped eyes, epicanthal folds, upslanting palpebral fissures, high nasal bridge, high-arched palate, crowded teeth, posteriorly rotated ears, micrognathia/retrognathia, and malar hypoplasia
Lathosterolosis	AR	Variable ID	Axial/appendicular skeletal anomalies	Y "SLOS-like"
Desmosterolosis	AR	Severe ID	Mild to severe arthrogryposis	Y

AR, Autosomal recessive; *ID*, intellectual disability; *"SLOS-like"*, Smith-Lemli-Opitz syndrome-like; *Y*, yes.

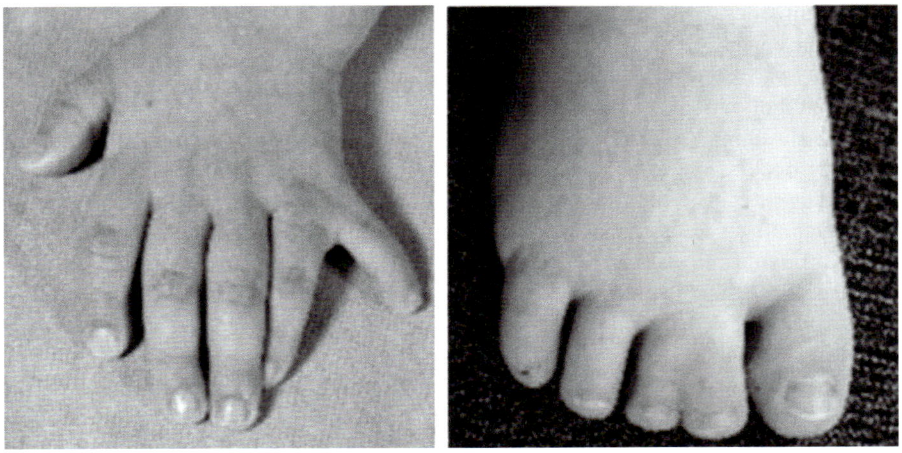

Fig. 36.7 Clinical findings of Smith-Lemli-Opitz syndrome. ***(Left)*** Patient at 1 year of age with microcephaly, bitemporal narrowing, broad nasal tip with anteverted nares, prominent glabella with long philtrum tented upper lip (cupid's bow or carp-shaped), and micrognathia; ***(middle)*** short, proximally placed thumb and ***(right)*** syndactyly of the second and third toes. (From Porter, F. D. [2008]. Smith-Lemli-Opitz syndrome: Pathogenesis, diagnosis and management. ***European Journal of Medical Genetics, 16***, 535–541.)

differences, to a severe lethal malformation syndrome. Those on the milder end of the spectrum are likely underdiagnosed.

Children with SLOS may present with microcephaly, dysmorphic features (narrow forehead, broad anteverted nares, micrognathia, a high-arched palate or cleft uvula, ptosis, cataracts, optic nerve hypoplasia/atrophy, syndactyly (especially digits 2 and 3 of the lower extremities) (Fig. 36.7), postaxial polydactyly, cardiac abnormalities, genitourinary anomalies (ambiguous genitalia, cryptorchidism, inguinal hernia, renal cysts), increased frequency of gastrointestinal anomalies (pyloric stenosis, gastroesophageal reflux disease, Hirschsprung disease, malrotation), adrenal abnormalities (both glucocorticoid and mineralocorticoid deficiencies), and brain malformations such as varied cerebellar abnormalities, ventricular dilation, myelination abnormalities, Dandy-Walker variant, and holoprosencephaly. The neurodevelopmental and behavioral profile is varied and can include intellectual disability (usually moderate to severe), autism, sensory hypersensitivity, irritability, language impairments, sleep-wake cycle disturbances, and self-injurious behaviors. Expressive language skills tend to be more impaired than receptive language, and gross motor skills tend to be more impaired than fine motor. Delayed attainment of gross motor milestones is nearly universal, but most children with SLOS learn to walk (Nowaczyk & Irons, 2012).

Current therapeutic approaches include dietary supplementation with cholesterol and, rarely, the administration of bile salts, with equivocal responses likely due to the inability of exogenous cholesterol to cross the blood-brain barrier. There are reports of patients supplemented with dietary cholesterol demonstrating improvements in alertness, socialization, hearing, and muscle tone and showing decreased tactile hypersensitivity, irritability, aggression, photosensitivity, and number of infections. These results have not been corroborated by any systematic investigations to date.

Cerebrotendinous Xanthomatosis

Cerebrotendinous xanthomatosis (CTX) is an autosomal recessive disorder caused by a deficiency of the CYP27A1 enzyme. The deficiency results in decreased synthesis of cholic acid and chenodeoxycholic acid and the accumulation of cholesterol metabolism intermediates in the blood, brain, and tissues throughout the body. CTX can be diagnosed with measurement of serum cholestanol and urine bile acids as well as other cholesterol intermediaries. Sign and symptoms may include infantile-onset diarrhea, childhood-onset cataracts, adolescent-onset tendinous xanthomas (Fig. 36.8), and adult onset neuropsychiatric disease, which can include dementia, neuropathy, Parkinsonism, seizures, pyramidal signs, cerebellar signs, and psychiatric disturbances. Childhood

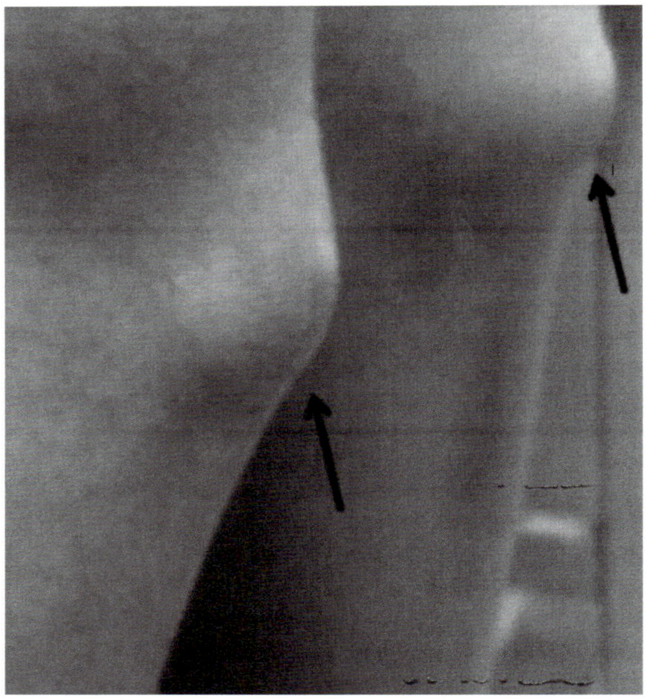

Fig. 36.8 Tendinous xanthomas below the knee in an individual with cerebrotendinous xanthomatosis. (From Pedroso, J. L. et al. [2012]. Early-onset epilepsy as the main neurological manifestation of cerebrotendinous xanthomatosis. ***Epilepsy & Behavior, 24***[3], 380–381.)

onset cataracts are the presenting feature in 75% of cases. Developmental delays, ADHD, and autism may be present early in life; however, most individuals with CTX do not show signs of intellectual impairment until puberty. Unlike other disorders of cholesterol metabolism, CTX is treatable with chenodeoxycholic acid, which prevents progression but does not reverse neurologic disease (Nie, Chen, Cao, & Zhang, 2014; Wong, Walsh, Hayden, & Eichler, 2018).

THERAPEUTICS

As mentioned in prior sections, the natural history and prognosis of many genetic and inherited metabolic diseases are rapidly changing as multiple different types of disease-modifying therapies become available. This section is intended to introduce different therapeutic strategies that have been used. Please refer to clinicaltrials.gov and primary literature sources for the most accurate and updated information regarding treatment options available for specific diseases. Though not revisited in this section, for many metabolic disorders, dietary and vitamin/supplement therapies (e.g., carnitine) remain the mainstay of treatment and will continue to remain of paramount importance for the foreseeable future.

In general, multiple factors, including the blood-brain barrier, narrow therapeutic windows, and (for many neurodevelopmental disorders) the appearance of disease manifestations *in utero*, make the development of efficacious therapeutic options for many of the central nervous system–related diseases discussed in this chapter particularly challenging. Additionally, many of these therapies also place significant economic burden on the health care system. Although individual genetic and metabolic diseases are extremely rare, they do in aggregate affect a significant fraction of the population. The hope is that as therapeutic advances are made, these will be applied to conditions that share similar fundamental mechanisms of disease to streamline the implementation process and decrease costs.

Gene and RNA-Based Therapies

The goal of gene therapy is to restore gene function through different approaches, depending on the consequences of the genetic mutation. Options include gene replacement, gene silencing, and mutation correction via gene editing. The foundation of gene replacement therapy relies on the introduction of a therapeutic gene into the patient's genome in a specific tissue using a modified viral vector. Current trials use adeno-associated virus (AAV), lentivirus, and adenovirus vectors. Nonviral vectors include synthetic delivery options.

Gene therapies may also use RNA as a therapeutic molecule to modulate gene expression. Examples include antisense oligonucleotides (ASOs) and small interfering RNA. ASOs are synthetic, short, single-stranded oligodeoxynucleotides that can alter complementary messenger RNA function and resultant protein expression through a variety of strategies that include targeted degradation, translational arrest, increased translation, RNA-binding protein inhibition, and splicing modulation. Small interfering RNAs are synthetic, double-stranded oligonucleotides that degrade target messenger RNA to decrease expression of a specific gene. That strategy may be used if an enzyme deficiency results in the accumulation of a toxic metabolite, and blocking another upstream enzyme results in the accumulation of a benign metabolite in lieu of the toxic metabolite.

Enzyme Replacement Therapies

Direct ERT is one of the most intuitive strategies used to treat inherited diseases in which the pathogenesis of disease-related symptoms arises directly from the deficiency of a specific enzyme. ERT has been successfully used in the amelioration of several non–central nervous system–mediated disorders such as nonneuronopathic Gaucher disease and Fabry disease. Both the use of modified ERT, in which the chemical structure and/or composition of the enzyme is modified to allow transfer across the blood-brain barrier, and direct intrathecal/intraventricular delivery remains under investigation for enzyme deficiencies that cause neurologic symptoms. Several have already been approved for clinical use.

Cell-Based Therapies

Cell-based therapy involves modifying a patient's own cells, or using exogenous wild-type cells from a donor, to correct a genetic/enzymatic problem and alleviate the metabolic disorder. Examples of exogenous cell sources include HSCT and solid organ transplant such as liver transplant. Cell-based therapy is currently used to treat many of the disorders discussed in this chapter, examples of which include severe organic acidemias, glycogen storage disorders, LSD such MPS I and XALD, and mitochondrial diseases such as mitochondrial neurogastrointestinal encephalopathy (MNGIE). Autologous HSCT may be combined with lentiviral vector-based *ex vivo* gene replacement therapy (e.g., with XALD).

A unique situation arises in conditions that are confined to a specific organ (e.g., the liver in the case of urea cycle disorders). In these situations solid organ transplantation essentially "cures" the individual of the genetic disorder but replaces it with the chronic morbidities and mortality risk associated with being a solid organ transplant recipient. In some cases gene replacement therapy may more safely and effectively replace organ transplantation in the future.

Small Molecule Therapies

Small molecule therapy uses both naturally occurring and synthetic low-mass chemical compounds that impact disease pathogenesis. An example is pharmacologic chaperones, which act at a protein level. Chaperones stabilize proteins carrying missense mutations that cause misfolding, and they restore the appropriate folding pattern to increase enzyme activity. These chaperone therapies are often mutation specific and work only for patients with specific genotypes. Some pathogenic variants in Fabry disease, for example, are amenable to chaperone therapy, migalastat (Galafold), while most Fabry mutations require enzyme replacement. Some small molecule therapies, such as tetrahydrobiopterin, act at the site of the interaction between an enzyme and its endogenous cofactor to increase enzymatic activity.

TABLE 36.9 Neurodevelopmental Profile for Inborn Errors of Metabolism by Presenting Feature and Most Common Age of Onset

	DD/ID									Disease Course		
	Speech	Motor	ASD	ADHD/Behavior Issues	Regression/Change in School Performance/Onset Psychiatric Symptoms/Dementia	Seizures	Movement Disorder/Ataxia	Spasticity	Hypotonia	Progressive	Episodic	Static
Neonatal	N/A	N/A	N/A	Ser (incessant crying and poor feeding)	N/A	PDE/PNPO GLUT-1 NKH GABA/Gln PBD ISOD/MoCD ***Menkes*** Mito GM3 ***CLN10*** UCD ***Alexanders*** ***Ser***		Ser	NKH ISOD/MoCD ETC PBD CDG UCD Menkes Alexanders	CLN10 Menkes ISOD/MoCD Alexanders Serine GM3	UCD	NKH CDG GABA/Gln
Early infancy 1–6 mo	CFD ***Alexanders*** Gaucher AADC GM1 MSD MLIV	TH CFD ***Tay-Sachs*** Canavan ***Alexanders*** Gaucher NPA AACD GM1 MSD MLIV	N/A	***Infantile Krabbe*** (extreme irritability) Serine	Tay-Sachs (loss visual attentiveness) Menkes (loss motor milestones) TH (progressive hypotonia and encephalopathy)	PDE/PNPO GLUT-1 NKH GABA/Gln PBD ISOD/MoCD Menkes Mito GM3 ***CLN1, CLN14*** UCD ***GAMT*** Infantile Krabbe Canavan Alexanders Serine	***AADC***	Infantile Krabbe Canavan Gaucher NPA GM1 Serine	NKH ISOD/MoCD ETC CLN1 PBD CDG UCD TH NPC ***Canavan*** Alexanders Gaucher NPA ***AADC*** ***GM1*** MSD MLIV ***Pompe***	CLN1, CLN14 ISOD/MoCD Infantile Krabbe Tay-Sachs Canavan Gaucher NPA GM1 MSD MLIV Serine GM3 Menkes	UCD AADC	NKH CDG NPC CFD PBD GAMT

Late infancy 6–12 mo	***CTD*** CFD ***Alexanders*** Gaucher AADC GM1 MSD MLIV	TH CFD LNS ***Tay-Sachs*** Canavan ***Alexan-ders*** Gaucher AACD GM1 MSD MLIV	N/A	***Infantile Krabbe***	Tay-sachs Menkes TH	PDE/PNPO GLUT-1 NKH GABA/Gln PBD ISOD/MoCD Menkes Mito GM3 UCD ***GAMT*** Infantile Krabbe Tay-Sachs Canavan Alexanders Gaucher	***AADC***	Infantile Krabbe NKH Canavan Gaucher GM1	NKH ISOD/ MoCD ETC PBD CDG UCD TH LNS NPC ***Canavan*** Alexan-ders Gaucher ***AADC*** MSD MLIV ***Pompe***	ISOD/ MoCD Infantile Krabbe Canavan Gaucher Tay-Sachs GM1 MLIV Alexanders Menkes	UCD AADC	NKH CDG LNS NPC PBD GAMT
Toddlerhood 12 mo–3 yr	***CLN2*** ***AGAT*** ***GAMT*** ***CTD*** CFD MPS2 MPS1 Tay-Sachs Gaucher MSD Cobalamin	CFD MPS1 Tay-Sachs Gaucher MLD MSD Cobalamin GM1	***AGAT*** ***GAMT*** ***CTD*** CFD MPS2	***GAMT*** ***CTD*** ***LNS*** ***MPS2***	CLN2 MPS1 MPS Tay-Sachs Gaucher MLD Krabbe GM1	CLN2 Late onset Krabbe Tay-Sachs Gaucher	TH GAMT ***LNS*** ***Tay-Sachs*** ***Late-GM1***	Late onset Krabbe ***Tay-Sachs*** Gaucher MLD Cobalamin	CLN2 Late onset Krabbe Gaucher MLD MSD	CLN2 MPS2 MPS1 (slow) Late onset Krabbe Tay-Sachs Gaucher MLD GM1 MSD	TH	LNS Cobalamin AGAT GAMT CTD CFD
Preschool 3–5 yr	***CLN2*** ***AGAT*** ***CTD*** CFD MPS2 ***MPS3*** MPS1 ***Alpha-Manno-sidosis*** Fucosidosis Cobalamin	CFD MPS1 MLD Alpha-manno-sidosis AGU ***Fucosis-dosis*** Cobalamin	***AGAT*** ***GAMT*** ***CTD*** CFD MPS2 MPS3	CLN5 ***GAMT*** ***CTD*** ***LNS*** ***MPS2*** MPS3 ***MLD***	CLN2, CLN3 ***CLN5*** MLD MPS2 MPS3 MPS1 MLD Krabbe	CLN2, CLN3 ***(vision loss)*** Krabbe	TH CFD ***LNS*** Cobalamin	Krabbe Cobalamin	CLN5 Krabbe MLD AGU	CLN2, CLN3, CLN5 MPS2 MPS3 MPS1 (slow) Krabbe MLD AGU (not until 3rd decade) Alpha-man-nosidosis (slow) Fucosidosis (slow)	TH	LNS Cobalamin AGAT CRTFCFD

(Continued)

TABLE 36.9 Neurodevelopmental Profile for Inborn Errors of Metabolism by Presenting Feature and Most Common Age of Onset—cont'd

	DD/ID									Disease Course		
	Speech	**Motor**	**ASD**	**ADHD/ Behavior Issues**	**Regression/ Change in School Performance/Onset Psychiatric Symptoms/ Dementia**	**Seizures**	**Movement Disorder/ Ataxia**	**Spasticity**	**Hypotonia**	**Progressive**	**Episodic**	**Static**
Early childhood 5–8 yr	***MPS3*** Alexanders ***Alpha-mannosidosis*** AGU Hcy Cobalamin	MPS3 Krabbe ***Alexanders*** MLD Alpha-mannosidosis AGU Hcy Cobalamin	MPS3	CLN5 Late-onset UCD XALD MPS3 Krabbe ***MLD***	***CLN5*** CLN3, CLN8 Late-onset UCD ***XALD*** MLD Krabbe	CLN3, ***CLN8*** XALD Hcy	GLUT-1 PDH TH ***GTPCH-1*** ***Hcy*** Cobalamin	Cobalamin	Krabbe MLD AGU	CLN5 XALD MPS3 Krabbe MLD Alpha-mannosidosis Alexanders AGU (not until third decade)	Late-onset UCD GLUT-1 PDH TH GTPCH-1	Hcy Cobalamin
Middle childhood 8–11 yr	Alexanders ***Alpha-mannosidosis*** ***HcY***	MPS3 Krabbe ***Alexanders*** Alpha-mannosidosis Hcy	MPS3	Late-onset UCD XALD MPS3 Krabbe	***CLN12*** Late-onset UCD ***XALD*** ***NPC*** ML1 MPS3	XALD NPC Hcy	CLN12 GLUT-1 PDH TH ***NPC*** ***GTPCH-1*** ***ML1*** ***Hcy***			CLN12 XALD Krabbe Alexanders Alpha-mannosidosis (slow) MPS3 NPC Krabbe ML1	Late-onset UCD GLUT-1 PDH TH GTPCH-1	Hcy
Early adolescence 11–14 yr	Alexanders ***Alpha-mannosidosis*** Beta-mannosidosis	***Alexanders*** Alpha-mannosidosis		Late onset UCD ***Beta-mannosidosis*** ***Wilsons***	Late onset UCD NPC Wilsons ***CTX*** ***NPC*** ML1	NPC	GLUT-1 PDH TH ***NPC*** ***GTPCH-1*** ***ML1***	***Wilsons***		Alexanders Alpha-mannosidosis (slow) Beta-mannosidosis NPC ML1	Late onset UCD GLUT-1 PDH TH GTPCH-1	
Adolescence	Beta-mannosidosis			Tay-Sachs ***Beta-mannosidosis*** ***Wilsons*** ***Cobalamin***	***NPC*** ML1		Tay-Sachs ***ML1***	Tay-Sachs ***Wilsons***		NPC Tay-Sachs Beta-mannosidosis ML1 Cobalamin		

Adulthood	Beta-mannosidosis		Krabbe Tay-Sachs *Beta-mannosidosis* *Wilsons* *Cobalamin*	*CLN4, CLN11* *NPC* *MLD* ML1	*CLN4, CLN11*	Tay-Sachs *Alexanders* MLD *ML1*	Tay-Sachs *Alexanders* MLD *Wilsons*		CLN4, CLN11 NPC Krabbe Tay-Sachs Alexanders MLD ML1 Cobalamin Beta-mannosidosis

Note: Most common presentation italicized.

AADC, Aromatic L-amino acid decarboxylase deficiency; ***AGAT***, arginine:glycine amidinotransferase deficiency; ***ASU***, aspartylglucosaminuria; ***CDG***, congenital disorders of glycosylation; ***CFD***, cerebral folate deficiency; ***CLN***, neuronal ceroid lipofuscinosis 10; ***CTX***, cerebrotendinous xanthomatosis; ***ETC***, electron transport chain deficiencies; ***GABA/Gln***, disorders of GABA and glutamine metabolism; ***GAMT***, guanidinoacetate methyltransfer-ase deficiency; ***GLUT1w***, glucose transporter type 1 deficiency; ***GM1***, GM1 gangliosidosis; ***GM3***, GM3 synthase deficiency; ***Hcy***, homocystinuria; ***GTPCH-1***, GTP cyclohydrolase 1 deficiency; ***ISOD***, isolated sulfite oxidase deficiency; ***LNS***, Lesch-Nyhan syndrome; ***MLI***, mucolipidosis type I; ***MLIV***, mucolipidosis type IV; ***mito***, mitochondrial disease; ***MLD***, metachromatic leukodystrophy; ***MoCD***, molybdenum cofactor deficiency; ***MPS***, mucopolysacharridosis; ***MSD***, multiple sulfatase deficiency; ***NKH***, nonketotic hyperglycinemia; ***NPA***, Niemann-Pick A; ***NPC***, Niemann-Pick C; ***PBD***, peroxisome biogenesis disorders; ***PDE***, pyridoxine dependent epilepsy; ***PDH***, pyruvate dehydrogenase deficiency; ***PNPO***, pyridoxamine-phosphate oxidase deficiency; ***Ser***, serine deficiency; ***TH***, tyrosine hydroxylase deficiency; ***UCD***, urea cycle disorder; ***XALD***, X-linked adrenoleukodystrophy.

Substrate reduction therapy aims to reduce the amount of accumulated toxic metabolite to lessen disease burden. Miglustat (Zavesca), for example, inhibits the first step of the ganglioside biosynthetic pathway and in doing so lessens the downstream accumulation of glucocerebroside seen in individuals with Gaucher disease.

Other examples of small molecule therapies include read-through agents, which target genetic variants resulting in the generation of a premature stop codon. There are also small molecule proteostasis regulators and autophagy inducers. In addition to newly developed molecules, many researchers use broad libraries of existing US Food and Drug Administration–approved molecules to test cell- and animal-based disease models for potentially as-yet-undiscovered benefits. This method allows existing small molecule drugs to be quickly repurposed for rare diseases. Given their size, when combined with the correct chemical properties, some small molecule therapies may possess the unique capability of crossing the blood-brain barrier, making their future role in the treatment of central nervous system–related diseases promising.

CONCLUSION

Our understanding of the full phenotypic spectrum of IEMs is evolving as increasing numbers of patients are diagnosed via broad genetic testing. The initial symptoms of many IEMs may be behavioral or developmental concerns. An astute diagnostic evaluation at the time of the assessment for developmental manifestations may identify a disease that is amenable to disease-modifying therapies. The number of approved disease-modifying therapies for IEMs has increased dramatically in recent years.

In other cases improved treatment has significantly lengthened life expectancy for patients with many IEMs that were previously fatal early in life. Many of those patients surviving later into childhood and adolescence have developmental and behavioral manifestations of disease that require ongoing attention and management. Though not comprehensive, Table 36.9 offers a summary of the neurodevelopmental profiles of many IEMs.

REFERENCES

Andrade, F., Aldámiz-Echevarría, L., Llarena, M., & Couce, M. L. (2015). Sanfilippo syndrome: Overall review. *Pediatrics International*, *57*(3), 331–338.

Atwal, P. S., & Scaglia, F. (2016). Molybdenum cofactor deficiency. *Molecular Genetics and Metabolism*, *117*(1), 1–4.

Barca, E., Long, Y., Cooley, V., Schoenaker, R., Emmanuele, V., DiMauro, S., ... Hirano, M. (2020). Mitochondrial diseases in North America: An analysis of the NAMDC registry. *Neurology Genetics*, *6*(2).

Braverman, N. E., Raymond, G. V., Rizzo, W. B., Moser, A. B., Wilkinson, M. E., Stone, E. M., ... Bose, M. (2016). Peroxisome biogenesis disorders in the Zellweger spectrum: An overview of current diagnosis, clinical manifestations, and treatment guidelines. *Molecular Genetics and Metabolism*, *117*(3), 313–321.

Chang, I. J., He, M., & Lam, C. T. (2018). Congenital disorders of glycosylation. *Annals of Translational Medicine*, *6*(24).

Claerhout, H., Witters, P., Régal, L., Jansen, K., Van Hoestenberghe, M. R., Breckpot, J., & Vermeersch, P. (2018). Isolated sulfite oxidase deficiency. *Journal of Inherited Metabolic Disease: Official Journal of the Society for the Study of Inborn Errors of Metabolism*, *41*(1), 101–108.

Clark, J. F., & Cecil, K. M. (2015). Diagnostic methods and recommendations for the cerebral creatine deficiency syndromes. *Pediatric Research*, *77*(3), 398–405.

Demirbas, D., Brucker, W. J., & Berry, G. T. (2018). Inborn errors of metabolism with hepatopathy: Metabolism defects of galactose, fructose, and tyrosine. *Pediatric Clinics of North America*, *65*(2), 337–352.

Erez, A., Nagamani, S. C. S., & Lee, B. (2011). Argininosuccinate lyase deficiency—Argininosuccinic aciduria and beyond. *American Journal of Medical Genetics Part C: Seminars in Medical Genetics*, *157*(1), 45–53.

Geberhiwot, T., Moro, A., Dardis, A., Ramaswami, U., Sirrs, S., Marfa, M. P., ... Patterson, M. (2018). Consensus clinical management guidelines for Niemann-Pick disease type C. *Orphanet Journal of Rare Diseases*, *13*(1), 1–19.

Gorman, G. S., Chinnery, P. F., DiMauro, S., Hirano, M., Koga, Y., McFarland, R., ... Turnbull, D. M. (2016). Mitochondrial diseases. *Nature Reviews Disease Primers*, *2*(1), 1–22.

Häberle, J., Burlina, A., Chakrapani, A., Dixon, M., Karall, D., Lindner, M., ... Dionisi-Vici, C. (2019). Suggested guidelines for the diagnosis and management of urea cycle disorders: First revision. *Journal of Inherited Metabolic Disease*, *42*(6), 1192–1230.

Jinnah, H. A. (2020). HPRT1 disorders. In M. P. Adam, H. H. Ardinger, R. A. Pagon, et al. (Eds.), *GeneReviews*. University of Washington–Seattle. https://www.ncbi.nlm.nih.gov/books/NBK1149/

Jinnah, H. A., De Gregorio, L., Harris, J. C., Nyhan, W. L., & O'Neill, J. P. (2000). The spectrum of inherited mutations causing HPRT deficiency: 75 new cases and a review of 196 previously reported cases. *Mutation Research/Reviews in Mutation Research*, *463*(3), 309–326.

Kanungo, S., Soares, N., He, M., & Steiner, R. D. (2013). Sterol metabolism disorders and neurodevelopment—An update. *Developmental Disabilities Research Reviews*, *17*(3), 197–210.

Lichter-Konecki, U., Caldovic, L., Morizono, H., et al. (2016). Ornithine transcarbamylase deficiency. In: M. P. Adam, H. H. Ardinger, R. A. Pagon, et al. (Eds.), *GeneReviews*. University of Washington–Seattle. https://www.ncbi.nlm.nih.gov/books/NBK154378/

Martinelli, D., Diodato, D., Ponzi, E., Monné, M., Boenzi, S., Bertini, E., ... Dionisi-Vici, C. (2015). The hyperornithinemia-hyperammonemia-homocitrullinuria syndrome. *Orphanet Journal of Rare Diseases*, *10*(1), 1–17.

Mastrangelo, M. (2020). Epilepsy in inherited neurotransmitter disorders: Spotlights on pathophysiology and clinical management. *Metabolic Brain Disease*, 1–15.

Matsumoto, S., Häberle, J., Kido, J., Mitsubuchi, H., Endo, F., & Nakamura, K. (2019). Urea cycle disorders—Update. *Journal of Human Genetics*, *64*(9), 833–847.

Mohamed, S., He, Q. Q., Singh, A. A., & Ferro, V. (2019). Mucopolysaccharidosis type II (Hunter syndrome): Clinical and biochemical aspects of the disease and approaches to its diagnosis and treatment. *Advances in Carbohydrate Chemistry and Biochemistry*, *77*, 71–117.

Mole, S. E., Anderson, G., Band, H. A., Berkovic, S. F., Cooper, J. D., Holthaus, S. M. K., ... Smith, A. J. (2019). Clinical challenges and future therapeutic approaches for neuronal ceroid lipofuscinosis. *The Lancet Neurology*, *18*(1), 107–116.

Morris, A. A., Kožich, V., Santra, S., Andria, G., Ben-Omran, T. I., Chakrapani, A. B., ... Chapman, K. A. (2017). Guidelines for the diagnosis and management of cystathionine beta-synthase deficiency. *Journal of Inherited Metabolic Disease*, *40*(1), 49–74.

Nie, S., Chen, G., Cao, X., & Zhang, Y. (2014). Cerebrotendinous xanthomatosis: A comprehensive review of pathogenesis, clinical manifestations, diagnosis, and management. *Orphanet Journal of Rare Diseases*, *9*(1), 1–11.

Nowaczyk, M. J., & Irons, M. B. (2012). Smith–Lemli–Opitz syndrome: Phenotype, natural history, and epidemiology. *American Journal of Medical Genetics Part C: Seminars in Medical Genetics*, *160*(4), 250–262.

Parikh, S., Goldstein, A., Koenig, M. K., Scaglia, F., Enns, G. M., Saneto, R., ... DiMauro, S. (2015). Diagnosis and management of mitochondrial disease: A consensus statement from the Mitochondrial Medicine Society. *Genetics in Medicine*, *17*(9), 689–701.

Patel, K. P., O'Brien, T. W., Subramony, S. H., Shuster, J., & Stacpoole, P. W. (2012). The spectrum of pyruvate dehydrogenase complex deficiency: Clinical, biochemical and genetic features in 371 patients. *Molecular Genetics and Metabolism*, *105*(1), 34–43. https://doi.org/10.1016/j.ymgme.2011.09.032

Platt, F. M., d'Azzo, A., Davidson, B. L., Neufeld, E. F., & Tifft, C. J. (2018). Lysosomal storage diseases. *Nature Reviews Disease Primers*, *4*(1), 1–25.

Porter, F. D. (2008). Smith-Lemli-Opitz syndrome: Pathogenesis, diagnosis and management. *European Journal of Medical Genetics*, *16*, 535–541.

Rahman, S. (2020). Mitochondrial disease in children. *Journal of Internal Medicine*, *287*(6), 609–633.

Regier, D. S., & Greene, C. L. (2017). Phenylalanine hydroxylase deficiency. In M. P. Adam, H. H. Ardinger, R. A. Pagon, et al. (Eds.), *GeneReviews*. University of Washington–Seattle. https://www.ncbi.nlm.nih.gov/books/NBK1504/

Schiff, M., Roda, C., Monin, M. L., Arion, A., Barth, M., Bednarek, N., ... De Lonlay, P. (2017). Clinical, laboratory and molecular findings and long-term follow-up data in 96 French patients with PMM2-CDG (phosphomannomutase 2-congenital disorder of glycosylation) and review of the literature. *Journal of Medical Genetics*, *54*(12), 843–851.

Schillaci, L. A. P., DeBrosse, S. D., & McCandless, S. E. (2018). Inborn errors of metabolism with acidosis: Organic acidemias and defects of pyruvate and ketone body metabolism. *Pediatric Clinics*, *65*(2), 209–230.

Sun, A., Crombez, E. A., & Wong, D. (2020). Arginase deficiency. In M. P. Adam, H. H. Ardinger, R. A. Pagon, et al. (Eds.), *GeneReviews*. University of Washington–Seattle. https://www.ncbi.nlm.nih.gov/books/NBK1159/

Turk, B. R., Theda, C., Fatemi, A., & Moser, A. B. (2020). X-linked adrenoleukodystrophy: Pathology, pathophysiology, diagnostic testing, newborn screening and therapies. *International Journal of Developmental Neuroscience*, *80*(1), 52–72.

Van Hove, J. L. K., Coughlin II, C., Swanson, M., et al. (2019). Nonketotic hyperglycinemia. In M. P. Adam, H. H. Ardinger, R. A. Pagon, et al. (Eds.), *GeneReviews*. University of Washington–Seattle. https://www.ncbi.nlm.nih.gov/books/NBK1357/

Wang, D., Pascual, J. M., & De Vivo, D. (2018). Glucose transporter type 1 deficiency syndrome. In M. P. Adam, H. H. Ardinger, R. A. Pagon, et al. (Eds.), *GeneReviews*. University of Washington–Seattle. https://www.ncbi.nlm.nih.gov/books/NBK1430/

Waterham, H. R., Ferdinandusse, S., & Wanders, R. J. (2016). Human disorders of peroxisome metabolism and biogenesis. *Biochimica Et Biophysica Acta (BBA)-Molecular Cell Research*, *1863*(5), 922–933.

Wilson, M. P., Plecko, B., Mills, P. B., & Clayton, P. T. (2019). Disorders affecting vitamin B6 metabolism. *Journal of Inherited Metabolic Disease*, *42*(4), 629–646.

Wong, J. C., Walsh, K., Hayden, D., & Eichler, F. S. (2018). Natural history of neurological abnormalities in cerebrotendinous xanthomatosis. *Journal of Inherited Metabolic Disease*, *41*(4), 647–656.

37

Prenatal Exposure of Alcohol, Tobacco, and Drugs

Carol Weitzman and Michele Ledesma

For additional material related to the content of this chapter, please see Chapters 38 and 53.

VIGNETTE

Connor is a loving, engaging 3-year-old boy, who has always been short. He presents to your office because his adoptive parents have concerns about hyperactivity and impulsivity. Connor tested positive for cocaine at birth and was placed with his adoptive parents shortly after. His birth mother also had a history of prenatal alcohol and drug use, although the timing and extent of use is unknown. Connor was a fussy, irritable baby with mild developmental delays. When he started preschool this year, his teachers reported that he is lagging behind peers and has intermittent trouble adjusting to the classroom. He is easily frustrated and frequently bolts from the classroom when he is upset. While he is friendly and social, he also misreads the cues of his peers and can be inappropriate or physically aggressive toward them. At home, his parents note that while he is affectionate, he becomes easily upset and has intense tantrums multiple times each week. He is highly impulsive and often darts across parking lots or engages in risky behaviors such as jumping from high heights. His parents fear for his safety.

INTRODUCTION

In the chapter-opening vignette much of Connor's birth history remains unknown. However, careful consideration of multiple potential influences, including prenatal exposures that may have contributed to his presentation, can help you to understand his complexity and to develop a multipronged approach to his care. This chapter reviews the effects of prenatal exposure to toxins, including alcohol, tobacco, and prescription, recreational, and illicit drugs, with an emphasis on developmental and behavioral outcomes. In general, susceptibility to prenatal exposures depends on the developmental stage at which the exposure occurs, the mechanism of action and target tissue of the drug, the dose of the drug, and the genotype of the conceptus. Discussion of environmental toxins is described in Chapter 38.

ALCOHOL

Syndromes Associated With Prenatal Alcohol Exposure

Fetal alcohol syndrome was first described in 1973 as a group of specific birth defects resulting from prenatal alcohol exposure (PAE). Since that time, PAE has been recognized as the most common preventable cause of intellectual and developmental disabilities in the United States. The disorders caused by PAE are grouped under the umbrella term *fetal alcohol spectrum disorders (FASDs)*, which in most classification systems does not designate a diagnostic term but a group of specific conditions with mild to severe phenotypes (Hagan et al., 2016; Hoyme et al., 2016). Other countries, including Canada and Australia, have adopted FASD as a diagnostic term. As listed in Table 37.1, in the United States the FASDs include:

- Fetal alcohol syndrome (FAS)
- Partial FAS (pFAS)
- Alcohol-related neurodevelopmental disorder (ARND)
- Neurobehavioral disorder associated with prenatal alcohol exposure (ND-PAE), also called neurodevelopmental disorder associated with PAE
- Alcohol-related birth defects (ARBD)

These diagnoses are differentiated based on the presence of absence of (1) documentation of PAE; (2) facial dysmorphology; (3) neurobehavioral impairment; (4) pre- and/or postnatal growth deficiency (5) evidence of deficient brain growth, abnormal morphogenesis, or abnormal neurophysiology; and (6) major malformations (see Table 37.1). This terminology continues to evolve; some diagnoses, such as ARND and ND-PAE, are similar but not fully overlapping. Although FAS may be the most recognizable of the FASDs due to the presence of facial dysmorphology, fewer than 20% of children with an FASD have FAS. Although many congenital anomalies and minor malformations may be seen in children with an FASD, the three sentinel features include short palpebral fissures, thin vermillion border, and a smooth philtrum. These features may become less recognizable after the onset of puberty.

Epidemiology of Prenatal Alcohol Use

Surveys completed between 2011 and 2013 have shown that approximately 1 in 10 pregnant women reported alcohol consumption in the past 30 days; 1 in 33 pregnant women

TABLE 37.1 Diagnoses Included Within the Fetal Alcohol Spectrum Disorders (FASDs)

FASD	Diagnostic Criteria
Fetal alcohol syndrome	• At least two sentinel facial features must be present • Growth deficiency • Structural, neurologic, or functional central nervous system (CNS) abnormalities • Neurobehavioral impairment characterized by cognitive impairment and/or behavioral impairment, and for younger children evidence of developmental delay • This diagnosis can be made in the absence of documented prenatal alcohol exposure
Partial fetal alcohol syndrome	**With documented prenatal alcohol exposure:** • At least two sentinel facial features • Neurobehavioral impairment characterized by cognitive impairment and/or behavioral impairment, and for younger children evidence of developmental delay
	Without documented prenatal alcohol exposure: • At least two sentinel facial features • Growth deficiency **or** structural, neurologic, or functional CNS abnormalities • Neurobehavioral impairment characterized by cognitive impairment and/or behavioral impairment, and for younger children evidence of developmental delay
Alcohol-related neurodevelopmental disorder	• Documented prenatal alcohol exposure • Neurobehavioral impairment characterized by cognitive impairment and/or behavioral impairment, and for younger children evidence of developmental delay • Cannot be definitively diagnosed in children <3 yr of age
Alcohol-related birth defects	• Documented prenatal alcohol exposure • At least one specific major malformation associated with prenatal alcohol exposure*

Neurobehavioral disorder associated with prenatal alcohol exposure	• Documented prenatal alcohol exposure
	• Neurobehavioral impairment characterized by impairment in the domains of:
	  • Neurocognitive deficits
	  • Impairment in self-regulation
	  • Impairment in adaptive functioning
	• Evidence of sentinel facial features, CNS or growth abnormalities is not required
	• Problems must cause functional impairment, be diagnosed in childhood, and are not better accounted for by other causes

*Includes specific cardiac, skeletal, renal, ocular malformations and hearing loss.

reporting binge drinking, defined as four or more drinks at one occasion (Green et al., 2016). In a metaanalysis of 24 studies with active case ascertainment the estimated global prevalence of FASD in the population of children age 0 to 16 years was 0.77% (95% confidence interval [CI] 0.5%–1.2%). Reports of alcohol consumption and binge drinking vary across regions of the world, likely due to differences in reporting, culture, and stigma (Lange et al., 2017). In a US study conservative prevalence estimates of FASDs were between 1% and 1.5% of all children (May et al., 2018).

Mechanisms of Prenatal Alcohol Effects

Alcohol's toxic effects are likely due to several mechanisms, including interference with neuronal migration, impaired development and function of neurotransmitter receptors, and neuronal necrosis (apoptosis). Brain abnormalities associated with PAE include reduced brain volume. Many areas of the brain potentially may be affected, including the frontal lobe, striatum and caudate nucleus, thalamus, hippocampus, and cerebellum; thinning of the corpus callosum is also seen. Alcohol can cause harmful effects to the developing fetus at all stages of gestation; exposure in the first trimester is most likely to be associated with facial anomalies and major structural abnormalities. The effects of PAE on the developing fetus are affected by many variables, including drinking patterns, maternal age and nutrition, other maternal substance use (including nicotine), and maternal and fetal genetics. Because of this variability, there is no known safe amount of alcohol consumption during pregnancy or when trying to become pregnant. The American Academy of Pediatrics (AAP), the American College of Obstetricians and Gynecologists (ACOG), and the Centers for Disease Control and Prevention (CDC) all advocate for complete abstention from alcohol consumption during pregnancy. In 2016 the National Institute of Alcohol Abuse and Alcoholism defined documented alcohol exposure as one of the following: six or more drinks per week for 2 or more weeks, three or more drinks per occasion on two or more occasions, documentation of alcohol use by a screening instrument during pregnancy, alcohol-related social or legal problems, or positive blood, breath, or urine alcohol testing (Hoyme et al., 2016). In adopted children, such as Connor in the vignette, the precise history of PAE is often unknown, although additional informative records can occasionally be obtained. It is common to obtain histories of polydrug abuse.

Heterogeneity in the presentation of FASD in children is due to the variability of PAE during pregnancy and the frequent cooccurrence of other risk factors, including other

TABLE 37.2 Prevalence of Developmental and Behavioral Problems Seen in Children With Fetal Alcohol Spectrum Disorders (FASDs)

Problem	Approximate % Affected	Increased Likelihood Compared With Non-FASD Children
Attention-deficit/hyperactivity disorder and executive functioning deficits	50	10
Intellectual disability	23	23
Learning disabilities (most commonly nonverbal skills and memory deficits)	20	2
Oppositional defiant disorder	16.3	4.9
Anxiety and depression	14.1	4-11.2
Psychotic disorders	12.3	24.5
Bipolar disorder	8.6	3.2
Posttraumatic stress disorder	6	1.5
Reactive attachment disorder	4.7	9.3

Adapted from Weyrauch, D., Schwartz, M., Hart, B., Klug, M. G., & Burd, L. (2017). Comorbid mental disorders in fetal alcohol spectrum disorders: A systematic review. *Journal of Developmental and Behavioral Pediatrics, 38*(4), 283–291. https://doi.org/10.1097/DBP.0000000000000440

ubstance abuse, maternal mental health issues, poverty, and other adverse psychosocial stressors. Children with FASDs often have a complex presentation (Table 37.2) (Weyrauch et al., 2017). Children with FASDs often have difficulties in adaptive functioning and may exhibit indiscriminate sociability. Connor's issues (in the vignette) emerged during infancy, and his clinical evaluation may lead to diagnosis. Children who go undiagnosed and untreated are at the highest risk for the poor outcomes, which include disrupted school experiences, accident and injury, problems with alcohol or drug abuse, and encounters with law enforcement, unemployment, homelessness, and premature death. Protective factors include diagnosis before age 6 years and a stable and consistent home environment (Streissguth et al., 2004).

NICOTINE

Prenatal exposure to nicotine can occur in several ways, including active maternal smoking, exposure of a pregnant woman to environmental tobacco smoke, and maternal use of nontobacco products such as nicotine replacement therapy or electronic nicotine delivery systems. Both nicotine and its major metabolite, cotinine, cross the placental barrier; cotinine measurements in amniotic fluid are higher than in maternal serum, indicating accumulation. Prenatal nicotine exposure has been associated with altered brain structure and function. The proposed mechanism is interference with signaling among progenitor cells during brain development. Recent studies have also suggested that epigenetic effects, carried through generations, may also play a part (Polli & Kohlmeier, 2020). Developmental and behavioral outcomes associated with prenatal nicotine exposure include attention-deficit/hyperactivity disorder, conduct problems, depression and anxiety, and neurosensorial hearing loss. It is important to note that many pre- and postnatal psychosocial factors often complicate these relations (Polli & Kohlmeier, 2020).

PRESCRIPTION MEDICATIONS AFFECTING DEVELOPMENT AND BEHAVIOR

Antiepileptic Drugs

Approximately 3 to 5 of every 1000 pregnancies are to women with epilepsy, and the majority of women on antiepileptic medications (AEDs) give birth to healthy, typically developing infants. However, some AEDs have been associated with fetal malformation and other abnormalities. The risk-benefit ratio must be carefully considered when prescribing these medications; poorly controlled seizures and use of selected antiepileptic drugs are both potential risks to the fetus (Nadebaum et al., 2012). Data from neuroimaging studies have found that brains of adults exposed to AEDs in utero show reduced gray matter volumes in the basal ganglia and hypothalamus (Ikonomidou et al., 2007); these findings are consistent with reports of attentional impairment that has been associated with prenatal AED exposure. Data from population-based studies have shown that exposure to AEDs in utero has also been associated with impaired fine motor skills at 6 months, impaired gross motor skills and autistic traits at 18 months, and poor gross motor skills, speech-language skills, and autistic traits at 36 months (Veiby et al., 2013). The risk of autistic traits may be mitigated by periconception folic acid supplementation (Bjork et al., 2018). Polytherapy carries a greater risk of impaired cognitive and behavioral outcomes than monotherapy, particularly when valproic acid is part of the regimen (Nadebaum et al., 2012). For monotherapy, risk estimates for lamotrigine, valproate, and carbamazepine were similar (Veiby et al., 2013).

Valproic Acid

Valproic acid is associated with developmental delays, particularly speech-language delays, and reductions in full-scale IQ with verbal skills more affected than nonverbal skills. Deficits in working memory and attention and an increased rate of autism spectrum disorders have been associated with prenatal valproate exposure (Nadebaum et al., 2012). Rarely, fetal valproate syndrome is seen, which includes neural tube and congenital heart defects, musculoskeletal abnormalities, distinctive facial features, and developmental delays (National Organization of Rare Disorder, n.d.).

Other Medications

Studies on the impact of prenatal carbamazepine exposure have been inconsistent with regard to early cognitive and motor development, IQ, educational achievement, and adaptive behavior (Nadebaum et al., 2012). Similarly, results from studies on prenatal phenytoin exposure have been inconsistent; some studies report improved cognitive outcomes, and other studies report delayed motor development and low IQs. Likewise, there is no consensus on the neurobehavioral effects of prenatal phenobarbital exposure. There are limited data for the newest medications, including ethosuximide, primidone, clonazepam, gabapentin, topiramate, vigabatrin, tiagabine, clobazam, oxcarbazepine, and levetiracetam.

Antineoplastic Agents

Approximately 1 to 2 in 2000 pregnancies are complicated by cancer, and maternal treatment may consist of chemotherapy, radiotherapy, and/or surgery; targeted therapy, which uses drugs that alter specific genes and proteins involved in the growth and survival of cancer cells, is generally avoided due to high fetal risks. Any adverse effects from medication add to the impact of the traumatic experience of a cancer diagnosis and associated maternal symptoms of anxiety and depression that have also been linked to externalizing behaviors in children (Betchen et al., 2020). Maternal malnutrition may also have consequences for fetal development (Vercruysse et al., 2016).

Radiotherapy

Ionizing radiation causes direct damage to DNA and other cell components. The developing brain is most sensitive to radiation at 8 to 25 weeks after conception, and even a low dose of ionizing radiation can interfere with neuronal migration and structural brain development. This cascade can result in a significant decrease in IQ, as has been seen in children who had been *in utero* during nuclear explosions. Exposure to radiation also increases the relative risk of childhood cancer and leukemia (Vercruysse et al., 2016).

Chemotherapy

Agents that cross both the placenta and the fetal blood-brain barrier can be neurotoxic. Chemotherapeutic drugs are aimed at the inhibition of cell division and can thus interfere with the process of neurogenesis as well as the development of the blood supply to the brain. Other mechanisms include direct neurotoxicity, oxidative stress, and modulation of the immune system. Overall, however, no major consequences on neurocognitive development have been found, though long-term follow-up is lacking (Vercruysse et al., 2016).

Anticoagulants

Anticoagulants have been postulated to have potential effects related to intracranial hemorrhage and resulting developmental sequelae. Guidelines recommend low-molecular-weight heparins and unfractionated heparins as the preferred anticoagulants in pregnancy as they do not cross the placenta. Coumarin, prescribed for women with prosthetic heart valves, carries an increased risk of minor neurologic dysfunction and low IQ (Wesseling et al., 2001).

Psychotropic Medication

Psychotropic drugs often cross the placenta and reach the fetal central nervous system. These features raise concerns regarding their potential impacts on fetal brain development, neonatal adaptation, and neurodevelopmental outcomes. Perinatal mental health treatment is important, as untreated or undertreated maternal psychiatric illness also can impart significant burdens on the mother, child, and family.

Selective Serotonin Reuptake Inhibitors

Selective serotonin reuptake inhibitors (SSRIs) appear to affect the hypothalamic-pituitary-adrenal axis in both animals and humans, and they potentially induce epigenetic changes. Neonatal adaptation syndrome (NAS) refers to signs exhibited by the newborn exposed to SSRIs *in utero*, such as low Apgar scores. There is no consensus definition for NAS. NAS has been hypothesized to be secondary to either effects or withdrawal and/or increased serotonergic tone. NAS appears to occur more commonly in infants exposed to paroxetine, venlafaxine, and fluoxetine than in infants exposed to other SSRIs (Betcher & Wisner, 2020). Other possible negative effects associated with SSRIs have been proposed, including lower psychomotor development scores and an increased risk of autism spectrum disorder (Boukhris et al., 2016), though studies have shown variable outcomes. Untreated maternal depression itself may negatively affect a child's development (Ornoy et al., 2017).

Antipsychotics

Antipsychotic medications block D_2 dopamine receptors, thereby reducing the effects of dopamine primarily in the mesolimbic system and prefrontal cortex. Data pertaining to the use of first-generation antipsychotics in pregnancy indicate that they are generally safe and have not been associated with an increase in the rate of major anomalies or neurodevelopmental problems. Data for newer antipsychotic medications are limited, but a few studies have suggested poor neonatal adaptation and withdrawal symptoms (Ornoy et al., 2017).

Tricyclic and Tetracyclic Antidepressants

Tricyclic antidepressants, such as clomipramine, nortriptyline, and imipramine, and tetracyclic antidepressants, such as mirtazapine, were widely used before the introduction of

SSRIs. They affect the serotonergic and noradrenergic systems by blocking transporters and increasing synaptic concentrations of neurotransmitters. Most studies have not shown an association with major structural anomalies or neurodevelopmental problems (Ornoy et al., 2017).

Mood Stabilizers

Lithium is used as a mood stabilizer. Lithium ions equilibrate across the placenta, which can lead to perinatal toxicity, including hypotonicity, heart failure, and nephrogenic diabetes insipidus. Prenatal exposure to lithium has been associated with major cardiac anomalies, specifically Ebstein anomaly, but long-term studies on neurodevelopmental outcomes are lacking (Ornoy et al., 2017). Antiepileptic medications are also used as mood stabilizers, and their effects are discussed earlier in this section.

Retinoids

Retinoids have long been recognized for their teratogenic potential, with the earliest research focusing on gross central nervous system malformations associated with maternal hypervitaminosis A such as neural tube defects and a "crowded brain" defect. More recent research, however, has focused on the effects on brain development; animal studies show that motor deficits result from altered cerebellar development and effects on corticocerebellar circuitry (Adams, 2010).

ILLICIT AND RECREATIONAL DRUGS

Recent survey data from the Substance Abuse and Mental Health Services Administration estimates that approximately 5.4% of pregnant women aged 14 to 44 years report illicit and recreational drug use. While rates of illicit drug use are declining, significant increases in marijuana use were observed (McCance-Katz, 2019). The use of multiple agents, including alcohol and nicotine, is common. Subsequent postnatal caregiver-child interactions often complicate the attribution of specific effects to a single substance. Both medical (physical and mental health of both the mother and the child) and psychosocial factors, such as poverty, malnutrition, and other stressors, also impact outcomes; as such, outcomes are rarely isolated neurodevelopmental insults. Results of studies must further be interpreted with caution as they often rely on interviewer or questionnaire recall of exposure, which may be inaccurate.

Cocaine

Cocaine causes peripheral vasoconstriction, which decreases blood flow to the placenta and consequently affects intrauterine growth; growth suppression may persist beyond infancy (Richardson et al., 2013). Prenatal cocaine exposure has also been associated with premature birth, though studies have failed to support the association between serious congenital malformations and medical complications (Bada et al., 2007).

Cocaine readily crosses the placenta. In the fetal brain it increases dopamine activity (Lambert & Bauer, 2012) and affects neuronal maturation. Fetal frontal lobes are particularly vulnerable, potentially disrupting the development of the infant's behavioral regulatory system (Lambert & Bauer, 2012). Neuroimaging evidence has shown differences in activation of the arousal regulation system, with stronger functional connectivity in the default mode network (DMN) at resting state, but less deactivation during a working memory task with emotional distracters (Li et al., 2011). Chronic prenatal cocaine exposure is also a potential intrauterine stressor, potentially disrupting the development of the infant's stress response physiology (Lambert & Bauer, 2012). Studies have demonstrated poor cognitive and speech-language skills (Lambert & Bauer, 2012) and increased learning disabilities, internalizing and externalizing behavior problems (Bada et al., 2007), and attention problems, even when controlling for confounders, including other drug use. In the case of Connor at the beginning of this chapter his challenges potentially can be related, in part, to prenatal cocaine exposure. However, studies also show significant interactions with caregiver psychological mental functioning (Bada et al., 2007) and document adverse sociodemographic characteristics in children exposed to cocaine (Lambert & Bauer, 2012).

Opioids

Opioids produce altered levels of neurotransmitters, particularly norepinephrine, dopamine, and serotonin. Neuroimaging studies have demonstrated altered neurogenesis in the somatosensory cortex (Nygaard et al., 2016). Morphologic effects include intrauterine growth restriction and small fetal head circumferences, prematurity, neural tube defects, and congenital heart defects (Larson et al., 2019; Patrick et al., 2015). Studies of neurobehavioral outcomes related to prenatal opioid exposure suggest delays in cognitive, motor and speech-language development, lower IQ scores and academic achievement, and increased attention and behaviors problems (Larson et al., 2019; Yeoh et al., 2019). However, it is difficult to attribute long-term effects solely to opioids due to the presence of multiple confounders, including other drug use, socioeconomic status, and epigenetic modifications. The use of tobacco (Patrick et al., 2015) or prescription sedatives (Huybrechts et al., 2017) may increase the risk and/or severity of neonatal opioid withdrawal.

Neonatal Opioid Withdrawal Syndrome

Previously called neonatal abstinence syndrome, neonatal opioid withdrawal syndrome (NOWS) refers to drug withdrawal that is primarily from *in utero* opioid exposure. With the progression of the opioid crisis in the 21st century, opioid use and opioid dependence among pregnant women also increased, and increases in maternal opioid use were accompanied by a parallel increase in NOWS. As with adults, opioid receptors are concentrated in the central nervous system and gastrointestinal tracts. Infants withdrawing from opioid exposure present with a syndrome consisting of dysregulated neurobehaviors, including excessive crying, poor sleep, a hyperactive Moro reflex, tremors and myoclonus, increased muscle tone, excoriation, mottling, fever, nasal stuffiness or sweating, difficulty breathing, poor feeding, vomiting and diarrhea, failure to thrive, and excessive irritability. The presentation and onset of these symptoms varies by opioid type, half-life of the opioid involved, and maternal drug history and metabolism. Nonpharmacologic care is tailored to the clinical, behavioral, and physiologic signs that the infant exhibits. The AAP calls for comprehensive care addressing medical and psychosocial needs of both mother and infant.

Cannabis

Cannabis, or marijuana, is the most frequently used recreational drug in the United States; 4.7% of pregnant women reported using marijuana in 2018 (McCance-Katz, 2019). ACOG anticipates an increase in marijuana use in pregnancy with the increasing legalization of marijuana across the United States. The psychoactive component of marijuana is delta-9-tetrahydrocannabinol (THC). Increasingly potent forms of marijuana containing increased concentrations of THC are becoming available. Cannabidiol, or CBD, is posited to be nonpsychoactive. There is limited literature on effects on the fetus and long-term consequences related to prenatal CBD exposure. The following discussion will focus on effects of THC as contained in marijuana, rather than on isolated CBD products.

Marijuana is thought to exert its action through potential interference with the endocannabinoid system and the dopaminergic pathways, which are involved in regulating pain, nausea, and appetite, as well as affecting placenta implantation and maintenance. It crosses the placenta and is increased in breastmilk. Lower birthweights have been associated with prenatal marijuana exposure; reported decrements are minimal, on the order of 100 g (Metz & Stickrath, 2015). Prenatal marijuana exposure has been associated with several findings: deficits in executive function (problem solving, sustained attention, short-term memory); poor academic achievement (Metz & Stickrath, 2015); increased hyperactivity, impulsivity, and inattention; increased delinquency, mediated by inattention (Goldschmidt et al., 2000); and higher levels of self-reported depressive symptoms (Gray et al., 2005).

Amphetamines

Methamphetamine exerts its neurotoxic effect on dopamine- and norepinephrine-containing cells and has been shown to affect areas of the brain associated with attention and behavior. Imaging studies from children exposed to methamphetamine *in utero* have shown neurochemical abnormalities in the frontal white matter and smaller subcortical volumes in the putamen, globus pallidus, and hippocampus (Kiblawi et al., 2013). Prenatal methamphetamine exposure has been linked to deficits in executive function, visual spatial performance, and math and language skills. In the Infant Development, Environment, and Lifestyle (IDEAL) study prenatal methamphetamine exposure was associated with subtle differences in continuous performance test measures relating to sustained attention and impulsivity at age 5 years (Kiblawi et al., 2013) and to increased externalizing, rule-breaking, and aggressive behaviors. The experience of early adversity, caregiver psychological problems, and quality of the home have been found to mediate the relationship between prenatal methamphetamine exposure and behavior problems (Chu et al., 2020; Eze et al., 2016).

Little is known about the effects of 3,4-methylenedioxy-methampentamine (MDMA or ecstasy) on the developing brain. A longitudinal study of 28 MDMA-exposed infants followed to 2 years of age showed motor impairment in the first 2 years of life; the amount of prenatal MDMA exposure was predictive of the motor deficits at 12 months of age. Animal studies have shown adverse effects on memory and learning following exposure to MDMA in the latter stages of pregnancy in rats (Broening et al., 2001).

SCREENING FOR EXPOSURE

It is important that clinicians evaluating a child for developmental, behavioral, academic, or mental health conditions obtain a thorough maternal history, including information on alcohol, tobacco, and drug use, both prescription and nonprescription, at multiple time points, including prepregnancy, before recognition of pregnancy, after recognition of pregnancy, and after the child's birth. ACOG recommends universal screening for substance use at the first prenatal visit, using validated tools (Table 37.3). The AAP suggests universal screening of all infants, children, and youth for PAE at initial pediatric visits and when developmental, behavioral, or emotional problems are detected (Turchi et al., 2018). As in the case of Connor, in the opening vignette, efforts to learn more about this child's exposures may help the clinician to develop a comprehensive evaluation and management plan. Knowing a child's prenatal exposures and associated neurodevelopmental

TABLE 37.3 Validated Tools for Screening Maternal History of Alcohol, Tobacco, and Drug Abuse

Tool	Description	Source
4 Ps: Parents, Partner, Past, and Present	Four questions with appropriate follow-up	https://www.ntiupstream.com/4psabout
NIDA drug screening tool	Four questions about the past 1 yr	https://archives.drugabuse.gov/nmassist/step/0
CRAFFT	Six basic questions, updated to include vaping	http://crafft.org/

NIDA, National Institute on Drug Abuse

outcomes allows clinicians to evaluate potential areas of challenge and implement evidence-based interventions early to address presenting signs and symptoms. Discussion of these issues with biological parents, especially mothers, may be likely difficult if the topic arouses grief, guilt, and defensiveness. In either case emphasis on the potential positive impacts of a warm and nurturing social environment with appropriate cognitive and academic stimulation may inspire parents to look forward to maximize their child's outcomes.

REFERENCES

Adams, J. (2010). The neurobehavioral teratology of retinoids: A 50-year history. *Birth Defects Research Part A Clinical and Molecular Teratology*, *88*(10), 895–905. https://doi.org/10.1002/bdra.20721.

American College of Obstetrics and Gynecology. (n.d.). Screening for opioid use and opioid use disorder in pregnancy. https://www.acog.org/Clinical-Guidance-and-Publications/Committee-Opinions/Committee-on-Obstetric-Practice/Opioid-Use-and-Opioid-Use-Disorder-in-Pregnancy.

Bada, H. S., Das, A., Bauer, C. R., Shankaran, S., Lester, B., LaGasse, L., … Higgins, R. (2007). Impact of prenatal cocaine exposure on child behavior problems through school age. *Pediatrics*, *119*(2), e348–e359. https://doi.org/10.1542/peds.2006-1404.

Betchen, M., Grunberg, V. A., Gringlas, M., & Cardonick, E. (2020). Being a mother after a cancer diagnosis during pregnancy: Maternal psychosocial functioning and child cognitive development and behavior. *Psychooncology*, *29*(7), 1148–1155. https://doi.org/10.1002/pon.5390.

Betcher, H. K., & Wisner, K. L. (2020). Psychotropic treatment during pregnancy: Research synthesis and clinical care principles. *Journal of Women's Health*, *29*(3), 310–318. https://doi.org/10.1089/jwh.2019.7781.

Bjork, M., Riedel, B., Spigset, O., Veiby, G., Kolstad, E., Daltveit, A. K., & Gilhus, N. E. (2018). Association of folic acid supplementation during pregnancy with the risk of autistic traits in children exposed to antiepileptic drugs in utero. *JAMA Neurology*, *75*(2), 160–168. https://doi.org/10.1001/jamaneurol.2017.3897.

Boukhris, T., Sheehy, O., Mottron, L., & Berard, A. (2016). Antidepressant use during pregnancy and the risk of autism spectrum disorder in children. *JAMA Pediatrics*, *170*(2), 117–124. https://doi.org/10.1001/jamapediatrics.2015.3356.

Broening, H. W., Morford, L. L., Inman-Wood, S. L., Fukumura, M., & Vorhees, C. V. (2001). 3,4-methylenedioxymethamphetamine (ecstasy)-induced learning and memory impairments depend on the age of exposure during early development. *Journal of Neuroscience*, *21*(9), 3228–3235.

Chu, E. K., Smith, L. M., Derauf, C., Newman, E., Neal, C. R., Arria, A. M., … Lester, B. M. (2020). Behavior problems during early childhood in children with prenatal methamphetamine exposure. *Pediatrics*, *146*(6). https://doi.org/10.1542/peds.2019-0270.

Eze, N., Smith, L. M., LaGasse, L. L., Derauf, C., Newman, E., Arria, A., … Lester, B. M. (2016). School-aged outcomes following prenatal methamphetamine exposure: 7.5-year follow-up from the Infant Development, Environment, and Lifestyle Study. *Journal of Pediatrics*, *170*, 34–38. https://doi.org/10.1016/j.jpeds.2015.11.070. e31.

Goldschmidt, L., Day, N. L., & Richardson, G. A. (2000). Effects of prenatal marijuana exposure on child behavior problems at age 10. *Neurotoxicology and Teratology*, *22*(3), 325–336. https://doi.org/10.1016/s0892-0362(00)00066-0.

Gray, K. A., Day, N. L., Leech, S., & Richardson, G. A. (2005). Prenatal marijuana exposure: Effect on child depressive symptoms at ten years of age. *Neurotoxicology and Teratology*, *27*(3), 439–448. https://doi.org/10.1016/j.ntt.2005.03.010.

Green, P. P., McKnight-Eily, L. R., Tan, C. H., Mejia, R., & Denny, C. H. (2016). Vital signs: Alcohol-exposed pregnancies—United States, 2011–2013. *Morbidity and Mortality Weekly Report*, *65*(4), 91–97.

Hagan, J. F., Balachova, T., Bertrand, J., Chasnoff, I., Dang, E., Fernandez-Baca, D., … Zubler, J. (2016). Neurobehavioral disorder associated with prenatal alcohol exposure. *Pediatrics*, *138*(4), e20151553. https://doi.org/10.1542/peds.2015-1553.

Hoyme, H. E., Kalberg, W. O., Elliott, A. J., Blankenship, J., Buckley, D., Marais, A. S., … May, P. A. (2016). Updated clinical guidelines for diagnosing fetal alcohol spectrum disorders. *Pediatrics*, *138*(2). https://doi.org/10.1542/peds.2015-4256.

Huybrechts, K. F., Bateman, B. T., Desai, R. J., Hernandez-Diaz, S., Rough, K., Mogun, H., … Patorno, E. (2017). Risk of neonatal drug withdrawal after intrauterine co-exposure to opioids and psychotropic medications: Cohort study. *BMJ*, *358*, j3326. https://doi.org/10.1136/bmj.j3326.

Ikonomidou, C., Scheer, I., Wilhelm, T., Juengling, F. D., Titze, K., Stover, B., … Kassubek, J. (2007). Brain morphology alterations in the basal ganglia and the hypothalamus following prenatal exposure to antiepileptic drugs. *European Journal of Paediatric Neurology*, *11*(5), 297–301. https://doi.org/10.1016/j.ejpn.2007.02.006.

Kiblawi, Z. N., Smith, L. M., LaGasse, L. L., Derauf, C., Newman, E., Shah, R., … Lester, B. (2013). The effect of prenatal methamphetamine exposure on attention as assessed by continuous performance tests: Results from the Infant Development, Environment, and Lifestyle Study. *Journal of Developmental and Behavioral Pediatrics*, *34*(1), 31–37. https://doi.org/10.1097/DBP.0b013e318277a1c5.

Lambert, B. L., & Bauer, C. R. (2012). Developmental and behavioral consequences of prenatal cocaine exposure: A review. *Journal of Perinatology*, *32*(11), 819–828. https://doi.org/10.1038/jp.2012.90.

Lange, S., Probst, C., Gmel, G., Rehm, J., Burd, L., & Popova, S. (2017). Global prevalence of fetal alcohol spectrum disorder among children and youth: A systematic review and meta-analysis. *JAMA Pediatrics*, *171*(10), 948–956. https://doi.org/10.1001/jamapediatrics.2017.1919.

Larson, J. J., Graham, D. L., Singer, L. T., Beckwith, A. M., Terplan, M., Davis, J. M., … Bada, H. S. (2019). Cognitive and behavioral impact on children exposed to opioids during pregnancy. *Pediatrics*, *144*(2). https://doi.org/10.1542/peds.2019-0514.

Li, Z., Santhanam, P., Coles, C. D., Lynch, M. E., Hamann, S., Peltier, S., & Hu, X. (2011). Increased "default mode" activity in adolescents prenatally exposed to cocaine. *Human Brain Mapping*, *32*(5), 759–770. https://doi.org/10.1002/hbm.21059.

May, P. A., Chambers, C. D., Kalberg, W. O., Zellner, J., Feldman, H., Buckley, D., … Hoyme, H. E. (2018). Prevalence of fetal alcohol spectrum disorders in 4 US communities. *JAMA*, *319*(5), 474–482. https://doi.org/10.1001/jama.2017.21896.

McCance-Katz. E. F. (2019). *The national survey on drug use and health: 2018*. Substance Abuse and Mental Health Services Administration. https://www.samhsa.gov/data/sites/default/files/nsduh-ppt-09-2018.pdf

Metz, T. D., & Stickrath, E. H. (2015). Marijuana use in pregnancy and lactation: A review of the evidence. *American Journal of Obstetrics and Gynecology*, *213*(6), 761–778. https://doi.org/10.1016/j.ajog.2015.05.025.

Nadebaum, C., Anderson, V., Vajda, F., Reutens, D., & Wood, A. (2012). Neurobehavioral consequences of prenatal antiepileptic drug exposure. *Developmental Neuropsychology*, *37*(1), 1–29. https://doi.org/10.1080/87565641.2011.589483.

National Organization of Rare Disorder. (n.d.). Fetal valproate syndrome. https://rarediseases.org/rare-diseases/fetal-valproate-syndrome/

Ornoy, A., Weinstein-Fudim, L., & Ergaz, Z. (2017). Antidepressants, antipsychotics, and mood stabilizers in pregnancy: What do we know and how should we treat pregnant women with depression. *Birth Defects Research*, *109*(12), 933–956. https://doi.org/10.1002/bdr2.1079.

Patrick, S. W., Dudley, J., Martin, P. R., Harrell, F. E., Warren, M. D., Hartmann, K. E., … Cooper, W. O. (2015). Prescription opioid epidemic and infant outcomes. *Pediatrics*, *135*(5), 842–850. https://doi.org/10.1542/peds.2014-3299.

Polli, F. S., & Kohlmeier, K. A. (2020). Prenatal nicotine exposure in rodents: Why are there so many variations in behavioral outcomes? *Nicotine and Tobacco Research*, *22*(10), 1694–1710. https://doi.org/10.1093/ntr/ntz196.

Richardson, G. A., Goldschmidt, L., Larkby, C., & Day, N. L. (2013). Effects of prenatal cocaine exposure on child behavior and growth at 10 years of age. *Neurotoxicology and Teratology*, *40*, 1–8. https://doi.org/10.1016/j.ntt.2013.08.001.

Streissguth, A. P., Bookstein, F. L., Barr, H. M., Sampson, P. D., O'Malley, K., & Young, J. K. (2004). Risk factors for adverse life outcomes in fetal alcohol syndrome and fetal alcohol effects. *Journal of Developmental and Behavioral Pediatrics*, *25*(4), 228–238. https://doi.org/10.1097/00004703-200408000-00002.

Turchi, R. M., Smith, V. C., & Committee on Substance Use and Prevention, & Council on Children with Disabilities. (2018). The role of integrated care in a medical home for patients with a fetal alcohol spectrum disorder. *Pediatrics*, *142*(4). https://doi.org/10.1542/peds.2018-2333.

Veiby, G., Engelsen, B. A., & Gilhus, N. E. (2013). Early child development and exposure to antiepileptic drugs prenatally and through breastfeeding: A prospective cohort study on children of women with epilepsy. *JAMA Neurology*, *70*(11), 1367–1374. https://doi.org/10.1001/jamaneurol.2013.4290.

Vercruysse, D. C., Deprez, S., Sunaert, S., Van Calsteren, K., & Amant, F. (2016). Effects of prenatal exposure to cancer treatment on neurocognitive development, a review. *Neurotoxicology*, *54*, 11–21. https://doi.org/10.1016/j.neuro.2016.02.013.

Wesseling, J., Van Driel, D., Heymans, H. S., Rosendaal, F. R., Geven-Boere, L. M., Smrkovsky, M., … Van der Veer, E. (2001). Coumarins during pregnancy: Long-term effects on growth and development of school-age children. *Journal of Thrombosis and Haemostasis*, *85*(4), 609–613.

Weyrauch, D., Schwartz, M., Hart, B., Klug, M. G., & Burd, L. (2017). Comorbid mental disorders in fetal alcohol spectrum disorders: A systematic review. *Journal of Developmental and Behavioral Pediatrics*, *38*(4), 283–291. https://doi.org/10.1097/DBP.0000000000000440.

Yeoh, S. L., Eastwood, J., Wright, I. M., Morton, R., Melhuish, E., Ward, M., & Oei, J. L. (2019). Cognitive and motor outcomes of children with prenatal opioid exposure: A systematic review and meta-analysis. *JAMA Network Open*, *2*(7), e197025. https://doi.org/10.1001/jamanetworkopen.2019.7025.

38

The Impact of Environmental Chemicals on the Developing Brain

Marissa Hauptman and Philip J. Landrigan

For additional material related to the content of this chapter, please see Chapter 37.

VIGNETTE

An 8-year-old nonverbal girl with severe autism spectrum disorder and persistent pica was tested for lead by her developmental pediatrician 2 years prior to the current evaluation. She was found to have an elevated blood lead level (BLL) of 25 mcg/dL. Her prior BLLs obtained during routine testing at 1 and 2 years of age were less than 5 mcg/dL. She had evidence of iron deficiency anemia on laboratory analysis and was prescribed iron supplementation. Her abdominal radiographs did not demonstrate retained foreign bodies, and she did not require whole bowel irrigation.

The family's home, built in 1930s, was found to have lead-based paint hazards. There was no history of occupational take-home lead exposure or use of lead-containing traditional medicines or lead-containing cosmetics. The family remediated the lead paint hazards identified in their home following state guidelines. Despite oversight by the state health department and the family's following all recommended procedures, the child developed a substantial increase in her BLL to 60 mcg/dL following the lead abatement, and she was admitted to our hospital for chelation therapy.

Our patient's persistent pica behavior places her at particularly high risk for continued lead exposure in any home or school environment, despite compliance with lead-safe regulations.

NEURODEVELOPMENTAL DISABILITIES CAUSED BY TOXIC CHEMICALS IN THE ENVIRONMENT

Toxic chemicals in the environment are important and potentially preventable causes of developmental and behavioral disorders in children and should always be considered in the differential diagnosis. Most neurodevelopmental disabilities caused by toxic chemicals are not distinct in their clinical presentation from disorders due to other causes. For this reason a diagnosis of chemical causation can easily be overlooked. Opportunities for prevention and treatment are then lost.

An environmental exposure history performed by an alert clinician with a high index of suspicion is the single most effective tool for the diagnosis of disease in children caused by toxic exposures in the environment (Miller, 2004). Such a history should enquire about both prenatal and postnatal exposures. It needs to be a routine component of the evaluation of every child with a neurodevelopmental disability. Suspicious findings elicited in the environmental history can trigger more detailed follow-up evaluation that may include laboratory testing or a home visit by an environmental specialist or staff from a pediatric environmental health specialty unit (PEHSU) (Paulson et al., 2009).

UBIQUITOUS NATURE OF ENVIRONMENTAL CHEMICALS

Children in today's world are surrounded by more than 120,000 manufactured chemicals. These are new synthetic materials that have been invented and produced in the past 75 years and never before existed on earth. They are incorporated into millions of consumer products that include foods and food packaging, clothing, building materials, electronics, cleaning materials, pesticides, cosmetics, toys, blankets, mattresses, and baby bottles. Global chemical manufacturing is increasing 3.5% per year and is on track to double by 2030 (Landrigan et al., 2018).

Children are especially at risk of exposure to more than 3000 chemicals produced in volumes exceeding 1 million pounds per year. These high-production volume chemicals have become widely distributed in the children's environments—in air, food, and drinking water. The Centers for Disease Control and Prevention (CDC) National Biomonitoring Survey routinely detects measurable quantities of more than 200 manufactured chemicals in blood and urine in virtually all Americans (CDC, 2021a). Elevated levels of high-production volume chemicals are found also in the breast milk of nursing mothers and cord blood of newborn infants.

The great majority of manufactured chemicals have never been tested for safety or toxicity (Landrigan & Goldman, 2011). Information is especially lacking on potential toxicity to prenatal and early childhood development. Chemicals are allowed to enter markets in most countries, including the United States, with little or no premarket safety assessments. Many manufactured chemicals have been found—sometimes only after years or even decades of use—to have caused grave damage to the environment and to human health. Historical examples include asbestos, tetraethyl lead, DDT, and the ozone-destroying chlorofluorocarbons. More recently developed chemicals such as phthalates, neonicotinoid insecticides, brominated flame retardants, and perfluorinated substances (PFAS) appear on track to repeat this dismal history. Failure to test chemicals for toxicity puts children at daily risk of exposures to materials of unknown hazard and at risk of previously unencountered disease.

CHILDREN'S UNIQUE VULNERABILITIES TO TOXIC CHEMICALS

Infants and young children are much more sensitive to toxic chemicals in the environment than adults. They are more heavily exposed per kilogram body weight because they eat more food, drink more water, and breathe more air than adults; in addition, they play close to the ground and display oral exploratory behavior. Children's sensitivity is further magnified during early development. Even brief low-level exposures to toxic chemicals during windows of exquisite vulnerability in early life can lead to lasting disability (Heindel et al., 2015). Because of the enormous complexity of its development the brain is at especially high risk (Grandjean & Landrigan, 2006).

Toddlers lack the cognitive abilities to discriminate food from nonfood items and frequently put nonfood items in the mouth, a behavior known as pica. The US Environmental Protection Agency (EPA) estimates that young children consume, on average, 200 to 800 mg of dirt daily (Binder, Sokal, & Maughan, 1986). If that dirt is contaminated with lead or other hazardous materials, as in the opening vignette, toxicity can result. Persistent pica behaviors are linked to certain medical conditions such as iron deficiency anemia and sickle cell disease. Children with developmental disorders such as autism and severe intellectual disability have a higher propensity for pica persisting into later childhood and even adolescence. A recent study reported that children 30 to 68 months of age with autism spectrum disorder and intellectual disability had a 28% prevalence of pica, compared to 14% in children with autism spectrum disorder without intellectual disability, 10% in children with nonautistic developmental delay and intellectual disability, and 3.5% in population-based controls (Fields et al., 2021).

FROM ACUTE TOXICITY TO SILENT TOXICITY

Developmental neurotoxicity in children exposed to toxic chemicals in the environment is typically first identified through recognition of clinically obvious symptoms such as obtundation, coma, and convulsions in children who have experienced high-dose exposures. Subsequent studies of children with lower-level exposures and no obvious symptoms have documented the presence of less striking but nonetheless serious functional deficits such as loss of IQ, shortening of attention span, and disruption of behavior. Prospective birth cohort epidemiologic studies of children exposed to neurotoxic chemicals in utero and in early postnatal life have been especially informative in elucidating these causal associations (Bellinger, Stiles, & Needleman, 1992; Lanphear et al., 2005).

This sequence of scientific discovery, which had its origins in studies of children with asymptomatic exposure to lead (Landrigan et al., 1975; Needleman et al., 1979), has led to the understanding that neurotoxic chemicals can exert a range of adverse effects—some are clinically evident, while others can be discerned only through special testing and are not evident on the standard examination; hence they are termed subclinical toxicity. The underlying concept is that there is a dose-dependent continuum of toxicity in which clinically obvious effects have their silent counterparts (Grandjean & Landrigan, 2006). Box 38.1 describes Dr. Herbert Needleman, a pioneer in this field.

The increasing application of prospective birth cohort studies in pediatric research has generated information on a series of previously unrecognized associations between toxic chemical exposures and neurodevelopmental disabilities in children (Table 38.1). A major unanswered question is whether there are additional chemicals in use today that can cause still undiscovered neurodevelopmental effects (Fig. 38.1).

TABLE 38.1 Chemicals Known and Suspected to Damage the Developing Human Brain
Lead
Methylmercury
Polychlorinated biphenyls (PCBs)
Arsenic
Manganese
Fluoride
Organic solvents (e.g., ethanol and toluene)
Organophosphate pesticides (chlorpyrifos)
Organochlorine pesticides
Phthalates
Bisphenol A
Brominated flame retardants
Polycyclic aromatic hydrocarbons

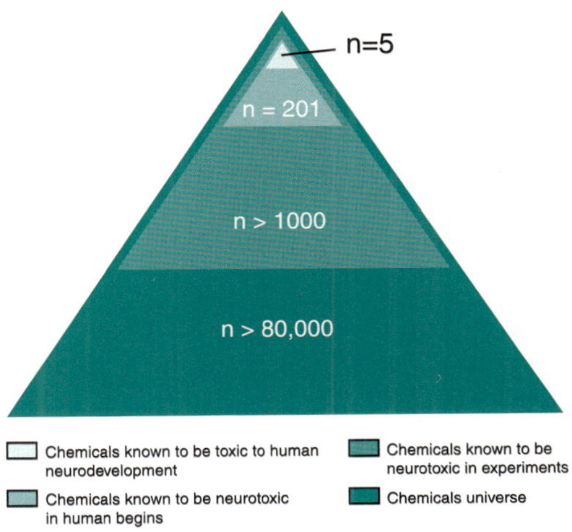

Fig. 38.1 Are there additional developmental toxicants not yet discovered?

BOX 38.1 Herbert L. Needleman, MD

Herbert L. Needleman, MD (1927–2017) (Fig. 38.2) was a pediatrician and child psychiatrist whose pioneering research established conclusively that lead and other chemicals in the environment can cause neurotoxicity in children even at low levels of exposure that produce no clinically evident symptoms. Dr. Needleman documented that the loss of intelligence, shortening of attention span, and disruption of behavior that result from subclinical lead poisoning are permanent, untreatable, and irreversible. He argued that the only rational approach to prevention of lead poisoning is to prevent exposure to lead.

Dr. Needleman's research provided the key impetus for nations around the world to remove lead from gasoline. In the United States, where approximately 100,000 tons of lead had been added to gasoline each year until the mid-1970s to increase automotive engine performance, the removal of lead from gasoline reduced children's blood lead levels by more than 90% and raised the average intelligence of all American children born since 1980 by an estimated 5 IQ points.

Because his discoveries threatened the lead industry and its markets, Dr. Needleman was subjected to vicious, prolonged, and highly personal attack. In the 1980s, two lead industry scientists who had visited his laboratory under the pretext that they wished to collaborate with him in research and without revealing their industry connections, claimed falsely that Dr. Needleman had committed scientific fraud. They demanded a full investigation of his work by the National Institutes of Health (NIH). This investigation was conducted over a painfully protracted 4-year period, and in this time Dr. Needleman was locked out of his laboratory. The investigation concluded that there was no evidence of misconduct, and Dr. Needleman was fully vindicated. Indeed, the industry scientists were criticized sharply by NIH for having filed false accusations.

Dr. Needleman's extraordinary contributions to children's health were recognized through multiple awards, among them the Charles A. Dana Award, the Heinz Award for the Environment, and the Prince Mahidol Medal presented by the King of Thailand. Dr. Needleman's scientific findings on subclinical lead poisoning have been validated by researchers in the United States, Europe, and Australia. He is a true hero of children's environmental health.

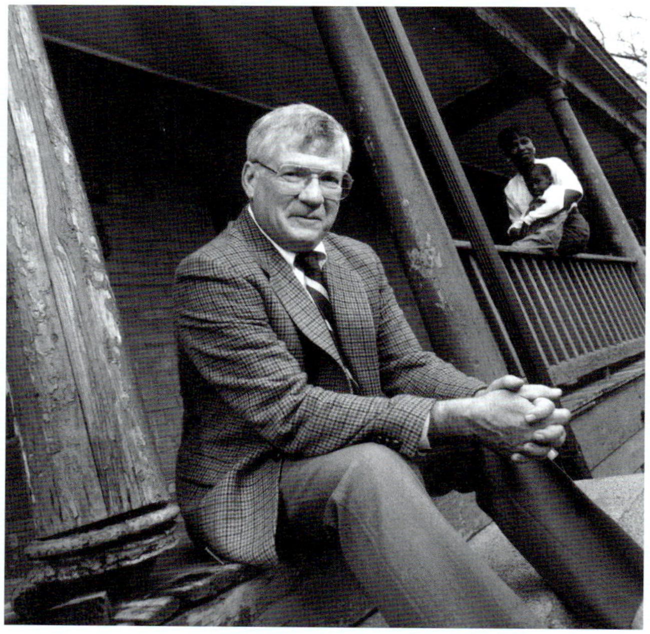

Fig. 38.2 Herbert L. Needleman, MD was a pioneer in research in environmental effects on the developing brain.

ENVIRONMENTAL INFLUENCES ON DEVELOPMENT

Lead

Exposure of children to lead in their environment continues to be an enormous public health issue that is global in scope. As many as 500,000 children ages 1 to 5 years in the United States have BLLs above the reference value of 5 mcg/dL set by the CDC (2021b). Lead is a known neurotoxin, able to produce metabolic and infrastructural perturbations at the molecular and cellular levels of the developing nervous system. Prospective longitudinal studies have demonstrated the long-lasting sequelae of lead exposure on intellectual and academic achievement later in childhood even after apparently low-level exposures with BLL less than 10 mcg/dL (Bellinger et al., 1992; Canfield et al., 2003). Neurologic outcomes include cognitive damage, hearing loss, visual effects, delayed speech acquisition, learning disabilities, lower reading and arithmetic skills, poor attention, deficits of other aspects of executive function, and other educational, behavioral, and emotional problems, which can persist into adolescence and adulthood.

Over the past 50 years, the United States has made extraordinary progress in reducing children's exposure to lead. In the early 1970s lead was ubiquitous in the American

TABLE 38.2 The Consequences of Removing Lead From Gasoline in the United States

95% reduction in blood lead levels in US children
95% reduction in incidence of lead poisoning
5-point gain in population mean IQ for all children born since 1980
$200 billion annual economic benefit to United States each year since 1980 through increased economic productivity of more intelligent and creative children

environment. It was marketed aggressively by the lead industry and used widely in paint and water pipes. At peak use in the early 1970s, more than 100,000 tons of lead were added each year to gasoline. The mean blood level in American children at that time was close to 20 mcg/dL, symptomatic lead poisoning with coma and convulsions was common, and the CDC reference level for intervening against lead poisoning was a concentration of lead in blood of 40 mcg/dL, a level below which produced no obvious symptoms.

Following the removal of lead from gasoline and paint that began in 1975, lead levels fell precipitously from 17 mcg/dL in 1976, to 4 mcg/dL in the early 1990s, to below 2 mcg/dL today, and the incidence of acute symptomatic lead poisoning plummeted (Table 38.2). At the same time, steady increases in knowledge of lead's toxicity at increasingly lower levels caused the CDC to repeatedly ratchet down its blood lead reference level: first to 25 mcg/dL, then to 10 mcg/dL, then to 5 mcg/dL in 2012 , and most recently to 3.5 mcg/dL in 2021. The CDC and the World Health Organization now state that any detectable level of lead is abnormal and that no level of lead in a child's blood is safe.

The source of lead for most children in the United States today with elevated BLLs is lead-laden dust and paint chips from deteriorating lead paint on interior surfaces.

Lead plumbing (Latin *plumbus*, "lead") has contaminated drinking water for centuries, especially if water has high acidity or low mineral content. This route of exposure was unfortunately exemplified most recently through an episode of drinking water contamination in Flint, Michigan. This community-wide contamination was caused by a change in water source that resulted in need for augmenting disinfection processes. Appropriate corrosion control procedures were not implemented following those changes, and thus the water's ability to leach lead from leaded and galvanized pipes, solder, and plumbing fixtures increased. A study conducted by Hanna-Attisha, LaChance, Sadler, & Champney Schnepp, (2016) and corroborated by Kennedy et al. (2016) identified a statistically significant increased odds of having an elevated BLL in the period following the switch in drinking water source for this community. The majority of elevated BLLs tested were in the range of 5 to 9 mcg/dL, although few children under 1 year of age were tested (Kennedy et al., 2016).

Mercury

Mercury exists in three forms: the metallic elemental form, inorganic form in mercurous or mercuric salts, and organic form (such as methylmercury and ethylmercury). Severe elemental mercury and inorganic mercury salt poisoning (responsible for pink disease, or acrodynia, from mercurous chloride teething lotions or diaper powder) has become rare. However, a more insidious concern is that of chronic exposure to organic mercurials, particularly methylmercury, resulting from contamination of the food chain, especially certain species of fish. Methylmercury is a potent neurotoxin, and the adverse effects of exposure of the developing fetus to methylmercury in utero have been well described. The consequences include dose-related reduction in IQ, shortening of attention span, and irreversible developmental and neurologic effects. Large outbreaks of high-dose prenatal methylmercury poisoning have occurred in Minamata Bay, Japan, from maternal consumption of fish contaminated by factory waste discharged into the bay, and in Iraq from consumption of contaminated bread baked from grain treated with a methylmercury fungicide (Schmid & Rotenberg, 2005). Severe central nervous system effects occurred in both instances, with a particular susceptibility noted in the fetuses of poisoned pregnant women (almost 30% of children born during the height of the Minamata Bay epidemic had moderate or severe developmental disabilities).

More recent concern has centered, as for lead, on more subtle neurocognitive effects that may be attributed to chronic low-level mercury exposure through consumption of fish or other contaminated food (Karagas et al., 2012; Schmid & Rotenberg, 2005). For example, a large study in the Faroe Islands identified deficits in pediatric cognitive function, particularly language, memory, and attention, occurring at levels of prenatal mercury exposure that were less than 3% of the toxic threshold suggested by the Iraq outbreak (Grandjean et al., 1997). In 2017 the US Food and Drug Administration (FDA) and the EPA issued revised advice regarding fish consumption for pregnant women or women who may become pregnant and individuals who are breastfeeding. The revised guidance, which was endorsed by the American College of Obstetrics and Gynecology (ACOG), recognizes that different fish species contain different mercury levels. It recommended eating two to three servings a week of a variety of fish, but consuming no more than one serving a week (≤6 oz) of certain predator fish such as albacore (white) tuna, swordfish, shark, king mackerel, and Spanish mackerel known to have the highest mercury concentrations (ACOG, 2020).

Organophosphate Pesticides

The organophosphates are a family of insecticides developed in Germany in the 1930s and deliberately designed to cause injury to the brain and nervous system by inhibiting activity of the enzyme acetylcholinesterase. Multiple organophosphates of varying potency are on the market today. Chlorpyrifos is the organophosphate most widely used in the United States. One of the most notorious members of the family is sarin, the highly potent chemical warfare agent used in the 1995 Tokyo subway attack.

Three recent prospective birth cohort studies provide strong evidence for the developmental neurotoxicity of chlorpyrifos. The first of these studies undertaken by a team from the University of California at Berkeley reports harmful effects on cognition with reductions in IQ scores among the children of agricultural workers exposed prenatally to chlorpyrifos and other pesticides in the Salinas Valley of California (Eskenazi et al., 2007). The second study undertaken at the Mount Sinai School of Medicine found similar effects in a New York City Latino population whose exposures to chlorpyrifos were residential and dietary (Engel et al., 2015). The third study, also conducted in New York City by investigators at Columbia University among a population of Black and Dominican children exposed residentially and through their mother's diet, found negative effects of prenatal chlorpyrifos exposure on children's brain development (Rauh et al., 2011).

In addition to damaging children's cognitive abilities, chlorpyrifos exposure during pregnancy is associated with changes in children's behavior and with developmental delays. Thus the Columbia University study found that children with higher prenatal exposures to chlorpyrifos were behind their peers from the same communities in motor and mental development by age 3 years. These children were also more likely than their peers to be diagnosed with autism spectrum disorder and to develop symptoms of attention-deficit/hyperactivity disorder (Rauh et al., 2011).

Another striking finding from the Columbia University study was that children born prior to a 2000 ban on residential application of chlorpyrifos tended to be smaller and to have poorer reflexes and smaller head circumference at birth than children in the same communities born after the ban. These changes were correlated with levels of prenatal exposure to chlorpyrifos (Rauh et al., 2011).

Most recently, a follow-up analysis within the Columbia University cohort used magnetic resonance imaging (MRI) to study brain development in 9- to 11-year-old children exposed prenatally to chlorpyrifos. It found that even low to moderate levels of prenatal chlorpyrifos exposure (i.e., levels below current EPA standards) were associated with persistent changes in brain structure and function (Rauh et al., 2012).

In late 2016 the EPA was on the verge of banning chlorpyrifos in the United States. This proposed ban was, however, rescinded by the incoming administration, and chlorpyrifos remained on the market in the United States from 2016 to 2021. Thousands of children were thus unnecessarily exposed to chlorpyrifos. In April 2021 a federal appeals court ruled the EPA must ban all uses of chlorpyrifos on food within 60 days or establish new standards for chlorpyrifos that are safe for children.

Additional Developmental Neurotoxicants

Leading scientific and medical experts and children's health advocates under the auspices of Project Targeting Environmental Neurodevelopmental Risks (TENDR) have identified a list of toxic chemicals and pollutants that on the basis of currently available epidemiologic, toxicologic, and mechanistic evidence appear to increase children's risks for neurodevelopmental disorders (Bennett et al., 2016). These include chemicals that are used extensively in consumer products and that have become widespread in the environment. In addition to lead, mercury, and organophosphate pesticides, this list includes air pollution (Clifford, Lang, Chen, Anstey, & Seaton,2016; Suades-González, Gascon, Guxens, & Sunyer, 2015), polybrominated diphenyl ethers (PBDEs), a class of industrial chemicals used as flame retardants (Lam et al., 2017), and polychlorinated biphenyls (PCBs) (Jacobson & Jacobson, 1996) (see Table 38.1).

The great majority of manufactured chemicals have never been tested for safety or toxicity, and because of this lack of toxicity testing data there is much we do not know in terms of the impact of toxic chemicals on our developing brains (Landrigan & Goldman, 2011). For example, several ongoing associations and causal relationships are being evaluated with additional chemicals such as fluoride and essential elements such as manganese, copper, and iron where both too little exposure or too much exposure may be associated with neurodevelopmental sequelae. Lastly, more research is needed to evaluate the impact of multiple environmental exposures as is often the case for many disadvantaged communities.

SPECIFIC DEVELOPMENTAL DISABILITIES: AUTISM SPECTRUM DISORDER

Concern about the possibility that toxic environmental exposures might contribute to the causation of autism spectrum disorder and other neurodevelopmental disabilities in children has increased in recent years. Proof of the principle that prenatal environmental exposures to neurotoxic hazards can cause autism spectrum disorder comes from earlier studies linking autism with exposures to certain medications, including thalidomide, misoprostol, and valproic acid as well as to first trimester rubella infection and from more recent studies linking autism to prenatal exposures to lead, chlorpyrifos, and traffic-related air pollution.

Childhood immunization has received much scrutiny as a potential environmental cause of autism spectrum disorder. Claims of a link between vaccines and autism first arose in the late 1990s in the United Kingdom, the United States, and other countries and were triggered by reports of onset of autism in the days immediately following vaccination. In the United Kingdom these claims focused on the measles-mumps-rubella vaccine; the British study that advanced that claim has since been dismissed as a scientific fraud and its author banned from medical practice. In the United States these concerns focused initially on thimerosal, a preservative containing ethylmercury, a preservative added to multidose vials of many vaccines to prevent microbial contamination and then focused later on the frequency and timing of childhood immunizations.

To address this issue, pediatric and public health researchers in the United States, the United Kingdom, Europe, and Japan have undertaken an extensive series of epidemiologic studies. None of these studies has found any evidence for a link between vaccines and autism (Landrigan, 2010).

Children with developmental disorders, such as autism spectrum disorder, who have persistent pica behaviors (ingestion of nonfood items) and/or poor cognitive discriminatory recognition, as in the opening vignette, remain at elevated risk of lead contamination and likely other environmental

TABLE 38.3 Taking an Environmental History

Medical History

Ask about:

- Symptoms
- Developmental history
- Mouthing activities
- Pica
- Previous blood lead level measurements
- Family/maternal history of exposures to lead

Environmental History

Paint and soil exposure:

- What year was the residence built?
- Does the family have any concerns with the condition of the residence?
- Is there evidence of chewed or peeling paint on woodwork, furniture, or toys?
- How long has the family lived at that residence?
- Have there been recent renovations or repairs in the house?
- Has the residence ever been inspected for lead-based paint or other environmental hazards?
- Are there other sites where the child spends significant amounts of time?
- What is the character of indoor play areas?
- Do outdoor play areas contain bare soil that may be contaminated?
- How does the family attempt to control dust/dirt?

Pests and pesticides:

- Does the family have any concerns with existing rodents/insects (mice, rats, cockroaches)?
- Does the family have concerns about pesticide, herbicide, insecticide exposure (e.g., pesticide use in the home, close proximity to agricultural sources of pesticide applications)?

Mold/water leaks:

- Does the family have any concerns water leaks/mold in the residence?

Water source:

- What is the primary water source of the home (municipal, well)?
- Has the water been tested or found to have elevated levels of lead, arsenic, or other water contaminants?

Safety:

- Does the home have a working smoke and carbon monoxide detector?
- Does the family have concerns about safely storing prescription medicines? Does the family know how to reach the regional poison control center? (If not, have them store 1-800-222-1222 in their phone)

Air pollution:

- Do household members smoke or vape? Do household members smoke or vape in the residence or car?
- Does the family have concerns about air pollution (e.g., local industrial sources, close proximity to major traffic sources or bus depots)?

Relevant Behavioral Characteristics of the Child

- To what degree does the child exhibit hand-to-mouth activity?
- Does the child exhibit pica?
- Are the child's hands washed before meals and snacks?

Exposures to and Behaviors of Household Members

- What are the occupations of adult household members? Are there any potential take-home occupational lead or other environmental exposures?
- What are the hobbies of household members? (Fishing, working with ceramics or stained glass, and hunting are examples of hobbies that involve risk for lead exposure.)
- Are painted materials or unusual materials burned in household fireplaces? Are cookstoves or ovens used as a heating source?

Miscellaneous Questions

- Does the home contain vinyl miniblinds made overseas and purchased before 1997?
- Does the child receive or have access to imported food, cosmetics, or ayurvedic or herbal supplements?
- Is food prepared or stored in imported pottery or metal vessels?
- Does the family have any other concerns about the child's/children's environment at home or school?

Nutritional History

- Take a dietary history with specific focus on fish and type of fish intake
- Evaluate the child's iron status using appropriate laboratory tests
- Ask about history of Special Supplemental Nutrition Program for Women, Infants, and Children program (WIC) participation

Physical Examination

- Pay particular attention to the neurologic examination and to the child's psychosocial and language development
- Pay particular attention to stigmata of anemia (e.g., conjunctival pallor and tachycardia)

Adapted from Hauptman, M., & Woolf, A. D. (2017). Childhood ingestions of environmental toxins: What are the risks? *Pediatric Annals, 46*(12), 1–6.

exposures as they grow into school age and adolescence, life stages in which children are not routinely tested for elevated BLLs (Hauptman, Stierman, & Woolf, 2019; Shannon & Graef, 1996). Because these older children and adolescents with continuing pica behaviors are taller and stronger than the toddlers more typically exposed to lead, they can access new surfaces and areas of households that may contain lead hazards not previously accessible to them at a younger age. A study that investigated epidemiologic characteristics of severe lead poisoning in New York City found a trend toward severe lead poisoning occurring at older ages in children with autism spectrum disorder compared to the cases without the disorder (5.99 years vs. 3.69 years, respectively) (Keller, Faciano, Tsega, & Ehrlich, 2017). Published reviews on the management of autism spectrum disorder often advise health care providers to monitor children with the disorder and pica behaviors for elevated BLL (Myers, Johnson, & American Academy of Pediatrics Council on Children With Disabilities, 2007) (Table 38.3).

Some children with autism spectrum disorder may have nutritional deficiencies in iron, calcium, magnesium, or vitamin D. Iron deficiency anemia is a known comorbidity of childhood lead poisoning as in the opening vignette, and may increase risk for pica. Such deficiencies may result in increased lead absorption through the intestinal wall active transport system for metals. Ensuring adequate dietary or supplemental intake of sources of iron, magnesium, calcium, and vitamin D is likely to help protect the child from lead absorption in the gastrointestinal tract. As evidenced by mouse studies, the presence of iron deficiency may enhance gastrointestinal uptake of lead, predisposing those with lead exposure to elevated BLLs (Elsenhans, Janser, Windisch, & Schümann, 2011).

Providers should be aware of the recommended universal or targeted lead screening guidelines in their locality and, at a minimum, adhere to these guidelines. Most children with autism spectrum disorder will require enhanced and extended monitoring for lead poisoning, especially if parents report persistent pica behaviors and the family lives in an older house.

The complexity of the medical needs of children with both autism spectrum disorder and an elevated BLL demands a thoughtful, comprehensive, coordinated, and multidisciplinary approach to their care. Social, educational, economic, housing, and occupational challenges confront their parents and guardians. The use of chelating agents to treat autism spectrum disorder in children who do not have documented lead poisoning is discouraged as a scientifically unfounded practice that may produce untoward consequences, neurotoxic adverse effects, or death (Brown, Willis, Omalu, & Leiker, 2008; James, Stevenson, Silove, & Williams, 2015). Federal policies and lead regulations in many states protect children under the age of 6 years from lead hazards in their environment, requiring hazard abatement if the child is found to have an elevated lead level and lead-contaminated surfaces are discovered at the time of inspection of their residence. These laws were designed with younger children in mind since they are most vulnerable to the deleterious effects of lead and explore their environment through pica and hand-to-mouth behaviors. However, both pica and oral exploratory habits may not end in the preschool years in children with autism spectrum disorder, as is the case in our clinical vignette, and instead persist throughout childhood and into adolescence. Laws regarding residential lead hazards are not adequately protective for children with autism spectrum disorder and persistent pica behaviors living in a contaminated environment.

ENVIRONMENTAL HEALTH DISPARITIES

Some subgroups of children are especially susceptible to exposures to environmental chemicals. Children living at or below the poverty line who live in older housing are disproportionately at greatest risk of lead poisoning (Vivier et al., 2011). For many known industrial chemicals such as lead, organophosphorus pesticides, PBDEs, and air pollution, communities of color, recent immigrants, and socioeconomically stressed communities face disproportionately high exposures and health impacts. Additionally, children of low socioeconomic status are at increased risk of nutritional deficiency such as iron deficiency, which has been associated with a four- to fivefold increase in baseline risk of lead poisoning due to increased absorption of lead by the divalent metal transporter in the gastrointestinal tract (Wright, Tsaih, Schwartz, Wright, & Hu, 2003).

CONCLUSION: ADVICE FOR DEVELOPMENTAL-BEHAVIORAL CLINICIANS

Pediatric health care clinicians play a pivotal role in educating parents about the hazards in the environment that confront their children and how best to avoid them. Developmental pediatricians need to be especially cognizant of the environmental hazards confronting older children and adolescents with autism spectrum disorder and intellectual impairment, as evidenced in the opening vignette. Clinicians need to ensure that if treatment of a hazardous environmental exposure is warranted, it is done safely and by health care professionals with expertise in toxicology or environmental medicine. As is often the case with environmental regulations, testing guidelines vary considerably by jurisdictions.

Clinicians with concerns about hazardous environmental exposures are strongly advised to consult their regional PEHSU (www.pehsu.net) or their city, county, or state health department to determine the appropriate follow-up steps in caring for a child with known or suspected environmental toxicant exposures.

At the national level, a new policy framework is badly needed to assess chemicals that have the potential to disrupt brain development and contribute to neurodevelopmental disorders and to prevent the introduction of these chemicals that may pose a risk in our environments (Landrigan & Goldman, 2011). This new policy will help to ensure that where our children live, learn, and play is as safe as possible for all children regardless of their development.

CONCLUSION

Pediatric health care clinicians play a pivotal role in educating parents about the hazards in the environment that confront their children and how best to avoid them. Developmental pediatricians need to be especially cognizant of the environmental hazards confronting older children and adolescents with autism spectrum disorder and intellectual impairment. Clinicians need to ensure that if treatment of a hazardous environmental exposure is warranted it is done safely and by health care professionals with expertise in toxicology or environmental medicine. As is often the case with environmental regulations, testing guidelines vary considerably by jurisdictions.

REFERENCES

American College of Obstetrics and Gynecology. (2020). *Update on seafood consumption during pregnancy*. https://www.acog.org/clinical/clinical-guidance/practice-advisory/articles/2017/01/update-on-seafood-consumption-during-pregnancy

Bellinger, D. C., Stiles, K. M., & Needleman, H. L. (1992). Low-level lead exposure, intelligence and academic achievement: A long-term follow-up study. *Pediatrics*, *90*(6), 855–861.

Bennett, D., Bellinger, D.C., Birnbaum, L.S., Bradman, A., Chen, A., Cory-Slechta, D.A., ... National Medical Association. (2016). Project TENDR: Targeting Environmental Neuro-Developmental Risks The TENDR Consensus Statement. Environmental Health Perspectives, 124(7), A118–A122.

Binder, S., Sokal, D., & Maughan, D. (1986). Estimating soil ingestion: The use of tracer elements in estimating the amount of soil ingested by young children. *Archives of Environmental Health*, *41*(6), 341–345.

Brown, M. J., Willis, T., Omalu, B., & Leiker, R. (2008). Deaths resulting from hypocalcemia after administration of edetate disodium: 2003–2005. *Pediatrics*, *118*, e534–e536.

Canfield, R. L., Henderson, C. R., Cory-Slechta, D. A., Cox, C., Jusko, T. A., & Lanphear, B. P. (2003). Intellectual impairment in children with blood lead concentrations below 10 µg per deciliter. *New England Journal of Medicine*, *348*(16), 1517–1526.

Centers for Disease Control and Prevention (CDC). (2021a). National Biomonitoring Program. https://www.cdc.gov/biomonitoring/index.html

Centers for Disease Control and Prevention (CDC). (2021b). *Lead*. https://www.cdc.gov/nceh/lead/

Clifford, A., Lang, L., Chen, R., Anstey, K. J., & Seaton, A. (2016). Exposure to air pollution and cognitive functioning across the life course—A systematic literature review. *Environmental Research*, *147*(5), 383–398.

Elsenhans, B., Janser, H., Windisch, W., & Schümann, K. (2011). Does lead use the intestinal absorptive pathways of iron? Impact of iron status on murine 210Pb and 59Fe absorption in duodenum and ileum in vivo. *Toxicology*, *284*, 7–11.

Engel, S. M., Bradman, A., Wolff, M. S., Rauh, V. A., Harley, K. G., Yang, J. H., ... Eskenazi, B. (2015). Prenatal organophosphorus pesticide exposure and child neurodevelopment at 24 months: An analysis of four birth cohorts. *Environmental Health Perspectives*, *124*, 822–830.

Eskenazi, B., Marks, A. R., Bradman, A., Harley, K., Barr, D. B., Johnson, C., ... Jewell, N. P. (2007). Organophosphate pesticide exposure and neurodevelopment in young Mexican-American children. *Environmental Health Perspectives*, *115*(5), 792–798.

Fields, V. L., Soke, G. N., Reynolds, A., Tian, L. H., Wiggins, L., Maenner, M., ... Schieve, L. A. (2021). Pica, autism and other disabilities. *Pediatrics*, *147*(2), e2020C462.

Grandjean, P., & Landrigan, P. J. (2006). Developmental neurotoxicity of industrial chemicals A silent pandemic. *Lancet*, *368*(9553), 2167–2178.

Grandjean, P., Weihe, P., White, R. F., Debes, F., Araki, S., Yokoyama, K., ... Jørgensen, J. (1997). Cognitive deficit in 7-year-old children with prenatal exposure to methylmercury. *Neurotoxicology and Teratology*, *19*, 417–428.

Hanna-Attisha, M., LaChance, J., Sadler, R. C., & Champney Schnepp, A. (2016). Elevated blood lead levels in children associated with the flint drinking water crisis: A spatial analysis of risk and public health response. *American Journal of Public Health*, *106*(2), 283–290.

Hauptman, M., Stierman, B., & Woolf, A. D. (2019). Children with autism spectrum disorder and lead poisoning: Diagnostic challenges and management complexities. *Clinical Pediatrics (Philadelphia)*, *58*(6), 605–612.

Hauptman, M., & Woolf, A. D. (2017). Childhood ingestions of environmental toxins: What are the risks? *Pediatric Annals*, *46*(12), 1–6.

Heindel, J. J., Balbus, J., Birnbaum, L., Brune-Drisse, M. N., Grandjean, P., Gray, K., ... Hanson, M. (2015). Developmental origins of health and disease: Integrating environmental influences. *Endocrinology*, *156*(10), 3416–3421.

Jacobson, J. L., & Jacobson, S. W. (1996). Intellectual impairment in children exposed to polychlorinated biphenyls in utero. *New England Journal of Medicine*, *335*(11), 783–789.

James, S., Stevenson, S. W., Silove, N., & Williams, K. (2015). Chelation for autism spectrum disorder (ASD). *Cochrane Database for Systematic Reviews*, *5*, CD010766.

Karagas, M. R., Choi, A. L., Oken, E., Horvat, M., Schoeny, R., Kamai, E., ... Korrick, S. (2012). Evidence on the human health effects of low-level methylmercury exposure. *Environmental Health Perspectives*, *120*(6), 799–806.

Keller, B., Faciano, A., Tsega, A., & Ehrlich, J. (2017). Epidemiologic characteristics of children with blood lead levels ≥45µg/dL. *Journal of Pediatrics*, *180*, 229–234.

Kennedy, C., Yard, E., Dignam, T., Buchanan, S., Condon, S., Brown, M. J., ... Breysse, P. (2016). Blood lead levels among children aged. *MMWR*, *65*(25), 650–654.

Lam, J., Lanphear, B. P., Bellinger, D., Axelrad, D. A., McPartland, J., Sutton, P., ... Woodruff, T. J. (2017). Developmental PBDE exposure and IQ/ADHD in childhood: A systematic review and meta-analysis. *Environmental Health Perspectives*, *125*(8), 086001.

Landrigan, P. J. (2010). What causes autism? Exploring the environmental contribution. *Current Opinions in Pediatrics*, *22*(2), 219–225.

Landrigan, P. J., Fuller, R., Acosta, N. J. R., Adeyi, O., Arnold, R., Basu, N. N., ... Zhong, M. (2018). The Lancet Commission on Pollution and Health. *Lancet*, *391*(10119), 462–512.

Landrigan, P. J., & Goldman, L. R. (2011). Children's vulnerability to toxic chemicals: A challenge and opportunity to strengthen health and environmental policy. *Health Affairs*, *30*(5), 842–850.

Landrigan, P. J., Whitworth, R. H., Baloh, R. W., Staehling, N. W., Barthel, W. F., & Rosenblum, B. F. (1975). Neuropsychological dysfunction in children with chronic low-level lead absorption. *Lancet*, *1*, 708–712.

Lanphear, B. P., Hornung, R., Khoury, J., Yolton, K., Baghurst, P., Bellinger, D. C., … Roberts, R. (2005). Low-level environmental lead exposure and children's intellectual function: An international pooled analysis. *Environmental Health Perspectives*, *113*, 894–899.

Miller, R. W. (2004). How environmental hazards in childhood have been discovered: Carcinogens, teratogens, neurotoxicants, and others. *Pediatrics*, *113*, 945–951.

Myers, S. M., Johnson, C. P., & American Academy of Pediatrics Council on Children With Disabilities. (2007). Management of children with autism spectrum disorders. *Pediatrics*, *120*, 1162–1182.

Needleman, H. L., Gunnoe, C., Leviton, A., Reed, R., Peresie, H., Maher, C., & Barrett, P. (1979). Deficits in psychologic and classroom performance of children with elevated dentine lead levels. *New England Journal of Medicine*, *300*, 689–695.

Paulson, J. A., Karr, C. J., Seltzer, J. M., Cherry, D. C., Sheffield, P. E., Cifuentes, E., … Amler, R. W. (2009). Development of the pediatric environmental health specialty unit network in North America. *American Journal of Public Health*, *99*(3), S511–S516.

Rauh, V., Arunajadai, S., Horton, M., Perera, F., Hoepner, L., Barr, D. B., & Whyatt, R. (2011). Seven-year neurodevelopmental scores and prenatal exposure to chlorpyrifos, a common agricultural pesticide. *Environmental Health Perspectives*, *119*(8), 1196–1201.

Rauh, V. A., Perera, F. P., Horton, M. K., Whyatt, R. M., Bansal, R., Hao, X., … Peterson, B. S. (2012). Brain anomalies in children exposed prenatally to a common organophosphate pesticide. *Proceedings of the National Academy of Science USA*, *109*(20), 7871–7876.

Schmid, C., & Rotenberg, J. S. (2005). Neurodevelopmental toxicology. *Neurology Clinics*, *23*, 321–336.

Shannon, M., & Graef, J. W. (1996). Lead intoxication in children with pervasive developmental disorders. *Journal of Toxicology: Clinical Toxicology*, *34*(2), 177–181.

Suades-González, E., Gascon, M., Guxens, M., & Sunyer, J. (2015). Air pollution and neuropsychological development: A review of the latest evidence. *Endocrinology*, *156*(10), 3473–3482.

Vivier, P. M., Hauptman, M., Weitzen, S. H., Bell, S., Quilliam, D. N., & Logan, J. R. (2011). The important health impact of where a child lives: Neighborhood characteristics and the burden of lead poisoning. *Maternal and Child Health Journal*, *15*(8), 1195–1202.

Wright, R. O., Tsaih, S. W., Schwartz, J., Wright, R. J., & Hu, H. (2003). Association between iron deficiency and blood lead level in a longitudinal analysis of children followed in an urban primary care clinic. *Journal of Pediatrics*, *142*(1), 9–14.

39

Cerebral Palsy and Other Motor Disorders

Kilby Mann, Joyce Oleszek, and Nancy Murphy

For additional material related to the content of this chapter, please see Chapter 89

VIGNETTE

Anna is a 13-year-old girl with spastic quadriplegic cerebral palsy (CP), Gross Motor Function Classification System (GMFCS) level IV. She was born preterm at 28 weeks of gestation, with the complication of bilateral grade III intraventricular hemorrhages. Upon discharge from the neonatal intensive care unit, she was enrolled in an early intervention program. Now as an adolescent, she enjoys being with her peers yet struggles to participate in social and recreational activities. She uses a manual wheelchair and a gait trainer, wears bilateral ankle-foot orthoses, and has a communication device. Anna works with school-based therapists. She has well-controlled seizures. Her spasticity is mostly well controlled on oral baclofen, and she occasionally receives botulinum toxin injections for focal tone management. Years ago she underwent surgery for hip dysplasia, and she and her family are now considering spine fusion for neuromuscular scoliosis. Anna has dysphagia yet takes 100% of her nutrition and hydration orally; she struggles to maintain a healthy weight, and gastrostomy tube placement is being considered. She has recently reached menarche, and periods seem to exacerbate her seizures and spasticity. Her family is considering menstrual suppression, but they worry about the potential impact on her bone health as she had a femoral insufficiency fracture a few years ago. Her family seeks guidance on how to best support her developing sexuality, her safe participation in community activities, and function and maximal independence as she approaches adulthood.

DEFINITION OF CEREBRAL PALSY

CP is the most common childhood physical disability worldwide, with an incidence in the United States of 2 to 3 per 1000 live births (Maenner et al., 2016). CP is "a group of permanent disorders of the development of movement and posture, causing activity limitation, that are attributed to non-progressive disturbances that occurred in the developing fetal or infant brain. The motor disorders of CP are often accompanied by disturbances of sensation, perception, cognition, communication and behaviour; by epilepsy, and by secondary musculoskeletal problems" (Rosenbaum et al., 2007, p. 9). Although CP is a permanent disorder with a nonprogressive structural brain abnormality, the clinical manifestations can change with growth and development.

Etiology

CP results from injury to the developing brain in the prenatal, perinatal, or postnatal periods, in both preterm and term infants (Box 39.1). Prematurity is the leading risk factor for CP, accounting for nearly half of all cases in high-income countries (see Chapter 34). The risk of CP in infants born before 28 weeks of gestation is approximately 50 times that of full-term births (Korzeniewski, Slaughter, Lenski, Haak, & Paneth, N. 2018). Chorioamnionitis, multiple births, and intrauterine growth restriction are additional risk factors.

More than 50% of infants with CP are born at or near term. CP in term infants is associated with placental abnormalities, fetal growth restriction, and (in low-income countries) kernicterus. Approximately, 10% to 15% of children with CP have a cortical brain malformation such as polymicrogyria, schizencephaly, or lissencephaly (Korzeniewski et al., 2018). Perinatal stroke accounts for up to half of all term infants with hemiplegic CP, whereas children with other subtypes of CP often have multifocal or more diffuse injuries (Korzeniewski et al., 2018).

Neurodegenerative, late onset, or atypical movement disorders such as hereditary spastic paraplegia, Rett syndrome, and Lesch-Nyhan syndrome can mimic CP (Pearson, Pons, Ghaoui, & Sue, 2019). Fluctuations in motor impairments or paroxysmal symptoms may suggest an underlying metabolic disorder, for which prompt diagnosis and treatment can improve outcomes (see Chapter 36). Ataxic CP is rare, and other disorders such as Friedreich ataxia or ataxia telangiectasia should be considered. Children with prolonged infantile generalized hypotonia should be evaluated for underlying neuromuscular disorders (see Chapter 30).

MAKING THE DIAGNOSIS

Early identification of motor delays allows for timely referral for developmental interventions, diagnostic evaluations, and treatment planning, which can optimize infant neuroplasticity,

BOX 39.1 Common Causes of Cerebral Palsy

Prenatal (AACPDM, 2017)	Perinatal (Ashwal et al., 2004; Jin et al., 2020; Springer et al., 2019)	Postnatal
Intrauterine strokes	Placental abruption	Central nervous system infections
TORCH (toxoplasmosis, rubella, cytomegalovirus, herpes simplex, other)	Cord prolapse	Cerebrovascular insults
Infections	Uterine rupture	Acquired brain injuries
Maternal toxemia	Kernicterus	Anoxic insults
Congenital brain malformations	Strokes	Progressive hydrocephalus

minimize complications, and enhance caregiver wellbeing. The American Academy of Cerebral Palsy and Developmental Medicine's (AACPDM) care pathway, *Early Detection of CP*, can guide providers in making the diagnosis (2017).

History

Making a diagnosis of CP requires a thorough family, birth, and developmental history. Children with CP must have delays in gross motor development and qualitative motor impairments. Feeding difficulties as well as vision and hearing impairments should be explored. It is crucial to identify developmental regression and distinguish CP from other degenerative conditions.

Physical Examination

The diagnosis of CP requires that a nonprogressive motor abnormality be present. Abnormalities in tone, posture, and motor control can accompany a weak cry, poor suck, tongue thrusting, and irritability during infancy. Children with CP demonstrate persistent or prolonged primitive reflexes, as well as pathologic or absent postural reactions. Serial neurologic exams are helpful in establishing the diagnosis.

Most children with CP have spasticity, dystonia, athetosis, chorea, and/or tremors (see Movement Disorders in Children With CP, later). Upper motor neuron findings, including increased muscle stretch reflexes, clonus, extensor plantar responses, crossed adductor responses, muscle weakness, and decreased selective motor control, are often present. Characteristic patterns of movement include lower extremity extension synergies (hip extension/adduction, knee extension, and ankle plantar flexion) and upper extremity flexion synergies (elbow flexion, wrist flexion, finger flexion, wrist pronation, and thumb adduction). Hypertonicity and impaired selective motor control limit reciprocal movements, contributing to floor mobility via commando crawling, bunny hopping, knee walking, and toe walking. Handedness prior to 1 year of age and asymmetries in movement, such as flexor posturing of an upper limb when walking, should raise suspicion for hemiplegic CP.

Neuroimaging

Neuroimaging can often confirm a clinical diagnosis of CP and provide information regarding etiology, prognosis, associated comorbidities, and treatment options. Cranial ultrasound (CUS) identifies periventricular leukomalacia (PVL) in preterm infants and predicts CP in preterm infants with high specificity. Sequential CUS is recommended as PVL can be missed by a single CUS performed at term equivalent age. Magnetic resonance imaging (MRI), preferred over computed tomography (CT), detects brain abnormalities in nearly 90% of children with CP, particularly in those with prematurity and PVL (Ashwal et al., 2004). Children with dyskinetic CP and no perinatal risk factors tend to have normal MRI (Springer et al., 2019). Children with GMFCS I and II have higher rates of focal vascular insults, whereas those at GMFCS V are more likely to show gray matter injuries and malformations.

Additional Investigations

Approximately, 10% to 15% of children with a clinical diagnosis of CP have a normal brain MRI (Ashwal et al., 2004; Springer et al., 2019). When brain MRI is normal in a child under 2 years of age, repeat imaging is recommended as subtle lesions can be missed at a young age. Currently, a genetic basis can be identified in 10% to 30% of individuals with CP related to either de novo or inherited variants (AACPDM, 2017). In the largest genetic study of CP to date 14% of all cases of CP were found to have a genetic etiology (see Chapter 24) (Jin et al., 2020).

Children with hemiplegic CP related to stroke should be evaluated for coagulopathies, including factor V Leiden mutation, antithrombin deficiency, and protein S deficiency, among others (Ashwal et al., 2004). Prothrombic states have been identified in up to 20% of children with acute ischemic strokes.

CLASSIFICATION OF CEREBRAL PALSY

Classification schemes provide a precise and robust description of children with CP, who historically have been described in terms of the quality and topography of their motor disorders (see Movement Disorders in Children With CP, later). Topography clarifies which limbs are affected: monoplegia involving one limb, diplegia involving both lower limbs, hemiplegia involving one side of the body, triplegia involving three limbs, and quadriplegia involving all four limbs. Because this traditional approach does not capture the functional heterogeneity of children with CP, functional classification schemes are used to standardize communications among families and providers, and to advance research (Table 39.1). These classification schemes are based on a child's usual performance (what is usually done) rather than capability (what the child is able to do).

TABLE 39.1 Cerebral Palsy Classification Schemes

	GMFCS	MACS	EDACS	VSS	FCCS	CFCS	VFCS
Level 1	Walks without limitations	Handles objects easily and successfully	Eats and drinks safely and efficiently	Speech is not affected by motor disorder	Effective communicator in most situations	Independently and effectively alternates between being a sender and receiver of information with most people in most environments	Uses visual function easily and successfully in vision-related activities
Level 2	Walks with limitations	Handles most objects but with some reduced quality and/or speed	Eats and drinks safely but with some limitations to efficiency	Speech is imprecise but usually understandable to unfamiliar listeners Loudness of speech is adequate for one-to-one conversation Voice may be breathy or harsh sounding but does not impair intelligibility Articulation is imprecise Speech is usually understandable to unfamiliar listeners out of context	Effective communicator in most situations, but needs some help	Independently alternates between being a sender and receiver with most people in most environments but the conversation may be slower	Uses visual function successfully but needs self-initiated compensatory strategies
Level 3	Walks using a handheld mobility device	Handles objects with difficulty—needs help to prepare and/or modify activities	Eats and drinks with some limitations to safety; maybe limitations to efficiency	Speech is unclear and not usually understandable to unfamiliar listeners out of context Difficulties controlling breathing for speech—is sometimes too loud or too quiet to be understood Voice may be harsh sounding; pitch may change suddenly Speech may be markedly hypernasal A very small range of consonants are produced Speech is difficult to understand out of context	An effective communicator in some situations Can communicate a small range of messages/topics to most familiar people	Usually communicates effectively with familiar communication partners, but not unfamiliar partners, in most environments	Uses visual function but needs some adaptations

(Continued)

TABLE 39.1 Cerebral Palsy Classification Schemes—cont'd

	GMFCS	MACS	EDACS	VSS	FCCS	CFCS	VFCS
Level 4	Self-mobility with limitations; may use powered mobility	Handles a limited selection of easily managed objects and always requires some help from others	Eats and drinks with significant limitations to safety	No understandable speech	Assistance is required in most situations, especially with unfamiliar people Communicates routine needs and wants with familiar people	Not always consistent at communicating with familiar communication partners	Uses visual function in very adapted environments but performs just part of vision-related activities
Level 5	Transported in a manual wheelchair	The child is not able to handle objects or to complete even simple actions with the hands	Unable to eat or drink safely—tube feeding may be considered to provide nutrition				

The Gross Motor Function Classification System (GMFCS) describes the gross motor abilities of children with CP, with revisions in 2008 to provide additional information by age group and incorporate environmental and personal factors in accordance with the International Classification of Functioning (ICF) and remains stable across time (Palisano, Rosenbaum, Bartlett, & Livingston, 2008). The Manual Ability Classification System (MACS, 2006) is a similar five-level classification scheme that describes how children with CP, ages 4–18 years, use their hands when handling objects in daily activities (Eliasson et al., 2006). The Eating and Drinking Ability Classification System (EDACS) classifies oral motor impairments in children with CP >3 years of age, with proven validity and reliability (Sellers, Mandy, Pennington, Hankins, & Morris, 2014). The Viking Speech Scale (VSS) classifies speech in children ≥4 years of age according to the degree of dysarthria and level of intelligibility to unfamiliar listeners (Pennington et al., 2013). The Functional Communication Classification System (FCCS) describes expressive communication abilities in children ≥4 years of age with CP in a variety of settings (Barty, Caynes, & Johnston, 2016). The Communication Function Classification System (CFCS) describes a child's ability to send and receive information, and to use augmentative and alternative communication (AAC) (Hidecker et al., 2011). Similar to the CFCS, VFCS incorporates adaptive strategies that children may use to support their vision (Baranello et al., 2020).

MOVEMENT DISORDERS IN CHILDREN WITH CP

Spasticity, defined as velocity-dependent resistance to passive range of motion, is the primary movement disorder in 85% of children with CP. Dyskinesia (including dystonia, chorea, or athetosis) is present in 7%. Dystonia involves involuntary sustained or intermittent muscle contractions cause twisting and repetitive movements, abnormal postures, or both. Spasticity and dystonia often coexist. A care pathway, *Dystonia in Cerebral Palsy*, is available to guide clinicians in management as current evidence is limited (AACPDM, 2017).

Managing muscle tone in children with CP is an art and a science. Interventions should be individualized to address each child's abilities and functional goals, with consideration of tone, strength, selective motor control, and balance (Novak et al., 2020). Goals are to maximize function, independence, comfort, and quality of life (QOL) while minimizing sedation and adverse effects (Table 39.2).

Systemic Medications

Although systemic medications can be useful in managing generalized hypertonia, their clinical use must balance functional benefits with adverse effects (Table 39.3).

Injections

Botulinum toxin (BoNT), from the bacteria *Clostridium botulinum*, is used to treat localized spasticity. BoNT binds to the neuromuscular junction and blocks presynaptic release of acetylcholine, thereby weakening targeted muscles. Onset of action is within 2 weeks of administration, duration is 3 to 6 months, and effects wane as the neuromuscular junction reestablishes its original function. Injections should be administered no more frequently than every 3 months to reduce neutralizing antibody formation, which occurs in 1% to 2% of treated individuals (Mathevon, Declemy, Laffont, & Perennou, 2019).

BoNT-A is a safe and effective tool in managing spasticity in children with CP. The most common adverse events include localized pain and weakness, unsteadiness and

TABLE 39.2 Tone Management Strategies

Rehabilitation Strategies	Enteral Medications* Spasticity	Enteral Medications* Dystonia	Injected Medications	Surgery
Therapies Stretching regimen Orthoses	Benzodiazepines Baclofen Clonidine Tizanidine Dantrolene	Benzodiazepines Baclofen Trihexyphenidyl	Botulinum toxin Phenol	Intrathecal baclofen pump Selective dorsal rhizotomy

*See Table 39.3 for dosing guidelines.

TABLE 39.3 Oral Medications for Tone Management in Children: Dosing Guidelines, Pharmacologic Actions, and Adverse Effects

Oral Medication Dosing Guidelines	Pharmacologic Action	Adverse Effects/Precautions
Baclofen **Range:** 0.125–1 mg/kg/day **>4 mo–<2 yr:** 10–20 mg/day divided q8h; max dose 40 mg/day **2–7 yr:** Start 2.5 mg tid; titrate to 20–40 mg/day; max dose 60 mg/day **8–12 yr:** Start 5 mg tid; titrate to 30–40 mg/day; max dose 60 mg/day **>12 yr:** May require q6h dosing; max dose 60–80 mg/day	• Centrally acting, structural analog of GABA • Binds to $GABA_B$ receptors causing presynaptic inhibition of mono/polysynaptic spinal reflexes • Rapid absorption, blood level peaks in 1 hr, half-life 4.5 hr • Renal (>70% unchanged) and feces excretion • Hepatic metabolism (15%)	• CNS effects • Nausea/vomiting • Headache • Hypotonia • Sialorrhea • Asthenia • Urinary retention Abrupt withdrawal may cause seizures, hallucinations, rebound spasticity, and hyperpyrexia Caution advised with renal impairment; dose reduction may be necessary

Diazepam (Novak et al., 2020)
6 mo–12 yr:
0.12–0.8 mg/kg/day PO divided q6-8h; max 10 mg/dose
>12 yr:
2–10 mg PO two to four times daily
Note: Starting a qhs dose only or proportionately larger dose at bedtime may limit excessive daytime sedation.
	• Centrally acting
	• Binds to $GABA_A$ receptors mediating presynaptic inhibition in brainstem reticular formation and spinal polysynaptic pathways
	• Rapid absorption, blood level peaks in 1 hr, half-life of 30–60 hr
		• CNS depression
		• US boxed warnings:
		  • Abuse, misuse, addiction
		  • Dependence and withdrawal reactions
		• Tolerance: long half-life
		• Paradoxic reaction
		• Hypotension
		• Respiratory depression
		• Asthenia
		Use with caution in renal and hepatic impairment

Dantrolene Sodium **>5 yr–adolescence:** Titration <50 kg: 0.5 mg/kg/dose qd-bid for 7 days, then 0.5 mg/kg/dose tid for 7 days, then 1 mg/kg/dose tid for 7 days, then 2 mg/kg tid; max dose 12 mg/kg/day or 400 mg/day Titration >50 kg: 25 mg qd for 7 days, then 25 mg tid for 7 days, then 50 mg tid for 7 days, then 100 mg tid; some patients may require qid dosing; max 400 mg/day	• Peripheral action • Blocking release of calcium from sarcoplasmic reticulum with uncoupling of nerve excitation and skeletal muscle contraction • Blood level peaks in 3–6 hr (active metabolite 4–8 hr) half-life 15 hr	• CNS depression • US boxed warning: • Hepatotoxicity • Nausea • Dysphagia • Muscle weakness Hepatotoxicity: baseline liver function tests MUST be obtained before initiation and monitored regularly but more frequently with dose changes. Discontinue promptly if liver enzymes become elevated.
Tizanidine (Novak et al., 2020) **2–10 yr:** Start 1 mg qhs; titrate to 0.3–0.5 mg/kg/day in three to four divided doses **>10 yr:** Start 2 mg qhs; titrate to 0.3–0.5 mg/kg/day in three to four divided doses; max dose 24 mg/day	• Centrally acting • Alpha-2 adrenoceptor agonist activity at spinal and supraspinal sites; prevents release of excitatory amino acids, facilitating presynaptic inhibition • Good oral absorption, blood level peaks in 1–2 hr, half-life 2.5 hr	• Drowsiness, dizziness • Visual hallucinations • Hypotension (although 10x less antihypertensive potency than clonidine) • Xerostomia • Asthenia Potential for hepatotoxicity: monitor liver function tests at baseline, 1, 3, 6 mo and periodically thereafter Avoid abrupt withdrawal

(Continued)

TABLE 39.3 Oral Medications for Tone Management in Children: Dosing Guidelines, Pharmacologic Actions, and Adverse Effects—cont'd

Oral Medication Dosing Guidelines	Pharmacologic Action	Adverse Effects/Precautions
Trihexyphenidyl ***Children and adolescents:*** Start 0.1–0.2 mg/kg/day in two to three divided doses for 7 days; then titrate every 1–2 wk as tolerated by 0.15 mg/kg/day or by 10%–20%; max dose 0.75 mg/kg/day in three divided doses or 2.6 mg/kg/day in three divided doses	• Selective muscarinic acetylcholine receptor antagonist, blocks cholinergic activity centrally and peripherally; increases the availability of dopamine • Onset of action within 1 hr of oral administration; peak effect 2–3 hr; duration of action 6–12 hr	• CNS effects • Ocular effects: blurred vision; may precipitate angle closure with an increase in intraocular pressure • Anticholinergic effects • Anhidrosis/hyperthermia

bid, Twice a day; *CNS*, central nervous system; *GABA*, gamma-amino butyric acid; *PO*, per os; *tid*, three times a day.

increased falls, fatigue, urinary incontinence, and dysphagia. Systemic adverse effects can occur in up to 3.6% of children with CP receiving BoNT-A, and those with a history of dysphagia and/or aspiration pneumonia are at increased risk (Paget, Swinney, Burton, Bau, & O'Flaherty, S. J., 2018). The US Food and Drug Administration (FDA) requires black box labeling on BoNT products cautioning of a rare but potentially life-threatening complication of BoNT effects spreading beyond the injection site.

Phenol neurolysis nonselectively denatures proteins, thereby interfering with nerve conduction. Phenol injections typically target nerves to large proximal muscles (musculocutaneous, obturator, and sciatic nerves), and the duration of effect may be longer than BoNT. Although the evidence on the use of phenol in children with CP is limited, a few small studies demonstrate its safety and efficacy, with adverse effects including pain, swelling and inflammation, and dysesthesias.

Surgical Management

Surgical management of spasticity can be considered for children with suboptimal tone management despite optimized habilitative and medical interventions.

Intrathecal baclofen (ITB) is FDA approved to treat spasticity of cerebral origin. This route of delivery yields much higher local concentrations in the cerebrospinal fluid at a fraction of the equivalent oral dose of baclofen, thereby minimizing the central nervous system depressive effects (Buizer et al., 2019). Intrathecal catheter tips are typically positioned at C5-T2 but can be placed intraventricularly for severe dystonia. ITB pumps require refills at 2- to 6-month intervals and replacement at 5 to 7 years. In children with CP ITB effectively reduces spasticity and dystonia, and it improves the ease of care and QOL (Buizer et al., 2019).

Nearly 25% of patients encounter ITB complications; most frequent are infections (9%), cerebrospinal fluid leaks (5%), catheter problems (15%), and pump-related problems (1%) (Motta & Antonello, 2014). ITB withdrawal is a medical emergency and must be identified and managed quickly. Symptoms include fever, altered mental status, exaggerated rebound spasticity, and muscle rigidity that, in rare cases, can advance to rhabdomyolysis, multiorgan system failure, and death. Families and health care providers need to be informed of the early symptoms of ITB withdrawal and the critical importance of regular monitoring, refilling, and oversight when this therapy is chosen.

Selective dorsal rhizotomy (SDR) is a neurosurgical procedure that treats muscle spasticity by sectioning hyperexcitatory sensory nerve rootlets that innervate the lower extremities. The procedure involves single or multilevel laminectomies exposing the L2-S1 nerve roots and selective sectioning of sensory rootlets using intraoperative electromyography. Although there is no international consensus regarding the selection of patients for SDR, ideal candidates are children 3 to 8 years of age with spastic diplegic CP, minimal upper limb involvement, good selective motor control, adequate strength to rise from the floor independently, minimal contractures, and good cognitive skills. Adults with CP who underwent SDR as children report higher levels of function, decreased gross motor decline with age, and similar prevalence of pain and fatigue as those who did not undergo SDR (Daunter, Kratz, & Hurvitz, 2017).

Adverse events after SDR include bladder or bowel dysfunction, sensory dysesthesias, and back pain; these occur infrequently and are mostly transient. Although approximately 30% of children with CP develop scoliosis after SDR (Wheelwright et al., 2020), the risk for spinal deformity after SDR has not been established as higher than that in those who have not undergone SDR.

ORTHOPEDIC ISSUES IN CP

Children with CP are at risk of musculoskeletal complications, including contractures, bony deformities, malalignment, hip displacement, and scoliosis. Orthopedic interventions must be individualized to the functional level and goals of each child.

Contractures

Contractures are common in children with CP, particularly in muscles that cross two joints such as the gastrocnemius, rectus femoris, and biceps brachii. In children with GMFCS IV and V, spasticity and postural asymmetry can lead to windswept hips, pelvic obliquity, and joint contractures. Avoidance of contractures begins with regular programs of stretching, strengthening, and positioning. When contractures are mild, serial casting can be effective, often in combination with BoNT therapy (Novak et al., 2020). Fixed contractures may require surgical correction, including multilevel orthopedic surgeries that address hip, knee, and ankle dynamics (Amirmudin, Lavelle, Theologis, Thompson, & Ryan, 2019). Surgical interventions should align with child and family goals and expectations.

Scoliosis

Children with CP are at an increased risk for neuromuscular scoliosis with a prevalence of nearly 30% (Novak et al., 2020). Spasticity, axial hypotonia, and impaired trunk control contribute to scoliosis, which is strongly associated with GMFCS levels. The incidence of neuromuscular scoliosis at GMFCS I and II is similar to that of idiopathic scoliosis in typical children but increases significantly with severity of CP. The risk for severe scoliosis before 16 years of age is highest for those with GMFCS IV and V, female sex, epilepsy, and limited knee extension at the age of 5 years (Pettersson et al., 2020). Scoliosis surveillance for children with CP is indicated from a young age and into adulthood at a frequency determined by risk and rate of progression.

The evidence for managing scoliosis with postural seating systems and bracing is limited. Bracing does not prevent the long-term progression of neuromuscular scoliosis and is often poorly tolerated. Spinal fusion is typically performed when curves exceed 50 degrees, with the goals of reducing curves and pelvic obliquity, and improving child and family QOL and comfort. However, complication rates are moderately high. The decision to proceed with spinal fusion requires thoughtful individualized assessments of risk and benefit, with a preoperative assessment of each child's overall health and medical stability.

Spastic Hip Dysplasia

Children with CP can develop spastic hip displacement with progressive femoral head subluxation and dislocation associated with pain, decreased function, difficulty with positioning, and reduced QOL. Monitoring for hip subluxation is essential throughout childhood as described in the *Hip Surveillance in Cerebral Palsy* care pathway (AACPDM, 2017). Hip subluxation refers to partial femoral head displacement out of the acetabulum, and dislocation refers to its complete displacement. Children at GMFCS I have a low risk of hip displacement, while those with GMFCS V have a 68% to 90% risk (Miller et al., 2017). *Hip Surveillance in Cerebral Palsy* recommends clinical and baseline AP pelvis radiographic examinations at 2 years of age, followed by intervals tailored to individual risk factors (age, GMFCS levels, rate of migration progression) (AACPDM, 2017). Hip displacement progresses after skeletal maturity, particularly in those with neuromuscular scoliosis, pelvic obliquity, leg length discrepancies, and GMFCS III through V.

EVALUATION AND MANAGEMENT OF PAIN

Pain warrants regular attention in individuals with CP. Pain can originate from multiple sites, yet cognitive and communication impairments can limit description of symptoms (see Chapters 64 and 78). Both acute and chronic pain can negatively impact function and QOL (see Life Expectancy and Quality of Life, later). Nearly 70% of children with CP reported acute pain, and 42% reported both acute and chronic pain; children reported that pain interfered with sleep, attention, and play (Ostojic, Paget, Kyriagis, & Morrow, 2020). Acute pain can be associated with iatrogenic interventions, including splinting, serial casting, and BoNT injections. Clinicians must consider how well-intended interventions might contribute to pain. Pain management in children with CP can include over-the-counter analgesics, muscle relaxants, reflux medications, and laxatives as spasticity, gastroesophageal reflux disease (GERD), and constipation are common sources of pain.

BONE HEALTH EVALUATION AND MANAGEMENT

Children with CP are at risk for impairments of growth and nutrition. The consequences of restricted growth and suboptimal nutrition are significant, including reduced bone mineral density (BMD), muscle mass, function, and overall wellbeing.

Bone modeling and remodeling is a dynamic process that begins *in utero*, continues into adolescence, and peaks in early adulthood. Muscle activity and mechanical stresses upon the growing skeleton stimulate bone deposition. Variations in muscle tone, strength, and weight-bearing status can greatly influence bone development in children with CP. Delayed puberty and sexual maturation can reduce the peak strength and load-bearing capacity of bone. Children with CP are threatened by immobility, both chronically and during acute phases of casting or postoperative healing. Immobilization reduces muscle bulk, mechanical forces on bones, and ultimately bone quality.

Prevention of osteoporosis involves ensuring appropriate intake of calcium, phosphorus, vitamin D, zinc, and magnesium. Certain medications can negatively impact bone density. Anticonvulsants, chronic steroids, antidepressants, proton pump inhibitors, and medroxyprogesterone acetate can negatively affect bone health.

Assessing bone density is an important step in diagnosing osteoporosis, planning surgeries, and monitoring responses to bisphosphonate therapy. The current gold standard is dual-energy x-ray absorptiometry (DXA). However, DXA can be limited by contractures, artifacts from indwelling devices (orthopedic hardware, ITB pumps, feeding tubes, shunts), and the availability of pediatric reference values. Ambulatory status, physical development, gender, and pubertal status are important considerations in the interpretation of results.

CP is the most prevalent childhood condition associated with low BMD. Although low BMD is asymptomatic, painful fragility fractures can occur with little or no trauma. They most frequently occur in the distal femur and are 20% more common in nonambulatory children (Ozel, Switzer, Macintosh, & Fehlings, 2016). Fracture risk in children with CP nearly doubles per year after the first fracture. A few small and uncontrolled studies suggest benefits of static standing on bone health.

Bisphosphonates are often used to treat osteoporosis in children. They are not recommended for prevention because of uncertainty about long-term impacts on growing bones. Close monitoring for acute phase reaction (fever, bone pain, nausea, vomiting), hypocalcemia, and hypophosphatemia is necessary. Osteonecrosis of the jaw and atypical femur fractures are rarely seen in adults but not yet reported in children. Overall there is probable evidence for bisphosphonates, possible evidence for vitamin D/calcium, and insufficient evidence for weight-bearing activities as effective interventions to improve low BMD in children with CP. There is possible evidence for bisphosphonates in reducing fragility fractures. The care pathway, *Osteoporosis in Cerebral Palsy*, offers guidance to health care providers (AACPDM, 2017).

GROWTH

Growth charts are the gold standard by which pediatricians monitor the overall health of children. These charts are suboptimal in assessing the growth of children with CP, thus CP-specific growth charts have been developed, stratified by GMFCS (Brooks, Day, Shavelle, & Strauss, 2011). Knee height, upper arm length, midupper arm muscle area, triceps skinfold, and subscapular skinfold thickness are used to assess growth and body composition but can be inaccurate due to joint contractures, scoliosis, and involuntary movements. Weight for height and body mass index measures do not accurately reflect fat stores in nearly half of all children with CP, who tend to have adequate fat but low muscle mass.

Children with CP often have impaired nutritional intake and growth. Despite gastrostomy tube feedings, most children with CP remain small. Growth is driven by nutritive and nonnutritive factors as evidenced in the side-to-side differences in limb length and muscle bulk characteristics of children with hemiplegic CP. There are also clear relationships between low weights, number of associated chronic conditions, and increased risk of death (Brooks et al., 2011). Even well-nourished children with CP show a decline in growth with age and often lack the pubertal growth spurt characteristic of typically growing adolescents. The nutritional status of children with CP is best assessed longitudinally, following trends over time with multifaceted indices and in regular consultation with dieticians.

Puberty

Puberty begins earlier and ends later for children with moderate to severe CP and can be confused with premature adrenarche. Anticipatory guidance regarding sexuality and puberty is often sparse or nonexistent. Parents often seek information on menstrual management from other parents, schools, and informal social groups. Pediatric providers can be a source of sexuality education and advocacy for safety and abuse prevention for children with CP and their families.

Menarche can be a challenging time for girls with CP. Hormonal cycles may bring mood fluctuations, pain and spasticity changes, and catamenial seizures. Although the onset of puberty tends to be early, menarche occurs later in girls with CP. Initially, menstrual cycles can be quite irregular for 2 to 3 years. Menstrual management should be tailored to the needs of each child and family. Depot medroxyprogesterone acetate is less often recommended as it contributes to low bone density. The American Academy of Pediatrics clinical report on menstrual management for adolescents with disabilities is a ready resource (Quint, O'Brien, Committee on Adolescence, & The North American Society for Pediatric and Adolescent Gynecology, 2016).

As part of guiding adolescents from childhood to adulthood it is essential to address issues of sexuality. Pregnancy prevention, protection against sexually transmitted infections, and issues of sexual violence and abuse should be openly discussed with confidential, developmentally appropriate approaches (see Chapter 74).

Growth Attenuation

In 2006 a case report of growth attenuation with high-dose estrogen for a child with severe, permanent disability brought widespread attention to a common and complex problem (Gunther & Diekema, 2006). As children with CP grow, families can be challenged by the physical demands of caregiving. High-dose estrogen stimulates early closure of growth plates, reduces overall stature, and can sustain care at home. Naturally occurring precocious puberty can also lead to short stature, and nontreatment is an acceptable decision. Overall, growth attenuation is a sufficiently safe therapy that offers the possibility of an improved QOL for nonambulatory children with profound cognitive disability. Pediatric endocrinologists report that families often request growth attenuation therapy (see Chapter 111).

Gastrointestinal and Nutrition Issues

Many children with CP have dysphagia and require assistance with feeding. In contrast to swallowing, feeding is influenced by child and caregiver interactions, as well as child behaviors (see Chapter 65). Impaired swallowing can threaten lung health (see Pulmonary Concerns, later), and impaired feeding skills can detract from nonfeeding activities and threaten adequacy of intake. It is estimated that 50% of children with CP have swallowing problems, and 54% have feeding problems, with direct correlations with GMFCS levels (Speyer et al., 2019). When evaluating swallowing and feeding issues, goals of care must be explored. In some instances oral feeding is deemed a key part of QOL, and families might decline enteral feeding regardless of risk. Other families may perceive the need for a feeding tube as a parenting failure. Even with dysphagia, most children can safely receive tastes of food for pleasure and inclusion in family meals.

Constipation affects 25% to 74% of children with CP and is one of the leading reasons for hospitalization (Vande Velde, Van Renterghem, Van Winkel, De Bruyne, & Van Biervliet,, 2018). Severity of constipation is associated with severity of CP, as well as the use of antiepileptic medications, benzodiazepines, and proton pump inhibitors. Management includes dietary changes, adequate hydration, and medications. Constipation can exacerbate spasticity and dystonia and warrants prompt identification and management.

PULMONARY CONCERNS

Respiratory disease is a major cause of morbidity and mortality for people with CP. Aspiration, nutritional status, airway clearance, upper airway function, and scoliosis can impact lung function. Children with CP are at increased risk of hospitalization for respiratory compromise if they have GMFCS V, at least one hospital admission for respiratory illness in the previous year, oropharyngeal dysphagia, active seizures, frequent respiratory symptoms, GERD, at least two courses of antibiotics for respiratory infection in the past year, mealtime respiratory symptoms, and nightly snoring (Box 39.2) (Gibson et al., 2021). Aspiration can occur because of dysphagia (see Gastrointestinal and Nutrition Issues, earlier) and/or saliva, either overtly or silently. The care pathway, *Sialorrhea in Cerebral Palsy*, offers strategies for evaluation and management (AACPDM, 2017).

Sleep disorders occur in approximately 20% of children with CP (see Chapter 70) (Horwood, Mok, Li, Oskoui, Shevell, & Constantin, 2018). Poor sleep impacts both the child's and family's physical and mental health (Horwood, Mok, Li, Oskoui, Shevell, & Constantin,, 2019). Additionally, 10% to 25% of children with CP have sleep-disordered breathing, particularly those who are older and those with higher GMFCS levels, multiple comorbidities including seizures, and auditory, visual, and cognitive impairments (Horwood et al., 2019). Environmental factors (bed-sharing, caregiver sleep issues, nocturnal orthoses) can affect sleep.

GYNECOLOGIC AND UROLOGIC ISSUES

Mature bladder and bowel continence requires close integration of the autonomic and somatic nervous systems, with complex control at the level of the brain and spinal cord (see Chapter 68). Children with CP achieve daytime and nighttime bladder and bowel continence more slowly and less completely than typical children, with 61% being continent by day and 55% by night at the age of 17 years. The majority (88%) of children with CP GMFCS I and II attain daytime and nighttime continence by 5.5 years of age. GMFCS level and intellectual ability are strongly associated with continence, and those at GMFCS V are not likely to attain continence (Wright, Fletcher, Scrutton, & Baird, 2016).

BOX 39.2 Prevention and Management of Respiratory Disease in Children With Cerebral Palsy (CP) (Gibson et al., 2021)

Recognizing and Managing Risks to Prevent Respiratory Illness in Children With CP

Consensus-Based Recommendations

- Discuss increased risk with any child with GMFCS V*
- Discuss increased risk with any child with EDACS III, IV, or V*
- Manage comorbidities that increase aspiration risk (dysphagia, uncontrolled seizures, reflux, sialorrhea)
- Provide techniques that optimize cough and manage secretions
- Optimize positioning for lung expansion
- Refer to specialists as needed for evaluation of apnea and snoring
- Consider therapies that optimize chest wall mobility; regularly assess and manage scoliosis
- Optimize nutrition
- Regular dental care to decrease bacterial burden that can cause respiratory disease
- Yearly flu vaccine for children and their family members
- Avoid tobacco exposure

Practice Points

- Promote physical activity

Assessment of Respiratory Health in Children With CP

Consensus-Based Recommendations

- Multidisciplinary assessment
- Obtain detailed history, including GMFCS, EDACS, epilepsy, GERD, drooling, aspiration, wheezy or noisy breathing
- Obtain history of respiratory illness in the past year, including antibiotic use, hospital admissions, and need for noninvasive ventilatory support
- Baseline physical exam, including assessment of breathing pattern, respiratory rate, work of breathing, chest wall shape, palpation, auscultation, tonsils, oxygen saturation; assess nutritional status and aspiration risk; evaluate for skeletal deformities
- Order studies as indicated, including VFSS to evaluate aspiration, sleep study, and chest imaging to help guide treatment

Treatment of Respiratory Illness in CP

Consensus-Based Recommendations

- Low threshold for treatment of respiratory illness
- Ensure nutrition adequate to promote healing
- Consider referral to PT for positioning strategies that optimize lung function
- Consider chest physiotherapy, suctioning, airway clearance regimen in appropriate patients**
- Reassess dysphagia when sick and consider alternate route of nutrition

EDACS, Eating and Drinking Ability Classification System; *GERD*, gastroesophageal reflux disease; *GMFCS*, Gross Motor Function Classification System; *PT*, physical therapy; *VFSS*, videofluoroscopic swallowing study.

*See Classification of Cerebral Palsy for more information on GMFCS and EDACS.

**No consensus reached on use of mechanical assistive devices to help with airway clearance.

Children with CP often have detrusor sphincter dyssynergia and impairments of upper motor neuron control. Vesicoureteral reflux and hydronephrosis are infrequent complications, and routine screening is not necessary unless there are issues of retention, urinary tract infection, stones, or other symptoms. With communication, mobility, and environmental modifications, many children with CP can attain continence in adulthood (see Chapter 69).

Sexual Health

The experience of intimate and sexual relationships is an integral element of human development. Teens with physical disabilities tend to become less socially active and more isolated with age, whereas those without disabilities become more socially active. Young adults with CP have less experience with romantic relationships and sexual activities. Most describe physical problems with sex related to CP itself, emotional barriers to intimacy, and the need for more information on sexuality and reproduction. For people with CP, functional limitations are perceived barriers to dating and are strongly influenced by environmental (family, peers, attitudes, accessibility, transportation) and personal factors (psychological adaptation, self-efficacy, sexual self-esteem). Open discussions are needed to inform and support this important and often overlooked element of human development across the life span (see Chapter 74).

VISION AND HEARING ISSUES

CP is "often accompanied by disturbances of sensation," including vision, hearing, and other sensory modalities (Rosenbaum et al., 2006). Vision impairments can be peripheral and/or central, and 60% to 70% of children with CP have cortical visual impairment (Fazzi et al., 2012). Children with quadriplegic CP tend to have more severe visual impairments when compared to those with diplegic CP. It is important for children with CP to undergo regular eye exams. The impact of visual impairment on visual ability can be classified using the Visual Function Classification Scale (VFCS) (see Table 39.2) (Baranello et al., 2020). Approximately, 8% of children with CP have hearing loss, and those with higher GMFCS levels or dyskinetic or hypotonic CP are most likely to be affected (see Chapters 42 and 43).

MENTAL HEALTH CONSIDERATIONS

Mental health symptoms affect nearly one-third of children with CP, and 20% have a clinically diagnosed psychiatric illness (Downs et al., 2018). Limited physical activity and the presence of pain contribute to depression (see Chapters 49 and 51). Autism spectrum disorders and attention-deficit/hyperactivity disorder affect up to 30% of children with CP (see Chapters 46 and 54).

Mothers of children with CP are 2.5 times more likely to experience depression than are mothers of typical children (Barreto et al., 2020). Depression in mothers of children with CP is associated with higher GMFCS levels, poor sleep, and greater time spent providing care for their child (Barreto et al., 2020). At the time of diagnosis, parents often mourn the loss of a typically developing child and grapple with the uncertainties of CP.

LIFE EXPECTANCY AND QUALITY OF LIFE

QOL is an individual's perception of one's position in life, in the context of the culture and value systems in which the person lives and in relation to the person's goals, expectations, standards, and concerns. Although teens with CP report their QOL to be similar to that of the general population, parents perceive the QOL of their children with CP to be lower. Parents have difficulties interpreting the world through the eyes of their children, and providers can share with parents an optimistic view of the self-reported QOL of children with CP (Boldyreva, Streiner, Rosenbaum, & Ronen, 2020).

Persons with CP have life expectancies similar to that of the general population. Updated life expectancy calculations take mobility and feeding status into consideration. For example, the life expectancy of a female with CP who is enterally fed and dependent for mobility is 28 years, that of a female with CP who eats and ambulates independently is 70 years, and that of the general female population is 80 years (Strauss, Brooks, Rosenbloom, & Shavelle,, 2008). Similarly, the health-related QOL of young adults with CP is comparable to that of the general population. While physical health is better in individuals with GMFCS I and II, mental health is poorer (Jacobson, Löwing, & Tedroff, 2020). Young adults with CP describe fatigue, pain, and anxiety that occur daily and interfere with sleep, work, and daily functioning. Many lack adult health care services and opportunities to engage in meaningful and appropriate employment and social activities. Although CP is a nonprogressive neurologic condition, adults with CP experience an age-related premature decline in mobility and function. Opportunities to exercise, socialize, and stay strong benefit persons with CP across the life span.

REHABILITATION THERAPIES

A key benefit of an early diagnosis of CP is early initiation of therapies (see Chapters 103, 106–110), which is associated with improved outcomes. Early intervention services (see Chapter 103), schools, home health agencies, or outpatient centers provide therapeutic options. Bimanual training, constraint-induced movement therapy, goal-directed training, and occupational therapy post-BoNT are effective interventions (Novak et al., 2020). Active therapies are more beneficial than passive modalities. Hippotherapy, dance, and aquatic therapies can improve posture, balance, and overall fitness.

Participation

Children with CP may need accommodations to promote active and full participation in various aspects of their lives. A creative new framework called *F-Words* characterizes the

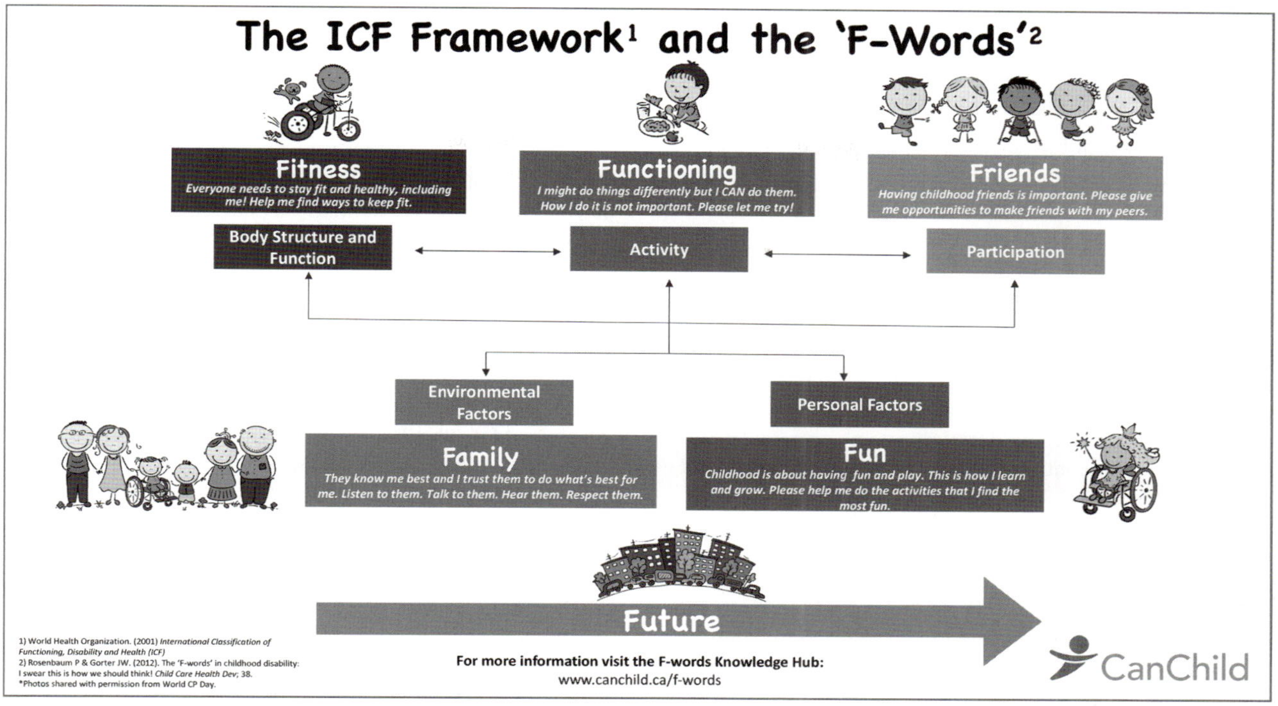

Fig. 39.1 International Classification of Functioning (ICF) framework and the F-Words. (From CanChild. https://www.canchild.ca/en/research-in-practice/f-words-in-childhood-disability)

function and participation of children with disabilities, placing a strong emphasis on children's capabilities rather than their impairments (Fig. 39.1) (Rosenbaum & Gorter, 2012).

Orthoses and Durable Medical Equipment

Children with CP often benefit from orthoses to maintain range of motion and improve function, and adaptive equipment to promote mobility and participation. Children with CP GMFCS III through V navigate with the support of mobility devices such as gait trainers, walkers, crutches, adaptive strollers, manual wheelchairs, and power wheelchairs. Other devices to consider are standers, overhead lift systems, bath equipment, hospital beds, and home modifications. While durable medical equipment is often covered by insurance, home modifications and vehicle modifications usually require additional sources of funding.

CONCLUSION

Thinking back to our case study of Anna, a 13-year-old girl with spastic quadriplegic CP GMFCS IV, we see key points on the topic of CP emerge. Her diagnosis is consistent with her history and neuroimaging, and she has benefited from early intervention, educational programs, and adaptive equipment as well as medical and surgical treatments for her musculoskeletal and associated conditions of dysphagia, seizures, dysmenorrhea, and osteopenia. With goal-directed care that includes Anna, her family, interdisciplinary health care providers, and community programs, she can continue to enjoy QOL and the approach of adulthood in good health and optimal functions.

REFERENCES

AACPDM: Care Pathways. (2017). AACPDM Care Pathways. https://www.aacpdm.org/publications/care-pathways

Amirmudin, N. A., Lavelle, G., Theologis, T., Thompson, N., & Ryan, J. M. (2019). Multilevel Surgery for Children With Cerebral Palsy: A Meta-analysis. *Pediatrics*, *143*(4). https://doi.org/10.1542/peds.2018-3390

Ashwal, S., Russman, B. S., Blasco, P. A., Miller, G., Sandler, A., Shevell, M., & Stevenson, R. (2004). Practice parameter: diagnostic assessment of the child with cerebral palsy: report of the Quality Standards Subcommittee of the American Academy of Neurology and the Practice Committee of the Child Neurology Society Quality Standards Subcommittee of the American Academy of, N., & Practice Committee of the Child Neurology, S. *Neurology*, *62*(6), 851–863. https://doi.org/10.1212/01.wnl.0000117981.35364.1b

Baranello, G., Signorini, S., Tinelli, F., Guzzetta, A., Pagliano, E., Rossi, A., … Group, V. S. (2020). Visual Function Classification System for children with cerebral palsy: development and validation. *Developmental Medicine and Child Neurology*, *62*(1), 104–110. https://doi.org/10.1111/dmcn.14270

Barreto, T. M., Bento, M. N., Barreto, T. M., Jagersbacher, J. G., Jones, N. S., Lucena, R., & Bandeira, I. D. (2020). Prevalence of depression, anxiety, and substance-related disorders in parents of children with cerebral palsy: a systematic review 2020-02-01. *Developmental Medicine & Child Neurology*, *62*(2), 163–168. https://doi.org/10.1111/dmcn.14321

Barty, E., Caynes, K., & Johnston, L. M. (2016). Development and reliability of the Functional Communication Classification System for children with cerebral palsy. *Developmental Medicine and Child Neurology*, *58*(10), 1036–1041. https://doi.org/10.1111/dmcn.13124

Boldyreva, U., Streiner, D. L., Rosenbaum, P. L., & Ronen, G. M. (2020). Quality of life in adolescents with epilepsy, cerebral palsy, and population norms 05. *Developmental Medicine and Child Neurology*, *62*(5), 609–614. https://doi.org/10.1111/dmcn.14450

Brooks, J., Day, S., Shavelle, R., & Strauss, D. (2011). Low Weight, Morbidity, and Mortality in Children With Cerebral Palsy: New Clinical Growth Charts 2011-08-01. *Pediatrics*, *128*(2), e299–e307. https://doi.org/10.1542/peds.2010-2801

Buizer, A. I., Martens, B. H. M., Grandbois van Ravenhorst, C., Schoonmade, L. J., Becher, J. G., & Vermeulen, R. J. (2019). Effect of continuous intrathecal baclofen therapy in children: a systematic review. *Developmental Medicine and Child Neurology*, *61*(2), 128–134. https://doi.org/10.1111/dmcn.14005

Daunter, A. K., Kratz, A. L., & Hurvitz, E. A. (2017). Long-term impact of childhood selective dorsal rhizotomy on pain, fatigue, and function: a case-control study. *Developmental Medicine and Child Neurology*, *59*(10), 1089–1095. https://doi.org/10.1111/dmcn.13481

Downs, J., Blackmore, A. M., Epstein, A., Skoss, R., Langdon, K., Jacoby, P., … Glasson, E. J. (2018). The prevalence of mental health disorders and symptoms in children and adolescents with cerebral palsy: a systematic review and meta-analysis 2018-01-01. *Developmental Medicine & Child Neurology*, *60*(1), 30–38. https://doi.org/10.1111/dmcn.13555

Eliasson, A. C., Krumlinde-Sundholm, L., Rosblad, B., Beckung, E., Arner, M., Ohrvall, A. M., & Rosenbaum, P. (2006). The Manual Ability Classification System (MACS) for children with cerebral palsy: scale development and evidence of validity and reliability. *Developmental Medicine and Child Neurology*, *48*(7), 549–554. https://doi.org/10.1017/S0012162206001162

Fazzi, E., Signorini, S. G., La Piana, R., Bertone, C., Misefari, W., Galli, J., … Bianchi, P. E. (2012). Neuro-ophthalmological disorders in cerebral palsy: ophthalmological, oculomotor, and visual aspects 2012-08-01. *Developmental Medicine & Child Neurology*, *54*(8), 730–736. https://doi.org/10.1111/j.1469-8749.2012.04324.x

Gibson, N., Blackmore, A. M., Chang, A. B., Cooper, M. S., Jaffe, A., Kong, W. R., … Wilson, A. C. (2021). Prevention and management of respiratory disease in young people with cerebral palsy: consensus statement 2021-02-01. *Developmental Medicine & Child Neurology*, *63*(2), 172–182. https://doi.org/10.1111/dmcn.14640

Gunther, D. F., & Diekema, D. S. (2006). Attenuating Growth in Children With Profound Developmental Disability 2006-10-01. *Archives of Pediatrics & Adolescent Medicine*, *160*(10), 1013. https://doi.org/10.1001/archpedi.160.10.1013

Hidecker, M. J., Paneth, N., Rosenbaum, P. L., Kent, R. D., Lillie, J., Eulenberg, J. B., … Taylor, K. (2011). Developing and validating the Communication Function Classification System for individuals with cerebral palsy. *Developmental Medicine and Child Neurology*, *53*(8), 704–710. https://doi.org/10.1111/j.1469-8749.2011.03996.x

Horwood, L., Li, P., Mok, E., Shevell, M., & Constantin, E. (2019). A systematic review and meta-analysis of the prevalence of sleep problems in children with cerebral palsy: how do children with cerebral palsy differ from each other and from typically developing children? *Sleep Health*, *5*(6), 555–571. https://doi.org/10.1016/j.sleh.2019.08.006

Horwood, L., Mok, E., Li, P., Oskoui, M., Shevell, M., & Constantin, E. (2018). Prevalence of sleep problems and sleep-related characteristics in preschool- and school-aged children with cerebral palsy. *Sleep Medicine*, *50*, 1–6. https://doi.org/10.1016/j.sleep.2018.05.008

Jacobson, D. N. O., Löwing, K., & Tedroff, K. (2020). Health-related quality of life, pain, and fatigue in young adults with cerebral palsy. *Developmental Medicine and Child Neurology*, *62*(3), 372–378. https://doi.org/10.1111/dmcn.14413

Jin, S. C., Lewis, S. A., Bakhtiari, S., Zeng, X., Sierant, M. C., Shetty, S., … Kruer, M. C. (2020). Mutations disrupting neuritogenesis genes confer risk for cerebral palsy. *Nature Genetics*, *52*(10), 1046–1056. https://doi.org/10.1038/s41588-020-0695-1

Korzeniewski, S. J., Slaughter, J., Lenski, M., Haak, P., & Paneth, N. (2018). The complex aetiology of cerebral palsy. *Nature Reviews Neurology*, *14*(9), 528–543. https://doi.org/10.1038/s41582-018-0043-6

Maenner, M. J., Blumberg, S. J., Kogan, M. D., Christensen, D., Yeargin-Allsopp, M., & Schieve, L. A. (2016). Prevalence of cerebral palsy and intellectual disability among children identified in two U.S. National Surveys, 2011–2013 2016-03-01. *Annals of Epidemiology*, *26*(3), 222–226. https://doi.org/10.1016/j.annepidem.2016.01.001

Mathevon, L., Declemy, A., Laffont, I., & Perennou, D. (2019). Immunogenicity induced by botulinum toxin injections for limb spasticity: A systematic review. *Annals of Physical and Rehabilitation Medicine*, *62*(4), 241–251. https://doi.org/10.1016/j.rehab.2019.03.004

Miller, S. D., Juricic, M., Hesketh, K., Mclean, L., Magnuson, S., Gasior, S., … Mulpuri, K. (2017). Prevention of hip displacement in children with cerebral palsy: a systematic review. *Developmental Medicine and Child Neurology*, *59*(11), 1130–1138. https://doi.org/10.1111/dmcn.13480

Motta, F., & Antonello, C. E. (2014). Analysis of complications in 430 consecutive pediatric patients treated with intrathecal baclofen therapy: 14-year experience. *Journal of Neurosurgery: Pediatrics*, *13*(3), 301–306. https://doi.org/10.3171/2013.11.PEDS13253

Novak, I., Morgan, C., Fahey, M., Finch-Edmondson, M., Galea, C., Hines, A., … Badawi, N. (2020). State of the Evidence Traffic Lights 2019: Systematic Review of Interventions for Preventing and Treating Children with Cerebral Palsy 2020-02-01. *Current neurology and neuroscience reports*, *20*(2). https://doi.org/10.1007/s11910-020-1022-z

Ostojic, K., Paget, S., Kyriagis, M., & Morrow, A. (2020). Acute and Chronic Pain in Children and Adolescents With Cerebral Palsy: Prevalence, Interference, and Management. *Archives of Physical Medicine and Rehabilitation*, *101*(2), 213–219. https://doi.org/10.1016/j.apmr.2019.08.475

Ozel, S., Switzer, L., Macintosh, A., & Fehlings, D. (2016). Informing evidence-based clinical practice guidelines for children with cerebral palsy at risk of osteoporosis: an update. *Developmental Medicine and Child Neurology*, *58*(9), 918–923. https://doi.org/10.1111/dmcn.13196

Paget, S. P., Swinney, C. M., Burton, K. L. O., Bau, K., & O'Flaherty, S. J. (2018). Systemic adverse events after botulinum neurotoxin A injections in children with cerebral palsy. *Developmental Medicine and Child Neurology*, *60*(11), 1172–1177. https://doi.org/10.1111/dmcn.13995

Palisano, R. J., Rosenbaum, P., Bartlett, D., & Livingston, M. H. (2008). Content validity of the expanded and revised Gross Motor Function Classification System. *Developmental Medicine and Child Neurology*, *50*(10), 744–750. https://doi.org/10.1111/j.1469-8749.2008.03089.x

Pearson, T. S., Pons, R., Ghaoui, R., & Sue, C. M. (2019). Genetic mimics of cerebral palsy. *Movement Disorders*, *34*(5), 625–636. https://doi.org/10.1002/mds.27655

Pennington, L., Virella, D., Mjoen, T., da Graca Andrada, M., Murray, J., Colver, A., … de la Cruz, J. (2013). Development of The Viking Speech Scale to classify the speech of children with cerebral palsy. *Research in Developmental Disabilities*, *34*(10), 3202–3210. https://doi.org/10.1016/j.ridd.2013.06.035

Pettersson, K., Wagner, P., & Rodby-Bousquet, E. (2020). Development of a risk score for scoliosis in children with cerebral palsy. *Acta orthopaedica*, *91*(2), 203–208. https://doi.org/10.1080/17453674.2020.1711621

Quint, E. H., O'Brien, R. F., ADOLESCENCE, C. O., & Gynecology, N. A. S. f P. a A. (2016). Menstrual Management for Adolescents With Disabilities. *Pediatrics*, *138*(1). https://doi.org/10.1542/peds.2016-0295

Rosenbaum, P., & Gorter, J. W. (2012). The 'F-words' in childhood disability: I swear this is how we should think! Child: Care 2012-07-01. *Health and Development*, *38*(4), 457–463. https://doi.org/10.1111/j.1365-2214.2011.01338.x

Rosenbaum, P., Paneth, N., Leviton, A., Goldstein, M., Bax, M., Damiano, D., … Jacobsson, B. (2007). A report: the definition and classification of cerebral palsy April 2006. *Developmental Medicine and Child Neurology. Supplement*, *109*, 8–14. https://www.ncbi.nlm.nih.gov/pubmed/17370477

Sellers, D., Mandy, A., Pennington, L., Hankins, M., & Morris, C. (2014). Development and reliability of a system to classify the eating and drinking ability of people with cerebral palsy. *Developmental Medicine and Child Neurology*, *56*(3), 245–251. https://doi.org/10.1111/dmcn.12352

Speyer, R., Cordier, R., Kim, J. H., Cocks, N., Michou, E., & Wilkes-Gillan, S. (2019). Prevalence of drooling, swallowing, and feeding problems in cerebral palsy across the lifespan: a systematic review and meta-analyses , 2019-11-01. *Developmental Medicine & Child Neurology*, *61*(11), 1249–1258. https://doi.org/10.1111/dmcn.14316

Springer, A., Dyck Holzinger, S., Andersen, J., Buckley, D., Fehlings, D., Kirton, A., … Shevell, M. (2019). Profile of children with cerebral palsy spectrum disorder and a normal MRI study. *Neurology*, *93*(1), e88–e96. https://doi.org/10.1212/WNL.0000000000007726

Strauss, D., Brooks, J., Rosenbloom, L., & Shavelle, R. (2008). Life expectancy in cerebral palsy: an update. *Developmental Medicine and Child Neurology*, *50*(7), 487–493. https://doi.org/10.1111/j.1469-8749.2008.03000.x

Vande Velde, S., Van Renterghem, K., Van Winkel, M., De Bruyne, R., & Van Biervliet, S. (2018). Constipation and fecal incontinence in children with cerebral palsy. Overview of literature and flowchart for a stepwise approach. *Acta Gastro-Enterologica Belgica*, *81*(3), 415–418. https://www.ncbi.nlm.nih.gov/pubmed/30350531

Wheelwright, M., Selvey, P. J., Steinbok, P., Singhal, A., Ibrahim, G., Fallah, A., … Tu, A. (2020). Systematic review of spinal deformities following multi-level selective dorsal rhizotomy. *Child's Nervous System*, *36*(5), 1025–1035. https://doi.org/10.1007/s00381-019-04375-x

Wright, A. J., Fletcher, O., Scrutton, D., & Baird, G. (2016). Bladder and bowel continence in bilateral cerebral palsy: A population study. *Journal of pediatric urology*, *12*(6), 383. https://doi.org/10.1016/j.jpurol.2016.05.027. e381–383.e388.

40

Intellectual Disability

Sandra L. Friedman and Ellen Roy Elias

For additional material related to the content of this chapter, please see Chapters 25, 29, 34, 39, and 59.

VIGNETTE

A 6-year-old boy is seen in your office for concern that he lost developmental skills over the past year. He has displayed progressive difficulties moving, speaking, and caring for himself. He had mildly delayed early developmental milestones, for which he received early intervention services. He has had an individualized education plan (IEP) since preschool, providing him with language, motor, and early childhood special education services. Birth, medical, family medical, and social history were unremarkable.

On physical exam, his weight, height, and head circumference were all between the 5th and 10th percentile. He answered simple questions in phrases and short sentences, with moderately reduced speech intelligibility. On neurologic exam, he presented with mildly reduced axial and appendicular muscle tone, and his gait was ataxic. On cognitive testing, his full-scale IQ was 69, without a significant split between his verbal and nonverbal skills. His adaptive behavior composite standard score was 55, with social skills an area of relative strength and motor and daily living skills areas of relative weakness.

Chromosomal microarray analysis (CMA) and DNA testing for fragile X were unremarkable. Brain magnetic resonance imaging with axial T2-weighted images showed focal discrete bilaterally symmetric hyperintensity in the basal ganglia and brainstem. Serum lactate was elevated, and serum pyruvate was low in comparison to the lactate. Muscle biopsy was done to obtain respiratory chain enzymes in cultured fibroblasts, showing severe reduction in Complex IV activity, also known as cytochrome c oxidase (COX) or Leigh syndrome. This was followed by obtaining positive mitochondrial DNA consistent with this diagnosis.

INTELLECTUAL DISABILITY: EVOLUTION OF TERMINOLOGY

The history of disability is outlined in Chapter 1. Just as the conceptualization of people with disabilities, their rights to integrate within the community, and calls for self-determination have evolved over time, so has the terminology to reflect public perception and understanding of intellectual disability (ID). The American Association on Intellectual and Developmental Disabilities (AAIDD) is the oldest professional disability organization in the United States. In 1876 this organization was called the Association of Medical Officers of American Institutions for Idiotic and Feebleminded Persons; in 1906 the name was changed to the American Association for the Study of the Feebleminded, in 1933 to the American Association on Mental Deficiency, and in 1987 to the American Association on Mental Retardation. The AAIDD has been on the forefront of changing the terminology of mental retardation to intellectual disability and changed its name in 2007 (Schalock et al., 2010). Rosa's law (PL 111-256) was passed in 2010, changing the terminology to intellectual disability in all federal health, education, and labor policies.

AAIDD, the American Psychological Association (APA, 2013), and the World Health Organization (WHO, 2021) have all changed the terminology to intellectual disability. In these definitions several important factors need to be considered when diagnosing an individual with ID. Previously there was heavy reliance on cognitive testing (IQ scores). The cutoff for ID was an IQ score of 70. While currently there needs to be the presence of significant deficits in both cognitive and adaptive skills, an individual's adaptive abilities, how the person functions day to day, are considered to be more relevant than IQ scores alone. In addition, consideration of supports and opportunities needed to enhance a person's daily life in community settings, such as at work and school, are also considered. Unlike the AAIDD definition, severity scores continue to be used in the APA definition (Table 40.1).

In 2021 the AAIDD refined the definition of intellectual disability as follows: "ID is characterized by significant limitations, both in intellectual function and in adaptive behavior as expressed by conceptual, social, and practical adaptive skills. This disability originates during the developmental period, which is defined operationally as before the individual attains age 22" (Schalock, Luckasson, & Tasse, 2021). Systems of supports provide resources and strategies specific for an individual's needs, interests, and overall welfare. Like the medical home concept, these systems of support should be person centered, comprehensive, and coordinated. In addition, they should be outcome oriented. It is important to note that a person's functional level is not static and may change over time.

Despite the gains that have been made in the integration of individuals with ID into typical classroom settings, inclusive higher education, expanding employment opportunities, and residing in community settings, barriers continue to exist in multiple aspects of life. Of note are continued negative

TABLE 40.1 *DSM-5* Intellectual Disability Severity Level

Severity Category	Approximate Percent Distribution of Cases by Severity	*DSM-5* Criteria (Severity Classification From Daily Skills)
Mild	85%	Able to live independently with minimal level support
Moderate	10%	Independent living possible with moderate level support
Severe	3.5%	Requires daily assistance with self-care and safety supervision
Profound	1.5%	Requires 24-hr care

DSM-5, Diagnostic and Statistical Manual of Mental Disorders, Fifth Edition.
Adapted from National Academies of Sciences, Engineering, and Medicine. (2015). *Mental disorders and disabilities among low-income children.* The National Academies Press. https://doi.org/10.17226/21780

attitudinal barriers that affect how both the general public and the medical community conceptualizes people with ID. It has been shown, however, that the more direct contact neurotypical individuals have with individuals with ID, the more accepting they are of people with this disability (Morin, Valois, Crocker, Robitaille, & Lopes, 2018).

PREVALENCE

It is important to understand the prevalence of ID, as these numbers affect public health programs, policies, and allocated resources. The prevalence of ID often is cited to be approximately 1% to 3% of the worldwide population, although published prevalence rates vary based on disability definition and methods used to obtain data. There are multiple different surveillance projects that evaluate the prevalence of various developmental disabilities (DD) in children, although there are barriers to obtaining accurate data on adults with ID in the United States and a lack of distinction between ID and DD (Havercamp, Krahn, Larson, Weeks, & National Surveillance of IDD Workgroup, 2019). DD includes physical and cognitive disabilities that occur before adulthood and are often lifelong conditions. There is overlap, although these terms are not synonymous. For example, cerebral palsy (CP) is a developmental disability. Some individuals with CP have intellectual functioning within the average range while others may have ID.

Metaanalysis using 52 global studies indicated a global ID prevalence of 10.4 per 1000 people. There was rate variability based on income, age, and study design. The highest rates were seen in low- and middle-income countries, where resources to support people with ID are relatively less than in higher-income countries (Maulik, Mascarenhas, Mathers, Dua, & Saxena, 2011). Some of the discrepancy in determining an accurate prevalence rate relates to differences in terminology used in different countries.

The 2009–2016 National Health Interview Survey (NHIS) estimated the prevalence of ID to be 11.1 per 1000 children between the ages of 3 and 17 years in the United States. There were overall significant increases in the prevalence of any DD with one in six children with a DD. The prevalence of ID had been stable between 1997 and 2008, although it subsequently increased with the change of terminology from mental retardation to intellectual disability, suggesting people may be more comfortable endorsing the term intellectual disability. During this period the prevalence of ID increased from 0.9% to 1.2% (Zablotsky et al., 2019).

ETIOLOGIC FACTORS

With scientific advances, we better understand factors that contribute to the diagnosis of ID. These potential causative insults may be classified as genetic, metabolic, infectious, toxic, traumatic, environmental, or idiopathic. Other than genetic causes, these potential etiologic factors may occur in the pre-, peri-, or postnatal period. While there continue to be patients with ID for whom an etiology cannot be identified, the percentage of people in whom etiology is idiopathic has considerably decreased with the significant advances in genetic testing. We better understand metabolic mechanisms that contribute to development. We have prevented, and have better treatments for, certain infections associated with DD. We also have increased awareness of the effects of potential toxins and teratogenic agents on the developing brain. Environmental factors associated with ID have been better identified. While we know that significant physical brain trauma in early life may result in ID, we also note that emotional trauma, poverty, and nonstimulating environments, particularly in the absence of factors that support resilience, also affect cognitive development.

It is important to evaluate how environment and genetics interact. In a study of more than 1 million sibling pairs and 9000 twin pairs cognitive assessment was performed looking for the presence of ID. Both genetic and environmental factors were considered. It was determined that most individuals with ID had similar potential genetic and environmental etiologic factors to those with cognitive skills in the normal range; however, those with severe ID are more likely to have noninherited genetic causes. Examples of contributing etiology factors in severe ID include, although are not limited to, de novo point mutations, imprinting, and environmental factors (Reichenberg et al., 2015).

Genetics

There is a strong genetic influence of the presentation of ID that is complex and heterogeneous. Chromosomal abnormalities include aneuploidy, deletions, duplications, and unbalanced translocations. There also are single gene defects. Unless there is a definitive etiology, genetic testing is recommended in those who carry this diagnosis. With more precise testing available, the diagnostic yield has increased significantly. Genetic testing often is performed stepwise, with CMA, fragile X, autism spectrum disorder (ASD)/ID panels, and sometimes whole exome sequencing (WES). Karyotype screen also may be ordered if there is concern for unbalanced translocation, sometimes associated with a maternal history of multiple miscarriages. The diagnostic yield progressively increases when microarray and WES are included in the evaluation (Wang, Wang, Wang, Chen, & Sheng, 2020). Consideration of whole genome sequencing (WGS) as a first-line diagnostic test for unexplained DD has been suggested (Bowling, et al., 2017). While cost may be a concern, some contend that doing WES or WGS from the onset may be a more cost-effective or efficient way to identify a genetic etiology (Pekeles et al., 2019). Advances in genetic testing and changes in cost and test availability will continue to evolve and shape how children are assessed.

Metabolic

While inborn errors of metabolism (IEMs) are relatively infrequent, accounting for 1% to 5% of children with ID, they are an important diagnostic consideration in the medical workup (Moeschler, Shevell, & Committee on Genetics, 2014; van Karnebeek, Shevell, Zschocke, Moeschler, & Stockler, 2014). IEMs often are identified in the neonatal period with acute and life-threatening presentations. There are other IEMs triggered by illness or other types of increase in oxidative stress. They also may present with a loss of milestones as in the vignette, prolonged recovering form an acute illness, growth failure, protein avoidance, skin and hair disorders, among other symptoms. These types of occurrences often trigger the medical professional to consider initiating a metabolic workup. However, there also are IEMs whose primary presenting feature may be ID, for which potential treatments may improve development function, some behavioral difficulties, as well as neurologic and/or other presenting medical problems (van Karnebeek et al., 2014).

Infections

Congenital and perinatal infections have decreased significantly with the advent of maternal immunization and prepartum antibacterial treatment. These types of infections have been associated with developmental delays, ID, hearing and/or vision loss, epilepsy, and other developmental and medical morbidities. Some of the prenatal and perinatal viral infections include congenital toxoplasmosis, congenital rubella syndrome, congenital cytomegalovirus (CMV) infection, congenital herpes simplex virus infection, and congenital Zika syndrome, as well as other less common pathogens transmitted to the fetus (Ostrander & Bale, 2019).

Neonatal bacterial meningitis is most often caused by group B streptococci; this infection has decreased in neonates with use of intrapartum antibiotics (Gupta, 2018). *Escherichia coli* and *Listeria monocytogenes* are other bacterial pathogens that may cause neonatal bacterial meningitis. Bacterial meningitis during childhood, caused by *Hemophilus influenzae Neisseria meningitidis* and *Streptococcus pneumoniae* are life-threatening illnesses that are associated with significant developmental sequelae (Kaplan & DiPentima, 2019). While the mortality and morbidity rates for these infections have significantly decreased due to immunizations and prompt treatments with antimicrobials, they continue to pose threats to developmental outcomes around the world.

Trauma

Both physical and psychosocial trauma affect developmental outcomes. Other than elderly individuals, children less than 4 years of age have the highest rate of traumatic brain injury (TBI; Keenan, Presson, Clark, Cox, & Ewing- Cobbs, 2019). There are many factors that affect developmental outcome in the context of TBI, such as severity of the injury, other medical and/or developmental issues, and environmental factors. The more severe the injury, the more apt cognitive abilities and behavioral issues will persist. Older children and adolescents who experience TBI, particularly those with severe insults, also may experience long-term cognitive, executive function, and behavioral difficulties (see Chapter 32).

Prenatal and postpartum maternal stress and other adverse childhood experiences (ACEs), particularly in the absence of factors that foster resilience, have been shown to result in potential negative health-related and developmental outcomes. Poverty has been associated with structural brain changes in the frontal lobe, temporal lobe, and hippocampus with reduced gray matter volume and with negative effects on academic achievement (Hair et al., 2015). Children living in poverty, experiencing food insecurity, and exposure to other ACEs potentially may experience long-term health and cognitive problems.

Toxins

Lead and mercury are heavy metals associated with cognitive deficits. While there currently is less lead exposure than in the past, with the elimination of lead in paint and gasoline, there continues to be lead toxicity in children, particularly where lead paint exists in older buildings. Exposure to mercury, such as through prenatal consumption of fish with high mercury content, has been cited as contributing to developmental problems (Hauptman & Woolf, 2017).

Prenatal exposure to alcohol has long been identified as a contributor to a range of neurocognitive and behavioral disabilities, as well as a distinctive physical presentation (see Chapter 37). The impact of other environmental toxins on the brain is discussed in Chapter 38.

EVALUATION OF INTELLECTUAL DISABILITY

There are multiple factors to consider in the evaluation leading to the diagnosis of ID. A holistic approach considers biomedical, psychoeducational, sociocultural, and justice frameworks, using an integrative model. This model is informed by evidence-based practice, clinical judgment, and knowledge of community supports and family resources to develop a plan to best support an individual's needs and wishes (Schalock et al., 2021). Psychoeducational and adaptive skill assessments are presented in Chapters 85 through 88. The following addresses considerations for medical etiologic assessment for all children and youth with ID. This evaluation includes exploration for potential contributing factors occurring in the pre-, peri-, and postnatal periods. This information will guide plans for medical tests and/or procedures.

In exploring the prenatal period inquiry should be made about maternal age, illnesses, bleeding, fetal growth, medications, substance use, preterm labor, recurrent miscarriages, maternal obesity, issues with infertility, and other potential contributing factors. Perinatal questions should include information about gestational age, birthweight, Apgar scores, infection, oxygen use, need for intensive care, and treatments. Postnatal questions should focus on medical illnesses, treatments, hospitalization, growth, nutrition, and potential exposures to toxins and/or trauma. Developmental history should include assessment of age at milestone acquisition, as well as developmental trajectory, as regression or a long developmental plateau may signal need for specific medical tests or procedures. Ideally, a three-generation family medical history should be obtained, as well as a thorough social history.

Physical examination should assess for dysmorphic features, as the greater number of minor dysmorphic features, the greater the likelihood of a positive genetic finding. Growth parameters should be evaluated, including the proportion of head circumference to height. General physical examination should assess for positive findings in the different organ systems, such as neurocutaneous or other skin findings, organomegaly, and evaluation of fingers and toes. Neurologic examination should focus on presence or absence of primitive and protective reflexes in infants, as well as abnormalities and asymmetries in assessment of cranial nerves, other reflexes, muscle tone, strength, movement patterns, and sensory systems for all children and youth. It also may be important to gather information from other sources, such as teachers and/or therapists, from which formulation of the presenting issues is made, as well as medical and nonmedical recommendations.

Determination of medical tests ideally should be performed in a stepwise manner to avoid ordering unnecessary and costly tests yet ensure that potential etiologic factors are identified in a systematic fashion. Published guidelines that include algorithms provide this type of guidance (Moeschler et al., 2014; van Karnebeek et al., 2014). In essence, if history and examination suggest a specific diagnosis, testing for that specific diagnosis should first be performed. If that test is negative or if etiology is unknown, the first-line testing currently is CMA and fragile X. Some clinicians may obtain first-tier testing for IEMs at this point as well. If these tests are negative, additional tests of IEM, brain imaging, and other gene panels may be considered. Any time a test is positive, then counseling, management, and resources should be provided for that specific diagnosis. Even after extensive medical workup, etiology may not be identified, and therefore regular review should be considered as the sensitivity of diagnostic testing continues to improve.

COOCCURRING CONDITIONS

Individuals with ID often have cooccurring medical, behavioral, and emotional conditions that warrant evaluation and intervention. Treatment of some of these conditions may improve developmental function and/or quality of life, such as thyroid disease, significant anemia, depression, seizure disorders, hearing loss, vision loss, sleep disorders, and chronic constipation. The more significant the cognitive and adaptive skill impairments, the greater the likelihood of having additional chronic medical conditions (Friedman, 2010). The following sections discuss some of the conditions to consider when caring for an individual with ID.

Behavioral and Emotional

Children, youth, and adults with ID have higher rates of behavioral and emotional diagnoses compared to the general population. This cooccurrence is sometimes described as dual diagnoses (see Chapter 54). For children and youth, it is estimated that the prevalence of psychiatric disorders is three to four times higher than the general population; however, it is difficult to determine an exact prevalence due to differences in criteria for ID, severity of disability, sex, socioeconomic status, and other potential moderators of the relationship between ID and behavioral or emotional disorders (Munir, 2016). Some researchers estimate that between 30% and 50% of children and youth with ID have a cooccurring mental health diagnosis compared to an overall prevalence of 16.5% in the general population (Einfeld, Ellis, & Emerson, 2011). A prevalence rate of mental health disorders among adolescents and adults with ID was found to be 33.6%, using a systematic review and metaanalysis (Mazza, Rossetti, Crespi, & Clerici, 2020).

Seizures and Epilepsy

ID is a complex and heterogeneous neurologically based condition and therefore individuals with ID may have distinctive sensory, motor, movement, reflexive, neurodegenerative, and other manifestations that affect the nervous system. Overall, individuals with ID have an increased prevalence of seizures compared to the general population, with estimates of 20% to 30% in people with ID compared to up to 1% in the general population (van Ool et al., 2016). Seizures and/or epilepsy are frequent presentations in individuals with and without syndromic ID. A person is considered to have epilepsy when experiencing two or more seizures. Seizure frequency tends to increase with increasing severity of the ID. There are different types of seizures, and patients may have more than one type. It is important to recognize seizures, perform appropriate neurophysiologic studies to characterize the seizures, and control them as best as possible. There are times when seizures cannot totally be prevented, and there needs to be a balance between seizure control and medications affect on alertness that promotes interaction with others in the environment.

Certain types and frequency of seizures may be associated with specific genetic syndromes. For example, Strehlow et al. (2016) found that 10% of individuals with 22q11.2 deletion syndrome (DS), associated with hypocalcemia, mild to moderate ID, and neuropsychiatric disorders, had generalized and myoclonic seizures. Eaton et al. (2019) noted that children and youth with 22q11.2 DS may present with cognitive, psychiatric, and/or motor coordination problems, as well as a high likelihood for epilepsy. Many also may display seizures or seizure-like behaviors, which may be epilepsy, although this is not identified in routine clinical care. CDKL5 deficiency disorder, an X-linked gene disorder associated with significant delays, is characterized by early onset and often intractable seizures. Seizures have been noted to occur in up to 98% of patients with this disorder. These children most commonly present with epileptic spasms, frequently without hypsarrhythmia, and tonic seizures that tend to cluster together (Demarest et al., 2019).

While it is beyond the scope of the chapter to characterize seizures for multiple different genetic conditions, or management strategies with antiseizure medication, surgical, and nutritional interventions, it is important to be aware of the strong association of seizures and epilepsy in individuals with ID to ensure that appropriate diagnostic evaluation and interventions are taken to optimize seizure control. See Chapter 31 for more details.

Gastrointestinal

Individuals with ID are at increased risk for gastrointestinal issues, such as gastroesophageal reflux with and without esophagitis, constipation, delayed gastric emptying, and feeding problems with associated nutritional issues. As with other associated medical conditions, the more severe the ID, the more frequent are the gastrointestinal problems. See Chapter 59 for a more comprehensive discussion of the myriad issues seen in patients with medical complexity who frequently have concurrent ID. Other chapters in this book also address feeding disorders (Chapter 65) and their evaluation as well as nutritional concerns (Chapter 35).

Abnormalities in gut motility can contribute to constipation as well as feeding tolerance or gastroesophageal reflux, which in turn may lead to inflammation of the lower esophagitis and Barrett esophagitis. Eosinophilic esophagitis, often associated with aversion to oral intake and behavioral problems, also has been identified in individuals with ID and other DD.

Some children and youth with ID have feeding problems that may be exacerbated by motor, sensory, and behavioral challenges. Feeding evaluations and feeding therapy are often indicated. When nutritional intake is inadequate for growth, even after nutritional supplements, and/or aspiration of food into the lungs is occurring, placement of an enteral tube may be considered. This may be a difficult decision for parents, as they often want their child to experience the pleasures of eating. Feeding tubes may also be associated with problems such as granulomatous issue and infection about the site. Multidisciplinary assessment, including physicians, nutritionists, occupational therapists, speech and language pathologists, psychologists, and feeding specialists, may be necessary to determine that the benefits of improved nutrition outweigh the risks.

Orthopedic

Children with ID, particularly those with associated motor problems and CP, are at increased risk for orthopedic deformities. As with other medical issues present in individuals with ID, the more severe the ID, the more apt there are to be motor issues, which may involve problems with muscle tone, muscle strength, and movement patterns.

Children, youth, and adults with severe motor and intellectual disabilities are at increased risk for osteoporosis and associated bone fractures. Contributing factors are antiseizure medications and reduced weight bearing, which may result in reduced bone mass. It is important that vitamin D and calcium levels be monitored, as well as bone density. Children with neuromuscular diseases require additional evaluation and monitoring as discussed in Chapters 30 and 39.

Sensory

Children with ID have a greater prevalence of hearing and vision problems compared to the general population. Conductive, sensorineural, and mixed hearing losses are commonly seen in individuals with ID. Certain genetic syndromes are associated with hearing and/or vision loss. Children with Down syndrome primarily have conductive hearing loss due to increased risk of chronic middle ear effusions, although they also may present with sensorineural and mixed hearing loss (Kreicher, Weir, Nguyen, & Meyer, 2018). Children with Bardet-Biedl syndrome present with retinal abnormalities and delayed cognitive skills (Forsythe et al., 2018). Children with CDKL5 deficiency disorder often have cortical vision impairment and significant developmental delays (Demarest et al., 2019). There also are congenital infections associated with vision, hearing, and cognitive impairments such as congenital CMV and congenital rubella infections. For more information, see Chapter 43 regarding visual issues and Chapter 42 on hearing loss.

Any child with developmental delay, even after a normal neonatal hearing test, requires a reliable audiology assessment. Audiologic assessment may need to be modified based on the child's or youth's ability to participate in this testing. Sometimes auditory brainstem response testing needs to be done if there is no other way to obtain reliable assessment of hearing acuity through other testing means. Similarly, it is important to assess vision in children and youth with ID, often requiring an examination by an ophthalmologist familiar with examining children with developmental differences.

Sleep

Sleep problems may be caused by obstructive or central apnea, periodic limb movements, sleep disordered breathing, and parasomnias and thus affect sleep duration and quality of sleep. While sleep problems are common in the general population, reduced sleep duration and quality have been noted to frequently occur in individuals with ID. The mechanism that accounts for this increased frequency in the ID population is not clear (Surtees, Oliver, Jones, Evans, & Richards, 2018). Sleep disorders also occur with multiple syndromes that are associated with ID, such as Down syndrome, fragile X, William syndrome, and ASD (D'Souza, D'Souza, Horváthe, Plunkett, & Karmiloff- Smith, 2020).

Problems with sleep can negatively affect a person's behavior as well as quality of life for both the person with ID and the family. In addition to daytime sleepiness, poor sleep may negatively affect behavior, attention, learning, emotional regulation, and health (Dolan, Lane, Hillis, & Delanty, 2019). It is important to identity potential medical conditions that may reduce sleep quality, delay sleep onset, or interfere with sleep maintenance, such as obstructive sleep apnea or periodic limb movement. There may be problems with gastroesophageal reflux or other medical conditions causing pain or discomfort that require intervention. Even if there are identified medical contributing factors, frequently there also are learned components to sleep problems that can be addressed by improved sleep hygiene and behavioral interventions (see Chapter 70). At times, medical interventions such as use of nasal steroids, continuous positive airway pressure, iron supplementation, melatonin, and/or medications may be needed to improve sleep problems.

OUTCOMES AND DISPARITIES

Life Expectancy

People with ID are living longer with the advent of improved treatments for infections, aspiration, nutritional problems, hypoxemia, seizures, and other chronic conditions. These medical advances in the context of improved living conditions and community integration have resulted in life expectancy approaching that of the general population for most individuals with ID. The causes of death also are similar to those in the general population. However, those with more severe ID associated medical complexity, and individuals with Down syndrome, continue to have higher mortality rates (Dolan et al., 2019). End-of-life care for people with ID often may be an emotionally charged subject, as historically the lives of people with ID were devalued and their options for life-sustaining interventions were limited. There continues to be bias about whether life-sustaining treatment should be provided to people with significant disabilities. However, there has been significant advocacy to provide equal value to every life while honoring the wishes of individuals with ID and/or their designated stakeholders.

Guardianship and Supported Decision Making

Historically, parents, guardians, and even state officials obtained guardianship when an individual with ID reached 18 years of age. To obtain guardianship, the state court must receive documentation that the individual is not capable of making decisions to manage multiple areas of daily living, such as finances and medical care. Guardians are appointed by the court and most commonly are the individual's parents. The parents of some young adults may not obtain guardianship, although they may obtain legal documentation to have medical decision-making authority.

In lieu of guardianship there is now an emphasis on supported decision making, whereby an individual is entrusted with the responsibility to provide information to the individual with ID in a manner that is understandable, thus allowing the person with ID to make choices that reflect one's own wishes. Some US states have developed legislation with regard to supported decision making. Article 12 of the United Nation's Convention on the Rights of Persons with Disabilities protects the human rights and freedom of people with disabilities. It also indicates people with disabilities have the right to legal capacity, indicating they have the right to make their own decisions (Devi, 2014). There continue to be differences of opinion regarding application of the concepts of legal capacity, mental capacity, and supported decision making. Because everyone with ID presents with unique needs to make decisions in many aspects of life, a supported decision-making inventory (SDMI) was developed. This tool assists in identifying areas where an individual needs support of a close and reliable person to make decisions that reflect the preferences and wishes of the person with ID (Shogren, Wehmeyer, Uyanik, & Heidrich, 2017).

Advocacy and Self-Determination

People with ID have progressively become advocates for their own interests, rather than defer to the wishes of others. There are very active self-advocate organizations, such as Self-Advocates Becoming Empowered (SABE), and many disability organizations, councils, and federally funded grant programs require that voices of people with disability be included, acknowledging the significant value and insight people with disabilities provide.

People with ID historically have not had the same opportunities or supports to make decisions that affect their lives. Adolescents and adults with ID who engage in self-determination have been shown to have a higher quality of life and display higher academic achievement than peers who do not (Wehmeyer, 2020), although these skills are not often taught to youth while in school. Self-directed services for people with ID have been noted to result in increased satisfaction, outcomes, and savings. However, some state administrators have balanced these positive outcomes with the stewardship of public funds by using an approval process to prevent excessive spending of some goods and services leading to restrictions on spending flexibility (Bogenschutz, DeCarlo, Hall-Lande, & Hewitt, 2019).

Community Integration

The number of people with ID living in institutional and congregate care facilities has progressively and significantly decreased through the years. More individuals with disabilities reside in community settings, many with their families, although some now live in their own home with support provided as needed. Individuals with ID and significant medical complexity require more support. However, even those with complex needs can successfully reside in a community setting. In the past, there were reports that living in the community was associated with a higher mortality rate, which is no longer the case. Since that time, there have been more supports provided to people in the community, such as through the Medicaid Home and Community-Based Services (HCBS) 1915(c) Waiver Program, with improved quality of life reported for those living in the community.

Employment

In the past employment for adults with ID often focused on sheltered workshops with individuals frequently doing tasks that were tedious, did not interest them, and provided little satisfaction. There continues to be many barriers to employment, and those employed often receive subminimal wage. Assessment of data from 2015 to 2016 from the National Core Indicators Project revealed that 19% of working-age adults supported by state ID/DD agencies worked in one of three forms of integrated employment: group supported, individual supported, or competitive (in the regular workforce without supports); 12% worked in competitive or individual-supported employment, and 7% worked in group-supported employment (Hiersteiner, Bershadsky, Bonardi, & Butterworth, 2016). Others have found that employers are more comfortable hiring a person with a physical disability than someone with ID (Kocman, Fischer, & Weber, 2018).

There currently are national initiatives for competitive employment, as well as strong support for providing individuals with disabilities with at least minimal wages for the work that they do. By age 16, an individual with an IEP should have a transition plan that specifies goals for postsecondary education or employment. This plan may include supports by the Office of Vocational Rehabilitation. In general, having a meaningful job and contributing to the community are associated with increased happiness and self-esteem.

Postsecondary Education

There currently are multiple programs that allow individuals with ID to participate in inclusive higher education. They participate in classes with neurotypical peers and receive support from university faculty, staff, and peers. The courses are usually matched to the career interest and sometimes culminate in certificates of completion or degrees. These programs may occur at community colleges as well as state universities. This educational opportunity also supports an individual's ability to obtain employment and live more independently. With strong support and advocacy from parents, it has been demonstrated young adults with more significant disabilities and communication challenges have the potential to engage in meaningful postsecondary experiences (Rossetti, Lehr, Pelerin, Huang, & Lederer, 2016).

Sexuality

Sexual feelings and desires are part of the human experience for most people, including those with ID. Many people with ID are interested in having romantic and sexual relationships. People with ID also may be subject to exploitation because of lack of understanding of consent. It is important to provide sex education, including awareness of one's body, healthy relationships, reproduction, and avoidance of victimization. Medicaid HCBS waivers are rarely used for these types of services, and when they are used, it more frequently addresses interventions and plans to stop sexual behaviors (Friedman & Owen, 2017).

Some people with ID have their own children, making it important to provide them with practical, resource, and emotional support to care for their offspring. Mothers with ID have more serious health and economic problems than mothers without ID (Powell, Parish, & Akobirshoev, 2017). Some mothers with ID have been found to have more pre- and postnatal problems than the general population, although many of the causes for these problems are amenable to preventative measures (Fairthorne et al., 2020).

Poverty

Despite the numerous advances made in the areas of deinstitutionalization, education, medicine, living arrangements, and advocacy, most people with ID continue to live in poverty. Many individuals rely on Social Security benefits, Medicaid, and/or Medicare. Many adults with ID do not have adequate access to housing, transportation, and easily accessible health care. For those who work, wages are often below minimal wage. In the past there was a limit on how much a person could earn and save without losing federal benefits. However, in 2014 the Achieving a Better Life Experience (ABLE) Act became law. This law allows people with disabilities to save money in a tax-advantaged account without losing their federal benefits. Funds can be used for housing, transportation, education, and other disability-related expenses (National Disability Institute, 2019).

Diversity

Children, youth, and adults with ID from minoritized ethnic and/or racial groups experience significant disparity in the time of diagnosis of some DD, as well as access to a medical home and specialty care. There has been a recent movement to address issues related to diversity, equity, and inclusion in general, as well as for those with disability specifically. There also is a need to explore implicit bias toward people with ID, with more medical school curricula including experiences and education about DD.

PREVENTION

Immunizations

Vaccine use to prevent some viral and bacterial infections has significantly reduced the infectious causes of DD and ID. Prior to the measle-mumps-rubella vaccine, infants born with congenital rubella often were deaf, blind, and developmentally delayed. Although rare, latent measles infection may cause subacute sclerosing panencephalitis, a progressive neurologic disorder associated with deterioration of cognitive skills, motor impairment, seizures, and death. The diphtheria-pertussis-tetanus vaccine reduced the incidence of pertussis, with associated medical and developmental morbidity and mortality. Vaccines to prevent infection by *H. influenzae* type B, *N. meningitides*, and *S. pneumoniae* bacterial infections have been instrumental in significantly reducing meningitis from these bacteria, also associated with significant medical and developmental morbidity and increased mortality.

Nutritional

A complete and balanced diet is important for cognitive function. Severe malnutrition, chronic undernutrition, iron deficiency, and iodine deficiency have all be noted to negatively affect brain development. The children of women who received the Special Supplemental Nutrition Program for Women, Infants, and Children (WIC) during pregnancy had better cognitive and developmental outcome at age 2 years compared to matched controls who were not in the WIC program (Guan et al., 2021).

Safety Laws and Recommendations

Seat belt laws have reduced head injuries associated with motor vehicle crashes. Similarly, use of helmets while engaged in sport activities, such as bicycle riding and skateboarding, also has served to protect the brain from injury. Fencing around swimming pools has reduced drowning and near-drowning incidents. Carbon monoxide and fire monitors have reduced the morbidity and mortality associated with carbon monoxide poisoning and smoke inhalation that may be deadly or result in long-lasting cognitive deficits.

Environmental

Eliminating lead paint and leaded gasoline has significantly reduced the negative developmental and behavior sequelae of lead toxicity. Pregnant women are advised to avoid consumption of large quantities of fish containing mercury, which may negatively affect cognitive skills of offspring. Similarly, pregnant women are advised to not smoke cigarettes during pregnancy, as the smoke has been associated with behavioral and cognitive issues, in addition to small-for-gestational-age babies. Pregnant mothers also are advised to avoid cat feces, which may contain toxoplasmosis, as congenital toxoplasmosis is associated with cognitive and motor delays, as well as progressive vision and hearing loss. Prenatal exposure to alcohol, causing fetal alcohol spectrum disorders in approximately 11.1 to 50 per 1000 children in the United States (May et al., 2019), led to warning labels being placed on alcohol-containing beverages to dissuade pregnant women from drinking.

Neonatal Screening

Neonatal screening, currently performed in all US states, identifies conditions that can be treated to reduce morbidity, including IEMs and some endocrine, hematologic, and immunologic diseases (El-Hattab, 2018). ID can be prevented in IEMs such as phenylketonuria and the endocrinologic condition of congenital hypothyroidism by early identification and appropriate treatments.

Social Determinants of Health

The environment in which a child lives has long-lasting impact on physical, developmental, psychiatric, and behavioral outcomes. Exposure to ACEs (see Chapter 15) is associated with less favorable child outcomes. It is important to screen for ACEs in children and families. There also are factors that contribute to resilience in the presence of ACEs. It therefore is helpful to provide families with resources and support that may potentially serve as sources of strength. There are many local, state, and federal initiatives (e.g., addressing health delivery systems, building healthy neighborhoods, nutritional programs, payment reform linking health care to social needs) to counteract negative environmental factors (Heiman & Artiga, 2015).

RECENT AND FUTURE THERAPIES AND ADVANCES

We have a much greater understanding of the underlying causes of ID, although we still do not fully grasp all the underlying molecular and metabolic mechanisms affecting cognition. Clearly, advances in genetic testing have been significant, and the advent of techniques such as WES and WGS, which are currently not the first step in the workup, may ultimately be the first-line approach to etiologic evaluation (Vissers, Gilissen, & Veltman, 2016). The understanding of neuronal function on a cellular and intercellular level has advanced enormously. We now understand many of the genes controlling cortical development, which may lead to therapeutic interventions in the future (Oegema et al., 2020; Saillour & Chelly, 2016).

Once an underlying etiology is determined, interventions may someday be possible for either reducing or even eliminating the disabilities. From the interventions of the past, including detecting hypothyroidism or phenylketonuria with newborn screening and intervening with medication or special diets, we can now consider sophisticated medical, surgical, and genetic approaches. Medical and surgical advances have also been enormous and have led to survival and improved quality of life for children born severely premature or with life-threatening birth defects. Prenatal diagnoses and interventions are even possible in some cases to address life-threatening problems *in utero* or make diagnoses for which there are interventions that can be started soon after birth and improve cognitive outcome (Sparks et al., 2020). An example is prenatal surgery for fetuses with neural tube defects, which can lead to prevention of Chiari II defects and subsequent hydrocephalus, decreasing the risk of injury to the brain.

Understanding the molecular defects causing spinal muscular atrophy, for example, has led to the development of medical interventions to improve developmental progress and life span for this devastating disease. Gene modification using new modalities such as CRISPR-CAS9, currently not used in humans due to ethical and logistical concerns, may allow repair of pathologic genetic variations in the future. Enzyme replacement has been available for a few rare metabolic genetic disorders, although it may become available for many more disorders in the future. Currently, in research development interventions with pleuripotent cells show great promise for genetic interventions in the future.

RESOURCES

There are numerous local, state, national, and international disability organizations that provide different types of resources. In addition, there are condition-specific organization, such as for Rett syndrome, fragile X, Down syndrome, and organizations for rare diseases. This section provides a sample of organizations and resources that are available to patients, families, and professionals.

Parent Groups

- Family Voices (https://familyvoices.org/) is a national network that promotes family-centered care for children with special needs by supporting families to advocate for themselves and build partnerships between families and service providers.
- Parent to Parent USA (https://www.p2pusa.org/) has local groups in many states that provide emotional support to families by matching parents who have children with the same type of disability or special health care need to share information and provide support. Its mission is to support a national network of Parent to Parent programs to ensure access to quality emotional support for families of individuals with disabilities and/or special health care needs.

Advocacy Organizations

- The Arc of the United States (https://thearc.org/about-us/) is the largest national community-based organization advocating for people with ID and DD, with many local and state chapters throughout the country. The Arc provides resources for individuals with disabilities, is involved in advocacy and disability policy, and works to support full community participation.
- Self-Advocates Becoming Empowered (SABE) (https://www.sabeusa.org/) is a national organization of self-advocates that has representation in every US state. The organization is committed to empowering people with disabilities to receive the same treatment and opportunities as people without disabilities.

Youth and Adult Activities

- Special Olympics (https://www.specialolympics.org/) provides sport training and athletic competition for children and adults with ID, giving them continuing opportunities to improve their physical fitness, enhance their confidence, experience joy, and develop friendships.
- Best Buddies International (https://www.bestbuddies.org/) is an organization that promotes meaningful friendships between people 18 years of age and older with and without disabilities. The organization is also geared to support the integration of people with ID/DD into the community in areas such as employment and living arrangements. It also supports personal growth of people with ID/DD through advocacy and leadership development.

Employment

- National Organization on Disability (NOD) (https://www.nod.org/) is an organization for all people with disabilities, with a focus on full community participation, including improving employment opportunities for Americans with disabilities.
- Office of Disability Employment Policy (ODEP) (https://www.dol.gov/agencies/odep) is a nonregulatory federal agency that promotes policies, shares information about effective employment practices, and hires and retrains people with disabilities in the workforce.

Professional Organizations

- American Association on Intellectual and Developmental Disabilities (AAIDD) (www.aaidd.org) is the oldest interdisciplinary professional organization. It has been on the forefront of providing definitions of ID, which has evolved through the years, with its most recent update published in 2021. It provides resources on timely and relevant issues, such as the intersectionality of ID/DD with race and ethnicity, sexuality, poverty, health disparities, among other salient topics.
- Association of University Centers on Disability (AUCD) (www.aucd.org) provides support to university-based interdisciplinary programs across the United States and territories. The organization supports these centers to provide clinical services, training, research, advocacy, technical assistance to community and government partners, program evaluation, and dissemination of relevant information to individuals with disabilities and their families, as well as other professionals.

Diversity, Equity, and Inclusion

- The National Center for Cultural Competence (https://nccc.georgetown.edu/) has many resources and self-assessments, with resources relevant to people with disabilities.
- Diversity and Inclusion Toolkit, AUCD (https://www.aucd.org/itac/template/strategy.cfm?id=161) provides resources and strategies to promote diversity, equity, inclusion, and cultural and linguistic competence, with specific information geared to federal agencies, national organizations, and university-based centers and programs.

REFERENCES

American Psychiatric Association. (2013). *Diagnostic and statistical manual of mental disorders* (5th ed.). APA Publishing.

Bogenschutz, M. D., DeCarlo, M., Hall-Lande, J., & Hewitt, A. (2019). Fiscal stewardship, choice, and control: The context of self-directed services for people with intellectual and developmental disabilities (IDD) in the United States. *Intellectual and Developmental Disabilities*, *57*, 158–171.

Bowling, K. M., Thompson, M. L., Amaral, M. D., Finnila, C. R., Hiatt, S. M., et al. (2017). Genomic diagnosis for children with intellectual disability and/or developmental delay. *Genome Medicine*, *9*, 43. https://doi.org/10.1186/s13073-017-0433-1

Demarest, S. T., Olson, H. E., Moss, A., Pestana-Knight, E., Zhang, X., et al. (2019). CDKL5 deficiency disorder: Relationship between genotype, epilepsy, cortical visual impairment, and development. *Epilepsia*, *60*, 1733–1742.

Devi, N. (2014). Supported decision-making and personal autonomy for persons with intellectual disabilities: Article 12 of the UN Convention on the rights of persons with disabilities. *Journal of Law and Medical Ethics*, *41*, 792–806.

Dolan, E., Lane, J., Hillis, G., & Delanty, N. (2019). Changing trends in life expectancy in intellectual disability over time. *Irish Medical Journal, 112*, 1006. PMID:31651135.

D'Souza, D., D'Souza, H., Horváthe, K., Plunkett, K., & Karmiloff-Smith, A. (2020). Sleep is atypical across neurodevelopmental disorders in infants and toddlers: A cross-syndrome study. *Research in Developmental Disabilities, 97*, 135–149.

Eaton, C. B., Thomas, R. H., Hamandi, K., Payne, G. C., Kerr, M. P., Linden, D. E., et al. (2019). Epilepsy and seizures in young people with 22q11.2 deletion syndrome: Prevalence and links with other neurodevelopmental disorders. *Epilepsia, 60*, 818–829.

Einfeld, S. L., Ellis, L. A., & Emerson, E. (2011). Comorbidity of intellectual disability and mental disorder in children and adolescents: A systematic review. *Journal of Intellectual and Developmental Disability, 36*, 137–143. https://doi.org/10.1080/13668250.2011.572548

El-Hattab. A. W. (2018). Newborn screening: History, current status, and future directions. *Pediatric Clinics of North America, 65*, 389–405.

Fairthorne, J., Bourke, J., O'Donnell, M., Wong, K., de Klerk, N., et al. (2020). Pregnancy and birth outcomes of mothers with intellectual disability and their infants: Advocacy needed to improve well-being. *Disability and Health Journal, 13*, 100871.

Forsythe, R., Kenny, J., Bacchelli, C., & Beales, P. L. (2018). Managing Bardet–Biedl syndrome—Now and in the future. *Frontiers in Pediatrics, 6*, 23. https://doi.org/10.3389/fped.2018.00023

Friedman, S. L. (2010). Complex medical problems affecting life and lifespan in children. In S. L. Friedman & D. Helm (Eds.), *End-of-life care for children and adults with intellectual and developmental disabilities*. AAIDD Press.

Friedman, C., Owen. C. L. (2017). Sexual health in the community: Services for people with intellectual and developmental disabilities. *Disability and Health Journal, 10*, 387–393.

Guan, A., Hamad, R., Batra, A., Bush, N. R., Tylavsky, F. A., et al. (2021). The revised WIC food package and child development: A quasi-experimental study. *Pediatrics, 147*, e20201853.

Gupta, F. (2018). *Neonatal meningitis*. https://emedicine.medscape.com/article/1176960-overview

Hauptman, M., & Woolf, A. D. (2017). Childhood ingestion of environmental toxins: What are the risks? *Pediatric Annals, 46*, e466–e3471.

Havercamp, S. M., Krahn, G., Larson, S., Weeks, J. D., & National Surveillance of IDD Workgroup. (2019). *Working through the IDD data conundrum*. Administration on Intellectual and Developmental Disabilities.

Heiman, H. J., & Artiga, S. (2015, November). Beyond health care: The role of social determinants in promoting health and health equity. Kaiser Commission on Medicaid and Uninsured, Issue Brief.

Hiersteiner, D., Bershadsky, J, Bonardi, A, & Butterworth, J. (2016). Working in the community: The status and outcomes of people with intellectual and developmental disabilities in integrated employment—Update 2. NCI Data Brief, April. 2016. Human Services Research Institute.

Kaplan, S. L., & Di Pentima, C. (2019). Patient education: Meningitis in children (beyond the basics). *UpToDate*. https://www.uptodate.com/contents/meningitis-in-children-beyond-the-basics

Keenan, H. T., Presson, A. P., Clark, A. E., Cox, C. S., & Ewing-Cobbs, L. (2019). Longitudinal developmental outcomes after traumatic brain injury in young children: Are infants more vulnerable than toddlers? *Journal of Neurotrauma, 36*, 282–292.

Kocman, A., Fischer, L., & Weber, G. (2018). The employers' perspective on barriers and facilitators to employment of people with intellectual disability: A differential mixed-method approach. *Journal of Applied Research in Intellect Disabilities, 31*, 120–131.

Kreicher, K. L., Weir, F. W., Nguyen, S. A., & Meyer, T. A. (2018). Characteristics and progression of hearing loss in children with Down syndrome. *Journal of Pediatrics, 193*, 27–33.

Maulik, P. K., Mascarenhas, M. N., Mathers, C. D., Dua, T., & Saxena, S. (2011). Prevalence of intellectual disability: A meta-analysis of population-based studies. *Research in Developmental Disabilities, 32*, 419–436.

May, P. A., Chambers, C. D., Kalberg, W. O., et al. (2019). Prevalence of fetal alcohol spectrum disorders in 4 US communities. *JAMA, 319*, 474–482.

Mazza, M. G., Rossetti, A., Crespi, G., & Clerici, M. (2020). Prevalence of co-occurring psychiatric disorders in adults and adolescents with intellectual disability: A systematic review and meta-analysis. *Journal of Applied Research in Intellectual Disabilities, 33*, 126–138.

Moeschler, J. B., Shevell, M., & Committee on Genetics, (2014). Comprehensive evaluation of the child with intellectual disability or global developmental delays. *Pediatrics, 134*(3), e903–e918.

Morin, D., Valois, P., Crocker, A. G., Robitaille, C., & Lopes, T. (2018). Attitudes of health care professionals toward people with intellectual disability: A comparison with the general population. *Journal of Intellectual Disability Research, 62*, 746–758.

Munir, K. (2016). The co-occurrence of mental disorders in children and adolescents with intellectual disability/intellectual developmental disorder. *Current Opinion in Psychiatry, 29*, 95–102.

National Disability Institute. (2019). *ABLE*. https://www.nationaldisabilityinstitute.org/financial-wellness/able-accounts/

Oegema, R., Barakat, T. S., Wilke, M., Stouffs, K., Aronica, E., et al. (2020). International consensus recommendations on the diagnostic work-up for malformations of cortical development. *Nature Reviews Neurology, 16*, 618–635.

Ostrander, B., & Bale, J. F. (2019). Congenital and perinatal infections. In L. S. de VriesH. C. (2019). Glass (Eds.), *Handbook of clinical neurology: Neonatal neurology* (Vol. 162, 3rd series). Elsevier. https://doi.org/10.1016/B978-0-444-64029-1.00006-0

Pekeles, H., Accogli, A., Boudrahem-Addour, N., Russell, L., Parente, F., et al. (2019). Yield of intellectual disability gene panels. *Pediatric Neurology, 92*, 32–36.

Powell, R. M., Parish, S. L., & Akobirshoev, I. (2017). The health and economic well-being of US mothers with intellectual impairments. *Journal of Applied Research in Intellectual Disabilities, 30*, 456–468.

Reichenberg, A., Cederlöf, M., McMillan, A., Trzaskowski, M., Kapara, O., et al. (2015). Discontinuity in the genetic and environmental causes of the intellectual disability spectrum. *Proceedings of the National Academy of Sciences, 113*. e8549–e1103. https://doi.org/10.1073/pnas.1508093112

Rossetti, Z., Lehr, D., Pelerin, D., Huang, S., & Lederer, L. (2016). Parent involvement in meaningful post-school experiences for young adults with IDD and pervasive support needs. *Intellectual and Developmental Disabilities*, *54*, 260–272. https://doi.org/10.1352/1934-9556-54.4.260

Saillour, Y., & Chelly, J. (2016). Genetic causes of intellectual disability: The genes controlling cortical development. In C. Sala & C. Verpelli (Eds.), *Neuronal and synaptic dysfunction in autism spectrum disorder and intellectual disability*. Academic Press.

Schalock, R. L., Buntinx, W. H. E., Borthwick-Duffy, S., Bradley, V., Craig, E. M., et al. (2010). *Intellectual disability: Definition, classification, and system of supports* (11th ed.). American Association on Intellectual and Developmental Disabilities.

Schalock, R. L., Luckasson, R., & Tasse, M. (2021). *Intellectual disability: Definition, diagnosis, classification, and systems of support* (12th ed.). AAIDD.

Shogren, K. A., Wehmeyer, M. L., Uyanik, H., & Heidrich, M. (2017). Development of the supported decision-making inventor system. *Intellectual and Developmental Disabilities*, *55*, 432–439.

Sparks, T. N., Lianoglou, B. R., Adami, R. R., Pluym, I. D., Holliman, K., et al. (2020). Exome sequencing for prenatal diagnosis in nonimmune hydrops fetalis. *New England Journal of Medicine*, *383*, 1746–1756.

Strehlow, V., Swinkels, M. E., Thomas, R. H., Rapps, N., Syrbe, S., Dorn, T., et al. (2016). Generalized epilepsy, and myoclonic seizures in 22q11.2 deletion syndrome. *Molecular Syndromology*, *7*, 239–246.

Surtees, A. D. R., Oliver, C., Jones, C. A., Evans, D. L., & Richards, C. (2018). Sleep duration and sleep quality in people with and without intellectual disability: A meta-analysis. *Sleep Medicine Reviews*, *40*, 135–150.

van Karnebeek, C. D. M., Shevell, M., Zschocke, J., Moeschler, J. B., & Stockler, S. (2014). The metabolic evaluation of the child with an intellectual developmental disorder: Diagnostic algorithm for identification of treatable causes and new digital resource. *Molecular Genetics and Metabolism*, *111*, 428–438.

van Ool, J. S., Snoeijen-Schouwenaars, F. M., Schelhaas, H. J., Tana, I. Y., Aldenkamp, A. P., & Hendriksen, J. G. M. (2016). A systematic review of neuropsychiatric comorbidities in patients with both epilepsy and intellectual disability. *Epilepsy & Behavior*, *60*, 130–137.

Vissers, L. E., Gilissen, C., & Veltman, J. A. (2016). Genetic studies in intellectual disability and related disorders. *Nature Review Genetics*, *17*, 9–18.

Wang, J., Wang, Y., Wang, L., Chen, W. Y., & Sheng, M. (2020). The diagnostic yield of intellectual disability: Combined whole genome low coverage sequencing and medical exome sequencing. *BMC Medical Genomics*, *13*, 70. https://doi.org/10.1186/s12920-020-0726-x

Wehmeyer. M. (2020). Self-determination in adolescents and adults with intellectual and developmental disabilities. *Current Opinion in Psychology*, *33*, 81–85.

World Health Organization, Regional Office for Europe. (2021). *Definition: Intellectual disability*. https://www.euro.who.int/en/health-topics/noncommunicable-diseases/mental-health/news/news/2010/15/childrens-right-to-family-life/definition-intellectual-disability

Zablotsky, B., Black, L. I., Maenner, M. J., Schieve, L. A., Danielson, M. L., et al. (2019). Prevalence and trends of developmental disabilities among children in the United States: 2009–2017. *Pediatrics*, *14*(4), e20190811.

Autism Spectrum Disorder

Bibiana Restrepo, Janice Enriquez, and Robin L. Hansen

For additional material related to the content of this chapter, please see Chapters 40, 84, 94, 113, and 115.

VIGNETTE

Colin is a 24-month-old boy with an unremarkable past medical history. He was referred to an early intervention program at 15 months by his primary care provider because of speech delay. His parents remain concerned about his communication, as he is repeating phrases from his favorite videos but not using words or gestures to communicate his needs. He has frequent tantrums, which his parents describe as occurring at least every hour with screaming, hitting, and throwing, and he is very difficult to soothe. He prefers to play by himself, primarily with trains and trucks, which he lines up and rolls back and forth, and will usually tantrum if others try to engage him in play [video #1 intake visit].

Autism spectrum disorder (ASD) is a biologically based, highly heterogeneous neurodevelopmental disorder characterized by deficits in social communication and reciprocity as well as the presence of repetitive and restrictive patterns of behaviors that impact the daily life experiences of the individual as well as the family and community. Our understanding of the complexities underlying etiology, diagnosis, comorbidities, and empirically based interventions has advanced significantly over the past several decades as support for research has expanded to include basic and translational science, behavioral and biomedical intervention studies, and health services research across the life span to address gaps and disparities in services.

SIGNS AND SYMPTOMS OF AUTISM SPECTRUM DISORDER

Diagnostic criteria for ASD have undergone substantial change with each revision of the *Diagnostic and Statistical Manual of Mental Disorders*, currently in the fifth revision (*DSM-5*) (American Psychiatric Association [APA], 2013), although the diagnosis remains based on developmental and behavioral symptoms now conceptualized in two behavioral domains. In the social domain individuals with ASD show deficits in social communication and reciprocity, with impaired use of nonverbal behaviors such as eye contact, facial expression and gestures to initiate and regulate social interactions, decreased seeking to share interests and enjoyment, and difficulty developing age-appropriate symbolic play and relationships with others. Characteristics reflected in the repetitive and restrictive behavior domain include unusual and intense interests, stereotyped body movements and/or language use, inflexible adherence to nonfunctional routines, and atypical sensory responsiveness. The developmental course and severity of symptoms vary across individuals as well as across the life span.

EPIDEMIOLOGY

ASD occurs across all racial, ethnic, and socioeconomic groups, although cultural and economic factors influence access to diagnostic services and interventions. The prevalence of ASD in the United States has been monitored by the Centers for Disease Control and Prevention (CDC) at 11 sites across the nation through the Autism and Developmental Disabilities Monitoring (ADDM) Network, a tracking system that has been in place since 2000. The most recent (Maenner et al., 2020) ASD prevalence estimates are 18.5 per 1000 (1 in 54) children at 8 years of age, with rates in boys 4.3 times that of girls based on 2016 data. This reflects a continued increase in prevalence from previous reports using the same methodology and sites (1 in 59, 2014 data). Despite variability across sites, overall prevalence rates were not significantly different for non-Hispanic White, non-Hispanic Black, and Asian/Pacific Islander children but were lower for Hispanic children (15.4 per 1000). One-third of children with data on cognitive functioning were classified as having intellectual disability (girls 39% vs. boys 32%; see Chapter 40). The median age of ASD diagnosis is 51 months, similar by sex and racial/ethnic groups, although Black children with ASD were less likely than White children to have a first evaluation by 36 months.

Chiarotti & Venerosi (2020) reviewed ASD prevalence studies published since 2014 and found high variability in prevalence estimates worldwide, although longitudinal studies in countries other than the United States confirm similar ongoing increases in ASD prevalence, despite differences in methodologies, geographic, sociocultural, and socioeconomic factors.

ETIOLOGY

The etiology underlying ASD is as heterogeneous as the clinical presentation. Twin studies have long confirmed the high heritability of ASD, with concordance rates of 98% in monozygotic twins and 53% to 67% concordance in dizygotic twins in a meta-analysis of twin pairs (Tick, Bolton, Happé, Rutter, & Rijsdijk, 2016). Despite these high estimates of heritability, genetic testing in children with ASD currently yields diagnostic results in 5% to 14% using chromosomal microarray (CMA) and up to 20% using whole exome sequencing (WES) (Srivastava et al., 2019). Ongoing research has increasingly investigated etiologic

The stability of early ASD diagnosis is quite high. In a population-based study of toddlers diagnosed with ASD and retested each 12 months until age 3 years Pierce and colleagues (2019) found that diagnostic stability for ASD was 0.84 overall when evaluations were done by highly experienced clinicians, with stability of 0.79 at 14 months and 0.83 by 16 months. Nearly one-fourth (23.8%) of children with a non-ASD diagnosis at initial evaluation received a later diagnosis of ASD at 36 months, but only 1.8% of children with an earlier ASD diagnosis no longer met criteria by 3 years of age.

Although it is clear that a subset of children with ASD can be reliably diagnosed in the second year of life, young children with less severe phenotypes may not be recognized until they enter into group childcare or educational settings when social demands exceed their limited social and pragmatic language capacities, and difficulties with peer interactions, social-emotional reciprocity, and flexibility are apparent (Goodwin, Matthews, & Smith, 2019). A subset of children followed prospectively as part of infant sibling studies demonstrated very few or subthreshold symptoms when evaluated using best practice at 3 years of age, but were later diagnosed with ASD after age 5 years, suggesting the need for continued monitoring of high-risk children over time (see Screening/Assessment/Diagnostic Evaluation, later) (Ozonoff et al., 2018).

The developmental course of toddlers and young children with ASD is clearly impacted by interventions received, although individual response is difficult to predict and dependent on many factors. Based on a recent randomized multicenter study, the degree of developmental delay at the beginning of the treatment did not moderate the effect on progress in the areas explored, including communication and nonverbal abilities, and had only a moderate effect based on autism symptoms (Rogers et al., 2020). Growing evidence supports the effect of parent-mediated interventions focused on social communication in reducing autism severity and improving dyadic communication skills, although the magnitude of those improvements is variable and difficult to predict for individual children at the time of diagnosis (Pickles et al., 2016; Weitlauf et al., 2014). (See video vignettes 2–4 for examples of response to intervention with therapist and parent coaching. Video 2 is 6 weeks into intervention using the Early Start Denver Model; Colin continues to be quickly reactive to unexpected events or frustrations, but he also demonstrates rapid learning of activity routines, simple communication exchanges, and play actions. Video 3 shows Colin after 1 year of intervention, during which he has ceased having tantrums, has learned to use language and other strategies to wait, make alternative choices, and express his feelings verbally. Video 4 shows Colin at age 4, after 2 years of intervention. His developmental skills are within the average range in all areas, and play dates have been added to his intervention to prepare him for transition to typical preschool.)

School-Aged Children

Children who are initially diagnosed with ASD during school age or adolescence (5–18 years) have generally been found to have higher cognitive and language skills and lower severity levels of ASD symptoms (Goodwin et al., 2019). They may have been initially diagnosed with ADHD or other cooccurring disorders that delay ASD diagnosis. When compared to children who received a diagnosis of ASD at earlier ages, children diagnosed after starting school show slightly fewer but persistent social communication concerns at the time of their diagnosis and fewer historical symptoms reported for preoccupations, rituals, and mannerisms but no differences in their current symptom severity. They also presented with higher cognitive and language abilities than children diagnosed earlier, which may help mask challenges associated with ASD until school entry (Goodwin et al., 2019).

Despite interventions and developmental gains, school-aged children with ASD face increasing challenges related to social engagement and cognitive flexibility. Pragmatic language difficulties, including conversational reciprocity and narratives, as well as limited nonverbal communication skills, clearly influence their ability to develop and maintain relationships, often becoming increasingly problematic over time as social expectations increase. Repetitive behaviors, adherence to routines, sensory issues, and restrictive patterns of behaviors can also contribute to functional impairment during daily activities in school and relationships with peers.

Children with ASD without intellectual disability often have learning difficulties despite performing well on standardized measures of educational achievement. They may begin to have difficulty in the third or fourth grade when limited pragmatic language skills and social awareness affect reading comprehension and written expression (Solari, Grimm, McIntyre, Zajic, & Mundy, 2019). Children with ASD and learning difficulties can become frustrated and develop problem behaviors if the learning difficulties are not recognized and addressed.

Executive dysfunctions also interfere with academic success at these and subsequent grade levels and may predict academic progress in higher education as planning/organization, independence and self-determination skills become more important for adolescence and adulthood (Dijkhuis, de Sonneville, Ziermans, Staal, & Swaab, 2020). (Video 5 shows Colin at age 6 years, at follow-up assessment. At this point, he is enrolled in a general education classroom and functioning at or above grade level. However, he now demonstrates high levels of motor activity and difficulties with attention.)

Adolescents

Adolescence is a very crucial time in the developmental course of individuals with ASD as they are experiencing hormonal changes, rapid physical changes, self-discovery, and increasing social demands. There is growing recognition of the vulnerability of autistic adolescents for mental health problems to be exacerbated during this period due in part to the increasing difficulty in finding evidence-based supports both within and outside of educational settings, paired with more expectations for independence in the face of accumulating negative social experiences (e.g., isolation, marginalization, and bullying) and ongoing challenges with social communication and cognitive flexibility. Anxiety in autistic adolescents is a strong predictor of suicidal ideation, depression, bipolar disorder, and other psychiatric conditions in adulthood (Anderson, Liang, & Lord, 2014). The risk of substance use is higher among autistic individuals without intellectual disability (Castellanos, Carcache, & Ng, 2020) and those with low social support, social deficits, and weak executive functioning (Ressel et al., 2020). Transition planning for medical care transition, postsecondary education, vocational training, and employment goals, as well as planning related to decision-making authority after age 18, should start by 12 to 14 years of age and involve the adolescent, family, educational counselors, and health care providers in shared decision making. Therapeutic goals should align with family and educational goals to support social functioning, employment skills, community inclusion, and independent living.

Adults

Supportive services once individuals leave the education system are generally quite limited, contributing to isolation for adults with ASD and their families, increasing the risk for mental health issues. Although educational attainment has improved over the last few decades, community inclusion and employment rates do not match educational levels attained, with only 25% of autistic adults with cognitive skills in the average range living independently (Anderson et al., 2014) and only 58% employed (Roux, Shattuck, Rast, Rava, & Anderson, 2015).

Historically Understudied Populations

Girls and children from racially and ethnically diverse groups with limited English proficiency or low socioeconomic status are more likely to be diagnosed at later ages (Stahmer et al., 2019), and there is much less information about the impact of these factors on their developmental course and outcomes.

Girls generally have lower levels of repetitive and restrictive behaviors (Kaat et al., 2021), and their restricted interests tend to be more socially acceptable. There is emerging evidence supporting a different autistic social traits trajectory in females. Studies have reported improvement of autistic symptoms in girls across early childhood, but this pattern is no longer seen in midadolescence when both genders experienced similar challenges (Mandy, Pellicano, St, Pourcain, Skuse, & Heron, 2018). It has been proposed that autistic girls may be better at compensating or camouflaging their social deficits (Lai et al., 2019), and other authors have theorized that some autistic social traits in females present later in life when high social demands exceed their abilities, especially during adolescence (Mandy et al., 2018). Recent studies have reported increased symptoms of emotional reactivity in autistic girls from early childhood (Nordahl et al., 2020) and more symptoms of depression during adolescence compared to autistic males (Wieckowski et al., 2020).

The developmental trajectories of individuals from populations historically underrepresented in autism research are just beginning to be investigated and are critical to the field. Disparities in early identification of ASD and service provision exist for individuals based on race, culture, socioeconomic status, and geographic location (Daniels & Mandell, 2014). Although in 2020 the ADDM Network found no differences in identification of ASD of Black children as compared to White children by 8 years of age, significant disparities remain in early identification by race, with Black and Hispanic children receiving diagnoses at later ages than White children (Constantino et al., 2020; Daniels & Mandell, 2014). While families with lower socioeconomic resources or in rural areas may have more difficulty accessing early diagnostic and intervention systems, the findings to date about these populations are mixed largely due to study methods (Daniels & Mandell, 2014). Given the importance of the positive effects of early intervention on functional living skills for individuals with ASD, it is important to further understand and eliminate these disparities.

SCREENING/ASSESSMENT/DIAGNOSTIC EVALUATION

Surveillance and Screening

Routine developmental surveillance and screening is critical to the early identification of children with ASD and other neurodevelopmental disorders so that early and appropriate interventions and supports can be initiated. Surveillance strategies, such as asking caregivers about their developmental concerns for their child and developmentally informed behavioral observations, are important for early recognition. Resources such as the CDC "Learn the Signs/Act Early" (https://www.cdc.gov/ncbddd/actearly/) and Autism Navigator (www.autismnavigator.com), a video glossary of early ASD symptoms in toddlers, are aimed at increasing the awareness of parents to early signs of ASD. The American Academy of Pediatrics (AAP) Council on Children with Disabilities and Section on Developmental Behavioral Pediatrics recently updated recommendations for surveillance and screening, including information on both validated and promising ASD-specific screening tools for toddlers and young children (Lipkin, Macias, & Council on Children with Disabilities, Section on Developmental and Behavioral Pediatrics, 2020) as well as recommendations for identification, evaluation, and management of ASD (Hyman et al., 2020). Both have descriptions of validated ASD screening tools for infants, toddlers, and preschoolers, including parent-completed questionnaires and clinician observation tools.

Developmental screening for ASD at 18 to 24 months is currently recommended, and parent questionnaires are available in multiple languages that may be administered to screen for ASD. The most extensively studied tool for children 16 to 30 months of age is the M-CHAT family, the most recent revision of which is the Modified Checklist for Autism in Toddlers, Revised with Follow-up (MCHAT-R/F). It is available online (http://mchatscreen.com/) and has electronic health records (EHR) compatible forms. Robins et al. (2014) reported that universal screening using the MCHAT-R/F with timely referrals for screen positive children lowered the age of ASD diagnosis from the current average age of 51 months (Maenner et al., 2020) to closer to 24 months of age.

The Infant Toddler Checklist (ITC) is a parent-completed questionnaire for children age 6 to 24 months designed to identify language delays and ASD symptoms (https://brookespublishing.com/product/csbs-dp-itc/). It is a useful tool when ASD concerns arise through surveillance prior to 18 months of age. At the present time, there are no AAP recommendations for routine ASD screening for children older than 30 months; however, there are standardized caregiver measures, including the Social Communication Questionnaire (Rutter, Bailey, & Lord, 2003a) developed from the Autism Diagnostic Interview-Revised (Rutter, Le Couteur, & Lord, 2003b) intended to evaluate symptoms of ASD in individuals at least 4 years of age and the Social Responsiveness Scale, Second Edition (Constantino & Gruber, 2012), that are accessible and have acceptable validity.

Comprehensive Assessments and Multimodal Evaluation Methods

Comprehensive evaluation is warranted for individuals who fail the first level of screening or those who show symptoms or behaviors relatively specific for ASD, often referred to as red flags for ASD. Once concerns are raised, because of limited access and long wait lists for comprehensive evaluations, these children should also be referred for interventions while waiting for a full diagnostic evaluation (Hyman et al., 2020).

Essential components of the diagnostic evaluation include (1) a developmental history and interview with parents; (2) review of available records related to previous testing, intervention reports, medical conditions; (3) direct observation and interaction with the child; and oftentimes (4) standardized or semistructured evaluation measures. The interview with parents should elicit their concerns for their child and goals for the evaluation, as well as the child's developmental history, medical and mental health history, and any prior interventions. Particular attention should be paid to the child's developmental trajectory, with detailed information about social and language development, and current functional level. Family medical and psychosocial history, including history of trauma and other related adverse childhood experiences, are also important components in the assessment process. Behavioral observation of the child in various contexts is ideal, as are collateral interviews or standardized report measures from teachers or other caregivers if possible.

It is critical to assess cognitive development, if not done previously, to base behavioral observations and caregiver reports of ASD symptoms within the appropriate developmental context.

In addition to direct behavioral observation of a child, semistructured and standardized assessment measures are typically included within diagnostic evaluations for ASD. Play-based assessments, either in person, such as the Autism Diagnostic Observation Schedule, Second Edition (Lord et al., 2012), or via telehealth if accessible, are frequently included in assessing ASD in children. Caregiver-completed adaptive functioning measures are important to determine functional deficits in independent daily living skills. Additional broadband standardized measures or symptom-specific measures may also be included to determine or rule out comorbid behavioral or mental health conditions. More comprehensive assessment of neuropsychological functioning (attention, memory, executive function), language and pragmatic language, academic achievement, motor function, and sensory processing may be important for intervention planning for some children.

MEDICAL EVALUATIONS

A child diagnosed with ASD should have a detailed medical evaluation with the purpose of assessing potential etiologic factors and the cooccurrence of other conditions frequently associated with ASD, guiding treatment decisions and determining the need for further family assessment. A complete medical history, including prenatal, perinatal, postnatal, and early childhood history is important to assess risk factors such as maternal illness or exposure to teratogens during pregnancy, perinatal complications, congenital anomalies, or serious illnesses. A complete review of systems should be done, with attention to neurologic symptoms such as seizures, regression, gastrointestinal symptoms and dietary restrictions, sensory impairments, sleep disturbances, and growth. A three-generation detailed family history should be gathered, with particular focus on developmental, educational, and social difficulties as well as psychiatric disorders.

Careful physical and neurologic examination is critical to identify recognizable genetic syndromes highly associated with ASD, such as fragile X syndrome, tuberous sclerosis, 15q duplication syndrome, *PTEN* mutation, Rett, and other genetic syndromes, as well as to recognize abnormal neurologic findings suggestive of overt central nervous system insult or sensory impairment, such as hearing loss or visual abnormalities. Growth parameters should be carefully assessed, including head circumference trajectories.

A genetic workup using WES, if available, or CMA along with DNA analysis for fragile X are recommended unless findings on physical examination suggest a specific etiology (Srivastava et al., 2019). WES should include both parents when possible and other affected family members. Many labs increasingly include CMA and mitochondrial DNA as part of WES analysis. Genetic technology is advancing quickly, and in the near future whole genome sequencing is expected to supersede both WES and CMA in clinical testing as costs decrease. Parents should be offered genetic testing with the purpose of exploring an etiology that may have potential impact on treatment and prognosis, as well as assessing the risk for recurrence. Parents should be involved in the decision by providing counseling about the utility, long-term implications, and limitations.

Additional assessments should be based on history and exam. All children with speech delay and inconsistent responsiveness during social interaction should undergo formal audiology testing. Vision testing is frequently recommended if the child's presentation warrants concern about vision in addition to poor eye contact. An ophthalmologic evaluation should be considered in children with history of prematurity, or metabolic or genetic conditions associated with eye problems.

Lead testing is appropriate if environmental risk factors exist, particularly for children who persist in mouthing objects or with pica, as elevated levels are treatable, and environmental lead abatement would be critically important. Metabolic studies should be considered when indicated by history or exam such as cyclic vomiting, lethargy, or hypoglycemia associated with mild illness, unusual odors, organomegaly, poor growth and feeding, or progressive loss of developmental skills.

The need for neuroimaging or electroencephalography (EEG) is individually determined based on history or clinical findings. Magnetic resonance imaging is the most commonly used technology in cases where an underlying brain abnormality is suspected. Some indications include microcephaly, macrocephaly, or localized neurologic findings. EEG is indicated if there is a history suggestive of seizures. Abnormal EEGs occur in the absence of clinical seizures, although there is little evidence to support treatment of these abnormalities at the current time.

Differential Diagnosis Versus Comorbidities

ASD commonly cooccurs with other neurodevelopmental, behavioral, and mental health disorders, which may mimic or mask ASD symptomatology and need to be differentiated. It is especially important to carefully consider ASD symptoms at early ages, particularly within the context of other diagnostic concerns, such as language delay, motor difficulty, short attention span, cognitive delay, and other medical conditions; in some cases diagnostic overshadowing and borderline presentations in children evaluated prior to the age of 6 years may result in children receiving a later ASD diagnosis. Thus it is important that the assessment of children with behavioral or developmental concerns includes a thorough evaluation of ASD symptoms as well as other disorders that may have overlapping symptoms and/or cooccur with ASD (Lai et al., 2019). However, the *DSM-5* recognizes the complexity of the diagnosis and allows multiple diagnoses, including other neurodevelopmental disorders such as ADHD and mental health disorders.

Intellectual Disability

The assessment of cognitive abilities should be part of the ASD diagnostic assessment to identify children with global developmental delay or intellectual disability (see Chapter 40) whose communication and behavior symptoms are consistent with their developmental age and do not meet ASD criteria, as well as to specify the presence of global developmental delay or intellectual disability in children who do meet diagnostic criteria of ASD. Reevaluating cognitive skills in children with ASD periodically is important, as cognitive evaluations prior to school-aged years may not be predictive of later functioning, and changes in cognitive skill levels may occur over time.

Social Communication Disorder

Social communication disorder was specified as a neurodevelopmental disorder in the *DSM-5* for the first time and should be considered in those children with pragmatic communication deficits, including difficulties in the use of communication for social purposes (e.g., greeting or sharing information), impairment in the ability to adapt communication to match social context (e.g., playground vs classroom), difficulties following rules for conversation and/or storytelling, and deficits in understanding nonliteral or ambiguous use of language such as idioms, humor, and metaphors. These deficits affect communication in ways that impair functional communication and overlap with communication difficulties seen in ASD, but they are not associated with restricted, repetitive patterns of behavior, interests, or activities.

Selective Mutism

Selective mutism is an anxiety disorder characterized by failure to initiate speech or respond when spoken to in social situations such as childcare settings or school, which significantly impacts social communication, although some of these children may use nonverbal strategies to communicate and participate with peers. These children do speak at home and with immediate family members, although evaluating their speech and language skills can be quite challenging. Children with selective mutism may be excessively shy, socially isolated, and withdrawn with compulsive traits and temper tantrums that must be differentiated from the social deficits and behavioral difficulties seen in children with ASD.

Language Disorders

Autism concerns are sometimes raised in children with isolated speech and language delay (see Chapter 44) presenting with verbal communication deficits and behavioral concerns; however, other aspects of nonverbal communication should be at their age level. Children with isolated speech delay also have age-appropriate play and reciprocal peer social interactions.

Attention-Deficit/Hyperactivity Disorder

Difficulties with attention and activity are common in both ASD and ADHD, with ADHD estimated to occur in 50% to 80% of children with ASD (see Chapter 46) (Barbaresi et al., 2020). Sometimes ADHD may be the first diagnosis delaying the diagnosis of ASD (Barbaresi et al., 2020).

Anxiety Disorders

Anxiety is common in children with ASD, and many will meet criteria for an anxiety disorder (see Chapter 51). However, the differential diagnosis between anxiety disorders and ASD can be complex as some behaviors in young children with a history of trauma and/or anxiety disorders may mimic characteristics of autism in terms of social withdrawal, difficulty with change or transitions, and/or sensory reactivity.

Childhood Onset Schizophrenia

Prodromal symptoms of schizophrenia such as hallucinations, delusions, and disorganized speech and thoughts can be associated with the emergence of atypical interests and impairments in social interactions, although these symptoms generally do not appear until late adolescence or adulthood, after a prolonged period of typical development and behavior. Deterioration in functioning often associated with prodromal symptoms is rarely seen in children before early teen years.

Stereotypic Movement Disorder

The presence of repetitive and purposeless motor behaviors in children with appropriate social communication skills is the essential feature for stereotypic movement disorder (see Chapter 71). These motor behaviors are usually rhythmic and interfere with daily functioning. Although these behaviors may seem purposeless at times, they can be related to emotional states and attempts at self-regulation. These behaviors usually start in early life and improve with motor mastery.

Co-occurring Medical and Mental Health Conditions

It is estimated that approximately 70% of people with an ASD diagnosis have an associated cooccurring medical or mental health condition, and over 40% may have two or more co-occurring conditions, but prevalence may vary based on the population studied. These comorbidities are not part of the diagnostic criteria but can exacerbate difficulties in function for autistic individuals as well as put their health and safety at risk.

Medical Co-occurring Conditions

Seizures are common in ASD, with prevalence ranges from 6.6% to 24.6%, with higher rates of cooccurring seizure disorders in females and individuals with intellectual disability (Jokiranta et al., 2014). There are two peak risk periods for seizures, during early childhood and adolescence. All types of seizures occur in association with ASD, including major motor, myoclonic, and febrile seizures, but complex partial seizures are most frequently reported.

Restrictive food intake is a common problem reported by parents, which is often related to sensory issues. Preferences for high-carbohydrate foods with low nutritional value may contribute to higher obesity rates later in life. Pica has an estimated prevalence of 23.3% compared to 8.4% in children with other developmental disorders (Fields et al., 2021).

Gastrointestinal problems commonly reported in children with ASD include diarrhea and constipation, which may be exacerbated by both diet and pica as well as higher incidence of reflux esophagitis. The presence of more than one gastrointestinal symptom was associated with increased sleep disturbances, somatic complaints, and self-injurious behaviors (Restrepo et al., 2020), emphasizing the importance of evaluation and treatment of gastrointestinal symptoms in individuals with ASD consistent with standards of care for neurotypical individuals.

Sleep problems common in children with ASD include bedtime resistance, sleep anxiety, sleep-onset disturbances, frequent waking, restlessness, or abnormal sleep architecture. The incidence of sleep problems has been associated with an increased occurrence of aggression, anxiety/depression, and attention problems and increased autism symptom severity. It is important to obtain information about family bedtime routines, possible sleep associations, and sleep patterns (Williams Buckley et al., 2020). (See Chapter 70 for more information on sleep problems in children with ASD.)

Motor impairments are often found, which can clearly impact their daily functioning, socialization, academic function, and independence. Those motor challenges vary from delays in skill development to impaired postural control, imitation, and coordination. Commonly, these motor impairments are pervasive and largely unrecognized (Bhat, 2020).

Mental Health Co-occurring Conditions

Emotional and behavioral problems occur more frequently across the life span for autistic individuals than neurotypicals, and mental health concerns increase with age. Young children with ASD frequently experience challenges in emotional and behavioral regulation. Difficulties with self-regulation may be associated with externalizing behaviors, including tantrums, aggression, and self-injury. These emotional responses may lead to safety issues and may negatively impact a child's adaptive skills, school performance, and further compound challenges with peer interactions.

More than 50% of parents have reported elopement episodes at some point after the age of 4 years. This behavior places them in dangerous situations and at increased risk for accidents, which are the leading cause of death in children and autistic adults (Guan & Li, 2017). Overall, the risk for elopement is high in individuals with intellectual disability and increases with autism severity and in those with behavioral issues such as affective problems, anxiety, and ADHD (Wiggins et al., 2020).

Depression and other mood disorders are prevalent in adolescents and adults with ASD, particularly those without intellectual impairment (Kirsch et al., 2020). Suicidal risk is important to assess, as autistic adolescents and adults are at increased risk for suicidal behaviors, especially those with a dual diagnosis of ASD and ADHD (Hirvikoski et al., 2020) or mood disorders. The risk of substance use is higher among autistic individuals without intellectual disability (Castellanos et al., 2020) and those with low social support, social deficits, and weak executive functioning (Ressel et al., 2020).

Gender nonconformity as well as nonheterosexual sexual orientation is more common in autistic than nonautistic children, adolescents, and adults (see Chapter 76). This in combination with the underlying deficits in social communication and social interactions places autistic adolescents and young adults at increased risk for adverse sexual experiences and victimization.

INTERVENTIONS

Behavioral Interventions for Core Symptoms

Behavioral interventions are currently the only evidenced-based treatments that address the core symptoms of ASD. The National Research Council (2001) identified autism-specific, evidence-based intervention recommendations that include (1) the use of positive behavioral supports such as functional behavior analyses and development of positive teaching plans, (2) targeting increased communication, (3) engaging children in age-appropriate learning using naturalistic teaching methods or didactic methods, (4) well-developed and developmentally appropriate teaching lessons for children's functional skills delivered at a high frequency throughout the day and in multiple settings with measurable progress, (5) generalizability and ecologic validity of skills, and (6) inclusion of parents in shared decision making important for a child's development (Stansberry-Brusnahan & Collet-Klingenberg, 2010). More recent systematic reviews of evidence-based practices identified both comprehensive treatment models and focused intervention practices (Steinbrenner et al., 2020).

Comprehensive treatments include program models with practices that result in a developmental impact on the core ASD symptoms. Chapter 94 includes a comprehensive description of evidence-based applied behavioral analysis interventions for ASD, which include both comprehensive treatment models and focused intervention strategies for specific skills or challenging behaviors.

Children diagnosed with ASD younger than age 3 years qualify for early intervention through the Individuals with Disabilities Education Improvement Act of 2004 (IDEA) Part C services. These services may be offered in a variety of settings (e.g., home, school, community based), methods (e.g., therapist, parent or teacher mediated), or of various theoretical orientations (e.g., applied behavioral analysis, naturalistic developmental behavioral models [NDBIs]) and intensities. Children over age 3 years with ASD are further supported through public mandates IDEA Part B services, the No Child Left Behind Act of 2001 (P.L. 107-110), and its successor Every Student Succeeds Act of 2015 (P.L. 114-95).

In summary, current best practices for early intervention prior to age 3 years should include autism-specific developmental and behavioral interventions as soon as possible with measurable goals related to ASD symptoms, overall development and daily living skills, active involvement of caregivers/family members, and should consider the sociocultural beliefs and economic capability of the family in terms of moderating treatment impact and outcome. Accessible online evidence-based treatment resources are available for professionals and family members (Autism Focused Intervention Resources and Modules, https://afirm.fpg.unc.edu; Help is in your Hands, https://helpisinyourhands.org/course).

Treatment strategies for school-age children and adolescents are generally focused on treatments that are developmentally appropriate and integrate school-based strategies and other supportive services such as social skills and speech-language therapy (see Chapter 107) and/or occupational therapy (see Chapter 106), as described later.

Educational Supports

Children with a medically determined diagnosis of ASD may qualify for educational support through an individualized education plan or Section 504 of the Rehabilitation Act of 1973 through their school if functional impairments associated with ASD are negatively impacting them in their educational environment, warranting modifications or accommodations to their educational curriculum. Clinical providers can support parents in advocating for an inclusive educational setting and educational placement in a least restrictive environment, should this setting in their local school district support their child's needs. In addition to teacher-implemented curriculum strategies for children with autism, individuals may benefit from additional supportive services through their school, including social skills support, speech-language intervention, occupational therapy, or mental health services.

Speech and Language Therapy

Individuals with ASD may exhibit expressive and receptive language delays, for which speech-language therapy is indicated (see Chapter 107). Interventions specific to the communicative deficits in individuals with ASD generally fall into three categories, which overlap with evidence-based behavioral interventions for ASD: didactic, naturalistic, and developmental or pragmatic. Descriptions of didactic and applied behavioral analysis–based interventions that impact language skills are detailed in Chapter 94. Naturalistic approaches for individuals with ASD and verbal language may include rehearsing and practicing social scripts, as well as video modeling and role playing. Developmentally based pragmatic language approaches have been developed to target the difficulties verbal individuals with ASD may have with grammar, syntax, and narrative that impact social communication. Other effective social pragmatic approaches have been found to improve social communication, cognition and motivation, self-regulation, and provide transactional supports to children with ASD (Laugeson, 2013). Sandbank and colleagues (2020) found evidence that effects were largest for expressive and composite language outcomes, for children with initially higher language abilities, and for interventions implemented by clinicians or by caregivers and clinicians combined, although additional research is needed to better identify intervention effectiveness and corresponding moderators.

Some children with ASD and limited verbal language benefit greatly from alternative and augmentative communication strategies. Picture exchange communication systems involve an individual using a picture in exchange for a desired item and then using the pictures to create more complex sentence structures. Aided communication devices such as voice output communication devices can also be helpful for nonverbal individuals with ASD by incorporating technology for vocal output.

Occupational Therapy

There is limited evidence to support sensory-based strategies (see Chapter 45), such as Ayers Sensory Integration, for improving fine motor and sensory sensitivities, resulting in improved adaptive living skills (Schaaf, Dumont, Arbesman, & May-Benson, 2017), decreasing self-injurious, stereotyped, and maladaptive behaviors, and promoting positive social engagement and communication.

Behavioral and Mental Health Interventions

ASD frequently cooccurs with other behavioral and mental health concerns for which evidence-based interventions with adaptations for ASD have been found useful. Behavioral interventions such as Triple P Stepping Stones and Parent Child Interaction Therapy have been found to help decrease externalizing behaviors for children with ASD (see Chapter 93). These parent-implemented strategies equip caregivers with additional tools to help manage aggression or acting-out behaviors in a consistent manner. Evidence-based interventions using cognitive-behavioral therapy (CBT) and trauma-focused CBT have been adapted for children with ASD to address anxiety or depression and trauma symptoms (Chapter 98)

Medical Interventions

While behavioral treatments are currently the only evidence-based interventions to treat the core symptoms of ASD, psychopharmacologic agents can be considered as adjunct therapy to behavioral and psychotherapeutic interventions when services and accommodations have been maximized but the individual still presents with functional impairments or safety issues related to cooccurring symptoms such as inattention, hyperactivity, obsessive-compulsive behaviors, aggression, self-injury, irritability, and mood lability.

There are two medications approved by the US Food and Drug Administration (FDA) for the treatment of irritability associated with ASD (see Chapter 99). Risperidone, approved for children older than 5 years of age, and aripiprazole, approved for children 6 to 17 years of age, were approved based on results of multicenter clinical trials that found effectiveness in reducing irritability and, to a lesser degree, repetitive behaviors. These two atypical antipsychotic medications share similar safety profiles; the most common side effects include fatigue, increased appetite, gastrointestinal symptoms, hyperprolactinemia, weight gain, and sedation, and less commonly activation including restlessness and akathisia. They are also linked to more serious side effects, including dyslipidemia, hyperglycemia, metabolic syndrome, and extrapyramidal symptoms or drug-induced movement disorders. Therefore close clinical and laboratory monitoring is recommended. Given that the efficacy and safety of these medications have not been established for the long-term treatment of irritability in autistic individuals, it is important to periodically reevaluate the need for continuation of treatment.

There are other potential medications used to treat associated behavioral symptoms in autistic individuals, including selective serotonin reuptake inhibitors, alpha-2 agonists, stimulants, nonstimulants, mood stabilizers, and anticonvulsants (see Chapter 99). Individuals with ASD are often sensitive to medication effects and more likely to have adverse effects, so pharmacologic treatment should be started at lower doses and adjusted slowly. The autistic individual should be involved in the decision-making process as much as possible along with caregivers and be well informed about the rationale behind the treatment, including the symptoms or behaviors being targeted for treatment, potential risks and benefits, safety profile, and required monitoring over time. Obtaining objective targeted symptom measures at baseline and during treatment is key to objectively evaluating response to treatment. Ideally, information should be obtained from different sources to better assess the child's functioning and response to treatment in different settings.

There is some evidence suggesting low melatonin levels affecting the circadian rhythm in autistic children. In cases where behavioral and environmental interventions have been implemented for sleep disturbances, particularly sleep-onset issues but with limited response, clinicians may recommend the use of melatonin, which is usually well tolerated and has a low incidence of side effects. Usual starting doses are 0.5 to 2 mg, depending on age, increasing by 1 mg as needed to a maximum 10 mg. There is increasing evidence for the use of prolonged-release melatonin in autistic individuals, and this may be tried in cases with limited response to regular release formulations (Williams Buckley et al., 2020). Melatonin is an over-the-counter product that is not regulated by the FDA. When parents/caregivers purchase melatonin they should seek a formulation that contains melatonin as the only active ingredient.

Changes in severity of behavioral symptoms or the onset of new behaviors should prompt further history and examination to determine if new environmental stressors or health-related issues such as dental pain, ear or other infections, gastrointestinal disturbances, or unrecognized injuries are contributing to the behavioral changes before increasing or changing medications.

Cooccurring medical conditions in children with ASD are well documented, and emerging evidence suggests that autistic children have more unmet health care needs and more cooccurring conditions than either children with other special health care needs or those without, and adults with ASD have higher rates of adverse physical health outcomes (Bishop-Fitzpatrick & Kind, 2017). Unmet health care needs are particularly experienced by Hispanic and Black children, based on the National Autism Indicators Report (NAIR) on Health and Health Care (https://drexel.edu/autismoutcomes/publications-and-reports/publications/NAIRHealth/). The risk of premature death is up to 10-fold higher for autistic individuals compared to the general population, with an average age of death 35.8 years younger than the general population (Guan & Li, 2017). Medical providers should address disparities and barriers to receiving comprehensive medical care, including preventive services and identification and management of frequently cooccurring medical and mental health conditions.

Complementary and Alternative Therapies

The heterogeneity of clinical symptoms and of potential etiologic mechanisms in ASD has given rise to many poorly or unsubstantiated theories related to the underlying causes and treatments of ASD. The use of complementary and alternative medicine (CAM) therapy is very common in the United States generally, and up to 71% of the families of children with ASD have reported using CAM treatments (Black, Clarke, Barnes, Stussman, & Nahin, 2015) with the hope of improving their children's health, functional levels, and skills. It is challenging for providers to stay well informed with nonstandard interventions disseminated online and by family, friends, or celebrities. Hyman et al. (2020) present a thorough review of many currently popular CAM treatments disseminated as correcting various underlying biologic causes of ASD, but it is beyond the scope of this chapter. The National Center for Complementary and Integrative Health (https://nccih.nih.gov/health/autism) provides updated reviews of novel therapies for ASD. It is vital that providers routinely ask in a nonjudgmental fashion about the use of CAM, both at the time of diagnosis and at subsequent visits. Many parents feel desperate to try "anything" to help their child and have difficulty interpreting the validity of the evidence to support various CAM treatments. If parents are interested in initiating a CAM treatment, it is critical to openly discuss targeted symptom(s), the available evidence base related to efficacy, the potential risks relative to health and safety, and the needed resources in terms of finances and time commitment. If families choose to proceed with CAM interventions that do not pose a significant safety risk, clinicians can support the family by facilitating a trial that establishes a target symptom, a baseline assessment for that symptom prior to treatment, and periodic monitoring for therapeutic response as well as side effects in an objective and measurable fashion.

FAMILY-CENTERED, CULTURALLY AND LINGUISTICALLY COMPETENT AND EQUITABLE CARE

Families are at the center of support for their children; throughout each step of their journey, individuals with ASD and their caregivers benefit from family-centered, culturally and linguistically competent care, although they are less likely to receive it compared to children with other special health care needs (Bishop-Fitzpatrick & Kind, 2017). Families from racially and ethnically diverse groups, with limited English proficiency or with low socioeconomic status, experience more challenges in accessing diagnostic and intervention services and in navigating complex systems of care (Stahmer et al., 2019). Most families feel isolated after receiving an ASD diagnosis and face many new responsibilities, including facilitating a multidisciplinary and complex management team for their children. Many families have to deal with additional social and cultural stressors, including feeling judged by others about their parenting skills or blamed for their child's diagnosis. Connecting families with navigator programs, which assist them with accessing diagnostic evaluations, navigating intervention services, and accessing community resources such as parent support organizations (Stahmer et al., 2019), is recommended to foster social connectiveness and peer-to-peer support. Sibling support is another important aspect to consider in providing family-centered care.

Family-centered care that integrates the National Standards for Culturally and Linguistically Appropriate Services (CLAS; https://thinkculturalhealth.hhs.gov/clas) standards is particularly important for underrepresented children and their families who may have higher levels of mistrust, different cultural norms, cultural stigma, or self-blame associated with ASD diagnosis, which increase risk for miscommunication with providers and difficulties in collaborative relationship building and shared decision making (Stahmer et al., 2019). Families from underrepresented groups may also have additional barriers related to extra support needs (e.g., so they can continue to work), language, transportation, or immigration status, which result in further difficulty accessing information and understanding ASD as well as navigating complex systems.

Another aspect of providing culturally competent and equitable care includes recognizing an ongoing paradigm shift, largely led by autistic individuals, to redefine our conceptualization of neurodevelopmental disabilities to a perspective that embraces neurodiversity and reframes our understanding of neurocognitive functioning toward a strengths-based perspective. Fundamental principles of this paradigm shift include accepting neurodiversity as a natural and valuable form of human diversity and variation, and recognizing that current definitions of typical neurocognitive functioning and behavior are culturally constructed concepts that have a negative impact by marginalizing specific groups of people (Honeybourne, 2019). Neurodiversity recognizes the importance of honoring the culture of people with neurodivergent perspectives (Honeybourne, 2019). Individuals with ASD, or autistic individuals, as some prefer to be called, add to the diversity of our culture by their distinctive strengths, which are often unrecognized within traditional deficit-based models that focus on fixing or curing differences (Silberman, 2015). This movement prioritizes changing the environment to provide individualized supports for people who identify as neurodiverse, rather than changing the individual. It is important to highlight that individuals who identify as neurodiverse may also identify with multiple other cultural identities and linguistic capabilities. These intersecting identities may further marginalize neurodiverse individuals in our society, emphasizing the importance of recognizing and valuing the various permutations of neurodiversity to achieve a more fully inclusive society.

FUTURE DIRECTIONS

The interprofessional fields involved in autism care and research must continue working to address disparities in diagnosis and service delivery based on racial, cultural, linguistic, and socioeconomic backgrounds as well as gender. We must promote understanding and acceptance of the value of neurodiversity and build systems that support autistic individuals and their families emotionally, behaviorally, and medically in ways that are respectful to their individual, family, and cultural values to optimize outcomes across the life span.

In the face of a crisis generated by a global pandemic many clinicians shifted from in-person to remote services, including virtual assessments and therapy delivery. The evidence supporting these types of assessments and treatments prior to the pandemic was emerging but still limited. Well-designed studies are necessary to evaluate the opportunities and challenges of remote diagnostic assessment and service delivery and to evaluate possible impacts on health disparities.

Ongoing research directed at increasing our understanding of the genetic, environmental, and neurobiologic mechanisms underlying ASD promises the identification of specific early biomarkers and/or development of targeted treatments for specific etiologic or phenotypic subgroups of ASD that may be initiated prior to symptom emergence at a time of maximal neuroplasticity.

At the same time, research initiatives must focus on improving the quality of life and wellbeing for people on the autism spectrum across the life span. Multiple fields play vital roles in the lives of autistic individuals and their families; from the time of first diagnosis our therapeutic goals should focus on comprehensively addressing the complex conditions affecting the quality of life of autistic individuals and their families. We must build and evaluate comprehensive systems of multidisciplinary, collaborative, and family-centered care that optimize quality of life outcomes, empower autistic individuals to be valued for their individual strengths, and embrace the idea of autism as an identity and neurodiversity as a cultural value. The importance of embedding family-centered, culturally and linguistically competent care with antiracist strategies for individuals with ASD and their families must be addressed if we are to meaningfully change and provide service to all individuals with ASD and their families in the future.

REFERENCES

American Psychiatric Association. (2013). *Diagnostic and statistical manual of mental disorders* (5th ed.). APA. https://doi.org/10.1176/appi.books.9780890425596.

Anderson, D. K., Liang, J. W., & Lord, C. (2014). Predicting young adult outcome among more and less cognitively able individuals with autism spectrum disorders. *Journal of Child Psychology and Psychiatry, 55*(5), 485–494.

Barbaresi, W. J., Campbell, L., Diekroger, E. A., Froehlich, T. E., Liu, Y. H., O'Malley, E., … Chan, E. (2020). Society for developmental and behavioral pediatrics clinical practice guideline for the assessment and treatment of children and adolescents with complex attention-deficit/hyperactivity disorder. *Journal of Developmental & Behavioral Pediatrics, 41*, S35–S57.

Bhat, A. N. (2020). Is motor impairment in autism spectrum disorder distinct from developmental coordination disorder? A report from the SPARK study. *Physical Therapy, 100*(4), 633–644.

Bishop-Fitzpatrick, L., & Kind, A. J. (2017). A scoping review of health disparities in autism spectrum disorder. *Journal of Autism and Developmental Disorders, 47*(11), 3380–3391.

Black, L. I., Clarke, T. C., Barnes, P. M., Stussman, B. J., & Nahin, R. L. (2015). Use of complementary health approaches among children aged 4–17 years in the United States: National Health Interview Survey, 2007–2012. *National Health Statistics Reports, 78*, 1–19.

Castellanos, D., Carcache, L., & Ng, C. (2020). Substance use in youth with autism spectrum disorder. *Addictive Disorders & Their Treatment, 19*(2), 118–122.

Chiarotti, F., & Venerosi, A. (2020). Epidemiology of autism spectrum disorders: A review of worldwide prevalence estimates since 2014. *Brain Sciences, 10*(5). https://doi.org/10.3390/brainsci10050274.

Constantino, J. N., Abbacchi, A. M., Saulnier, C., Klaiman, C., Mandell, D. S., Zhang, Y., … Geschwind, D. H. (2020). Timing of the diagnosis of autism in African American children. *Pediatrics, 146*(3), e20193629. https://doi.org/10.1542/peds.2019-3629.

Constantino, J. N., & Gruber, C. P. (2012). *Social responsiveness scale: SRS-2*. Western Psychological Services.

Daniels, A. M., & Mandell, D. S. (2014). Explaining differences in age at autism spectrum disorder diagnosis: A critical review. *Autism, 18*(5), 583–597. https://doi.org/10.1177/1362361313480277.

Dijkhuis, R., de Sonneville, L., Ziermans, T., Staal, W., & Swaab, H. (2020). Autism symptoms, executive functioning and academic progress in higher education students. *Journal of Autism and Developmental Disorders, 50*(4), 1353–1363. https://doi.org/10.1007/s10803-019-04267-8.

Fields, V. L., Soke, G. N., Reynolds, A., Tian, L. H., Wiggins, L., Maenner, M., … Schieve, L. A. (2021). Pica, autism, and other disabilities. *Pediatrics, 147*, 1.

Goodwin, A., Matthews, N. L., & Smith, C. J. (2019). Parent-reported early symptoms of autism spectrum disorder in children without intellectual disability who were diagnosed at school age. *Autism, 23*(3), 770–782.

Guan, J., & Li, G. (2017). Injury mortality in individuals with autism. *American Journal of Public Health, 107*(5), 791–793.

Hirvikoski, T., Boman, M., Chen, Q., D'Onofrio, B. M., Mittendorfer-Rutz, E., Lichtenstein, P., … Larsson, H. (2020). Individual risk and familial liability for suicide attempt and suicide in autism: A population-based study. *Psychological Medicine, 50*(9), 1463–1474.

Honeybourne, V. (2019). *A practical guide to happiness in adults on the autism spectrum: A positive psychology approach*. Jessica Kingsley Publishers.

Hyman, S. L., Levy, S. E., Myers, S. M., & Council on Children with Disabilities, Section on Developmental and Behavioral Pediatrics. (2020). Identification, evaluation, and management of children with autism spectrum disorder. *Pediatrics, 145*(1). https://doi.org/10.1542/peds.2019-3447.

Jokiranta, E., Sourander, A., Suominen, A., Timonen-Soivio, L., Brown, A. S., & Sillanpää, M. (2014). Epilepsy among children and adolescents with autism spectrum disorders: A population-based study. *Journal of Autism and Developmental Disorders, 44*(10), 2547–2557. https://doi.org/10.1007/s10803-014-2126-6.

Kaat, A. J., Shui, A. M., Ghods, S. S., Farmer, C. A., Esler, A. N., Thurm, A., … Bishop, S. L. (2021). Sex differences in scores on standardized measures of autism symptoms: A multisite integrative data analysis. *Journal of Child Psychology and Psychiatry, and Allied Disciplines, 62*(1), 97–106. https://doi.org/10.1111/jcpp.13242.

Kirsch, A. C., Huebner, A. R., Mehta, S. Q., Howie, F. R., Weaver, A. L., Myers, S. M., … Katusic, S. K. (2020). Association of comorbid mood and anxiety disorders with autism spectrum disorder. *JAMA Pediatrics, 174*(1), 63–70.

Lai, M.-C., Kassee, C., Besney, R., Bonato, S., Hull, L., Mandy, W., … Ameis, S. H. (2019). Prevalence of co-occurring mental health diagnoses in the autism population: A systematic review and meta-analysis. *The Lancet Psychiatry, 6*(10), 819–829.

Laugeson, E. A. (2013). Review: Social skills groups may improve social competence in children and adolescents with autism spectrum disorder. *Evidence-Based Mental Health*, *16*(1), 11. https://doi.org/10.1136/eb-2012-100985.

Lipkin, P. H., Macias, M. M., & Council on Children with Disabilities, Section on Developmental and Behavioral Pediatrics. (2020). Promoting optimal development: Identifying infants and young children with developmental disorders through developmental surveillance and screening. *Pediatrics*, *145*(1). https://doi.org/10.1542/peds.2019-3449.

Lord, C., Rutter, M., DiLavore, P. C., Risi, S., Gotham, K., & Bishop, S. L. (2012). *Autism diagnostic observation schedule, (ADOS-2) modules 1-4*. Western Psychological Services.

Maenner, M. J., Shaw, K. A., Baio, J., EdS1, Washington, A., Patrick, M., DiRienzo, M., … Dietz, P. M. (2020). Prevalence of autism spectrum disorder among children aged 8 years—Autism and Developmental Disabilities Monitoring Network, 11 Sites, United States, 2016. *MMWR Surveillance Summaries*, *69*(4), 1–12. https://doi.org/10.15585/mmwr.ss6904a1.

Mandy, W., Pellicano, L., St, Pourcain, B., Skuse, D., & Heron, J. (2018). The development of autistic social traits across childhood and adolescence in males and females. *Journal of Child Psychology and Psychiatry, and Allied Disciplines*, *59*(11), 1143–1151. https://doi.org/10.1111/jcpp.12913.

Mazurek, M. O., Lu, F., Macklin, E. A., & Handen, B. L. (2019). Factors associated with *DSM-5* severity level ratings for autism spectrum disorder. *Autism*, *23*(2), 468–476. https://doi.org/10.1177/1362361318755318.

Miller, M., Musser, E. D., Young, G. S., Olson, B., Steiner, R. D., & Nigg, J. T. (2019). Sibling recurrence risk and cross-aggregation of attention-deficit/hyperactivity disorder and autism spectrum disorder. *JAMA Pediatrics*, *173*(2), 147–152. https://doi.org/10.1001/jamapediatrics.2018.4076.

Nordahl, C. W., Iosif, A. -M., Young, G. S., Hechtman, A., Heath, B., Lee, J. K., … Amaral, D. G. (2020). High psychopathology subgroup in young children with autism: Associations with biological sex and amygdala volume. *Journal of the American Academy of Child & Adolescent Psychiatry*, *59*(12), 1353–1363.

Ozonoff, S., & Iosif, A. -M. (2019). Changing conceptualizations of regression: What prospective studies reveal about the onset of autism spectrum disorder. *Neuroscience & Biobehavioral Reviews*, *100*, 296–304.

Ozonoff, S., Young, G. S., Brian, J., Charman, T., Shephard, E., Solish, A., & Zwaigenbaum, L. (2018). Diagnosis of autism spectrum disorder after age 5 in children evaluated longitudinally since infancy. *Journal of the American Academy of Child & Adolescent Psychiatry*, *57*(11), 849–857. e2. https://doi.org/10.1016/j.jaac.2018.06.022.

Pickles, A., Le Couteur, A., Leadbitter, K., Salomone, E., Cole-Fletcher, R., Tobin, H., … Byford, S. (2016). Parent-mediated social communication therapy for young children with autism (PACT): Long-term follow-up of a randomised controlled trial. *The Lancet*, *388*(10059), 2501–2509.

Pierce, K., Gazestani, V. H., Bacon, E., Barnes, C. C., Cha, D., Nalabolu, S., … Courchesne, E. (2019). Evaluation of the diagnostic stability of the early autism spectrum disorder phenotype in the general population starting at 12 months. *JAMA Pediatrics*, *173*(6), 578–587. https://doi.org/10.1001/jamapediatrics.2019.0624.

Ramirez-Celis, A., Becker, M., Nuño, M., Schauer, J., Aghaeepour, N., & Van de Water, J. (2021). Risk assessment analysis for maternal autoantibody-related autism (MAR-ASD): A subtype of autism. *Molecular Psychiatry*, 1–10.

Ressel, M., Thompson, B., Poulin, M.-H., Normand, C. L., Fisher, M. H., Couture, G., & Iarocci, G. (2020). Systematic review of risk and protective factors associated with substance use and abuse in individuals with autism spectrum disorders. *Autism*, *24*(4), 899–918.

Restrepo, B., Angkustsiri, K., Taylor, S. L., Rogers, S. J., Cabral, J., Heath, B., … Amaral, D. G. (2020). Developmental–behavioral profiles in children with autism spectrum disorder and co-occurring gastrointestinal symptoms. *Autism Research*, *13*(10), 1778–1789.

Robins, D. L., Casagrande, K., Barton, M , Chen, C. -M. A., Dumont-Mathieu, T., & Fein, D. (2014). Validation of the Mmodified Checklist for Autism in Toddlers, Revised with Follow-up (M-CHAT-R/F). *Pediatrics*, *133*(1), 37–45.

Rogers, S. J., Yoder, P., Estes, A., Warren, Z., McEachin, J., Munson, J., … Gardner, E. (2020). A multisite randomized controlled trial comparing the effects of intervention intensity and intervention style on outcomes for young children with autism. *Journal of the American Academy of Child & Adolescent Psychiatry*.

Roux, A. M., Shattuck, P. T., Rast, J. E., Rava, J. A., & Anderson, K. (2015). National Autism Indicators Report: Transition into young adulthood. *Autism Outcomes*. https://drexel.edu/autismoutcomes/publications-and-reports/publications/National-Autism-Indicators-Report-Transition-to-Adulthood/.

Rutter, M., Bailey, A., & Lord, C. (2003a). *SCQ. The social communication questionnaire*. Western Psychological Services.

Rutter, M., Le Couteur, A., & Lord, C. (2003b). Autism diagnostic interview-revised. *Western Psychological Services*, *29*(2003), 30.

Sandbank, M., Bottema-Beutel, K., Crowley, S., Cassidy, M., Feldman, J. I., Canihuante, M., & Woynaroski, T. (2020). Intervention effects on language in children with autism: A project AIM meta-analysis. *Journal of Speech, Language, and Hearing Research*, *63*(5), 1537–1560.

Schaaf, R. C., Dumont, R. L., Arbesman, M., & May-Benson, T. A. (2017). Efficacy of occupational therapy using Ayres sensory integration: A systematic review. *American Journal of Occupational Therapy*, *72*(1). 7201190010p1. https://doi.org/10.5014/ajot.2018.028431.

Silberman, S. (2015). *Neurotribes: The legacy of autism and the future of neurodiversity*. Penguin.

Solari, E. J., Grimm, R. P., McIntyre, N. S., Zajic, M., & Mundy, P. C. (2019). Longitudinal stability of reading profiles in individuals with higher functioning autism. *Autism: The International Journal of Research and Practice*, *23*(8), 1911–1926. https://doi.org/10.1177/1362361318812423.

Srivastava, S., Love-Nichols, J. A., Dies, K. A., Ledbetter, D. H., Martin, C. L., Chung, W. K., … NDD Exome Scoping Review Work Group. (2019). Meta-analysis and multidisciplinary consensus statement: Exome sequencing is a first-tier clinical diagnostic test for individuals with neurodevelopmental disorders. *Genetics in Medicine: Official Journal of the American College of Medical Genetics*, *21*(11), 2413–2421. https://doi.org/10.1038/s41436-019-0554-6.

Stahmer, A. C., Vejnoska, S., Iadarola, S., Straiton, D., Segovia, F. R., Luelmo, P., … Kasari, C. (2019). Caregiver voices: Cross-cultural input on improving access to autism services. *Journal of Racial and Ethnic Health Disparities*, *6*(4), 752–773. https://doi.org/10.1007/s40615-019-00575-y.

Stansberry-Brusnahan, L. L., & Collet-Klingenberg, L. L. (2010). Evidence-based practices for young children with autism spectrum disorders: Guidelines and recommendations from the National Resource Council and National Professional Development Center on Autism Spectrum Disorders. *International Journal of Early Childhood Special Education*, *2*(1).

Steinbrenner, J. R., Hume, K., Odom, S. L., Morin, K. L., Nowell, S. W., Tomaszewski, B., … Savage, M. N. (2020). *Evidence-based practices for children, youth, and young adults with autism spectrum disorder*. UNC.

Surén, P., Roth, C., Bresnahan, M., Haugen, M., Hornig, M., Hirtz, D., … Reichborn-Kjennerud, T. (2013). Association between maternal use of folic acid supplements and risk of autism spectrum disorders in children. *JAMA*, *309*(6), 570–577.

Tick, B., Bolton, P., Happé, F., Rutter, M., & Rijsdijk, F. (2016). Heritability of autism spectrum disorders: A meta-analysis of twin studies. *Journal of Child Psychology and Psychiatry, and Allied Disciplines*, *57*(5), 585–595. https://doi.org/10.1111/jcpp.12499.

Waye, M. M. Y., & Cheng, H. Y. (2018). Genetics and epigenetics of autism: A review. *Psychiatry and Clinical Neurosciences*, *72*(4), 228–244. https://doi.org/10.1111/pcn.12606.

Weitlauf, A. S., McPheeters, M. L., Peters, B., Sathe, N., Travis, R., Aiello, R., … Jerome, R. (2014). *Therapies for children with autism spectrum disorder*. Agency for Healthcare Research and Quality.

Wieckowski, A. T., Luallin, S., Pan, Z., Righi, G., Gabriels, R. L., & Mazefsky, C. (2020). Gender differences in emotion dysregulation in an autism inpatient psychiatric sample. *Autism Research*, *13*(8), 1343–1348.

Wiggins, L. D., DiGuiseppi, C., Schieve, L., Moody, E., Soke, G., Giarelli, E., & Levy, S. (2020). Wandering among preschool children with and without autism spectrum disorder. *Journal of Developmental and Behavioral Pediatrics: JDBP*, *41*(4), 251.

Williams Buckley, A., Hirtz, D., Oskoui, M., Armstrong, M. J., Batra, A., Bridgemohan, C., … Ashwal, S. (2020). Practice guideline: Treatment for insomnia and disrupted sleep behavior in children and adolescents with autism spectrum disorder: Report of the Guideline Development, Dissemination, and Implementation Subcommittee of the American Academy of Neurology. *Neurology*, *94*(9), 392–404. https://doi.org/10.1212/WNL.0000000000009033.

Wolff, J. J., & Piven, J. (2020). Predicting autism risk in infancy. *Journal of the American Academy of Child and Adolescent Psychiatry* S0890-8567(20)32061-X. Epub ahead of print. https://doi.org/10.1016/j.jaac.2020.07.910. PMID: 33161062.

42

Developmental Considerations in Deafness

Deborah Mood and Angela Yarnell Bonino

For additional material related to the content of this chapter, please see Chapters 44, and 107.

VIGNETTE

Charlie referred on newborn hearing screening for both ears. Auditory brainstem response (ABR) revealed bilateral moderate sensorineural hearing loss (SNHL). Diagnostic evaluation was consistent with congenital cytomegalovirus (CMV), resulting in a consultation with infectious disease and a course of valganciclovir. Magnetic resonance imaging (MRI) revealed several posterior white matter lesions. At 3 months, Charlie was fit with bilateral hearing aids, and he began early intervention services for deaf children, including American Sign Language (ASL) instruction. Vision services were added following diagnosis of cortical vision impairment, and Charlie's functional vision improved. Charlie walked at 30 months. At 36 months, he used 5 spoken words and 10 signs. Results of a multidisciplinary developmental evaluation indicated low average visual problem-solving skills and concerns for motor planning difficulties. Additional occupational therapy and targeted speech-language therapy intervention incorporating ASL and visual supports was recommended, resulting in reduced behaviors due to frustration. At 40 months, his parents noticed a decline in his vocalizations, and audiologic testing revealed a progression to profound SNHL bilaterally. Charlie received cochlear implants at 45 months. At age 6 years, Charlie continued to make slow consistent language gains with continued exposure to ASL and spoken language at home and school. He attends a center-based program for deaf children utilizing a total communication approach. In addition, with use of augmentative and alternative communication Charlie was able to make requests and engage with peers.

Charlie's case highlights the importance of early diagnosis, medical management, multidisciplinary teaming, and ongoing audiologic and developmental monitoring to identify progressive hearing loss and provide quality family-centered individualized intervention.

TERMINOLOGY

In medical textbooks, reduced hearing is commonly called "hearing impairment" and individuals have been referred to as "hearing impaired." Terms such as *deaf and hard of hearing* (DHH) emphasize audiologic functioning, distinguishing children who are deaf (i.e., profound hearing loss) from those with lesser degrees of hearing loss. Even the term *hearing loss* has been questioned as many are born with a congenital hearing difference that does not progress (i.e., they do not "lose" hearing) and do not experience hearing differences psychologically as a "loss." Terminology is important—particularly when referring to individuals from historically oppressed minority groups—and it is recommended to move from terms that emphasize hearing status to those that emphasize cultural identity. The Deaf community rejects medical terminology that they perceive as pathologizing (e.g., *impairment*) and instead adopts *Deaf* (indicated with a capital *D*) to celebrate the community's shared learned behaviors, values, rich traditions, and language (i.e., ASL in the United States). Individuals with reduced hearing of any severity who identify as culturally Deaf strongly prefer this term. The term *deaf* (lowercase *d*) is also preferred when referencing individuals with reduced hearing, regardless of the severity, when their cultural affiliation is unknown or in the case of children who are still developing their own identity. In addition, identity-centered language (e.g., *deaf children* or *Deaf children*) is preferred. Here we will use the identity-centered term *deaf children* unless specifically referencing individuals who align with Deaf culture or in specific instances when degree or type of hearing loss is relevant. Although imperfect, *hearing loss* is used to refer to type and degree of hearing levels.

Hearing loss can be described based on laterality, severity, and type. Hearing loss in one ear is a unilateral hearing loss, whereas hearing loss in both ears is a bilateral hearing loss. The severity of the hearing loss is often computed by averaging hearing thresholds in decibels hearing level (dB HL) at 500, 1000, and 2000 Hz. However, classification systems can include other frequencies or examine individual thresholds. The upper limit of normal hearing sensitivity for children is often set at 15 dB HL because a hearing loss greater than this can affect speech perception and language acquisition. The degree of hearing loss is defined as normal (≤15 dB HL), slight (16–25 dB HL), mild (26–40 dB HL), moderate (41–55 dB HL), moderately severe (56–70 dB HL), severe (71–90 dB HL), or profound (>90 dB HL).

Type of hearing loss is based on the affected part of the auditory system. Conductive hearing loss (CHL) results when the mechanical system (i.e., outer and middle ear) of the auditory system is impeded in its ability to transmit sound to the inner ear. Depending on the etiology, a CHL may resolve with time or be correctable. Sensorineural hearing loss is a permanent hearing loss resulting from dysfunction of the inner ear or difficulty transmitting the signal along the neural pathways to the auditory cortex. Mixed hearing loss describes CHL and SNHL in the same ear. Auditory neuropathy spectrum disorder (ANSD) is a neural hearing loss likely due to dysfunction in the ability to encode the signal in the transmission process between the auditory nerve and the auditory cortex. ANSD is typically bilateral (>90% of cases) and explains approximately 10% of newly identified cases of hearing loss in children (Madden et al., 2002). Auditory, speech, and language outcomes for this population are highly variable requiring close monitoring. Cortical deafness is rare but can occur in the context of diffuse brain damage and is associated with central-level difficulties perceiving or discriminating sounds.

EPIDEMIOLOGY

The prevalence of hearing loss increases from 2 to 3 per 1000 infants to 6 to 10 per 1000 school-age children. By the teenage years the prevalence rate of hearing loss has been reported to be as high as 22.5% based on national surveillance data in the United States (Su & Chan, 2017), but most of these cases were unilateral and slight in severity. Thus the incidence of hearing loss increases with age, and hearing should be monitored throughout childhood.

ETIOLOGY

Genetic

There are more than 400 genetic causes of hearing loss, which explain 30% to 50% of SNHL cases. Although it fails to capture gene-gene or gene-environment interactions, genetic causes of hearing loss are often classified as syndromic (i.e., associated with other congenital or developmental anomalies) or nonsyndromic. More than 70% of genetic causes of hearing loss are nonsyndromic and most commonly result from an autosomal recessive inheritance pattern. For example, 10% of all childhood hearing loss cases can be attributed to a nonsyndromic, autosomal recessive hearing loss due to a mutation of the *GJB2* gene. This mutation results in the inadequate production of a protein, Connexin 26, that is needed for the passage of ions in and out of cells and thus results in congenital or progressive SNHL.

Developmental Disabilities

Hearing loss co-occurs frequently in genetic causes of developmental disabilities. Estimates of hearing loss among children with Down syndrome range from 38% to 84%, with the most common type being CHL due to middle ear effusion as a result of the craniofacial characteristics in this population (Kreicher et al., 2018). Unlike CHL for typically developing children, children with Down syndrome tend to have persistent CHL; 2% to 5% of children with Down syndrome have a SNHL component to their hearing loss (De Schrijver et al., 2019). Estimates of hearing loss among individuals with Turner syndrome have been reported to be as high as 72.3% (Hamberis et al., 2020) and is most frequently CHL, followed by mixed hearing loss, and SNHL. Similarly, high rates of hearing loss (38%) have been reported among children with 22q11.2 deletion syndrome (Jiramongkolchai et al., 2016). In the case of hearing loss associated with 22q11.2, 68% of children had CHL, 14% had SNHL, and 18% had mixed hearing loss.

In addition to these genetic comorbidities we draw attention to increased risk for reduced hearing among three additional developmental disabilities. Estimates of hearing loss among individuals with intellectual disability range from 16% to 40% but vary based on the type and severity of intellectual disability (Hey et al., 2014). The prevalence estimates of co-occurring hearing loss in children with cerebral palsy range from 4% to 13% in population-based studies to 39% in clinical samples. In one clinical sample, 48% of children with cerebral palsy had CHL, 24% had mixed hearing loss, and 4% had SNHL (Weir et al., 2018). Third, hearing loss co-occurs with autism spectrum disorder (ASD) more frequently than expected in the general population, with prevalence estimates ranging from 2% to 7% (Szymanski et al., 2012). ASD occurs among children with all degrees and types of hearing loss, but some studies have described increased rates of ASD among children with more severe degrees of SNHL (Meinzen-Derr et al., 2014; Szymanski et al., 2012).

For children with developmental disabilities, hearing loss may be missed or overshadowed by complex medical conditions or developmental needs. However, co-occurring hearing loss, particularly when identified late or not managed appropriately, can significantly impact developmental outcomes. Children with developmental disabilities require closer monitoring for hearing loss across the life span, and surveillance should be tailored based on the common hearing profiles observed in particular populations.

Risk Factors for Childhood Hearing Loss

Table 42.1 outlines a variety of risk factors that have been associated with childhood hearing loss. Here we provide information on the most common risk factors and highlight the resulting hearing profile(s) that are commonly seen. Prenatal infections have been associated with hearing loss. The best known of these infections are referred to by the acronym TORCH (toxoplasma, rubella, CMV, and herpes simplex), but there are others, including syphilis, human immunodeficiency virus, viral hepatitis, and Zika. Infectious diseases are among the etiologies that change most rapidly, and providers should monitor for new infections that may cause hearing loss. For the United States and many other developed countries, the infection that is currently associated with the highest number of cases of hearing loss is congenital CMV (cCMV). It is estimated that 6.4 per 1000 infants are cCMV positive, with 90% being asymptomatic at birth. By 5 years of age the incident rate of SNHL is 34% to 41% for symptomatic and 7% to 11% for asymptomatic cases (Bartlett et al., 2017). Nearly half of the children with hearing loss will "pass" their newborn hearing screening, making cCMV the leading cause of postnatal-onset hearing loss.

Newborns admitted to the neonatal intensive care unit (NICU) for any reason for more than 5 days are at risk for permanent hearing loss with a prevalence rate of hearing loss nearly seven times higher than babies who did not require the NICU (Butcher et al., 2019). One notable risk factor for ANSD and SNHL in this population is hyperbilirubinemia. Approximately 6% of infants with hyperbilirubinemia do not

TABLE 42.1 **Risk Indicators Associated With Permanent Congenital, Delayed-Onset, or Progressive Hearing Loss in Childhood**

Stage of Development	Risk Factor Classification
Perinatal	Family history of permanent childhood hearing loss (early, progressive, or delayed onset)
	Neonatal intensive care of >5 days
	Hyperbilirubinemia with exchange transfusion
	Aminoglycoside administration for >5 days
	Asphyxia or hypoxic ischemic encephalopathy
	Extracorporeal membrane oxygenation
	In utero infections, including cytomegalovirus, herpes, rubella, syphilis, Zika, and toxoplasmosis
	Certain birth conditions or findings: craniofacial malformations, including microtia/atresia, ear dysplasia, oral facial clefting, white forelock, and microphthalmia; congenital microcephaly, congenital or acquired hydrocephalus; or temporal bone abnormalities
	Diagnosis of a syndrome associated with hearing loss
Perinatal or postnatal	Culture-positive infections associated with sensorineural hearing loss, including confirmed bacterial and viral (especially herpes viruses and varicella) meningitis or encephalitis
	Events associated with hearing loss, such as significant head trauma (especially basal skull/temporal bone fractures) or chemotherapy
	Caregiver concern regarding hearing, speech, language, developmental delay and/or developmental regression

Adapted from Joint Committee on Infant Hearing. (2019). Year 2019 position statement: Principles and guidelines for early hearing detection and intervention programs. *Journal of Early Hearing Detection and Intervention*, 4(2), 1–44.

pass their hearing screening. Regardless of NICU status, hearing should be monitored for children with a history of maternal drug use. Exposure to heroin, cocaine, alcohol, tobacco, and ototoxic prescription drugs have been linked to hearing loss or differences in auditory system functioning.

Established postnatal risk factors for childhood hearing loss are infection, exposure to an ototoxic medication, or accident. Aminoglycoside antibiotics and platinum-based neoplastics are the most commonly prescribed ototoxic medications. Careful and routine hearing monitoring, especially in the high frequencies, is recommended for children prescribed these drugs. Bacterial meningitis often results in a profound bilateral SNHL, and a cochlear implantation evaluation is recommended soon after recovery. Dramatic hearing loss can be the result of head trauma. In particular, temporal bone fractures: 82% of children developed a hearing loss after a fracture (Lee et al., 1998). Another cause of late-onset hearing loss is noise exposure, which can damage the auditory system through direct mechanical trauma (e.g., blast trauma) and metabolic changes. Recommended safety levels are often exceeded by noise sources in the home (e.g., toys, sound machines), in agricultural or factory settings, or during recreational activities.

EVALUATION

Hearing Screening

Newborn hearing screening has become the standard of care in the United States and in many other countries. Current guidelines from the Joint Committee on Infant Hearing (JCIH, 2019) state that all infants receive a hearing screening by 1 month of age. The two available hearing screening technologies are otoacoustic emissions (OAEs) and automated auditory brainstem response (AABR). OAEs are a preneural measurement that tests the outer hair cell function within the cochlea, whereas AABR is a measure of the integrity of the auditory pathway from the cochlea to the brainstem. Babies in the well-baby nursery can be evaluated with OAEs, AABR, or both. AABR is the recommended procedure for screening in the NICU because OAEs are not a sensitive screener for ANSD. All states are required to have established systems and protocols in place for identifying, monitoring, tracking, and reporting data. In contrast there are no standardized protocols or systems at a state level for detecting postnatal-onset hearing loss. However, children commonly have their hearing screened by school-based health screening programs and the medical home.

Diagnostic Hearing Evaluation

A diagnostic evaluation is conducted by an audiologist with specialized equipment in a sound-treated booth, including both physiologic and behavioral measures of hearing. Based on the child's developmental age, the test battery components and testing procedures change.

The gold standard of diagnostic care is behavioral testing, resulting in the audiogram. Behavioral testing evaluates the entire auditory system, requires the listener to provide a response, and determines the type and severity of hearing loss across a range of frequencies. The behavioral testing method used to obtain the audiogram is based on the child's developmental abilities. Visual reinforced audiometry (VRA) requires the child to make a head-turn response toward a reinforcer (e.g., mechanical toy), whereas conditioned play audiometry (CPA) requires a child to make a play-based motor response when the signal is detected. These procedures correspond to a developmental age of 6 to 24 months and 2 to 5 years for VRA and CPA, respectively. For children under 6 months or if behavioral data cannot be obtained, diagnostic ABR testing is used to determine the type and severity of hearing loss.

Thresholds are expected to be cross-checked with other tests. Common physiologic tests include tympanometry, OAEs, and acoustic reflexes. Tympanometry tests the status of the middle ear to detect possible middle ear pathologies. Absent OAEs suggest that the cochlea may not be functioning properly, but obtaining a response is dependent on the absence of middle ear pathology. Acoustic reflexes test the pathways used in the stapedial reflex and can be used to verify type and severity of hearing loss or to screen for ANSD. For older children, behavioral speech testing may be performed.

Medical Evaluation

As clearly outlined by the American Academy of Pediatrics (AAP, 2010), the role of the medical home is critical for the diagnosis and management of childhood hearing loss. This section addresses monitoring for hearing loss by the medical home and the initial medical workup after a child receives a hearing loss diagnosis.

Surveillance of hearing happens across the life span. For newborns, the medical home should ensure that a hearing screening and any recommended follow-up testing are completed. Even if newborn hearing screening is passed, when infants have risk factors for hearing loss, JCIH (2019) recommends a diagnostic hearing evaluation at 9 months. Regardless of previous hearing screening outcomes or risk factors, it is recommended that the medical home provides ongoing hearing surveillance based on the periodicity schedule (Bright Futures/AAP, 2020). For children under 4 years, monitoring is often accomplished by caregiver report, but OAE screening protocols can be used. Starting at 4 years it is recommended that the medical home performs behavioral hearing screenings. Appearance of behaviors associated with typical hearing (e.g., turning to a sound) is not sufficient for ruling out hearing loss. A referral for a diagnostic hearing evaluation with an audiologist should be initiated if there is caregiver concern regarding hearing or communication development, or if a child does not pass a hearing or speech-language screener.

All infants and children should undergo an extensive medical evaluation outlined in the JCIH (2019) after the initial diagnosis of permanent or chronic hearing loss. The goal of the evaluation is to establish an etiology for the hearing loss and identify associated problems that may affect developmental or health outcomes. Evaluation should include a case history; physical examination to identify syndromic features, associated ear-specific disorders, and anatomic situations that negatively impact communication; radiographic imaging; and additional laboratory testing based on the suspected etiology.

Completion of the medical evaluation typically involves the following specialties: otolaryngology, ophthalmology, nephrology, cardiology, and genetics. Every infant identified with hearing loss should be referred to an otolaryngologist to assess middle ear function, identify any structural abnormalities, and evaluate for any surgically correctable causes of hearing loss. All families of children with confirmed hearing loss should be offered a genetics evaluation and counseling. Due to high rates of co-occurring vision loss, an ophthalmologic evaluation is strongly recommended. Children with external ear abnormalities (e.g., microtia, ear pits) should be referred to nephrology for a renal ultrasound. For newborns identified with hearing loss, a cCMV evaluation should be considered. When a congenital or acquired infection is suspected, children should be referred to an infectious disease specialist. In the absence of an alternative identified cause of hearing loss, electrocardiograms are recommended to identify a long QT interval, which can be fatal if undetected and is commonly associated with Jervell and Lange-Nielsen syndrome (JCIH, 2019).

For children newly diagnosed with hearing loss, radiologic imaging is an important aspect of the medical assessment. High-resolution computed tomography (HRCT) and/or MRI is used to complete an anatomic assessment of the temporal bones; auditory, vestibular, and facial nerves; and the brain. These results help determine the etiology of the child's hearing loss, identify anatomic characteristics that may predict progressive loss, establish candidacy for listening devices, and identify lesions of the central nervous system that require medical intervention.

Developmental Evaluation

A child's hearing status in and of itself does not necessarily have a negative impact on development when hearing loss is identified early, and early and consistent access to communication is established. However, establishing early and consistent access to communication to prevent negative developmental, academic, and social outcomes associated with poor language skills requires a coordinated effort between medical professionals, interventionists, and the family. Furthermore, without continued coordinated effort, the gains made during early intervention may not be maintained throughout childhood. For example, deaf children whose language scores approximate typically hearing peers at 3 years can academically and socially struggle in elementary school, and the gap widens by high school (Meinzen-Derr et al., 2018). Furthermore, graduation (high school and college) and employment rates for deaf adults are lower than for peers with typical hearing. These findings, coupled with consistent reports that up to 40% of deaf children have an additional developmental disability, support the need for developmental monitoring across the lifespan for all deaf children.

Physicians are familiar with developmental monitoring for young children, including screening of attainment of developmental skills, within the medical home according to the pediatric periodicity schedule (Bright Futures/AAP, 2020). When children do not pass these screenings they should be referred for developmental assessment in the areas of concern.

Physicians can also review developmental assessments completed by early intervention or school teams to assist with developmental monitoring. Formal clinical evaluation with a licensed psychologist may be warranted if concerns are raised regarding global developmental delays, if there are indications of potential comorbid developmental disabilities (e.g., ASD, attention-deficit/hyperactivity disorder [ADHD]), or if mental health concerns are suspected. An aspect of developmental surveillance that is unique to deaf children is the need to monitor language access. Monitoring language access includes establishing routine pediatric audiology care, determining consistency of listening device use, monitoring middle ear status, determining whether the child has access to visual language, and ensuring the family has resources for learning visual language. In addition, medical providers should refer for routine language evaluations, which should include comprehensive evaluation of the child's receptive and expressive language skills in the child's preferred language, including acquisition of phonologic, morphologic, semantic, syntactic, and pragmatic skills (Meinzen-Derr et al., 2011; Toe et al., 2020). Language development in ASL should be monitored as closely as spoken language development. Resources for assessment of ASL are provided (in the resource list). In the absence of many standardized assessments of ASL development, some have recommended use of dynamic assessment in which response to explicit language instruction is assessed to measure what the child can learn and what instructional strategies are most effective rather than how much a child knows.

Lack of assessments standardized for use with deaf children significantly complicates developmental assessment. Special consideration must be given to the deaf child's receptive and expressive language skills to ensure they have appropriate access to presented materials and can demonstrate their skills, especially when they communicate using a language other than the language reflected in the normative data. In addition, symptoms of mental health disorders and developmental disabilities (e.g., ASD) can be difficult to distinguish from symptoms of sensory and language deprivation (de Vaan et al., 2016; Szarkowski et al., 2014). Valid assessment is most likely to be carried out by Deaf or deafness trained professionals, who can select, administer, and interpret assessments fairly. State schools for the deaf are often valuable resources for either conducting these evaluations or referring to appropriately trained providers.

Medical providers should cautiously interpret results of intelligence tests that were administered by providers not familiar with working with deaf children. In the absence of additional developmental disabilities, deaf children tend to perform within the low average to average range on measures of visual perceptual reasoning abilities (Krouse & Braden, 2011). Use of verbal IQ or verbal subtests factoring into a full-scale IQ may not be a fair and valid estimate of cognitive ability (Reesman et al., 2014). Nonverbally administered assessments of cognitive ability are preferred, although these tools are not entirely free of language and should be interpreted cautiously with children who have not had consistent language access (Henner et al., 2019). For individuals who communicate using sign language, use of available psychological rating scales that have been translated to ASL may reduce risk of misdiagnosis (e.g., Mini International Neuropsychiatric Interview and the Strengths and Difficulties Questionnaire; Niclasen & Dammeyer, 2016; Øhre et al., 2014).

DEVELOPMENTAL AND BEHAVIORAL OUTCOMES

Auditory Development

Although the cochlea is mature at the time of full-term birth, the development of central auditory pathways and listening strategies extends well into adolescence and is dependent on access to auditory input. The course of development for the central auditory system can be affected by permanent hearing loss due to auditory deprivation or the provision of a degraded representation of sound from the impaired peripheral auditory system. One clinical implication is that children who are implanted early (<3.5 years) are more likely to develop typical central auditory pathways than those children who have prolonged auditory deprivation. Another clinical implication is that deaf children often have difficulty performing in noisy listening environments (e.g., classrooms) despite early access to listening devices.

Speech Development

The effects of hearing loss on speech development are most noticeable in children whose hearing loss has been present from birth or early childhood. Children with severe to profound congenital hearing loss may not follow the typical developmental patterns for acquiring speech, and their progress may plateau. Technology advancements have led to improved speech intelligibility outcomes. For example, children who are implanted early have a high likelihood of achieving fully intelligible speech. As a general rule, speech outcomes reflect the amount of residual hearing. Other factors that affect outcomes include age when listening devices were obtained, cognitive skills, communication mode, access to appropriate intervention, and the quality of family support.

Language Development

Communication options for deaf children have been described in several ways. These options fall into the following general categories: spoken language without supportive signs (e.g., auditory-oral auditory-verbal approaches), naturally emerging signed languages (e.g., ASL), spoken language supported with signs (e.g., simultaneous communication, total communication), manually coded English (e.g., systems such as Signed Exact English, which represent the grammar and syntax of English visually), and Cued Speech (a visual representation of spoken language at the phonetic level). Of these, only the first two represent naturally emerging complete language systems; the others were developed in an effort to make the spoken language more visually accessible. There has been much debate about the utility and outcomes associated with each of these approaches. Moreover, it has often been argued that the use of ASL or sign supports could interfere with acquiring a spoken language, despite the lack of research to support this claim (Hall et al., 2019). Rather, access to a natural sign language may enable neurologic structures for learning language in deaf children, ultimately facilitating learning a spoken language (Davidson et al., 2014).

Deaf children are at significant risk for language delays compared to hearing peers. Although early identification of hearing loss and access to intervention services are associated with improved language development for deaf children (Yoshinaga-Itano et al., 1998), delays in language have continued to be documented (Meinzen-Derr et al., 2018). It is of critical importance that deaf children have appropriate access to language to achieve mastery of a first language: a key predictor of overall child development. Appropriate language access is achieved when the child has access to high-quality language input that the child is able to fully receive.

Cognitive Development

Broadly speaking, deaf children have equal cognitive potential as hearing children. As a group, deaf children outperform hearing children on particular cognitive tasks (e.g., mental rotation tasks, visual spatial tasks) (Marschark et al., 2015). In some instances, where cognitive deficits for deaf children have been implied, differences are associated with reduced language access (as in the case of measures of auditory working memory) or language proficiency. For example, in both hearing and deaf children, language delays are associated with executive functioning deficits. Specifically for deaf children, these difficulties have been attributed to poor language (whether signed or spoken) rather than reduced hearing—(Hall et al., 2018). The clinical implication of this is that one must first consider language access and language fluency when considering whether a deaf child has ADHD. Having said this, many etiologies of hearing loss have known impact on the developing brain and place children at greater risk for executive functioning difficulties.

Social and Emotional Development

Several studies have reported that on average deaf children have increased social/emotional and behavioral challenges, regardless of the severity or onset point for the hearing loss. Deaf children also frequently report peer isolation and bullying behavior (Fellinger et al., 2009a). Variability in social/emotional function has been attributed in part to reduced language access and proficiency, which can cause delays in theory of mind development. Other factors that may influence social-emotional functioning include the ability to communicate well with classmates (Fellinger et al., 2009b) and parental support (Hintermair, 2008). Deaf children with additional disabilities, particularly those with a visual loss, are up to three times more likely to have mental health disorders or psychosocial difficulties than typically developing deaf children (Dammeyer, 2011, 2012).

Academic

Historically, deaf children's academic skills have lagged significantly behind their same-age peers with typical hearing. For example, Qi and Mitchell (2012) found median reading levels of deaf children at deaf schools (age 15–18 years) fell between the third- and fourth-grade level equivalents. Similarly, deaf children have demonstrated gaps in math performance. A systematic review of math performance for children with greater than moderate hearing loss found that deaf children are 1 to 4 years behind normative data (Gottardis et al., 2011). Academic difficulty is not just limited to children with significant degrees of hearing loss. Deaf children, regardless of the degree of their hearing loss or laterality, often need additional supports at school to mitigate the effects of their reduced language access on their academic achievement.

MANAGEMENT

Family-Centered Early Intervention

JCIH guidelines and the Individuals with Disabilities Education Act (IDEA) mandate that audiologists refer to early intervention (Part C) services as soon as hearing loss is confirmed and inform the infant's medical home. Intervention services provide an opportunity to establish language access—through spoken or sign language—and to promote the implementation of language facilitation strategies in the home. Research has clearly shown that timely establishment of intervention leads to better linguistic, cognitive, and social/emotional outcomes of deaf children than seen if intervention is started after 6 months of age (Yoshinaga-Itano et al., 2000). To support families and minimize stress it is critical that intervention and medical providers adopt a family-centered, mutually respectful relationship. This family-centered relationship fosters the family's ability to adapt to their child's developmental needs (Pipp-Siegel et al., 2002), and in turn caregiver responsiveness and engagement lead to improved child language outcomes (Moeller, 2000). It is also important to connect children and their families with deaf/Deaf individuals. For many parents, the first deaf individual they encounter is their own child. Access to deaf/Deaf role models allows families to integrate a strength-based conceptualization of deafness rather than focusing on perceived limitations, provide practical insights into experiences of being deaf, share valuable community resources, and may help teach sign language and strategies for supporting visual communication if chosen by the family (Hamilton & Clark, 2020). A critical role of the medical home is to ensure that deaf children have been connected with early intervention services. Although early intervention systems vary across states, positive outcomes have been associated for early intervention services that are specific to deaf children.

Medical Management

Ongoing medical management is often needed for children with otitis media. Otitis media is a primary inflammation of the middle ear space, often the result of a bacterial or viral infection, commonly as a result of an age-dependent dysfunctional eustachian tube. APA (2004) guidelines for otitis media recommend a "wait and see" approach prior to considering other options. If the hearing loss does not resolve, a referral to an audiologist or otolaryngologist is warranted. In contrast to the APA's recommended course of management, a more aggressive approach is often needed for children who have communication delays, developmental disabilities, craniofacial disorders, or immune system disorders. For children with craniofacial differences, serial screening for a CHL component via otoscopy is recommended. Children at risk for delayed speech and language due to chronic middle ear conditions are also recommended to be evaluated for intervention services. If a CHL present at birth has not been resolved by 6 months of age, the child should be evaluated for listening devices and referred to early intervention. Children with craniofacial anomalies (e.g., cleft palate or Down syndrome) are at high risk for prolonged periods of time with compromised access to speech because of middle ear disease. Children with hearing aids may require changes in their programming to achieve appropriate access to auditory information. Otitis media in children with cochlear implants can lead to serious infections and to the extraction of the device or meningitis.

For children with permanent hearing loss it is important to screen for vestibular dysfunction. Estimates of vestibular dysfunction range from 18% to 96% of children with SNHL and 3% to 84% of children with cochlear implants (Ghai et al., 2019). Children whose etiology of hearing loss is enlarged vestibular aqueduct syndrome, Usher syndrome, cCMV, CHARGE syndrome, or bacterial meningitis are particularly at risk. Vestibular dysfunction may present as delays for motor milestones or poor balance that leads to falls, especially for activities that require high-level motor skills. A referral to a physical therapist and/or an audiologist with specialization in pediatric vestibular assessment may be warranted.

Approximately 20% of children with SNHL have inner ear malformations (Sennaroğlu & Bajin, 2017). It is more often seen in unilateral than bilateral hearing loss cases, and the loss is often progressive. Ultimately, many of these children receive a cochlear implant, but there are surgical challenges that need to be considered. Families should be counseled on strategies to prevent head injury to prevent shifts in hearing loss. For example, 34% of children with enlarged vestibular aqueduct had significant hearing changes after minor head trauma (Noordman et al., 2015). This population is at risk for meningitis and as a result should be vaccinated against it, and otitis media should be aggressively managed.

For children who use listening devices, the physician should inquire about daily usage and benefit from the devices. The recommended goal is to have children consistently wearing their devices all waking hours. For deaf children with additional disabilities who have device tolerance issues, it may be beneficial to refer them for support services to address their developmental or behavioral needs. If a child is not making appropriate developmental gains, the listening devices and communication access may need to be reevaluated.

Audiological Management

Regular audiological management is critical for deaf children, especially those who use listening devices and/or a spoken language. After diagnosis, hearing should continue to be reevaluated on a regular basis (6–12 months) to monitor for shifts in hearing. One of the primary audiology management goals is to select and fit appropriate listening devices. Children using listening devices will require ongoing care, but infants or children who recently received their devices will require frequent visits for programming and support to establish full-time consistent usage of the devices.

There are a variety of listening device options that are appropriate to use for deaf children. The three main categories of listening devices are traditional air conduction hearing aids, bone conduction hearing devices, and cochlear implants. These devices differ based on how they transmit the auditory signal as well as their candidacy requirements (e.g., hearing type and severity, medical factors, and age). Initially, most children will be fit with traditional behind-the-ear (BTE) hearing aids. This is the primary choice of hearing aid for children because of flexibility in the fitting of the device, safety features, and durability. Although many children with permanent CHL successfully use traditional hearing aids, there are listening devices (surgical and nonsurgical) that transmit the sound via bone conduction. This technology may be the best option for children with abnormal outer ear structures, chronic drainage, or a maximum CHL.

Children with SNHL or ANSD who show little benefit from traditional hearing aids may be evaluated for a cochlear implant. A cochlear implant involves an external processor and a surgically implanted, internal component. The external processor is worn on the child and includes a microphone, sound processor, and transmitter system. The internal component includes the receiver and the electrode array (located in the cochlea), which generates electrical currents to represent the auditory signal. The US Food and Drug Administration (FDA) recently lowered the minimum age limit from 12 to 9 months, as earlier implantation results in speech and language advantages. FDA guidelines require a bilateral profound hearing loss for children 9 to 24 months or a severe to profound bilateral hearing loss for children 2 to 17 years. A unilateral and asymmetric hearing loss can qualify, assuming one ear has a profound SNHL, in children over 5 years. As a general rule, deaf children with developmental disabilities are candidates. Although outcomes may be more variable in this population, families' criteria for success may include sound awareness, increased personal and social interactions, increased connectivity to the environment, and higher quality of life and satisfaction. The data are limited and highly variable for the development of oral communication in this population (Meinzen-Derr et al., 2011).

Developmental Interventions

Children typically acquire language through regular exposure to multiple users of the language. However, for deaf children, intentional intervention is required that promotes language access to ensure appropriate language development. The needs of children and families are somewhat different based on the modality of the language being learned and are discussed separately. In reality, this distinction is not clear cut for many families because it is common to change modality over time or to use both.

Most deaf children have hearing parents who use a spoken language and will require support to access ASL instruction and exposure to the Deaf community in addition to environmental modifications that support visual access. Children acquiring a spoken language require access to audiological management, and their families need support designed to promote audition, speech, and language skills in their children. Learning a spoken language for most deaf children often requires the use of listening devices to obtain appropriate auditory access. For children who wear hearing aids both the quality of the fitting and the duration of daily wear time contributes to language outcomes (Tomblin et al., 2015). In addition to audiologic care, developing a spoken language requires habilitative services from therapists with expertise in speech and language development in deaf children. Unfortunately there is a lack of well-controlled studies comparing specific approaches for deaf children.

Regardless of the modality, establishing fluent language is critical to lay the foundation for academic and social development. When fluent language has not been established, intervention and communication approaches should be revisited, and additional support for learning language such as the use of technology-assisted speech-language therapy may be helpful (Meinzen-Derr et al., 2021). For deaf children with an additional developmental disability known to impact language development (e.g., apraxia or ASD) evidence-based interventions targeting the comorbid disability should also be used. For example, children with apraxia may benefit from PROMPT, a tactile-kinesthetic speech/language approach (Namasivayam et al., 2020). Children with ASD often benefit from the use of picture exchange communication systems (PECS) or alternative and augmentative communication (AAC), as well as approaches and interventions based in applied behavior analysis (ABA). Individualized intervention is often required for deaf learners because of reduced language access coupled with tremendous diversity and individual variability among the population (Marschark & Knoors, 2019).

Education

IDEA mandates that supports are provided to allow children to receive a free and appropriate public school education in their least restrictive environment. For deaf children, determining accessible education requires consideration of how a child accesses communication (e.g., through audition, visual access to language), how the child communicates most effectively, and opportunity for social interaction with deaf peers. Many states require that deaf children have a communication plan as part of their individualized education plan (IEP), which outlines how the educational placement will support these needs. Educational settings for deaf children may include general education classrooms, center-based resource programs for deaf children, day programs, or residential schools for the deaf. For deaf children with co-occurring developmental disabilities, educational placement and programming must be highly individualized to ensure accessible communication while meeting their developmental needs. Whether the educational environment appropriately fits the child's needs should be considered when evaluating behavioral, mental health, or learning concerns.

Sign language interpreters or cued speech transliterators may be appropriate if the child has the ability to effectively utilize the service. This can be difficult for young children, children who have not yet developed fluent ASL skills, and children who have difficulty shifting their attention between the teacher and interpreter. For these children, direct communication with a teacher of the deaf, or use of an ASL-fluent language mediator (who modifies instruction to match the child's comprehension level) is preferable. Care must also be taken to ensure that the skill level of an interpreter is sufficient to adequately communicate both the academic and social content. In addition to traditional support services tailored to the child's individualized needs, specialized support services may include an educational audiologist, instruction from a teacher of the deaf, and speech-language therapy. For children with dual hearing and vision loss, support from a teacher of the visually impaired and/or orientation and mobility specialist may be indicated. For a useful resource regarding educational accommodations, see the Hands and Voices IEP checklist. In addition, some school districts adopt an expanded core curriculum for deaf children to address functional educational needs unique to this population (e.g., self-advocacy, technology, communication).

Assistive Technology, Transition Services, Vocational Planning

Assistive technology, transition services, and vocational planning promote independence skills. Common forms of hearing assistive technology include remote-microphone systems (e.g., FM systems and induction loops) used to improve the signal-to-noise ratio to overcome the poor acoustics of everyday listening environments, closed captioning, and telecommunication services. Captioning services are appropriate for individuals who have a high reading proficiency and are commonly requested for secondary or college students. These should support, not replace, access to sign language and interpretation services when appropriate. Adapted warning devices (e.g., vibrating alarm clocks and flickering lights for the doorbell) provide access to the environment and promote independence and safety. Transition planning is mandated by IDEA to be in effect in the first IEP after the child turns 16 years old. Traditional transition programs often assume that individuals have language and reading proficiency, and content may need to be modified for deaf young adults particularly if they have not achieved fluent language. Young deaf adults may require specific transition services (e.g., advocacy and training in disability disclosure, communication strategies, mentoring regarding career opportunities). Integration of vocational rehabilitation services prior to exiting the public school system is strongly recommended.

CONCLUSION

Adoption of universal newborn infant hearing screening in the United States has lowered the age of identification and intervention for hearing loss, contributing to improved outcomes.

To prevent the risks of unidentified hearing loss, screening for hearing loss across the life span, particularly among at-risk groups, is strongly recommended. Promoting successful outcomes for deaf children requires careful attention to establishing early and consistent communication access, ongoing medical management of hearing loss and associated medical concerns, identification of and access to appropriate intervention, and close developmental monitoring.

ACKNOWLEDGMENTS

Preparation of this chapter was facilitated by a research grant from the National Institute on Deafness and Other Communication Disorders of the National Institutes of Health (R21DC018656) and Leadership Education in Neurodevelopmental Disabilities Audiology Supplement under Award (T73MC11044) from the Health Resources and Services Administration of the US Department of Health and Human Services. Views expressed here do not reflect the funding source.

REFERENCES

American Academy of Pediatrics. (2010). Early hearing detection and intervention (EHDI) guidelines for pediatric medical home providers. https://www.aap.org/en-us/advocacy-and-policy/aap-health-initiatives/PEHDIC/Documents/Algorithm1_2010.pdf

American Academy of Pediatrics Subcommittee on Management of Acute Otitis Media. (2004). Diagnosis and management of acute otitis media. *Pediatrics, 113*(5), 1451–1465.

Bartlett, A. W., McMullan, B., Rawlinson, W. D., & Palasanthiran, P. (2017). Hearing and neurodevelopmental outcomes for children with asymptomatic congenital cytomegalovirus infection: A systematic review. *Reviews in Medical Virology, 27*, e1938.

Bright Futures/American Academy of Pediatrics. (2020). Recommendations for preventive pediatric health care. https://downloads.aap.org/AAP/PDF/periodicity_schedule.pdf

Butcher, E., Dezateux, C., Cortina-Borja, M., & Knowles, R. L. (2019). Prevalence of permanent childhood hearing loss detected at the universal newborn hearing screen: Systematic review and meta-analysis. *PloS One, 14*(7), e0219600.

Dammeyer. J. (2011). Mental and behavioral disorders among people with congenital deafblindness. *Research in Developmental Disabilities, 32*(2), 571–575.

Dammeyer. J. (2012). Children with Usher syndrome: Mental and behavioral disorders. *Behavioral and Brain Functions, 8*, 16.

Davidson, K., Lillo-Martin, D., & Chen Pichler, D. (2014). Spoken English language development among native signing children with cochlear implants. *Journal of Deaf Studies and Deaf Education, 19*(2), 238–250.

De Schrijver, L., Topsakal, V., Wojciechowski, M., Van de Heyning, P., & Boudewyns, A. (2019). Prevalence and etiology of sensorineural hearing loss in children with Down syndrome: A cross-sectional study. *International Journal of Pediatric Otorhinolaryngology, 116*, 168–172.

de Vaan, G., Vervloed, M., Peters-Scheffer, N. C., van Gent, T., Knoors, H., & Verhoeven, L. (2016). Behavioural assessment of autism spectrum disorders in people with multiple disabilities. *Journal of Intellectual Disability Research, 60*(2), 101–112.

Fellinger, J., Holzinger, D., Beitel, C., Laucht, M., & Goldberg, D. P. (2009b). The impact of language skills on mental health in teenagers with hearing impairments. *Acta Psychiatrica Scandinavica, 120*(2), 153–159.

Fellinger, J., Holzinger, D., Sattel, H., Laucht, M., & Goldberg, D. (2009a). Correlates of mental health disorders among children with hearing impairments. *Developmental Medicine and Child Neurology, 51*(8), 635–641.

Ghai, S., Hakim, M., Dannenbaum, E., & Lamontagne, A. (2019). Prevalence of vestibular dysfunction in children with neurological disabilities: A systematic review. *Frontiers in Neurology, 10*, 1294.

Gottardis, L., Nunes, T., & Lunt, I. (2011). A synthesis of research on deaf and hearing children's mathematical achievement. *Deafness & Education International, 13*(3), 131–150.

Hall, M. L., Eigsti, I.-M., Bortfeld, H., & Lillo-Martin, D. (2018). Executive function in deaf children: Auditory access and language access. *Journal of Speech, Language, and Hearing Research, 61*(8), 1970–1988.

Hall, M. L., Hall, W. C., & Caselli, N. K. (2019). Deaf children need language, not (just) speech. *First Language, 39*(4), 367–395.

Hamberis, A. O., Mehta, C. H., Dornhoffer, J. R., & Meyer, T. A. (2020). Characteristics and progression of hearing loss in children with Turner's syndrome. *The Laryngoscope, 130*(6), 1540–1546.

Hamilton, B., & Clark, M. D. M. (2020). The deaf mentor program: Benefits to families. *Psychology, 11*(05), 713–736.

Henner, J., Novogrodsky, R., Caldwell-Harris, C., & Hoffmeister, R. (2019). The development of American Sign Language-based analogical reasoning in signing deaf children. *Journal of Speech, Language, and Hearing Research, 62*(1), 93–105.

Hey, C., Fessler, S., Hafner, N., Lange, B. P., Euler, H. A., & Neumann, K. (2014). High prevalence of hearing loss at the special olympics: Is this representative of people with intellectual disability? *Journal of Applied Research in Intellectual Disabilities, 27*(2), 125–133.

Hintermair. M. (2008). Self-esteem and satisfaction with life of deaf and hard-of-hearing people—a resource-oriented approach to identity work. *Journal of Deaf Studies and Deaf Education, 13*(2), 278–300.

Jiramongkolchai, P., Kumar, M. S., Chinnadurai, S., Wootten, C. T., & Goudy, S. L. (2016). Prevalence of hearing loss in children with 22q11.2 deletion syndrome. *International Journal of Pediatric Otorhinolaryngology, 87*, 130–133.

Joint Committee on Infant Hearing. (2019). Year 2019 position statement: Principles and guidelines for early hearing detection and intervention programs. *Journal of Early Hearing Detection and Intervention, 4*(2), 1–44.

Kreicher, K. L., Weir, F. W., Nguyen, S. A., & Meyer, T. A. (2018). Characteristics and progression of hearing loss in children with Down syndrome. *The Journal of Pediatrics, 193*, 27–33.e2.

Krouse, H. E., & Braden, J. P. (2011). The reliability and validity of WISC-IV scores with deaf and hard-of-hearing children. *Journal of Psychoeducational Assessment, 29*(3), 238–248.

Lee, D., Honrado, C., Har-El, G., & Goldsmith, A. (1998). Pediatric temporal bone fractures. *The Laryngoscope, 108*(6), 816–821.

Madden, C., Rutter, M., Hilbert, L., Greinwald, J. H., Jr, & Choo, D. I. (2002). Clinical and audiological features in auditory neuropathy. *Archives of Otolaryngology—Head & Neck Surgery, 128*(9), 1026–1030.

Marschark, M., & Knoors, H. (2019). Sleuthing the 93% solution in deaf education. In H. Knoors & M. Marschark (Eds.), *Evidence-based practices in deaf education* (pp. 1–29). Oxford University Press.
Marschark, M., Spencer, L. J., Durkin, A., Borgna, G., Convertino, C., Machmer, E., … Trani, A. (2015). Understanding language, hearing status, and visual-spatial skills. *Journal of Deaf Studies and Deaf Education, 20*(4), 310–330.
Meinzen-Derr, J., Sheldon, R., Altaye, M., Lane, L., Mays, L., & Wiley, S. (2021). A technology-assisted language intervention for children who are deaf or hard of hearing: A randomized clinical trial. *Pediatrics, 147*(2), e2020025734.
Meinzen-Derr, J., Sheldon, R., Grether, S., Altaye, M., Smith, L., Choo, D. I., & Wiley, S. (2018). Language underperformance in young children who are deaf or hard-of-hearing: Are the expectations too low? *Journal of Developmental and Behavioral Pediatrics, 39*(2), 116–125.
Meinzen-Derr, J., Wiley, S., Bishop, S., Manning-Courtney, P., Choo, D. I., & Murray, D. (2014). Autism spectrum disorders in 24 children who are deaf or hard of hearing *International Journal of Pediatric Otorhinolaryngology, 78*(1), 112–118. doi:10.1016/j.ijporl.2013.10.065.
Meinzen-Derr, J., Wiley, S., Grether, S., & Choo, D. I. (2011). Children with cochlear implants and developmental disabilities: A language skills study with developmentally matched hearing peers. *Research in Developmental Disabilities, 32*(2), 757–767. doi: 10.1016.j.ridd.2010.11.004.
Moeller. M. P. (2000). Early intervention and language development in children who are deaf and hard of hearing. *Pediatrics, 106*(3), e43.
Namasivayam, A. K., Huynh, A., Granata, F., Law, V., & van Lieshout, P. (2020). PROMPT intervention for children with severe speech motor delay: A randomized control trial. *Pediatric Research.* https://doi.org/10.1038/s41390-020-0924-4.
Niclasen, J., & Dammeyer, J. (2016). Psychometric properties of the strengths and difficulties questionnaire and mental health problems among children with hearing loss. *Journal of Deaf Studies and Deaf Education, 21*(2), 129–140.
Noordman, B. J., van Beeck Calkoen, E., Witte, B., Goverts, T., Hensen, E., & Merkus, P. (2015). Prognostic factors for sudden drops in hearing level after minor head injury in patients with an enlarged vestibular aqueduct: A meta-analysis. *Otology & Neurotology, 36*(1), 4–11.
Øhre, B., Saltnes, H., von Tetzchner, S., & Falkum, E. (2014). Psychometric properties of a sign language version of the Mini International Neuropsychiatric Interview (MINI). *BMC Psychiatry, 14*, 148.
Pipp-Siegel, S., Sedey, A. L., & Yoshinaga-Itano, C. (2002). Predictors of parental stress in mothers of young children with hearing loss. *Journal of Deaf Studies and Deaf Education, 7*(1), 1–17.
Qi, S., & Mitchell, R. E. (2012). Large-scale academic achievement testing of deaf and hard-of-hearing students: Past, present, and future. *Journal of Deaf Studies and Deaf Education, 17*(1), 1–18.
Reesman, J. H., Day, L. A., Szymanski, C. A., Hughes-Wheatland, R., Witkin, G. A., Kalback, S. R., & Brice, P. J. (2014). Review of intellectual assessment measures for children who are deaf or hard of hearing. *Rehabilitation Psychology, 59*(1), 99–106.
Sennaroğlu, L., & Bajin, M. D. (2017). Classification and current management of inner ear malformations. *Balkan Medical Journal, 34*(5), 397–411.
Su, B. M., & Chan, D. K. (2017). Prevalence of hearing loss in US children and adolescents: Findings from NHANES 1988-2010. *JAMA Otolaryngology-Head & Neck Surgery, 143*(9), 920–927.
Szarkowski, A., Mood, D., Shield, A., Wiley, S., & Yoshinaga-Itano, C. (2014). A summary of current understanding regarding children with autism spectrum disorder who are deaf or hard of hearing. *Seminars in Speech and Language, 35*(4), 241–259.
Szymanski, C. A., Brice, P. J., Lam, K. H., & Hotto, S. A. (2012). Deaf children with autism spectrum disorders. *Journal of Autism and Developmental Disorders, 42*(10), 2027–2037.
Toe, D., Mood, D., Most, T., Walker, E., & Tucci, S. (2020). The assessment of pragmatic skills in young deaf and hard of hearing children. *Pediatrics, 146*(3), S284–S291.
Tomblin, J. B., Harrison, M., Ambrose, S. E., Walker, E. A., Oleson, J. J., & Moeller, M. P. (2015). Language outcomes in young children with mild to severe hearing loss. *Ear and Hearing, 36*(1), 76S–91S.
Weir, F. W., Hatch, J. L., McRackan, T. R., Wallace, S. A., & Meyer, T. A. (2018). Hearing loss in pediatric patients with cerebral palsy. *Otology & Neurotology, 39*(1), 59–64.
Yoshinaga-Itano, C., Coulter, D., & Thomson, V. (2000). The Colorado Newborn Hearing Screening Project: Effects on speech and language development for children with hearing loss. *Journal of Perinatology, 20*, S132–S137.
Yoshinaga-Itano, C., Sedey, A. L., Coulter, D. K., & Mehl, A. L. (1998). Language of early- and later-identified children with hearing loss. *Pediatrics, 102*(5), 1161–1171.

RESOURCES

American Academy of Pediatrics (2010) EHDI Guidelines for Medical Providers: https://tinyurl.com/y5zzowco
American Sign Language assessments: http://signlang-assessment.info/
Centers for Disease Control and Prevention DC Hearing Loss: https://www.cdc.gov/ncbddd/hearingloss/data.html
Genetic causes of hearing loss: https://hereditaryhearingloss.org/
Hands and Voices educational accommodations: https://www.handsandvoices.org/pdf/IEP_Checklist.pdf
Joint Committeession Infant Hearing: http://www.jcih.org/
National Deaf Center adaptive technology: https://www.nationaldeafcenter.org/topics/assistive-technology
Newborn Infant Hearing Screening: http://www.infanthearing.org

43

Blindness and Visual Impairment

Michael A. Puente, Tanni L. Anthony, and Robert W. Enzenauer

For additional material related to the content of this chapter, please see Chapters 25, 32, 34, and 36.

VIGNETTE

Henry C. is a 3.5-year-old boy with the diagnoses of spastic quadriplegia and moderately severe cognitive impairments associated with prematurity. After being born at 24 weeks weighing just 670 g, Henry survived a stormy 6-month hospitalization requiring mechanical ventilation for 3 months, complicated by bilateral moderately severe proliferative retinopathy of prematurity (ROP), grade 3, zone 2, treated with laser photocoagulation. Head ultrasound was remarkable for a cerebellar bleed. Upon discharge, the family returned to a small town 6 hours away from the major medical center. The child's mother was concerned by several visual behaviors, including chaotic eye movements and squeezing of the eyelids from photophobia. Henry's mother also noted that after locating an object visually, Henry would turn his head and his eyes in the opposite direction during the act of reaching for the object. She sought consultation by a pediatric ophthalmologist, who first saw him at 17 months of age.

The ophthalmologist diagnosed marked amblyopiagenic myopia, and spectacles were prescribed. The pediatric ophthalmologist also felt that the child had cortical visual impairment. Henry was referred for a functional visual assessment at a local center for children with low vision to facilitate early interventions to nurture the child's emotional, social, and intellectual skills. Henry had strabismus surgery at 2 years of age for exotropia. By 3 years of age he had marked pathologic myopia with astigmatism, which would have resulted in his innate focus without glasses to be less than 4 inches from his face. However, with glasses and personalized educational and developmental supports, Henry's visual function and learning were greatly enhanced.

CAUSES OF BLINDNESS AND VISUAL IMPAIRMENT

There are countless reasons a child may have impaired vision. Ophthalmologic (pregeniculate) causes of visual impairment include abnormalities of all parts of the visual axis from front to back: corneal opacities, anterior segment abnormalities, cataracts, and glaucoma, along with retinal anomalies and dystrophies and optic nerve pathologies. Reduced visual function may also be secondary to postgeniculate causes such as delayed visual maturation and cerebral visual impairment. The following sections will discuss important causes of visual dysfunction in developmentally delayed children.

Among 200 developmentally delayed children who received routine eye examinations, it was found that there was a high incidence of ocular defects. These defects included refractive error (98 children), strabismus (74 children), and nystagmus (15 children), along with cataract, retinopathy, and optic atrophy. This high incidence of ocular defects emphasized the need for the routine ophthalmic examination of children with disabilities to detect and treat ocular conditions, which might otherwise have gone undetected, and enable the visual sense of these children to be evaluated in relationship to their general development (Bankes, 1975).

Diseases of the Orbit

Craniosynostosis Syndromes

Craniosynostosis is a condition characterized by premature fusion of one or more cranial sutures. It is the second most common craniofacial anomaly after orofacial clefts. Craniosynostosis can be isolated or part of a genetic syndrome. There are over 100 described synostosis syndromes, and the most common include Crouzon, Pfeiffer, Apert, Saethre-Chotzen, and Muenke syndromes. Associated abnormalities in these patients include midface hypoplasia with shallow orbits and various ocular abnormalities, including strabismus, high refractive error, proptosis, corneal exposure, papilledema, and eventual optic atrophy. Prevalence of strabismus ranges from 39% to 91% in Crouzon, Apert, Pfeiffer, and Saethre-Chotzen syndromes. Absence of multiple extraocular muscles is also not uncommon in craniosynostosis, with absence of the cyclovertical muscles especially prevalent (i.e., obliques and vertical recti).

For all syndromic and nonsyndromic craniosynostoses, papilledema and secondary optic atrophy are major concerns. Regular ophthalmologic evaluation is warranted to assess optic nerve status and to monitor for strabismus, refractive error, and amblyopia. Abducens nerve palsy has developed following expansion cranioplasty with distraction osteogenesis (Yoo, Chung, & Yoon, 2014). Periocular asymmetry is very common in infants with plagiocephaly, with pseudoptosis most commonly identified. The majority of patients with plagiocephaly present with vertical strabismus, though horizontal strabismus is also very common, particularly V-pattern exotropias (referring to an exotropia that is most pronounced in up-gaze and least pronounced in down-gaze). Fortunately, ocular misalignment is rarely surgically induced in primary position by craniofacial surgery but can result from cranial nerve palsies.

Other Orbital Syndromes

Pierre-Robin sequence is classically defined as a triad of congenital anomalies, including micrognathia, glossoptosis, and upper airway obstruction. The incidence of Pierre-Robin sequence is estimated to be 1 in 5600 to 14,000 live births, with a mortality rate reported in the range of 10% to 30%. The sequence has a strong correlation with craniofacial syndromes that are associated with ocular anomalies, including Stickler syndrome caused by mutations in collagen 2, velocardiofacial syndrome caused by deletions in chromosome 22q11, and Treacher-Collins syndrome. Pierre-Robin anomaly has been associated with a variety of ocular conditions, including myopia, strabismus, glaucoma, microphthalmos, cataract, retinal detachment, and nasolacrimal duct obstruction.

Treacher-Collins syndrome is thought to affect approximately 1 in 50,000 live births. About 40% of patients will have a hereditary form, while the other 60% result from de novo mutations. It is an autosomal dominant disorder with a gene mutation found on the *TCOF1* gene, though two other genes commonly involved include the *POLTRIC* and *POLRID* genes. Ophthalmologic anomalies in Treacher-Collins syndrome include downward slanting of the palpebral fissures due to absence of the lateral orbital walls, lower eyelid colobomas or pseudocolobomas, absence of the eyelashes in the medial aspect of the lower eyelids, nasolacrimal duct obstruction, and ptosis (Fisher, 2011). Decreased vision is present in 37% of patients, most often secondary to significant refractive error and amblyopia (Hertle, Zylan, & Katowitz, 1993). Strabismus is present in 37% of patients, with exotropia more common than esotropia. Patients with significant lid dystopia may develop corneal exposure, optic atrophy, and papilledema.

Frontonasal dysplasia, also known as median cleft syndrome or frontonasal dysostosis, is a congenital condition resulting in malformation of the forehead and midface. In 2004 mutations in a receptor tyrosine kinase protein encoded by the *EFNB1* gene were found to be causative. Like most craniofacial syndromes, the most common ophthalmic abnormality is strabismus, along with ametropia with astigmatism, which may result in amblyopia. Patients also frequently have nystagmus. Other ocular manifestations include optic nerve anomalies, such as morning glory disc, along with colobomas of the iris, choroid, or retina and ptosis. Less commonly associated findings include cataract, nystagmus, anophthalmia, and microphthalmia.

Ocular Abnormalities

Microphthalmia

Some children are born with grossly maldeveloped and small eyes, leading to lifelong visual impairment in the affected eye or eyes, a condition referred to as microphthalmia. While microphthalmia is often sporadic and unilateral, it can sometimes represent a component of a systemic syndrome, such as Lenz microphthalmia syndrome. Children with this condition typically demonstrate bilateral microphthalmia, microcephaly, intellectual disability, and dental and skeletal anomalies. Microphthalmia may also be seen in children with trisomy or other chromosomal anomalies, as well as in fetal alcohol syndrome (Chambers et al., 2018).

Cornea

The cornea is the anterior-most aspect of the eye. It is designed to be transparent to allow light to enter the eye and is responsible for approximately two-thirds of the eye's focusing power. Corneal opacities may lead to reduced vision due to impaired ability of light to enter the eye, while some corneal disorders may cause blurred vision due to abnormalities in the focusing power of the eye.

Peters anomaly refers to opacification of the corneal stroma due to a congenital defect of the corneal endothelium, often associated with other developmental anomalies of the front of the eye. While affected children often have no other systemic abnormalities, patients with biallelic mutations of the *B3GLCT* gene may develop Peters-plus syndrome, a constellation of Peters anomaly, short limbs, craniofacial anomalies, and intellectual disability. Nearly 80% of children with Peters-plus syndrome have developmental delay, with intellectual disability ranging from mild to severe (Lesnik et al., 2007).

Corneal visual impairment can also be seen in children with some metabolic disorders. For example, children with mucopolysaccharidosis type 1H (Hurler syndrome) typically suffer from severe intellectual impairment with corneal haze secondary to accumulation of dermatan and heparan sulfate. The corneal clouding in some patients is severe enough to require corneal transplant surgery. Likewise, patients with tyrosinemia type II may develop corneal opacification due to corneal ulcers and scarring. Some patients may also develop seizures and mental impairment, though visual symptoms are often the first manifestation of their disease (Macsai et al., 2001).

Some congenital infections may also cause visual impairment from corneal pathology. Neonatal infection with herpes simplex virus (HSV) can lead to disseminated disease with the potential for severe neurologic morbidity and permanent visual impairment, which may be secondary to corneal scarring, cataracts, or retinal involvement. Corneal involvement in congenital syphilis may not manifest until late childhood or adolescence. Such children may develop rapidly progressive bilateral corneal edema with neovascularization resulting in potential vision loss from corneal opacification (Hariprasad, Moon, Allen, & Wilhelmus, 2002).

Aside from corneal opacity, some children with corneal disease may suffer vision loss from abnormalities in the cornea's refractive (or focusing) power. One such condition is keratoconus, a disorder characterized by progressive corneal thinning and a gradual shift in the shape of the cornea from a relatively spherical form to a protruding conical shape. Affected children experience potentially severe blurring of their vision due to myopia and astigmatism, which may not be amenable to improvement with glasses. Severe keratoconus may even require corneal transplant surgery. Keratoconus typically begins to develop in adolescence and is especially prevalent in patients with trisomy 21, with some studies estimating that approximately one-third of patients with Down syndrome meet diagnostic criteria for keratoconus (Imbornoni, Wise, Taravella, Hickey, & McCourt, 2020).

Anterior Segment

The iris is the colored tissue in the anterior segment of the eye, sitting just posterior to the cornea and just anterior to the lens. Children with aniridia are born with hypoplastic irides, presenting with a seemingly dilated or irregular pupil. The condition also typically includes irregularities of multiple other components of the eye, including the cornea, lens, and retina, all of which are vital for clear vision. Some children also go on to develop vision-threatening glaucoma due to dysgenesis of the anterior segment of the eye. While the majority of cases of aniridia are not associated with systemic disease, aniridia in some patients is a component of the systemic disease called WAGR syndrome, caused by a contiguous mutation of the *PAX6* and *WT1* genes on chromosome 11. The syndrome's name refers to the tetrad of Wilms tumor, aniridia, genitourinary anomalies, and retardation (i.e., intellectual disability).

Lens

Disorders of the lens include anomalies of lens clarity, size, shape, or location. Such lens pathology is seen in many developmental disorders and can be responsible for significant visual impairment.

A cataract refers to a clouding of the normally clear lens. Pediatric cataracts may be congenital or acquired, and they are responsible for 5% to 20% of childhood blindness globally (Sheeladevi et al., 2016). While unilateral congenital cataracts are typically unrelated to systemic disease, congenital cataracts related to systemic disease are most commonly bilateral. A wide variety of systemic diseases and syndromes have been associated with pediatric cataracts (Table 43.1). Visually significant cataracts require surgical removal, with bilateral congenital cataracts ideally removed between 6 and 8 weeks of age. Later removal predisposes children to developing nystagmus or amblyopia, which may limit postsurgical visual improvement. Potential complications of pediatric cataract surgery include postoperative glaucoma and an increased risk of retinal detachment, with the risk of retinal detachment especially high in children with intellectual disability and self-injurious behavior (Haargaard et al., 2014).

Some children may have lens-related visual impairment caused by lens dislocation, as may be seen in Marfan syndrome, homocystinuria, Weill-Marchesani syndrome, and sulfite oxidase deficiency. Homocystinuria, caused by an autosomal recessive mutation in the gene for cystathionine beta-synthase, is characterized by homocysteine accumulation in the blood and urine. Affected patients classically present with inferior subluxation of the lens, which typically develops in children from 3 to 10 years of age. Many patients also present with seizures and intellectual disability. Though surgical extraction of the dislocated lens may be necessary, children with homocystinuria are at an increased risk of deep venous thrombosis during general anesthesia. The rare metabolic disorder sulfite oxidase deficiency may also cause lenticular displacement; but this is dwarfed in significance by the generally severe neurologic impairment in affected children, with most patients dying in early childhood (Claerhout et al., 2018).

TABLE 43.1 Systemic Conditions Associated With Pediatric Cataracts

Chromosomal abnormalities
Trisomies 21, 18, 13
Other translocations, deletions, and duplications
Congenital infection
Toxoplasmosis
Rubella
Cytomegalovirus
Herpes simplex
Varicella zoster
Syphilis
Metabolic disorders
Galactosemia
Wilson disease
Diabetes mellitus
Cerebrotendinous xanthomatosis
Craniofacial syndromes
Rubinstein-Taybi
Smith-Lemli-Opitz
Nance-Horan
Musculoskeletal disorders
Conradi-Hünermann syndrome
Myotonic dystrophy
Renal syndromes
Alport syndrome
Lowe syndrome
Trauma (including abusive head trauma)

From Hered, R. W., et al. (2019). *Basic and clinical science course: Pediatric ophthalmology and strabismus, 2019–2020*. American Academy of Ophthalmology.

Glaucoma

Pediatric glaucoma refers to the condition of progressive damage to a child's eye and optic nerve caused by elevated intraocular pressure. Pediatric glaucoma may be a primary condition isolated to the eye, but in some cases it is secondary to systemic disease. The underlying cause of elevated intraocular pressure in young children is most commonly maldevelopment of the drainage pathway of the aqueous humor in the anterior segment of the eye, and such dysgenesis may be seen in any congenital disorder affecting the anterior segment of the eye (corneal disorders, aniridia, lens dislocation, etc.). Pediatric glaucoma generally requires surgical management. If left untreated, affected eyes may go completely blind.

One of the most common systemic conditions associated with childhood glaucoma is encephalotrigeminal angiomatosis, or Sturge-Weber syndrome. Children with this condition develop capillary vascular malformations of the brain, skin, and periocular tissues, and children with a so-called port-wine stain near the eye are predisposed to developing glaucoma. Though the pathogenesis of glaucoma in these children has not been definitively determined, it is thought to be potentially secondary to increased episcleral venous pressure inhibiting the egress of aqueous humor from the eye (Javaid,

Ali, Jamal, & Butt, 2018). Pediatric glaucoma may also be seen in children with neurofibromatosis type I, Lowe syndrome, congenital rubella, and homocystinuria.

Retina/Vitreous

In middle- and high-income countries retinal disease is the most common cause of pediatric blindness (Kong, Fry, Al-Samarraie, Gilbert, & Steinkuller, 2012).

One of the most important retinal diseases seen in children is retinopathy of prematurity, which is a vasoproliferative disorder of the retina seen in children who are born long before retinal vascularization has completed (see Chapter 34 for further discussion). Children most at risk for this potentially blinding disease are those who were born at or before 30 weeks of gestation, 1500 g or less at birth, or premature neonates outside those criteria with a particularly unstable postnatal clinical course. The patient in the chapter-opening vignette is a good example of this concern. Advanced ROP may be blinding due to the development of retinal detachments; but even children with milder ROP may eventually develop visually significant sequelae such as amblyopia, strabismus, unusual refractive error, glaucoma, and even retinal detachments years after birth. Many patients born premature enough to develop ROP also suffer from concomitant cerebral visual impairment related to their prematurity. In fact, visual impairment in premature children is more commonly caused by damage to the brain than ROP (Dutton, 2013).

Similar retinal vascular pathology to ROP may also be seen in female children with incontinentia pigmenti, a rare X-linked dominant condition that is usually lethal to males *in utero* and causes characteristic skin findings, including bullae and reticular hyperpigmentation. Affected females may suffer vision loss from retinal detachments and commonly also demonstrate some degree of intellectual disability. Another X-linked condition causing visual impairment is Norrie disease, which is due to an X-linked recessive mutation in the *NDP* gene and causes blindness from birth, sensorineural hearing loss, and cognitive impairment. Due to its X-linked recessive nature, the most severe visual deficits are seen in males, while female carriers may have only mild, visually insignificant retinal changes.

Retinal pathology is also commonly seen in many metabolic disorders, especially mucopolysaccharidosis (MPS) syndromes. Children with these conditions have enzyme deficiencies leading to accumulation of glycosaminoglycans in various tissues, including ocular tissues and the central nervous system. Patients with MPS types I, II, and III may develop a pigmentary retinal degeneration as well as atrophy of the optic nerve. Retinal involvement can cause progressive death of retinal photoreceptors, leading to potentially severe visual loss (Ferrari et al., 2011). Intellectual and behavioral impairment are common in these disorders, and few children with MPS III live beyond their teenage years.

Intrauterine or perinatal infections may also cause retinal disease. Cytomegalovirus is the most common congenital infection globally. Extensive systemic manifestations may be seen, including sensorineural hearing loss, microcephaly, and ocular involvement (most classically bilateral necrotizing retinitis). Similar retinal necrosis and central nervous system involvement may also be seen in children with congenital HSV infections, as well as in young children infected with lymphocytic choriomeningitis virus from exposure to infected mice or hamsters. Congenital toxoplasmosis infection is also recognized as an important cause of retinal scarring in children, though long-term visual prognosis is good if the condition is promptly diagnosed and treated.

Aicardi syndrome is a rare X-linked dominant disorder characterized by the triad of infantile spams, agenesis of the corpus callosum, and scattered round punched-out retinal lacunae. Good visual acuity is usually maintained if retinal involvement spares the fovea, but foveal involvement may cause significant visual limitations. Given its X-linked dominant inheritance, the condition is generally lethal to males in utero. Affected females commonly have marked developmental delay (Aicardi, 2005).

Neuroophthalmologic Causes of Blindness and Visual Impairment

Optic Nerve

A variety of disorders of the optic nerve can also cause visual impairment in children, the most common of which is optic nerve hypoplasia (ONH). The condition may be unilateral or bilateral, and vision can range from 20/20 to no light perception (NLP). Children with ONH may have associated neuroanatomic anomalies, including absence of the septum pellucidum, agenesis of the corpus callosum, schizencephaly, and white matter hypoplasia (Garcia-Filion & Borchert, 2013). Such children also commonly have pituitary gland abnormalities with various associated hormone deficiencies.

Another important congenital optic nerve abnormality is morning glory disc anomaly, which refers to embryologic maldevelopment of the junction of the distal optic nerve with the posterior sclera. Associated neurologic abnormalities include moyamoya disease (carotid circulation abnormalities), basal encephalocele, and PHACE syndrome (posterior fossa malformations, hemangiomas, arterial lesions, cardiac and eye anomalies). A similar optic nerve deformity is an optic nerve coloboma, referring to incomplete closure of an embryonic fissure at the junction of the optic nerve with the posterior aspect of the eye. This anomaly is associated with a number of systemic conditions, most notably CHARGE syndrome (coloboma, heart defects, choanal atresia, growth retardation, genitourinary abnormalities, and ear abnormalities).

The most severe congenital optic nerve anomaly is optic nerve aplasia, a rare condition characterized by complete absence of optic nerve axons and retinal blood vessels. Patients thus have no light perception, and bilateral involvement is usually associated with further central nervous system anomalies (Ghassemi et al., 2015).

Other children born with normal optic nerves may experience progressive vision loss secondary to optic nerve atrophy, which can be caused by a wide variety of neuroophthalmologic pathologies. Some such conditions are autosomally inheritered, such as Behr syndrome, which is caused by a biallelic mutation of the *OPA1* gene and is associated with optic atrophy, intellectual disability, ataxia, and pyramidal signs (Marelli et al., 2011). Optic atrophy may also develop after prolonged increased intracranial pressure, which may be caused by a myriad of systemic and neurologic conditions. Optic atrophy may also develop secondary to optic neuritis, as may be seen in multiple sclerosis or neuromyelitis optica.

Abusive Head Trauma

An unfortunately frequent cause of visual impairment in children is abusive head trauma. One metaanalysis estimate found that retinal hemorrhages were present in approximately 78% of cases of likely abusive head trauma in young children, with many of these children also suffering substantial neurologic injuries (Maguire et al., 2013). Blindness may occur in approximately 15% of survivors, with nearly half of all survivors experiencing some degree of visual impairment (Chevignard & Lind, 2014). Visual sequelae may range from cortical blindness to visual field loss, visual acuity loss, or ocular motility deficits. Most visual impairment in these children is thought to be secondary to neurologic injury rather than injury of the eye itself.

Cortical/Cerebral Visual Impairment

Cerebral (cortical) visual impairment (CVI) is the leading cause of pediatric vision impairment in developed countries and refers to bilateral decrease in vision attributable to neurologic rather than ocular pathology, generally with a preserved pupillary light response. CVI comprises visual malfunction due to retrochiasmal pathology, which can be isolated or accompany anterior visual pathway dysfunction, with affected children often also manifesting strabismus, optic atrophy, refractive error, or photophobia. Visual deficits can range from altered visual fields to difficulty with visual object recognition, visual-spatial skills, or face and letter recognition. It is a major cause of low vision in children in the developed and developing world due to increasing survival in pediatric and neonatal intensive care.

There are multiple causes of CVI, and it is common in children with cerebral palsy and survivors of extreme prematurity, especially those affected by periventricular leukomalacia. Neonatal brain lesions are the main cause of CVI in infancy. Most children with CVI have moderate to severe lesions of the optic radiations, the periventricular white matter surrounding the posterior horns, or less frequently to the visual cortex (Philip, Guzzeta, Chorna, & Gole, 2020). The most common cause of CVI is hypoxic-ischemic encephalopathy, particularly in premature children.

CVI is also associated with other neurologic (hydrocephalus), posttraumatic (traumatic brain injury and shaken baby syndrome), metabolic (Tay-Sachs, Leigh disease), chromosomal, genetic, syndromic, and infectious entities (cytomegalovirus, Zika) in children.

Looking at CVI from the other side of the equation, the prevalence of visual impairments in people with severe and profound multiple disabilities (SPMD) is as high as 92%, with the severity of the visual impairment related to the severity of the intellectual disability. In addition to the problem of decreased acuity, there may also be impairments in the visual field, contrast sensitivity, binocular functioning, or ability to visually follow objects of interest. It is important to recognize that while visual problems are relatively common in children with SPMD, such problems may be easily overlooked as the focus may be on other aspects of health and management.

Although frequently associated with cerebral palsy and intellectual disability, CVI can also occur in isolation. CVI can be cryptic in children with mild visual impairment, as may be the case in children born prematurely or suffering perinatal hypoxia. It is important to identify children whose principal visual disability is visuoperceptual in nature. For example, children with lower visual field impairment may be thought to be misbehaving when they refuse to jump off a low bench (because they cannot see the ground) or jump into a swimming pool. Those with optic ataxia can be considered clumsy, and those with simultanagnostic and attentional problems can be deemed to be careless because they miss what they do not see, which leads to "careless mistakes." They also can become distressed in crowded situations and react with "bad behavior." Children who cannot interpret facial expressions (due to low acuity, low-contrast sensitivity, dyskinetopsia, prosopagnosia, or a combination) can be labeled as having atypical autism spectrum disorder (ASD) on account of their failure to engage socially. The children who cannot identify their friends on the playground tend to play alone and can be thought of as being aloof, and this may compound the impression of autistic behavior. While ASD is a well-recognized complication of premature birth, atypical presentations warrant reevaluation for evidence of such visual dysfunctions (Dutton, 2013). Severe early onset visual dysfunction accords the greatest risk of impairment of cognitive, motor, and social development that resemble ASD. Therefore the development of assessment tools that include the type and level of visual impairment and validation testing in a larger population sample are needed to confirm the diagnosis of ASD in visually impaired children (Fazzi et al., 2019).

Most children with CVI have at least some residual vision, and many children share similar adaptive behaviors. They commonly see better in familiar environments, where they understand what to look for and where to look for it. They also often rely on touch or other senses to help identify objects. Children with restricted visual fields may look side to side to orient themselves to the surroundings of their object of regard (Jan, Groenveld, Skyanda, & Hoyt, 1987).

Vestibular-ocular reflexes (VORs) are commonly impaired in children with CVI. For example, one study found the doll's head maneuver failed to substantially overcome the deviated eye position in 62% of children with conjugate gaze deviation, suggesting these children may lack important visual compensatory mechanisms to stabilize gaze during head movements (Mansukhani, Ho, & Brodsky, 2020). According to Salati et al. (2002) CVI patients commonly demonstrate paroxysmal ocular deviations (78%), variable angle strabismus (86%), and defective coordination of saccades (93%). Exploration of the environment and fixation were also impaired (88% and 84%, respectively). These abnormalities likely characterize lack of gaze coordination found in children with brain damage (Salati, Borgatti, Giammari, & Jacobson, 2002).

Additionally, children with developmental coordination disorder (DCD) and cerebral palsy are much more likely to also suffer from CVI, so while DCD and cerebral palsy can be the visible deficit, potential underlying CVI is invisible and often goes unnoticed in these children, who grow up unaware that their vision is defective (Chockron & Dutton, 2016).

PEDIATRIC SCREENING RESPONSIBILITIES

Vision screening begins the process of identifying pediatric vision problems. However, unlike universal newborn hearing screening, there is not a universal or mandated vision screening process for infants (Pellegrino, 2019). Consensus, however, is that early identification of vision problems or impairments is critical for purposes of possible medical treatment to reverse or mitigate vision loss and/or for prompt referral for early intervention or education supports (Anthony, 2016; Pellegrino, 2019).

Early vision screening is conducted with young children through pediatric checkups with medical personnel such as pediatricians, family practice physicians, or nursing staff. Vision screening is conducted to identify young children within the educational system through the federally required early intervention and school-based Child Find programs, which are required to locate and identify children ages birth through 21 with disabilities who may benefit from special education services and supports. Unlike medical practitioners who may use an ophthalmoscope to discern a red reflex as a component of a vision screening protocol, education-based vision screening procedures typically include data collection on the following:

- Family and child medical history
- External inspection of the appearance of the eyes
- Pupillary responses to bright light
- Functional vision responses specific to eye alignment, visual acuity, and ocular binocularity and motility tasks of fixation, tracking, convergence
- Notation of usual behaviors such as squinting, frowning, closing eye(s), and/or head postures during viewing tasks

Photoscreeners, which involve a special camera that can automatically detect refractive errors and other eye abnormalities, are used both in medical and educational settings. These cameras can be used with very young children and are especially helpful with older children with disabilities who are nonverbal. Standard acuity cards or charts, such as the LEA or Lighthouse visual acuity symbols, can be used successfully with children by 3 years of age. Parent questionnaires are key to eliciting information about a child's visual appearance of the eyes, behavior, and complaint data that are useful for highlighting risk factors for ocular, cortical, and cerebral visual impairment. Such questionnaires were used effectively during the COVID-19 pandemic to gather information about a child's visual functioning status when in-person vision screening could not be conducted (Colorado Department of Education, 2020). Box 43.1 details early warning signs of visual problems or ocular-/brain-based visual impairment that should be built into the parent questionnaire and/or vision screening protocol procedures. Early referral to an eye care specialist following a failed vision screening is critical to next steps of further evaluation.

BOX 43.1 Warning Signs of a Visual Problem/Impairment

- Abnormal appearance of eye(s): structure, shape, size, and symmetry
- Drooping eyelid(s)
- Involuntary shaking movement of eyes
- Extreme redness of eye(s)
- Poor eye alignment (occasional or steady eye[s] turning in, out, up, or down)
- Excessive eye blinking, tearing, and/or mattering
- Shows extreme sensitivity to light and/or gazes at a light source for long periods
- Covers or closes one eye while looking at a person or object
- Rubs eyes frequently (beyond when tired)
- Tilts head, frowns, and/or squints while looking at a person or object
- Has a consistent inaccurate visual-reach for objects that is not tied to motor challenges
- Positions self unusually close to view objects/brings objects very near to eyes to view
- Notices pets or people only when they are moving
- Inconsistent visual abilities (across day, from day-to-day)
- Stumbles frequently over objects in travel path or bumps into walls
- Hesitates frequently when there is a change in ground surface (stair, curb, tile to carpet)

Many children with neurodevelopmental disabilities have deficits in their senses, with vision impairment being potentially the most limiting to successful participation in life. Several studies have found that vision care represents one of the greatest unmet needs for children with special health care needs. The American Academy of Pediatrics has published a report and policy statement that provide guidance on how to evaluate and when to refer children for full ophthalmologic evaluation (Donahue et al., 2016). It is possible for pediatricians to screen children with neurodevelopmental disabilities for vision problems, but it may be challenging due to cognitive impairment, inability to cooperate, multiple sensory deficits, processing delays, and expressive language delay. Pediatricians should have a low threshold for sending a child with a neurodevelopmental disability for full ophthalmologic evaluation if there are any concerns about vision or if the child has a medical condition with a significant risk of ocular abnormalities.

Structured questionnaires have proven to be successful screening tools for children with cerebral visual impairment, especially among extremely preterm born children, while a multidisciplinary pediatric assessment involving a comprehensive neurodevelopmental assessment evaluation is the starting point for habilitation and interventions (Ortibus,

Fazzi, & Dle, 2019). Several clinical practice guidelines have been proposed to provide a systematic approach for examining the visual functions of a child with special needs (Swaminathan, Jayaraman, & Jacob, 2019). Visual acuity testing is of benefit in children with special needs to both their parents and ophthalmologist, providing quantitative information about visual impairment and reducing stress experienced by parents.

In much of the world the major barrier to accessing eye care services for infants is the absence of trained personnel who can diagnose a problem early. Developed countries have established referral systems; however, pediatric eye care centers are rare in developing countries. There are financial and geographic barriers for many parents from poorer communities. Diagnostic, curative, and rehabilitative services may not be available in the region. Pediatric eye care interventions are also more expensive than adult treatment. Another significant barrier is the lack of knowledge on the part of health care providers, who often ask parents to wait until the child is older before any treatment can be given, at which point the appropriate referral may be too late to be effective.

The pediatrician is essential for the early detection of children who are visually impaired. Studies clearly indicate that the earlier the child is identified, and the earlier intervention is begun, the less limited will be the child's overall interaction with the environment and ability to learn. Increasingly sophisticated early detection screening devices are available and should be used by pediatricians. Nevertheless, it is equally important to regard the wise and continuous observations of the parents carefully, which probably are the best guide to detecting the child at risk for visual impairment.

CHARACTERISTICS AND DEFINITIONS OF BLINDNESS AND VISUAL IMPAIRMENT

Visual impairment may manifest in poor visual acuity, reduced visual field, photophobia, poor depth perception, or poor binocular function and deficient ocular motility. The extent of these difficulties is highly individualized and tied to the actual diagnosis. A child may have a permanent visual impairment, yet still may benefit from prescriptive lenses to correct a concomitant refractive error.

For the pediatric age group, and especially for nonverbal children, there is no universally acceptable definition of the term *blindness*. Legal blindness refers to best corrected distance visual acuity in the better eye of 20/200 or less or a visual field in the better eye of less than 20 degrees, or both. These criteria, originally established as governmental guidelines in determining eligibility for disability services in adults, are used for children, but they often do not translate effectively when applied to the unique medical and developmental circumstances of infants and children with visual difficulties. Students with low vision have best corrected visual acuities in the 20/70 to 20/200 range, and although not considered legally blind meet eligibility requirements for special education services within a public school setting. Ascertainment of visual acuity is often difficult in young children, and criteria for impairment solely on acuity neglect the importance of other determinants of visual function.

Approximately 75% of legally blind children have some remaining vision that is functional and can provide for the foundation for individually tailored learning plans, including environmental and curricular adaptations at home and school. Ultimately, the most important criteria for provision of services specific to blindness or visual impairment at home and school should be based on how the child is actually functioning, not solely on the basis of visual acuity measurements. To qualify for such services within a public school setting, a child must have a diagnosis that results in uncorrectable diminished visual acuity or visual field or the confirmation of a degenerative visual condition and show an educational need for the special education services.

OPHTHALMOLOGIC INTERVENTIONS AND MANAGEMENT

Most children with complex and even routine neurodevelopmental disability deserve evaluation and possible intervention by a pediatric ophthalmologist. As noted in the disease-specific discussions, perhaps as many as 50% of these at-risk children may have significant refractive errors. However, it is a clinical judgment as to what refractive errors might benefit from spectacle correction. For example, 2 diopters of astigmatism could be expected to reduce uncorrected visual acuity to 20/40; however, if a child's visual potential is 20/200 at best, then the treating eye specialist could determine that spectacle correction might not be indicated. Low vision aid evaluation should be part of the routine ophthalmic care of all children with subnormal vision (Tongue, 1980).

Unless a child has NLP vision, surgical correction of strabismus can often be beneficial for children with neurodevelopmental disability, as surgery has been shown to result in rapid improvement in motor development of gross motor milestones (Drover, Stager, Morale, Leffler, & Birch, 2008). In CVI patients with improving visual behavior and a stable angle of strabismus strabismus surgery should be considered.

DEVELOPMENTAL AND EDUCATIONAL IMPLICATIONS OF PEDIATRIC BLINDNESS/ VISUAL IMPAIRMENT

Early onset blindness/visual impairment is likely to impact the rate and sequence of some developmental domains; the biggest challenges occur with developmental areas dependent or significantly linked to vision, such as concept and motor development. The impact will be highly individualized based on the age of onset, severity of the vision loss, presence of concomitant conditions, and family support systems. Developmentally appropriate and family-centered practices will be critical to early intervention supports provided to families of infants and toddlers with blindness/visual impairments. As the child becomes school age there will be significant educational considerations specific to specially designed instruction and equipment needs. Across the age range of learning, blindness/visual impairment is best addressed through strategies to equalize accessibility to visually based information.

Research supports variability in developmental trajectories as the child with blindness/visual impairment navigates the world unique to the child's available senses. The variable that seems to make the most profound difference in the early development of children with blindness/visual impairment will be the presence of additional disabilities (Ferrell, 1998), often stemming from premature birth, neurologic insult, and/or syndromes with a constellation of conditions that include blindness/visual impairment or deaf-blindness (e.g., Down, CHARGE, Usher, and Treacher-Collins syndromes).

Understanding the role of vision across developmental domains will inform support strategies in the early years for young children with blindness/visual impairment with or without additional disabilities. The role of vision in the early development of a very young child is indisputable. Vision is the main avenue for learning in the first years of life, as well as being the leading sense to invite a child's curiosity, integrate information, and entice exploration. As one of two primary near and distance learning senses, the influence on vision upon development is paramount for physical, cognitive, neurologic, and emotional development.

Much of what is learned in the early years and throughout one's lifetime is through incidental learning or being able to observe one's environment, its contents, and the activities occurring away from one's body. Incidental learning undergirds much of a young child's understanding about people, objects, settings, and events and fuels a more meaningful understanding of the words assigned to objects in view, and, as such, bolsters background knowledge for later reading comprehension (Anthony, Yoshinaga-Itano, & Wiggin, 2015). Children with significant visual impairment lose untold hours of incidental learning and opportunities for learning from visual imitation of others. A continual goal across the early years and beyond is to provide concrete experiences to mitigate the restrictions in the range and variety of experiences that may occur due to blindness. Without support, the child is at risk for missed, fragmented, and/or misunderstood information. The child with blindness or significant vision impairment learns through meaningful listening and tactile experiences, which will require ample opportunities for meaningful exploration to make sense of a world of sounds and blurred or absent visual images.

Articulation and speech development are not areas of typical concern with young children who are blind/visually impaired. Care should be taken to assist with the understanding of pronouns and words with multiple meanings (e.g., the bark of a tree and the bark of a dog). Verbal descriptions of settings and activities around the child are key to both concept and language development, in addition to providing information about social cues in preschool settings (e.g., "Your friends Diana and Jose are playing at the water table. Would you like to join them to help fill up a bucket of water for watering the plants?"). It is important not to inundate the child with a steady stream of auditory information but to allow time for the child to listen, understand, and respond. There may be times when the child becomes still and quiet to concentrate on auditory information; this stilling is parallel to a sighted person's stare, where information is being absorbed and processed. Finally, all young children should be screened for any hearing concerns, but this is especially important for the child with blindness/visual impairment who will rely on optimal auditory clarity. Communication and language acquisition will be more affected by additional disabilities, including deaf-blindness; some learners will need assistive or augmentative supports or devices to support expressive and receptive communication and will benefit from the services of a speech language pathologist and, if deaf/hard of hearing, from a teacher trained in deaf education.

Strategies to support learning will be tied to the child's sensory abilities and may include postural or sensory supports for children with vestibular or proprioceptive needs; customized visual displays to address ocular or cortical visual impairment needs for color, contrast, lighting, complexity, novelty, etc.; and tactile supports of real objects or meaningful tactile symbols. Defined work or play spaces give boundaries to play areas and contain dropped toys for easier visual or tactile retrieval. The use of hand-under-hand guidance (the adult's hands under the child's hands) facilitates guided discovery of actions and new objects.

Motor development is often affected by early onset blindness or severe visual impairment. Movement-based milestones, such as crawling or independent walking, tend to occur later than the range of sighted norms. Several factors can influence the gross and fine motor skills of a child with early-onset blindness/visual impairment. Three possible single or overlapping challenges include (1) the lack or reduction of visual reinforcement for movement, (2) hypotonia or low muscle tone, and (3) the role of object permanence in the ambulation skills of a child who is blind or has significant visual impairment. The team of parents, the teacher of students with visual impairments, the orientation and mobility specialists, the occupational therapist, and the physical therapist can address these factors to support high-quality motor skill acquisition of the child. The orientation and mobility specialist will be critical to the introduction and training support for adapted or wearable mobility devices and/or the long cane in the early years (Sapp & Anthony, in press).

School-Age Children and Adolescents

At 3 years of age, children with blindness/visual impairment can enter public school if they meet eligibility criteria for special education services and supports. These criteria must align with the federal Individuals with Disabilities Education Act (IDEA) but are also specific to each individual state. In general, the criteria involve confirmation of a condition of blindness/visual impairment, usually confirmed by eye exam report from the ophthalmologist, and evidence of educational impact tied to the disability that requires specially designed instruction. The latter finding comes from results of educational evaluation and not medical evaluation. The role of the eye doctor is not to make educational recommendations. Specially designed instruction means "adapting, as appropriate to the needs of an eligible child ... the content, methodology, or delivery of instruction" (US Department of Education, 2021). For the student with blindness/visual impairment it will likely require the expertise of both a teacher of students with visual impairments and an orientation mobility specialist.

Instructional strategies will continue to include direct teaching and modeling of skills most often learned through incidental learning (shaking hands, turning to a speaker, independent living tasks), as well as providing the student with audio description of the environment and events. The latter skills should be taught and used by classroom teachers and sighted peers. A focus on unifying experiences is key to assist the learner in gaining a totality of experience such as cooking, which involves meal planning, grocery shopping, meal preparation, and cleanup (Holbrook & Rosenblum, 2017). The depth of detail includes location of items in the grocery store, which items are in the refrigeration/freezer section, how to open jars and cans, the use of the stove and dishwasher, etc. In the classroom, for example, a unifying teaching approach will address full part-whole exploration of the needed materials to be a full participant in a science experience.

Students with blindness/visual impairments will benefit from real objects whenever possible, as well as adapted materials such as scale models and tactile graphics. The American Printing House for the Blind and other vendors provide specialized equipment that may be as low tech as bold lined paper or as sophisticated as braille technology, including manual braille writers, refreshable braille displays (devices with small pins that electronically move up and down through six holes representing a braille cell), braille notetakers (portable devices with refreshable braille displays that connect to the internet and have word processing applications), and braille embossers.

Screen reading software will provide access to digitized text. Some students, including those who are dual media learners (print and braille), require screen enlargement software, video magnification (formerly called closed circuit televisions), and low vision magnification near and distance tools.

In addition to supporting access to the general education curriculum, a student who is blind/visually impaired will also benefit from the expanded core curriculum (ECC) for students who are blind/visually impaired, including those with deaf-blindness and additional disabilities. The ECC provides the specific skill set needed to address vision loss that is foundational for other learning. It consists of nine components, including (1) compensatory access, (2) sensory efficiency skills, (3) assistive technology skills, (4) orientation and mobility, (5) independent living skills, (6) social interaction skills, (7) recreation and leisure skills, (8) career educational skills, and (9) self-determination skills. As such, students who are blind/visually impaired "will receive instruction in two equally essential and interrelated curricula" (Holbrook & Rosenblum, 2017, p. 204). It is important to also note that while the ECC was created as a curricular focus for school-age students, all nine of the components have roots in the early childhood years, and early intervention programs will view and teach the ECC from a developmental perspective.

While the focus will be on each grade level, the educational team should work continually with the student to prepare for postschool life. Secondary transition starts formally at age 16 and involves specific postsecondary goals in the student's IEP. This timeframe is especially important for students with blindness or visual impairments to participate in structured activities that will help them to develop their career and life plans. The use of role models is especially important during this time, as are job preparation and employment experiences. Wolffe (2014) has designed a transition competencies checklist specific to the needs of students with blindness/visual impairments to prepare for postsecondary educational or vocational training.

CONCLUSION AND RECOMMENDATIONS

The identification of and medical and educational supports to children and youth with blindness/visual impairment requires and benefits from a collaborative team approach.

The team should work together to provide a thorough cross-discipline, medical, developmental, and academic evaluation of each student. Each discipline will have a unique and connected role. Communication of evaluation findings assists in every person's understanding of the child's abilities and needs. The child and family should always be central in the determination of next steps, be they medically or educational based.

Individualized and tailored care will be the goal for each child with blindness/visual impairment. These features should include the following:

- Provide emotional supports and help parents understand their child's medical diagnosis and corresponding treatment options. Family support services are crucial, particularly in the weeks and months following the child's diagnosis of blindness/visual impairment.
- Direct families to local, state, and national parent groups and organizations to link new and veteran parents together for purposes of support, networking, and training (see Resources).
- Partner with families to assist and support them in their advocacy for their child.
- Upon medical diagnosis, promptly refer to early intervention services specializing in blindness/visual impairments. If the child is older than 3 years, refer to the local school district's Child Find program or directly to the director of special education.
- Encourage families to keep a folder of medical and educational records.
- Encourage discussion of the child's developmental and academic status with a focus on strengths and areas upon which to build. Listen to families and contribute to identification of the child's preferences, interests, and abilities.
- Explore the emotional impact of the child's disability on siblings.
- Include the child in age-appropriate discussions about the disability, strengths, and needs. Encourage the child to be involved in the IEP meetings. Start early with career

exploration, including home chores and responsibilities that build early employment concepts and skills.

- Become knowledgeable regarding school-based services for students with blindness/visual impairments. Contact your state department of education for guidance. Not every state education agency has an assigned state consultant on blindness/visual impairment, but many do.
- Support the family with training on individual family service plans for the birth to 2-year-old services and IEPs from age 3 to 21 years.
- Help families prepare for major transitions as their child leaves the Part C program for public school, changes schools, and/or prepares to graduate from public school.
- Seek out training on specialized strategies from state departments of education, agencies of the blind, national, and state professional organizations, and parent organizations.
- Seek out publications on general child development and topics specific to blindness/visual impairment. Take time to be informed on the expanded core curriculum (see Resource list).
- Link students and families to role models who are blind/visually impaired or deaf-blind.
- Remember that all children need love, attention, opportunities, practice, friends, recreation and leisure, and support. Not every challenge will be tied to the child's blindness/visual impairment. Many will be just age-appropriate struggles.

REFERENCES

Aicardi, J. (2005). Aicardi syndrome. *Brain and Development*, *27*(3), 164–171.

Anthony, T. L. (2016). Early childhood. In S. Z. Sacks & M. Zatta (Eds.), *Keys to educational success: Teaching students with visual impairments and multiple disabilities* (pp. 487–528). American Foundation for the Blind.

Anthony, T. L., Yoshinaga-Itano, C., & Wiggin, M. (2015). Strategies for infants and toddlers with sensory disabilities. In S. A. Raver & D. Childress (Eds.), *Family-centered early intervention: Supporting infants & toddlers in natural environments* (pp. 216–254). Paul Brookes Publishing.

Bankes, J. L. (1975). The ophthalmologist's role in multidisciplinary assessment of developmentally handicapped children. *Child: Care, Health and Development*, *1*(5), 325–333.

Chambers, T. M., et al. (2018). Epidemiology of anophthalmia and microphthalmia: Prevalence and patterns in Texas, 1999–2009. *American Journal of Medical Genetics*, *176*(9), 1810–1818.

Chevignard, M. P., & Lind, K. (2014). Long-term outcome of abusive head trauma. *Pediatric Radiology*, *44*, 548–558. https://doi.org/10.1007/s00247-014-3169-8

Chockron, S., & Dutton, G. N. (2016). Impact of cerebral visual impairments on motor skills: Implicaions for developmental coordination disorders. *Frontiers in Psychology*, *7*, 1471. https://doi.org/10.3389/fpsyg.2016.01471

Claerhout, H., Witters, P., Régal, L., et al. (2018). Isolated sulfite oxidase deficiency. *Journal of Inherited Metabolic Disease*, *41*, 101–108. https://doi.org/10.1007/s10545-017-0089-4

Colorado Department of Education. (2020). *Vision screening parent questionnaire for children ages birth through five*. http://www.cde.state.co.us/cdesped/sped_data

Donahue, S. P., Baker, C. N., & Committee on Practice and Ambulatory Medicine, Section on Ophthalmology, American Association of Certified Orthoptists, American Association for Pediatric Ophthalmology and Strabismus, & American Academy of Ophthalmology. (2016). Visual system assessment in infants, children, and young adults by pediatricians. *Pediatrics*, *137*(1), e20153596. https://doi.org/10.1542/peds.2015-3596

Drover, J. R., Stager, D. R., Morale, S. E., Leffler, J. N., & Birch, E. E. (2008). Improvement in motor development following surgery for infantile esotropia. *Journal of the American Association for Pediatric Ophthalmology and Strabismus*, *12*, 136–140.

Dutton, G. N. (2013). The spectrum of cerebral visual impairment as a sequel to premature birth: An overview. *Documenta Ophthalmologic*, *127*(1), 69–78.

Fazzi, E., Micheletti, S., Galli, J., Rossi, A., Gitti, F., & Molinaro, A. (2019). Autism in children with cerebral and peripheral visual impairment: Fact or artifact? *Seminars in Pediatric Neurology*, *31*, 57–67. https://doi.org/10.1016/j.spen.2019.05.008

Ferrari, S., Ponzin, D., Ashworth, J. L., et al. (2011). Diagnosis and management of ophthalmological features in patients with mucopolysaccharidosis. *British Journal of Ophthalmology*, *95*, 613–619.

Ferrell, K. A. (1998). *Project PRISM: A longitudinal study of the developmental patterns of children who are visually impaired: Executive summary: CFDA 84.0203C: Field-initiated research HO23C10188*. University of Northern Colorado.

Fisher, E. (2011). Exploring the genetic origins of Treacher Collins syndrome. *Clinical Genetics*, *79*, 330–332.

Garcia-Filion, P., & Borchert, M. (2013). Optic nerve hypoplasia syndrome: A review of the epidemiology and clinical associations. *Current Treatment Options in Neurology*, *15*(1), 78–89.

Ghassemi, F., Bazvand, F., Hosseini, S. S., Karkhaneh, R., Ebrahimiadib, N., & Shekarchi, B. (2015). Optic nerve aplasia: Case report and literature review. *Journal of Ophthalmic and Vision Research*, *10*(2), 187–192. https://doi.org/10.4103/2008-322X.163779

Haargaard, B., et al. (2014). Risk of retinal detachment after pediatric cataract surgery. *Investigative Ophthalmology & Visual Science*, *55*, 2947–2951.

Hariprasad, S. M., Moon, S. J., Allen, R. C., & Wilhelmus, K. R. (2002). Keratopathy from congenital syphilis. *Cornea*, *21*(6), 608–609.

Hered, R. W., et al. (2019). *Basic and clinical science course: Pediatric ophthalmology and strabismus, 2019–2020*. American Academy of Ophthalmology.

Hertle, R. W., Zylan, S., & Katowitz, J. A. (1993). Ophthalmic features and visual prognosis in Treacher-Collins syndrome. *British Journal of Ophthalmology*, *77*, 642–645.

Holbrook, M. C., & Rosenblum, L. P. (2017). Planning instruction in unique skills. In M. C. Holbrook, T. McCarthy, & C. Kamei-Hannan (Eds.), *Foundations of education: Vol 2: Instructional strategies for teaching children and youths with visual impairment* (3rd ed., pp. 203–230). AFB Press.

Imbornoni, L. M., Wise, R. E., Taravella, M. J., Hickey, F., & McCourt, E. A. (2020). Keratoconus and corneal morphology in patients with Down syndrome at a pediatric hospital. *Journal of the American Association for Pediatric Ophthalmology and Strabismus*, *24*(3), 140.e1–140.e5. https://doi.org/10.1016/j.jaapos.2020.02.004

Jan, J. E., Groenveld, M., Skyanda, A. M., & Hoyt, C. S. (1987). Behavioral characteristics of children with permanent cortical visual impairment. *Developmental*

Medicine and Child Neurology, *29*(5), 571–576. https://doi.org/10.1111/j.1469-8749.1987.tb08498.x

Javaid, U., Ali, M. H., Jamal, S., & Butt, N. H. (2018). Pathophysiology, diagnosis, and management of glaucoma associated with Sturge–Weber syndrome. *International Ophthalmology*, *8*, 409–416.

Kong, L., Fry, M., Al-Samarraie, M., Gilbert, C., & Steinkuller, P. G. (2012). An update on progress and the changing epidemiology of causes of childhood blindness worldwide. *Journal of the American Association for Pediatric Ophthalmology and Strabismus*, *16*(6), 501–507.

Lesnik Oberstein, S. A. J., Ruivenkamp, C. A. L., & Hennekam, R. C. (2007). Peters plus syndrome. In M. P. Adam, H. H. Ardinger, R. A. Pagon, S. E. Wallace, L. J. H. Bean, G. Mirzaa, & A. Amemiya (Eds.), *GeneReviews*. University of Washington. PMID: 20301637.

Macsai, M. S., et al. (2001). Tyrosinemia type II: Nine cases of ocular signs and symptoms. *American Journal of Ophthalmology*, *132*(4), 522–527.

Maguire, S., Watts, P., Shaw, A., et al. (2013). Retinal haemorrhages and related findings in abusive and non-abusive head trauma: A systematic review. *Eye*, *27*, 28–36. https://doi.org/10.1038/eye.2012.213

Mansukhani, S. A., Ho, M.-L., & Brodsky, M. C. (2020). Abnormal vestibular-ocular reflexes in children with cortical visual impairment. *Journal of Neuroophthalmology*. https://doi.org/10.1097/WNO.0000000000000999

Marelli, C., et al. (2011). Heterozygous *OPA1* mutations in Behr syndrome. *Brain*, *134*(1–2), e169.

Ortibus, E., Fazzi, E., & Dle, N. (2019). Cerebral visual impairment and clinical assessment: The European perspective. *Seminars in Pediatric Neurology*, *31*, 15–24.

Pellegrino, L. (2019). The senses, the world we see, hear, and feel. In M. L. Batshaw, N. J. Roizen, & L. Pellegrino (Eds.), *Children with disabilities* (8th ed., pp. 99–117). Paul Brookes Publishing Company.

Philip, S. S., Guzzeta, A., Chorna, O., & Gole, G. (2020). Relationship between brain structure and cerebral visual impairment in children with cerebral palsy. A systematic review. *Research in Developmental Disabilities*, *99*, 130580.

Salati, R., Borgatti, R., Giammari, G., & Jacobson, L. (2002). Oculomotor dysfunction in cerebral visual impairment following perinatal hypoxia. *Developmental Medicine and Child Neurology*, *44*(8), 542–550.

Sapp, W. K., & Anthony, T. L. (in press). Orientation and mobility in the early childhood years. In W. R. Wiener, R. L. Welsh, & R. Wall (Eds.), *Foundations of orientation and mobility, Vol. II: Instructional strategies and practical applications* (4th ed.). APH Press.

Sheeladevi, S., Lawrenson, J., Fielder, A., et al. (2016). Global prevalence of childhood cataract: A systematic review. *Eye*, *30*, 1160–1169. https://doi.org/10.1038/eye.2016.156

Swaminathan, M., Jayaraman, D., & Jacob, N. (2019). Visual function assessment, ocular examination, and intervention in children with developmental delay: A systematic approach. Part 1. *Indian Journal of Ophthalmology*, *67*, 196. https://doi.org/10.4103/ijo.IJO_524_18

Tongue, A. C. (1980). Low vision examination in children with visual impairment. *Journal of Pediatric Ophthalmology and Strabismus*, *17*(3), 175–179.

United States Department of Education. (2021b). *Individuals with Education Act, Section 300.39 Special Education*. https://sites.ed.gov/idea/regs/b/a/300.39

Wolffe, K. E. (2014). Career education. In C. B. Alman & S. Lewis (Eds.), *ECC essentials: Teaching the expanded core curriculum to students with visual impairments* (pp. 411–469). AFB Press.

Yoo, H., Chung, S. A., & Yoon, S. H. (2014). Abducents nerve palsy following expansion cranioplasty with distraction osteogenesis. *Neuro-Ophthalmology*, *38*(6), 326–330.

RESOURCES

American Association for Pediatric Ophthalmology and Strabismus: http://aapos.org

American Foundation for the Blind: www.afb.org

American Printing House for the Blind: www.aph.org

Blind Babies Foundation: http://blindbabies.typepad.com/resources

Early Support. (n.d.). *Helping every child succeed. Developmental journal for babies and children with visual impairment*. DCSF Publications. www.dcsf.gov.uk/everychildmatters/earlysupport

Levin, A. V., & Enzenauer, R. W. (Eds.). (2017). *The eye in pediatric systemic disease*. Springer International Publishing.

National Association of Parents of Children with Visual Impairments (NAPVI): http://www.spedex.com/napvi/index.html

National Federation of the Blind: www.nfb.org

Perkins School for the Blind: www.perkins.org

Southwell, C., & Haigh, K. (2010). *Visual impairment and physioltherapy. The best of both: Working together to support children with visual impairment and additional complex needs*. RNIB.

Texas School for the Blind and Visually Impaired: http://www.tsbvi.edu

44

Language and Speech Disorders

Heidi M. Feldman and Cheryl Messick

For additional material related to the content of this chapter, please see Chapter 107.

> **VIGNETTE**
>
> *Travis was a handsome, social 24-month-old child whose language skills lagged far behind those of his older sister when she was that age. His primary care clinician wanted to begin an evaluation and intervene. His mother insisted on waiting because, she reasoned, boys develop more slowly than girls, he had had multiple bouts of otitis media, and his chatty sister frequently spoke for him. However, 2 months later, Travis began to tantrum when he was not understood. His mother then arranged an audiologic assessment and accepted the referral to an early intervention program. Travis's hearing, assessed via sound field, was found to be adequate for speech perception. The speech-language pathologist confirmed that his expressive language skills were at the 14-month age level, although receptive and symbolic play skills were near age level. He was enrolled in a toddler communication group, 2 hours/session, two sessions/week, with a parent-training component. His pace of language learning increased. By 36 months his vocabulary was greater than 300 words, and he was speaking in up to four-word phrases. At age 48 months, he had residual speech-sound immaturities but had caught up in language skills. At age 7 years, his second-grade teacher called his parents in for a conference because his reading skills were below age expectations.*

DEFINITIONS

Language is the distinctly human communication system through which humans share ideas, thoughts, emotions, and beliefs. Language is symbolic; meaning is conveyed through arbitrary sounds and words, which have no direct connection to their referents. Language is systematic; rules govern the placement of sounds in words and words in sentences, which cannot be altered without changing meaning or violating rules. Using arbitrary signs and combinatory rules, humans can create and understand an infinite number of messages, not only about the here and now but also about the past and future, the abstract, hypothetical, or imagined. Speech refers specifically to the oral or verbal output of language. Speech results from a complex interaction of the respiratory system, larynx, pharynx, mouth structures, and nose. Alternative outputs of the language system are sign language and written language.

Language and speech are subdivided into components, described in Tables 44.1 and 44.2, respectively. Receptive language refers to the ability to understand, and expressive language refers to the ability to produce words, sentences, discourse, and conversation. Comprehensive evaluations typically assess many of these features of language and speech (see Chapter 107).

NORMAL DEVELOPMENT

Newborns show the social and auditory building blocks for language development. At birth, they prefer the human face and human voice over other visual or auditory stimuli. Infants can discriminate similar speech sounds (*/ba/* vs. */pa/*). They use the statistical properties of sound cooccurrences in continuous streams of speech to group syllables into wordlike units (Saffran, Johnson, Aslin, & Newport, 1999). These perceptual mechanisms assist children in parsing the continuous sound stream into recognizable chunks.

The language the infant hears refines innate speech perception mechanisms. By about 9 months of age, infants show greater precision in differentiating the phonemes of their native language than phonemes from other languages. American and Japanese infants younger than 6 months old are equally accurate at discriminating between /r/ and /l/, but 9-month-old Japanese infants lose that ability because /r/ and /l/ are used interchangeably in Japanese (Kuhl, 2004). At approximately 9 months of age, infants learn to produce actions in response to verbal commands ("wave bye-bye") and to comprehend common words such as *no, mama*, and *daddy*.

For most children, language learning proceeds in a predictable, orderly fashion. During the first year of life, infants learn to produce the sounds of their native language (Table 44.3). By their first birthday, they produce a repertoire of consonants and chains of syllables with the intonation patterns of sentences (i.e., jargon) and they typically convey meaning with nonverbal methods, such as pointing, shrugging, nodding, and iconic gestures. At age 1 year, they begin to produce words. From 12 to 18 months, they learn a handful of words every month; between 12 and 18 months, they begin to learn a handful of words every day. The rapid increase in vocabulary typically coincides with their ability to make two-word phrases. By age 3 years, children produce simple complete sentences. By age 4 to 5 years, they have mastered the rules of language, participating in conversations and constructing narrative discourse. Despite residual immaturities in speech sound production, their speech is nearly 100% intelligible to

TABLE 44.1 Components of Language

Term	Definition	Examples
Phoneme	Smallest unit of the sound system that can change meaning	*/p, b, i, a, t,* and *n/* differentiate the meaning of ***pit, bit, pat,*** and ***pan***
Phonology	Inventory of phonemes within a language and the rules for combining them	In English: */st/* and */fr/* can occur sequentially, */sht/* or */bt/* cannot
Morpheme	Smallest unit of meaning in a language, including words and word parts	Prefixes ***(un-, dis-)***, suffixes ***(-ly, -ness)***, grammatical markers (plural ***-s***, past tense -***ed***), articles (***a, the***)
Lexicon (vocabulary)	Inventory of words	Early words: ***mama, bye, more*** Late words: adverbs
Syntax (grammar), also known as morphosyntax	Rules for combining words and morphemes	"The cat is eating" is a sentence (but "cat the eating is" is not)
Semantics	The meaning of words and sentences	Early meanings: attribution ("big ball"), possession ("my ball"), and agent + action + object ("daddy throw ball")
Pragmatics	Social aspects of language use that affect the effectiveness of communication	Intonation, politeness, appropriateness, turn-taking, and communicative functions

TABLE 44.2 Elements of Normal and Disordered Speech

Element	Definition
Speech sound inventory	Set of phonemes used by the speaker in total and as a function of placement within a syllable (initial vs. final)
Articulation errors	Speech sound errors based on incorrect motor patterns (e.g., */sh/ for /s/* in syllable initial and final positions)
Phonologic errors	Speech sound errors based on inappropriate use of language rules, such as reducing consonant clusters ("tick" for *stick* and "boom" for *broom*) and deleting the final consonants ("da" for *dog*)
Intelligibility	Understandability of speech, which can be measured as the percent of words understood by the listener
Stimulability	Ability to imitate sounds correctly in a hierarchy of increasing linguistic complexity (e.g., sound level */s/*; syllable level */sa/, /su/*; single syllable word *sit;* multisyllabic word *sucker;* phrase *sit down*)
Fluency	Flow of language. Dysfluency can be erratic pacing or stuttering
Voice and resonance	Vocal quality of speech sounds, including characteristics of hoarseness, breathiness, and hyponasality or hypernasality

TABLE 44.3 Stages in the Development of Speech Sounds in the First Year of Life

Stage (Age)	Type of Vocalization	Description
Stage 1 (birth–1 mo)	Vegetative and reflexive vocalizations	Crying, fussing, coughing, and burping Normal phonation, limited resonance Vocalizations with closed or nearly closed small mouth
Stage 2 (2–3 mo)	Cooing	Sounds produced in the back of the mouth Primitive consonant-vowel syllables without timing of articulatory gestures for adult consonants
Stage 3 (4–6 mo)	Vocal play	Experimentation with sounds, including repetition of vowel-like elements Squeals, yells, raspberries, and clicks Adult-like vowels and consonant-vowel syllables without regular-syllable timing
Stage 4A (6–8 mo)	Canonical or reduplicated babbling	Strings of repeated true consonant-resonant vowel sequences *(/bababa/, /dididi/)*
Stage 4B (8–12 mo)	Variegated babbling	Large variety of consonants and vowels within a single utterance Sentence-like intonation (jargon)

TABLE 44.4 Receptive Language Development: Average Age of Acquisition and Age Indicating Significant Delay or Red Flag

Receptive Language Milestones	Average Age of Acquisition	Significant Delays and Red Flags
Alerts or quiets to sound	Birth–1 mo	2 mo
Turns to the source of sound	Birth–1 mo, then again 3–5 mo	6 mo
Responds to own name	6–8 mo	10 mo
Follows verbal routines ("Wave bye-bye")	8–10 mo	12 mo
Understands simple questions ("Where's mommy?")	9–11 mo	15 mo
Stops when told "No"	9–10 mo	15 mo
Understands at least three different words	10–13 mo	15 mo
Points to three different body parts	12–16 mo	18 mo
Follow simple commands ("Show me the ball" or "Get your shoes")	12 mo	18 mo
Follows two-part commands ("Get your shoes and give them to Dad")	24 mo	30 mo
Answers simple questions ("Who is that?" or "What are you doing?")	24–30 mo	36 mo

TABLE 44.5 Expressive Language Development: Average Age of Acquisition and Age Indicating Significant Delay or Red Flag

Expressive Language Milestones	Average Age Range	Significant Delays and Red Flags
Cooing	2–3 mo	6 mo
Babbling	6–8 mo	10 mo
Nonverbal purposeful messages (requests with reach; shows objects)	9–10 mo	12 mo
Pointing	10–11 mo	14 mo
Says three different spontaneous words	12–15 mo	16 mo
Vocabulary at least 35–50 words	18–22 mo	24 mo
Production of two-word phrases ("Mommy sock"; "No water")	18–22 mo	24 mo
Simple sentences ("I want juice"; "Where's my ball?")	24–30 mo	36 mo
Intelligibility to unfamiliar adult at >50%	30–36 mo	42 mo
Able to tell about a past event with parent asking questions (personal narrative)	24–30 mo	36 mo
Able to tell or retell a familiar story	36–48 mo	54 mo
Fully intelligible to an unfamiliar adult (despite some immature sounds, such as consonant clusters or */r/* and */l/*)	48–54 mo	60 mo
Fully mature speech sounds	Up to 72 mo	>72 mo

unfamiliar people. Tables 44.4 and 44.5 describe key steps in receptive and expressive language, respectively, including red flags (i.e., signs that development is delayed or atypical, warranting a comprehensive speech-language assessment).

DEVELOPMENTAL VARIATIONS

The rate of language and speech development varies widely, even among children who ultimately exhibit normal skills. Many children build a vocabulary of object names (*ball*, *dog*, and *shoe*) and progress from a one- to two-word phase ("Mommy shoe"). Other children first learn social expressions ("thank you," "gimmedat," or "whazat"), using language to express needs or to interact with others. These early stylistic differences do not seem to predict important differences in later development (Bates et al., 1994).

The mother in the opening vignette offered many possible explanations for her son's early delays. Though these notions are commonly held, none should postpone evaluation and treatment of delays. Studies document that girls are ahead of boys during the early stages of language development. However, delays in the vocabulary size and grammar of boys are minor, equivalent to about 1 to 2 months of developmental progress (Fenson et al., 1994). Moreover, boys are more likely than girls to develop language disorders. Minor stylistic differences may be found in the language development of first-born versus later-born children. These differences are likely related to differences in the environments of children of different birth orders (Hoff-Ginsburg, 1998). However, children usually find great utility in speaking for themselves rather than letting an older sibling guess what they want. Children in bilingual households may show language mixing in their early language development. As they acquire more language skills they segregate the two languages into separate systems. Their developmental rate should not be delayed if the accomplishments in both languages are added together (Pearson, Fernandez, & Oller, 1993). Early delays in language or speech development are often attributed to chronic otitis media. However, randomized clinical trials of tympanostomy tubes for persistent middle ear effusion found that prompt tube insertion did not improve language or speech outcomes up to middle childhood (Paradise et al., 2007), suggesting otitis media does not cause language delay.

Rates of vocabulary and syntactic development are associated with the amount and quality of child-directed language. The term *language nutrition* is used to capture the environmental features that support language development. On average, parents in lower socioeconomic classes provide less child-directed language than middle-class parents (Hart & Risley, 1995). As a group, children from the lower socioeconomic classes show slower language development, reduced vocabulary, and less developed syntax than children from middle-class families (Dollaghan et al., 1999). Randomized clinical studies document that children who received enhanced language nutrition show improvements in child language skills, suggesting that environmental features play a causative role in language development (Ramírez, Lytle, & Kuhl, 2020). Many community-based public health programs are designed to improve language nutrition in groups at risk for delays as strategy for primary prevention of disorders.

DEVELOPMENTAL DELAY

A child's communication may be considered delayed when it is noticeably behind age-matched peers. No single criterion has been established as clinically significant. For some purposes, the criterion for language delay is performance at least 1.5 to 2 SD below the population mean on standardized tests of speech or language. In some states a developmental delay of at least 25% in one or more domains of functioning, calculated from the ratio of developmental age to chronologic age, renders the child eligible for early intervention services. Using this latter definition, a 24-month-old who is functioning below the 18-month age level in at least one aspect of language development has a significant delay.

It is difficult to predict which children who show initial delays are destined to develop language disorders. Approximately half of children delayed at 2 years of age catch up to peers by 3 years of age. Resolution of the delays has been weakly associated with good receptive language and mature symbolic play skills, as found in the child in the opening vignette. Assessment of language in toddlers should include an evaluation of comprehension and play. Language is used for a variety of purposes, including expressing wants and needs, greeting others, describing objects or actions, and answering questions. If the range of communicative functions and social skills is restricted, the child may have a language disorder. The more components of language affected and the greater the severity of deficit, the higher the likelihood that the child will have long-term communication deficits.

EVALUATION PROCEDURES

Screening

Screening establishes whether asymptomatic children are at high risk for language or speech impairment. Screening procedures rely heavily on parent reports or interviews because direct assessment of children at young ages is time consuming and unreliable. Validated developmental screening tools are currently available in the United States and internationally (see Chapter 81).

Diagnostic Testing

Diagnostic testing establishes strengths and weaknesses in multiple aspects of communication. The purposes of assessment are to explain developmental, social, academic, social, or communication difficulties; to identify children in need of therapeutic and support services; and to establish specific targets for intervention. Assessments serve as baseline measures for monitoring progress and may prove useful for educating parents about strategies for facilitating communication development. Diagnostic testing is typically in the purview of the speech-language therapist (see Chapter 107).

Accurate assessment of infants and toddlers is challenging because of the low frequency of verbal output and the difficulty that young children have in cooperating with clinicians. Informal observations, parent interview tools, and natural assessments play an important role in the evaluation of young children. Formal assessments become more central to evaluation as the child reaches preschool age and beyond. Chapter 107 includes measures commonly used.

Observational and Interview Assessment Strategies

Conversation sampling assesses functional communication in a naturalistic setting. Speech-language pathologists may transcribe and analyze the conversation in real time or may create audio- or videotapes for subsequent detailed analysis. Conversation analysis allows multiple components of the child and parent communication to be assessed concurrently. Observation is ideal for assessing pragmatic behaviors (e.g., topic maintenance) and to assessing connected discourse (e.g., telling or retelling stories, describing pictures). Conversation sampling is often used in conjunction with standardized measures for a comprehensive assessment.

Parent report inventories and interviews circumvent challenges of conversational analysis and have proven to be valuable tools, particularly for evaluating children in the birth through 36-month age range. They tap into parents' extensive knowledge and frequent observations of their child's abilities. Parent report inventories that ask about current skills as opposed to past skills or age of acquisition have been shown to have good to excellent reliability and concurrent validity, although accuracy may vary by age and social class (Feldman et al., 2000). Direct child observation is another strategy of evaluation for young children.

Norm-Referenced Formal Measures

Norm-referenced measures require standardized procedures for administration and scoring to generate age-adjusted standard scores. They are often used to qualify a child as eligible for early intervention services or other supports and to compare the relative level of language skills in relation to other abilities, such as cognition or motor skills. Norm-referenced formal measures play an increasingly prominent role in the evaluation of children as they enter school age and their skills become increasingly differentiated. Receptive and expressive skills and specific language skills may be evaluated comprehensively or in separate tests or subtests.

Criterion-Referenced Measures

Criterion-referenced tests measure what skills the child has mastered from either a development sequence or a curriculum used to treat children who are delayed in development. Criterion-referenced measures allow adjustment in the administration of items for children with sensory or motor impairments and emphasize the specific behaviors that have been mastered, rather than relative standing in reference to the group. They can be used to compare children with themselves, allowing longitudinal tracking of changes in development. That makes these measures useful for planning interventions and monitoring progress during treatment. Many federally funded early intervention programs use these types of measures to determine if children qualify for services, to generate the objectives on the individualized family service plans (IFSP), and to monitor progress.

Assessment of Speech

Tests are available to assess speech sound development. These tests typically assess speech sound production in single words but not in connected discourse. They may overestimate the child's overall speech abilities and level of intelligibility for speech. Conversational analysis is a useful adjunct to identify children with a few selected articulation problems or to characterize the speech problems that emerge as words and sentences increase in length.

LANGUAGE DISORDERS

Epidemiology

Disorders of language and speech are highly prevalent. Approximately 16% of children show clinically significant delays at age 2; approximately half of those children remain delayed to kindergarten entry. Speech and language impairment is the most common condition in preschool years establishing eligibility for special education services. Language and speech disorders may occur in isolation, together, and in conjunction with other delays or disorders.

Known Causes

Table 44.6 summarizes the requirements for normal language development. Children need to interact with responsive adults, ideally in an unstressed environment. They must hear an ample corpus of language, using cognitive and neural processes to derive meaning from sound and to learn the combinatorial rules for sounds, words, and sentences. They must be able to organize their pharynx, tongue, mouth, and breathing apparatus to produce speech quickly and accurately. Table 44.6 also provides examples of known causes of language delays and disorders within the social environment, verbal environment, hearing apparatus, cognitive/neurologic system, and speech production mechanisms. These conditions constitute the differential diagnosis of language and speech disorders.

Unresponsive Social Environment and Impoverished Language Environment

Children raised in orphanages typically experience language and speech disorders. A randomized trial found that transfer of children from orphanages to foster care before age 24 months dramatically improved outcomes, demonstrating that the enhanced environment caused the gains (Windsor et al., 2011). Children who have experienced child abuse and child neglect also frequently develop language disorders. For children living in poverty, language delays may be related to poor language nutrition (Hart & Risley, 1995) and other challenges, such as poor nutrition (see Chapter 66) and high levels of stress (see Chapter 15) (Hurt & Betancourt, 2016).

TABLE 44.6 Causes of Delays and Disorders in Language and Speech as a Function of Fundamental Requirements

Requirements	Social Interactions	Verbal Input	Hearing	Neural Processing	Speech Apparatus
Normal	Responsive	Adequate	Threshold <20 dB	Intact neural pathways	Intact oral and respiratory mechanisms
Causes of delays and disorders	Unresponsive social interactions Psychosocial deprivation Child abuse and neglect Toxic stress	Impoverished verbal input	Hearing loss Auditory neuropathy Auditory processing disorder	Cognitive impairment Chromosomal or genetic disorder Neural injury Seizure disorders Autism Specific language impairment Dysarthria Childhood apraxia of speech	Cleft lip and cleft palate Velopharyngeal insufficiency Anatomic disorders of any structure within the speech system Oral motor dysfunction

Hearing Loss

Normal conversation averages 40 to 60 dB in intensity in the range of 500 to 2000 Hz in frequency. Vowels and high-energy/low-frequency consonants, such as /*m*, *n*, and *b*/, are relatively easy to hear. Low-energy/high-frequency consonants, such as /*s*, *f*, and *th*/, are relatively difficult to hear. The degree of hearing loss and the range of frequencies affected determine the amount of speech readily perceived (see Chapter 42). In mild hearing loss the quietest sound that a person can hear is 25 to 40 dB; high-frequency speech sounds may be difficult to detect or distorted, especially in background noise. In moderate hearing loss the quietest sound that a person can hear is 40 to 60 or 70 dB; most conversations are difficult to detect without amplification. In severe and profound hearing loss the quietest sound that a person can hear is greater than 70 dB; language cannot be reliably perceived without amplification. Therefore individuals with profound hearing loss may be candidates for cochlear implantation (Papsin & Gordon, 2007).

Children with mild to severe hearing loss are at increased risk for delays in language development. Outcomes are more favorable if hearing loss is detected early through universal newborn hearing screening (Kennedy et al., 2006) and children receive hearing aids before age 6 months and use hearing aids consistently (Tomblin et al., 2015). The nature of the language environment unsurprisingly also impacts outcomes; children with hearing impairment whose mothers have high levels of education have better outcomes than children of mothers with limited education.

For children with severe to profound hearing loss, the most effective therapy is debated. The oral approach focuses on listening and speaking with the goal of facilitating spoken language and social engagement with hearing peers. The manual approach focuses on sign language with the goal of facilitating communication and allowing engagement with deaf peers. Total communication is a combination. A meta-analysis comparing oral and manual methods concluded that the data are not sufficiently strong to conclude which method is better (Fitzpatrick et al., 2016). Informed families should participate in decision making about therapeutic approaches.

Cognitive Impairment

Language delays are often the presenting complaint for children with mild to moderate overall cognitive impairment or mild intellectual disability (see Chapter 40). These children usually progress in their speech and language skills in the typical sequence but at a slow rate. Vocabulary and grammar are typically affected; pragmatic skills may be preserved. Abstract language concepts may present severe challenges. Parents of children who function in the range of mild intellectual disability are more likely to have cognitive impairments than parents of children of normal intelligence, and they may not provide stimulating verbal input, adding environmental factors to genetic contributions to the language disorder. Early intervention services may improve the quality and quantity of language input to children with mild cognitive disability, directing services to both the parents and/or the children.

In moderate, severe, and profound intellectual disability the prognosis for language skills depends on the cause and is less favorable than for mild intellectual disability. Social interactions with typically developing peers and speech-language therapy may improve functional communication. Treatment typically focuses on promoting communication skills in different environments (e.g., at home, at school) and on improving effectiveness of nonverbal communication for children with poor speech. Low-technology alternative or augmentative means may be incorporated to help improve communication. A child might be trained to hit a switch as a means of activating a tape recorder to offer a social greeting. This approach provides a method for teaching cause-effect relationships and for motivating communication.

Chromosomal and Genetic Causes of Cognitive Impairment

Some chromosomal and genetic conditions with associated cognitive impairment have distinctive behavioral phenotypes in terms of language. Children with Down syndrome (see Chapter 27) typically show more significant impairments in speech and language than would be predicted on the basis of their cognitive abilities or receptive language skills. Grammatical skills are particularly weak. They may also often have poor speech skills and dysfluency. Boys with fragile X syndrome (see Chapter 28) typically show vocabulary and grammatical skills consistent with their level of nonverbal intelligence. Frequent rapid bursts of language and phonologic disorders may make them unintelligible to unfamiliar listeners. Boys with fragile X syndrome also exhibit echolalia, or repetition of words, especially at the end of sentences, interfering with completing sentences. They have poor pragmatic skills and inability to stay on topic, associated with poor eye-to-eye gaze and heightened anxiety. Children with Williams syndrome show better expressive language skills than would be expected from their cognitive abilities. They may be quite delayed initially in language abilities; however, they often eventually develop language and social skills at a faster rate than visuospatial skills. Fluent conversational abilities often mask difficulties in abstract language, grammatical knowledge, and language comprehension.

Autism

Autism is characterized by qualitative impairments of communication (as discussed in Chapter 41) and should be considered in the differential diagnosis for children with primary language delays or regression of skills in the language and social domains. In the severe cases of autism children lack a means of symbolic communication, including verbal language, sign language, or gestures. They rely on nonsymbolic communication, such as leading a parent to a desired object. They may eventually learn rudimentary language, but social interactions focus on making requests or demands. In moderately severe cases children with autism may show limited vocabulary and grammar skills; poor pragmatic skills; and stereotyped, repetitive, or idiosyncratic uses of language. At the mild end of the spectrum, children may have difficulty initiating or sustaining a conversation and maintaining the topic of conversation. Poor communication compromises their social interactions, limiting their ability to develop peer friendships or social relationships.

The prognosis for language and communication for children with autism is evolving as the definition of the disorder changes and intensive early intervention services become routine. In adults with autism who have become successful communicators pragmatic skills typically remain underdeveloped. They have difficulties understanding humor or metaphor, reading the social cues of their listener, modifying the topics of communication, and engaging in social interactions. Intonation often remains flat or unchanging.

Neurologic Conditions

Distinctive patterns of language use have been associated with specific neurologic conditions. Hydrocephaly, the abnormal accumulation of the cerebrospinal fluid, is associated with "cocktail party chatter." These children develop diverse vocabularies and appropriate syntax but show difficulties with semantics and pragmatics, verbosity, and superficiality. They may not understand the meaning of figurative language such as idioms, may be weak at drawing inferences, and may show difficulty with reading comprehension.

Landau-Kleffner syndrome is a rare, acquired seizure disorder that manifests with an abrupt disruption of receptive language in a child who had previously displayed normal language development. The abnormalities on electroencephalography vary. Although the prognosis for seizures is generally favorable, the long-term outcomes of cognition and language are highly variable. Electric status epilepticus in slow-wave sleep or continuous spike and wave in slow-wave sleep is another rare, acquired seizure disorder that affects language functioning. Age of onset is typically 5 to 7 years. Atrophy and neural injuries on imaging are more likely than in Landau-Kleffner syndrome, and affected individuals may have memory disturbances and behavioral disorders of varying severity.

Children with traumatic brain injuries often show persistent speech and language disorders (see Chapter 32). Children with focal left hemisphere injuries show less severe disturbances in language functioning than adults with comparable injuries (Levine, Beharelle, Demir, & Small, 2016). Functional imaging of children with early left hemisphere injury typically shows that language processing occurs in the right hemisphere and in healthy areas of the left hemisphere, indicative of the plasticity of the nervous system for language and speech.

Specific Language Impairment

Specific language impairment (SLI), also known as developmental language disorder, refers to impairments in language skills in children despite normal intelligence, hearing, neurologic functioning, and oral mechanisms and the absence of any known causes. Although a heterogeneous disorder, most children with SLI have greater difficulty with expressive than receptive skills, especially in morphology and syntax. Some children also have difficulty with the phonologic rules of language, resulting in decreased intelligibility of speech. They may also have significant comprehension deficits resulting in pragmatic irregularities, in addition to grammatical deficits. The prevalence of SLI among children in kindergarten was found to be 7.4% (Tomblin et al., 1997). Children with SLI and those whose early delays in language and speech apparently resolve during preschool may show reading difficulties at school age, as occurred with Travis in the opening vignette.

Genetic contributions to SLI are assumed based on high rates of disorders within families, high concordance among twins, and high estimates of heritability (Rice, Taylor, Zubrick, Hoffman, & Earnest, 2020). The specific genetic basis is unknown. Genetic variations likely shape neural structures that support language skills and then lead to a wide spectrum in speech and language ability. SLI resembles complex genetic disorders, such as asthma and diabetes; these conditions run in families but their inheritance pattern is not dominant or recessive. A continuous distribution of multiple genetic and environmental causes and a heritable deficiency in verbal traits most likely underlie developmental speech and language disorders. One exception to that general finding of unknown genetic causes comes from a large multigeneration family, called the KE family, in whom impairments in the ability to sequence verbal movements were found to be inherited as an autosomal dominant trait. Genetic analysis determined that the affected members of this family had a point mutation on chromosome 7 in the *FOXP2* gene, a transcriptional factor (Lai et al., 2001).

Genetic and environmental factors likely contribute to characteristics of underlying processing mechanisms that give rise to normal development or SLI. One major theory is that the language deficits are secondary to more fundamental auditory perceptual processes that affect nonlinguistic and linguistic stimuli. A related theory is that these children have difficulty in processing rapid or brief stimuli, whether in the auditory or other sensory systems (Tallal, 2004). The results of this processing issue would be most dramatic in speech because within speech, discriminations require perception of multiple and rapidly changing stimuli.

Genetic and environmental factors may also impact neural systems. An expanding set of electrophysiologic, functional neuroimaging, and advanced structural imaging studies of auditory perception and language processing in humans have suggested that two pathways arise from primary auditory cortex: a ventral stream, which is involved in mapping sound onto meaning, and a dorsal stream, which is involved in mapping sound onto articulatory-based representations. The ventral stream projects toward the inferior posterior temporal cortex and ultimately links to widely distributed conceptual representations. The dorsal stream connects posteriorly via the inferior parietal lobe to the frontal lobes, including Broca's area. Each pathway is sensitive to different characteristics of the signal and different modes of processing. Differences in the relative balance of information processing between the two streams or differences in the maturity or health of neural circuitry connecting these regions may explain phenomena of SLI (Vydrova et al., 2015). In adults regions and circuits of the left hemisphere are more important for language processing than homologous regions of the right hemisphere. However, the role of laterality in children with SLI is subject to ongoing debate. Children with SLI generally show gradual improvement over time, although language processing, reading, and writing may remain areas of relative weakness as they age.

Management of Language Disorders

The treatment of language disorders is predicated primarily on the child's language profile and level of communication skill, regardless of etiology. Speech and language pathologists play an essential role in treatment (see Chapter 107) as therapists and consultants to the interdisciplinary team. An initial step in management is to create an optimal language learning environment. A warm, responsive, and nurturing environment is a prerequisite for learning language. Parents can be shown how to expand a child's utterances, slow their own rate of speech, use exaggerated intonation patterns, and articulate their own language clearly.

The overall goal of therapy is to improve functional communication; specific goals may be increasing vocabulary, varying sentence structure, lengthening conversations, or maintaining topics of conversation. Techniques typically involve direct engagement with the child to facilitate learning and assume that children with disorders require a high level of exposure to learn. Modeling and imitation are useful strategies. The speech-language pathologist provides systematic opportunities for the child to use what they are learning frequently in the clinic and in other environments (i.e., classroom, playground, and home) to encourage generalization of new abilities to everyday situations.

The outcome of therapy varies. Children with mild to moderate disorders are more likely to resolve difficulties than children with severe disorders. Metaanalyses find that many interventions are highly successful in improving expressive and receptive language skills (Law, Garrett, & Nye, 2003; Roberts & Kaiser, 2011). Research is necessary to link disorders, methods, and outcomes.

SPEECH SOUND DISORDERS

A speech sound disorder represents impairment in the ability to produce sounds of the words of the language. A primary symptom of speech impairment may be unintelligible speech. Speech disorders are described in terms of the characteristics of the speech sound errors or the cause of the problem. Often an underlying cause for the speech sound disorder cannot be identified.

Articulation Disorders

The inability to produce speech sounds correctly is referred to as an articulation disorder. Children with articulation disorders typically exhibit errors on a small subset of sounds (e.g., */r, l, s/*). In most cases the cause of an articulation disorder is unknown; they are presumed to be the result of mislearning. An articulation error may occur in all contexts (e.g., at the beginning, middle, or end of a word) or in a single position (e.g., at the end of a word). Children with articulation disorders may have mild to moderate deficits, and most of their speech may be intelligible to unfamiliar listeners despite errors. However, articulation disorders can be severe.

One known cause of articulation disorders is permanent bilateral mild to moderate hearing loss. These children may benefit considerably from amplification with hearing aids. They also may benefit from speech therapy to correct inaccurate speech sound productions. Children with severe to profound hearing losses have severe speech sound errors.

Phonologic Disorders

When a child shows speech errors based on patterns or implicit rules despite the ability to produce the same sounds correctly in other contexts, the condition is labeled a phonologic disorder. The child says "pi" for *pig*, despite being able to say "go" or "tuh" for *tub*, although capable of pronouncing "bee." These are examples of final consonant deletion. The child is applying an incorrect rule (e.g., it is permissible to drop the last sound of a word) rather than showing an inability to produce the sound correctly. When asked to imitate nonsense syllables (e.g., "mib," "bup"), the child may not use the rule and thereby produce the syllable correctly. When asked to imitate real words (e.g., *mob, beep*), the child applies the rule and, in this case, drops the final consonant. Commonly, children continue to follow a rule that was appropriate at an earlier time. However, they may produce errors atypical within normal development (e.g., deletion of initial consonants). Children with phonologic errors typically have moderate to severe deficits in speech skills. Research has suggested that children with phonologic disorders need 21 to 42 sessions to advance from being understood by unfamiliar listeners less than 50% of the time to being understood 75% of the time (Campbell, 1999).

Anatomic Disorders

Ankyloglossia, or tongue tie, is a common congenital anomaly that has been assumed to affect speech. However, ankyloglossia does not typically cause speech impairment. While tongue tie may be significant at birth, its severity decreases over time as oral structures grow. Moreover, speech sounds can be produced with minimal tongue elevation. Cutting the tongue frenulum typically does not improve speech. An exception may be children with cerebral palsy whose ankyloglossia is related to neurologic impairments.

Children with cleft palate are at high risk for phonologic disorders and language deficits. Even after repair of an isolated cleft palate, they may exhibit unusual or idiosyncratic patterns of articulation. Velopharyngeal structures function abnormally, resulting in an inability to generate adequate intraoral air pressure for the production of consonants. They may produce consonants made in the back of the mouth (e.g., */k, g, u/*) or use consonants that do not appear in English (e.g., pharyngeal fricatives and nasal snorts).

Some children have isolated velopharyngeal insufficiency for unknown reasons. These children are at risk for speech sound disorders similar to those of children with cleft palate. The velum is supported in early childhood by the adenoids.

As the adenoids shrink with age, the speech disorder may become more severe. Velopharyngeal insufficiency is not amenable to the usual articulation therapy and may require surgical correction. Adenoidectomy might exacerbate speech problems in children with velopharyngeal insufficiency. For that reason, otolaryngologists should attempt to evaluate the velum before adenoidectomy.

Neurologic Disorders

Dysarthria is a speech disorder associated with neuromotor disorders, such as cerebral palsy. High muscle tone, poor coordination of motor movements, and poor coordination of respiration and sound production result in slow muscular movements and limited range of motion. Dysarthric speech has a slurred and strained quality, affecting accuracy of speech sound production, rate, pitch, and intonation. Speech therapy for such children can help them to slow the pace of speaking, improve respiratory control for phrase production, and improve their intelligibility. If speech intelligibility is severely compromised despite intact language, an assistive or augmentative communication device, such as a picture exchange system or a computer, may improve functional communication.

Childhood apraxia of speech, known previously as developmental verbal apraxia or dyspraxia, is a condition in which children have difficulty with the controlled production of speech sounds. The presumed etiology is neurologic in origin, although anatomic lesions are not usually found. Delay in expressive language is an early but nondiagnostic finding. As expressive language emerges, speech may consist of primarily vowel sequences, with few consonants, even in babbling. Children make errors in producing vowels and consonants and show enormous variability in how they produce phonemes and in loudness. The inconsistency in production and in errors makes interpretation of their speech very challenging. When they produce a sound correctly in a single word (e.g., /m/ in *mom*), they may not be able to produce the same sound in other words, longer words (e.g., *mama, moon, broom*). Childhood apraxia of speech may be an isolated or may be associated with cognitive, learning, motor, or social-emotional abnormalities.

Intensive levels of treatment are needed to help children with childhood apraxia of speech learn to produce sounds in syllables of increasing complexity. Research has suggested that children with apraxia needed on average 144 to 168 sessions to move from 50% of their speech being understood by unfamiliar listeners to 75% of their speech being understood, fivefold more sessions than needed for a phonologic disorder (Campbell & Dollaghan, 1995). In the initial phases of treatment each phoneme, in increasing levels of complexity, must be taught because the child may have no ability to generalize production of the sound in one syllable to varied syllables. Treatment integrates motor learning, strategies with multimodality input, and language enrichment. However, limited studies are available to guide treatment strategies or frequency (Morgan, Murray, & Liegeois, 2018). Many affected children have residual speech sound errors and exhibit difficulties in comprehension and narrative skills in school-age years.

Stuttering

Dysfluency is a disruption in the flow of speech. Children age 3 to 4 years old frequently show developmental dysfluency, often repeating whole words or phrases, as they try to put complex meanings into long sentences. Fluency in typically developing children improves at age 4. Adults may display dysfluency when trying to explain difficult material or speaking under stress.

Stuttering is the most common cause of significant dysfluency, manifested by repetition of sounds and syllables and prolongation of vowels or consonants made with a continuous airflow (e.g., */s, f/*). Stuttering is often accompanied by inappropriate pauses, repetitive facial expressions, or other behavioral routines (i.e., arm jerks or knee slapping). Approximately 1% of adults stutter. The degree of stuttering varies across individuals, ranging from mild annoyances to severe disruptions of speech. The degree of stuttering also varies within individuals, subsiding in relaxed conversation and flaring on the telephone or during public speaking. Stuttering disorders may cooccur with speech sound disorders or language disorders or both. They also are common in children and adults with developmental disabilities owing to cognitive impairments.

Stuttering is now considered a neurodevelopmental disorder, characterized by atypical development of neural networks involved in speech motor planning and execution. Stuttering runs in families, suggestive of genetic contributions. Differences can be found in multiple neural pathways, comparing adults who do and do not stutter (Kronfeld-Duenias, Civier, Amir, Ezrati-Vinacour, & Ben-Shachar, 2018). A multifactorial dynamic approach may link specific factors to specific neural pathways within individual children who stutter (Smith & Weber, 2017). Stuttering is exacerbated by anxiety, but anxiety is not currently considered a primary cause.

Speech therapy has been shown to improve true stuttering, especially if started early. Therapy can be started in preschool if the child meets criteria for true stutter. If stuttering is accompanied by behavior routines, treatment is indicated as soon as possible. Treatment has several goals: increasing fluency, reducing the negative impacts of speaking difficulties, and improving overall communication. Therapy may also be directed at parents and community to support the child with stuttering.

Voice and Resonance

Voice disorders are abnormalities in the production of vocal tone. They include abnormalities in the volume of the voice (inordinate loudness or softness) and abnormalities of the vibratory quality of the vocal cords (hoarseness, harshness or aphonia, the lack of sound). Voice depends on the vibratory characteristics of the vocal folds, setting the air above the level of the larynx into vibrations. The intonation and stress patterns of conversation and connected discourse require rapid changes in the delicate laryngeal musculature.

TABLE 44.7 **Evaluation of a Preschool Child With Delayed Language or Speech**

Evaluation	Proposed Evaluator(s)	Areas and Techniques of Assessment	Follow-up of Abnormal Findings
Hearing	Audiologist for children <4 yr Physician, SLP, or school nurse conducts hearing screening for children >4 yr	Do not rely on newborn screen OAE and ABR for infants Visual reinforcement, conditioned play, or conventional audiometry for children >1 yr	Audiologist for amplification Genetic evaluation for cause ENT evaluation for structural abnormalities or evaluation for cochlear implants
Developmental status	Primary care clinician Early intervention Psychologist Developmental-behavioral pediatrician	Social skills Cognition/problem-solving/play skills Adaptive skills	Early intervention, special education, and occupational therapy, as indicated
Medical and neurologic issues	Primary care clinician Developmental-behavioral pediatrician Child neurologist Geneticist	Family history General health Growth parameters Dysmorphic features Skin Neurologic examination	Subspecialty follow-up, as indicated Laboratory and neuroimaging evaluations, as indicated Medical intervention for primary issues (e.g., repair of cleft palate) or associated issues (e.g., management of anxiety)
Psychosocial conditions—quality of social interaction; amount of verbal input	All evaluators Social workers	Quality and quantity of verbal input Quality of social interactions, including warmth, responsivity, reciprocity, and safety Quality and type of stressful environmental conditions	Education about importance of verbal input Parent-to-parent support Enrollment in high-quality educational setting Social service, as indicated Child Protective Services, as indicated

ABR, Auditory brainstem response; *ENT*, ear, nose, and throat; *OAE*, otoacoustic emission; *SLP*, speech-language pathologist.

A common voice problem seen in children is due to stress on the laryngeal tissues from excessive screaming and shouting. Loudness can be generated without damage, as in the case of actors or opera singers. In young untrained children the effect may be edema and inflammation of the vocal cords. Over the long term, such vocal abuse can cause polyps, requiring surgical intervention. Referral of a child with a voice disorder to an otolaryngologist can determine the etiology of the disorder and the appropriate course of treatment. Voice therapy can reeducate children to vary their voice patterns to prevent these complications.

Management of Speech Sound Disorders

Speech therapy plays a key role in the management of speech sound disorders (see Chapter 107). Regardless of the nature of the disorder, speech therapy is particularly useful in helping affected children to identify and practice the mature patterns of speech. The ultimate goal is always improvements in functional communication. Children and adults with speech disorders often experience embarrassment and poor self-esteem. Therapy also serves to reduce the negative psychological consequences of the disorder.

Augmentative and alternative communication (AAC) becomes an option for children who cannot master intelligible speech. Augmentative communication supplements oral speech (e.g., sign language, pictures, or a letter board) to make the communication clearer to the listener. Alternative communication offers different modalities as the sole method (e.g., sign language, speech generating devices, applications on mobile electronic devices). Speech generating systems may use a text-based system, requiring the user to know how to read and spell or may use pictures or symbols for users who cannot read. Use of AAC often brings users a sense of independence and increased social engagement. However, it may prove isolating to users if members of the user's social environment are not patient and supportive.

CONCLUSION

Most children acquire mastery of language by age 5 years and speech by age 7 years, though variation is high. Delays at age 2 years represent a risk factor for speech and/or language disorders. Language and speech sound disorders are prevalent and can adversely affect other domains of functioning. Therapy is often useful in improving outcomes and increasing functional communication.

Travis, in the opening vignette, warrants a prompt assessment though he is a second-born boy with frequent ear infections. Table 44.7 provides an approach to the assessment of a child with language and speech delays. Therapy is predicated primarily on the level of functioning across domains and the specific diagnosis. Early treatment provides children with the best opportunities for normalization of language and speech. Close monitoring of functional improvement is important to refine management, combat poor self-esteem, and provide alternative communication strategies if verbal language does not develop. Ongoing monitoring can detect complications, such as academic difficulties. Neuroscience and genetics are contributing to the understanding of normal speech and language development and disorders and may bring new assessment procedures or treatment approaches in the future.

REFERENCES

Bates, E., Marchman, V., Thal, D., et al. (1994). Developmental and stylistic variation in the composition of early vocabulary. *Journal of Child Language*, *21*, 85–123.

Campbell, T. F. (1999). Functional treatment outcomes in young children with motor speech disorders. In A. J. Caruso & E. A. Strand (Eds.), *Clinical management of motor speech disorders in children* (pp. 385–396). Thieme.

Campbell, T. F., & Dollaghan, C. A. (1995). Speaking rate, articulatory speed, and linguistic processing in children and adolescents with severe traumatic brain injury. *Journal of Speech, Language and Hearing Research*, *38*, 864–875.

Dollaghan, C. A., Campbell, T. F., Paradise, J. L., et al. (1999). Maternal education and measures of early speech and language. *Journal of Speech, Language and Hearing Research*, *42*, 1432–1443.

Feldman, H. M., Dollaghan, C. A., Campbell, T. F., et al. (2000). Measurement properties of the Macarthur communicative development inventories at ages one and two years. *Child Development*, *71*, 310–322.

Fenson, L., Dale, P. S., Reznick, J. S., et al. (1994). Variability in early communicative development. *Monographs of the Society for Research in Child Development*, *59*, 1–173, discussion 174–185.

Fitzpatrick, E. M., Hamel, C., Stevens, A., Pratt, M., Moher, D., Doucet, S. P., … Na, E. (2016). Sign language and spoken language for children with hearing loss: A systematic review. *Pediatrics*, *137*(1).

Hart, B., & Risley, T. R. (1995). *Meaningful differences in the everyday*. Paul H. Brookes.

Hoff-Ginsburg, E. (1998). The relation of birth order and socioeconomic status to children's language experience and language development. *Applied Psychology*, *19*, 603–629.

Hurt, H., & Betancourt, L. M. (2016). Effect of socioeconomic status disparity on child language and neural outcome: How early is early? *Pediatric Research*, *79*(1), 148–158.

Kennedy, C. R., McCann, D. C., Campbell, M. J., et al. (2006). Language ability after early detection of permanent childhood hearing impairment. *New England Journal of Medicine*, *354*, 2131–2141.

Kronfeld-Duenias, V., Civier, O., Amir, O., Ezrati-Vinacour, R., & Ben-Shachar, M. (2018). White matter pathways in persistent developmental stuttering: Lessons from tractography. *Journal of Fluency Disorders*, *55*, 68–83.

Kuhl, P. K. (2004). Early language acquisition: Cracking the speech code. *Nature Reviews Neuroscience*, *5*, 831–843.

Lai, C. S., Fisher, S. E., Hurst, J. A., et al. (2001). A forkhead-domain gene is mutated in a severe speech and language disorder. *Nature*, *413*, 519–523.

Law, J., Garrett, Z., & Nye, C. (2003). Speech and language therapy interventions for children with primary speech and language delay or disorder. *Cochrane Database of Systematic Reviews*, *3*, CD004110.

Levine, S. C., Beharelle, A. R., Demir, Ö. E., & Small, S. L. (2016). Perinatal focal brain injury: Scope and limits of plasticity for language functions. In: *Neurobiology of language* (pp. 969–983). Academic Press.

Morgan, A. T., Murray, E., & Liegeois, F. J. (2018). Interventions for childhood apraxia of speech. *Cochrane Database of Systematic Reviews*, 5.

Papsin, B. C., & Gordon, K. A. (2007). Cochlear implants for children with severe-to-profound hearing loss. *New England Journal of Medicine*, *357*(23), 2380–2387.

Paradise, J. L., Feldman, H. M., Campbell, T. F., Dollaghan, C. A., Rockette, H. E., Pitcairn, D. L., … Pelham, W. E., Jr (2007). Tympanostomy tubes and developmental outcomes at 9 to 11 years of age. *New England Journal of Medicine*, *356*(3), 248–261. PMID: 17229952.

Pearson, B. Z., Fernandez, S. C., & Oller, D. K. (1993). Lexical development in bilingual infants and toddlers: Comparison to monolingual norms. *Language Learning*, *43*, 93–120.

Ramírez, N. F., Lytle, S. R., & Kuhl, P. K. (2020). Parent coaching increases conversational turns and advances infant language development. *Proceedings of the National Academy of Sciences*, *117*(7), 3484–3491.

Rice, M. L., Taylor, C. L., Zubrick, S. R., Hoffman, L., & Earnest, K. K. (2020). Heritability of specific language impairment and nonspecific language impairment at ages 4 and 6 years across phenotypes of speech, language, and nonverbal cognition. *Journal of Speech, Language, and Hearing Research*, *63*(3), 793–813.

Roberts, M. Y., & Kaiser, A. P. (2011). The effectiveness of parent-implemented language interventions: A meta-analysis. *American Journal of Speech-Language Pathology*, *20*(3), 180–199.

Saffran, J. R., Johnson, E. K., Aslin, R. N., & Newport, E. L. (1999). Statistical learning of tone sequences by human infants and adults. *Cognition*, *70*, 27–52.

Smith, A., & Weber, C. (2017). How stuttering develops: The multifactorial dynamic pathways theory. *Journal of Speech, Language, and Hearing Research*, *60*(9), 2483–2505.

Tallal, P. (2004). Improving language and literacy is a matter of time. *Nature Reviews Neuroscience*, *5*, 721–728.

Tomblin, J. B., Harrison, M., Ambrose, S. E., Walker, E. A., Oleson, J. J., & Moeller, M. P. (2015). Language outcomes in young children with mild to severe hearing loss. *Ear and Hearing*, *36*(1), 76S.

Tomblin, J. B., Records, N. L., Buckwalter, P., et al. (1997). Prevalence of specific language impairment in kindergarten children. *Journal of Speech, Language and Hearing Research*, *40*, 1245–1260.

Vydrova, R., Komarek, V., Sanda, J., Sterbova, K., Jahodova, A., Maulisova, A., … Kyncl, M. (2015). Structural alterations of the language connectome in children with specific language impairment. *Brain and Language*, *151*, 35–41.

Windsor, J., Benigno, J. P., Wing, C. A., Carroll, P. J., Koga, S. F., Nelson, C. A., III, … Zeanah, C. H. (2011). Effect of foster care on young children's language learning. *Child Development*, *82*(4), 1040–1046.

45

Sensory Processing Disorders

Karen Ratliff-Schaub and Sara O'Rourke

For additional material related to the content of the chapter, please see Chapters 41, 80, and 106.

VIGNETTE

Mornings tend to be stressful for the Towson family. Although 4-year-old Bethany is often the first to awaken, getting dressed tends to be a battle because she prefers to stay in her soft nightgown and refuses to don her preschool clothes, which feel "scratchy." Despite her mother using softeners to make new clothes more acceptable to her, Bethany has a dresser full of clothes that she refuses to wear. She does not wear socks with seams; clothes that are stiff, textured, or rough; or shirts with tags. She refuses to wear clothes washed in "smelly" (fragrant) detergent. Breakfast also is a struggle because Bethany rejects the foods that the other family members enjoy. She prefers totally bland and soft foods, stating that other foods "do not feel right" or "smell yucky." Although Bethany's parents do their best to accommodate her pickiness, she often arrives late at school, hungry, and wearing her outfit from the previous day.

Sensory processing disorder (SPD), sometimes termed sensory integration dysfunction or sensory integrative problems, refers to children with problems in somatosensory and vestibular system processing and integration. Children with SPD also may have secondary problems in visual perception or auditory processing without impairment of hearing or visual acuity. Because SPD cannot be directly observed, the condition is identified through atypical behavioral patterns or performance deficits. This chapter focuses on children whose difficulty with sensory processing causes behavioral or performance problems that limit or disrupt participation in everyday life activities or school performance.

TYPES OF SENSORY PROCESSING DISORDER

Sensory processing problems can be categorized into three groups: (1) sensory modulation disorders (SMDs), (2) sensory-based motor disorders (SBMD), and (3) sensory discrimination disorders (SDDs) (Miller et al., 2007). Prevalence estimates vary from 5% to 16% in typically developing children and 30% to 80% in children with specific diagnoses (Pfeiffer et al., 2018a). One study suggests that Black children were 2.5 to 3 times more likely than White children to meet criteria for SMD, although environmental factors, stressors, toxins, and poverty may play a role (Reynolds et al., 2008). Because SPD is conceptualized as a continuum from severe (i.e., causing serious behavioral or performance dysfunction) to mild (i.e., causing behavioral quirks or minor difficulty in everyday life), published estimates should be viewed with caution. Many children with mild symptoms are not diagnosed, which clouds our understanding of prevalence. The different categories of SPD are described with examples in the following sections.

Sensory Modulation Disorder

Sensory modulation refers to the ability to regulate the degree, intensity, and nature of responses to sensory input. This basic physiologic ability allows individuals to respond appropriately and adaptively to the sensory experiences of everyday life. Ability to modulate falls on a continuum of overresponsiveness (hypersensitivity) to underresponsiveness (hyposensitivity), with most individuals functioning in a midrange. In children with SMD their sensitivity is beyond the normal range such that they have difficulty adapting to the sensations of everyday activities. Most children with SMD are overreactive, underreactive, or both to more than one sensory modality (e.g., smells, sounds, and touch). These children have difficulty modulating, organizing, or making meaning of sensory input. As a result, sensory input, which typically produces pleasure in children, is experienced as aversive, uncomfortable, or even painful.

Overresponsiveness is generally heightened when the child is tired, when the input is unexpected, or when stimulation is repeated. Children with SMD who are overreactive may show difficulty with common everyday experiences. Dunn (2001) characterized these children as overaroused. The overaroused child tends to become quickly disorganized and anxious and has difficulty calming and reorganizing. Because the hypersensitive child is motivated to avoid sensory input, the child may resist transitions, have a temper tantrum in the grocery store, refuse to dress or brush teeth, or refuse to eat certain foods. Bethany described in the chapter-opening vignette demonstrates many characteristics of sensory hypersensitivity. When possible, providing opportunities for a child like Bethany to remove herself from the overstimulating environment or tasks may help her to calm and reorganize.

Understanding of the causes of sensory overresponsiveness is still emerging. There is evidence that tactile and auditory overresponsiveness are heritable (Keuler et al., 2011). There are studies of patterns of behavior of sensory modulation and their relationship with physiologic measures that have found differences in sympathetic reactivity to activity, sound, and engagement (Chang et al., 2012; Reynolds et al., 2015).

Children who are underresponsive need more intense sensory stimulation to show an adaptive response. They may appear either (1) lethargic and unresponsive or (2) hyperactive and sensory seeking. The lethargic and unresponsive child is passive, sedentary, difficult to engage, and needs intensive support to participate in activities (Parham & Mailloux, 2005). These children typically go undetected in infancy or toddlerhood, labeled as a "good baby" because they demand little from their caregiver.

Sensory-seeking children are very active and crave intensive sensory experiences to maintain arousal. These children may run into others, stomp instead of walk, chew on inedible objects, purposely fall, play overly rough, or frequently rock. Their behaviors can be disruptive or inappropriate in social situations. In extreme cases safety is a concern. If unstructured, additional sensory input may result in even more unorganized behavior. However, specific, goal-orientated and directed types of sensory input can have an organizing effect (Miller et al., 2007). Atypical behavioral responses to sensory input can negatively impact participation in daily activities. Table 45.1 outlines some of the potential impacts of sensory modulation dysfunction.

Sensory-Based Motor Disorders

SBMDs can be categorized as (1) vestibular-based postural disorders (children with balance and postural deficits) and (2) dyspraxia (children with motor planning problems). Both groups of children may exhibit discrimination deficits in perception of vestibular, proprioceptive, and tactile input such that feedback from movement and touch is less accurately interpreted. With limited perception of somatosensory feedback, manipulating objects or moving through the environment becomes slower and less precise. Sensory memories of movements are less reliable when the same or a similar task is presented to the child, slowing development of skill. In vestibular-based postural disorders children show balance problems and postural instability. They often exhibit bilateral coordination delays and ocular motor deficits. In dyspraxia children exhibit motor planning problems with delays in skillful movement and learning of multistep complex movements.

Vestibular-Based Postural Disorders

A child with vestibular-based postural disorder tends to have poor awareness of where their own body is in space. The child has difficulty when asked to perform a dynamic balancing task (e.g., walking heel to toe or walking on a line). With immature balance mechanisms, the child's movements appear awkward or rigid. Reciprocal and coordinated movements of arms and legs may be delayed or impaired (e.g., a 6-year-old child not able to perform jumping jacks or a hop-skip-jump sequence). The child may be fearful on unstable surfaces or high surfaces or be hesitant and slow when descending stairs. The child often overuses the visual system to compensate for lack of specific information from the vestibular-proprioceptive systems. Some children with postural disorders may avoid movement. Postural disorders are differentiated from avoidance of movement (overresponsivity) by observing if the child is unstable/fearful in challenging positions (postures) or has an adverse response to movement (overresponsive) (Miller-Kuhaneck et al., 2006).

Dyspraxia

Children with dyspraxia or motor planning problems generally have concurrent deficits in somatosensory discrimination.

TABLE 45.1 Problems for Children With Sensory Modulation Disorder

Issue	Behavior	Impact
Limited sensory registration	• Does not notice touch, pain, movement, smell, sights, sounds • May not notice physical injury • Potential for self-injury	• Limited participation due to lack of awareness of people, objects, and sensations
Tactile defensiveness	• Discomfort or irritation with light touch, physical proximity to people • Anxiety, anger, aggression, distress, and fear response to stimuli	• Stress and anxiety during daily routines • Limited participation in activities such as dressing and grooming
Gravitational insecurity	• Aversive response to movement, being on unstable surface • Fear of common movements such as tilting head backward • Fear of even slight heights	• Reluctance to explore environment • Passive, sedentary • Limited participation in games with peers, refusal to ascend stairs, distress being lifted into car
Auditory/visual/olfactory and gustatory defensiveness	• Avoids certain tastes, smells, bright lights, loud sounds	• Mealtimes may be limited by smells/tastes of food • Limited participation in cafeteria and community events (birthday parties, fairs)

Adapted from O'Brien, J. C., & Kuhaneck, H. (Eds.). (2020). *Case-Smith's occupational therapy for children and adolescents* (8th ed., Table 20.1). Mosby/Elsevier.

A child with dyspraxia has difficulty recognizing shapes or textures by touch and manipulation alone and seems to receive less accurate feedback from fine movements. The child generally has average range intelligence and achieves motor milestones at typical ages; however, skilled manipulation and complex multistep movements are limited, and achievement of activities of daily living, such as dressing, buttoning, and shoe tying, is delayed. Teachers often note that the child's drawing and writing are immature.

Children with dyspraxia have been shown to be more introverted and to have fewer social interactions in environments where motor skill is the focus of interaction (e.g., on the playground) (Smyth & Anderson, 2000); however, others have found that some of these children are highly creative and verbal, preferring fantasy games to reality (Miller, 2007). Table 45.2 lists secondary issues associated with SBMDs.

Sensory Discrimination Disorder

SDD is characterized by difficulty interpreting the qualities of sensory input with difficulty perceiving similarities and differences. For example, a child may not be able to distinguish the shape of an object through touch alone (Miller et al., 2007; O'Brien & Kuhaneck, 2020). SDD can be observed in only one system (e.g., a visual discrimination disorder but good discrimination in all other sensory systems; Miller, 2007). Children with sensory modulation difficulties may also show difficulties with discrimination. For example, defensive reactions may make it challenging to attend to the details of some stimuli and impede perception (O'Brien & Kuhaneck, 2020). Table 45.3 provides more descriptions of sensory discrimination issues and their impact on participation.

ASSESSMENT

Evidence that SPD has an impact on a child's performance or behavior problems can be extracted from a detailed history and parent interview. Referral to an occupational therapist (see Chapter 106) for detailed assessment of occupational performance can confirm the diagnosis. Table 45.4 lists commonly used assessment tools and a variety of neurologic soft signs that may be evident on examination.

History

The parent's history of the child's birth and developmental milestones often reveals an unremarkable birth and typical achievement of motor milestones in the first years of life. The parents of children with SMD may describe them as difficult, irritable, and anxious infants, and defiant, stubborn, or rigid toddlers. Sleeping and eating problems are common. When asked about antecedent factors, patterns emerge suggesting that the child's behaviors are associated with specific sensory experiences. Conversely, parents of children with SMD may describe a passive child who seems reluctant to try new activities and who struggles to learn new skills.

Some children become less reactive to various sensations as they mature; however, their negative and defiant behaviors may persist when these are reinforced by adult attention or parents' emotional responses. The interview may reveal that sensory processing problems in infants become behavioral problems in preschoolers that are self-sustaining because of the reactions from others (see Chapter 93).

INTERVENTION

Occupational therapists are typically the professionals who focus on the treatment of SPD. Services are directed to the child, the family, and other adults who teach or care for the child. A priority goal of intervention is to improve the child's adaptive and organized responses to sensory input (McIntosh et al., 1999). Equally important goals are to help the child learn to compensate for SPD, to help parents understand and reframe the problem, and to modify the child's environments

TABLE 45.2 Problems for Children With Sensory-Based Motor Disorders

Issue	Behavior	Impact
Vestibular-postural disorder	• Poor balance • Postural instability • "Floppy" movement • Slouched posture • Frequent tripping or falling • Hesitancy when leaning or reaching	• Delays in bilateral coordination • Difficulty pedaling a bike or tying shoes • Difficulty participating in activities such as sports, dance, or play • Loses place when copying from board, with impact on academic performance
Dyspraxia	• Poor motor planning with novel tasks • Decreased bilateral coordination and sequenced actions • Lack of ideas of new ways to use a toy • Imitates rather than initiating something new • Poor handwriting • Delays in activities of daily living • Difficulty with complex motor actions • Difficulty performing action sequence	• Resistant to attempting novel tasks • Poor skills in ball play, jumping rope, other sports, or games • Limited participation in sports • Poor self-esteem associated with repeated failure (Miller et al., 2007) • Grades suffer due to poor handwriting, trouble keeping up with work

Adapted from O'Brien, J. C., & Kuhaneck, H. (Eds.). (2020). *Case-Smith's occupational therapy for children and adolescents* (8th ed., Table 20.3). Mosby/Elsevier.

TABLE 45.3 Problems for Children With Sensory Discrimination Disorder

Issue	Behavior	Impact
Tactile	• Difficulty localizing touch • Difficulty with stereognosis • Visual perception and motor planning problems	• Struggles with activities requiring precise hand movements • Difficulty using spoon, controlling pencil, or doing fasteners • Fine motor tasks more stressful because require visual guidance
Proprioceptive	• Appears clumsy/awkward • Relies on movement to guide movement • May seek excessive input (pushing, pulling, throwing, jumping) • Breaking toys, bumping into others, poor sense of personal space	• Decreased participation with peers because behavior seen as deliberately disruptive • Decreased participation in movement or sports-related activities
Visual	• May affect grasp and balance • Difficulty with visual perception/spatial/construction/motor tasks	• Decreased participation in play skills such as puzzles, blocks, crafts • Decreased academic performance due to difficulty with handwriting, construction projects
Auditory	• Unable to locate origin of a sound • Difficulty following directions • Difficulty with conversation • Decreased focus on words when there is background noise	• Decreased social play • Difficulty understanding spoken directions and cues leading to decreased participation in activities

Adapted from O'Brien, J. C., & Kuhaneck, H. (Eds.). (2020). ***Case-Smith's occupational therapy for children and adolescents*** (8th ed., Table 20.2). Mosby/Elsevier.

TABLE 45.4 Evaluations to Identify and Analyze Sensory Processing Problems

Evaluation Method	Diagnostic Tests/Scales
Standardized assessments	• Sensory Integration and Practice Tests (SIPT) (Ayres, 1989) • Bruininks Oseretsky Test of Motor Proficiency (2nd ed.) (BOT-2) (Bruininks & Bruininks, 2006) • Motor Assessment Battery for Children (MABC) (Henderson & Sudgen, 1992) • The Evaluation in Ayres Sensory Integration (EASI) (Mailloux et al., 2018)
Parent/caregiver report or questionnaires	• Sensory Profile (Dunn, 1999) • Sensory Processing Measure (Parham et al., 2007)
Teacher report	• Sensory Processing Measure Main Classroom Form (Miller-Kuhaneck et al., 2006)
Neurologic soft signs	• Running/walking gait • Skipping, hopping • Standing on one foot • Stressed walking • Right-left discrimination • Hand/foot/eye dominance • Synkinesia (abnormal mirror movements/overflow of finger movements) • Diadochokinesia (ability to perform rapid alternating movements, such as rapid pronation/supination)

and routines to improve overall performance. The intervention plan should consider the child's multiple environments (e.g., home and school) and should emphasize caregivers' understanding of the problem such that they learn to accommodate the child's sensory needs (Bundy & Koomar, 2001). Children with significant SPD may receive occupational therapy services at school and in a clinic. Generally these services complement each other.

In 2018 the American Occupational Therapy Association (AOTA, 2018) recommended occupational therapy practitioners avoid using sensory interventions with their clients unless there is a specific assessment of sensory function completed that indicates sensory integration/processing difficulties. Interventions should link directly to assessment results and focus on Ayres Sensory Integration (ASI; see later), sensory-based strategies and environmental changes, cognitive and occupation-based interventions, and parent-teacher education and coaching (Miller-Kuhaneck & Watling, 2018).

The ASI intervention is designed to help a child gain skills and confidence in performing everyday activities in multiple environments by presenting individualized challenges that improve sensory integration capacities (O'Brien & Kuhaneck, 2020). Sensory environmental modifications apply sensory stimuli as the intervention, which may include a weighted vest, deep pressure, changing the texture of clothing, and the brightness of lights among others (Bodison & Parham, 2018). These techniques can sometimes be used throughout the day to create a sensory diet. This diet helps the child's arousal and organization throughout the day and generally includes activities that provide deep pressure, heavy work, linear vestibular input, and sometimes rhythmic movement such as bouncing. The goals of these activities vary with the child's symptoms and may include increasing arousal, calming, helping organize, increasing attentiveness or alertness, and decreasing activity level (Koomar & Bundy, 2002). Sensory diets should be closely monitored and modified over time; they should fit easily into the family's daily routine.

Occupational therapy–based interventions include the use of daily activities to improve participation, quality of life and wellbeing, with cognitive interventions focused on teaching processing strategies to improve self-regulation and achieve successful performance (Pfeiffer et al., 2018a). Parent or teacher education and coaching interventions empower parents and teachers to design their own solutions to meet the child's needs through a collaborative process with the therapist (Miller-Kuhaneck & Watling, 2018). Resources for parents are provided in Box 45.1.

OUTCOMES OF SENSORY INTEGRATION INTERVENTION

The effectiveness of sensory-based intervention across various domains has been demonstrated (Miller-Kuhaneck & Watling, 2018). There is strong evidence that ASI intervention demonstrates positive outcomes in improving individualized goals of functioning and participation among children with autism spectrum disorder. There is moderate evidence

BOX 45.1 Resources for Parents

Biel, L., & Peske, N. (2004). *Raising a sensory smart child: The definitive handbook for helping your child with sensory integration issues.* Penguin Books.

Kranowitz, C. S. (2004). *The goodenoughs get in sync.* Sensory Resources.

Kranowitz, C. S. (2005). *The out-of-sync child: Recognizing and coping with sensory integration dysfunction.* Penguin Group.

Miller, L. J. (2006). *Sensational kids: Hope and help for children with sensory processing disorder.* Penguin Group.

The Star Institute. https://www.spdstar.org/.

Data from https://sensoryhealth.org/basic/books-products-and-online-tools

supporting improvements in autistic behaviors and skills-based outcomes, reducing caregiver assistance with self-care activities (Schaaf et al., 2018), and moderate support for specific types of cognitive- and occupation-based interventions to support self-regulation (Pfeiffer et al., 2018a). Miller-Kuhaneck and Watling (2018) found that it is likely that parent training and coaching will be an effective method for improving specific child and parent outcomes, and that parents can be trained to provide specific interventions with fidelity. While outcomes vary, research on the effectiveness of interventions that address problems with integrating and processing sensory input is improving in rigor and quality (Pfeiffer et al., 2018b).

In two qualitative studies (Cohn, 2001a, 2001b) parents whose children received sensory integration intervention expressed that their children's participation in a range of activities had increased, and the child's perception of self-worth seemed to improve. Equally important outcomes for parents were (1) increased understanding of their children, (2) increased ability to establish expectations for their children, (3) validation of their parenting experiences, and (4) learning strategies for supporting and advocating for their children.

CONCLUSION

Children with SPD present with a range of behavioral presentations and participation consequences. Identification requires history and examination, and when suspected SPD should be confirmed by standardized sensory-motor-perceptual scales administered by an occupational therapist. Essential elements of intervention include psychoeducation of family members, modifications of the child's environment and routines, accommodations to meet the child's sensory processing needs, and teaching the child methods to maintain optimal levels of arousal, attentiveness, organized behavior, and skillful performance. For Bethany described at the beginning of this chapter, the intervention would likely include sensory environmental modifications within her morning routine, and cognitive- and occupational therapy–based interventions to improve her self-regulation when encountering a noxious stimuli within an activity such as dressing or eating. Parent education and coaching would be utilized so that her family could understand and meet Bethany's needs, as well as generalize strategies learned in therapy to new challenges

REFERENCES

American Occupational Therapy Association (AOTA). (2018). Five things patients and providers should question. https://www.choosingwisely.org/societies/american-occupational-therapy-association-inc/.

Ayres. J. (1989). *Sensory integration and praxis tests.* Western Psychological Services

Bodison, S. C., & Parham, L. D. (2018). Specific sensory techniques and sensory environmental modifications for children and youth with sensory integration difficulties: A systematic review. *American Journal of Occupational Therapy, 72,* 7201190040. https://doi.org/10.5014/ajot.2018.029413.

Bruininks, R., & Bruininks, B. (2006). *Bruninks Oseretsky Test of Motor Proficiency* (2nd ed.). AGS Publishing.

Bundy, A., & Koomar, J. A. (2001). Orchestrating intervention: The art of practice. In A. C. Bundy, S. J. Lane, & E. A. Murray (Eds.), *Sensory integration: Theory and practice* (2nd ed., pp. 242–259). FA Davis.

Chang, M. C., Parham, L. D., Blanche, E. I., Schell, A., Chou, C. P., Dawson, M., & Cark, F. (2012). Autonomic and behavioral responses of children with autism to auditory stimuli. *American Journal of Occupational Therapy, 66*, 567–576. https://doi.org/10.5014/ajot.2012.004242.

Cohn. E. S. (2001a). From waiting to relating: Parents' experiences in the waiting room of an occupational therapy clinic. *American Journal of Occupational Therapy, 55*, 167–174.

Cohn. E. S. (2001b). Parent perspectives of occupational therapy using a sensory integration approach. *American Journal of Occupational Therapy, 55*, 285–294.

Dunn. W. (1999). *The sensory profile: Examiner's manual.* The Psychological Corporation.

Dunn. W. (2001). The sensations of everyday life: Empirical, theoretical, and pragmatic consideration. *American Journal of Occupational Therapy, 44*, 608–620.

Henderson, S. E., & Sugden, D. A. (1992). *Movement assessment battery for children manual.* Psychological Corporation.

Keuler, M. M., Schmidt, N. L., Van Hulle, C. A., Lemery-Chalfant, K., & Goldsmith, H. H. (2011). Sensory overresponsivity: Prenatal risk factors and temperamental contributions. *Journal of Developmental and Behavioral Pediatrics, 32*(7), 533–541. https://doi.org/10.1097/DBP.0b013e3182245c05.

Koomar, J. A., & Bundy, A. C. (2002). Creating direct intervention from theory. In A. C. Bundy, S. J. Lane, & E. A. Murray (Eds.), *Sensory integration: Theory and practice* (2nd ed., pp. 261–308). FA Davis.

Mailloux, Z., Parham, D., Smith Roley, S., Ruzzano, L., & Schaaf, R. (2018). Introduction to the Evaluation in Ayres Sensory Integration® (EASI). *American Journal of Occupational Therapy, 72*(1), 7201195030p1–7201195030p7. https://doi.org/10.5014/ajot.2018.028241.

McIntosh, D., Miller, L. J., Shyu, V., & Hagerman, R. (1999). Sensory modulation disruption, electrodermal responses, and functional behaviors. *Developmental Medicine and Child Neurology, 41*, 608–615.

Miller. L. J. (2006). *Sensational kids: Hope and help for children with sensory processing disorder.* Penguin Group.

Miller, L. J., Anzalone, M. E., Lane, S. J., Cermak, S. A., & Osten, E. T. (2007). Concept evolution in sensory integration: A proposed nosology for diagnosis. *American Journal of Occupational Therapy, 61*(2), 135–140.

Miller-Kuhaneck, H., & Watling, R. (2018). Parental or teacher education and coaching to support function and participation of children and youth with sensory processing and sensory integration challenges: A systematic review. *American Journal of Occupational Therapy, 72*, 7201190030p1-7201190030p11. https://doi.org/10.5014/ajot.2018.029017.

Miller-Kuhaneck, H., Henry, D. A., & Glennon, T. J. (2006). *Sensory processing measure main classroom form.* Western Psychological Services.

O'Brien, J. C., & Kuhaneck, H. (Eds.). (2020). *Case-Smith's occupational therapy for children and adolescents* (8th ed.). Mosby/Elsevier.

Parham, L. D., & Mailloux, Z. (2005). Sensory integration. In J. Case-Smith (Ed.), *Occupational therapy for children.* Mosby.

Parham, L. D., Ecker, C., Miller-Kuhaneck, H., Henry, D. A., Glennon, T. J. (2007). *Sensory Processing Measure Manual.* Western Psychological Services.

Pfeiffer, B., Frolek Clark, G., & Arbesman, M. (2018a). Effectiveness of cognitive and occupation-based interventions for children with challenges in sensory processing and integration: A systematic review. *American Journal of Occupational Therapy, 72*, 7201190020. https://doi.org/10.5014/ajot.2018.028233.

Pfeiffer, B., May-Benson, T. A., & Bodison, S. C. (2018b). Guest editorial—State of the science of sensory integration research with children and youth. *American Journal of Occupational Therapy, 72*, 7201170010. https://doi.org/10.5014/ajot.2018.721003.

Reynolds, S., Costanza, S., Odom, M., Lane, S., Meeley, L., Owen, A., Pepe, G., Chinn, M., Davis, D., & Wilson, L. (2015). Effect of engagement in sensory-based tasks on autonomic nervous system activity and attention. *American Journal of Occupational Therapy, 69*(Suppl 1), W6911520072. https://doi.org/10.5014/ajot.2015.69S1-RP101B.

Reynolds, S., Shepherd, J., & Lane, S. (2008). Sensory modulation disorders in a minority Head Start population: Preliminary prevalence and characterization. *Journal of Occupational Therapy, Schools, & Early Intervention, 1*(3–4), 186–198. https://doi.org/10.1080/19411240802589031.

Schaaf, R. C., Dumont, R. L., Arbesman, M., & May-Benson, T. A. (2018). Efficacy of occupational therapy using Ayres Sensory Integration: A systematic review. *American Journal of Occupational Therapy, 72*, 7201190010. https://doi.org/10.5014/ajot.2018.028431.

Smyth, M. M., & Anderson, H. I. (2000). Coping with clumsiness in the school playground: Social and physical play in children with coordination impairments. *British Journal of Developmental Psychology, 18*, 389–413.

46

Attention-Deficit/Hyperactivity Disorder (ADHD)

William J. Barbaresi and Jason M. Fogler

For additional material related to the content of this chapter, please see Chapters 47, 86, 93, 99, and 114.

VIGNETTE

When David was 3.5 years old his parents noted that he was the one child in preschool who could never stay in the circle during an activity. This behavior persisted through kindergarten and first grade, but his teachers and paternal grandparents reassured his parents that "he is a boy and will grow out of it. Dad and his brother were the exact same way as children, and they turned out fine." When David still had trouble staying at the dinner table and his desk in second grade and was sanctioned for "not listening" at every extracurricular activity he attended, his parents brought him to his pediatrician for evaluation. He was prescribed stimulant medication, which helped him to sit still and focus in school but did not improve his study habits, organizational skills, or emotional reactivity. In middle school, he reacted aggressively to bullies and was suspended for fighting. Now at age 16, David has a recurring problem with forgetting to turn in his homework assignments; he is in danger of failing this semester and is dreading midterms. He skips classes to vape with his peers and gets angry when friends and family ask him where he is thinking of applying for college. David can play videogames or sculpt for hours but cannot sustain his attention to read more than a paragraph for school. He wants to drive but has been dragging his heels on taking the permit test, and his parents secretly worry that he will get into an accident due to distracted driving.

WHAT IS ADHD?

ADHD is often mistakenly described as a constellation of annoying, typical childhood behaviors that have been medicalized, leading to unnecessary psychopharmacologic treatment. However, decades of research have clearly demonstrated that ADHD is a common, chronic, neurodevelopmental disorder that is often accompanied by other mental health and neurodevelopmental conditions and is associated with impairment and adverse long-term outcomes in virtually all key functional domains, including educational, vocational, interpersonal, and health (Harstad, Katusic, Sideridis, Weaver, Voigt, & Barbaresi, 2020). This chapter is therefore informed by a life-course perspective with a focus on information required to support diagnostic and treatment approaches aimed not at simple reduction in core ADHD symptoms of inattention, hyperactivity, and impulsivity but at improving short- and long-term function for affected children, adolescents, and ultimately adults.

The prevalence of ADHD among US children ages 2 to 17 years based on parent-reported diagnosis is 8.4% (Danielson et al., 2016), with prevalence more than twice as high among boys versus girls. Population-based estimates of the cumulative incidence of ADHD through age 19 are 7.5% to 9.4% (Barbaresi, Colligan, Weaver, Voigt, Killian, & Katusic, 2002). Children with higher IQs are just as likely as those with average IQ to have ADHD (Katusic, Voigt, Colligan, Weaver, & Barbaresi, 2011), whereas those with IQ in the borderline to mild intellectual disability range are up to six times more likely to also have ADHD (Voigt, Barbaresi, Colligan, Weaver, & Katusic, 2006). The recently published Society for Developmental and Behavioral Pediatrics (SDBP) practice guideline focused on complex ADHD, defined in part by the presence of coexisting conditions (Barbaresi et al., 2020). From an epidemiologic perspective, coexisting neurodevelopmental and mental health conditions are the rule, rather than the exception, in children and adolescents with ADHD. Specific learning disabilities in reading, writing, and math (see Chapter 47) occur in approximately one-half to two-thirds of children and adolescents with ADHD, while coexisting mental health disorders also occur in one-half to two-thirds. ADHD may cooccur with autism spectrum disorder, as well as with genetic disorders such as Down syndrome. Of particular concern is the significant increase in risk for the development of substance use disorders, with rates approximately six times greater than adolescents without ADHD (nearly one-quarter of boys, and 10%–15% of girls with ADHD). Rates are highest among boys who do not receive treatment for ADHD. Along with increased risk for use of alcohol, marijuana, and other drugs, adolescents with ADHD also have higher rates of smoking compared to peers without ADHD.

The *Diagnostic and Statistical Manual of Mental Disorders,* fifth edition (*DSM-5*) specifies that a diagnosis of ADHD requires a child to exhibit six of nine symptoms of inattention and/or six of nine symptoms of hyperactivity/

TABLE 46.1 Attention-Deficit/Hyperactivity Disorder

Attention-Deficit/Hyperactivity Disorder

Diagnostic Criteria

A A presistent pattern of inattention and/or hyperactivity-Impulsivity that interferes with functioning or development, as characterized by (1) and/or (2)

1. **Inattention:** Six (or more) of the following symptoms have persisted for at least 6 months to a degree that is inconsistent with developmental level and that negatively impacts directly on social and academic/occupational activities

   Note: The symptoms are not solely a manifestation of oppositional behavior, defiance, hostility, or failure to understand tasks or Instructions For older adolescents and adults (age 17 and older), at least five symptoms are required.

   a Often fails to give close attention to details or makes careless mistakes in schoolwork, at work, or during other activities (e g, overlooks or misses details, work is inaccurate)

   b Often has difficulty sustaining attention in tasks or play activities (e.g, has difficulty remaining focused during lectures, conversations, or lengthy reading)

   c Often does not seem to listen when spoken to directly (e g., mind seems elsewhere, even in the absence of any obvious distraction)

   d Often does not follow through on instructions and fails to finish schoolwork, chores, or duties in the workplace (e g., starts tasks but quickly loses focus and is easily sidetracked)

   e Often has difficulty organizing tasks and activities (e g, difficulty managing sequential tasks, difficulty keeping materials and belongings in order, messy, disorganized work; has poor time management, fails to meet deadlines)

   f Often avoids, dislikes, or is reluctant to engage in tasks that require sustained mental effort (e g, schoolwork or homework, for older adolescents and adults, preparing reports, completing forms, reviewing lengthy papers).

   g Often loses things necessary for tasks or activities (e p., school materials, pencils, books, tools, wallets, keys, paperwork, eyeglasses, mobile telephones)

   h Is often easily distracted by extraneous stimuli (for older adolescents and adults, may include unrelated thoughts)

   i Is often forgetful in daily adtivities (e g, doing chores, running errands, for older adolescents and adults, returning calls, paying bills, keeping appointments)

2. **Hyperactivity and impulsivity:** Six (or more) of the following symptoms have persisted for at least 6 months to a degree that is inconsistent with developmental level and that negatively impacts directly on social and academic/occupational activities
   Note: The symptoms are not solely a manifestation of oppositional behavior, defiance, hostility, or a failure to understand tasks or instructions For older adolescents and adults (age 17 and older), at least five symptoms are required

   a Often fidgets with or taps hands or feet or squirms in seat

   b Often leaves seat in situations when remaining seated is expected (e g, leaves his or her place in the classroom, in the office or other workplace, or in other situations that require remaining in place)

   c Often runs about or climbs in situations where it is inappropriate (**Note:** In adolescents or adults, may be limited to feeling restless)

   d Often unable to play or engage in leisure activities quietly

   e Is often "on the go," acting as if "driven by a motor" (e g, Is unable to be or uncomfortable being still for extended time, as in restaurants, meetings, may be experienced by others as being restless or difficult to keep up with)

   f Often talks excessively

   g Often blurts out an answer before a question has been completed (e g, completes people's sentences; cannot wait for turn in conversation)

   h Often has difficulty waiting his or her turn (e.g, while waiting in line)

   i Often interrupts or intrudes on others (e g, butts into conversations, games, or activities, may start using other people's things without asking or receiving permission, for adolescents and adults, may intrude into or take over what others are doing).

B Several inattentive or hyperactive-impulsive symptoms were present prior to age 12 years.

C Several inattentive or hyperactive-impulsive symptoms are present in two or more settings (e g, at home, school, or work, with friends or relatives, in other activities)

D There is clear evidence that the symptoms interfere with, or reduce the quality of, social, academic, or occupational functioning

E The symptoms do not occur exclusively during the course of schizophrenia or another psychotic disorder and are not better explained by another mental disorder (e g, mood disorder, anxiety disorder, dissociative disorder, personality disorder, substance intoxication or withdrawal)

From American Psychiatric Association. (2013). *Diagnostic and statistical manual of mental disorders* (5th ed.).

impulsivity at a sufficient level to cause functional impairment in two or more settings (Table 46.1); even with significant advances in neuroscience, behavioral genetics, and epidemiology, however, the precise etiology of ADHD has remained somewhat elusive.

Inattention is something of a misnomer in that people with ADHD can easily become distracted and fail to listen to instructions, but some may also hyperfocus on preferred activities and media. Rather than an absolute absence of attention, the inattentive component of ADHD might better be thought of as an attention deployment problem: Interesting topics or activities may have an all-consuming quality, whereas boring activities are either tuned out or experienced as unbearably tedious.

Hyperactivity is perhaps best captured in the symptom of often being on the go, acting as if begin driven by a motor, and may include fidgeting, pacing, restless, bouncing legs, finger tapping and drumming on desks, or incessant humming and singing when quiet is required. Impulsivity can lead to intrusive and dysfunctional social interactions or poor decision making. It can take overtly emotional forms (e.g., overreacting to a minor frustration) or fit under the broad category of bad judgment (i.e., the decisions made without considering their long-term consequences).

The argument is often made that some degree of inattention, hyperactivity, and impulsivity are normal and, by extension, ADHD is not a real disorder. However, this assertion ignores the functional impact of impairing degrees of these symptoms. ADHD is not unlike other medical conditions such as hypertension; blood pressure at a certain level only defines hypertension because that blood pressure is associated with impairment of bodily function (e.g., renal, cardiac). Similarly, ADHD is diagnosed when core symptoms are present to a degree that leads to impairment. Some children have severe neurobiologic deficits that will lead to impairing symptoms of ADHD even in optimal or near optimal environments. Others may have neurobiologic vulnerabilities that may only manifest as impairing symptoms of ADHD in certain environments (e.g., those that demand greater attentional and impulse control, task persistence, and executive function [EF]). This notion is supported by large-scale genetic studies that have found relationships between genetics and the degree of ADHD symptoms (Faraone & Larsson, 2019). The focus of this chapter is on symptoms that cause significant functional impairment in multiple domains, thereby constituting the neurodevelopmental disorder ADHD. Furthermore, our particular focus is on aspects of ADHD that may be of greatest relevance to clinicians who provide subspecialty level care to children and adolescents with complex ADHD as defined in recent practice guidelines (Barbaresi et al., 2020).

UNDERSTANDING ADHD

Historical Perspective

Among the many misconceptions about ADHD is the notion that it is a creation of the late 20th century, an idea that contributes to a failure to understand its neurobiologic basis. A diagnosis of ADHD depends on interpretation of behaviors and their context, as opposed to a biologic marker for the disorder, potentially reinforcing the impression that ADHD is a more subjective perception than biologically based reality. This impression is further reinforced by the many revisions in diagnostic criteria for ADHD over the past 50 years. However, the symptoms and behaviors we currently describe as ADHD have been documented in both medical and nonmedical literature over many centuries: Depictions of inattentive, hyperactive, and impulsive behavior may be found in the writings of Hippocrates and Shakespeare, while colorful descriptions of such behaviors fill stories such as "Slovenly Peter, Straw Peter" and "Fidgety Philip" and "Johnny Look-in-the-air" by early 19th-century German psychiatrist Heinrich Hoffmann (Martinez-Badía & Martinez-Raga, 2015). The earliest medical texts to describe ADHD symptoms include the work of Melchior Adam Weikard and Sir Alexander Crichton, both published in the late 18th century. Weikard's text on mental illness included the chapter "Attention Deficit," and Crichton's 1798 work included the chapter "On Attention and Its Diseases" (Mahone & Denckla, 2017). Nineteenth-century medical writers, including Benjamin Rush and William James, also wrote about disorders of attention and impulse control. It was not, however, until the publication of George F. Still's 1902 lecture, "Some Abnormal Psychical Conditions in Children: The Goulstonian Lectures," that the modern concept of what we now call ADHD is generally considered to have been introduced. Parents are typically surprised to learn of the first published report of stimulant medication's positive effect on ADHD symptoms was in 1937.

The Evolving Understanding of the Fundamental Nature of ADHD

Neurobiology

The past 50 years have been marked by literally thousands of studies that have described the epidemiology, diagnosis, treatment, and outcomes of ADHD. During this same period our understanding of the fundamental neurobiologic, neuropsychological, and genetic basis of ADHD has evolved. Advances in neurobiology and neuropsychology have occurred in parallel and may generally be described as moving from a focus on frontostriatal circuits and response inhibition to a much more complex view of widely distributed, interconnected brain regions and nuanced understanding of EF as well as newer neuropsychological theories (see Chapter 87).

Studies of brain structure and function in persons with ADHD have primarily described findings at the group as opposed to the individual level. Therefore while this research has provided insight into the underlying changes in brain morphology and function associated with ADHD, studies such as magnetic resonance imaging (MRI), functional MRI, positron emission tomography, and electroencephalography do not provide clinically meaningful information about individual persons with ADHD, either with respect to diagnosis or response to treatment. Furthermore, most available studies have used small sample sizes, often producing contradictory findings. Nevertheless, increasingly sophisticated approaches and pooled data from large studies continue to demonstrate that the neurobiology of ADHD is far more complex than was initially believed.

Shaw et al. (2007) compared growth trajectories in the brains of 223 children with ADHD and 223 typically developing (TD) children, reporting a median 3-year delay in the age to attain peak cortical thickness in prefrontal regions in children with ADHD (10.5 years vs. 7.5 years, respectively). This finding has been replicated in adolescent samples (in regard to gyrification; Shaw, Malek, Watson, Sharp, Evans, & Greenstein, 2012); and the term minus 33%, referring to this delay or brain immaturity, is gaining traction in popular media surrounding ADHD (e.g., Barkley, 2014). This finding on the developmental nature of differences in brain volume parallels studies that have clearly demonstrated developmental changes in ADHD symptom profiles. Shaw, Lerch, and Greenstein (2006) suggested that greater reduction in the thickness of medial prefrontal cortex may be associated with a more unfavorable course of ADHD and that treatment with methylphenidate may be associated with a reduction in cortical thinning over time (Shaw, Sharp, & Morrison, 2009). Volumetric studies have demonstrated differences in specific regions beyond the frontal lobe, including the basal ganglia, amygdala, hippocampus, and cerebellum (in particular, the cerebellar vermis).

Recently, large-scale, longitudinal studies have provided additional evidence that differences in intracranial volume and subcortical volumes are found in children but not adolescents or adults with ADHD. A large study found that children with ADHD had lower cortical surface area overall as well as in the frontal, cingulate, and temporal regions (Hoogman, Bralten, & Hibar, 2017). Cortical thickness was reduced among children with ADHD in the fusiform gyrus and temporal pole. Interestingly, these reductions in cortical surface area and thickness were not found in adolescents or adults with ADHD. The same consortium of researchers found that subcortical volumes were also lower in children with ADHD in the accumbens nucleus, amygdala, caudate, hippocampus, and putamen, as well as in overall intracranial volume. As with studies of cortical thickness and surface area, these differences were not seen in adolescents or adults. It has been clearly shown that ADHD symptoms change with increasing age and, in some individuals, symptoms no longer rise to a diagnostic threshold. Thus changes in cortical thickness with age may correlate with, or possibly help to explain, these behavioral changes.

Neurophysiology

Advances in neuroimaging have permitted studies of brain activation both in the resting state and while subjects are asked to perform tasks that require attention or inhibition. Findings from these studies, consistent with morphologic studies, demonstrate hypoactivity in the frontal region (dorsolateral prefrontal, inferior prefrontal, and orbitofrontal), anterior cingulum, superior parietal region, caudate nucleus, and thalamus (Kasparek, Theiner, & Filova, 2015). Impairments have also been demonstrated in connectivity between key brain regions (e.g., frontoparietal, frontocerebellar) in both resting state and functional paradigms.

Dopamine (DA) and norepinephrine (NE) play important roles in the pathophysiology of ADHD, exerting modulatory influence over frontostriatal-cerebellar circuits (Del Campo, Chamberlain, Sahakian, & Robbins, 2011; Faraone, 2018). Furthermore, stimulant medications used to treat ADHD such as methylphenidate and amphetamine act to increase the availability of DA and NE in these brain regions, providing additional evidence for the central role of these neurotransmitters in ADHD. Methylphenidate primarily acts to block reuptake of DA and NE, while amphetamine both decreases reuptake and increases release of these neurotransmitters (Del Campo et al., 2011). Functional imaging studies have shown that methylphenidate and amphetamine increase the availability of DA and NE in multiple brain regions, including not only frontostriatal circuits but also the cerebellum and amygdala (Fig. 46.1). Furthermore, other neurotransmitters, including serotonin, acetylcholine, opioid, and glutamate pathways, have also been linked to ADHD (Faraone, 2018). Pharmacogenetic studies have identified multiple genetic variants with small effect sizes on the efficacy of methylphenidate. Future studies are likely to provide additional information that may ultimately inform medication choice and dosing on an individualized basis.

Neuropsychological Foundations

EF skills involved in supporting strategic, goal-directed behavior mature during different developmental periods (Diamond, 2013). Modal periods of development have been identified for four key EFs: Capacities for behavioral control and updating information in working memory tend to be consolidated by roughly age 8 years in TD children, and capacities for future goal setting and seamless set shifting (i.e., multitasking) tend to be consolidated by the middle teens (Anderson, 2002). These capacities are likely to be delayed by 3 to 5 years in children diagnosed with ADHD, which can understandably lead to considerable frustration in parents who see their children with ADHD lagging behind same-aged or younger peers.

Several researchers have posed the idea that ADHD may be better understood as dimensional extremes in two distinct inattention and hyperactivity/impulsivity factors, each mediated by different aspects of EF and each corresponding to different types of cooccurring developmental psychopathology (Barkley, 1997; Miyake & Friedman, 2012; Nigg, 2017a). For example, inattention may be more strongly associated with problems in set shifting, rumination, and internalizing symptoms, whereas hyperactivity/impulsivity may be more strongly associated with problems in behavioral inhibition and externalizing behaviors. Before advances in neuroimaging, performance on standardized neuropsychological tests came closest to capturing how the brain functioned and solved problems in real time. Different tests place different levels of demand on functions such as set shifting, working memory, and response inhibition. Classic tasks include Trails A and B (a proxy for cognitive flexibility and set shifting), the Stroop Test (measuring response inhibition for the prepotent, automatic response of reading), and the Wisconsin Card Sort Task, wherein participants must infer the changing rules of

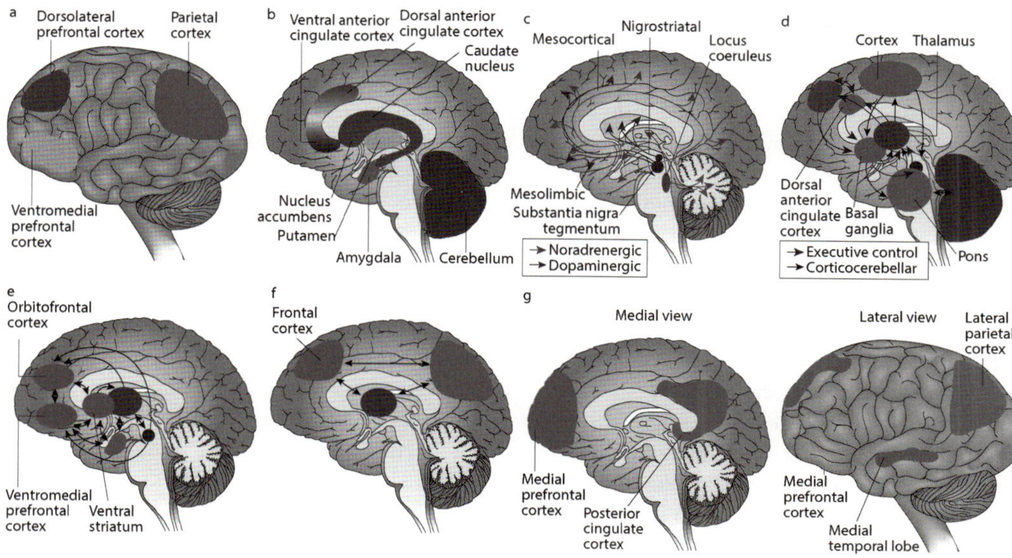

Fig. 46.1 Brain Mechanisms in ADHD*. (a) The cortical regions (lateral view) of the brain have a role in attention-deficit/hyperactivity disorder (ADHD). The dorsolateral prefrontal cortex is linked to working memory, the ventromedial prefrontal cortex to complex decision making and strategic planning, and the parietal cortex to orientation of attention. (b) ADHD involves the subcortical structures (medial view) of the brain. The ventral anterior cingulate cortex and the dorsal anterior cingulate cortex subserve affective and cognitive components of executive control. Together with the basal ganglia (comprising the nucleus accumbens, caudate nucleus, and putamen), they form the frontostriatal circuit. Neuroimaging studies show structural and functional abnormalities in all of these structures in patients with ADHD, extending into the amygdala and cerebellum. (c) Neurotransmitter circuits in the brain are involved in ADHD. The dopamine system plays an important part in planning and initiation of motor responses, activation, switching, reaction to novelty, and processing of reward. The noradrenergic system influences arousal modulation, signal-to-noise ratios in cortical areas, state-dependent cognitive processes, and cognitive preparation of urgent stimuli. (d) Executive control networks are affected in patients with ADHD. The executive control and cortico-cerebellar networks coordinate executive functioning (i.e., planning, goal-directed behavior, inhibition, working memory, and the flexible adaptation to context). These networks are underactivated and have lower internal functional connectivity in individuals with ADHD compared with individuals without the disorder. (e) ADHD involves the reward network. The ventromedial prefrontal cortex, orbitofrontal cortex, and ventral striatum are at the center of the brain network that responds to anticipation and receipt of reward. Other structures involved are the thalamus, the amygdala, and the cell bodies of dopaminergic neurons in the substantia nigra, which, as indicated by the arrows, interact in a complex manner. Behavioral and neural responses to reward are abnormal in ADHD. (f) The alerting network is impaired in ADHD. The frontal and parietal cortical areas and the thalamus intensively interact in the alerting network (indicated by the arrows), which supports attentional functioning and is weaker in individuals with ADHD than in controls. (g) ADHD involves the default-mode network (DMN). The DMN consists of the medial prefrontal cortex and the posterior cingulate cortex (medial view) as well as the lateral parietal cortex and the medial temporal lobe (lateral view). DMN fluctuations are 180° out of phase with fluctuations in networks that become activated during externally oriented tasks, presumably reflecting competition between opposing processes for processing resources. Negative correlations between the DMN and the frontoparietal control network are weaker in patients with ADHD than in people who do not have the disorder.
S.V. Faraone, P. Asherson, T. Banaschewski, J. Biederman, J.K. Buitelaar, J.A. Ramos-Quiroga, et al. Attention-deficit/hyperactivity disorder. *Nat. Rev. Dis. Primers*, 1(2015), p. 15020.

a card game without any guidance from the examiner other than whether their choices were correct or incorrect. The marshmallow test of delayed gratification (Tobin & Graziano, 2009) and computer-administered gambling tasks (Brand, Recknor, Grabenhorst, & Bechara, 2007) have allowed for assessment not only of the so-called cold EFs (e.g., attention, problem solving, working memory) associated with academic performance but also the so-called hot EFs (emotional regulation) implicated in problems with impulse control (Chan et al., 2008; Zimmerman, Ownsworth, O'Donovan, Roberts, & Gullo, 2016). Neuroimaging later validated which areas of the brain were most or least active during different tasks; however, recent findings suggest that there might even be heterogeneity in what areas of the brain are active during the same task (Sanfratello et al., 2014).

With so many areas of the brain identified as having significant changes in structure and function in persons with ADHD, and with changes in these brain regions over development, it is not surprising that a wide range of EFs (e.g., emotional regulation, time management, motor coordination and planning, discovery of salience) are thought to be impacted by ADHD. Nevertheless, three EF domains commonly emerge in the literature as deficient or inconsistently functioning in ADHD: response inhibition, set shifting, and the maintenance of information in working memory (Friedman, Miyake, & Altamirano, 2016), although there are variable estimates of the relative importance or clinical utility of these factors (Roberts, Martel, & Nigg, 2017). Response inhibition refers to the ability to control and direct one's impulses (e.g., refraining from blurting an answer in the classroom or resisting being provoked by a peer into an inappropriate response). Set shifting refers to the ability to flexibly shift one's attention serially between different tasks, from a conversation with a peer back to one's work for example. Working memory refers to the ability to hold and manipulate information in mind; examples include following a multistep command and performing mental arithmetic in class.

Nigg (2017b) reports the strongest empirical support for ADHD-related deficits in response inhibition, spatial working memory, and alertness/vigilance to continuous performance tasks; less robust, but still compelling metaanalytic support exists for deficiencies in verbal working memory, set shifting on tasks such as the Wisconsin Card Sort, planning, impulsive preference for short-term rewards over longer-term but larger rewards, motor control, and temporal processing (time sense). These latter functions resonate with the complaints of ADHD-diagnosed college students that it takes them longer and requires more effort to complete assignments (Lewandowski, Lovett, Codding, & Gordon, 2008) and with parents' complaints about their ADHD-affected child's lack of motivation and sense of responsibility to initiate and complete tasks.

While compelling from a research perspective, neuropsychological test performance (Barkley & Murphy, 2010) or imaging of regions of interest in areas of the brain hypothesized to be associated with ADHD have not led to the development of clinically useful diagnostic tests for ADHD. Hence, views on the relative importance of executive dysfunction in ADHD vary widely from conceptualizing it as the essential core of the disorder (e.g., Barkley, 1997) and seeing it as an interesting covariate of ADHD symptoms (e.g., Mahone et al., 2002) to an inconsequential distraction to effective assessment and treatment of ADHD (e.g., Alloway, Gathercole, Holmes, Place, Elliott, & Hilton, 2009). Recently, EF dysfunction, especially when it translates to poor study skills or problems in academic or work performance, has emerged as an important treatment target (Evans et al., 2016; Sibley et al., 2016).

Genetics

The genetic basis of ADHD has been well established, including twin studies that demonstrate heritability in the 70% to 80% range and a 5- to 10-fold increase in risk for ADHD among first-degree relatives (Faraone et al., 2015). Early genetic studies focused on candidate genes related to dopamine and other neurotransmitters implicated in ADHD, with results consistently showing small effect sizes and frequent failure to replicate findings across studies (Del Campo et al., 2011). More recently, the availability of large, pooled samples has permitted genome-wide association studies. These studies focus on common genetic variants (i.e., affecting >1% of the population) and have identified the regulation of neurotransmitter release (especially dopamine) as well as neurite growth and axon guidance as etiologic factors for ADHD. Another important theme is that multiple, common genetic variants with small effect sizes likely act together to increase genetic risk for ADHD, suggesting that ADHD is a polygenic disorder. It has even proven possible to utilize polygenic liability scores to predict the occurrence of ADHD symptoms in the general population. A recent genome-wide association study used a pooled sample of 55,374 individuals (Demontis, Walters, & Martin, 2019). This study identified 12 independent loci associated with ADHD, and findings were consistent with the notion that clinically diagnosed ADHD is a polygenic disorder with significant genetic overlap with commonly cooccurring conditions (e.g., depression), representing an extreme expression of heritable traits. Studies of ADHD among persons with rare disorders such as tuberous sclerosis and fragile X syndrome have provided additional insights, amplified by studies of rarer copy number variants that are beginning to implicate other pathways that may be relevant to the etiology and/or treatment of ADHD (e.g., ion channelopathies and regulation of oxidative stress; Demontis et al., 2019). Over the past 10 years, studies have also demonstrated that shared genetic factors account for the cooccurrence of neurodevelopmental (autism spectrum disorder, intellectual disability) and psychiatric disorders (internalizing and externalizing disorders) with ADHD.

Other Etiologic Factors. Although ADHD is most commonly genetic in origin there are many other factors that increase risk for the development of ADHD. Prematurity as well as late preterm birth are associated with increased risk for ADHD (Harris et al., 2013). Increased risk for ADHD is also noted among infants with prenatal alcohol exposure and maternal smoking. In general, prenatal factors associated with structural and/or functional brain damage can be expected to manifest as increased risk for the expression of ADHD symptoms. This is not surprising given the widely distributed brain regions and neural networks that are now understood to influence the expression of ADHD symptoms and executive dysfunction. Ultimately research that more precisely defines the relationships between etiologic factors and ADHD symptoms, coexisting conditions, and response to treatment may permit more precise, individualized prediction of developmental trajectory, response to treatment, and outcome.

THE IMPACT OF ADHD

Health Disparities and Socioeconomic Costs

Health disparities are a concern for children and adolescents with ADHD, with the most recent data suggesting slightly higher prevalence among Black children and lower prevalence among Hispanic/Latino children (Danielson, Bitsko, Ghandour, Holbrook, Kogan, & Blumberg, 2018). Children living in poverty, having public insurance, or residing in the Midwest or South also have higher reported prevalence of ADHD. Compared to White children, Black children are somewhat more likely to receive behavioral treatment and Hispanic children are more likely to receive medical treatment for ADHD. The reasons for these ongoing disparities are complex and beyond the scope of this chapter, including issues such as disparities in rate of diagnosis as well as variability in findings across studies; nevertheless, clinicians should be alert to these disparities, and future research is required to better understand and address factors contributing to them.

Due to its high prevalence, the costs attributable to ADHD in the health care system and in society in general are considerable, with total costs estimated to be several hundred billion dollars per year, primarily attributable to lost productivity and income among adults with ADHD (Doshi et al., 2012). Health care costs and utilization are considerably higher for children with ADHD compared to their peers.

Persistence Into Adulthood

Recent studies have reinforced our understanding of ADHD as a truly neurodevelopmental disorder, just as neurobiologic studies have begun to describe developmental changes in the brain among persons with ADHD. Among children ages 3 to 7 years diagnosed with ADHD on the basis of a comprehensive, interdisciplinary, developmental, and psychological assessment, 70% continued to meet diagnostic criteria for ADHD at a mean age of 12 years, with higher rates of persistence among children with psychiatric comorbidities, family history of psychopathology, and exposure to childhood adversity (Law, Sideridis, Prock, & Sheridan, 2014). Prevalence of ADHD increases with increasing age, at least through middle childhood. ADHD has been shown to persist from childhood into adulthood for approximately 30% to 40% of affected children, and adult prevalence is 4% (Barbaresi et al., 2013). It is possible that in some cases of ADHD may not present until late adolescence or early adulthood, presumably when persons with less severe neurobiologic vulnerability encounter environments that exceed the functional capacity of the affected person such that symptoms of ADHD lead to impaired function.

Functional Impairment in Children and Adolescents

By definition the diagnosis of ADHD requires that symptoms cause impairment in two or more settings. Children and adolescents with ADHD typically experience functional impairment in home, school, and community settings, and with peers.

Poor school function is a common presenting concern and is often focused on disruptive classroom behaviors, especially among boys. Virtually all indicators of academic achievement and school function are significantly worse on average, including increased rates of absenteeism, grade retention, school dropout before high school graduation, and lower rates of completion of postsecondary education. Children and adolescents with ADHD often have challenging behaviors, including oppositionality and more serious disruptive behaviors. Interactions with peers are often unsatisfactory, with disrupted friendships and increased rates of bullying and victimization. ADHD is also associated with increased risk for driving violations and accidents, other types of accidents and injuries, and emergency room visits. These functional impairments are broad and go far beyond the impact of core ADHD symptoms. Despite the high population level of risk for adverse function among children and adolescents with ADHD, it is important for clinicians not to lose sight of the unique strengths and potential of each affected child.

Medical Comorbidities

Children with ADHD have also been found to be at increased risk for certain other medical conditions. The association between ADHD and tics/tic disorders is well established, with rates of up to 25% for chronic tics in children with ADHD and rates of ADHD of 50% or more in children and adolescents with Tourette syndrome (see Chapter 71). Children with ADHD have also been found to have higher rates of epilepsy and elimination disorders; girls with ADHD have increased obesity rates. Some studies have suggested that there may be increased rates of other medical conditions in children with ADHD, but it is uncertain whether these findings reflect a true increase in rate of occurrence or increased likelihood of diagnosis in children who have more frequent medical visits.

Adult Outcomes

A comprehensive understanding of ADHD must be based on a life-course perspective, as the challenges will vary over time as they did for David, described in the chapter-opening vignette. Among adults with a history of childhood ADHD, rates of other mental health conditions (e.g., anxiety, depression, substance use disorders) are over 50%; rates are even higher among those whose ADHD persists into adulthood (Barbaresi et al., 2013). Children with ADHD have been found to have increased rates of adverse adult outcomes in a wide array of domains, including lower educational attainment, unstable employment, and significantly lower income; decreased likelihood of marriage, earlier age of initiation of sexual activity, and higher rates of single parenthood; increased rates of driving violations and driving under the influence; increased rates of legal problems and criminality; and higher rates of substance use disorder as well as having received treatment for substance use (Harstad et al., 2020). Importantly, individual increased risk for adverse adult outcomes crosses these domains, highlighting the importance of a broad approach to prevention and amelioration of risk for adverse long-term outcomes in all children with ADHD.

COMPLEX ADHD AS A CONCEPT AND FOCUS ON IMPROVING FUNCTIONAL OUTCOMES

The recent SDBP practice guidelines on ADHD, as well as the most recent ADHD practice guidelines from the American Academy of Pediatrics, provide detailed information on approaches to diagnosis and treatment (Wolraich et al., 2019). The SDBP guidelines define complex ADHD based on age (<4 years or >12 years at the time of initial presentation), presence of coexisting mental health, neurodevelopmental or other factors (medical, psychosocial adversity), degree of functional impairment, diagnostic uncertainty, or inadequate response to the treatment that would typically be provided in a general pediatric setting (Barbaresi et al., 2020). From an epidemiologic perspective, coexisting neurodevelopmental and mental health conditions are the rule rather than the exception in children and adolescents with ADHD. While the diagnosis of ADHD requires the documentation of core symptoms, the approach to diagnosis and treatment for complex ADHD depends on the identification and treatment of sources of functional impairment to improve short-term function and long-term outcomes.

Diagnosis and Nomenclature

The diagnostic criteria for ADHD have evolved over time, reflecting many of the advances in our understanding of the neurobiology and neuropsychology of ADHD summarized earlier in this chapter. The constellation of symptoms now called ADHD was previously described with the term minimal brain dysfunction; interestingly, as it has become apparent that ADHD symptoms reflect differences in structure and function of multiple neural networks, that term, although nonspecific, may not be entirely inaccurate. The current diagnostic criteria and terminology in the *DSM-5* have replaced earlier concepts of ADHD "subtypes" (combined, inattentive, and hyperactive/impulsive) with the term "presentations", to reflect the fact that individual symptom profiles are not stable over time (American Psychiatric Association, 2013). ADHD is also now appropriately categorized as a neurodevelopmental disorder. The *DSM-5* diagnostic criteria were revised from *DSM-IV* to allow for age of onset prior to age 12 years, reflecting growing understanding of the different ways that ADHD may manifest over time; this change is in contrast to the *International Classification of Diseases*, tenth revision (*ICD-10*) requirement for onset prior to age 7 years. While not a topic of this chapter, the *DSM-5* has, consistent with recent research, specified a lower symptom number threshold for diagnosis of ADHD in adults than the *ICD-10*.

ASSESSMENT

The diagnosis of ADHD begins with documentation of symptoms sufficient in number and type to be consistent with the *DSM-5* diagnostic criteria. Accuracy and precision in this step are dependent on obtaining information from multiple sources and settings (typically home, school, and community) by way of standardized, ADHD-specific rating scales such as the Vanderbilt Assessment Scales (https://www.nichq.org/sites/default/files/resource-file/NICHQ_Vanderbilt_Assessment_Scales.pdf). Compared to paper versions of rating scales, newer, electronic approaches offer much higher rates of success in obtaining initial and follow-up ratings to guide both diagnostic and treatment decisions.

The diagnosis of ADHD is not complete after one obtains a checklist of ADHD symptoms, nor should one stop the search if the symptom count falls short of six in each domain. The threshold of six symptoms must be reached based on the total number of symptoms reported across settings (e.g., home and school) and does not require that six symptoms or more are noted in every setting. It is also important to note that there are often discrepancies between symptoms reported by parents and teachers, sometimes complicating the diagnostic process. The next step should include a comprehensive history focusing on function in the home, school, and community, and review of information from sources such as school records, report cards, special educational evaluations and individualized education plans (IEPs), and school or private psychological and educational assessments. Clinical judgment and discussion with parents and the affected child or adolescent are central to the assessment of function, given (a) the limited standardized measures available for this purpose and (b) the frequent need to reconcile discrepant ratings between parents and teachers (who might observe different aspects of ADHD in their respective settings). Assessment of the degree and scope of functional impairment is important not only for the diagnostic assessment but also for treatment planning.

Since there are as yet no definitive biomarker-based diagnostic tools, and since it is not uncommon for there to be discrepancies between parents' and teachers' symptom ratings, the diagnosis of ADHD requires careful consideration of alternative explanations for observed ADHD symptoms. These can include hearing or vision impairment, varying degrees of intellectual disability, other neurodevelopmental disorders such as autism spectrum disorder, language and learning disorders, medical conditions (e.g., epilepsy, lead poisoning, sleep disorders), mental health disorders such as anxiety or depression, and environmental factors (e.g., psychosocial adversity, poor school environment). A thorough physical and neurologic examination, as well as hearing and vision testing, should be completed. Importantly, these alternative potential causes of ADHD symptoms are also conditions and factors that commonly cooccur in children and adolescents with ADHD, greatly increasing the complexity of the diagnostic process. In preschool-age children and adolescents this assessment is even more complicated, thus the SDBP practice guideline notes that the assessment and treatment of children with complex ADHD requires either subspecialty training or equivalent experience.

The extremely high rates of coexisting developmental and mental health conditions that accompany ADHD require a careful consideration of these conditions as a core component of the diagnostic assessment for every child. It may be possible to complete this portion of the diagnostic assessment by using the results of previously obtained psychological testing (either through school or private testing); however, it is often necessary to include psychological testing as part of the diagnostic assessment to obtain this critically important information. Thus an interdisciplinary approach is required, incorporating the expertise of psychologists and often others such as educational specialists or speech-language pathologists for more complicated cases. To complete a thorough diagnostic assessment, direct interaction is essential with the diagnosing clinician for a sufficient amount of time to complete a thorough history and physical examination along with time to review rating scales and relevant information from other sources. For children who require psychological or other testing, several additional hours are required to complete an assessment. Unfortunately, despite the strong evidence base for this careful approach, particularly for children with complex ADHD, multiple factors (e.g., communication, availability of clinicians, insurance reimbursement) often create barriers to comprehensive diagnostic assessments for many children and their families.

TREATMENT

Decades of research studies have clearly demonstrated that pharmacologic treatment with stimulant medications is associated with short-term improvement in core ADHD symptoms (Greenhill, Kollins, & Abikoff, 2006; MTA Cooperative Group, 1999) and with improved short-term function in domains of school performance, behavior, peer interactions, and reduced risk for accidents (Chang, Lichtenstein, D'Onofrio, Sjölander, & Larsson, 2014; Froehlich, Fogler, Barbaresi, Elsayed, Evans, & Chan, 2018). However, evidence for improved long-term outcomes in adulthood with pharmacologic treatment is limited. It is inherently difficult to conduct research examining the impact of childhood treatment on adult outcomes, although some studies have reported associations between stimulant treatment and longer-term school outcomes and reduced risk for substance use disorder. Similarly, psychosocial/behavioral treatments have been shown to improve short-term school performance, behavior, peer interactions, and family function, while the impact of psychosocial treatment on long-term adult outcomes is also limited. Nevertheless, given the importance of focusing on improvement in short- and long-term function, and the direct relationship between psychosocial intervention and key functional domains, current guidelines emphasize that psychosocial interventions are foundational (i.e., they should be implemented for all children and adolescents with ADHD and given first consideration in treatment). However, considerations such as severity of impairment, urgency of a child's particular situation (e.g., threatened school expulsion or daycare exclusion), parental choice, and the availability of psychosocial treatment may require pharmacologic treatment before or concurrent with initiation of psychosocial treatment. Ultimately, children and adolescents with ADHD should all receive multimodal, multiple-setting treatment to address their unique needs.

Psychoeducation and Psychosocial Interventions

The first step in treatment for ADHD is psychoeducation about the disorder for parents/caregivers and the affected child or adolescent, depending on age and developmental level. There are many excellent sources of information available from books, professional organizations, and advocacy groups; clinicians should provide guidance about accurate sources of information, particularly since misleading or inaccurate information about ADHD is so readily available via the Internet and in the media. To support shared decision making, parents/caregivers and their children/adolescent need accurate information. Furthermore, since there are no definitive treatments that universally lead to improved short- and long-term outcomes, treatment decisions require ongoing assessment of risks and benefits of recommended approaches.

Among psychosocial treatments for ADHD, behavioral management, taught directly to parents for home application (i.e., parent training in behavioral management) or delivered in school or recreational settings (i.e., contingency management, usually documented on daily report cards) has the strongest evidence base (Evans, Owens, Wymbs, & Ray, 2018; also see Chapter 93 for further discussion). These forms of treatment are optimally targeted toward preschool- through elementary school-age children. In adolescence the small prizes (sticker charts) and positive attention technique ("catch them being good") commonly used in these interventions begin to lose their luster (Chan, Fogler, & Hammerness, 2016). Therefore for adolescents, these techniques require greater creativity on the part of parents and educators, and additional motivational enhancement techniques on the part of clinicians. A second category of psychosocial treatment (skills training) usually in study and organizational skills, has also been found to be effective at improving functional outcomes in older school-age children and adolescents with ADHD; this tends to require a more intensive laboratory classroom setting, however, with highly trained personnel, often bolstered by contingency management at home (Chan, Fogler, & Hammerness, 2016). Skills training delivered at lower intensity (e.g., through school consultation) has to date produced much more modest outcomes. Other forms of electronic "brain training" through computerized tasks or some form of direct stimulation to the parts of the brain implicated in attention seem to confer improvements that are specific to the electronic tasks themselves and not to the kinds of generalizable functional outcome improvements commonly sought by parents (i.e., school performance, reduced parent-child conflict). Far less effective are office-based treatments that require the child with ADHD to apply something that has been discussed in the abstract (e.g., social skills) to an in vivo experience.

The overlay of cooccurring conditions for children and adolescents with complex ADHD often requires additional modalities. Examples include techniques from cognitive-behavioral therapy (see Chapter 98) such as behavioral activation and mindfulness-based self-soothing for depression and generalized anxiety, exposure-based and interoceptive therapies for panic and anxiety disorders with a classically phobic presentation, exposure and response prevention for obsessive-compulsive disorder, and multisystemic therapies for conduct and oppositional-defiant disorder. Thoughtful and comprehensive assessment will help in the prioritization of treatment targets, but broadly speaking, treating ADHD and nascent coexisting conditions earlier in the life span confers greater chance of positive long-term outcomes.

The best empirically supported interventions for school settings include techniques that support more attentive and less disruptive classroom participation and techniques that aim to improve academic performance (Harrison, Bunford, Evans, & Owens, 2013). Contingency management and judiciously applied movement breaks are better at supporting classroom engagement, whereas skills training (with a highly responsive teacher offering frequent opportunities to respond) is better at improving academic outcomes. Broadly speaking, strategies implemented by the teacher within the regular classroom fall under the category of a 504 plan; and interventions requiring time spent with specialists outside the classroom fall under the category of an IEP (see Chapter 113). School teams commonly offer extra time to complete assignments and tests in the classroom and at home, but this may not be sufficient without additional opportunities to respond along with frequent prompting and training to check one's work.

Recent research highlights the importance of sequencing psychosocial and pharmacologic treatment for ADHD: When compared to those receiving medication as the first-line treatment, children receiving low-intensity psychosocial treatment as their first-line option (1) showed significantly better reductions in ADHD symptoms and observed problematic behavior and significantly better increases in academic and sports skill acquisition; and (2) required lower doses of psychostimulant medication to achieve optimal outcomes (for review, see Pelham & Altzsuler, 2020). Medications were found to be effective in reducing problem behavior but not in skill acquisition. Furthermore, caregivers whose children received medication as the first-line treatment, compared to psychosocial treatment-first families, were less engaged in psychosocial treatment when it was offered later.

Pharmacotherapy

A detailed consideration of the many US Food and Drug Administration (FDA)–approved medications for ADHD is beyond the scope of this chapter, and additional information about medication is provided in Chapter 99. However, there are several general principles that should be considered for each child for whom pharmacologic treatment is prescribed.

Psychoeducation

Each class of FDA-approved medication for ADHD (stimulants, norepinephrine reuptake inhibitors, and alpha-2 adrenergic agonists) has a unique set of potential risks and benefits that should be considered and discussed with parents/caregivers and their child or adolescent. This process should provide adequate time for parents to make a decision; depending on the unique circumstances of the child, some families may require a considerable amount of time to reach a decision about whether to initiate pharmacologic treatment.

Special attention should be given to a discussion about what medication can and cannot do, both with regard to core ADHD symptoms and function. For example, families may not understand that improvement of ADHD symptoms will not necessarily lead to improved academic performance, particularly for a child with a coexisting specific learning disorder.

Caregivers also should be provided with information about ways in which their child's longstanding behaviors may change; for example, a child who is overtly hyperactive, talkative, and impulsive may seem "abnormal" if, with pharmacologic treatment, the child is able to be calm, quiet, and attentive during tasks.

Medication Choice

Unfortunately, there is limited information about the comparative effectiveness of different medications within medication classes or across classes. Based on the many decades of research demonstrating the safety and efficacy of stimulant medications, they should be considered the first-line pharmacologic treatment for core ADHD symptoms. It is not possible to predict which stimulant medication is likely to be most effective for a specific child, and a child who responds poorly to one stimulant may respond well to another in the same or different class (i.e., methylphenidate or amphetamine). Similarly, there are multiple preparations of stimulant medications with varying modes of administration (oral, dermal patch), preparation (pills, capsules that can be swallowed whole or whose contents can be sprinkled into food, chewable tablets, and liquids), and duration of action (short, intermediate, long acting). Nonstimulant medications are often considered safer by the general public because of inaccurate perceptions about stimulant medication side effects and the fact that they are not controlled substances. However, these medications also have side effects, and in general they do not seem to be as effective as stimulants in clinical practice. Medication choice requires an examination of the ways in which ADHD symptoms are impairing for a particular child, including setting, activities, functional domains that are disrupted (school, home, community), and timing of troublesome symptoms (morning, school day, evening). Pharmacogenomic research aimed at more precisely identifying genetic factors that influence response to specific medications or doses of medication may ultimately provide information that facilitates the process of medication selection.

Continuous Versus Intermittent Treatment

In the past it was common to recommend pharmacologic treatment with stimulant medications only on school days because of concern about adverse impact on growth (for review, see Swanson et al., 2017), as well as lack of appreciation of the impact of ADHD beyond school function. While some studies have suggested potential small decreases in adult height on the order of 1 cm, long-term studies have not consistently found that treatment with stimulant medication is associated with significant reduction in long-term growth as reflected in adult height (Harstad et al., 2014). ADHD symptoms clearly do impact function outside of school; hence treatment should typically be continuous, throughout the week, both during and outside of the school year.

When to Consider Stopping Medication

The decision to stop pharmacologic treatment is as nuanced as the decision to initiate treatment. Ongoing monitoring of target symptoms of ADHD and coexisting conditions may suggest diminution of functional impairment over time and thus consideration of changes or discontinuation of medication. However, given that ADHD generally persists throughout childhood and adolescence, caution should be exercised when considering discontinuation of treatment. If a decision is made to stop medication, special attention should be given to monitoring for recurrence of impairing symptoms of ADHD and coexisting conditions. Historically, the failure to appreciate that ADHD is a chronic, neurodevelopmental disorder has likely led to premature discontinuation of treatment to the detriment of affected children and adolescents.

Fostering Understanding and Adherence

In other chronic health conditions such as diabetes efforts are made to provide education to the affected child from the very beginning, to foster increased understanding of the health condition and, over time, increased adherence to recommended treatment. The same approach should be taken with pharmacologic and psychosocial treatment for ADHD, with ongoing discussion between the child, family, and clinician aimed at improving the child's understanding of ADHD as well as the benefits of treatment (Fogler, Burke, Lynch, Barbaresi, & Chan, 2017). It is not appropriate to wait to begin this process until early adolescence, at which time many patients begin to question or even refuse treatment.

TREATMENT ACROSS THE LIFE SPAN

By definition, a majority of children and adolescents will have one or more coexisting conditions, and nearly all who have complex ADHD will have coexisting conditions. Treatment in these cases requires careful consideration of the primary source of impairment. For example, an adolescent with ADHD and an anxiety disorder may have severe, impairing symptoms of ADHD and relatively mild anxiety symptoms, in which case the ADHD symptoms should be the primary target of treatment. The extent to which specific symptoms lead to impairment is likely to change over time, requiring ongoing consideration of treatment targets, with corresponding adjustments in treatment modalities and approach. This approach is consistent with a parsimonious consideration of pharmacologic treatment deemed appropriate because of the still limited evidence for treatment with varying combinations of medication from different classes.

There is limited evidence for what constitutes appropriate, let alone optimal, frequency of follow-up for children and adolescents with ADHD. By convention and expert consensus, those who are receiving medication should be seen every 3 to 4 months. The option to conduct virtual visits may represent a more efficient and accessible approach to follow-up for some children, in combination with in-person visits. Even for children who are not receiving medication, follow-up at times of transition is recommended, including the transition from preschool to school, elementary to middle school, middle school to high school, and high school to postsecondary education or employment. In addition to increasing academic demands in higher grades, children with ADHD are also at risk to encounter increasing levels of social difficulties, including bullying (Fogler, Weaver, Katusic, Voigt, & Barbaresi, 2020).

As described earlier in this chapter, we now understand that ADHD persists into adulthood for many affected adolescents, and that even for those whose ADHD does not persist, other mental health conditions and functional imparaments are often encountered. It is therefore essential to facilitate the transfer of care to the adult health care system for adolescents and young adults with ADHD. The precise timing of this transfer will depend on the circumstance for the adolescent and logistical considerations on the part of the clinician (e.g., training and experience, availability of appointments for older patients). Unfortunately, there are at present an inadequate number of clinicians who have the training and experience to provide care for the estimated 4% of the US adult population who have ADHD.

CONCLUSION

As is apparent throughout this chapter, while ADHD has been the subject of extensive research over decades, approaches to diagnosis and treatment still depend far too much on clinical experience, common sense, and consensus opinion. Future research on evidence-based approaches to diagnosis and treatment is especially needed for those who have ADHD and coexisting mental health disorders, as well as for preschool-age children and transition-age adolescents Similarly, additional research is needed on psychosocial treatments, particularly for adolescents, as well as for multimodal treatment approaches, optimal treatment monitoring, prevention of substance use and substance use disorders, and treatment that leads to the ultimate goal of improved long-term outcomes. The complexity of ADHD, including its neurologic basis, broad impact on function, diagnostic challenges, frequency of coexisting conditions, and impact at the individual and societal level are daunting. Ultimately it is likely that the development of more precise, individualized, evidence-based approaches will require new approaches that allow for clinical research that is incorporated into clinical care at multiple sites, with careful approaches to the collection of structured data to inform our understanding of these critically important issues.

ADHD is the most common neurodevelopmental disorder in childhood; it is a chronic condition that often persists into adulthood and is frequently associated with other conditions that complicate and compound the impact of ADHD on function across all domains of daily life. The impact of ADHD at the individual and societal level is significant. While ADHD is now understood to be neurologically based and primarily genetic in origin, much is still unknown about the precise ways in which differences in brain structure and function contribute to the development of ADHD and its coexisting conditions. Approaches to diagnosis and treatment have been refined over time and are supported by well-reasoned practice guidelines; however, treatment is still often based on consensus expert opinion rather than evidence, highlighting the need for additional research. Children and adolescents with ADHD are at high risk for a broad array of adverse short- and long-term outcomes, requiring careful, ongoing monitoring and treatment aimed at supporting each child based on unique strengths and challenges.

REFERENCES

Alloway, T. P., Gathercole, S. E., Holmes, J., Place, M., Elliott, J. G., & Hilton, K. (2009). The diagnostic utility of behavioral checklists in identifying children with ADHD and children with working memory deficits. *Child Psychiatry & Human Development*, *40*(3), 353–366. https://doi.org/10.1007/s10578-009-0131-3

American Psychiatric Association. (2013). *Diagnostic and statistical manual of mental disorders* (5th ed.).

Anderson, P. (2002). Assessment and development of executive function (EF) during childhood. *Child Neuropsychology*, *8*(2), 71–82. https://doi.org/10.1076/chin.8.2.71.8724

Barbaresi, W. J., Campbell, L., Diekroger, E. A., Froehlich, T. E., Liu, Y. H., O'Malley, E., ...Chan, E. (2020). Society for Developmental and Behavioral Pediatrics clinical practice guideline for the assessment and treatment of children and adolescents with complex attention-deficit/hyperactivity disorder. *Journal of Developmental & Behavioral Pediatrics*, *41*(2), S35–S57. https://doi.org/10.1097/DBP.0000000000000770

Barbaresi, W. J., Colligan, R. C., Weaver, A. L., Voigt, R. G., Killian, J. M., & Katusic, S. K. (2013). Mortality, ADHD, and psychosocial adversity in adults with childhood ADHD: A prospective study. *Pediatrics*, *131*(4), 637–644. https://doi.org/10.1542/peds.2012-2354

Barbaresi, W. J., Katusic, S. K., Colligan, R. C., Pankratz, V. S., Weaver, A. L., Weber, K. J., … Jacobsen, S. J. (2002). How common is attention-deficit/hyperactivity disorder? Incidence in a population-based birth cohort in Rochester, Minn. *Archives of Pediatric Adolescent Medicine*, *156*(3), 217–224. https://doi.org/10.1001/archpedi.156.3.217

Barkley, R. A. (1997). Behavioral inhibition, sustained attention, and executive functions: Constructing a unifying theory of ADHD. *Psychological Bulletin*, *121*(1), 65–94. https://doi.org/10.1037/0033-2909.121.1.65

Barkley, R. (2014). *The 30 essential ideas you should know about ADHD*. https://www.youtube.com/watch?v=BzhbAK1pdPM

Barkley, R. A., & Murphy, K. R. (2010). Impairment in occupational functioning and adult ADHD: The predictive utility of executive function (EF) ratings versus EF tests. *Archives of Clinical Neuropsychology*, *25*(3), 157–173. https://doi.org/10.1093/arclin/acq014

Brand, M., Recknor, E. C., Grabenhorst, F., & Bechara, A. (2007). Decisions under ambiguity and decisions under risk: Correlations with executive functions and comparisons of two different gambling tasks with implicit and explicit rules. *Journal of Clinical and Experimental Neuropsychology*, *29*(1), 86–99. https://doi.org/10.1080/13803390500507196

Chan, E., Fogler, J., & Hammerness, P. (2016). Treatment of attention-deficit hyperactivity disorder in adolescents and transitional-age youth: A systematic review. *JAMA*, *315*(18), 1997–2008. https://doi.org/10.1001/jama.2016.5453

Chang, Z., Lichtenstein, P., D'Onofrio, B. M., Sjölander, A., & Larsson, H. (2014). Serious transport accidents in adults with attention-deficit/hyperactivity disorder and the effect of medication: A population-based study. *JAMA Psychiatry*, *71*(3), 319–325. https://doi.org/10.1001/jamapsychiatry.2013.4174

Chan, R. C., Shum, D., Toulopoulou, T., & Chen, E. Y. (2008). Assessment of executive functions: Review of instruments and identification of critical issues. *Arch Clin Neuropsychol*. 2008 Mar;23(2):201–16. doi: 10.1016/j.acn.2007.08.010. Epub 2007 Dec 21. PMID: 18096360.

Danielson, M. L., Bitsko, R. H., Ghandour, R. M., Holbrook, J. R., Kogan, M. D., & Blumberg, S. J. (2016). Prevalence of ADHD among Black Youth Compared to White, Latino and Asian Youth: A Meta-Analysis, 2016. *Journal of Clinical Child & Adolescent Psychology*, *47*(2), 199–212. https://doi.org/10.1080/15374416.2022.2051524

Del Campo, N., Chamberlain, S. R., Sahakian, B. J., & Robbins, T. W. (2011). The roles of dopamine and noradrenaline in the pathophysiology and treatment of attention-deficit/hyperactivity disorder. *Biological Psychiatry*, *69*(12), e145–e157. https://doi.org/10.1016/j.biopsych.2011.02.036

Demontis, D., Walters, R. K., Martin, J., Mattheisen, M., Als, T. D., Agerbo, E., … Engel, M. (2019). Discovery of the first genome-wide significant risk loci for attention deficit/hyperactivity disorder. *Nature Genetics*, *51*(1), 63–75. https://doi.org/10.1038/s41588-018-0269-7. Epub 2018 Nov 26. PMID: 30478444; PMCID: PMC6481311.

Diamond, A. (2013). Executive functions. *Annual Review of Psychology*, *64*, 135–168. https://doi.org/10.1146/annurev-psych-113011-143750

Doshi, J. A., Hodgkins, P., Kahle, J., Sikirica, V., Cangelosi, M. J., Setyawan, J., … Neumann, P. J. (2012). Economic impact of childhood and adult attention-deficit/hyperactivity disorder in the United States. *Journal of the American Academy of Child & Adolescent Psychiatry*, *51*(10), 990–1002. e2. https://doi.org/10.1016/j.jaac.2012.07.008

Evans, S. W., Langberg, J. M., Schultz, B. K., Vaughn, A., Altaye, M., Marshall, S. A., & Zoromski, A. K. (2016). Evaluation of a school-based treatment program for young adolescents with ADHD. *Journal of Consulting & Clinical Psychology*, *84*(1), 15–30. https://doi.org/10.1037/ccp0000057

Evans, S. W., Owens, J. S., Wymbs, B. T., & Ray, A. R. (2018). Evidence-based psychosocial treatments for children and adolescents with attention deficit/hyperactivity disorder. *Journal of Clinical Child & Adolescent Psychology*, *47*(2), 157–198. https://doi.org/10.1080/15374416.2017.1390757

Faraone, S. V., Asherson, P., Banaschewski, T., Biederman, J., Buitelaar, J. K., Ramos-Quiroga, J. A., . . . Franke, B. (2015). Attention-deficit/hyperactivity disorder. *Nat Rev Dis Primers* Aug 6;1:15020. doi: 10.1038/nrdp.2015.20. PMID: 27189265.

Faraone, S. V. (2018). The pharmacology of amphetamine and methylphenidate: Relevance to the neurobiology of attention-deficit/hyperactivity disorder and other psychiatric comorbidities. *Neuroscience and Biobehavioral Reviews*, *87*, 255–270. https://doi.org/10.1016/j.neubiorev.2018.02.001

Faraone, S. V., & Larsson, H. (2019). Genetics of attention deficit hyperactivity disorder. *Molecular Psychiatry*, *24*(4), 562–575. https://doi.org/10.1038/s41380-018-0070-0

Fogler, J. M., Burke, D., Lynch, J., Barbaresi, W. J., & Chan, E. (2017). Topical review: Transitional services for teens and young adults with attention-deficit hyperactivity disorder: A process map and proposed model to overcoming barriers to care. *Journal of Pediatric Psychology*, *42*(10), 1108–1113. https://doi.org/1093/jpepsy/jsx102

Fogler, J. M., Weaver, A. L., Katusic, S., Voigt, R. G., & Barbaresi, W. J. (2020). Recalled experiences of bullying and victimization in a longitudinal, population-based birth cohort: The influence of ADHD and co-occurring psychiatric disorder. *Journal of Attention Disorders* 1087054720969981. https://doi.org/10.1177/1087054720969981. Epub ahead of print.

Friedman, N. P., Miyake, A., Altamirano, L. J., Corley, R. P., Young, S. E., Rhea, S. A., & Hewitt, J. K. (2016). Stability and change in executive function abilities from late adolescence to early adulthood: A longitudinal twin study. *Developmental Psychology*, *52*(2), 326–340. https://doi.org/10.1037/dev0000075

Froehlich, T., Fogler, J., Barbaresi, W., Elsayed, N., Evans, S., & Chan, E. (2018). Using ADHD medications to treat children with co-existing ADHD and reading disorders: A systematic review. *Clinical Pharmacology & Therapeutics, 104*(4), 619–637. https://doi.org/10.1002/cpt.1192

Greenhill, L., Kollins, S., Abikoff, H., McCracken, J., Riddle, M., Swanson, J., ... Cooper, T. (2006). Efficacy and safety of immediate-release methylphenidate treatment for preschoolers with ADHD. *Journal of the American Academy of Child & Adolescent Psychiatry, 45*, 1284–1293. https://doi.org/10.1097/01.chi.0000235077.32661.61

Harris, M. N., Voigt, R. G., Barbaresi, W. J., Voge, G. A., Killian, J. M., Weaver, A. L., ... Slavica K. Katusic, S. K. (2013). ADHD and learning disabilities in former late preterm infants: A population-based birth cohort. *Pediatrics, 132*(3), e630–e636. https://doi.org/10.1542/peds.2012-3588

Harrison, J. R., Bunford, N., Evans, S. W., & Owens, J. S. (2013). Educational accommodations for students with behavioral challenges: A systematic review of the literature. *Review of Educational Research, 83*(4), 551–597. https://doi.org/10.3102/0034654313497517

Harstad, E. B., Katusic, S., Sideridis, G., Weaver, A. L., Voigt, R. G., & Barbaresi, W. J. (2020). Children with ADHD are at risk for a broad array of adverse adult outcomes that cross functional domains: Results from a population-based birth cohort study. *Journal of Attention Disorders*. 1087054720964578.

Harstad, E. B., Weaver, A. L., Katusic, S. K., Colligan, R. C., Kumar, S., Chan, E., . . . Barbaresi, W. J. (2014). ADHD, stimulant treatment, and growth: A longitudinal study. *Pediatrics, 134*(4), e935–e944. https://doi.org/10.1542/peds.2014-0428

Hoogman, M., Bralten, J., Hibar, D. P., Mennes, M., Zwiers, M. P., Schweren, L. S. J., ... Franke, B. (2017). Subcortical brain volume differences in participants with attention deficit hyperactivity disorder in children and adults: A cross-sectional mega-analysis. *Lancet Psychiatry, 4*(4), 310–319. https://doi.org/10.1016/S2215-0366(17)30049-4

Kasparek, T., Theiner, P., & Filova, A. (2015). Neurobiology of ADHD from childhood to adulthood: Findings of imaging methods. *Journal of Attention Disorders, 19*(11), 931–943. https://doi.org/10.1177/1087054713505322

Katusic, M. Z., Voigt, R. G., Colligan, R. C., Weaver, A. L., & Barbaresi, W. J. (2011). Attention-deficit/hyperactivity disorder in children with high IQ: Results from a population-based study. *Journal of Developmental & Behavioral Pediatrics, 32*, 103–109.

Law, E. C., Sideridis, G. D., Prock, L. A., & Sheridan, M. A. (2014). Attention-deficit/hyperactivity disorder in young children: Predictors of diagnostic stability. *Pediatrics, 133*(4), 659–667. https://doi.org/10.1542/peds.2013-3433

Lewandowski, L. J., Lovett, B. J., Codding, R. S., & Gordon, M. (2008). Symptoms of ADHD and academic concerns in college students with and without ADHD diagnoses. *Journal of Attention Disorders, 12*(2), 156–161. https://doi.org/10.1177/1087054707310882

Mahone, E. M., & Denckla, M. B. (2017). Attention-deficit/hyperactivity disorder: A historical neuropsychological perspective. *Journal of the International Neuropsychological Society, 23*(9-10), 916–929. https://doi.org/10.1017/S1355617717000807

Mahone, E. M., Hagelthorn, K. M., Cutting, L. E., Schuerholz, L. J., Pelletier, S. F., Rawlins, C., Denckla, M. B. (2002). Effects of IQ on executive function measures in children with ADHD. *Child Neuropsychology, 8*(1), 52–65. https://doi.org/10.1076/chin.8.1.52.8719

Martinez-Badía, J., & Martinez-Raga, J. (2015). Who says this is a modern disorder? The early history of attention deficit hyperactivity disorder. *World Journal of Psychiatry, 5*(4), 379–386. https://doi.org/10.5498/wjp.v5.i4.379

Miyake, A., & Friedman, N. P. (2012). The nature and organization of individual differences in executive functions: Four general conclusions. *Current Directions in Psychological Science, 21*(1), 8–14. https://doi.org/10.1177/0963721411429458

The MTA Cooperative Group. (1999). A 14-month randomized clinical trial of treatment strategies for attention-deficit/hyperactivity disorder. *Archives of General Psychiatry, 56*(12), 1073–1086. https://doi.org/10.1001/archpsyc.56.12.1073

Nigg, J. T. (2017a). Annual research review: On the relations among self-regulation, self-control, executive functioning, effortful control, cognitive control, impulsivity, risk-taking, and inhibition for developmental psychopathology. *Journal of Child Psychology & Psychiatry, 58*(4), 361–383. https://doi.org/10.1111/jcpp.12675

Nigg, J. (2017b). Attention-deficit/hyperactivity disorder. In T. P. Beauchaine & S. P. Hinshaw (Eds.), *Child and adolescent psychopathology* (3rd ed., pp. 407–448). Wiley.

Pelham, W. E., Jr., & Altszuler, A. R. (2020). Combined treatment for children with attention-deficit/hyperactivity disorder: Brief history, the multimodal treatment for attention-deficit/hyperactivity disorder study, and the past 20 years of research. *Journa of Developmental & Behavioral Pediatrics, 41*(2), S88–S98. https://doi.org/10.1097/DBP.0000000000000777

Roberts, B. A., Martel, M. M., & Nigg, J. T. (2017). Are there executive dysfunction subtypes within ADHD? *Journal of Attention Disorders, 21*(4), 284–293. https://doi.org/10.1177/1087054713510349

Sanfratello, L., Caprihan, A., Stephen, J. M., Knoefel, J. E., Adair, J. C., Qualls, C., ... Aine, C. J. (2014). Same task, different strategies: How brain networks can be influenced by memory strategy. *Human Brain Mapping, 35*(10), 5127–5140. https://doi.org/10.1002/hbm.22538

Shaw, P., Eckstrand, K., Sharp, W., Blumenthal, J., Lerch, J. P., Greenstein, D., ... Rapoport, J. L. (2007). Attention-deficit/hyperactivity disorder is characterized by a delay in cortical maturation. *Proceedings of the National Academy of Science U.S.A., 104*(49), 19649–19654. https://doi.org/10.1073/pnas.0707741104

Shaw, P., Lerch, J., Greenstein, D., Sharp, W., Clasen, L., Evans, A., ... Rapoport, J. (2006). Longitudinal mapping of cortical thickness and clinical outcome in children and adolescents with attention-deficit/hyperactivity disorder. *Archives of General Psychiatry, 63*(5), 540–549. https://doi.org/10.1001/archpsyc.63.5.540

Shaw, P., Malek, M., Watson, B., Sharp, W., Evans, A., & Greenstein, D. (2012). Development of cortical surface area and gyrification in attention-deficit/hyperactivity disorder. *Biological Psychiatry, 72*(3), 191–197. https://doi.org/10.1016/j.biopsych.2012.01.031

Shaw, P., Sharp, W. S., Morrison, M., Eckstrand, K., Greenstein, D. K., Clasen. L. S., ... Rapoport, J. L. (2009). Psychostimulant treatment and the developing cortex in attention deficit hyperactivity disorder. *American Journal of Psychiatry, 166*(1), 58–63. https://doi.org/10.1176/appi.ajp.2008.08050781

Sibley, M. H., Graziano, P. A., Kuriyan, A. B., Coxe, S., Pelham, W. E., Rodriguez, L., ... Ward, A. (2016). Parent-teen behavior therapy + motivational interviewing for adolescents with

ADHD. *Journal of Consulting & Clinical Psychology*, *84*(8), 699–712. https://doi.org/10.1037/ccp0000106

Swanson, J. M., Arnold, L. E., Molina, B. S. G., Sibley, M. H., Hechtman, L. T., Hinshaw, S. P., … MTA Cooperative Group. (2017). Young adult outcomes in the follow-up of the multimodal treatment study of attention-deficit/hyperactivity disorder: symptom persistence, source discrepancy, and height suppression. *Journal of Child Psychology & Psychiatry*, *58*(6), 663–678. https://doi.org/10.1111/jcpp.12684

Tobin, R. M., & Graziano, W. G. (2009). Delay of gratification: A review of fifty years of regulation research. In R. H. Hoyle (Ed.), *Handbook of personality and self-regulation* (pp. 47–83). John Wiley & Sons.

Voigt, R. G., Barbaresi, W. J., Colligan, R. C., Weaver, A. L., & Katusic, S. K. (2006). Developmental dissociation, deviance, and delay: occurrence of attention-deficit-hyperactivity disorder in individuals with and without borderline-to-mild intellectual disability. *Developmental Medicine & Child Neurology*, *48*(10), 831–835.

Wolraich, M. L., Hagan, J. F., Allan, C., Chan, E., Davison, D., Earls, M., … Zurhellen, W. (2019). Clinical practice guideline for the diagnosis, evaluation, and treatment of attention-deficit/hyperactivity disorder in children and adolescents. *Pediatrics*, *144*(4).

Zimmerman, D. L., Ownsworth, T., O'Donovan, A., Roberts, J., & Gullo, M. J. (2016). Independence of hot and cold executive function deficits in high-functioning adults with autism spectrum disorder. *Frontiers of Human Neuroscience*, *10*(24). https://doi.org/10.3389/fnhum.2016.00024

47

Learning Disabilities

Nadine Gaab, Marie Reilly, and Eric Tridas

For additional material related to the content of this chapter, please see Chapters 46, 86, and 113.

VIGNETTE

Lucas is a 9-year-old boy who was born after an uncomplicated, full-term pregnancy and delivery. He has experienced no health problems. Lucas lives at home with his parents and three siblings. His parents completed high school. His mother is a schoolbus driver and his father works for a landscaping company. There is no known diagnosis of a learning disability in his family, but his father had an individualized education plan (IEP) for part of his K-12 education through which he received reading support.

Lucas presents with a longstanding history of challenges with reading. His parents first became concerned about his development in preschool when his teacher noted that while he had a firm grasp of prenumeric concepts, he had difficulty learning the alphabet and its associated letter sounds. As a result, his parents continued to monitor his development closely. In kindergarten Lucas' parents noted deficits in phonological awareness skills despite ongoing work to strengthen these skills in school and at home. Due to these challenges, as well as concerns regarding immaturity, Lucas was retained in kindergarten.

In the first grade Lucas began receiving response to intervention (RTI) reading support, with which he made modest progress. Due to concerns about inattention in the school setting, his pediatrician also started Lucas on extended-release methylphenidate; while this has improved his focus, to some degree, his parents report that Lucas' reading skills remain below grade level.

Lucas parents question whether Lucas has a learning disability and how they can best advocate for him in the school setting. A friend has recommended vision training, so his family would also like a referral to a provider who can address eye tracking.

BACKGROUND, DEFINITIONS, AND SYMPTOMATOLOGY OF LEARNING DISORDERS

Education attainment, which is highly dependent on proficiency in reading, writing, and/or mathematics, is a strong predictor of overall health and longevity (Johnston, 2019; Sanfilippo et al., 2020). These basic academic skills are recognized determinants of health outcomes and have been linked to mental health and indices of educational, vocational, economic, and social success (Irwin, Siddiqi, & Hertzman, 2007). Learning disorders/disabilities (LDs) are commonly referred to as a category of disorders that affect the acquisition, understanding, and/or retention of information taught in formal education settings and can affect both verbal and nonverbal information. This chapter will provide an overview about LDs, including definitions, epidemiology, etiology, coexisting conditions, treatment, prevention, laws impacting a child's education, and the transition to postsecondary education and adult life.

Unfortunately, among the various stakeholders working with individuals with LDs there are numerous different labels in use for the identification and classification of the various LDs. Furthermore, research studies often use a variety of different labels, and therefore the behavioral characteristics/symptomatology of the research participants is often unclear. For the purposes of this chapter, we will use the *Diagnostic and Statistical Manual of Mental Disorders*, fifth edition (*DSM-5*; American Psychiatric Association [APA], 2013) nosology, but Table 47.1 gives an overview of the various labels used to characterize/categorize a child's struggle in the domain of learning. In addition, for the purposes of this chapter we will use the terms *learning disorder* and *learning disability* interchangeably.

The *DSM-5* classifies specific LDs as neurodevelopmental disorders, defined as "a group of conditions with onset in the developmental period" that result in impairment in "personal, social academic, or occupational functioning" (APA, 2013, p. 7). LDs have a neurobiological etiology and are heritable; however, behavioral/psychosocial and environmental factors can significantly influence their clinical manifestation. Children are not diagnosed with LD if their learning challenges are caused by intellectual impairment, sensory deficits, or lack of instruction. To fulfill all of the diagnostic criteria, the symptoms that define LD must be present for more than 6 months despite academic interventions. LD can be classified by impairment in reading, writing, and/or mathematics.

Specific Learning Disorder/Disability With Impairment in Reading

Specific LD with impairment in reading (LD-R) is the most common type, accounting for 80% of LDs (Shaywitz, 2004). Despite its neurobiological etiology, reading is not a typical biological process; it must be taught explicitly. Reading can be generally described as the ability to perceive a series of written symbols and decode their meaning. Gough and Tunmer

TABLE 47.1 Common Labels for Children and Adults With Learning Disabilities

SLD With Impairment in Reading (*DSM-5*)	SLD with Impairment in Written Expression (*DSM-5*)	SLD With Impairment in Mathematics (*DSM-5*)
Note use the term *disability* and *disorder* interchangeably.		
Word reading Accuracy/developmental dyslexia	Spelling	Numerosity, memorization of arithmetic facts, accurate or fluent calculation Developmental dyscalculia
• Word reading deficit • Word blindness • Word-level reading disability • Alexia		• SLD in arithmetic calculation • Acalculia
Reading rate or fluency	Grammar and punctuation accuracy, clarity, or organization	Accurate math reasoning
Reading comprehension	• Specific learning disorder in written expression • Specific written expression disability	
• Specific reading comprehension deficit • Reading difficulty • Reading disorder		
	Developmental coordination disorder	
	• Dysgraphia • Agraphia	

DSM-5, Diagnostic and Statistical Manual of Mental Disorders, fifth edition; *SLD*, specific learning disability.

(1986) summarized the process of successful reading development with a mathematical formula called the Simple View of Reading. This formula describes the required functions for reading. The equation reads as follows: $D \times LC = R$. In this formula, D indicates decoding; LC, linguistic comprehension; R, reading. Decoding can be described as the mechanics of reading and requires a variety of skills such as phonological/phonemic awareness, which is the ability to manipulate sounds of the language of instruction (e.g., deciding whether two words rhyme, deleting a phoneme, or blending phonemes), grapheme-phoneme correspondence, and the recognition of sight words. Over the time course of learning to read, these mechanics of learning to read become increasingly automatic, leading to reading fluency. However, a child who has mastered the mechanics of reading can still struggle with reading fluency and comprehension due to inadequate language skills. To comprehend the decoded words and to read sentences fluently, vocabulary, listening comprehension, and other language skills are required. These oral language skills are critical for successful reading development and become increasingly strategic over the developmental time course. This concept of two essential strands important for successful reading development has been outlined by Scarborough's (2001) reading rope (Fig. 47.1).

TABLE 47.2 US Organizational Resources for Learning Disability for Clinicians, Educators, and Families

Organization	Website
The National Joint Committee on Learning Disabilities	www.NJCLD.org
The International Dyslexia Association	www.dyslexiaida.org
Learning Disability Association of America	www.ldaamerica.org
National Center for Learning Disabilities	www.NCLD.org
National Center on Improving Literacy	www.improvingliteracy.org
National Center for Intensive Intervention	www.intensiveintervention.org

Furthermore, there are numerous international and country-specific organizations.

Children who are struggling with reading are broadly classified under LD-R. Among these, developmental dyslexia affects the mechanics of reading and is characterized by difficulties with accurate and/or fluent word reading, as well as

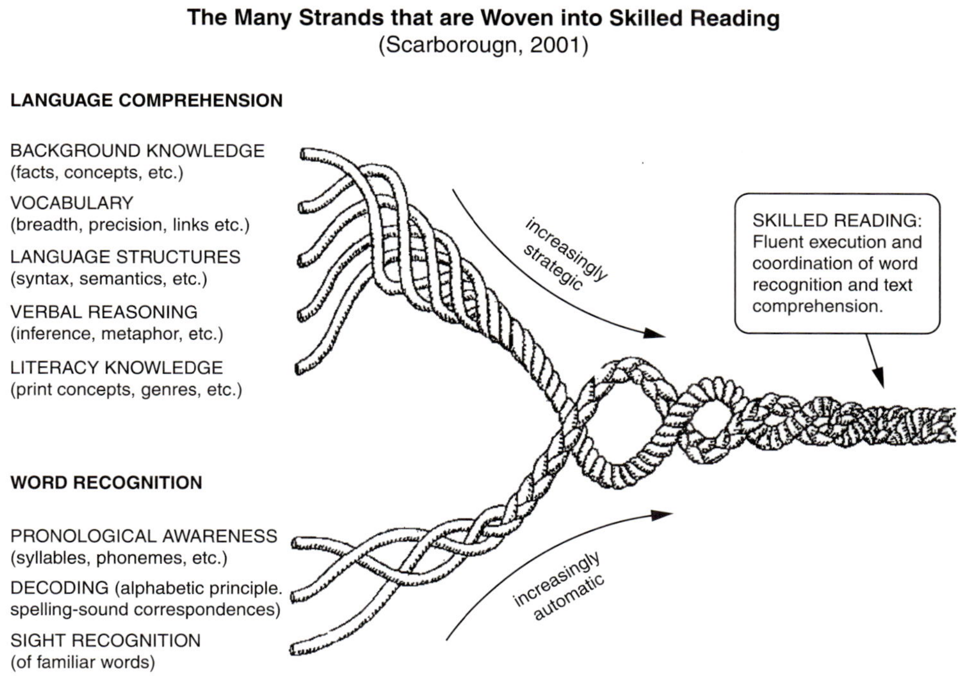

Fig. 47.1 The Scarborough reading rope.

poor spelling and decoding abilities (International Dyslexia Association, 2002). Children who show average word reading abilities but struggle with reading fluency or reading comprehension are usually not considered as having a diagnosis of developmental dyslexia, but they certainly fit the criteria for LD-R. However, children with dyslexia can show secondary deficits in fluency and comprehension that primarily stems from their underlying word reading deficits. Furthermore, dyslexia or LD-R cannot be explained by vision or hearing deficits, lack of motivation, or educational opportunities.

Specific Learning Disorder/Disability With Impairment in Written Expression

Children can also suffer from LD with impairment in written expression (LD-W), characterized by specific deficits in spelling accuracy, grammar and punctuation accuracy, and clarity or organization of written expression. Like reading disorders, children with LD-w can manifest impairment at the word level (spelling), at the content/language level (generating text), or both. Children with difficulty in spelling are likely to experience difficulties with word attack skills as they require similar skills. Spelling (encoding) and word attack skills (decoding) are two sides of the same coin, and they are usually present together in individuals diagnosed with dyslexia. Handwriting difficulties may also impact written output in children with LD-W. Although such children would more appropriately be classified as having a developmental coordination disorder, they are also often diagnosed with dysgraphia. A child who is experiencing difficulties with language skills will likely have challenges with written expression skills (e.g., semantics, general and topical knowledge, and genre and text structure).

Specific Learning Disorder/Disability With Impairment in Mathematics

Children who are exhibiting an LD with impairment in mathematics (LD-M) can be broadly characterized as having difficulties with the mechanics of mathematical skills, namely computational skills (arithmetic) and/or problem-solving abilities (mathematics). The latter tends to be strongly associated with difficulties in language and executive functioning (Bull & Lee, 2014). As with other LDs, *DSM-5* categorizes LD-M by the impairment associated with specific functions such as number sense (numerosity), memorization of math facts, accurate or fluent calculation, and accurate mathematical reasoning. The skill deficits in mathematics disorders can impact computation (e.g., numerosity, memorization, and fluency) and the application of those skills. Numerosity, or number sense, allows us to quantify elements in our environment without counting, estimate, and understand concepts such as more or less, big and small, etc. (De Smedt, Noël, Gilmore, & Ansari, 2013). Developmental dyscalculia is a specific mathematics LD, which mainly affects the acquisition of grade-level arithmetic skills (computation). It is defined as an impairment in learning basic arithmetic facts and performing accurate and fluent arithmetic operations (Kucian & von Aster, 2015). Cognitive difficulties may further include visual-spatial deficits or deficits in working memory or attention. It is important to note that language and reading skills are also strongly linked to academic performance in arithmetic and mathematics (e.g., for word problems or for understanding instructions) and can affect the acquisition of these skills (Moll, Landerl, Snowling, & Schulte-Körne, 2019).

In the past LDs were diagnosed in the context of a discrepancy model. For dyslexia this required that the assessed reading ability be at least 1 SD below a child's general cognitive ability index (e.g., IQ). A similar model was in place for dyscalculia. However, research has shown that dyslexia can occur independently of general cognitive abilities and that the discrepancy model should not be considered when making diagnostic decisions.

Furthermore, there is a misconception that individuals with LDs all exhibit certain strengths unique to individuals with LDs (such as entrepreneurship, above-average visuospatial skills). There is no evidence for such a common shared strength, and this myth can significantly exacerbate social-emotional problems (e.g., "I am not even good at having an LD"). It is important to emphasize that all children are unique and all have their individual strengths and weaknesses.

Nonverbal Learning Disability

The diagnosis of a nonverbal LD is used to describe a developmental profile that is notable for deficits in social interactions, nonverbal problem solving, visuospatial skills, motor coordination, reading comprehension, and math skills (Handler & Fierson, 2011). Individuals with nonverbal LDs often have strengths in their verbal abilities (Handler & Fierson, 2011). Of note, nonverbal LD is not included in the *DSM-5* and is therefore often not recognized in the same way as specific LDs are recognized; however, clinicians in developmental-behavioral pediatrics should be familiar with the general developmental profile associated with a nonverbal LD. At the time of this publication there is some controversy within the field as to the validity and merit of a nonverbal LD as a discrete entity.

EPIDEMIOLOGY AND ETIOLOGY

The National Center for Learning Disabilities (2017) estimates that roughly one in five children are suffering from LD. The National Assessment of Educational Progress (2019) indicated that approximately 60% of US fourth and eighth graders performed below proficient in reading and mathematics skills, but not all of these children meet criteria for a diagnosis of LD. Reading, arithmetic, and writing skills serve many everyday functions and provide a foundation for learning more advanced competencies. LDs are a widely recognized determinant of health and, if untreated, are likely to persist into adulthood. Individuals with LD-R, LD-W, or LD-M are less likely to enroll in college or other postsecondary education programs, have an increased risk of unemployment, and are more likely to be incarcerated. Furthermore, these individuals are at a greater risk for developing internalizing symptoms and externalizing behaviors (Hendren, Haft, Black, White, & Hoeft, 2018). LD-R and LD-M can even influence medical decision making, as comprehending written materials related to an individual's care or understanding of basic arithmetic concepts is often required to make informed decisions (e.g., percentage of risk, calculating medication doses) (Johnston, 2019). In summary, reading, writing, and arithmetic skills have a significant effect on individuals' wellbeing, education, and vocation and are crucial skills for functioning in modern society.

It has been estimated that 7% to 10% of children have dyslexia (Grigorenko et al., 2020). It is important to note that the prevalence of dyslexia is lower for languages that have a higher orthographic transparency (e.g., Spanish and Italian). The prevalence of dyscalculia has been reported to be 3% to 6% (Kaufmann & von Aster, 2012). While some studies claim that more boys are affected by reading disorders, the opposite has been claimed for dyscalculia. However, these gender differences remain controversial, and opposite findings have also been reported. The prevalence of LD-W has been estimated at 6% to 14%, but this is strongly influenced by the different labels and their characterizing symptomatology (Slavica, Katusic, Colligan, Weaver, & Barbaresi, 2009), and the prevalence in boys has been reported to be two to three times higher than for girls.

Learning disabilities are heritable, with a risk of reoccurrence of up to 50% to 60% in families with an affected member (first degree) (Willcutt et al., 2010). Several dyslexia susceptibility genes have been identified, but this remains an active area of research (Grigorenko et al., 2020). Multivariant genetic studies indicate high correlations between reading and arithmetic skills among twins, suggesting a substantial overlap between genes associated with these two skills (Daucourt, Erbeli, Little, Haughbrook, & Hart, 2020). For example, in a sample of twins in which at least one experienced an LD-R, 68% of monozygotic twins and 40% of dizygotic twins showed LD-R in one twin and LD-M in the other twin (Light & DeFries, 1995).

It is important to note that despite the heritability of LDs, their etiology is multifaceted and includes genetic, perceptual, cognitive, neurobiological, and environmental factors (Ozernov-Palchik, Yu, Gaab, & Wang, 2016). Various studies have reported atypical brain characteristics in individuals with dyslexia and/or dyscalculia. For instance, functional MRI (fMRI) studies have indicated that reading is primarily supported by a left hemispheric brain network that includes the inferior frontal, superior temporal, temporoparietal, and occipitotemporal cortices (Ozernov-Palchik & Gaab, 2016; Ozernov-Palchik et al., 2016). As a group, individuals with dyslexia and/or LD-R show structural and functional atypicalities in the reading network. This includes reports of reduced gray matter volume, alterations in white matter tracts, hypoactivation in response to prereading- and reading-related fMRI tasks, and reduced functional connectivity between key areas of the reading network (see Ozernov-Palchik et al., 2016 for a summary). Importantly, these differences in brain structure and function characteristic of LD-R and dyslexia can be observed before the start of formal reading instruction in educational contexts, indicating that at least some of these brain atypicalities are not a result of struggling with learning to read but rather represents a biological disposition (Ozernov-Palchik & Gaab, 2016; Ozernov-Palchik et al., 2016). In other words children are entering their first day of school with a brain that is less equipped to learn to read, which underlines the importance of early identification and intervention to prevent long-term reading impairments. Furthermore, several studies have reported unique brain atypicalities in children with specific reading comprehension deficits (a deficit within the LD-R category) suggesting unique and shared etiologies between specific word reading and specific reading comprehension difficulties (Bailey, Hoeft, Aboud, & Cutting, 2016).

Studies examining the brain characteristics of LD-M and dyscalculia have shown unique alterations in the brain networks supporting numeric cognition and arithmetic. Activation in bilateral regions of the intraparietal sulcus has been shown to be a key neural correlate of numeric cognition, which has been reported as early as infancy and preschool years (Hyde & Spelke, 2011). Furthermore, studies comparing typically developing children and children with LD-M and dyscalculia during arithmetic performance reported differences in parietal, prefrontal, and occipital-temporal regions with activation patterns modulated by notation, task complexity, and operation (addition vs. subtraction) (Ashkenazi, Rosenberg-Lee, Tenison, & Menon, 2012). Structural imaging studies suggest children with dyscalculia and LD-M have characteristic reductions in gray matter volume in a variety of brain regions, including the parietal cortex, inferior frontal, and parahippocampal gyrus (Matejko & Ansari, 2015), as well as alterations in white matter tracts (Matejko, Price, Mazzocco, & Ansari, 2013). Unfortunately, the neural correlates of LD-W are currently understudied.

COEXISTING CONDITIONS

Children with LD are also at risk for a number of coexisting conditions ranging from attention-deficit/hyperactivity disorder (ADHD) to mental health concerns to a second or third LD. There is significant comorbidity of LD-M with language disorders (25%), dyslexia (30%–70%), and ADHD (18%) (McGrath, Peterson, & Pennington, 2020). Given evidence that reading and arithmetic skills are strongly linked at cognitive, genetic, and neurocognitive levels, it is not surprising that LD-M and LD-R tend to cooccur, and the rates of cooccurrence seem to increase with age and grade level (Moll et al., 2019). Because of the increased risk of various coexisting conditions, it is critical that clinicians assess conditions with LD for these conditions and intervene quickly when they present additional challenges and impairments.

Attention-Deficit/Hyperactivity Disorder

ADHD is a developmental disorder that is notable for impairment related to inattention and/or hyperactivity impulsivity typically at both home and school (see Chapter 46). The connection between ADHD and LD is well established. Recent studies suggest that 20% to 40% of children with ADHD also have dyslexia, and a combination of shared and distinctive brain alterations between dyslexia and ADHD have been identified (Langer, Benjamin, Becker, & Gaab, 2019). Coexisting ADHD is also common with disorders of written expression. It is important to note that a child experiencing ADHD-related impairment in the school setting may experience academic difficulties across multiple subjects and settings, whereas a child with LD might present with an isolated deficit in reading, writing, or math. However, diffuse academic impairment across subjects can also be seen in children with multiple LDs. Nevertheless, inadequate control of ADHD symptoms during the school day should also enter diagnostic consideration.

Lucas, from the chapter-opening vignette, has an undiagnosed LD that may be either causing or contributing to his reported symptoms regarding inattention during the school day. It is important to recognize that undiagnosed or undertreated LDs can result in inattention, causing some to think that ADHD may also be present. It is certainly possible, and perhaps likely, that Lucas may also have ADHD given that they often coexist. Therefore a next clinical step might be to obtain parents' and teachers' reports of ADHD symptoms to clarify his profile.

Speech and Language Disorders

Children with speech and language disorders are at high risk of developing LDs, like LD-R/dyslexia and LD-W (see Chapter 44). The underlying mechanisms are thought to stem from factors related to a common etiology as well as neurocognitive differences. There is significant overlap between children with language disorders and children with dyslexia such that approximately half of children with dyslexia have a cooccurring language disorder and half of children with a language disorder have cooccurring dyslexia. It is also important to note that academic instruction is largely language mediated, which may exacerbate the vulnerabilities experienced by individuals with speech and language disorders. Furthermore, children who are dialect speakers or who are still learning the language of instruction (Hoff, 2013) have an increased risk for developing reading difficulties. This should be strongly considered in the process of early identification, diagnoses, and interventions.

Other Specific Learning Disorders

As mentioned, the presence of one LD does not preclude the possibility of another. In fact, children with dyscalculia and LD-W are more likely to have coexisting dyslexia than children without either of these conditions (Moll et al., 2019). Further, 30% to 47% of children with writing challenges also experience reading challenges (Chung, Patel, & Nizami, 2020). As previously discussed, children with dyslexia may experience math-related challenges due to difficulty reading word problems. This impairment alone would not be consistent with the presence of a coexisting LD in math; rather, this scenario is more indicative of the wide-reaching nature of reading and/or oral language impairment on a child's school functioning.

Autism Spectrum Disorder

Children with an autism spectrum disorder have been reported to be at increased risk of dyslexia. In the author's clinical experience children with autism can also experience deficits in reading comprehension related to challenges consistently understanding what a character might be feeling or what their motivation may be (e.g., social pragmatics). This likely stems from deficits in theory of mind and pragmatic language skills related to their diagnosis of autism (see Chapter 41). Writing has also been identified as an area in which individuals with autism spectrum disorders are at risk (Chung et al., 2020).

Similar to the diagnostic process associated with ADHD and learning, children with autism may experience learning challenges related to the presence of a comorbid LD or the presence of impairing behaviors that interfere with the process of learning. A careful history elucidating behavioral functioning and need for supports in the school setting may help clarify this potential concern.

Developmental Coordination Disorder

Developmental coordination disorder (DCD) is a condition that is characterized by deficits in motor skills that can result in impairment in areas such as academics (see Chapter 71). These deficits can include motor incoordination, impaired motor planning, and poor handwriting. Around half of children with DCD experience impaired writing skills (Chung et al., 2020). Further, up to 85% of children with dyspraxia/LD-W/DCD also have dyslexia (Pauc, 2005).

Mental Health Conditions

LDs can negatively impact mental health beginning at a young age. Children with dyslexia may be perceived as "lazy" or "stupid" when, in truth, their reading difficulties stem from an underlying disorder. Analogously, children with LD report experiencing lower self-esteem than their peers without LDs (Stein, Blum, & Barbaresi, 2011). Adolescents with LDs are also at increased risk of depression, suicidal ideation and attempts, and general risk-taking behavior (Stein et al., 2011). In general, children with dyslexia have been found to be at increased risk of both generalized anxiety and depression (Hendren et al., 2018). Externalizing conditions that may occur with dyslexia include conduct disorder and oppositional defiant disorder. Congruently, children who are more skilled at reading are less likely to be incarcerated (Cree, Kay, & Steward, 2012). Failure to recognize psychiatric comorbidity and to address coexisting mental health concerns can significantly worsen learning outcomes (Hendren et al., 2018).

Social Impairment

Qualitative studies of individuals with LD have been notable for self-reported social challenges related to factors that include "feeling different" or having "an invisible disability" (Stein et al., 2011). It is also important to recall that children with developmental differences in general are at higher risk of being bullied than their typical peers. Reported bullying rates among children with developmental differences are likely underestimates for a number of reasons, including those related to shame, difficulty perceiving bullying, and challenges with expressive language. Many children may be hesitant to disclose being bullied unless specifically asked.

Genetic Disorders

Well-described genetic syndromes such as Turner syndrome, Klinefelter syndrome, and neurofibromatosis type 1 can also be associated with LD (Karipidis & Hong, 2020).

DIAGNOSTIC APPROACH

Clinicians working with children should be alert to signs of learning challenges at various ages. In very young children signs concerning for emerging learning challenges include developmental language delays, delayed letter or number recognition, failure to acquire letter-sound correspondence or phonological processing skills, and difficulty counting with one-to-one correspondence. School-age children with LDs may present with signs of increased learning effort, school distress, or school failure (Rimrodt & Lipkin, 2011). Examples of increased learning effort can include complaints that school is boring, school anxiety, class clown behavior, or requiring more time than their peers to complete academic tasks (Rimrodt & Lipkin, 2011). Children experiencing school distress may present with failing grades, frequent school absences/detentions/suspensions, social disengagement, or bullying. Lastly, signs of school failure include grade retention, expulsion, and/or dropping out (Rimrodt & Lipkin, 2011).

Lucas, in the vignette, demonstrated early challenges with letter recognition and phonological processing, which were unaddressed and led to grade retention.

Medical Assessment of Learning Disability

The medical assessment of a child with a potential LD should begin with a detailed developmental history that includes timing of acquisition of developmental milestones, current school day routines (homework, sleep schedule, possible ADHD symptoms, current learning impairment), and a past school history (grade retention, behavioral challenges in the school setting, teacher feedback, and academic progress over time).

A careful past medical history should query prenatal and birth history, potential genetic disorders, sensory deficits, seizures, chronic conditions that may affect school attendance, and medications that can impact cognitive functioning. In addition to obtaining a social history, the family history should assess parental level of education and relatives with learning challenges that can range from grade retention to academic failure.

The family history from the vignette does not include a frank diagnosis of dyslexia but is highly suggestive of this condition. Given the challenges detecting LDs, especially in those who attended school many years ago, information regarding need for school supports and persistent reading challenges in adulthood can be informative.

The physical exam of a child presenting with learning challenges should include close observation of growth parameters or phenotypic differences that might be suggestive of an underlying genetic syndrome that is known to be associated with LD. Clinicians should also rule out vision and hearing deficits and mental health problems (e.g., anxiety or mood disorders) as potential causes of learning impairment.

Psychological Assessment of Learning Disability

The diagnosis of LD in a medical setting usually includes assessment of a child's intellectual and academic functioning by a psychologist using standardized, individually administered measures (see Chapters 85 and 86).

TREATMENT

Educational intervention of LD can be divided into three main approaches: remediation, accommodations, and modifications. Remediation is intended to reduce the performance gap in basic academic skills between the students diagnosed with LD and their peers by strengthening their weaknesses. This is typically provided through specialized instruction taught by special education teachers, certified therapists, speech-language pathologists, and tutors. Other services, including occupational, and physical therapy, are also part of this approach. Most students receiving this type of intervention have an Individualized Educational Plan (IEP) or are receiving services through a multitier system of support (MTSS). Accommodations are intended to prevent discrimination by providing equal access to educational activities (Dragoo & Cole, 2019). Some accommodations may include extended time, preferential sitting, adaptive equipment (text-to-speech/speech-to-text software, keyboarding, graphic organizers, etc.), and individual support (reading or scribing). These accommodations are often provided under Section 504 of the Rehabilitation Act of 1973 and Title II of the Americans with Disabilities Act (Dragoo & Cole, 2019). However, Section 504 also requires the provision of free and appropriate education (FAPE) in K-12 public schools (Barnes, 2021). Finally, schools can provide modifications, such as reducing the volume of work (e.g., the number of math homework problems or books to read). These are typically offered in the elementary and secondary settings but not in postsecondary facilities as they can impact diploma requirements.

The common tenets of effective intervention can be applied to all LDs, but content will vary depending on the type of impairment (reading, writing, or math). The child's RTI will determine how individualized, comprehensive, differentiated, and intense the instruction must be to address all the contributing factors, including coexisting conditions, impacting a specific skill development (Grigorenko et al., 2020).

Dyslexia and Reading Disorders

The treatment of children with dyslexia centers upon early recognition of the disability and the delivery of evidence-based reading intervention. High-quality, evidence-based reading interventions focus on intensive and explicit instruction in areas of reading, including phoneme awareness, the alphabetic principle and phonics, word analysis, fluency, and reading comprehension (Peterson, Pennington, & McGrath, 2018). The International Dyslexia Association coined the term *structured literacy* to refer to this approach to reading instruction. This type of evidence-based teaching requires systematic, explicit instruction (International Dyslexia Association, n.d.). Structured literacy integrates listening, speaking, reading, and writing. It emphasizes the structure of language, including phonology (speech sound system), orthography (writing system), syntax (sentence structure), morphology (meaningful parts of words), semantics (relationships among words), and discourse (organization of spoken and written language). When describing this integrated approach to instruction, the importance of simultaneously addressing content and methodology is stressed. Thus reading interventions should include the foundational skills necessary for reading along with language skills such as vocabulary and comprehension strategies (Peterson et al., 2018). Lovett et al. (2017) demonstrated that the effects of early intervention (first and second grade) resulted in gains that were double when compared with students who began to receive services in the third grade. Older students with reading problems respond best to remediation that emphasizes language and cognitive skills such as vocabulary and comprehension strategies (Peterson et al., 2018). However, they may still benefit from instruction in basic reading mechanics (e.g., phonics and fluency) if they lack these skills.

Visual impairment can certainly affect learning and academic progress. In addition, conditions such as strabismus, amblyopia, convergence and/or focusing deficiencies, and refractive errors can similarly impact learning (Handler & Fierson, 2011). However, there is no evidence to support the theory that eye problems either cause or increase the severity of LDs in general or dyslexia in particular (Handler & Fierson, 2011). There is also no evidence of treatment benefits for recommendations or techniques involving special balancing exercises, fish oils, vision therapy or glasses with tinted lenses, inner ear–improving medications, or the training of primitive reflexes.

Dyscalculia and Math Disorders

Intervention for children with dyscalculia focuses on the delivery of a research-supported math curriculum. These interventions include explicit instruction, skill modeling, practice, and corrective feedback in arithmetic/computational and mathematics skills, such as problem-solving strategies (Peterson et al., 2018). Typical and LD-M students benefit from this approach to instruction, but the child with LD-M requires greater instructional intensity. Children with dyscalculia often benefit from explicit teacher-led instruction coupled with peer-assisted learning (Soares et al., 2018). In addition, they may benefit from elements of teaching such as controlling task difficulty, more intensive elaboration on some topics, and instruction in the small group setting (Soares et al., 2018). The use of manipulatives, computer-based lessons, videos, and hands-on projects have also been found to support math instruction in this population.

Dysgraphia and Writing Disorders

Remediation of writing deficits can vary depending on the age of the child (Chung et al., 2020). For example, intervention for the early school-age child with dysgraphia may focus on development of fine motor skills, including hand coordination, strength, grip control, and writing posture (Chung et al., 2020). These strategies are thought to be most effective in remediating writing challenges when taught in conjunction with orthographic tasks (Chung et al., 2020). Older children and teens with dysgraphia often benefit from explicit instruction in aspects of writing such as planning, drafting, and revising (Chung et al., 2020). In addition to these remedial strategies, students with dysgraphia can benefit from writing accommodations, including keyboarding, spellcheck, and voice-to-text technology as well as writing modifications such as the ability to produce a shorter written product or adjusted grading expectations (Chung et al., 2020).

Children with LD-W can benefit from structured literacy instruction to address their spelling difficulties. Similarly, explicit and systematic instruction in written expression is helpful in addressing these challenges. Reading and writing foundational skills are derived from oral language skills. Strategies that facilitate the development of written expression include structured language activities that are applicable at the word, sentence, and paragraph level (Haynes, Smith, & Laud, 2019). As with other LD interventions, emphasis is placed on developing basic skills combined with higher-level reasoning linguistic concepts (e.g., vocabulary development, syntax, discourse) (Haynes et al., 2019).

LAWS IMPACTING SPECIAL EDUCATION

For more information on the ways that laws impact special eduation, see Chapter 113.

The Individuals With Disabilities Education Act (IDEA)

IDEA is a law that makes a free appropriate public education available to eligible children with disabilities and ensures special education and related services to those children. IDEA regulates the way states and public agencies provide early intervention, special education, and related services. It requires that the local educational agencies (1) evaluate and identify students with LD to ascertain eligibility for services, (2) convene a team, including the parents of the student, to develop an IEP detailing the specific special education and related services to ensure FAPE, and (3) the right to appeal the placement and determination of services through an administrative hearing. In summary, IDEA regulates the educational services provided for eligible students with disabilities and their families and establishes age limits (birth–21 years) (Dragoo & Cole, 2019).

Section 504 of the Rehabilitation Act of 1973

Section 504 provides a broad spectrum of antidiscrimination measures for any qualified individual with a disability, which includes individuals with LD. Thus for students enrolled in K-12 public schools, Section 504 requires that those identified as having a disability are provided with regular and special education services to meet their individual educational needs as adequately as those of typical students. Furthermore, Section 504 provides regulations to ensure adherence to procedures that guarantee FAPE (Barnes, 2021).

Title II of the Americans With Disabilities Act of 1990 (ADA)

ADA provides protection from discrimination similar to Section 504, but unlike Section 504, which applies only to entities receiving federal funds, ADA prohibits discrimination in public and private settings (Dragoo & Cole, 2019). It ensures (1) the provision of accessible facilities and transportation services, (2) delivery of effective communication for persons with disabilities equal to what is provided to the nondisabled population, and (3) available "auxiliary aids and services," such as alternative communication format materials (e.g., braille, sign language interpreters), and assistive technology.

These three laws ensure robust protections and rights for students with disabilities. The major difference between them is that Section 504 and ADA Title II are laws that prohibit the discrimination by ensuring equal access to individuals with disabilities of all ages. In addition, Section 504 ensures that students deemed disabled in K-12 public schools are guaranteed FAPE, procedural safeguards to protect them, and the proper assessment and evaluations to ascertain their disability to develop an educational plan (504 plan, not an IEP). IDEA mandates the provision of special education services (e.g., remediation) to individuals with disabilities from birth through 21 years through an IEP.

PREVENTION

In addition to the neurobiological factors that have been suggested to contribute to the etiology of LDs (see earlier), research studies have focused on the perceptual, language, and cognitive precursors of LDs.

Various longitudinal studies have linked dyslexia to early (and persisting) deficits in phonological and/or phonemic awareness (the ability to manipulate the sounds of language; see earlier). Other identified predictors include mapping sounds onto letters/letter combinations and vice versa (grapheme-phoneme mapping), pseudoword repetition (the ability to repeat orally presented nonsense words), and rapid automatized naming (the ability to quickly retrieve and name a series of highly familiar stimuli arranged in the reading direction), which has been shown to be a strong predictor of later reading fluency (Norton & Wolf, 2012). Furthermore, deficits in oral language comprehension and receptive and expressive vocabulary have been identified as strong predictors of subsequent reading outcomes. These precursors have been detected even before the onset of formal reading instruction (see Ozernov-Palchik & Gaab [2016] for an overview).

Dyscalculia has been related to a core deficit in processing numerosity, but the etiology of dyscalculia has been debated. Similar to dyslexia, several studies suggest a multifactorial approach and not one single cognitive deficit. Precursors of subsequent weaknesses in number recognition and arithmetic have been identified, but these are far less studied than precursors in the domain of reading. These precursors include precision of the approximate number system (ANS), difficulty learning to count, number knowledge, poor memory for numbers, and difficulties with organizing shapes. The ANS has been described as the ability to identify quantities rapidly (e.g., larger/smaller set) (Peterson et al., 2018). Preschoolers' precision of the ANS predicts later school mathematics performance (Mazzocco, Feigenson, & Halberda, 2011), but 6-year-old's number knowledge and not the precision of the ANS has been shown to be the best longitudinal predictor of mathematics performance 1 year later (Göbel, Watson, Lervåg, & Hulme, 2014). A recent metaanalysis reported consistent predictive value for the knowledge of symbolic numbers, but the findings for nonsymbolic formats were very inconsistent (De Smedt et al., 2013). This suggests that the predictive value of the number sense changes over the developmental time course.

It is important to note that a weakness in any of these tasks indicates an increased probability of subsequently developing LDs. Unfortunately, precursors of LD-W have not been reliably identified yet. The fact that longitudinal research studies have identified reliable precursors of LD as early as preschool and the evidence that the brain characteristics of LDs predate the onset of formal education has strong implications for the early identification and prevention of LDs. While most school districts and pediatricians currently operate under a "wait to fail" or "reactive approach" when it comes to learning disabilities (often referred to as the "dyslexia paradox" in the domain of reading), the evidence speaks for a preventive model where children at risk for LDs are identified early and intervention provided during a time of heightened brain plasticity for some of these skills with goal of preventing LDs or decreasing the severity of symptoms (Ozernov-Palchik et al., 2016; Wanzek & Vaughn, 2007).

These approaches have been shown to be successful for the prevention of reading disabilities. For example, using a metaanalytic approach, Wanzek et al. (2013) reported that word reading interventions were significantly more effective for improving reading outcomes when administered in kindergarten and first grade than when they were when administered during later elementary grades. Furthermore, when at-risk beginning readers receive intensive instruction, 56% to 92% of these children across six studies reached the range of average reading ability (Torgesen, 2004). Overall, converging research points to the importance of early and (often) individualized interventions for at-risk students for improving the effectiveness of remediation (Catts, Nielsen, Bridges, Liu, & Bontempo, 2015).

To move from a reactive to a proactive model when it comes to the early identification of children at risk for learning disabilities, it has been suggested that an effective screening approach followed by evidence-based early intervention is the best prevention method (Ozernov-Palchik et al., 2016; Wanzek & Vaughn, 2007). However, while primary care clinicians often screen for ADHD and autism, they usually do not screen for LDs (Sanfilippo et al., 2020). This approach has been justified by the fact that ADHD and autism often require medical interventions, while LDs require interventions in educational settings. However, given the fact that children with LDs have an increased risk for developing internalizing and externalizing problems and show higher incidences of anxiety, depression, and suicidal thoughts, screening in primary care settings should be strongly considered. Furthermore, the early precursors of a reading disability are primarily related to oral language (which includes phonological awareness), and therefore a referral to a speech-language pathologist can be highly effective in aiding the early intervention approach.

It is important to note that numerous states now have legislation that is directly related to the prevention of LDs. For instance, in 2020 over 35 US states had laws that mandate the screening for language-based LDs as early as kindergarten. For an overview of these laws, consult the National Center on Improving Literacy (NCIL). The advocacy and legislative map for the prevention of developmental dyscalculia is years behind that of developmental dyslexia. While a few screeners exist, the screening for developmental dyscalculia is scarce or even nonexistent to date.

It is also of great importance to include individuals who are bilingual or are still learning the language of their formal instruction (e.g., English language learners) in the screening and early identification process since these children are often overlooked (Hoff, 2013). Children are often not identified early since educators may think that it is their English proficiency that causes their reading problems rather than suspecting a language-based LD.

Response to Intervention

With the reauthorization of IDEA in 2004, funding was provided with the goal of offering early intervention services for students at risk of LD. Response to intervention (RTI) has been the predominant approach used to address assessment, instruction, and intervention services of students considered at risk for LD. RTI offers three tiers of educational support to students experiencing reading and other academic difficulties, assigns school personnel to provide the tiered educational support services, and collects and analyzes data to guide intervention and other educational decisions. An MTSS is more comprehensive in scope than RTI as it provides tiered academic, social, and behavioral supports. RTI's primary focus is the tiered provision of academic support services and can be implemented as a component of MTSS. The RTI model of LD identification involves universal screening of all young students for risk factors that predict academic skill failure. This is then followed by the provision of effective, evidence-based academic intervention to those students who are identified as being at risk. This approach requires repeated brief assessments (progress monitoring) over time to gauge the student's response to the intervention. An RTI model bases the identification of LD on a lack of response to evidence-based instruction/intervention as part of a tiered education/intervention approach. Students whose rate of progress over time is unsatisfactory and who fail to meet grade- or age-level expectations despite increasingly intensive instruction through a tiered system (often referred as unexpected underachievement) can be identified as or suspected of having an LD. For example, Miciak and Fletcher (2020) proposed a "hybrid dyslexia identification process" implemented through the MTSS process. Their model recommends collecting data using reading and spelling as specific markers for dyslexia in combination with insufficient response to evidence-based interventions. Thus a student who has reading and spelling challenges and who fails to respond to evidence-based intervention can be classified as having dyslexia. A comprehensive LD evaluation within an RTI model should also rule out other factors as the primary reason for a student's unsatisfactory response. These factors include irregular school attendance, limited English language proficiency, intellectual disability, vision/hearing/motor disabilities, classroom behavioral difficulties, or other environmental, economic, and/or cultural factors. Poor instruction or lack of instruction should also be ruled out prior to determining a student has an LD.

While in theory the approach of RTI as it is proposed offers a practical approach to early identification and intervention of students at risk for LD, the way that it is being currently implemented in the United States is not demonstrating a measurable difference. A report on a study published in 2015 revealed that first-grade students assigned to schools providing RTI services showed a worse academic performance than those in schools not using RTI (Balu et al., 2015). Analysis of the data revealed that many schools are not implementing RTI with the necessary fidelity or "in a manner supported by research and policy" (Fuchs & Fuchs, 2017). Thus using progress monitoring when the instruction is not delivered with sufficient intensity or fidelity may lead to the erroneous interpretation that a student's lack of progress is due to LD when it may be the result of poor instruction and remediation, one of the exclusion criteria as listed earlier.

TRANSITION TO POSTSECONDARY EDUCATION AND ADULT LIFE

Postsecondary Education

Every year thousands of students with LDs graduate from high school. As the job requirements of the US economy are increasingly becoming knowledge based, and the possibility of a higher earning potential increases with the person's educational level, pursuing a postsecondary education has become more crucial. The National Longitudinal Transition Study-2 (NLTS2) by the National Center for Education Statistics (NCES, 2011) reported that most young adults with disabilities (60%) continued to postsecondary education. These findings are comparable to those of their non-LD peers (67%) in the general population. The same study revealed that of those diagnosed with LD, 44% attended community colleges, 32% business or technical school, and 19% 4-year colleges and universities. The completion of postsecondary education was lower for students with LD (41%) than for those in the general population (52%). While 57% completed technical, business, or vocational school programs, 41% completed 2-year college programs. Approximately one-third of students with LD finished their 4-year college/university programs within 8 years of graduating from high school, in contrast with 62% of young adults in the general population (NCES, 2019). Studies indicate that students with LD who spent more time in general education classrooms and participated in career and technical education courses in secondary school had higher rates of on-time graduation, college attendance, and employment than students who did not spend as much time in similar school settings (Joshi & Bouck, 2017). When reviewing these data it is important to consider that in 2018 the NCES reported that of the 203,805 students identified as having LD, 14% dropped out of secondary education and only 79% obtained a regular high school diploma (NCES, 2019).

The postsecondary educational environment that students with disabilities will encounter is dramatically different from the primary and secondary (K-12) setting. For example, students with LD in a postsecondary setting who elect to request accommodations will be required to disclose their disability and provide the necessary documentation to the institution's disability services office. These requirements vary from one institution to another. As such, the young adult with LD must become familiar with the types of support services offered by each institution and the specific documentation requirements. For many of these students, this will be the first time that they must advocate for themselves while transitioning into a new environment with unfamiliar systems and supports. Postsecondary institutions are prohibited by law to inquire about any disability or a student's need for accommodations. As such, it is essential for the students and their parents or guardians to understand the legal and practical considerations to access those services and whether the student will choose to disclose a disability. Some of these considerations include where to find information on services for students with disabilities, what accommodations they may be eligible for, and what documentation is needed.

The laws that apply to students with disabilities in postsecondary education are different from those that regulate education at the elementary and secondary level. Section 504 and ADA Title II continue to prohibit discrimination on the basis of a student having a disability. In contrast, IDEA and Section 504 requirements related to providing special education and a free and appropriated education do not apply in postsecondary educational settings. Thus postsecondary educational institutions must offer appropriate accommodations to guarantee equal access to the content material. There are no legal mandates for them to provide modifications regarding course content or work expectations as might be in an IEP. For example, college students with LD may be allowed assistive technology accommodations such as recorded books and voice-to-text technology; however, they are still expected to read the same number of books and write as many papers as their classmates. Changing these requirements would be considered curriculum modifications. It is critical for students to understand they cannot circumvent academic requirements that the institution deems essential to a specific program by using modifications. In short, postgraduate educational settings will make accommodations, but they will not change expectations.

Employment

The NLTS2 showed that most young adults (63%) with LD were likely to be employed (NCES, 2011). However, their employment status varied depending on their highest level of educational attainment. Those who completed postsecondary education were more likely to be employed (99%) when compared with those who did not finish it (78%) or only completed high school requirements (89%). Most of the young adults with LD work close to 40 hours per week and their wages are comparable to those of their peers in the general population (NCES, 2011). Less than 5% required accommodations by their employers and most (94%) reported being satisfied with their jobs (NCES, 2011).

Criminal Justice System and Learning Disability

It is difficult to obtain prevalence data on children and adults in the criminal justice system diagnosed with LD. However, studies have estimated the rates of LD in the population in juvenile detention facilities as ranging from 13% to 41% (Grigorenko et al., 2015). It is important to remember that 43 million Americans in the general population (21%) are unable to identify information in prose text, follow simple written instructions, or locate numbers to perform simple math operations (NCES, 2019). There are multiple factors beyond LD that can impact literacy, including genetic, environmental (home, school, community), socioeconomic, social competencies, and health problems, and these must be considered when reviewing the statistics.

PRIMARY CARE PROVIDER ROLE AND ESTABLISHING PARTNERSHIPS

Primary care providers (PCPs) are usually the first professionals that parents will consult when their children are experiencing learning problems. Even though learning challenges may seem out of the realm of the traditional PCP role, they can play a significant part in the early identification and management of LD. Health care providers can offer advice to parents/caregivers about further diagnostic and therapeutic measures that may be needed. They can evaluate and manage medical factors that could affect learning such as chronic health conditions, sleep challenges, and common cooccurring conditions (e.g., encopresis and enuresis, ADHD, anxiety, depression). Often, PCPs have established long-term relationships with their patients and their families, which allows them to have a good understanding of the home environment and the community schools that may impact their patients. They can serve in an advocacy role for their patients and their families and assist them in the development of an intervention plan, including the identification of diagnostic and therapeutic measures that may be indicated in addressing the student's needs. To fulfill this role, PCPs should become familiarized with the steps needed to obtain educational support and assessment services through the school system. By developing relationships with key individuals within the local schools, PCPs can establish effective channels of communication to help diagnose and address their patients' learning challenges. Furthermore, such relationships can facilitate the coordination and implementation of the multimodal interventions that many students with LD require. Health care providers should identify other professionals in their community (e.g., psychologists, neuropsychologists, speech-language pathologists, behavior specialists, well-trained tutors, and reading therapists) that can assist with diagnostic, educational, and mental health intervention services that their patients may require.

CONCLUSION

Lucas, the patient in the vignette, presented with a history of early markers of LD including his difficulties learning letter names and sounds. However, his early mathematical skills were developing typically. Additionally, Lucas has a family history of learning difficulties. Lucas was prescribed stimulant medication to address his attention problems. While the attentional symptoms have improved, he continues to struggle with word reading. His history describes classical early markers of LD-R and ADHD. His pediatric practitioner can play a critical role pursing further assessment of Lucas' attention challenges and referring him for evaluation of his learning difficulties. This would identify the skills and functions that may require academic remediation, conduct a more thorough ADHD assessment, and identify potential emotional cooccurring conditions such as anxiety. This approach will ensure the most appropriate intervention. In the vignette it is noted that a friend of Lucas' family recommended vision therapy as an option for treatment of his difficulties. It is important that the pediatric practitioner provides the family information regarding evidence-based interventions for dyslexia and other learning disorders to prevent them from implementing costly and unproven interventions such as vision therapy. The Joint Technical Report on Learning Disabilities, Dyslexia and Vision by Handler and Fierson (2011) is an excellent resource for providers when questioned about vision therapy. Table 47.2 provides a list of US-based organizations that offer information for clinicians, educators, and families on the most appropriate ways to address challenges similar to those described in the vignette.

REFERENCES

American Psychiatric Association. (2013). *Diagnostic and statistical manual of mental disorders*. APA.

Ashkenazi, S., Rosenberg-Lee, M., Tenison, C., & Menon, V. (2012). Weak task-related modulation and stimulus representations during arithmetic problem solving in children with developmental dyscalculia. *Developmental Cognitive Neuroscience*, *2*(1), S152–S166.

Bailey, S., Hoeft, F., Aboud, K., & Cutting, L. (2016). Anomalous gray matter patterns in specific reading comprehension deficit are independent of dyslexia. *Annals of Dyslexia*, *66*(3), 256–274.

Balu, R., Zhu, P., Doolittle, F., Schiller, E., Jenkins, J., & Gersten, R. (2015). *Evaluation of response to intervention practices for elementary school reading*. https://files.eric.ed.gov/fulltext/ED560820.pdf

Barnes, J. (2021). *Section 504: The tool that should be in every advocate's toolkit*. Learning Disabilities Association of America. https://ldaamerica.org/lda_today/section-504-the-tool-that-should-be-in-every-advocates-toolkit/

Bull, R., & Lee, K. (2014). Executive functioning and mathematics achievement. *Child Development Perspectives*, *8*(1), 36–41. https://doi.org/10.1111/cdep.12059

Catts, H. W., Nielsen, D. C., Bridges, M. S., Liu, Y. S., & Bontempo, D. E. (2015). Early identification of reading disabilities within an RTI framework. *Journal of Learning Disabilities*, *48*(3), 281–297. https://doi.org/10.1177/0022219413498115

Chung, P. J., Patel, D. R., & Nizami, I. (2020). Disorder of written expression and dysgraphia: Definition, diagnosis, and management. *Translational Pediatrics*, *9*(1), S46–S54.

Cree, A., Kay, A., & Steward, J. (2012). *The economic and social cost of illiteracy: A snapshot of illiteracy in a global context*. World Literacy Foundation. https://worldliteracyfoundation.org/wp-content/uploads/2015/05/The-Economic-Social-Cost-ofIlliteracy.pdf

Daucourt, M. C., Erbeli, F., Little, C. W., Haughbrook, R., & Hart, S. A. (2020). A meta-analytical review of the genetic and environmental correlations between reading and attention-deficit/hyperactivity disorder symptoms and reading and math. *Scientific Studies of Reading*, *24*(1), 23–56. https://doi.org/10.1080/10888438.2019.1631827

De Smedt, B., Noël, M. P., Gilmore, C., & Ansari, D. (2013). How do symbolic and non-symbolic numerical magnitude processing skills relate to individual differences in children's mathematical skills? A review of evidence from brain and behavior. *Trends in Neuroscience and Education*, *2*(2), 48–55. https://doi.org/10.1016/j.tine.2013.06.001

Dragoo, K. E., & Cole, J. P. (2019). Laws affecting students with disabilities: Preschool through postsecondary education. *Congressional Research Service*. https://files.eric.ed.gov/fulltext/ED597875.pdf

Fuchs, D., & Fuchs, L. S. (2017). Critique of the national evaluation of response to intervention: A case for simpler frameworks. *Exceptional Children*, *83*(3), 255–268. https://doi.org/10.1177/0014402917693580

Göbel, S. M., Watson, S. E., Lervåg, A., & Hulme, C. (2014). Children's arithmetic development: It is number knowledge, not the approximate number sense, that counts. *Psychological Science*, *25*(3), 789–798. https://doi.org/10.1177/0956797613516471

Gough, P. B., & Tunmer, W. E. (1986). Decoding, reading, and reading disability. *Remedial and Special Education*, *7*, 6–10. https://doi.org/10.1177/074193258600700104

Grigorenko, E. L., Compton, D. L., Fuchs, L. S., Wagner, R. K., Willcutt, E. G., & Fletcher, J. M. (2020). Understanding, educating, and supporting children with specific learning disabilities: 50 years of science and practice. *American Psychologist*, *75*(1), 37–51. https://doi.org/10.1037/amp0000452

Grigorenko, E. L., Macomber, D., Hart, L., Naples, A., Chapman, J., Geib, C. F., … Wagner, R. (2015). Academic achievement among juvenile detainees. *Journal of Learning Disabilities*, *48*(4), 359–368. https://doi.org/10.1177/0022219413500991

Handler, S. M., & Fierson, W. M. (2011). Learning disabilities, dyslexia, and vision. *Pediatrics*, *127*(3). https://doi.org/10.1542/peds.2010-3670

Haynes, C. W., Smith, S. L., & Laud, L. (2019). Structured literacy approaches to teaching written expression. *Perspectives on Language and Literacy*, *45*(3), 22–28.

Hendren, R. L., Haft, S. L., Black, J. M., White, N. C., & Hoeft, F. (2018). Recognizing psychiatric comorbidity with reading disorders. *Frontiers in Psychiatry*, *9*(MAR). https://doi.org/10.3389/fpsyt.2018.00101

Hoff, E. (2013). Interpreting the early language trajectories of children from low-SES and language minority homes: Implications for closing achievement gaps. *Developmental Psychology*, *49*(1), 4–14.

Hyde, D. C., & Spelke, E. S. (2011). Neural signatures of number processing in human infants: Evidence for two core systems underlying numerical cognition. *Developmental Science*, *14*(2), 360–371. https://doi.org/10.1111/j.1467-7687.2010.00987.x

International Dyslexia Association. (n.d.). *Structured literacy: Effective instruction for students with dyslexia and related reading difficulties*. https://dyslexiaida.org/structured-literacy-effective-instruction-for-students-with-dyslexia-and-related-reading-difficulties/

International Dyslexia Association. (2002). *Definition of dyslexia*. https://dyslexiaida.org/definition-of-dyslexia/

Irwin, L. G., Siddiqi, A., & Hertzman, C. (2007). *Early child development: A powerful equalizer*. Human Early Learning Partnership (HELP).

Johnston, R. (2019). Poor education predicts poor health—a challenge unmet by American medicine. *NAM Perspectives* https://doi.org/10.31478/201904a.

Joshi, G. S., & Bouck, E. C. (2017). Examining postsecondary education predictors and participation for students with learning disabilities. *Journal of Learning Disabilities*, *501*(1), 3–13.

Karipidis, I. I., & Hong, D. S. (2020). Specific learning disorders in sex chromosome aneuploidies: Neural circuits of literacy and mathematics. *American Journal of Medical Genetics, Part C: Seminars in Medical Genetics*, *184*(2), 518–530. https://doi.org/10.1002/ajmg.c.31801

Kaufmann, L., & von Aster, M. (2012). Diagnostik und intervention bei Rechenstörung. *Deutsches Arzteblatt International*, *109*(45), 767–778. https://doi.org/10.3238/arztebl.2012.0767

Kucian, K., & von Aster, M. (2015). Developmental dyscalculia. *European Journal of Pediatrics*, *174*(1), 1–13. https://doi.org/10.1007/s00431-014-2455-7

Langer, N., Benjamin, C., Becker, B. L. C., & Gaab, N. (2019). Comorbidity of reading disabilities and ADHD: Structural and functional brain characteristics. *Human Brain Mapping*, *40*(9), 2677–2698.

Light, J. G., & DeFries, J. C. (1995). Comorbidity of reading and mathematics disabilities: Genetic and environmental etiologies. *Journal of Learning Disabilities*, *28*(2), 96–106. https://doi.org/10.1177/002221949502800204

Lovett, M. W., Frijters, J. C., Wolf, M., Steinbach, K. A., Sevcik, R. A., & Morris, R. D. (2017). Early intervention for children at risk for reading disabilities: The impact of grade at intervention and individual differences on intervention outcomes. *Journal of Educational Psychology*, *109*(7), 889–914.

Matejko, A. A., & Ansari, D. (2015). Drawing connections between white matter and numerical and mathematical cognition: A literature review. *Neuroscience and Biobehavioral Reviews*, *48*, 35–52. https://doi.org/10.1016/j.neubiorev.2014.11.006

Matejko, A. A., Price, G. R., Mazzocco, M. M. M., & Ansari, D. (2013). Individual differences in left parietal white matter predict math scores on the Preliminary Scholastic Aptitude Test. *NeuroImage, 66*, 604–610. https://doi.org/10.1016/j.neuroimage.2012.10.045

Mazzocco, M. M., Feigenson, L., & Halberda, J. (2011). Impaired acuity of the approximate number system underlies mathematical learning disability (dyscalculia). *Child Development, 82*(4), 1224–1237. https://doi.org/10.1111/j.1467-8624.2011.01608.x

McGrath, L. M., Peterson, R. L., & Pennington, B. F. (2020). The multiple deficit model: Progress, problems, and prospects. *Scientific Studies of Reading, 24*(1), 7–13. https://doi.org/10.1080/10888438.2019.1706180

Miciak, J., & Fletcher, J. M. (2020). The critical role of instructional response for identifying dyslexia and other learning disabilities. *Journal of Learning Disabilities, 53*(5), 343–353. https://doi.org/10.1177/0022219420906801

Moll, K., Landerl, K., Snowling, M. J., & Schulte-Körne, G. (2019). Understanding comorbidity of learning disorders: Task-dependent estimates of prevalence. *Journal of Child Psychology and Psychiatry and Allied Disciplines, 60*(3), 286–294. https://doi.org/10.1111/jcpp.12965

National Assessment of Educational Progress. (2019). *NAEP report card: 2019 NAEP reading assessment.* National Center for Education Statistics. https://www.nationsreportcard.gov/highlights/reading/2019/

National Center for Education Statistics. (2019). *Fast facts.* US Department of Education. https://nces.ed.gov/programs/digest/d19/tables/dt19_219.90.asp

National Center for Learning Disabilities. (2017). *The state of LD: Introduction.* https://www.ncld.org/research/state-of-learning-disabilities

National Center for Special Education Research. (2011). *The post-high school outcomes of young adults with disabilities up to 8 years after high school: A report from the National Longitudinal Transition Study-2 (NLTS2).* US Department of Education.

Norton, E. S., & Wolf, M. (2012). Rapid automatized naming (RAN) and reading fluency: Implications for understanding and treatment of reading disabilities. *Annual Review of Psychology, 63*, 427–452. https://doi.org/10.1146/annurev-psych-120710-100431

Ozernov-Palchik, O., & Gaab, N. (2016). Tackling the early identification of dyslexia with the help of neuroimaging. *Perspectives on Language and Literacy, 42*, 11–17.

Ozernov-Palchik, O., Yu, X., Gaab, N., & Wang, Y. (2016). Lessons to be learned: How a comprehensive neurobiological framework of atypical reading development can inform educational practice. *Current Opinion in Behavioral Sciences, 10*, 45–58. https://doi.org/10.1016/j.cobeha.2016.05.006.Lessons

Pauc, R. (2005). Comorbidity of dyslexia, dyspraxia, attention deficit disorder (ADD), attention deficit hyperactive disorder (ADHD), obsessive compulsive disorder (OCD) and Tourette's syndrome in children: A prospective epidemiological study. *Clinical Chiropractic, 8*(4), 189–198.

Peterson, R. L., Pennington, B. F., & McGrath, L. M. (2018). *Diagnosing learning disorders: From science to practice.* The Guilford Press.

Rimrodt, S. L., & Lipkin, P. H. (2011). Learning disabilities and school failure. *Pediatrics in Review, 32*(8), 315–324.

Sanfilippo, J., Ness, M., Petscher, Y., Rappaport, L., Zuckerman, B., & Gaab, N. (2020). Reintroducing dyslexia: Early identification and implications for pediatric practice. *Pediatrics, 146*(1). https://doi.org/10.1542/peds.2019-3046

Scarborough, H. S. (2001). Connecting early language and literacy to later reading (dis)abilities: Evidence, theory and practice. In S. Neumann & D. Dickinson (Eds.), *Handbook for research in early literacy.* Guilford Publications.

Shaywitz, S. E. (2004). Overcoming dyslexia: A new and complete science-based program for reading problems at any level. A.A. Knopf.

Slavica, K., Katusic, M. D., Colligan, R. C., Weaver, A. L., & Barbaresi, W. J. (2009). The forgotten learning disability—Epidemiology of written language disorder in a population-based birth cohort (1976–1982), Rochester, Minnesota. *Pediatrics, 123*(5), 1306–1313.

Soares, N., Evans, T., & Patel, D. R. (2018). Specific learning disability in mathematics: A comprehensive review. Translational Pediatrics, 7(1), 48–62.

Stein, D. S., Blum, N. J., & Barbaresi, W. J. (2011). Developmental and behavioral disorders through the life span. *Pediatrics, 128*(2), 364–373. https://doi.org/10.1542/peds.2011-0266

Torgesen, J. K. (2004). *Avoiding the devastating downward spiral: The evidence that early intervention prevents reading failure.* American Federation of Teachers. https://www.aft.org/periodical/american-educator/fall-2004/avoiding-devastating-downward-spiral

Wanzek, J., & Vaughn, S. (2007). Research-based implications from extensive early reading interventions. *School Psychology Review, 36*(4), 541–561.

Wanzek, J., Vaughn, S., Scammacca, N. K., Metz, K., Murray, C. S., Roberts, G., & Danielson, L. (2013). Extensive reading interventions for students with reading difficulties after grade 3. *Review of Educational Research, 83*, 163–195.

Willcutt, E. G., Pennington, B. F., Duncan, L., Smith, S. D., Keenan, J. M., Wadsworth, S., … Olson, R. K. (2010). Understanding the complex etiologies of developmental disorders: Behavioral and molecular genetic approaches. *Journal of Developmental and Behavioral Pediatrics, 31*(7), 533–544. https://doi.org/10.1097/DBP.0b013e3181ef42a1

48

Talent and Giftedness

Mary C. Kral

For additional material related to the content of this chapter, please see Chapters 8, and 18.

> **VIGNETTE**
>
> *Sally is a bright 13-year-old with a history of academic excellence and musical talent. She was placed in a gifted and talented program beginning in the third grade and attained the A/B Honor Roll throughout elementary school. Her academic success came rather easily to her, freeing up time after school to pursue cello lessons and participate in a community orchestra. With the transition to middle school, Sally demonstrated an unexpected decline in academic achievement that perplexed her parents and teachers. Her parents have been advised to consult with an expert to determine the source of her academic struggles and solutions for success.*

DEFINITIONS

Youth who are gifted and talented comprise 5% to 20% of the general school-age population, depending on how the term *gifted* or *talented* is defined or the criteria used to identify these students (Worrell, Subotnik, Olszewski-Kubilius, & Dixson, 2019). Some equate giftedness with high intelligence, others with high academic achievement. Still others highlight the domain-specific mastery characteristic, for example, of musically or artistically talented youth. What constitutes gifted and talented in terms of cognitive abilities, talents, personality traits, or environmental contributions is the source of ongoing investigation and public debate. Researchers and educators alike differ in how they define gifted and talented, and the empiric literature is characterized by the absence of a common vocabulary or universally defined terms, making comparisons across studies difficult. Within the realm of education there is no federal definition recognized by all states or universally implemented programs for students who are gifted and talented.

Gifted and Talented as Ability

Historically, giftedness has been equated with high intellectual functioning. In the early 20th century Lewis defined gifted as an IQ at or above 150 on the Stanford-Binet Intelligence Scale (Terman, Baldwin, & Bronson, 1926) Subsequently, the 98th percentile (IQ = 130) has commonly been used as the cutoff for giftedness. More recently, some school districts recognize students with IQs of 120 or above as eligible to receive gifted programming. The problem with viewing exceptionally high IQ as synonymous with gifted is that a fixed proportion of the population is always selected (e.g., top 3%–5%) (Renzulli, 2005). Research suggests that heritability accounts for most of the variance in IQ among youth in middle and upper socioeconomic classes. However, for youth from low-resource backgrounds or minoritized groups, environment (not genes) makes a bigger difference (Turkheimer et al., 2003). As such, use of an IQ cutoff as the criterion for gifted will underidentify youth from low-resource backgrounds. An additional problem with use of intelligence test scores to define giftedness is the limited predictive utility of these scores. IQ correlates only modestly with academic achievement, and noncognitive factors also account for a significant proportion of variance in academic attainment, including but not limited to motivation, interest, self-efficacy, and self-regulation skills. In addition, intelligence test scores are poor predictors of real-world functioning such as job performance (Neisser et al., 1996). Finally, IQ scores do not capture the range of cognitive abilities or talent. Therefore classifications that emphasize IQ for placement will miss those youth with uneven giftedness (e.g., nonverbal intelligence > verbal intelligence) (Lubinski, 2009). For all these reasons, IQ cutoff criteria frequently result in underidentification of gifted youth.

Gifted and Talented as Multifactorial

Joseph Renzulli's (2016) enrichment triad model introduced an alternative, multifactorial definition, emphasizing that a confluence of several factors is important in defining talent and giftedness. In his model Renzulli suggested that creative-productive people possess an interaction among three basic traits: (1) above-average ability, defined as high general intellectual functioning or well above average domain-specific performance, such as general verbal ability; (2) high levels of task commitment, defined as perseverance, hard work, intrinsic motivation, and self-confidence; and (3) high levels of creativity, or original, unconventional, ingenious thinking. These three factors interact with personality and environmental variables (e.g., educational opportunities) to give rise to gifted and talented performance.

Modern-day conceptualizations also recognize that giftedness and talent are not unitary constructs. For example, Howard Gardner's (1999) multiple intelligences highlight the multifactorial nature of giftedness and talent by defining eight domain-specific intelligences: linguistic, logical-mathematical, musical, bodily-kinesthetic, spatial, interpersonal, intrapersonal, and naturalistic. Similarly, Robert Sternberg (2005) asserts that gifted and talented individuals are characterized by three interrelated qualities: a synthesis of wisdom (balancing intrapersonal, interpersonal, short- and long-term goals), practical intelligence (ability to adapt to one's environment and to learn from experience), and creativity (applying and balancing innovative, analytic, and practical abilities).

Gardner's and Sternberg's models have led to talent searches that, for example, characterize some magnet schools of the performing and visual arts. These models differ from the ability/intelligence model in that they recognize talent and giftedness are based on potential that must be developed rather than static intelligence. These models apply to both academic and nonacademic domains that require cultivation of both ability and nonintellective factors (e.g., motivation, creativity, accelerative opportunities) to produce exceptional competencies (Gagné, 2018).

DEVELOPMENTAL CONCERNS

Cognitive Development

The terms *gifted* and *talented* often spark the nature-nurture debate. Those assuming the nature side of the argument emphasize the inborn, heritable ability and intrinsic drive of gifted and talented youth (e.g., high IQ). Those assuming the nurture side of the argument, however, suggest that giftedness and talent are the products of hard work or deliberate practice. According to modern-day theorists, as detailed previously, high ability is a necessary but not sufficient component of giftedness and talent. Opportunity also plays a large role and includes factors such as family support, societal and cultural values, educational opportunities, and resources. A developmental systems approach focuses on developmental processes rather than individual traits. For example, gifted and talented youth, as compared to their typically developing peers, excel at higher-order reasoning, independent solution of abstract problems, and transfer of skills to novel situations. Gifted and talented youth also are characterized by an intrinsic drive to master specific domains of interest. Signs of giftedness may emerge early in development, including early onset of language, excellent memory, intense curiosity, long attention span when engaged in activities of high interest, metacognitive awareness of problem-solving strategies, and efficient use of learning strategies. Many youth who are gifted acquire reading skills before entering kindergarten, demonstrate facility with numbers, and/or excel at abstract problem solving. While many gifted and talented youth demonstrate evenly developed intellectual functioning, others evidence domain-specific gifts in language or nonverbal/quantitative reasoning and acquisition of cognitive skills and talents in advance of social and emotional development (Dai, 2019).

Social-Emotional Development

Contrary to myths promoted by the media, most gifted and talented youth are socially and emotionally well adjusted (Neihart, Pfeiffer, & Cross, 2016). For example, a population-based study that included 2736 sixth graders found that gifted students enjoyed higher levels of social acceptance and nominations as friends when compared to their average-ability counterparts, as rated by teachers and peers (Verschueren, Lavrijsen, Weyns, Ramos, & De Fraine, 2019). In a metaanalysis internalizing symptoms (e.g., depression and anxiety), externalizing behavior problems, and adaptive behavioral functioning did not differ between gifted and nongifted students according to teacher report, and gifted students in fact demonstrated higher levels of self-confidence (Martin, Burns, & Schonlau, 2010). Similarly, Bain and Bell (2004) reported that the majority of gifted elementary and middle school students reported high self-concept and tended to attribute social success to ability and effort (internal locus of control) rather than to luck or task difficulty.

A number of steps have been suggested for the promotion of healthy cognitive, social, and emotional development among youth who are gifted and talented. First, the importance of the family cannot be overstated. Three family characteristics have been shown to facilitate social and emotional resilience among gifted youth: (1) parents who have high expectations of their gifted youth and model high achievement, (2) parents who give their youth more independence, and (3) parents who provide stimulation and nurturance (Winner, 2000). Moreover, families and mentors who teach psychosocial facilitators, including social skills (e.g., empathy, communication, problem solving, and cooperation) and emotional regulation (e.g., tolerance for ambiguity, managing setbacks, perseverance) help nurture the noncognitive qualities essential to high potential (Olszewski-Kubilius, Subotnik, Davis, & Worrell, 2019). Second, Eklund and colleagues (2015) suggest that the social-emotional functioning of students should receive attention equal to their academic performance from educators. Specifically, a prevention-oriented multitiered system is recommended that incorporates regular assessment of the social, emotional, and behavioral functioning of gifted and talented youth that might address need for early access to mental health–related supports.

EDUCATIONAL IDENTIFICATION AND PROGRAMMING

At the federal level, although specific legislation recognizes the unique educational needs of youth who are identified as gifted and talented (e.g., the Jacob K. Javits Gifted and Talented Students Education Act, reauthorized in 2015 as part of the Every Student Succeeds Act), the federal government does not mandate gifted and talented programs. Rather, the majority of programs and services that youth receive are determined by state laws and policies and funded at the state and local levels. State laws that define gifted and talented programming and teacher training requirements, along with available funding for gifted and talented education, vary widely. A searchable directory of state-specific definitions and mandates for identifying gifted and talented youth may be obtained in the "State of the States in Gifted Education Report" on the website of the National Association for Gifted Children: https://www.nagc.org/information-publications/gifted-state.

Most researchers agree that cognitive ability tests should constitute part but not all of the identification process and that other indicators of potential also should be used in the identification process. These other indicators should be given equal consideration in selecting those youth eligible for special services, and in the final analysis the informed judgment of educators should prevail over strict cutoff scores on psychometric instruments. Despite these ideals, in this era of high-stakes testing, identification of youth eligible for special programs typically relies on test scores (i.e., intelligence test cutoffs, performance on academic achievement tests, and talent searches).

CURRICULUM ALTERNATIVES

Research suggests that gifted and talented youth benefit from a differentiated curriculum that addresses their learning needs to maintain academic interest and high levels of achievement. The following is a brief introduction to the various curriculum alternatives for gifted and talented education.

Ability Grouping

Ability grouping refers to the practice of using ability test scores or measures of achievement to assign students to an educational program. This practice may involve part-time assignment to both regular and special classes or full-time grouping with students of similar abilities. Magnet schools are an example of ability grouping for students who are gifted and talented or students with special interest areas (e.g., science and math or the arts). Critics of ability grouping contend that this practice contributes to achievement gaps, inequities in educational opportunities, and adverse psychosocial outcomes. However, a meta-analysis of research studies on ability grouping reported that gifted students who received a differentiated curriculum through flexible grouping practices evidenced higher academic achievement at all grade levels compared with those students who do not receive a differentiated curriculum (Steenbergen-Hu, Makel, & Olszewski-Kubilius, 2016).

Acceleration

Acceleration is a placement, not an educational program. Accelerated programs are based on the notion that gifted and talented youth acquire knowledge and skills at a faster rate than their age-mates and involve methods that move students through a curriculum at a faster pace. For example, accelerated programs may include early entrance into kindergarten, grade advancement, early entry into college, dual enrollment in high school and college, and combined undergraduate and graduate degree programs. Curriculum compacting is another example of accelerated programming whereby a number of courses are compressed into one or students are exempt from instruction in an area in which they demonstrate mastery. Opponents of acceleration suggest that this form of educational programming is detrimental to the social, emotional, or physical development of gifted youth, and accelerated programs are not commonly used by most public schools. However, research reveals positive outcomes for exceptionally gifted and talented youth who are permitted radical acceleration (i.e., early entry into college), including sustained interest and involvement in academic activities, high levels of academic success, and transition into high status careers. Moreover, there is no evidence for social or emotional maladjustment when exceptionally gifted and talented students participated in well-planned acceleration procedures. Positive outcomes for youth who participate in radical acceleration procedures include high achievement motivation, persistence, effective study skills, and involvement in educational decision making (Assouline, Colengelo, Van Tassel-Baska, & Lupkowski-Shoplik, 2015; Steenbergen-Hu et al., 2016).

Enrichment

Enrichment refers to additional or new curricular material not delivered in regular education or instructional strategies that supplement what is taught in the regular education classroom (e.g., pull-out programs). Examples include advanced placement courses, part-time college courses, and summer enrichment programs. Gifted students report an increase in social self-concept when they participate in summer enrichment programs (Rinn, 2006). However, pull-out programs have been criticized for not providing appropriate educational programming throughout the school day or across all subject areas. In the Study for Mathematically Precocious Youth (SMPY), Wai and colleagues (2010) demonstrated that youth who received a greater dosage of enrichment opportunities (i.e., precollegiate advanced/enriched educational experiences) in science, technology, engineering, and mathematics (STEM) demonstrated greater subsequent accomplishments in these fields (e.g., acquisition of PhDs and publications in peer-refereed journals).

SPECIAL CONSIDERATIONS

Identification of Underrepresented Groups

According to the National Research Center on the Gifted and Talented, youth from low-resource families or minoritized groups are underidentified and underrepresented in gifted and talented educational programs. Moreover, a disproportionate number of gifted and talented youth who drop out of school are from lower socioeconomic backgrounds or had reduced access to educational opportunities or technology. Contributing factors include biased identification methods and systemic racism, leading to an achievement gap. For those living in communities with high rates of poverty the cultivation of giftedness and talent may be complicated by inequities in educational access, quality education, and enrichment programs; biases in educator expectations; and negative cultural and peer influences (Subotnik, Olszewski-Kubilius, & Worrell, 2011). Moreover, many gifted and talented youth from low-resource families or minoritized groups experience a stereotype threat when they perceive that the expression of their giftedness or talent would be in conflict with or not valued by members of their cultural group. Withdrawal from academic pursuits is a common reaction to the cognitive dissonance that occurs when a student first becomes aware of this conflict, usually during adolescence. For example, gifted

Black students may experience peer pressure to underachieve for fear of acting White (Ford, Grantham, & Whiting, 2008).

In a review of the literature Moore and colleagues (2005) reported that noncognitive factors more effectively predict persistence among academically gifted and talented Black youth than achievement and performance variables (e.g., tests and grades). These noncognitive factors include self-confidence, realistic self-appraisal, understanding of and ability to cope with racism, preference for long-range goals over more immediate short-term goals, support of academic pursuits from others, successful leadership experience, community service, and knowledge acquired in a field. Similarly, in a 3-year study of 35 economically disadvantaged, ethnically diverse, academically gifted high school students, Reis and associates (2005) reported that the presence of at least one supportive adult, peer support, and involvement in productive after-school or summer activities distinguished those youth who excelled academically.

Mentoring or coaching has been promoted as one strategy to cultivate academic giftedness and talent among youth from low-resource families or minoritized groups. Callahan and Kyburg (2005) suggest that the greater a gifted student's distance from that expected in terms of the stereotypical professional, the greater the need for role models who are closely matched to the student in terms of attitude, values, lifestyle, background experience, race, and gender. Often gifted students from low-income families or minoritized groups must master code switching, a process of deliberately changing behaviors to accommodate the expectations of different environments (Neihart, 2006). As such, at-risk gifted and talent youth need cultural brokers or caring adults who understand gender, class, racial, or ethnic factors and can identify these factors in a variety of contexts, mediate potential conflict, and build bridges. Finally, coaching may provide direct instruction in the social skills necessary for leadership in a variety of cultural contexts, including authority, self-control, and conflict resolution. For instance, in some cultures, behaviors that are encouraged in accelerated educational programs (e.g., questioning authority, critical thinking) are discouraged at home because they are perceived as disrespectful of authority.

The Underachieving Gifted and Talented Child

Gifted and talented youth who do not evidence ability-consistent academic achievement or talent represent one of the most frustrating dilemmas for clinicians and parents alike. Gifted underachievement, most commonly defined as a severe and persistent discrepancy between a student's academic performance and actual ability, represents a significant problem for some youth. In a review of the research on gifted underachievement Reis and colleagues (2005) reported that the beginning stages of academic underachievement among gifted and talented youth occur in elementary school, perhaps because of an unchallenging curriculum. Subsequently, underachievement appears to be periodic and episodic, occurring in some years and not others and in some academic subject areas but not others. Eventually, increasing episodes of underachievement will result in a more chronic pattern for some youth.

Gifted underachievement is often a complex problem involving multiple factors, including underchallenging educational programming (Reis & McCoach, 2000, 2002), peer pressure (Winner, 2000), certain parenting styles, and child-related factors. Parenting factors associated with underachievement include parents with less positive affect, disinterest toward education, overly strict or overly lenient parenting, and family conflict (Rimm, 1995). Child-related factors associated with underachievement include depression, anxiety, perfectionism, low motivation, and/or low self-confidence. A growing literature suggests that a focus on the child's strengths and interests is critical to reversing the pattern of underachievement (Baum, Renzulli, & Hébert, 1995; Dole, 2000; Reis et al., 2005). In addition, interventions that target family, child, peer, and academic factors are recommended. Academic interventions should include curricular changes that tap areas of talent and giftedness and that establish clear academic goals and objectives with rewards for attainment of these goals. There is some evidence that more rigorous academic challenges may actually have a positive impact on underachievement. Finally, peer groups that support achievement can be an important part of preventing and reversing underachievement. In this regard busier adolescents who are involved in clubs, extracurricular activities, sports, and religious activities are less likely to underachieve in school (Baum et al., 1995; Callahan & Kyburg, 2005).

Identification of Twice Exceptional Students

Gifted and talented youth who also possess a second exceptionality, referred to as twice exceptional, are frequently misunderstood and often do not receive appropriate educational programming that addresses the range of their needs. For example, education personnel are less likely to refer students with learning disabilities or emotional/behavioral disorders to gifted and talented programs. However, the unidentified second exceptionality often impedes the academic success of the gifted or talented student. Because some gifted and talented youth who are underachieving may suffer from an undiagnosed condition, it is important to consider that a second exceptionality is responsible for the student's underachievement. A review of several twice exceptional circumstances follows.

In a longitudinal study conducted by Antshel and colleagues (2007) gifted students with comorbid attention-deficit/hyperactivity disorder (ADHD) demonstrated similar functional impairments to students of average ability with ADHD, including academic underachievement, increased incidence of grade retention, and social-emotional difficulties. The researchers reported that these struggles emerged at a later age among the gifted cohort, suggesting that high ability may have served to mask functional impairments at a younger age. Sally, the child referenced in the introductory vignette, is a good example of this pattern. Early identification and treatment of ADHD are important to help prevent academic underachievement in gifted and talented youth. Identification of functional impairments in social and adaptive behavior domains may need to be established at an early age, considering that many schools only acknowledge functional impairment in the academic domain.

Gifted and talented youth with high functioning autism spectrum disorder (ASD) often encounter difficulties with executive functioning (organization, cognitive flexibility), expressive language skills, sustained attention, and fine motor skills that impede their academic success. Research suggests that the challenges and talents of these twice exceptional youth are often not adequately addressed (Cain, Kaboski, & Gilger, 2019). Intervention should include a differentiated curriculum that provides both enrichment and instructional supports. For example, a 504 plan may be required to help the gifted and talented student with ASD compensate for everyday behaviors associated with executive dysfunction.

That gifted and talented youth may also possess a learning disability has become widely recognized over the years (Brody & Mills, 1997). However, often these youth are not identified and are underserved. In a qualitative review of research studies examining gifted and talented youth with learning disabilities Lovett and Sparks (2011) found an IQ achievement model most commonly utilized to identify a learning disability and an IQ cutoff utilized to identify giftedness. These identification criteria, commonly utilized in the public school system, perpetuate underidentification. For example, one exceptionality often overshadows the other; the student's giftedness may mask the learning disability when the student demonstrates average achievement and remains served in the regular education classroom without services addressing either exceptionality. Gifted and talented youth with learning disabilities are best served by comprehensive assessment that may reveal an uneven pattern of cognitive functioning (e.g., spatial abilities > verbal abilities) and individualized education programming that addresses both strengths and needs.

Several key components that foster resilience among twice exceptional youth have been highlighted: early identification of both exceptionalities, educational programming that targets strengths and weaknesses (i.e., enrichment and remediation), direct instruction in compensatory strategies, and provision of accommodations at an early age to promote academic success. Twice exceptional youth also may benefit from psychological interventions that address their unique emotional needs, assist in the development of awareness about their strengths and weaknesses, and promote realistic goal setting. Finally, supportive adults and extracurricular activities that showcase strengths are needed among twice exceptional youth (Baum, 1990; Dole, 2000).

CONCLUSION

Current conceptualizations of giftedness and talent highlight the cognitive and noncognitive components necessary for exceptional competencies, including, for example, high intellectual ability, creativity, persistence and motivation, and self-efficacy. Although youth who are gifted represent a heterogeneous group from diverse backgrounds, those factors that promote healthy cognitive, social, and emotional development are largely the same and include supportive families that set high expectations for academic achievement; individualized, accelerative educational programs that address areas of strength and weakness; and opportunities to interact with peers who have similar abilities, interests, and motivation. Clinicians involved in the care of children are in an ideal position to guide parents of gifted and talented youth by first recognizing the signs early in development. They may provide families with guidance regarding developmentally appropriate expectations for behavior and effective parenting strategies. Finally, these clinicians may be the first to identify potential social or emotional problems among youth who are gifted and talented and direct families to appropriate interventions or mentoring.

Because identification of youth eligible for gifted and talented educational programming may vary from school district to school district, the clinicians working with this group are advised to become familiar with the policies relevant to the state in which they work. A searchable directory of state-specific information about gifted and talented educational programming can be found on the website of the National Association for Gifted Children (http://www.nagc.org). Consultation with district school psychologists may provide information about the identification process and programming unique to a given school.

REFERENCES

Antshel, K. M., Faraone, S. V., Stallone, K., Nave, A., et al. (2007). Is attention deficit hyperactivity disorder a valid diagnosis in the presence of high IQ? Results from the MGH longitudinal family studies of ADHD. *Journal of Child Psychology and Psychiatry*, *48*, 687–694.

Assouline, S. G., Colengelo, N., Van Tassel-Baska, J., & Lupkowski-Shoplik, A. (Eds.). (2015). *A nation empowered: Evidence trumps the excuses holding back America's brightest students*. IQ: Acceleration Institute.

Bain, S. K., & Bell, S. M. (2004). Social self-concept, social attributions, and peer relationships in fourth, fifth, and sixth graders who are gifted compared to high achievers. *Gifted Child Quarterly*, *48*, 166–178.

Baum, S. M. (1990). *Gifted but learning disabled: A puzzling paradox*. Council for Exceptional Youth, ERIC Digest No. E479.

Baum, S. M., Renzulli, J. S., & Hébert, T. P. (1995). Reversing underachievement: Creative productivity as a systematic intervention. *Gifted Child Quarterly*, *39*, 224–235.

Brody, L. E., & Mills, C. J. (1997). Gifted children with learning disabilities: A review of the issues. *Journal of Learning Disabilities*, *30*, 282–296.

Cain, M. K., Kaboski, J. R., & Gilger, J. W. (2019). Profiles and academic trajectories of cognitively gifted children with autism spectrum disorder. *Autism*, *23*, 1663–1674.

Callahan, C. M., & Kyburg, R. M. (2005). Talented and gifted youth. In D. L. DuBois & M. Karcher (Eds.), *Handbook of youth mentoring* (pp. 424–439). Sage.

Dai, D. Y. (2019). New directions in talent development research: A developmental systems perspective. In R. F. Subotnik, S. G. Assouline, et al. (Eds.), The future of research in talent development: promising trends, evidence, and implications of

innovative scholarship for policy and practice. *New Directions for Child and Adolescent Development, 168*, 177–197.
Dole, S. (2000). The implications of the risk and resilience literature for gifted students with learning disabilities. *Roeper Review, 23*, 91–96.
Eklund, K., Tanner, N., Stoll, K., & Anway, L. (2015). Identifying emotional and behavioral risk among gifted and non-gifted children: A multi-gate, multi-informant approach. *School Psychology Quarterly, 30*, 197–211.
Ford, D. T., Grantham, T. C., & Whiting, G. W. (2008). Another look at the achievement gap: Learning from the experience of gifted Black students. *Urban Education, 43*, 216–238.
Gagné, F. (2018). Academic talent development: Theory and best practice. In S. I. Pfeiffer, F. Shaunessy-Dedrick, & M. Foley-Nicpon (Eds.), *APA handbook of giftedness and talent* (pp. 163–183). American Psychological Association.
Gardner, H. (1999). *Intelligence reframed: Multiple intelligences for the 21st century*. Basic Books.
Lovett, B. J., & Sparks, R. L. (2011). The identification and performance of gifted students with learning disability diagnoses: A quantitative synthesis. *Journal of Learning Disabilities, 46*, 304–316.
Lubinski, D. (2009). Exceptional cognitive ability: The phenotype. *Behavioral Genetics, 39*, 350–358.
Martin, L. T., Burns, R. M., & Schonlau, M. (2010). Mental disorders among gifted and non-gifted youth: A selected review of the epidemiologic literature. *Gifted Child Quarterly, 54*, 31–41.
Moore, J. L., Ford, D. Y., & Milner, R. (2005). Recruitment is not enough: Retaining African American students in gifted education. *Gifted Child Quarterly, 49*, 51–67.
Neihart, M. (2006). Dimensions of underachievement, difficult contexts, and perceptions of self. *Roeper Review, 28*, 196–202.
Neihart, M., Pfeiffer, S. I., & Cross, T. L. (2016). *The social and emotional development of the gifted child: What do we know?* (2nd ed.). Prufrock Press.
Neisser, U., Boodoo, G., Bouchard, T. J., et al. (1996). Intelligence: Knowns and unknowns. *American Psychologist, 51*, 77–101.
Olszewski-Kubilius, P., Subotnik, R. F., Davis, L. C., & Worrell, F. C. (2019). Benchmarking psychosocial skills important for talent development. In R. F. Subotnik, S. G. Assouline, et al. (Eds.), The future of research in talent development: Promising trends, evidence, and implications of innovative scholarship for policy and practice. *New Directions for Child and Adolescent Development, 168*, 161–176.
Reis, S. M., Colbert, R. D., & Hébert, T. P. (2005). Understanding resilience in diverse, talented students in an urban high school. *Roeper Review, 27*, 110–120.
Reis, S. M., & McCoach, D. B. (2000). The underachievement of gifted students: What do we know and where do we go? *Gifted Child Quarterly, 44*, 152–170.
Reis, S. M., & McCoach, D. B. (2002). Underachievement in gifted and talented students with special needs. *Exceptionality, 10*, 113–125.
Renzulli, J. (2005). The three-ring conception of giftedness: A developmental model for promoting creative productivity. In R. J. Sternberg & J. E. Davidson (Eds.), *Conceptions of giftedness* (2nd ed., pp. 246–279). Cambridge University Press.
Renzulli, J. S. (2016). The enrichment triad model: A guide for developing defensible programs for the gifted and talented. In S. M. Reis (Ed.), *Reflections on gifted education: Critical works by Joseph Renzulli and colleagues* (pp. 193–210). Prufrock Press.
Rimm, S. (1995). *Why bright kids get poor grades and what you can do about it*. Crown Trade Paperbacks.
Rinn, A. N. (2006). Effects of a summer program on the social self-concepts of gifted adolescents. *Journal of Secondary Gifted Education, 17*, 65–75.
Steenbergen-Hu, S., Makel, M. C., & Olszewski-Kubilius, P. (2016). What one hundred years of research says about the effects of ability grouping and acceleration in K-12 students' academic achievement: Findings of two second-order meta-analyses. *Review of Educational Research, 86*, 849–899.
Sternberg, R. J. (2005). The WICS model of giftedness. In R. J. Sternberg & J. E. Davidson (Eds.), *Conceptions of giftedness* (2nd ed., pp. 327–342). Cambridge University Press.
Subotnik, R. F., Olszewski-Kubilius, P., & Worrell, F. C. (2011). Rethinking giftedness and gifted education: A proposed direction forward based on psychological sciences. *Psychological Science in the Public Interest, 12*, 3–54.
Terman, L. M., Baldwin, B. T., & Bronson, E. (Eds.), (1926). *Genetic studies of genius: Mental and physical traits of a thousand gifted youth* (2nd ed.). Stanford University Press.
Turkheimer, E., Haley, A., Waldron, M., et al. (2003). Socioeconomic status modifies heritability of IQ in young youth. *Psychological Science, 14*, 623–628.
Verschueren, K., Lavrijsen, J., Weyns, T., Ramos, A., & De Fraine, B. (2019). Social acceptance of high-ability youth: Multiple perspectives and contextual influences. In R. F. Subotnik, S. G. Assouline, et al. (Eds.), The future of research in talent development: Promising trends, evidence, and implications of innovative scholarship for policy and practice. *New Directions for Child and Adolescent Development, 168*, 27–46.
Wai, J., Lubinski, D., Benbow, C. P., & Steiger, J. H. (2010). Accomplishment in science, technology, engineering, and mathematics (STEM) and its relation to STEM educational dosage: A 25-year longitudinal study. *Journal of Educational Psychology, 102*, 860–871.
Winner, E. (2000). The origins and ends of giftedness. *American Psychologist, 55*, 159–169.
Worrell, F. C., Subotnik, R. F., Olszewski-Kubilius, P., & Dixson, D. D. (2019). Gifted students. *Annual Review of Psychology, 70*, 551–576.

49

Mood Disorders in Children and Adolescents

Musa Yilanli and Mary A. Fristad

For additional material related to the content of this chapter, please see Chapters 98, and 99.

DEPRESSIVE SPECTRUM DISORDERS

VIGNETTE

Until high school, Elizabeth, age 15, was outgoing, academically successful, and had many friends. However, midway through her sophomore year, finding motivation for schoolwork has been almost impossible, and academic performance has suffered. Elizabeth considers herself a failure and makes frequent negative comments about her future. On weekends, she stays in her room. Elizabeth's parents requested that she see her school counselor, and when her symptoms did not improve after a few sessions they sought treatment from her pediatrician. At that visit, Elizabeth denied suicidal ideation, appetite problems, or sleep disturbance, although she frequently stays up late then struggles with waking up in time for school. After completing a physical exam to rule out medical causes for her symptoms and confirming separately with Elizabeth and her parents that there was no suspicion of drug use, Elizabeth's pediatrician diagnosed her with persistent depressive disorder (PDD) and suggested an antidepressant in addition to more intensive outpatient psychotherapy. The pediatrician gave the family a fact sheet about adolescent depression, including warning signs for suicide. Elizabeth was hesitant to try medication due to potential side effects; however, she began outpatient cognitive-behavioral therapy (CBT). Although she made some progress, Elizabeth's grades continued to suffer. At the pediatric follow-up visit 2 months later, Elizabeth was open to trying medication and was placed on fluoxetine, a low-dose selective serotonin reuptake inhibitor (SSRI). Elizabeth and her parents noticed additional improvement within several weeks, especially in school performance and motivation. After also completing 16 sessions of CBT, Elizabeth appeared back on track.

BRIEF OVERVIEW

Depressive disorders are some of the most common psychiatric disorders that cause significant health burdens for children and adolescents (Avenevoli et al., 2015). Depressive disorders in children are associated with increased mortality and morbidity (Dwyer & Bloch, 2019). Early identification and treatment play significant roles in improving children's functional development and wellbeing (National Institute for Health and Care Excellence [NICE], 2019). Effective treatment of depressive disorders can decrease risk of suicidal behaviors and other comorbid psychiatric disorders, such as substance abuse, anxiety, and oppositional defiant disorder (ODD) (Avenevoli, Swendsen, He, Burstein, & Merikangas, 2015).

Box 49.1 lists depressive disorders included in the *Diagnostic and Statistical Manual of Mental Disorders*, fifth edition (*DSM-5*) (American Psychiatric Association [APA], 2013). *DSM-5* criteria for major depressive disorder (MDD) are similar to those in DSM-IV except for bereavement, which is no longer an exclusion criterion. *DSM-5* does describe the difference between the pain of grief and pathologic grief (APA, 2013).

EPIDEMIOLOGY

Nearly one in seven adolescents (13.3%, 3.2 million youth) has experienced at least one episode of MDD, and a majority of these (71%) report severe impairment (https://www.nimh.nih.gov/health/statistics/major-depression.shtml#part_155031). Past year prevalence in adolescents is 20% for girls and 6.8% for boys; risk increases with age (12-year-olds, 4.8%; 17-year-olds, 18.5%). Tragically, over half of youth with MDD (60.1%) do not receive any treatment. Although the gender ratio is well balanced during childhood, after puberty, females have a two- to threefold higher risk for developing depression (APA, 2013). Point prevalence estimates for PDD range from 0.6% to 4.6% in children and 1.6% to 8% in adolescents (Nobile, Cataldo, Marino, & Molteni, 2003). The prevalence of other depressive disorders is not well studied in children and adolescents.

CLINICAL PRESENTATION

Depression occurs on a continuum, from subsyndromal to severe with psychotic features. Course specifiers include with anxious distress, mixed features (subthreshold manic symptoms), melancholic features (e.g., anhedonia, profound moroseness, severe neurovegetative symptoms), atypical features (e.g., increased sleep/appetite, sensitivity rejection), mood-congruent psychotic features, mood-incongruent psychotic features, catatonia (markedly altered movement), peripartum onset, and seasonal pattern (*DSM-5*). While diagnostic criteria are the same regardless of age (except that irritable mood can substitute for dysphoric mood in youth), there are some developmental differences in symptom manifestation. Depressed children are often cranky and irritable (APA, 2013), with low frustration tolerance, and are more likely to express distress via somatic symptoms.

BOX 49.1 Depressive Disorders in *DSM-5*

1. Major depressive disorder: Persistent mood disturbance (depressive mood and/or loss of pleasure in activities) lasting ≥2 wk + a total of ≥5 symptoms, which can include weight loss or gain, insomnia or hypersomnia, psychomotor agitation or retardation, low energy or fatigue, feeling worthless or guilty, poor concentration or indecisiveness, thoughts of suicide or suicidal behaviors.
2. Persistent depressive disorder: Persistent dysphoric mood lasting ≥1 yr (≥2 yr for adults) + ≥ 2 associated symptoms: weight loss or gain, insomnia or hypersomnia, low energy or fatigue, low self-esteem, poor concentration or indecisiveness, hopelessness.
3. Disruptive mood dysregulation disorder: Severe, recurrent verbal and/or behavioral outbursts, ≥3/wk + persistently irritable or angry mood (most of the day, near daily, observable in ≥2 settings: home, school, peers) lasting ≥1 yr without a break in symptoms of ≥3 mo. Symptoms must begin by age 10; diagnosis should not be made before age 6 or after age 18. Must not have had >1 day of (hypo)mania.
4. Premenstrual dysphoric disorder: Episodic mood changes during the final week before most menses, improve within days of menses onset, dissipate in the week postmenses. Marked change in mood (lability, irritability, dysphoria, or anxiety) + ≥5 symptoms: mood changes; decreased interest, concentration, or energy; appetite changes/cravings; sleep disturbance; feeling overwhelmed; physical changes (breast tenderness, joint/muscle pain, bloating/weight gain).
5. Substance/medication-induced depressive disorder: Dysphoria and/or anhedonia; develops during/after medication exposure or substance intoxication/ withdrawal.
6. Depressive disorder due to another medical condition: Dysphoria and/or anhedonia that develops secondary to pathophysiologic consequences of a medical condition.
7. Other specified depressive disorder: Presenting symptoms do not meet full criteria for any other depressive disorder but they cause clinically significant distress or impaired functioning in different settings.
8. Unspecified depressive disorder: Depressive symptoms that do not meet full criteria for the abovementioned disorders and/or there is limited information to make a more specific diagnosis (e.g., in an emergency room setting).

DSM-5, Diagnostic and Statistical Manual of Mental Disorders, fifth edition.

PDD combines the *DSM-IV*–defined chronic MDD with *DSM-IV* dysthymic disorder to decrease confusion about the two almost identical conditions. While MDD requires more symptoms than PDD, PDD ultimately causes more functional impairment due to the longevity of symptoms (APA, 2013).

Disruptive mood dysregulation disorder (DMDD) is new to *DSM-5*. DMDD was added in an attempt to reduce overdiagnosis of childhood bipolar disorder and the overmedication of children. However, reliability of the diagnosis has been called into question (Fristad, 2021). The *International Classification of Diseases and Related Health Problems*, 11th edition (*ICD-11*) has chosen to place this clinical profile within its existing category of ODD with a severity modifier ("with chronic irritability-anger") (Fristad, 2021).

Various medical conditions (e.g., hypothyroidism, chronic fatigue syndrome, anemia, and cancers) may also either co-occur or mimic depressive symptoms (APA, 2013). Standard medical screenings that should be considered include a complete blood count to rule out anemia or infection; serum iron and ferritin levels for iron deficiency anemia (especially in pubertal girls); thyroid-stimulating hormone for patients with symptoms of hypothyroidism (e.g., recent weight gain, constipation, abnormal menstrual bleeding, fatigue); electrolytes, creatinine level, and blood urea nitrogen if there is a clinical concern about possible underlying kidney disease (e.g., symptoms of pale skin, edema, fever, rash, decreased or increased urine output); and liver function tests to consider hepatitis (e.g., symptoms of fatigue, dark urine, jaundice, abdominal pain, unexplained weight loss) (APA, 2013).

Certain medications, including steroids, antihypertensives, and hormonal contraceptives, may also induce depressive symptoms (APA, 2013). Determining onset, offset, and duration of symptoms in relation to medical history and treatments is essential to determine what is a primary psychiatric condition versus depression secondary to other medical concerns.

COMORBID CONDITIONS

Comorbidity is the rule, not the exception. Nearly two-thirds (63.7%) of youth with depression also experience behavioral, anxiety, and/or substance use disorders (Avenevoli et al., 2015). Girls are at greater risk for comorbid anxiety or attention-deficit/hyperactivity disorder (ADHD) compared to boys. MDD can cooccur with PDD; this is known as double depression (APA, 2013). Medical and neurologic conditions can also cooccur (APA, 2013).

SCREENING AND ASSESSMENT

Frequent depression screening is recommended (Box 49.2). Children age 3 years and older can be reliably screened if there is a concern for emotional or behavioral changes (Silver et al., 2021). The American Academy of Child and Adolescent Psychiatry supports routine screening for depression in children age 8 years and older, while the US Preventive Services Task Force recommends screening for MDD in adolescents age 12 to 18 years. Screening tools in the public domain with widespread use include the Patient Health Questionnaire-9, modified for adolescents (PHQ-A) and the Short Mood and Feelings Questionnaire (SMFQ) (Liu & Adrian, 2019). The Preschool Feelings Checklist (PFC) has been developed for 3- to 6-year-old children; high scores reflect broad transdiagnostic liability for psychopathology and impairment (Silver et al., 2021). Reliable change scores have been calculated for the SMFQ-C/P and the PHQ-9A, making them user friendly for monitoring treatment response.

BOX 49.2 Self-Report Measures for Screening and Measurement-Based Care[a]

Measure	PFC[b]	SMFQ-C[c]	SMFQ-P[d]	PHQ-9A[e]
Age	3–6 yr	6–17 yr	6–17 yr	12–18 yr
Informant	Parent	Child	Parent	Adolescent
Number of items	16	13	13	9
Time frame	–	Past 2 wk	Past 2 wk	Past 2 wk
Score range	0–16	0–26	0–26	0–27
Reliable change score	–	6	8	7
Screening cutoff score	<3: Below cutoff ≥3: Above cutoff	<8: Below cutoff 8–11: Above cutoff ≥12: Well above cutoff	<8: Below cutoff 8–11: Above cutoff ≥12: Well above cutoff	≤4: No/minimal symptoms 5–9: Mild symptoms 10–14: Moderate symptoms 15–19: Moderately severe symptoms 20–27: Severe symptoms

[a]Liu, F. F., & Adrian, M. C. (2019). Is treatment working? Detecting real change in the treatment of child and adolescent depression. *Journal of the American Academy of Child and Adolescent Psychiatry, 58*(12), 1157–1164.
[b]Preschool Feelings Checklist (Silver, J., Olino, T. M., Luby, J., Hawes, M. H., Carlson, G. A., & Klein, D. N. [2021]. Reliability and validity of preschool feelings checklist. *Research on Child and Adolescent Psychopathology*. https://doi.org/10.1007/s10802-020-00746-0)
[c]Short Mood and Feelings Questionnaire-Child Report
[d]Short Mood and Feelings Questionnaire-Parent Report
[e]Patient Health Questionnaire-9 Item Adolescent Form

Youth who score above a screening cutoff should receive a comprehensive diagnostic evaluation. If not depressed there is a high likelihood they have another psychiatric condition that warrants clinical attention. No biomarkers or brain imaging tests are currently available to diagnose depression. Key considerations for evaluation include importance of good rapport with the youth and parent; awareness of the child's stage of development, including normative adolescent issues (e.g., moodiness, increased interaction with peers, decreased interaction with parents; NICE, 2019); cultural and religious background, race, sex, and other environmental factors (NICE, 2019); and careful clinical observation. Interviewing parent(s) and child together and separately is recommended (NICE, 2019).

Suicidal and homicidal ideation are common in children and adolescents with depressive symptoms; these should be monitored throughout treatment (NICE, 2019). Nonsuicidal self-harm behaviors, which commonly involve self-cutting, scratching, and burning, often present in youth who are attempting to diminish negative emotions (e.g., anger, anxiety), increase positive emotions (e.g., feeling alive), receive positive social reinforcement (e.g., get attention), or escape negative social reinforcement (e.g., avoid an unwanted event) (Brown & Plener, 2017) (see Chapter 50 for more on this topic).

When assessing a first episode of depression it is important to consider the possibility that symptoms could represent unipolar depression or the first episode of bipolar disorder. A known family history of bipolar disorder, psychotic symptoms, atypical depressive symptoms, or medication-induced manic episodes increases the likelihood of a potential bipolar disorder (Diler & Birmaher, 2019). Taking a careful history to ascertain presence or absence of current or past mixed or subclinical hypomanic/manic symptoms is essential.

TREATMENT

Treating depression in youth can include multiple components and will vary based on severity of illness. Psychoeducation should always be included as it plays a vital role in treatment adherence (Zalpuri & Singh, 2019). Symptom recognition is critical in helping youth and parents understand what is part of a treatable condition rather than an unpleasant aspect of the child's personality or behavior. Understanding risk of recurrence is important when active treatment comes to an end so that the family can return to treatment before any relapse or recurrence becomes severe. Family involvement is integral for maintaining safety, treatment adherence, and monitoring clinical progress (Zalpuri & Singh, 2019).

In cases of mild depression psychotherapy is a recommended first treatment option, although adjunctive medication may also be required (Zalpuri & Singh, 2019). Lifestyle issues should also be considered—evidence supports the importance of regular aerobic exercise, adequate and regular sleep, healthful nutrition, prayer/meditation, and prosocial activity such as volunteering (Dickstein & Croarkin, 2019).

Psychotherapeutic Interventions

There are three evidenced-based, effective psychotherapeutic treatment options for depressed adolescents: CBT, dialectic behavioral therapy for adolescents (DBT-A), and interpersonal therapy for adolescents (IPT-A) (Clark, Ragan, & Berk, 2019; Santamarina & Packer, 2019). Psychotherapy for depression in children is less well studied; however, there is also limited evidence for CBT, DBT, and IPT in this age group (Santamarina & Packer, 2019). Integrating parents into treatment appears to be increasingly important with younger-aged youth. See Chapters 96 through 98 for more on psychotherapeutic interventions.

CBT, which focuses on connecting the relationship between thoughts, feelings, and behaviors, targets behavioral activation and challenging distorted cognitive patterns. CBT has a higher response rate when combined with medication, particularly fluoxetine, than when used alone; it also confers specific benefits, including reduced risk of suicide-related outcomes (Kim, Gandhi, & Cullen, 2019).

IPT strives to help youth improve communication and problem solving within significant relationships (e.g., peers, parents) by focusing on one or two of four problem areas (i.e., role disputes, role transitions, interpersonal deficits, grief) (Santamarina & Packer, 2019). IPT is recommended for youth with severe depressive symptoms, comorbid anxiety, and high levels of conflict with parents and peers (Santamarina & Packer, 2019).

DBT targets treatment engagement, reduction of self-harm and suicide attempts, and the learning/application of skills to enhance emotion regulation, distress tolerance, and build a life worth living (Asarnow, Berk, Bedics, Adrian, & McCauley, 2021). DBT decreases recurrent suicide attempts and self-harm in highly suicidal, self-harming adolescents (Asarnow et al., 2021).

Family therapy has some evidence of efficacy for treating depression in youth, while psychodynamic therapy and play therapy currently lack evidence for efficacy (Santamarina & Packer, 2019).

Pharmacotherapy

Although psychotherapy can be sufficient to treat mild to moderate depression in youth, medications also can be beneficial, particularly in combination with psychotherapy for moderate to severe depression (Box 49.3). The US Food and Drug Administration (FDA) has approved escitalopram and fluoxetine for pediatric depression (Kim et al., 2019). Sertraline has evidence of efficacy in two multicenter, double-blind, placebo-controlled studies (Kim et al., 2019). Citalopram should be prescribed cautiously due to its ability to increase the electrocardiogram QT interval that may lead to arrhythmia (Kim et al., 2019). Paroxetine and fluvoxamine lack efficacy in this age group (Kim et al., 2019). See Chapter 99 for more on psychopharmacology.

Antidepressants should be started at a low dose, with titration planned for every 2 to 3 weeks until a clinical effective dose is reached. Children may have a higher risk of withdrawal symptoms due to high drug metabolism rates. Twice-daily dosage may be used if necessary, to avoid experiencing daytime withdrawal symptoms (Cheung et al., 2018; Kim et al., 2019). Side effects are mostly dose dependent and may improve over time.

Serotonin reuptake inhibitors (SNRIs) have similar effectivity as SSRIs for treatment-resistant depression. However, SNRIs may increase blood pressure (Dwyer & Bloch, 2019). Duloxetine, an SNRI, has been used for adolescents with depression and comorbid pain (Dwyer & Bloch, 2019). There is little evidence supporting the use of bupropion, although it is sometimes used for patients with comorbid ADHD or for those committed to smoking cessation (Dwyer & Bloch, 2019). The immediate release form of bupropion is associated with seizures, especially when doses exceed 400 mg/day (Singh, 2019).

Tricyclic antidepressants (TCAs) are a last treatment option due to lack of efficacy compared to placebo, higher side effects, and overdose lethality concerns (Kim et al., 2019).

The FDA (2004) defined emergence or worsening of suicidal ideation as a serious adverse effect for antidepressants, indicating that patients being treated with antidepressants should be monitored closely especially in the first few months after initiating treatment or when dose adjustments occur (Ho, 2012). Since then, there have been conflicting studies about these potential risks (Cheung et al., 2018; Kim et al., 2019). In clinical practice suicidal risk should not be underestimated; patients should contact their providers immediately if suicidal ideation occurs (NICE, 2019).

PREVENTION

Prevention encompasses avoiding initial onset of depression and curtailing recurrent episodes. Addressing risk factors and treating prodromal depressive symptoms are important. Risk factors may include parental depression, prior depressive episodes, comorbidities, poor peer relations, psychosocial stressors, and subsyndromal symptoms (Hafeman & Spada, 2019). Most studies of depression prevention are CBT or IPT based; programs for at-risk populations appear to be more effective than universal programs (i.e., programs

BOX 49.3 Dosing of Antidepressants and Adverse Effects

Medication	Starting Dose (mg/day)	Dose Range (mg/day)	Maximum Dose (mg/day)	Common Side Effects
Citalopram	10	20–40	40	Headache, gastrointestinal (GI) upset, insomnia/sedation, QT prolongation
Fluoxetine	10–20	20–60	80	Headache, GI upset, insomnia, rash, anxiety
Sertraline	25–50	100–200	200	Headache, GI upset, insomnia/sedation
Escitalopram	5–10	10–20	20	Headache, GI upset, insomnia
Bupropion	100	150–300	300	Irritability, headache, dizziness, insomnia
Duloxetine	30	30–60	120	GI upset, headache, dry mouth, dizziness, appetite changes

Based on the US Food and Drug Administration (FDA) data. Retrieved from https://www.accessdata.fda.gov/scripts/cder/daf/index.cfm

that target the general public regardless of clinical status) (Hafeman & Spada, 2019).

SUICIDE IN CHILDREN AND ADOLESCENTS

Background

In the United States suicide is the second leading cause of death among 15- to 24-year-olds and the third leading cause of death in youth age 10 to 14 years (Clark et al., 2019). Half of completed suicides are the result of first attempts; 86% of adolescents with suicidal ideation will attempt within 1 year's time (Clark et al., 2019). Suicide risk significantly increases with age, particularly during the transition to adolescence. This increase may be related to hormonal shifts, a developmental transition to the importance of peers along with decreased interactions with parents, cognitive maturity to develop suicidal plans and preparation, and overall increased psychopathology during adolescence. Completed suicides are more common in males, whereas females show higher rates of suicidal ideation (Tondo & Baldessarini, 2021).

Suicidal behavior in children and adolescents may be seen with a variety of psychiatric disorders, including ADHD, conduct, anxiety, posttraumatic stress disorder (PTSD), eating, psychotic, and sleep disorders (Clark et al., 2019). Frequency and severity of suicidal ideation should be evaluated. More severe ideation, prior attempt, stronger intent, nonsuicidal self-injury, nonheterosexual orientation, childhood maltreatment, family history of suicide, and contagion (e.g., a suicide at the same school) are all significant risk factors for completed suicide (Clark et al., 2019). The Ask Suicide Screening Questions (ASQ) (Horowitz et al., 2012) is a four-item public domain screening instrument designed to identify risk of suicide in youth. The ASQ is considered positive for elevated suicide risk if a patient answers "yes" to any of the following questions:

1. In the past few weeks have you felt that you or your family would be better off if you were dead?
2. In the past few weeks have you wished you were dead?
3. In the past week have you been having thoughts about killing yourself?
4. Have you ever tried to kill yourself?

Treatment

Depression treatment alone may not be sufficient to reduce suicide risk; additional intervention may be needed (Clark et al., 2019). DBT-A is effective in treating highly suicidal, self-harming adolescents, making it a vital treatment component for high-risk youth (Asarnow et al., 2021). In a randomized controlled trial comparing DBT-A to individual and group supportive therapy adolescents treated with DBT-A had improved emotion regulation at the end of treatment and at 12-month follow-up. This improved emotion regulation mediated other substantive outcomes, including substance misuse, externalizing symptoms, and total problems posttreatment and at a 6-month follow-up, and externalizing symptoms at 12-month follow-up (Asarnow et al., 2021).

While there is no pharmacologic treatment for suicidal ideation or intent, lithium and clozapine may decrease suicidal ideation by increasing emotional regulation (Tondo & Baldessarini, 2021). Safety planning, means restriction, minimizing risk factors, and inpatient hospitalization or crisis stabilization are considered best practices for acute suicide prevention (Clark et al., 2019; NICE, 2019). See Chapter 50 for more information about this topic.

BIPOLAR SPECTRUM DISORDER

VIGNETTE

Rebecca, a bright 12-year-old middle school student, presented to her pediatrician's office with complaints of severe mood swings and irritability. Her parents describe Rebecca's recent behavior as "being on an emotional roller coaster." Rebecca can become very upset and irritable without any visible trigger. At times she starts laughing at almost everything. When in this up-mood, Rebecca talks excessively and hops around from topic to topic. These up-moods rarely last more than a day or two at a time, but the down-moods can go on for several weeks. Rebecca denied any sleep problems except for having vivid dreams; however, her mother mentioned that on her up-mood days Rebecca stays up extra late in her bedroom (not very quietly) yet has plenty of energy the next day.

Rebecca was diagnosed with ADHD around age 6 years and was prescribed methylphenidate for 2 years but discontinued it as her parents were concerned about chronic use of medication at a young age. Rebecca's father reported that he is prescribed lithium for his bipolar disorder, which he and Rebecca's mother agreed appears to be effective at managing his symptoms. After the clinical interview, the pediatrician diagnosed Rebecca with other specified bipolar and related disorders (OSBARD) and referred the family to the local mental health clinic. Rebecca saw a child and adolescent psychiatrist who started her on lithium and referred the family to a family psychoeducation plus skill-building group.

BRIEF OVERVIEW

Bipolar spectrum disorder (BPSD) (Box 49.4) is characterized by recurrent episodes of emotionally high states (i.e., mania, hypomania) and low states (i.e., depression) that often can lead to academic, social, and psychological impairment (Carvalho, Firth, & Vieta, 2020). Earlier onset BPSD is associated with poorer prognosis, including more severe depressive episodes and higher comorbidity rates (Carvalho et al., 2020). Family history of BPSD is the strongest risk factor for diagnosis (APA, 2013). BPSD onset is not associated with nationality or financial status (Van Meter, Moreira, & Youngstrom, 2019).

BOX 49.4 *DSM-5* Bipolar and Related Disorders

1. Bipolar I disorder (BP1): ≥1 manic episode (elevated, expansive, and/or irritable mood with increased activity) lasting ≥7 days (any duration if hospitalization is necessary) + ≥3 (4 if mood is only irritable) symptoms: grandiosity, increased energy and activity, decreased need for sleep, distractibility, racing thoughts, pressured speech, and increased involvement in activities characterized by poor judgment. M (+ D)
2. Bipolar II disorder (BP2): ≥1 major depressive episode (see Box 49-1) + ≥1 hypomanic episode (same as above) lasting ≥4 days + ≥3 (4 if mood is only irritable) symptoms (same as above). m + D
3. Cyclothymic disorder (CYC): Hypomanic + depressive symptoms that do not meet criteria for hypomanic or major depressive episodes lasting ≥1 yr (≥2 yr for adults) with no symptom-free period of ≥2 mo. Symptoms are impairing and not due to a medical condition or substance. m + d
4. Substance/medication-induced bipolar and related disorders: Elevated, expansive, and/or irritable mood with or without depressed mood or severe loss of interest/pleasure in most activities. Pronounced symptoms develop during or after medication exposure or intoxication/withdrawal from a substance known to cause such effects.
5. Bipolar and related disorders associated with another medical condition: Elevated, expansive, and/or irritable mood and increased energy with or without depressed mood or severe loss of interest/pleasure in most activities. Pronounced symptoms develop secondary to pathophysiologic consequences of another medical condition.
6. Other specified bipolar and related disorders (OSBARD): Presenting symptoms do not meet full criteria for any of the above, but do cause clinically significant distress or functional impairment. The most common cause in youth is recurrent short-duration hypomania (e.g., 1–3 days), alternating with MDD.
7. Unspecified bipolar and related disorders: Bipolar symptoms are present but do not meet full criteria for abovementioned disorders; most commonly diagnosed when limited information is available (e.g., in an emergency room setting).

DSM-5, Diagnostic and Statistical Manual of Mental Disorders, fifth edition.

A comprehensive clinical assessment (often with longitudinal follow-up) is necessary to differentiate unipolar depression from BPSD (Carvalho et al., 2020). Common symptom progression includes anxiety and sleep problems followed by recurrent depressive episodes and ultimately BPSD (Diler & Birmaher, 2019). Early intervention may prevent progression and long-term consequences (Hafeman & Spada, 2019).

EPIDEMIOLOGY

Prevalence of bipolar 1 (BP1) disorder in youth is 0.6%, while BPSD estimates range from 2.5% to 3.9% (Merikangas et al., 2011; Van Meter et al., 2019). A majority (90%) of those diagnosed report severe impairment (National Institute of Mental Health [NIMH], 2019). Rates are higher for girls (3.3%) than boys (2.6%), and risk increases with age: 1.9% for 13- to 14-year-olds, 3.1% for 15- to 16-year-olds, and 4.3% for 17- to 18-year-olds (NIMH, 2019).

CLINICAL PRESENTATION

BPSD can occur even in preschool years, although this is rare (McClellan, Kowatch, & Findling, 2007) and should be approached with extreme caution. Children with BPSD are more likely to present with OSBARD, while BP1 and BP2 are more likely to appear in adolescence (Hafeman & Spada, 2019). Despite BPSD significantly impacting normal development and psychosocial functioning and being associated with highly comorbid conditions, including suicide, substance abuse, and psychosis, a 7- to 10-year delay has been documented in correctly identifying mania in clinical settings (Diler & Birmaher, 2019; Miklowitz, 2019).

Symptoms that best differentiate BPSD from other psychiatric diagnoses are those not common to other diagnoses. Decreased need for sleep over repeated days is a clear indicator. This change in sleep should present a significant change from baseline (i.e., a difference of several hours) that is not due to environmental explanations (e.g., studying for final exams) with the individual feeling well rested the next day. Other hallmark symptoms include uncharacteristic grandiosity and hypersexuality. Irritability and psychomotor agitation are not specific to BPSD; these symptoms should only count toward a diagnosis if they only occur, or are clearly exacerbated, during a manic episode. Chronic irritability also is not an indicator of BPSD (Fristad, 2021). A key consideration when diagnosing a hypomanic or manic episode is that there is a clearly observable change in mood associated with accompanying excessive displays of energy, speech, or abnormal thought patterns, decreased judgment, or lack of insight. Again, these symptoms should not be in reaction to an environmental trigger. A longitudinal perspective is essential.

Numerous medical conditions can either exacerbate or mimic BPSD (Box 49.5). Also, illicit drugs, dopaminergic agents, corticosteroids, and anabolic androgens have potential to induce manic symptoms, while SSRIs, TCAs, SNRIs, monoamine oxidase inhibitors, and light therapy can induce mania in patients with strong genetic susceptibility for BPSD (Vieta et al., 2018).

When diagnosing a child or adolescent with BPSD, developmental level must be taken into consideration. A firm understanding of typical behavior is critical. Depressive episodes are the most common initial presentation for BPSD in youth (Diler & Birmaher, 2019). Recurrent episodes after the index episode are most commonly depressive (60%; hypomanic, 21%; manic, 15%) (Diler & Birmaher, 2019). Patients with bipolar depression, compared to those with unipolar depression, are more likely to have greater severity, more mixed features, and more comorbidity (Diler & Birmaher, 2019). Finally, course specifiers (same as for depression) also indicate important clinical features of BPSD.

BOX 49.5 Medical Conditions That Mimic Bipolar Disorder

Clinical Observations	Clinical Assessments
Autoimmune Encephalitis • Mood disturbances, including depression and mania • Catatonia • Perceptual changes (hallucinations, illusions, delusions) • Agitation, aggression, impulsive behaviors • Altered mental status and cognitive changes can be seen	Lab work: • Cerebrospinal fluid (CSF) shows pleocytosis (white blood cell count of >5 cells/mm) with elevated protein and normal glucose • Minimal elevation of inflammatory markers (e.g., erythrocyte sedimentation rate [ESR], C-reactive protein, serum antibody titers) Imaging/other studies: • Magnetic resonance imaging (MRI) may show enhanced temporal lobe/basal ganglia • Electroencephalography (EEG) generally shows nonspecific findings, including intermittent delta waves, epileptiform changes; extreme delta brush in NMDA-R encephalitis • Systemic body imaging (chest, abdomen, pelvis) to assess for presence of teratoma
Hyperthyroidism • Anxiety, mood lability, depression, insomnia are commonly seen • Manic, mixed episodes, and hallucinations are rare	Lab work: • Low thyroid-stimulating hormone level • Elevated plasma levels of T4 and/or T3 Physical exam: • Tremor • Hyperreflexia • Tachycardia • Frequent bowel movements • Enlarged thyroid gland (goiter) • Exophthalmos • Proximal muscle weakness/myopathy
Temporal Lobe Epilepsy • Stereotypic brief paroxysmal behavioral changes (e.g., olfactory hallucination, déjà vu, depersonalization, and/or derealization) • Interictal depression occurs in >30% of temporal lobe epilepsy patients	• EEG shows temporal lobe epileptiform activity • Brain MRI can identify possible structural causes of epilepsy (e.g., mesial temporal sclerosis, cortical dysplasia, low-grade gliomas, or cavernous angiomas)
Head Trauma • Aggression and irritability are common following injury • Delirium-associated mood disturbances, posttraumatic apathy, and/or personality change may occur • Pathologic laughter and crying (pseudobulbar affect) can be seen without pervasive mood alteration	• Head computed tomography, especially in acute settings—check for fractures, vascular injuries, cerebrovascular fluid leakage • MRI may be needed to detect presence of blood, nonhemorrhagic contusions, brainstem or axonal injuries
Multiple Sclerosis (MS) • Symptoms of depression, anxiety, euphoria, and/or psychosis • Bipolar disorder itself is rare in patients with MS	Lab work: • Increased oligoclonal bands in CSF • IgG index (comparison of IgG to albumin ratio in serum and CSF) is elevated Imaging/other studies: • MRI shows dissemination of white matter lesions across both space (location) and time (from baseline to subsequent studies) • Abnormal results on visual evoked potentials and optic coherence tomography in patients with optic neuritis Physical exam: • Positive findings on comprehensive neurologic exam

(Continued)

BOX 49.5 Medical Conditions That Mimic Bipolar Disorder—Cont'd

Clinical Observations	Clinical Assessments
Systemic Lupus Erythematosus (SLE)	
• Manic episode could be the first manifestation of SLE	Lab work: • Complete blood count may show anemia, leukopenia, or thrombocytopenia • ESR is elevated • Antinuclear antibody test is positive • Comprehensive metabolic panel, including kidney and liver function tests, can be abnormal • Urinalysis may show increased protein level or red blood cells Imaging/other studies: • Chest X-ray may reveal patchy areas of increased opacity • Echocardiogram may show acquired structural cardiac abnormalities
Alcohol-Related Neurodevelopmental Disorder	
• Can present with various mood disorders (MDD, 44%; PDD, 4%; BP1, 20%)	• Facial dysmorphism • Growth retardation • Central nervous system abnormalities • Cognitive and functional deficits
Wilson Disease	
• Depression, irritability • Poor school performance • Impulsivity, hyperactivity • Inappropriate behaviors • Frequent loss of emotional control, loss of sexual inhibition	Physical exam: • Abnormal comprehensive neurologic exam (e.g., dysarthria, dystonia, seizures, tremor) • Kayser-Fleischer rings in ocular slit-lamp examination supports the diagnosis Lab work: • Elevated liver function tests • Low serum ceruloplasmin • Elevated copper fraction • Elevated 24-hr urinary copper excretion

BP1, Bipolar type 1; *MDD*, major depressive disorder; *PDD*, persistent depressive disorder.

COMORBID CONDITIONS

BPSDs are highly complex and present heterogeneously. Epidemiologic studies have indicated that medical and psychiatric comorbid disorders are common in BPSD (APA, 2013). Anxiety disorders (54%), ADHD (48%), disruptive behavior disorders (31%), and substance use disorders (31%) are the most common, with pervasive developmental disorders being reported in 19% of youth with BPSD (Frías, Palma, & Farriols, 2015). ADHD is more common in childhood onset compared to adolescent onset BPSD, whereas substance use disorder is more common in adolescents than children. Notably, substance use disorder is more common in youth with comorbid BPSD and PTSD (Frías et al., 2015). Presence of any comorbid disorders negatively affects clinical outcome (Azzopardi-Larios & Galanter, 2019), therefore clinical assessments should be comprehensive and should address other possible comorbid conditions.

SCREENING AND ASSESSMENT

Measurement-based care can be used to efficiently screen for psychopathology, enhance clinical evaluation, monitor treatment progress, and aid in treatment planning (Singh, 2019). Important features of screening instruments include brevity, ease of scoring, availability in the public domain, and demonstration of strong psychometric properties. The Brief Child Mania Rating Scale (BCMRS) is a 10-item self-report instrument with youth (for age ≥12 years) and parent versions (Singh, 2019). Two additional optional questions allow for indicating whether symptoms have occurred at the same time and if any family member has ever been diagnosed with mania/BPSD (https://www.nationwidechildrens.org/specialties/behavioral-health/for-providers/psychological-measures).

Key elements in diagnosing BPSD are to assess behavior over time, in a developmental context, with a longitudinal perspective. Symptom onset, offset, and duration should be assessed in relation to the child's social history, physical, and mental health treatment history, and functioning at home, in school, and with peers should be ascertained.

Interviewing the parent(s), obtaining a family history, and observing and interviewing the child are essential. It is also critical to determine the child's baseline characteristic features and symptoms to evaluate whether episodic mood changes occur (Singh, 2019). The intensity, frequency, duration, and number of manic and depressive symptoms should be assessed, with careful consideration of both comorbid conditions and differential diagnoses. Drug screening may be needed to clarify substance-induced symptoms, particularly in emergency room settings

Structured interviews (e.g., the NIMHealth Diagnostic Interview Schedule for Children, Version IV, DISC-IV) and semistructured interviews (e.g., the Kiddie Schedule for Affective Disorders and Schizophrenia for School Age Children, Present and Lifetime Version, KSADS-PL) provide a comprehensive framework to aid diagnosis. The KSADS Mania Rating Scale (KMRS) is a clinical rating scale that focuses specifically on rating severity of manic symptoms. Finally, mood diaries may be useful to monitor treatment response over time as well as to obtain additional information about course of illness and episode triggers (Diler & Birmaher, 2019).

TREATMENT OF BIPOLAR DISORDER

Acute Manic/Mixed Mania

Pharmacotherapy is the primary treatment for BPSD (Box 49.6). The FDA has approved eight medications: seven second-generation antipsychotics (SGAs; risperidone, aripiprazole, olanzapine, olanzapine/fluoxetine combination, quetiapine, lurasidone, and asenapine) and one mood stabilizer (lithium) to treat acute mania and/or mixed mania in youth (Patino & DelBello, 2019).

Monotherapy is advised as the first step. Medication choice should be based on evidence of effectiveness, presence of comorbid conditions, possible side effects, disorder subtype, and the patient's and family members' prior medication treatment responses. As a general rule, prescribers should begin with the lowest therapeutic dose, then gradually increase unless the patient is severely manic, psychotic, extremely agitated, or suicidal. In those circumstances starting at a higher dose is justified. If this is insufficient, initiate another SGA option while tapering down the first medication. Lithium can be used as combination treatment if the patient is not responsive to multiple trials of antipsychotic medication.

If a patient does not tolerate or respond to the initial monotherapy (either SGA or mood stabilizer), the dose should be adjusted. A switch to another medication within the same class (i.e., SGA or mood stabilizer) can also be considered. If additional modifications are needed to achieve treatment response, the second class of medication could be added (e.g., combining an SGA with a mood stabilizer). During the acute phase of treatment, benzodiazepines may be utilized to manage severe agitation or sleep problems; melatonin and antihistamines such as diphenhydramine and hydroxyzine can also be used for insomnia. Beyond these concerns, it is important to prioritize stabilization of acute mania over treatment of a comorbid condition.

Patients and parents should be informed of possible short- and long-term effects of any medication prior to its initiation. Due to high teratogenic potential, a pregnancy test should be ordered for female adolescents, and psychoeducation should be provided regarding potential risks of being pregnant while on antimanic medications. In some cases urine toxicology screening may be helpful to detect possible triggers of a current episode (e.g., alcohol, stimulant abuse [including prescribed ADHD medication, cocaine, amphetamine, opioids, benzodiazepines]).

Bipolar Depression

Two FDA-approved interventions for youth aged 10 to 17 years with bipolar depression are lurasidone and an olanzapine plus fluoxetine combination, although treatment-emergent hyperlipidemia is common in the latter (Patino & DelBello, 2019). Other commonly used medications for bipolar depression are lithium, lamotrigine, valproate, cariprazine, lurasidone, and a combination of SGAs and antidepressants (Patino & DelBello, 2019). While effective for adults with bipolar depression, quetiapine has not proven to be effective for youth with bipolar depression (Patino & DelBello, 2019).

Antidepressant use carries risk of triggering mania/hypomania. Rates of activation secondary to SSRI treatment are higher in children compared to adolescents (Perlis et al., 2010). Omega-3 fatty acids are linked with improvement, but not amelioration, of symptoms in youth with bipolar depression (Patino & DelBello, 2019). Light therapy has limited evidence (Hirakawa, Terao, Muronaga, & Ishii, 2020).

Maintenance

There are two FDA-approved maintenance medications (lithium and quetiapine) for adults with BPSD, but limited data are found in youth. In general, treatments that have been effective in the acute phase should be continued, if possible, in maintenance treatment (Patino & DelBello, 2019). If mood symptoms increase, the overall treatment plan should be reviewed to determine if pharmacologic or nonpharmacologic components need to be intensified.

Treating Comorbid Conditions

Comorbid conditions may impact treatment success. Evidence-based guidelines are limited to ADHD; current data suggest that stabilization of BPSD should be prioritized before initiation of stimulant treatment for comorbid ADHD (Azzopardi-Larios & Galanter, 2019).

Specific Medication Considerations

Second-Generation Antipsychotics

Although effective, SGAs also have frequent side effects (see Box 49.6) that can pose concern, especially if used over an extended period of time. Clozapine is indicated in adults for resistant cases but requires very careful monitoring due to potentially serious side effects, including agranulocytosis, myocarditis, and seizures (McClellan et al., 2007).

One major consideration is the risk for metabolic changes and weight gain. Lurasidone and ziprasidone are associated with the least weight gain, while olanzapine and risperidone carry the highest risk. Consultation with a nutritionist and referral to a weight management clinic may be discussed with the family for anyone at risk of metabolic syndrome. Adjunctive metformin, in addition to lifestyle modifications, may be helpful (Diler & Birmaher, 2019; Zheng et al., 2019). Extrapyramidal symptoms must be monitored, as

BOX 49.6 Medications for Pediatric Bipolar Spectrum Disorder

Medication	Dosage	Side Effects	Clinical Notes
Second-Generation Antipsychotics (SGAs)			
Risperidone	Initial dose 0.5 mg qhs; titrate up to 6 mg/day. May be more effective in divided doses (2–3×/day)	Sedation, GI upset, weight gain, prolaction elevation, EPS	• Lower doses (0.5–2.5 mg) have better benefit-risk ratio than higher doses • Long-acting injection available
Quetiapine	Initial dose 25 mg qhs; titrate ≤400–600 mg/day	Headache, sedation, orthostasis, weight gain, GI upset, EPS	• Improves sleep quality • Extended-release formulation is available
Olanzapine	Initial dose 2.5–5 mg qhs; titrate ≤10–20 mg/day	Weight gain, dyslipidemia, sedation, EPS	High metabolic syndrome risk
Asenapine	Initial dose 2.5 mg 2× daily; titrate ≤10 mg 2× daily	Somnolence, sedation, dizziness, headache	• Avoid food and water for 10 min postadministration • Oral paresthesia secondary to sublingual administration
Lurasidone	Initial dose 20 mg; titrate ≤80 mg/day	Nausea, somnolence, akathisia, parkinsonism	• Minimal QTc prolongation • Must take with food (≥350 calories) to facilitate absorption
Aripiprazole	Initial dose 2 mg; titrate ≤30 mg/day	EPS, tardive dyskinesia, dystonia, parkinsonism, hyperglycemia, erythema multiforme	• Less sedating • Minimal EPS risk • Akathisia common
Mood Stabilizers			
Lithium	• Initial dose 30/mg/kg/day in divided doses (2×/day) • Target serum lithium level: • 0.8–1.2 mEq/L in acute mania • 0.6–0.8 mEq/L in maintenance	• GI distress, sedation, tremor, enuresis, weight gain, alopecia, acne • May induce hypothyroidism, diabetes insipidus, polyuria, renal disease	• Protects against suicide • Monitor lithium serum concentrations, blood urea nitrogen, creatinine, TFT every 6 mo
Sodium divalproex/ valproic acid	• Initial dose 10–15 mg/kg/day in divided doses • Target serum valproic acid level 50–125 mcg/mL	• Sedation, platelet dysfunction, liver disease, alopecia, weight gain • May induce elevated liver enzymes, bone marrow suppression, polycystic ovarian syndrome, risk of NTD to offspring if used in pregnant patients	• May be useful for externalizing behaviors • Highly teratogenic • Mostly adjunctive medication with SGA or lithium • Monitor LFTs and CBC
Carbamazepine	• Initial dose 15 mg/kg/day in divided doses • Target serum carbamazepine level 7–10 mcg/L	• Mild hepatic enzyme elevations, neurologic symptoms (drowsiness, diplopia, ataxia), erythema multiforme • May induce aplastic anemia, thrombocytopenia • Hyponatremia	• May decrease blood concentration of other medications • High risk for Stevens-Johnson syndrome with specific HLA antigen alleles (e.g., HLA-B*1502)
Oxcarbazepine	• Initial dose 8–10 mg/kg/day in divided doses • Does not require plasma level monitoring	• Similar but milder side effects than carbamazepine • Hyponatremia (increased risk in first 3 mo)	• Fewer interactions with other medications • High risk for Stevens-Johnson syndrome with specific HLA antigen alleles (e.g., HLA-B*1502)
Lamotrigine	Initial dose 25 mg/day; titrate ≤200 mg/day	Nausea, dyspepsia, erythema multiforme, leukopenia, sedation, or insomnia	• Less sedating than others in category • Significant risk of erythema multiforme major (Stevens-Johnson) • Requires slow titration (25 mg/week)

AP, Antipsychotics; *EPS*, extrapyradimal symptoms; *LFT*, liver function tests; *NTD*, neural tube defect; *qhs*, nightly at bedtime; *SGA*, second-generation antipsychotics; *TFT*, thyroid function test.

tardive dyskinesia and neuroleptic malignant syndrome can occur. Prior to treatment with SGAs, a baseline electrocardiogram should be considered, especially for patients with a family history of cardiac abnormalities or with a risk for QT prolongation.

Mood Stabilizers

Lithium treatment has some advantages, including being associated with fewer lifetime anxiety episodes, lowered suicide risk, and decreased need for antidepressant treatment when compared with other mood stabilizers (Hafeman et al., 2020). Due to a narrow therapeutic window, adjusting lithium doses should be made cautiously. As lithium is a salt, patients and parents should be mindful to avoid dehydration during intensive exercise and in hot weather.

Each mood stabilizer has unique effectivity and side effect profiles, requiring careful clinical monitoring (see Box 49.6). Lamotrigine has less robust evidence in treating pediatric BPSD (Patino & DelBello, 2019). It is primarily used to manage bipolar depression without causing manic mood shifts and tends to be well tolerated with a low risk of weight gain. Topiramate has very limited efficacy data and is linked to cognitive side effects, upper respiratory infections, paresthesia, and diarrhea (Patino & DelBello, 2019).

Antidepressants

Any antidepressant intervention runs the risk of triggering a switch to mania or initiating disinhibition. Disinhibition fades when medication is discontinued, whereas a switch to mania can lead to the need for increased antimanic intervention. The risk of increased suicidal ideation should be discussed with the family when prescribing an SSRI. A possible acute increase in agitation and emergence of serotonin syndrome (particularly for patients receiving lithium in addition to other serotonergic agents) should also be discussed. When indicated, most commonly to address accompanying anxiety symptoms or to decrease depressive symptom severity, SSRIs should be started at the lowest dose after stabilizing the manic episode; TCAs are not effective and should not be used (Patino & DelBello, 2019).

Electroconvulsive Therapy

Electroconvulsive therapy (ECT) should be considered if the patient is experiencing severe mania or depression and is nonresponsive to mood stabilizers and antipsychotic treatments. ECT can be a first-line treatment for urgent presentations, including severe suicidality or psychosis, malignant catatonia, or manic delirium.

Psychotherapeutic Interventions

Psychoeducation plays a significant role in treating BPSD (Fristad, 2016). Families and patients should be informed about possible causes/triggers, the nature of the disease, treatment options, and possible short- and long-term side effects of prescribed medications. The importance of treatment adherence, sleep hygiene, possible consequences of nonadherence, and risks of sleep deprivation should be stressed. Family-based psychoeducation plus skill building is a well-established class of psychosocial intervention for youth with BPSD and their families. Multiple randomized controlled trials by different investigators show improved mood regulation, overall functioning, and treatment adherence (Fristad, 2016). It may also help to prevent future episodes (Miklowitz, 2019). Three examples include family-focused therapy (FFT), child- and family-focused CBT (CFF-CBT), and psychoeducational psychotherapy (PEP). These treatments provide psychoeducation on symptoms and their management, plus skill building in emotion regulation, communication, and problem solving (Miklowitz, 2019).

Two other promising psychosocial interventions are DBT and interpersonal and social rhythm therapy (IPSRT). While less extensively studied, DBT has demonstrated decreased suicidal ideation among youth with BPSD (Miklowitz, 2019). IPSRT is effective in improving circadian rhythms and social routines, which can lower risk of new mood episodes (Miklowitz, 2019). Finally, additional evidence-based psychosocial interventions can be included to address comorbid conditions, including anxiety disorder and substance use disorders. Treating these conditions utilizing psychosocial rather than pharmacologic interventions lessens risks related to polypharmacy.

PREVENTION

Offspring of parents with BPSD and youth with subsyndromal symptoms of mania and depression are at increased risk to develop BP1 (Hafeman & Spada, 2019). Clinical staging models suggest that individuals with mild or nonspecific mood symptoms might benefit from family psychoeducation as well as evidence-based psychotherapy (Hafeman & Spada, 2019). Three studies provide preliminary evidence suggestive of preventive effects for youth at high risk for developing BP1, including FFT for high-risk youth (FFT-HR), IPSRT, and multifamily PEP (MF-PEP) (Miklowitz, 2019).

Choosing preventive pharmacotherapy for at-risk individuals is challenging. Small-sized studies have suggested the possible benefit of quetiapine and aripiprazole, while lithium and divalproex did not appear beneficial (Hafeman & Spada, 2019).

Nutritional supplements might offer some benefit. Folic acid may help to delay the initiation of mood disorders (Sharpley, Hockney, McPeake, Geddes, & Cowen, 2014). A broad-spectrum nutrient has been demonstrated in an open-label trial to improve mood in at-risk youth (Frazier, Fristad, & Arnold, 2012). Omega-3 fatty acids may provide some improvement in depressive and subthreshold manic symptoms (Fristad, 2016). However, considerably more research is needed to firmly establish what interventions will successfully delay or prevent BP1 in at-risk youth.

CONCLUSION

Depressive disorders are relatively frequent, and BPSD is not rare in youth. Comorbidity with other medical and psychiatric disorders that also require intervention is common. Accurate diagnosis and treatment planning require an understanding of typical development as well as the youth's baseline functioning, family and other environmental influences, and psychosocial stressors. Early intervention can play a critical role in reducing morbidity and mortality. Combination pharmacotherapy and psychotherapy is recommended for moderate to severe depression and BPSD. Psychoeducation about the diagnosis and treatment, including possible risks and benefits of interventions, should be provided for patients and their parents.

REFERENCES

American Psychiatric Association. (2013). *Diagnostic and statistical manual of mental disorders* (5th ed.). APA.

Asarnow, J. R., Berk, M., Bedics, J., Adrian, M., & McCauley, E. (2021). Dialectical behavior therapy for suicidal self-harming youths: Emotion regulation mechanisms, and meditators. *Journal of the American Academy of Child & Adolescent Psychiatry*. https://doi.org/10.1016/j.jaac.2021.01.016.

Avenevoli, S., Swendsen, J., He, J. P., Burstein, M., & Merikangas, K. R. (2015). Major depression in the National Comorbidity Survey—Adolescent supplements: Prevalence, correlates, and treatment. *Journal of the American Academy of Child & Adolescent Psychiatry*, *54*(1), 37–44.

Azzopardi-Larios, D., & Galanter, C. A. (2019). Management of common co-occurring conditions in pediatric mood disorders. In M. K. Singh (Ed.), *Clinical handbook for the diagnosis and treatment of pediatric mood disorders*. American Psychological Association.

Brown, R. C., & Plener, P. L. (2017). Non-suicidal self-injury in adolescence. *Current Psychiatry Reports*, *19*(3), 20.

Carvalho, A. F., Firth, J., & Vieta, E. (2020). Bipolar disorder. *New England Journal of Medicine*, *383*(1), 58–66.

Cheung, A. H., Zuckerbrot, R. A., Jensen, P. S., Laraque, D., Stein, R. E., & Glad-PC Steering Group. (2018). Guidelines for adolescent depression in primary care (GLAD-PC): Part II. Treatment and ongoing management. *Pediatrics*, *141*(3).

Clark, S., Ragan, E., & Berk, M. (2019). Management of suicidal youth. In M. K. Singh (Ed.), *Clinical handbook for the diagnosis and treatment of pediatric mood disorders*. American Psychological Association.

Dickstein, D. P., & Croarkin, P. E. (2019). Preventative and emerging pharmacological and nonpharmacological treatments. In M. K. Singh (Ed.), *Clinical handbook for the diagnosis and treatment of pediatric mood disorders*. American Psychological Association.

Diler, R. S., & Birmaher, B. (2019). Longer-term management of mood disorders in youth. In M. K. Singh (Ed.), *Clinical handbook for the diagnosis and treatment of pediatric mood disorders*. American Psychological Association.

Dwyer, J. B., & Bloch, M. H. (2019). Antidepressants for pediatric patients. *Current Psychiatry*, *18*(9), 26.

Frazier, E. A., Fristad, M. A., & Arnold, L. E. (2012). Feasibility of a nutritional supplement as treatment for pediatric bipolar spectrum disorders. *Journal of Alternative and Complementary Medicine*, *18*(7), 678–685. https://doi.org/10.1089/acm.2011.0270

Frías, Á., Palma, C., & Farriols, N. (2015). Comorbidity in pediatric bipolar disorder: Prevalence, clinical impact, etiology and treatment. *Journal of Affective Disorders*, *174*, 378–389.

Fristad, M. A. (2016). Evidence-based psychotherapies and nutritional interventions for children with bipolar spectrum disorders and their families. *Journal of Clinical Psychiatry*, *77*(3), Se04.

Fristad, M. A. (2021). Commentary: Irritability is everywhere—A commentary on Evans et al. (2021). Diagnostic classification of irritability and oppositionality in youth: A global field study comparing *ICD-11* with *ICD-10* and *DMS-5*. *Journal of Child Psychology and Psychiatry*, *62*(3), 313–315. https://doi.org/10.1111/jcpp.13354

Hafeman, D. M., Rooks, B., Merranko, J., Liao, F., Gill, M. K., Goldstein, T. R., … Birmaher, B. (2020). Lithium versus other mood-stabilizing medications in a longitudinal study of youth diagnosed with bipolar disorder. *Journal of the American Academy of Child Adolescent Psychiatry*, *59*(10), 1146–1155.

Hafeman, D. M., & Spada, M. (2019). Assessment, prognosis, and treatment of subthreshold mood symptoms. In M. K. Singh (Ed.), *Clinical handbook for the diagnosis and treatment of pediatric mood disorders*. American Psychological Association.

Hirakawa, H., Terao, T., Muronaga, M., & Ishii, N. (2020). Adjunctive bright light therapy for treating bipolar depression: A systematic review and meta-analysis of randomized controlled trials. *Brain and Behavior*, *10*(12), e01876.

Ho, D. (2012). Antidepressants and the FDA's black-box warning: Determining a rational public policy in the absence of sufficient evidence. *Virtual Mentor*, *14*(6), 483–488.

Horowitz, L. M., Bridge, J. A., Teach, S. J., Ballard, E., Klima, J., Rosenstein, D. L., … Pao, M. (2012). Ask suicide-screening questions (ASQ): A brief instrument for the pediatric emergency department. *Archives of Pediatrics and Adolescent Medicine*, *166*(12), 1170–1176.

Kim, G.-M., Gandhi, R., & Cullen, K. R. (2019). Pharmacotherapy for pediatric depression. In M. K. Singh (Ed.), *Clinical handbook for the diagnosis and treatment of pediatric mood disorders*. American Psychological Association.

Liu, F. F., & Adrian, M. C. (2019). Is treatment working? Detecting real change in the treatment of child and adolescent depression. *Journal of the American Academy of Child and Adolescent Psychiatry*, *58*(12), 1157–1164.

McClellan, J., Kowatch, R., & Findling, R. L. (2007). Practice parameter for the assessment and treatment of children and adolescents with bipolar disorder. *Journal of the American Academy of Child & Adolescent Psychiatry*, *46*(1), 107–125.

Merikangas, K. R., Jin, R., He, J. P., Kessler, R. C., Lee, S., Sampson, N. A., … Zarkov, Z. (2011). Prevalence and correlates of bipolar spectrum disorder in the World Mental Health survey initiative. *Archives in General Psychiatry*, *68*(3), 241–251.

Miklowitz, D. M. (2019). Evidence-based psychotherapies for pediatric bipolar disorder. In M. K. Singh (Ed.), *Clinical handbook for the diagnosis and treatment of pediatric mood disorders*. American Psychological Association.

National Institute for Health and Care Excellence. (2019). *Depression in children and young people: Identification and management*. www.nice.org/uk/guidance/ng134

National Institute of Mental Health. (2019). *Prevalence of bipolar disorder in adolescents*. https://www.nimh.nih.gov/health/statistics/bipolar-disorder.shtml#part_155460

Nobile, M., Cataldo, G. M., Marino, C., & Molteni, M. (2003). Diagnosis and treatment of dysthymia in children and adolescents. *CNS Drugs*, *17*(13), 927–946.

Patino, L. R., & DelBello, M. P. (2019). Pharmacotherapy for pediatric bipolar disorders. In M. K. Singh (Ed.), *Clinical handbook for the diagnosis and treatment of pediatric mood disorders*. American Psychological Association.

Perlis, R. H., Ostacher, M. J., Goldberg, J. F., Miklowitz, D. J., Friedman, E., Calabrese, J., & Sachs, G. S. (2010).

Transition to mania during treatment of bipolar depression. *Neuropsychopharmacology*, *35*(13), 2545–2552.

Santamarina, P., & Packer, M. M. (2019). Evidence-based psychotherapies for pediatric depressive disorders. In M. K. Singh (Ed.), *Clinical handbook for the diagnosis and treatment of pediatric mood disorders*. American Psychological Association.

Sharpley, A. L., Hockney, R., McPeake, L., Geddes, J. R., & Cowen, P. J. (2014). Folic acid supplementation for prevention of mood disorders in young people at familial risk: A randomized, double-blind, placebo-controlled trial. *Journal of Affective Disorders*, *167*, 306–311.

Silver, J., Olino, T. M., Luby, J., Hawes, M. H., Carlson, G. A., & Klein, D. N. (2021). Reliability and validity of preschool feelings checklist. *Research on Child and Adolescent Psychopathology* https://doi.org/10.1007/s10802-020-00746-0.

Singh, M. K. (2019). *Clinical handbook for the diagnosis and treatment of pediatric mood disorders*. American Psychological Association.

Tondo, L., & Baldessarini, R. J. (2021). Suicide in psychiatric disorders: rates, risk factors, and therapeutics. In G. H. Vazuez, C. A. Zarate, & E. M. Brietzke (Eds.), *Ketamine for treatment-resistant depression: Neurobiology and applications*. Academic Press.

Van Meter, A., Moreira, A. L. R., & Youngstrom, E. (2019). Updated meta-analysis of epidemiologic studies of pediatric bipolar disorder. *Journal of Clinical Psychiatry*, *80*(3).

Vieta, E., Berk, M., Schulze, T. G., Carvalho, A. F., Suppes, T., Calabrese, J. R., … Grande, I. (2018). Bipolar disorders. *Nature Reviews Disease Primers*, *4*(1), 1–16.

Zalpuri, I., & Singh, M. K. (2019). Principles of treatment of mood disorders across development. In M. K. Singh (Ed.), *Clinical handbook for the diagnosis and treatment of pediatric mood disorders*. American Psychological Association.

Zheng, W., Zhang, Q. E., Cai, D. B., Yang, X. H., Ungvari, G. S., Ng, C. H., … Xiang, Y. T. (2019). Combination of metformin and lifestyle intervention for antipsychotic-related weight gain: A meta-analysis of randomized controlled trials. *Pharmacopsychiatry*, *52*(1), 24–31.

50

Suicide Prevention Care in the Pediatric Setting: A Trauma-Informed Approach

Lucas Zullo, Brooks Keeshin, and Joan Asarnow

For additional material related to the content of this chapter, please see Chapters 49, and 99.

VIGNETTE

Carlos is a 15-year-old boy who moved from Mexico to the United States with his family when he was 8 years old. During the clinical visit, Carlos is visibly down. When you ask him about how things are going, he reports that he has been struggling with bullying from peers at school who have been telling him to "go home to Mexico." He reports frequently having thoughts about wanting to go to sleep and not waking up so that he can avoid the bullying. Carlos also shares that after he told his parents about the bullying, his father has begun to hit him during "boxing practice" to "toughen him up" because Carlos does not "fight back" against the bullies. Carlos reports that after these instances of "boxing practice" he often thinks of stealing his father's handgun to kill himself.

In this chapter we discuss the management of suicide and self-harm in youth through a trauma-informed lens. We will follow the case example of Carlos throughout this chapter to illustrate the application of an approach to screening, triage, and brief intervention for youth at risk for self-harm, including suicide attempts. To provide a context for this case illustration and discussion, we begin with an overview of the epidemiology and presentation of suicidal and self-harm behavior in youth, followed by discussion of links between suicidal and self-harm behavior and trauma, adversity, and social determinants of health (SDOH). We then return to Carlos to illustrate a care process model for screening, evaluation, risk management, and care.

EPIDEMIOLOGY AND PRESENTATION OF SUICIDE RISK

Suicide is currently the second leading cause of death among youth ages 10 to 24 in the United States, responsible for more deaths than any single major medical illness (Centers for Disease Control and Prevention [CDC], 2019). From 2007 to 2017, youth suicide rates increased by 56% (from 6.8 per 100,000 to 10.6 per 100,000) (Curtin & Heron, 2019). Indeed, in a recent national survey of high school–aged youth 32% endorsed experiencing persistent feelings of sadness, 17% reported seriously considering attempting suicide, 14% made a plan for suicide, 7% made a suicide attempt, and 2% were injured in a suicide attempt (Kann et al., 2018). Other self-harm, including nonsuicidal self-harm such as cutting without suicidal intent, is a strong predictor of future fatal and nonfatal suicide attempts, frequently cooccurs with suicidal ideation, and is associated with significant psychosocial impairment (Asarnow et al., 2011).

In this chapter we attend to overall self-harm, including suicide attempts, unclear self-harm, and nonsuicidal self-harm. Contact with the health care system is common prior to deaths by suicide, with a 10-year longitudinal study identifying an 83% rate of contact with any health service within 1 year of death by suicide (Ahmedani et al., 2014). The same study found that on average, 45% of those who died by suicide had contact with primary care providers within 1 month of death, marking the pediatric setting as a clear priority for suicide risk screening and potential intervention.

FACTORS INCREASING SUICIDE AND SELF-HARM RISK

The most powerful predictor of future suicide attempts and deaths by suicide is previous self-harm behavior, including suicide attempts and nonsuicidal self-injury (NSSI) (Ribeiro et al., 2016). While not all individuals who die by suicide have histories of psychiatric disorder, some psychological autopsy data suggest that over 90% of individuals who died by suicide showed signs of a psychiatric disorder prior to their death (O'Connor & Nock, 2014).

TRAUMATIC STRESS, ADVERSITY, AND SOCIAL DETERMINANTS OF HEALTH

SDOH, adverse childhood experiences (ACEs), and trauma are all associated with risk of suicidality and self-harm (Asarnow, Goldston, Tunno, Inscoe, & Pynoos, 2020). For the acutely suicidal youth, it is critical to address proximate and malleable risk factors to keep the youth safe and protected (e.g., access to firearms, hunger), while more chronic factors of SDOH (e.g., community violence, poverty) are more challenging to change and outside the control of the adolescent and many pediatric and developmental-pediatric practices.

However, with youth who are not acutely suicidal or as a preventative measure for higher-risk youth, it is important to recognize that many of the fundamental concepts that foster safe and supportive families address known suicidal risk factors. Additionally, when specific SDOH factors impair access to appropriate and evidence-based therapies and other interventions intended to reduce risk of suicide, it is critical that those be identified and mitigated, even if those mitigation strategies are only able to be maintained temporarily during the youth's highest risk period of suicidality.

In addition to SDOH, there exists a continuum of stresses and adversities that impact suicidality among youth. Of course, not all ACEs are equal, with some childhood traumas found to have stronger associations with suicidality. For instance, sexual assault has been linked to a 10-fold increase in risk and physical assault associated with a 4-fold increase in risk (Ivey-Stephenson et al., 2020). A range of stressors common in childhood are also associated with suicidal ideation and behavior, including bullying, substance use, dating violence victimization, a history of running away from home, lack of parental connectedness, parent divorce, and poor academic functioning (Bruffaerts et al., 2010; Taliaferro & Muehlenkamp, 2014). See Chapters 15, 49, 56, and 95 for related content.

CARE PROCESS MODEL FOR SCREENING, EVALUATION, AND MANAGEMENT OF SUICIDE/SELF-HARM RISK AND TRAUMATIC STRESS

Next we transition to presenting a practical evidence-based and trauma-informed care process model for evaluating and caring for youth presenting with suicide/self-harm risk. This approach begins with screening, followed by further evaluation of youth with positive screens, risk stratification and triage to appropriate care strategies based on risk stratification, and treatment and management strategies within pediatric care and other treatment or service settings as indicated.

This care process model is summarized using the acronym ABCD (assess, build hope, connect, develop plan). The SAFETY-Acute (A) approach (originally known as the Family Intervention for Suicide Prevention [FISP] approach) addresses each of the steps in the care process model using a therapeutic assessment model, which provides intervention elements designed to pull for or drag out protective processes that are incompatible with suicidal behavior. We proceed to describe each of the ABCD steps, followed by a broader discussion of the SAFETY-A approach.

Screening for Suicide/Self-Harm Risk—Assess (A)

The ask suicide-screening questions (ASQ) developed by Lisa Horowitz and a team at the National Institute of Mental Health has been widely tested and has strong evidence for reliability, validity, and feasibility of integrating within quality improvement programs (Aguinaldo et al., 2021; Horowitz & Mournet, 2021). The ASQ includes four brief questions that can be quickly administered and uses language appropriate for ages as low as age 8: "In the past few weeks, have you wished you were dead?" and "In the past few weeks, have you felt that you or your family would be better off if you were dead?" These questions are followed by a question assessing acute versus nonacute risk for youth endorsing any of the initial questions: "Are you having thoughts of killing yourself right now?" This approach allows for risk stratification, and the developers have enhanced the value of the tool by developing clinical pathways with clear clinical action steps for youth assessed as showing acute and nonacute risk (e.g., acute risk screen leads to a STAT safety and mental health evaluation, and patient is in sight and closely monitored to ensure safety). These resources can be found online: https://www.nimh.nih.gov/research/research-conducted-at-nimh/asq-toolkit-materials/.

Another frequently used screener is the Columbia Suicide Severity Rating Scale (C-SSRS) (Posner et al., 2008). The C-SSRS is developed in multiple formats, with both brief self-report and longer interview options, and has been widely used in both research and practice settings, with several major hospital systems, including the C-SSRS within developed clinical guidance (https://intermountainhealthcare.org/ckr-ext/Dcmnt?ncid=526742474; https://www.chop.edu/clinical-pathway/suicide-risk-assessment-and-care-planning-clinical-pathway). Questions begin by asking about passive suicidal thoughts ("Have you wished you were dead or wished you could go to sleep and not wake up?") and progress to questions on specific plan and intent ("Have you started to work out or worked out the details of how to kill yourself? Do you intend to carry out this plan?"). The C-SSRS has been developed with clear guidance regarding stratification of risk levels based on youth response, with actionable clinical steps for providers to follow at each risk level (The Columbia Lighthouse Project, https://cssrs.columbia.edu/), and there are data supporting validity for use with both adolescents and adults (Posner et al., 2011). Some organizations use specific responses to a depression screener such as the last question of the PHQ-9/PHQ-A to identify youth for further suicide risk screening such as the C-SSRS ("Over the last 2 weeks, how often have you been bothered by thoughts that you would be better off dead or hurting yourself in some way?"; https://intermountainhealthcare.org/ckr-ext/Dcmnt?ncid=526742474). However, this approach is likely to miss a subgroup of youth who do not endorse thoughts of death or suicide on the PHQ-9, but do on the ASQ (Horowitz et al., 2021).

While the ASQ and C-SSRS both emphasize screening for suicidal ideation and behavior, the heterogeneity of youth presenting with suicide/self-harm risk and diversity of risk factors and pathways has led to efforts to develop screeners that assess a broader range of risk factors using more complex measurement models. The Computerized Adaptive Screen for Suicidal Youth (CASSY) developed from the ED-STARS project represents one example of this approach (King et al., 2021), as well as the Behavioral Health Screen (BHS; Diamond et al., 2010).

Screening for Traumatic Stress—Assess (A)

Most youth will experience at least one potentially traumatic experience before the age of 18 (Turner, Finkelhor, &

Ormrod, 2010), so it is often necessary to identify, among all potentially trauma-exposed youth, which youth continue to experience the impacts of the trauma. One proposed mechanism that may clearly link potentially traumatic experiences such as physical abuse with suicidality is the presence of traumatic stress. Keeshin and colleagues (2020) developed the Care Process Model for Pediatric Traumatic Stress (CPM-PTS) (https://intermountainhealthcare.org/ckr-ext/Dcmnt?ncid=529796906). The CPM-PTS is a quick and easy way for frontline pediatric settings to identify youth who are at risk for prolonged and functionally impairing traumatic stress through a process that captures both potentially traumatic events and trauma symptoms (Keeshin et al., 2020, Giles, Shepard, Keeshin, & Asarnow, in press). The CPM-PTS can be used both as universal screening for all youth over 5 years of age receiving care in pediatric settings or can be used in a targeted fashion for mental/behavioral health or other high-risk visits. Importantly, the CPM-PTS incorporates the two-tiered screening approach described in this chapter for attending to both risk associated with trauma and risk for suicide and self-harm.

As a trauma-informed approach that addresses suicide risk in pediatric settings, the CPM-PTS addresses both traumatic stress, an important threat to child safety and risk factor for suicide/self-harm, and other indicators of potential suicide/self-harm risk. First, by systematically capturing potentially traumatic experiences, providers can explore with the family whether those prior experiences continue to pose a current risk to the youth. When a youth or youth's family continues to be physically at risk of violence and/or harm (i.e., severe domestic violence, ongoing physical abuse), a plan that includes approaches for mitigating risk and enhancing the safety of the family is critical to addressing the underlying distress that may drive the youth's suicidality and increase risk for potentially lethal self-harm. Secondly, the CPM-PTS captures important traumatic stress symptom data that can inform elements of the safety plan as well as ongoing treatment recommendations. For more trauma-related content, see Chapters ··.

The CPM-PTS can be viewed at https://intermountainhealthcare.org/ckr-ext/Dcmnt?ncid=529796906 and includes a guide on interpreting level of trauma symptom severity (low, medium, and high risk for PTS). Additionally, the CPM-PTS has a simple three-step method to inform the management of traumatic stress: (1) report if required, (2) respond to suicide risk, and (3) stratify treatment approach. Stratification is informed by the administration of the Pediatric Traumatic Stress Screening Tool, which assists in clarification of traumatic stress symptom severity (https://intermountainhealthcare.org/ckr-ext/Dcmnt?ncid=529795302).

From the perspective of suicide risk evaluation and management, it is also important to consider the influence of a variety of actions that could lead to events that may be experienced as traumatic to youth in crisis. These include events such as transportation to an emergency room in handcuffs, involuntary hospitalization, and separation from one's family.

SAFETY-A/FISP OVERVIEW AND EMPIRICAL SUPPORT

The SAFETY-Acute (A) (or FISP) intervention (https://www.sprc.org/resources-programs/family-intervention-suicide-prevention-fisp) is recognized in the National Registry of Evidence Based Practices and the Suicide Prevention Resource Center. This intervention can be feasibly adapted for pediatric or developmental-behavioral pediatric services due to its flexible approach and goals of enhancing youth safety and improving linkage to needed follow-up care and continuity of care. These are critical treatment goals when working with suicidal youth as rates of follow-up treatment among these youth are low, which is concerning due to the high-risk nature of this population. The importance of establishing continuity of care for youth at risk for suicide has been recognized in the National Strategy for Suicide Prevention, Objective 8.4 (US Department of Health and Human Services, 2012).

SAFETY-A can be used effectively when time is limited and can be completed in 20 to 60 minutes (Asarnow, Berk, & Baraff, 2009; Asarnow et al., 2020). When time constraints require a briefer (e.g., 20 minutes) intervention, some components are selected for abbreviation or omission to best meet the needs of the youth and family and ensure that the youth is appropriately triaged to the appropriate level of care. SAFETY-A offers a secondary assessment (step A in the ABCD approach) and focuses on the steps of B (building hope and reasons for living), C (strengthening connections), and D (developing a safety plan and plan for follow-up care (Fig. 50.1).

The SAFETY-A intervention includes five therapeutic tasks to be completed with the youth and three tasks to be completed with the caregiver. As SAFETY-A is a therapeutic assessment, the goal of each task is to gather information on the current level of suicide risk versus safety as well as to provide a brief therapeutic intervention dose to mitigate this risk, thus an element of A (assess) is woven throughout the process. The five youth tasks are (1) eliciting three self-strengths from the youth and strengths about the family and/or environment (i.e., B: build hope and reasons for living); (2) utilizing an emotional thermometer to help youth understand their emotional reactions (the first phase in D: developing a safety plan); (3) continuing to develop a safety plan (D) by engaging the youth in identifying behaviors, thoughts, and interpersonal strategies (e.g., go to Mom, call a friend) that can be used instead of self-harm; (4) listing at least three people who are able to support the youth in staying safe during a future crisis (prioritizing responsible adults in the safety plan [D] and step C: connect); and (5) eliciting a commitment from the youth to use skills from the safety plan as opposed to self-harm behavior when experiencing distress (D). Psychoeducation is also provided on lethal means restriction and the potential disinhibiting effects of substance use, as appropriate and needed.

Tasks to be conducted with the parent or caregiver are designed to assess and enhance the ability of the parent/caregiver to keep the youth safe. These tasks include (1) eliciting three strengths about the youth and strengths about the family

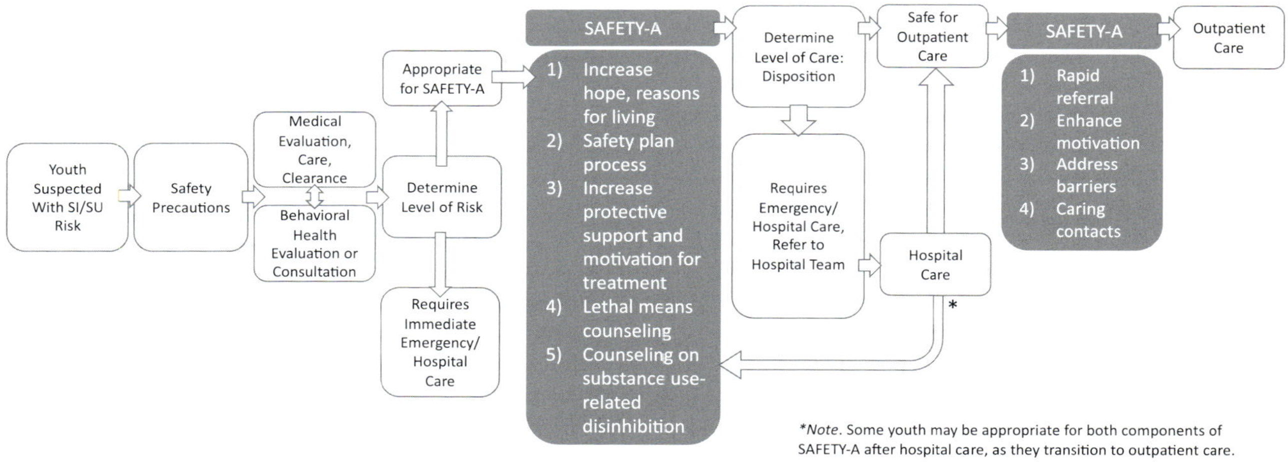

Fig. 50.1 SAFETY-A care process model.

and/or environment (step B: building hope and reasons for living); (2) explaining the importance of lethal means restriction (e.g., securing firearms) and identifying immediate steps that can be taken to establish safety, including increasing protective monitoring and supervision (step D: develop a plan for increasing youth safety); and (3) working with parent/caregiver to support youth in using the developed safety plan and managing stress that could increase suicide/self-harm risk (D). These tasks can be completed with the parent and/or other supportive adults when parent involvement is contraindicated (e.g., abuse), there are other key caregivers, and/or parent(s) are unavailable.

These steps with parents/caregivers parallel the ABCD steps taken with youth. Specifically, these SAFETY-A parent/caregiver action items are vital for assessing and ensuring that the youth can safely return to the home environment, building hope for the youth, connecting the youth to protective adults, and developing a plan for increasing youth safety.

In regard to outcomes, SAFETY-A has the strongest scientific support for effective linkage to care (Asarnow et al., 2011). There is also evidence of early postintervention clinical benefits of SAFETY-A, with the collective data supporting the value of SAFETY-A for stabilizing youth after an acute suicidal episode, enhancing safety, increasing linkage to follow-up care, and the value of SAFETY-A in combination with evidence-based follow-up treatment for reducing suicide attempt risk over a 3-month follow-up interval—the period associated with the greatest suicide attempt risk (Zullo et al., 2020).

SAFETY-A AND ABCD CASE ILLUSTRATION WITH CARLOS

Assess

We now return to Carlos. You have seen Carlos as a patient for the past several years and he typically presents as bright and cheerful. When you see Carlos today he is notably quiet and sad. He informs you that he is being bullied at school, and this makes him feel like he wants to go to sleep and not wake up to get away from the bullying. On screening, Carlos receives a PHQ-9 score of 17, consistent with moderately severe depression, and endorses thoughts of death or suicide. Per your clinic protocol, you administer the ASQ to clarify level of current suicidal thoughts. Carlos indicates "yes" to the question, "In the past week, have you been having thoughts about killing yourself?" but he answers "no" to the question, "Are you having thoughts of killing yourself right now?" (This indicated a nonacute positive screen based on ASQ.) You also administer the Pediatric Traumatic Stress Screening Tool, and he scores in the moderate range. You know now that Carlos needs your help today and you let him know that you also would like to talk to his mother about supporting him. Carlos' risk stratification can be viewed in Fig. 50.2.

Build Hope and Reasons for Living

To assess how Carlos is currently viewing himself and to learn about his strengths that may be harnessed for building hope and safety planning, the provider (hereafter you) begins by asking Carlos to share three strengths about himself and his life that he would like to share with you. When you ask this question, after a brief pause, Carlos tells you that he has been doing well on the soccer team this semester and his mood brightens as he describes a recent game. In addition, he mentions that he doesn't lash out against the bullies because he knows that

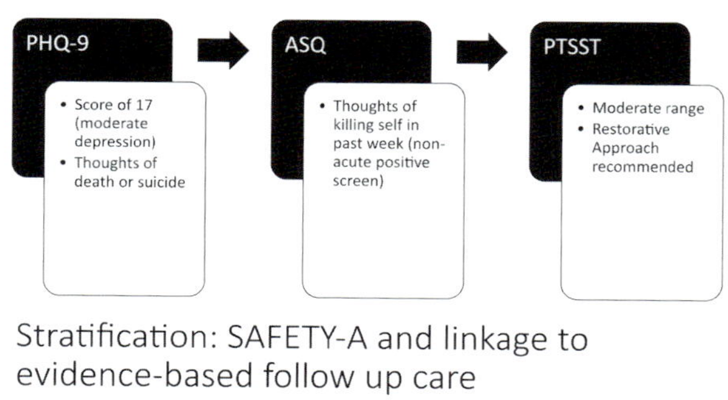

Fig. 50.2 Risk stratification example.

would make the situation worse and that he has been focusing on his schoolwork instead, which has allowed him to keep his grades up. You next ask Carlos to list three strengths about his family, and his eyes quickly begin to tear up and he starts to cry.

Connect

Seeing Carlos crying, you hand him a box of tissues and give him a few moments to blow his nose and dry his eyes. He shares with you that he has told his parents about the bullying and that while his mother was supportive and wants to speak to the school, his father became angry and has been trying to toughen Carlos up by hitting him in "boxing practice" and telling Carlos to "fight back" against the bullies. Carlos became tearful when describing the pressure he feels from his father as well as the bullies. You thank Carlos for his honesty in describing the situation and note that you are here to help him today and that no one deserves to be bullied. You also remind Carlos that you are his doctor and that you and the clinic staff are here for him and he can always call the office, strengthening the connection between Carlos and you and the broader clinic staff. Next, you highlight that you're glad his mother came with him for today's appointment as you'd like to talk with her about how she can work with the school to support Carlos in stopping the bullying and finding the best way to make the home a safe place for Carlos while he is having a hard time.

A key component of a trauma-informed approach is to know when and how to ask more about traumatic events. In this example you gently note that you want to make sure that Carlos is safe and protected, and ask what he means by his dad "hitting him in boxing practice." Carlos continues to look sad and indicates that his dad sees him as weak and he wants him to learn how to box. On further inquiry, Carlos indicates that his dad bought him boxing gloves and is pushing him to "be a fighter." He also notes that his father has never physically hurt him but tears up in discussing the pressure he feels. At this point, there is no indication that the "hitting" requires reporting to Child Protective Services; however, this is clearly a stressor that needs continued monitoring.

Develop Plan

To inform safety planning you proceed to an assessment of how Carlos experiences his emotions and situational triggers of suicidal thoughts and urges, using an emotional thermometer activity. You start by explaining that you want to understand what thoughts, feelings, and behaviors are associated with his emotions at different levels of intensity. Starting with the lowest level of distress (a zero on the emotion thermometer), you ask Carlos to describe a situation in which he would be feeling most comfortable and relaxed. Carlos explains that he loves to play soccer, and when he is playing with his friends he doesn't think about the bullying at all and is able to enjoy being outdoors. When asked about the opposite end of the thermometer, a rating of highest distress (a 10), Carlos explains that this would be when he has been bullied at school and when his father pushes him to "fight back" against the bullies. Carlos shares that one evening last week after a particularly bad time at school, he had thoughts of wanting to steal his father's handgun to kill himself due to his hopelessness about the future.

You thank Carlos for being so open during today's visit and let him know that your goal is to work with him to help him to stay safe so that he can have the kind of life he wants to have and that you want to continue to see him. To do that, you ask Carlos if he would be willing to work with you to develop a plan for what he can do to get through rough times. For example, times when his distress is high on the emotional thermometer and/or something happens that leads him to have thoughts of hurting himself. You hand him a piece of paper that has the headings "Warning Signs," "What I Can Do to Stay Safe," "What I Can Think to Stay Safe," and "Whom I Can Talk To" (Fig. 50.3). Beginning with "Warning Signs," Carlos tells you that before having thoughts of suicide he often isolates in his bedroom, feels completely hopeless about the future, and feels overwhelming anger toward himself for not being able to fix the situation. Moving on to "What I Can Do to Stay Safe," Carlos notes that he can go for a run, play with his dog, or look through old pictures of himself with his friends. For "What I Can Think to Stay Safe," Carlos shares that he can think about playing soccer with his friends the next day, remind himself that while the bullying is bad he still

PERSONAL PLAN

Warning Signs

1. __________
2. __________
3. __________

What I can do to stay safe:

1. __________
2. __________
3. __________

What I can think to stay safe:

1. __________
2. __________
3. __________

Whom I can talk to:

1. __________
2. __________
3. __________
4. **Call National Lifeline: 1-800-273-8255 (available 24 hr/day)**

If you are in immediate danger, go to the nearest Emergency Room or call 911

Fig. 50.3 Safety plan.

has many friends who support him, and that he's been coping with the bullying until now and it's worthwhile to keep himself safe until the bullying stops. In the final step of "Whom I Can Talk To" Carlos lists his mother, his soccer coach, and his math teacher as adults he can go to for support when his distress is high.

You ask Carlos if he can commit to using the steps on his plan for staying safe instead of doing something to hurt himself. Carlos indicates that he can and that he could get help from his mother if he had trouble using the other strategies on his plan to stay safe. You explain that since his mother is here today, it would be helpful to review this safety plan with her so that she can support Carlos in staying safe. Before switching to meeting with his mother, you provide brief psychoeducation on the dangers of substance use at this time, indicating that drugs and alcohol can make it hard to be in control and that would be dangerous for him now when he is having a hard time. Carlos denies any use. You also mention that you will be talking to his mother about making the home safe. It should be noted that teens typically do not object to including parents in these types of conversations, and if they do it is important to explore why. If there is fear of potential retaliation you may need to take additional steps to include a trusted adult.

When meeting alone with Carlos' mother, Gloria, she quickly tells you that she has been worried about how Carlos has been doing lately and informs you of the bullying at school and Carlos' father's efforts to "toughen him up." She shares that she is completely overwhelmed, is frightened because he has talked about suicide and wanting to die, and she doesn't know what to do to support her son right now. Gloria explains that her husband is old-fashioned in his views of mental health and "being a man" and he has confided in her that he is angry and frustrated at the bullying situation, which she realizes can be tough for Carlos, although she is sure that Carlos knows that his father loves him. To capitalize on her willingness to support Carlos at this time, you begin by asking Gloria what some of Carlos' strengths are and what some of the family strengths are. She tells you how Carlos is a thoughtful, caring, and smart boy who has been doing his best in this very difficult situation. In terms of family strengths, Gloria tells you that the family likes to cook together, that she and her husband always attend Carlos' soccer games, and they go to church together every Sunday.

As mentioned earlier, Carlos obtained a score of "moderate" on the Pediatric Traumatic Stress Screening Tool. Your recommendation is to connect with a therapist as consistent with the CPM-PTS recommended risk stratification, which emphasizes a "restorative approach" (see Fig. 50.2) with this level of risk and includes referral to a behavioral health provider. Given the moderate level of PTS symptoms that Carlos endorses, in conjunction with the ongoing traumatic stress he is experiencing with the bullying, referral to a provider who can deliver evidence-based trauma-informed suicide prevention care is optimal. Stabilization and ensuring safety, however, is clearly the highest priority given Carlos' significant suicidal ideation and intense feelings of hopelessness about his situation at times. Moreover, further assessment of the bullying and efforts to ensure safety and stabilize the school situation is indicated (e.g., providing a safe haven at school with a teacher, perhaps the soccer coach), as Carlos has tried and been unable to improve this situation on his own.

Next, you turn to the issue of limiting access to potentially lethal and dangerous methods of self-harm and mention that a key component of making the home environment safe for Carlos is to lock up anything that could be used for self-harm. You give examples of knives, sharps, ropes, cords, medications, and firearms. Gloria says she is willing to secure these items, but that her husband has a loaded firearm in the bedside table to protect the family and that he is likely unwilling to remove this from the home. You provide psychoeducation on how firearms are the most lethal means that a youth can use for a suicide attempt and that the firearm doesn't have to be completely removed from the house, options like a home safe are also possible and storing ammunition separately from the firearm. When hearing about the danger of firearms, Gloria looks distressed. You offer to speak with her husband, and Gloria texts him and you arrange to speak with him later that day. You also briefly provide psychoeducation on the dangers of substance use at this time, and Gloria assures you that Carlos has never engaged in substance use. Additionally, you explain the importance of staying with Carlos and engaging in pleasant activities with him such as cooking together or walking the dog together, which also provides opportunities for her to monitor him in a positive way for protection. You also explain that you and Carlos have developed a safety plan that he can use on days where he feels very upset, such as on days when the bullying occurs, and now as the session comes to an end you are going to bring Carlos back into the session so that he can share with her how she can help him in using the safety plan.

Carlos is lucky to have such a supportive mother. In the event that a parent is not present it would be important to identify a supportive adult if possible. One of the main goals of SAFETY-A and the ABCD approach is to establish short-term safety to promote effective linkage to care. Since teens can respond to strong emotions in dangerous ways such as self-harm or substance use, it is important to have the support of a responsible adult to encourage use of the safety plan in times of heightened distress and to provide protective support. If Carlos' mother was not able to provide the needed protection, you could have asked about extended family or family friends who might be able to function in this role and you could help Carlos and his mother to reach out to others who can provide support. Alternatively, if your assessment raises concerns about Carlos' safety in his current environment, a decision to step up care and send Carlos to emergency services for further evaluation may be indicated.

When bringing Carlos and Gloria together, you start by asking Gloria to share what she views as Carlos' strengths with him. After hearing these statements from his mother, Carlos begins to tear up and shares with her his thoughts of wanting to kill himself using his father's handgun on some days. Gloria expresses how glad she is that he was able to share this and asks for a separate referral so that Carlos can start to see an individual therapist. She also mentions that she will be asking for an emergency meeting with the school tomorrow to address the bullying. Together you review the safety plan with Carlos and his mother and discuss how Gloria can support him in using the plan to stay safe.

After providing Gloria with referral information for outpatient behavioral treatment, you obtain her commitment to schedule these appointments. At the end of the session, your evaluation is that Carlos is safe to return home. However, due to his level of risk, you arrange for a follow-up call from your office to check on Carlos' status and his mother's success in scheduling a behavioral appointment. You also schedule a follow-up visit within the next 2 weeks and let his mother and Carlos know that they should call in the event that he is feeling worse or they would like to speak with you. You send a note to behavioral services through the electronic health record indicating that you are concerned regarding suicidal ideation, and your assessment is that Carlos needs an appointment as soon as possible. Based on Gloria' information that her husband is available, you contact Carlos' father and share your concerns about Carlos' suicidal thoughts, level of stress, and the importance of ensuring that he can't access potentially deadly methods of self-harm during this time. You note that you have referred Carlos for treatment for these problems. You also note that access to firearms can lead to death, and ask the father to consider a plan for temporarily limiting access while Carlos is at risk and struggling, indicating that this is your recommendation as you want to help Carlos and the family get through this period safely.

CLINICAL IMPLICATIONS AND CONCLUSIONS

In some instances pediatric and developmental-behavioral pediatric practices may have access to integrated or embedded behavioral clinicians who can support suicide risk evaluation and management and conduct SAFETY-A and some follow-up care. However, the ABCD approach and a brief form of SAFETY-A can be used by developmental-behavioral pediatricians and other pediatric clinicians, and we note that youth tend to view primary care clinicians as among the most trusted adults who they can turn to for help, placing these clinicians in an excellent position to deliver and support suicide prevention care. Thus pediatric and developmental-behavioral pediatricians and other primary care clinicians are well positioned to function as a safety net for youth at risk for suicide, traumatic stress, or other adverse behavioral health outcomes due to their regular contact and familiarity with youth. It was our goal in this chapter to describe a usable care process model that can complement the care that is already provided in pediatrics and developmental-behavioral pediatrics. The main takeaway that we wish to emphasize is to stress the importance of assessment and linkage to needed evidence-based follow-up care after a youth is determined to be at risk and the role a developmental-behavioral pediatrician and other medical providers can play in this linkage and continuing monitoring. The Substance Abuse and Mental Health Services Administration (SAMHSA, 2020) has released a report on effective treatments for youth with suicidal or self-harm behavior, which can provide a guide in considering behavioral referrals or in embedding or integrating behavioral health care within medical practices.

Access to critical suicide prevention and behavioral health care will be improved with increased availability of colocated behavioral health and medical care, integrated care, collaborative care, and pediatric patient-centered medical home models (Asarnow et al., 2015; McDaniel et al., 2014; Stancin & Perrin, 2014). Through a systematic approach to screening, evaluation, and brief intervention (such as our ABCD model and SAFETY-A), pediatric and developmental-behavioral pediatric services can fill the critical need for regular monitoring and follow-up, alert caregivers to potential concerns, and link youth to behavioral health care as indicated. Next steps for the field may be to further develop models, such as the pediatric patient-centered medical home, which offer opportunities to integrate evidence-based behavioral health and suicide prevention care within pediatric and developmental-behavioral pediatric practice (Asarnow, Kolko, Miranda, & Kazak, 2017).

REFERENCES

Aguinaldo, L. D., Sullivant, S., Lanzillo, E. C., Ross, A., He, J. P., Bradley-Ewing, A., Bridge, J. A., Horowitz, L. M., & Wharff, E. A. (2021). Validation of the ask suicide-screening questions (ASQ) with youth in outpatient specialty and primary care clinics. *General Hospital Psychiatry*, *68*, 52–58.

Ahmedani, B. K., Simon, G. E., Stewart, C., Beck, A., Waitzfelder, B. E., Rossom, R., Lynch, F., Owen-Smith, A., Hunkeler, E. M., Whiteside, U., Operskalski, B. H., Coffey, J., & Solberg, L. I. (2014). Health care contacts in the year before suicide death. *Journal of General Internal Medicine*, *29*(6), 870–877.

Asarnow, J. R., Berk, M. S., & Baraff, L. J. (2009). Family Intervention for Suicide Prevention: A specialized emergency department intervention for suicidal youths. *Professional Psychology: Research and Practice*, *40*(2), 118.

Asarnow, J. R., Goldston, D. B., Tunno, A. M., Inscoe, A. B., & Pynoos, R. (2020). Suicide, self-harm, & traumatic stress exposure: A trauma-informed approach to the evaluation and management of suicide risk. *Evidence-Based Practice in Child and Adolescent Mental Health*, *5*(4), 483–500.

Asarnow, J. R., Hoagwood, K. E., Stancin, T., Lochman, J. E., Hughes, J. L., Miranda, J. M., Wysocki, T., Portwood, S. G., Piacentini, J., Tynan, D., Atkins, M., & Kazak, A. E. (2015). Psychological science and innovative strategies for informing health care redesign: A policy brief. *Journal of Clinical Child & Adolescent Psychology*, *44*(6), 923–932.

Asarnow, J. R., Kolko, D. J., Miranda, J., & Kazak, A. E. (2017). The pediatric patient-centered medical home: Innovative models for improving behavioral health. *American Psychologist*, *72*(1), 13.

Asarnow, J. R., Porta, G., Spirito, A., Emslie, G., Clarke, G., Wagner, K. D., Vitiello, B., Keller, M., Birmaher, B., McCracken, J., Mayes, T., Berk, M., & Brent, D. A. (2011). Suicide attempts and nonsuicidal self-injury in the treatment of resistant depression in adolescents: Findings from the TORDIA study. *Journal of the American Academy of Child & Adolescent Psychiatry, 50*(8), 772–781.

Bruffaerts, R., Demyttenaere, K., Borges, G., Haro, J. M., Chiu, W. T., Hwang, I., Karam, E. G., Kessler, R. C., Sampson, N., Alonso, J., Andrade, L. H., Angermeyer, M., Benjet, C., Bromet, E., de Girolamo, G., de Graaf, R., Florescu, S., Gureje, O., Horiguchi, I., … Nock, M. (2010). Childhood adversities as risk factors for onset and persistence of suicidal behaviour. *The British Journal of Psychiatry, 197*(1), 20–27.

Centers for Disease Control and Prevention. (2019). *Ten leading causes of death and injury charts*. https://www.cdc.gov/injury/wisqars/LeadingCauses.html

Curtin, S. C., & Heron, M. (2019). *Death rates due to suicide and homicide among persons aged 10–24: United States, 2000–2017*. National Center for Health Statistics. NCHS Data Brief, no 352.

Diamond, G., Levy, S., Bevans, K. B., Fein, J. A., Wintersteen, M. B., Tien, A., & Creed, T. (2010). Development, validation, and utility of internet-based, Behavioral Health Screen for adolescents. *Pediatrics, 126*(1), e163–e170.

Giles, L., Shepard, L., Keeshin, B. R., & Asarnow, J. R. (In press). Implementation of a trauma-informed suicide prevention intervention for youth presenting to the emergency department in crisis. *Evidence-Based Practice in Child and Adolescent Mental Health*.

Horowitz, L., & Mournet, A. (2021). Implementing suicide risk screening in pediatric medical patients: Feasible quality improvement projects that can save lives. *Evidence-Based Practice in Child and Adolescent Mental Health, 6*(3), 307–315.

Horowitz, L. M., Mournet, A. M., Lanzillo, E., He, J. P., Powell, D. S., Ross, A. M., Wharff, E. A., Bridge, J. A., & Pao, M. (2021). Screening pediatric medical patients for suicide risk: Is depression screening enough? *Journal of Adolescent Health, 68*(6), 1183–1188.

Ivey-Stephenson, A. Z., Demissie, Z., Crosby, A. E., Stone, D. M., Gaylor, E., Wilkins, N., Lowry, R., & Brown, M. (2020). Suicidal ideation and behaviors among high school students—youth risk behavior survey, United States, 2019. *MMWR Supplements, 69*(1), 47.

Kann, L., McManus, T., Harris, W. A., Shanklin, S. L., Flint, K. H., Queen, B., Lowry, R., Chyen, D., Whittle, L., Thornton, J., Lim, C., Bradford, D., Yamakawa, Y., Leon, M., Brener, N., & Ethier, K. A. (2018). Youth risk behavior surveillance—United States, 2017. *MMWR Surveillance Summaries, 67*(8), 1.

Keeshin, B., Byrne, K., Thorn, B., & Shepard, L. (2020). Screening for trauma in pediatric primary care. *Current Psychiatry Reports, 22*(11), 1–8.

King, C. A., Brent, D., Grupp-Phelan, J., Casper, T. C., Dean, J. M., Chernick, L. S., Fein, J., Mahabee-Gittens, E.M., Patel, S., Mistry, R., Duffy, S., Melzer-Lange, M., Rogers, A., Cohen, D., Keller, A., Shenoi, R., Hickey, R., Rea, M., Cwik, M., … Gibbons, R., (2021). Prospective development and validation of the Computerized Adaptive Screen for Suicidal Youth. *JAMA Psychiatry, 78*(5), 540–549.

McDaniel, S. H., Grus, C. L., Cubic, B. A., Hunter, C. L., Kearney, L. K., Schuman, C. C., Karel, M. J., Kessler, R. S., Larkin, K. T., McCutcheon, S., Miller, B. F., Nash, J., Qualls, S. H., Connolly, K. S., Stancin, T., Stanton, A. L., Sturm, L. A., & Johnson, S. B. (2014). Competencies for psychology practice in primary care. *American Psychologist, 69*(4), 409.

O'Connor, R. C., & Nock, M. K. (2014). The psychology of suicidal behaviour. *The Lancet Psychiatry, 1*(1), 73–85.

Posner, K., Brent, D., Lucas, C., Gould, M., Stanley, B., Brown, G., Fisher, P., Zelazny, J., Burke, A., Oquendo, M., & Mann, J. (2008). *Columbia-suicide Severity Rating Scale (C-SSRS)* (p. 10). Columbia University Medical Center.

Posner, K., Brown, G. K., Stanley, B., Brent, D. A., Yershova, K. V., Oquendo, M. A., Currier, G., Melvin, G., Greenhill, L., Shen, S., & Mann, J. J. (2011). The Columbia–Suicide Severity Rating Scale: Initial validity and internal consistency findings from three multisite studies with adolescents and adults. *American Journal of Psychiatry, 168*(12), 1266–1277.

Ribeiro, J. D., Franklin, J. C., Fox, K. R., Bentley, K. H., Kleiman, E. M., Chang, B. P., & Nock, M. K. (2016). Self-injurious thoughts and behaviors as risk factors for future suicide ideation, attempts, and death: A meta-analysis of longitudinal studies. *Psychological Medicine, 46*(2), 225–236.

Stancin, T., & Perrin, E. C. (2014). Psychologists and pediatricians: Opportunities for collaboration in primary care. *American Psychologist, 69*(4), 332.

Substance Abuse and Mental Health Services Administration (SAMHSA). (2020). *Treatment for suicidal ideation, self-harm, and suicide attempts among youth*. SAMHSA Publication No. PEP20-06-01-002. National Mental Health and Substance Use Policy Laboratory. Substance Abuse and Mental Health Services Administration.

Taliaferro, L. A., & Muehlenkamp, J. J. (2014). Risk and protective factors that distinguish adolescents who attempt suicide from those who only consider suicide in the past year. *Suicide and Life-Threatening Behavior, 44*(1), 6–22.

Turner, H. A., Finkelhor, D., & Ormrod, R. (2010). Poly-victimization in a national sample of children and youth. *American Journal of Preventive Medicine, 38*(3), 323–330.

US Department of Health and Human Services. (2012). *2012 national strategy for suicide prevention: Goals and objectives for action*. US Department of Health and Human Services.

Zullo, L., Meza, J. I., Rolon-Arroyo, B., Vargas, S., Venables, C., Miranda, J., & Asarnow, J. R. (2020). Enhancing safety: Acute and short-term treatment strategies for youths presenting with suicidality and self-harm. *The Behavior Therapist, 43*(8), 300–305.

51

Anxiety Disorders in Children and Adolescents

Rebecca A. Hazen and Marie A. Clark

For additional material related to the content of this chapter, please see Chapters 49, 98, and 99.

VIGNETTE

Paul is an 8-year-old boy who has always been described as shy and "slow to warm" to unfamiliar persons. He tends to be quiet and stays near his parents when he goes out of the house. He previously attended preschool and elementary school at a small private school near the family's home with a number of family friends' children. Although he had difficulty separating from his mother at the beginning of each school year, the number of familiar individuals was reassuring to him. However, this year Paul's prior school closed, and he must transfer to a new school further from home where he does not know anyone. In the weeks leading up to the start of school Paul becomes increasingly more anxious and begs his mother not to make him go to school there. He cries every day and begins screaming when his mother tells him he must try the new school. He also tells his mother that he is worried that something bad will happen to her when he is at school. On the first day, he refuses to leave his room to attend school.

Paul's mother is very upset and does not know what to do. She panics, imagining that he will never agree to go to school and that they will be reported for truancy. She remembers that Paul's pediatrician has told her to let him know if Paul has any difficulty with the new school. She contacts the office for advice. Paul's mother reports her concerns and asks if Paul should be prescribed medication. The pediatrician assesses Paul and refers to a local therapist for treatment. The pediatrician also writes a letter to the school describing Paul's school avoidance and recommending that the school work with the family on a plan to introduce Paul gradually to the school. He also begins a conversation with Paul's mother about whether anxiety has been a problem for her in the past. When she agrees that it has been troublesome for her throughout her life, he provides her with some recommendations for an adult psychotherapist.

INTRODUCTION

Anxiety is one of the most common mental health problems in childhood and adolescence. Symptoms of anxiety may be readily apparent to parents and health care clinicians, but it is also possible that other behaviors may mask underlying anxiety. There are effective treatments for anxiety, which may involve behavioral therapy and/or medication. It is important that clinicians are familiar with the different ways anxiety may present and the available treatments.

Symptoms of anxiety can be typical of certain developmental stages and may even be adaptive at times. Infants can be easily startled by noises. It is also appropriate for them to develop stranger anxiety at around 8 to 9 months of age as they begin to develop a strong preference for familiar faces and become distressed by those who are unfamiliar. Preschoolers may have fears about strangers and being separated from their caregivers. School-age children may worry about natural disasters or injuries. Adolescents most often have fears about social status, performance, and health.

Anxiety is the brain's response to danger and thus may be adaptive, helping the individual to avoid that danger. However, anxiety can become maladaptive when fears or worries that are irrational cause significant distress and interference in life. Other concerns may occur when the type of anxiety is not typical for the child's developmental level. Care must be given to characterize expressions of anxiety in terms of what is most appropriate given the child's level of cognitive, language, and social-emotional development.

There are several specific anxiety disorders, which this chapter will explore in detail. These encompass a range of symptom expressions. The *Diagnostic and Statistical Manual of Mental Disorders*, fifth edition (*DSM-5*), denotes the following anxiety disorders: separation anxiety disorder, generalized anxiety disorder (GAD), specific phobia, social anxiety disorder, panic disorder and agoraphobia, and selective mutism (American Psychiatric Association [APA], 2013). Although obsessive-compulsive disorder (OCD) is no longer classified as an anxiety disorder in the *DSM-5* due to the presence of anxiety in OCD and previous research on anxiety disorders that included it in the category of anxiety disorders, OCD and its treatment will be reviewed in the current chapter.

Up to 20% of individuals will experience an anxiety disorder during childhood and adolescence, with a higher prevalence of anxiety disorders in females (Lewinsohn et al., 2008). An analysis of the 2016 National Survey of Children's Health (NSCH) found that 7.1% of children ages 3 to 17 had current problems with anxiety (Ghandour et al., 2019). Of the children surveyed, non-Hispanic White children were more likely to be affected when compared with children of other racial/ethnic backgrounds. Rates of anxiety were also higher among the adolescent age range (ages 12–17) as compared to younger children.

The natural history of anxiety disorders usually begins with a history of anxiousness and overadaptation in childhood. Disorders begin to develop and peak most often at age 20 to 30, sometimes triggered by adverse life events. The course of anxiety disorders is often chronic with residual symptoms and mild impairment over a period of years. The severity and duration of symptoms, as well as comorbid depression, predict a more chronic course (Angst & Vollrath, 1991). An adolescent diagnosis of anxiety has been strongly associated with adult anxiety (Pine et al., 1998). The same study found a similar association between adolescent depression and adult anxiety and with adolescent anxiety and adult depression.

Because of their chronic course, anxiety disorders result in a cost to society related to the impact of the individuals' loss of productive functioning when affected. There are also related health care costs. A systematic review of cost of illness studies found that anxiety disorders were associated with a low proportion of health care costs on the population level; however, health care costs on the individual level were significantly increased for those with anxiety disorders compared with healthy controls (Konnopka & König, 2020). Chisholm et al. (2016) proposed a global investment case for treatment of anxiety and depression, which would result in a return of $4 for every $1 invested in scaling up treatment for depression and anxiety.

Treatment may ameliorate the burden of childhood anxiety, helping to prevent long-term consequences. Follow-up of youth in a treatment study found those with clinically meaningful improvement after 12 weeks of treatment were more likely to be in remission and had less severe anxiety and better functioning as compared to those with minimal or no initial improvement (Ginsburg et al., 2014). The authors suggest that early clinical improvement may provide protection against reoccurrence of anxiety disorders and associated disability. Given the high prevalence of anxiety, the associated negative consequences, and the efficacy of treatment, it is essential that health care clinicians are able to recognize childhood anxiety and treat or refer for treatment as necessary.

CORRELATES AND RISKS FACTORS

Temperament

Temperament is thought to be constitutionally based and stable over time (Rothbart, 1989). Research on temperament has focused on observation of behavior, physiologic reactions in toddlers/young children when confronted with particular situations, and parent-report measures of temperament. There are several theories and models of temperament that are proposed to relate to anxiety. A few of the most studied aspects of temperament will be highlighted.

The role of behavioral inhibition and anxiety has been extensively studied. Behavioral inhibition is typically measured as a categorical construct, with children in the behaviorally inhibited category being characterized as having negative reactivity and uncertainty and/or avoidance of novel situations/stimuli (Kagan, 1997). In the chapter-opening vignette Paul has the long-standing tendency to be "slow to warm up"; this could be indicative of behavioral inhibition. Longitudinal research supports the link between behavioral inhibition at a young age and the development of anxiety disorders, particularly social anxiety disorder, during later childhood and adolescence (Buzzell et al., 2017).

Rothbart (1989) conceptualized temperament as representing both a reactivity component and a self-regulatory component. The reactivity component of temperament includes both positive emotionality and negative emotionality. Similar to the concepts of positive and negative emotionality, neuroticism and negative affect are dimensional constructs that are characterized by a tendency toward distress and negative emotions, with both being associated with risk for anxiety and depression (Anthony et al., 2002). Research supports the stability of negative affect and indicates that children with high levels of negative affect are at greater risk for anxiety (Anthony et al., 2002). However, it is important to consider the self-regulatory aspects of temperament that may also impact the development of anxiety.

Self-regulatory aspects of temperament include attentional shifting, inhibition of behavior, and self-soothing (Rothbart, 1989). Effortful control is a self-regulatory aspect of temperament that is important in understanding anxiety. For example, children with high levels of effortful control are likely to be able to use self-regulatory process in the face of an anxiety-provoking situation despite a predisposition toward negative emotions. Lower levels of effortful control have been associated with higher levels of anxiety, and research indicates that the impact of tendencies toward negative emotionality may be buffered by effortful control (Muris, 2006).

Genetics

Research supports genetics as a significant predictor of the development of anxiety disorders. Paul's mother admits to his pediatrician that she also has anxiety. Perhaps there are other family members who share similar traits. Like many mental health disorders, there is not a singular gene that has been implicated for anxiety disorders but rather polygenetic and epigenetic models have the most support to date. It is important to note that familial aggregation of anxiety disorders can be due to multiple pathways and/or gene × environment interactions. For example, as will be discussed later, parents who are anxious may model anxious behavior and/or be motivated to utilize parenting strategies to reduce anxiety (Meier & Deckert, 2019), both of which may contribute to the development of anxiety in children.

A metaanalysis of genetics studies indicated that first-degree relatives of those with an anxiety disorder were four to six times more likely to develop an anxiety disorder (Hettema et al., 2001), and results of twin studies indicate heritability estimates of 30% to 50% (Meier & Deckert, 2019). Although there are differences in heritability estimates for different anxiety disorders, there is significant overlap in anxiety symptoms across anxiety disorders, and evidence suggests that anxiety disorders may share a common genetic basis (Eley et al., 2015). Furthermore, there is evidence suggesting that anxiety and depression may also share a common genetic basis, with some studies that support a more general tendency toward neuroticism as a genetic contribution to both anxiety and depression (Gottschalk & Domschke, 2017). However, additional research is needed to better understand the polygenetic and epigenetic influences on the development of anxiety disorders.

Societal Factors

There are societal factors that influence the prevalence of anxiety. Poverty has been shown to be associated with increased anxiety. In the NSCH the prevalence of anxiety was greater among children with public insurance as compared to those with private insurance. A longitudinal study of children from 4000 families followed from birth to adolescence found that living with poverty during the first 5 years predicted a small but significant increase in the risk of anxiety in adolescence (Spence et al., 2002). An analysis of data from the Fragile Families and Child Well-Being Study indicated that children who experienced both food insecurity and housing instability during early childhood had an increased risk of anxiety in adolescence (Hatem et al., 2020).

Another important societal risk factor that deserves further study is the experience of racism. A review of the literature conducted by Pachter and Coll (2009) found an association between self-reported discrimination and expectations of discrimination with depressive symptoms, low self-esteem, and anxiety in adolescents and preadolescents. Even parental experiences of racism can impact child anxiety. One of the studies reviewed by Pachter and Coll (2009) found that racial discrimination experienced by the parents of Black adolescents was associated with general anxiety and depression, independent of whether the child had experienced racial discrimination.

Parenting and Family Relationships

Parenting and family factors related to the development of maintenance of anxiety disorders have been the focus of study for decades. Parental overprotection has been implicated in the development of anxiety in children (Rapee, 2012). Specifically, parental attempts to control their child's choices and shield their children from potentially anxiety-producing situations may impact children's perceptions of threat, increase anxiety, and contribute to avoidance of those situations, which may then further increase and maintain anxiety once it has developed. It should also be noted that parental anxiety may lead to overprotective parenting, which then may impact child anxiety. In the case of Paul his mother panicked when he refused to go to school, rendering her ineffective in responding to his needs during that moment. It is possible that Paul's mother was also anxious about the new school, something that Paul perceived and that may have increased his own anxiety about the situation. In this case it was very helpful that the pediatrician had built a rapport with Paul's mother and could inquire about her mental health as part of his assessment of Paul's situation. Clinicians may find it helpful to assess family history of anxiety and the possible role of parental anxiety in parent-child interaction. Finally, although there is evidence for the causal role of parental overprotection in development and childhood anxiety, the relationship is best viewed as bidirectional, as parenting attempts to protect their child can also increase in response to high levels of child anxiety (Rapee, 2012).

There are more mixed results for the relationship between child anxiety and the more general aspects of parenting (Rapee, 2012). There is some evidence that higher levels of parental rejection are associated with higher levels of anxiety in children; however, effect sizes have been small (McLeod et al., 2007; Rapee, 2012). Many studies on parenting focus on mothers, but a metaanalysis by Möller and colleagues (2016) indicated that paternal negative interactions with children may explain more of the variance in anxiety. Inconsistencies in the literature may be partially due to other factors that may interact with parenting (e.g., family stressors, temperament) in predicting child anxiety.

It is known that parental modeling can have a significant impact on children's behaviors and emotional states. Given the familial aggregation of anxiety disorders, it is not surprising that anxious parents may model anxious responses and behaviors that contribute to the development of anxiety and anxious avoidance in their children (Fisak & Grills-Taquechel, 2007). Avoidance of anxiety-provoking situations is a key component in the diagnosis of many anxiety disorders (Table 51.1). Psychological treatments for anxiety in children frequently involve guidance for parents on how to model appropriate approach behaviors for their children (Higa-McMillan et al., 2016).

Stressors and Adverse Childhood Experiences

Multiple aspects of the environment may impact the development of anxiety. Stressful life events and adverse childhood experiences (ACEs) have been found to impact the development of anxiety (Elmore & Crouch, 2020; Hyland et al., 2016). ACEs can entail a range of negative experiences during childhood that have the potential to negatively impact brain development and future mental and physical health (Elmore & Crouch, 2020). These experiences may include such events as child abuse, parental divorce, frequent family moves, witnessing domestic violence, and a parent losing a job. The relationship between ACEs and health outcomes during adulthood has been extensively studied, with studies suggesting a significant impact on adults' psychological functioning and health status. Although there has been relatively less research in children, the presence of a higher number of ACEs has been associated with greater risk for anxiety during childhood (Elmore & Crouch, 2020). However, research also suggests that some ACEs (e.g., child abuse, witnessing domestic violence) may have a greater impact on the development of anxiety (Elmore & Crouch, 2020; Hyland et al., 2016).

Comorbidities

Anxiety disorders are frequently comorbid with each other and with other mental health and developmental disorders. Research indicated that at least 14% of children have two or more anxiety disorders, with higher rates among treatment-seeking youth (Freidl et al., 2017), with GAD, separation anxiety disorder, and social anxiety disorder frequently being

TABLE 51.1 *Diagnostic and Statistical Manual of Mental Disorders* Criteria for Anxiety Disorders and Obsessive Compulsive Disorder

Disorder	Symptoms/Diagnostic Criteria
Separation anxiety disorder	Three or more of the following: 1. Recurrent and excessive fear of separation from home or major attachment figures 2. Worry about losing or harm coming to major attachment figures 3. Worry about negative events (e.g., being kidnapped, having an accident) resulting in separation 4. Reluctance or refusal to leave house for school, work, or other activities 5. Fear or reluctance about being alone or being without major attachment figure 6. Reluctance or fear of sleeping away from home or without being near major attachment figure 7. Nightmares related to separation 8. Physical symptoms with separation or anticipated separation 9. Significant impairment or distress. Duration: at least 4 wk in children/adolescence
Social anxiety disorder	1. Fear or anxiety about at least one situation in which there is possible scrutiny 2. Fears that will act in a way or show anxiety that will be negatively evaluated 3. Social situation almost always provokes fear 4. Social situations avoided or endured with intense fear/anxiety 5. Fear or avoidance is out of proportion to danger 6. Significant impairment or distress 7. Fear or avoidance not due to substance or medical condition 8. Not better accounted for by other mental disorder 9. If medical condition, fear or avoidance is unrelated or excessive. Duration: at least 6 mo
Specific phobia	1. Fear about specific object or situation. In children, may be crying, tantrums, freezing, or clinging 2. Object or situation almost always provokes immediate anxiety 3. Object or situation is avoided or endured with fear/anxiety 4. Fear is out of proportion to actual danger 5. Cause significant impairment or distress 6. Not better accounted for by other anxiety disorder, obsessions, or reminders of trauma. Duration: At least 6 mo
Generalized anxiety disorder	1. Excessive anxiety or worry about a number of events or activities 2. Difficult to control worry 3. At least one (3 for adults) or more of 6 symptoms: restlessness or feeling keyed up or on edge; easily fatigued; difficulty concentrating or mind going blank; irritability; muscle tension; sleep disturbance 4. Significant distress or impairment 5. Not attributable to substance or other medical condition 6. Not better accounted for by other mental disorder. Duration: at least 6 mo
Selective mutism	1. Consistent failure to speak in social situations despite talking in other situations 2. Interferes with educational or occupational achievement or social communication 3. Not attributed to lack of knowledge or comfort with spoken language 4. Not better accounted for by communication disorder and not exclusively during course of autism, schizophrenia/psychotic disorder. Duration: at least 1 mo (not first month of school)
Panic disorder	1. Recurrent unexpected panic attacks 2. At least one panic attack followed by 1 mo of at least one of: worry about more panic attacks or maladaptive changes in behavior related to panic attacks 3. Not better accounted for by other anxiety disorder, obsessions, or reminders or trauma
Panic attack (symptom presentation and not diagnosis)	Abrupt surge or intense fear or discomfort that reaches peak within minutes with at least four of: palpitations; pounding heart or accelerated heart; sweating, trembling or shaking; feeling short of breath or smothering; feelings of choking, chest pain or discomfort; nausea or abdominal distress, feeling dizzy, unsteady, light-headed, or faint; chills or heat sensation; numbness or tingling sensation; derealization or depersonalization; fear of losing control; fear of dying

(Continued)

TABLE 51.1 *Diagnostic and Statistical Manual of Mental Disorders* Criteria for Anxiety Disorders and Obsessive Compulsive Disorder—Cont'd

Disorder	Symptoms/Diagnostic Criteria
Agoraphobia	1. Anxiety about 2 or more of 5 situations: public transportation; open spaces; being in enclosed places; standing in line or being in crowd; being outside of home alone 2. Fear or avoids situations due to thoughts that escape may be difficult or help may not be available or other incapacitating or embarrassing symptoms 3. Situation almost always provokes fear 4. Feared situation actively avoided, require presence of companion, or endured with intense anxiety 5. Fear is out of proportion to danger 6. Causes significant impairment or distress 7. If other medical condition (e.g., irritable bowel disease), avoidance or fear is excessive 8. Not better accounted for by other mental disorder. Duration: At least 6 mo
Obsessive-compulsive disorder	Presence of obsessions, compulsions, or both. Obsessions defined by both of the following: 1. Recurrent and persistent thoughts, urges, or images that are intrusive and inappropriate; cause marked anxiety and distress 2. Attempts to suppress or ignore such thoughts, impulses, or images or neutralize them with some other thought or action. Compulsions defined by both of the following: 1. Behaviors that the individual feels compelled to perform in response to obsession or rules that the individual thinks must be adhered to 2. Repetitive behaviors or mental acts are done to prevent or reduce anxiety or distress, or to prevent dreaded event/situation. Behaviors or mental acts are not realistically connected or are clearly excessive. Obsessions or compulsions must be time consuming Not duec to physiologic condition and not better explained by another mental disorder

*Change can be from calm or anxious state

From American Psychiatric Association. (2013). *Diagnostic and statistical manual of mental disorders* (5th ed.). https://doi.org/10.1176/appi.books.9780890425596

comorbid with each other. With regard to mood disorders, 10% to 15% of children with an anxiety disorder also have a depressive disorder (Cummings et al., 2014). Other common comorbidities include attention-deficit/hyperactivity disorder (ADHD), substance abuse disorder, bipolar disorder, OCD, eating disorders, and autism spectrum disorder (Walter et al., 2020). Children with OCD frequently have comorbid anxiety disorders as well as ADHD and tic disorders (APA, 2013). Given the high rate of comorbid conditions, Paul's pediatrician could also consider using a behavioral health screening tool to assess for other comorbidities in relationship with his anxiety.

There are several pediatric chronic medical conditions that increase risk for an anxiety disorder. These conditions include but are not limited to asthma, diabetes, congenital heart disease, epilepsy, inflammatory bowel disease, juvenile idiopathic arthritis, and sickle cell disease. Additionally, in a national sample 28% of parents who rated their child's health as fair or poor also reported that their child had been diagnosed with anxiety (Ghandour et al., 2019).

TYPES OF ANXIETY DISORDERS

The following section summarizes the different types of anxiety disorders diagnosed in children and adolescents and is based on diagnostic criteria from the *DSM-5*. Additional details regarding *DSM-5* criteria may be found in Table 51.1.

Separation Anxiety Disorder

Children with separation anxiety disorder experience excessive anxiety about separation from parents and/or major attachment figures to a degree that is not typical for their age. Symptoms of separation anxiety disorder may include but are not limited to fear when anticipating or experiencing separation from parents or attachment figures, worry about harm coming to parents when not with them, refusal to go places (e.g., school) due to worry about being away from parents, nightmares about losing a parent, and experiencing anxiety when not with their parents (APA, 2013) (see Table 51.1). Children with separation anxiety may be overly clingy with parents, and for younger children this may also include clingy behaviors toward their teacher. The median age of onset of separation anxiety disorder is 7 years (Freidl et al., 2017). The prevalence decreases as children reach adolescence, but it is the most commonly diagnosed anxiety disorder in children less than 12 years of age (Ehrenreich et al., 2008). The lifetime prevalence of separation anxiety disorder in childhood/adolescence is approximately 7.6% (Freidl et al., 2017). Separation anxiety may develop after stressful life events or trauma, has a high heritability estimate, and is more common in females (APA, 2013).

Social Anxiety Disorder

Symptoms of social anxiety disorder include heightened fear or anxiety in social situations in which there is the potential for scrutiny/criticism by others. This may include talking with unfamiliar people, being observed, and/or performing in front of others (see Table 51.1). Fear of negative evaluation is accompanied by avoidance of feared social situations, and it may reflect anxiety when interacting with others outside of the household and/or anxiety about performing in front of others (e.g., reading, singing). Children with social anxiety disorder will attempt to avoid interacting in social situations in which they feel uncomfortable. Although this may include social interactions with peers and/or adults, a diagnosis in children is only made if the fear is present in situations with peers. The median age of onset is 13 years (Freidl et al., 2017), and prevalence rates range from 5% to 15% (Kashdan & Herbert, 2001).

Generalized Anxiety Disorder

GAD is characterized by frequent and difficult-to-control worries about a range of topics (e.g., grades, family members, the future), with frequent worries being problematic for at least 6 months (APA, 2013) (see Table 51.1). In addition to excessive worry, children with a diagnosis of GAD experience at least one of the following: restlessness, fatigue, difficulty concentrating, irritability, muscle tension, and sleep disturbance. Children with GAD may report thoughts consistent with perfectionism, and parents and children may report that they worry about "everything." The median age of onset of GAD is 11 years, with a lifetime prevalence during childhood/adolescence of 2.2% (Freidl et al., 2017).

Specific Phobias

Specific phobias represent fears about specific objects or situations that elicit high levels of distress, which are more than expected based on the child's developmental level. Many children experience common fears during childhood (e.g., darkness, loud noises, insects). However, children who meet the *DSM-5* criteria for a specific phobia have a significant level of fear that leads to attempts to avoid the feared situation or stimuli or intense fear if having to be in the situation (see Table 51.1). Children with specific phobia may cry, cling, freeze up, or throw tantrums when confronted with their fears. Prevalence increases with childhood, with rates up to 16% in 13- to 17-year-olds (APA, 2013). The *DSM-5* groups specific phobias into the categories of animal (e.g., dogs), natural environment (e.g., heights, thunderstorms), blood-inject-injury, situational (e.g., airplanes), and other (e.g. costumed characters/mascots) (APA, 2013). Specific phobias are frequently comorbid with other anxiety disorders, and many specific phobias during childhood go untreated and frequently persist into adulthood (Pine et al., 1998).

Selective Mutism

Children with selective mutism do not speak in specific situations (e.g., classroom) but speak in other social situations (e.g., when with friends outside of school). To meet the *DSM-5* diagnostic criteria (see Table 51.1), the symptoms must be present for at least 1 month and cause interference with aspects of functioning (e.g., school, social communication). The *DSM-5* stipulates that a communication disorder should not better account for the symptoms, and they should not be exclusively related to the course of autism or psychotic conditions. The average age of onset has been identified as 2.7 to 4.6 years (Driessen et al., 2020). It is a rare disorder, with prevalence rates up to 1% (APA, 2013). Selective mutism has a high level of comorbidity with social anxiety disorder (Driessen et al., 2020). Selective mutism can cause significant problems at school, as children may not ask for help or express their needs at school. In addition, peer relationships can be significantly impacted for those children who will not speak with peers at school.

Panic Disorder and Agoraphobia

Although panic disorder is more common in adults, children and adolescents can also be diagnosed with panic disorder. The *DSM-5* diagnostic criteria for panic disorder include recurrent and unexpected panic attacks. Panic attacks are characterized by intense fear or discomfort that is accompanied by four or more symptoms, such as sweating, pounding heart, shaking, or chest pain (see Table 51.1 for complete list). A diagnosis of panic disorder includes the presence of either worry about having additional panic attacks/their consequences or changes in behavior related to the panic attacks (e.g., avoidance of unfamiliar situations). The median age of onset for panic disorder is 20 to 24 years (Freidl et al., 2017), and the prevalence among children and adolescents is estimated to have a mean of 0.4% for children and 2% to 3% in adolescents and adults (APA, 2013). Although panic disorder is rare in children, children with other anxiety disorders may experience panic attacks in the feared situations. Panic attacks only within the context of feared situations/stimuli would not meet the diagnostic criteria for panic disorder due to the fact that they do not occur out of the blue (APA, 2013).

Panic disorder may also be comorbid with agoraphobia, which is defined as significant fear or anxiety in two or more of five situations: using public transportation, being in open spaces (e.g., parking lots), being in enclosed spaces (e.g., move theater), standing in line or being in a crowd, and being outside of the home without others (APA, 2013). The anxiety is associated with avoidance of situations due to fear of not being able to escape or get help. Similar to panic disorder, it is rare during childhood but has a prevalence of 1.7% in adolescents and adults (APA, 2013). It should be noted that agoraphobia can occur in the absence of panic disorder.

OBSESSIVE-COMPULSIVE DISORDER

OCD is characterized by the presence of obsessions, compulsions, or both obsessions and compulsions. Obsessions are defined in the *DSM-5* as recurrent or persistent thoughts, urges, or images that are intrusive and unwanted and usually cause anxiety and distress. In addition, to be classified as an obsession there must be attempts to ignore or suppress the thoughts and urges or to neutralize with a compulsive behavior. Compulsions are repetitive behaviors (e.g., checking or counting things, putting objects in a specific order) that the person feels compelled to perform in response to an obsession or because of perceptions that rules need to be rigidly applied. Compulsions require that the behaviors or mental acts are done to prevent or reduce anxiety or distress or prevent a distressing situation. The diagnostic criteria require that the compulsions are time consuming or cause significant distress or impairment. OCD can be difficult to diagnose, particularly in young children, as they may not have the insight or have difficulty expressing the purpose of their compulsive behaviors. Rates of OCD are higher in males during childhood but are more common in females during adulthood. It is reported that 25% of cases start by age 14 years, and onset is more likely to be gradual versus having an acute onset (APA, 2013).

Assessment

Assessment of anxiety can occur through a variety of modalities. Much of the research on treatment for anxiety disorders uses validated semistructured diagnostics interviews administered to parents and/or children to assess symptoms of specific anxiety disorders. In typical medical practice it may not be feasible to administer semistructured diagnostic interviews. There are several well-validated self- and parent/proxy-report measures of anxiety that can assist in the evaluation of anxiety within the medical setting (Freidl et al., 2017). Given that anxiety is an internal feeling that may not be apparent to others, for children who are able to complete anxiety rating scales it is typically recommended that child-report measures are included in anxiety assessment. In addition to parent report, it can be useful to get reports from teachers, particularly if there is anxiety that is causing distress or difficulties at school. With regard to OCD, parent and child rating scales specific to OCD can be used when OCD is suspected or to monitor progress throughout the course of treatment.

There are also more general screening measures of behavioral and emotional problems that can be used in pediatric practice to identify youth who may be experiencing high levels of internalizing symptoms that warrant further evaluation. In the case of Paul, from the vignette, a screening instrument used by his pediatrician's office routinely may have picked up on concerns related to internalizing symptoms prior to the school refusal. A high score on internalizing problems would warrant further assessment, which could include specific anxiety rating scales. Rating scales are available for children, parents, and teachers (see Chapters 76, 81, and 82 for additional information regarding general assessment and screening instruments).

Observations during the office visit should also be considered when assessing anxiety. This may include behaviors such as fidgeting when asked questions, looking to the parent to answer questions for them, avoiding eye contact, and getting upset if there is a brief separation from their parent. These behaviors could be indicative of other difficulties but may be possible signs of anxiety. As discussed later, there is also symptom overlap across developmental and mental health disorders that should be considered when interpreting observations of behaviors in the office.

Differential Diagnosis

Many symptoms of anxiety disorders show commonalities with symptoms of other childhood mental health conditions. For example, difficulty focusing and restlessness can occur with anxiety (e.g., GAD) and with ADHD. Determining whether the inattention is related to internal versus external stimuli can help to delineate whether the symptoms are due to anxiety versus ADHD. Restlessness across situations and regardless of anxiety is more likely to be a symptom of ADHD. Children with autism and social anxiety disorder may exhibit poor eye contact and impaired social interactions, and it can be challenging to determine the cause of these difficulties. It is important to obtain a full developmental history, assess the onset of symptoms (typically earlier for autism), and consider whether language impairment is present. Anxiety and depression may also pose diagnostic challenges due to similarities in symptoms and/or cognitions. When assessing for depression and anxiety, the clinician should consider whether the child exhibits low levels of positive affect or anhedonia (Freidl et al., 2017). Assessment for possible OCD can be complicated by the presence of autism, and they can be comorbid. Children with autism but not OCD are more likely to have multiple repetitive behaviors that are not tied to an attempt to reduce anxiety about a specific stimuli/situation.

In addition to distinguishing symptoms of anxiety from symptoms of other mental health problems, medical causes for potential anxiety symptoms need to be ruled out (Walter et al., 2020). For example, physiologic manifestations of anxiety (e.g., racing heart, difficulty breathing, feeling tired) can also be signs of cardiovascular and pulmonary conditions. There are several other medical conditions that should also be considered when evaluating anxiety, such as thyroid disorders, epilepsy, gastrointestinal disorders, and diabetes (Walter et al., 2020).

TREATMENTS

Behavior Therapy

Behavioral treatments for anxiety, particularly specific phobias, have a broad body of literature that supports their efficacy (Böhnlein et al., 2020). Current behavioral approaches frequently include graduated/gradual exposure to fear situations (e.g., heights, dogs). The rationale for these treatments focuses on decreasing avoidance of the feared stimuli so that children can experience a decline in their anxiety after exposure. In addition to more gradual exposure, some behavioral treatments use a flooding approach in which the child is exposed to highly anxiety-provoking situations.

Cognitive-Behavioral Therapy

Cognitive-behavioral therapy (CBT) is one of the most researched psychological interventions for children and adults with anxiety disorders. CBT focuses on the interplay between thoughts, feelings, and behaviors. CBT includes commonalities with behavior therapy (e.g., exposure to feared stimuli) but the role of cognitions is key to CBT. There are a number of manualized CBT treatments, with Kendall's Coping Cat (Kendall, 1994) being the first and highly researched manualized treatment. There is support for delivering CBT in a variety of modalities (e.g., individual, group, family based, virtual), and CBT can be adapted to specific symptom presentations and family needs (Freidl et al., 2017). There is a substantial body of research to support CBT for anxiety disorders in children and adolescents, and CBT is considered the most evidence-based psychological treatment for childhood anxiety disorders (Higa-McMillan et al., 2016).

Cognitive restructuring is an essential component of CBT, and a variety of specific strategies may be used, but the basis for the strategies is that anxiety is associated with irrational beliefs and thoughts. By identifying and addressing maladaptive thoughts, anxiety can be reduced. For example, in the vignette Paul is worried that something bad will happen to his mother while he is at school (separation anxiety). Paul's therapist may help him to identify the evidence for the thought that something bad will happen to his mother and coach him in developing alternative thoughts and coping strategies when confronted with the thought in the future.

The link between physiologic sensations and feelings of anxiety is a key concept integrated into CBT. Children are encouraged to become aware of how their physiologic sensations relate to their feelings of anxiety. Children may be asked to draw a picture of themselves and identify changes in their body that they notice when they are feeling anxious. The therapist teaches the child about the relationship between physiologic symptoms and anxiety, as well as how to use relaxation strategies (e.g., diaphragmatic breathing, progressive muscle relaxation) (see Chapter 98).

As discussed earlier, parents can play a key role in the CBT strategies outside of the office. This is particularly relevant for younger children. The role of parents may include supporting the child in practicing exposure exercise, providing praise/positive reinforcement for practicing strategies at home, and modeling approach behaviors in anxiety-provoking situations. Paul's mother could be guided in these methods to support him through future anxiety-provoking encounters.

Exposure and Response Prevention

Exposure and response prevention is a key component of CBT that has a substantial amount of support for the treatment of OCD (Geller & March, 2012). This strategy involves working on gradual exposures to anxiety-provoking stimuli/situations and then preventing compulsive behaviors in response to the stimuli/situation. For example, a child with anxiety about germs could be asked to touch a surface that may have germs on it but then be asked to prevent oneself from engaging in hand washing in response to touching the surface. By preventing the compulsive behavior, the child's anxiety will go down over time because the perceived importance of the compulsive behavior will be diminished (i.e., child was okay despite getting germs on the hands and not washing the hands repeatedly). Parents can be an important part of this treatment as they may be asked to help their child to stop engaging in the compulsive behavior at home despite experiencing intrusive thoughts.

Psychopharmacology

Pharmacologic treatments are an important consideration in the treatment of childhood anxiety. Several classes of medication are used by clinicians to treat anxiety, including antidepressant medication such as selective serotonin reuptake inhibitors (SSRIs) and tricyclic antidepressants (TCAs), benzodiazepines, buspirone, guanfacine, and hydroxyzine (Table 51.2). The 2020 update of the clinical practice guideline of the American Academy of Child and Adolescent Psychiatry (AACAP) recognizes that there is significant evidence-based support for the use of both CBT and SSRIs as first-line treatment options for anxiety in children and adolescents (Walter et al., 2020). Many clinicians will begin treatment with medication and behavioral therapy when anxiety significantly limits function at initial presentation or when augmentation is desired for behavioral treatments in cases where impairment began as mild or moderate. Paul's pediatrician has elected to begin with behavioral therapy, likely given the new onset of his presentation (see vignette). If he persists in refusing to attend school despite working with a therapist and the school, a trial of medication could be considered.

A systematic review and metaanalysis of childhood anxiety treatments found that SSRIs, a similar antidepressant class of medication called serotonin and norepinephrine reuptake inhibitors (SNRIs), and CBT were each effective in the reduction of anxiety symptoms (Wang et al., 2017). Use of SSRIs and SNRIs was associated with adverse events that were generally not serious. The authors concluded that when deciding among these options, decisions should be based on a family's values, preferences, availability of services, and side effect profile. We review various medication options and considerations later. An overview is provided here, with more detail available in Chapter 99.

Antidepressant Medications

The most commonly used medications to treat childhood anxiety are the SSRIs. Use of SSRIs in patients 6 to 18 years of age with social anxiety, generalized anxiety, separation anxiety, or panic disorder is endorsed with confidence in the AACAP clinical practice guideline (Walter et al., 2020). In the Wang et al.'s (2017) systemic review and metaanalysis medications in the SSRI class improved primary anxiety symptoms as reported by parent and clinician, response to treatment, remission of disorder, and global functioning.

The class of SSRI medications functions in the inhibition of the reuptake of serotonin in brain synapses, increasing the amount of serotonin available in the synaptic cleft. Serotonin plays a role in the brain's response to and ability to process fears and stress. The most studied SSRIs are fluoxetine, fluvoxamine, paroxetine, and sertraline.

Side effects across these medications are similar and may be noted within the first several weeks after beginning

TABLE 51.2 Medications Commonly Used to Treat Childhood Anxiety

Class	Medication	Side Effects	Dosage	FDA-Approval Status for Pediatric Anxiety Disorders or OCD
Selective serotonin reuptake inhibitors	Sertraline Fluoxetine Paroxetine Fluvoxamine	Common or notable: insomnia, sedation, agitation, tremors, headache, dizziness, gastrointestinal, sexual dysfunction, treatment emergent activation syndrome Severe: seizures, induction of mania, suicidality	25–200 mg/day 10–80 mg/day 10–60 mg each morning 25–200 mg/day	OCD: age ≥6 yr OCD: age ≥7 yr No OCD: age ≥8 yr
Serotonin and norepinephrine reuptake inhibitors (SNRIs)	Venlafaxine	Common or notable: insomnia, sedation, agitation, tremors, headache, dizziness, gastrointestinal, sexual dysfunction, treatment emergent activation syndrome, increase in blood pressure Severe: seizures, hyponatremia, induction of mania, suicidality	37.5–225 mg/day	No
SNRIs	Duloxetine	Common or notable: insomnia, sedation, agitation, tremors, headache, dizziness, gastrointestinal, sexual dysfunction, treatment emergent activation syndrome, increase in blood pressure, urinary retention Severe: seizures, induction of mania, suicidality	30–60 mg once daily	Generalized anxiety: ages 7–17
Nonbenzodiazepine anxiolytic	Buspirone	Common or notable: dizziness, drowsiness, nausea, headache, insomnia, impaired concentration, xerostomia Severe: serotonin syndrome, akathisia, extrapyramidal symptoms, tardive dyskinesia, dystonia	15–60 mg/day divided twice daily	No
Alpha-2 agonist	Guanfacine	Common or notable: sedation, dizziness, abdominal pain, hypotension, dry mouth Severe: sinus bradycardia	1–4 mg daily (may increase up to 7 mg for adolescents)	No
First-generation antihistamine; nonbenzodiazepine anxiolytic	Hydroxyzine	Common or notable: xerostomia, drowsiness, dizziness, ataxia, weakness, headache Severe: hypersensitivity reaction, dyspnea, seizures, heat stroke, QT prolongation	2 mg/kg/day in divided doses or 50–100 mg divided four times per day in older children/adolescents	Anxiety

FDA, US Food and Drug Administration; *OCD*, obsessive-compulsive disorder.

treatment. Common side effects reported include dry mouth, gastrointestinal effects such as nausea and diarrhea, headache, sleep disturbance (somnolence or insomnia), dizziness, change in appetite that may lead to weight loss or gain, and tremors. More rare but concerning side effects are suicidal thoughts and behaviors, activation syndrome (a state of restlessness, agitation, and anxiety), mania, serotonin syndrome, and seizures.

The US Food and Drug Administration (FDA) applied a boxed warning to SSRI medications due to the noted increase in suicidal thoughts and behaviors. A metaanalysis of 27 trials involving use of SSRI medications to treat pediatric depression, OCD, and anxiety disorders found a small but increased risk of treatment-emergent suicidal ideation/suicide attempt for each indication with pooled random effects risk differences of less than 1% (Bridge et al., 2007). Specifically for anxiety, the number needed to harm was 143, compared to the number needed to treat (3), thus indicating many more individuals would benefit from treatment than the few who might develop suicidal ideation related to treatment. No completed suicides were noted in the literature. Recommendations to address the risk of suicidality include starting at low doses and increasing the dose gradually. Clinicians should also monitor patients closely at the onset of medication use.

Use of the SNRIs is becoming more common. The AACAP suggests the use of SNRIs, indicating some greater uncertainty in their use given less available evidence (Walter et al., 2020). The SNRI mechanism of action is similar to the SSRI class, with medications blocking reuptake of norepinephrine in addition to serotonin at the synaptic cleft leading to greater neurotransmission. Duloxetine and venlafaxine are two SNRIs that have been studied in the pediatric population. The side effect profile is similar to that of the SSRI medications.

TCAs were utilized more commonly in the past. However, as other medications such as SSRIs have increased in usage, rates of usage of TCAs have fallen given their more significant side effect profile. Anticholinergic side effects such as dry mouth and constipation are common. Patients should have a cardiac risk screening assessment, including an electrocardiogram, prior to commencing therapy. TCAs are included in the FDA boxed warning about increased risk of suicidality.

Benzodiazepines

Due to their addictive nature and side effect profile, benzodiazepines such as lorazepam or clonazepam are not recommended as first-line medications for childhood anxiety. There is little evidence to support their use in children. The rapid onset of action as compared to the SSRI medications may make these medications seem a desirable choice. The risk of abuse and addiction should be strongly weighed against potential benefits until additional evidence to support their use in children is available.

Other Medications

Buspirone is a nonbenzodiazepine anxiolytic that binds to serotonin and dopamine D2 receptors. It is approved for use to treat anxiety in adults. Common side effects include dizziness, drowsiness, insomnia, headache, and nausea. There is little in the published literature to support the use of buspirone in pediatric anxiety disorders.

Guanfacine is an alpha-2 agonist used in treatment of pediatric ADHD. Guanfacine is generally well tolerated, but there is little evidence to support its use in pediatric anxiety. Side effects include headache, somnolence, and dizziness.

Hydroxyzine is an older medication, noted primarily for its antiitch properties, which can also be effective in treating anxiety. It has a relatively safe side effect profile and is generally well tolerated. It is approved for use in pediatric anxiety and can be useful for episodic anxiety.

Medication for OCD

Treatment for OCD can be very effective, with about 70% of patients experiencing relief with pharmacologic treatment. SSRIs are the most effective agents, although they are used at higher doses and for more prolonged periods than for other disorders. Second-line agents include the tricyclic antidepressant clomipramine and augmentation with neuroleptic medications (Geller & March, 2012).

Other Treatments

There are additional treatments for anxiety disorders that have less support than CBT and pharmacologic treatment but should be considered as a primary or adjunctive treatment, particularly for those who do not respond to CBT or are not interested in CBT (Freidl et al., 2017). Examples of such treatments with research support include hypnosis, biofeedback, stress inoculation therapy, and mindfulness.

Combined Treatments

The combination of CBT and medication is generally recommended for more severe presentations or for children who have not responded adequately to monotherapy. The Child/Adolescent Anxiety Multimodal Treatment Study (CAMS) compared CBT, pharmacotherapy with sertraline, a combination of CBT and sertraline, and placebo. The study included 488 youth with separation anxiety disorder, GAD, and social phobia. A study comparing remission rates after 12 weeks of treatment found that both CBT alone and sertraline alone had significantly higher remission rates than placebo, but the combination therapy group had significantly higher rates than all the study arms (Ginsburg et al., 2011)

CONCLUSION AND CLINICAL IMPLICATIONS

Anxiety disorders are common during childhood and adolescence, and early treatment is important in reducing long-term impairment. In the case of Paul, described in the vignette, there are multiple factors (e.g. temperament, parental reactions) that can contribute to anxiety in children. Treatment should be individualized to specific circumstances, such as Paul's treatment was. CBT and pharmacotherapy have a strong evidence base that supports their use as first-line treatments. Additional research is needed on predictors of response to treatment and alternative treatments for anxiety disorders. Screening and assessment of anxiety by medical professionals are key for identifying anxiety and making referrals for evidence-based treatments.

REFERENCES

American Psychiatric Association. (2013). *Diagnostic and statistical manual of mental disorders* (5th ed.). https://doi.org/10.1176/appi.books.9780890425596

Angst, J., & Vollrath, M. (1991). The natural history of anxiety disorders. *Acta Psychiatrica Scandinavica, 84*(5), 446–452.

Anthony, J. L., Lonigan, C. J., Hooe, E. S., & Phillips, B. M. (2002). An affect-based, hierarchical model of temperament and its relations with internalizing symptomatology. *Journal of Clinical Child and Adolescent Psychology, 31*, 480–490.

Böhnlein, J., Altegoer, L., Muck, N. K., Roesmann, K., Redlich, R., Dannlowski, U., & Leehr, E. J. (2020). Factors influencing the success of exposure therapy for specific phobia: A systematic review. *Neuroscience & Biobehavioral Reviews, 108*, 796–820.

Bridge, J. A., Iyengar, S., Salary, C. B., Barbe, R. P., Birmaher, B., Pincus, H. A., Ren, L., & Brent, D. A. (2007). Clinical response and risk for reported suicidal ideation and suicide attempts in pediatric antidepressant treatment: A meta-analysis of randomized controlled trials. *JAMA, 297*(15), 1683–1696.

Buzzell, G. A., Troller-Renfree, S. V., Barker, T. V., Bowman, L. C., Chronis-Tuscano, A., Henderson, H. A., Kagan, J., Pine, D. S., & Fox, N. A. (2017). A neurobehavioral mechanism linking behaviorally inhibited temperament and later adolescent social anxiety. *Journal of the American Academy of Child and Adolescent Psychiatry, 56*(12), 1097–1105. https://doi.org/10.1016/j.jaac.2017.10.007

Chisholm, D., Sweeny, K., Sheehan, P., Rasmussen, B., Smit, F., Cuijpers, P., & Saxena, S. (2016). Scaling-up treatment of depression and anxiety: A global return on investment analysis. *The Lancet Psychiatry, 3*(5), 415–424.

Cummings, C. M., Caporino, N. E., & Kendall, P. C. (2014). Comorbidity of anxiety and depression in children and adolescents: 20 years after. *Psychological Bulletin, 140*(3), 816–845. https://doi.org/10.1037/a0034733

Driessen, J., Blom, J. D., Muris, P., Blashfield, R. K., & Molendijk, M. L. (2020). Anxiety in children with selective mutism: A meta-analysis. *Child Psychiatry & Human Development, 51*(2), 330–341.

Ehrenreich, J. T., Santucci, L. C., & Weiner, C. L. (2008). Separation anxiety disorder in youth: Phenomenology, assessment, and treatment. *Behavioral Research, 16*(3), 389–412. https://doi.org/10.1901/jaba.2008.16-389

Eley, T. C., McAdams, T. A., Rijsdijk, F. V., Lichtenstein, P., Narusyte, J., Reiss, D., Spotts, E. L., Ganiban, J. M., & Neiderhiser, J. M. (2015). The intergenerational transmission of anxiety: A children-of-twins study. *American Journal of Psychiatry, 172*(7), 630–637.

Elmore, A. L., & Crouch, E. (2020). The association of adverse childhood experiences with anxiety and depression for children and youth, 8 to 17 years of age. *Academic Pediatrics, 20*(5), 600–608. https://doi.org/10.1016/j.acap.2020.02.012

Fisak, B., & Grills-Taquechel, A. E. (2007). Parental modeling, reinforcement, and information transfer: Risk factors in the development of child anxiety? *Clinical Child and Family Psychology Review, 10*(3), 213–231.

Freidl, E. K., Stroeh, O. M., Elkins, R. M., Steinberg, E., Albano, A. M., & Rynn, M. (2017). Assessment and treatment of anxiety among children and adolescents. *Focus, 15*(2), 144–156.

Geller, D. A., & March, J. (2012). Practice parameter for the assessment and treatment of children and adolescents with obsessive-compulsive disorder. *Journal of the American Academy of Child & Adolescent Psychiatry, 51*(1), 98–113.

Ghandour, R. M., Sherman, L. J., Vladutiu, C. J., Ali, M. M., Lynch, S. E., Bitsko, R. H., & Blumberg, S. J. (2019). Prevalence and treatment of depression, anxiety, and conduct problems in US children. *The Journal of Pediatrics, 206*, 256–267.

Ginsburg, G. S., Becker, E. M., Keeton, C. P., Sakolsky, D., Piacentini, J., Albano, A. M., Compton, S. N., Iyengar, S., Sullivan, K., Caporino, N., Peris, T., Birmaher, B., Rynn, M., & Kendall, P. C. (2014). Naturalistic follow-up of youths treated for pediatric anxiety disorders. *JAMA Psychiatry, 71*(3), 310–318.

Ginsburg, G. S., Kendall, P. C., Sakolsky, D., Compton, S. N., Piacentini, J., Albano, A. M., Walkup, J. T., Sherrill, J., Coffey, K. A., Rynn, M. A., Keeton, C. P., McCracken, J. T., Bergman, L., Iyengar, S., Birmaher, B., & March, J. (2011). Remission after acute treatment in children and adolescents with anxiety disorders: Findings from the CAMS. *Journal of Consulting and Clinical Psychology, 79*(6), 806–813.

Gottschalk, M. G., & Domschke, K. (2017). Genetics of generalized anxiety disorder and related traits. *Dialogues in Clinical Neuroscience, 19*(2), 159–168.

Hatem, C., Lee, C. Y., Zhao, X., Reesor-Oyer, L., Lopez, T., & Hernandez, D. C. (2020). Food insecurity and housing instability during early childhood as predictors of adolescent mental health. *Journal of Family Psychology, 34*(6), 721–730.

Hettema, J. M., Neale, M. C., & Kendler, K. S. (2001). A review and meta-analysis of the genetic epidemiology of anxiety disorders. *American Journal of Psychiatry, 158*(10), 1568–1578.

Higa-McMillan, C. K., Francis, S. E., Rith-Najarian, L., & Chorpita, B. F. (2016). Evidence base update: 50 years of research on treatment for child and adolescent anxiety. *Journal of Clinical Child and Adolescent Psychology, 45*(2), 91–113. https://doi.org/10.1080/15374416.2015.1046177

Hyland, P., Shevlin, M., Elklit, A., Christoffersen, M., & Murphy, J. (2016). Social, familial and psychological risk factors for mood and anxiety disorders in childhood and early adulthood: A birth cohort study using the Danish Registry System. *Social Psychiatry and Psychiatric Epidemiology, 51*(3), 331–338. https://doi.org/10.1007/s00127-016-1171-1

Kagan, J. (1997). Temperament and the reactions to unfamiliarity. *Child Development, 68*, 139–143.

Kashdan, T. B., & Herbert, J. D. (2001). Social anxiety disorder in childhood and adolescence: Current status and future directions. *Clinical Child and Family Psychology Review, 4*(1), 37–61.

Kendall, P. C. (1994). Treating anxiety disorders in children: Results of a randomized clinical trial. *Journal of Consulting and Clinical Psychology, 62*(1), 100–110. https://doi.org/10.1037/0022-006X.62.1.100

Konnopka, A., & König, H. (2020). Economic burden of anxiety disorders: A systematic review and meta-analysis. *Pharmacoeconomics, 38*(1), 25–37.

Lewinsohn, P. M., Holm-Denoma, J. M., Small, J. W., Seeley, J. R., & Joiner, T. E., Jr (2008). Separation anxiety disorder in childhood as a risk factor for future mental illness. *Journal of the American Academy of Child & Adolescent Psychiatry, 47*(5), 548–555.

McLeod, B. D., Wood, J. J., & Weisz, J. R. (2007). Examining the association between parenting and childhood anxiety: A meta-analysis. *Clinical Psychology Review, 27*(2), 155–172.

Meier, S. M., & Deckert, J. (2019). Genetics of anxiety disorders. *Current Psychiatry Reports, 21*(3), 1–8.

Möller, E. L., Nikolić, M., Majdandžić, M., & Bögels, S. M. (2016). Associations between maternal and paternal parenting behaviors, anxiety and its precursors in early childhood: A meta-analysis. *Clinical Psychology Review, 45*, 17–33. https://doi.org/10.1016/j.cpr.2016.03.002

Muris, P. (2006). Unique and interactive effects of neuroticism and effortful control on psychopathological symptoms in non-clinical adolescents. *Personality and Individual Differences, 40*(7), 1409–1419.

Pachter, L. M., & Coll, C. G. (2009). Racism and child health: A review of the literature and future directions. *Journal of Developmental and Behavioral Pediatrics, 30*(3), 255–263.

Pine, D. S., Cohen, P., Gurley, D., Brook, J., & Ma, Y. (1998). The risk for early-adulthood anxiety and depressive disorders in adolescents with anxiety and depressive disorders. *Archives of General Psychiatry, 55*(1), 56–64.

Rapee, R. M. (2012). Family factors in the development and management of anxiety disorders. *Clinical Child and Family Psychology Review*, *15*(1), 69–80.

Rothbart, M. K. (1989). Temperament and development. In G. A. Kohnstamm, J. E. Bates, & M. K. Rothbart (Eds.), *Temperament in childhood* (pp. 59–73), John Wiley and Sons.

Spence, S. H., Najman, J. M., Bor, W., O'Callaghan, M. J., & Williams, G. M. (2002). Maternal anxiety and depression, poverty and marital relationship factors during early childhood as predictors of anxiety and depressive symptoms in adolescence. *Journal of Child Psychology and Psychiatry*, *43*(4), 457–469.

Walter, H. J., Bukstein, O. G., Abright, A. R., Keable, H., Ramtekkar, U., Ripperger-Suhler, J., & Rockhill, C. (2020). Clinical practice guideline for the assessment and treatment of children and adolescents with anxiety disorders. *Journal of the American Academy of Child & Adolescent Psychiatry*, *59*(10), 1107–1124.

Wang, Z., Whiteside, S. P., Sim, L., Farah, W., Morrow, A. S., Alsawas, M., Barrionuevo, P., Tello, M., Asi, N., Beuschel, B., Daraz, L., Almasri, J., Zaiem, Z., Larrea-Mantilla, L., Ponce, O. J., LeBlanc, A., Prokop, L. J., & Murad, M. H. (2017). Comparative effectiveness and safety of cognitive behavioral therapy and pharmacotherapy for childhood anxiety disorders: A systematic review and meta-analysis. *JAMA Pediatrics*, *171*(11), 1049–1056.

52

Psychotic-Spectrum Disorders in Children and Adolescents

Sarah A. Hamilton, Craig J. Parris, Nicholas J.K. Breitborde, and Walter H. Stearns

For additional material related to the content of this chapter, please see Chapter 99.

Psychosis is a disturbance of the brain that impairs an individual's ability to discern reality. Psychosis and psychotic symptoms occur on a continuum of severity—from aspects of normal development to chronic, prolonged, and debilitating—with the most marked being a primary psychotic disorder such as schizophrenia. Although the typical age of onset of psychosis is late teens to early 20s, with onset skewing later in age for women (Jongsma et al., 2018), it is not uncommon to have individuals experiencing an onset of psychotic symptoms in their early to midteens or, more rarely, prior to age 13. Thus, within the field of child and adolescent psychiatry, there is growing interest in the study and treatment of psychotic disorders, given the typical emergence of these symptoms and their putative early warning signs (i.e., clinical high-risk [CHR] states) in childhood and adolescence. This chapter will delve further into these two clinical categories to highlight important diagnostic and treatment considerations relevant to pediatric clinicians.

CLINICAL HIGH-RISK STATES FOR PSYCHOSIS

VIGNETTE

Josh is a 15-year-old male who presents to establish care with a primary care clinician after his family's relatively recent move. Over the past year, Josh reports onset of mood and anxiety symptoms. In the past 6 months he reports development of intermittent perceptual disturbances, such as seeing shadowy figures and movement in his peripheral vision, as well as hearing a static noise and footsteps when no one is home. These experiences intrigue him though he recognizes that they are not real. His teachers report that he has seemed more mistrustful and suspicious of classmates lately, leading to more behavioral escalations with peers along with school avoidance. Josh reports feeling sad on most days and feels anxious at school. Parents note that he spends most of his time playing videogames and researching conspiracy theories on the Internet. Family history is significant for a maternal uncle with bipolar disorder. Josh is referred for further psychiatric evaluation, where he is diagnosed with having depression, anxiety, and attenuated psychotic symptoms (APS). He is enrolled into a specialty clinic serving individuals with first-episode psychosis and those at CHR for psychosis, where he receives individual therapy and psychoeducation. Josh is not prescribed medication, but he remains in the clinic for weekly therapy appointments learning cognitive-behavioral therapy techniques and methods to reduce stress and manage mood and anxiety concerns. After 1 year of treatment, Josh voices improvement in mood and anxiety symptoms. He denies any further perceptual disturbances and has fewer behavioral issues at school. He is referred back to his primary care clinician to resume ongoing, routine preventative care.

CLINICAL DESCRIPTION

A prodromal or CHR phase prior to the development of a primary psychotic disorder has been often recognized retrospectively. It is defined as the period between one's departure from premorbid levels of functioning and the onset of psychosis. The word *prodrome* (from the Greek meaning "forerunner") is reserved to describe this period in hindsight only after a first episode of frank psychotic symptoms has already occurred with certainty. CHR is used to describe the group of individuals who are demonstrating increased risk to develop psychosis. The duration of a prodrome spans an average of 1 to 2 years (Woods, Miller, & McGlashan, 2001), and the most vulnerable ages are 12 to 25 years old.

In an attempt to identify this population more accurately, diagnostic criteria that are predictive of the development of psychosis have been described. The Criteria of Prodromal States (COPS) defines three CHR subtypes (Miller et al., 2003):

- *Attenuated psychotic symptoms:* The experience of thoughts (i.e., overvalued ideas) or perceptual disturbances that deviate from normal phenomena but are not frankly psychotic. Although potentially distressing or perplexing, individuals will typically maintain insight into the nonreality basis of these experiences.
- *Brief intermittent psychotic syndrome:* The experience of transitory psychotic symptoms lasting less than a week that self-resolve without treatment.
- *Genetic risk and functional decline:* Concurrent genetic predisposition for psychosis, either by having a first-degree relative with a psychotic disorder or by having schizotypal personality disorder, along with functional deterioration within the past year.

DIFFERENTIAL DIAGNOSIS

Experiences that may appear similar to psychosis may present commonly in the general population without a person going on to develop frank psychosis, with an estimated 7.5% to 17% prevalence in the general population of children and adolescents reporting nonclinically relevant psychotic symptoms (Kelleher et al., 2012). Psychotic risk states can also be challenging to differentiate from nonpsychotic disorders such as obsessive-compulsive disorder (OCD), autism spectrum disorders (ASDs), severe personality disorder/traits, and posttraumatic stress disorder (PTSD), which can present in children and adolescents with similar diagnostic features.

Psychotic-Like Experiences

Psychotic and psychotic-like experiences in children younger than age 13 are common and usually not pathologic. Features of psychotic experiences that are less likely to be representative of risk for psychotic disorder include absence of premorbid difficulties, auditory hallucinations that are nonbizarre and related to stressors, absence of delusions, perceptual disturbances that have less prominent or intrusive impact on behavior, and maintaining of social and academic functioning despite mental health concerns (Abidi, 2013).

Obsessive-Compulsive Disorder

In adults the intrusive thoughts and compulsive behaviors that characterize OCD can often be differentiated from psychosis as, in most cases, the patient maintains insight with regard to their mental health challenges. In children and adolescents, where cognitive abilities are still maturing, these thoughts may be described as "voices" and may comprehend the experience as being external to the self (Abidi, 2013).

Autism Spectrum Disorder

ASD is characterized by social, emotional, and communication challenges (as opposed to social withdrawal or poverty of speech in psychosis), including lack of emotional reciprocity, misreading of social queues, restricted or flattened affect, and language delay that may be misinterpreted as negative symptoms of psychosis. Thought content can present in a somewhat similar fashion with perseveration and concrete thinking, though individuals with ASD often have restricted interests, including preoccupation with fantastical or magical ideals/beliefs (Chandrasekhar, Copeland, Spanos, & Sikich, 2020) (see Chapter 41).

Posttraumatic Stress Disorder and Personality Disorders

Psychotic-like symptoms associated with PTSD and severe personality disorders differ from primary psychotic disorders, typically in the more transient nature of the psychosis along with a propensity to dissociation and a lack of a thought disorder (Cavelti, Thompson, Chanen, & Kaess, 2021; O'Conghaile & DeLisi, 2015). Higher rates of trauma are associated with higher psychosis risk and greater symptom frequency and severity (Croft et al., 2019) (see Chapter 56).

ASSESSMENT

It is not uncommon for children and adolescents to report psychotic-like symptoms. A metaanalysis from almost 30,000 youth from community samples found nearly 10% of participants reported experiencing perceptual disturbances (Healy et al., 2019). When interviewing children and adolescents, it is important to create a linear narrative of symptom onset focusing on developmental milestones, affective/behavioral responses, medical history, genetic risk, social functioning, cultural implications, and cognitive abilities. Therefore it is prudent to involve a patient's caregiver(s) and teachers whenever possible to collect history. Perceptual disturbances in a youth may indicate normal development, a schizophrenia spectrum disorder, a CHR for psychosis state, or another primary mental health disorder.

To mitigate the risk of false positives and improve interrater reliability, Miller et al. (2003) devised the structured interview for psychosis-risk syndromes (SIPS). The SIPS is a semistructured interview that helps to assess for CHR states of psychosis and frank psychotic symptoms. The SIPS has been validated for persons 10 to 45 years old. The patient must have a minimum IQ of 70, absence of traumatic brain injury, and be without complicating neurologic conditions to participate in the SIPS.

COURSE AND PROGNOSIS

Among individuals at CHR for psychosis, available data suggest that 36% will experience the onset of a psychotic disorder within 3 years (Fusar-Poli et al., 2012). Variables that were most likely to indicate transition are discussed later in this chapter. The potential influence of factors, such as childhood trauma, migration status, urbanicity, and perceived discrimination, have been studied, though research is still needed to draw conclusions. Neuroimaging has revealed potential structural brain changes, notably increased rate of gray matter loss and changes in thalamic connectivity, that may play a role in transition to psychosis (Nelson & McGorry, 2020).

TREATMENT

With the increased ability to reliably identify individuals at elevated risk states for developing psychotic disorders, there has been a growing interest in developing specialized interventions targeted to this population. Such interventions seek to address the mental health and functional concerns experienced by individuals at CHR for psychosis with the ultimate goal of reducing rates of transition to frank psychotic disorders among this population.

Pharmacologic Interventions

Early treatment studies among individuals at CHR for developing a psychotic disorder focused primarily on investigating the use of antipsychotic medications to prevent conversion to frank psychotic disorder (McGlashan et al., 2006; McGorry et al., 2002). Ultimately, these studies suggested that the benefits of antipsychotic medication in preventing the onset of psychotic disorders were limited, whereas the side effects of the medication (e.g., weight gain) were oftentimes severe. Consequently, antipsychotics are currently considered an inappropriate first-line treatment during the CHR phase and should be reserved for people at the highest severity of APS and/or distress (Fusar-Poli et al., 2013). Interestingly, several studies have suggested that selective serotonin reuptake inhibitors (SSRIs) may reduce rates of transition to a frank psychotic disorder (Cornblatt et al., 2007; Fusar-Poli et al., 2015). This research is intriguing given the better side effect profile and lower perceived stigma associated with SSRIs relative to antipsychotic medications (Fusar-Poli, Valmaggia, & McGuire, 2007).

Psychosocial Interventions

Given the challenges associated with antipsychotic treatment during the CHR phase, growing attention has been directed toward investigating the potential benefits of psychosocial interventions during this phase of illness. To date, several psychosocial interventions have shown promise in addressing the symptomatic and/or functional challenges experienced by individuals at CHR for psychosis, including cognitive-behavioral therapy (Devoe, Farris, Townes, & Addington, 2020), cognitive remediation (Glenthøj, Hjorthøj, Kristensen, Davidson, & Nordentoft, 2017), and family psychoeducation (Miklowitz et al., 2014).

Multicomponent Interventions

Ultimately, no single psychosocial or pharmacologic intervention has been shown to help address all of the clinical concerns experienced by individuals at CHR for psychosis (Addington, Piskulic, Devoe, Santesteban-Echarri, & Stowkowy, 2020). Consequently, clinical services for individuals at CHR for psychosis have begun organizing themselves around providing multidisciplinary, multiintervention care for individuals at CHR for psychosis (Addington, Devoe, & Santesteban-Echarri, 2019). For example, within the United States, the Substance Abuse and Mental Health Services Administration (SAMHSA) recently funded the launch of 21 clinical centers designed to provide multiintervention care to individuals at CHR for psychosis using a step-based model of care (Breitborde et al., 2020). Within this care delivery model, individuals initially participate in interventions that are low intensity, nonpsychosis specific, and more benign (e.g., fewer side effects). When individuals do not show adequate response to these treatments based on a priori response criteria, they proceed onto treatments that are psychosis specific with increased potential for side effects (e.g., antipsychotic medication).

PSYCHOTIC-SPECTRUM DISORDERS IN CHILDREN AND ADOLESCENTS

VIGNETTE

Three years after resuming care with his primary care clinician, Josh is referred back to the specialty clinic serving individuals at CHR for psychosis as well as those with first-episode psychosis. Per history obtained in referral, following transition back to routine care, Josh continued to do well, graduated high school, and began attending college several hours from his home. While at school he started using marijuana with his roommates at parties. His grades fell in several classes, and his roommates noticed odd behaviors, including writing various Bible verses on the walls of his room and frequently calling them to ask their whereabouts and questioning whether they were safe living in their dorm. Upon interview, Josh noted that a few months prior, he began feeling that pedestrians outside of his building were government agents in disguise, his parents were members of a secret society, and he found passages in the Bible referencing him being "the chosen one." A few weeks prior to the interview, he began hearing the voice of God providing instructions to prevent the apocalypse. Josh denied any suicidal or homicidal ideation and demonstrated no dangerous behaviors, but he acknowledged feeling fearful and distressed by these occurrences. Although he did not feel these were symptoms of an illness, he was agreeable to using medication in an attempt to feel better. He was started on a low-dose antipsychotic and, with strong encouragement, stopped using cannabis. He also began participating in weekly cognitive-behavioral therapy sessions focused on addressing his psychotic symptoms. After several months of treatment and with sustained sobriety, these symptoms lessened and eventually resolved, after which he demonstrated good insight into the bizarre nature of these experiences.

CLINICAL DESCRIPTION

Psychosis is a disturbance of the brain that impairs an individual's ability to discern reality. Psychosis and psychotic symptoms occur on a continuum of severity—from aspects of normal development to chronic, prolonged, and debilitating—with the most marked being a primary psychotic disorder. Some common examples of psychosis include hallucinations and delusions. Hallucinations are perceptions, experienced by the individual, in the absence of a stimulus, such as hearing voices or seeing things. A delusion is a disturbance of thought content with a false belief that the person holds true, despite evidence to the contrary. Common delusional themes are persecutory (belief that an individual, group, or organization intends ill will or harm toward oneself) and referential (belief that gestures, comments, or environmental cues are directed at oneself), though numerous others exist (Table 52.1).

TABLE 52.1 Common Symptoms of Psychosis

Positive Symptoms		Negative Symptoms	
Delusions	Fixed false beliefs that are unmoving despite conflicting evidence, the most common being persecutory (~50%)	**Blunting of affect**	Diminished emotional expression, including reductions in the expression of emotions in the face, eye contact, intonation of speech, and movements of the hand, head, and face that normally give an emotional emphasis to speech
Hallucinations	Perception-like experiences that occur without an external stimulus	**Alogia**	Diminished speech output
	May occur in any sensory modality but auditory hallucinations are the most common in schizophrenia (~80%)	**Avolition**	Decrease in motivated self-initiated purposeful activities
Disorganized thinking/ speech	Derailment or loosening of associations (abrupt switching from one topic to another), tangentiality (answering questions obliquely or unrelated to the question asked), or "word salad" (incomprehensible) (~65%)	**Anhedonia**	Inability to experience or anticipate pleasure from positive stimuli
Disorganized behavior	Ranging from child-like silliness to unpredictable agitation to hypoactive catatonia (marked negativism and stupor) (~50%)	**Asociality**	Reduced social interactions
Cognitive			
Varying degrees of impairment from minimal to marked deficits in listed domains with potential for up to 2SD drop from premorbid IQ		**Attention** **Executive function** **Processing speed**	**Episodic and working memory** **Language skills** **Crystallized knowledge**

Psychosis can present in a variety of ways and as symptoms of various mental health disorders. Psychotic and psychotic-like experiences in young children are common, and many are not pathologic. Nonpathologic psychotic-like experiences are typically transient, often perceived as positive, nonthreatening, and nondistressing, usually experienced as less dangerous and more controllable and, by definition, are not associated with functional impairment (Tyson, House, & Donovan, 2020). Despite the potential benign nature of these occurrences, however, the presence of psychotic-like experiences in childhood, even among community samples, is associated with a threefold risk of any mental health disorder and fourfold risk of a psychotic disorder (Healy et al., 2019).

What we call psychotic disorders are in fact syndromes, constellations of symptoms with varying severity, responses to treatment, and overall prognosis. Schizophrenia, the most common primary psychotic disorder, is a chronic and potentially significantly disabling illness with a lifetime prevalence of approximately 0.7% (Saha, Chant, Welham, & McGrath, 2005). Typical age of onset of psychosis is late teens to early 20s, with onset skewing later in age for women (Jongsma et al., 2018). With that being the case, it is not uncommon to have individuals presenting in their early to midteens or even very rarely prior to age 13 (childhood onset). The course of schizophrenia can be quite variable depending on the severity and disabling nature of symptoms, but early and intensive intervention can improve outcomes (Kane et al., 2016). Schizophrenia is associated with increased mortality related to both physical and mental health outcomes, with a life expectancy 15 years less than typical or average and a suicide rate of approximately 5% (Hjorthøj, Stürup, McGrath, & Nordentoft, 2017; Hor & Taylor, 2010).

PSYCHOTIC-SPECTRUM DISORDERS

Schizophrenia, the prototypical psychotic-spectrum disorder, is marked not only by positive symptoms, those most easily observed and commonly considered in a psychotic disorder, but an array of other neuropsychiatric symptoms. As per the *Diagnostic and Statistical Manual of Mental Disorders*, fifth edition (*DSM-5*) (American Psychiatric Association, 2013), a diagnosis requires two or more key symptoms (i.e., delusions, hallucinations, disorganized speech, disorganized or catatonic behavior, and negative symptoms) with 1 month of active symptoms and 6 months of functional impairment to meet criteria for diagnosis. Common symptoms associated with schizophrenia in children and adolescents are highlighted in Table 52.1 (Harvey & Isner, 2020; Stentebjerg-Olesen, Pagsberg, Fink-Jensen, Correll, & Jeppesen, 2016).

Individuals with childhood-onset schizophrenia (COS) meet diagnostic criteria for schizophrenia before age 13. This is an extremely rare condition with a prevalence of <0.04%. By the nature of its rarity, it should be considered a diagnosis of exclusion, commonly misdiagnosed in the setting of affective psychosis, organic psychosis, ASD, or atypical psychosis-associated multidimensional impaired group (transient psychosis, lability, interpersonal problems, cognitive deficits). More than 50% of individuals with COS have social, language, and/or academic difficulties, with 44% also exhibiting motor difficulties. These individuals tend to have marked genetic loading with more clear pathophysiologic detriment on neuroimaging, strong family history of psychotic illness and generally a worse prognosis, typically responding only to treatment with clozapine as opposed to alternative antipsychotic treatments (Driver, Thomas, Gogtay, & Rapoport, 2020).

Individuals with early-onset schizophrenia (EOS) meet diagnostic criteria for schizophrenia before age 18, and those meeting criteria after this point are considered adult-onset (AOS). There is limited literature specific to EOS compared to AOS, as much of the literature base for schizophrenia includes an age range down to ~15 years.

Schizophreniform Disorder

This disorder is characterized by the presence of the symptoms of schizophrenia but is distinguished by its shorter duration, in which symptoms are present for at least 1 month but less than 6 months.

Schizoaffective Disorder

A diagnosis of schizoaffective disorder requires an uninterrupted period of illness meeting primary criterion for schizophrenia with concurrent periods of major mood symptoms (either manic or depressive episodes) present for a majority of the total duration of active and residual portions of illness. Schizoaffective disorder is delineated from depressive or bipolar disorder with psychotic features based on the presence of psychotic symptoms for at least 2 weeks in the absence of a major mood episode.

Affective Disorders With Psychosis

Affective disorders with psychosis are distinguished from primary psychotic disorders by the temporal relationship between the mood disturbance and psychosis. If delusions or hallucinations occur exclusively during a major depressive episode, the diagnosis is major depressive disorder with psychotic features. In bipolar disorder, as in the case of major depressive disorder with psychotic features, delusions or hallucinations occur exclusively during a depressive or manic episode.

Unspecified Schizophrenia

This diagnosis applies to presentations in which symptoms characteristic of schizophrenia spectrum cause clinically significant distress or impairment predominate but do not meet full criteria for any of the disorders in the schizophrenia spectrum. This diagnosis is often used in situations in which the clinician chooses not to specify the reason criteria are not met and includes presentations in which there is insufficient information to make a more specific diagnosis (e.g., diagnosis made in the emergency room).

Delusional Disorder

This illness is characterized by 1 month of delusions with absence of other psychotic symptoms. Delusions are fixed, false beliefs based on inaccurate inference about reality that persist despite evidence to the contrary. In individuals with delusional disorder cognition and reality testing otherwise remain intact as do other psychosocial abilities. If hallucinations occur, they are specific to the delusional belief.

Brief Psychotic Disorder

A sudden onset of psychotic behavior that lasts less than 1 month followed by complete remission with possible future relapses. It is differentiated from schizophreniform disorder (>1 month but <6 months) and schizophrenia (>6 months) by the duration of psychosis. Can occur as a response to a specific trigger (i.e., stressor or trauma) or in the absence of any clear inciting event.

Other Disorders With Psychosis in Children and Adolescents

Substance-Induced Psychosis

This type of psychosis involves the presence of delusions or hallucinations that developed during or soon after substance intoxication or withdrawal or after exposure to a medication and resolves within 1 month of last exposure to the substance. Substance-induced psychosis often features a later age of onset, increased insight into symptoms of psychosis, fewer or less severe negative symptoms, and a weaker family history of psychosis compared to primary psychotic disorders (Beckmann et al., 2020). Substance-induced psychosis is associated with the development of severe mental illness. Larger registry studies have found that 24% to 32% of individuals with a diagnosis of substance-induced psychosis subsequently developed a schizophrenia spectrum or bipolar disorder (Starzer, Nordentoft, & Hjorthøj, 2018).

Psychosis Associated With a General Medical Condition

A wide variety of medical illnesses can present with hallucinations/delusions or psychotic-like symptoms. Some possible illnesses include (Freudenreich, Brown, & Holt, 2016) (1) central nervous system disorders (epilepsy, head trauma, migraine), (2) demyelinating diseases (multiple sclerosis, metachromatic leukodystrophy), (3) autoimmune disorders (systemic lupus erythematosus, rheumatic fever, myasthenia gravis), (4) infections (HIV, viral encephalitis), (5) endocrinopathies (hypoglycemia, Addison disease, Cushing disease, thyroid disease), (6) sleep disorders (narcolepsy, hypnagogic and hypnopompic hallucinations), (7) nutritional deficiencies (magnesium, vitamins A, D, B_1, B_3, B_{12}), (8) metabolic disorders (Wilson disease, porphyria, amino acid aberrations), and (9) chromosomal abnormalities.

Factors increasing suspicion for an underlying organic cause include acute or subacute onset of psychotic symptoms, symptoms accompanied by regression (behavioral or cognitive), or symptoms associated with apparent triggers (infection, medication, etc.). Additionally, the presence of unique physical symptoms (i.e., seizures, dysmorphic facies, and malar rash) or psychiatric symptoms (i.e. confusion and catatonia) raises suspicion for a psychosis associated with a somatic disorder. Identification is crucial as this will determine the appropriate treatment approach and course (Benjamin, Lauterbach, & Stanislawski, 2013).

DIFFERENTIAL DIAGNOSIS

Similar to psychotic risk states, EOS can be challenging to differentiate from nonpsychotic disorders such as ASD, PTSD, OCD, and severe personality disorder/traits, which can present in children and adolescents. An example of this might be schizotypal personality disorder, which typically presents in early adulthood and is a pervasive pattern of social and interpersonal deficits and reduced capacity for close relationships as well as cognitive and perceptual distortions characterized by odd beliefs or magical thinking, ideas of reference, paranoid or suspicious ideation, lack of close friendships outside of relatives, unusual perceptual experiences, and peculiar behavior or appearance (American Psychiatric Association, 2013). Considerations noted previously for differentiating CHR states from these nonpsychotic disorders can also be applied to help differentiate these conditions from frank psychotic symptoms in children and adolescents.

NEUROBIOLOGIC AND GENETIC RISK FACTORS

Schizophrenia is thought to be neurodevelopmental in origin for the vast majority of people (Murray, Bhavsar, Tripoli, & Howes, 2017). Expression of the illness is determined by epigenetics, the interaction between genes and the environment, likely with the pathophysiologic process occurring long before overt clinical symptoms manifest. On the basis of twin and family studies, heritability is estimated to explain 80% of the risk for schizophrenia in the general population (Forsyth & Asarnow, 2020). Many of the genes that are identified in genome-wide association and gene-expression profiling studies implicate pathways associated with the immune system, cytoskeletal development, and synaptic plasticity and function (Bennett, 2011; Radhakrishnan, Kaser, & Guloksuz, 2017). Environmental factors include pre- and perinatal complications (e.g., maternal infection, smoking during pregnancy, and obstetric complications leading to fetal hypoxia), early-life adversity, childhood residence in urban areas, isolation from those of similar ethnic or minority group (first-generation immigrant status), as well as strong associations with substance use (Davies et al., 2020; Selten, van der Ven, & Termorshuizen, 2020). Imaging studies reveal an overall decrease in gray matter and fraying of white matter tracts, further pointing to the neurodevelopmental and neurodegenerative aspects of the illness (Bakhshi & Chance, 2015).

COURSE AND PROGNOSIS

The course of schizophrenia is quite variable, with some individuals manifesting only mild symptoms without significant functional impairment while others develop marked symptoms and loss of independence. Negative prognostic factors include poor premorbid functioning, lower IQ, substance use, family history, age of onset, male gender, longer duration of untreated psychosis, negative symptoms, lack of precipitating factors, treatment-resistant positive symptoms, and multiple relapses (Díaz-Caneja et al., 2015). Many of these factors are not modifiable, making it paramount to address those that are, including shortening duration of untreated psychosis, maintaining compliance with treatment as a means of preventing relapse, abstaining from substance use, and encouraging or facilitating psychosocial and family support.

TREATMENT

Pharmacologic Treatment

At the point in the illness process when symptom severity is functionally distressing, sometimes before the onset of fully formed psychosis, the use of antipsychotic medication becomes a crucial part of treatment. There are a host of antipsychotic medications, some approved in a younger population, all with a similar mechanism of action (dopamine blockade) and efficacy in this age range (<18 years of age) but with varying side effect profiles (Howes & Kapur, 2009). The one exception is clozapine, which has a more marked side effect profile, but greater efficacy and is the only antipsychotic shown to be more effective when other antipsychotics fail (McEvoy et al., 2006). This efficacy has been repeatedly demonstrated in adult populations but also is true for EOS and COS, who might have even a greater response to clozapine (Schneider, Corrigall, Hayes, Kyriakopoulos, & Frangou, 2014).

In early illness the response to medication is generally more robust and less variable. As a result of this responsiveness, it is advised to utilize treatment that has the lowest side effect burden (Emsley, Rabinowitz, & Medori, 2006). Side effects among antipsychotic agents differ largely, with the most common, metabolic and extrapyramidal effects, being most severe in younger age people (Stroup & Gray, 2018). In addition, the response time to medication when one is first treated should be approached in terms of months rather than days or weeks, as is commonly the case with older, more chronic populations and for much of general medicine (Derks et al., 2010; Pagsberg et al., 2017). Yet, some individuals, even in their first episode, will exhibit signs of treatment refractory illness and should be tried on a subsequent medication, ideally one that might have some increased efficacy, although it is debatable in this patient population which agent that might be (Agid et al., 2011). If this second option is also unsuccessful, a trial of clozapine is warranted, given evidence that additional nonclozapine treatments are unlikely to be impactful, and delays in initiating clozapine (when appropriate) are associated with worse outcomes (Kahn et al., 2018; Üçok et al., 2015).

Even in the adult population, about 20% to 30% of people with a primary psychotic disorder warrant a clozapine trial, and those percentages are likely even higher with a younger age of onset (Demjaha et al., 2017). Individuals with EOS, especially COS, commonly need clozapine; therefore use of clozapine in this population should be considered almost an expectation rather than an anomalous event (Driver et al., 2020). Clozapine is also the only antipsychotic that has demonstrated reduction in suicidality, for which it holds a US Food and Drug Administration indication—a key concern among individuals with psychotic disorders (Hor & Taylor, 2010) (see Chapter 99).

Psychosocial Interventions

To date, numerous evidence-based psychosocial interventions have been identified for the treatment of psychotic disorders. Although investigations with regard to these interventions among specifically children and adolescents with psychotic disorders, are limited relative to studies in adult populations, available data suggest that these treatments are effective in younger populations (Breitborde & Moe, 2019). Moreover, similar to pharmacologic treatments, available data suggest that the potency of these treatments may be maximized by providing them as soon as possible following the initial onset of psychotic symptoms (e.g., McFarlane, 2002). Cognitive-behavioral therapy for psychosis (CBT-p), which aims to help clients understand and cope with symptoms, prevent relapse, and identify and work toward meaningful goals, has been shown to be effective in reducing positive symptoms of psychosis (Turner, van der Gaag, Karyotaki, & Cuijpers, 2014). Cognitive remediation produces meaningful improvements in cognitive functioning among individuals with psychosis and, when paired with concurrent psychiatric rehabilitation services, facilitates downstream benefits on psychosocial functioning (Wykes, Huddy, Cellard, McGurk, & Czobor, 2011). Family psychoeducational interventions providing education on psychotic disorders and problem-solving support facilitate reduced rates of symptomatic relapse among individuals with psychosis and may also lead to improved well-being among caregiving relatives (Claxton, Onwumere, & Fornells-Ambrojo, 2017). Social skills training is an evidence-based intervention that focuses on helping individuals learn and practice skills involved in social interactions and is the most potent psychosocial intervention with regard to treating negative symptoms (Turner et al., 2014).

Multicomponent Interventions

Similar to intervention for individuals at CHR for psychosis, no single pharmacologic or psychosocial intervention is effective in addressing all of the challenges experienced by children and adolescents with psychosis. Consequently, there is growing interest in the development of multiintervention treatment programs designed to simultaneously address the multiple negative consequences associated with psychotic disorders (Breitborde & Moe, 2017). For example, within the United States, there has been a recent and rapid dissemination of coordinated specialty care (CSC) programs offering a treatment package comprised of case management, family support/education, medication management, psychotherapy, and supported employment/education (Azrin, Goldstein, & Heinssen, 2015). Compared to usual care, CSC has been shown to facilitate improved outcomes with regard to symptomatology and quality of life among individuals early in the course of a psychotic disorder (Kane et al., 2016).

Of note, the addition of family involvement within CSC has helped improve patient outcomes and engagement. Families can feel isolated, distraught, and confused regarding how to help their loved one who is experiencing psychosis. Caregivers may experience difficulty in managing medications and appointments, providing increased supervision at home, balancing outside work/school expectations, and coping with their own fears about their loved one's prognosis as well as their own genetic risk to develop a similar illness. In fact, available data have shown that stressful aspects of the caregiving experience can have deleterious effect on the physical and mental health of caregiving relatives of individuals with psychotic disorders (Breitborde, Lopez, & Kopelowicz, 2010). CSC programs will usually offer regular meetings for family members and other natural supports that provide education, support, and hope for recovery.

SUBSTANCE USE AND PSYCHOSIS

Cannabis is the most commonly used illicit drug worldwide, and its use has increased over the last few decades, with 18.4% of adolescents and 32.6% of college students in North America reporting cannabis use in the past 30 days (Wright, Cather, Gilman, & Evins, 2020). Cannabis-induced psychosis is associated with the highest risk for severe mental illness, with about 46% of patients subsequently developing schizophrenia, and studies showing a 50% to 200% increase in risk for participants who used most heavily (Wright et al., 2020). Moreover, persistent cannabis use after the first episode of schizophrenia has been associated with a 2.2-fold increased risk for relapse, even after controlling for confounding factors, including medication adherence, and discontinuation of cannabis use after first-episode psychosis significantly reduces relapse risk to the level of nonusers, improving both symptoms and functioning (Wright et al., 2020). Given this association and the association of substance use with primary psychotic disorders, the legalization of recreational marijuana use is of concern and should prompt clinicians to regularly counsel those they are caring for as to the potential dangers of even legal substance use.

Amphetamine and other stimulant-induced psychoses tend to resolve within days, although some research suggests psychotic symptoms may persist for years. Starzer and colleagues (2018) found that 32.3% of individuals diagnosed with substance-induced psychosis related to amphetamine use were later diagnosed with either schizophrenia or bipolar disorder, a high proportion but less than that seen with cannabis.

Daily tobacco use is associated with an earlier age at onset of psychotic illness, and individuals who use cigarettes during adolescence have an increased risk for subsequent psychotic experiences. Patients with first-episode psychosis tend to have smoked for years before the onset of psychosis, have high prevalence of tobacco use at the time of treatment, and are more likely to smoke than age-matched individuals (Gurillo, Jauhar, Murray, & MacCabe, 2015).

CONCLUSION

Psychotic disorders are serious mental illnesses that are associated with significant morbidity and mortality. As prognosis is impacted by several unmodifiable factors, it is imperative to search for strategies that can meaningfully influence change. At present, the modifiable factor that most clearly shapes the course and prognosis of psychotic disorders in children and adolescents is the time between the onset of psychotic symptoms and the receipt of evidence-based care. Reducing this duration of untreated psychosis is critical in promoting positive clinical and functional outcomes. At the current time there is no clear "silver bullet" with regard to newer medications or psychosocial treatments on the horizon although clear efforts are being made to optimize care both at the patient and the system level, via federal and state government funding. More recently, efforts to develop specialized treatment strategies targeted toward people demonstrating the early warning signs of a burgeoning psychotic disorder offer hope for the identification of preventative strategies for these challenging disorders.

REFERENCES

Abidi. S. (2013). Psychosis in children and youth: Focus on early-onset schizophrenia. *Pediatrics in Review*, *34*(7), 296–305.

Addington, J., Devoe, D. J., & Santesteban-Echarri, O. (2019). Multidisciplinary treatment for individuals at clinical high risk of developing psychosis. *Current Treatment Options in Psychiatry*, *6*(1), 1–16.

Addington, J., Piskulic, D., Devoe, D. J., Santesteban-Echarri, O., & Stowkowy, J. (2020). Indicated prevention in psychosis risk—psychological approaches. In A. D. Thompson & M. R. Broome (Eds.), *Risk factors for psychosis: Paradigms, mechanims, and prevention*. Academic Press.

Agid, O., Arenovich, T., Sajeev, G., Zipursky, R. B., Kapur, S., Foussias, G., & Remington, G. (2011). An algorithm-based approach to first-episode schizophrenia: Response rates over 3 prospective antipsychotic trials with a retrospective data analysis. *Journal of Clinical Psychiatry*, *72*(11), 1439–1444.

American Psychiatric Association. (2013). *Diagnostic and statistical manual of mental disorders* (5th ed.). American Psychiatric Publishing.

Azrin, S. T., Goldstein, A. B., & Heinssen, R. K. (2015). Early intervention for psychosis: The recovery after an initial schizophrenia episode project. *Psychiatric Annals*, *45*(11), 548–553.

Bakhshi, K., & Chance, S. (2015). The neuropathology of schizophrenia: A selective review of past studies and emerging themes in brain structure and cytoarchitecture. *Neuroscience*, *303*, 82–102.

Beckmann, D., Lowman, K. L., Nargiso, J., McKowen, J., Watt, L., & Yule, A. M. (2020). Substance-induced psychosis in youth. *Child and Adolescent Psychiatric Clinics of North America*, *29*(1), 131–143.

Benjamin, S., Lauterbach, M. D., & Stanislawski, A. L. (2013). Congenital and acquired disorders presenting as psychosis in children and young adults. *Child and Adolescent Psychiatric Clinics of North America*, *22*(4), 581–608.

Bennett, M. (2011). Schizophrenia: Susceptibility genes, dendritic-spine pathology and gray matter loss. *Progress in Neurobiology*, *95*(3), 275–300.

Breitborde, N. J. K., Guirgis, H., Stearns, W., Carpenter, K. M., Lteif, G., Pine, J. G., … Moe, A. M. (2020). The Ohio State University Early Psychosis Intervention Center (EPICENTER) step-based care programme for individuals at clinical high risk for psychosis: Study protocol for an observational study. *BMJ Open*, *10*, e034031.

Breitborde, N. J. K., Lopez, S. R., & Kopelowicz, A. (2010). Expressed emotion and health outcomes among Mexican-Americans with schizophrenia and their caregiving relatives. *Journal of Nervous and Mental Disease*, *198*(2), 105–109.

Breitborde, N. J. K., & Moe, A. M. (2017). Early intervention in psychosis in the United States: From science to policy reform. *Policy Insights from the Brain and Behavioral Sciences*, *4*(1), 1–9.

Breitborde, N. J. K., & Moe, A. M. (2019). Optimizing mental health treatment for emerging adults with first-episode psychosis. *Evidence-Based Practice in Child and Adolescent Mental Health*, *4*(2), 157–169.

Cavelti, M., Thompson, K., Chanen, A., & Kaess, M. (2021). Psychotic symptoms in borderline personality disorder: Developmental aspects. *Current Opinion in Psychology*, *37*, 26–31.

Chandrasekhar, T., Copeland, J. N., Spanos, M., & Sikich, L. (2020). Autism, psychosis, or both? Unraveling complex patient presentations. *Child and Adolescent Psychiatric Clinics of North America*, *29*(1), 103–113.

Claxton, M., Onwumere, J., & Fornells-Ambrojo, M. (2017). Do family interventions improve outcomes in early psychosis? A systematic review and meta-analysis. *Frontiers in Psychology*, *8*, 371.

Cornblatt, B. A., Lencz, T., Smith, C. W., Olsen, R., Auther, A. M., Nakayama, E., … Correll, C. U. (2007). Can antidepressants be used to treat the schizophrenia prodrome? Results of a prospective, naturalistic treatment study of adolescents. *Journal of Clinical Psychiatry*, *68*(4), 546–557. https://doi.org/10.4088/jcp.v68n0410

Croft, J., Heron, J., Teufel, C., Cannon, M., Wolke, D., Thompson, A., … Zammit, S. (2019). Association of trauma type, age of exposure, and frequency in childhood and adolescence with psychotic experiences in early adulthood. *JAMA Psychiatry*, *76*(1), 79–86. https://doi.org/10.1001/jamapsychiatry.2018.3155

Davies, C., Segre, G., Estradé, A., Radua, J., De Micheli, A., Provenzani, U., … Fusar-Poli, P. (2020). Prenatal and perinatal risk and protective factors for psychosis: A systematic review and meta-analysis. *Lancet Psychiatry*, *7*(5), 399–410. https://doi.org/10.1016/S2215-0366(20)30057-2

Demjaha, A., Lappin, J., Stahl, D., Patel, M., MacCabe, J., Howes, O., … Lomas, B. (2017). Antipsychotic treatment resistance in first-episode psychosis: Prevalence, subtypes and predictors. *Psychological Medicine*, *47*(11), 1981–1989. https://doi.org/10.1017/S0033291717000435

Derks, E. M., Fleischhacker, W. W., Boter, H., Peuskens, J., Kahn, R. S., & Group, E. S. (2010). Antipsychotic drug treatment in first-episode psychosis: should patients be switched to a different antipsychotic drug after 2, 4, or 6 weeks of nonresponse? *Journal of Clinical Psychopharmacology, 30*(2), 176–180.

Devoe, D. J., Farris, M. S., Townes, P., & Addington, J. (2020). Interventions and transition in youth at risk of psychosis: A systematic review and meta-analyses. *Journal of Clinical Psychiatry, 81*(3), 17r12053.

Díaz-Caneja, C. M., Pina-Camacho, L., Rodríguez-Quiroga, A., Fraguas, D., Parellada, M., & Arango, C. (2015). Predictors of outcome in early-onset psychosis: A systematic review. *NPJ Schizophrenia, 1*(1), 1–10.

Driver, D. I., Thomas, S., Gogtay, N., & Rapoport, J. L. (2020). Childhood-onset schizophrenia and early-onset schizophrenia spectrum disorders: An update. *Child and Adolescent Psychiatric Clinics of North America, 29*(1), 71–90.

Emsley, R., Rabinowitz, J., & Medori, R. (2006). Time course for antipsychotic treatment response in first-episode schizophrenia. *American Journal of Psychiatry, 163*(4), 743–745.

Forsyth, J. K., & Asarnow, R. F. (2020). Genetics of childhood-onset schizophrenia 2019 update. *Child and Adolescent Psychiatric Clinics of North America, 29*(1), 157–170.

Freudenreich, O., Brown, H. E., & Holt, D. J. (2016). Psychosis and schizophrenia. In T. A. Stern, M. Fava, T. E. Wilens, & J. F. Rosenbaum (Eds.), *Massachusetts General Hospital comprehensive clinical psychiatry* (2nd ed., pp. 307–323). Elsevier.

Fusar-Poli, P., Bonoldi, I., Yung, A. R., Borgwardt, S., Kempton, M. J., Valmaggia, L., ... McGuire, P. (2012). Predicting psychosis: Meta-analysis of transition outcomes in individuals at high clinical risk. *Archives of General Psychiatry, 69*(3), 220–229. https://doi.org/10.1001/archgenpsychiatry.2011.1472

Fusar-Poli, P., Borgwardt, S., Bechdolf, A., Addington, J., Riecher-Rössler, A., Schultze-Lutter, F., ... Yung, A. (2013). The psychosis high-risk state: A comprehensive state-of-the-art (Review). *JAMA Psychiatry, 70*(1), 107–120. https://doi.org/10.1001/jamapsychiatry.2013.269

Fusar-Poli, P., Frascarelli, M., Valmaggia, L., Byrne, M., Stahl, D., Rocchetti, M., ... McGuire, P. (2015). Antidepressant, antipsychotic and psychological interventions in subjects at high clinical risk for psychosis: OASIS 6-year naturalistic study. *Psychological Medicine, 45*(6), 1327–1339. https://doi.org/10.1017/S003329171400244X

Fusar-Poli, P., Valmaggia, L., & McGuire, P. (2007). Can antidepressants prevent psychosis? *Lancet, 370*(9601), 1746–1748.

Glenthøj, L. B., Hjorthøj, C., Kristensen, T. D., Davidson, C. A., & Nordentoft, M. (2017). The effect of cognitive remediation in individuals at ultra-high risk for psychosis: A systematic review. *NPJ Schizophrenia, 3*(1), 1–8.

Gurillo, P., Jauhar, S., Murray, R. M., & MacCabe, J. H. (2015). Does tobacco use cause psychosis? Systematic review and meta-analysis. *Lancet Psychiatry, 2*(8), 718–725.

Harvey, P. D., & Isner, E. C. (2020). Cognition, social cognition, and functional capacity in early-onset schizophrenia. *Child and Adolescent Psychiatric Clinics, 29*(1), 171–182.

Healy, C., Brannigan, R., Dooley, N., Coughlan, H., Clarke, M., Kelleher, I., & Cannon, M. (2019). Childhood and adolescent psychotic experiences and risk of mental disorder: A systematic review and meta-analysis. *Psychological Medicine, 49*(10), 1589–1599.

Hjorthøj, C., Stürup, A. E., McGrath, J. J., & Nordentoft, M. (2017). Years of potential life lost and life expectancy in schizophrenia: A systematic review and meta-analysis. *Lancet Psychiatry, 4*(4), 295–301.

Hor, K., & Taylor, M. (2010). Suicide and schizophrenia: A systematic review of rates and risk factors. *Journal of Psychopharmacology, 24*(4), S81–S90.

Howes, O. D., & Kapur, S. (2009). The dopamine hypothesis of schizophrenia: version III—the final common pathway. *Schizophrenia Bulletin, 35*(3), 549–562.

Jongsma, H. E., Gayer-Anderson, C., Lasalvia, A., Quattrone, D., Mulè, A., Szöke, A., ... European Network of National Schizophrenia Networks Studying Gene-Environment Interactions Work Package 2 (EU-GEI WP2) Group. (2018). Treated Incidence of Psychotic Disorders in the Multinational EU-GEI Study. *JAMA Psychiatry, 75*(1), 36–46. https://doi.org/10.1001/jamapsychiatry.2017.3554

Kahn, R. S., Winter van Rossum, I., Leucht, S., McGuire, P., Lewis, S. W., Leboyer, M., ... OPTiMiSE Study Group. (2018). Amisulpride and olanzapine followed by open-label treatment with clozapine in first-episode schizophrenia and schizophreniform disorder (OPTiMiSE): A three-phase switching study. *Lancet Psychiatry, 5*(10), 797–807. https://doi.org/10.1016/S2215-0366(18)30252-9

Kane, J. M., Robinson, D. G., Schooler, N. R., Mueser, K. T., Penn, D. L., Rosenheck, R. A., Addington, J., Brunette, M. F., Correll, C. U., Estroff, S. E., Marcy, P., Robinson, J., Meyer-Kalos, P. S., Gottlieb, J. D., Glynn, S. M., Lynde, D. W., Pipes, R., Kurian, B. T., Miller, A. L., Heinssen, R. K. (2016). Comprehensive versus usual community care for first-episode psychosis: 2-year outcomes from the NIMH RAISE Early Treatment Program. *American Journal of Psychiatry, 173*(4), 362–372. https://doi.org/10.1176/appi.ajp.2015.15050632

Kelleher, I., Connor, D., Clarke, M. C., Devlin, N., Harley, M., & Cannon, M. (2012). Prevalence of psychotic symptoms in childhood and adolescence: A systematic review and meta-analysis of population-based studies. *Psychological Medicine, 42*(9), 1857–1863.

McEvoy, J. P., Lieberman, J. A., Stroup, T. S., Davis, S. M., Meltzer, H. Y., Rosenheck, R. A., ... CATIE Investigators. (2006). Effectiveness of clozapine versus olanzapine, quetiapine, and risperidone in patients with chronic schizophrenia who did not respond to prior atypical antipsychotic treatment. *American Journal of Psychiatry*, 163(4), 600–610. https://doi.org/10.1176/appi.ajp.163.4.600

McFarlane, W. R. (2002). *Multifamily groups in the treatment of severe psychiatric disorders*. Guilford.

McGlashan, T. H., Zipursky, R. B., Perkins, D., Addington, J., Miller, T., Woods, S. W., ... Breier, A. (2006). Randomized, double-blind trial of olanzapine versus placebo in patients prodromally symptomatic for psychosis. *American Journal of Psychiatry, 163*(5), 790–799. https://doi.org/10.1176/ajp.2006.163.5.790

McGorry, P. D., Yung, A. R., Phillips, L. J., Yuen, H. P., Francey, S., Cosgrave, E. M., ... Jackson, H. (2002). Randomized controlled trial of interventions designed to reduce the risk of progression to first-episode psychosis in a clinical sample with subthreshold symptoms. *Archives of General Psychiatry, 59*(10), 921–928. https://doi.org/10.1001/archpsyc.59.10.921

Miklowitz, D. J., O'Brien, M. P., Schlosser, D. A., Addington, J., Candan, K. A., Marshall, C., ... Cannon, T. D. (2014). Family-focused treatment for adolescents and young adults at high risk for psychosis: Results of a randomized trial. *Journal of the American Academy of Child and Adolescent Psychiatry, 53*(8), 848–858. https://doi.org/10.1016/j.jaac.2014.04.020

Miller, T. J., McGlashan, T. H., Rosen, J. L., Cadenhead, K., Cannon, T., Ventura, J., ... Woods, S. W. (2003). Prodromal assessment with the structured interview for prodromal syndromes and the scale of prodromal symptoms: predictive validity, interrater reliability, and training to reliability. *Schizophrenia Bulletin, 29*(4), 703–715. https://doi.org/10.1093/oxfordjournals.schbul.a007040

Murray, R. M., Bhavsar, V., Tripoli, G., & Howes, O. (2017). 30 years on: How the neurodevelopmental hypothesis of schizophrenia morphed into the developmental risk factor model of psychosis. *Schizophrenia Bulletin, 43*(6), 1190–1196.

Nelson, B., & McGorry, P. (2020). The prodrome of psychotic disorders: Identification, prediction, and preventive treatment. *Child and Adolescent Psychiatric Clinics of North America, 29*(1), 57–69.

O'Conghaile, A., & DeLisi, L. E. (2015). Distinguishing schizophrenia from posttraumatic stress disorder with psychosis. *Current Opinion in Psychiatry, 28*(3), 249–255.

Pagsberg, A. K., Tarp, S., Glintborg, D., Stenstrøm, A. D., Fink-Jensen, A., Correll, C. U., & Christensen, R. (2017). Acute antipsychotic treatment of children and adolescents with schizophrenia-spectrum disorders: A systematic review and network meta-analysis. *Journal of the American Academy of Child & Adolescent Psychiatry, 56*(3), 191–202.

Radhakrishnan, R., Kaser, M., & Guloksuz, S. (2017). The link between the immune system, environment, and psychosis. *Schizophrenia Bulletin, 43*(4), 693–697.

Saha, S., Chant, D., Welham, J., & McGrath, J. (2005). A systematic review of the prevalence of schizophrenia. *PLoS Medicine, 2*(5), e141.

Schneider, C., Corrigall, R., Hayes, D., Kyriakopoulos, M., & Frangou, S. (2014). Systematic review of the efficacy and tolerability of clozapine in the treatment of youth with early onset schizophrenia. *European Psychiatry, 29*(1), 1–10.

Selten, J.-P., van der Ven, E., & Termorshuizen, F. (2020). Migration and psychosis: A meta-analysis of incidence studies. *Psychological Medicine, 50*(2), 303–313.

Starzer, M. S. K., Nordentoft, M., & Hjorthøj, C. (2018). Rates and predictors of conversion to schizophrenia or bipolar disorder following substance-induced psychosis. *American Journal of Psychiatry, 175*(4), 343–350.

Stentebjerg-Olesen, M., Pagsberg, A. K., Fink-Jensen, A., Correll, C. U., & Jeppesen, P. (2016). Clinical characteristics and predictors of outcome of schizophrenia-spectrum psychosis in children and adolescents: A systematic review. *Journal of Child and Adolescent Psychopharmacology, 26*(5), 410–427.

Stroup, T. S., & Gray, N. (2018). Management of common adverse effects of antipsychotic medications. *World Psychiatry, 17*(3), 341–356.

Turner, D. T., van der Gaag, M., Karyotaki, E., & Cuijpers, P. (2014). Psychological interventions for psychosis: A meta-analysis of comparative outcome studies. *American Journal of Psychiatry, 171*(5), 523–538.

Tyson, J. W., House, E. M., & Donovan, A. L. (2020). Assessing youth with psychotic experiences: A phenomenological approach. *Child and Adolescent Psychiatric Clinics of North America, 29*(1), 1–13.

Üçok, A., Çikrikçili, U., Karabulut, S., Salaj, A., Öztürk, M., Tabak, Ö., & Durak, R. (2015). Delayed initiation of clozapine may be related to poor response in treatment-resistant schizophrenia. *International Clinical Psychopharmacology, 30*(5), 290–295.

Woods, S. W., Miller, T. J., & McGlashan, T. H. (2001). The "prodromal" patient: Both symptomatic and at-risk. *CNS Spectrums, 6*(3), 223–232.

Wright, A., Cather, C., Gilman, J., & Evins, A. E. (2020). The changing legal landscape of cannabis use and its role in youth-onset psychosis. *Child and Adolescent Psychiatric Clinics of North America, 29*(1), 145–156.

Wykes, T., Huddy, V., Cellard, C., McGurk, S. R., & Czobor, P. (2011). A meta-analysis of cognitive remediation for schizophrenia: Methodology and effect sizes. *American Journal of Psychiatry, 168*(5), 472–485.

53

Substance Use Disorders and Other Risk-Taking Behaviors in Youth

Kevin M. Simon, Marianne Pugatch, and John R. Knight

For additional material related to the content of this chapter, please see Chapters 9.

VIGNETTE

Cameron (who prefers Cam) is a 15-year-old high school sophomore with attention-deficit/hyperactivity disorder (ADHD)–combined type, whom you have treated since fourth grade with extended-release methylphenidate. He also received classroom accommodations and was doing well until about 6 months ago when his grades fell from A-B to C-D. Teachers' ratings on the National Institute for Children's Health Quality (NICHQ) Vanderbilt scales suggested Cam's ADHD symptoms were not well controlled, so you adjusted his medication. Today Cam's parents make an urgent care appointment because he came home last night "looking high." They say he has repeatedly stayed out late and slept over at friends' houses on short notice. He has become irritable and sullen during family dinners and more reclusive when home. His mother searched his room this morning and found a small plastic bag with what looked like a USB memory stick and cartridges that an Internet search indicated were vaping "pods." They ask you to perform a drug test to "see what the problem is."

INTRODUCTION

The use of substances (tobacco, alcohol, cannabis, and other drugs) among adolescents is one of our nation's most serious public health problems. Treatment of associated medical and psychosocial problems places a considerable burden on time and health care costs and inflicts considerable pain and suffering on individual users and their family members. Pediatric care providers can help adolescents avoid substance use and related harms through early identification and intervention.

ADOLESCENT DEVELOPMENT

Puberty refers to the physiologic changes that occur between late childhood and young adulthood, including rapid acceleration in linear growth, gametogenesis, and development of secondary sexual characteristics. Brain development, including the formation of critical pathways through pruning, myelination, and interconnectivity, continues through age 25, as does maturation of the prefrontal cortex, responsible for future planning, impulse control, and problem solving (Jordan & Andersen, 2017). Early exposures to drugs of abuse in susceptible individuals increase the risk of developing addictive disorders. Adolescence describes the accompanying psychosocial changes required to become an independent adult. To accomplish this, adolescents engage in behavioral strategies that include experimentation, risk taking, limit testing, and questioning of established rules and authority. While these strategies are often functional, they can lead to severe injury and illness when combined with substance use. In social relationships there is movement from predominant family influence (preconformist), to peer influence (conformist), to independent thinking (postconformist) (Daniels, Saracino, Fraley, Christian, & Pardo, 2018). Cognitively, the development of formal operations (age ≥12 years) leads to the ability to think abstractly (Dulit, 1972). This allows for propositional logic (i.e., forming hypotheses and considering possible solutions), which is essential for establishing therapeutic relationships and for counseling interventions such as cognitive-behavioral therapy.

SUBSTANCE USE

Epidemiology

According to the 2020 Monitoring the Future Study, 6 of 10 students began to drink by the end of high school, 2 of 5 students got drunk at least once, 2 of 5 tried an illicit drug, but less than 1 in 4 students tried an illicit drug other than marijuana. Rises in usage of specific drugs can be predicted by two factors: an increase in the perceived availability of the drug, and a decrease in the perceived risk of harm associated with use of the drug. Data show a significant rise over the past 5 years in e-cigarette (i.e., vaping) use of nicotine and marijuana pods. The 2020 data indicate that any illicit drug use has remained steady for the last decade, but use of prescription drugs (including narcotic analgesics, stimulants, and tranquilizers) has declined.

Tobacco

Tobacco use remains the leading cause of preventable death in the United States, and over 95% of adult smokers began during adolescence (Russell, McKeganey, Dickson, & Nides, 2018). Fortunately, prevalence has dropped at least fourfold since the mid-1990s and is at or near historic lows. However, recent years have seen a rapid rise in adolescent use of e-cigarettes, which deliver nicotine in high doses. From 2017 to 2019, past

12-month usage roughly doubled for 8th graders from 7.5% to 16.5%, for 10th graders from 15.8% to 30.7%, and for 12th graders from 18.8% to 35.3%. E-cigarettes are increasingly the initial form of exposure for adolescents to nicotine, and evidence is mounting that ever using an e-cigarette predicts future cigarette smoking (Chadi, Schroeder, Jensen, & Levy, 2019).

Alcohol

Alcohol use in 2019–2020 (12 months) leveled off from its historical gradual decline. In 2019 24.6% of 14- to 15-year-olds reported having at least one drink in the past 12 months (National Institute on Alcohol Abuse and Alcoholism [NIAAA], n.d.). Most concerning is the prevalence of heavy episodic drinking, defined as five or more drinks for boys and four or more drinks for girls in about 2 hours (White, Tapert, & Shukla, 2018). The prevalence of past-30-days heavy episodic drinking was 13.5% among high school students in 2019 (Redfield et al., 2020). While heavy episodic drinking is slightly more prevalent among boys than girls, in recent years girls have been catching up. Drinking alcohol is illegal for individuals under age 21 years, as is driving after drinking any alcohol. Despite this, in 2017, 24% of drivers aged 15 to 20 who were killed in fatal motor vehicle crashes had been drinking (National Highway Traffic Safety Administration, US Department of Transportation, 2017).

Cannabis

Cannabis sativa (tall, narrow-leaf varieties of cannabis) and *indica* (stout, broad-leaf plants), also known as marijuana, continue to be the most commonly used drug among US adolescents and the leading reason for entering substance use treatment (Johnson, 2018). In 2019 15.2% of 8th graders, 34% of 10th graders, and 43.7% of 12th graders had ever tried cannabis. During recent years most states have legalized marijuana for medical purposes, and a growing number have legalized it for adult recreational use. This has created widespread availability of edible products, concentrates, and vaping pods containing high levels of marijuana's primary psychoactive ingredient, delta-9-tetrahydrocannabinol (THC). In 2019 past-30-day prevalence of THC vaping was reported by 3.9% of 8th graders, 12.6% of 10th graders, and 14% of 12th graders (Miech, Patrick, O'Malley, Johnston, & Bachman, 2020). There is a significant increase in the odds of using cannabis among youth who have used e-cigarettes (Chadi et al., 2019).

Illicit Drugs

Illicit drugs are substances that either stimulate (e.g., cocaine, methamphetamine) or depress (e.g., heroin, benzodiazepines) the central nervous system or cause hallucinogenic effects (i.e., peyote, psilocybin, lysergic acid diethylamide) and whose use has been made illegal. In 2019 15% of high school students reported having ever used an illicit drug. Another class, volatile inhalants, are found in many common household products (e.g., solvents, glue, and aerosols) readily available to young people. This is the only class of substance with use highest among eighth graders, the youngest group surveyed; in 2019, 12.5% of eighth graders have tried some form of inhalant.

Prescription Drugs

The national survey also asks about the use of any prescription drug "without a doctor telling you to use them." Among high school seniors, lifetime misuse of amphetamines (e.g., dexamphetamine, mixed salt-amphetamine) is 7.3%, opioids (e.g., oxycodone, hydrocodone) is 2.4% and 1.2%, respectively, and tranquilizers (e.g., clonazepam) is 7%.

Substance Use Progression

Substance use during adolescence exists on a developmental spectrum ranging from abstinence to experimentation, recurrent use, problematic use, and mild, moderate, or severe substance use disorder (SUD) as defined by the *Diagnostic and Statistical Manual of Mental Disorders*, fifth edition (American Psychiatric Association, 2013) and categorized by each specific substance (Fig. 53.1).

Associated Problems

Evidence suggests 37% to 80% of adolescents with SUD have at least one other mental disorder (Heradstveit, Skogen, Hetland, Stewart, & Hysing, 2019). ADHD, mood and anxiety disorders, and psychosis significantly increase the risk of adolescent substance use (Gray & Squeglia, 2018). ADHD and SUD involve disinhibition, which suggests an underlying vulnerability shared by both disorders. Alternatively, features of ADHD, such as impulsivity, may increase the risk of initiating substance use. Children with ADHD are significantly more likely to try a range of substances during their lifetime compared with non-ADHD counterparts (Harstad et al., 2014). Adolescent substance use also increases the risk of school dropout, trauma exposure, suicidal behavior, high-risk sexual behaviors, and sexually transmitted infections (Wasserman & McReynolds, 2011; Yonek et al., 2019)

Prevention

Risk Factors

Genetic predictors of SUDs have been found in both twin and adoption studies (Meyers & Dick, 2010). However, this risk is compounded by age at first use. Those who engage in substance use during their preteen years are more likely to develop an SUD later in life compared to those who delay initial use until college. Having friends who use substances is an important determinant for initiation of substance use among adolescents (Ramirez, Hinman, Sterling, Weisner, & Campbell, 2012). However, peer influences do not predict the development of substance use problems or disorders. Family history of SUD and lack of parental involvement in the activities of their children increase risk (Acheson, Vincent, Cohoon, & Lovallo, 2018). Personality characteristics associated with substance use include low assertiveness, low self-esteem, low self-efficacy, low self-confidence, low social confidence, and external locus of control (Habersaat et al., 2018). Persons who engage in

<table>
<tr><th></th><th>DSM-5 Substance Use Disorder—Criteria</th><th></th></tr>
<tr><td>1.</td><td>[Substance] are often taken in larger amounts or over a longer period than was intended.</td><td rowspan="11">The essential features are the same for most of the categories. A problematic pattern of use leading to clinically significant impairment or distress, as manifested by at least two of the following, occurring within a 12-month period:
The presence of at least 2 of these symptoms indicates a [substance] use disorder (SUD). The severity of the SUD is defined as:
Mild:
The presence of 2–3 symptoms
Moderate:
The presence of 4–5 symptoms
Severe:
The presence of 6 symptoms</td></tr>
<tr><td>2.</td><td>There is a persistent desire or unsuccessful efforts to cut down or control [substance].</td></tr>
<tr><td>3.</td><td>A great deal of time is spent in activities necessary to obtain the [substance], use the [substance], or recover from its effects.</td></tr>
<tr><td>4.</td><td>Craving, or a strong desire or urge to use [substance].</td></tr>
<tr><td>5.</td><td>Recurrent [substance] use resulting in a failure to fulfill major role obligations at work, school, or home.</td></tr>
<tr><td>6.</td><td>Continued [substance] use despite having persistent or recurrent social or interpersonal problems caused or exacerbated by the effects of [substance].</td></tr>
<tr><td>7.</td><td>Important social, occupational, or recreational activities are given up or reduced because of [substance] use.</td></tr>
<tr><td>8.</td><td>Recurrent [substance] use in situations in which it is physically hazardous.</td></tr>
<tr><td>9.</td><td>Continued [substance] use despite knowledge of having a persistent or recurrent physical or psychological problem that is likely to have been caused or exacerbated by the substance.</td></tr>
<tr><td>10.</td><td>Tolerance, as defined by either of the following:
a. A need for markedly increased amounts of opioids to achieve intoxication or desired effect.
b. A markedly diminished effect with continued use of the same amount of an [substance].
Note: This criterion is not considered to be met for those taking opioids solely under appropriate medical supervision.</td></tr>
<tr><td>11.</td><td>Withdrawal, as manifest by either of the following:
a. The characteristic [substance] withdrawal syndrome (refer to criteria A and B of the criteria set for [substance] withdrawal).
b. [Substance] (or a closely related substance) are taken to relieve or avoid withdrawal symptoms.</td></tr>
</table>

Fig. 53.1 Substance use disorder criteria. (Adapted from American Psychiatric Association. [2013]. *Diagnostic and statistical manual of mental disorders* [*DSM-5*; 5th ed.]. Author.)

substance use tend to have lower religiosity (Miller, Davies, & Greenwald, 2000).

Social determinants of health (SDOH) contribute substantially to an individual's overall physical and mental health and can have a deleterious effect on health outcomes. SDOH disproportionally affect vulnerable populations, such those with SUD by influencing both substance use behaviors and the health consequences of use (Galea & Vlahov, 2002). To improve the health outcomes of adolescents with substance use, attempts to moderate SDOH should be prioritized (Compton, Gfroerer, Conway, & Finger, 2014).

Principles of Effective Prevention

Effective prevention programs include components that target the adolescent's family, school, and community, and include strategies to bolster protective factors and reduce risk factors. Increased parental supervision, high levels of parental support, absence of parental substance use, higher levels of parental involvement, and better family communication are protective for initiation of substance use (Allen et al., 2016). School-based programs may include the provision of psychoeducation regarding the effect of adolescent substance use on the developing brain, support the development of positive communication between parents/caregivers and adolescents, and help caregivers establish and enforce family rules against underage drinking with clear "no use" messages regarding drugs. For adolescents who have started to use substances, targeting and engaging families in prevention interventions have been shown to reduce negative behavioral symptoms (Connell, Dishion, Yasui, & Kavanagh, 2007).

Principles of Effective Parent Guidance

Pediatric primary care settings are often the first and only contact that adolescent patients have with the health care system and hold promise for prevention and treatment of addiction. Parent guidance visits are clinical encounters that offer support tailored to the age and development of the adolescent as well as biopsychosocial factors and family dynamics. Supporting the quality of relationship between the parent and teen is achieved through accessing the family's strengths, supporting parents in authoritative parenting, and improving communication (Kuppens & Ceulemans, 2019). For adolescents who are actively using substances, guidance includes supporting parents to establish clear boundaries that target teens' access to substances and substance-using peers (e.g., cash, credit cards, car, computer, cellphone). As the adolescent remains drug and alcohol free, parents may return privileges one at a time. Parents may also remove or limit access to alcohol in their home for at least a time. Another key aspect of all parent guidance, and family work, is geographic proximity of all treatment and support services. Because implementing principles of parent guidance can be challenging, requiring a tailored approach, compassionate and coordinated support of providers, paraprofessionals, and peers is essential.

SCREENING AND ASSESSMENT

The American Academy of Pediatrics and the American Academy of Child and Adolescent Psychiatry recommend annual screening of all adolescents for substance use. The most effective method of screening is a confidential history, taken without parents in the room. Adolescents should be told that "anything you tell me will be kept confidential unless I think there is a risk to your safety, or someone else's safety. Should that happen, I will let you know, and you and I together will figure out how to tell your parents."

You tell Cam's parents you would first like to talk with Cam in private. After explaining the ground rules of confidentiality, his parents leave the room. You ask Cam how things are going at school and home. "School is boring and stupid except for my friends. I hate homework. I don't care about grades. I'm not going to college. I want to get a job and earn money. My parents are annoying. I can't believe my Mom searched my room. She had no right! As soon as I've got enough money for my own place, I'm moving out."

Begin the interview with an initial inquiry about the adolescent's current life circumstances. Ask about school, home, and activities. Then move to questions about the use of legitimate substances (e.g., prescribed medications), those that are socially tolerated (e.g., tobacco, alcohol, cannabis) to those that are illegal (e.g., cocaine, heroin, lysergic acid diethylamide). With younger adolescents, first ask a question about use among school peers, then friends' use, and finally personal use. The interview style should be nonjudgmental, using open-ended questions and concentrating on what the effects have been of alcohol or drug use.

Screening Tools

The ideal screening tool is brief, easy to administer and score, sensitive and specific for identifying SUD and related problems, and can guide assessment and intervention when needed. Several brief screeners are designed specifically for adolescents, backed by empirical evidence and free of charge (Fig. 53.2).

CRAFFT

CRAFFT is a mnemonic acronym created from the first letters of key words in its six questions: car, relax, alone, forget, family, and trouble. Like all four screens, CRAFFT begins with three items asking for the number of days during the past 12 months of using (1) alcohol, (2) marijuana, (3) anything else "to get high" (drug, prescription medication, inhalant), and the CRAFFT-N has (4) nicotine products. If the responses to items 1 through 3 are all zero, they answer the "car" question only. If any days of use are reported on items 1 through 3, they answer six CRAFFT questions. Each "yes" answer receives 1 point, and a total score of 2 or more indicates high risk. CRAFFT is available as a self-report questionnaire or an interview, but most adolescents prefer questionnaires to interviews and will respond more honestly. For information and free download of all versions, visit www.crafft.org. See Cam's completed CRAFFT+N interview in Fig. 53.3.

NIAAA

The National Institute of Alcohol Abuse and Alcoholism measure is a two-question screen with different versions based on age group (elementary, middle, and high school age), designed to identify the level of risk for alcohol-related problems. The past-year frequency item (number of days of drinking) had the best performance in predicting any past-year alcohol use disorder in a large, nationally representative sample of adolescents aged 12 to 18 (Spirito et al., 2016). However, optimal cut points for number of drinking days were found to vary by age and gender, resulting in different thresholds for moderate and high risk across age-gender groups (NIAAA, 2015).

S2BI

The Screening-to-Brief Intervention (S2B1) tool has demonstrated high sensitivity and specificity for identifying substance use and SUD (Levy et al., 2014). The instrument begins by asking about frequency of use of tobacco, alcohol, and/or marijuana in the past year (never, once or twice, monthly, weekly or more). If the patient endorses past-year use of any of the three substances, then follow-up questions are posed about use of prescription drugs, illegal drugs, inhalants, and herbs or synthetic drugs. Adolescents who report "once or twice" in the past year are unlikely to have a SUD, those who report "monthly" are likely to meet criteria for a mild

Tool	Questions	Description	Cutoff	Psychometrics
CRAFFT 2.1	4–9	Asks past-12-month number of days of use of alcohol, marijuana, and other drugs, and asks about problems associated with use	2 yes responses on six CRAFFT items	Sensitivity: 0.91 Specificity: 0.93
NIAAA	2	Alcohol only: Screens for friends' use and for days of personal use in past 12 months in children and adolescents (9–18yo)	Age 15 or under: 1+ days in past 12 months Age 16–17: 6+ days in past 12 months Age 18+: 12+ days in past 12 months	Sensitivity: 0.89 Middle School Sensitivity: 0.88 High School Specificity: 0.91 Middle School Specificity: 0.81 High School
S2BI	3–7	Asks frequency of use in past year of tobacco, alcohol, marijuana, and other drugs	Monthly single past year frequency question from the S2BI was sensitive and specific for discriminating among 4 categories of substance use experience (no past-year use, use without a SUD, mild or moderate SUD, and severe SUD) for each substance.	Sensitivity: 1.00 Specificity: 0.94
BSTAD	6–36	Asks past-12-month days of tobacco, alcohol, marijuana or other substance use by person and their friends	Tobacco 6days Alcohol 2days Marijuana 2	Sensitivity: 0.95 Specificity: 0.97 Sensitivity: 0.96 Specificity: 0.85 Sensitivity: 0.80 Specificity: 0.93

Abbreviations: BSTAD, Brief Screening for Alcohol, Tobacco, and other Drugs; CRAFFT, Car, Relax, Alone, Friends/Family, Forget, Trouble; NIAA, National Institute of Alcohol Abuse and Alcoholism; S2BI, Screening to Brief Intervention.

Fig. 53.2

or moderate SUD, and those who report "weekly or more" a severe SUD (Subramaniam & Volkov, 2014).

BSTAD

The Brief Screener for Tobacco, Alcohol, and other Drugs (BSTAD) is a web-based and well-validated instrument for identifying substance use and substance use disorder (Kelly et al., 2014). BSTAD asks a single frequency question for past year use of each of the three substances most commonly used by adolescents: tobacco, alcohol, and marijuana (Teens Screening Tool, n.d.). The measure triages adolescents (ages 12–17) into three levels of risk for SUD based on their report of past year use: no reported use, lower risk, and higher risk. Consistent with the NIAAA instrument, for those aged 12 to 14, "friends" questions are asked first; if aged 15 to 17, "personal use" questions are asked first. Each risk level maps onto suggested clinical actions, summarized on the results screen.

The CRAFFT+N Interview

To be verbally administered by the clinician

Begin: *"I'm going to ask you a few questions that I ask all my patients. Please be honest. I will keep your answers confidential."*

Part A

During the PAST 12 MONTHS, on how many days did you:

1. Drink more than a few sips of beer, wine, or any drink containing **alcohol**? Say "0" if none. — **20** # of days
2. Use any **marijuana** (cannabis, weed, oil, wax, or hash by smoking, vaping, dabbing, or in edibles) or "**synthetic marijuana**" (like "K2," "Spice")? Say "0" if none. — **50** # of days
3. Use **anything else to get high** (like other illegal drugs, pills, prescription or over-the-counter medications, and things that you sniff, huff, vape, or inject)? Say "0" if none. — **0** # of days
4. Use a **vaping device* containing nicotine and/or flavors,** or use any **tobacco products†?** Say "0" if none. — **25** # of days
   **Such as e-cigs, mods, pod devices like JUUL, disposable vapes like Puff Bar, vape pens, or e-hookahs. †Cigarettes, cigars, cigarillos, hookahs, chewing tobacco, snuff, snus, dissolvables, or nicotine pouches.*

If the patient answered...

"0" for all questions in Part A	"1" or more for Q. 1, 2, or 3	"1" or more for Q. 4
↓	↓	↓
Ask 1st question only in Part B below, then STOP	Ask all 6 questions in Part B below	Ask all 10 questions in Part C on next page

Part B

		Circle one	
C	Have you ever ridden in a **CAR** driven by someone (including yourself) who was "high" or had been using alcohol or drugs?	No	**[Yes]**
R	Do you ever use alcohol or drugs to **RELAX**, feel better about yourself, or fit in?	No	**[Yes]**
A	Do you ever use alcohol or drugs while you are by yourself, or **ALONE**?	No	**[Yes]**
F	Do you ever **FORGET** things you did while using alcohol or drugs?	**[No]**	Yes
F	Do your **FAMILY** or **FRIENDS** ever tell you that you should cut down on your drinking or drug use?	No	**[Yes]**
T	Have you ever gotten into **TROUBLE** while you were using alcohol or drugs?	**[No]**	Yes

Two or more YES answers in Part B suggest a serious problemthatneedsfurther assessment. See Page 3 for further instructions. →

NOTICE TO CLINIC STAFF AND MEDICAL RECORDS:
The information on this page is protected by special federal confidentiality rules (42 CFR Part 2), which prohibit disclosure of this information unless authorized by specific written consent.

Fig. 53.3

Part C

"The following questions ask about your use of any ***vaping devices containing nicotine and/or flavors****, or use of any* ***tobacco products.****"*

	Circle one	
1. Have you ever tried to QUIT using, but couldn't?	Yes	No
2. Do you vape or use tobacco NOW because it is really hard to quit?	Yes	No
3. Have you ever felt like you were ADDICTED to vaping or tobacco?	Yes	No
4. Do you ever have strong CRAVINGS to vape or use tobacco?	Yes	No
5. Have you ever felt like you really NEEDED to vape or use tobacco?	Yes	No
6. Is it hard to keep from vaping or using tobacco in PLACES where you are not supposed to, like school?	Yes	No
7. When you HAVEN'T vaped or used tobacco in a while (or when you tried to stop using)…		
a. did you find it hard to CONCENTRATE because you couldn't vape or use tobacco?	Yes	No
b. did you feel more IRRITABLE because you couldn't vape or use tobacco?	Yes	No
c. did you feel a strong NEED or urge to vape or use tobacco?	Yes	No
d. did you feel NERVOUS, restless, or anxious because you couldn't vape or use tobacco?	Yes	No

One or more YES answers in Part C suggest a serious problem with nicotine that needs further assessment. See Page 3 for further instructions. ⟶

**References:*

Wheeler, K. C., Fletcher, K. E., Wellman, R. J., & DiFranza, J. R. (2004). Screening adolescents for nicotine dependence: the Hooked On Nicotine Checklist. *J Adolesc Health*, *35*(3), 225–230;

McKelvey, K., Baiocchi, M., & Halpern-Felsher, B. (2018). Adolescents' and young adults' use and perceptions of pod-based electronic cigarettes. *JAMA Netw Open*, *1*(6), e183535.

NOTICE TO CLINIC STAFF AND MEDICAL RECORDS:
The information on this page is protected by special federal confidentiality rules (42 CFR Part 2), which prohibit disclosure of this information unless authorized by specific written consent.

Fig. 53.3 cont'd

CRAFFT Score Interpretation

Probability of a *DSM-5* Substance Use Disorder by CRAFFT score*

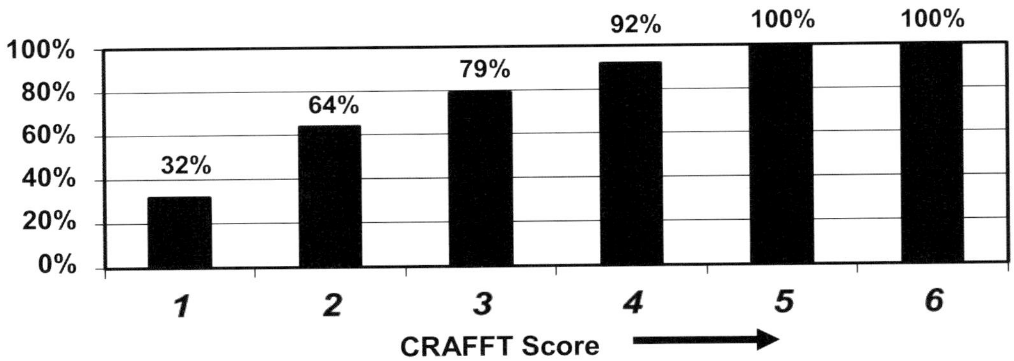

*Data source: Mitchell SG, Kelly SM, Gryczynski J, Myers CP, O'Grady KE, Kirk AS, & Schwartz RP. (2014). The CRAFFT cut-points and DSM-5 criteria for alcohol and other drugs: a reevaluation and reexamination. Substance Abuse, 35(4), 376–80.

Use the 5 R's talking points for brief counseling.

1. **REVIEW** screening results.
   For each "yes" response: *"Can you tell me more about that?"*

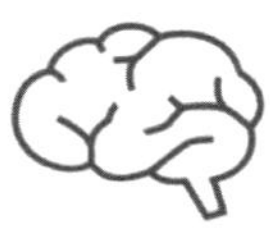

2. **RECOMMEND** not to use.
   "As your doctor (nurse/health care provider), my recommendation is not to use any alcohol, nicotine, marijuana or other drug because they can: 1) Harm your developing brain; 2) Interfere with learning and memory, and 3) Put you in embarrassing or dangerous situations."

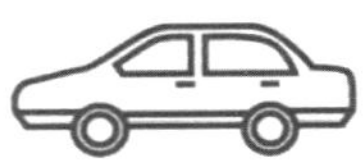

3. **RIDING/DRIVING** risk counseling.
   "Motor vehicle crashes are the leading cause of death for young people. I give all my patients the Contract for Life. Please take it home and discuss it with your parents/guardians to create a plan for safe rides home."

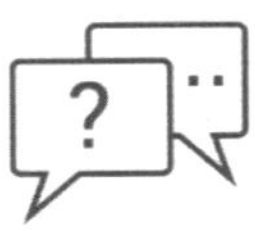

4. **RESPONSE** elicit self-motivational statements.
   Non-users: *"If someone asked you why you don't drink, vape, or use tobacco or drugs, what would you say?"* Users: *"What would be some of the benefits of not using?"*

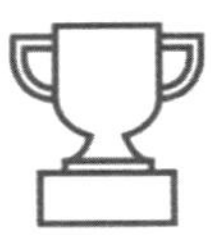

5. **REINFORCE** self-efficacy.
   "I believe you have what it takes to keep substance use from getting in the way of achieving your goals."

Give patient Contract for Life. Available at www.crafft.org/contract

---

crafft@childrens.harvard.edu www.crafft.org

For more information and versions in other languages, see www.crafft.org.

Fig. 53.3 cont'd

After assuring Cam that his responses will be confidential, you ask him the CRAFFT+N interview questions (see Fig. 53.3*). He reports multiple days of use for alcohol, marijuana (THC vaping), and tobacco (nicotine vaping). Reviewing parts A and B, his CRAFFT total score is 4, which correlates to a 92% risk for SUD; additionally, he answers "yes" to more than one answer in part C, which suggests a serious problem that needs further assessment. You review his positive responses beginning with the usage items by saying, "Can you tell me more about that?" He tells you that he began drinking at weekend parties about 6 months ago, usually two or three beers per occasion. He then tried vaping nicotine with a friend, thought it was "cool," and bought his own vaping pen. A week later, he tried vaping THC at a party, enjoyed it, and bought a few THC pods. "car": He does not yet have his license but rides home from parties with friends who have been drinking and vaping. "relax": Vaping helps "calm my mind" when stressed by school and makes playing videogames more fun. It helps him fit in at parties, especially talking with girls. "alone": He vapes at home once or twice a week but doesn't drink alone. "family": "They're the only reason I came today. I don't have a problem with weed. My parents are the problem." Currently he seldom vapes nicotine but keeps "a few pods around in case my parents get suspicious."*

Assessment

The assessment interview with the adolescent should include age at first use; current pattern of use (quantity and frequency); impact on physical and emotional health, school, and family; and negative consequence from use (e.g., accidents or injuries). A parent interview may be included as part of a substance use assessment, although parents typically underestimate the severity of use of their child (Curtis, Ashford, Rosenbach, Stern, & Kirby, 2019). Parents are good sources for their child's past medical and psychiatric history, hospitalizations and surgeries, and past or present symptoms of mood and anxiety disorders, trauma, suicidal ideation and attempts, social, developmental and educational history, and the family's medical and psychiatric history.

A physical examination should include a full set of vital signs and mental status exam. When performing the eye examination, note pupil size. Nasal mucosa should be examined for inflammation or erosion characteristic of drug insufflation (snorting). Liver and spleen should be palpated. A skin examination may reveal needle marks, although this finding is quite uncommon in adolescents. Abnormal breath sounds (e.g., wheezing) may be found in patients who are smoking/vaping tobacco, cannabis, cocaine, or heroin.

In regard to laboratory testing, avoid performing drug tests at the request of parents or legal authorities. First, explain the potential risks, benefits, and limitations of testing to the patient and their parents. Most adolescents use drugs sporadically, making laboratory testing unreliable for purposes of screening. Serum half-lives of most substance are brief, so urine testing reflects drug use only within the last 24 to 48 hours. A notable exception is THC; its carboxylic acid metabolite may be detected in the urine for several weeks after discontinuation of daily use (Hadland & Levy, 2016). Therefore when drug testing for THC is being done as part of a monitoring plan, serial urine specimens must include quantitative THC and creatinine determinations. Abstinence is supported by a finding of successive decrease in the THC:creatinine ratio over time. By contrast, alcohol has a very brief window of detection in urine. One of its metabolites, ethyl glucuronide, may be detected in urine for 3 to 5 days following an episode of drinking; however, low levels can also be produced after exposure to ethanol-based handwash and metered-dose inhalers that use ethanol as a propellant. Laboratory toxicologists and certified medical review officers are good sources of information before ordering any laboratory testing. Urine specimens must be collected by direct observation or according to the mandatory guidelines for federal drug testing programs (https://www.transportation.gov/sites/dot.gov/files/docs/Urine_Specimen_Collection_Guidelines_July3_2014_A.pdf). Urine specific gravity and creatinine levels should always be measured because urine concentration directly affects the validity of the test. Urine testing is a two-tiered procedure that begins with a rapid radioimmunoassay screen for a limited number of commonly used drugs (THC, heroin, cocaine, amphetamine, and barbiturates). Testing for synthetic opioids such as oxycodone or hydrocodone may require a specific order. Any positive screen result must be confirmed by gas chromatography and mass spectrometry before reporting to the adolescent or family members that a test is positive.

Cam does not want to have a urine drug test and says he will not cooperate with donating a sample today under any conditions.

INTERVENTIONS

Tobacco/Nicotine Dependence

Nicotine replacement therapy is an agonist-based harm reduction approach, which may be the treatment of choice for tobacco use disorder (Hammond & Gray, 2016). Results of the few controlled trials of smoking cessation pharmacotherapies in adolescents suggest that nicotine transdermal patches offer at least short-term benefits. Other psychopharmacologic agents may be considered, specifically bupropion SR and varenicline. However, both come with a US Food and Drug Administration (FDA) label warning of potential adverse psychiatric side effects, including increase in suicidal ideation. Analyses of controlled trials and large-scale observational studies in adults do not confirm causal associations between these medications and serious psychiatric adverse events, but cautious and careful monitoring are warranted, especially when prescribing for adolescents.

1.	Adolescent substance use needs to be identified and addressed as soon as possible.
2.	Adolescents can benefit from a drug abuse intervention even if they are not addicted to a drug.
3.	Routine annual medical visits are an opportunity to ask adolescents about drug use.
4.	Legal interventions and sanctions or family pressure may play a role in getting adolescents to enter, stay in, and complete treatment.
5.	Substance use disorder treatment should be tailored to the unique needs of the adolescent.
6.	Treatment should address the needs of the whole person rather than just focusing on his or her drug use.
7.	Behavioral therapies are effective in addressing adolescent drug use.
8.	Families and the community are important aspects of treatment.
9.	Effectively treating substance use disorders in adolescents requires also identifying and treating any other mental health conditions they may have.
10.	Sensitive issues such as violence and child abuse or risk of suicide should be identified and addressed.
11.	It is important to monitoring drug use during treatment.
12.	Staying in treatment for an adequate period of time and continuity of care afterward are important.
13.	Testing adolescents for sexually transmitted diseases like HIV, as well as hepatitis B and C, is an important part of drug treatment.

Fig. 53.4

Substance Use Disorder Treatment

Research and best practices indicate that SUD treatment plans for adolescents should include (1) motivation and engagement; (2) family involvement to improve supervision, monitoring, and communication between parents and children; (3) improved problem-solving skills, social skills, and relapse prevention; (4) simultaneous treatment of comorbid psychiatric disorders through psychosocial therapies and/or medication(s); (5) interventions that increase prosocial behaviors, peer relationships, and academic functioning; and (6) adequate duration of treatment, including provision of follow-up care following acute treatment (National Institute on Drug Abuse, n.d.). Self-help support groups can be encouraged as adjuncts to these modalities (Fig. 53.4).

The treatment of adolescents with SUD can take place in school-based groups offering targeted interventions or more sustained outpatient care (e.g., "Sober Schools"), intensive outpatient interventions such as partial hospitalization programs, and residential treatment of variable duration. Factors affecting the level of care include the following: (1) the need to provide a safe substance-free environment and the ability of the adolescent to care for oneself; (2) motivation and willingness of the adolescent and family to engage in treatment, including close geographic proximity; (3) the least restrictive environment that can accommodate the adolescent's current need for structure, limit setting, and safety; (4) the existence of cooccurring medical or psychiatric conditions that require availability of high-level professional staff; (5) the availability of treatment settings caring only for adolescents or where they are separated from adult treatment; (6) the adolescent and family preference for a particular setting; and (7) treatment failure in a less restrictive setting or level of care. Many parents' initial question to pediatric clinicians is, "What's the best program for our child?" This may reflect a desire for the so-called geographic cure. They may have heard about programs in other states, including wilderness settings and boot camps that helped another child. However, such programs may or may not be licensed or inspected, have staff with any formal training or certification, have high costs that insurance does not cover, preclude family involvement in treatment until a predischarge "family weekend," and lack any evidence of effectiveness other than testimonials.

Brief Interventions

Motivational interviewing (MI) (Miller & Rollnick, 2012) is a nonjudgmental, supportive, and nonconfrontational conversation style (D'Amico et al., 2018) often integrated throughout standardized cognitive-behavioral therapy in substance use treatment. MI can also be used as an effective brief single-session, stand-alone intervention for adolescents who present or screen positive for problematic substance use or substance-related medical problems in medical office-based or hospital settings (Neighbors, Barnett, Rohsenow, Colby, & Monti, 2010). While a full discussion goes beyond the scope of this chapter, its key strategies are embodied in the DARES acronym: develop a discrepancy between current behavior and important goals or values, avoid arguing, roll with resistance, empathy as a counseling style, and support self-efficacy.

You use the CRAFFT guide (see Fig. 53.3) for a brief therapeutic intervention. You elect not to show Cam the CRAFFT score graphic because feedback to those at high risk can lead to arguing. Instead, you say, "As your doctor, I am concerned about the effects of THC on your developing brain, its interference with learning and memory, and that it can put you at risk from unsafe car rides. You told me that it relaxes you, makes it easier to talk with girls, and makes videogames more fun. But what about the cost? How much do you spend each week? Far more important: your grades have fallen, you've given up on attending college, and your parents are really upset with you." You ask whether he has enough control to stop for a few weeks—if he wanted to. He replies tentatively, "Of course, I could." Then you ask, "What would be some of the benefits of not using?" He thinks for a while, then replies, "It'd get my parents off my back. I guess I could save a little money to buy something else." "Sounds great," you reply, "let's tell your parents you've decided to stop for now and follow up with me in a couple of weeks. Stopping may be hard, but I think you have what it takes to do it. One longer-term benefit to keep in mind," you add with a smile, "is that once you get your license, they'll trust you enough to drive their car."

Treatment Options

Adolescents who are not willing or able to engage in a brief intervention should be referred either to an allied mental health professional (e.g., social worker, psychologist, or other counselor) or to an adolescent substance abuse treatment program for further support. Pediatric clinicians need to learn about treatment resources in their own community and establish referral patterns to specific programs or professionals who provide adolescent SUD treatment.

Psychosocial/Behavioral Interventions

These are considered first-line treatment for adolescents with SUD. Both group and individual cognitive-behavioral therapy have been shown to be efficacious for the treatment of SUD and associated problems in adolescents (Hendriks, van der Schee, & Blanken, 2011; Macgowan & Engle, 2010). Evidence-based family therapies include multidimensional family therapy (Rigter et al., 2013), functional family therapy (Waldron & Turner, 2008), brief strategic family therapy (Henderson, Dakof, Greenbaum, & Liddle, 2010), and adolescent community reinforcement approach (Robbins et al., 2011). These interventions focus on improving (1) adolescent functioning in family and social contexts, (2) parental monitoring skills and functioning in other adult roles, (3) communication between family and social systems (e.g., schools), and (4) improving adolescents' coping, communication, decision-making skills, and problem-solving skills to avoid drug use.

Medical/Psychiatric Interventions

In general, treatment programs fall into one of the following categories: detoxification, residential treatment, and outpatient treatment, which are potentially combined with psychopharmacologic management.

Detoxification

Detoxification programs are relatively short-term inpatient programs, whose goal is the medical management of physiologic withdrawal symptoms. Traditionally these programs have concentrated on alcohol use disorders because withdrawal symptoms can be life threatening. Detoxification is also appropriate to safely stabilize withdrawal from opioids, heroin, barbiturates, and sedatives. Most adolescents do not require detoxification because physiologic dependence is relatively uncommon. When it is necessary, detoxification should be viewed as a first step in treatment and always followed by long-term counseling and support.

Medication-Assisted Treatment

Four medications that target the mu-opioid receptor have been approved by the FDA for the treatment of opioid use disorders (OUD) in adults: methadone (full agonist), buprenorphine (partial agonist), buprenorphine/naloxone combination (a nonorally available antagonist added to reduce abuse potential), and naltrexone (antagonist) (Hammond & Gray, 2016). Options for adolescents with OUD are more limited (e.g., methadone maintenance is unavailable to patients <18 years of age), and fewer controlled studies have been conducted in this age group. Early research and our own clinical experience support induction and maintenance therapy with buprenorphine for adolescents with OUD for 6 to 12 months or until a substantial period of monitored, stable sobriety is achieved. While buprenorphine maintenance for adults is recommended for life, too little is known about the impact of long-term maintenance on adolescents' neurodevelopment (Hagman, 1994). Medication-assisted treatment may be most effective when combined with outpatient counseling, group therapy, educational and vocational assistance, and psychosocial support (Pugatch, Knight, Mcguiness, Sherritt, & Levy, 2014; Woody & Fishman, 2020).

Acute Residential Treatment

Acute residential treatment may be available through a general psychiatric program for children and adolescents.

Treatment for SUD may be included on a limited basis, but this option is safer than placing adolescents in adult addiction-treatment programs where they are exposed to behaviors associated with high-severity chronic use and can be targeted by older patients.

Long-Term Residential Treatment

Long-term residential treatment includes highly structured programs lasting 30 to 90 days, but some last up to 12 months that may be based on self-help or 12-step principles, often staffed by persons in recovery and designed to remove the adolescent with SUD from the toxic environment. These programs are best reserved for those adolescents for whom outpatient treatment has failed or who have a high degree of antisocial behaviors associated with their substance use.

Outpatient Treatment

Most adolescents receive SUD treatment as outpatients in settings that range from hospital-based day treatment to varying combinations of individual counseling, family therapy, group therapy, cognitive-behavioral therapy, in person or via telehealth (Molfenter, Brown, O'neill, Kopetsky, & Toy, 2018), and monitoring through random urine drug testing. Referral to 12-step support groups, such as Alcoholics Anonymous or Narcotics Anonymous, may also be useful. Twelve-step groups are developmentally challenging for adolescents and will often not work without an interested recovering person who acts as initial liaison or "temporary sponsor." Participation in 12-step fellowships is associated with improved abstinence after treatment (Kelly, Dow, Yeterian, & Kahler, 2010).

Pediatric Clinicians

Pediatric clinicians can provide important support to adolescents in treatment by scheduling follow-up visits at regular intervals. "So tell me, have you joined an AA group? Have you found a sponsor yet? Which of the 12 steps are you working on now?" Never hesitate to tell recovering adolescents how proud you are of them. The process of recovery is difficult and poses special challenges for teens (e.g., need to change friends, accepting of their "chronic" disease).

Family

Family members should be encouraged to participate in treatment with the child. They may benefit from individual counseling and participation in 12-step fellowships such as Al-Anon. Parents should not become overly restrictive; they must be encouraged to adopt a firm, yet reasonable position with their child. In the most severe cases parents may need the support of the clinician in taking a very difficult stance (e.g., informing a teenager who continues to use that he or she must either go into treatment or find another place to live) in order to protect other children or themselves. On occasion, clinicians will encounter parents who are either unwilling or unable to assist in treatment. For example, they may refuse to eliminate alcohol or other drugs from the house, or because they have a substance use problem of their own.

ADHD, Psychostimulants, and Substance Use

Misuse, including overuse and nonprescribed use of stimulant medications intended for the treatment of ADHD, has increased markedly in recent years (Bavarian, Flay, Ketcham, & Smit, 2015). Amphetamine or methylphenidate derivate-based stimulants in tablet form can be ground up and then self-administered by nasal insufflation ("snorting") or dissolved and injected. Like cocaine, this can potentially lead to sudden cardiac arrhythmia and death. Children with ADHD are at increased risk for developing a SUD during adolescence and as adults (Chang et al., 2014). However, appropriate treatment with stimulant medications appears to be protective (McCabe, Dickinson, West, & Wilens, 2016). Because there is significant cooccurrence of ADHD and substance use, patients with ADHD will benefit from regular anticipatory guidance and substance use screening. Because prescription diversion is a risk, parents or other responsible adults should be counseled to provide supervision of medication storage and administration when treating high-risk youth (Mcguier et al., 2020).

You meet with Cam and his parents and tell them you see no reason for a drug test today. "Cam and I had an open and honest discussion about his vaping. He's decided to stop at least for now, so that we can all be assured that he hasn't lost control and needs a higher level of care. We'll schedule another visit in 2 to 3 weeks to discuss how this is working. In the meantime, I'd like you to see our social worker for a more complete assessment and to begin family counseling." You then hand Cam and his parents the Contract for Life. "This is a document developed by Students Against Destructive Decisions. Teens agree not to drive after using a substance or accept a ride from someone who has. Instead, they agree to call their parents for a safe ride home. Parents agree to provide safe and sober transportation home and postpone any discussion until the next day when it can be done calmly. Please take this home, discuss it, and let me know if you have any questions." You also recommend that Cam continue his stimulant medication, but that his parents oversee storage and monitoring of the prescription bottle.

Intoxication and Withdrawal

Adolescent patients may present with symptoms of acute or pathologic intoxication, and less commonly with acute withdrawal. Fig. 53.5 lists the signs, symptoms, and treatment options for common substance of use.

PARENTS/CAREGIVERS WHO USE ALCOHOL AND OTHER SUBSTANCES

There are an estimated 8.5 million children and adolescents in the United States who have a parent with SUD, or one of every eight children, and one of every two children is exposed to alcohol abuse or dependence in the family (Fewell Huff, 2020). Children of alcoholics are at risk for being born with

A. Alcohol

Names/Preparations	Intoxication		Withdrawal	
	Signs and Symptoms	Treatment	Signs and Symptoms	Treatment
Beer Wine Hard liquor	**Mild-Mod:** ↓ level of consciousness, poor coordination, ataxia, nystagmus, conjunctival injection, slurred speech, orthostatic hypotension	Observation and supportive care, protect airway, position on side to avoid aspiration	**Mild-Mod:** restlessness, agitation, coarse tremor, ↑ sensitivity to sensory input, nausea, vomiting, anorexia, autonomic hyperactivity (tachycardia, hypertension, hyperthermia), anxiety/depression, headache, insomnia	Thiamine 100 mg PO or IM daily, folate 1 mg PO daily, multivitamins 1 daily Benzodiazepine taper over 3-7 days (chlordiazepoxide 25-50 mg q6h ¥ 24 hrs., then 25 mg q6h ¥ 48 hrs.; or diazepam, clonazepam, oxazepam)
	Severe: Sluggish pupillary response, respiratory depression, stupor, coma, death (Chronic: pancreatitis, cirrhosis, but rare in adolescents.)	Ventilatory support, intensive care	**Severe:** seizures, hallucinations, delirium, death	**Seizures:** benzodiazepines (lorazepam 0.1-0.2 mg/kg/dose IV or PR, repeat 0.05 mg/kg q5 minutes if needed; usual max. dose = 4 mg but larger doses may be needed) **Hallucinations:** haloperidol
	Pathological: belligerent, excited, combative, psychotic state (even after small amount in susceptible person)	Physical restraint, low dose benzodiazepine (lorazepam 1-5 mg PO as needed), or haloperidol 1-5 mg q4-8 hrs. IM or 1-15 mg/dose PO		

B. Cannabis

Names/Preparations	Intoxication		Withdrawal	
	Signs and Symptoms	Treatment	Signs and Symptoms	Treatment
Marijuana, *Pot, herb, grass, weed, dope, sinsemilla, Thai sticks* THC edibles, pods for vaping Hashish Hashish oil	**Acute:** euphoria, sensory stimulation, pupillary constriction, conjunctival injection, photophobia, nystagmus, diplopia, ↑ appetite, autonomic dysfunction (tachycardia, hypertension, orthostatic hypotension) temporary bronchodilatation	Reassurance and observation.		
	Chronic: decreased learning, memory, gynecomastia, weight gain, lethargy, amotivational syndrome	Discontinuation of use, symptomatic treatment/care (bronchodilators for wheezing)	**Chronic users**: mild irritability, agitation, insomnia, EEG changes	Reassurance, symptoms disappear in 3-4 days
	Pathological: panic, delirium, psychosis, risk of violence, suicide	**Psychosis:** neuroleptic medication		

C. Hallucinogens

Names/Preparations	Intoxication		Withdrawal	
	Signs and Symptoms	Treatment	Signs and Symptoms	Treatment
Phencyclidine (PCP), *angel dust, super grass, peace weed* Ketamine, *Special K* Lysergic acid diethylamide (LSD), *acid, blotters, sunshine, microdots* Mescaline, *mesc* Peyote, *buttons, cactus* Psilocybin, *magic mushrooms, shrooms* Jimson weed, *locoweed* Nightshade	**Acute:** perceptual (visual, auditory) distortion and hallucinations, nystagmus, feelings of depersonalization, nausea, tremors, tachycardia, hypertension, hyperreflexia	Reassurance and observation. (For anticholinergics, i.e., Jimson weed, nightshade, symptoms are more severe and may require gastric lavage, benzodiazepine sedation and hospitalization.)	Psychological	Reassurance
	Chronic: flashbacks	Discontinuation of use		
	Pathological: panic, paranoia, psychosis	**Psychosis:** close observation in a quiet room Benzodiazepines (lorazepam 1-5 mg PO). Use of neuroleptic medication is controversial		

D. Inhalants

Names/Preparations	Intoxication		Withdrawal	
	Signs and Symptoms	Treatment	Signs and Symptoms	Treatment
Nitrous oxide, *laughing gas, whippets* Amyl Nitrite, *poppers, snappers* Butyl Nitrate, *rush, bullet, climax* Chlorohydrocarbons, *aerosol spray cans* Hydrocarbons, *gasoline, glue, solvents, White-out (typewriter correction fluid)*	**Acute:** euphoria, disorientation, sedation, loss of consciousness and traumatic injury, conjunctival injection, damage to CNS, liver, kidneys **Nitrates:** sudden hypoxemia, hypotension	Symptomatic medical management	Psychological Physiological - unknown	Reassurance, support
	Chronic: peripheral nerve, CNS, liver, & kidney damage Leaded Gasoline (not in US): plumbism	Discontinuation of use, supportive therapies (dialysis, etc.) **Plumbism:** chelation therapy		
	Pathological: cardiac arrhythmia and arrest	Resuscitation, hospitalization		

Fig. 53.5

E. Stimulants

Names/Preparations	Acute Intoxication		Withdrawal	
	Signs and Symptoms	**Treatment**	**Signs and Symptoms**	**Treatment**
Cocaine, *coke, snow, flake, blow, nose candy* Crack, *freebase, rocks* Amphetamines, *speed, black beauties* Methamphetamine, *crank, crystal meth, ice* Methylphenidate, *ritalin* "Legal speed," *OTC diet or stay awake pills*	**Acute:** exhilaration, euphoria, restlessness, irritability, insomnia, pupillary dilatation, tachycardia, arrhythmia, chest pain, hypertension, anorexia, hyperpyrexia, hyperreflexia	Reassurance and observation Symptomatic care **Agitation:** high dose benzodiazepines (Diazepam 10-25 mg.) Tachycardia, HTN: (controversial, see below) **Hyperthermia:** external cooling		
	Chronic: ("snorting": inflamed nasal mucosa, septal erosion or perforation), confusion, sensory hallucinations, paranoia, depression	Discontinuation of use, symptomatic treatment/care. Psychosis: neuroleptic medication	**Chronic users:** severe depression with suicidal/homicidal ideation, exhaustion, prolonged sleep, voracious appetite	Close observation, reassurance, symptoms disappear in 3-4 days
	Pathological: sudden cardiac arrest, hypertensive crisis, seizures	Resuscitation, hospitalization HTN crisis: beta-blockers, phentolamine, nitroprusside Seizures: IV diazepam, (see alcohol section above), or phenytoin 15-20 mg/kg slow IV push with cardiac monitor		

Miscellaneous Information: While use of cocaine and crack has declined somewhat in recent years, amphetamines have become more popular. Methamphetamine is more commonly available in California, the West and Southwest. With the increased public awareness of ADHD and the popularity of stimulant medications to treat it, methylphenidate has become a drug of abuse among some adolescents. It can be ground up and "snorted" and has been implicated in reports of sudden cardiac arrest and death. So-called "legal speed", OTC preparations which are available in pharmacies and through mail order houses, can cause toxicity similar to more potent stimulants when taken in high doses. Kratom is legal in many states and sold in health and convenience stores.

F. Depressants

Names/Preparations	Intoxication		Withdrawal	
	Signs and Symptoms	**Treatment**	**Signs and Symptoms**	**Treatment**
Benzodiazepines, *valium, "V's", librium, serax, klonopin, tranxene, xanax, halcion, rohypnol, "Ruffies"*	**Mild-Mod:** CNS sedation, pupillary constriction, disorientation, slurred speech, staggering gait	Observation and supportive care, protect airway, position on side to avoid aspiration	**Mild-Mod**: restlessness, anxiety, agitation, tremor, abdominal cramps, nausea, vomiting, hyperreflexia, hypertension, headache, insomnia	Gradual reduction of the drug of dependency, or phenobarbital substitution (calculate phenobarbital equivalent of daily dose, or give 3-4 mg/kg/day ÷ q8h) with gradual taper. Or change short-acting benzodiazepine to longer-acting benzodiazepine and then taper
Barbiturates, *nembutal, seconal, amytal, tuinal, downers, barbs, blue devils, red devils, yellows, yellow jackets*	**Severe:** respiratory depression, hypothermia, coma, death	**Acute OD:** gastric lavage. Supportive: ventilator, warming blanket, ICU care	**Severe:** seizures, delirium, hyperpyrexia, hallucinations, death.	Seizures: diazepam Hallucinations: haloperidol (see alcohol section above for doses)
Methaqualone, *quaaludes, ludes, sopors*	**Pathological:** paradoxical disinhibition, hyperexcitability	Symptoms pass in a matter of hours. Physical restraint, low dose benzodiazepine rarely needed		

Miscellaneous Information: These compounds are all similar to alcohol in effect and highly addictive. Withdrawal symptoms are severe, and may begin 12-16 hours after last dose, or may be delayed for up to a week.

G. Narcotics

Names/Preparations	Intoxication		Withdrawal	
	Signs and Symptoms	**Treatment**	**Signs and Symptoms**	**Treatment**
Heroin, *smack, horse, junk, brown sugar, Big H, mud* Opium Rx narcotics *Morphine, meperidine fentanyl, oxycodone, hydrocodone, codeine darvon, etc.*	**Acute:** euphoria, pupillary constriction, depression of respirations and gag reflex, bradycardia, hypotension, constipation	Airway protection, naloxone with careful monitoring (See Misc. Information below.)		**Acute medical management:** Methadone (PO) 0.7 mg/kg/day ÷ q4-6 hrs. with slow taper. Buprenorphine (SL) 2 mg. q1-2 hrs. until symptoms abate, then 8-16 mg. QAM or BID Clonidine (PO) 5-7 mcg/kg/day ÷ q6-12 hrs. (max = 0.9 mg/day)
	Chronic: complications of IV use include Hepatitis B, HIV/AIDS, SBE, brain abscesses	Discontinuation of use, targeted medical care for infectious complications	**Chronic users:** restlessness, lacrimation, yawning, pupillary dilatation, rhinorrhea, sniffing, sneezing, sweating, flushing, tachycardia, hypertension, muscle cramps, abdominal cramps, nausea, vomiting, diarrhea	
	Pathological: acute OD may cause respiratory arrest and death	Intubation and ventilation, naloxone (IV, IM, SC, ETT): children <20 kg: 0.1 mg/kg/dose q2-3 hrs. children >20 kg: 2-5 mg/dose		**Long-term treatment:** medication-assisted Treatment with either methadone (specialized clinics only) or buprenorphine. Naltrexone may also be considered

Miscellaneous Information: Individuals who abuse narcotics seldom seek treatment for intoxication. They are more often found semi-comatose and brought to the hospital by friends or the EMS. When treating an overdose, remember that naloxone has a shorter duration of action than most narcotic drugs, and doses therefore need to be repeated at fairly frequent intervals. These patients may require lengthy (12-24 hrs.) periods of observation in hospital.

Acknowledgment: Michael Shannon MD MPH (Toxicology Program) & Brigid Vaughan MD (Department of Psychiatry) at Children's Hospital, Boston assisted with preparation of this table.

Fig. 53.5 cont'd

serious medical problems, including fetal alcohol spectrum disorder (Ross, Graham, Money, & Stanwood, 2015). Having an alcoholic parent is associated with higher health care costs, decreased appetite, gastrointestinal distress, musculoskeletal complaints, vascular and migraine headaches, chronic fatigue, and sleep disturbance. Witnessing parents drink is associated with higher odds of adolescents' use of alcohol and heavy drinking (Cox, Janssen, Lopez-Vergara, Barnett, & Jackson, 2018). Having a parent with SUD is also associated with mood and anxiety disorders, including posttraumatic stress disorder (Smith & Wilson, 2016), language-based learning difficulties, poor attention, school suspensions, truancy, absenteeism, and grade retention; yet they have fewer educational services than other children with special needs (Smith & Wilson, 2016). In addition, children of parents with some drug use disorders may be passively exposed to smoked drugs and chemicals used to manufacture drugs, accidental ingestions, and chaos within the home from illegal activity surrounding the acquisition, sale, and use of illicit substances. Having a parent with SUD may adversely affect a child's self-esteem and self-efficacy. Avoid labeling them and always mention their relative strengths, resilience, and supports within the home and at school.

Pediatric clinicians have an opportunity to ask about parental/caregiver use of alcohol and drugs with the use of the AUDIT and DAST screening tools (Frank et al., 2008; Ghitza et al., 2013). If the clinician is intimately involved with the family and has knowledge of family history and current family functioning, then a brief screener such as the AUDIT-C may be sufficient (Wilson et al., 2008). However, if the clinician is not aware of genetic history, family strengths, and problems, then the full version of screening tools is recommended; they include questions about psychosocial functioning that can help facilitate a referral to the parent's own doctor or another evaluation resource while maintaining the therapeutic alliance. Parents with lower odds of hazardous drinking were more likely to enforce rules regarding adolescents' drinking, delivered more frequent messaging about the risks of drinking, and were more likely to apply negative consequences for adolescent drinking behavior (Cox et al., 2018). For those parents who continue unhealthy drug or alcohol use or lose custody, an interdisciplinary team can work together across specialties to support the child, maintain safe contact with the parent(s), and offer them emotional support and resources. Family-based interventions that include skills training in alcohol-specific parenting practices and reducing parental alcohol use at home are recommended (Cox et al., 2018). Because health care providers are mandated reporters, understanding state-specific requirements and how to file a report with child protective services is key (Croft & Parish, 2013). If an adolescent asks about a parent's SUD, provide age-appropriate information to assure the child that the parent's issues are not anyone's fault and that recovery is possible. Alternatively, individual and family counseling through a referral, including to child-centered support groups (e.g., Alateen, Alatot), may be helpful.

CONCLUSION

Substance use and substance use disorders are a leading cause of morbidity and mortality for adolescents in the United States. Pediatric clinicians should routinely screen all teenagers and view use of alcohol and drugs on a spectrum from the high-prevalence, low-severity phenomenon of experimentation through the low-prevalence, high-severity use disorders. For low-severity cases, brief office interventions are appropriate. Once a teenager has progressed to disorder, referral to specialty treatment is needed. Clinicians should be familiar with treatment resources in the local community and provide follow-up during the process of recovery. More research is needed on what constitutes effective treatment. All health care providers should also be aware that children may be affected by substance use and substance use disorders on the part of their parents. Questions about parental use of alcohol and drugs should be part of a family screening. When problems are identified, clinicians should refer parents to adult mental health professionals for formal evaluation and treatment and insist on being a part of continuing family health care.

REFERENCES

Acheson, A., Vincent, A. S., Cohoon, A. J., & Lovallo, W. R. (2018). Defining the phenotype of young adults with family histories of alcohol and other substance use disorders: Studies from the family health patterns project HHS Public Access. *Addictive Behaviors*, *77*, 247–254. https://doi.org/10.1016/j.addbeh.2017.10.014

Allen, M. L., Garcia-Huidobro, D., Porta, C., Curran, D., Patel, R., Miller, J., & Borowsky, I. (2016). Effective parenting interventions to reduce youth substance use: A systematic review. *Pediatrics*, *138*(2). www.aappublications.org/news

American Psychiatric Association. (2013). *Diagnostic and statistical manual of mental disorders* (5th ed.). Author. https://doi.org/10.1176/appi.books.9780890425596.x00diagnosticclassification

Bavarian, N., Flay, B. R., Ketcham, P. L., & Smit, E. (2015). The illicit use of prescription stimulants on college campuses: A theory-guided systematic review. *Health Education and Behavior*, *42*(6), 719–729. https://doi.org/10.1177/1090198115580576

Chadi, N., Schroeder, R., Jensen, J. W., & Levy, S. (2019). Association between electronic cigarette use and marijuana use among adolescents and young adults: A systematic review and meta-analysis. *JAMA Pediatrics*, *173*(10). https://doi.org/10.1001/jamapediatrics.2019.2574

Chang, Z., Lichtenstein, P., Halldner, L., D'Onofrio, B., Serlachius, E., Fazel, S., & Larsson, H. (2014). Stimulant ADHD medication and risk for substance abuse. *Journal of Child Psychology and Psychiatry and Allied Disciplines*, *55*(8), 878–885. https://doi.org/10.1111/jcpp.12164

Compton, W. M., Gfroerer, J., Conway, K. P., & Finger, M. S. (2014). Unemployment and substance outcomes in the United States 2002–2010. *Drug and Alcohol Dependence*, *142*, 350–353. https://doi.org/10.1016/j.drugalcdep.2014.06.012

Connell, A. M., Dishion, T. J., Yasui, M., & Kavanagh, K. (2007). An adaptive approach to family intervention: Linking engagement in family-centered intervention to reductions in adolescent problem behavior. *Journal of Consulting and Clinical Psychology*, *75*(4), 568–579. https://doi.org/10.1037/0022-006X.75.4.568

Cox, M. J., Janssen, T., Lopez-Vergara, H., Barnett, N. P., & Jackson, K. M. (2018). Parental drinking as context for parental socialization of adolescent alcohol use. *Journal of Adolescence*, *69*, 22–32. https://doi.org/10.1016/j.adolescence.2018.08.009

Croft, B., & Parish, S. L. (2013). Care integration in the patient protection and affordable care act: Implications for behavioral health. *Administration and Policy in Mental Health and Mental Health Services Research*, *40*(4), 258–263. https://doi.org/10.1007/s10488-012-0405-0

Curtis, B., Ashford, R., Rosenbach, S., Stern, M., & Kirby, K. (2019). Parental identification and response to adolescent substance use and substance use disorders. *Drugs: Education, Prevention and Policy*, *26*(2), 175–183. https://doi.org/10.1080/09687637.2017.1383973

D'Amico, E. J., Parast, L., Shadel, W. G., Meredith, L. S., Seelam, R., & Stein, B. D. (2018). Brief motivational interviewing intervention to reduce alcohol and marijuana use for at-risk adolescents in primary care. *Journal of Consulting and Clinical Psychology*, *86*(9), 775–786. https://doi.org/10.1037/ccp0000332

Daniels, D., Saracino, T., Fraley, M., Christian, J., & Pardo, S. (2018). Advancing ego development in adulthood through study of the enneagram system of personality. *Journal of Adult Development*, *25*(4), 229–241. https://doi.org/10.1007/s10804-018-9289-x

Dulit, E. (1972). Adolescent thinking ála Piaget: The formal stage. *Journal of Youth and Adolescence*, *1*(4), 281–301. https://doi.org/10.1007/BF01537818

Fewell Huff, C. (2020). Young children of parents with substance use disorders (SUD): A review of the literature and implications for social work practice: Neta Peleg-Oren and Meir Teichman. In *Impact of substance abuse on children and families* (pp. 66–78). Routledge. https://doi.org/10.4324/9780203462638-7

Frank, D., DeBenedetti, A. F., Volk, R. J., Williams, E. C., Kivlahan, D. R., & Bradley, K. A. (2008). Effectiveness of the AUDIT-C as a screening test for alcohol misuse in three race/ethnic groups. *Journal of General Internal Medicine*, *23*(6), 781–787. https://doi.org/10.1007/s11606-008-0594-0

Galea, S., & Vlahov, D. (2002). Social determinants and the health of drug users: Socioeconomic status, homelessness, and incarceration. In *Public health reports* (Vol. 117, pp. S135). Sage Publications. /pmc/articles/PMC1913691/?report=abstract

Ghitza, U. E., Gore-Langton, R. E., Lindblad, R., Shide, D., Subramaniam, G., & Tai, B. (2013). Common data elements for substance use disorders in electronic health records: The NIDA Clinical Trials Network experience. *Addiction*, *108*(1), 3–8. https://doi.org/10.1111/j.1360-0443.2012.03876.x

Gray, K. M., & Squeglia, L. M. (2018). Research review: What have we learned about adolescent substance use? *Journal of Child Psychology and Psychiatry and Allied Disciplines*, *59*(6), 618–627. https://doi.org/10.1111/jcpp.12783

Habersaat, S., Ramain, J., Mantzouranis, G., Palix, J., Boonmann, C., Fegert, J. M., … Urben, S. (2018). Substance-use disorders, personality traits, and sex differences in institutionalized adolescents. *American Journal of Drug and Alcohol Abuse*, *44*(6), 686–694. https://doi.org/10.1080/00952990.2018.1491587

Hadland, S. E., & Levy, S. (2016). Objective testing: Urine and other drug tests. *Child and Adolescent Psychiatric Clinics of North America*, *25*(3), 549–565. https://doi.org/10.1016/j.chc.2016.02.005

Hagman, G. (1994). Methadone maintenance counseling. Definition, principles, components. *Journal of Substance Abuse Treatment*, *11*(5), 405–413. https://doi.org/10.1016/0740-5472(94)90093-0

Hammond, C. J., & Gray, K. M. (2016). Pharmacotherapy for substance use disorders in youths. *Journal of Child and Adolescent Substance Abuse*, *25*(4), 292–316. https://doi.org/10.1080/1067828X.2015.1037517

Harstad, E., Levy, S., Ammerman, S. D., Gonzalez, P. K., Ryan, S. A., Siqueira, L. M., … Crumley, K. (2014). Attention-deficit/hyperactivity disorder and substance abuse. *Pediatrics*, *134*(1). https://doi.org/10.1542/peds.2014-0992

Henderson, C. E., Dakof, G. A., Greenbaum, P. E., & Liddle, H. A. (2010). Effectiveness of multidimensional family therapy with higher severity substance-abusing adolescents: Report from two randomized controlled trials. *Journal of Consulting and Clinical Psychology*, *78*(6), 885–897. https://doi.org/10.1037/a0020620

Hendriks, V., van der Schee, E., & Blanken, P. (2011). Treatment of adolescents with a cannabis use disorder: Main findings of a randomized controlled trial comparing multidimensional family therapy and cognitive behavioral therapy in The Netherlands. *Drug and Alcohol Dependence*, *119*(1–2), 64–71. https://doi.org/10.1016/j.drugalcdep.2011.05.021

Heradstveit, O., Skogen, J. C., Hetland, J., Stewart, R., & Hysing, M. (2019). Psychiatric diagnoses differ considerably in their associations with alcohol/drug-related problems among adolescents. A Norwegian population-based survey linked with National Patient Registry data. *Frontiers in Psychology*, *10*. https://doi.org/10.3389/fpsyg.2019.01003

Johnson, J. K. (2018). Elucidating the impact of adolescent marijuana use. *Journal of Adolescent Health*, *63*(2), 129–130. https://doi.org/10.1016/j.jadohealth.2018.06.002

Jordan, C. J., & Andersen, S. L. (2017). Sensitive periods of substance abuse: Early risk for the transition to dependence. *Developmental Cognitive Neuroscience*, *25*, 29–44. https://doi.org/10.1016/j.dcn.2016.10.004

Kelly, J. F., Dow, S. J., Yeterian, J. D., & Kahler, C. W. (2010). Can 12-step group participation strengthen and extend the benefits of adolescent addiction treatment? A prospective analysis. *Drug and Alcohol Dependence*, *110*(1–2), 117–125. https://doi.org/10.1016/j.drugalcdep.2010.02.019

Kelly, S. M., Gryczynski, J., Mitchell, S. G., Kirk, A., O'Grady, K. E., & Schwartz, R. P. (2014). Validity of brief screening instrument for adolescent tobacco, alcohol, and drug use. *Pediatrics*, *133*(5), 819–826. https://doi.org/10.1542/peds.2013-2346

Kuppens, S., & Ceulemans, E. (2019). Parenting styles: A closer look at a well-known concept. *Journal of Child and Family Studies*, *28*(1), 168–181. https://doi.org/10.1007/s10826-018-1242-x

Levy, S., Weiss, R., Sherritt, L., Ziemnik, R., Spalding, A., Van Hook, S., & Shrier, L. A. (2014). An electronic screen for triaging adolescent substance use by risk levels. *JAMA Pediatrics*, *168*(9), 822–828. https://doi.org/10.1001/jamapediatrics.2014.774

Macgowan, M. J., & Engle, B. (2010). Evidence for optimism: Behavior therapies and motivational interviewing in adolescent substance abuse treatment. *Child and Adolescent Psychiatric Clinics of North America*, *19*(3), 527–545. https://doi.org/10.1016/j.chc.2010.03.006

McCabe, S. E., Dickinson, K., West, B. T., & Wilens, T. E. (2016). Age of onset, duration, and type of medication therapy for attention-deficit/hyperactivity disorder and substance use during adolescence: A multi-cohort national study. *Journal of the American Academy of Child and Adolescent Psychiatry*, *55*(6), 479–486. https://doi.org/10.1016/j.jaac.2016.03.011

McGuier, E. A., Kolko, D. J., Joseph, H. M., Kipp, H. L., Lindstrom, R. A., Pedersen, S. L., … Molina, B. S. G. (2020). Use of stimulant diversion prevention strategies in pediatric primary care and associations with provider characteristics. *Journal of Adolescent Health*, 1–8. https://doi.org/10.1016/j.jadohealth.2020.12.006

Meyers, J. L., & Dick, D. M. (2010). Genetic and environmental risk factors for adolescent-onset substance use disorders. *Child and Adolescent Psychiatric Clinics of North America*, *19*(3), 465–477. https://doi.org/10.1016/j.chc.2010.03.013

Miech, R. A., Patrick, M. E., O'Malley, P. M., Johnston, L. D., & Bachman, J. G. (2020). Trends in reported marijuana vaping among US adolescents, 2017–2019. *JAMA*, *323*(5), 475–476. https://doi.org/10.1001/jama.2019.20185

Miller, L., Davies, M., & Greenwald, S. (2000). Religiosity and substance use and abuse among adolescents in the national comorbidity survey. *Journal of the American Academy of Child and Adolescent Psychiatry*, *39*(9), 1190–1197. https://doi.org/10.1097/00004583-200009000-00020

Miller, W. R., & Rollnick, S. (2012). Meeting in the middle: Motivational interviewing and self-determination theory. *International Journal of Behavioral Nutrition and Physical Activity*, *9*. https://doi.org/10.1186/1479-5868-9-25

Molfenter, T., Brown, R., O'neill, A., Kopetsky, E., & Toy, A. (2018). Use of telemedicine in addiction treatment: Current practices and organizational implementation characteristics. *International Journal of Telemedicine and Applications*, *2018*. https://doi.org/10.1155/2018/3932643

Neighbors, C. J., Barnett, N. P., Rohsenow, D. J., Colby, S. M., & Monti, P. M. (2010). Cost-effectiveness of a motivational intervention for alcohol-involved youth in a hospital emergency department. *Journal of Studies on Alcohol and Drugs*, *71*(3), 384–394. https://doi.org/10.15288/jsad.2010.71.384

National Highway Traffic Safety Administration, US Department of Transportation. (2017). *2017 data: Young drivers*. www.cdc.gov/injury/wisqars/fatal.html

National Institute on Alcohol Abuse and Alcoholism (NIAAA). (n.d.). *Underage drinking*. https://www.niaaa.nih.gov/publications/brochures-and-fact-sheets/underage-drinking

National Institute on Alcohol Abuse and Alcoholism (NIAAA). (2015). *Alcohol screening and brief intervention for youth*. Author.

National Institute on Drug Abuse (NIDA). (n.d.). *Principles of adolescent substance use disorder treatment*. https://www.drugabuse.gov/publications/principles-adolescent-substance-use-disorder-treatment-research-based-guide/principles-adolescent-substance-use-disorder-treatment

Pugatch, M., Knight, J. R., Mcguiness, P., Sherritt, L., & Levy, S. (2014). A group therapy program for opioid-dependent adolescents and their parents. *Substance Abuse*, *35*(4), 435–441. https://doi.org/10.1080/08897077.2014.958208

Ramirez, R., Hinman, A., Sterling, S., Weisner, C., & Campbell, C. (2012). Peer influences on adolescent alcohol and other drug use outcomes. *Journal of Nursing Scholarship*, *44*(1), 36–44. https://doi.org/10.1111/j.1547-5069.2011.01437.x

Redfield, R. R., Bunnell, R., Greenspan, A., Kent, C. K., Leahy, M. A., Martinroe, J. C., … Bobb Swanson, M. (2020). *Morbidity and Mortality Weekly Report, 69*. https://www.cdc.gov/healthyyouth/data/yrbs/index.htm

Rigter, H., Henderson, C. E., Pelc, I., Tossmann, P., Phan, O., Hendriks, V., … Rowe, C. L. (2013). Multidimensional family therapy lowers the rate of cannabis dependence in adolescents: A randomised controlled trial in Western European outpatient settings. *Drug and Alcohol Dependence*, *130*(1–3), 85–93. https://doi.org/10.1016/j.drugalcdep.2012.10.013

Robbins, M. S., Feaster, D. J., Horigian, V. E., Rohrbaugh, M., Shoham, V., Bachrach, K., … Szapocznik, J. (2011). Brief strategic family therapy versus treatment as usual: Results of a multisite randomized trial for substance using adolescents. *Journal of Consulting and Clinical Psychology*, *79*(6), 713–727. https://doi.org/10.1037/a0025477

Ross, E. J., Graham, D. L., Money, K. M., & Stanwood, G. D. (2015). Developmental consequences of fetal exposure to drugs: What we know and what we still must learn. *Neuropsychopharmacology*, *40*(1), 61–87. https://doi.org/10.1038/npp.2014.147

Russell, C., McKeganey, N., Dickson, T., & Nides, M. (2018). Changing patterns of first e-cigarette flavor used and current flavors used by 20,836 adult frequent e-cigarette users in the USA. *Harm Reduction Journal*, *15*(1). https://doi.org/10.1186/s12954-018-0238-6

Smith, V. C., & Wilson, C. R. (2016). Families affected by parental substance use. *Pediatrics*, *138*(2). https://doi.org/10.1542/peds.2016-1575

Spirito, A., Bromberg, J. R., Casper, T. C., Chun, T. H., Mello, M. J., Dean, J. M., & Linakis, J. G. (2016). Reliability and validity of a two-question alcohol screen in the pediatric emergency department. *Pediatrics*, *138*(6). https://doi.org/10.1542/peds.2016-0691

Subramaniam, G. A., & Volkov, N. D. (2014). Substance misuse among adolescents: To screen or not to screen? *JAMA Pediatrics*, *168*(9), 798–799. https://doi.org/10.1001/jamapediatrics.2014.958

Teens Screening Tool. (n.d.). https://www.drugabuse.gov/ast/bstad/#/

Waldron, H. B., & Turner, C. W. (2008). Evidence-based psychosocial treatments for adolescent substance abuse. *Journal of Clinical Child and Adolescent Psychology*, *37*(1), 238–261. https://doi.org/10.1080/15374410701820133

Wasserman, G. A., & McReynolds, L. S. (2011). Contributors to traumatic exposure and posttraumatic stress disorder in juvenile justice youths. *Journal of Traumatic Stress*, *24*(4), 422–429. https://doi.org/10.1002/jts.20664

White, A. M., Tapert, S., & Shukla, S. D. (2018). Binge drinking. *Alcohol Research: Current Reviews*, *39*(1), 1–3. https://doi.org/10.7748/phc.15.6.8.s9

Wilson, C. R., Harris, S. K., Sherritt, L., Lawrence, N., Glotzer, D., Shaw, J. S., & Knight, J. R. (2008). Parental alcohol screening in pediatric practices. *Pediatrics*, *122*(5). https://doi.org/10.1542/peds.2008-1183

Woody, G. E., & Fishman, M. (2020). Medication treatment for opioid-addicted youth: What are we waiting for? *Journal of Adolescent Health*, *67*(1), 9–10. https://doi.org/10.1016/j.jadohealth.2020.04.002

Yonek, J. C., Dauria, E. F., Kemp, K., Koinis-Mitchell, D., Marshall, B. D. L., & Tolou-Shams, M. (2019). Factors associated with use of mental health and substance use treatment services by justice-involved youths. *Psychiatric Services*, *70*(7), 586–595. https://doi.org/10.1176/appi.ps.201800322

54

Dual Diagnosis of Mental Health and Developmental Disorders in Developmental-Behavioral Pediatrics

Shalonda Brooks and Eric M. Butter

For additional material related to the content of this chapter, please see Chapter 40.

VIGNETTE

A 13-year-old boy with borderline intellectual functioning, specific cognitive impairments, and autism spectrum disorder (ASD) was referred because of irritable and aggressive behavior. At school, he had an individualized education plan and attended both inclusion and special education classes daily. He had been doing very well at school until recently, when he became aggressive with a teacher after being embarrassed when he couldn't answer a question she posed, and was subsequently suspended for similar incidents. Upon assessment, a pattern of increasingly avoidant behavior, lower self-esteem, and social withdrawal was noted as well. During a suicide risk assessment, he struggled answering some questions literally, such as "Have you ever thought you'd be better off dead?" He replied, "Off, like a light switch?" Ultimately, with careful interviewing, suicidal ideation was confirmed and a safety plan developed. The completed diagnostic assessment demonstrated he met criteria for major depressive disorder. He was treated with a selective serotonin reuptake inhibitor (SSRI) initially and supportive counseling that included modified cognitive-behavioral therapy. Within 2 months he recovered and returned to increased social and educational engagement.

Dual diagnosis, in the context of developmental-behavioral pediatrics (DBP), refers to the study and treatment of mental health problems and psychiatric disorders in people with developmental disabilities. Though historically experts argued that people with impaired and low intellectual functioning could not experience anxiety, depression, or other psychopathologies, it is now generally accepted that people with intellectual disabilities experience the full range of mental health expressions. Further, it has long been recognized that individuals with intellectual and developmental disabilities (IDD) are at both increased risk for emotional disturbance and suffer the decreased opportunity for adequate treatment (Schlauch, Gordon, & Schmidt, 2016). These factors complicate and exacerbate the impact of psychiatric disorders among those with developmental disorders.

PREVALENCE AND EPIDEMIOLOGY

The exact prevalence of the cooccurrence of IDD and mental health disorders is unknown, but it is generally estimated that 35% to 40% of individuals with IDD also experience a psychiatric condition. The most commonly cooccurring disorders—attention-deficit/hyperactivity disorder (ADHD, 9%) and anxiety (9%)—are often a focus of clinical assessment and intervention (Witwer, Lawton, & Aman, 2014). Conduct problems are reported at relatively high levels (25%) but are often associated with the irritable and aggressive behaviors directly related to the cognitive, communication, and adaptive skill deficits among those with IDD. All types of mental health disorders have been described, and there is no evidence of occurrence of disorders unique to this population.

There are important disparities associated with IDD and dual diagnoses. For example, rates of identification for Black and Hispanic children compared to non-Hispanic White children with IDD and ASD have been documented. Children from racial and ethnic minority groups and children from low-income families diagnosed with ASD and/or IDD experience disparities for access to routine and acute care, number of service hours, specialized educational and community services, and overall quality of care (Smith, Gehricke, Iadarola, Wolfe, & Kuhltau, 2020). Sex-based disparities have also been identified revealing that girls with ASD are at greater risk for most comorbid mental health conditions than boys (Rodgaard, Jensen, Miskowiak, & Mottron, 2021).

DIAGNOSTIC CONSIDERATIONS

Diagnostic criteria used to diagnose psychiatric disorders in those with typical intellectual functioning can be used to diagnose individuals with IDD. However, comorbid mental health disorders among those with IDD often go unrecognized and undiagnosed. A phenomenon known as diagnostic overshadowing, a confirmation bias in medical decision making where a clinician favors the original or prevailing diagnosis when considering emerging behaviors and symptoms, is a significant concern in the management of youth with IDD. The clinician's tendency to overlook the presence of mental disorders in these patients is associated with attributing challenging or unusual behaviors observed in the child to the IDD exclusively while ignoring the possibility of a cooccurring psychiatric condition.

DIAGNOSTIC ASSESSMENT

Diagnostic assessments may be a more complicated and longer process with dual diagnoses. The clinical assessment is done in the context of the total clinical picture, including developmental levels in various domains, associated disabilities, and psychosocial factors. Detailed history is essential, and multiple informants (such as parents, teachers, and therapists) provide better description of the problem than a single observer. The patient should have a recent, comprehensive medical review to rule out comorbid medical disorders. In children and adolescents who do not have communicative language pain or discomfort from an undiagnosed medical condition is a frequent cause of a behavioral change. The comprehensive clinical interview and observation of a child's behavior is key (see Chapter 77).

Rating Instruments

Broadband rating scales developed for general child and adolescent populations can be used. Measures such as the Achenbach System of Empirically Based Assessment (ASEBA; Achenbach, 2015), the Behavior Assessment Scale for Children (BASC-3; Reynolds & Kamphaus, 2015), and the Conners Comprehensive Behavior Rating Scales (Conners, 2019) prove useful in understanding parent/caregiver and teacher experiences of the child's emotional and behavioral adjustment. Specific symptom rating scales, such as Conners-3 Rating Scales for ADHD (Conners, 2015), the Aberrant Behavior Checklist (ABC; Aman, Singh, Stewart, & Field, 1985), the Autism Spectrum Rating Scales (ASRS; Goldstein & Naglieri, 2013), and the Revised Children's Anxiety and Depression Scale (Weiss & Chorpita, 2011), may supplement the clinical observations. More recently, transdiagnostic, symptom-specific inventories have been suggested to have significant utility to track clinical outcomes. The Emotion Dysregulation Inventory (EDI; Mazefsky, Lan, & Pilkonis, 2020) is one such rating scale that may be useful in guiding treatment decisions and monitoring response to treatment. An important caution is that some rating scales may not have been normed on individuals with IDD, and therefore interpretation of the results may be difficult (see Chapter 82 for more on use of behavior rating scales).

DIAGNOSIS OF SPECIFIC MENTAL DISORDERS

Autism Spectrum Disorder

ASD is a neurodevelopmental disability with specific impairments in social-communication skills and the presence of restricted and repetitive behaviors. Intellectual disability is a common comorbidity with ASD, thus these diagnoses are not mutually exclusive for many children. Therefore the more accurate diagnostic question is often whether the child who has an ASD comorbid with IDD has other cooccurring concerns (e.g., anxiety, ADHD, depression). Similarly, children with ASD who have typical cognitive abilities are also at risk for a cooccurring psychiatric disorder. Children with significant IDD alone usually are able to develop social interaction, although their patterns of relating and social communication are immature for their chronologic age, and prolonged observation may be required to recognize it. It is important to note that the diagnosis of intellectual disability is often a strong indicator that a specific etiologic factor underlies the diagnosis of ASD (Thurm, Farmer, Salzman, Lord, & Bishop, 2019). ASD is discussed in detail in Chapter 41.

Attention-Deficit/Hyperactivity Disorder

ADHD is one of the most common cooccurring mental health conditions among children with IDD, and possibly ASD. Notably, hyperactivity symptoms are more commonly observed earlier in development for children dually diagnosed with IDD and ADHD (Siegel et al., 2020). Treatment for ADHD symptoms should be multimodal, including behavioral intervention, parent training, classroom and educational modifications, and possibly medication. The approach to prescribing ADHD medications (e.g., methylphenidate, amphetamine, atomoxetine, and guanfacine) for children with IDD is not dissimilar to the approach for children diagnosed only with IDD. There are concerns that these medications seem less effective and may cause more side effects in children with IDD and/or ASD than when used to treat ADHD alone (Siegel et al., 2020). Thus there is increased value in using parent training and other behavioral interventions for children dually diagnosed even if attempting pharmacologic interventions for ADHD symptoms (Handen et al., 2015) (see Chapter 46).

Anxiety

Anxiety as a cooccurring condition in IDD and/or ASD is a significant and common concern, and left untreated can lead to negative outcomes, including greater social isolation, avoidance of school, and limited community and family integration. Anxiety is associated with learning failure and limitations on adaptive behavior as well as increased parenting stress and family dysfunction. Even more seriously, in a sample of 329 children with ASD, nearly 16% of youth with ASD spoke of harming or killing self at clinically meaningful levels (Mayes, Calhoun, Baweja, & Mahr, 2015). In another study 11% of children with ASD and comorbid anxiety between the ages of 7 and 16 years reported suicidal thoughts and behavior (Storch et al., 2013). Yet, anxiety is particularly difficult to assess in children with IDD. Children with language impairments or who are minimally verbal and/or who are cognitively delayed may not have the ability, insight, or vocabulary to report fears or worries. Similarly, parents and caregivers may not endorse that their children "worry" or complain of things that scare them although symptom-specific measures (e.g., the SCARED or the Parent Rated Anxiety Scale-ASD

[PRAS-ASD]) are available (Scahill et al., 2019). Parents often report that their children express anxiety through emotional outbursts, tantrums, and noncompliance (see Chapter 51).

Mood Disorders

All types of mood disorders can be seen in individuals with IDD, but the diagnosis of depression in persons with IDD is often missed, especially when individuals are ignored because they may be quiet and do not disturb their caregivers. Clinical manifestations of mood disorders may be modified by a person's level of cognitive skills, language, and experiences; verbal productions cannot be used to assess affective state if the individual has limited or no language. However, most of the diagnostic criteria for mood disorders in the *Diagnostic and Statistical Manual of Mental Disorders*, fifth edition (American Psychiatric Association, 2013) can be satisfied on the basis of observations made by others (such as caregivers). These include observations of vegetative signs (sleeping and eating disorders), psychomotor impairments, agitation or aggressive behaviors, withdrawal, anhedonia, tearfulness, irritability, and general appearance of sadness. The individual may be described as refusing to engage in previously preferred activities. Often individuals with IDD and limited language skills can provide useful information about their feelings and mood, although they are likely to use concrete and simple descriptions, such as stating that they feel sick rather than depressed (Siegel et al., 2020).

Bipolar and related disorders (BD) are also a distinctive consideration for comorbidity among patients with IDD. There is thought to be common vulnerability genes shared between ASD and BD, for example. Longitudinal research suggests that youth with BD+ASD are likely to experience typical BD symptoms but with earlier onset, mixed symptom presentation, and increased functional impairments than peers not dually diagnosed. Early identification and evidence-based intervention and medicine have been associated with successful management of clinical symptoms over time and improved clinical outcomes (Borue et al., 2016) (see Chapter 49 for more on mood disorders).

Suicide and Suicide Risk Assessment

Suicidal ideation among youth diagnosed with IDD is not rare. Research has suggested that 63% of parents indicate that their child "talks about death or suicide" in regular and persistent ways (Horowitz et al., 2018). Rates of suicidal ideation among youth age 10 to 18 years with IQs below 70 are nearly identical to youth without IDD. Research by Baer et al. (2018) suggests that children 8 years or younger is the most commonly reported age of onset for both passive ideation (28.7%) and active ideation (33.9%). Parents whose children had tried to end their lives reported the onset of these suicidal behaviors as young as 5 years. Importantly, these data suggest that clinicians must routinely assess suicide risk, suicidal ideation, and the presence of suicidal behaviors in children with IDD. Assessment strategies should account for the patient's language, social cognitive, and generalized cognitive impairments. Vocabulary deficits and a penchant for literal meaning and interpretations of metaphoric language should be considered, and clinicians should check patient's understanding of standard suicide risk questions. It is important to use concrete language. Safety planning is best supported using visualizations of warning signs and feeling states, cognitive distortions, and coping strategies. Family and friends should be an active part of safety planning processes, and steps for careful physical monitoring should be taken (see Chapter 50 for more on suicide prevention).

Gender Diversity and Gender Dysphoria

A growing body of research is observing a link between gender diversity and gender dysphoria with ASD. Gender diversity, and to a greater extent gender dysphoria, includes consistent rejection of typical, culturally congruent gender behavior thought to be associated with one's sex assigned at birth, feelings of embarrassment about one's body, or expressions of rejection as puberty-related body changes occur. Youth expressing such gender diversity may experience stigmatization, bullying by peers, and rejection by parents or other family members. Youth with IDD and/or ASD expressing gender diversity or experiencing gender dysphoria may be less inclined than same-age typically developing peers to discuss, share, or seek help for the feelings and thoughts they have around this topic. Gender-affirming approaches to treatment, support for parents/caregivers to support their child, and referral to interdisciplinary gender care clinics represent current best practice approaches. It is important to recognize that treatment at the intersection of gender identity and ASD and/or IDD is complex due to the cognitive and social-cognitive differences among youth with these diagnoses (Glidden, Bouman, Jones, & Arcelus, 2016) (see Chapter 76 for more on gender variations).

Conduct Problems and Aggression

Disruptive behavior disorders, including oppositional defiant disorder (ODD) and conduct disorder (CD) are distinctive clinical diagnoses that should be considered carefully in individuals with IDD (Siegel et al., 2020). Though distinct, symptoms associated with IDD and CD or ODD are likely to exacerbate the other and should be considered in that intersecting context. Cooccurring diagnoses of CD and ODD are often less helpful than considering any severe and challenging behaviors, often in the form of aggression toward others, as relatively common among children and adolescents with IDD. Noncompliance and patterns of defiance among youth with IDD are often associated with cognitive delays, communication impairments, and limitations in adaptive behavior, emotional regulation, and autonomy. Behavioral parent training, classroom behavior management supports, and self-management strategies are typically effective first-level interventions. Physical harm toward others and property destruction can escalate situations for our patients. Most often the severe behavior is shown to be consistent with impairments associated with their IDD, ineffective management of frustration and negative affect, and poor environmental supports for the youth. In many of these circumstances the diagnostic criteria for CD or the criminal threshold for delinquency are not met and are not warranted (see Chapter 55).

Trauma and Posttraumatic Stress Disorder

The role of adverse experiences and possibility of significant traumatic events underlying acute and persistent behavioral changes among youth with IDD should be considered. Specifically, the possibility of traumatic stress disorders should be kept in mind in any assessment of persons with IDD and otherwise unexplained history of behavior change. Traumatic stress disorders are frequently unnoticed, including trauma associated with childhood sexual abuse because the patients might be unable to report traumatic events (Norris, Cunningham, & Butter, 2016). Symptoms such as distressing flashbacks, dreams, avoidance of places and activities related to the trauma, and hypervigilance may be seen, as well as behavioral changes seen in abused children (mood changes, irritability, sleep disorder, sexualized behaviors). When trauma is identified, trauma-informed care will be critically important and should influence the application and adaptation of behavioral interventions, psychotherapeutic treatments, and educational approaches. Families will need to be supported with practical solutions to promote healing and foster resiliency (see Chapter 56 for more on stress disorders).

Schizophrenia Spectrum and Other Psychotic Disorders

Schizophrenia spectrum and other psychotic disorders may be difficult to diagnose accurately in individuals who have significant IDD because, in the absence of language, recognition of hallucinations, delusions, and thought disorder may not be possible. In such patients the less specific diagnosis of unspecified schizophrenia spectrum and other psychotic disorder might have to be made on the basis of behavioral changes compared with premorbid behavior. In particular, the appearance of symptoms of social or affective withdrawal, bizarre behaviors not seen before, and deterioration in the level of functioning may suggest such a diagnosis. On the other hand, psychosis should not be diagnosed in a person with significant IDD merely on the basis of self-stimulatory or aggressive behavior. In adolescents who have 22q11.2 deletion syndrome (which may also be associated with IDD) there is an increased prevalence of psychosis and psychotic symptoms (26.7%) as well as ASD (50%) (Vorstman, Morcus, & Duijff, 2006) (see Chapter 52).

Catatonia is relatively more common in individuals with IDD and/or ASD, although symptoms, including a range of motor, speech, and behavioral impairments, often are unrecognized and undiagnosed. Most problematically associated with catatonia is severe self-injury. Treatment is difficult, and a small subset of patients are at risk for neuroleptic malignant syndrome or related conditions. Psychiatric and neurology consultations are often necessary to make a diagnosis and to develop a treatment plan. Electroconvulsive therapy can be helpful for some patients with IDD and catatonia but must be evaluated and monitored under highly controlled conditions by specifically credentialed psychiatrists (Luiselli, Bird, & Wachtel, 2021).

Stereotypic Movement Disorder

Stereotypic movement disorder is characterized by nonfunctional motor behaviors, such as persistent rocking, hand shaking, and self-biting that are repetitive, are driven, and result in significant functional impairment, including academic and/or social functioning (Machalicek et al., 2016). A specifier "with self-injurious behavior" is added if the behavior (such as self-hitting, head banging) results in an injury requiring medical care. Serious damage may result from these behaviors, such as retinal detachment and blindness. Often the individual may switch from one type of behavior to another. Self-injurious behavior is more common when the IDD is severe and in certain IDD-associated syndromes such as Lesch-Nyhan and Cornelia de Lange. Treatment is multifocal, depending on causative factors that are involved. It may include behavioral modification (such as rewards for positive behavior and teaching replacement, competing, or alternate behaviors), milieu manipulation (e.g., proper education or work placement, reduction of unnecessary stimulation), and teaching of alternative communication skills (if needed). Psychotropic drugs (antipsychotics and SSRIs) may have an important role. In any case a combination of measures rather than a single intervention is needed (Fischer et al., 2020) (see Chapter 71 for more on movement disorders).

Pica

Pica is the persistent and compulsive eating of nonnutritional, nonfood substances (e.g., dirt, clay, or paint). Pica diagnoses could be present for many years and have periods of time when compulsive eating is exacerbated and worsened. When evaluating for pica, it is important to assess for related medical etiologies and complications such as anemia, infectious diseases, blood toxicities, and intestinal blockages. Expanded lab order sets may be helpful to evaluate hematologic parameters regarding iron, zinc, and other trace elements and heavy metals as well as monitoring liver and kidney status over time. Interventions for pica often require highly individualized and carefully monitored behavioral interventions that incorporate response prevention, differential reinforcement of other alternate and competing behaviors, and significant stimulus control and stimulus-shaping behavioral interventions. The support of a cotreating psychologist or behavior analyst is usually most helpful (see Chapters 93 and 94).

EVALUATION AND TREATMENT OF MEDICAL CONDITIONS

When youth with IDD present for concerns related to mental health symptoms, it is most often because of distinct behavior change and disruption. It is important to consider possible contributions of an underlying medical condition that could also be acutely associated with the presenting behavior change. The clinician should optimize objective data related to physical health status given that the subjective nature of the data used to assist in making a mental health diagnosis is highly limited by parent and self-report. Across the life span, individuals with IDD have shorter life expectancies and higher mortality risk compared to neurotypical populations (Ng, Wallen, & Ahlstrom, 2017). The differences in longevity, vitality, and resilience are greatly attributable to physical health conditions such as diabetes, hypertension, hyperlipidemia, and other respiratory, circulatory, and central nervous system conditions. Undiagnosed pain or gastrointestinal conditions could also present as the primary factor related to acute behavioral changes. Further, effective medical management of associated physical health conditions can reduce rates of self-injurious behavior, improve mood stability, and limit or avoid acute psychiatric hospitalizations. Medications used for many chronic medical conditions do have central nervous system effects that remain largely unclarified in improving or complicating mental health disorders. Finally, addressing sleep problems, obesity, and sedentary patterns of activity can also help to mitigate the impact of dual diagnoses on patient and family quality of life as well as help manage subclinical levels of psychiatric symptoms (Siegel et al., 2020).

TREATMENT

Treatment Planning

Clinicians should resist the temptations and pressure to immediately prescribe medications for challenging behaviors before the total clinical picture and potentially explanatory factors involved are understood.

Psychotherapies and Psychological Interventions

There has been a growing literature base on the utility of psychotherapy and psychological interventions for individuals with IDD, ASD, and mental health concerns. Behavioral skills training, behavioral parent training, social skills training, and direct social-communication skills and adaptive skills teaching, as well as other forms of direct interventions using behavior therapy approaches, are the most common and effective forms of psychological intervention for patients with IDD. Traditional one-to-one psychotherapy with individuals who have IDD may be effective as well. The prerequisite is that the therapist be well trained and experienced with this population. Evidence-based psychotherapeutic treatments developed for psychiatric disorders without a sensitivity for youth with IDD will require skillful adaptation to be effective for children with dual diagnoses.

As one example, dialectical behavior therapy (DBT) has been adapted for use with patients with dual diagnoses, such as borderline or mild intellectual disability and ASD, trauma, and mood and anxiety disorders. DBT uses principles of mindfulness, emotion regulation, distress tolerance, and interpersonal effectiveness to help patients cope with chronic relationship and emotional problems. Adaptations for youth with IDD, ASD, and other mental health disorders include the use of concrete, clear, and brief descriptions of the therapeutic tools in DBT as well as the use of multiple facilitators for DBT groups and carefully developed discussion questions and therapeutic metaphors (Hartmann, Urbano, Manser, & Okwara, 2012). Similar modifications and approaches have been made with other cognitive-behavioral therapies (see Chapter 98).

Psychological interventions may be designed to support and/or supplement other treatments such as psychopharmacologic interventions. For instance, patients with IDD and a dual diagnosis may be prescribed medications, yet they may have no experience swallowing pills. A behavioral shaping intervention protocol for pill swallowing may be necessary. Additionally, many psychosocial treatment packages, such as behavioral parent training, have been shown to enhance the effects of medication interventions (Aman et al., 2009). There is value to starting with a psychological intervention prior to beginning medication treatment or starting a psychological intervention at the same time as a needed medication is prescribed. Though medications may be helpful in creating emotional and behavioral stability, behavioral and psychological interventions will expand adaptive behavior, teach coping skills, and enhance quality of life in ways that pharmacologic agents cannot. Psychotherapy and other psychological interventions are further discussed in Section 9 of this text.

Psychotropic Medications

The use of these medications is described in detail in Chapter 99. In using psychotropic medications physicians must follow the same principles of evidence-based treatment as they would with patients who do not have IDD. The primary approach is to use medications in the lowest effective dose and to use follow-up data to monitor effectiveness. The use of multiple medications should be avoided (adding one drug after another if the previous one is not effective, rather than discontinuing the ineffective one), unless a combination is clearly proved to be effective. These drugs should be prescribed (as any other drug is) by a physician who is thoroughly familiar with them. Medications should be a part of a comprehensive treatment program, not a substitute for it. Various treatment modalities, such as psychotherapy, milieu therapy, and behavior modification, have a synergistic effect with the medications. As much as possible, medications should be used for their designated action in specific disorders. For example, antipsychotics should be used primarily for treatment of psychotic disorder and not as a nonspecific "major tranquilizer." Whereas they are often prescribed "for aggression," there is really no specific antiaggression drug. Aggressive behavior may be caused by psychosis, depression, a painful condition, anger, or reaction to environmental conditions, each of which requires quite different interventions. High doses of an antipsychotic drug might suppress any aggressive behavior, but the cost of side effects and suppression of the person's general functioning should be carefully monitored.

Another caveat in the use of drugs in this population concerns side effects (Siegel et al., 2020). Children and adolescents who do not have verbal skills may have considerable difficulty in reporting side effects. They should be monitored carefully, according to predetermined criteria and baseline data. Some side effects may mimic original symptoms; for example, akathisia resulting from a too rapid withdrawal of an antipsychotic, particularly a first-generation one, may look like an increase in preexisting agitation, especially if the patient cannot describe how he or she feels. The involuntary movements of tardive dyskinesia may be difficult to differentiate from preexisting stereotypies. Videotaping of the patient's behavior before the drug is started may help in this differentiation.

Prescribing medications among patients with IDD and co-occurring mental health disorders is a complicated endeavor and requires attention to many nuances. Analysis of national prescribing patterns for dual diagnoses suggests that there is great variability and transiency in the use of prescription medications (Feroe et al., 2021). The importance of early and persistent monitoring of patients with IDD, ASD, and cooccurring psychiatric disorders can help guide medical management. A general strategy for prescribing psychotropic medications for dual diagnoses is outlined in Table 54.1. In addition to the protocol suggested there, prescribers should consider consolidating any medications with sedative effects and be conservative with medications that lower seizure thresholds. Also, dose schedules may be nuanced. For instance, instead of prescribing medications "two times daily," which is often applied as morning and bedtime, it may be more advantageous to specify times to optimize medication efficacy during daytime hours.

TABLE 54.1 Approach to Prescribing Psychotropic Medications for Patients With Intellectual Disability and Other Mental and Behavioral Health Disorders

1. Document baseline functioning	Start by assessing the patient's current level and best level of functioning
2. Current assessment	Observe, interview, and quantify changes from baseline and/or best prior levels of functioning as well as type of and response to prior treatments
3. Alternatives or parallel interventions	Consider role of nonpharmacologic treatments or changes to current nonpharmacologic treatments to optimize effectiveness of comprehensive treatment plan
4. Informed, conservative prescribing	Use best practice guidelines for prescribing for nonintellectually disabled patients but with cautious, rational adjustments where needed
5. Adjust with standardized data	Use multiinformant, multisetting approach to collecting standardized rating forms related to treatment targets
6. Adjust based upon systematic caregiver observations	Use data gathered by caregivers that quantify symptoms over time
7. Monitor all necessary labs and side effects	Obtain baseline labs and side effect reviews prior to starting medications and follow all relevant standard monitoring protocols
8. Consider treatment synergies	Consider adjustments based on the progress and impact from related psychotherapy, supportive, and educational interventions
9. Avoid clinical inertia	Use expected outcomes and dose response to titrate medications to establish appropriate targets such that medication is escalated to achieve treatment goals
10. Consider decreasing or discontinuing medication treatments	Plan for and monitor conditions when decreasing dose or discontinuing medications for dual diagnoses would be appropriate (e.g., stable for 6–12 mo)

CARE COORDINATION AND CONSULTATION

Patients with IDD and behavioral health disorders often utilize multiple physicians, psychologists, therapists, and community and school resources, and care plans can quickly become disjointed, duplicative, and even counterproductive. Care coordination is one strategy to increase the effective treatment of patients with dual diagnoses. Care coordination is the deliberate organization of patient care activities among all relevant clinicians involved to facilitate the appropriate delivery of health care services through the exchange of information among participants responsible for different aspects of care (Agency for Healthcare Research and Quality, 2014). Care coordination for dually diagnosed youth reflects interprofessional collaboration across a health system as well as interagency collaboration that brings together multiple professionals from across systems and organizations beyond the health system, including schools, community mental health centers, and other community facing agencies (McClain, Shahidullah, & Mezher, 2020).

Consultation is another critical professional activity when caring for children with dual diagnoses. Consultation can be bidirectional. Often, the developmental specialist benefits from consultation from child psychiatrists in managing symptoms and prescribing unfamiliar medications and navigating higher intensity levels of care and hospitalizations. At other times, the DBP as specialist is assisting a child psychiatrist who may have less experience with the complexities and implications of IDD and development in general. Similarly, DBP clinicians consult with primary care physicians to support the medical home and to help in managing aspects of dual diagnosis care when specialty care is not needed. Referral for child psychiatric consultation is indicated if the child's disturbance is pervasive, there is a potential for danger to the child or others, and first-line treatment by a nonpsychiatrist has not been successful. In a formal way Project ECHO (Extensions for Community Health Outcomes) offers case-based learning in a virtual, online community around specific patient populations. ECHO Autism and pediatric behavioral health ECHOs have proliferated and are increasingly supporting best practice care models for children with IDD and mental health disorders (Sohl, Mazurek, & Brown, 2017).

CONCLUSION

In summary, the treatment of mental health disorders alongside cooccurring developmental disorders is complicated. Effective treatment requires a multidisciplinary team with complementary expertise and careful care coordination. The independent occurrence of a mental health disorder in the context of an intellectual developmental disorder or other neurodevelopmental condition is to be carefully screened for, assessed, treated, and monitored. Treatment plans are most effective when pharmacological and psychological, behavioral, and psychosocial interventions are integrated into treatment and treatment response is viewed with interactive complexity. Careful consideration, assessment, and adaptation of the capacity of the family and caregiving environments as well as school and community environments should be made and ongoing. In the vignette that opened this chapter, a 13-year-old boy with mild intellectual deficits and autism spectrum disorder presented with a recent, escalating pattern of behavior harmful to others, including his teachers. Careful assessment revealed symptoms consistent with depression and suicidal ideation. Evaluation and treatment needed to be carefully adapted in the context of his intellectual and developmental disabilities, and when done so, the patient responded well and was returned with a quality of life and social engagement no longer impacted by symptoms of depression.

REFERENCES

Achenbach, T. M. (2015). Developmental psychopathology. In T. P. Beauchaine & S. P. Hinshaw (Eds.), *The Oxford handbook of externalizing spectrum disorders* (pp. 488–512). Oxford University Press.

Agency for Healthcare Research and Quality. (2014). *Care coordination and quality improvement*. https://www.ahrq.gov/ncepcr/care/coordination.html

Aman, M. G., McDougle, C. J., Scahill, L., Handen, B., Arnold, L. E., Johnson, C., … for the Research Units on Pediatric Psychopharmacology Autism Network. (2009). Medication and parent training in children with pervasive developmental disorders and serious behavior problems; results from a randomized trial. *Journal of the American Academy of Child and Adolescent Psychiatry*, *48*(12), 1143–1154.

Aman, M. G., Singh, N. N., Stewart, A. W., & Field, C. J. (1985). The Aberrant Behavior Checklist: A behavior rating scale of the assessment of treatment effects. *American Journal of Mental Deficiency*, *89*(5), 485–491.

American Psychiatric Association. (2013). *Diagnostic and statistical manual of mental disorders* (5th ed.). Author.

Baer, B. L., Law, J. K., Kalb, L., Marvin, A. R., Vasa, R. A., Wilcox, H. C., & Lipkin, P. H. (2018). Suicidal ideation and behaviors in children, youth, and young adults with autism spectrum disorder (ASD): Rates & outcomes based on parent-report of 992 individuals with ASD. Poster presentation at the Annual Meeting for the International Society for Autism Research, Rotterdam, Netherlands.

Borue, X., Mazefsky, C., Rooks, B. T., Strober, M., Keller, M. B., Hower, H., … Birmaher, B. (2016). Longitudinal course of bipolar disorder in youth with high-functioning autism spectrum disorder. *Journal of the American Academy of Child & Adolescent Psychiatry*, *55*(12), 1064–1072.

Conners, C. K. (2015). *Conners third edition: DSM-5 update*. Multi-Health Systems.

Conners, C. K. (2019). *Conners fourth edition: DSM-5 update*. Multi-Health Systems.

Feroe, A. G., Uppal, N., Gutierrez-Sacristan, A., Mousavi, S., Greenspun, P., Surati, R., … Avillach, P. (2021). Medication use in the management of comorbidities among individuals with autism spectrum disorder from a large nationwide insurance database. *JAMA Pediatrics*. https://doi.org/10.1001/jamapediatrics.2021.1329.

Fischer, J., Mainka, T., Worbe, Y., Pringsheim, T., Bhatia, K., & Ganos, C. (2020). Self-injurious behaviour in movement disorders: Systematic review. *Journal of Neurology, Neurosurgery & Psychiatry*, *91*, 712–719.

Glidden, D., Bouman, W. P., Jones, B. A., & Arcelus, J. (2016). Gender dysphoria and autism spectrum disorder: A systematic review of the literature. *Sexual Medicine*, *4*(1), 3–14.

Goldstein, S., & Naglieri, J. A. (2013). *Autism spectrum rating scales: ASRS*. MHS.

Handen, B. L., Aman, M. G., Arnold, L. E., Hyman, S. L., Tumuluru, R. V., Lecavalier, L., … Smith, T. (2015). Atomoxetine, parent training, and their combination in children with autism spectrum disorder and attention-deficit/hyperactivity disorder. *Journal of the American Academy of Child and Adolescent Psychiatry*, *54*(11), 905–915.

Hartmann, K., Urbano, M., Manser, K., & Okwara, L. (2012). Modified dialectical behavioral therapy to improve emotion regulation in autism spectrum disorders. *Autism Spectrum Disorders*, 43–72.

Horowitz, L. M., Thurm, A., Framer, C., Mazefsky, C., Lanzillo, E., & Bridge, J. A. (2018). Talking about death or suicide: Prevalence and clinical correlates in youth with autism spectrum disorder in psychiatric inpatient setting. *Journal of Autism and Developmental Disorder*, *48*, 3702–3710.

Luiselli, J. K., Bird, F., & Wachtel, L. E. (2021). Electroconvulsive therapy (ECT) for autism spectrum disorder associated with catatonia and self-injury: A clinical review. *Advances in Neurodevelopmental Disorders*, *5*, 117–125.

Machalicek, W., Raulston, T., Knowles, C., Ruppert, T., Carnett, A., & Alresheed, F. (2016). Challenging behavior. In J. L. Matson (Ed.), *Comorbid conditions among children with autism spectrum disorder* (pp. 137–170). Springer.

Mayes, S. D., Calhoun, S. L., Baweja, R., & Mahr, F. (2015). Suicide ideation and attempts in children with psychiatric disorders and typical development. *Crisis*, *36*(1), 55–60.

Mazefsky, C. A., Lan, Y., & Pilkonis, P. A. (2020). Psychometric properties of the emotion dysregulation inventory in a nationally representative sample of youth. *Journal of Clinical Child &*

Adolescent Psychology. https://doi.org/10.1080/15374416.2019.1703710.

McClain, M. B., Shahidullah, J. D., & Mezher, K. R. (Eds.). (2020). *Interprofessional care coordination for pediatric autism spectrum disorder: Translating research into practice*. Springer.

Ng, N., Wallen, E. F., & Ahlstrom, G. (2017). Mortality patterns and risk among older men and women with intellectual disability: a Swedish national retrospective cohort study. *BMC Geriatrics*, *17*(269), 1–13.

Norris, M., Cunningham, N., & Butter, E. M. (2016). Sexual trauma in children and adolescents with IDD. In J. R. Lutzker, K. Guastaferro, & M. L. Benka-Coker (Eds.), *Maltreatment of people with intellectual and developmental disabilities* (pp. 83–108). American Association on Intellectual and Developmental Disabilities.

Reynolds, C. R., & Kamphaus, R. W. (2015). *Behavior assessment system for children* (3rd ed.). Pearson.

Rodgaard, E. M., Jensen, K., Miskowiak, K. M., & Mottron, L. (2021). Autism comorbidities show elevated female-to-make odds rations and are associated with age of first autism diagnosis. *Acta Psychiatrica Scandanavica*. https://doi.org/10.1111/acps.13345.

Scahill, L., Lecavalier, L., Schultz, R. T., Evans, A. N., Maddox, B., Pritchett, J., … Edwards, M. C. (2019). Development of the parent-rated anxiety scale for youth with autism spectrum disorder. *Journal of the American Academy of Child and Adolescent Psychiatry*, *58*(9), 887–896.

Schlauch, R. C., Gordon, K. H., & Schmidt, N. B. (2016). The assessment, diagnosis, and treatment of psychiatric disorders in individuals with a dual diagnosis: The co-occurrence of developmental disorders and psychiatric disorders. In J. D. Buckner, Y. Castro, & N. Ellis (Eds.), *Mental health care for people of diverse backgrounds: The epidemiologically based needs assessment reviews* (vol. 1, pp. 101–120). Taylor & Francis/CRC Press.

Siegel, M., McGuire, K., Veenstra-VandeWeele, J., Statigos, K., King, B., & the American Academy of Child and Adolescent Psychiatry Committee on Quality Issues. (2020). Practice parameter for the assessment and treatment of psychiatric disorders in children and adolescents with intellectual disability. *Journal of the American Academy of Child and Adolescent Psychiatry*, *59*(4), 468–496.

Smith, K. A., Gehricke, J. G., Iadarola, S., Wolfe, A., & Kuhltau, K. A. (2020). Disparities in service use among children with autism. *Pediatrics*, *145*(1), S35–S46.

Sohl, K., Mazurek, M. O., & Brown, R. (2017). ECHO autism: Using technology and mentorship to bridge gaps, increase access to care, and bring best practice autism care to primary care. *Clinical Pediatrics*, *56*(6), 509–511.

Storch, E. A., Sulkowski, M. L., Nadeau, J., Lewin, A. B., Arnold, E. B., Mutch, P. J., … Murphy, T. K. (2013). The phenomenology and clinical correlates of suicidal thoughts and behaviors in youth with autistic spectrum disorders. *Journal of Autism and Developmental Disorder*, *43*, 2450–2459.

Thurm, A., Farmer, C., Salzman, E., Lord, C., & Bishop, S. (2019). State of the field: Differentiating intellectual disability from autism spectrum disorder. *Frontiers in Psychiatry*, *10*(526), 1–10.

Vorstman, J. A. S., Morcus, M. E. J., Duijff, S. N., et al. (2006). The 22q11.2 deletion in children: High rate of autistic disorders and early onset of psychotic symptoms. *Journal of the American Academy of Child and Adolescent Psychiatry*, *45*, 1104–1113.

Weiss, D. C., & Chorpita, B. F. (2011). *Revised children's anxiety and depression scale*. UCLA Child First.

Witwer, A. N., Lawton, K., & Aman, M. G. (2014). Intellectual disability. In E. J. Mash & R. A. Barkley (Eds.), *Child psychopathology* (pp. 593–624). Guilford Press.

55

Aggression and Disruptive Behavior Disorders

Stephen S. Leff, Christine Waanders, and Sandhyaa Iyengar

For additional material related to the content of this chapter, please see Chapters 8, and 99.

The writing of the manuscript was supported, in part, by a National Institute of Child Health and Human Development (NICHD; 1R01HD094833-01A1) award to Stephen Leff, PhD.

VIGNETTE

The mother of 8-year-old James gets tears in her eyes as she describes his frequent aggression to their health care provider. He pushes and hits his 6-year-old brother on a daily basis. This tends to happen when James's brother interrupts something he is doing or when he won't do what James tells him to do. James is quick to anger, easily frustrated, and tends not to talk about his feelings—lashing out physically instead. He recently got in trouble at school when he hit a peer who he thought was laughing at him. James is also aggressive toward his parents at times, pushing them or throwing his videogame controller at them when they ask him to stop playing and come to dinner. He rarely complies with their instructions or requests. The clinician listens sympathetically, and then asks some clarifying questions to assess for the frequency, duration, and seriousness of James's behavior problems.

INTRODUCTION

In this case example, James presents with significant aggression toward his sibling and other peers, resulting from his poor emotion regulation and low frustration tolerance. His aggression is also directed toward his parents during transitions and in response to their requests. Aggression and persistent noncompliance have led James's parents to seek help from a clinician. Clinicians, including general pediatricians and subspecialists such as developmental-behavioral pediatricians (DBPs), are often first in line to discuss behavioral concerns with parents. They have the unique advantage of building a relationship of trust and communication over the course of a child's development, allowing parents to feel comfortable confiding these details. Discussing children's behavioral challenges is complex because parents may be fearful that the issues reflect poorly on their own behavior or parenting ability. The stress associated with children's externalizing behaviors often leads to parents' own frustration, anxiety, and anger. This highlights the need for pediatric health providers to develop the clinical acumen to elicit relevant behavioral information in an empathetic way and to engage parents so that they can direct them to appropriate further care as well as to implement positive behavioral strategies.

Disruptive, oppositional, and aggressive behaviors can take various forms and present as part of several different developmental disorders. In this chapter we discuss differential diagnosis for patients like James and outline the approach clinicians can take to help determine the suitable next steps in his care. Without appropriate intervention, disruptive behavior disorders (DBDs) can negatively impact children's academic outcomes, family functioning, and social relationships. Fortunately there are several effective treatment models available; and when clinicians provide brief behavioral counseling and/or refer a child with disruptive behavior for supportive therapeutic services at an early age, it lowers the chance of long-term negative sequelae from aggression and general disruptive behavior.

DEFINING DISRUPTIVE BEHAVIOR DISORDERS

Starting in early childhood, many children engage in occasional mild aggression and defiant behavior. When these behaviors occur with greater intensity and frequency at home and at school, however, the child may meet criteria for diagnosis with a DBD. DBDs are a group of disorders involving externalizing behaviors such as hyperactivity, noncompliance, anger outbursts, physical aggression and destruction of property. This category includes attention-deficit/hyperactivity disorder (ADHD), oppositional defiant disorder (ODD), and conduct disorder (CD). (Note: ADHD is addressed separately and more fully in Chapter 46.)

The DBDs involve a sustained pattern of externalizing behaviors, which impair the child's social and/or academic functioning in a significant way. In ODD and CD, children and youth act out their frequent frustration, anger, and irritability by refusing to comply with adult requests, arguing repeatedly with peers and adults, blaming others for their own misbehavior, and often acting in a vindictive manner. When a young child has ODD (see Table 55.1), the argumentativeness, defiance, and aggression tend to manifest daily. For older children, these behaviors occur at minimum several times per week. Children and adolescents with CD (see Table 55.2), which is considered the most serious of the DBDs, are also significantly oppositional; in addition, they tend to act indifferent or hostile toward other people and engage in more severe antisocial

TABLE 55.1 ***Diagnostic and Statistical Manual of Mental Disorders,*** **Fifth Edition, Diagnostic Criteria for Oppositional Defiant Disorder (Interntional Classification of Diseases, Tenth Revision, Code F91.3)**

A. A pattern of angry/irritable mood, argumentative/defiant behavior, or vindictiveness lasting at least 6 mo as evidenced by at least four symptoms from any of the following categories, and exhibited during interaction with at least one individual who is not a sibling.

Angry/Irritable Mood

1. Often loses temper
2. Is often touchy or easily annoyed
3. Is often angry and resentful

Argumentative/Defiant Behavior

4. Often argues with authority figures or, for children and adolescents, with adults
5. Often actively defies or refuses to comply with requests from authority figures or with rules
6. Often deliberately annoys others
7. Often blames others for his or her mistakes or misbehavior

Vindictiveness

8. Has been spiteful or vindictive at least twice within the past 6 mo

Note: The persistence and frequency of these behaviors should be used to distinguish a behavior that is within normal limits from a behavior that is symptomatic. For children <5 yr, the behavior should occur on most days for a period of at least 6 mo unless otherwise noted. For individuals ≥5 yr, the behavior should occur at least once per week for at least 6 mo, unless otherwise noted. While these frequency criteria provide guidance on a minimal level of frequency to define symptoms, other factors should also be considered, such as whether the frequency and intensity of the behaviors are outside a range that is normative for the individual's developmental level, gender, and culture.

B. The disturbance in behavior is associated with distress in the individual or others in his or her immediate social context (e.g., family, peer group, work colleagues), or it impacts negatively on social, educational, occupational, or other important areas of functioning.

C. The behaviors do not occur exclusively during the course of a psychotic, substance use, depressive, or bipolar disorder. Also, the criteria are not met for disruptive mood dysregulation disorder.

Specify current severity:

Mild: Symptoms are confined to only one setting (e.g., at home, at school, at work, with peers). Moderate: Some symptoms are present in at least two settings.

Severe: Some symptoms are present in three or more settings.

or covert rule-breaking behavior, including lying, stealing, destruction of property, and proactive planned aggression toward animals or people. The CD diagnosis is generally given only after a longstanding pattern of callous and/or delinquent behavior has been established and once other disorders have been ruled out (see Table 55.2).

PREVALENCE

In the United States and other countries around the world, ODD and CD are diagnosed in 3% to 5% of children and youth (Canino et al., 2010; Maughan et al., 2004). There is notable comorbidity between ADHD, ODD, and CD. Comorbidity rates vary, but approximately 40% to 50% of children with ADHD have ODD, and approximately 15% of children with ADHD have CD (Azeredo, Moreira, & Barbosa, 2018; MTA Cooperative Group, 1999). ODD is generally thought of as a precursor to CD; however, ODD does not necessarily develop into CD. There are gender differences in the prevalence of the DBDs. Some studies have found that boys are 1.5 to 3 times as likely as girls to have a DBD diagnosis (Canino, Polanczyk, Bauermeister, Rohde, & Frick, 2010; Demmer et al., 2017), possibly due to biologic differences in brain development between the sexes. However, it is also possible that the diagnostic criteria outlined for ADHD and ODD in the *Diagnostic and Statistical Manual of Mental Disorders*, Fifth Edition (American Psychiatric Association, 2013) may cause a portion of girls with the disorder to be missed. For example, there are girls who are functionally impaired by their disruptive behavior, but whose disruptive behavior is qualitatively different from boys, possibly due to engaging in more relational aggression (e.g., excluding peers or taking actions that harm others' social status and reputation) than physical aggression (Crick & Grotpeter, 1995). These girls might not be diagnosed with a DBD unless they are compared against an all-female sample of their agemates. Another issue is that the onset of antisocial behavior in boys more often occurs in early to middle

TABLE 55.2 *Diagnostic and Statistical Manual of Mental Disorders*, Fifth Edition, Diagnostic Criteria for Conduct Disorder (International Classification of Diseases, Tenth Revision, Codes F91.1 and F91.2)

A. A repetitive and persistent pattern of behavior in which the basic rights of others or major age-appropriate societal norms or rules are violated, as manifested by the presence of at least 3 of the following 15 criteria in the past 12 mo from any of the categories below, with at least 1 criterion present in the past 6 mo:

Aggression to People and Animals

1. Often bullies, threatens, or intimidates others
2. Often initiates physical fights
3. Has used a weapon that can cause serious physical harm to others (e.g., a bat, brick, broken bottle, knife, gun)
4. Has been physically cruel to people
5. Has been physically cruel to animals
6. Has stolen while confronting a victim (e.g., mugging, purse snatching, extortion, armed robbery)
7. Has forced someone into sexual activity

Destruction of Property

8. Has deliberately engaged in fire setting with the intention of causing serious damage
9. Has deliberately destroyed others' property (other than by fire setting)

Deceitfulness or Theft

10. Has broken into someone else's house, building, or car
11. Often lies to obtain goods or favors or to avoid obligations (i.e., "cons" others)
12. Has stolen items of nontrivial value without confronting a victim (e.g., shoplifting, but without breaking and entering; forgery)

Serious Violations of Rules

13. Often stays out at night despite parental prohibitions, beginning <13 yr old
14. Has run away from home overnight at least twice while living in the parental or parental surrogate home, or once without returning for a lengthy period
15. Is often truant from school, beginning <13 yr old

B. The disturbance in behavior causes clinically significant impairment in social, academic, or occupational functioning.

C. If the individual is age ≥18 yr, criteria are not met for antisocial personality disorder.

Specify whether:

312.81 (F91.1) Childhood-onset type: Individuals show at least one symptom characteristic of conduct disorder prior to age 10 yr

312.82 (F91.2) Adolescent-onset type: Individuals show no symptom characteristic of conduct disorder prior to age 10 yr

childhood, while girls' antisocial behaviors develop in adolescence, which helps to account for the prevalence discrepancy often seen in childhood (Demmer et al., 2017). ODD and CD are more commonly diagnosed in youth of lower socioeconomic status, but additional research is needed to more fully understand the different factors that determine this discrepancy (Pliszka & AACAP Work Group on Quality Issues, 2007).

ROLE OF AGGRESSION IN DISRUPTIVE BEHAVIOR DISORDERS

Aggression is one of the defining diagnostic criteria for CD, and although it is not a diagnostic criterion for ADHD or ODD, it is commonly associated with all three of the DBDs (Pliszka & AACAP Work Group on Quality Issues, 2007). In the following section we review the most common subtypes or forms of aggressive behavior, as well as differentiating the primary functions of reactive and proactive aggression.

Forms of Aggression

For many decades the study, understanding, and treatment of aggression focused on the overt forms of the behavior, comprised of physical and verbal aggressive behaviors related to physical dominance (e.g., hitting, pushing, verbal threats). While overt aggression is most common among males expressing their anger or annoyance toward others, it has not accounted for the most common way in which females express their aggression toward others (Crick & Grotpeter, 1995). Over the past few decades, research has demonstrated that

BOX 55.1 Sample Parent Interview Questions for Disruptive Behavior

- When did the child start having episodes of disruptive behavior/aggression/tantrums?
- How often do these episodes occur?
- Does aggression occur only with tantrums or does it occur when the child is calm?
- What does the disruptive episode look like (e.g., hitting, throwing, screaming)?
- How long do the disruptive episodes typically last?
- How do the episodes usually come to an end (e.g., redirection, suddenly "snapping out of it," gradually calming down when left alone, use of time-out)?
- What are the specific triggers (e.g., transitions, denied access to something, communication frustration)?
- Where/to whom is aggression directed?
- What have you tried to address the behaviors, and how successful has this been?
- Where do these outbursts occur (e.g., home, school, extracurricular activities, public places like grocery or park, extended family members' homes)?
- What happens afterwards (e.g., child resumes activity with others or remains upset for a while)?
- Are there any changes going on in the child's life (e.g., a residential move, illness in the family)?
- Are there any medical issues that could be exacerbating the disruptive behavior (e.g., constipation, infection)?

aggressive behaviors can be more subtle and indirect, taking the form of relational aggression. These behaviors, such as spreading rumors and using social exclusion when angry, are related to manipulating one's social dominance or social standing within the peer group. Relationally aggressive behaviors are the ones by which young females most frequently harm their peers, and they have been related to a range of problem-solving and emotion regulation deficits, internalizing symptoms such as anxiety, depression, and loneliness, and with academic challenges (see Leff et al., 2010). Recent longitudinal research has shown a bidirectional relationship between relational aggression and the development of symptoms of ODD and CD: Boys and girls who engaged in relational aggression at age 10 showed an increase in ODD and CD symptoms by age 16; likewise, youth with symptoms of ODD and CD at age 10 showed increased relational aggression by age 16 (Aizpitarte et al., 2017).

Over the past 15 years, cyberaggression has become more prevalent as almost all youngsters have ready access to mobile phones, tablets, computers, and videogame systems where they can talk with other players. Cyberaggression is often relational aggression carried out using an electronic modality. Victims of cyberaggression are at heightened risk for internalizing problems such as anxiety, loneliness, and depression, with some studies suggesting that these youth also are at higher risk for suicidal ideation and behaviors (Massing-Schaffer & Nesi, 2020). Perpetrators of cyberaggression are at risk for externalizing problems, including hyperactivity and physical aggression, as well as social difficulties (Sourander et al., 2010).

Functions of Aggression

When evaluating a patient with aggressive behavior and screening for DBDs, it is helpful to differentiate between two primary functions of their aggression, reactive and proactive. Proactive aggression consists of strategic and goal-directed aggressive behaviors that are used to help the aggressor achieve a purpose or objective. Proactive aggression is thought to be associated with delinquency and rule breaking, which in turn is associated with adolescent substance abuse and later antisocial behaviors (see Fite et al., 2008). A pattern of repeated proactive aggression can be a symptom of CD. An example of proactive aggression would be when one child pushes or intimidates another to obtain a desired toy or prize. In contrast, reactive aggression is typically viewed as an aggressive behavior occurring in response to another individual's behavior, which was experienced as being intentional and mean. For example, a child may respond aggressively after being pushed or teased by peers. Reactive aggression is associated with emotional regulation difficulties, peer relationship problems (e.g., peer rejection), and higher levels of social isolation (see Rieffe et al., 2016); some have posited that it may be associated with ODD.

How Bullying Relates to Disruptive Behavior Disorders

In discussing aggression and disruptive behavior with the clinician, parents may report that their child bullies peers. Bullying is a form of aggression where someone repeatedly aggresses toward a less powerful person, using verbal, social, cyber, or physical means. Rates of peer bullying vary from 5% to 13%, and victimization ranges from 10% to 33% of youth depending on the study (see Hymel & Swearer, 2015). Children with DBDs are even more prone to engaging in bullying, which may be attributed to difficulty managing emotions and impulses within social interactions (Fite et al., 2014). The clinician should assess for bullying as an additional risk factor for aggression and violence in the patient with ODD or CD.

ETIOLOGY OF AGGRESSION AND DISRUPTIVE BEHAVIORS

Research related to better understanding the genetics of ODD and CD has yielded mixed results, although most studies suggest that temperamental factors, such as negative affectivity, extreme reactive responding, and rigidity, are associated with the development of DBDs (Sanson & Prior, 1999). Genetic studies have shown that the vulnerability to DBDs is highly heritable, although environmental and social factors influence the severity of the behavioral difficulties. Some studies have suggested that aggressive delinquent youth with ODD have preexisting physiologic underarousal. In addition, biologic factors, including exposure to toxins in utero, and prenatal deficiencies in vitamins and nutrition may have an impact on the expression of ODD. Other studies have found that prefrontal cortex abnormalities in children with ODD may influence neurotransmitter and hormone function, especially related to lower levels of serotonin, noradrenaline, dopamine, and cortisol, and high testosterone levels (see Pliszka & AACAP Work Group on Quality Issues, 2007).

Although not specifically focused on ODD or CD, there is a substantial body of literature aimed at explaining the development of aggressive behavior and violence. Most theorists agree that disruptive, aggressive behavior and violence are multidetermined and quite complex. As a result, no one etiologic theory is thought to fully explain why youth act in aggressive ways. At the same time there is much to be learned by considering important characteristics and phenomena associated with aggression and delinquent behavior from the perspective of sociobiologic, psychological, developmental, and ecologic theories.

Biologic Theories

Biologic theories of aggression have focused on a range of biologic variables, including genes, neurotransmitters, and hormones, to help explain aggression and violence. Genetic research has also been used to try to explain why men are more likely to be physically aggressive and violent than women. Having an extra Y chromosome (XYY trisomy) increases the probability that one will exhibit aggressive behavior. In addition, Klinefelter syndrome (i.e., having XXY chromosomes) has been explored for its negative association with aggression, as these males are somewhat passive and withdrawn though frequently exhibit antisocial actions, including estimates that 30% of incarcerated males have Klinefelter syndrome.

Neurotransmitters in the brain are also thought to play a role in supporting or maintaining aggressive behavior. A number of neurotransmitters such as serotonin, the catecholamines, acetylcholine, and gamma-aminobutyric acid are thought to be involved in the regulation of aggressive behavior as result of their influence on the central nervous system and structures of the limbic system (Garaigordobil, 2014).

Neuroendocrinologic theories have suggested that aggressiveness is influenced by levels of androgens, estrogens, and/or other hormones (Garaigordobil, 2014). The body's rapid response to a perceived threat, often termed the fight-or-flight response, involves the hypothalamic-pituitary-adrenal (HPA) axis in the brain, which secretes epinephrine, norepinephrine, adrenaline, and cortisol. The release of these hormones readies the mind and body to respond in stressful or dangerous situations that require a quick reaction. Increasing numbers of researchers are examining how chronic and toxic stress related to poverty, discrimination, and high levels of community violence impacts neurocognitive functioning. A high allostatic load, (i.e., the negative impact of chronic stress on the brain and body) causes an overactivation of the HPA axis and an overreactivity to cortisol, which over time appears to lead to higher rates of aggressive behavior ((Rocque et al., 2015). This illustrates how biologic research is being integrated with our more longstanding psychological theories of aggression (see later) to create a fuller understanding of the development of aggressive behavior.

Social Learning Theories

For many years social learning theorists have suggested that aggression is a learned behavior that is heavily influenced by environmental experiences as opposed to being primarily innate or genetic. Individuals can learn aggressive behavior through classical conditioning, where a stimulus is paired with another variable that incites aggression inherently. Over time, certain provocations serve as prompts for aggressive actions. For example, when an individual becomes frustrated, aggression is triggered. The learning of aggression can also occur through operant conditioning, such as when one is rewarded for aggressive behavior, which then increases the likelihood of future aggression. Finally, social learning theorists have suggested that children learn aggressive behaviors by observing others who act aggressively and are positively reinforced for this behavior (Bandura, 1973). Thus aggression is thought to occur because it is modeled or reinforced again and again.

Social Information Processing

The social-Information processing model of aggression posits that the way in which individuals process and respond to a series of sequential social cues will impact how they eventually respond in different social situations (Crick & Dodge, 1994). Physically aggressive youth are thought to be deficient at a number of sequential social cognitive steps starting with how they encode social cues, access their social goals (e.g., to be dominant, to be affiliative), attribute intent to others, make and evaluate their response options and choices, and ultimately behave. Social information models have been especially helpful for intervention planning, informing a problem-solving approach to helping aggressive youth more accurately encode social cues, more accurately attribute others' intentions, and make choices that take into consideration the social context and how others might respond to them (e.g., see Leff et al., 2018).

Developmental/Ecologic Theories

Developmental/ecologic theories of aggression suggest that behavioral patterns are heavily influenced by the ongoing interactions that individuals have with others in their social environments (Bronfenbrenner, 1986). Thus an individual's biology, combined with interactions within the family (parents, siblings), the school (peers and teachers), community (neighbors, schoolmates), and broader cultural context, all influence their behavior as they mature. Relatively recently, Swearer and Hymel (2015) have extended this developmental/ecologic theory into a socioecologic diathesis-stress model to help explain aggression and bullying behaviors. The premise is that the interaction between one's biologic and cognitive vulnerabilities and stressful life events (such as aggression and victimization) serves as a catalyst for the development of psychological problems and difficulties. There is corresponding research in the area of DBDs that shows living in a high-risk neighborhood confers additional stresses that alter a child's developmental trajectory from simply having inattention and hyperactivity to engaging in oppositional and aggressive behavior associated with ODD and CD (Galán et al., 2020).

This overview of the myriad factors involved in aggressive and disruptive behavior highlights the complexity of the phenomenon and our as-yet incomplete understanding of the causes. However, recent work integrating social, psychological, and biologic causes represents a promising new direction in this research.

As the clinician discusses James's behavioral challenges with his family, they share that he has frequent frustration, anger, and irritability and often refuses to comply with adult requests. His parents describe how he has started to argue with them more frequently within the past year and that his aggression seems vindictive—he admits to trying to get back at his brother for things that anger him. The clinician makes a diagnosis of ODD and also completes an evaluation for ADHD. Then the family is coached through some foundational positive behavior management strategies and referred for intensive and ongoing behavioral supports. At subsequent visits, the clinician notes that James is responding well to his parents' new strategies and that his relationship with his sibling has improved as a result.

ASSESSMENT OF DISRUPTIVE BEHAVIOR

When meeting patients with significant disruptive and aggressive behavior, clinicians should be aware of the importance of building a strong alliance with both the patient and the family. This is best begun by validating the challenges faced by both parent and child and expressing understanding of the anger and frustration experienced by the child, without endorsing the child's defiant or aggressive behavior (Pliszka & AACAP Work Group on Quality Issues, 2007). Interviewing the parents about their use of behavioral management strategies will give the provider a sense of the parents' skill level and need for further psychoeducational support. Asking about the child's response to both positive and negative parenting practices will give a sense of the severity of the disruptive symptoms and the need for individual versus group or family treatment.

Another role of the pediatric clinician is providing diagnostic clarity, including the delineation of any possible comorbidities. As disruptive behavior can be a presenting symptom of several developmental conditions, clinicians should also regularly screen patients for behaviors such as rigidity, tantrums, aggression, bullying, and mood dysregulation. They may choose to do so via an informal review of behavioral symptoms, or they may use parent-completed or teacher-completed rating scales such as the Child Behavior Checklist (CBCL) (Achenbach, 2009) or the DBD Rating Scale (DBDRS; Pelham et al., 1992). It is also important to remember that a psychosocial history update can lend insight into the presentation of disruptive behaviors related to stresses, such as the birth of a new sibling or a move to a new school.

Finally, it is important to recognize that oppositional and aggressive behavior can manifest as a part of several disorders other than ODD or CD, which would require a different treatment approach. For example, many children with autism spectrum disorder, anxiety, and/or sensory integration dysfunction demonstrate rigid or oppositional behavior, likely out of a striving for control over their own environments or experiences (Pliszka & AACAP Work Group on Quality Issues, 2007). They may exhibit difficulty with transitions between activities at school or at home, or resistance to completion of nonpreferred or anxiety-provoking tasks. Furthermore, the stresses of daily life can cause irritability in anxious children, which can lead to poorer cooperation overall. Children on the autism spectrum may also use aggression to avoid demands or communicate frustration. Youth who are undergoing stressful or traumatic life experiences (including physical or sexual abuse) may also present with frequent, severe angry outbursts, which can be attributed to their distress over their circumstances (Carliner et al., 2017) as opposed to a primary DBD. All of these examples underscore the need for careful history-taking and evaluation of the function served by the oppositional, angry, or aggressive behavior before diagnosing a child or adolescent with a DBD.

TREATMENT OF DISRUPTIVE BEHAVIOR DISORDERS

Pediatric practices and hospitals have created a range of innovative solutions to address challenging behaviors in the patients they care for (e.g., having a social worker who is available during clinical encounters to meet with families and explain a referral process, attending collaborative office rounds with psychologists and/or psychiatrists to discuss patient cases, or hosting a parent information workshop about behavioral strategies for reducing disruptive behavior). Clinicians should be prepared to have a discussion with families about the etiology of aggressive or disruptive behaviors and the need for a comprehensive behavioral subspecialty evaluation and treatment. In many cases referral to a behavioral specialist is indicated. The treatment of aggressive and disruptive behavior typically involves addressing symptoms directly with a positive behavioral management plan. Other aspects of treatment include working toward the creation of coping skills, emotional regulation, and prosocial skills.

Because DBDs involve biologic, psychological, family, and social dynamics, multimodal treatment is likely to be the most effective. Parental responses can play a role in maintaining or exacerbating oppositional behavior: When parents of typically developing young children are able to respond calmly and consistently, the child's disruptive behavior usually decreases over time; however, children with disruptive behavioral tendencies may respond poorly to many parenting strategies, refusing to comply with aspects of the normal daily routine, and creating extra parenting stress and family conflict. For this reason, parent training and family therapy are often the best treatment options for preventing and treating ODD and CD.

Lifestyle Interventions

Clinical observation may show that lifestyle factors, such as sleep and nutrition, are exacerbating disruptive behavior in children. Poor sleep has been linked to poorer behavioral adjustment in preschool and aggressive behavior across the life span (Kamphuis et al., 2012). A helpful intervention is to provide recommendations and guidance related to regular nighttime routines and good sleep hygiene practices. Another part of the holistic management of disruptive behaviors (though an area with less of an evidence base) is to discuss with parents the importance of well-balanced dietary intake to generally reduce behavioral issues such as tantrums and aggression. There is some evidence that malnutrition or a "few foods diet" in childhood is associated with externalizing/disruptive behaviors and hyperactivity (Pelsser et al., 2017).

The pediatric clinician should base treatment recommendations on the availability of different treatment resources, the age of the child, the family's level of emotional and physical resources, and the severity of the symptoms. Several empirically validated child and family treatments exist for ODD and CD, which are outlined later. Clinicians may consult this resource from the Substance Abuse and Mental Health Services Administration (SAMHSA) describing therapeutic interventions with moderate to strong empirical support: https://www.samhsa.gov/resource/ebp/interventions-disruptive-behavior-disorders-evidence-based-practices-ebp-kit. This kit also includes information to help clinicians choose the most appropriate treatment for the patient, given age, family circumstances, and cultural background.

Empirically Supported Parent Training and Family Therapies for Disruptive Behavior Disorders

Parent-Child Interaction Therapy (PCIT)

PCIT is a dyadic approach to therapy for families with young children (ages 2–7) who are exhibiting oppositional and aggressive behavior (Eyberg & Calzada, 1998; Shuhman et al., 1998). Parents receive live coaching and instruction in applying play therapy techniques and effective behavior management strategies (with an emphasis on positive reinforcement) to reduce disruptive behavior and enhance compliance. Treatment is often carried out in a playroom with an observation area behind a one-way mirror to foster the parents' authority and sense of confidence in carrying out these techniques. In multiple studies with predominantly White participants, PCIT has demonstrated significant reductions in children's behavior problems at home and in school, and improvements in parents' interaction style when compared to control group participants (SAMHSA, 2011) (see Chapter 93 for more on PCIT).

Collaborative and Proactive Solutions (CPS)

Ross Greene et al.'s (2004) book, *The Explosive Child*, is very helpful reading for parents, teachers, and providers working with children with DBDs. Greene's therapeutic approach, CPS, is designed for children ages 4 to 12. CPS helps adults reframe their view of the child's difficult behavior as resulting from a developmental delay or skills deficit. He outlines a problem-solving approach for the therapist to guide the family, teaching the parent and child how to prioritize and communicate effectively about the issues contributing to the child's noncompliance. This therapeutic approach is somewhat newer than the others described here and less well studied; however, several rigorous studies of CPS with majority White participants have demonstrated its effectiveness in reducing oppositional and disruptive behavior, and in alleviating parental stress (e.g., Ollendick et al., 2015).

Multisystemic Treatment (MST)

MST is a form of intensive family and community treatment (Henggeler et al., 1997) designed for aggressive and delinquent teens (ages 12–17). MST involves multiple clinicians working together to strengthen individual, family, and community systems to reinforce the child/teen for decreasing their delinquent or disruptive behavior and to support the parents to handle behavioral challenges effectively via frequent sessions or supportive telephone consultations. At the core of this treatment is the clinicians' focus on repairing and enhancing close, positive relationships between parents and children. Home visits allow the clinicians to provide the most relevant, supportive therapy during parenting challenges and behavioral crises. This widely studied therapeutic approach has established effectiveness with Black and White families. Its significant impacts include decreased arrests and rearrests, increased school attendance, decreased behavior problems, decreased substance use, and improved family relations (SAMHSA, 2011).

The Coping Power Program

The Coping Power Program offers an integrated group treatment for children and youth (ages 8–14) who are exhibiting aggressive and disruptive behavior and their parents (Lochman & Wells, 2002). This manualized treatment targets youth social cognitions, problem-solving skills, and anger management skills, among other issues. The parent group teaches strategies and skills for setting clear expectations and using effective, positive parenting practices to prevent and respond to children's problem behaviors. In White and Black samples, Coping Power has been shown to significantly reduce aggressive and disruptive behavior and to prevent substance abuse in the years following program completion (SAMHSA, 2011).

Medication

For patients with ODD and CD, medication may be a helpful adjunct to therapy, reducing the frequency and intensity of disruptive behaviors. It should not be used alone, given the child's or adolescent's need for additional problem-solving skills, and the benefit to parents of behavioral parent training. There are several medication options that clinicians can consider. Stimulants can be used to reduce impulsive acting out or aggressive behavior in children with ODD and comorbid ADHD (MTA Cooperative Group, 1999). There is evidence that atypical antipsychotics are an effective adjunctive treatment method for DBDs (Khan et al., 2019). In the Treatment of Severe Childhood Aggression (TOSCA) Study of children with ADHD and ODD/CD receiving multimodal treatments, risperidone led to improvements in reactive aggression (Gadow et al., 2016). The atypical antipsychotics require close monitoring for side effects related to weight gain and metabolic and neurologic changes. Less frequently, clinicians may also use an alpha-agonist trial, such as guanfacine or clonidine, to target hyperactive and impulsive behaviors in the context of disruptive behavior.

Wraparound or Behavioral Health Rehabilitative Services (BHRS)

While not empirically validated, many communities offer BHRS for youth with disruptive behavior, delivered by a team that includes a behavior specialist who performs a functional behavior analysis, develops a behavioral treatment plan, and supervises therapeutic support staff to deliver behavior management strategies at school, at home, or in the community, according to the treatment plan. If needed, there is a mobile therapist to provide therapy directly to the child. This treatment is Medicaid-funded and available to children and youth up to age 21 in most states. The quality of these services varies widely, but they can serve as a valuable support for distressed families. A major benefit of this model is that children with behavioral challenges can receive support in their existing environment without requiring exclusion from their activities, a more restrictive placement, or additional burden on the family to seek intensive outpatient care.

OUTCOMES

The urgency for clinicians to address persistent disruptive behavior and aggression in children and adolescents is directly related to its impact on future functioning. Studies have shown that children exhibiting disruptive and aggressive behavior have worse outcomes later in life, including poorer mental health, school performance, employment status, and more challenging interpersonal relationships. DBDs can be considered a major public health concern due to their impact on societal and individual outcomes (Burke, Rowe, & Boylan, 2014).

There are well-defined longitudinal predictive links between childhood aggression and health risks, such as dropping out of school, early and single childbearing, and living in poverty. A strong body of evidence shows additional links with risky behaviors such as dangerous driving and smoking. The long-term outcomes, typically by age 25, of conduct problems have been shown to include increased risk of crime, mental health problems (defined by depression/anxiety disorder, personality disorder, or suicide attempt), substance dependence, and relationship/parenthood issues (defined by early age of becoming a parent, intimate-partner violence, or multiple sex partners) (Fergusson et al., 2009). Regarding physical health outcomes, childhood aggressive behaviors directly and positively predict medical service usage, lifestyle-related medical illnesses (e.g., obesity, type 2 diabetes, ulcers, alcoholism, and substance abuse), and injuries (Temcheff et al., 2011).

There is evidence that the age of diagnosis is a critical aspect to consider. Children who receive a later aggression-related diagnosis (i.e., ADHD, ODD, CD) experience more negative outcomes, specifically criminal records and lower personal incomes. Other outcomes of suicide risk and school performance are not related to age of diagnosis. These relationships hold for all youth when controlling for family and neighborhood variables, using a population registry (Campbell, Lundstrom, Larsson, Lichtenstein, & Lubke, 2019). Given the severity of the negative sequelae of DBDs, early identification and treatment planning for aggressive and/or disruptive behaviors is of the utmost importance. It is possible that proactive management by clinicians and other health care and mental health providers can influence the developmental trajectory of individuals experiencing DBDs, and this will play a role in improved individual and societal outcomes.

CONCLUSION

Aggression and other disruptive behaviors are a challenging aspect of children's development and are a critical concern for general and developmental-behavioral clinicians to address. While a certain degree of aggression and defiance may occur in the normal course of typical development for both boys and girls, it is important to identify and help parents recognize when these behaviors are more serious or frequent than normal. When the clinician notes that a child's oppositional or aggressive behavior is more persistent or more serious than the average child's, they should evaluate for a DBD. In fact, the DBDs are the most common reason for mental health referrals, and clinicians should be prepared to counsel and guide parents toward the most effective treatments.

In many communities, pediatric health providers have long been concerned about limited resources for mental and behavioral health, and they have taken an informed and proactive role in this area. In our vignette with James, his clinician thoughtfully addresses the parents' complaints by asking appropriate details about the nature of the behaviors. This conversation starts by acknowledging the real impact disruptive behaviors have on a child, and often on family functioning. These behaviors can also extend into the school setting, impacting academic achievement or peer relationships, and requiring additional investigation about that setting. By employing an empathic and evidence-based approach, clinicians can engage patients and families and play a vital role in connecting them with appropriate treatments for children's disruptive behaviors.

REFERENCES

Achenbach, T. M. (2009). *The Achenbach system of empirically based assessment (ASEBA): Development, findings, theory, and applications.* University of Vermont Research Center for Children, Youth, & Families.

American Psychiatric Association (2013). *Diagnostic and statistical manual of mental disorders* (5th ed).

Aizpitarte, A., Atherton, O., & Robins, R. (2017). The co-development of relational aggression and disruptive behavior symptoms from late childhood through adolescence. *Clinical Psychological Science*, *5*(5), 866–873.

Azeredo, A., Moreira, D., & Barbosa, F. (2018). ADHD, CD, and ODD: Systematic review of genetic and environmental risk factors. *Research in Developmental Disabilities*, *82*, 10–19. https://doi.org/10.1016/j.ridd.2017.12.010

Bandura, A. (1973). *Aggression: A social learning analysis*. Prentice-Hall.

Bronfenbrenner, U. (1986). Ecology of the family as a context for human development: Research perspectives. *Developmental Psychology*, *22*(6), 723.

Burke, J. D., Rowe, R., & Boylan, K. (2014). Functional outcomes of child and adolescent oppositional defiant disorder symptoms in young adult men. *Journal of Child Psychology and Psychiatry*, *55*(3), 264–272. https://doi.org/10.1111/jcpp.12150

Campbell, I., Lundstrom, S., Larsson, H., Lichtenstein, P., & Lubke, G. (2019). The relation between the age at diagnosis of problem behaviors related to aggression and distal outcomes in Swedish children. *European Child & Adolescent Psychiatry*, *28*, 899–911. https://doi.org/10.1007/s00787-018-1250-9

Canino, G., Polanczyk, G., Bauermeister, J. J., Rohde, L. A., & Frick, P. J. (2010). Does the prevalence of CD and ODD vary across cultures? *Social Psychiatry and Psychiatric Epidemiology*, *45*(7), 695–704. https://doi.org/10.1007/s00127-010-0242-y

Carliner, H., Gary, D., McLaughlin, K. A., & Keyes, K. M. (2017). Trauma exposure and externalizing disorders in adolescents: Results from the National Comorbidity Survey Adolescent Supplement. *Journal of the American Academy of Child Adolescent Psychiatry*, *56*(9), 755–764.

Crick, N. R., & Dodge, K. A. (1994). A review and reformulation of social information-processing mechanisms in children's social adjustment. *Psychological Bulletin*, *115*(1), 74.

Crick, N. R., & Grotpeter, J. K. (1995). Relational aggression, gender, and social psychological adjustment. *Child Development*, *66*(3), 710–722. https://doi.org/10.1111/j.1467-8624.1995.tb00900.x

Demmer, D. H., Hooley, M., Sheen, J., McGillivray, J. A., & Lum, J. A. G. (2017). Sex differences in the prevalence of oppositional defiant disorder during middle childhood: A meta-analysis. *Journal of Abnormal Child Psychology*, *45*(2), 313–325. https://doi.org/10.1007/s10802-016-0170-8

Eyberg, S. M., & Calzada, E. J. (1998). *Parent-child interaction therapy: Procedures manual*. University of Florida.

Fergusson, D. M., Boden, J. M., & Horwood, L. J. (2009). Situational and generalised conduct problems and later life outcomes: Evidence from a New Zealand birth cohort. *Journal of Child Psychology and Psychiatry*, *50*(9), 1084–1092. https://doi.org/10.1111/j.1469-7610.2009.02070.x

Fite, P. J., Colder, C. R., Lochman, J. E., & Wells, K. C. (2008). Developmental trajectories of proactive and reactive aggression from fifth to ninth grade. *Journal of Clinical Child & Adolescent Psychology*, *37*(2), 412–421.

Fite, P. J., Evans, S. C., Cooley, J. L., & Rubens, S. L. (2014). Further evaluation of associations between attention-deficit/hyperactivity and oppositional defiant disorder symptoms and bullying-victimization in adolescence. *Child Psychiatry & Human Development*, *45*(1), 32–41.

Gadow, K. D., Brown, N. V., Arnold, L. E., Buchan-Page, K. A., Bukstein, O. G., Butter, E., … Aman, M. G. (2016). Severely aggressive children receiving stimulant medication versus stimulant and risperidone: 12-month follow-up of the TOSCA trial. *Journal of the American Academy of Child and Adolescent Psychiatry*, *55*(6), 469–478. https://doi.org/10.1016/j.jaac.2016.03.014

Galán, C. A., Wang, F. L., Shaw, D. S., & Forbes, E. E. (2020). Early childhood trajectories of conduct problems and hyperactivity/attention problems: Predicting adolescent and adult antisocial behavior and internalizing problems. *Journal of Clinical Child & Adolescent Psychology*, *49*(2), 200–214. https://doi.org/10.1080/15374416.2018.1534206

Garaigordobil, M. (2014). Psychology of hatred and violence: Definition, explanatory theories, cognitive-emotional factors and prevention strategies. In A. M. Columbus (Ed.), *Advances in psychology research* (pp. 47–69). Nova Science Publishers, Inc.

Greene, R. W., Ablon, J. S., Goring, J. C., Raezer-Blakely, L., Markey, J., Monuteaux, M. C., … Rabbitt, S. (2004). Effectiveness of collaborative problem solving in affectively dysregulated children with oppositional-defiant disorder: Initial findings. *Journal of Consulting and Clinical Psychology*, *72*(6), 1157–1164.

Henggeler, S. W., Melton, G. B., Brondino, M. J., Scherer, D. G., & Hanley, J. H. (1997). Multisystemic therapy with violent and chronic juvenile offenders and their families: The role of treatment fidelity in successful dissemination. *Journal of Consulting and Clinical Psychology*, *65*, 821–833.

Hymel, S., & Swearer, S. M. (2015). Four decades of research on school bullying: An introduction. *American Psychologist*, *70*(4), 293.

Kamphuis, J., Meerlo, P., Koolhaas, J. M., & Lancel, M. (2012). Poor sleep as a potential causal factor in aggression and violence. *Sleep Medicine*, *13*(4), 327–334. https://doi.org/10.1016/j.sleep.2011.12.006

Khan, S., Down, J., Aouira, N., Bor, W., Haywood, A., Littlewood, R., … McDermott, B. (2019). Current pharmacotherapy options for conduct disorders in adolescents and children. Expert Opinion Pharmacotherapy. *Expert Opinion Pharmacotherapy*, *20*(5), 571–583. doi:10.1080/14656566.2018.1561862

Leff, S. S., Waasdorp, T. E., & Crick, N. R. (2010). A review of existing relational aggression programs: Strengths, limitations, and future directions. *School Psychology Review*, *39*(4), 508–535.

Leff, S. S., Waasdorp, T. E., & Mehari, K. R. (2018). An updated review of existing relational aggression programs. In S. M. Coyne & J. M. Ostrov (Eds.), *The development of relational aggression* (pp. 283–317). Oxford University Press.

Lochman, J. E., & Wells, K. C. (2002). Contextual social-cognitive mediators and child outcome: A test of the theoretical model in the Coping Power Program. *Development and Psychopathology*, *14*, 945–967.

Massing-Schaffer, M., & Nesi, J. (2020). Cybervictimization and suicide risk in adolescence: An integrative model of social media and suicide theories. *Adolescent Research Review*, *5*, 49–65. https://doi.org/10.1007/s40894-019-00116-y

Maughan, B., Rowe, R., Messer, J., Goodman, R., & Meltzer, H. (2004). Conduct disorder and oppositional defiant disorder in a national sample: Developmental epidemiology. *Journal of Child Psychology and Psychiatry*, *45*(3), 609–621.

MTA Cooperative Group. (1999). A 14-month randomized clinical trial of treatment strategies for attention-deficit/hyperactivity disorder. Multimodal treatment study of children with ADHD. *Archives of General Psychiatry*, *56*(12), 1073–1086. https://doi.org/10.1001/archpsyc.56.12.1073

Ollendick, T. H., Greene, R. W., Austin, K. E., Fraire, M. G., Halldorsdottir, T., Allen, K. B., . . . Wolff, J.C. (2015). Parent management training and collaborative & proactive solutions: A randomized control trial for oppositional youth. *Journal of Clinical Child and Adolescent Psychology*, *45*(5), 591–604. https://doi.org/10.1080/15374416.2015.1004681

Pelham, W. E., Gnagy, E. M., Greenslade, K. E., & Milich, R. (1992). Teacher ratings of DSM-III-R symptoms for the disruptive behavior disorders. *Journal of the American Academy of Child and Adolescent Psychiatry*, *31*(2), 210–218.

Pelsser, L. M., Frankena, K., Toorman, J., & Rodrigues Pereira, R. (2017). Diet and ADHD, reviewing the evidence: A systematic review of meta-analyses of double-blind placebo-controlled trials evaluating the efficacy of diet interventions on the behavior of children with ADHD. *PLoS ONE*, *12*(1), e0169277. https://doi.org/10.1371/journal.pone.0169277

Pliszka, S., & AACAP Work Group on Quality Issues. (2007). Practice parameter for the assessment and treatment of children and adolescents with attention-deficit/hyperactivity disorder. *Journal of the American Academy of Child & Adolescent Psychiatry*, *46*(7), 894–921.

Rieffe, C., Broekhof, E., Kouwenberg, M., Faber, J., Tsutsui, M. M., & Güroğlu, B. (2016). Disentangling proactive and reactive aggression in children using self-report. *European Journal of Developmental Psychology*, *13*(4), 439–451. https://doi.org/10.1080/17405629.2015.1109506

Rocque, M., Posick, C., & Felix, S. (2015). The role of the brain in urban violent offending: Integrating biology with structural theories of 'the streets. *Criminal Justice Studies*, *28*(1), 84–103. https://doi.org/10.1080/1478601X.2014.1000006

Sanson, A., & Prior, M. (1999). Temperament and behavioral precursors to oppositional defiant disorder and conduct disorder: *In Handbook of disruptive behavior disorders* (pp. 397–417). Springer.

Shuhman, E. M., Foote, R. C., Eyberg, S. M., Boggs, S., & Algina, J. (1998). Efficacy of parent child interaction therapy: Interim report of a randomized trial with short term maintenance. *Journal of Clinical Child Psychology*, *27*(1), 34–45. https://doi.org/10.1207/s15374424jccp2701_4

Sourander, A., Brunstein Klomek, A., Ikonen, M., Lindroos, J., Luntamo, T., Koskelainen, M., … Helenius, H. (2010). Psychosocial risk factors associated with cyberbullying among adolescents a population-based study. *Archives of General Psychiatry*, *67*(7), 720–728. https://doi.org/10.1001/archgenpsychiatry.2010.79

Substance Abuse and Mental Health Services Administration (SAMHSA). (2011). *Interventions for disruptive behavior disorders: Evidence-based and promising practices.* Center for Mental Health Services, Substance Abuse and Mental Health Services Administration, US Department of Health and Human Services. HHS Pub. No. SMA-11-4634.

Swearer, S. M., & Hymel, S. (2015). Understanding the psychology of bullying: Moving toward a social-ecological diathesis–stress model. *American Psychologist*, *70*(4), 344–353. https://doi.org/10.1037/a0038929

Temcheff, C. E., Serbin, L. A., Martin-Storey, A., Stack, D. M., Ledingham, J., & Schwartzman, A. E. (2011). Predicting adult physical health outcomes from childhood aggression, social withdrawal and likeability: A 30-year prospective, longitudinal study. *International Journal of Behavioral Medicine*, *18*(1), 5–12. https://doi.org/10.1007/s12529-010-9082-0

56

Acute Stress Disorder and Posttraumatic Stress Disorder in Youth

Jason M. Fogler, Amanda Van Scoyoc, Melissa Marquardt, and Randall Phelps

For additional material related to the content of this chapter, please see Chapter 15.

VIGNETTES

1. Single Trauma Incident

Forrest, an 8-year-old boy, and his father sustained minor injuries in an automobile crash (e.g., rubbing marks from the seatbelt, bruises); they were taken to the emergency department by ambulance and released shortly after. Forrest did not report any pain and is medically healthy with no developmental concerns, prior behavioral concerns, or previous traumatic experiences. Forrest does well in school and parents state he is typically a "happy kid." Since the accident, Forrest says that he frequently thinks about the car crash and becomes upset despite trying not to. When he rides in a car he reports a sense that it is going to crash. He often asks his parents if they think they will get in another crash and avoids getting in the car as much as possible, even if it means skipping activities he enjoys. When his parents drive him to school, they avoid the turn where the crash occurred because Forrest starts to cry when they pass that intersection.

2. Complex Trauma

Antonia is an 8-year-old girl removed from her foster home due to experiencing sexual abuse. She disclosed the abuse at school. Antonia had lived with this foster family for 4 months, and her foster father occasionally came into her bedroom and touched her privates. Antonia's biological mother struggled with addiction since before Antonia was born and used methamphetamine while pregnant. Biological father is unknown. Antonia had neonatal abstinence syndrome at birth and spent 2 weeks in the neonatal intensive care unit. Her mother entered a treatment center that allowed Antonia to live with her. Antonia was removed from mother's care at the age of 2.5 years after a neighbor called child welfare. At the welfare check, Antonia was found alone, underweight, in an overly dirty diaper, and in an unsanitary apartment. Antonia was placed in foster care. Since then, she has lived in six foster homes. At one home she was hit repeatedly with a belt. She has been removed from other homes due to disruptive behaviors (e.g., hitting, biting, or destroying objects when upset). At school, she has difficulty paying attention and at times becomes aggressive toward other children, particularly when she feels that she is not being treated fairly. Antonia often delays falling asleep at night and wakes up frequently.

The idea that profoundly disturbing events, particularly war, can fundamentally shudder one's sense of self and felt security in the world was documented as early as the times of ancient Greece and William Shakespeare (Brown, 2020; Sofranac, 2011). War neurosis, or shell shock (renamed "combat stress reaction" after World War II), was the prevailing paradigm for the first half of the 20th century (Linden & Jones, 2014); and the hollow-eyed soldier remains an enduring archetype of psychological trauma through the present. Posttraumatic stress disorder (PTSD) was formally codified in the third edition of the *Diagnostic and Statistical Manual of Mental Disorders* (*DSM-3*; American Psychiatric Association [APA], 1980), and most of our empirical knowledge about this disorder and its treatment came from large-scale studies of Vietnam veterans (e.g., King, King, Foy, Keane, & Fairbank, 1999). Acute stress disorder (AStD), used to describe traumatic stress symptoms (TSS) that last from 3 days to 1 month after an index traumatic event, was codified in 1994 (APA, 1994).

One might reasonably ask how it came to be that a psychiatric condition that was discovered and studied in adult soldiers would become so core to our understanding of child development and societal health. After decades of research we now understand that traumatic experiences in childhood can have a profound impact on development, with pervasive effects on physical and mental health. This is particularly true with repeated traumas or when trauma occurs in the absence of a supportive, nurturing environment (Finkelhor, Ormrod, & Turner, 2007; Herman, 1992a; Terr, 1991). Conversely, the ability to overcome trauma is a remarkable ability that humans possess; but the resources and evidence-based supports that facilitate this process are not equitably distributed. BIPOC (Black, Indigenous, People of Color) communities are more likely to experience recurring trauma and to have relatively fewer resources to support recovery.

AN INTENTIONALLY CIRCUMSCRIBED OVERVIEW

Our chapter reflects this textbook's intentional compartmentalization of reactions to potentially traumatic events (and more broadly, adverse childhood experiences [ACEs]) into three domains: the pervasive and disruptive effects of toxic stress on development and lifelong health (e.g., neighborhood violence, impaired and unpredictable parenting; see Chapters 13–15), the relatively short-lived psychological effects of adjusting to acute

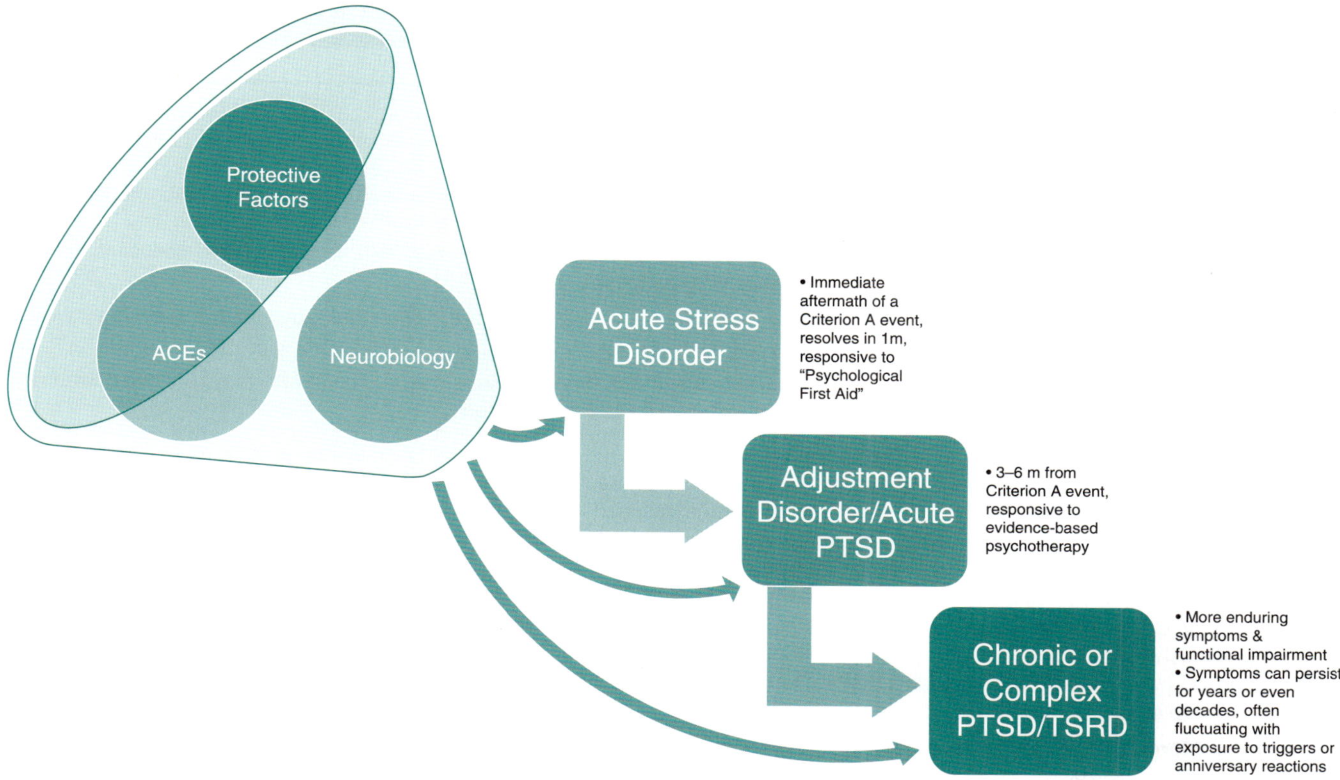

Fig. 56.1 Conceptual model of the relationship between risk and protective factors and different manifestations of acute stress disorder, adjustment disorder, and posttraumatic stress sisorder based on chronicity and severity.

and temporary stressors (see Chapter 57), and our discussion of a thoroughly studied but by no means universal psychobiologic reaction to horrific events, namely PTSD and AStD. Although widespread events, such as war and natural disaster, certainly increase one's risk for developing the characteristic symptoms of PTSD (See Chapter 22), PTSD is only one of many possible responses; recovery and resilience are far more common (Bonnano & Mancini, 2008). Fig. 56.1 offers a conceptual map for how these related phenomena fit together, with three categories of trauma and stressor-related disorders (TRSD: AStD, adjustment disorder/acute PTSD, and chronic or complex PTSD) being differentiated by duration and severity of symptoms—and all three are moderated by the presence or absence of protective factors, ACEs (see Chapter 15), and genetic and neurobiologic vulnerabilities (see Pharmacotherapy for Traumatic Stress [later] and McCullough and Ressler [2018] for an excellent review). We concede that this figure in no way can do justice to the relative strength of each factor's effect—alone or in moderated/mediated relationships with other factors—and complicated gene × environment interactions that go into this illustrated funnel of cascading developmental trajectories.

PHENOMENOLOGY

Since PTSD was first codified based on epidemiologic and psychometric research with samples of combat veterans and survivors of car accidents and single-event natural disasters (Breslau, 2001), three core symptom clusters have held constant through three editions of the *DSM* (Table 56.1): (1) reexperiencing in the form of nightmares, flashbacks, and intrusive memories; (2) avoidance of traumatic reminders and emotional numbing; and (3) exaggerated startle and hypervigilance. A new symptom cluster, dysphoric mood and negative sense of self and the future, was added in *DSM-5* based on psychometric evidence from large-scale confirmatory factor analyses (Friedman, Resick, Bryant, & Brewin, 2011).

AStD is conferred when any nine symptoms of the four symptom clusters (plus a fifth, dissociation, essentially a psychic disconnection from one's lived experience that is also exhibited in cases of PTSD) occur for 3 days to 1 month following an index traumatic event (Table 56.2). Adjustment disorder is conferred when very similar symptoms persist for 6 months following a stressful event that is not deemed to be traumatic (i.e., life threatening, such as parental divorce or moving to a new community) (see Chapter 57).

PTSD, AStD, and the family of TSRD by extension are distinguished from all other mental health conditions by the requirement of a "burden of proof" or clearly defined index event: the criterion A traumatic stressor. Once strictly defined as an event that needed to happen to the person directly, such as war or violent crime, the definition has been extended to include traumatic events that are more likely to happen to children: separation from an attachment figure, witnessed harm to another person, and inappropriate touching by an adult. More so, the criteria are more relevant to children in that they no longer require the ability to clearly articulate a

TABLE 56.1 Acute Stress Disorder

Diagnostic Criteria **308.3**

A. Exposure to actual or threatened death, serious injury, or sexual violence in one (or more) of the following ways

1. Directly experiencing the traumatic event(s)
2. Witnessing, in person, the event(s) as it occurred to others
3. Learning that the event(s) occurred to a close family member or close friend **Note:** In cases of actual or threatened death of a family member or friend, the event(s) must have been violent or accidental
4. Experiencing repeated or extreme exposure to aversive details of the traumatic event(s) (e g , first responders collecting human remains, police officers repeatedly exposed to details of child abuse).

Note: This does not apply to exposure through electronic media, television, movies, or pictures, unless this exposure is work related.

B. Presence of nine (or more) of the following symptoms from any of the five categories of intrusion, negative mood, dissociation, avoidance, and arousal, beginning or worsening after the traumatic event(s) occurred

Intrusion Symptoms

1. Recurrent, involuntary, and intrusive distressing memories of the traumatic event(s) **Note:** In children, repetitive play may occur in which themes or aspects of the traumatic event(s) are expressed
2. Recurrent distressing dreams in which the content and/or affect of the dream are related to the event(s) **Note:** In children, there may be frightening dreams without recognizable content
3. Dissociative reactions (e.g , flashbacks) in which the individual feels or acts as if the traumatic event(s) were recurring (Such reactions may occur on a continuum, with the most extreme expression being a complete loss of awareness of present surroundings) **Note:** In children, trauma-specific reenactment may occur in play
4. Intense or prolonged psychological distress or marked physiological reactions in response to internal or external cues that symbolize or resemble an aspect of the traumatic event(s)

Negative Mood

5. Persistent inability to experience positive emotions (e g , inability to experience happiness, satisfaction, or loving feelings)

Dissociative Symptoms

6. An altered sense of the reality of one's surroundings or oneself (e g , seeing oneself from another's perspective, being in a daze, time slowing).
7. Inability to remember an important aspect of the traumatic event(s) (typically due to dissociative amnesia and not to other factors such as head injury, alcohol, or drugs)

Avoidance Symptoms

8. Efforts to avoid distressing memories, thoughts, or feelings about or closely associated with the traumatic event(s)
9. Efforts to avoid external reminders (people, places, conversations, activities, objects, situations) that arouse distressing memories, thoughts, or feelings about or closely associated with the traumatic event(s)

Arousal Symptoms

10. Sleep disturbance (e.g , difficulty falling or staying asleep, restless sleep).
11. Irritable behavior and angry outbursts (with little or no provocation), typically expressed as verbal or physical aggression toward people or objects.
12. Hypervigilance
13. Problems with concentration
14. Exaggerated startle response.

C. Duration of the disturbance (symptoms in Criterion B) is 3 days to 1 month after trauma exposure

Note: Symptoms typically begin immediately after the trauma, but persistence for at least 3 days and up to a month is needed to meet disorder criteria

D. The disturbance causes clinically significant distress or impairment in social, occupational, or other important areas of functioning

E. The disturbance is not attributable to the physiological effects of a substance (e g, medication or alcohol) or another medical condition (e g , mild traumatic brain injury) and is not better explained by brief psychotic disorder

sense of overwhelming horror as a consequence of the event (Friedman et al., 2011).

Exposure to traumatic stress in childhood leads to a wide range of reactions. The traumatic experience itself can be identified as an experience that leads to a sense of helplessness, loss of control, inability to manage the overwhelming emotional response, and dysregulation leading to changes in thinking, feeling, and acting (Epstein et al., 2017). The experience of trauma is common with most children encountering a potentially traumatic event by the age of 18 (Felitti et al., 1998). In a cross-sectional survey designed to estimate youth exposure to trauma in the United States 60%

TABLE 56.2 Posttraumatic Stress Disorder

Diagnostic Criteria **309.81**

Posttraumatic Stress Disorder

Note: The following criteria apply to adults, adolescents, and children older than 6 years For children 6 years and younger, see corresponding criteria below

A. Exposure to actual or threatened death, serious injury, or sexual violence in one (or more) of the following ways
   1. Directly experiencing the traumatic event(s).
   2. Witnessing, in person, the event(s) as it occurred to others
   3. Learning that the traumatic event(s) occurred to a close family member or close friend In cases of actual or threatened death of a family member or friend, the event(s) must have been violent or accidental
   4. Experiencing repeated or extreme exposure to aversive details of the traumatic event(s) (e g , first responders collecting human remains; police officers repeatedly exposed to details of child abuse)

      Note: Criterion A4 does not apply to exposure through electronic media, television, movies, or pictures, unless this exposure is work related

B. Presence of one (or more) of the following intrusion symptoms associated with the traumatic event(s), beginning after the traumatic event(s) occurred
   1. Recurrent, involuntary, and intrusive distressing memories of the traumatic event(s)

      Note: In children older than 6 years, repetitive play may occur in which themes or aspects of the traumatic event(s) are expressed
   2. Recurrent distressing dreams in which the content and/or affect of the dream are related to the traumatic event(s)

      Note: In children, there may be frightening dreams without recognizable content
   3. Dissociative reactions (e g , flashbacks) in which the individual feels or acts as if the traumatic event(s) were recurring (Such reactions may occur on a continuum, with the most extreme expression being a complete loss of awareness of present surroundings)

      Note: In children, trauma-specific reenactment may occur in play
   4. Intense or prolonged psychological distress at exposure to internal or external cues that symbolize or resemble an aspect of the traumatic event(s)
   5. Marked physiological reactions to internal or external cues that symbolize or resemble an aspect of the traumatic event(s)

C. Persistent avoidance of stimuli associated with the traumatic event(s), beginning after the traumatic event(s) occurred, as evidenced by one or both of the following
   1. Avoidance of or efforts to avoid distressing memories, thoughts, or feelings about or closely associated with the traumatic event(s)
   2. Avoidance of or efforts to avoid external reminders (people, places, conversations, activities, objects, situations) that arouse distressing memories, thoughts, or feelings about or closely associated with the traumatic event(s)

D. Negative alterations in cognitions and mood associated with the traumatic event(s), beginning or worsening after the traumatic event(s) occurred, as evidenced by two (or more) of the following
   1. Inability to remember an impdrtant aspect of the traumatic event(s) (typically due to dissociative amnesia and not to other factors such as head injury, alcohol, or drugs)
   2. Persistent and exaggerated negative beliefs or expectations about oneself, others, or the world (e g, "I am bad," "No one can be trusted," "The world is completely dangerous," "My whole nervous system is permanently ruined").
   3. Persistent, distorted cognitions about the cause or consequences of the traumatic event(s) that lead the individual to blame himself/herself or others
   4. Persistent negative emotional state (e g , fear, horror, anger, guilt, or shame)
   5. Markedly diminished interest or participation in significant activities.
   6. Feelings of detachment or estrangement from others
   7. Persistent inability to experience positive emotions (e g , inability to experience happiness, satisfaction, or loving feelings)

E. Marked alterations in arousal and reactivity associated with the traumatic event(s), beginning or worsening after the traumatic event(s) occurred, as evidenced by two (or more) of the following.
   1. Irritable behavior and angry outbursts (with little or no provocation) typically expressed as verbal or physical aggression toward people or objects
   2. Reckless or self-destructive behavior
   3. Hypervigilance
   4. Exaggerated startle response
   5. Problems with concentration
   6. Sleep disturbance (e g , difficulty falling or staying asleep or restless sleep)

TABLE 56.2 Posttraumatic Stress Disorder —Cont'd

Diagnostic Criteria **309.81**

F. Duration of the disturbance (Criteria B, C, D, and E) is more than 1 month
G. The disturbance causes clinically significant distress or impairment in social, occupational, or other important areas of functioning
H. The disturbance is not attributable to the physiological effects of a substance (e g , medication, alcohol) or another medical condition

Specify whether

With dissociative symptoms: The individual's symptoms meet the criteria for post-traumatic stress disorder, and in addition, in response to the stressor, the individual experiences persistent or recurrent symptoms of either of the following

1. **Depersonalization:** Persistent or recurrent experiences of feeling detached from, and as if one were an outside observer of, one's mental processes or body (e g , feeling as though one were in a dream, feeling a sense of unreality of self or body or of time moving slowly).
2. **Derealization:** Persistent or recurrent experiences of unreality of surroundings (e g , the world around the individual is experienced as unreal, dreamlike, distant, or distorted)

Note: To use this subtype, the dissociative symptoms must not be attributable to the physiological effects of a substance (e g , blackouts, behavior during alcohol intoxication) or another medical condition (e g., complex partial seizures).

Specify if

With delayed expression: If the full diagnostic criteria are not met until at least 6 months after the event (although the onset and expression of some symptoms may be immediate).

Posttraumatic Stress Disorder for Children 6 Years and Younger

A. In children 6 years and younger, exposure to actual or threatened death, serious injury, or sexual violence in one (or more) of the following ways
   1. Directly experiencing the traumatic event(s)
   2. Witnessing, in person, the event(s) as it occurred to others, especially primary care givers

      Note: Witnessing does not include events that are witnessed only in electronic media, television, movies, or pictures
   3. Learning that the traumatic event(s) occurred to a parent or caregiving figure

B. Presence of one (or more) of the following intrusion symptoms associated with the traumatic event(s), beginning after the traumatic event(s) occurred.
   1. Recurrent, involuntary, and intrusive distressing memories of the traumatic event(s)

      Note: Spontaneous and intrusive memories may not necessarily appear distressing and may be expressed as play reenactment
   2. Recurrent distressing dreams in which the content and/or affect of the dream are related to the traumatic event(s)

      Note: It may not be possible to ascertain that the frightening content is related to the traumatic event
   3. Dissociative reactions (e g , flashbacks) in which the child feels or acts as if the traumatic event(s) were recurring. (Such reactions may occur on a continuum, with the most extreme expression being a complete loss of awareness of present surroundings) Such trauma-specific reenactment may occur in play
   4. Intense or prolonged psychological distress at exposure to internal or external cues that symbolize or resemble an aspect of the traumatic event(s)
   5. Marked physiological reactions to reminders of the traumatic event(s)

C. One (or more) of the following symptoms, representing either persistent avoidance of stimuli associated with the traumatic event(s) or negative alterations in cognitions and mood associated with the traumatic event(s), must be present, beginning after the event(s) or worsening after the event(s)

   Persistent Avoidance of Stimuli

   1. Avoidance of or efforts to avoid activities, places, or physical reminders that arouse recollections of the traumatic event(s)
   2. Avoidance of or efforts to avoid people, conversations, or interpersonal situations that arouse recollections of the traumatic event(s)

   Negative Alterations in Cognitions

   3. Substantially increased frequency of negative emotional states (e g , fear, guilt, sadness, shame, confusion)
   4. Markedly diminished interest or participation in significant activities, including constriction of play
   5. Socially withdrawn behavior.
   6. Persistent reduction in expression of positive emotions

(*Continued*)

TABLE 56.2 Posttraumatic Stress Disorder—Cont'd

Diagnostic Criteria	**309.81**
D. Alterations in arousal and reactivity associated with the traumatic event(s), beginning or worsening after the traumatic event(s) occurred, as evidenced by two (or more) of the following 1. Irritable behavior and angry outbursts (with little or no provocation) typically expressed as verbal or physical aggression toward people or objects (including extreme temper tantrums) 2. Hypervigilance 3. Exaggerated startle response 4. Problems with concentration 5. Sleep disturbance (e.g , difficulty falling or staying asleep or restless sleep) F. The duration of the disturbance is more than 1 month G. The disturbance causes clinically significant distress or impairment in relationships with parents, siblings, peers, or other caregivers or with school behavior. H. The disturbance is not attributable to the physiological effects of a substance (e g , medication or alcohol) or another medical condition *Specify whether* **With dissociative symptoms:** The individual's symptoms meet the criteria for posttraumatic stress disorder, and the individual experiences persistent or recurrent symptoms of either of the following 1. **Depersonalization:** Persistent or recurrent experiences of feeling detached from, and as if one were an outside observer of, one's mental processes or body (e g , feeling as though one were in a dream; feeling a sense of unreality of self or body or of time moving slowly) 2. **Derealization:** Persistent or recurrent experiences of unreality of surroundings (e g , the world around the individual is experienced as unreal, dreamlike, distant, or distorted) **Note:** To use this subtype, the dissociative symptoms must not be attributable to the physiological effects of a substance (e g , blackouts) or another medical condition (e g., complex partial seizures) *Specify* if **With delayed expression:** If the full diagnostic criteria are not met until at least 6 months after the event (although the onset and expression of some symptoms may be immediate).	

of children and adolescents had experienced a traumatic incident in the past year, with approximately 10% experiencing a form of child maltreatment, 6% experiencing a sexual victimization, and 46% experiencing a physical assault (Finkelhor, Turner, Ormrod, & Hamby, 2009).

In many instances children recover well from potentially traumatic experiences, and the experience of an event alone does not necessitate diagnosis or the need for treatment. After identifying that a child or adolescent has experienced a trauma, one should identify how recently the incident occurred and whether the child has a history of experiencing chronic or repeated exposure to environmental stress or has had a more discrete traumatic incident. Posttraumatic reactions can be thought of as occurring in three phases. Initially there is the acute phase in the immediate aftermath (hours) after the incident has occurred. Next is the peritraumatic phase lasting for the first few weeks, followed by the posttraumatic phase.

During the acute phase, children respond in many different ways to the experience of being overwhelmed. Some children scream, cry, cling to their parents, or otherwise display strong emotions. Other children may seem particularly calm or withdrawn. Although their behavior may be less visible, children who respond with decreased emotional reactivity and avoidance are also having traumatic stress reactions and may require supportive treatment. During the acute phase, intervention focuses on stabilization and meeting logistical needs for families and children in crisis (Epstein, Hahn, Berkowitz, & Marans, 2017).

After the immediate aftermath of the incident is the peritraumatic period, which lasts for the first few weeks. During this period of time, posttraumatic symptoms are often very prominent and can cause dramatic changes in how a child is thinking, feeling, and behaving. Fortunately, during the peritraumatic period, symptoms are also more flexible, and interventions can be particularly effective at decreasing posttraumatic reactions (Berkowitz, Stover, & Marans, 2011).

In the posttraumatic phase, with greater time since the traumatic incident, symptoms have become solidified; and prolonged traumatic stress reactions have likely had a much stronger impact on development, adaptive functioning, sense of self, personality, and engagement in the world. Posttraumatic challenges often require more intensive interventions that also consider how the trauma experience has impacted beliefs about the self, world, and future.

Some children experience a single acute trauma, as in the opening vignette about Forrest (e.g., dog bite, car accident, wildfire), in the context of developing in an otherwise supportive environment. However, in cases of complex trauma represented by Antonia's vignette, children grow up in the context of multiple or ongoing traumatic experiences that lead to wide-ranging developmental and interpersonal challenges. For example, children who are in foster care may have grown up in a household where they witnessed domestic violence, substance abuse, and inconsistent caregiving due to mental illness. While in the foster care system, they may also have to manage the trauma of multiple caregiver transitions and intermittent exposure to unstable birth parents. These types of ongoing experiences can disrupt their ability to form a secure attachment with their caregivers and ultimately prevent expected developmental trajectories by undermining the development of self-regulation skills and formation of interpersonal relatedness (Cook et al., 2017). With these impaired capacities for self-regulation and relationships, children with complex trauma often meet criteria for other diagnoses, including depression, attention-deficit/hyperactivity disorder (ADHD), oppositional defiant disorder (ODD), anxiety disorders, and conduct disorder (see Differential Diagnosis, later).

CONCEPTUALIZATION AND ASSESSMENT

History of PTSD Diagnostic Conceptualization

When PTSD was first officially introduced into the *DSM-3*, it was conceptualized within the framework of anxiety and fear, falling under the "anxiety disorder" category, and remained under that classification until the publication of the *DSM-5* in 2013. As such, early conceptualizations of PTSD revolved around a fear-based understanding of trauma and TSS (DiMauro, Carter, Folk, & Kashdan, 2014). As conceptualization of PTSD progressed, Keane and Barlow (2002) proposed a triple vulnerability model to explain the development of PTSD based on the presence of preexisting psychological variables, preexisting biologic variables, and the experience of a traumatic event.

Within the triple vulnerability model, someone who has such preexisting vulnerabilities and is then exposed to a traumatic event is more susceptible to the classical conditioning process thought to be responsible for TSS. The traumatic event is considered to be a true alarm that triggers a fear response in the individual. Under the principles of classical conditioning, this fear response is then extended to learned events. Fear becomes associated with stimuli that were present during the actual trauma, such as certain smells or sounds, as well as through stimulus generalization, which broadens the scope of stimuli that elicits the fear response (Keane, Marshall, & Taft, 2006). For example, a child who was in a car that crashed may find himself fearful not only of being in moving vehicles but may also have a fear response when playing with toy cars or even reading books about automobiles. While preexisting variables were considered, they were not strongly emphasized in the conceptualization of PTSD, and the emphasis was on the learned fear response and symptoms that appeared clearly related to the triggering event.

This framework of PTSD is consistent with the conceptualization of how a fear response develops in anxiety disorders such as specific phobias. With phobias, the etiology is often a negative experience with the phobic object or experience (e.g., loud barking dog), which leads to the continued fear response toward the object (e.g., fear of dogs). Thus it is easy to understand how PTSD was classified under the umbrella of "anxiety disorders" in earlier versions of the DSM. However, rather than developing from an association with a perceived threat, as is the case with other anxiety disorders, experience of an actual threat (criterion A) is central to the diagnosis of PTSD.

Trauma reactions in children often vary from this fear-based conceptualization and include withdrawal, avoidance, irritability, clinginess, or even truancy (Van der Kolk, 2005). While a learning-based model provides a strong conceptualization for the trauma response in certain acute cases of PTSD, particularly with a singular traumatic event as in the case of Forrest, this model does not provide a strong conceptualization for many of the traumatic experiences that children have (e.g., loss of relationship with caregiver, witnessing domestic violence, fear of neighborhood violence). A separate conceptualization of PTSD and the trauma response was needed to account for the larger array of traumatic stress reactions, particularly in children who experienced repeated traumas in their childhood that impacted the course of their development. In recognition that not all traumatic stress responses involve a fear-based style of responding, the *DSM-5* broadened the definition of PTSD to include emotional reactions to trauma.

Among practitioners, attempts have been made to categorize traumatic responses based on the nature of the trauma experienced. Conceptually, two main trauma types have been discussed in the literature (Terr, 1991). Type I trauma maps onto the description of acute trauma described earlier in the chapter and occurs from a single-incident event. A type I trauma may lead to development of AStD rather than PTSD, especially when intervention happens in the peritraumatic period. PTSD that develops subsequent to a type I trauma is often easier for practitioners to identify, and many individuals may have presented for care knowing their symptoms are related to the specific traumatic event.

Type II trauma is the result of longstanding or repeated traumatic events, is usually interpersonal in nature, and often involves significant betrayal of trust within the primary caregiving relationship. Type II trauma has also been referred to as complex trauma, leading to complex PTSD (C-PTSD)—not a formal diagnostic term in the *DSM-5* (Herman, 1992b). Symptoms of C-PTSD extend beyond the primary symptoms observed in PTSD and include difficulty in emotion regulation, changes in the perception of reality, changes in self-perception (e.g. shame, guilt, helplessness, difference from others), preoccupation with revenge, isolation, withdrawal, and persistent distrust, and a loss of faith and/or sense of hopelessness. Van der Kolk (2005) extended this conceptualization into a developmental framework, introducing the term developmental trauma disorder (see Chapter 15 for details). It is important to note, however briefly, that this conceptualization emerged alongside the ACEs study, which has played a significant role in advancing our understanding of how common ACEs are and their widespread consequences for physical and mental health (Centers for Disease Control and Prevention, 2020). C-PTSD may be harder to identify than acute PTSD, given the wider range of symptom presentation. Further, an individual may be less aware that the experiences count as a trauma and may seek care for other concerns such as learning or attentional difficulties (Prock & Fogler, 2018).

Conceptualization of PTSD also advanced alongside studies focused on the complex neurobiologic impact of trauma, including alterations in both the central and autonomic nervous systems (De Bellis, 2005; also refer to Pharmacotherapy for Traumatic Stress [later] for more in-depth discussion). Of particular note, neurobiologic research has identified that trauma is often associated with alterations in the hypothalamic-pituitary-adrenal (HPA) axis, suggesting substantial impact on how individuals respond to stress, among other effects. Trauma interferes with the ability to integrate sensory, emotional, and cognitive information. When these systems are altered it is common to see increased physiologic arousal, disrupted sleep, and difficulties with emotion and behavior regulation. Research suggests that these neurobiologic changes help explain the wide array of TSS, especially in individuals with C-PTSD (Kuhlman, Vargas, Geiss, & Lopez-Duran, 2015). Antonia, from the second vignette, is an example of a child who was exposed to ongoing trauma early in her childhood. Her behaviors are not fully explained by a more traditional fear-based conceptualization of trauma. Rather, her behaviors map onto likely alterations in her neurobiology as a result of her early history.

The triple vulnerability model in many ways laid the foundation for the now generally accepted notion that preexisting psychological and biologic variables contribute to how likely an individual is to develop PTSD. As in Fig. 56.1 (earlier), the impact of ACEs research and the general acceptance of C-PTSD further expands on this conceptualization by identifying the impact of environmental factors as either risk or protective factors for a traumatic stress response. Growing evidence implicates physical proximity to the trauma, previous trauma exposure, biologic factors, sociocultural factors, parental trauma history, and parental trauma-related distress as risk factors in not only the development of PTSD and AStD but also the severity and duration of the traumatic stress response (American Academy of Child and Adolescent Psychiatry, 1998).

Diagnosis

While establishing whether a traumatic event (criterion A) occurred can be straightforward in the case of someone presenting for care after experiencing a discrete traumatic event, as in the case of Forrest in the first vignette, identifying or being cognizant to explore a possible criterion A event can be more complicated in cases of C-PTSD; a thorough developmental history and trauma interview is often needed (Prock & Fogler, 2018). Antonia, in the second vignette, presents as a combination of these two scenarios: her disclosed abuse at school constitutes a clear criterion A event, but without a complete developmental history, a clinician would have been unaware of either the full extent of her trauma history or her biologic vulnerability.

Once criterion A has been established, diagnosis of PTSD or AStD relies on the presence of symptoms within the symptom clusters summarized in Tables 56.1 and 56.2: reexperiencing symptoms (criterion B), avoidance of reminders of the trauma (criterion C), alterations in cognitions or mood (criterion D), and physiologic arousal symptoms (criterion E). To meet diagnostic criteria for PTSD, symptoms must be present from each of the symptom clusters for greater than 1 month after the experience of the traumatic event and must result in functional impairment. Acute stress responses immediately following a traumatic event often present in diverse ways. To account for this variation in experience, an individual must display at least 9 of 14 symptoms (from any of the four PTSD symptom clusters) to meet criteria for AStD; there is no requirement for symptoms to be present within each cluster, as is required for a diagnosis of PTSD. Symptoms must be present for 3 days to 1 month after the traumatic event and cause functional impairment.

In some cases of acute trauma TSS may be fairly straightforward. However, as previously discussed, TSRDs vary based on a number of different aspects, including whether a child experienced a single traumatic event or has a history of complex trauma. In addition, traumatic stress reactions differ based on the developmental stage of the child. Understanding the wide spectrum of reactions that children can have is a starting point for assessment as well as differential diagnosis. For some children, diagnosis may focus on whether reactions to a single trauma are leading to significant challenges in everyday life in the context of an otherwise unremarkable developmental trajectory. For a child with a history of complex trauma, assessment may identify traumatic stress reactions to the most recent or worst trauma (Prock & Fogler, 2018) or may consider the ways that living within the context of ongoing multiple traumas impacted key aspects of development, as in the case for Antonia.

For children whose developmental trajectories are altered by ongoing overwhelming experiences, challenges across many areas of functioning can lead to difficulties with differential diagnosis. For example, a child who did not learn to manage overwhelming emotional states due to growing up in the context of unsupportive caregiving relationships or ongoing trauma (e.g., domestic violence, physical abuse) may in adolescence present with difficulties related to the underdeveloped capacity to self-regulate. When a child with this difficulty experiences overwhelming emotions (e.g., when angered by a teacher at school), rather than seeking support from others or having the ability to self-soothe, this child may act out in anger and frustration leading to consequences at school (e.g., detention or expulsion) and a diagnosis of ODD or conduct disorder. In many instances the experience of early trauma may explain the etiology of complex challenges and multiple diagnoses related to poorly developed regulatory skills. Thus it is particularly important when conducting an assessment to carefully consider differential diagnosis of PTSD or AStD and common comorbid diagnoses.

Differential Diagnosis

Aside from differentiating PTSD or AStD from other TSRD it is important to be aware of the overlap between PTSD symptoms in children and other common childhood disorders. While information in this section is provided to help with differentiating between PTSD and other common childhood disorders, it is important to note that there is a high rate of co-occurrence between PTSD and other psychological disorders. For this reason, using the phrase "differential diagnosis" may be a bit misleading. Comorbidity is common with PTSD and other psychological conditions, with rates estimated to be as high as 80% to 90% (Scheeringa, Zeanah, Myers, & Putnam, 2003). Thus it is important for clinicians to be aware of the most common comorbid diagnoses to help guide a comprehensive assessment and accurate diagnosis. In preschool-aged children the most common comorbidity is with ODD and separation anxiety disorder. Other psychological disorders that are often either comorbid or commonly misdiagnosed among the pediatric population with PTSD include ADHD and autism spectrum disorder (Famularo, Fenton, Kinscherff, & Augustyn, 1996). Please refer to the online supplemental material for a summary of symptom overlap and/or differential diagnosis considerations between PTSD and common comorbid or misdiagnosed disorders.

Assessment

Children at different ages express trauma-related distress and dysregulation in different ways based on their stage of development. At all ages, it is important to consider that the traumatic experience often leads to changes in routines and relationships, and that these changes can be particularly disruptive for children. Indeed, such changes as removal from a primary care provider or no longer being allowed to leave home due to parents' fear of danger may have as significant an impact on a child as the traumatic experience itself.

For babies and young toddlers, distress signals following a traumatic incident often include changes to eating, sleeping, fussiness, and withdrawal, which serve as general indicators of self-regulation at this age. For these very young children, the connection to a safe, stable, and nurturing caregiver with whom they can form an attachment is key to healthy development. When early life stress disrupts this relationship (e.g., caregiver is less engaged due to own mental health struggles, complete disruption due to caregiver death), infants demonstrate disruptions in their regulation. Research suggests that even moderate early life stress can impact infants' brain development and emotional reactions (Graham, Pfeifer, Fisher, Carpenter, & Fair, 2015). Older toddlers and young preschoolers are more independent and understand themselves as being separate from their caregiver. At this age, common traumatic stress reactions include increased fussiness, clinginess to caregivers, skill regression (e.g., having more toileting accidents, no longer sleeping through the night), withdrawal, increased tantrums, and increased fear.

In preschoolers and beyond screening should consider traumatic stress reactions in the following areas: behavioral challenges (including aggression), interpersonal challenges, irritability, physiologic hyperarousal, intrusive thoughts (e.g., thinking about the incident when not wanting to), and avoidance (e.g., school refusal if the incident occurred at school, avoiding thinking or talking about the event). In preschoolers and early grade school children also often express trauma reactions with increased clinginess to caregivers. They may also express worries and fears, report nightmares, have tantrums, demonstrate decreased ability to sustain attention, exhibit irritability and regressed behaviors, complain of physical pain, or withdraw socially from friends and/or family. For some children, school or preschool teachers may notice differences in the classroom, and it is often helpful to ask for input from these care providers.

In older grade school and high school changes in school performance, school refusal, or lack of interest in activities or hobbies can often be notable. Mood changes can include increased anxiety, depression, anger, irritability, or anhedonia. As discussed, these challenges, unless considered in the context of the traumatic experience, can look quite similar to such diagnoses as ADHD, depression, anxiety, ODD, or conduct disorder. Unless teachers have an understanding of the impact of trauma, children's challenges may be compounded by teachers' negative responses to poor behavior in the classroom (Szarkowski & Fogler, 2020). In adolescence challenges can also include problematic and unsafe behaviors, including lying, stealing, truancy, engaging in unsafe sexual encounters, physical fighting, and substance use. This can lead to significant difficulties at home, in school, and with the justice system, especially in BIPOC communities where people disproportionately experience both higher rates of ACEs and bias in the justice system in a terrible feedback loop.

When identifying the way that a child is responding to a traumatic incident, it is important to first have the child's stage of development in mind. Questions are best asked of both the parent and the child (once the child is developmentally able to respond to questions). A good first interview question can be to ask if the caregiver has noticed any differences in how the child is thinking, feeling, and acting. Follow-up questions can consider more specific reactions (see, for example, NCTSN.org). When talking with parents and children about the child's reactions, it is important to specifically inquire about typical TSS, which (1) helps identify whether the child is having trauma reactions while (2) supporting the caregiver in noticing these behavioral changes (and understanding that they are related to the traumatic experience). Interviewing also helps the child/teenager to begin to organize the dysregulated experience and TSS in relation to the traumatic event.

As previously discussed, determining the criterion A traumatic event can be a critically helpful step when identifying whether a child is having specific traumatic stress reactions, but this may not always be possible. In some instances the traumatic event may be readily apparent and perhaps part of the reason for the referral. Even when the recent traumatic event is identified, completing a trauma history is a best practice to identify whether the child has experienced multiple traumas and has a history suggestive of complex trauma. Even when trauma is not a part of the referral, frequently children present with TSS, necessitating a differential diagnosis that considers PTSD/AStD. Questionnaires are helpful both when asking about the child's trauma history and when identifying whether a child is having specific traumatic stress reactions (see online supplemental material). When identifying whether the child has a trauma history, if there is a history of conflict or perpetration of abuse between the parent and child, it is very important that they are separated when these questions are asked. In most instances it is helpful to hear the child's and parents' perspectives, even when there is a supportive relationship. The child may have had experiences that have not been shared with the parent or, alternatively, the child may not be aware of one's own experiences in early childhood.

It is important to note that during the screening for posttraumatic reactions this is not an opportunity to ask the child for a narrative of the traumatic experience. Having a child recount the incident will often lead to an increase in TSS with accompanied distress, which in turn increases challenges with engagement in sessions. Instead, more detailed information about the incident can be provided by the parents or other adults, and complete details may not be necessary to begin treatment. If a child begins to tell the trauma narrative, it is important to contain the story, listening but letting the child know that you do not need to know the details but that you would like to know how the experience is currently impacting the child. With many therapies the child will eventually develop a trauma narrative, but only after first developing significant coping skills and being slowly exposed to thinking about the traumatic event in a safe, containing environment that is simultaneously buffered and titrated.

TREATMENT

Until recently (APA, 2013), PTSD was clustered with the anxiety disorders and treated accordingly through a rigorous form of systematic desensitization known as flooding, later to be administered in a more graduated manner under the name *prolonged exposure*. Combat veterans might be asked to recount the story of witnessed violent deaths in excruciating detail while recordings of helicopters and bombs played in the background. Our understanding of TSRD, and more humane ways to treat it, has evolved considerably in the last 40 years. These methods include using distraction to make the experiential exposure more bearable, as in the case of eye movement desensitization and response (EMDR; Bradley et al., 2005); using meditation-based grounding techniques, as in the case of dialectical behavior therapy for traumatic stress (Ritschel, Lim, & Stewart, 2015); and orienting one's life toward preferred values, such as community, forgiveness, or love, despite traumatic experiences (as in the case of acceptance and commitment therapy; McMackin, Newman, Fogler, & Keane, 2012). Nonetheless, nonresponse and dropout from treatment remain longstanding challenges, in part because of the stress and psychological discomfort inherent in these treatments (Schottenbauer, Glass, Arnkoff, Tendick, & Hafter Gray, 2008).

Overall Approach: Support Emotional Regulation

In the acute phase if (1) the trauma is ongoing (e.g., a painful medical treatment, being removed from parents) or happened within the last few hours, or (2) children are expressing strong emotional reactions or appear in distress, it can be helpful to (3) name for them what you see (e.g., I see that you are crying) and (4) provide skills to calm the physiologic reactions that they are experiencing. The immediate goal is stabilization of symptoms. General coregulation strategies that can be helpful include doing simple drawing exercises together (e.g., drawing a spiral), taking deep breaths together, or having them focus on their senses like the coolness of an offered drink or the way that their body is feeling. Asking a symptomatic child to discuss the traumatic incident is likely to increase symptoms and lead to further destabilization.

In the immediate aftermath of a potentially traumatic event children may be worried about their own safety and their future. It can be helpful to remind them that they are safe now, describe immediately pertinent logistics (e.g., your aunt is on the way to the hospital and will take you back to her house tonight), and ask if the child has any questions. Questions should be answered truthfully, considering the child's developmental level, and in a way that continues to help establish a sense of trust, transparency, and safety. For example, in the immediate aftermath of a fire if a child asked if his house burned down, one might say, "We don't know yet, but the firemen will go and check when it is safe enough. Tonight, you will go to a shelter with your mom and dad. There will be clothes for you there and a bed for you to sleep in. Do you have any other questions or things that you are worrying about?" Following a potentially traumatic incident, parents sometimes struggle to talk with their children about difficult truths and may avoid having challenging conversations. It can be helpful to suggest wording to parents about how to talk with their child about what happened or offer to have that conversation together with the child.

Psychosocial Treatments for Traumatic Stress

It is much more common to provide care after a traumatic incident has occurred. In the peritraumatic period traumatic stress reactions are often particularly high but also more likely to decrease rapidly with intervention. For this reason, if a child is experiencing traumatic stress reactions, it is ideal to refer the child for trauma-informed treatment by a care provider who has experience working with children during the peritraumatic period and who has immediate openings for care. The reader is referred to the online supplemental material for a sampling of key evidence-based psychotherapies for pediatric TSRD, but it is offered with an important caveat: this level of detail can lead to difficulties when identifying appropriate services for specific children. In many areas of the country, particularly more rural areas, it may not be realistic to identify a provider who is trained in the ideal intervention for a particular client. Even when there are multiple specialized providers in an urban area there may still be barriers to accessing care (e.g., financial, transportation, linguistic, or access to culturally competent or BIPOC providers). Accessing care may be particularly challenging for individuals seeking a provider that shares or is knowledgeable about their ethnic background, cultural background, or sexual/gender orientation.

With the proliferation of specific interventions there is a siloing of knowledge and a lack of practitioners trained to deliver specific evidence-based interventions that directly match client experience (Chorpita et al., 2011). This problem is exacerbated by the fact that intervention targets have become quite specific, while training in evidence-based intervention is often labor intensive. Researchers, noting this challenge, have identified the need to consider effective common elements and processes to develop protocols that target a much broader spectrum of patients (Layne et al., 2011). Despite the differences between interventions, the core elements of trauma-focused therapy are often relatively consistent and include the following key areas of intervention: psychoeducation about posttraumatic stress reactions, developing stronger coping skills, maintaining adaptive routines, parenting support, teaching safety skills, and developing a trauma narrative. In an ideal world children would be matched to interventions with a strong evidence base matched to their own characteristics, but it is important to remember that the key elements of trauma therapy are generally shared. Furthermore, research on the effectiveness of therapy in general suggests that different models of therapy tend to be similarly effective, perhaps due to shared experiences (e.g., the therapeutic relationship, engagement in self-expression, increased understanding of one's experience) (Luborsky et al., 2002).

Pharmacotherapy for Traumatic Stress

Pharmacologic Prevention of PTSD Onset in Children

There is less evidence in the literature for pharmacologic prevention of PTSD by treatment shortly following trauma for children as compared to adults. In a retrospective chart review of children (pediatric burn patients), randomized for propranolol within the first 10 days of burn and treatment sustained for 1 month, no benefit was observed with respect to development of subsequent AStD (Sharp, Thomas, Rosenberg, Rosenberg, & Meyer, 2010). In a second retrospective study of pediatric burn patients a 7-day course of imipramine versus chloral hydrate ($n = 25$) showed benefits of imipramine as compared to chloral hydrate (Robert, Blakeney, Villarreal, Rosenberg, & Meyer, 1999). Children who developed PTSD at 3 months received less morphine than those who did not (Saxe et al., 2001; Stoddard et al., 2009).

Pharmacologic Treatment of PTSD Symptoms in Children With PTSD

The bulk of PTSD psychopharmacologic treatment literature relates not to prevention of the development of PTSD in people who have experienced trauma but to treatment of associated symptoms in people diagnosed with PTSD. In children the only randomized controlled trials (RCTs) for treatment of PTSD in the literature investigate the use of selective serotonin reuptake inhibitors (SSRIs). There are RCTs of the use of fluoxetine and of sertraline in children with PTSD, and these studies indicate statistically significant benefits of these agents (see online supplement Table S56.1). There are no RCTs for citalopram, but open-label studies provide some evidence for benefits in the treatment of symptoms associated with PTSD (Seedat, Lockhat, Kaminer, Zungu-Dirwayi, & Stein, 2001).

There are no other RCTs for other classes of medications that investigate the treatment of PTSD in children. RCTs and other studies of psychopharmacologic treatment of adults are summarized in supplemental materials. Small open-label studies and case reports indicate some benefit of classes of medications such as antipsychotics, anticonvulsants, and adrenergics for the treatment of symptoms associated with PTSD in children; details on these studies are summarized in the supplemental materials.

Practical Considerations in Psychopharmacologic Treatment of PTSD

Data are still rather meager, with few RCTs and small RCTs, and so we still must rely heavily on practical clinical experience. Neurotransmitter changes that have been found to be associated with PTSD notwithstanding, clinical guidelines of psychopharmacologic management of PTSD are organized around the identification of treatable symptom clusters in individual patients, not around the management of neurotransmitter levels per se (Cohen et al., 2001; Donnelly, 2003). In other words although psychopharmacologic management of PTSD entails the administration of medications that modify neurotransmitter levels and/or affinity for their receptors, that knowledge has little direct clinical application. In practice, the goal is to treat each patient with PTSD as an individual, to identify sets of behavioral symptoms that are known to respond to different classes of psychotropics, and to balance these considerations with risks and side effects specific to the patient. Medication management is not the center of PTSD treatment; it is merely a bridge to participation in effective behavioral therapy by reducing behavioral symptoms, which otherwise interfere with the family's ability to really engage in therapy and to benefit from it.

As PTSD is associated with anxiety and activation, psychotropics known to be clinically effective in treating such symptoms might be anticipated to be helpful for many children with PTSD (Cohen, Mannarino, & Rogal, 2001). The RCTs and other evidence in the literature cited earlier bear this out. However, best practice is still to treat individual children as individual children. If a child diagnosed with PTSD has a behavioral presentation in which inattentive or hyperactive/impulsive symptoms predominate, that child may benefit most from solid evidence-based psychopharmacologic management of the ADHD symptoms, such as the use of stimulants. Thus stimulants are not well supported as a primary treatment for PTSD and should be used with some caution given the risk of increased activation and/or preoccupation with intrusive trauma-related memories and thoughts. Nevertheless, if a specific patient presents with ADHD, that child may still benefit from treating the ADHD symptoms to improve overall functioning, even if the ADHD symptoms exist in the larger context of PTSD. If stimulants are not well tolerated, alpha-adrenergics can have the double benefit of treating impulsivity and hyperarousal. The prescriber should also bear in mind a higher than usual rate of adverse reactions and proceed accordingly, with extra care in monitoring of response (Donnelly, 2003). The prescriber should also consider the possibility that fidgetiness and distractibility in the context of PTSD may reflect underlying anxiety and targeting anxiety accordingly for psychopharmacologic intervention. Although practitioners of psychopharmacology should endeavor to keep medication regimens as simple as possible to minimize side effects and to improve adherence, children with comorbid conditions such as ADHD in addition to PTSD may require simultaneous treatment of core ADHD symptoms and underlying anxiety.

It is similarly crucial to treat associated somatic symptoms related to comorbid health issues, such as elimination disorders (constipation, stool withholding, encopresis, and enuresis). Sleep disorders, whether secondary to PTSD or just associated, are both common and important to treat to promote overall function and ultimately greater prognosis.

As is always true when embarking on psychopharmacologic intervention, the goal of alleviation of behavioral symptoms must be balanced with risk of side effects. For example, children who have experienced trauma may have such explosive, disruptive behavior that a provider may feel inclined to trial an antipsychotic medication or mood stabilizer; children in foster care have much higher rates of multiple antipsychotic prescriptions for this reason. It should be borne in mind, though, that these medications may have only transient benefits while the side effects can be quite substantial, may persist, or be irreversible (Siegel & Beaulieu, 2012). Treatment of the underlying anxiety may have less dramatic or less rapid initial benefits with regard to explosive or disruptive behavior, but this is likely to have more sustained benefit and fewer and milder long-term side effects. Alternatively, the alpha-adrenergic agonists, such as guanfacine, are milder with less risk of serious side effects and thus are prudent to try before the riskier antipsychotic class of medications. SSRIs and adrenergics also have the advantage over antipsychotic medication of not needing to obtain regular screening laboratories, which may be especially challenging for children with PTSD. It is with good reason that Child Protective Services issues balancing tests for their wards, to ascertain that prescribers are indeed balancing these considerations. These balancing tests should be taken seriously, and even if such paperwork is not required in a given clinical situation, prescribers should balance costs and benefits and describe these clearly in detailed, thoughtful, and balanced informed consent discussions with children, adolescents, and their parents/guardians. Within this collaborative partnership, treating common cooccurring conditions of PTSD, such as ADHD and anxiety, can help to reduce stress in the home, improve that child's success and self-esteem, and encourage productive engagement in family therapy.

CONCLUSIONS, IMPLICATIONS, AND FUTURE DIRECTIONS

The conceptualization of TSRD, exemplified but not solely represented by PTSD and AStD, has evolved considerably in the last 40 years, informed by breakthroughs in biologic psychiatry, neuroimaging, and latent variable modeling. Once categorized and treated as an anxiety disorder, our field has cultivated a greater appreciation of the heterogeneity and complexity of this diagnostic taxon, with assessment and treatment accordingly becoming more sophisticated. Perhaps one of the most important breakthroughs has been a greater appreciation of the impact of trauma, biologic and psychological, on a developing child as opposed to an adult soldier or civilian. We have evolved from moral judgments about soldiers' cowardice or lack of moral fiber to withstand the horrors of war, and Freud's profoundly destructive "blame the victim" stance toward sexual assault and dissociative "hysteria," to viewing psychological trauma as a public health threat that can be every bit as neurotoxic as lead paint and other environmental pollutants. Although it has yet to be formally codified in our diagnostic system, the concept of developmental trauma, bolstered by 2 decades of published research on toxic stress and ACEs, endures as an important heuristic and guiding principle in our work. The rise and growing influence of such organizations as the National Child Traumatic Stress Network, Center on the Developing Child, and Trauma and Learning Policy Initiative underscore an increasing focus on our youngest and most vulnerable survivors of traumatic events.

Another important area of consideration is focusing on engaging families in trauma-focused therapy. As previously described, therapy is particularly effective during the peritraumatic period, soon after a potentially traumatic experience. However, even when families are seeking treatment, it can be difficult to find a therapist with specialization in treating childhood trauma and availability to immediately initiate services. Rates in urban communities of treatment disengagement and early termination of treatment are notably high, with one study identifying that half of child therapy appointments are missed and a third of families that request services never begin treatment (McKay et al., 2001). In addition, families where trauma is ongoing (e.g., domestic violence) may be particularly unlikely to seek out services due to concerns about child welfare involvement or challenges with meeting the logistical demands of bringing a child in for treatment. For families where parents are experiencing trauma reactions, TSS can directly lead to avoidance of treatment. The thought of reaching out for trauma treatment may in and of itself increase parent symptomatology, leading families to avoid seeking care. Given these challenges it is important to consider strategies to engage families impacted by trauma into treatment, including families that do not seek out services.

One way to increase engagement in services is to consider different access points. Children who have experienced a potentially traumatic event may require services in the emergency department (e.g., following a car crash or other accident, or suspected nonaccidental injury), may receive services through the police department (e.g., after witnessing or experiencing violence), or may be identified as in need of services at school or during a visit to the pediatrician. Thus the emergency department, police department, school, primary care office, and other community supports (e.g., church, homeless shelter) create important access points for identifying families in need of services and beginning the process of engagement in trauma-focused services. This scaling-up of public health and emergency service infrastructure to become more (psychologically) trauma informed requires a significant investment of resources and even greater prioritization by our elected officials than already exists. Model programs currently exist but more often than not only through extramural grant funding and therefore discouragingly short lived. There is a call for policy change that prioritizes funding programs that include a multisystemic approach to treating childhood trauma. For example, the Families First Protection Act could be an avenue to fund such initiatives (Bosk et al., under review).

Despite the significant impact that trauma can have on children's psychological well-being, there are many options for effective treatment, and children demonstrate a remarkable resilience in the face of trauma, which is only enhanced when provided with therapeutic support (Masten, 2001). Current guidelines recommend primarily psychosocial, trauma-focused treatments, possibly augmented by medication to help alleviate specific symptoms (e.g., agitation, sleep disturbance) and improve functioning rather than try to target the etiology. These treatments have evolved to become more principle than technique driven, though some version of experiential exposure remains the gold standard for managing TSS arising from a very specific traumatic memory that the survivor is able to verbalize. This demand for narrative (i.e., being able to tell the trauma story in painful detail) obviously has its limitations when trauma is experienced preverbally, even in utero in the case of a pregnant woman enduring domestic violence and other traumatic events. Perhaps for this reason, among others, many of the advances in trauma theory, research, and treatment have focused on the mind-body connection and other things unspoken (e.g., Solomon & Siegel, 2003; Van der Kolk, 2015). At the time of this writing, these emerging interventions have yet to accrue the evidence needed to be considered recommended evidence-based treatments for PTSD/AStD (see online supplement).

Conclusion

This chapter provides an overview of the diagnosis, conceptualization, and treatment of PTSD and AStD as well as the state of the current research in these areas. While the impact of childhood trauma can be profound, potentially traumatic experiences are common, and for many children they are a normative aspect of development. The deleterious effects of PTSD/AStD can be successfully mitigated with appropriate evidence-based treatment. Careful consideration of traumatic experiences, ACEs, and caregiving environments when conceptualizing and treating childhood psychopathology increases the chances of children receiving the most appropriate treatment, supporting their optimal development. With increased access to evidence-based treatment for childhood trauma we have the tools to support positive developmental trajectories for all children and to ultimately bolster the health and productivity of society. Literature should of course help to inform our clinical decisions, but population-based evidence does not always apply to specific scenarios. Children, youth, and families may have their own experiences, preferences, and idiosyncratic reactions, and all of this must take precedence in collaborative, client-centered care.

REFERENCES

American Academy of Child and Adolescent Psychiatry (AACAP). (1998). Practice parameters for the assessment and treatment of children and adolescents with posttraumatic stress disorder. *Journal of the American Academy of Child & Adolescent Psychiatry*, S4–S26.

American Psychiatric Association (APA).(1980). *Diagnostic and statistical manual of mental disorders* (3rd ed.). Author.

American Psychiatric Association (APA).(1994). *Diagnostic and statistical manual of mental disorders* (4th ed.). Author.

American Psychiatric Association (APA).(2013). *Diagnostic and statistical manual of mental disorders* (5th ed.). Author.

Berkowitz, S. J., Stover, C. S., & Marans, S. R. (2011). The Child and Family Traumatic Stress Intervention: Secondary prevention for youth at risk of developing PTSD. *Journal of Child Psychology & Psychiatry*, *52*(6), 676–685. https://doi.org/10.1111/j.1469-7610.2010.02321.x

Bonnano, G. A., & Mancini, A. D. (2008). The human capacity to thrive in the face of potential trauma. *Pediatrics*, *121*, 369–375. https://doi.org/10.1542/peds.2007-1648

Bosk, E., Van Scoyoc, A., Mihalec-Adkins, B, et al. (under review). Integrating responses to caregiver substance misuse, intimate partner violence and child maltreatment: Initiatives and policies that support families at risk for entering the child welfare system.

Bradley, R., Greene, J., Russ, E., Dutra, L., & Westen, D. (2005). A multidimensional meta-analysis of psychotherapy for PTSD. *American Journal of Psychiatry*, *162*, 214–227.

Breslau, N. (2001). The epidemiology of posttraumatic stress disorder: What is the extent of the problem? *Journal of Clinical Psychiatry*, *62*(17), S16–S22.

Brown, E. (2020). *The hidden evidence of PTSD in the ancient world*. https://medium.com/lessons-from-history/the-hidden-evidence-of-ptsd-in-the-ancient-world-eb83752b7d4e

Centers for Disease Control and Prevention (CDC). (2020). https://www.cdc.gov/violenceprevention/aces/resources.html

Chorpita, B. F., Rotheram-Borus, M. J., Daleiden, E. L., et al. (2011). The old solutions are the new problem: How do we better use what we already know about reducing the burden of mental illness? *Perspectives on Psychological Science*, *6*(5), 493–497. https://doi.org/10.1177/1745691611418240

Cohen, J. A., Mannarino, A. P., & Rogal, S. (2001). Treatment practices for childhood posttraumatic stress disorder. *Child Abuse & Neglect*, *25*, 123–135.

Cook, A., Spinazzola, J., Ford, J., Lanktree, C., Blaustein, M., Cloitre, M., … van der Kolk, B. (2017). Complex trauma in children and adolescents. *Psychiatric Annals*, *35*(5), 390–398. https://doi.org/10.3928/00485713-20050501-05

De Bellis, M. D. (2005). The psychobiology of neglect. *Child Maltreatment*, *10*(2), 150–172.

De Bellis, M. D., Lefter, L., Trickett, P. K., et al. (1994b). Urinary catecholamine excretion in sexually abused girls. *Journal of the American Academy of Child and Adolescent Psychiatry*, *33*, 320–327.

DiMauro, J., Carter, S., Folk, J. B., & Kashdan, T. B. (2014). A historical review of trauma-related diagnoses to reconsider the heterogeneity of PTSD. *Journal of Anxiety Disorders*, *28*(8), 774–786. https://doi.org/10.1016/j.janxdis.2014.09.002

Donnelly, C. L. (2003). Pharmacologic treatment approaches for children and adolescents with posttraumatic stress disorder. *Child and Adolescent Psychiatric Clinics of North America, 12*(2), 251–269. https://doi.org/10.1016/S1056-4993(02)00102-5

Epstein, C., Hahn, H., Berkowitz, S., & Marans, S. (2017). The Child and Family Traumatic Stress Intervention: In *Evidence-based treatments for trauma related disorders in children and adolescents* (pp. 145–166). Springer.

Famularo, R., Fenton, T., Kinscherff, R., & Augustyn, M. (1996). Psychiatric comorbidity in childhood posttraumatic stress disorder. *Child Abuse & Neglect, 20*(10), 953–961.

Felitti, V. J., Anda, R. F., Nordenberg, D., Williamson, D. F., Spitz, A. M., Edwards, V., … Marks, J. S. (1998). Relationship of childhood abuse and household dysfunction to many of the leading causes of death in adults. The Adverse Childhood Experiences (ACE) Study. *American Journal of Prevention Medicine, 14*(4), 245–258. https://doi.org/10.1016/s0749-3797(98)00017-8

Finkelhor, D., Ormrod, R. K., & Turner, H. A. (2007). Poly-victimization: A neglected component in child victimization. *Child Abuse & Neglect, 31*, 7–26.

Finkelhor, D., Turner, H., Ormrod, R., & Hamby, S. L. (2009). Violence, abuse, and crime exposure in a national sample of children and youth. *Pediatrics, 124*(5), 1411–1423. https://doi.org/10.1542/peds.2009-0467

Friedman, M. J., Resick, P. A., Bryant, R. A., & Brewin, C. R. (2011). Considering PTSD for DSM-5. *Depression & Anxiety, 28*(9), 750–769. https://doi.org/10.1002/da.20767

Graham, A. M., Pfeifer, J. H., Fisher, P. A., Carpenter, S., & Fair, D. A. (2015). Early life stress is associated with default system integrity and emotionality during infancy. *Journal of Child Psychology & Psychiatry, 56*(11), 1212–1222. https://doi.org/10.1111/jcpp.12409

Herman, J. L. (1992a). *Trauma and recovery*. Basic Books.

Herman, J. L. (1992b). Complex PTSD: A syndrome in survivors of prolonged and repeated trauma. *Journal of Traumatic Stress, 5*(3), 377–391.

Keane, T. M., & Barlow, D. H. (2002). Posttraumatic stress disorder. In D. H. Barlow (Ed.), *Anxiety and its disorders: The nature and treatment of anxiety and panic* (2nd ed., pp. 418–453). Guilford Press.

Keane, T. M., Marshall, A. D., & Taft, C. T. (2006). Posttraumatic stress disorder: Etiology, epidemiology, and treatment outcome. *Annual Review of Clinical Psychology, 2*, 161–197.

King, D. W., King, L. A., Foy, D. W., Keane, T. M., & Fairbank, J. A. (1999). Posttraumatic stress disorder in a national sample of female and male Vietnam veterans: Risk factors, war-zone stressors, and resilience-recovery variables. *Journal of Abnormal Psychology, 108*(1), 164–170. https://doi.org/10.1037/0021-843X.108.1.164

Kuhlman, K. R., Vargas, I., Geiss, E. G., & Lopez-Duran, N. L. (2015). Age of trauma onset and HPA axis dysregulation among trauma-exposed youth. *Journal of Traumatic Stress, 28*(6), 572–579.

Layne, C. M., Ippen, C. G., Strand, V., et al. (2011). The core curriculum on childhood trauma: a tool for training a trauma-informed workforce. *Psychological Trauma: Theory. Research, Practice, and Policy, 3*(3), 243–252.

Linden, S. C., & Jones, E. (2014). "Shell shock" revisited: An examination of the case records of the National Hospital in London. *Medical History, 58*(4), 519–545. https://doi.org/10.1017/mdh.2014.51

Luborsky, L., Rosenthal, R., Diguer, L., et al. (2002). The dodo bird verdict is alive and well—Mostly. *Clinical Psychology: Science and Practice, 9*(1), 2–12. https://doi.org/10.1093/clipsy.9.1.2

Masten, A. S. (2001). Ordinary magic. *Resilience processes in development. American Psychologist, 56*(3), 227–238. https://doi.org/10.1037//0003-066x.56.3.227

McCullough, J. M., & Ressler, R. J. (2018). Posttraumatic stress disorder: From neurobiology to cycles of violence. In J. M. Fogler & R. A. Phelps (Eds.), *Trauma, autism, and neurodevelopmental disorder: Integrating research, practice, and policy* (pp. 19–54). Springer Nature.

McKay, M. M., Pennington, J., Lynn, C. J., & McCadam, K. (2001). Understanding urban child mental health service use: Two studies of child, family, and environmental correlates. *Journal of Behavioral Health Services and Research, 28*, 475–483.

McMackin, R. A., Newman, E., Fogler, J. M., & Keane, T. M. (Eds.), (2012). *Trauma therapy in context: The science and craft of evidence-based practice*. American Psychiatric Press. https://doi.org/10.1037/13746-000

Perry, B. D. (1994). Neurobiological sequelae of childhood trauma: PTSD in children (pp. 233–255). *American Psychiatric Press.*

Prock, L., & Fogler, J. (2018). Trauma and neurodevelopmental disorder: Assessment, treatment and triage. In J. M. Fogler & R. A. Phelps (Eds.), *Trauma, autism, and neurodevelopmental disorders: Integrating research practice, and policy* (pp. 55–71). Springer Nature.

Ritschel, L. A., Lim, N. E., & Stewart, L. M. (2015). Transdiagnostic applications of DBT for adolescents and adults. *American Journal of Psychotherapy, 69*(2), 111–128.

Robert, R., Blakeney, P. E., Villarreal, C., Rosenberg, L., & Meyer, W. J., III. (1999). Imipramine treatment in pediatric burn patients with symptoms of acute stress disorder: A pilot study. *Journal of the American Academy of Child and Adolescent Psychiatry, 38*(7), 873–882.

Saxe, G., Stoddard, F., Courtney, D., et al. (2001). Relationship between acute morphine and the course of PTSD in children with burns. *Journal of the American Academy of Child and Adolescent Psychiatry, 40*(8), 915–921.

Scheeringa, M. S., Zeanah, C. H., Myers, L., & Putnam, F. W. (2003). New findings on alternative criteria for PTSD in preschool children. *Journal of the American Academy of Child & Adolescent Psychiatry, 42*(5), 561–570.

Schottenbauer, M. A., Glass, C. R., Arnkoff, D. B., Tendick, V., & Hafter Gray, S. (2008). Nonresponse and outcome rates in outcome studies on PTSD: Review and methodological considerations. *Psychiatry, 71*(2), 134–168.

Seedat, S., Lockhat, R., Kaminer, D., Zungu-Dirwayi, N., & Stein, D. J. (2001). An open trial of citalopram in adolescents with posttraumatic stress disorder. *International Clinical Psychopharmacology, 16*(1), 21–25.

Sharp, S., Thomas, C., Rosenberg, L., Rosenberg, M., & Meyer, W., III. (2010). Propranolol does not reduce risk for acute stress disorder in pediatric burn trauma. *Journal of Trauma, 68*(1), 193–197.

Siegel, M., & Beaulieu, A. A. (2012). Psychotropic medications in children with autism spectrum disorders: A systematic review and synthesis for evidence-based practice. *Journal of Autism and Developmental Disorders, 42*(8), 1592–1605.

Sofranac, M. (2011). Traumatizing memories and memorizing trauma—Hamlet and the Macbeths. *Linguistics and Literature, 9*(1), 47–52.

Stoddard, F. J., Jr., et al., Sorrentino, E. A., Ceranoglu, T. A., et al. (2009). Preliminary evidence for the effects of morphine on posttraumatic stress disorder symptoms in one- to four-year-olds with burns. *Journal of Burn Care & Research: Official Publication of the American Burn Association*, *30*(5), 836–843.

Szarkowski, A., & Fogler, J. (2020). Supporting students with disabilities in trauma-sensitive schools. *Educational Leadership*, *78*(2), 64–68.

Terr, L. C. (1991). Childhood traumas: An outline and overview. *American Journal of Psychiatry*, *148*, 10–20.

Van der Kolk, B. (2001). The psychobiology and psychopharmacology of PTSD. *Human Psychopharmacology:Clinical & Experimental*, *16*, S49–S64. https://doi.org/10.1002/hup.270

Van der Kolk, B. A. (2005). Developmental trauma disorder: Toward a rational diagnosis for children with complex trauma histories. *Psychiatric Annals*, *35*(5), 401–408.

57

Adjustment and Adjustment Disorders in Developmental-Behavioral Pediatrics

Kathryn Mancini and Robert Needlman

For additional material related to the content of this chapter, please see Chapters 12, 92, and 110.

> **VIGNETTE**
>
> *Luis, a 12-year-old boy in seventh grade, is displaying irritability, sleepiness, and fighting with his siblings. Previously a B-C student, his grades are dropping because he refuses to complete homework. He claims that everything is stupid and that nobody likes him. Although once an avid soccer player, now he spends most of his time in his room on his tablet. His mother says he is "sad," although he seemed happy when given a new videogame. On detailed questioning, his mother describes that Luis current problems developed after transitioning to remote schooling in 2020 during the COVID-19 pandemic.*

INTRODUCTION

Cases like Luis raise a number of questions. Assuming his maladaptive behaviors and emotions are a response to his schooling change, how are the event and the child's functioning actually linked? Why has this child not been able to cope more effectively? What diagnosis does his current status suggest? How can the clinician differentiate a temporary downswing from an adjustment disorder from an incipient emotional or behavioral disorder? What interventions are likely to help? What is the prognosis?

This chapter discusses adjustment and adjustment disorders. Adjustment is a broad concept dealing with how a child responds to stress. Stress refers to internal or external factors that challenge a child's wellbeing. Coping is a concept that focuses on the moment-to-moment stress response. Adjustment refers to the child's responses to stress over weeks and months. At this most general level, a certain circularity is unavoidable: Adjustment is an adaptive response to stress, whereas stress is anything that requires the child to make an adjustment.

Children cope with stress every day. A child wakes up and cannot find a clean shirt to put on; she gets teased on the bus; she struggles on a math test; she does not get a part in the school play. The classic children's book *Alexander and the Terrible, Horrible, No Good, Very Bad Day* by Judith Viorst (1974) portrays the universal experience of disappointment and frustration. Children cope in various ways. They encourage and console themselves; they seek distractions; they complain to friends or family members. If their distress rises to the point of being noticed, it may alert a support system that includes siblings, parents, and teachers. If these corrective processes fail, the child may come to medical attention.

CONCEPTS OF STRESS AND ADJUSTMENT

Stress Response Systems

Stressors are internal or external factors that threaten to disrupt an organism's physical or psychological homeostasis. In children homeostasis includes expected physical growth and psychological development, as well as current wellbeing. Stressors can be physiologic (e.g., illness, injury) or psychosocial (e.g., loss and threatened loss of security, relationships, or stature) and are positive, tolerable, or toxic in nature. Positive stress is low intensity, manageable stress that results in positive outcomes or growth. For example, many youth experience stress about taking tests or giving presentations at school. This stress is temporary and typically yields a positive outcome, such as learning something new. Developmental challenges such as toilet training are also considered positive stress. Tolerable stress is moderate-intensity stress that may or may not resolve quickly, but the child has the resources and support necessary to manage the stress. Toxic stress is high-intensity, persistent or recurrent stress, and the child does not have the resources or support to manage it. Toxic stress is linked to a variety of negative and chronic health conditions and mental health disorders, including systemic inflammation, poor insulin responsivity, cardiovascular disease, substance use disorders, and anxiety and depression (Garner et al., 2012; Shonkoff, Boyce, Levitt, Martinez, & McEwen, 2021) (see also Chapters 15, 19, 22, and 56). Research into the psychobiology of stress further demonstrates connections between the physiologic and psychological dimensions of stress and adjustment.

Stress activates two major neuroendocrine systems. The sympathetic-adrenal-medullary (SAM) system provides a rapid, short-lived response transmitted through the sympathetic nervous system and mediated by serum catecholamines. SAM system activation is characterized by increased heart rate, blood pressure, and muscle tension and redistribution of blood flow to striated muscle. This is the well-known fight-or-flight response. The hypothalamic-pituitary-adrenal (HPA) axis provides a longer-term response. Serum cortisol rises approximately 20 to 30 minutes after a stressor, followed by increases in blood glucose concentration, decreased immune responsiveness, and emotional distress. The balance between the SAM and HPA systems influences the effects of a particular stressor on the individual's physical and emotional (Bauer, Quas, & Boyce, 2002).

Sympathetic nervous system responses are counterbalanced by activation of the parasympathetic nervous system, the main fibers of which travel along the vagus nerve. Vagal outputs regulate heart rate, and vagal tone can be gauged by measuring variability of heart rate in response to respiration, a value termed respiratory sinus arrhythmia. Higher vagal tone has been associated with greater ability to withstand stress and to self-regulate emotional responses to stressors (Porges, 2007). Vagal tone can be measured in early infancy, implying that the stress response early on is influenced by genetics and the intrauterine environment. As the child grows, additional experiences may alter or interact with vagal tone. For instance, in a longitudinal study school-age children with lower vagal tone showed more behavior problems in the presence of parental problem drinking (El-Sheikh, 2005).

There are individual differences in sensitivity to stress. Although stress sensitivity is a continuous and complex process, broadly, people can be more or less reactive to stress. Boyce, Levitt, Martinez, McEwen, and Shonkoff (2021) described individual children as either "orchids" (highly sensitive to stress but capable of excellence under optimal conditions) or "dandelions" (less sensitive to stress but also less responsive to optimal rearing) (Ellis, Essex, & Boyce, 2005). More recently, Lionetti et al. (2018) have proposed three distinct sensitivity profiles in children: high, medium, and low. Here sensitivity is characterized by ease of excitation, aesthetic awareness, and sensory threshold. Highly sensitive individuals are typically easily excited, highly aware of their environments, and respond to a lower threshold of stimuli. They also have additional genetic, physiologic, and psychological factors ("plasticity factors") that make them more malleable and more vulnerable to their surroundings, both to positive and negative events (Belsky & Pluess, 2009). Low-sensitive individuals tend to be less reactive and appear to remain stable regardless of context; medium-sensitive individuals cope well with certain stressors or in certain situations but not in others.

Imagine three children sitting in their classroom as a fire alarm goes off. The highly sensitive child experiences palpitations (increased heart rate), shows signs of distress, looks to an adult for help, and remains distressed for the rest of the morning; the medium-sensitivity child jumps in his chair at first, scrambles to complete the drill, but then goes about his day; the low-sensitivity child laughs with her friends, mimics the sound of the alarm, and carries on unfazed. Differential susceptibility to stress explains how the same event may have very different effects, depending on the child.

A person's sensitivity to stress develops at or before conception and changes over time. Genetic predisposition and certain gene variants interact with environmental factors *in utero*; bidirectional interactions later occur among neural, immune, and metabolic systems to influence sensitivity to stress. During certain sensitive developmental periods, environmental factors are particularly impactful. These interactions are broadly labeled gene-environment-time interactions (Shonkoff et al., 2021) and occur continuously across development, affecting both sensitivity to stress and the nature of the physical response (Boyce et al., 2021; Garner et al., 2012).

Resilience

Resilience is the ability to adapt successfully to stress and to function well despite stress. Like vulnerability, resilience is dynamic and can be traced to genetic, physiologic, psychological, contextual, and systemic factors (Masten, 2014). For example, in her classic longitudinal study of children growing up in poverty on the island of Kauai Werner (1992) found that children who thrived tended to be physically attractive, temperamentally easy, and to have at least one adult mentor. Positive temperament and supportive social environments may have transactional as well as additive effects. For instance, individual resources such as self-efficacy, self-esteem, and hopefulness provide protective mechanisms that interact with social environments to enhance the development of resilience during adolescence (Olsson, Bond, Burns, Vella-Brodrick, & Sawyer, 2003). Similarly, social resources, such as loving and supportive relationships, buffer against the negative impacts of stress (Shonkoff et al., 2021).

Ecologic and Cultural Perspectives

The specific behaviors that characterize stress response, adjustment, and resilience are determined by the lived experiences of people in the context of family values, community expectations, and cultural norms. Culture influences whether specific experiences are stressful and how those stresses are expressed. Stress and adjustment are ongoing bidirectional transactions between a person and their surroundings (Moos, 2002). Multiple factors come into play, including the individual's cognitive abilities, social skills, and capacity for coping; the social climate and available resources; life events (particularly, earlier experiences of stress or trauma); and the cultural and societal milieu.

Of particular relevance to adjustment disorders is the observation that in many cultures people experience stress physically rather than psychologically. Thus a stressed child may present with stomachaches rather than sadness. Conversely, symptoms that in the industrialized West are understood to be manifestations of organic dysfunction may in other cultures be considered evidence of spiritual derangement. In *The Spirit Catches You and You Fall Down* Anne Fadiman (1997) describes how a young child's seizure disorder is understood differently by her Cambodian family and by her American physicians, with tragic consequences.

Children are inducted into cultural norms implicitly through social learning and explicitly through direct education. What is stressful in one community may be normative in another. Even within families, what is stressful for one family member may not bother another. Cultures have both characteristic responses to stress and characteristic approaches to adjustment. Specific aspects of culture impact how caregivers teach their children about emotions, how children experience emotions, and what outcomes occur (Raval & Walker, 2019). For example, some cultures promote discussion of problems; others encourage repression or meditation.

Individual, community, and cultural differences add to the complexity of stress and adjustment. Importantly, the focus is not on the stressor or the stressful event itself, but on the individual's stress response systems and capacity for adjustment and resilience in the context of family and community.

ADJUSTMENT DISORDERS

Adjustment encompasses responses to developmentally normative challenges such as toilet training or dating, as well as responses to upsetting or traumatic events. The diagnosis of adjustment disorder attempts to designate a group of psychiatric diagnoses that occupy an intermediate ground between reactions that are merely concerning and those severe enough to merit major psychiatric diagnoses. Although fraught with theoretical and practical difficulties, the diagnosis of adjustment disorder remains important for its prevalence and its association with sometimes serious outcomes (Bachem & Casey, 2018; Carta, Balestrieri, Murru, & Hardoy, 2009).

At their core, adjustment disorders are disorders of the stress response systems. As defined in the *Diagnostic and Statistical Manual of Mental Disorders,* fifth edition (*DSM-5*), the diagnosis of adjustment disorder requires four features: (1) emotional or behavioral symptoms that arise within 3 months of the onset of an identified stressor, (2) the symptoms are out of proportion to the severity of the stressor and cause significant impairment, (3) the symptoms do not meet the criteria for another mental disorder and are not an exacerbation of a preexisting disorder, and (4) the symptoms resolve within 6 months after the cessation of the stressor (American Psychiatric Association, 2013). In addition, *DSM-5* excludes bereavement. The *International Classification of Diseases,* eleventh revision (*ICD-11*) criteria are similar but structured differently to include broad preoccupation with the stressor and failure to adapt, which interferes with everyday functioning (World Health Organization, 2022). The timing outlined in the *ICD-11* is also slightly different than the *DSM-5*, stating that the reaction occurs within 1 month after exposure to the stressor.

An obvious difficulty with the *DSM-5* diagnosis is that although it calls for the existence of "symptoms," it does not specify their precise nature or number. In this respect, adjustment disorder differs from many other *DSM-5* diagnoses (e.g., major depressive disorder). A rough indication of the kinds of symptoms that compose adjustment disorder is apparent from the six subtypes: adjustment disorder with depressed mood; with anxiety; with mixed anxiety and depressed mood; with disturbance of conduct; with mixed disturbance of emotions and conduct; and unspecified. These similarities raise the question of how the adjustment disorders are differentiated from their corresponding major mood and behavior disorders. Presumably in adjustment disorder the symptoms are fewer in number or lesser in magnitude because otherwise another diagnosis would supersede the diagnosis of adjustment disorder. Thus, for example, an adolescent might experience symptoms, including sadness, tearfulness, and anhedonia; if the symptoms were sufficient to merit the diagnosis of major depressive disorder, then that would be the diagnosis rather than adjustment disorder with depressed mood.

For differential diagnosis of adjustment disorder, the provider must consider (1) the possibility that symptoms represent a normative stress response and that no psychiatric diagnosis is present, (2) the possibility that the patient meets criteria for another mood or behavior disorder such as major depressive disorder or oppositional defiant disorder, (3) whether the stress response is so significant that it is better captured by acute stress disorder, and (4) whether there are underlying medical problems such as substance use or accidental exposure to substances, sleep apnea or other sleep disorder, or chronic medical condition.

Adjustment disorder can be diagnosed in addition to another disorder as long as the adjustment disorder cannot be accounted for by the other diagnosis. For example, a child with dysthymia could merit an additional diagnosis of adjustment disorder with anxiety if the anxiety symptoms arose in response to an identified stressor. Adjustment disorders share some characteristics with acute stress disorder and posttraumatic stress disorder. However, in adjustment disorder the stress response is typically less extreme, and core features of posttraumatic stress disorder, such as nightmares, flashbacks, and behavioral avoidance, are absent.

By definition, adjustment disorders are time limited. When symptoms persist well beyond the original stressor, the diagnosis must change. However, there is no sure way to distinguish ahead of time between cases of adjustment disorder that are destined to resolve and those that mark the beginning of more chronic psychiatric conditions. Therefore it is unclear whether the adjustment disorder turns into another disorder (usually with the "unspecified" modifier) or whether the child had that disorder all along. Moreover, the time frame of 6 months appears arbitrary and does not take the patient's age into account.

The 6-month time limit begins after the inciting stressor ends. If the stressor persists over time, then the adjustment disorder can be prolonged indefinitely, becoming chronic adjustment disorder. An example of a time-limited stressor might be the breakup of an adolescent romance; examples of persisting stressors include a chronic medical illness such as sickle cell disease, the multiple ongoing stresses subsumed under the headings of poverty and racism, and a parent's chronic psychiatric illness. Often, children are exposed to a mixture of acute and chronic stressors that change over time, and it may be difficult to define a precise beginning and end. The existence of apparent stress-related responses that begin later than 3 months after the stressor and last longer than 3 months suggests a degree of arbitrariness in the diagnostic criteria (Bachem & Casey, 2018).

The diagnosis of adjustment disorder relies on a presumed connection between a stressor and subsequent symptoms; however, both stressors and symptoms are common and therefore may arise together by coincidence. In the diagnosis of adjustment disorders, therefore, special care should be taken to consider alternative explanations, including potentially treatable medical conditions such as hyperthyroidism and hypothyroidism, whose symptoms can mimic those of psychological distress. Given the difficulties enumerated, it is not surprising that the reliability of the diagnosis is relatively low compared with other diagnoses (Patra & Sarkar, 2013).

Prevalence

The prevalence of adjustment disorders is 1% to 2% in the general population and between 2.9% and 18.9% in clinical or high-risk samples. According to *DSM-IV*, adjustment disorder was the primary diagnosis for 5% to 20% of individuals receiving outpatient psychotherapy. Adjustment disorders are highly prevalent in consultation liaison hospital settings, with rates ranging from between 15% and 19% to 35% in samples of oncology patients (O'Donnell, Agathos, Metcalf, Gibson, & Lau, 2019). In children adjustment disorder is the most common diagnosis (Carta et al., 2009).

Adjustment Disorders and Medical Illness

Adjustment disorders are common among children and adolescents with chronic medical conditions. A review of studies of survivors of childhood cancer, for example, found frequent behavioral and emotional difficulties, including problems of depression, anxiety, stressed peer relations, and poor school and work performance. These problems may be expected, given the enormous strains on personal, spiritual, family, school, and community systems that accompany a diagnosis of cancer. Nonetheless, the majority of childhood cancer survivors are psychologically well, perhaps due to protective effects of family support. A recent metaanalysis indicated that greater family cohesion, expressiveness, and support and lower family conflict were related to more positive outcomes for children with cancer (Van Schoors et al., 2017).

Adjustment disorders are also frequently diagnosed in children with type 1 diabetes, particularly during the initial time of adaptation to the diagnosis. In turn, higher stress is linked to worse glycemic control, creating a positive-feedback loop (Delamater, de Wit, McDarby, Malik, & Acerini, 2014). The accommodation to a new diagnosis of type 1 diabetes or any chronic medical condition demands changes in multiple people and systems in a child's life. If any of these adaptations goes awry, it places additional emotional or physical strains on the child, whose subsequent diagnosis of adjustment disorder expresses the dysfunction of the wider system.

Adjustment Disorders and Psychosocial Stressors

As noted, adjustment disorders arise in response to common problems in school, at home, and with peers, particularly boyfriend or girlfriend problems, bullying, and family stresses such as divorce or separation. Community-wide stressors, such as endemic racism and gun violence, can also lead to adjustment problems. Hidden stressors, such as sexual abuse or parental alcoholism, may surface only after careful investigation, if at all.

Adjustment disorders have been diagnosed more frequently during the COVID-19 pandemic than in prior years (Imran, Aamer, Sharif, Bodla, & Naveed, 2020). As a result of enforced quarantine and school closures, school-age children reported isolation, social exclusion, fear, difficulty concentrating, restlessness, and worrying; children aged 3 to 6 years were more likely to be clingy and irritable. Still, even with the most severe stressors, such as wars, earthquakes, and other catastrophes, the incidence is lower than 100%. Symptoms typically emerge when there is a convergence of temperamental and environmental risk.

Prevention and Treatment

The goals of treatment are to reduce stress and promote healthy adjustment. Little has been written that explicitly addresses the prevention of adjustment disorders in children and adolescents. However, a number of principles can be gleaned from the literature (Table 57.1). Primary prevention entails building resiliency within children, families, and larger systems. Pediatric preventive initiatives aimed at promoting physical and psychological wellbeing may play a role in the prevention of adjustment problems.

One promising target for such intervention might be language development. Young children use language to self-regulate their emotions and behavior, and language delays are associated with preschool behavior problems. Primary care interventions, such as Reach Out and Read, that promote early reading aloud have been associated with increased child language competence in high-risk populations (Zuckerman, 2009). To encourage adjustment to stress, children can be taught a vocabulary to describe their stress and their reaction to it. They then have tools for engaging their social support network. They can also read or be read stories that illustrate resilience in the face of comparable stresses.

A second promising intervention might be promoting close, supportive, and loving relationships. A supportive relationship can significantly reduce stress intensity, rendering potentially toxic stress tolerable (Shonkoff et al., 2021). It is possible to nurture and support these beneficial relationships in the context of traditional pediatric well-child care. For instance, the Video Interaction Project brings in child development specialists to work with parents and young children during well-child visits, strengthening parenting skills and the parent-child relationship. A wide range of positive results, including improved school readiness and overall resilience, have been reported (Canfield, Roby, & Mendelsohn, 2020).

Preventative guidance might be especially important for children with temperamental traits that may make them more vulnerable to the effects of stress (e.g., children judged to be low in adaptability, "slow to warm up," or "difficult"). Such children may have medium-sensitivity or high-sensitivity profiles, as described earlier, and may be particularly likely to benefit from preventative guidance.

Secondary prevention would target children known to be at risk for the development of an adjustment disorder. A limited body of research has evaluated specific strategies. For example, a randomized prospective trial employed

TABLE 57.1 Examples of Preventative Mechanisms for Adjustment Disorder

Intervention Type	Goal	Example	Mechanism
Primary prevention	Build resilience and promote wellbeing for all children	Universal implementation of program to improve literacy and language development	Give children vocabulary to express themselves and self-regulate emotions and behavior
Secondary prevention	Target children known to be at risk for adjustment disorder	Have nurses visit children recently diagnosed with chronic medical issues	Nurses show emotional support and meet individualized needs, reduce stigma, and improve day-to-day experience
Tertiary prevention	Ameliorate effects of diagnosed adjustment disorders	Cognitive-behavioral therapy	Parent training and cognitive and behavioral coping skills reduce the frequency and intensity of adjustment disorder symptoms

nurse home visiting in 332 children aged 4 to 16 years with chronic medical issues. The intervention sought to raise family wellbeing and parental competence and to lower parental stress. The nurse visitors forged relationships with families, providing emotional support and individualized information. Concerns about the child's behavior or school functioning, parenting, and family relationships were common. Parent ratings of behavior problems did not change in response to the intervention, but parent-rated psychosocial adjustment was better in the intervention group, as was child-reported positive self-concept (Pless et al., 1994).

Tertiary prevention would be aimed at ameliorating the effects of identified adjustment disorders, speeding the resolution of symptoms, and reducing the incidence of later psychiatric diagnoses. Nonpharmacologic approaches that support self-control and enhanced coping strategies might include relaxation–mental imagery, cognitive-behavioral therapy, creative expression, family counseling, and parent guidance. Where adjustment disorders are linked to stressors in the school, interventions to ameliorate the stressors might prove effective, such as working with teachers and staff to eliminate bullying and support positive peer interactions (Gaffney, Farrington, & Ttofi, 2019). Similarly, when stressors are identified at home, parental guidance (or, for example, marital therapy) may prove the most effective. In cases in which impairment is severe pharmacologic treatments might provide rapid relief. The choice of medication would presumably follow from treatments for related internalizing and externalizing disorders. However, studies evaluating specific therapies in children diagnosed with adjustment disorders are lacking.

CONCLUSION

Returning to our example of Luis from the beginning of the chapter, it is likely that Luis' mood and behavior changes are best explained by an adjustment disorder. With cognitive-behavioral therapy and loving and supportive relationships, it is likely that these symptoms are temporary and Luis will improve.

Taken together, adjustment disorders are a common, clinically useful yet scientifically understudied set of disorders. Adjustment disorders are disorders of the stress response system and represent a significant and distressing failure to cope with and adapt to stress. Prevalence, treatment, and prognosis appear unpredictable and variable based on disorder subtype as well as individual, family, community, and cultural factors. Future clinicians and scientists are encouraged to further examine the subtypes of adjustment, protective factors, and treatment options.

REFERENCES

American Psychiatric Association. (2013). *Diagnostic and statistical manual of mental disorders* (5th ed.). Author.

Bachem, R., & Casey, P. (2018). Adjustment disorder: A diagnosis whose time has come. *Journal of Affective Disorders, 227*, 243–253.

Bauer, A. M., Quas, J. A., & Boyce, W. T. (2002). Associations between physiological reactivity and children's behavior: Advantages of a multisystem approach. *Journal of Developmental & Behavioral Pediatrics, 23*(2), 102–113.

Belsky, J., & Pluess, M. (2009). Beyond diathesis stress: Differential susceptibility to environmental influences. *Psychological Bulletin, 135*(6), 885.

Boyce, W. T., Levitt, P., Martinez, F. D., McEwen, B. S., & Shonkoff, J. P. (2021). Genes, environments, and time: The biology of adversity and resilience. *Pediatrics.*

Canfield, C., Roby, E., & Mendelsohn, A. (2020). The video interaction project (VIP). In E. T. Gershoff & S. J. Lee (Eds.), *Ending the physical punishment of children: A guide for clinicians and practitioners* (pp. 73–80). American Psychological Association.

Carta, M. G., Balestrieri, M., Murru, A., & Hardoy, M. C. (2009). Adjustment disorder: Epidemiology, diagnosis and treatment. *Clinical Practice and Epidemiology in Mental Health, 5*(1), 1–15.

Delamater, A. M., de Wit, M., McDarby, V., Malik, J., & Acerini, C. L. (2014). Psychological care of children and adolescents with type 1 diabetes. *Pediatric diabetes, 15*(20), S232–S244.

El-Sheikh, M. (2005). Stability of respiratory sinus arrhythmia in children and young adolescents: A longitudinal examination. *Developmental Psychobiology, 46*(1), 66–74.

Ellis, B. J., Essex, M. J., & Boyce, W. T. (2005). Biological sensitivity to context: II. Empirical explorations of an evolutionary–developmental theory. *Development and Psychopathology, 17*(2), 303–328.

Fadiman, A. (1997). *The spirit catches you and you fall down: A Hmong child, her American doctors, and the collision of two cultures*. Farrar, Straus, and Giroux.

Gaffney, H., Farrington, D. P., & Ttofi, M. M. (2019). Examining the effectiveness of school-bullying intervention programs globally: A meta-analysis. *International Journal of Bullying Prevention, 1*(1), 14–31.

Garner, A. S., Shonkoff, J. P., Siegel, B. S., Dobbins, M. I., Earls, M. F., McGuinn, L., ... & Committee on Early Childhood, Adoption, and Dependent Care. (2012). Early childhood adversity, toxic stress, and the role of the pediatrician: Translating developmental science into lifelong health. *Pediatrics, 129*(1), e224–e231.

Imran, N., Aamer, I., Sharif, M. I., Bodla, Z. H., & Naveed, S. (2020). Psychological burden of quarantine in children and adolescents: A rapid systematic review and proposed solutions. *Pakistan Journal of Medical Sciences, 36*(5), 1106.

Lionetti, F., Aron, A., Aron, E. N., Burns, G. L., Jagiellowicz, J., & Pluess, M. (2018). Dandelions, tulips and orchids: Evidence for the existence of low-sensitive, medium-sensitive and high-sensitive individuals. *Translational Psychiatry, 8*(1), 1–11.

Masten, A. S. (2014). Global perspectives on resilience in children and youth. *Child Development, 85*(1), 6–20.

Moos, R. H. (2002). 2001 Invited address: The mystery of human context and coping: An unraveling of clues. *American Journal of Community PsychologyAmerican, 30*(1), 67–88.

O'Donnell, M. L., Agathos, J. A., Metcalf, O., Gibson, K., & Lau, W. (2019). Adjustment disorder: Current developments and future directions. *International Journal of Environmental Research and Public Health, 16*(14), 2537.

Olsson, C. A., Bond, L., Burns, J. M., Vella-Brodrick, D. A., & Sawyer, S. M. (2003). Adolescent resilience: A concept analysis. *Journal of Adolescence, 26*(1), 1–11.

Patra, B. N., & Sarkar, S. (2013). Adjustment disorder: current diagnostic status. *Indian Journal of Psychological Medicine, 35*(1), 4–9.

Pless, I. B.Dougherty, G., Willard, B., Feeley, N., Gottlieb, L., & Rowat, K., A randomized trial of a nursing intervention to promote the adjustment of children with chronic physical disorders. *Pediatrics, 94*(1), 70–75.

Porges, S. W. (2007). The polyvagal perspective. *Biological Psychology, 74*(2), 116–143.

Raval, V. V., & Walker, B. L. (2019). Unpacking "culture": Caregiver socialization of emotion and child functioning in diverse families. *Developmental Review, 51*, 146–174.

Shonkoff, J. P., Boyce, W. T., Levitt, P., Martinez, F. D., & McEwen, B. (2021). Leveraging the biology of adversity and resilience to transform pediatric practice. *Pediatrics.*

Van Schoors, M., Caes, L., Knoble, N. B., Goubert, L., Verhofstadt, L. L., & Alderfer, M. A. (2017). Systematic review: Associations between family functioning and child adjustment after pediatric cancer diagnosis: A meta-analysis. *Journal of Pediatric Psychology, 42*(1), 6–18.

Viorst, J. (1974). *Alexander and the terrible, horrible, no good, very bad day*. Atheneum Books.

Werner, E. E. (1992). The children of Kauai: Resiliency and recovery in adolescence and adulthood. *The Journal of Adolescent Health, 13*(4), 262–268.

World Health Organization. (2022). *International classification of diseases* (11th revision). Author.

Zuckerman, B. (2009). Promoting early literacy in pediatric practice: Twenty years of reach out and read. *Pediatrics, 124*(6), 1660–1665.

58

Impact of Hospitalization and Acute Medical Care on Children and Families

Gayle Chesley and Paul M. Robins

For additional material related to the content of this chapter, see Chapters 2, 51, and 56.

VIGNETTE

Jamir is a 13-year-old Black boy with cerebral palsy and mild cognitive impairment who is cared for by a single mother, Eve. At a medical visit, it was discussed that Jamir needs hamstring lengthening surgery to address his crouched gait. Eve has not agreed with this recommendation during past visits, and Jamir's gait has increasingly worsened. A social worker met with the family as part of the medical visit and further explored concerns. Eve reported that Jamir had "bad experiences" with surgeries and subsequent hospitalizations in early childhood, including screaming with IV sticks, prolonged pain, and distress with bed restriction. She recalled one incident in which Jamir was in surgery for much longer than anticipated, and she became increasingly frantic in the waiting room, worried that he had died. Eve noted she had nightmares for many months after this experience. She stated that she realized it was her duty to protect Jamir from harm, and she continues to try to shield him from danger. Jamir has frequently been told by Eve how lucky he is that he was young enough to forget these experiences. When the social worker talked with Jamir, Jamir informed her that he does not want the surgery because it is frightening, but he has trouble identifying specific reasons.

Each year, many children experience an acute medical problem requiring hospitalization. There were nearly 5.9 million hospital stays for children in the United States in 2012 (Witt, Weiss, & Elixhauser, 2014). Hospitalization may significantly impact a child due to exposure to potentially painful and invasive procedures, loss of control, separation from family, and an unfamiliar environment. Additionally, parental impact is significant and occurs both vicariously (e.g., exposure to their child undergoing painful experience) and directly (e.g., loss of control). It is important to understand these reactions to provide timely and needed care at the optimal level of intervention.

IMPACT OF HOSPITALIZATION ON CHILD AND CAREGIVER FUNCTIONING

Several studies have examined the impact of hospitalization on youth. Jepsen, Haahr, Eg, & Jorgensen, (2019) conducted a qualitative meta-synthesis of existing literature to examine the impact of hospitalization; all studies involved observation or interview of the child. The most frequent challenge identified was the "unfamiliar," including the child's role as a patient, limited bodily functioning, and pain and discomfort. Children experienced novel machine noises and medical language, unusual and unclear routines, and uncertainty about treatment and discharge plans. Thus it is not surprising that state anxiety has been found to be significantly higher in hospitalized children compared to nonhospitalized children (Delvecchio, Salcuni, Lis, Germani, & Di Riso, 2019). Hospital-based fears were found to be common among previously hospitalized children, with the most frequently reported fears being injections and the hospital environment (Ozturk & Topan, 2019). Based on semistructured interviews with hospitalized children, fears and concerns included separation from family, friends, and life at home (e.g., food, routine); possibility of pain, impairment, or death with procedures; and loss of independence (e.g., access to food, sleep schedule) (Coyne, 2006). Children who were younger, more severely medically ill, and exposed to higher numbers of procedures demonstrated increased medical fears and posttraumatic stress symptoms 6 months postdischarge (Rennick, Johnston, Dougherty, Platt, & Ritchie, 2002).

The impact of hospitalization is not limited to children; caregivers also experience difficulty. A longitudinal study found that 3 months after discharge of their child from intensive care, parents were experiencing the following rates of symptomatology: Posttraumatic stress disorder (PTSD), 23%; moderate-severe anxiety, 41%; moderate-severe depression, 7%. These rates remained comparable at 6-month follow-up (Rodriguez-Rey, Alonso-Tapia, & Colville, 2019). Other studies examining parents' functioning after their child's acute hospitalization found rates of acute traumatic stress, depression, and anxiety in parents were high (Bronner et al., 2009;

Muscara et al., 2015) and similar across illness type (Muscara et al., 2015). Parental posttraumatic symptoms at 3 months postintensive care discharge, particularly hyperarousal and avoidance, predicted prolonged PTSD (Bronner et al., 2010). In a review of insurance claim data 9.5% of parents received a new mental health diagnosis 6 months after their child's intensive care stay, representing a 110% increase compared to 6 months prior (Logan, Sahrmann, Gu, & Hartman, 2020); mothers were two times more likely than fathers to receive a diagnosis. Other factors associated with increased parental symptomatology risk included presence of economic difficulties, history of mental health difficulties, and single parenting (Rodriguez-Rey et al., 2019).

CONCEPTUAL MODELS

Bioecologic Systems Theory

The impact of childhood hospitalization is influenced by factors at multiple system levels. Bronfenbrenner (1979) describes these systems in the bioecologic systems theory (BST) as "a set of nested structures, each inside the next" (p. 3), with each level existing with a complex network of interconnections (see Chapter 2). One's adaptation to a new role and environment depends on influences spanning from the personal to the larger culture, and the interactions between these influences. Individual factors impacting response to hospitalization likely include developmental or cognitive level, preexisting emotional and behavioral functioning, and physiologic functioning.

Based on BST, the impact of hospitalization will be determined by the interaction of the individual with larger systems: The microsystem, mesosystem, exosystem, and macrosystem. The microsystem is comprised of the child's immediate environment. For the hospitalized child, family functioning is an important microsystem factor. Premorbid family system organization, adaptability of the family system to shift in response to hospitalization, and family roles influence the impact of hospitalization on children and their caregivers (Robins & Rourke, 2012). The mesosystem involves interrelations between microsystem settings. Within the mesosystem, interactions between patients, caregivers, and hospital providers will affect the hospital experience. For example, does the clinician account for developmental, cognitive, and cultural considerations when choosing language to discuss a new diagnosis? Important exosystem considerations, involving social systems that the child does not directly interact with, include community social support and parental employment flexibility. Larger system considerations at the macrosystem level encompass policies and legal safeguards (e.g., Family Medical Leave Act), availability of health insurance, and cultural attitudes toward illness and impairment. Macrolevel issues include institutionalized inequalities for socially and economically disenfranchised groups; these inequalities are associated with medical mistrust (Jaiswal & Halkitis, 2019). Chronosystem, individual and environmental changes over time, was later added to the BST model (Bronfenbrenner, 1986). For example, previous negative experience with hospitalization at a young age may influence reaction to hospitalization in adolescence. Taken together, these interacting systems help explain how past experiences and the current environment impact a child's response to hospitalization.

One experience that may have lasting biologic and psychosocial impacts is childhood surgery. There has been concern that exposure to anesthesia in young children may have neurotoxic effects and may be associated with an increased risk of neurocognitive deficits, particularly if the exposure was prolonged (see Lin, Lee, Lee, Deng, & Loepke, 2017 for a review of preclinical and clinical studies) or occurred over the course of multiple surgeries (Kobayashi et al., 2020). However, there are also studies that suggest more limited effects on isolated neurodevelopmental domains, particularly motor functioning (Walkden et al., 2020). Caregivers' emotional reaction when recalling the child's surgery can in turn impact the child's response to further medical care. Thus individual factors such as cognition and emotion, and microsystem factors, including caregiver past and current coping, are important components to understand potential impact of an upcoming surgery. In the vignette Jamir's recurrent observations of his mother's anxiety related to his past surgeries and hospitalizations likely contributed to his view of procedures as a danger to be feared and avoided. Eve's efforts to protect Jamir from danger are negatively impacting Jamir's ability to receive needed medical care.

Pediatric Psychosocial Preventative Health Model

Whereas the BST model focuses on larger system influences on an individual, the pediatric psychosocial preventative health model (PPPHM) incorporates a social ecologic framework to stratify level of psychosocial risk for medically ill children and their families (Kazak, 2006). In this model three tiers of risk are depicted in a pyramid format. Universal, the largest tier, is at the base. Families in the Universal category experience typical distress associated with the onset or worsening of a pediatric medical condition, and in the short term they adequately respond using available resources. The middle tier of the pyramid, Targeted, includes families that are at greater risk for ongoing difficulties. Increased risk may be due to premorbid difficulties at the level of the individual (e.g., history of parental mental health difficulties), family system (e.g., child-parent discord), social system (e.g., limited school resources), and community (e.g., environment unfavorable to child's disability). The smallest tier, Clinical/Treatment, encompasses families with the greatest risk for prolonged distress. Here, risk is exacerbated by challenges at multiple system levels and their interaction with one another. For example, a parent with premorbid ongoing mental health difficulties dealing with stressors related to a child's prolonged hospitalization might be unable to access typical mental health care due to the child's hospitalization. It is anticipated that families in this tier will have heightened and persistent distress without intervention. Using this model, service intensity and resources can be matched to family need. In the case of Jamir and Eve the family is at risk due to previous "bad experiences" with surgery and hospitalization, so earlier identification of these Targeted needs and related interventions may have reduced delay in Jamir's needed surgery. The family has now moved to the Clinical/Treatment tier, where intervention is likely necessary to address family dynamics and emotional distress that are barriers to medical care.

INTERVENTION

These conceptual models can help clinicians better identify intervention scope, targets, and timing. Intervention for hospitalized children may occur at any level of the child's system, could involve all children in a population or a small number, and could occur at multiple points in time. The focus of the intervention can range from reducing the likelihood that a problem will occur (i.e., prevention based) to resolving a crisis. Matching the right intervention to the right time can save time and resources, and can direct care to where it is most needed.

One such model incorporating matching system level, scope, and intervention was developed by Carter et al. (2018) to guide inpatient psychological prevention and intervention. The authors combined the BST and PPPHM models, noting that clinicians may intervene at each level of the PPPHM, which may have an impact at the various BST system levels. At the Universal level, interventions may focus on prevention and education, and span the range of system levels. For example, staff may develop educational handouts with coping tips to be provided to all inpatients (individual system) and their parents (microsystem) on common adaptive coping techniques. Education may be provided to schools to help increase understanding of the reintegration needs of children with medical conditions in general (exosystem). Research and advocacy efforts may focus on interventions for children with a specific medical condition (macrosystem). At the Targeted level, at-risk families may receive more specific education and potentially short-term, individualized intervention. Hospital staff may meet with parents and school personnel upon the discharge of an at-risk child with a newly acquired impairment to provide recommendations for school accommodations (mesosystem). At the Clinical/Treatment level, interventions typically include direct work with the child and family to address ongoing or escalating difficulties. Families may be referred to clinicians to teach specific coping strategies (microsystem). Interventions at this level are more likely to be focused on the individual and family system.

Most research on intervention targets for hospitalized children focus on the individual or family. Spirito, Stark, & Tyc, (1994) compared coping strategies used by acutely ill and chronically ill hospitalized children, and found that acutely ill children were more likely to use avoidant coping strategies such as self-blame and wishful thinking. Avoidant coping strategies are generally associated with worse outcomes; active and approach strategies, such as information seeking and problem solving, are associated with more positive outcomes (Clavé et al., 2019; Enlow et al., 2019; Greer et al., 2018). Play is often provided as a universal intervention by pediatric hospitals, through introduction of developmentally appropriate materials or play rooms, and has been shown to be helpful (Jepsen et al., 2019). The potential benefits of play include distraction, fun, and with medical play an opportunity to make sense of the unfamiliar environment.

Individual and family strategies have also been employed to reduce acute and posttraumatic stress symptomatology, with mixed results. When Kramer and Landolt (2011) conducted a metaanalysis to examine if early psychological intervention after medical trauma could impact outcome, they found that interventions focused on the individual and family could be helpful. It was recommended that interventions include age-appropriate psychoeducation, support for individual coping skills, parent involvement, and possibly trauma exposure therapy. The authors later studied a targeted, two-session early intervention for at-risk children who experienced a serious physical injury. They found that intervention with school-aged children was effective in reducing internalizing problems, but not with preschool-aged children (Kramer & Landolt, 2014). Berkowitz, Stover, & Marans, (2011) found that a brief intervention for at-risk youth who recently experienced a potentially traumatic event, targeting caregiver-child communication and behavioral skills, resulted in significantly lower posttraumatic and anxiety scores in an intervention group compared to a supportive comparison control group. Alternatively, an early intervention aimed at reducing medical posttraumatic stress in school-aged children was not found to be effective in preventing later symptoms in a randomized trial (Kassam-Adams et al., 2011).

Many interventions have been developed to help caregivers or family of the hospitalized child directly, rather than as an adjunct to child treatment, with the added benefit that improved parental and family functioning may positively impact the child. For example, Burns-Nader, Hernandez-Reif, & Porter, (2014) found that the number of coping strategies used by mothers of hospitalized children was related to diminished anxiety in the child. Brief therapy targeting parents of hospitalized children was shown to be effective in reducing trauma symptoms in fathers and adolescents (Kazak et al., 2004). Problem-focused parental coping was found to be associated with improved caregiver adjustment to a child's hospitalization, and interventions targeting improved parental problem-focused coping and sense of control were recommended (Wartella, Auerbach, & Ward, 2009). During a child's hospitalization, such interventions could include involving caregivers in bathing and feeding, offering choice in routine when available, and shared medical decision making. The Creating Opportunities for Parent Empowerment (COPE) intervention is a preventative education-based model aimed at caregivers. Mothers of hospitalized children were provided education about typical reactions and ways to promote adaptive coping at three time points: during intensive care admission, following discharge to a pediatric floor, and soon after discharge. In a randomized control the intervention was found to be associated with reduced maternal stress and depression, fewer posttraumatic stress symptoms, and increased caretaking for the child's physical and emotional needs compared to a control group (Melnyk et al., 2004).

Family interventions can be further refined by targeting the type of family organization or structural problem. Robins and Rourke (2012) identified aspects of the family system that may impact response to hospitalization and matched strategies (Table 58.1) that could be used during a child's hospitalization to help support families experiencing difficulties in this area.

As evidenced by Table 58.1, interventions focusing on the health care team can be helpful in supporting positive child and family adjustment. The Universal tier is an ideal level to intervene, as intervention will impact all families. As a Universal strategy, clinical practice guidelines were created to outline best practices to support families in a patient-centered intensive care unit. Recommendations for unit staff include clear and consistent family messaging, consistent staff assignments, a shared medical decision-making model, and availability of staff support for caregivers (Davidson et al., 2007). Educational programs have helped to prepare hospital staff to care for children with autism spectrum disorder (Lucarelli et al., 2018).

In the vignette, intervention for Eve at the time of Jamir's initial surgeries may have prevented later challenge. Improved communication during an unexpectedly prolonged surgery may have prevented fear of his death and subsequent post-traumatic stress symptoms. Upfront education to families about anticipated pain and ways to promote adaptive coping, such as ways parents can help manage their child's pain, may have increased Eve's sense of efficacy. Additionally, education about common shifts in family roles due to medical needs and strategies to promote adaptive family functioning may have reduced her protective response that impeded care. She may have learned to protect Jamir through implementation of adaptive pain management and other coping strategies, rather than protection through medical care refusal. Now that Jamir and Eve's fears about surgery are identified, a Clinical/Treatment tier intervention can be applied. A clinician can help Jamir and Eve identify the source of their anxieties and impact on family functioning and implement specific, individualized strategies to address hospital-related fears for Jamir to obtain needed medical care. At all points of care, the cultural context should be considered, including the possibility

TABLE 58.1 Interventions Targeting the Family of a Hospitalized Child

Family System Challenge	Interventions to Consider
Family's developmental level: Normative phases of a family's development over time	• Normalize the ways in which the demands of illness are often inconsistent with what a child needs developmentally • Partner with family to identify developmentally appropriate roles a child and parent can take • Help family develop new routines, with care to soothe worry, support growth, and avoid judgment and punishment • Coach children and parents through fears in developmentally appropriate ways ("I know this is hard/scary, but you can do it, and there is a team to support you"); avoid overindulging or overprotecting the family
Organization/hierarchy: Roles and leadership positions developing within and between family members	• Assign family members roles and responsibilities consistent with an appropriate place in the hierarchy • Identify a staff member to partner with the family, to provide resources that will support the newl assigned roles • Treat the parent and child as competent and convey your confidence that they will be able to shift their roles • Connect families to groups of other families managing similar conditions, which can offer positive role models and peers
Adaptability: Flexibility in leadership, roles, and relationship rules	• Help families understand typical hospital routines to provide a sense of predictability when possible (e.g., meals, rounding) • Provide families with access to clear information, including upfront education to expect multiple changes, and timely information about changes when they occur • Encourage families to develop a routine to care for their own needs (e.g., bedside schedule, cafeteria trips for their own meals, frequency of communication with family and friends)
Cohesion: Emotional bonds between family members	• Educate families that each member's reactions to hospitalization are likely to be different; this information can help caregivers and children recognize these differences, rather than assuming others are coping similarly • Develop age-appropriate tasks and roles for parents and for patients, and support families in carrying these out • Assist parents and children with staying connected to roles and important family and friends outside of the hospital • Encourage children to engage in developmentally appropriate hobbies and interests

Based on Interventions from Robins & Rourke, 2012. Robins P. & Rourke M. (2012). Psychological Reactions to Critical Care Events. In Abend N. & Helfaer M., *Neurocritical Care*. Springer Publishing, pp. 443–454.

of Eve experiencing medical mistrust given historical and ongoing racist practices and policies in medical institutions.

CONCLUSION

Childhood hospitalization is frequent and can have a significant and negative impact on child and caregiver functioning, including mood and posttraumatic stress symptoms. Conceptual frameworks are presented to help illuminate challenges to hospitalized children and their families on multiple levels. Adaptation to hospitalization can be considered on interrelated system levels, from the individual to the macrosystem level. The impact of hospitalization can also be considered by risk stratification, from focus on a population to targeting those children and families that have clinically significant difficulties. These models can help guide prevention and intervention strategies. Effective intervention strategies may focus on the child, caregivers, or health care team to improve outcomes.

REFERENCES

Berkowitz, S., Stover, C., & Marans, S. (2011). The child and family traumatic stress intervention: Secondary prevention for youth at risk of developing PTSD. *Journal of Child Psychology and Psychiatry*, *52*(6), 676–685.

Bronfenbrenner, U. (1979). *The ecology of human development*. Harvard University Press.

Bronfenbrenner, U. (1986). Ecology of the family as a context for human development: Research perspectives. *Developmental Psychology*, *22*(6), 723–742.

Bronner, M., Kayser, A., Knoester, H., Bos, A., Last, B., & Grootenhuis, M. (2009). A pilot study on peritraumatic dissociation and coping styles as risk factors for posttraumatic stress, anxiety and depression in parents after their child's unexpected admission to a pediatric intensive care unit. *Child and Adolescent Psychiatry and Mental Health*, *3*, 33.

Bronner, M., Peek, N., Knoester, H., Bos, A., Last, B., & Grootenhuis, M. (2010). Course and predictors of posttraumatic stress disorder in parents after pediatric intensive care treatment of their child. *Journal of Pediatric Psychology*, *35*(9), 966–974.

Burns-Nader, S., Hernandez-Reif, M., & Porter, M. (2014). The relationship between mothers' coping patterns and children's anxiety about their hospitalization as reflected in drawings. *Journal of Child Health Care*, *18*(1), 6–18.

Carter, B., Kronenberger, W., Scott, E., Kullgren, K., Piazza-Waggoner, C., & Brady, C. (2018). Inpatient pediatric consultation-liaison. In M. Roberts & R. Steele (Eds.), *Handbook of pediatric psychology* (5th ed.). The Guilford Press.

Clavé, S., Tsimaratos, M., Boucekine, M., Ranchin, B., Salomon, R., Dunand, O., … Berbis, J. (2019). Quality of life in adolescents with chronic kidney disease who initiate haemodialysis treatment. *BMC Nephrology*, *20*(1), 163.

Coyne, I. (2006). Children's experiences of hospitalization. *Journal of Children's Health Care*, *10*(4), 326–336.

Davidson, J., Powers, K., Hedayat, K., Tieszen, M., Kon, A., Shepard, E., … Armstrong, D. (2007). Clinical practice guidelines for support of the family in the patient-centered intensive care unit: American College of Critical Care Medicine Task Force 2004–2005. *Critical Care Medicine*, *35*(2), 605–622.

Delvecchio, E., Salcuni, S., Lis, A., Germani, A., & Di Riso, D. (2019). Hospitalized children: Anxiety, coping strategies, and pretend play. *Frontiers in Public Health*, *7*, 250.

Enlow, P. T., Brown Kirschman, K. J., Mentrikoski, J., Szabo, M. M., Butz, C., Aballay, A. M., & Duncan, C. L. (2019). The role of youth coping strategies and caregiver psychopathology in predicting posttraumatic stress symptoms in pediatric burn survivors. *Journal of Burn Care Research*, *40*(5), 620–626.

Greer, J. A., Jacobs, J. M., El-Jawahri, A., Nipp, R. D., Gallagher, E. R., Pirl, W. F., … Temel, J. S. (2018). Role of patient coping strategies in understanding the effects of early palliative care on quality of life and mood. *Journal of Clinical Oncology*, *36*(1), 53–60.

Jaiswal, J., & Halkitis, P. N. (2019). Towards a more inclusive and dynamic understanding of medical mistrust informed by science. *Behavioral Medicine*, *45*(2), 79–85.

Jepsen, S., Haahr, A., Eg, M., & Jorgensen, L. (2019). Coping with the unfamiliar: How do children cope with hospitalization in relation to acute and/or critical illness? A qualitative metasynthesis. *Journal of Child Health Care*, *23*(4), 534–550.

Kassam-Adams, N., Garcia-Espana, J., Marsac, M., Kohser, K., Baxt, C., Nance, M., & Winston, F. (2011). A pilot randomized controlled trial assessing secondary prevention of traumatic stress integrated into pediatric trauma care. *Journal of Traumatic Stress*, *24*(3), 252–259.

Kazak, A. (2006). Pediatric Psychosocial Preventative Health Model (PPPHM): Research, practice, and collaboration in pediatric family systems medicine. *Families, Systems & Health*, *24*(4), 381–395.

Kazak, A., Alderfer, M., Streisand, R., Simms, S., Rourke, M., Barakat, L., … Cnaan, A. (2004). Treatment of posttraumatic stress symptoms in adolescent survivors of childhood cancer and their families: A randomized clinical trial. *Journal of Family Psychology*, *183*, 493–504.

Kobayashi, Y., Tokuda, N., Adachi, S., Takeshima, Y., Hirose, M., Shima, M., & Japan Environment and Children's Study (JECS) Group. (2020). Association between surgical procedures under general anesthesia in infancy and developmental outcomes at 1 year: The Japan Environment and Children's Study. *Environmental Health and Preventive Medicine*, *25*(1), 32.

Kramer, D., & Landolt, M. (2011). Characteristics and efficacy of early psychological interventions in children and adolescents after single trauma: A meta-analysis. *European Journal of Psychotraumatology*, *2*, 7858.

Kramer, D., & Landolt, M. (2014). Early psychological intervention in accidentally injured children ages 2–16: A randomized controlled trial. *European Journal of Psychotraumatology*, *5*, 24402.

Lin, E. P., Lee, J. R., Lee, C. S., Deng, M., & Loepke, A. W. (2017). Do anesthetics harm the developing human brain? An integrative analysis of animal and human studies. *Neurotoxicology and Teratology*, *60*, 117–128.

Logan, G., Sahrmann, J., Gu, H., & Hartman, M. (2020). Parental mental health care after their child's pediatric intensive care hospitalization. *Pediatric Critical Care Medicine*, *21*(11), 941–948.

Lucarelli, J., Welchons, L., Sideridis, G., Sullivan, N. R., Chan, E., & Weissman, L. (2018). Development and evaluation of an educational initiative to improve hospital personnel preparedness to care for children with autism spectrum disorder. *Journal of Developmental Behavioral Pediatrics*, *39*(5), 358–364.

Melnyk, B. M., Alpert-Gillis, L., Feinstein, N. F., Crean, H. F., Johnson, J., Fairbanks, E., … Corbo-Richert, B. (2004). Creating opportunities for parent empowerment: Program effects on the mental health/coping outcomes of critically ill young children and their mothers. *Pediatrics*, *113*(6), e597–e607.

Muscara, F., McCarthy, M., Woolf, C., Hearps, S., Burke, K., & Anderson, V. (2015). Early psychological reactions in parents of children with a life threatening illness within a pediatric hospital setting. *European Psychiatry*, *30*, 555–561.

Ozturk, S., & Topan, A. (2019). Investigation of the fear of 7–18-year-old hospitalized children for illness and hospital. *Journal of Religion and Health*, *58*(3), 1011–1023.

Rennick, J., Johnston, C., Dougherty, G., Platt, R., & Ritchie, J. (2002). Children's psychological responses after critical illness and exposure to invasive technology. *Journal of Developmental and Behavioral Pediatrics*, *23*(3), 133–144.

Robins, P., & Rourke, M. (2012). Psychological reactions to critical care events. In N. Abend, & M. Helfaer (Eds.), *Neurocritical care* (pp. 443–454). Springer Publishing.

Rodriguez-Rey, R., Alonso-Tapia, J., & Colville, G. (2019). Prediction of parental posttraumatic stress, anxiety and depression after a child's critical hospitalization. *Journal of Critical Care*, *45*, 149–155.

Spirito, A., Stark, L., & Tyc, V. (1994). Stressors and coping strategies described during hospitalization by chronically ill children. *Journal of Clinical Child Psychology*, *23*(3), 31.

Walkden, G. J., Gill, H., Davies, N. M., Peters, A. E., Wright, I., & Pickering, A. E. (2020). Early childhood general anesthesia and neurodevelopmental outcomes in the Avon Longitudinal Study of parent and children birth cohort. *Anesthesiology*, *133*, 1007–1020.

Wartella, J. E., Auerbach, S. M., & Ward, K. R. (2009). Emotional distress, coping and adjustment in family members of neuroscience intensive care unit patients. *Journal of Psychosomatic Research*, *66*(6), 503–509.

Witt, W., Weiss, A., & Elixhauser, A. (2014). *Overview of hospital stays for children in the United States, 2012. HCUP Statistical Brief No. 187*. Agency for Healthcare Research and Quality. http://www.hcup-us.ahrq.gov/reports/statbriefs/sb187-Hospital-Stays-Children-2012.pdf

59

Children with Chronic Illness and Medical Complexity

Kourtney Santucci and Ellen Roy Elias

For additional material related to the content of this chapter, see Chapters 11, 23, 31, 34, 35, 39 and 63.

VIGNETTE

Hannah is a 16-year-old girl being seen in clinic for follow-up of symptoms stemming from hypermobile Ehlers-Danlos syndrome (hEDS). This connective tissue disorder is associated with abnormal skin integrity, joint laxity, chronic pain, gastrointestinal dysfunction, and neurologic symptoms. Today, she is most troubled by frequent migraine headaches, which are triggered by instances of presyncope. She has a long history of joint subluxation with minor activities and experiences chronic musculoskeletal pain. For 3 years, she has suffered chronic nausea, gastroparesis, alternating diarrhea and constipation, and intermittent ability to gain weight despite nasogastric feedings. She is again losing weight. Her skin bruises easily, though she's not had abnormal bleeding. She is struggling with anxiety and depression. Hannah's vital signs reveal orthostasis. The management of headache is Hannah's primary need today. You realize that management of orthostasis could help with headache prevention. Getting her joint pain and intestinal symptoms under control would also aid her quality of life and may curb weight loss. Her evaluation and management plan are complex and will need to involve care with a multidisciplinary team of specialists and therapists, including attention to her mental health.

DEFINITIONS OF CHRONIC ILLNESS AND MEDICAL COMPLEXITY

Chronic illnesses in childhood include a wide variety of health conditions, from asthma and juvenile-onset diabetes, which are relatively common, to genetic disorders, neural tube defects such as spina bifida, cardiac malformations, autoimmune diseases, epilepsy, and malignant neoplasms, which are relatively rare. Individually, any chronic illness diagnosis may be very rare, but grouped together chronic illnesses present health challenges for a substantial percentage of youth. Approximately 15% of American children have a diagnosis of a chronic illness, and for epidemiologic purposes they are regarded as children and youth with special health conditions (CYSHC). Due in large part to advances in neonatal care and pediatric complex medical care in general, this group is growing; the proportion of children with a chronic condition that interferes with daily activities has increased by over 400% since the 1960s, and approximately 20% of US households are home to a CYSHC. Chronic illnesses impact physical, emotional, and/or developmental health and, in general, are not anticipated to resolve.

Fortunately, consensus guidelines for management of many conditions have been developed. The American Academy of Pediatrics, and its journal *Pediatrics*, has regularly updated clinical care guidelines for children with many chronic conditions, including asthma, attention-deficit/hyperactivity disorder (ADHD), and Down syndrome, allowing parents and practitioners to stay apprised of recent updates. While there are still the challenges of maintaining care of the chronic condition in addition to all the typical challenges of raising a child, the presence of a roadmap for good care alleviates much anxiety for parents and medical providers.

Of the total number of CYSHC, a subset has particularly complex illnesses impacting on various body systems, needing care from a team of subspecialists (and coordinated by a primary health care provider), and possessing a high degree of dependence on medications or medical technology and community supports. These children with medical complexity (CMC) represent between 1% and 6% of the US pediatric population (depending on the precise definitions used in population studies). However, their intense care needs require considerable resources. In 2012 CMC were estimated to account for about one-third of all child health care costs.

For CMC, care is not straightforward. The condition may be exceedingly rare, sometimes identified in only a small handful of patients; understanding the condition and how best to treat it may be yet evolving, as is the case for the EDS, referenced in the vignette. The simultaneous presence of many diagnoses complicates what might be clearcut care plans had each condition occurred in isolation. This situation is confusing and exhausting for parents and children to navigate. It is crucial that a primary health care clinician be available to the family to help coordinate care plans and ensure communication among specialists. Some families, due to the rare nature of their child's condition, may live at a great distance from specialists with the necessary experience, and thus may travel often for care. For these families, it is crucial that communications back to the local primary care provider be prompt and informative. If possible, having a specialty pediatrician at the tertiary care center (such as an experienced pediatrician in complex care clinics at many pediatric tertiary care centers) can be very helpful to consolidate the care plan and offer a go-to provider at the tertiary center for the local clinician when issues arise.

ETIOLOGY

CMC, by definition, present with multiple, complex, and concurrent problems. The underlying etiology of the child's issues may be clear, such as documented anoxia at birth, closed head trauma, or a confirmed genetic disorder. Often an underlying etiology for the child's medical and developmental problems is elusive. For example, intellectual disability and cerebral palsy are descriptive terms that can serve as unifying diagnoses, although neither is an etiologic diagnosis (i.e., the root, underlying cause of the child's health condition). Intellectual disability means that the child has significant limitation in intellectual functioning (often measured as a full-scale IQ <70), significant limitations in adaptive behavior, and onset before age 18 (see Chapter 40). Cerebral palsy implies that the child has a nonprogressive (static) disorder of movement and posture caused by abnormal development of or damage to the motor cortex (see Chapter 39). In recent years science has advanced the level to which we can understand the etiology of conditions such as intellectual disability and cerebral palsy, and other conditions such as neural tube defects, structural brain malformations, and metabolic disorders. The astute clinician should no longer be satisfied with a diagnosis such as intellectual disability or cerebral palsy. Evaluating for etiology has implications not only for proper treatment of the child affected but also for counseling of parents and siblings. Certain genetic diagnoses carry with them known associated medical problems that may develop in the future, and having that diagnosis allows the clinician to prognosticate accurately and intervene at an earlier stage when those problems do develop. The etiologic diagnosis may allow for specific, effective, and appropriate medical interventions. Even for diagnoses as common as Down syndrome or spina bifida, many families are unaware of their recurrence risks, of available means of prenatal detection in future pregnancies, or of the possibilities of interventions to reduce the recurrence risk, such as folic acid supplementation to reduce the risk of neural tube defects.

When caring for CMC, if there is no clear etiologic diagnosis, or the suggested etiology is inconsistent with the history or progress of the child over time, the clinician should be suspicious. A genetic evaluation or consultation is appropriate for any child with dysmorphic features or known birth defects. Metabolic testing should be considered for a child with a history of decline in neurologic status or loss of milestones, or a change in developmental status associated with intercurrent illnesses. The pediatrician should obtain a good family history: Are there other individuals in the family with similar symptoms, or a history of consanguinity, infertility, fetal loss, or death during early infancy? If the child has atypical head circumference with no history of brain injury, then a brain imaging study such as magnetic resonance imaging (MRI) may be appropriate to look for central nervous system dysgenesis (see Chapter 89). The more severe the disabilities and medical problems, the more likely that an etiology will be found. See Chapter 23 for a detailed approach to the workup of a child with disabilities, and Chapter 36 for a detailed discussion of the workup of inborn errors of metabolism.

COMPLEXITY OF DIAGNOSES AND MANAGEMENT

A major challenge of caring for CMC is caring for multiple diagnoses simultaneously. Often, in addition to the difficulty of managing conditions that impact physical health, managing behavioral or psychiatric diagnoses occurring in the same child present challenges for parents and clinicians. More than half of children with cerebral palsy have cognitive disabilities. Children with cerebral palsy also may have sensory deficits, including poor vision or hearing impairment. A child might have more than one sensory impairment. A child with CHARGE syndrome (coloboma, heart disease, atresia choanae, genital hypoplasia, and ear anomalies) may have visual impairment secondary to retinal colobomas and congenital sensorineural hearing loss (see Chapter 24). The importance of understanding these associations cannot be overemphasized because the comprehensive evaluation of the child, management plan, and referrals for appropriate therapeutic and educational services are contingent on recognizing that more than one condition may coexist.

Children with cognitive disabilities may display various mental health issues, including significant depression, ADHD, aggression, and obsessive-compulsive disorder, any of which may be more functionally disabling than the underlying physical or cognitive problems. Children with intellectual disability (see Chapter 40) at the more severe end of the spectrum may present with extremely challenging self-stimulatory and self-injurious behaviors that further compromise functional skills and significant sleep problems that have a negative impact on learning (see Chapter 70). Finding mental health providers who are knowledgeable and skilled in the behavioral management of and psychopharmacology for children with intellectual disability is often quite difficult.

Coordinating the Care Team

In Hannah, from the vignette, with EDS we see an example of coexisting physical and mental health diagnoses, impacting on one another. EDS involves a group of connective tissue disorders, impacting the structure and function of the proteins that comprise ligaments, tendons, vessel walls, viscera, and skin. There are 14 types of EDS, per the most recent classification system in 2017, with hypermobile EDS (hEDS) being the most common. The causative genes for this form of EDS are not known.

Caring for the whole child with hEDS requires addressing both complex physical and mental health needs. Connective tissue is ubiquitous and affects every part of the body. Therefore symptoms of dysfunction range broadly: Joints may be hypermobile, with subluxations or frank dislocations of joints, and pain. Skin is stretchy and heals poorly from injury. Vessel walls are fragile, giving easy bruising and bleeding. We are just beginning to understand the mechanisms by which tissue fragility in the viscera impacts gut function, but patients with hEDS commonly experience constipation, irritable bowel syndrome, and may develop severe intestinal dysmotility and malabsorption. Less well understood is the impact of atypical connective tissue on the nervous system, but these nervous system impacts may be the etiology of the very common struggles with migraine headaches, abnormal proprioception, cognitive dysfunction, atypical neurodevelopment, and sensory processing difficulties seen in these patients. Another complex system impacted is the immunologic system. Patients with hEDS can experience a broad range of multiple food and drug allergies or sensitivities, and commonly have atopy.

Hypermobile EDS is a good example of invisible CMC and disability, in which the patient may appear outwardly healthy (without dysmorphic features or visible structural malformations and with normal cognitive function). It may appear as though "nothing is wrong," yet, with such far-reaching symptoms resulting from their connective tissue disorder, "everything is wrong." This situation is very difficult for the patients and their families, who often meet with disbelief from medical clinicians or teachers who do not see the issues that impact the children's everyday functioning. The situation may be particularly challenging prior to the diagnosis of hEDS being made.

A patient, like Hannah, who has not yet been given an etiologic diagnosis such as hEDS, may have had evaluations by physical therapists (for joint laxity and pains), orthopedists (for joint injury), neurologists (for headache or cognitive symptoms), gastroenterologists (for intestinal symptoms and constipation), allergists (for atopic symptoms), and mental health professionals (for anxiety and depression). Yet without the unifying diagnosis, these many providers are treating the individual symptoms without understanding how they are connected. This situation is reminiscent of the famous story that describes six blindfolded people all trying to identify the animal they are examining, which is an elephant. The one grasping the tail states, "It is a thin, snakelike creature, smallish, tubelike and flexible!" The one holding the ear states, "No! It is a rather large but thin, floppy, and leathery creature!" The one touching the high, broad flank states, "No! It is a massive creature and must be fierce!" The person holding the trunk has yet another opinion and thinks the others are all crazy. Of course, these examiners are all correct and yet incorrect at the same time. Only by removing the blindfolds can they discover that the animal simply has many different physical aspects, all connected and part of the same creature. This analogy serves well to describe the plight of the care team working without an etiologic diagnosis. We still have our blindfolds on.

The role of the general pediatrician, developmental pediatrician, or geneticist involved in the care of CMC, particularly with a rare or poorly understood diagnosis, is to continually try to remove the blindfolds for ourselves and our colleagues and for the extended care team of therapists, educators, social workers, coaches, and family members. Helping the team to understand the connections between aspects of a complex illness and continually looking for opportunities to streamline the care plan for the patient are key to good care.

At a visit for complex care coordination, time should be spent reviewing the impressions and recommendations of specialists, rooting out gaps in data, redundancies in interventions, or misunderstandings on the part of the clinicians or family. Discussions with individual specialists, or scheduling care conferences bringing the family and care team together, are often needed. This team approach can help to guide decisions about which medications to trial and in what order, how diagnostic procedures might be combined to reduce anesthetic exposures, approaches to improve developmental standing and mental health of the child, and to reach agreement (including the family's) about prioritizing goals of care. As a rule of thumb, "make one change at a time, and observe carefully for response" serves well to reduce confounding variables and polypharmacy interactions.

Intensity of Care Needs From Medical Clinicians

Caring for CMC can provide great satisfaction to the pediatrician and care team. However, there are clearly extraordinary demands for attention, time, and care coordination for these children, and any single clinician, including the primary care clinician, is challenged to accommodate all the demands. Visits are more frequent, need to last longer, and must address more complex issues than for children without medical complexity. CMC also require hospitalizations at a much higher rate than other children, including admission to regular pediatrics services and to the intensive care unit. During hospitalizations, it is often crucial for the physician who knows the child and family best to be available for difficult discussions about goals of care or end-of-life issues (see Chapter 63), or for care conferences to help plan future medical interventions.

Not only are visits, hospitalizations, and care conferences lengthy, time consuming, and often difficult to schedule, they also are poorly reimbursed. Many children with CMC have Medicaid insurance. Regardless of payer, the reimbursement to clinicians in the United States for these services has been insufficient. For this reason many physicians have made a conscious decision not to care for CMC, often leaving families searching for providers who are knowledgeable and willing to accept them as patients. Fortunately, at this writing, selected state Medicaid programs are beginning to offer reimbursement adjusted to account for the level of complexity of the patient. This issue must be addressed so that the child can flourish even in the context of multiple, complex medical, developmental, and mental health conditions.

Although CMC constitute an ever-increasing proportion of hospitalized children, few pediatric training programs in the United States offer a dedicated curriculum for trainee education of issues specific to care of CMC. Family medicine, internal medicine, nurse practitioner, and physician assistant trainees receive even less training in the management of patients with CMC than pediatricians, yet in large areas of the United States these professionals are the primary care clinicians available to patients. Many CMC who use medical technology (often referred to as technology assistance) such as ventilators and feeding tubes are entering the public school system, and pediatricians or other physicians are being asked to assist the schools in their management. The role of the developmental pediatric consultant in the management of CMC has become even more crucial for these patients.

AN APPROACH TO THE CHILD WITH MEDICAL COMPLEXITY

In the beginning of an assessment of the CMC it is important to get to know them as individuals and members of their families, schools, and communities. Parents report it is refreshing when a new clinician on their child's care team asks for a description of the child on his or her "best days." Placing focus on the child's abilities, rather than disabilities, and inquiring about the child's preferences and favorite activities can frame the clinician's impression through a "whole child" lens. It is also important to understand the family dynamics, as family circumstances have implications for what types of school and therapy plans might be feasible and beneficial. For example, for a family who have several other children, in-home physical or speech therapy might reduce transit time and give the therapist a window into the physical, social, and emotional space in which the child functions. If a family has several children enrolled at a neighborhood school, and options exist for their CMC to attend that same school and receive therapy services there, versus attending a more specialized school, the family may rightly opt for their children to be together for myriad practical and social reasons.

The clinician should also establish what agenda is most important to the parent, and if the child can participate, to the child. Again, parents of CMC are typically no strangers to medical appointments and care plans. They are also typically juggling many demands. Therefore making sure that the most pressing needs are addressed during visits is important. Setting agenda by inquiring, "What do you most want to discuss at our visit today?" near the beginning of the visit helps to ensure that time is spent on the issues most helpful to the family and that "housekeeping" issues (such as refills of chronic medications and preparing letters of medical necessity for any equipment or therapy referrals needed) are handled efficiently.

The discrete medical diagnoses present in CMC are intertwined. Feeding problems can be difficult to manage and lead to failure to thrive, behavior exacerbations, and/or respiratory compromise. In turn, respiratory issues leading to chronic lung disease also are quite common, sometimes stemming from neuromotor tone and coordination deficits. Comorbid neurologic conditions, particularly seizures, are common and often require medication management. Severe neuromotor disabilities generally impact on orthopedic development (e.g., neuromuscular hip dysplasia or scoliosis in children with limited ability to ambulate).

How can the coordinating clinician begin to untangle these issues and conceive of a management plan to foster improvement? An organized survey of all bodily systems can address the medical management of CMC. Many of these topics are covered in greater detail in separate chapters, but an overall approach to the medical evaluation of CMC is presented here. The systems approach begins with developmental and growth concerns. We then focus on issues regarding the nutrition and gastrointestinal and respiratory systems.

Developmental Concerns

CMC routinely have many developmental issues and needs. Developmental delays noted in the first 3 years of life are particularly amenable to early intervention therapies, including physical, therapy, speech-language, and general developmental therapy. In the United States these services are typically administered by the state of residence via a state-run early intervention program (see Chapter 103). After age 3 years, many children transition to having their local school district provide for ongoing therapy as an appropriate component of their educational program (see Chapter 104). For some patients, therapy services within the health care setting may be indicated for medical purposes that are not appropriate for early intervention or special education. For example, the physical therapist in the medical setting may provide interventions to maintain normal range of motion of joints and to prevent or respond to hip dysplasia and scoliosis (see Chapter 106). Occupational therapists in the medical setting may focus on activities of self-care involving the upper extremities and hands and may supervise feeding therapy (see Chapter 106). Addressing the current therapy team and educational plan for the patient, as well as advocating to resolve any gaps in that plan, is an important job for the pediatric clinician.

Growth Issues

Concerns about growth in CMC include short stature, poor weight gain, overgrowth, and obesity. A reduced body mass index (BMI), 20th to 50th percentile for age, is ideal for children with mobility impairments. If a child's linear growth is faltering, growth hormone deficiency or hypothyroidism might be suspected, and appropriate referrals and laboratory investigations should be done. If weight is excessive for height, excessive food intake for energy expenditure is likely. In such cases treatment of obesity is important. Children with severe mobility impairment and profound cognitive disability may present a particular challenge for caregiving, and in a few specific cases hormonal growth attenuation therapy can be considered (supervised by a pediatric endocrinologist with experience with this therapy) (see Chapter 111). Once linear growth is completed and BMI is healthy, the goal is weight maintenance, as obesity can present a further restriction to mobility.

Nutritional Problems and Gastrointestinal issues

Nutritional concerns may rank high on the visit agenda for the parent of CMC. Following the child's growth curve over time is important. The pediatric clinician should be alert to the existence of specialized growth curves for children with specific genetic diagnoses, including trisomy 21 (Down syndrome), Noonan syndrome, Cornelia de Lange syndrome, and achondroplasia. Children with these syndromes are best tracked using the condition-specific curves. Underweight and overweight on these curves should be managed in the same ways as they are for children without specific genetic conditions.

Feeding disorders, in which the child is unable to safely and efficiently consume adequate nourishment and hydration for good health, have many underlying causes (see Chapters 35, 55, and 56). Table 59.1 summarizes several commonly used methods to support the nutritional needs of CMC.

TABLE 59.1 **Overview of Frequently Used Feeding Technologies**

Category	Specific Options	Key Points
Oral feeding	Thickening of liquids by mouth	Any of these options may suffice for mild-moderate dysphagia Should be supervised by a pediatric speech or feeding therapist
	Specialized feeding vessel/nipple	
	Pacing/careful selection of solid food consistencies	
Tube feeding	Nasogastric (NG) tube feedings	Caregiver may replace at home May be used for bolus feedings Generally used <6 mo
	Nasojejunal (NJ) tube feedings	Must be replaced with radiology confirmation Bypass the stomach Can only be used for slow-paced, "continuous" feedings
	Gastrostomy (GTube) button	Tract mature after 2 mo First tube exchange should be done by surgeon Thereafter, caregiver may change tube in home every 3 mo Can be used for bolus or continuous feedings
	Gastrojejunostomy (GJ) button	Allows direct access from "button" on abdominal wall to the jejunum for long-term transpyloric feeding access Allows simultaneous venting of stomach (via G port) and feeding (via J port) Must be replaced with Radiology confirmation

Reasons for trouble with feeding and swallowing include oromotor dyscoordination, low muscle tone, and anatomic abnormalities of the palate or airway or both. Often problems of oromotor coordination stem from delayed introduction of oral feeding because of early medical problems or anatomic abnormalities. Feeding therapy offered by either an occupational therapist or speech therapist may be invaluable in these patients.

Dysphagia

Dysphagia is an abnormality of the coordination and control of swallowing, which results in incomplete clearing of food/liquid contents from the mouth with swallowing and/or aspiration of swallowed contents into the airway. Infants with a history of traumatic birth, structural brain malformation, or brain injury may show signs of dysphagia, such as choking with feedings, color change of the skin around the eyes or on the face with feeding, coughing after swallowing, or refusal of feeding beginning after age 6 months. Symptoms of dysphagia should prompt a formal evaluation of swallowing (with either a fluoroendoscopic evaluation of swallowing or modified barium swallow). Some children may do well with thickened liquids, until developmentally based feeding issues improve or resolve. However, some children with a neurologic etiology of their dysphagia may never be able to achieve the necessary calories and hydration by mouth, even with thickening. In the case of severe dysphagia, particularly with associated poor growth, a feeding tube should be considered.

Many types of feeding tubes are available for children with dysphagia. Some are temporary, such as nasogastric tubes, which can be safely placed by the trained caregiver at home. Other types require medical intervention, such as nasojejunal tubes, placed with the assistance of fluoroscopy, and gastrostomy and jejunostomy tubes, which require surgical placement. The type of tube most appropriate should be decided based on knowledge of the child's underlying diagnosis, prognosis, and specific feeding and nutritional needs. Table 59.1 provides more details about feeding tubes.

Many formulas are available for children who require caloric supplementation. Several special formulas developed in the last 10 years address the common issue of chronic constipation, more common in nonambulatory children. In general, these formulas use whole-food ingredients and provide adequate nutrients, fluids, and dietary fiber. A registered dietician familiar with CMC may be helpful for devising the feeding plan and monitoring for growth adequacy.

Gastrointestinal Complications

Gastrointestinal issues outside of dysphagia are common and may significantly complicate feedings. When obtaining history during a visit, one should include questions about feeding volumes, timing, and nature of problematic symptoms such as those discussed next.

Gastroesophageal reflux disease. Gastroesophageal reflux disease (GERD) is extremely common in children with abnormal muscle tone (spasticity and hypotonia) and in those who are not yet ambulatory. Symptoms include gagging, retching, and vomiting. If chronic, patients may develop esophagitis, a painful condition that may lead to food refusal. The mainstay of treatment for GERD is suppression of gastric acid production. Two main classes of medications used are histamine type 2 receptor antagonists and proton pump inhibitors. Some children also need help with foregut motility, and promotility medications such as erythromycin or cyproheptadine may be used (typically with supervision by a pediatric gastroenterologist).

If GERD is severe enough to affect weight gain and quality of life of the child, and medical management is ineffective, a surgical fundoplication may be indicated. Fundoplication is not necessary for every patient and may be associated with complications. The decision for surgical fundoplication should be made on an individual basis by providers experienced in caring for patients with CMC and severe feeding disorders.

Gastritis. Irritation of the gastric mucosa is often seen in children with gastrostomy tubes. This irritation can evolve into a frank ulcer with gastrointestinal bleeding. The parents may notice "coffee-ground" gastrostomy tube drainage, or melanotic stools. Acute treatment with sucralfate is often helpful. Consultation with a pediatric gastroenterologist is advised.

Constipation. Constipation (long periods between stool output and firm consistency of the stool) is common in children with motor disabilities, especially children with low muscle tone, and is associated with spina bifida. When protracted, constipation can lead to food refusal and feeding intolerance. Milder cases often can be managed with dietary modifications, increased fiber intake, and increased fluid intake. Severe cases may require treatment with stool softening (e.g., polyethylene glycol) or stimulant laxatives (e.g., bisacodyl or sennasides). Intractable constipation among children with severe motor disturbances may require temporary use of enemas or suppositories. Surgical interventions such as a cecostomy to allow for anterograde enema flushes of the colon or administration in the operating room of botulinum toxin (Botox) to the perianal muscles to aid defecation may be required.

Respiratory Issues

Respiratory issues also are common among CMC. Table 59.2 summarizes several commonly used types of respiratory technology assistance used by CMC. Multiple etiologies include abnormalities of swallowing and secretion handling, and malformations of the airway and diseases of the lung. A child might have more than one respiratory problem. Elements of the history suggestive of respiratory problems include need for respiratory support (supplemental oxygen daytime and nighttime), need for help with secretion handling, and interval changes in color, fatigue, or tone.

TABLE 59.2 Overview of Frequently Used Technologies for Respiratory Insufficiency

Intervention	Key Points
Supplemental oxygen (by nasal cannula or simple facemask)	Commonly needed for months following hospital discharge in premature babies with bronchopulmonary dysplasia Can be supplied from a home oxygen concentrator or portable oxygen tanks
Noninvasive positive pressure ventilation	May include continuous positive airway pressure, biphasic positive airway pressure, or average volume assured pressure support modalities Should be supervised by a pediatric pulmonologist
Tracheostomy	May be used simply to bypass an upper airway malformation (i.e., Pierre-Robin sequence) or to allow chronic ventilation for chronic lung disease (in conjunction with long-term home ventilation)

Abnormalities of the Airway

The most serious of the anatomic airway abnormalities manifest at birth and may require immediate interventions, including intubation and tracheostomy. These include tracheal stenosis, some tracheoesophageal fistulas, and diaphragmatic hernias. Airway malformations may be part of an underlying syndrome. For example, Pierre-Robin sequence is the association of cleft palate, micrognathia, and glossoptosis, leading to airway obstruction. Pierre-Robin may be associated with an underlying genetic disorder, such as a collagen-2 mutation. Choanal atresia is another anomaly of the airway that requires intervention at birth and is associated with underlying genetic conditions, including CHARGE association and certain craniosynostosis disorders.

Subtle airway issues may develop over time. Children with midface hypoplasia (e.g., Down syndrome and achondroplasia) are prone to the development of upper airway obstruction from adenoidal and tonsillar hypertrophy. The symptoms include noisy breathing or snoring at night, often with restless sleep. Evaluation with a sleep study is indicated. Treatment may include removal of the enlarged tonsils and adenoids.

Laryngomalacia and tracheomalacia are common airway abnormalities in children with abnormal muscle tone, particularly hypotonia. These conditions may be seen commonly in infants born preterm, who required long-term intubation in the neonatal intensive care unit. Symptoms of laryngo- or tracheomalacia include noisy breathing that is positional, worse in supine and better in prone. Typically, the sound is noted with the inspiratory phase. Anatomic abnormalities (e.g., laryngeal clefts) of the lower airway may mimic the symptoms of laryngo- or tracheomalacia and require evaluation by an ear, nose, and throat surgeon.

Lung Diseases

Diseases of the lung can cause significant respiratory issues. Recurrent aspiration pneumonia is prevalent in children with feeding/swallowing dysfunction. The right upper or middle lobe is particularly affected in cases of aspiration pneumonia because of the lower angle of takeoff of the bronchus to those lobes. Evaluation with a modified barium swallow is indicated for a child who has experienced aspiration pneumonia.

Children born prematurely also are at risk for chronic lung disease. Difficulty tolerating upper respiratory infections is more common in former preterm newborns, and many of these patients require consultation by a pulmonologist and long-term therapy with nebulized saline, bronchodilators, and inhaled steroids. Premature infants, particularly those living at high altitudes, may require supplemental oxygen via nasal cannula for months after hospital discharge or may require intermittent oxygen use in association with intercurrent illness. Children with congenital heart disease and respiratory symptoms may require diuretic treatment in addition to pulmonary medications and oxygen.

Ventilatory Support

In the case of obstructive sleep apnea tonsillectomy and adenoidectomy are often first-stage interventions. Dental interventions, such as palatal expansion, may also be tried. See Table 59.2 for information regarding other forms of ventilatory support, including noninvasive positive-pressure ventilation in sleep (continuous positive airway pressure or biphasic positive airway pressure), and invasive sleep ventilation via tracheostomy with ventilator support, which may be necessary in severe cases.

Anatomic anomalies of the airway, often identified at birth, require tracheostomy on an emergent basis. In many CMC, however, airway issues develop insidiously; the decision for tracheostomy may be elective. For example, a child with severe brain injury may develop significant upper airway obstruction and frequent respiratory infections over time. This patient should be evaluated by specialists, including ear, nose, and throat surgeons and pulmonologists, to assess whether the airway obstruction is severe enough to merit surgical intervention.

The decision to perform a tracheostomy is a major one, which should be made after careful consideration of the child's medical status and prognosis. Having a tracheostomy significantly complicates the level of home medical care that the child requires. Because of the shortage of qualified home care personnel, much of the daily care of a CMC with a tracheostomy falls to the parents. Parents need to learn how to suction the tracheostomy, change the tracheostomy, and assess symptoms indicative of worsening status.

Other forms of ventilatory support include suctioning, chest physiotherapy, and vibratory physiotherapy vests. A vibratory physiotherapy vest is a mechanical device that is worn (like a scuba vest) around the chest. This vibration helps lower airway thick, viscous secretions to mobilize, making the secretions easier for the child to cough up. Used for many years in children with chronic respiratory diseases such as cystic fibrosis, the technology has recently become available for CMC. Use should be supervised by a pediatric pulmonologist.

OTHER SPECIALIZED MEDICAL TECHNOLOGIES

Jane, the patient with spina bifida, is a classic example of a CMC, requiring a multidisciplinary approach to medical and surgical management, ongoing therapy, and educational and community support. Table 59.3 reviews care team needs. A child with spina bifida requires neurosurgical closure of the open back lesion at birth. Ongoing management includes monitoring and treating hydrocephalus, which includes placement of an intraventricular shunt in 85% of cases. The child with spina bifida also has many orthopedic concerns, including management of foot deformities, hip dysplasia, and scoliosis. If neurogenic bowel and bladder are present, the child may require specialized management by a urologist and sometimes a gastroenterologist or colorectal specialist.

The role of the primary care clinician in the management of a child with spina bifida is crucial. This clinician needs to have a basic understanding of the surgical interventions that the child has undergone and when to contact surgical specialists should complications arise. The primary care clinician is a member of the team who can assess the child's overall state of health, including nutritional status, particularly if the child has feeding problems related to an Arnold-Chiari II malformation. The primary care clinician also is often required to play an important role in the assessment of therapeutic interventions and specialized classroom supports for the child with spina bifida,

VIGNETTE

Jane is a 12-year-old girl with a history of myelomeningocele, or spina bifida, of the lumbar region, treated with closure surgery at birth and placement of a ventriculoperitoneal (VP) shunt. She has an individualized education plan at school to support learning disabilities. She is being seen in clinic today for fever. She has a history of recurrent urinary tract infections and requires cecostomy flushes to pass bowel movements. Evaluation of fever requires the clinician to consider the possibilities of infection of the indwelling hardware (VP shunt), bladder, or other routine viral illness. Urinalysis is suggestive of infection in the office, and a culture sample is collected. Empiric antibiotic selection is guided by her prior urine culture results.

TABLE 59.3 Care Team Considerations for Patients With Neural Tube Defects

Body System	Specialists	Interventions
Central nervous system	Neurosurgery Neurology (if seizures present)	Spinal/skin defect closure May need ventriculoperitoneal shunt May need tethered cord release Treat seizures (if present)
Urologic	Urology Physical therapy	Treat neurogenic bladder May need bladder augmentation
Gastrointestinal	Pediatrician Gastroenterology Colorectal surgery	Relieve constipation Monitor weight closely May need enemas or cecostomy
Orthopedic	Physical therapist Orthopedist	Monitor for joint alignment Monitor for hip dysplasia and scoliosis

who may have associated learning disabilities. Comorbid diagnoses such as seizures are common. Additionally, the child with spina bifida has a risk of developing latex sensitivity, owing to repeated exposure to latex in the medical environment, a preventable complication.

The primary care clinician also should be aware of the genetic implications of this diagnosis and understand the recurrence risk in future pregnancies (5% for the patient, 2%–3% for the parents, and 1%–2% for the siblings) and the importance of folate prophylaxis to reduce this risk. When taken by the woman for a minimum of 3 months before conception and during the first month of pregnancy, an appropriate dose of folic acid can reduce the recurrence risk by more than 50%. Although folate supplementation has been available in foods in the United States for decades, this public health measure has not eradicated the incidence of neural tube defects, and many underlying genetic factors may be at play (see Chapter 23). Neural tube defects may also occur as part of an underlying genetic syndrome or as a teratogenic consequence of maternal alcohol abuse or valproic acid use during pregnancy. Referral to a geneticist may be indicated in certain cases.

Patients with neural tube defects are often diagnosed prenatally on ultrasound. With the advent of prenatal maternal serum screening, the presence of spina bifida can be prenatally suspected due to an elevated maternal serum alpha-fetoprotein and confirmed with ultrasound. Prenatal detection of a neural tube defect may offer the opportunity to treat the child prenatally with fetal surgery to close the defect, which is an innovation available at a few pediatric tertiary care centers. Prenatal surgical intervention may decrease the development of Chiari II malformation and hydrocephalus, although it increases the risk of premature delivery. Prenatal diagnosis may allow the delivery to occur at a larger medical center so that immediate neurosurgical care can be offered to the newborn. Children with spina bifida are often followed in a multidisciplinary clinic, where the pediatrician and surgical subspecialists see the child during one clinic session, usually several times a year. This model has been used for many years and is often appreciated by the families.

Ventriculoperitoneal Shunts

Approximately 85% of children with spina bifida and some children with other disorders, such as multiple suture craniosynostosis syndromes, and congenital hydrocephalus require shunt placement. In children the most common form of shunt is the VP shunt. A recent development in shunt technology is the programmable shunt. This type of shunt allows the degree of shunt drainage to be regulated (increasing or decreasing as needed) via a magnet, without requiring an additional surgical procedure.

The major complications of shunts are malfunction and infection. The symptoms of shunt malfunction are related to increased intracranial pressure and include severe headache, vomiting, and lethargy. Evaluation of possible shunt malfunction generally includes a head computed tomography scan to evaluate the size of the ventricles, and a shunt series (x-rays to look for discontinuity in the tubing). Intermittent shunt malfunction also may occur and be associated with a worsening in school performance or personality changes.

Shunt infection often manifests with similar symptoms to shunt malfunction, plus fever. A shunt tap may be required to analyze cerebrospinal fluid (CSF) for possible infection. The typical bacteria causing shunt infection are skin flora, such as *Staphylococcus epidermitis*. Treatment of shunt infection generally requires removing the old shunt hardware and tubing and replacing with a completely new system after the CSF has been sterilized.

Urologic Procedures in Children With Neurogenic Bowel and Bladder

For patients with spina bifida and other anatomic abnormalities associated with a neurogenic bowel and bladder, achieving continence is an important goal, allowing the patient to get out of diapers and have an age-appropriate social experience. Fully emptying the bladder and bowel are also critical to maintenance of a healthy urologic and gastrointestinal tract.

To achieve bladder emptying, many patients require clean intermittent catheterization, a simple procedure that can be easily taught to the primary caregivers. By early elementary school age, most children can learn to catheterize themselves independently. Urinary tract infections are common in patients with neurogenic bladders and can manifest as fever, gastrointestinal symptoms such as vomiting or diarrhea, or a change to the color or odor of the urine.

Many children with spina bifida undergo continence surgical procedures to enhance bladder capacity aid in management of constipation from neurogenic bowel. The Mitrofanoff procedure is an operation in which the appendix is used to create a conduit between the skin surface and the urinary bladder. This conduit allows children with neurogenic bladders to avoid transurethral catheterization. The ACE procedure brings the appendix to the surface of the abdominal wall and creates a conduit through which stool softening medication can lead to evacuation of the colon from above.

Orthopedic Procedures in CMC

Children with spinal cord defects and congenital paralysis may develop club foot deformities from decreased fetal movement and malpositioning of the foot *in utero*. After birth, these deformities may be treated with serial casting to bring the foot position gradually into normal alignment. Surgical intervention is frequently required, however, if casting is not fully successful.

Many assistive devices promote the upright, weight-bearing position of children who are nonambulatory. Devices may be as minimal as walking sticks or canes, or as supportive as motorized wheelchairs. Devices typically require careful measurements by trained physiotherapists and equipment vendors to ensure the equipment fits the child, and medical orders from the physician for these pieces of durable medical equipment.

Scoliosis is a common complication in children with vertebral anomalies or tone abnormalities. In contrast to idiopathic scoliosis, which generally starts in the teenage years and is more common in girls, the neuromuscular scoliosis may be seen at a very young age and equally in boys and girls. Conservative management with physical therapy and the use of spinal orthoses are often part of the initial management. Surgical intervention is often required, however, with spinal rod fixation.

CONCLUSION

Caring for CMC requires great dedication, compassion, and specialized areas of knowledge. The CMC and family require the support of a primary care clinician who can see the big picture, prioritize interventions, evaluate the recommendations of multiple consultants, and help the family make informed and reasonable decisions. This clinician begins by appreciating the child's distinct personality, preferences, and contributions; then must assess the basic needs of the child, including adequacy of nutrition, growth, and respiratory function, always cognizant of associated comorbid conditions and other treatments. A thoughtful assessment of the underlying etiologic diagnosis should be made so that appropriate medical care and counseling to the family can be offered. All of this coordination is essential though challenging, especially given insufficient time to address multiple problems during clinic sessions and inadequate reimbursement for activities such as care coordination.

As in the vignettes, the care for CMC requires the support of numerous pediatric and surgical subspecialists, each expert in a domain of medical treatment, therapeutic potential, and/or technology assistance for the child. The child may use multiple pieces of medical equipment, may receive special education and rehabilitation therapies, and may require home care nursing. The child may be on multiple medications. All of these are necessary interventions, although their use can be remarkably stressful for the parents and primary caregivers to handle.

Given the growing number of CMC, we recommend that pediatric and family medicine postgraduate training programs include specific training of residents to care for this population of children. We encourage advanced practice nurses and physician assistants to consider specialized training for this population as well. We know that more pediatric subspecialists are needed to meet the needs of this group than are currently available. As more clinicians learn the skills necessary to care for CMC in the future, we anticipate that access will improve, and children and their families will have their medical, rehabilitative, educational, and social needs adequately met.

REFERENCES

Adams, S., Nicholas, D., Mahant, S., Weiser, N., et al. (2019). Care maps and care plans for children with medical complexity. *Child Care Health Development*, *45*(1), 104–110.

Bergman, D. A., Keller, D., Kuo, D. Z., Lerner, C., Mansour, M., Stille, C., Richardson, T., Rodean, J., Hudak, M. (2020). Costs and use for children with medical complexity in a care management program. *Pediatrics*, *145*(4).

Cohen, E., Berry, J. G., Camacho, X., Anderson, G., et al. (2012). Patterns and costs of health care use of children with medical complexity. *Pediatrics*, *130*(6).

Cohen, E., Berry, J., Sanders, L., Schor, E., & Wise, P. H. (2018). Status complexicus? The emergence of pediatric complex care. *Pediatrics*, *141*(3), S202–S211.

Houtrow, A., Murphy, N., & American Academy of Pediatrics Council on Children with Disabilities. (2019). Prescribing physical, occupational and speech therapy services for children with disabilities. *Pediatrics*, *143*(4).

Kuo, D. Z., Houtrow, A., & American Academy of Pediatrics Council on Children with Disabilities. (2016). Recognition and management of medical complexity. *Pediatrics*, *138*(6).

RESOURCES

American Academy of Pediatrics: www.medicalhomeinfo.org

American Association on Intellectual and Developmental Disabilities: https://www.aaidd.org

National Information Center for Children and Youth with Disabilities: www.nichcy.org

Spina Bifida Association: https://www.spinabifidaassociation.org

60

Survivors of Childhood Brain Tumors: Developmental and Behavioral Considerations

Emily K. Shabason, May V. Albee, and Matthew C. Hocking

For additional material related to the content of this chapter, please see Chapters 41, 46, 58, 87, and 105.

VIGNETTE

Charlie is an 18-year-old male, who is getting ready to graduate high school. He previously had medulloblastoma at age 3, which was treated with surgery, chemotherapy, and cranial radiation. His parents would like him to attend college, but Charlie struggled academically throughout school so it is unclear whether he will be accepted to a college. Charlie also has difficulty making new friends and independently performing his activities of daily living. He worries about the prospect of moving out of his parents' home and living on his own. Charlie also has some ongoing medical issues, including hypothyroidism, hearing loss, difficulty sleeping, and seizures. He has been followed by a multidisciplinary survivorship clinic, and his family is now facing the challenge of transitioning his care to adult providers. Charlie and his family are working hard to plan for success as he transitions into the next stage of his life.

Childhood is a time of tremendous, intricate neurologic growth, necessary for attainment of complex developmental milestones. Unfortunately, however, childhood is also a time when abnormal cellular growth can occur in children's brains, leading to malignant and nonmalignant tumors. Such neurologic disease and related treatments, including surgical resection, chemotherapy, and radiation therapy, can have long-lasting impacts on children's developmental and behavioral trajectories. Brain and central nervous system (CNS) tumors are the most common solid tumors in children. Increasing survival rates have reinforced the importance of addressing developmental and behavioral sequelae to optimize survivors' long-term outcomes. Note: Throughout this chapter, the term *survivors* will refer specifically to survivors of pediatric brain tumors, unless otherwise specified.

PEDIATRIC BRAIN TUMORS

Types and Frequency

In children ages 0 to 14 years the brain and CNS are the most common sites for tumors (both malignant and nonmalignant), with an average annual age-adjusted incidence rate of 5.74 per 100,000 population based on the Central Brain Tumor Registry of the United States for diagnosis years 2012 to 2016. The average age-adjusted mortality rate is 0.72 per 100,000, and it is the most common cause of cancer-related death in this age group. The 5-year survival rate for children has increased over the past few decades, now at 74.7% for malignant and 97.2% for nonmalignant brain and CNS tumors (Ostrom et al., 2019).

The most common histology is glioma (51.6%), followed by pilocytic astrocytoma (17.8%), glioma malignant, not otherwise specified (14.0%), and embryonal tumors (13.1%), of which medulloblastoma is the most common type. The most common tumor locations are in the cerebellum (15.2%) and brainstem (13.3%) (Ostrom et al., 2019).

In adolescents (ages 15–19) brain and CNS tumors have an average annual age-adjusted incidence rate of 6.98 per 100,000 population. Pituitary tumors increase in incidence for children 14 and older, becoming the most common histology for children ages 15 to 19 (30.8%). Gliomas as a group account for approximately 31% of tumors, of which pilocytic astrocytoma is the most common (8.3%). The most common tumor location is in the pituitary and craniopharyngeal duct (33.5%), followed by 19.9% of tumors occurring in the frontal lobe, temporal lobe, occipital lobe, and parietal lobe, combined (Ostrom et al., 2019).

Clinical Suspicion of a Brain Tumor

The clinical presentation of a brain tumor can depend on the tumor location and extent of tumor involvement. Presenting symptoms typically include morning headaches, nausea, and lethargy, which are related to increased intracranial pressure from obstructing hydrocephalus. Vision changes can present with optic pathway gliomas. Supratentorial tumors are more likely to be associated with seizures, and infratentorial tumors are more likely to be associated with balance and cranial nerve deficits (Mulhern & Butler, 2004).

Brain tumors should also be suspected in children presenting with sudden changes in behavior or unusual presentations of otherwise common behavioral disorders. For example, case reports have described two patients who were both diagnosed with attention-deficit/hyperactivity disorder (ADHD) at 7 years of age and found to have brain tumors in their frontal lobes at age 10. Following surgical resection, both patients had behavioral improvements, suggesting that at least some of the ADHD symptoms were related to the tumors. Further, a patient diagnosed with autism spectrum disorder at 45 months of age based on the Autism Diagnostic Observation Schedule and Autism Diagnostic Interview-Revised who had a right temporal lobe tumor has been described. Video electroencephalography showed ictal-like patterns originating from the right temporal region. Following surgical resection, the patient showed near resolution of the autism-related symptoms (Hrdlicka et al., 2019).

Tumor Treatments

Brain and CNS tumors are typically treated with various combinations of surgery, chemotherapy, and radiation therapy. Chemotherapy may be administered systemically or via intrathecal administration to bypass the blood-brain barrier. Radiation can be delivered via different modalities, with newer types aiming to maximize treatment to the tumor tissue while limiting toxicity to normal brain tissue. Photon radiation (x-rays) delivers more radiation to surrounding tissues, in contrast to proton radiation, which is able to spare more of the surrounding tissues. Radiation can lead to both acute and late effects, the latter of which are usually permanent and progressive, such as hearing loss, neurocognitive deficits, and neuroendocrine dysfunction (Denunzio & Yock, 2020).

More recently, there have been advances in targeted molecular therapies and immunotherapy to provide as precise and accurate a treatment as possible while limiting toxicities, such as with MEK inhibitors for low-grade gliomas (Duke & Packer, 2020).

LATE EFFECTS OF BRAIN TUMORS AND THEIR TREATMENT

Late effects describe the long-term sequelae that survivors experience, and they can be observed in multiple domains, including medical, neurocognitive, and psychosocial domains. Such late effects can be interrelated, impacting a child's developmental trajectory and family system as a whole (Turner et al., 2009). Survivors are less likely to be married or to have completed secondary education, and they are more likely to be unemployed than peers (Schulte et al., 2019).

Specific late effects will be discussed later, many of which Charlie is experiencing, as described in the vignette. In general, survivors have more impaired functional status (e.g., needing assistance with personal care needs and daily routines, and difficulty maintaining a job or attending school), more activity limitations, and more adverse general health when compared to their siblings (Hudson et al., 2003).

Mechanisms of Injury

Late effects may relate to neurologic damage to the developing brain from the tumor itself, as well as from related surgery, chemotherapy-related toxicity, and radiation toxicity. For example, a frontal tumor mass can cause direct disruption of frontal lobe functioning or disconnection from subcortical afferents, thus leading to attention impairment and behavioral disorders (Messina et al., 2014). Damage from radiation and chemotherapy can cause neurocognitive impairment through disruption of neural progenitor cells, which then impacts adult hippocampal neurogenesis and subcortical white matter integrity (Monje & Dietrich, 2012).

MEDICAL LATE EFFECTS

Physical Changes

Survivors can have changes to their physical appearances, such as scars from craniotomies or previous central lines, alopecia from cranial radiation or chemotherapy, and/or short stature related to radiation and/or hypothalamic-pituitary axis dysfunction (Turner et al., 2009). Survivors of brain tumors are more likely to have cosmetic changes, such as facial disfigurement, compared to other cancer survivors (Mulhern, Hancock, Fairclough, & Kun, 1992).

Sensory Impairment: Vision and Hearing

Survivors are at increased risk of neurosensory impairment, estimated to occur in 17% of survivors. Impairments may include hearing loss, legal blindness in one or both eyes, and/or double vision. There is increased likelihood of hearing impairment in survivors who received radiation to their posterior fossa (Packer et al., 2003).

Neurologic Dysfunction: Seizures, Strokes, Balance Impairment

Survivors are at increased risk of late-occurring strokes ($\geq$5 years after cancer diagnosis). One large study identified stroke in 6.3% of survivors, with a mean interval of 13.9 years from cancer diagnosis, and a relative risk of 29.0 compared to siblings. Survivors previously treated with cranial radiation were at higher risk of stroke than those who did not receive cranial radiation, with an even greater risk if they had received both radiation and an alkylating chemotherapy agent (Bowers et al., 2006).

Seizure disorders have been described in 25% of survivors, and they can present as late-effect seizure disorders that occur 5 or more years after diagnosis (6.5% of survivors). There is an increased risk of seizures in those who received radiation to cortical segments of their brain (Packer et al., 2003).

Balance impairment is also a common late effect, found in 48% of adult survivors of pediatric CNS tumors, with an increased risk in those with infratentorial tumors, shunt placement, hearing loss, peripheral neuropathy, flexibility limitations, and cognitive deficits. Balance impairment may be associated with limitations in mobility and physical performance (Varedi et al., 2020).

Endocrine Dysfunction

Survivors are at increased risk of having at least one endocrine condition (estimated in 43% of survivors), such as hypothyroidism, growth hormone deficiency, and/or requiring medication to induce puberty (Gurney et al., 2003).

Sleep Disorders

Sleep disturbance is common in survivors and likely related to multiple factors, including neuroinflammation and disruption of the hypothalamic-pituitary-adrenal axis (Mogavero,

Bruni, Delrosso, & Ferri, 2020). Nearly half of survivors who have neurocognitive impairment have been identified as having sleep problems, including difficulty initiating and maintaining sleep and excessive somnolence, with increased risk in those with emotional problems and/or hyperactivity/inattention. Such sleep problems are associated with worse parent-reported executive functioning (van Kooten et al., 2019).

Secondary Malignancy

The strongest risk factor for a secondary malignancy is prior treatment with radiation, which can cause a new primary CNS tumor that is distinct from the original tumor. Gliomas and meningiomas are the most common secondary malignancies, typically occurring 9 and 17 years postdiagnosis, respectively. Sarcomas can also develop and are associated with poor prognosis (Turner et al., 2009).

NEUROPSYCHOLOGICAL LATE EFFECTS

Neurocognitive Late Effects

Neurocognitive late effects may include lower IQ, lower academic achievement, and impairment in executive function skills, such as difficulty with attention, processing speed, working memory, and psychomotor and visual-spatial skills (Mulhern & Butler, 2004). Difficulties with neurocognitive functioning are progressive in nature. Additionally, deficits are developmental, as they may not become apparent until years after treatment when survivors reach an age at which they would otherwise be expected to demonstrate a particular skill. Survivors typically make gains in skills, but not at the same rates as their peers (Conklin et al., 2012). Cognitive deficits can have wide-ranging implications, including having a negative impact on social functioning (Willard, Allen, Hardy, & Bonner, 2017), health-related quality of life (Netson et al., 2016), educational attainment, and employment.

IQ, Working Memory, and Processing Speed

Survivors have been identified as having more impaired functioning in cognitive ability, verbal intelligence, nonverbal intelligence, visual-spatial skills, and academic achievement in reading, math, and spelling, with a large metaanalysis showing that effect sizes range from small to large depending on the study (Robinson et al., 2010). Another metaanalysis showed that full-scale IQ scores are commonly below average and that lower intellectual functioning is associated with a history of cranial radiation, chemotherapy, and a longer time since diagnosis. Tumor location and age at diagnosis were not found to predict intellectual function, though the authors posit that effects of age at diagnosis may be more apparent with longer follow-ups (De Ruiter, Van Mourik, Schouten-Van Meeteren, Grootenhuis, & Oosterlaan, 2013). Other studies have identified younger age at diagnosis as a risk factor for more severe neurocognitive late effects (Mulhern & Butler, 2004).

Compared to siblings and to survivors of other solid tumors, survivors of childhood brain tumors have more impairment in working memory, which is correlated with lower IQ. Those who have been treated with cranial radiation perform worse on working memory tasks compared to survivors who did not receive cranial radiation. Working memory deficits may contribute to survivors' declines in intellectual functioning, as the gap widens between survivors' intellectual abilities and their typical peers over time (Conklin et al., 2012).

Processing speed deficits are also increased in survivors, primarily in those who received either focal or cranial-spinal radiation. However, a little over one-third of survivors who have not received radiation still show deficits on at least one measure of processing speed. There is also increased risk of impairment in processing speed in survivors with seizures and with shunts (Brinkman et al., 2016).

These neurocognitive impairments have a significant impact on adult function, as those with these difficulties have lower educational attainment, higher rates of unemployment, and are less likely to live independently (Brinkman et al., 2016).

Attention

Impairments in attention, with or without diagnoses of ADHD, are increased in survivors compared to the general population. A study of survivors tested between ages 12 and 17 years using a computerized performance measure of attention and a diagnostic interview identified primary or secondary ADHD in 10%, and even more had clinical elevations of inattention on rating scales but without meeting *Diagnostic and Statistical Manual of Mental Disorders,* fourth edition, diagnostic criteria (American Psychiatric Association, 1994; Kahalley et al., 2011). This is generally consistent with a study that found that 13.1% of survivors had a clinical diagnosis of ADHD, and another reported that almost 20% had ADHD-related symptoms, with an association between ADHD and younger age at tumor diagnosis and supratentorial tumor location (Shabason et al., 2019). Higher rates of ADHD symptoms have been reported in children referred for neuropsychological testing (Hardy, Willard, Gioia, Sharkey, & Walsh, 2018).

Interventions for Neurocognitive Functioning

There are a number of interventions aimed at optimizing survivors' neurocognitive functioning, including school supports, cognitive remediation programs, and medications.

School supports, such as through individualized education plans, offer tailored supports and accommodations to address learning, cognitive, and psychosocial difficulties. School reentry programs may be offered by hospitals to assist the patient, family, and teachers with the transition back into school. However, there is still significant work to be done to optimize survivors' transitions back to school following treatments, as one survey of parents identified that half of them did not feel adequately prepared for school reentry. Parents had particular concerns related to neuropsychological testing, resources related to learning impairments, educational terms, and legal rights related to school services (Ruble, Pare-Blagoev, Cooper, Martin, & Jacobson, 2019). To aid with this, the Children's Oncology Group maintains a website with resources on school supports for families and teachers (www.childrensoncologygroup.org/index.php/school-support). Furthermore, ongoing monitoring and evaluation of survivors is important, as neurocognitive deficits can arise or become progressively worse over time. Survivors are recommended to have a comprehensive neuropsychological assessment after the end of treatment, with a reassessment 2 to 3 years after treatment, or sooner if monitoring suggests significant changes (Annett, Patel, & Phipps, 2015).

The use of computerized cognitive remediation programs has increased in popularity given their relative ease of access. One such program has been shown to improve working memory and math skills in survivors upon program completion and at 6-month follow-up, though it is unclear how that may translate into academic outcomes (Carlson-Green, Puig, & Bendel, 2017). Additionally, there are feasibility concerns with these interventions in survivors who have more problems with attention and working memory (Hocking, Paltin, Quast, & Barakat, 2019).

Stimulant medications typically used to treat ADHD have been shown to enhance attention based on a measures of sustained attention, as well as parent-, teacher- and self-reported ratings of attention, though without observed gains in academic skills (Conklin et al., 2010).

Modafinil, a commonly used medication for narcolepsy, is currently being studied to treat memory and attention problems in children treated for brain tumors (NCT01381718). It has been studied in adult patients with brain tumors with mixed results (Gehring et al., 2012).

Physical exercise is gaining interest for addressing cognitive deficits (Cox et al., 2020; Sharma, Allison, Tucker, Mabbott, & Timmons, 2020). There are also studies underway looking at prevention of cognitive late effects, including with memantine (NCT03194906, NCT04217694) and metformin (NCT02040376).

Neurobehavioral Late Effects

Survivors may experience a variety of neurobehavioral changes upon treatment completion and into survivorship, which can be interrelated with neurocognitive and social difficulties. Survivors may have elevated levels of internalizing symptoms, such as anxiety and depression, though the data show mixed results and may depend on the informant of parent- versus self-report (Fuemmeler, Elkin, & Mullins, 2002). Fatigue is also commonly seen, and it may include general fatigue, sleep/rest fatigue, and cognitive fatigue. Fatigue has been shown to be inversely related to health-related quality of life in survivors, including in survivors who completed their treatment over 1 year prior (Meeske, Katz, Palmer, Burwinkle, & Varni, 2004). Modafinil and stimulants have been shown to improve fatigue and mood in adult patients with brain tumors (Gehring et al., 2012).

Social Competence

Survivors of childhood brain tumors have been identified as having more difficulties in social functioning compared to survivors of other cancers (Hocking et al., 2015). Compared to healthy controls, survivors are more likely to have fewer close friends, lower rates of peer acceptance, and greater social isolation (Barrera, Shaw, Speechley, Maunsell, & Pogany, 2005; Vannatta, Gartstein, Short, & Noll, 1998). Additionally, survivors of childhood brain tumors are also less likely to be able to name a friend compared to survivors of other cancer types (Hocking et al., 2020a).

Survivors may have trouble recognizing facial expressions, even when controlling for IQ. Furthermore, those with more difficulty recognizing facial expressions are rated by their parents as having more social problems and are less likely to be able to name a friend (Bonner et al., 2008; Hocking et al., 2020a).

Based on a study of social attention using eye tracking technology, survivors demonstrated eye gaze patterns and social attention that was more comparable to children with autism spectrum disorder than to typically developing youth. Among survivors, those who had received multimodal tumor-directed therapy had less gaze preference for faces (Hocking et al., 2020b).

Medical factors associated with poorer social adjustment in survivors include younger age at diagnosis, a history of radiation therapy, tumors located outside of the third ventricle, increased abnormal brain volume, and more severe cosmetic and functional impairment (Bonner et al., 2008; Carpentieri, Mulhern, Douglas, Hanna, & Fairclough, 1993; Mulhern, Carpentieri, Shema, Stone, & Fairclough, 1993). Deficits in social functioning have also been associated with more attention problems, slower processing speed, and poorer facial recognition (Willard et al., 2017).

Interventions for Social Skills

Various social skills interventions have been studied, many of which target a common set of skills, including assertiveness, making new friends, responding to teasing/bullying, empathy, conflict resolution, and cooperation. While results overall indicate some success with such interventions, the level of benefit varies, with more benefit in those who had poorer baseline functioning prior to intervention (Willard, 2018). Additional social skills interventions and longitudinal follow-up are needed to better understand the best ways to support survivors.

SURVIVORSHIP CARE

Survivorship care is paramount as patients transition from cancer diagnosis and tumor-directed therapy to the management of late effects. In 2005 the Institute of Medicine (now named, National Academy of Medicine) published recommendations for enhancing survivorship care, including that awareness be increased about the needs of survivors, that survivors have clear written plans that include a comprehensive care summary and follow-up plan, that late effects be managed with evidence-based clinical practice guidelines, that there be assessment tools and screening instruments, and that the effects of cancer on employment be studied (Hewitt, Greenfield, & Stovall, 2006).

A comprehensive evidence-based compilation of the psychosocial standards of cancer survivorship care were published in a supplement issue of *Pediatric Blood and Cancer* in December 2015. The standards are also available online through the Mattie Miracle Cancer Foundation, whose advocacy had helped lead to their creation (www.mattiemiracle.com/standards). While some progress has since been made, there are still many areas that warrant continued attention to support survivors' success.

Comprehensive survivorship care is also essential for children previously treated for other cancer types, too. For example, children previously treated for leukemia may also experience neurocognitive and psychosocial impairments, particularly if they were treated with cranial-spinal radiation and/or intrathecal chemotherapy (Stefanski et al., 2021).

As discussed in the vignette, Charlie is grappling with many late effects that are commonly seen in survivors of brain tumors, including medical issues, neurocognitive and academic impairments, and psychosocial difficulties. While his family's goals include having him attend college and living independently, Charlie, his parents, and his educational team should discuss his interests and the options for vocational training, postsecondary education, or employment consistent with his goals and skills. Regardless of what his specific next academic and/or vocational step is though, he will require continued supports through a multifaceted approach to help optimize his long-term success.

REFERENCES

American Psychiatric Association. (1994). *Diagnostic and statistical manual of mental disorders* (4th ed.). Author.

Annett, R. D., Patel, S. K., & Phipps, S. (2015). Monitoring and assessment of neuropsychological outcomes as a standard of care in pediatric oncology. *Pediatric Blood & Cancer, 62*(5), S460–S513. https://doi.org/10.1002/pbc.25749

Barrera, M., Shaw, A. K., Speechley, K. N., Maunsell, E., & Pogany, L. (2005). Educational and social late effects of childhood cancer and related clinical, personal and familial characteristics. *Cancer, 104*(8), 1751–1760.

Bonner, M. J., Hardy, K. K., Willard, V. W., Anthony, K. K., Hood, M., & Gururangan, S. (2008). Social functioning and facial expression recognition in survivors of pediatric brain tumors. *Journal of Pediatric Psychology, 33*(10), 1142–1152.

Bowers, D. C., Liu, Y., Leisenring, W., McNeil, E., Stovall, M., Gurney, J. G., … Oeffinger, K. C. (2006). Late-occurring stroke among long-term survivors of childhood leukemia and brain tumors: A report from the childhood cancer survivor study. *Journal of Clinical Oncology, 24*(33), 5277–5282. https://doi.org/10.1200/JCO.2006.07.2884

Brinkman, T. M., Krasin, M. J., Liu, W., Armstrong, G. T., Ojha, R. P., Sadighi, Z. S., … Krull, K. R. (2016). Long-term neurocognitive functioning and social attainment in adult survivors of pediatric CNS tumors: Results from the St Jude lifetime cohort study. *Journal of Clinical Oncology, 34*(12), 1358–1367. https://doi.org/10.1200/JCO.2015.62.2589

Carlson-Green, B., Puig, J., & Bendel, A. (2017). Feasibility and efficacy of an extended trial of homebased working memory training for pediatric brain tumor survivors: A pilot study. *Neuro-Oncology Practice, 4*(2), 111–120. https://doi.org/10.1093/nop/npw015

Carpentieri, S. C., Mulhern, R. K., Douglas, S., Hanna, S., & Fairclough, D. L. (1993). Behavioral resiliency among children surviving brain tumors: A longitudinal study. *Journal of Clinical Child Psychology, 22*, 236–246.

Conklin, H. M., Ashford, J. M., Howarth, R. A., Merchant, T. E., Ogg, R. J., Santana, V. M., … Xiong, X. (2012). Working memory performance among childhood brain tumor survivors. *Journal of the International Neuropsychological Society, 18*(6), 996–1005. https://doi.org/10.1017/S1355617712000793

Conklin, H. M., Reddick, W. E., Ashford, J., Ogg, S., Howard, S. C., Morris, E. B., … Khan, R. B. (2010). Long-term efficacy of methylphenidate in enhancing attention regulation, social skills, and academic abilities of childhood cancer survivors. *Journal of Clinical Oncology, 28*(29), 4465–4472. https://doi.org/10.1200/JCO.2010.28.4026

Cox, E., Bells, S., Timmons, B. W., Laughlin, S., Bouffet, E., de Medeiros, C., … Mabbott, D. J. (2020). Corrigendum to "A controlled clinical crossover trial of exercise training to improve cognition and neural communication in pediatric brain tumor survivors." *Clinical Neurophysiology, 131*(7), 1533–1547. https://doi.org/10.1016/j.clinph.2020.06.002

De Ruiter, M. A., Van Mourik, R., Schouten-Van Meeteren, A. Y. N., Grootenhuis, M. A., & Oosterlaan, J. (2013). Neurocognitive consequences of a paediatric brain tumour and its treatment: A meta-analysis. *Developmental Medicine and Child Neurology, 55*(5), 408–417. https://doi.org/10.1111/dmcn.12020

Denunzio, N. J., & Yock, T. I. (2020). Modern radiotherapy for pediatric brain tumors. *Cancers, 12*(6), 1–16. https://doi.org/10.3390/cancers12061533

Duke, E. S., & Packer, R. J. (2020). Update on pediatric brain tumors: The molecular era and neuro-immunologic beginnings. *Current Neurology and Neuroscience Reports, 20*(8). https://doi.org/10.1007/s11910-020-01050-6

Fuemmeler, B. F., Elkin, T. D., & Mullins, L. L. (2002). Survivors of childhood brain tumors: Behavioral, emotional, and social adjustment. *Clinical Psychology Review, 22*(4), 547–585. https://doi.org/10.1016/S0272-7358(01)00120-9

Gehring, K., Patwardhan, S. Y., Collins, R., Groves, M. D., Etzel, C. J., Meyers, C. A., & Wefel, J. S. (2012). A randomized trial on the efficacy of methylphenidate and modafinil for improving cognitive functioning and symptoms in patients with a primary brain tumor. *Journal of Neuro-Oncology, 107*(1), 165–174. https://doi.org/10.1007/s11060-011-0723-1

Gurney, J. G., Kadan-Lottick, N. S., Packer, R. J., Neglia, J. P., Sklar, C. A., Punyko, J. A., … Study, C. C. S. (2003). Endocrine and cardiovascular late effects among adult survivors of childhood brain tumors. *Cancer, 97*(3), 663–673. https://doi.org/10.1002/cncr.11094

Hardy, K. K., Willard, V. W., Gioia, A., Sharkey, C., & Walsh, K. S. (2018). Attention-mediated neurocognitive profiles in survivors of pediatric brain tumors: Comparison to children with neurodevelopmental ADHD. *Neuro-Oncology, 20*(5), 705–715. https://doi.org/10.1093/neuonc/nox174

Hewitt, M., Greenfield, S., & Stovall, E. (2006). *From cancer patient to cancer survivor: Lost in transition*. National Academies Press.

Hocking, M. C., McCurdy, M., Turner, E., Kazak, A. E., Noll, R. B., Phillips, P., & Barakat, L. P. (2015). Social competence in pediatric brain tumor survivors: Application of a model from social neuroscience and developmental psychology. *Pediatric Blood & Cancer, 62*(3), 375–384. https://doi.org/10.1002/pbc.25300

Hocking, M. C., Paltin, I., Quast, L. F., & Barakat, L. P. (2019). Acceptability and feasibility in a pilot randomized clinical trial of computerized working memory training and parental problem-solving training with pediatric brain tumor survivors. *Journal of Pediatric Psychology, 44*(6), 669–678. https://doi.org/10.1093/jpepsy/jsz015

Hocking, M. C., Noll, R. B., Kazak, A. E., Brodsky, C., Phillips, P., & Barakat, L. P. (2020a). Friendships in pediatric brain tumor survivors and non-central nervous system tumor survivors. *Journal of Pediatric Psychology, 45*(2), 194–202. https://doi.org/10.1093/jpepsy/jsz101

Hocking, M. C., Parish-Morris, J., Schultz, R. T., Minturn, J. E., Brodsky, C., Shabason, E. K., & Herrington, J. D. (2020b). Diminished social attention in pediatric brain tumor survivors:

Using eye tracking technology during naturalistic social perception. *Neuropsychology*, *34*(3), 350–358. https://doi.org/10.1037/neu0000623

Hrdlicka, M., Kudr, M., Krsek, P., Tichy, M., Kyncl, M., Zamecnik, J., … Dudova, I. (2019). Recovery from autism after successful surgery for a benign brain tumor associated with epilepsy. *Journal of Autism and Developmental Disorders*, *49*(12), 5100–5104. https://doi.org/10.1007/s10803-019-03935-z

Hudson, M. M., Mertens, A. C., Yasui, Y., Hobbie, W., Chen, H., Gurney, J. G., … Oeffinger, K. C. (2003). Health status of adult long-term survivors of childhood cancer: A report from the Childhood Cancer Survivor Study. *JAMA*, *290*(12), 1583–1592. https://doi.org/10.1001/jama.290.12.1583

Kahalley, L. S., Conklin, H. M., Tyc, V. L., Wilson, S. J., Hinds, P. S., Wu, S., … Hudson, M. M. (2011). ADHD and secondary ADHD criteria fail to identify many at-risk survivors of pediatric ALL and brain tumor. *Pediatric Blood and Cancer*, *57*(1), 110–118. https://doi.org/10.1002/pbc.22998

Meeske, K., Katz, E. R., Palmer, S. N., Burwinkle, T., & Varni, J. W. (2004). Parent proxy-reported health-related quality of life and fatigue in pediatric patients diagnosed with brain tumors and acute lymphoblastic leukemia. *Cancer*, *101*(9), 2116–2125. https://doi.org/10.1002/cncr.20609

Messina, R., Cefalo, M. G., Secco, D. E., Cappelletti, S., Rebessi, E., Carai, A., … Mastronuzzi, A. (2014). Behavioral disorders as unusual presentation of pediatric extraventricular neurocytoma: Report on two cases and review of the literature. *BMC Neurology*, *14*(1), 1–7. https://doi.org/10.1186/s12883-014-0242-8

Mogavero, M. P., Bruni, O., Delrosso, L. M., & Ferri, R. (2020). Neurodevelopmental consequences of pediatric cancer and its treatment: The role of sleep. *Brain Sciences*, *10*(7), 1–15. https://doi.org/10.3390/brainsci10070411

Monje, M., & Dietrich, J. (2012). Cognitive side effects of cancer therapy demonstrate a functional role for adult neurogenesis. *Behavioural Brain Research*, *227*(2), 376–379. https://doi.org/10.1016/j.bbr.2011.05.012

Mulhern, R. K., & Butler, R. W. (2004). Neurocognitive sequelae of childhood cancers and their treatment. *Pediatric Rehabilitation*, *7*(1), 1–14. Discussion 15–16. https://doi.org/10.1080/13638490310001655528

Mulhern, R. K., Carpentieri, S., Shema, S., Stone, P., & Fairclough, D. (1993). Factors associated with social and behavioral problems among children recently diagnosed with brain tumor. *Journal of Pediatric Psychology*, *18*(3).

Mulhern, R., Hancock, J., Fairclough, D., & Kun, L. (1992). Medical and pediatric oncology: Neuropsychological status of children treated for brain tumors: A critical review and integrative analysis. *Medical and Pediatric Oncology*, *20*, 181–191. http://www.ncbi.nlm.nih.gov/pubmed/15237199

Netson, K. L., Ashford, J. M., Skinner, T., Carty, L., Wu, S., Merchant, T. E., & Conklin, H. M. (2016). Executive dysfunction is associated with poorer health-related quality of life in pediatric brain tumor survivors. *Journal of Neuro-Oncology*, *128*(2), 313–321. https://doi.org/10.1007/s11060-016-2113-1

Ostrom, Q. T., Cioffi, G., Gittleman, H., Patil, N., Waite, K., Kruchko, C., & Barnholtz-Sloan, J. S. (2019). CBTRUS statistical report: Primary brain and other central nervous system tumors diagnosed in the United States in 2012–2016. *Neuro-Oncology*, *21*, V1–V100. https://doi.org/10.1093/neuonc/noz150

Packer, R. J., Gurney, J. G., Punyko, J. A., Donaldson, S. S., Inskip, P. D., Stovall, M., … Robison, L. L. (2003). Long-term neurologic and neurosensory sequelae in adult survivors of a childhood brain tumor: Childhood cancer survivor study. *Journal of Clinical Oncology*, *21*(17), 3255–3261. https://doi.org/10.1200/JCO.2003.01.202

Robinson, K., Kuttesch, J., Champion, J., Andreotti, C., Hipp, D., Bettis, A., … Compas, B. (2010). A quantitative meta-analysis of neurocognitive sequelae in survivors of pediatric brain tumors. *Pediatric Blood & Cancer*, *55*, 525–531.

Ruble, K., Pare-Blagoev, J., Cooper, S., Martin, A., & Jacobson, L. (2019). Parent perspectives on oncology team communication regarding neurocognitive impacts of cancer therapy and school reentry. *Pediatric Blood & Cancer*, *66*(1), e27427.

Schulte, F., Kunin-Batson, A. S., Olson-Bullis, B. A., Banerjee, P., Hocking, M. C., Janzen, L., … Krull, K. R. (2019). Social attainment in survivors of pediatric central nervous system tumors: A systematic review and meta-analysis from the Children's Oncology Group. *Journal of Cancer Survivorship*, *13*(6), 921–931. https://doi.org/10.1007/s11764-019-00808-3

Shabason, E. K., Brodsky, C., Baran, J., Isaac, L., Minturn, J. E., Ginsberg, J. P., . . . Hocking, M. C. (2019). Clinical diagnosis of attention-deficit/hyperactivity disorder in survivors of pediatric brain tumors. *Journal of Neuro-Oncology*, *143*, 305–312. https://doi.org/10.1007/s11060-019-03165-4

Sharma, B., Allison, D., Tucker, P., Mabbott, D., & Timmons, B. W. (2020). Exercise trials in pediatric brain tumor: A systematic review of randomized studies. *Journal of Pediatric Hematology/Oncology*. https://doi.org/10.1097/MPH.0000000000001844

Stefanski, K. J., Anixt, J. S., Goodman, P., Bowers, K., Leisenring, W., Baker, K., … Recklitis, C. (2020). Long-term neurocognitive and psychosocial outcomes after acute myeloid leukemia: A Childhood Cancer Survivor Study Report. *Journal of the National Cancer Institute*, *113*(4), 481–495.

Turner, C. D., Rey-Casserly, C., Liptak, C. C., & Chordas, C. (2009). Late effects of therapy for pediatric brain tumor survivors. *Journal of Child Neurology*, *24*(11), 1455–1463. https://doi.org/10.1177/0883073809341709

van Kooten, J. A. M. C., Maurice-Stam, H., Schouten, A. Y. N., van Vuurden, D. G., Granzen, B., Gidding, C., … Grootenhuis, M. A. (2019). High occurrence of sleep problems in survivors of a childhood brain tumor with neurocognitive complaints: The association with psychosocial and behavioral executive functioning. *Pediatric Blood & Cancer*, *66*(11), e27947. https://doi.org/10.1002/pbc.27947

Vannatta, K., Gartstein, M. A., Short, A., & Noll, R. B. (1998). A controlled study of peer relationships of children surviving brain tumors: Teacher, peer, and self ratings. *Journal of Pediatric Psychology*, *23*(5), 279–287.

Varedi, M., Lu, L., Phillips, N. S., Partin, R. E., Brinkman, T. M., Armstrong, G. T., … Ness, K. K. (2020). Balance impairment in survivors of pediatric brain cancers: Risk factors and associated physical limitations. *Journal of Cancer Survivorship*. https://doi.org/10.1007/s11764-020-00932-5

Willard, V. W. (2018). Social skills interventions for survivors of pediatric brain tumors: A review and reformulation. *Pediatric Blood & Cancer*, *65*(12), 1–10. https://doi.org/10.1002/pbc.27434

Willard, V. W., Allen, T. M., Hardy, K. K., & Bonner, M. J. (2017). Social functioning in survivors of pediatric brain tumors: Contribution of neurocognitive and social-cognitive skills. *Children's Health Care*, *46*(2), 181–195. https://doi.org/10.1080/02739615.2015.1124769

61

Neurodevelopment in Children With Congenital Heart Disease

David C. Bellinger and Leonard A. Rappaport

For additional material related to the content of this chapter, please see Chapters 29, 79, 87, and 105.

VIGNETTE

Joshua is a 7-year-old boy referred to you for consultation due to attentional issues, social issues with his classmates, and difficulty learning the alphabet. His medical history is remarkable for d-transposition of the great arteries (d-TGA) with a ventricular septal defect (VSD) discovered by prenatal ultrasound. He was delivered at 37 weeks of gestation at a major medical center and was seen by cardiology immediately after birth. Cardiac echo confirmed the diagnosis. He was scheduled for the Switch operation and repair of the VSD, which went without complications except for a brief clinical seizure in the cardiac intensive care unit that never recurred without treatment. Developmental milestones were on the late side, but within normal limits. He was enrolled in early intervention, which he received until 3 years of age with a qualifying diagnosis of language delay. When he turned 3 years old, Joshua was tested by his local school system but did not qualify for preschool special education services. He went to a private nursery school where he was happy but had minor difficulties making friends. When he started attending public kindergarten, his parents were told by his kindergarten teacher at their first conference that he was having trouble with his early preacademic skills, was avoiding all fine motor activities such as writing and drawing, except for Legos, and was overly active. The pediatrician solicited teacher and parent Vanderbilt forms, which were consistent with the diagnosis of attention-deficit/hyperactivity disorder (ADHD) combined type, and referred Joshua for a neuropsychological screening, which revealed a full-scale IQ score of 97. He was started on stimulant medication with a good response, verified on follow-up Vanderbilt forms. However, he continued to have social problems with peers, deficits in executive functions and fine motor skills, and difficulties with early reading mechanics.

Congenital heart disease (CHD) is the most common birth defect, affecting approximately 1% of children. Each year, approximately 40,000 children require corrective or palliative cardiac surgery. With advances in surgical and medical management, up to 90% of children with critical CHD now survive to adulthood. This growing population is increasingly recognized to be at elevated risk of lifelong cognitive and behavioral deficits that can impair quality of life.

ETIOLOGY OF NEURODEVELOPMENTAL DEFICITS IN CHD

The etiology of the deficits is multifactorial. A myriad of prenatal, preoperative, operative, postoperative, and childhood conditions and events related to CHD potentially contribute to the risk of impaired neurodevelopment (Fig. 61.1). About one-third of children with CHD have a chromosomal abnormality (trisomy, microdeletion, duplication), and unbiased screening methods, such as whole exome sequencing, hold promise of identifying many more pathogenic variants that contribute to CHD risk. A congenital cardiac malformation can be a feature of many recognized genetic syndromes (e.g., Alagille, VACTERL, Jacobsen 22q11 microdeletion, Williams, CHARGE, Noonan, Down, Turner), and CHD patients with a genetic syndrome are at greatly increased risk of neurodevelopmental impairment.

Several decades ago it was hypothesized that increased risk resulted from the dramatic medical interventions that patients with CHD undergo. Randomized trials and observational studies evaluated the impact of intraoperative factors, such as the vital organ support strategy, acid-base management, and degree of hemodilution. Unfortunately, the results suggested modest impact, if any, of these factors on neurodevelopmental risk. The studies did, however, identify selected medical factors that place a child at increased risk, including single ventricle physiology (Wernovsky et al., 2000) and perioperative seizures (Rappaport et al.,1998).

A major development in the field came in the early 2000s when it became apparent that some of the morbidities of children with CHD originate prior to birth. Fetuses with CHD show reductions in the rate of maturation in brain development, particularly in the third trimester. At term, their brains correspond in volume to the brain of a 36-week fetus (Limperopoulos et al., 2010). They also show slower increases over gestation in aspects of brain metabolism (e.g., NAA:choline ratio). Even before surgery, their brains show reduced regional functional connectivity (De Asis-Cruz, Donofrio, Vezina, & Limperopoulos, 2017). These changes are thought to be the result of hemodynamic compromise, specifically reduced cerebral perfusion with oxygen (Marelli,

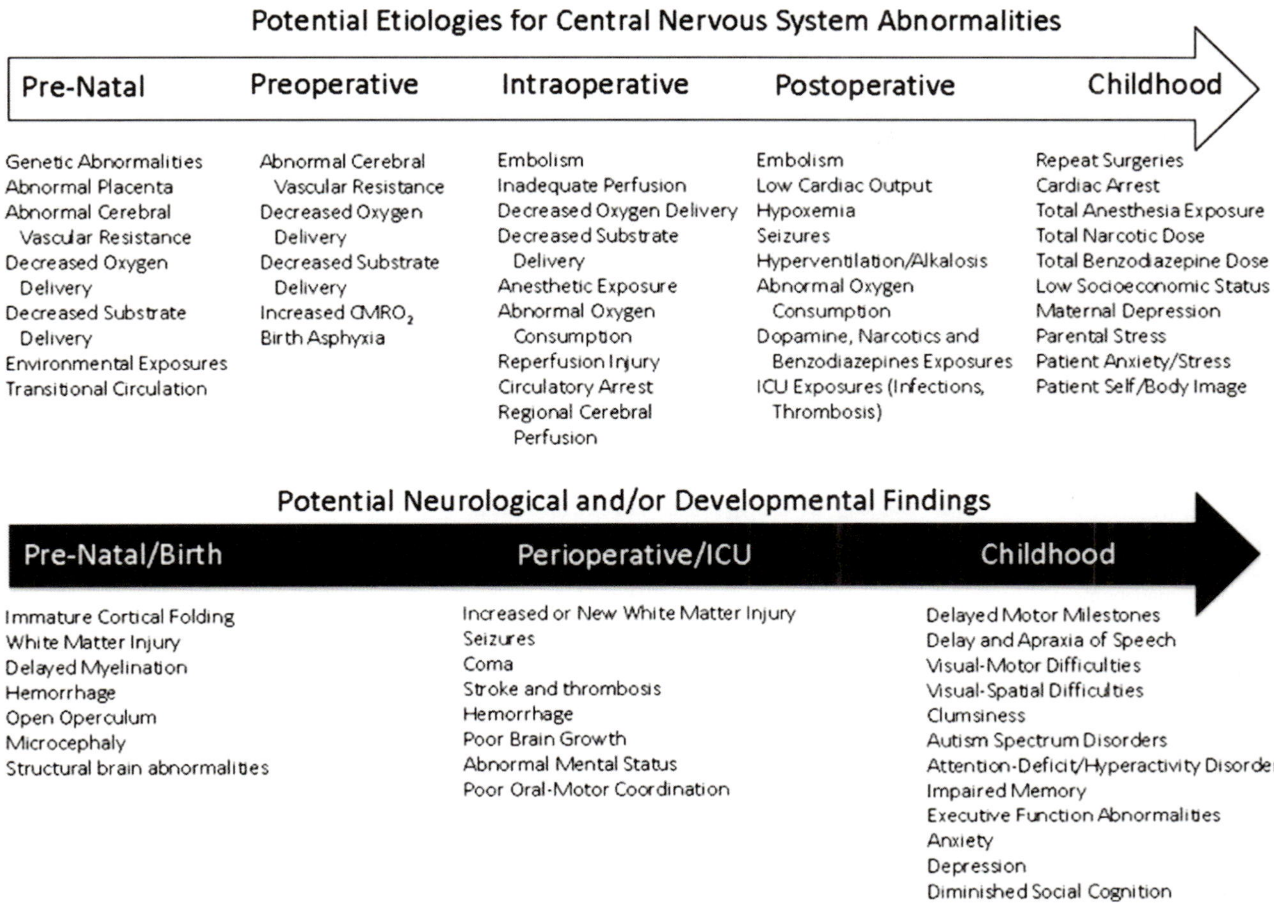

Fig. 61.1 Potential and accumulating factors leading to central nervous system abnormalities in children with congenital heart disease and neurologic and developmental findings. (From Wernovsky, G., & Licht, D. J. [2016]. Neurodevelopmental outcomes in children with congenital heart disease—What can we impact? *Pediatric Critical Care Medicine, 17*[8 Suppl 1], 232–242.)

Miller, Marino, Jefferson, & Newburger, 2016). The characteristic pattern of injury involves white matter, similar to the pattern observed in preterm infants, whereby oligodendrocyte progenitor cells fail to differentiate into mature, myelin-producing oligodendrocytes with resulting injury or dysmaturity.

NEURODEVELOPMENT IN CHILDREN WITH CHD

As a group, children with CHD are at increased risk of neurodevelopmental deficits. Greater complexity of CHD is associated with a greater likelihood of impairment (Fig. 61.2). In many children deficits are evident in multiple domains and may become more prominent over time. In a cohort of children with d-TGA the percentage of children with an impairment in one or more neurodevelopmental domains was twice as high at 8 to 14 years (55%) as it had been at age 5 years; at the older age, 7% of children showed impairment in all domains assessed (cognitive, language, speech, academic, neurologic) (Hovels-Gurich et al., 2002). Whether these findings reflect a true worsening of deficits or are, in part, an artifact of the greater sensitivity of assessments conducted at older ages is not clear. However, the findings point to the need for ongoing developmental surveillance after infancy when, as in the opening vignette, neurodevelopmental issues may emerge.

Intelligence

Although the distribution of IQ scores in cohorts of children with CHD tends to be shifted toward lower scores, they are not strikingly lower than scores for children in the general population. The dispersion of scores (i.e., standard deviation) is greater than expected, however, reflecting the presence of a subset of children scoring well below normative values. In many cases, these are children with complications, such as seizures or stroke. A surveillance strategy limited to the assessment of IQ is insufficient insofar as it would fail to identify many children who are at substantial risk of neurodevelopmental impairment, such as Joshua in the vignette.

Speech and Language

A delay in early expressive language development is a common early sign of impairment. One reason is likely to be oromotor dyscoordination; in a cohort of children with d-TGA, one-fourth of children had oromotor apraxia at 4 years of age (Bellinger et al., 1999) and 13% still met criteria at age 8 years (Bellinger, Bernstein, Kirkwood, Rappaport, & Newburger, 2003a). Oromotor apraxia likely also underlies the frequent early feeding difficulties of infants with CHD.

As children with CHD get older, they continue to show difficulties in many aspects of speech and language, including receptive skills, auditory analysis, phonologic awareness,

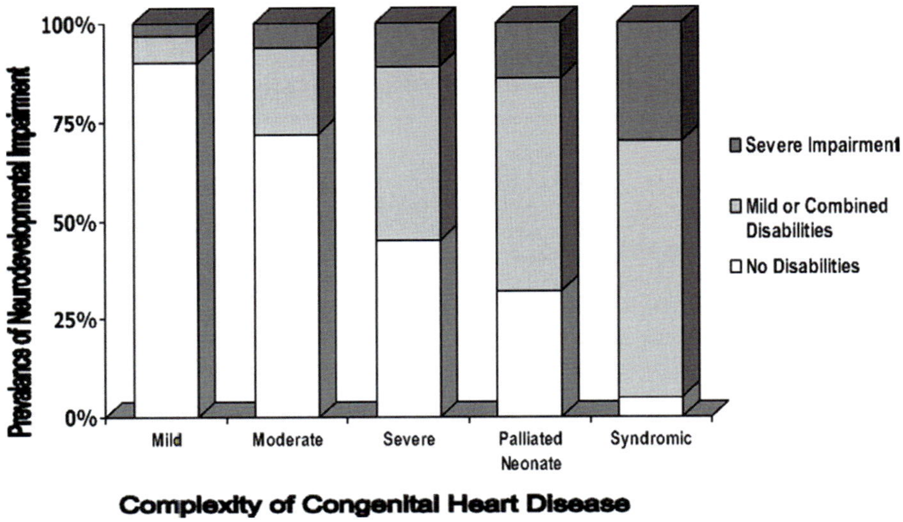

Fig. 61.2 Prevalence of neurodevelopmental disorders as related to the complexity of congenital heart disease. (From Marino, B. S., Lipkin, P. H., Newburger, J. W., Peacock, G., Gerdes, M., Gaynor, J. W., et al. [2012]. Neurodevelopmental outcomes in children with congenital heart disease: Evaluation and management: A scientific statement from the American Heart Association. *Circulation, 126*[9], 1143–1172.)

fluency, and complex syntactic skills. By early school age, pragmatic language skills involving higher-order discourse and narrative skills put in the service of social communication may also be weak (Bellinger, 2008).

Visual-Spatial Skills

Children with CHD are consistently reported to have difficulty on design-copying tasks. Children with d-TGA, administered the Rey-Osterrieth Complex Figure task at 8 years, created copies that were very poorly organized. The children tended to focus on the parts of the figure ("part-oriented" strategy) rather than the whole ("configurational" strategy) (Bellinger et al., 2003b). Children who produced the least organized copies were approximately six times more likely to require remedial services in school than children who produced the best copies.

Executive Function

Difficulties with executive functions (i.e., metacognitive and self-regulatory capacities) are especially marked in children with CHD and tend to become increasing problematic over time. These weaknesses are expressed as difficulties with time management, planning and organizing, seeing the big picture without getting lost in details, cognitive flexibility (e.g., multitasking), working memory, impulse control, and anticipating future consequences. That these problems increase with age is likely the result of the increasing demands placed on children for self-regulation and other organizational skills, especially in the school setting. In a study of adolescents with tetralogy of Fallot a subset of whom had an identified genetic syndrome, the Behavior Rating Inventory of Executive Function (BRIEF) was completed by teachers, parents, and the adolescents themselves (Bellinger et al., 2015a). According to parents, 27% of adolescents without a genetic/phenotypic syndrome had a score 65 or above ("potential clinical significance"), compared to 48% of adolescents with a syndrome. According to teachers, the rates were slightly higher, 36% and 50%, respectively. According to adolescents' self-reports, however, only 12% and 11% of scores were in the range of concern. The same pattern was observed in a cohort of patients with single ventricle physiology (Bellinger et al., 2015b).

Social Cognition

Children and adolescents with CHD, like Joshua in the vignette, have poorer social cognition skills than their peers (Bellinger, 2008). Such skills enable one to read the thoughts and emotions of other people from facial expression, body language, and paralinguistic cues. These deficits persist, and have also been reported in adults with CHD (Chiavarino et al., 2015). Individuals with poor social cognition skills can have difficulty establishing and sustaining satisfying social relationships. Someone with deficits in cognitive processing, executive functions (specifically in working memory and cognitive flexibility), emotion recognition, and pragmatic language skills are likely to find the fast-paced, coded interactions typical of adolescence to be challenging, potentially interfering with social development and peer group acceptance.

The presence of social cognition deficits in children with CHD has led to studies to determine if the prevalence of an autism spectrum disorder is increased in this patient group. Although studies suggest a modest association, it remains unclear whether this finding reflects overlap between the behavioral phenotypes of children with CHD and autism spectrum disorder.

Approximately half of children with complex CHD require one or more remedial academic services (e.g., special education, tutoring, early intervention, occupational therapy). It is important to note, however, that in the absence of a history of seizures, stroke, or other significant medical factors, the strongest predictors of variance in neurodevelopmental outcomes are the same as those observed in children without CHD, including family socioeconomic status, parental intelligence, and the availability of learning opportunities.

Many neurodevelopmental deficits, first detected in childhood, are present in adolescence or adulthood, often becoming more pronounced. Concern has been raised about whether CHD increases the risk of dementia later in life. Individuals with CHD are at increased risk of developing conditions associated with reduced cerebral blood flow and reduced brain volume, including arrhythmias, heart failure, hypertension, coronary artery disease, and diabetes mellitus. A nationwide (Denmark), population-based cohort study of more than 10,000 individuals with CHD found a 4% cumulative incidence of dementia; compared to controls, a hazard ratio of 1.6 (95% confidence interval: 1.3–2.0). The hazard ratio was greater for severe CHD compared to mild or moderate CHD and greater for early-onset dementia than late-onset dementia (Bagge et al., 2018).

PSYCHIATRIC OUTCOMES AND QUALITY OF LIFE

In a systematic review Clancy et al. (2020) found that the most consistent finding among studies of young children with CHD was what they described as a "high prevalence of low-severity emotional and behavioral dysregulation." Like the neurocognitive challenges faced by children with CHD, the behavioral challenges tend to become more apparent with age. By school age, both parents and teachers rate their behavior as more problematic, particularly in terms of internalizing behaviors (namely anxiety and depression) (Bellinger et al., 2009). By the time children with CHD reach adolescence, clinicians rate them as having poorer global psychosocial status than peers, with a substantial subgroup, especially those with more complex disease, manifesting ratings in the range of clinical concern. Among adolescents with single ventricle CHD who underwent the Fontan procedure, the lifetime prevalence of psychiatric disorder, as determined using a clinician-rated structured interview, was 65%, three times greater than among controls; anxiety disorder and ADHD were the most common diagnoses (DeMaso et al., 2017). Just as adolescents' self-reports about their executive functioning tend to be rosier than reports from parents and teachers, children tend to view their quality of life more positively than their parents do (Drakouli et al., 2015). A study by Wang, Hay, Clarke, & Menahem, (2014) suggested targets for intervention, as adolescents' health-related quality of life was found to positively correlate with knowledge about their cardiac condition, feelings of optimism, adequate social support, and a strong sense of coherence.

GUIDELINES FOR NEURODEVELOPMENTAL SCREENING AND EVALUATION

In 2012 the American Heart Association published guidelines for the evaluation and management of neurodevelopmental outcomes in children with CHD (Marino et al., 2012) (Fig. 61.3). It included a strategy for risk stratification and an algorithm for surveillance, screening, evaluation, diagnosis, and management of developmental disabilities. The following groups were considered to be at the greatest risk of neurodevelopmental disabilities:

- Neonates or infants requiring open heart surgery (cyanotic and acyanotic types): hypoplastic left heart syndrome, interrupted aortic arch, pulmonary atresia with intact ventricular septum, truncus arteriosis, total anomalous pulmonary venous connection, transposition of the great arteries, tetralogy of Fallot, tricuspid atresia
- Children with cyanotic heart lesions not requiring open heart surgery during the neonatal or infant period: tetralogy of Fallot with pulmonary atresia and major aortopulmonary collateral arteries, tetralogy of Fallot with shunt without use of cardiopulmonary bypass, Ebstein anomaly
- Any combination of CHD and certain comorbidities: prematurity (<37 weeks), developmental delay recognized in infancy, suspected genetic abnormality or syndrome associated with developmental delay, history of mechanical support (extracorporeal membrane oxygenation; ventricular assist device), heart transplantation, cardiopulmonary resuscitation at any point, prolonged hospitalization (postoperative length of stay >2 weeks), perioperative seizures related to CHD surgery, microcephaly or significant abnormalities on neuroimaging, other conditions determined at the discretion of the medical home providers

The algorithm for managing neurodevelopmental risk in patients with CHD is presented in Fig. 61.2. The recommendations begin with the American Academy of Pediatrics developmental surveillance guidelines, then adapted in light of what is known about the needs of children with CHD.

IMPACT OF CHD ON THE FAMILY

How a child with CHD affects other members of the family is understudied. In a large prospective Norwegian cohort CHD in a child accounted for nearly 40% of distress reported by mothers (Landolt, Ystrom, Stene-Larsen, Holmstrom, & Vollrath, 2014). A systematic review found that up to 30% of parents show symptoms consistent with posttraumatic stress disorder, more than 80% manifest clinical symptoms of trauma, and 25% to 50% report clinically significant signs and symptoms of depression and/or anxiety (Woolf-King, Anger, Arnold, Weiss, & Teitel, 2017). Factors that influence family wellbeing include parents' perceived level of social support, parental coping strategies, and family cohesion (Jackson, Higgins, Frydenberg, & Liang, 2018). A study to identify the needs of parents of a young child with CHD found that, in effect, parents wanted to be empowered to meet their child's needs and to be effective advocates for their child. They expressed a desire for interventions that would promote self-care, facilitate communication with their child's clinicians, provide anticipatory guidance about their child's development, and assist parents in securing social supports (Gramszlo et al., 2020). Although most studies have focused on mothers' needs in families that include a child with CHD, there is evidence that fathers of children with CHD respond to the stresses differently than mothers, and some report feeling excluded as a partner in the child's care and a lack of supports for the unique challenges that fathers face. Very limited data are available on the impact of having a sibling with CHD.

TRANSITION TO ADULT CARE

Ensuring a smooth transition between pediatric and adult care for individuals with CHD is critical. The transition should begin during early adolescence and focus, at least, on fostering self-knowledge about a patient's CHD, self-care skills, and self-advocacy skills. Significant patient knowledge gaps have been reported. In a sample of adolescents (mean age of 17 years), only 61% knew the name of their cardiac condition, 22% were aware of the recommendations for follow-up care, and only 13% of females knew to have their heart condition checked before becoming pregnant (Ladouceur et al., 2017). In another survey adolescents (median age 17 years) demonstrated only moderate knowledge of critical information, such as the follow-up schedules, medication regimens, the implications of CHD for occupational and sexual

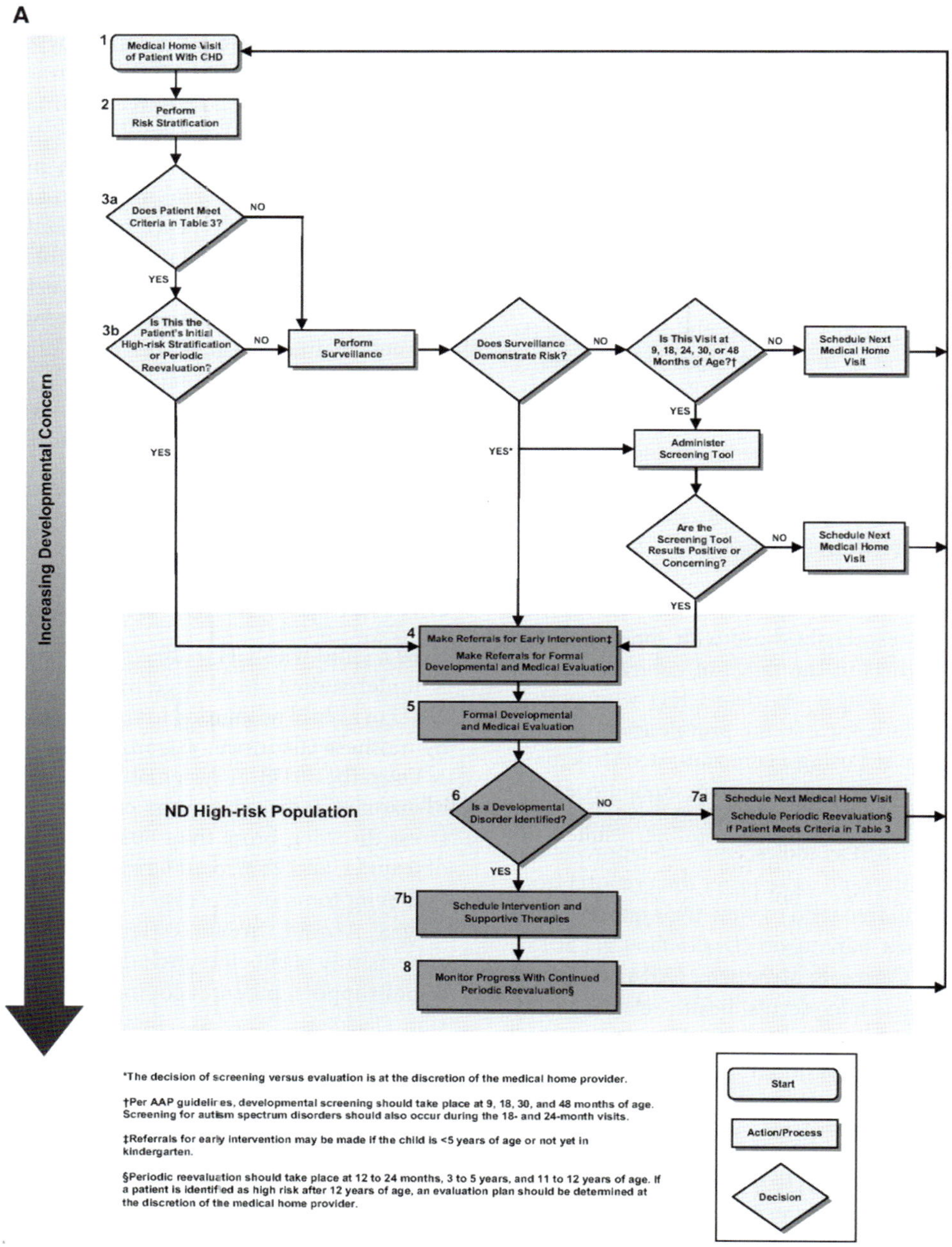

Fig. 61.3 Milder forms of congenital heart disease (CHD) include atrial septal defect or ventricular septal defect, and isolated semilunar valve disease. Moderate forms of CHD include two-ventricle CHD (coarctation of the aorta, complex semilunar valve disease, atrioventricular septal defect, ventricular septal defect with comorbidities, tetralogy of Fallot, total anomalous pulmonary venous connection.) Severe forms of CHD include palliated single-ventricle CHD, transposition of the great arteries, truncus arteriosus, interrupted aortic arch, tetralogy of Fallot/pulmonary atresia with major aortopulmonary collateral arteries, pulmonary atresia with intact ventricular septum, hypoplastic left heart syndrome, and tricuspid atresia. CHD associated with genetic disorders or syndromes (e.g., Down syndrome, 22q11 deletion, Noonan syndrome, Williams syndrome) and multiple congenital anomalies (e.g., CHARGE syndrome) are nearly always associated with developmental disorders. (Adapted from Wernovsky, G. [2006]. Current insights regarding neurological and developmental abnormalities in children and young adults with complex congenital cardiac disease. *Cardiology in the Young, 16*[1], S92–S104.)

activities, symptoms that indicate possible deterioration of their condition, the effects of smoking and alcohol on their condition, and issues relating to pregnancy (Van Deyk et al., 2010). Fostering awareness of the psychosocial implications of having a chronic disease is also important in the transition process, as mood and anxiety disorders are prevalent among adults with CHD (Kovacs and Bellinger, 2020).

The American Heart Association also published a scientific statement in 2011 outlining best practices for the management of adolescents transitioning to adult CHD (ACHD) care (Sable et al., 2011). It underscores the fact that neurodevelopmental deficits can impact patients' capabilities for both learning and developing self-management skills required to assume responsibility for their health care management. Adults with CHD and advanced heart failure are typically asked to attend frequent clinic appointments, restrict fluids and sodium, manage complicated medication regimens, and watch for symptoms that warrant urgent medical attention. Cognitive deficits, especially those involving executive functioning, increase the difficulty of maintaining good adherence to these practices.

THERAPEUTIC INTERVENTIONS

Limited information is available regarding interventions that improve the neurodevelopmental outcomes of children with CHD. Although many aspects of surgical and medical management have improved in recent decades, pooled analyses indicate that the scores of children with CHD increased only modestly over the period of 1996 to 2009 after adjustment for patient factors such as illness severity (Gaynor et al., 2015). McCusker et al. (2012) found that an intervention focused on parenting skills in families with 4- to 5-year-old children with CHD significantly improved maternal mental health and family functioning but had only modest impact on children's outcomes. Calderon et al. (2020) reported the results of a pilot randomized controlled trial in adolescents that suggested that a 6-week program of working memory training resulted in significant benefits. The persistence of the benefits, and their transfer to related skills that were not targeted by training, is uncertain.

CONCLUSION

Improvements in survival of individuals with CHD through biomedical and surgical advances have been truly fantastic. However, these individuals are at high risk for impairments in neurodevelopment, psychiatric disorders, family stress, and reduced quality of life. Historically, the neurodevelopmental challenges of children and adults with CHD have been underrecognized. Patients and parents were not necessarily provided appropriate anticipatory guidance about what to expect with regard to the possible emergence of problems. One favorable product of the burgeoning research has been the establishment of multidisciplinary hospital programs that focus solely on diagnosing and managing neurodevelopmental morbidities in children with CHD. Currently, more than 40 such cardiac neurodevelopment programs exist in the United States, organized under the rubric of the Cardiac Neurodevelopment Outcomes Collaborative (www.cardiacneuro.org). Coincident with this newfound appreciation has been the recognition that many of these patients will require varying intensities of lifelong assistance to maximize their quality of life even if they survive to old age.

REFERENCES

Bagge, C. N., Henderson, V. W., Laursen, H. B., Adelborg, K., Olsen, M., & Madsen, N. L. (2018). Risk of dementia in adults with congenital heart disease: Population-based cohort study. *Circulation*, *137*(18), 1912–1920.

Bellinger, D. C. (2008). Are children with congenital cardiac malformations at increased risk of deficits in social cognition. *Cardiology in the Young*, *18*, 3–9.

Bellinger, D. C., Wypij, D., duPlessis, A. J., Rappaport, L. A., Wernovsky, G., & Newburger, J. W. (2003a). Neurodevelopmental status at eight years in children with dextro-transposition of the great arteries: The Boston Circulatory Arrest Trial. *Journal of Thoracic and Cardiovascular Surgery*, *126*, 1385–1396.

Bellinger, D. C., Bernstein, J. H., Kirkwood, M. W., Rappaport, L. A., & Newburger, J. W. (2003b). Visual-spatial skills in children after open-heart surgery. *Journal of Developmental and Behavioral Pediatrics*, *24*(3), 169–179.

Bellinger, D. C., Newburger, J. W., Wypij, D., Kuban, K. C., duPlesssis, A. J., & Rappaport, L. A. (2009). Behaviour at eight years in children with surgically corrected transposition: The Boston Circulatory Arrest Trial. *Cardiology in the Young*, *19*(1), 86–97.

Bellinger, D. C., Rivkin, M. J., DeMaso, D., Robertson, R. L., Stopp, C., Dunbar-Masterson, C., . . . Newburger, J. W. (2015a). Adolescents with tetralogy of Fallot: Neuropsychological assessment and structural brain imaging *Cardiology in the Young*, *25*(2), 338–347.

Bellinger, D. C., Watson, C. G., Rivkin, M. J., Robertson, R. L., Roberts, A. E., Stopp, C., . . . Newburger, J. W. (2015b). Neuropsychological status and structural brain imaging in adolescents with single ventricle who underwent the Fontan procedure. *Journal of the American Heart Association*, *4*(12), e002302.

Bellinger, D. C., Wypij, D., Kuban, K. C., Rappaport, L. A., Hickey, P. R., Wernovsky, G., . . . Newburger, J. W. (1999). Developmental and neurologic status of children at 4 years of age after heart surgery with hypothermic circulatory arrest or low-flow cardiopulmonary bypass. *Circulation*, *100*, 526–532.

Bellinger, D. C., Wypij, D., Rivkin, M. J., DeMaso, D. R., Robertson, R. L., Dunbar-Masterson, C., ... Newburger, J. W. (2011). Adolescents with d-transposition of the great arteries corrected with the arterial switch procedure: Neuropsychological assessment and structural brain imaging. *Circulation*, *124*(12), 1361–1369.

Calderon, J., Wypij, D., Rofeberg, V., Stopp, C., Roseman, A., Albers, D., ... Bellinger, D. C. (2020). Randomized controlled trial of working memory intervention in congenital heart disease. *Journal of Pediatrics*, *227*, 191–198. e3.

Chiavarino, C., Bianchino, C., Brach-Prever, C., Riggi, C., Palumbo, L., Bara, B. G., & Bosco, F. M. (2015). Theory of mind deficit in adult patients with congenital heart disease. *Journal of Health Psychology*, *20*(10), 1253–1262.

Clancy, T., Jordan, B., de Weerth, C., & Muscara, F. (2020). Early emotional, behavioural and social development of infants and young children with congenital heart disease: A systematic review. *Journal of Clinical Psychology in Medical Settings*, *27*(4), 686–703.

De Asis-Cruz, J., Donofrio, M. T., Vezina, G., & Limperopoulos, C. (2017). Aberrant brain functional connectivity in newborns with congenital heart disease before cardiac surgery. *Neuroimage: Clinical*, *17*, 31–42.

DeMaso, D. R., Calderon, J., Taylor, G. A., Holland, J. E., Stopp, C., White, M. T., … Newburger, J. W. (2017). Psychiatric disorders in adolescents with single ventricle congenital heart disease. *Pediatrics*, *139*(3), e20162241.

Drakouli, M., Petsios, K., Giannakopoulou, M., Patiraki, E., Voutoufianaki, I., & Matziou, V. (2015). Determinants of quality of life in children and adolescents with CHD: A systematic review. *Cardiology in the Young*, *25*(6), 1027–1036.

Gaynor, J. W., Stopp, C., Wypij, D., Andropoulos, D. B., Atallah, J., Atz, A. M., ... International Cardiac Collaborative on Neurodevelopment (ICCON) Investigators. (2015). Neurodevelopmental outcomes after cardiac surgery in infancy. *Pediatrics*, *135*(5), 816–825.

Gramszlo, C., Karpyn, A., Demianczyk, A. C., Shillingford, A., Riegel, E., Kazak, A. E., & Sood, E. (2020). Parent perspectives on family-based psychosocial interventions for congenital heart disease. *Journal of Pediatrics*, *216*, 51–57.

Hovels-Gurich, H. H., Konrad, K., Wisner, M., Minkenberg, R., Herpertz-Dahlman, B., Messmer, B. J., & von Bernuth, G. (2002). Long term behavioural outcome after neonatal arterial switch operation for transposition of the great arteries. *Archives of Disease in Children*, *87*, 506–510.

Jackson, A. C., Higgins, R. O., Frydenberg, E., & Liang, R. P. (2018). Parents' perceptions on how they cope with the impact on their family of a child with heart disease. *Journal of Pediatric Nursing*, *40*, e9–e17.

Kovacs, A. H., & Bellinger, D. C. (2020). Neurocognitive and psychosocial outcomes in adult congenital heart disease: A lifespan approach. *Heart*. https://doi.org/heartjnl-2016-310862

Ladouceur, M., Calderon, J., Traore, M., Cheurfi, R., Pagnon, C., Khraiche, D., … Bonnet, D. (2017). Educational needs of adolescents with congenital heart disease: Impact of a transition intervention programme. *Archives of Cardiovascular Disease*, *110*(5), 317–324.

Landolt, M. A., Ystrom, E., Stene-Larsen, K., Holmstrom, H., & Vollrath, M. E. (2014). Exploring causal pathways of child behavior and maternal mental health in families with a child with congenital heart disease: A longitudinal study. *Psychological Medicine*, *44*(16), 3421–3433.

Limperopoulos, C., Tworetzky, W., McElhinney, D. B., Newburger, J. W., Brown, D. W., Robertson, R. L., & duPlessis, A. J. (2010). Brain volume and metabolism in fetuses with congenital heart disease: Evaluation with quantitative magnetic resonance imaging and spectroscopy. *Circulation*, *121*(1), 26–33.

Marelli, A., Miller, S. P., Marino, B. S., Jefferson, A. L., & Newburger, J. W. (2016). Brain in congenital heart disease across the lifespan: The cumulative burden of injury. *Circulation*, *133*(20), 1951–1962.

Marino, B. S., Lipkin, P. H., Newburger, J. W., Peacock, G., Gerdes, M., Gaynor, J. W., … Mahle, W. T. (2012). Neurodevelopmental outcomes in children with congenital heart disease: Evaluation and management: A scientific statement from the American Heart Association. *Circulation*, *126*(9), 1143–1172.

McCusker, C. G., Doherty, N. N., Molloy, B., Rooney, N., Mullholland, C., Sands, A., … Casey, F. (2012). A randomized controlled trial of interventions to promote adjustment in children with congenital heart disease entering school and their families. *Journal of Pediatric Psychology*, *37*(10), 1089–1103.

Rappaport, L. A., Wypij, D., Bellinger, D. C., Helmers, S. L., Holmes, G. L., Barnes, P. D., … Newburger, J. W. (1998). Relation of seizures after cardiac surgery in early infancy to neurodevelopmental outcome. Boston Circulatory Arrest Study Group. *Circulation*, *97*(8), 773–779.

Sable, C., Foster, E., Uzark, K., Bjornsen, K., Canobbio, M. M., Connolly, H. M., … Williams, R. G. (2011). Best practices in managing transition to adulthood for adolescents with congenital heart disease: The transition process and medical and psychosocial issues: A scientific statement from the American Heart Association. *Circulation*, *123*(13), 1454–1485.

Van Deyk, K., Pelgrims, E., Troost, E., Goossens, E., Budts, W., & Gewillig Moons, P. (2010). Adolescents' understanding of their congenital heart disease on transfer to adult-focused care. *American Journal of Cardiology*, *106*(12), 1803–1807.

Wang, Q., Hay, M., Clarke, D., & Menahem, S. (2014). Associations between knowledge of disease, depression and anxiety, social support, sense of coherence and optimism with health-related quality of life in an ambulatory sample of adolescents with heart disease. *Cardiology in the Young*, *24*(1), 126–133.

Wernovsky, G., Stiles, K. M., Gauvreau, K., Gentles, T. L., duPlessis, A. J., Bellinger, D. C., … (2000). Cognitive development after the Fontan operation. *Circulation*, *102*(8), 883–889.

Woolf-King, S. E., Anger, A., Arnold, E. A., Weiss, S. J., & Teitel, D. (2017). Mental health among parents of children with critical congenital heart defects: A systematic review. *Journal of the American Heart Association*, *6*(2), e004862.

Medications With Developmental and Behavioral Side Effects

Sonia A. Monteiro and Robert G. Voigt

For additional material related to the content of this chapter, please see Chapters 31 and 34.

VIGNETTE

Leah is an 8-year-old girl presenting for an evaluation of attention-deficit/hyperactivity disorder (ADHD). She was diagnosed with epilepsy (simple focal seizures) when she was 3 years old, and she has been treated with several antiepileptic drugs (AEDs) over the past 5 years. She has been taking her current anticonvulsant medication, oxcarbazepine, for the past year. Her parents report that third grade has been very challenging for Leah; her grades have fallen over the past 6 months. Leah has previously been determined by her school district to qualify for an individualized education plan (IEP) under the categorical label "specific learning disability" and "other health impairment" (given her history of epilepsy). Her current special educational supports include pullout resource room remedial instruction for language arts and reading three times per week for 45-minute sessions. She also receives accommodations when taking tests, and her classwork in selected areas is modified. Both her third-grade teacher and special education teacher report that Leah has difficulty remaining focused and requires frequent reminders to stay on task. Her mother describes Leah as a "daydreamer"; Leah's parents have to frequently repeat directions at home. Her father has been reading online about the various side effects of AEDs and questions whether Leah's symptoms are a side effect of her treatment with oxcarbazepine. He also reports a personal history of ADHD. Leah is evaluated by a neurologist every 3 months, and she has not had a seizure in 6 months. While talking with Leah in the exam room, you notice that she talks excessively and frequently goes off on tangents during conversations. During the neurodevelopmental examination, Leah requires frequent redirection to complete tasks. On standardized developmental testing, Leah's academic abilities score within a first- to second-grade range. What do you recommend?

INTRODUCTION

Children presenting with concerns about their development or behavior may have additional medical diagnoses for which they are being treated with medication. It is thus particularly important to obtain a history of all current and prior medications that a child has been taking, as many medications have a direct impact on a child's behavior or development. In this chapter we review the adverse developmental and behavioral effects of AEDs, first- and second-generation antihistamines, and corticosteroids.

ANTIEPILEPTIC DRUGS (ANTICONVULSANTS)

Seizure disorders affect between 0.5% and 1% of children and are the most common neurologic disorder in children (see Chapter 31) (Aaberg et al., 2017). Neurodevelopmental comorbidities in children with epilepsy are extremely common. In terms of cognitive impairment, a population-based cohort of school-aged children reported intellectual disability in 40% and borderline intelligence in 15% of children with epilepsy (Reilly et al., 2014). Between 5% and 46% of children with autism spectrum disorder have epilepsy, with increased prevalence in those with severe intellectual disability (Nickels et al., 2016). ADHD has been reported in 12% to 50% of children with epilepsy, with higher rates in those who are intellectually disabled; the primarily inattentive subtype is most common (Cohen et al., 2013; Williams et al., 2016). Increased rates of cooccurring anxiety (15%–20%) and depression (23%–26%) are also encountered in children and adolescents with epilepsy (Schraegle & Titus, 2017). The overall frequency of psychiatric comorbidities is significantly higher in children with epilepsy than in the general population, and these comorbidities have been shown to have a greater impact on both parent- and child-reported quality of life than indicators of seizure severity or frequency (Baca, Vickrey, Caplan, Vassar, & Berg, 2011). Given this array of neurodevelopmental and neurobehavioral morbidity that complicates the lives of children and adolescents with epilepsy, the goal of therapy with medical management is to reduce seizures without worsening any underlying comorbid developmental, cognitive, learning, or neurobehavioral disorders.

Many AEDs have cognitive and behavioral side effects (Tables 62.1 and 62.2). These side effects can occur when initiating a new medication, titrating the dose of an existing medication, or adding a new medication to the anticonvulsant regimen. Side effects for many AEDs are dose dependent; increased rates of cognitive impairment have been reported for some AEDs with increasing dosage (Moavero et al., 2017). When adjusting the dose of an AED, titrating up too rapidly can increase the risk of adverse events. For many children, multiple medications are required to achieve seizure control,

TABLE 62.1 Classical/Older Antiepileptic Drugs: Cognitive and Behavioral Effects

Medication Name	Seizures Treated	Cognitive Effect	Behavioral Effect
Phenobarbital	Infantile seizures Generalized partial or febrile	Negative effect on cognition, attention, memory	Hyperactivity, withdrawal, sedation, sleep disturbances
Phenytoin	Broad spectrum	Negative effect on memory, attention, mental speed	Schizophrenic-like psychosis at high doses
Ethosuximide	Generalized absence	Inconclusive	Inconclusive/possible psychosis
Carbamazepine	Complex partial	Neutral effects	Neutral effects

Adapted from Halma, E., de Louw, A. J., Klinkenberg, S., Aldenkamp, A. P., IJff, D. M., & Majoie, M. (2014). Behavioral side-effects of levetiracetam in children with epilepsy: A systematic review. *Seizure, 23*(9), 685–691. https://doi.org/10.1016/j.seizure.2014.06.004; Moavero, R., Santarone, M. E., Galasso, C., & Curatolo, P. (2017). Cognitive and behavioral effects of new antiepileptic drugs in pediatric epilepsy. *Brain & Development, 39*(6), 464–469. https://doi.org/10.1016/j.braindev.2017.01.006; Watkins, L. V., Pickrell, W. O., & Kerr, M. P. (2019). Treatment of psychiatric comorbidities in patients with epilepsy and intellectual disabilities: Is there a role for the neurologist? *Epilepsy & Behavior, 98*(Pt B), 322–327. https://doi.org/10.1016/j.yebeh.2018.09.010

an additional risk factor for cognitive and behavioral adverse events, especially when AEDs with similar adverse event profiles are used in conjunction. Prior to initiating an AED trial, thorough developmental, medical, and family histories must be obtained, and the child's baseline cognitive and behavioral functioning should be assessed to identify any preexisting developmental or behavioral comorbidity. Such assessment should continue throughout treatment to assess for any adverse cognitive or behavioral sequelae of the AED treatment itself.

Previous research on both older AEDs (see Table 62.1) and newer AEDs (see Table 62.2) has limitations, with limited data on the efficacy and safety in children for newer AEDs. However, studies suggest an overall decrease in adverse events associated with the use of newer AEDs compared to older AEDs. Many studies assessing the cognitive and behavioral effects of AEDs have included individuals without epilepsy, so these studies may not accurately reflect the potential side effects for individuals with epilepsy and other comorbid conditions. Research on adverse events in individuals with epilepsy and intellectual disability has been limited, which is particularly concerning given the association between polypharmacy and intellectual disability (Reilly et al., 2014). Additionally, the time span over which studies are conducted is typically much shorter than the period of time that many children require AED treatment. These studies may not reflect the cumulative developmental and behavioral effects that may occur. Ideally, data on adverse cognitive and behavioral effects would come from randomized controlled trials with monotherapy; however, this research strategy is difficult due to many patients requiring multiple AEDs to adequately control their seizures. Tables 62.1 and 62.2 compare the adverse cognitive and behavioral effects of old and new AEDs, respectively.

TABLE 62.2 Newer Antiepileptic Drugs: Cognitive and Behavioral Effects

Medication Name	Seizures Treated	Cognitive Effect	Behavioral Effect
Lamotrigine (Lamictal)	Effective for most seizure types	Potential benefit on cognitive	Potential improvement in attention Insomnia Anxiety
Levetiracetam (Keppra)	Used for partial-onset seizures and adjunctive for myoclonic seizures	No substantial effect on cognition	Increased irritability, aggression, depression, hostility, and hyperexcitability
Topiramate (Topamax)	Partial-onset and generalized-onset seizures	Some reports of mental slowing/memory difficulties and verbal fluency	Increased rates of behavioral problems reported in children with intellectual disability Psychosis Depression
Oxcarbazepine (Tegretol)	Monotherapy or adjunctive therapy in partial/secondarily generalized seizures	No evidence for cognitive impact	No data
Zonisamide (Zonegran)	Adjunctive in refractory partial seizures	Cognitive slowing/difficulties with concentration	Limited data

Adapted from Moavero, R., Santarone, M. E., Galasso, C., & Curatolo, P. (2017). Cognitive and behavioral effects of new antiepileptic drugs in pediatric epilepsy. *Brain & Development, 39*(6) 464–469. https://doi.org/10.1016/j.braindev.2017.01.006; Watkins, L. V., Pickrell, W. O., & Kerr, M. P. (2019). Treatment of psychiatric comorbidities in patients with epilepsy and intellectual disabilities: Is there a role for the neurologist? *Epilepsy & Behavior, 98*(Pt B), 322–327. https://doi.org/10.1016/j.yebeh.2018.09.010

Leah's parents and teacher complete standardized behavioral ratings scales. The results are consistent with ADHD, inattentive subtype, which is a common comorbidity of both Leah's epilepsy and learning disability and possibly related to her family history. Leah and her parents begin behavioral therapy. After further discussion with both her parents and treating neurologist, Leah is started on a trial of extended-release methylphenidate. Her parents are advised to closely monitor for any new seizure activity. When Leah returns for follow-up, they report an improvement in her focus and school performance and in Leah's attitude about school.

ANTIHISTAMINES

Antihistamines are recommended for many conditions, such as allergic conditions and urticaria. However, off-label usage of antihistamines has increased over time compared to other classes of medications. Higher rates of off-label ordering have been observed in children with chronic medical conditions who are on multiple medications (Hoon et al., 2019). Given the widespread availability of antihistamines and over-the-counter access, the possibility for both self-medication and for parents administering these medications to their children without first seeking advice from their physician is high. Many parents may be unaware of the potential risks and side effects of antihistamines. Developmental-behavioral clinicians should take a careful history of prescribed and over-the-counter medications.

First-Generation Antihistamines (Diphenhydramine, Hydroxyzine, and Cyproheptadine)

On-label treatment with first-generation antihistamines for adults and older pediatric patients with symptoms of allergies has been extensively studied; however, clinical trials, including younger children, have been limited (Motola et al., 2017). First-generation antihistamines are commonly used off-label by parents as a sleep aid for their children. Despite the popularity of this treatment, studies investigating the effectiveness of antihistamines in aiding sleep have been mixed, depending on the age of the child being treated. One study demonstrated no difference between diphenhydramine and placebo in reducing nighttime awakenings or in improving overall parental happiness in infants from 6 to 15 months of age, while another study reported decreased sleep onset latency, a reduction in nighttime awakenings, and longer sleep duration in children from 2 to 12 years of age (Merenstein et al., 2006; Russo et al., 1976). Given these conflicting data, and given that children may experience paradoxic behavioral excitation with the use of first-generation antihistamines (see later), despite their easy availability, first-generation antihistamines are not recommended as a first-line treatment of pediatric insomnia (see Chapter 70).

The cognitive and behavioral side effects of first-generation antihistamines are a result of their poor selectivity for H1 receptors, which leads to antimuscarinic, antiadrenergic, and antiserotoninergic side effects, including visual changes, confusion, and dry mouth. First-generation antihistamines have a direct effect on cognition and behavior through their ability to cross the blood-brain barrier into the central nervous system resulting in sedation, drowsiness, and sleep disruptions. First-generation antihistamines may also negatively impact learning through decreased cognitive processing (Ng et al., 2004). Additionally, these medications pose the risk for a range of cognitive, behavioral, and motor side effects opposite to what would be expected (drowsiness/sedation), also known as paradoxic central excitation. These side effects can range from restlessness, behavioral changes, nervousness, and insomnia progressing to hallucinations, seizures, and movement disorders (Blaiss, 2004). These side effects are primarily observed with overdosage but have also been reported when these medications are given to children and adolescents at the recommended dosage. The short half-life of first-generation antihistamines necessitates multiple daily doses, thus increasing the risk for these adverse events.

Second-Generation Antihistamines (Cetirizine, Loratadine, Fexofenadine)

In the 1980s second-generation antihistamines were developed that have greater specificity for the H1 receptor and are lipophobic, resulting in poor penetration of the blood-brain barrier and reduced risk for sedation and cognitive impairment. These medications have been studied in children as young as 6 months of age and have demonstrated efficacy in the treatment of allergic rhinitis; cetirizine has been found to be more efficacious than loratadine (Nayak et al., 2017; Phan et al., 2009). Cetirizine has been shown to have a higher risk for sedation compared to loratadine and fexofenadine, but the degree of sedation is still less than what is seen with first-generation antihistamines (Blaiss, 2004).

While antihistamines, especially the first-generation antihistamines, have potential cognitive and behavioral side effects, it has also been shown that untreated allergic rhinitis is associated with impairments in daytime attention, decreased concentration, and fatigue secondary to poor sleep, all of which negatively impacts a child's ability to learn and to function at school. Studies investigating the impact on learning for school-aged children with allergic rhinitis who are treated with second-generation antihistamines are limited. One study from 2001 showing no difference in learning for children treated with either loratadine or placebo and another study from 2010 showing higher conceptual knowledge scores in children treated with loratadine compared to both treatment with diphenhydramine and placebo (Bender, McCormick, & Milgrom, 2001; Church et al., 2010). More research on this condition and its treatment should be a high priority, given the high prevalence of allergy among children.

CORTICOSTEROIDS (PREDNISONE, DEXAMETHASONE, BETAMETHASONE, METHYLPREDNISOLONE)

Despite their widespread use for a variety of pediatric medical conditions, research on the neurobehavioral side effects of corticosteroids in children has been limited primarily to

TABLE 62.3 Cognitive and Behavioral Side Effects of Corticosteroid Use in Specific Conditions

Condition	Steroid Used	Indication/Duration of Treatment	Cognitive/Behavioral Side Effects
Asthma and croup	Prednisolone	Short course (3–5 days) for exacerbation	Behavioral changes (4%): anxiety, depressive symptoms, aggressive (especially at higher doses) Sleep disturbance in 4%
Inflammatory bowel disease Ulcerative colitis (UC) and Crohn disease	Prednisone Prednisolone Methylprednisolone	UC: Long course (4–12 wk) Crohn: 10–14 days for flareup	Irritability/insomnia/depressive Rare case reports of psychosis Limited cognitive impact
Duchenne muscular dystrophy	Prednisone	Long course: >12 mo to improve muscle strength	Behavioral changes
Nephrotic syndrome	Prednisone Prednisolone	Long course: 12 wk	Anxiety, depression, increased aggression, attention problems

Adapted from Abrams, E. M., Becker, A. B., & Szefler, S. J. (2018). Use of oral corticosteroids in the wheezy toddler. *Journal of Pediatrics, 201,* 16–20. https://doi.org/10.1016/j.jpeds.2018.06.011; Gloss, D., Moxley III, R. T., Ashwal, S., & Oskoui, M. (2016). Practice guideline update summary: Corticosteroid treatment of Duchenne muscular dystrophy: Report of the Guideline Development Subcommittee of the American Academy of Neurology. *Neurology, 86*(5), 465–472. https://doi.org/10.1212/WNL.0000000000002337; Kim, J. W., Kang, K. S., & Kang, N. R. (2020). Steroid-induced psychosis in adolescent patient with Crohn's disease. *Soa—ch'ongsonyon chongsin uihak (Journal of Child & Adolescent Psychiatry), 31*(3), 161–164. https://doi.org/10.5765/jkacap.200022; Mrakotsky, C., Forbes, P. W., Bernstein, J. H., Grand, R. J., Bousvaros, A., Szigethy, E., & Waber, D. P. (2013). Acute cognitive and behavioral effects of systemic corticosteroids in children treated for inflammatory bowel disease. *Journal of the International Neuropsychological Society, 19*(1), 96–109. https://doi.org/10.1017/S1355617712001014; Upadhyay, A., Mishra, O. P., Prasad, R., Upadhyay, S. K., & Schaefer, F. (2016). Behavioural abnormalities in children with new-onset nephrotic syndrome receiving corticosteroid therapy: Results of a prospective longitudinal study. *Pediatric Nephrology (Berlin, Germany), 31*(2), 233–238. https://doi.org/10.1007/s00467-015-3216-1

case reports and case series, with few large-scale, prospective studies. Rates of behavioral changes have been reported to be higher in long-course compared to short-course corticosteroid treatment. In the adult population side effects have been well described and can range from depressive symptoms and mild cognitive effects to psychosis. In children side effects of a short course of corticosteroid treatment may include sleep disturbances (insomnia or fatigue) and behavioral changes. Mood changes, including irritability, anxiety, depression, hyperactivity, and aggression, are associated with high doses. Steroid-induced psychosis is seen more frequently in adults than children, but it has been reported to occur in children receiving steroid treatment for asthma, autoimmune disease, and cancer (Hodgins et al., 2018). For some parents, these behaviors may go unreported, depending on severity, and may be considered to be normal childhood behaviors, such as tantrums or aggression. Thus inquiring about preexisting mood or behavioral symptoms prior to initiation of medication, counseling on these potential side effects, and close monitoring over the course of treatment are recommended. The treatment of these adverse cognitive and behavioral effects in children and adolescents includes cessation of treatment or dose reduction. For some medical conditions, where the treatment cannot be stopped or the dose cannot be reduced, of treatment of cognitive and behavioral side effects with benzodiazepines or antipsychotic medications symptoms have been reported to counteract the side effects of corticosteroids (Drozdowicz & Bostwick, 2014).

Corticosteroid Usage in Specific Pediatric Medical Conditions

Table 62.3 details specific cognitive and behavioral side effects of specific corticosteroid treatment in specific pediatric medical conditions, including asthma, croup, inflammatory bowel disease (ulcerative colitis, Crohn disease), Duchenne muscular dystrophy (see Chapter 39), and nephrotic syndrome. Corticosteroids are also given repeatedly over the course of treatment for acute lymphoblastic leukemia (ALL), with dexamethasone becoming the preferred corticosteroid in the past 20 years, given its increased efficacy and decreased risk for relapse. However, in a randomized controlled trial of 1600 children and adolescents with ALL 6% of children treated with dexamethasone experienced behavioral changes (including mood swings, severe depression, and increased violence directed toward self and others) compared to only 1% in children treated with prednisolone (Mitchell et al., 2005). A recent systematic review of randomized controlled trials did not find clinically meaningful differences in rates of behavioral change among children treated with dexamethasone versus prednisone (Warris et al., 2014).

Corticosteroid Usage in Preterm and Low Birthweight Infants

Given their established role in increasing survival and reducing morbidity through their antiinflammatory effects, corticosteroids are routinely administered to preterm or low birthweight infants for various conditions, including bronchopulmonary dysplasia, congenital heart defects, and congenital adrenal hyperplasia (see Chapter 34) (Drozdowicz & Bostwick, 2014). Reports of neurodevelopmental outcomes for former low birthweight infants who received dexamethasone treatment have ranged from increased risk for gross and fine motor incoordination to increased risk for cerebral palsy and cognitive impairment (Kutschera et al., 2005; O'Shea et al., 2007). This important topic requires further research, given the high prevalence of prematurity and the long-term effects of early treatments (see Chapter 3).

CONCLUSION

As illustrated, medications that are prescribed or taken to treat a variety of nonbehavioral or developmental conditions have the risk of behavioral and cognitive side effects. These effects should not be overlooked or misattributed. Stopping medications, especially for conditions that are not indicated, such as antihistamines for sleep, or adjusting dosage for indicated medications, such as AEDs for seizures, could result in improved functioning. Physicians prescribing or caring for children taking these medications should be cognizant of their side effects and provide education to caregivers about their potential negative behavioral or developmental impacts. Developmental-behavioral clinicians should take a careful history of all medications used by the children and adolescents whom they evaluate.

REFERENCES

Aaberg, K. M., Gunnes, N., Bakken, I. J., Lund Søraas, C., Berntsen, A., Magnus, P., ... Surén, P. (2017). Incidence and prevalence of childhood epilepsy: A nationwide cohort study. *Pediatrics, 139*(5), e20163908. https://doi.org/10.1542/peds.2016-3908

Abrams, E. M., Becker, A. B., & Szefler, S. J. (2018). Use of oral corticosteroids in the wheezy toddler. *Journal of Pediatrics, 201*, 16–20. https://doi.org/10.1016/j.jpeds.2018.06.011

Baca, C. B., Vickrey, B. G., Caplan, R., Vassar, S. D., & Berg, A. T. (2011). Psychiatric and medical comorbidity and quality of life outcomes in childhood-onset epilepsy. *Pediatrics, 128*(6), e1532–e1543. https://doi.org/10.1542/peds.2011-0245

Bender, B. G., McCormick, D. R., & Milgrom, H. (2001). Children's school performance is not impaired by short-term administration of diphenhydramine or loratadine. *Journal of Pediatrics, 138*(5), 656–660. https://doi.org/10.1067/mpd.2001.112647

Blaiss, M. (2004). Current concepts and therapeutic strategies for allergic rhinitis in school-age children. *Clinical Therapeutics, 26*(11), 1876–1889. https://doi.org/10.1016/j.clinthera.2004.11.003

Church, M. K., Maurer. M., Simons, F. E., Bindslev-Jensen, C., van Cauwenberge, P., Bousquet, J., ... Global Allergy and Asthma European Network. (2010). Risk of first-generation H(1)-antihistamines: A GA(2)LEN position paper. *Allergy, 65*(4), 459–466. https://doi.org/10.1111/j.1398-9995.2009.02325.x

Cohen, R., Senecky, Y., Shuper, A., Inbar, D., Chodick, G., Shalev, V., & Raz, R. (2013). Prevalence of epilepsy and attention-deficit hyperactivity (ADHD) disorder: A population-based study. *Journal of Child Neurology, 28*(1), 120–123. https://doi.org/10.1177/0883073812440327

Drozdowicz, L. B., & Bostwick, J. M. (2014). Psychiatric adverse effects of pediatric corticosteroid use. *Mayo Clinic Proceedings, 89*(6), 817–834. https://doi.org/10.1016/j.mayocp.2014.01.010

Gloss, D., Moxley, III, R. T., Ashwal, S., & Oskoui, M. (2016). Practice guideline update summary: Corticosteroid treatment of Duchenne muscular dystrophy: Report of the Guideline Development Subcommittee of the American Academy of Neurology. *Neurology, 86*(5), 465–472. https://doi.org/10.1212/WNL.0000000000002337

Halma, E., de Louw, A. J., Klinkenberg, S., Aldenkamp, A. P., IJff, D. M., & Majoie, M. (2014). Behavioral side-effects of levetiracetam in children with epilepsy: A systematic review. *Seizure, 23*(9), 685–691. https://doi.org/10.1016/j.seizure.2014.06.004

Hodgins, G. E., Saltz, S. B., Gibbs, E. P., Gonzalez, R., Regan, J., & Nemeroff, C. (2018). Steroid-induced psychosis in the pediatric population: A new case and review of the literature. *Journal of Child and Adolescent Psychopharmacology, 28*(5), 354–359. https://doi.org/10.1089/cap.2018.0017

Hoon, D., Taylor, M. T., Kapadia, P., Gerhard, T., Strom, B. L., & Horton, D. B. (2019). Trends in off-label drug use in ambulatory settings: 2006–2015. *Pediatrics, 144*(4), e20190896. https://doi.org/10.1542/peds.2019-0896

Kim, J. W., Kang, K. S., & Kang, N. R. (2020). Steroid-induced psychosis in adolescent patient with Crohn's disease. *Soa—ch'ongsonyon chongsin uihak (Journal of Child & Adolescent Psychiatry), 31*(3), 161–164. https://doi.org/10.5765/jkacap.200022

Kutschera, J., Tomaselli, J., Maurer, U., Mueller, W., & Urlesberger, B. (2005). Minor neurological dysfunction, cognitive development, and somatic development at the age of 3 to 7 years after dexamethasone treatment in very-low birth-weight infants. *Early Human Development, 81*(3), 281–287. https://doi.org/10.1016/j.earlhumdev.2004.07.004

Merenstein, D., Diener-West, M., Halbower, A. C., Krist, A., & Rubin, H. R. (2006). The trial of infant response to diphenhydramine: The TIRED study—a randomized, controlled, patient-oriented trial. *Archives of Pediatrics and Adolescent Medicine, 160*(7), 707–712. https://doi.org/10.1001/archpedi.160.7.707

Mitchell, C. D., Richards, S. M., Kinsey, S. E., Lilleyman, J., Vora, A., Eden, T. O., & Medical Research Council Childhood Leukaemia Working Party. (2005). Benefit of dexamethasone compared with prednisolone for childhood acute lymphoblastic leukaemia: Results of the UK Medical Research Council ALL97 randomized trial. *British Journal of Haematology, 129*(6), 734–745. https://doi.org/10.1111/j.1365-2141.2005.05509.x

Moavero, R., Santarone, M. E., Galasso, C., & Curatolo, P. (2017). Cognitive and behavioral effects of new antiepileptic drugs in pediatric epilepsy. *Brain & Development, 39*(6), 464–469. https://doi.org/10.1016/j.braindev.2017.01.006

Motola, D., Donati, M., Biagi, C., Calamelli, E., Cipriani, F., Melis, M., ... Ricci, G. (2017). Safety profile of H1-antihistamines in pediatrics: An analysis based on data from VigiBase. *Pharmacoepidemiology and Drug Safety, 26*(10), 1164–1171. https://doi.org/10.1002/pds.4246

Mrakotsky, C., Forbes, P. W., Bernstein, J. H., Grand, R. J., Bousvaros, A., Szigethy, E., & Waber, D. P. (2013). Acute cognitive and behavioral effects of systemic corticosteroids in children treated for inflammatory bowel disease. *Journal of the International Neuropsychological Society*, *19*(1), 96–109. https://doi.org/10.1017/S1355617712001014

Nayak, A. S., Berger, W. E., LaForce, C. F., Urdaneta, E. R., Patel, M. K., Franklin, K. B., & Wu, M. M. (2017). Randomized, placebo-controlled study of cetirizine and loratadine in children with seasonal allergic rhinitis. *Allergy and Asthma Proceedings*, *38*(3), 222–230. https://doi.org/10.2500/aap.2017.38.4050

Ng, K. H., Chong, D., Wong, C. K., Ong, H. T., Lee, C. Y., Lee, B. W., & Shek, L. P. (2004). Central nervous system side effects of first- and second-generation antihistamines in school children with perennial allergic rhinitis: A randomized, double-blind, placebo-controlled comparative study. *Pediatrics*, *113*(2), e116–e121. https://doi.org/10.1542/peds.113.2.e116

Nickels, K. C., Zaccariello, M. J., Hamiwka, L. D., & Wirrell, E. C. (2016). Cognitive and neurodevelopmental comorbidities in paediatric epilepsy. *Nature Reviews: Neurology*, *12*(8), 465–476. https://doi.org/10.1038/nrneurol.2016.98

O'Shea, T. M., Washburn, L. K., Nixon, P. A., & Goldstein, D. J. (2007). Follow-up of a randomized, placebo-controlled trial of dexamethasone to decrease the duration of ventilator dependency in very low birth weight infants: Neurodevelopmental outcomes at 4 to 11 years of age. *Pediatrics*, *120*(3), 594–602. https://doi.org/10.1542/peds.2007-0486

Phan, H., Moeller, M. L., & Nahata, M. C. (2009). Treatment of allergic rhinitis in infants and children: Efficacy and safety of second-generation antihistamines and the leukotriene receptor antagonist montelukast. *Drugs*, *69*(18), 2541–2576. https://doi.org/10.2165/9884960-000000000-00000

Reilly, C., Atkinson, P., Das, K. B., Chin, R. F., Aylett, S. E., Burch, V., … Neville, B. G. (2014). Neurobehavioral comorbidities in children with active epilepsy: A population-based study. *Pediatrics*, *133*(6), e1586–e1593. https://doi.org/10.1542/peds.2013-3787

Russo, R. M., Gururaj, V. J., & Allen, J. E. (1976). The effectiveness of diphenhydramine HCI in pediatric sleep disorders. *Journal of Clinical Pharmacology*, *16*(5–6), 284–288. https://doi.org/10.1002/j.1552-4604.1976.tb02406.x

Schraegle, W. A., & Titus, J. B. (2017). The relationship of seizure focus with depression, anxiety, and health-related quality of life in children and adolescents with epilepsy. *Epilepsy & Behavior*, *68*, 115–122. https://doi.org/10.1016/j.yebeh.2016.12.009

Upadhyay, A., Mishra, O. P., Prasad, R., Upadhyay, S. K., & Schaefer, F. (2016). Behavioural abnormalities in children with new-onset nephrotic syndrome receiving corticosteroid therapy: Results of a prospective longitudinal study. *Pediatric Nephrology (Berlin, Germany)*, *31*(2), 233–238. https://doi.org/10.1007/s00467-015-3216-1

Warris, L. T., van den Heuvel-Eibrink, M. M., den Hoed, M. A., Aarsen, F. K., Pieters, R., & van den Akker, E. L. (2014). Does dexamethasone induce more neuropsychological side effects than prednisone in pediatric acute lymphoblastic leukemia? A systematic review. *Pediatric Blood & Cancer*, *61*(7), 1313–1318. https://doi.org/10.1002/pbc.24988

Watkins, L. V., Pickrell, W. O., & Kerr, M. P. (2019). Treatment of psychiatric comorbidities in patients with epilepsy and intellectual disabilities: Is there a role for the neurologist? *Epilepsy & Behavior*, *98*(Pt B), 322–327. https://doi.org/10.1016/j.yebeh.2018.09.010

Williams, A. E., Giust, J. M., Kronenberger, W. G., & Dunn, D. W. (2016). Epilepsy and attention-deficit hyperactivity disorder: Links, risks, and challenges. *Neuropsychiatric Disease and Treatment*, *12*, 287–296. https://doi.org/10.2147/NDT.S81549

63

Palliative Care for Children With Medical Complexity

Irene Cihon Dietz and Ishani Sandesara

For additional material related to the content of this chapter, please see Chapters 11, 59, 64, and 109.

> **VIGNETTE**
>
> *Joe is a 17-year-old male with moderate autism (deficits in social communication, level 2) and moderate intellectual disability as assessed using a nonverbal IQ test and a comprehensive functional assessment. His medical history is significant for seizures, and he is on anticonvulsant medications. Over 18 months, he has had an increase in seizures, change in medication, deteriorating behavioral regulation, and increased aggressive tantrums. Moreover, his communication has regressed. He previously had a handful of words that he used primarily to request wants or needs; he could reliably select between two presented options. Now, he uses only an iPad for augmentative communication to provide answers to yes-no questions and to ask for desired foods. Parents have noted intermittent coughing with oral intake, but this symptom has never been worked up. During a hospitalization for medication titration, he underwent a video swallow study, which demonstrated aspiration of liquids of all consistencies. The hospital team recommended he discontinue oral feeding and initiate nasogastric (NG) feeds. They made plans for percutaneous gastrostomy placement once his seizures were under good control. Joe has become very agitated since NG tube placement. He has pulled out the NG tube multiple times, resulting in the addition of neuroleptic medications to reduce his behavioral dysregulation. At the urging of a family member, his parents requested involvement of the palliative care team at the hospital for decisional support surrounding feeding and for discussion of long-term goals regarding where he should live in the future.*

Palliative care starts with plans that honestly discuss the goals of care, options to treat the underlying condition, possible outcomes with each modality, and evaluations of pain and suffering. Cures may not always be possible; clinicians need to openly look at the total picture, including psychosocial and emotional components. This chapter outlines steps a primary care provider can take with the subspecialist team to identify goals of care, recognize sources of pain or suffering, and frame or reframe goals as often as needed based on the patient's health trajectory toward improvement or decreased health. Techniques for evaluation of pain and feeding intolerance and techniques for team interaction and setting goals of care are discussed. We hope this chapter will prepare team members for difficult and essential conversations for patients and/or families with children who have medical complexity.

OVERVIEW

In 2002 the World Health Organization (WHO) defined palliative care as an approach to care that seeks to improve the quality of life of patients with life-limiting conditions and their families (World Health Organization, 2002). However, over time, the scope of practice of palliative care has expanded. Palliative care is increasingly implemented earlier in the trajectory of life-threatening illness or highly complex health conditions. A 2020 consensus study arrived at the following definition: "palliative care is the active holistic care of individuals across all ages with serious health-related suffering due to severe illness and especially of those near the end of life" (Radbruch et al., 2020). Practically, palliative care medicine is a discipline practiced where interdisciplinary clinicians seek to identify the goals of care, assess pain and suffering, and provide emotional and physical wellbeing to support an individual with serious and complex illness and that person's entire family in reaching the goals of care.

Palliative care is distinct from hospice care. In palliative care there is no obligation to forgo or disregard specific therapies. Additionally, when conversations regarding goals of care are initiated, it is with the focus on specific family values and decision-making support, rather than with the purpose of promoting a specific decision.

The opening vignette is a clinical scenario in which palliative care interventions might proceed along with general medical treatment to support Joe and his family. The adolescent has complex medical care needs (see Chapter 59). As with many other patients, his interventions—medications, surgeries, and therapies—are designed to address troubling symptoms and yet are not curative. With each intervention comes possible improvements and also risks for complications. In Joe's case the placement of an NG tube to avoid aspiration and pneumonia led to many behavioral problems and occasioned the start of a major psychoactive medication. The palliative care approach can be utilized at this point in his course. Conversations surrounding goals of care can occur in conjunction with other disease-directed or life-prolonging therapies. Many families appreciate the validation that the medical team is thinking of and willing to engage in conversations regarding the same "what-ifs" and worries that the family has been considering in private.

Relationship to Primary Care and Developmental-Behavioral Pediatrics

Children with complex medical needs and their families often interact with large teams of clinicians across multiple disciplines, including medical subspecialties (e.g., neurology and genetics), developmental-behavioral pediatrics, psychology, psychiatry, and primary care. These teams must not only provide medical and health care but also ensure clear communication across subspecialties and consistency in communications between the team and the family. Existing team members, such as the developmental-behavioral pediatrician or primary care clinician, can initiate palliative care principles, particularly if these clinicians have a trusting relationship with the patient and family. Regardless of training, for example, they can begin the conversations about treatment options, including interventions designed to cure a condition, modify the disease, prolong life, or provide comfort. Palliative care specialists may join the team if their expertise would be valued by patient, family, or other team members. Unfortunately, the number of palliative care specialists is limited compared to the needs. Therefore the principles of palliative care must be understood by clinicians who specialize in other areas of health care.

Palliative care specialists, when they are available, are often invited to join the care team when individuals are in severe pain or showing feeding intolerance. Under those circumstances, training and experience may expand the options that the team, patient, and family consider. The palliative care team uses a standardized approach to symptom assessment and management. They engage in family-centered communication surrounding goals of care and complex medical decision making. This chapter is a primer for those approaches, with emphasis on the management of pain, feeding intolerance, and having difficult conversations with children or adolescents and their families.

PAIN

Pain is a common and underdiagnosed experience of children and adults with medical complexity (see Chapter 64). Pain may cause significant distress to children with medical complexity and to their caregivers. In addition to pain, discomfort may be associated with nausea, vomiting, significant upper airway secretions and respiratory distress, dyspnea, insomnia or otherwise dysregulated sleep, constipation, urinary retention, among others. In the medically complex patient pain perception is often increased compared to pain perception in healthy individuals. Heightened pain may be related to neuronal excitability, central neuropathic pain, autonomic dysfunction, sensitization to pain due to early traumatic experiences, and a diminished ability to understand and cope with painful stimuli.

Identifying the source of pain in children with medical complexity may present significant challenges to providers, related to the child's inability to reliably localize pain or provide details of pain quality. Unfortunately, acute and chronic pain are both common and distressing occurrences in this population. Pain assessment is further confounded by an incorrect but prevailing belief (Hauer, 2018) that children with medical complexity experience less or no pain compared to other children. The Guidelines for Ruling Out and Assessing Source of Pain (GRASP) tool (Fig. 63.1) has been recently validated for use in children with complex medical needs admitted for pain of unknown etiology. The tool is adapted for multiple providers and specifically suggests educating family to identify and record signs and symptoms of pain in a conclusive way that guides history and workup. The algorithm and differential diagnosis list also suggest endpoints around the medical workup and/or tests. The tool was developed to assist clinicians and may be able to save time and admissions; prevent unnecessary painful, stressful, expensive, or futile workup; and identify reasons for admission (Morse, Solodiuk, Greco, Mauskar, & Hauer, 2020).

Signs of Pain

Common signs of pain (sometimes referred to as pain behaviors) include changes in mental status, increased or decreased vocalization (e.g., crying, moaning), changes in facial expression (e.g., grimacing, furrowed brow), autonomic instability, inconsolable crying, increased or decreased movement or activity, arching, diaphoresis, tachycardia, and even self-injurious behavior (Hauer, 2013). The constellation of findings is unique to each child. Caregivers are often finely attuned to subtle changes in a child's behavior and may identify these behaviors immediately when they occur. However, for many it is still difficult to perceive and identify pain. Health care clinicians must rely on physical assessment and caregiver reports to assess pain in a nonverbal patient. The primary care clinician, urgent care or emergency room physicians, and the hospitalist teams should all be familiar with use of the GRASP tool (see Fig. 63.1) to guide them through a long differential diagnosis and to describe acute changes in patient wellbeing, including new fever, feeding intolerance, increased seizures, or pain behaviors (Morse et al., 2020). If possible, the clinicians should then rate pain intensity. Conversation about ability to decrease pain versus completely resolve pain is also highly appropriate.

Pain Assessment Tools

Multiple pain assessment tools have been studied and validated across pediatric and adult patient populations, including patients with medical complexity and those who are otherwise unable to communicate. It is important for the caregivers and the health care team to be aware of and familiar with typical and atypical pain behaviors that are unique to each child. Caregivers who are most familiar with their children should be empowered to serve as a proxy in the assessment process and to advocate on behalf of their children when they note pain behaviors. One simple assessment tool is the Wong-Baker FACES, in which the patient or caregiver chooses the face corresponding to the pain experience of the patient (Fig. 63.2) (Wong-Baker FACES Foundation, 2020). Pediatric nurses often use the revised FLACC scale, which looks at a child's face, legs, arms, cry, and consolability (Fig. 63.3) (Malviya, Vopel-Lewis, Burke Merkel, & Tait, 2006). Parental report can also be assessed using the Individualized Numeric Rating Scale (INRS) (Fig. 63.4) (McCaffery et al., 1989; Myles, Troedel, Boquest, & Reeves, 1999).

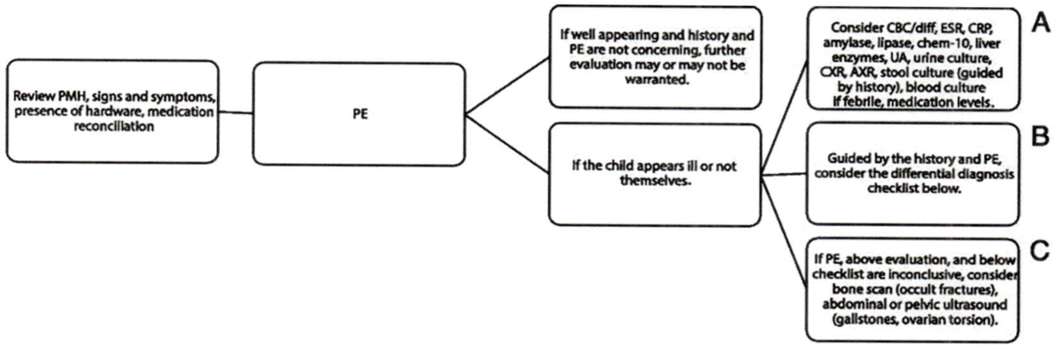

Differential Diagnoses	History, Signs, Symptoms	Further Evaluation
	Neurologic	
VP shunt malfunction	Δ in mental status, nausea and/or vomiting, fever, abdominal pain	Shunt series, head CT scan and/or MRI
↑ tone and spasticity	spasticity	Response to treatment
↑ seizures	recent Δ in antiepileptic drug regimen	EEG, check drug interactions
Neuropathic pain	Recurrent pain behaviors; may be triggered by GI or bladder distention	Response to gabapentin
	Infectious	
Meningitis	Δ in baseline temperature, mental status Δ, headache	Lumbar puncture
Sinusitis	Δ in baseline temperature, cough, nasal symptoms >10 days, face swelling	Sinus CT
Otitis media	Δ in baseline temperature, ↓ hearing, positive otoscopic examination results	*No further evaluation suggested*
Dental Abscess	Δ in baseline temperature, onset of symptoms, recent dental work	Consult dentist, dental radiograph
Tracheitis	Barking cough after respiratory infection, inspiratory stridor	Sputum culture, neck film
Pneumonia and/or pulmonary embolism	Δ in baseline temperature, aspiration, Δ in feeding, respiratory distress, secretions	Sputum cultures, venous blood gasses
Chronic aspirations	Choking, cough, color Δ with feeds, feeding refusal	Swallow study
Endocarditis	History of cardiac disease, fever, diaphoresis	ECG, echocardiogram
Urinary tract infection	Δ in baseline temperature, dysuria	Renal ultrasound`
***Clostridium difficile*, GI infection**	Δ in baseline temperature, antibiotic use, diarrhea, blood and/or mucus in stool	Stool culture
Cellulitis, infected implants	Δ in baseline temperature, √ implants: baclofen pump, rods, vagal nerve stimulator	Pro calcitonin, CK level, consult specialist
Osteomyelitis	Δ in baseline temperature, guarding or localized pain	Bone scan, imaging of suspected bone(s)
	Respiratory	
Pneumothorax	↑ WOB, respiratory distress	Venous blood gasses
	Gastrointestinal	
Appendicitis	Δ in baseline temperature, anorexia, vomiting	Ultrasound, CT of abdomen
Bowel obstruction	Vomiting, abdominal distention, diarrhea, constipation	CT of abdomen
Gastritis, esophagitis, and/or PUD	Vomiting, Δ in feeding, worsening symptoms after feeds, asthma, chronic cough, pneumonia, need to position during or after feeds	Gastric pH and occult blood, upper GI radiograph series
Constipation	Δ in stool patterns, consistency	Response to treatment
Pancreatitis	Vomiting, risk factors, including valproic acid and hypothermia (fever)	Ultrasound, CT scan, or MRI of abdomen
Cholecystitis	Vomiting, Δ in baseline temperature	Ultrasound, HIDA scan, MRCP, CT scan of abdomen
GI dysmotility	Unspecified GI symptoms	Gastric emptying, motility studies
Small-bowel overgrowth	Dysmotility, flatulence, √ for fecal fat, KUB displays air	Stool sample for *C difficile*, fecal fat
G/J tube issues (malposition, erosion)	Localized pain	G/J tube study
Visceral hyperalgesia	Pain triggered by distention, vomiting	Response to gabapentin
	Genitourinary	
Urinary retention	Incomplete voiding, long periods without voiding	Bladder scan >100 mL, urodynamic studies
Bladder rupture	Hematuria, suprapubic tenderness, distention, peritoneal signs	retrograde cystogram
Kidney stones	History of renal stones or UTIs, vomiting, hematuria, dysuria, genitourinary U structural abnormalities, ketogenic diet, medications associated with stone formation	UA for stones, CT scan of abdomen, ultrasound of kidney
Testicular torsion	Sudden onset of pain, nausea or vomiting, testicular tenderness, erythema, edema	Ultrasound of testicles
Ovarian Torsion	Sudden onset of pain, nausea, vomiting	Ultrasound of ovaries
Dysmenorrhea	Vomiting, diarrhea, headache, dizziness, pain around menstruation	Response to NSAID and/or oral contraceptive
Pregnancy	Morning vomiting, abdominal distention, amenorrhea	HCG test
	Musculoskeletal	
Fractures (femur, spine)	Sudden onset of pain with movement	Skeletal radiograph, bone scan
Hip subluxation	Sudden onset of pain and with movement	Consult orthopedics
Scoliosis (worsening)	Pain with position change, improved with repositioning	Radiograph
	Other	
Corneal abrasion or glaucoma	Tearing and redness of 1 eye	Fluorescein dye
Medication reactions or interactions	Serotonin or neuroleptic malignant syndrome, Δ in medications (last 3 months; ie, SSRI, tramadol, trazadone, risperidone, linezolid, metoclopramide)	Improvement when drug(s) discontinued
Rheumatologic	Joint swelling, change in mobility	Rheumatology evaluation
Social concerns	Psychosocial challenges, PMH of trauma	Interviews with close or trusted contacts

Fig. 63.1 Guidelines for Ruling Out and Assessing Source of Pain (GRASP). (Brenna L. Morse et al. Initial Validation of GRASP: A Differential Diagnoses Algorithm for Children With Medical Complexity and an Unknown Source of Pain. *Hosp Pediatr.* (2020) 10(8):633–640. https://doi.org/10.1542/hpeds.2019-0322)

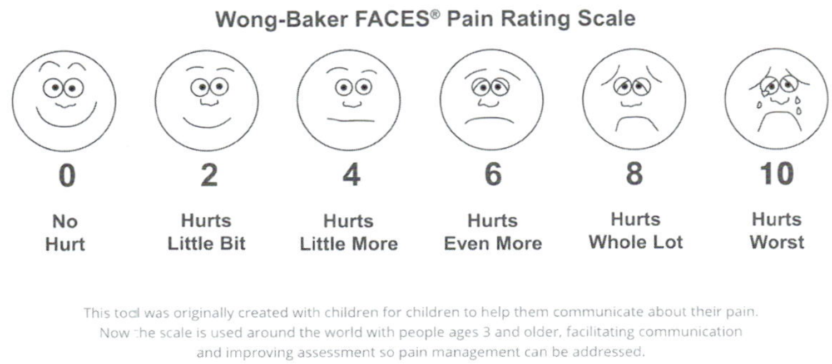
Wong-Baker FACES® Pain Rating Scale
0
No Hurt
2
Hurts Little Bit
4
Hurts Little More
6
Hurts Even More
8
Hurts Whole Lot
10
Hurts Worst
This tool was originally created with children for children to help them communicate about their pain.
Now the scale is used around the world with people ages 3 and older, facilitating communication
and improving assessment so pain management can be addressed.

Fig. 63.2 Wong-Baker FACES pain rating scale for quantification of pain. (From Wong-Baker FACES Foundation. http://www.WongBakerFACES.org)

(REVISED) **FLACC Scale** **SCORING**			
Categories	**0**	**1**	**2**
Face	No particular expression or smile.	Occasional grimace or frown, withdrawn, disinterested, **Sad, appears worried.**	Frequent to constant quivering chin, clenched jaw, **distressed looking face, expression of fright/panic.**
Legs	Normal position or relaxed; **usual tone and motion to limbs.**	Uneasy, restless, tense, **occasional tremors.**	Kicking, or legs drawn up, **marked increase in spasticity, constant tremors, jerking.**
Activity	Lying quietly, normal position, moves easily, **regular, rhythmic respirations.**	Squirming, shifting back and forth, tense, **tense/guarded movements, mildly agitated, shallow/ splinting respirations, intermittent sighs.**	Arched, rigid or jerking, **severe agitation, head banging, shivering, breath holding, gasping, severe splinting.**
Cry	No cry (awake or asleep).	Moans or whimpers: occasional complaint, **occasional verbal outbursts, constant grunting.**	Crying steadily, screams or sobs, frequent complaints, **repeated outbursts, constant grunting.**
Consolability	Content, relaxed.	Reassured by occasional touching, hugging, or being talked to: distractible.	Difficult to console or comfort, **pushing caregiver away, resisting care or comfort measures.**
Each of the five categories (**F**) Face; (**L**) Legs; (**A**) Activity; (**C**) Cry; (**C**) Consolability is scored from 0 to 2, which results in a total score between 0 and 10.			
References: Merkel, S. et al. The FLACC: A Behavioural Scale for Scoring Postoperative Pain in Young Children, Pediatric Nurse 23(3): 293-297, 1997. Copyright: Jannetti Co. University of Michigan Medical Centre. **Malviya, S., Vopel-Lewis, T. Burke, Merkel, S., Tait, A.R. (2006). The revised FLACC Observational Pain Tool: Improved Reliability and Validity for Pain Assessment in Children with Cognitive Impairment. (Pediatric Anesthesia 16: 258-265).**			

Fig. 63.3 Revised FLACC scale, which looks at the patient's face, legs, arms, cry, and consolability as a method for objectively evaluating pain.

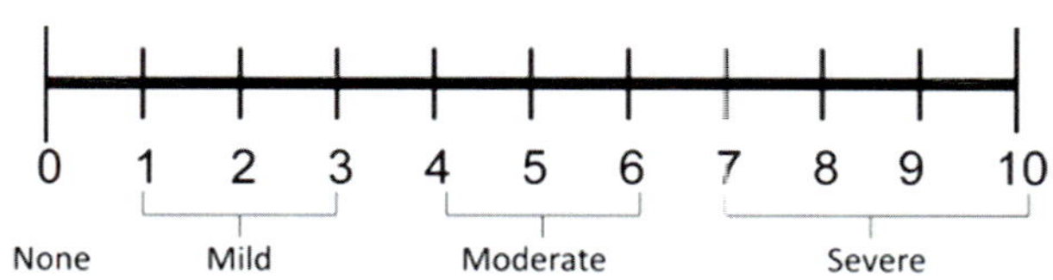

Fig. 63.4 The Individualized Numeric Rating Scale instructions. General information: The patient is asked to make three pain ratings, corresponding to current, best, and worst pain experienced over the past 24 hours. The average of the three ratings is used to represent the patient's level of pain over the previous 24 hours. (From McCaffery, M., Beebe, A., et al. [1989]. *Pain: Clinical manual for nursing practice*. Mosby.)

Approach to Treatment

When considering an approach to pain and use of analgesics, drug-drug interactions and sedation must be considered. The patient's airway and respiratory status must be considered especially when using benzodiazepines and high doses of opioids. Children with intellectual disability may respond with excitation to diphenhydramine and with increased agitation to benzodiazepines. The Neonatal Pain, Agitation, and Sedation Scale (N-PASS) (Hummel et al., 2008) has been validated to assess pain in infants (Fig. 63.5).

BEHAVIOR INDICATORS	SEDATION SCORING	SEDATION		NORMAL/ PAIN	PAIN/AGITATION		PAIN/ AGITATION SCORING
		-2	-1	0/0	1	2	
Crying Irritability		No cry with painful stimuli	Moans or cries minimally with painful stimuli	Appropriate crying Not irritable	Irritable or crying at intervals; Consolable	High-pitched or silent-continuous cry; Inconsolable	
Behavior State		No arousal to any stimuli; No spontaneous movement	Arouses minimally to stimuli; Little spontaneous movement	Appropriate for gestational age	Restless, squirming; Awakens frequently	Arching, kicking; Constantly awake or Arouses minimally no movement (not sedated)	
Facial Expression		Mouth is lax; No expression	Minimal expression with stimuli	Relaxed appropriate	Any pain expression, intermittent	Any pain expression, continual	
Extremities Tone		No grasp reflex; Flaccid tone	Weak grasp reflex; decreased muscle tone	Relaxed hands and feet Normal tone	Intermittent clenched toes, fists or finger splay; Body is not tense	Continual clenched toes, fists, or finger splay; Body is tense	
Vital Signs HR, RR, BP, SaO_2		No variability with stimuli; Hypoventilation or apnea	Less than 10% variability from baseline with stimuli	Within baseline or normal for gestational age	Increase 10-20% from baseline; SaO_2 76-85% with stimulation – quick increase	Increase greater than 20% from baseline; SaO_2 less than or equal too 75% with stimulation – slow increase; Out of sync/ fighting vent	
Gestation/ Corrected age	N/A						
TOTAL SEDATION SCORE	/-10					TOTAL PAIN/ AGITATION SCORE	/13

Fig. 63.5 Neonatal Pain, Agitation, and Sedation Scale (N-PASS). (From Hummel, P., Puchalsik, M., Creech, S. D., & Weiss, M. G. [2008]. Clinical reliability and validity of the N-PASS: Neonatal pain, agitation and sedation scale with prolonged pain. *Journal of Perinatology, 28*, 55–60.)

Once a diagnosis is obtained, disease-directed or curative interventions may be prioritized in the hopes that cure will alleviate pain. However, pain management is often complicated in medically complex children by a lack of awareness of available treatment modalities. Many clinicians also report discomfort prescribing or managing pain given their fear of harm or adverse effects of balancing symptom management with continued interventions. Both clinicians and families/caregivers describe worries that an added focus on comfort may hint at a shift in goals; they experience anxiety about "giving up too soon" when an underlying diagnosis is not being actively treated.

Medication options can be guided by the WHO (2021) pain management ladder (Fig. 63.6). Medication options include gabapentinoids, tricyclic antidepressants, opioids, benzodiazepines, alpha-2 antagonists, anticholinergics, serotonin-norepinephrine reuptake inhibitors, and cannabinoids. WHO recommendations include adjuvant therapies. Review of this document as well as consultation of pharmacology is highly recommended for patients on multiple medications to avoid serious drug-drug interaction.

Trials of empirical symptom management early in the process of workup and investigation can often be beneficial. It is also important to set reasonable expectations on the possible outcomes with initiation of new medications that are being utilized for other symptom management. Patients and/or caregivers can certainly be encouraged to maintain hope while also preparing for a wide range of results. In addition to pharmacologic interventions, complementary alternative therapies contribute a great deal to comfort in this population. They include strategies such as cuddling, repositioning (including supportive equipment), warm baths, weighted blankets, massage, vibratory stimulation (like high-frequency chest wall oscillation), venting the gastrostomy tube, and adjustments to the feeding regimen. Information on the benefit of aromatherapy and acupuncture is limited, though anecdotal accounts are promising. Many families also already integrate a variety of complementary and alternative medications (CAM) (see Chapter 109), such as herbs, high doses of vitamins, probiotics, nutraceuticals, and heavy metals (e.g., silver, gold) for chronic pain. The clinician needs to be very open to discussion around CAM while simultaneously considering adverse side effects and drug interactions when addressing symptoms and symptom control. To reduce the degree of opioid use, insurance providers such as Medicaid now will often cover therapeutic options such as acupuncture and chiropractic services when performed by a qualified chiropractor within the scope of practice for either low back pain or migraine. Providers need to familiarize themselves regularly with current evidence for adjuvant therapies (Williamson, Alikhan, Greene, Becker, & Tewarson, 2020).

FEEDING INTOLERANCE

Feeding intolerance is defined as an inability to tolerate a calculated volume of nutrition and fluids. It is often a significant source of distress for families because it can limit tolerance of tube feeds and result in prolonged hospitalizations. Medications may confer limited benefit; however, children may not improve despite medical optimization. The failure to improve may reflect progressive changes in the central nervous system (CNS), affecting intestinal motility and the vomiting center of the brain. Moreover, decreased metabolism commonly occurs in children with decreased mobility, exacerbated by visceral hyperalgesia, medication side effects, and decreased activity. It is often upsetting for families to watch a child who is unable to tolerate feeds because they think that providing adequate nutrition and hydration are central to the human experience and to the personal perceptions of being

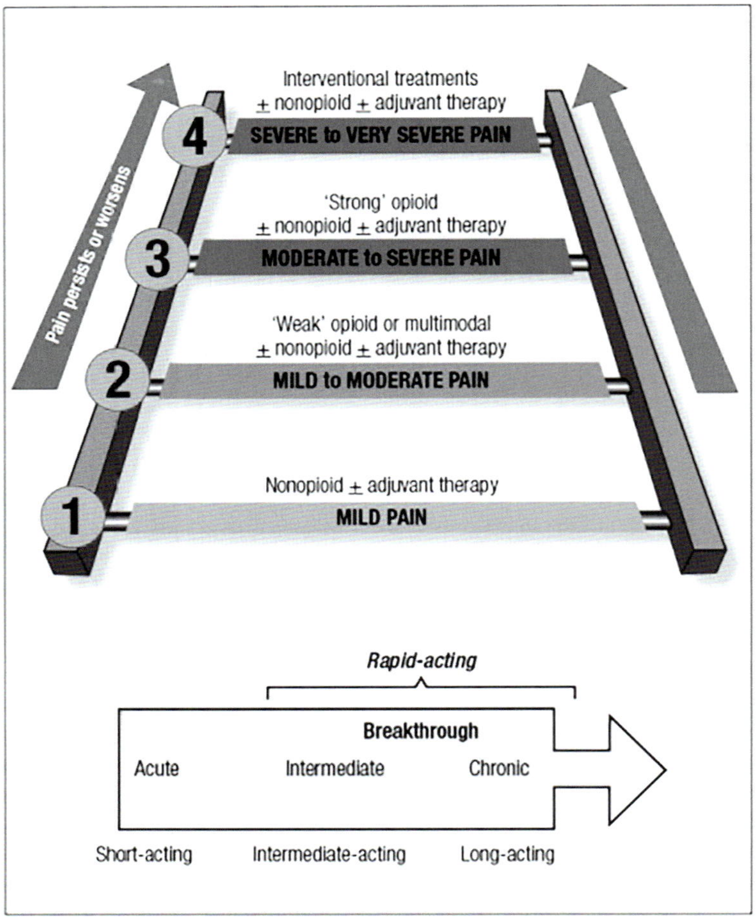

Figure 3. An updated version of the 1986 WHO pain ladder. Persistent and chronic pain syndromes should be treated with long-acting opioids; rapid-onset opioids are appropriate for breakthrough pain. A fourth step has been added for "very severe" pain that can be treated with peripheral nerve blockade.

A

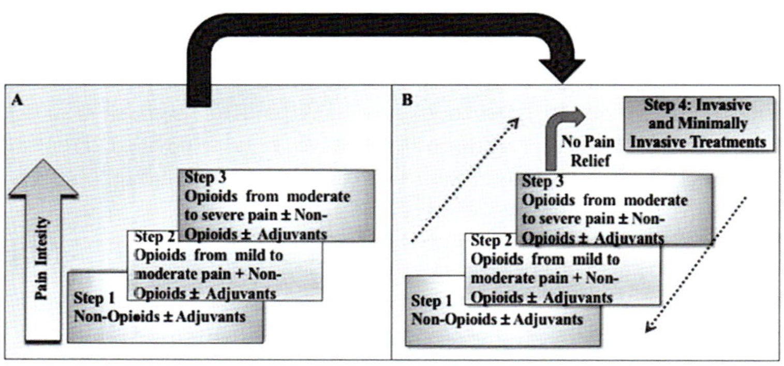

Transition from the original WHO three-step analgesic ladder (**A**) to the revised WHO fourth-step form (**B**). The additional step 4 is an "interventional" step and includes invasive and minimally invasive techniques. This updated WHO ladder provides a bidirectional approach.

B

Fig. 63.6 World Health Organization analgesic ladder offers a systematic approach to pain management. (A) The pain ladder suggests use of opioid and nonopioid medications as a function of pain severity. (B) Modified analgesic ladder adds a fourth step to the original ladder. (A, From Pergolizzi Jr, J. V., & Raffa, R. B. [2015]. The WHO pain ladder: Do we need another step? *Practical Pain Management, 14*[1]; B, Anekar, A. A., & Cascella, M. [2021]. *WHO analgesic ladder*. StatPearls Publishing. https://www.ncbi.nlm.nih.gov/books/NBK554435/)

a "good parent." It can be reassuring to families to emphasize that therapeutic decreases in feeding volume would be beneficial for children in a number of clinical scenarios, such as cardiac dysfunction, and thus allowing children to take in less food and fluid may be a reasonable option in their children without causing starvation or dehydration.

Despite evaluation, treatment, and management of all reversible sources of discomfort and feeding intolerance, clinicians should remember that children with medical complexity and severe neurologic impairment may experience a slow, progressive, and irreversible decline, reflected in decreased oral intake. The changes are likely related to ongoing CNS and autonomic functional decline in peristalsis. Medication side effects must also always be considered as the cause of apparent feeding intolerance.

A palliative care approach would help the family and health care team to understand that starvation is the withholding of food from a patient that experiences hunger and the desire to eat. In an acute medical setting persons with severe medical illness and feeding intolerance are most often not experiencing hunger. Forcing additional enteral calories and fluids can also be a source of discomfort for some patients experiencing this decline. In various juridictions forgoing enteral nutrition may be limited by state law. It may also be unacceptable in various cultural and community belief systems. Inadequate nutrition can lead to long-term complications such as loss of subcutaneous fat stores and increased risk for decubitus ulcers.

For Joe, eating by mouth was one of the few daily routines that was enjoyable for him. The team's decision to withhold oral intake, while potentially avoiding life-threatening chronic aspiration pneumonia, led to the need for gastrostomy surgery, increased medication, and possible placement in a care setting where none of the residents take food by mouth. The palliative care team encourages the medical team, family, and patient to consider new questions: Is it possible for Joe to have pleasurable tastes? What strategies could possibly improve oral feeding safety, including feeding therapy, textural changes in the food, or adjusting the timing of means and size of the bolus? What supports could keep Joe from pulling out his own NG tube or feeding tube? The family also wanted to consider whether Joe could return to his home and prior feeding regimen despite the newly identified risks. Their questions resulted not only in a palliative care consult but also in involvement of the ethics committee and opinions from the hospital legal team.

DIFFICULT CONVERSATIONS

The integration of palliative care conversations into standard care, including disease-directed therapies and life-prolonging measures, has proven beneficial for medically complex children and their support systems. Despite these data, referral to palliative care is often deferred until late in the course of disease (if at all), reducing the benefits families may experience.

Responsibility for initiating Palliative Care

Advanced care planning conversations can be initiated in the outpatient setting by any clinician who is a part of a child's care team. Clinicians indicate that it is more comfortable and easier to elicit and integrate goals and values into an acceptable care plan when a child is clinically stable rather than critically ill, when decisions may need to be made urgently. Qualitative studies have demonstrated that families often perceive that the goals of care conversations are introduced far too late in the disease process; they often feel rushed or forced to make difficult decisions. Starting these conversations early in the disease course, using a calm manner, allows the patient and family to consider their options, make wise choices, and fully utilize resources and services that they might find helpful.

Recommendations for Positive Difficult Conversation

Team Coordination

Prior to any meetings between the health care team and the family it is often useful to have a discussion among only the members of the health care team. The purpose is to arrive at a common understanding of the patient's condition and prognosis, to anticipate or reduce conflict among team members, and to provide consistent information and recommendations that represent the mutually agreed upon suggestions of all the subspecialists caring for the child. In a well-functioning team mutual trust among collaborators allows dissent and health team problem solving. Team discussions may lead to a reevaluation of clinical goals and recommendations.

Within the team meeting it may become important to step back from the current clinical scenario and think about the big picture: What was the child's previous baseline? How do we expect any particular treatment to help the patient? Will the current approach maintain, reduce, or improve the patient's quality of life? What is the family expecting or hoping for? How will family life be affected by our recommendations?

Sharing Serious News as a Team

It is important to plan which members of the team will attend a planned meeting. It may be worthwhile to consider and assign discrete roles to team members. The roles include information giver, facilitator, emotional supporter, and spiritual supporter. The meeting should be uninterrupted to the extent possible, with no distractions from pagers and phones. Sufficient time should also be allotted.

Shared Mental Model

To the extent possible, it is critical to know the patient's or family's understanding of the illness, the patient's and family's beliefs, and their values. Patients and families may have a belief that the introduction of palliative care heralds a rapid decline in status or imminent death. Therefore making clear what palliative care, that it is distinct from hospice care and is specifically to improve quality of individual and family life, is essential. A back-and-forth dialogue is evidence that the team members are listening and not just talking. Often obtaining each member of the family's input ensures that everyone has had a chance to express their opinion. It is also important to allow patients and families sufficient time for decision making around the team's recommendations. It is unrealistic for the family to agree fully to a new plan at the first discussion of that plan, unless the situation is urgent. The goal of the conversation is shared decision making.

Methods

A useful method for teams to consider when initiating care planning and the difficult conversation is SPIKES (setting, perception, invitation, knowledge, emotion, and summarize) (Fig. 63.7) (Baile et al., 2000; Kaplan, 2010). The goal is to foster an environment where conversations can take place. Caregivers may need to step away from their child so they may participate in discussions. They may want to identify trusted supporters to be with them, such as friends, family, primary care physicians, social workers, or spiritual counselors. In the current era use of virtual methods may allow distant family or friends to attend a meeting even when the available space is limited. It is important to position the family at the head of a long or oblong table rather than across from a large team so they recognize their influence in the discussion. Here are additional recommendations:

- Pace the delivery of information to avoid overwhelming the family.
- Avoid medical jargon.
- Take cues from the questions being asked and body language to appropriately provide updates.
- Ascertain how families prefer to receive information: Studies indicate that many parents express a desire for complete and honest information, but preferences vary by gender and location of care.
- Use person-first language.
- Avoid expressions such as "needing" a specific surgery or procedure. Replace them with realistic thoughts such as "we can consider or offer" an intervention.
- Present risks and benefits for each intervention, including the possibility of a poor outcome. Present the risks and benefits of not doing a suggested recommendation as well.

Understanding Legal and Institutional Policies

The team presenting the difficult conversation to the patient and family needs a comprehensive understanding of the institution's policies and procedures. It is also helpful to have a good understanding of local or state laws. For example, in some institutions and states there are specific policies regarding "unilateral do not resuscitate (DNR)" where two physicians can determine the futility of ongoing aggressive care. Ideally, any decisions about discontinuation of care are arrived at via ethical and shared decision making.

Team Flexibility

There is often a good reason to maintain hope for a cure or return to baseline function. Teams should support families in hopeful thinking. However, patients may experience a gradual decline of function and quality of life despite best medical interventions and state-of-the-art care. Families need to be presented with realistic outcomes when being offered interventions and procedures to prolong their loved one's life. The family may bring up information not previously known or understood by the team. The willingness of the team to pause and to amend or pause making recommendations may be helpful to families, particularly as they adjust to a deterioration in an individual's functioning.

There may be times when the team and family cannot come to consensus. Mediators may be necessary. They may include members of the clergy, mental health professionals, and other trusted people.

Barriers to Successful Difficult Conversations

Multiple identified barriers reduce clinicians' ability to break bad news and discuss goals of care conversations. These obstacles are individual, systemic, team level, and familial.

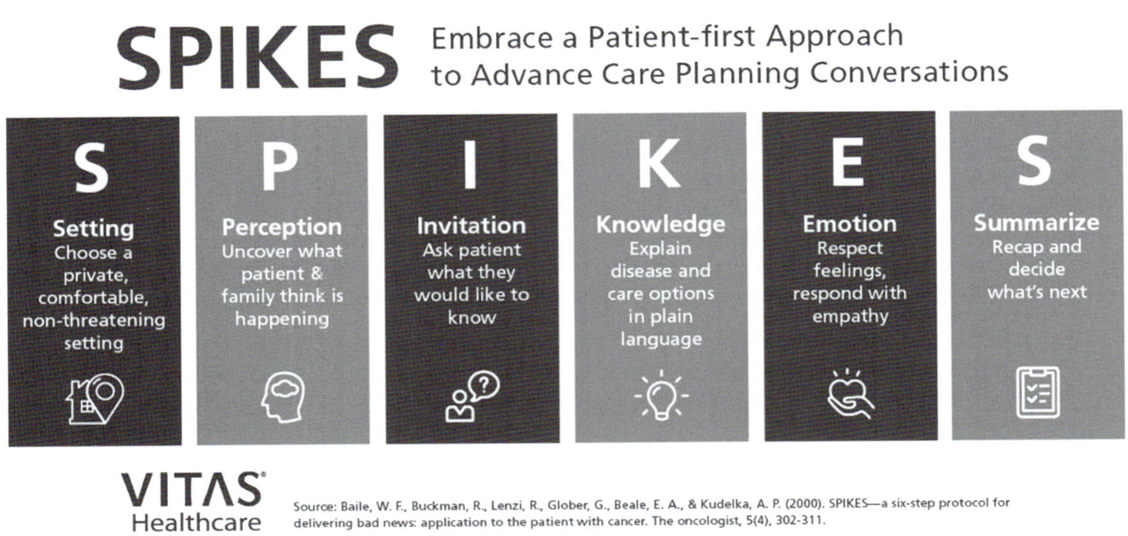

Fig. 63.7 SPIKES provides a systematic, patient-centered approach to advanced care planning. (From Baile, W. F., Buckman, R., Lenzi, R., Glober, G., Beale, E. A., & Kudelka, A. P. [2000]. SP KES—A six-step protocol for delivering bad news: Application to the patient with cancer. *The Oncologist, 5*[4], 302–311.)

Caregiver Barriers

In neonatology perceived parental distress influences the delivery of information. Parents may ask questions that seem unreasonable based on the clinical status of their child. There is a benefit of eliciting information from parents to allow the team to ascertain the parents' comprehension of their child's illness. This dialogue ensures a common understanding and enhances subsequent communication.

Parents often have strongly held beliefs that can be gently confronted during conversations. Two common beliefs are that the care for their child with medical complexity is their life's commitment and that the situation cannot change. The goal of the conversation may be to allow parents to understand that planning for a reduction in support or end-of-life care can be evidence of their deep love for the child. They can also be informed that palliative care can be integrated seamlessly into the medical care their child is already receiving. The additional goals may include symptom control, family support, and child comfort.

The trajectory of disease severity is often unpredictable and waxes and wanes unexpectedly. Parents may have experienced instances where caregivers were told that their child was not expected to recover but then the child survived. The uncertainty becomes particularly thorny as life-sustaining medical therapies and interventions advance and become more accessible. If this pattern of inaccurate prediction has been repeated, families may lose faith in prognostication. Then they have motivation for postponing discussions, particularly surrounding end-of-life care (Drach, Hansen, King, & Sibinga, 2020).

Parental values concerning quality of life for their child are unique to every family and must be directly discussed. For children with medical complexity or technology dependence, families often describe a sense of loss of agency, isolation, and powerlessness. Parents often perceive that the discussions about treatments are inclined toward aggressive interventions. Parents may recognize that their personal values are at odds with those of the clinicians regarding quality of life and that clinicians' personal values are influencing care practices and recommendations. Under other circumstances, parents may be included to choose aggressive interventions while clinicians want to withdraw support. Families often interpret that physicians' personal values surrounding quality of life direct their practice and recommendations. They may experience the clinicians as having undue influence.

Clinician Barriers

Many factors are obstacles to clinicians initiating difficult conversations. They include the following:

- Team hierarchy and variations in beliefs, values, and experience across the members
- Desire to avoid criticizing colleagues, especially in public situations
- Structural challenges to private conversation with families with ample time allotted
- Group norms in favor of restorative goals
- Diffusion of responsibilities so that no one assumes the role of initiator
- Inhibited expressions of sorrow and norms about maintaining composure and avoiding significant expressions of sorrow in front of patients
- Lack of social support for clinicians who feel sorrow, depression, or burnout
- Reinforcement of labeling and conflict

Clinicians often treat reactions of anger or insistence for aggressive treatment as fixed, unchangeable traits inherent to families, instead of a reaction to stress, a coping style, or a current belief. Families may undergo gradual transitions among sets of goals or reactions.

Negative beliefs regarding families may result in self-fulfilling prophecies, particularly if the clinicians expect an individual to be hostile. Clinicians may end up issuing ultimatums to families or conducting insensitive communication based on their expectations about the individual or family rather than based on the actual conversation. In severe cases the conflict between clinicians and family becomes the central focus instead of the child's needs.

As clinicians, we need to be aware of our own beliefs, unconscious biases, and discomfort surrounding difficult conversations about outcomes and goals of care. We may have different assumptions regarding what constitutes an acceptable baseline quality of life than patients and families have. The medical culture often undervalues the quality of life for those with severe cognitive disabilities (Graham et al., 2005). Health care providers also struggle with uncertainty; this struggle has been associated with the excessive ordering of tests, withholding of information, and premature closure in the informed-consent or decision-making process. We must always remind ourselves that the definitions of an acceptable quality of life are not universal or constant and will constantly evolve over the course of a child's lifetime.

It is common for clinicians to experience feelings of failure and distress in this context. Most clinicians chose their career to promote healing or to cure. Acknowledging the emotions when healing and cure become elusive and confronting the uncertainty inherent to the care of children with medical complexity is reassuring for both the clinicians and the families under their care. Many team members have been important in the lifelong support and goals of care for the child, especially those acting as the primary care provider, and they experience personal attachment and fear of perceived abandonment of this role. Many clinicians also have limited communication training and suffer time pressures.

Health System Barriers

Surveys have demonstrated that many health care providers, regardless of the site of care or training, cite a lack of instruction and comfort as a significant barrier to having goals-of-care conversations. Pediatricians, in particular, often lack training and experience with these difficult conversations, even though they are caring for children with chronic health conditions. There may be a tension between life-sustaining technology/disease-directed therapies and a willingness to integrate palliative care, often related to misconceptions surrounding palliative medicine. Despite increased awareness and availability of palliative care services, there remains a common understanding that palliative medicine can only be introduced if and when there are no further interventions or therapies left to offer.

Clinicians may present an aggressive treatment by saying that the patient "needs" the specific procedure. Discussion of significant intervention, such as a feeding tube, baclofen infusion pump, orthopedic surgery, or tracheostomy, may occur without allowing families to fully understand the implications of the procedures and to get the necessary support to participate in shared decision making. It is important for patients and families to be aware if life-sustaining interventions may in fact prolong suffering and/or reduce the child's and family's overall quality of life. An alternative approach that may overcome these barriers to palliative care is discussing any potential interventions as "options."

Regoaling

Regoaling is a term coined by Dr. Chris Feudtner to describe the process of transitioning from one set of goals to another (Hill et al., 2014). Multiple factors may either promote or inhibit regoaling. It is important to note that medical clinicians must also undergo regoaling to provide optimal care to patients as their clinical status and goals of care evolve.

Caregiver Regoaling

As a child's condition changes, familial hopes and goals will likely change. Sometimes, families are faced with the conclusion that their initial goals are no longer realistic or possible. They have two paths going forward: They may persist in their pursuit of these initial goals or they may yield those goals and pursue a set of new goals. These new goals may include limiting interventions based on risk or benefit, maintaining quality of life, or minimize pain or suffering. This second option is regoaling.

Factors that affect regoaling include the ability to disengage from the original goals related to how they respond to treatment failure or clinical decline. Negative affect is a response to perceived failure that results in caregiver anxiety, despair, or dysphoria. Negative affect can initially lead to increase efforts to meet initial goals; however, after repeated poor outcomes, negative affect may lead to disengagement from goals. There are scant goal disengagement studies, but initial data indicate that families of children with serious illness who disengage with early goals and engage with new goals have better long-term outcomes related to parents' ability to define their own high-priority goals and relinquish lower priority goals. Negative affect may serve as an alarm when repeated efforts to achieve initial goals are unsuccessful. Disengagement is more likely to occur when there is a high level of certainty that the initial goal is unattainable and that continued efforts may lead to negative consequences, harm, or suffering. The presence of reasonable alternatives to initial goals increases the likelihood of disengagement.

Disengagement may be hindered by positive illusions, which are objectively unrealistic beliefs that positive outcomes may occur or that negative events will not. In most contexts positive illusions are adaptive and protective, allowing parents to persist and cope with negative situations. In extremes they are maladaptive and can be harmful. Another factor inhibiting disengagement is perceived sunk costs, as families may often continue with aggressive treatment because refocusing goals would acknowledge that efforts and suffering to this point may have been seemingly for nothing. As we know, caregivers with medically complex children often describe feeling exhausted both physically and emotionally. This fatigue often interferes with their ability to self-regulate and reexamine their initial goals.

Clinician and Health System Regoaling

To effectively assist each family, clinicians and health systems must similarly undergo regoaling and reframe their own perspectives on a patient's care, reconciling their own beliefs with the care plan going forward. Inhibitors to regoaling include avoidance of criticizing subspecialist colleagues, structural communication challenges, medical norms in favor of disease-directed and life-sustaining therapies, and norms of maintaining composure and avoiding significant expressions of sorrow. This last factor makes it difficult for individual team members to seek support when coping with negative emotions, subsequently increasing risk for burnout. Another factor is the varying assumptions regarding what constitutes an acceptable quality of life; studies show that those in medical culture often undervalue the quality of life for those with severe cognitive disabilities (Graham et al., 2005). Physicians also struggle with uncertainty, which is associated with an excessive ordering of tests and the withholding of information. As patient care evolves away from disease-directed or life-sustaining therapies, health care providers often experience feelings of failure and distress.

Factors that facilitate regoaling include a shared mental model among the entire team, including premeetings without family present and frequent sharing of information. This reduces mixed messages and ensures delivery of consistent information and recommendations to the family. Additionally, mutual trust and respect among team members and specialists are important to encourage dissent and discussion. Teams must also frequently and consistently step back from the clinical scenario and reevaluate the big picture to contextualize the current situation in the setting of previous baseline, treatment objectives, and the family's hopes and goals.

CONCLUSION

Palliative care is an active and holistic approach to care of individuals with serious health-related suffering due to severe illness and especially of those near the end of life. Palliative care can be offered by many members of the team caring for children with complex medical conditions. Recently, specialized teams have been constructed. Their focus is often on managing pain, treating feeding intolerance, and participating in difficult conversations, especially when goals need to be reconsidered or care withheld. To the extent possible, the goal is to make decisions with full participation of the individual, to the extent possible, and the family. The palliative care principles become increasingly important as medical treatments extend life without necessarily improving function or quality of life.

REFERENCES

Anekar, A. A., & Cascella, M. (2021). *WHO analgesic ladder*. StatPearls Publishing. https://www.ncbi.nlm.nih.gov/books/NBK554435/

Baile, W. F., Buckman, R., Lenzi, R., Glober, G., Beale, E. A., & Kudelka, A. P. (2000). SPIKES—A six-step protocol for delivering bad news: Application to the patient with cancer. *The Oncologist*, *5*(4), 302–311. https://doi.org/10.1634/theoncologist.5-4-302

Drach, L. L., Hansen, D. A., King, T. M., & Sibinga, E. M. S. (2020). Communication between neonatologists and parents when prognosis is uncertain. *Journal of Perinatology*, *40*(9), 1412–1422. https://doi.org/10.1038/s41372-020-0673-6

Graham, R. J., & Robinson, W. M. (2005). Integrating palliative care into chronic care for children with severe neurodevelopmental disabilities. *Journal of Developmental and Behavioral Pediatrics*, *26*(5), 361–365. https://doi.org/10.1097/00004703-200510000-00004

Hauer, J. M. (2013). *Caring for children who have severe neurologic impairment*. The Johns Hopkins University Press.

Hauer, J. (2018). Feeding intolerance in children with severe impairment of the central nervous system: Strategies for treatment and prevention. *Children (Basel)*, *5*(1), 1. https://doi.org/10.3390/children5010001

Hill, D. L., Miller, V., Walter, J. K., et al. (2014). Regoaling: A conceptual model of how parents of children with serious illness change medical care goals. *BMC Palliative Care*, *13*, 9. https://doi.org/10.1186/1472-684X-13-9

Kaplan, M. (2010). SPIKES: A framework for breaking bad news to patients with cancer. *Journal of Clinical Oncology*, *14*(4), 514–516. https://doi.org/10.1188/10.CJON.514-516

Malviya, S., Vopel-Lewis, T., Burke Merkel, S., & Tait, A. R. (2006). The revised FLACC observational pain tool: Improved reliability and validity for pain assessment in children with cognitive impairment. *Pediatric Anesthesia*, *16*, 258–265.

McCaffery, M., Beebe, A., et al. (1989). *Pain: Clinical manual for nursing practice*. Mosby.

Morse, B. L., Solodiuk, J. C., Greco, C. D., Mauskar, S., & Hauer, J. (2020). Initial validation of GRASP: A differential diagnoses algorithm for children with medical complexity and an unknown source of pain. *Hospital Pediatrics*, *10*(8), 633–640. https://doi.org/10.1542/hpeds.2019-0322

Myles, P. S., Troedel, S., Boquest, M., & Reeves, M. (1999). The pain visual analog scale: Is is linear or nonlinear? *Anesthesia & Analgesia*, *89*(6), 1517. https://doi.org/10.1213/00000539-199912000-00038

Pergolizzi, J. V., & Raffia, R. B. (2015). The WHO pain ladder: Do we need another step? *Practical Pain Management*, *14*(1).

Radbruch, L., De Lima, L., Knaul, F., Wenk, R., Ali, Z., Bhatnaghar, S., … Pastrana, T. (2020). Redefining Palliative Care-A New Consensus-Based Definition. *Journal of pain and symptom management*, *60*(4), 754–764. https://doi.org/10.1016/j.jpainsymman.2020.04.027

Walter, J. K., Hill, D. L., DiDomenico, C., Parikh, S., & Feudtner, C. (2019). A conceptual model of barriers and facilitators to primary clinical teams requesting pediatric palliative care consultation based upon a narrative review. *BMC Palliative Care*, *18*(1), 116. https://doi.org/10.1186/s12904-019-0504-8

Williamson, K., Alikhan, S., Greene, K., Becker, M., & Tewarson, H. (2020). *Expanding access to non-opioid management of chronic pain: Considerations for governors*. National Governors Association Center for Best Practices.

Wong-Baker FACES Foundation. (2020). *Wong-Baker FACES pain rating scale*. http://www.WongBakerFACES.org. [Originally published in *Whaley & Wong's Nursing Care of Infants and Children*].

World Health Organization. (2002). *National cancer control programmes: Policies and managerial guidelines* (2nd ed). https://www.who.int/health-topics/palliative-care

World Health Organization. (2021). *WHO guidelines on the management of chronic pain in children executive summary*. Author.

64

Chronic Pain

Caitlin B. Murray and Tonya M. Palermo

For additional material related to the content of this chapter, please see Chapters 2, 70, 92, 98, and 100.

> **VIGNETTE**
>
> *Ashley is a 16-year-old girl who has had almost constant abdominal pain for the past 6 months. She has already been evaluated by gastroenterology, and there are no red flags in her history or diagnostic tests that suggest an underlying organic disease process. Ashley's pain has begun to interfere significantly with several aspects of her life. She misses at least 3 days of school each week. She was previously active in basketball but is no longer participating. She describes a high level of general worry. She is usually a high-achieving student and describes feeling stressed about being behind on schoolwork. It is taking Ashley several hours to fall asleep at bedtime, which is interfering with waking in the morning for school. She worries a lot about her pain and whether it will ever improve. Her parents feel overwhelmed with anxiety about her health and wellbeing and want to pursue any treatment that can provide their daughter relief from abdominal pain.*

Pain is common in childhood. Pain that recurs or persists beyond the expected time of healing from injury, illness, or surgical procedures—typically for longer than 3 months—is termed chronic pain. As described for Ashley in the opening vignette, chronic pain in childhood can be a significant clinical problem. It is an important public health problem because of the substantial burden and individual impact, including physical limitations, social impairment, psychological distress, and lost school and work productivity. Chronic pain affects an estimated 1.7 million children in the United States and is one of the most costly chronic health conditions in childhood, with economic expenditures estimated at around $19.5 billion annually (Groenewald et al., 2014).

Pain accounts for 20% to 40% of pediatric primary care visits, and around one in four of these youth experience significant functional impairment (Holm et al., 2012). Evaluating children with chronic pain often starts with the primary care clinician, yet this task can be quite daunting and complex. Several barriers can impede pain management, including a clinician's lack of formal education on the assessment and treatment of chronic pain, the short length of the care visit, the multifactorial etiology of pediatric pain, and the high levels of distress experienced by children and parents. Irrespective of whether a child's pain is a symptom of a medical condition or a primary diagnosis, the evaluation and management can be challenging for the treating clinician.

The purpose of this chapter is to describe the significance of the problem of chronic pain in childhood, including the prevalence, impact, and long-term course of pain, as well as to review evidence-based assessment and treatment using the widely adopted biopsychosocial model (see Chapter 2) of pediatric pain as a guiding framework.

THE SIGNIFICANCE OF CHILDHOOD CHRONIC PAIN

Definitions and Common Childhood Pain Conditions

Chronic pain affects a large percentage of children worldwide. Epidemiologic research indicates that between 11% and 38% of children report chronic pain (King et al., 2011) and 5% and 8% report moderate to severe disabling chronic pain (Huguet & Miro, 2008). The incidence of chronic pain peaks during adolescence, likely due to the numerous biologic, emotional, and social changes that characterize this developmental stage. Children may experience chronic or recurrent pain associated with an active underlying disease process (e.g., arthritis, inflammatory bowel disease), including life-limiting and/or life-threatening medical conditions (e.g., cancer, end stage, and palliative conditions), or may experience chronic pain as the primary condition or disease (e.g., functional abdominal pain disorder [FAPD], complex regional pain syndrome [CRPS]). The most frequent forms of chronic pain in childhood are primary pain conditions, specifically musculoskeletal (MSK) pain, abdominal pain, and headache (King et al., 2011). Although space limitations preclude a comprehensive review, we briefly describe these three common pain conditions next.

Chronic Musculoskeletal Pain

MSK pain is common in the general pediatric population, with prevalence estimates up to 40% in children and adolescents (King et al., 2011). The global impact of MSK pain in youth is primarily due to back and neck pain, which are the most common types of MSK pain and among the top 10 leading causes of years lived with disability in the world for adolescents (Kyu et al., 2016). Less common, noninflammatory MSK pain conditions include juvenile fibromyalgia and CRPS type 1. Juvenile fibromyalgia occurs in 2% to 6.1% of children and adolescents and is characterized by chronic diffuse/widespread MSK pain and several associated symptoms, including difficulties sleeping, fatigue, and mood concerns (Wolfe et al., 2010). CRPS is a fairly rare neuropathic pain condition (incidence of 1.2 in 100,000 children) characterized by severe neuropathic pain, allodynia, and vasomotor instability in a localized part of the body (usually one or both extremities) (Abu-Arafeh & Abu-Arafeh, 2016). While MSK pain remits for most youth, research suggests approximately 30% experience persistent pain several months to several years later (Holley et al., 2017).

Functional Abdominal Pain Disorder

FAPD is one of the most common pain conditions in childhood, affecting 10.5% to 16.8% of children and adolescents worldwide (Korterink et al., 2015). Similar to adults, FAPD is subclassified according to Rome IV criteria and characterized by persistent abdominal pain (with or without other gastrointestinal symptoms) after medical evaluation determines the symptoms cannot be attributed to another medical condition (Hyams et al., 2016). Subclassifications according to Rome IV criteria include abdominal migraine, irritable bowel syndrome, functional dyspepsia, and functional abdominal pain not otherwise specified. Symptoms of FAPD commonly emerge in early adolescence and are more common in females than males (Korterink et al., 2015).

Headache

Headache is a frequently reported recurrent pain problem among children and adolescents. The International Classification of Headache Disorders (ICHD) criteria classifies headaches as primary (not associated with an underlying medical condition) or secondary (comorbid with injury, disease, or disorder [e.g., brain tumor]) (Olesen, 2018). Primary headaches in childhood and adolescence are most often tension-type and migraine headaches, with prevalence rates of 31% and 9.1%, respectively (Wöber-Bingöl, 2013). Tension-type headache (TTH) is characterized by mild to moderate bandlike pain or pressure lasting 30 minutes to several days. Migraine headache (with or without aura) is characterized by episodes of moderate to severe head pain with a pulsating or sharp quality that worsens with physical activity and can be accompanied by nausea, vomiting, photophobia (light sensitivity), and/or phonophobia (sensitivity to sound). Chronic daily headache (CDH) is defined as a headache that recurs at least 15 days per month and is often viewed as the most debilitating form of recurrent headache. Current estimates indicate that CDH affects between 1% and 2% of children, with the most common being chronic TTH (Wang et al., 2006). Across these pediatric headache diagnoses, children show differences by sex, with more girls than boys affected.

Impact of Chronic Pain on Children and Families

An estimated 5% to 8% of children with chronic pain experience significant impact or disability related to pain across multiple areas of life, including poor physical functioning, psychological difficulties, school impairment, sleep deficiency, and family disruption (Huguet & Miro, 2008). Pain can interfere with a child's ability to participate in regular physical activities (e.g., sports, hobbies, walking), including vigorous physical activities and activities of daily living. Pain can also lead to significant emotional distress, and children with chronic pain often present with comorbidities, including depression and anxiety. Sleep deficiency is also common in children with chronic pain, characterized by difficulty falling asleep, maintaining sleep, and short sleep duration with many meeting diagnostic criteria for insomnia (Palermo et al., 2012). Within the child's social context, pediatric pain often leads to impairments in school and peer functioning. In particular, the experience of chronic pain often makes it difficult for children and adolescents to attend school and maintain friendships. Children with chronic pain report reduced school attendance, missed schoolwork, poorer academic performance, fewer friends, and are perceived to be more socially isolated relative to their peers (Forgeron et al., 2010).

The experience of chronic pain may also affect the entire family system. Compared to families of otherwise healthy children, families of children with chronic pain experience greater conflict and poorer communication (Lewandowski et al., 2010). Moreover, it is well appreciated that parenting a child with chronic pain can lead to high parental burden and distress. Parents experience significant direct and indirect costs related to the evaluation and management of chronic pain. Direct costs of pain treatment include emergency room visits and hospitalizations, visits to multiple physicians, and costs of diagnostic procedures and medications. Indirect costs include parental time off work, transportation costs, childcare, and incidental costs. Importantly, research has revealed the bidirectional relationship between children's pain experience and parent and family factors, such that children's pain may both influence and be influenced by family and parent processes (Palermo et al., 2014). We discuss the role of parent and family influences on children's pain and disability within the context of a biopsychosocial framework in greater detail later.

Long-Term Course and Outcomes of Childhood Chronic Pain

Unfortunately, many children do not simply outgrow pain. Chronic or recurrent pain persists well into young adulthood for up to 50% of children (Walker et al., 2010). Moreover, childhood pain can increase the risk for other adverse outcomes in adulthood, including the onset of new types of chronic pain, anxiety, and depressive disorders (e.g., see Noel et al., 2016). History of childhood chronic pain is also associated with decrements in educational and vocational functioning (e.g., a lower likelihood for obtaining a high school and a college degree) (Murray et al., 2020). Therefore further research is critical to identify vulnerabilities that maintain pain and disability as well as resiliencies that resolve pain during childhood through to adulthood. This will then give rise to the development of effective preventative and intervention strategies (Palermo, 2020) and may be critical for interrupting long-term trajectories of pain and disability.

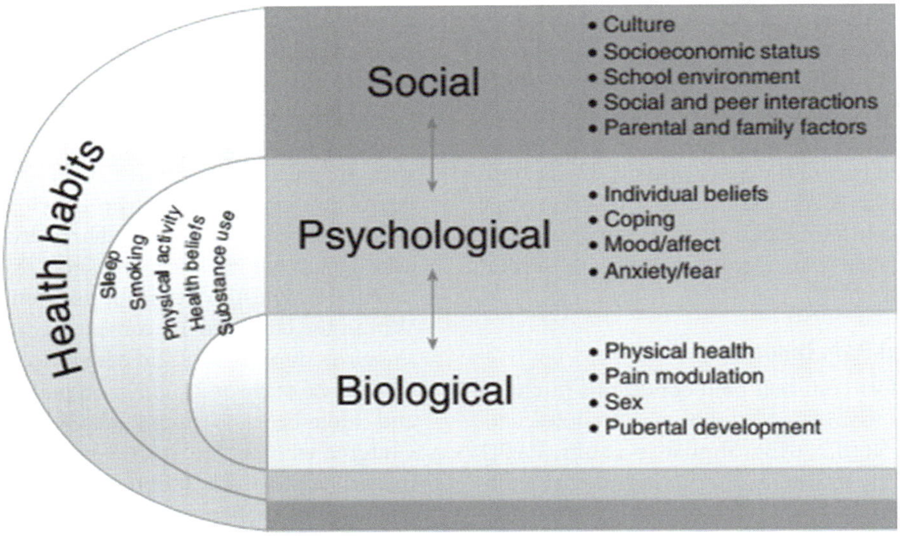

Fig. 64.1 Biopsychosocial framework for understanding pediatric chronic pain. (From Palermo, T. M. (2012). *Cognitive-behavioral therapy for chronic pain in children and adolescents.* Oxford University Press.).

UNDERSTANDING CHRONIC PAIN: A BIOPSYCHOSOCIAL FRAMEWORK

Central to contemporary models of chronic pain are the interrelationships among physical, cognitive, affective, and social factors that influence pain and disability, which are commonly referred to as the biopsychosocial model of pain (Fig. 64.1) (Palermo, 2012). This model has been used to understand and identify factors that contribute to the development of pain or that maintain pain and disability to better focus assessment and treatment strategies. Here we discuss developmental, biologic, psychological, and social factors to help with understanding children's pain from a multidimensional perspective.

Developmental

It is important to recognize that across childhood, adolescence, and young adulthood there is tremendous variability in neurocognitive development, physiology, and behavioral and emotional maturation that contribute to individual differences in the experience of pain. Within this context there are distinct developmental differences with respect to pain etiology, impact, and treatment response. For example, young children may rely more on parents for understanding their pain and offering pain management strategies. At the other end of the pediatric age spectrum, adolescents seek more autonomy with pain management and have emerging unique psychological and behavioral vulnerabilities, including increases in depressive symptoms, negative health behaviors (e.g., smoking, substance use), and declines in physical activity, all of which have the potential to impact the onset and maintenance of chronic pain.

Biologic

Current conceptualizations of chronic pain implicate central and peripheral nervous system mechanisms (Ji et al., 2018). Processes of central sensitization and deficiencies in endogenous pain modulation are proposed to underlie persistent pain. For example, impairment in inhibitory pain modulation measured by psychophysical pain testing has been found to predict the transition from acute to chronic MSK pain in children (Holley et al., 2017). More recently, neuroimmune and neuroendocrine interactions have been investigated to extend our understanding of chronic pain conditions. For example, research highlights the involvement of the brain-gut axis in functional abdominal pain syndromes and the structural and functional brain changes that occur in CRPS (Powell et al., 2017).

The influences of sex have also been highlighted. Population-based research indicates that chronic pain is more common in girls than boys, especially around the time of puberty (King et al., 2011), and that girls generally report higher pain intensity, longer-lasting, and more frequent pain than boys. In line with this research female sex has been identified as a prognostic factor for the transition from acute to persistent MSK pain in children and adolescents, where females have increased likelihood of developing persistent MSK pain (Holley et al., 2017). Although there is a large body of evidence showing sex differences in pediatric pain, the nature of these differences is not yet clear. Several underlying mechanisms have been considered, including differences in hormones, pain central sensitization, and coping styles.

Psychological

Emotional vulnerabilities, including anxiety and depression, are contributing factors and consequences of chronic pain in childhood. Symptoms of depression and anxiety are associated with increased pain and may exacerbate school impairment (Kashikar-Zuck et al., 2010) and sleep disturbances in children (Palermo et al., 2012). Moreover, maladaptive beliefs and coping related to the child's pain have been shown to amplify pain and disability, most notably pain-specific anxiety (e.g., fear of pain), and pain catastrophizing (e.g., thoughts of helplessness and inability to cope with pain). Recent evidence further suggests that the experience of adverse childhood events and stressful life events may be related to the occurrence of chronic pain in childhood (Groenewald et al., 2020).

Social

Chronic pain should also be viewed from a broad social context in which family plays a central role. Research on parent and family factors has examined individual parent characteristics and behaviors (e.g., parent distress and parental protective behaviors; see Donnelly et al. [2020] for a systematic review and metaanalysis), dyadic factors (e.g., parent-child conflict), and family-level factors (e.g., family conflict and cohesion; see Lewandowski et al., 2010) related to the child's experience of pain and disability. For example, high levels of parental distress have been linked to increased pain and disability in children, although the temporal nature of these effects is likely bidirectional child pain also contributing to parent distress.

Moreover, exposure to a parent with chronic pain in childhood is a risk factor for pain and adverse mental and physical health outcomes. In one study having a parent with irritable bowel syndrome placed children at a twice greater risk for developing a diagnosis of FAPD (Aguas et al., 2011) compared to children of parents without the syndrome. Current conceptual models for the transmission of risk for chronic pain from parents to offspring (Stone & Wilson, 2016) highlight the potential contribution of biologic and social mechanisms, including genetics, alterations in early neurobiologic development, pain-specific social learning, general parenting, family health, and exposure to a stressful environment. Pain-specific social learning has been the most well studied. Solicitous or protective parental reactions to children's expressions of discomfort and maternal modeling of illness behavior contribute to a greater focus on somatic sensations, leading to illness behaviors and increased disability in children. Parent protective behavior has also been associated with decreased school functioning in children with chronic pain (Donnelly et al., 2020).

ASSESSMENT OF CHRONIC PAIN IN CHILDREN

Consistent with the biopsychosocial model of pediatric pain, a standard evaluation should include not only a child's medical history and physical examination, but also information on the history and functional impact of pain. The majority of information on pain history and impact may be elicited with clinical interview supplemented by questionnaire measures as needed.

Pain History

Accurate assessment of children's pain includes asking questions about the timing and specific characteristics of their pain, including quality, intensity, and location(s). Using the acronym QuILT can be a helpful way to ascertain pain history

TABLE 64.1 Gathering Pain History Using the QuILT Acronym

QuILT Domain	Example Interview Probes
Quality	• How would you describe your pain (e.g., shooting, burning, tingling, electric shock)?
Intensity	Measure using single-item self-report measures asking about average and worst pain intensity (see Birnie et al., (2019) for a systematic review of measures) • Older children ages 8–18: 10-point numeric rating scale (0–10; 0="no pain" to 10="worst pain imaginable") • Young children ages 6–8: FACES Pain Scale-Revised
Location	• What areas of your body do you have pain? • Where are you most bothered by pain?
Timing	Onset: • When did your pain first start? • How has it changed since it first began? Frequency: • How many times have you had pain over the last week? Duration: • How long does your pain usually last?

Adapted from Sickkids online education module (see Table 64.3 for Internet link).

(Table 64.1). Moreover, the physician should identify and investigate any red flags or clinical indicators of pathologic findings indicative of a specific, underlying disease (e.g., bone pain, joint swelling, etc.).

Pain Impact

While assessment of pain is important, assessment of the functional impact of pain on key aspects of a child's life is equally critical. It can be communicated to families that evaluating the child's functioning is an essential part of a comprehensive pain assessment. At a minimum, six key questions can be used in the routine assessment as outlined in a recent comprehensive review of pediatric pain (Eccleston et al., 2021):

1. What impact does pain have on your life?
2. What is the typical day like for you when you have pain?
3. What would you be doing if your pain was lessened?
4. What are the things you do that make your pain better, and things you do that make your pain worse?
5. What are your concerns and worries about your pain?
6. How would you know that a pain treatment was working for you? What would be a meaningful change for you?

These key questions can serve to elicit the child's narrative about pain and reveal important information about perceptions of disability due to pain. Further prompts and targeted questions (Table 64.2) can then be used to provide a comprehensive assessment of the individual impact of pain on the

TABLE 64.2 Assessment of Pediatric Chronic Pain Impact: Examples of Interview Questions and Measures by the Domain

Domain	Example Interview Probes	Example Measures
Physical	• What kinds of things are hard for you to do because of pain? • Are you able to participate in hobbies or sports?	• Functional Disability Inventory (Walker & Greene, 1991) • Child Activity Limitations Interview (Palermo et al., 2004) • PROMIS Pediatric Pain Interference Scale (Varni et al., 2010)
Emotional	• Tell me about your mood. • Are you feeling sad or down? • How has pain affected your mood?	• Child Depression Inventory (Helsel & Matson, 1984) • PROMIS Anxiety and Depression (Schalet et al., 2016)
School/Work	• How often do you miss school (or work) due to pain? Do you stay at school (or work) for the whole day? • Are you able to stay on top of homework (tasks at work)?	• Pediatric Quality of Life Inventory 4.0—school subscale (Varni et al., 2001)
Sleep	• How long does it take you to fall asleep? Do you wake up during the night? • Do you think that you sleep well?	• PROMIS sleep disturbance (Bevans et al., 2019) • Adolescent Sleep Wake Scale (Essner et al., 2015)

Adapted from Palermo, T. M. (2012). *Cognitive-behavioral therapy for chronic pain in children and adolescents.* Oxford University Press.

child's life, and treatment strategies can then be targeted to improve the child's functioning in these areas. For example, depression and anxiety often cooccur with chronic pain. As described in Ashley's case example, if a child describes high levels of general worry and significant emotional distress due to pain, further interview questions and questionnaire measures (as described later) may be useful to determine the clinical severity of the child's psychological symptoms, with subsequent referral to a mental health professional for further evaluation and treatment as appropriate.

As recommended by expert consensus per the Pediatric Initiative on Methods, Measurement, and Pain Assessment in Clinical Trials (Ped-IMMPACT) (McGrath et al., 2008), several core domains are critical to evaluate in children with chronic pain. This includes but is not limited to assessment of physical, emotional, role (e.g., school) functioning, and sleep, although the specific areas addressed will largely depend on the child's unique needs and presenting concerns. Applying a developmental perspective can guide evaluation of the most relevant and clinically meaningful areas of chronic pain impact. For example, there are a number of studies that have described the negative impact of chronic pain on school functioning and academic achievement in adolescents with chronic pain, which may impede future educational and vocational goals during the transition to young adulthood (Murray et al., 2020). Moreover, insomnia and mood disorders peak during adolescence. Thus evaluation of emotional functioning and sleep may be important areas to evaluate in the adolescent age group, particularly as these comorbidities can interfere with treatment response.

Information on key domains of chronic pain impact can be gathered using a combination of clinical interview questions and standardized self-report measures. We list example clinical interview questions and commonly used validated measures in Table 64.2. In particular, Patient-Reported Outcomes Measurement Information System (PROMIS) measures have been recommended as targeted, readily available, well-validated assessment tools that span several domains of functioning, including pain interference, depression, anxiety, and sleep. Importantly, PROMIS measures include scoring guidelines and clinical cutoffs that are useful to integrate with clinical evaluation and treatment recommendations. Finally, in addition to the questionnaires listed in Table 64.2, clinicians may consider multidimensional measures that assess the broad impact of chronic pain on the child, parent, and family (e.g., Pediatric Quality of Life Inventory [PedsQL]; Varni, Seid et al., 2001).

CHRONIC PAIN MANAGEMENT IN CHILDREN

Counseling Families

Families look to their primary care clinicians to evaluate and treat their child's chronic pain, yet providers may feel unsure about how to manage pain and make appropriate referrals. In some cases there may be a diagnosis evident from the exam and evaluation, and clear next steps to take with further diagnostic evaluation or initiation of treatment. However, for the majority of youth, medical evaluation and diagnostic testing may indicate that painful symptoms are not attributed to a clear underlying disease process. The lack of clarity around a diagnosis and explanation for their child's pain can create considerable frustration and distress for families, especially if they fear that a medical diagnosis has been missed.

As such, the initial discussions and explanations about chronic pain are critical and should be approached with sensitivity and clear communication. A focus on rapport building through acknowledging the family's frustration and providing reassurance and validation of the child's chronic pain is imperative. It is particularly important for the provider to be aware of how language about pain has often been pejorative and reductionistic, and that the field has more recently advocated for changes in terminology. Previously, the term "functional pain" was used when pain occurred in the absence of identifiable organic disease; however, this led to widespread misunderstanding that the etiology of this pain was solely psychological (see Schechter (2014) for a useful discussion of pain terminology). This misunderstanding can lead to considerable frustration for the patient and family and an unsuccessful approach to treatment. Instead, "primary pain disorder" has been promoted as a more useful term to categorize pain that is not associated with a disease causing tissue damage, but rather that pain itself is the chronic disease.

The primary care provider plays an important role in educating children and families about the etiology of chronic pain, setting collaborative goals for treatment, and coordinating treatment with an interdisciplinary team of health professionals. Chronic pain can be described in contrast to acute pain: While acute pain acts as the body's alarm system to protect the child, with chronic pain the alarm system stays turned on or is easily triggered to stay on. It becomes a false alarm, like a fire alarm going off without a fire. Highlighting this key difference between acute and chronic pain can help clinicians guide the family toward the understanding that chronic pain does not respond to the same treatments as acute pain (e.g., rest or opioid pain medications). Instead, because of the multidimensional nature of chronic pain, effective management may require multimodal treatment to effectively change the way the child's body, brain, and nervous system are responding. To help generate appropriate goals and expectations for treatment it is critical to set the expectation that the overarching goal of chronic pain treatment is not total pain relief but to help children restore function despite having pain. Examples of realistic goals include attending school more frequently despite the pain and increasing the number of strategies the child uses to manage pain. Along with coordination of treatment with other health professionals (including psychologists, physical therapists, or providers of complementary and alternative medicine [CAM]), routine follow-up is essential to encourage the child's participation in therapies and to provide feedback on progress toward goals.

Treatment of Chronic Pain in Children

Dedicated pediatric pain treatment facilities remain limited, with most centers located in major cities. Even when pediatric pain experts and resources are available, a child's ability to participate in treatment may be limited by time, expense, insurance, or system barriers. If experts in chronic pain cannot be located, the primary care or developmental-behavioral pediatrics clinician can assemble a team of knowledgeable professionals, educate the team on chronic pain, and establish a treatment plan with other providers. These clinicians should be kept informed of treatment progress. See Table 64.3 for a list of additional pediatric pain assessment and treatment resources.

We broadly review the evidence base for chronic pain treatment in children, for which the primary goals are to reduce pain-related disability and improve their pain experience. Depending on the type and severity of a child's pain, a combination of interventions can be used. including psychological treatments, physical therapy, pharmacologic strategies, CAM treatments, and telehealth and digital health interventions.

Psychological Interventions

The overarching goal of psychological treatment is to teach the child to cope more effectively with pain and increase participation in normal activities. Compared to physical and pharmacologic treatments, psychological interventions have the most robust evidence base for reducing pain and disability in children and adolescents with chronic pain (see Fisher et al.. 2019). The most common psychological treatment for pediatric chronic pain is cognitive-behavioral therapy (CBT; see Chapter 98). CBT targets maladaptive cognitions, behaviors, emotions, and contextual factors (e.g., family, school) that play a role in the maintenance and exacerbation of pain and disability. CBT typically includes multiple components: pain education, relaxation skills, cognitive strategies, behavioral strategies, and parent training. Briefly, pain education teaches children and parents about the biopsychosocial model and neurophysiology of chronic pain. Relaxation skills (e.g., deep breathing, progressive muscle relaxation) decrease physiologic arousal and emotional distress. Cognitive strategies target maladaptive thoughts related to pain and teach children to reframe or replace them with more adaptive thoughts. Behavioral strategies focus on reengaging children in activities (e.g., school, hobbies). One example is activity pacing, which helps children gradually build participation in activity over time by alternating active periods with rest breaks. Parents may also be taught strategies for decreasing their own worries, modifying unhelpful beliefs about pain, and encouraging their child's adaptive behaviors (e.g., school attendance) using praise and rewards. For a detailed CBT protocol for pediatric chronic pain management, see Palermo (2012).

Most children with chronic pain will benefit from referral to psychological interventions. Instead of a last resort effort, making referrals early and as part of routine care may be better received and accepted by families. Few psychologists in the community have received specific training in psychological treatment for pain management. However, referrals to mental health providers with experience in CBT and/or working with children with chronic conditions may be appropriate. Moreover, there has been growing interest in integrating psychologists within primary care settings, who can work alongside medical providers to identify and treat chronic pain. Treatment interventions for other conditions delivered in an integrated primary care setting have shown great promise, providing accessible, evidence-based care while reducing health care costs. Such innovative treatment models have the potential to overcome large gaps in clinical care for youth with chronic pain, as the vast majority of families experience significant barriers to accessing specialized pain care.

TABLE 64.3 Pediatric Chronic Pain Resources

International Association for the Study of Pain (IASP)
- IASP website: www.iasp-pain.org
- IASP Special Interest Group on Pain in Childhood: http://childpain.org/
- International directory of Pediatric Chronic Pain Programs: http://childpain.org/wp-content/uploads/2021/01/Pediatric-Chronic-Pain-Programs-2021-Update.pdf
  - List of dedicated pediatric chronic pain programs in the United States, Canada, and internationally has been developed and maintained since 2012 by Tonya Palermo, PhD.

Pediatric Pain Listserv
- International Internet forum for informal discussion of any topic related to pain in children, including but not limited to clinical problems or questions, announcements of meetings, and political or administrative aspects of children's pain management. The list is open to any professional with interest or expertise in the area.
- To subscribe to the list, send a message to LISTSERV@lists.dal.ca with the following in the first line of the body of the message: SUB PEDIATRIC-PAIN your-first-name your-last-name.

SickKids Online Pediatric Pain Curriculum
- Website: https://www.sickkids.ca/en/care-services/centres/pain-centre/#oppc
- Aimed at health care professionals and includes a variety of topics, such as a section on chronic pain ("Chronic Pain Management: Special Considerations").

SKIP (Solutions for Kids in Pain)
- Website: https://www.kidsinpain.ca/
- SKIP is aimed at improving children's pain management in Canada and around the world. See the Pain Management Apps & Online Resources Page on their site, which can be printed for families.

PROMIS Measures
- Website: https://www.healthmeasures.net/explore-measurement-systems/promis/obtain-administer-measures
- PROMIS measures are available for free and include child self-report (ages 8–17) and parent proxy report (ages 5–17) across multiple domains of functioning relevant to children with chronic pain (see Table 64.2 for examples of appropriate PROMIS measures).

Lancet Child & Health Commission on Pediatric Pain*

Outlines strategic path for the field of pediatric pain organized under four transformative goals: (1) make pain better, (2) make pain understood, (3) make pain visible, and (4) make pain better. Provides an up-to-date and comprehensive review of the literature on pediatric pain.

*See Eccleston, C., Fisher, E., Howard, R. F., Slater, R., Forgeron, P., Palermo, T. M., Birnie, K. A., et al. (2021). Delivering transformative action in paediatric pain: A Lancet Child & Adolescent Health Commission. *The Lancet Child & Adolescent Health, 5*(1), 47–87.

Physical Interventions

Physical interventions are an important aspect of chronic pain treatment and may include therapeutic exercises to address impairments in body functions or structures (e.g., endurance training, range of motion) as well as specific self-management techniques to alleviate pain and stiffness (e.g., massage, applying heat or cold). The majority of studies describing the unique effects of physical interventions have focused on therapeutic exercise, including neuromuscular exercise training and aerobic exercise (see Birnie et al., 2020 for a useful review of current evidence gaps). Other research has examined exercise training within the context of intensive inpatient or outpatient pain treatment programs (Simons et al., 2018). Combined interventions integrating CBT with therapeutic exercise have also shown promising results. For example, a novel pilot intervention integrating CBT and specialized neuromuscular training in adolescents with juvenile fibromyalgia showed enhanced efficacy compared to those receiving CBT alone (Kashikar-Zuck et al., 2018). Combined physical and psychological treatment packages may serve to strengthen treatment benefit in children with chronic MSK pain, although more research in this area is needed.

Pharmacologic Treatments

The goal of pharmacologic treatments is to provide pain relief and improve function. Over-the-counter analgesics are commonly used for many types of pain (e.g., nonsteroidal anti-inflammatory drugs are helpful for pain resulting from tissue inflammation from injuries or arthritis). Adjuvant medications, including anticonvulsants (e.g., gabapentin, pregabalin) and antidepressants (e.g., amitriptyline, duloxetine), have also been used in the treatment of pediatric chronic pain. Opioid medications (e.g., codeine, morphine, oxycodone) are used less frequently and are not generally indicated for chronic noncancer pain. A recent overview of systematic reviews found low-quality evidence for pharmacologic treatments for children with chronic pain, primarily due to the lack of data and the low number of randomized controlled trials (RCTs) (Eccleston et al., 2019). At present there is insufficient support for the efficacy and safety of any pharmacologic treatments to routinely recommend them for chronic pain.

CAM Therapies

CAM therapies encompass medical practices and products that are not commonly considered to be part of conventional medicine, often categorized as alternative medicine systems/ energy healing therapies (e.g., acupuncture), mind-body practices (e.g., biofeedback, yoga), manipulative/ body-based therapies (chiropractic, massage), and biologically based therapies (e.g., special diets, herbal supplements). Epidemiologic evidence indicates one in five children with chronic pain use CAM strategies, most commonly biologically based and body-based therapies (Groenewald et al., 2017). However, the evidence base on the potential therapeutic benefits of CAM is limited, with only a few RCTs conducted to date (Snyder & Brown, 2012). Large-scale RCTs are needed to better understand which CAM therapies may provide therapeutic benefit for pediatric pain management.

Interdisciplinary Pediatric Pain Treatment Programs

Typically housed within tertiary care medical centers, interdisciplinary pediatric pain clinics provide intensive multimodal treatment (e.g., physical, psychological, CAM therapies) through outpatient and/or inpatient services. These programs have demonstrated efficacy in improving pain, pain-related disability, and school absenteeism in children with complex and disabling chronic pain (Simons et al., 2018). Unfortunately, the availability of these programs is extremely limited. For an online listing of pediatric pain programs in the United States, Canada, and internationally, please see Table 64.3.

Telehealth and Digital Health Interventions

Access to specialized pain care remains a substantial challenge for children due to the scarcity of interdisciplinary pain management programs, long wait times, large geographic distances, and health care policy and reimbursement barriers. Remote delivery of treatment using telehealth and digital health technologies has the potential to address barriers and improve access to high-quality, evidence-based treatment. Remote interventions offer several potential advantages, including more rapid availability, the ability to reach children on a larger scale, and cost effectiveness. Moreover, pediatric health interventions delivered through Internet-based and smartphone platforms are appealing to children and adolescents, who are "digital natives" to these technologies. Due to restrictions placed on face-to-face or in-person health care visits during the COVID-19 pandemic, the importance of leveraging digital approaches to optimize pain treatment delivery in children has been underscored. At this time, the majority of evidence for digital health interventions is for psychological treatments in pediatric chronic pain (Fisher et al., 2019). However, the scalability and accessibility of digital health interventions remain a challenge, as those that are tested for efficacy are often difficult to implement. For a resource page on digital health tools for pediatric pain assessment and management available to families, see the Solutions for Kids in Pain (SKIP) in Table 64.3. See also a systematic review of researcher-led digital health tools for pediatric pain assessment and management and availability of tools for end users (Higgins et al., 2018).

CONCLUSION

Children and adolescents commonly present to primary care with pain complaints, and families often look to their primary care clinicians to evaluate and treat their child's chronic pain. While interdisciplinary intensive pain clinics offer comprehensive evaluation and multimodal treatment, their availability is unfortunately very limited. However, primary care or developmental and behavioral pediatric clinicians can play a significant role in evaluation and treatment even when they do not have substantial expertise in pediatric chronic pain. Consistent with the biopsychosocial model of pediatric pain, a standard evaluation includes not only a child's medical history and physical examination but also information on the history and functional impact of pain. Under the guiding principle of an interdisciplinary, rehabilitative care approach, children benefit most when multiple modalities are used, including psychological, physical, and CAM treatments. The child's physician can assemble a team of knowledgeable health professionals, establish an interdisciplinary treatment plan, and provide follow-up and feedback on progress toward treatment goals. The provision of care for children with chronic pain can be challenging. However, primary care clinicians are often first in line to identify and treat pain, and they have great potential to make a significant impact on the lives of children with chronic pain and their families.

REFERENCES

Abu-Arafeh, H., & Abu-Arafeh, I. (2016). Complex regional pain syndrome in children: Incidence and clinical characteristics. *Archives of Disease in Childhood*, *101*, 719–723.

Aguas, M., Garrigues, V., Bastida, G., Nos, P., Ortiz, V., Fernandez, A., & Ponce, J. (2011). Prevalence of irritable bowel syndrome (IBS) in first-degree relatives of patients with inflammatory bowel disease (IBD). *Journal of Crohn's and Colitis*, *5*, 227–233.

Bevans, K. B., Meltzer, L. J., De La Motte, A., Kratchman, A., Viél, D., & Forrest, C. B. (2019). Qualitative development and content validation of the PROMIS pediatric sleep health items. *Behavioral Sleep Medicine*, *17*, 657–671.

Birnie, K. A., Hundert, A. S., Lalloo, C., Nguyen, C., & Stinson, J. N. (2019). Recommendations for selection of self-report pain intensity measures in children and adolescents: A systematic review and quality assessment of measurement properties. *Pain*, *160*, 5–18.

Birnie, K. A., Ouellette, C., Do Amaral, T., & Stinson, J. N. (2020). Mapping the evidence and gaps of interventions for pediatric chronic pain to inform policy, research, and practice: A systematic review and quality assessment of systematic reviews. *Canadian Journal of Pain*, *4*, 129–148.

Donnelly, T. J., Palermo, T. M., & Newton-John, T. R. O. (2020). Parent cognitive, behavioural, and affective factors and their relation to child pain and functioning in pediatric chronic pain: A systematic review and meta-analysis. *Pain*, *161*, 1401–1419.

Eccleston, C., Fisher, E., Cooper, T. E., Grégoire, M. -C., Heathcote, L. C., Krane, E., ... Anderson, B. (2019). Pharmacological interventions for chronic pain in children: An overview of systematic reviews. *Pain*, *160*, 1698–1707.

Eccleston, C., Fisher, E., Howard, R. F., Slater, R., Forgeron, P., Palermo, T. M., ... Crombez, G. (2021). Delivering transformative action in paediatric pain: A Lancet Child & Adolescent Health Commission. *The Lancet Child & Adolescent Health*, *5*, 47–87.

Essner, B., Noel, M., Myrvik, M., & Palermo, T. (2015). Examination of the factor structure of the Adolescent Sleep-Wake Scale (ASWS). *Behavioral Sleep Medicine*, *13*, 296–307.

Fisher, E., Law, E., Dudeney, J., Eccleston, C., & Palermo, T. M. (2019). Psychological therapies (remotely delivered) for the management of chronic and recurrent pain in children and adolescents. *Cochrane Database of Systematic Reviews*, *4*, CD011118.

Forgeron, P. A., King, S., Stinson, J. N., McGrath, P. J., MacDonald, A. J., & Chambers, C. T. (2010). Social functioning and peer relationships in children and adolescents with chronic pain: A systematic review. *Pain Research and Management*, *15*, 27–41.

Groenewald, C. B., Beals-Erickson, S. E., Ralston-Wilson, J., Rabbitts, J. A., & Palermo, T. M. (2017). Complementary and alternative medicine use by children with pain in the United States. *Academic Pediatrics*, *17*, 785–793.

Groenewald, C. B., Essner, B. S., Wright, D., Fesinmeyer, M. D., & Palermo, T. M. (2014). The economic costs of chronic pain among a cohort of treatment-seeking adolescents in the United States. *Journal of Pain*, *15*, 925–933.

Groenewald, C. B., Murray, C. B., & Palermo, T. M. (2020). Adverse childhood experiences and chronic pain among children and adolescents in the United States. *Pain Reports*, *5*(5), e839.

Helsel, W. J., & Matson, J. L. (1984). The assessment of depression in children: The internal structure of the Child Depression Inventory (CDI). *Behaviour Research and Therapy*, *22*, 289–298.

Higgins, K. S., Tutelman, P. R., Chambers, C. T., Witteman, H. O., Barwick, M., Corkum, P., ... Robins, S. (2018). Availability of researcher-led eHealth tools for pain assessment and management: Barriers, facilitators, costs, and design. *Pain Reports*, *3*, e686.

Holley, A., Lewandowski, A., Wilson, C., & Palermo, T. M. (2017). Predictors of the transition from acute to persistent musculoskeletal pain in children and adolescents: A prospective study. *Pain*, *158*, 794.

Holm, S., Ljungman, G., & Söderlund, A. (2012). Pain in children and adolescents in primary care; chronic and recurrent pain is common. *Acta Paediatrica*, *101*, 1246–1252.

Huguet, A., & Miro, J. (2008). The severity of chronic pediatric pain: An epidemiological study. *Journal of Pain*, *9*, 226–236.

Hyams, J. S., Di Lorenzo, C., Saps, M., Shulman, R. J., Staiano, A., & van Tilburg, M. (2016). Childhood functional gastrointestinal disorders: Child/adolescent. *Gastroenterology*, *150*, 1456–1468.

Ji, R. R., Nackley, A., Huh, Y., Terrando, N., & Maixner, W. (2018). Neuroinflammation and central sensitization in chronic and widespread pain. *Anesthesiology*, *129*, 343–366.

Kashikar-Zuck, S., Black, W. R., Pfeiffer, M., Peugh, J., Williams, S. E., Ting, T. V., ... Myer, G. D. (2018). Pilot randomized trial of integrated cognitive-behavioral therapy and neuromuscular training for juvenile fibromyalgia: The FIT Teens Program. *Journal of Pain*, *19*, 1049–1062.

Kashikar-Zuck, S., Johnston, M., Ting, T. V., Graham, B. T., Lynch-Jordan, A. M., Verkamp, E., ... Spalding, S. (2010). Relationship between school absenteeism and depressive symptoms among adolescents with juvenile fibromyalgia. *Journal of Pediatric Psychology*, *35*, 996–1004.

King, S., Chambers, C. T., Huguet, A., MacNevin, R. C., McGrath, P. J., Parker, L., & MacDonald, A. J. (2011). The epidemiology of chronic pain in children and adolescents revisited: A systematic review. *Pain*, *152*, 2729–2738.

Korterink, J. J., Diederen, K., Benninga, M. A., & Tabbers, M. M. (2015). Epidemiology of pediatric functional abdominal pain disorders: A meta-analysis. *PLoS One*, *10*, e0126982.

Kyu, H. H., Pinho, C., Wagner, J. A., Brown, J. C., Bertozzi-Villa, A., Charlson, F. J., ... Ferrari, A. J. (2016). Global and national burden of diseases and injuries among children and adolescents between 1990 and 2013: Findings from the global burden of disease 2013 study. *JAMA Pediatrics*, *170*, 267–287.

Lewandowski, A. S., Palermo, T. M., Stinson, J., Handley, S., & Chambers, C. T. (2010). Systematic review of family functioning in families of children and adolescents with chronic pain. *Journal of Pain*, *11*, 1027–1038.

McGrath, P. J., Walco, G. A., Turk, D. C., Dworkin, R. H., Brown, M. T., Davidson, K., ... PedIMMPACT. (2008). Core outcome domains and measures for pediatric acute and chronic/recurrent pain clinical trials: PedIMMPACT recommendations. *Journal of Pain*, *9*, 771–783.

Murray, C. B., Groenewald, C. B., de la Vega, R., & Palermo, T. M. (2020). Long-term impact of adolescent chronic pain on young adult educational, vocational, and social outcomes. *Pain*, *161*, 439–445.

Noel, M., Groenewald, C. B., Beals-Erickson, S. E., Gebert, J. T., & Palermo, T. M. (2016). Chronic pain in adolescence and internalizing mental health disorders: A nationally representative study. Pain, *157*(6), 1333–1338.

Olesen, J. (2018). International classification of headache disorders. *The Lancet Neurology*, *17*, 396–397.

Palermo, T. M. (2012). *Cognitive-behavioral therapy for chronic pain in children and adolescents*. Oxford University Press.

Palermo, T. M. (2020). Pain prevention and management must begin in childhood: The key role of psychological interventions. *Pain*, *161*(1), S114–S121.

Palermo, T. M., Law, E., Churchill, S. S., & Walker, A. (2012). Longitudinal course and impact of insomnia symptoms in adolescents with and without chronic pain. *Journal of Pain*, *13*, 1099–1106.

Palermo, T. M., Valrie, C. R., & Karlson, C. W. (2014). Family and parent influences on pediatric chronic pain: A developmental perspective. *American Journal of Psychology*, *69*, 142–152.

Palermo, T. M., Witherspoon, D., Valenzuela, D., & Drotar, D. D. (2004). The child activity limitations interview: A measure of pain-related functional impairment in school-age children and adolescents. *Pain*, *109*, 461–470.

Powell, N., Walker, M. M., & Talley, N. J. (2017). The mucosal immune system: Master regulator of bidirectional gut–brain communications. *Nature Reviews Gastroenterology & Hepatology*, *14*, 143–159.

Schalet, B. D., Pilkonis, P. A., Yu, L., Dodds, N., Johnston, K. L., Yount, S., ... Cella, D. (2016). Clinical validity of PROMIS depression, anxiety, and anger across diverse clinical samples. *Journal of Clinical Epidemiology*, *73*, 119–127.

Schechter, N. L. (2014). Pain terminology—Reply. *JAMA Pediatrics*, *168*, 1168.

Simons, L. E., Sieberg, C. B., Conroy, C., Randall, E. T., Shulman, J., Borsook, D., ... Logan, D. E. (2018). Children with chronic

pain: Response trajectories after intensive pain rehabilitation treatment. *Journal of Pain, 19*, 207–218.
Snyder, J., & Brown, P. (2012). Complementary and alternative medicine in children: An analysis of the recent literature. *Current Opinion in Pediatrics, 24*, 539–546.
Stone, A. L., & Wilson, A. C. (2016). Transmission of risk from parents with chronic pain to offspring: An integrative conceptual model. *Pain, 157*, 2628.
Varni, J. W., Seid, M., & Kurtin, P. S. (2001). PedsQL™ 4.0: Reliability and validity of the Pediatric Quality of Life Inventory™ Version 4.0 Generic Core Scales in healthy and patient populations. *Medical Care, 39*, 800–812.
Varni, J. W., Stucky, B. D., Thissen, D., DeWitt, E. M., Irwin, D. E., Lai, J. -S., … DeWalt, D. A. (2010). PROMIS Pediatric Pain Interference Scale: An item response theory analysis of the pediatric pain item bank. *Journal of Pain, 11*, 1109–1119.
Walker, L. S., Dengler-Crish, C. M., Rippel, S., & Bruehl, S. (2010). Functional abdominal pain in childhood and adolescence increases risk for chronic pain in adulthood. *Pain, 150*, 568–572.
Walker, L. S., & Greene, J. W. (1991). The functional disability inventory: Measuring a neglected dimension of child health status. *Journal of Pediatric Psychology, 16*, 39–58.
Wang, S.-J., Fuh, J.-L., Lu, S.-R., & Juang, K.-D. (2006). Chronic daily headache in adolescents: Prevalence, impact, and medication overuse. *Neurology, 66*, 193–197.
Wöber-Bingöl, Ç. (2013). Epidemiology of migraine and headache in children and adolescents. *Current Pain and Headache Reports, 17*, 1–11.
Wolfe, F., Clauw, D. J., Fitzcharles, M. A., Goldenberg, D. L., Katz, R. S., Mease, P., … Yunus, M. B. (2010). The American College of Rheumatology preliminary diagnostic criteria for fibromyalgia and measurement of symptom severity. *Arthritis Care Research (Hoboken), 62*, 600–610.

65

Feeding and Swallowing Disorders

Laura Pickler, Kaitlyn Cavanaugh, and Holly Knotowicz

For additional material related to the content of this chapter, please see Chapters 59, and 63.

VIGNETTE

RD is a 15-month-old boy with a significant past history for trisomy 21. During his 12-month primary care appointment concerns regarding growth and feeding were identified. His primary care provider has performed all necessary laboratory studies to investigate reasons for failure to thrive without discovering any etiology for these issues. He is referred to you for further evaluation and management. Upon meeting RD, his mother reports delays in all areas of development, but he is making progress with current early intervention services that include physical therapy, occupational therapy, and speech-language therapy all once weekly. None of his therapists are currently working on feeding skills specifically. You perform an observation of feeding and discover that RD has significant oral motor and oral sensory dysfunction that limit his intake to liquids and purees. He frequently coughs and chokes with both consistencies. He has good head control, but hypotonia is noted that limits his other motor skills, in particular sitting in the highchair his family usually uses. What are your next steps? How will you intervene to support feeding and growth?

INTRODUCTION

Patients with Down syndrome offer an excellent example of where feeding, swallowing, and developmental considerations all are present and may present to the clinician in developmental pediatrics due to challenges with growth, overall health, or just "not making progress as expected" despite having available therapeutic support. In this chapter we explore feeding and swallowing development in typical children and provide examples of how feeding is impacted in children with structural, physiologic, or experiential challenges. Our opinion is that both feeding and swallowing are best assessed in a multidisciplinary fashion, which is also consistent with literature in the field (Arvedson & Brodsky, 2017; Gosa, Dodrill, Lefton-Greif, & Silverman, 2020). The point of a multidisciplinary evaluation is to fully understand all the contributing factors to a feeding or swallowing problem and then design an intervention strategy that addresses complex problems.

There is a wealth of information on feeding, in particular, available in the lay press. Some resources are reputable; however, unfortunately the volume of distracting and even harmful information can complicate even a typically developing child's progress with eating a wide variety of nutritious foods that support optimal growth. We recommend a cautious approach when applying treatment principles for a child with feeding difficulties if the underlying contributing factors are not well understood. Feeding difficulties often coexist with other difficulties in physiologic and psychological domains that may complicate assessment (Zucker et al., 2015). Before diving into some common problems, it is first necessary to understand typical development as it relates to feeding skills.

TYPICAL FEEDING DEVELOPMENT

Successful development of feeding skills is multifactorial and dependent upon musculoskeletal, cardiovascular, pulmonary, nervous, and gastrointestinal (GI) systems. In addition, children require positive experiences and opportunities for learning. Every infant's feeding development varies; however, there is a typical developmental pattern that we utilize as a guideline (Dwyer, 2018). Table 65.1 summarizes typical feeding development.

Eating is a developmental skill, one that requires modeling, interaction, and support. It is important for a caregiver to recognize the infant's cues to foster a healthy feeding relationship from an early age. This is referred to as cue-based feeding. Cue-based feeding is a technique that was developed for infants born prematurely and was first used in hospital-based settings. However, the message and ideology apply to all infants. It speaks to identifying the infant's cues (e.g., what are this infant's cues for hunger?). The clinician may also instruct caregivers to watching the infant's cues for feeding challenges: Is the rate of flow from breast or bottle too fast, is it dripping out of the sides of the mouth? Is it too slow? What are the cues of being full? Pulling off the nipple? Turning the head away? By helping caregivers identify and respond to cues, they engage in a process commonly referred to as baby-led feeding (Shaker, 2013).

Feeding development begins before birth (Wick, 2018). Swallowing and sucking skills both begin developing while in

TABLE 65.1 Infant Feeding Milestones

Age	Positioning	Skill	Texture
0–4 mo	Fully supported head, neck, and body; slightly reclined Caregiver present providing support *Avoid bottle propping with pillow	Infant brings one or both hands/bottle to mouth while being held 0–3 mo reflex sucking 3–4 mo sucking becomes volitional	Liquid
4–6 mo	Sitting with caregiver support or supported in a highchair	Introduce spoon feeding/fed by caregiver Improved hand/eye coordination Holds objects and brings to the mouth	Cereal, smooth purees (similar to stage 1 baby foods)
6–8 mo	Sitting in highchair with tray and foot support	Opens mouth in anticipation of food Holds bottle with both hands Suckle transit pattern is used to swallow purees	Cereal, smooth purees, variety of pureed foods similar to stage 2 baby foods
8–10 mo	Sitting in highchair with tray and foot support	Infant holds and bangs spoon Can bring small pieces of food to mouth with a fisted grasp; uses fingers to help keep food in mouth Primarily fed by caregiver Emerging vertical (up/down) chewing pattern	Pureed foods, dissolvable solids, very soft solids
10–12 mo	Sitting in highchair with tray and foot support	Can bring food to mouth with finger grasp, reaches for spoon; introduce open, sipper, and/or straw cup for practice Controlled biting off pieces of food Tongue lateralization of bolus to the molars observed Vertical (up/down) chewing pattern	Pureed foods, dissolvable solids, soft solids
12–14 mo	Sitting in highchair with tray with foot support or in highchair without tray at the table with foot support	Beginning self-feeding with a spoon, gains skill with an open, sipper, and/or straw cup with two hands Vertical (up/down) chewing pattern	Pureed foods, dissolvable solids, soft solids, some solids
15–18 mo	Sitting in booster or highchair at the table with foot support	Child scoops food and brings spoon to mouth with some loss, continues skill development with cup drinking (open, sipper, and/or straw cup) Emerging rotary (circular) chewing pattern with open mouth	Pureed foods, dissolvable solids, soft solids, solids
18–24 mo	Sitting in booster chair at the table	Child feeds self with a spoon, uses cup independently Rotary (circular) chewing pattern present with intermittent open/closed mouth	Pureed foods, dissolvable solids, soft solids, solids, some mixed textures
24–36 mo	Sitting in a child size chair or a booster chair at the table	Child feeds self with little to no spilling, child uses a fork to spear food One-handed cup holding Rotary (circular) chewing pattern present with closed mouth	Pureed foods, dissolvable solids, soft solids, solid, mixed textures

utero by 7 to 8 weeks gestational age. Infants swallow amniotic fluid, and some infants begin sucking hands or fingers by 21 weeks of gestation.

For infants aged 0 to 3 months, sucking is reflexive. Sucking becomes volitional around age 3 to 4 months. You may begin to see signs of hunger by mouthing on fists or sucking on a pacifier. You will also see infants bring one or both hands to the bottle or to the breast while being held and fed. They need their head, neck, and body in a fully supported position, slightly reclined with the head higher than the body. The caregiver is present, providing the support and practicing cue-based feeding.

For infants aged 4 to 6 months, smooth purees by spoon can be offered. Determination of which month to specifically begin spoon feedings for infants is dependent on their current motor development and ability to control/support the head. Spoon feedings can begin when infants can sit in a supported seating system that provides head, body, and foot support without easily falling to the side and when independent head control is consistent. Even if infants cannot sit on their own, if they have good head control it is safe to begin offering smooth purees while seated in a supportive seating system such as a high chair. Caregivers should continue to follow cue-based feeding and never force-feed infants. When infants are enjoying feedings, they will look at the caregiver and open the mouth in anticipation of the spoon.

For infants aged 6 to 8 months, the clinician will begin to note increased interest in feeding. For bottle-fed infants, they may begin to hold their own bottle with both hands for the majority of the feeding with continued positioning support. They may begin to sit more independently; however, they continue to require support from a highchair. For infants aged 8 to 10 months, more active participation in the mealtime is typical. Positioning continues to be important throughout the infant's development. Infants should continue to be in a highchair with a tray and adequate foot, head, and body support. They will begin to reach for the spoon, holding it and banging it on the tray. They will begin to use a fisted/raking grasp, bringing small pieces of food to the mouth. For infants aged 10 to 12 months, you will begin to see improved hand-eye coordination during feedings. They will bring food to the mouth with a finger/pincer grasp and will continue to reach for the spoon. They can begin to hold the spoon and feed themselves while the caregiver remains the primary feeder with another spoon. For toddlers age 12 to 14 months, they become more efficient with self-feeding by spoon with less spillage at this age. Finger feeding continues to be the primary method for self-feeding. Straw drinking will develop and continued desire for independence during the mealtime is observed.

At age 15 to 18 months, toddlers will begin to scoop food with a spoon and bring it to their mouth with some loss. The caregiver should continue to offer a variety of purees, dissolvable solids, and soft solids five times per day. Some solid foods can be offered at this age as chewing patterns advance from a vertical (up/down) to an emerging rotary (circular) chewing pattern with an open mouth.

At age 18 to 24 months, chewing will be more consistent and will present as a rotary (circular) chewing pattern with a closed mouth. Cup use will be independent at this age, and efficiency with spoon feeding will have improved. The caregiver may begin to introduce mixed textures and consistencies, and the child's chewing will be able to support more advanced textures. Examples of food textures in each category are included in Table 65.2.

TABLE 65.2 Food Texture Examples

Liquids
Breast milk
Formula
Milk
Water
Purees (Smooth Purees Without Lumps or Bumps)
Stage 1 and 2 infant purees
Infant cereal
Smooth yogurt
Hummus
Dissolvable Solids (Foods That Can Melt in the Mouth and Do Not Require Chewing)
Infant puffs
Baby Mum mums
Bambas
Butter cookies/crackers
Soft Solids (Foods That Are Easy to Chew and Have a Consistent Texture)
Soft fruits (bananas, avocados, or canned fruits)
Cooked vegetables (carrots, sweet potatoes, peas)
Pancakes with butter and syrup
Cooked fish (not fish sticks)
Solids (Foods That Require Thorough Chewing)
Most meats (bacon, sausage, hot dogs, chicken, steak)
Fresh fruits (apple, pear, grapes, raisins, pineapple)
Nuts (cashew, peanut, almond, hazelnut, pistachios)
Breads, including waffles, bagels
Mixed Textures (Foods That Have More Than One Consistency)
Pizza
Lasagna
Soups (not pureed)
Sandwiches

At ages 24 to 36 months, children will begin to be independent using a spoon and spearing food with a fork. Full transition off breast and bottle to open, sipper, or straw cup should be complete.

SWALLOWING DISORDERS

Anatomy and Physiology of Swallowing

Swallowing is the semiautomatic motor action of the muscles of the respiratory and GI tracts that propels and transports food from the oral cavity, through the pharynx and esophagus, to the stomach. Swallowing includes not only food placement in the mouth and transport to the stomach but also allows for clearing the mouth and pharynx of secretions, mucus, and possible regurgitated stomach contents. Swallowing is complex in nature and requires coordination of 31 muscles, 6 cranial nerves, and multiple levels of the central nervous system, including the brainstem and cerebral cortex (Arvedson & Brodsky, 2017). The nasal, oral, and pharyngeal cavities as well as the larynx make up the upper aerodigestive tract and swallowing mechanism. These structures all work together in a well-coordinated manner to support normal respiration and swallowing. A detailed description of the anatomy for successful swallowing is out of the scope of this text; however, the reader is referred to excellent work on the subject collated by the Dysphagia Research Society.

Swallowing is divided into three distinct phases: oral phase (includes both oral preparatory and oral transit), pharyngeal phase, and esophageal phase. The oral phase is a voluntary phase in which an individual manipulates and prepares food or liquid to form a cohesive bolus that is propelled to the pharynx. The pharyngeal phase begins with the initiation of a voluntary swallow that propels the bolus through the pharynx. The exact anatomic location of where initiation of the swallow varies and can occur at the anterior tonsillar pillars, the base of the tongue, valleculae, or the pyriform sinuses. This phase is critical as the potential for aspiration is greatest in this phase of swallowing as precise timing and coordination of laryngeal closure is needed. Involuntary peristaltic contractions in the esophagus aid with transporting the bolus through the pharynx into the esophagus. The esophageal phase is also involuntary and involves movement of the bolus through the esophagus to the stomach via peristalsis. Once the bolus has moved through the esophagus it will reach the lower esophageal sphincter that must relax to allow food to pass through to the stomach. This sphincter will close once the bolus enters the stomach to prevent reflux or stomach contents coming back up when oral feedings are finished.

Dysphagia and Aspiration

Dysphagia is the impaired swallowing of liquids, solids, or even saliva secondary to dysfunction in the oral, pharyngeal, and/or esophageal phases. When dysphagia occurs, the precisely timed, coordinated, and synchronized series of events the body must perform to ensure a safe swallow are disrupted (Arvedson & Brodsky, 2017). This disruption significantly increases the potential for aspiration. For individuals with dysphasia there can be varying degrees of laryngeal penetration, and as a result the potential for aspiration also varies.

Aspiration is the inhalation of foreign material into the lower airway, which can be an acute event or a chronic recurrent syndrome and may occur during oral feeding as a result of dysphagia, after feeding during episodes of gastroesophageal reflux, or with insufficient management of nasal/oral secretions (Gosa et al., 2020). Chronic and recurrent aspiration can have devastating effects on lung development and pulmonary health. As noted in the chapter-opening vignette, coughing and choking when swallowing, wheezing, laryngeal gurgling/wetness, and recurrent pneumonias are strong clinical indicators of aspiration (Arvedson & Brodsky, 2017). However, for many patients, like RD, aspiration can occur without signs or symptoms (silent aspiration), and diagnostic evaluation is needed to further assess swallow function. Instrumental evaluation may be conducted to determine the nature of a swallowing disorder and to guide intervention, which may include possible modification of food and liquid consistencies or positioning. A videofluoroscopic swallow study (VFSS) or fiberoptic endoscopic evaluation of swallowing (FEES) is an instrumental assessment utilized to evaluate swallow function.

Instrumental Assessments to Evaluate Swallow Function

A VFSS is an instrumental assessment that provides visualization of the oral, pharyngeal, laryngeal, and upper esophageal structures through the use of dynamic video recording while swallowing barium contrast (Dodrill & Gosa, 2015). This assessment also provides information about the function and integration of all areas during the dynamic process of swallowing. The goal of a VFSS is to document whether aspiration is occurring, to determine the physiologic cause of dysphagia symptoms (aspiration or laryngeal penetration, nasopharyngeal backflow, swallow trigger, and pharyngeal residue), and then identify the most appropriate compensatory and treatment strategies to improve swallow function and ensure the safest feeding plan (Dodrill & Gosa, 2015). The limitations of a VFSS include small sample of oral feeding, which may impact generalizability, inability to identify structural abnormalities well, and need for barium contrast, which alters taste and is not always easily accepted.

A FEES is a procedure in which a clinician passes a fiberoptic endoscope through the nose into the pharynx so that the larynx, pharynx, and upper esophageal opening can be viewed directly from above. This also allows for visualization of the tongue base and soft palate; however, it does not provide visualization of the oral phase of swallowing. FEES provides information about events that occur just before and immediately after the swallow. Pharyngeal management of secretions and saliva can also be assessed. In addition, swallow function can be assessed with and without the presentation of liquids or solid foods as well as without the need for radiation exposure.

The esophagram or upper GI is a radiologic instrumental assessment used to evaluate the structure and function of the esophagus, stomach, and duodenum. Swallow function cannot be adequately assessed with the use of an esophagram or upper GI as this is not representative of a child's typical feeding. During this study children are positioned supine, and rapid ingestion is encouraged but limited swallows are actually observed.

The International Dysphagia Diet Standardization Initiative

Texture-modified foods and thickened liquids are utilized to reduce the risk of choking and aspiration for the approximately 8% of the world's population that experience dysphagia. "The International Dysphagia Diet Standardization Initiative (IDDSI) was founded with the goal of developing globally standardized terminology and definitions for texture-modified foods and liquids applicable to individuals with dysphagia of all ages, in all care settings, and all cultures" (Cichero et al., 2017, p. 293). The IDDSI framework consists of a continuum of eight levels (0–7), where drinks are measured from levels 0 to 4, and foods are measured from levels 3 to 7. The IDDSI framework provides a common terminology to describe food textures and drink thickness (IDDSI.org). Gravity flow testing with a 10-mL syringe is an objective measure that can be utilized to confirm the flow or textural characteristics of a particular liquid.

Management Tips

When a child is experiencing oral feeding difficulties as a result of dysphagia, intervention may be warranted. Intervention approaches may consist of environmental modifications, direct therapeutic techniques, or indirect therapy to support feeding as well as improve safety and efficiency. Postural or positional changes (head and body positioning, external support) may be one strategy used. Another strategy is diet modification, which involves altering the viscosity, texture, temperature, or taste of foods and liquids. Use of adaptive or assistive equipment and utensils can also support children with safety, efficiency, and independence when eating. Direct feeding therapy can provide specific oral motor treatment and help implement cue-based feeding or provide parent support for use of pacing strategies. Children may also need direct therapy to address sensory processing difficulties that impact safety, awareness, and efficiency when eating. For some children, behavioral therapy support may also be necessary to facilitate learning and implementation of strategies utilized in feeding therapy. Due to the complex interaction between dysphagia and oral feeding, it is important for there to be collaboration between a child's primary medical team and feeding specialists to ensure that a safe and successful feeding plan is established and that appropriate treatment and management approaches are utilized.

COMMON PROBLEMS

Feeding dysfunction is recognized in multiple medical diagnoses and has three broad causes: structural, physiologic, and experiential. Efficient eating requires coordination of multiple organ systems as well as positive experiences for learning in order to develop normally. It is important to remember that eating is reflexive at birth; however, subsequent learning must occur to replace integrated reflexes that usually extinguish within the first 6 months of life. (See Table 65.1 for a summary of feeding milestones.) This section is not intended to be a complete discourse on all the conditions when feeding and/or swallowing can be interrupted or impaired; however, the examples provided should prompt the reader to look for feeding and/or swallowing dysfunction in any child with medical complexity. Selective eating may occur with any of the conditions or experiences noted (Table 65.3).

TABLE 65.3 Impacts of Structure, Physiology, and Experiences

	Structure	Physiology	Experiences
Examples	Cleft lip and palate Micrognathia Dental malocclusion Esophageal stricture Esophageal atresia Tracheoesophageal fistula Pyloric stenosis Short bowel syndrome Congenital heart disease Tracheomalacia Laryngomalacia	Reflux Eosinophilic esophagitis Constipation Delayed gastric emptying Bronchopulmonary dysplasia Congestive heart failure Renal disease Liver disease Allergy	Lack of schedule and routine with eating Forced feeding Physical abuse Fear during mealtime Lack of control Food insecurity Sensory processing differences Missed opportunities due to medical or behavioral complexity
Problem	Inability to coordinate breathing with eating Inability to efficiently chew Coughing, regurgitation, or pain with swallowing Aspiration of liquids Need for surgical intervention	Aspiration of liquids Pain/discomfort Lack of hunger/satiety cues Inability to support needs for growth Allergic reaction	Meals are not predictable with a routine and clear roles Negative reinforcement at mealtimes Lack of experience
Outcome	Work of eating is too hard, uncomfortable, or impossible; selective eating develops, learning does not occur	Work of eating is too hard, uncomfortable, or impossible; selective eating develops, learning does not occur	Eating is seen as a negative experience to be avoided; selective eating develops, learning does not occur

FUTURE DIRECTIONS

International Association for Pediatric Feeding and Swallowing

In response to a desire for increased collaboration, raised awareness, and academic rigor in the field of feeding and swallowing disorders, the International Association for Pediatric Feeding and Swallowing was formed. This organization is unique in that from its inception a multidisciplinary approach was valued. While professionals from several different disciplines within health care frequently participate in the diagnosis and treatment of feeding and swallowing disorders, until recently there was not a professional organization that fostered collaboration between physicians and other clinicians. Further information can be obtained by visiting www.iapfs.org.

Video Appointments

The COVID-19 pandemic has challenged our health care system on many levels; however, concerns about infectious disease transmission spawned innovation in the field of feeding. Eating with others has been identified as a high-risk activity (Centers for Disease Control and Prevention, 2019). While data are just beginning to be published, families are willing to access care using telehealth, and there is evidence to support this treatment model (Clark, Fischer, Lehman, & Bloomfield, 2019). For some families, telehealth is preferred and even provides better service than in-person appointments. Telehealth eliminates the burden of travel, especially for families that live in rural areas (Pickler, 2021 unpublished data). We do have concerns about health disparities and whether the use of technology to provide care is burdensome for families who experience financial stress or lack access to adequate Internet service. Further research is needed to better understand the benefits and challenges of telehealth and how to eliminate the impact on patients whose families experience health disparities.

Research

Research in the field of feeding and swallowing is growing but lacks rigor. There are many unanswered questions with regard to assessment and treatment methods for both feeding and swallowing disorders. The heterogeneity of the patient population adds to difficulty when trialing interventions. In addition, many papers and readily available trainings focus on supporting best practice in the field that is primarily expert opinion and not based on modern accepted research methods. The formation of professional organizations such as IAPFS and the Dysphagia Research Society provide opportunities for clinicians to engage in interdisciplinary research and opportunities for presenting to multidisciplinary audiences. The translation of research into clinical practice will require improved funding so that collaborative efforts between researchers can progress.

CONCLUSION

Feeding and swallowing disorders represent heterogeneous types of dysfunction with many factors that contribute to challenges in these areas. Both feeding and swallowing problems in children can be thought of as symptoms of underlying pathology rather than pathology in their own right. In this chapter we have attempted to summarize normal development as it relates to feeding and to provide a framework for understanding where pathology can arise in structural, physiologic, and experiential ways while fully acknowledging that some patients will have challenges in all three areas that complicate developing skills for eating and drinking by mouth. Swallowing disorders frequently cooccur in children with feeding problems, and the clinician should be familiar with red flags that suggest when an instrumental evaluation of swallow function should be performed. Due to the complexity of issues in pediatric feeding and swallowing disorders, a multidisciplinary team approach is best for assessment and intervention.

REFERENCES

Arvedson, J. C., & Brodsky, L. (2017). *Pediatric swallowing and feeding: Assessment and management* (3rd ed.). Plural Publishing, Incorporated.

Centers for Disease Control and Prevention. (2019). *Activities and gatherings*. https://www.cdc.gov/coronavirus/2019-ncov/daily-life-coping/personal-social-activities.html#restaurant

Cichero, J. A. Y., Lam, P., Steele, C. M., Hanson, B., Chen, J., Dantas, R. O., … Stanschus, S. (2017). Development of international terminology and definitions for texture-modified foods and thickened fluids used in dysphagia management: The IDDSI framework. *Dysphagia*, *32*, 293–314.

Clark, R. R., Fischer, A. J., Lehman, E. L. & Bloomfield, B.S. (2019). Developing and implementing a telehealth enhanced interdisciplinary pediatric feeding disorders clinic: A program description and evaluation. *Journal of Developmental and Physical Disabilities*, *31*, 171–188. https://doi.org/10.1007/s10882-018-9652-7.

Dodrill, P., & Gosa, M. (2015). Pediatric dysphagia: Physiology, assessment, and management. *Annals of Nutrition and Metabolism*, *66*(5), S24–S31. https://doi.org/10.1159/000381372.

Dwyer, J. (2018). The Feeding Infants And Toddlers Study (FITS) 2016: Moving forward. *Journal of Nutrition*, *148*(3), S1575–S1580.

Gosa, M. M., Dodrill, P., Lefton-Greif, M., & Silverman, A. (2020). A multidisciplinary approach to pediatric feeding disorders: Roles of the speech-language pathologist and behavioral psychologist. *American Journal of Speech-Language Pathology*, *29*(2), 956–966. https://doi.org/10.1044/2020_AJSLP-19-00069.

International Dysphagia Diet Standardization Initiative. (2019). *The IDDSI framework*. https://iddsi.org/Framework

Shaker, C. (2013). Cue based feeding in the NICU: Using the infant's communication as a guide. *Neonatal Network*, *32*(6), 404–408.

Wick, M. J. (2018). *Mayo Clinic guide to a healthy pregnancy*. Mayo Foundation for Medical Education and Research.

Zucker, N., Copland, W., Franz, L., Carpenter, K., Keeling, L., Angold, A., & Egger, H. (2015). Psychological and psychosocial impairment in preschoolers with selective eating. *Pediatrics*, *136*(3), e582–e590.

66

Growth Faltering

Jennifer M. Rathbun, Annelise Brochier, and Deborah A. Frank

For additional material related to the content of this chapter, please see Chapters 15, 35, 59, and 65.

VIGNETTE

At age 14, Lisa lost her mother to breast cancer. At 17, she ran away from an emotionally abusive aunt and met Joe. She became pregnant by Joe delivering vaginally at 37 weeks, a 2.55-kg baby boy they named John. Lisa breastfed and was discharged with WIC (Special Supplemental Nutrition Program for Women, Infants, and Children) to a teen mother shelter. At 6 months, she "lost her milk," bought cheap formula, and diluted it. John became "congested" and "spitty" with itchy skin. Joe noticed that at 10 months of age, John was not bearing weight on his legs and brought him to the hospital. In the emergency room John weighed 3.86 kg, appearing cachectic. When Lisa heard "admission," she picked up John and ran. Joe and security stopped her.

Lisa stayed with John in the hospital living on juice and crackers available in the inpatient unit until the hospital's Grow Program consult team offered meal vouchers, starting a rapprochement between mother and staff. John was diagnosed with severe malnutrition, cow's milk protein allergy, atopic dermatitis, anemia, and biochemical rickets. Nutrition instituted extensively hydrolyzed formula, advanced to 28 calories/ounce with prescribed vitamin D and iron. Catchup growth was 60 g/day. At discharge, the Grow Program physician coordinated primary care, allergy, and endocrine clinics; monitored labs; and referred the family to WIC and early intervention. A social worker and nutritionist visited the shelter frequently with baby food, baby books, diapers, and a listening ear.

With monthly clinic visits, after John's body mass index (BMI) reached the 10th percentile he transitioned slowly to 20 calories/ounce formula, then to whole milk. Parents delighted in his walking, chortling, and mischief. He "graduated" from Grow Program at 22 months. Lisa said, "I thought people were trying to make me feel bad, but now I know you ask me what I think."

MEDICAL

Failure to thrive (FTT) is a commonly used but outdated term referring to young children whose growth is faltering. FTT is not a diagnosis but a symptom complex, the quintessential biopsychosocial challenge to developmental-behavioral practitioners. Assessment draws on all aspects of expertise in fields ranging from diverse medical and genetic conditions, subtle neurologic variations, nutritional assessment and intervention, developmental risk, and many psychosocial dimensions, ranging from social determinants of health (SDH) to parent-child interactions and mental health concerns. Focus on a single dimension is not sufficient to guide optimal diagnosis and treatment. Since no one provider can offer proficiency in all these domains, multidisciplinary team management is essential—whether from a dedicated expert team designed to focus on many children and families facing this problem such as the Grow Program described in the vignette or an ad hoc group of providers put together for an individual patient and family.

Historically, growth faltering was considered a manifestation of maternal deprivation, with little recognition of medical, nutritional, developmental-behavioral, or psychosocial contexts. The myth of maternal deprivation led to the classic but unhelpful organic-nonorganic dichotomy, which assumed that, lacking a major medical disorder, a child whose growth was faltering was by definition "neglected" with a subtext of blaming parents (usually mothers). It is now recognized that effective management requires evaluation and treatment along four dimensions: medical, nutritional, developmental-behavioral, and social-emotional. Many current authorities (Tang, Adolphe, Rogers, & Frank, 2021) replace the potentially pejorative diagnostic FTT label with growth faltering, which will be used throughout the current chapter. Similarly, rather than referring to multidisciplinary teams caring for children with growth faltering as FTT programs, we will use Grow Programs.

Though specialized clinics for addressing growth faltering exist under many names across the United States, they are not ubiquitous; thus the child's clinicians may need to assemble an ad hoc team to provide comprehensive care to patients whose growth is faltering. Evaluation should be conceptualized as a team effort from the first contact with the family. Joint interviews by two professionals (e.g., medical and social work or nutrition, or nutrition and social work) can be efficient if the number of providers in the room does not overwhelm the adults bringing the child to care. The first visit may take several hours. Families should be reassured that the interviewer will not disclose information to most external institutions such as Immigration and Customs Enforcement or to other family members or school systems without explicit parental permission. Information will be shared with other members of the Grow Program, and no secrets will be kept from other team clinicians. It is important to reassure family members that in the event reporting to a child protection system is legally mandated, such report will be promptly disclosed and discussed with the caregiver.

Families working with a multidisciplinary team may not direct disclosures to the professional in whose field the topic ostensibly belongs. Symptoms of allergic reactions or aspiration may first be reported to the nutritionist. Similarly, medically important information may first come to the attention of the social worker or mental health professional, while the medical provider may learn of stressors critical to the mental health clinicians. Close and ongoing communication between all team members will assure thorough information gathering and, ultimately, effective, coordinated care.

Growth faltering is a nonspecific indicator of almost every serious pediatric somatic health condition: congenital, acute, or chronic. The story of John illustrates common somatic health issues in a context of inequitable social conditions. The first task of the medical provider is to ensure meticulous review of the child's health history from the prenatal period to the current visit, including previous laboratory and diagnostic procedures. Boxes 66.1 to 66.3 summarize the key items of prenatal and postnatal history and physical exam that should be assessed and documented. Psychosocial issues potentially contributing to the child's growth faltering may emerge during the medical evaluation. These include illnesses of other family members, which may create an overwhelming caregiving burden in the home, jeopardizing the growth of the index child. In the same routine tone as the interviewer inquires about family history of celiac disease or early cardiac problems, the interviewer can ascertain a family history of substance use and mental health disorders and, as in the vignette earlier, document deaths of important family members from violence, accident, or medical causes. Traumatic losses during the caregiver's childhood and recent loss (especially during the pregnancy and life of the identified child and around the time of the onset of growth faltering) may elucidate possible triggers that contribute to the child's growth faltering.

Many common pediatric conditions may contribute to growth faltering, particularly if children do not have consistent access to attentive medical management. It is important for medical providers to be aware of the infection malnutrition cycle. Malnutrition increases children's susceptibility to infection and the severity of infections. Symptoms of infection (vomiting, diarrhea, loss of appetite, fever) accelerate weight loss. Inflammation associated with infection impedes efficient utilization of nutrients (Bourke, Berkley, & Prendergast, 2016). Immune recovery takes longer than nutritional recovery so that children who have resumed growth may relapse after developing another infection (Chevalier et al., 1998). Other common conditions such as asthma, enlarged tonsils and adenoids, food allergies, dental caries, human immunodeficiency virus (HIV) infection, cystic fibrosis, celiac disease, and sickle cell disease are also associated with growth faltering (Shahrin, Chisti, & Ahmed, 2015). The medical provider from the Grow Program needs to coordinate closely with the child's primary care provider and other subspecialists. It is critical that nutritional and medical recommendations from all health professionals are consistent. Assistance may be needed to facilitate access to health insurance and health care as well as transportation to appointments for the child and family.

BOX 66.1 Pregnancy and Delivery

Mother's Reproductive History and The Neonatal Course

Age
Gravidity/parity/abortions (spontaneous or induced), stillbirths
History of pregnancy with identified patient
Conception planned or unplanned
- Difficulties with fertility
- Conceived while mother using contraception
- Abortion considered

Mother's nutritional status during pregnancy
- Weight at conception
- Pregnancy weight gain
- WIC
- Hyperemesis

Mother's health habits during pregnancy
- Cigarette packs/day
- Alcohol
- Prescribed drug use (particularly anticonvulsants)
- Illicit drug use
- X-rays
- Occupational exposure

Complications of pregnancy
- Infections/high fevers
- Bleeding
- Toxemia
- Violence or trauma

Labor and delivery
Vaginal or cesarean
Anesthesia
Maternal complications
Neonatal status
Gestational age
Apgar scores
Birthweight, length, head circumference (parameters and percentiles for gestational age)
Mother and child separation
- Need for special care
- Duration of hospitalization for mother and child

Complications: Jaundice, respiratory, CNS, sepsis, necrotizing enterocolitis, neonatal opiate withdrawal syndrome
Early feeding difficulties
Transfusions
Eye examination
Hearing examination

CNS, Central nervous system; *WIC*, Special Supplemental Nutrition Program for Women, Infants, and Children.
Adapted from Frank, D. A., Blenner, S., Wilbur, M. A., Black, M. M., & Drotar, D. (2009). Failure to thrive. In R. M. Reece, & C. W. Christian (Eds.), *Child abuse: Medical diagnosis and management* (3rd ed., pp. 465–512). American Academy of Pediatrics.

BOX 66.2 Child's Family and Postneonatal Health History

Midparental height
Consanguinity
Heritable conditions
Immunizations
Allergies
Surgeries
Hospitalizations
Current medications
Review of systems
Timing of onset of growth faltering
- Weight loss
- Diarrhea/vomiting
- Dysphagia/choking
- Snoring, difficulty with tonsils or adenoids
- Recurring pneumonia, otitis, or sinusitis
- Painful teeth
- Loss of previously acquired milestones, seizures
- Thrush/recurrent monilial rash
- Atopic dermatitis, hives

Pets
Travel or immigration
Passive tobacco exposure

Adapted from Frank, D. A., Blenner, S., Wilbur, M. A., Black, M. M., & Drotar, D. (2009). Failure to thrive. In R. M. Reece, & C. W. Christian (Eds.), *Child abuse: Medical diagnosis and management* (3rd ed., pp. 465–512). American Academy of Pediatrics.

BOX 66.3 Physical Examination

Vital signs: Blood pressure if >2 yr old, temperature, pulse, respirations
Anthropometry
General appearance: Activity, affect, posture
Skin: Hygiene, rashes, trauma (bruises, burns, scars)
Head: Hair whorls, color and pluckability of hair, occipital alopecia, fontanelle size and patency, frontal bossing, sutures, shape, facial dysmorphisms
Eyes: Ptosis, strabismus, funduscopic where possible, palpebral fissures, conjunctival pallor
Ears: External form, rotation, tympanic membranes
Mouth, nose, throat: Hydration, dental eruption and hygiene, caries, glossitis, cheilosis, gum bleeding
Neck: Hairline, masses, lymphadenopathy
Abdomen: Protuberance, hepatosplenomegaly, masses
Genitalia: Malformations, hygiene, trauma
Rectum: Fissures, trauma, hemorrhoids
Extremities: Edema, dysmorphisms, rachitic changes, nails and nail beds
Neurologic: Cranial nerves, reflexes, tone, retention of primitive reflexes, quality of voluntary movement

Adapted from Frank, D. A., Blenner, S., Wilbur, M. A., Black, M. M., & Drotar, D. (2009). Failure to thrive. In R. M. Reece, & C. W. Christian (Eds.), *Child abuse: Medical diagnosis and management* (3rd ed., pp. 465–512). American Academy of Pediatrics.

A number of rare conditions, which are addressed elsewhere in this book, may emerge during the history and physical of a child presenting for growth faltering and will not be discussed in detail here. This is not to suggest that children and families experiencing these conditions do not warrant careful multidisciplinary assessment and care. The diagnostic, therapeutic, and prognostic issues of growth faltering, which these less frequent conditions pose, are well covered by others. They include genetic disorders and other chromosomal conditions (see Chapters 24–28), congenital infections (see Chapter 33), inborn errors of metabolism (see Chapter 36), fetal alcohol spectrum disorder (see Chapter 37), cerebral palsy (see Chapter 39), and autism spectrum disorder (see Chapter 41), among others.

Anthropometric Evaluation: Objective Identification of Growth Faltering

The most important tools for identifying growth faltering are growth charts for weight, length/height (height when child is over age 2 years), BMI (weight/length squared), and head circumference appropriate for the child's age, biologic sex, and gestational age. Accurate anthropometric technique is essential for informed diagnosis. Under 2 years of age, children should be weighed naked or in a dry diaper; above 2 years clothing should be light, and shoes should be off. A length board (rather than paper and pencil) should be used under age 2 years for length, and a calibrated stadiometer should be used for older children (Conkle, Ramakrishnan, Flores-Ayala, Suchdev, & Martorell, 2017). Sequential observations displayed on growth charts are optimal for diagnosis since they elucidate current growth parameters and allow evaluation of rate of growth. If there is weight loss or slowed weight gain, interventions can be initiated before the child's growth has deteriorated below some arbitrary cutoff. Growth charts should be requested from referring providers at the time of intake for care. Single measurements can be used for initial triage followed by ongoing documentation of progress by repeated measurements displayed on a growth chart. While traditionally percentile cutoffs have been used to identify growth faltering, the modern practice is to use standard deviation units (Z scores), according to the criteria of the American Society for Parenteral and Enteral Nutrition (ASPEN). ASPEN defines malnutrition as "imbalance between nutrient requirements and intake that results in cumulative deficits of energy, protein, or micronutrients that may negatively affect growth, development, and other relevant outcomes" (Mehta et al., 2013). The vast majority of children presenting for growth faltering are suffering from either primary or secondary malnutrition (Shahrin et al., 2015). Use and interpretation of growth parameters are dealt with in detail elsewhere in this volume (see Chapter 35).

Complex Consideration in Addressing Growth Faltering Following Low Birthweight

Unless specifically excluded, children born too early (<37 weeks) or born with low birthweight (LBW; <2500 g) are overrepresented in clinical populations of children referred for growth faltering. In Massachusetts with a LBW rate of approximately 7%, a statewide network of Growth and Nutrition Clinics found that of 2915 children presenting with known birthweights who enrolled from January 2011 to December 2020, 829 (28.4%) had birthweight below 2500 g, 260 (8.9%) had very low birthweight (<1500 g), and 145 (5%) had extremely low birthweight (<1000 g) (Massachusetts Department of Public Health, 2021).

In evaluating growth of children born preterm it is critical that the former preterm infant's growth be evaluated using corrected (postmenstrual) rather than postnatal age to avoid overdiagnosis of growth faltering. If growth faltering is noted after appropriate correction for prematurity, these children should be evaluated and never be dismissed as "just born small." Children who were born premature or small for gestational age (SGA; birthweight <10th percentile for gestational age), particularly those who were both premature and SGA and whose growth subsequently falters in extrauterine life, have less optimal developmental and behavioral outcomes than those who show anthropometric recovery (Casey, 2008). However, optimal rate of postnatal catchup growth is controversial for infants with LBW, whether preterm or SGA. The concern is balancing growth goals to enhance cognitive outcomes with the long-term cardiovascular risk of overfeeding and obesity. Sustained deterioration in growth velocity is always a matter of concern, and in the first year of life it has been linked to suboptimal cognitive performance in the short and long term (Belfort, Gillman, Buka, Casey, & McCormick, 2013). The long-term developmental-behavioral risks associated with preterm birth are addressed elsewhere (see Chapter 34). Monitoring growth of these formerly preterm infants requires transition between growth charts. Recently developed extrauterine growth charts for preterm infants, including the INTERGROWTH-21st Preterm Postnatal Growth Standard, can be used until 64 weeks postmenstrual age (6 months corrected age), at which time anthropometric parameters should be assessed on the World Health Organization (WHO) growth standards with continued correction for postmenstrual age until the child is 2 to 3 years old (Villar et al., 2018).

Laboratory Assessment

Laboratory assessment should be judicious, guided by identifying indicators of nutritional status and the few occult causes of growth faltering not evident on history or physical. Review of mother's prenatal labs and neonatal screening results can indicate need for further assessment of rare conditions such as inborn errors of metabolism, hemoglobinopathy, neonatal hypothyroidism, and cystic fibrosis. If the child was not born in a US hospital, these may need to be ruled out at initial evaluation. At presentation, routine evaluation may include the following: complete blood count with differential for anemia and other rare abnormalities such as immunodeficiency and malignancy; iron studies as iron deficiency is common in children with poor growth; chemistry panel to assess for problems, including renal tubular acidosis; celiac evaluation, including total immunoglobulin A (IgA) and tissue transglutaminase IgA in children old enough to have been introduced to grains, as celiac disease is increasing in prevalence and can present with only growth faltering; urine tests if there is concern for infection, glycosuria, or renal pathology; stool studies for giardia for children who are homeless or in congregate childcare and screening for a broader array of parasites in children from endemic areas outside the United States. In areas where elevated lead or decreased vitamin D levels are endemic these parameters should also be assessed. Untargeted screening for food allergy is not necessary (Tang et al., 2021).

NUTRITIONAL

The first intervention is to ensure access to foods for the child's medical condition as well as the whole family's consistent access to nutritious food. Box 66.4 outlines the initial concepts that should guide nutritional history and feeding observations. In all but the most straightforward cases of mild malnutrition a nutritionist experienced in pediatric care should be actively involved in evaluation and ongoing treatment. Breastfed infants with growth faltering should be seen by a trained lactation consultant. For older children, simple advice to prepare formula properly, schedule feedings (for toddlers roughly every 2.5 hours), discontinue distractions such as screens, limit duration of feedings to 15 to 20 minutes (since forcing a child to sit for hours "until she eats" is counterproductive), discontinue constant sipping on milk, and remove nutrient-poor beverages from the diet are important first steps. If these interventions do not rapidly restore growth, a nutritionist should be consulted. Home or virtual visits to observe feedings directly are very helpful and if recorded can be reviewed with parents as a way of coaching more responsive feeding behaviors (Black, Tilton, Bento, Cureton, & Feigelman, 2016). Home visits often also expand the clinician's understanding of the family's food resources and facilities for food storage and preparation and facilitate engagement of other household members in implementing enhanced care of the child. Home visits as occurred for John are often instrumental in building rapport and delivering concrete supports, including food, highchairs, measuring cups, and feeding supplies, which are often not otherwise available in the most impoverished households. When possible in-person or virtual visits to observe feeding should also be made to other locations where children routinely are fed, including households of relatives and home- or center-based daycare (Wasser et al., 2013).

Assessment should be sensitive to cultural variations in preferred diet and in expected age of emergence of independent feeding skills in young children, with particular care in counseling families who have recently immigrated to the United States. The goal is not to convert families from other cultures to a Western diet but to help them adapt their traditional practices and available and preferred foods to meet the child's current nutritional needs (Tang et al., 2021).

While prepackaged calorically dense liquids, widely advertised directly to parents, can sometimes be helpful, they should only be implemented after careful consultation with a nutritionist. Unless they are funded by health insurance they may be prohibitively expensive. Even if available on prescription their

BOX 66.4 Nutritional Evaluation Protocol

Interview

Feeding history adjusted for age
- Breast or formula
- Age solids introduced
- Age switched to whole milk
- Food allergy or intolerance
- Vitamin or mineral supplements
- Complementary or alternative dietary supplements

Current feeding behaviors
- Difficulties with sucking, chewing, or swallowing
- Frequency of feeding
- Who feeds
- Where fed (alone or held, with or separate from family, lap or high chair)
- Finickiness, negativism
- Perceived appetite
- Pica

Caretaker's nutrition knowledge
- Difficulties with English or literacy
- Religious or cultural beliefs influencing feeding
- Adequacy of developmentally appropriate nutrition information
- Unusual dietary belief (food fad constraints on permitted foods): Are some foods perceived as dangerous?

Adequacy of financial resources for food purchase
- Supplemental Nutrition Assistance Program (SNAP, formerly Food Stamps): How much/month for how many people?
- Special Supplemental Nutrition Program for Women, Infants and Children
- Adequacy of earned income
- Benefits: TANF, SSI
- Recent change in food budget (cuts or increases in benefits, new mouths to feed, job gain or loss)
- Family's knowledge of how to budget food purchasing

Material resources for food preparation and storage
- Refrigeration
- Cooking facilities
- Running water

Food frequency, 24-hour dietary recall: Was yesterday typical?

SSI, Supplemental Security Income; *TANF*, Transitional Aid to Needy Families; *WIC*, Special Supplemental Nutrition Program for Women, Infants and Children.

Adapted from Frank, D. A., Blenner, S., Wilbur, M. A., Black, M. M., & Drotar, D. (2009). Failure to thrive. In R. M. Reece, & C. W. Christian (Eds.), *Child abuse: Medical diagnosis and management* (3rd ed., pp. 465–512). American Academy of Pediatrics.

use should be as a scheduled supplement after meals rather than a meal replacement or appetite may be further suppressed. A multivitamin with iron and zinc should be prescribed routinely. If indicated by deficiencies noted in laboratory measures, therapeutic (rather than maintenance) doses of iron and vitamin D should be provided, as in the case of John. Diagnosing and treating feeding difficulties, including aspiration, neuromotor or neurosensory dysfunction, or behavioral manifestations, are covered elsewhere in this text (see Chapter 65).

The goals of nutritional intervention are first catchup growth (gains in weight, length, and weight/length or BMI at a rate faster than that expected for chronologic age) and then maintenance of an age-appropriate growth trajectory on an obtainable diet once the child is adequately nutritionally replete to reach the potential for linear growth and sustain immune function, bone health, and cognitive and academic outcomes. Studies have shown immune function may not fully recover in formerly malnourished children until weight/length or BMI approximates the 10th percentile (Z score −1.28) (Chevalier et al., 1998). The anthropometric threshold for developmental-behavioral recovery is not known.

DEVELOPMENTAL-BEHAVIORAL DYSFUNCTION

Growth faltering can be simultaneously a cause and a consequence of developmental-behavioral dysfunction. Among children with developmental disorders there is a high incidence of feeding disorders and slow weight gain. Primary developmental factors such as sensorimotor oral dysfunction and neurologic conditions such as cerebral palsy may cause difficulty coordinating breathing, sucking, and swallowing, resulting in suboptimal nutrition intake (Malone, Sharif, & Glennon-Slattery, 2016). Conversely, growth faltering can result in developmental delays. When identified with growth faltering, children often show lags in motor and verbal domains, but it is important not to make predictions about long-term outcomes until reassessment after nutritional and health status has improved.

Research on chronic nutritional deprivation (stunting) in low- and middle-income countries (LMIC) indicates that height-for-age Z scores (HAZ) during the first 2 years of life are positively associated with gross motor scores and cognitive scores among children less than 12 years of age (Sudfeld et al., 2015). Early nutritional deprivation (<5 years of age) has the most profound and lasting effects on physical development, literacy/numeracy development, and learning (Perkins et al., 2017). Though larger in LMIC, residual IQ differences between children with and without growth faltering are small; however, in both settings early life malnutrition has a demonstrated impact on socioemotional development (Larson-Nath & Biank, 2016), including increasing the risk for attention-deficit/hyperactivity disorder, behavioral difficulties, and other outcomes (e.g., depression and school failure). Evidence suggests that these problems may persist through adolescence and adulthood (Galler et al., 2012a, 2012b; Waber et al., 2011).

While many children make remarkable developmental progress with growth recovery, medical/nutritional interventions are usually necessary but not sufficient; involvement of sustained, age-appropriate developmental-behavioral interventions, whether offered through home visits or center-based sessions, are critical to enhance the child's capacity to reach developmental potential (Grantham-McGregor et al., 2020; Hurley, Yousafzai, & Lopez-Boo, 2016). Early nutritional supplementation linked with developmental interventions improves trajectories of motor, cognitive, and psychosocial development, and children able to recover from growth delays experience smaller cognitive deficits in adolescence than those for whom growth faltering persists (Fink & Rockers, 2014; Perkins et al., 2017).

Even children who make good progress may remain at increased risk of developmental-behavioral challenges when they encounter the structured demands of formal education. Children who experienced growth faltering in early life should be reassessed at school entry to identify whether there are special education needs, which may be less attributable to IQ differences than to attention, behavioral modulation, and affect (Larson-Nath & Biank, 2016).

SOCIAL-EMOTIONAL

Social Determinants of Health in Growth Faltering

Not all children with growth faltering are from impoverished families, but poverty is the greatest psychosocial predictor of growth faltering. Multiple hardships stress caregivers in poverty and impede their emotional wellbeing and pragmatic access to resources for meeting their child's needs. SDH, defined as the conditions in which people are born, live, grow, and age (WHO, 2010), are often crucial risks for growth faltering. Adverse SDH include food insecurity, housing instability, and energy insecurity, which are often manifestations of more distal factors, including underemployment and structural racism. These may cause or interact with other etiologies of FTT to exacerbate children's growth faltering. Rapidly addressing food insecurity, an issue that has become ever more salient with the COVID-19 crisis, is often a crucial prerequisite to successful treatment of growth faltering. Other areas of deprivation must also be addressed.

Effectively addressing growth faltering demands first identifying any social risks a family experiences through systematic SDH screening and/or social work assessments. Second, clinical care teams must partner with families to address their priorities; engaging and involving families in decisions about their child's care boosts self-efficacy and facilitates social needs–informed care.

Clinical care teams, of which community navigators may be invaluable members, should identify resources at multiple levels and support families in accessing them. Nutritional resources include government-level nutrition assistance programs, such as the Supplemental Nutrition Assistance Program (SNAP) and WIC—both of which are associated with improved growth and development of young children (Ettinger de Cuba et al., 2019). Other programs include the National School Lunch Program and School Breakfast Program, as well as national, state, and local organizations offering services such as food vouchers and food pantries. Some medical centers provide their own food pantries or raise charitable dollars for supermarket vouchers.

Other social risks particularly relevant to growth faltering include housing instability, energy insecurity, parents' underemployment, and multiple demands on mothers' caregiving who, in addition to caring for a child with growth faltering, might also care for other children, partners, or older family members. Each of these social risks contributes to family stress and financial strain, which in turn may exacerbate growth problems in children. Enrollment in rental assistance programs through the Department of Housing and Urban Development (HUD), including subsidized housing, public housing, and the housing choice voucher program (Section 8), may provide lasting housing stability. The Low Income Home Energy Assistance Program (LIHEAP) as well as local and national organizations (faith-based and otherwise) help low-income families pay for winter heat, summer cooling, and electricity. Head Start and Early Head Start programs, administered through by the Department of Health and Human Services, provide quality childcare and nutrition to income-eligible families. Among young children, housing insecurity is associated with lower HAZ and higher developmental risk (Cutts et al., 2011); however, children of low-income families receiving public housing subsidies have demonstrably higher HAZ compared to those not receiving housing subsidies (Meyers et al., 2005). Additionally, children in households receiving assistance from LIHEAP are at decreased risk of undernutrition (Frank et al., 2006). The reduction in families' financial strain and corresponding positive impact of these government programs on children's growth is only experienced by families able to enroll in them; the support of clinical care teams in linking families to adequate resources is imperative. Notably, the complex relationships between food, housing, and energy security indicate holistic interventions aimed at addressing multiple types of economic hardship may be most effective (Lee, Zhao, Reesor-Oyer, Cepni, & Hernandez, 2021).

In the vignette John's improved medical and nutritional outcomes might have been fleeting if not for concomitant intervention on the social dimensions of his case. Rather than merely identifying John's allergy to cow's milk protein, the Grow Program facilitated Lisa's reenrollment in WIC with appropriate substitutions for a milk-free diet. The social worker helped her enroll in SNAP and apply for subsidized housing so that she could transition out of the shelter and secure more stable housing for her family. John was enrolled on a waiting list for Early Head Start and provided Early Intervention visits.

Child Protection Considerations in Growth Faltering and Indications for Hospitalization

Inability of parents to provide children with adequate nutrition as a result of poverty should not be conflated with child neglect or abuse (Black et al., 2006). Child abuse, including medical child abuse by food withholding, is a rare but potentially lethal cause of growth faltering (Kellogg & Lukefahr, 2005; Mash, Frazier, Nowacki, Worley, & Goldfarb, 2011). Other clinical concerns that may necessitate the involvement of Child Protective Services in the treatment of growth faltering include nonaccidental trauma or situations in which caregivers cannot provide or sustain needed outpatient interventions for their children because of untreated severe psychiatric illness, including substance use disorders or profound cognitive disability without adequate supports (Tang et al., 2021).

While hospitalization is indicated if the severity of malnutrition or associated medical conditions warrants, hospitalization for the purposes of comparing preadmission weight gain to in-hospital weight gain should not be used as a diagnostic method to determine whether growth faltering reflects neglect. One prospective study of children hospitalized for growth faltering found that most children, whether or not they had a serious organic condition, displayed improved weight gain. In-hospital weight gain has not been found to be specific for differentiating neglect from other etiologies (Larson-Nath, St. Clair, & Goday, 2018; Puls et al., 2018).

Psychiatry/Mental Health Support

With today's nuanced understanding of the many mental health factors contributing to growth faltering, mental health professionals (psychiatrists, psychologists, and psychiatric social workers) play vital roles on the treatment team. Key assessments include parents' mental health and family history of major mental illness, including substance use and eating disorders such as avoidant/restrictive food intake disorder (ARFID; in *Diagnostic and Statistical Manual of Mental Disorders,* fifth edition) (American Psychiatric Association, 2013; Chatoor, Begtrup, & Lucarelli, 2020; Katzman, Norris, & Zucker, 2019). Careful attention should be paid to psychosocial history of loss and trauma, current marital discord, multiple caregiving burdens, and the parents' level of trust in professional health providers. It is important to acknowledge the child's role in maladaptive interactions, exacerbated by the central nervous system impact of malnutrition and the discomfort of complicating medical conditions, including blunted responsiveness, lethargy, irritability, behavioral feeding disorder, and bonding difficulties. Selma Fraiberg wrote of "ghosts in the nursery," referring to memories/traumas in the caregiver that consciously or unconsciously affect the parents' interactions with their infant (Fraiberg, 1980; Fraiberg, Adelson, & Shapiro, 1975). Fraiberg asked parents, in their infant's presence, what their infant's cries, resistance to feeding, or other caretaking demands brought up for them. She worked with parents to first identify their ghosts, then own them and focus on meeting their infant's needs.

Formal psychiatric evaluation of parents, siblings, and the parent-child dyad may be necessary if complex mental health issues emerge that exceed the capacity of the core team to elucidate and treat. There may also be others in the family network whose mental health condition is disrupting the care of the identified patient. To provide this evaluation, mental health professionals should be rapidly available on site, and in coscheduled appointments with the Grow Program. They should be introduced to parents as integral members of the clinical team.

Mental health experts can offer critical support to the team as well. Helping children and families under great stress is emotionally depleting and often overwhelming. Progress may be slow and difficult, triggering distressing responses in the professionals involved. Case meetings with mental health consultants can offer time for the team to reassess and review, heal disagreements, and emotionally refuel.

CONCLUSION

Weight faltering, formerly termed "Failure to Thrive," is not a diagnosis but a symptom, the final common pathway of complex interactions among medical, developmental-behavioral, nutritional, and psychosocial factors (including social determinants of health and family medical and mental health conditions). The organic/not organic dichotomy is not useful. Effective diagnostic and therapeutic approaches are multidisciplinary, allied with families, and sustained over time.

REFERENCES

American Psychiatric Association. (2013). *Diagnostic and statistical manual of mental disorders* (5th ed.). https://doi.org/10.1176/appi.books.9780890425596

Belfort, M. B., Gillman, M. W., Buka, S. L., Casey, P. H., & McCormick, M. C. (2013). Preterm infant linear growth and adiposity gain: Trade-offs for later weight status and intelligence quotient. *Journal of Pediatrics, 163*(6), 1564–1569.e2. https://doi.org/10.1016/j.jpeds.2013.06.032

Black, M. M., Dubowitz, H., Casey, P. H., Cutts, D., Drewett, R. F., Drotar, D., ... Wright, C. M. (2006). Failure to thrive as distinct from child neglect. *Pediatrics, 117*(4), 1456–1458. Author reply 1458-1459. https://doi.org/10.1542/peds.2005-3043

Black, M. M., Tilton, N., Bento, S., Cureton, P., & Feigelman, S. (2016). Recovery in young children with weight faltering: Child and household risk factors. *Journal of Pediatrics, 170*, 301–306. https://doi.org/10.1016/j.jpeds.2015.11.007

Bourke, C. D., Berkley, J. A., & Prendergast, A. J. (2016). Immune dysfunction as a cause and consequence of malnutrition. *Trends in Immunology, 37*(6), 386–398. https://doi.org/10.1016/j.it.2016.04.003

Casey, P. H. (2008). Growth of low birth weight preterm children. *Seminars in Perinatology, 32*(1), 20–27. https://doi.org/10.1053/j.semperi.2007.12.004

Chatoor, I., Begtrup, R., & Lucarelli, L. (2020). Avoidant/restrictive food intake disorder is more than one disorder: Diagnosis and treatment of three subtypes from infancy to adolescence. *Journal of the American Academy of Child & Adolescent Psychiatry, 59*(10), 353–354. https://doi.org/10.1016/j.jaac.2020.07.871

Chevalier, P., Sevilla, R., Sejas, E., Zalles, L., Belmonte, G., & Parent, G. (1998). Immune recovery of malnourished children takes longer than nutritional recovery: Implications for treatment and discharge. *Journal of Tropical Pediatrics, 44*(5), 304–307. https://doi.org/10.1093/tropej/44.5.304

Conkle, J., Ramakrishnan, U., Flores-Ayala, R., Suchdev, P. S., & Martorell, R. (2017). Improving the quality of child anthropometry: Manual anthropometry in the Body Imaging for Nutritional Assessment Study (BINA). *PLoS One, 12*(12), e0189332. https://doi.org/10.1371/journal.pone.0189332

Cutts, D. B., Meyers, A. F., Black, M. M., Casey, P. H., Chilton, M., Cook, J. T., ... Frank, D. A. (2011). US housing insecurity and the health of very young children. *American Journal of Public Health, 101*(8), 1508–1514. https://doi.org/10.2105/AJPH.2011.300139

Ettinger de Cuba, S. A., Bovell-Ammon, A. R., Cook, J. T., Coleman, S. M., Black, M. M., Chilton, M. M., ... Frank, D. A. (2019). SNAP, young children's health, and family food security and healthcare access. *American Journal of Preventive Medicine, 57*(4), 525–532. https://doi.org/10.1016/j.amepre.2019.04.027

Fink, G., & Rockers, P. C. (2014). Childhood growth, schooling, and cognitive development: Further evidence from the Young Lives study. *The American Journal of Clinical Nutrition*, *100*(1), 182–188. https://doi.org/10.3945/ajcn.113.080960

Fraiberg, S. (1980). Infant-parent psychotherapy on behalf of a child in a critical nutritional state. In S. Fraiberg (Ed.), *Clinical studies in infant mental health: The first year of life*. Basic Books, Inc.

Fraiberg, S., Adelson, E., & Shapiro, V. (1975). Ghosts in the nursery: A psychoanalytic approach to the problems of impaired infant-mother relationships. *Journal of the American Academy of Child Psychiatry*, *14*(3), 387–421. https://doi.org/10.1016/S0002-7138(09)61442-4

Frank, D. A., Neault, N. B., Skalicky, A., Cook, J. T., Wilson, J. D., Levenson, S., … Berkowitz, C. (2006). Heat or eat: The Low Income Home Energy Assistance Program and nutritional and health risks among children less than 3 years of age. *Pediatrics*, *118*(5), e1293–e1302. https://doi.org/10.1542/peds.2005-2943

Galler, J. R., Bryce, C. P., Waber, D. P., Hock, R. S., Harrison, R., Eaglesfield, G. D., & Fitzmaurice, G. (2012). Infant malnutrition predicts conduct problems in adolescents. *Nutritional Neuroscience*, *15*(4), 186–192. https://doi.org/10.1179/1476830512Y.0000000012

Galler, J. R., Bryce, C. P., Zichlin, M. L., Fitzmaurice, G., Eaglesfield, G. D., & Waber, D. P. (2012). Infant malnutrition is associated with persisting attention deficits in middle adulthood. *The Journal of Nutrition*, *142*(4), 788–794. https://doi.org/10.3945/jn.111.145441

Grantham-McGregor, S., Adya, A., Attanasio, O., Augsburg, B., Behrman, J., Caeyers, B., … Vats, K. (2020). Group sessions or home visits for early childhood development in India: A cluster RCT. *Pediatrics*, *146*(6). https://doi.org/10.1542/peds.2020-002725

Hurley, K. M., Yousafzai, A. K., & Lopez-Boo, F. (2016). Early child development and nutrition: A review of the benefits and challenges of implementing integrated interventions. *Advances in Nutrition*, *7*(2), 357–363. https://doi.org/10.3945/an.115.010363

Katzman, D. K., Norris, M. L., & Zucker, N. (2019). Avoidant restrictive food intake disorder. *The Psychiatric Clinics of North America*, *42*(1), 45–57. https://doi.org/10.1016/j.psc.2018.10.003

Kellogg, N. D., & Lukefahr, J. L. (2005). Criminally prosecuted cases of child starvation. *Pediatrics*, *116*(6), 1309–1316. https://doi.org/10.1542/peds.2004-2616

Larson-Nath, C., & Biank, V. F. (2016). Clinical review of failure to thrive in pediatric patients. *Pediatric Annals*, *45*(2), e46–e49. https://doi.org/10.3928/00904481-20160114-01

Larson-Nath, C., St. Clair, N., & Goday, P. (2018). Hospitalization for failure to thrive: A prospective descriptive report. *Clinical Pediatrics*, *57*(2), 212–219. https://doi.org/10.1177/0009922817698803

Lee, C. Y., Zhao, X., Reesor-Oyer, L., Cepni, A. B., & Hernandez, D. C. (2021). Bidirectional relationship between food insecurity and housing instability. *Journal of the Academy of Nutrition and Dietetics*, *121*(1), 84–91. https://doi.org/10.1016/j.jand.2020.08.081

Malone, C., Sharif, F., & Glennon-Slattery, C. (2016). Growth and nutritional risk in children with developmental delay. *Irish Journal of Medical Science*, *185*(4), 839–846. https://doi.org/10.1007/s11845-015-1377-3

Mash, C., Frazier, T., Nowacki, A., Worley, S., & Goldfarb, J. (2011). Development of a risk-stratification tool for medical child abuse in failure to thrive. *Pediatrics*, *128*(6), e1467–e1473. https://doi.org/10.1542/peds.2011-1080

Massachusetts Department of Public Health. (2021). Internal Bureau of Family Health and Nutrition Growth and Nutrition Program report. Unpublished.

Mehta, N. M., Corkins, M. R., Lyman, B., Malone, A., Goday, P. S., Carney, L. N., … Schwenk, W. F. (2013). Defining pediatric malnutrition: A paradigm shift toward etiology-related definitions. *Journal of Parenteral and Enteral Nutrition*, *37*(4), 460–481. https://doi.org/10.1177/0148607113479972

Meyers, A., Cutts, D., Frank, D. A., Levenson, S., Skalicky, A., Heeren, T., … Zaldivar, N. (2005). Subsidized housing and children's nutritional status: Data from a multisite surveillance study. *Archives of Pediatrics & Adolescent Medicine*, *159*(6), 551–556. https://doi.org/10.1001/archpedi.159.6.551

Perkins, J. M., Kim, R., Krishna, A., McGovern, M., Aguayo, V. M., & Subramanian, S. V. (2017). Understanding the association between stunting and child development in low- and middle-income countries: Next steps for research and intervention. *Social Science & Medicine (1982)*, *193*, 101–109. https://doi.org/10.1016/j.socscimed.2017.09.039

Puls, H. T., Plencner, L., Krager, M., Frazier, T. N., Hall, M., & Bettenhausen, J. L. (2018). The diagnostic accuracy of in-hospital weight gain for differentiating neglect from other failure to thrive etiologies. *Hospital Pediatrics*, *8*(10), 620–627. https://doi.org/10.1542/hpeds.2018-0035

Shahrin, L., Chisti, M. J., & Ahmed, T. (2015). 3.1 Primary and secondary malnutrition. *World Review of Nutrition and Dietetics*, *113*, 139–146. https://doi.org/10.1159/000367880

Sudfeld, C. R., McCoy, D. C., Danaei, G., Fink, G., Ezzati, M., Andrews, K. G., & Fawzi, W. W. (2015). Linear growth and child development in low- and middle-income countries: A meta-analysis. *Pediatrics*, *135*(5), e1266–e1275. https://doi.org/10.1542/peds.2014-3111

Tang, M. N., Adolphe, S., Rogers, S. R., & Frank, D. A. (2021). Failure to thrive or growth faltering: Medical, developmental/behavioral, nutritional, and social dimensions. *Pediatrics in Review*, *42*(11), 590–603. https://doi.org/10.1542/pir.2020-001883

Villar, J., Cheikh Ismail, L., Staines Urias, E., Giuliani, F., Ohuma, E. O., Victora, C. G., … Kennedy, S. H. (2018). The satisfactory growth and development at 2 years of age of the INTERGROWTH-21(st) Fetal Growth Standards cohort support its appropriateness for constructing international standards. *American Journal of Obstetrics and Gynecology*, *218*(2S), S841–S854.e2. https://doi.org/10.1016/j.ajog.2017.11.564

Waber, D. P., Eaglesfield, D., Fitzmaurice, G. M., Bryce, C., Harrison, R. H., & Galler, J. R. (2011). Cognitive impairment as a mediator in the developmental pathway from infant malnutrition to adolescent depressive symptoms in Barbadian youth. *Journal of Developmental and Behavioral Pediatrics*, *32*(3), 225–232. https://doi.org/10.1097/DBP.0b013e31820b7707

Wasser, H. M., Thompson, A. L., Siega-Riz, A. M., Adair, L. S., Hodges, E. A., & Bentley, M. E. (2013). Who's feeding baby? Non-maternal involvement in feeding and its association with dietary intakes among infants and toddlers. *Appetite*, *71*, 7–15. https://doi.org/10.1016/j.appet.2013.06.096

World Health Organization. (2010). *A conceptual framework for action on the social determinants of health: Debates, policy & practice, case studies*. http://apps.who.int/iris/bitstream/10665/44489/1/9789241500852_eng.pdf

67

Childhood Obesity

Carol Curtin, Sandra G. Hassink, Susan L. Hyman and Linda G. Bandini

For additional material related to the content of this chapter, please see Chapters 2, 13, 21, and 91.

VIGNETTE

A 13-year-old girl with current body mass index (BMI) in the 95th percentile takes sertraline for anxiety. She was a 1200-g, 29-week infant with a 2-month neonatal intensive care unit stay for "growing." She receives academic support at school for learning disabilities and prefers to play videogames indoors after school since being bullied by classmates. Her mother, who also has obesity, is concerned that the medication contributes to the teen's weight gain but feels it is helping the anxiety.

When the clinician discusses the teen's weight with her, she indicates that she would like to be healthier and agreed that she could try to drink flavored water rather than soda after school. She reports no opportunity for more outdoor exercise but was willing to try videogames that required movement before her next visit.

EPIDEMIOLOGY

As the vignette suggests, a child's weight status represents a complex interplay of predisposing factors—individual, familial, and social factors that need to be explored and understood by the clinician to provide helpful support and guidance to pediatric patients and their families. Awareness of the developmental tasks of childhood as they relate to food intake, physical activity, leisure-time pursuits, and the evolving role of parents and the child's growing autonomy over the cours of childhood and adolescence is key to providing appropriate guidance to children and families. Likewise, we must understand the social determinants of health and recognize that we now live in an obesogenic society—one that prompts food consumption and limits opportunities for physical activity, exerts strong forces on individuals, and contributes to the increased prevalence of obesity worldwide.

Obesity has become a highly prevalent condition in children and adolescents in both developed and developing countries. Over the past 40 years the prevalence of obesity has increased at least 10-fold worldwide (Larqué et al., 2019). In the United States recent estimates suggest that 9.2% of children younger than 2 years of age meet criteria for obesity, and the prevalence increases in older age groups, with nearly 14% of children ages 2 to 5 years meeting criteria for obesity, 19.3% of children ages 6 to 11 years, and 20.9% of adolescents ages 12 to 19 years having obesity (Ogden et al., 2020). Racial and ethnic disparities exist, with increased prevalence of obesity in Black and Hispanic children (Table 67.1). Race is often used to highlight differences in obesity prevalence between groups; however, a better way to identify obesity disparities is to identify the underlying social determinants of health, which drive inequities and obesity risk. These underlying factors include socioeconomic position (i.e., education, occupation, income, and wealth), health care access, physical environment, racism, disempowerment, stress, and cultural norms around lifestyle and health behaviors.

The etiology of obesity is multifactorial and complex. Obesity is a highly heritable condition, with estimates suggesting 40% to 70% heritability. Over 25 obesity susceptibility loci have been detected, containing genes that are implicated in the regulation of food intake, both via central nervous system action and in adipocyte function. Several gene polymorphisms have been shown to be associated with early onset of severe childhood obesity (Vogelezang et al., 2020). Parental obesity, particularly in mothers, is a risk factor for child obesity, likely through both shared genetics and a shared environment. Early risk factors include prematurity and low birthweight, gestational diabetes, the infant who is small for gestational age, and rapid infant growth (Larqué et al., 2019). Observational studies have suggested that breastfeeding is a significant protective factor for obesity in children (Yan, Liu, Zhu, Huang, & Wang, 2014). Poor sleep, including delayed sleep onset, reduced sleep duration, and poor sleep quality, has also been associated with obesity in children and adolescents (Kumar & Kelly, 2017). Of notable importance is the inverse relationship between childhood obesity and socioeconomic status, with higher rates of obesity in children growing up in low-income communities and in disadvantaged families (Baum & Ruhm, 2009).

Environmental changes over the past several decades have been proposed as contributory to the obesity epidemic. Shifts in dietary patterns, physical activity, and sedentary behavior have resulted in changes in energy balance, such that energy intake often exceeds energy expenditure, which over time yields excess adiposity. Increased consumption of sugar-sweetened beverages, more frequent snacking, more meals being eaten out of the home, and increased portion sizes are trends that appear to account for increased energy consumption in the population (Duffey & Popkin, 2013). At the same time, decreased participation in physical activity and

TABLE 67.1 The Prevalence of Obesity in US Children by Age and Race/Ethnicity from 2015 to 2018[a]

Age in Years	All Children (%)	Non-Hispanic White (%)	Non-Hispanic Black (%)	Hispanic (%)
<2 yr	9.2	8.8	10.2	11.3
2–5 yr	13.7	12.4	12.5	17.3
6–11 yr	19.3	15.5	22.7	28.2
12–19 yr	20.9	15.9	28.2	30.6

[a]For children <2 yr of age, obesity is defined as high weight for length. For children age ≥2 yr, obesity is based on body mass index percentile.

increased sedentary behavior, especially related to screen time (e.g., television or recreational computer use), have increased over time. A minority of children meet guidelines for physical activity engagement and recommended limits on screen time (Friel, Duran, Shechter, & Diaz, 2020).

Obesity in childhood is associated with obesity in adulthood. This association is greater when obesity is present in older children and adolescents. There are multiple physical, psychological, and psychosocial consequences of obesity in children and adolescents, including elevated blood pressure, insulin resistance and type 2 diabetes, nonalcoholic fatty liver disease, and polycystic ovary disease. Children and adolescents with obesity are also more likely to have elevated triglyceride levels and lower levels of high-density lipoprotein cholesterol. Obesity has been associated with early sexual development in girls and with musculoskeletal problems in both boys and girls, including joint pain, malalignment of the lower extremities, and slipped capital femoral epiphyses. The presence of acanthus nigricans, a darkening and softening of the skin and a marker of insulin resistance, is more common in children and youth with higher weight status. Childhood obesity is associated with anxiety, depression, lower quality of life, and poor self-image, and children with obesity are also often victims of discrimination, teasing, and bullying (Kumar & Kelly, 2017). The mental health sequelae of obesity are circular in nature, such that obesity is both a cause and a consequence of anxiety, depression, sleep disruption, being bullied or bullying others, and poor self-image.

ASSESSMENT

Screening and Classification

Classification of child weight status can be achieved by calculating body mass index as weight (kg)/height (m)^2. BMI measures are easy to obtain from children and adolescents and do not require specialized equipment. Although BMI is not a measure of adiposity, it is highly correlated with more direct measures of body fat in most individuals, although it is less useful in athletes who have increased muscle mass. Given the differences in weight and height among girls and boys throughout the child and adolescent period, sex-specific BMI-for-age percentiles are calculated relative to the 2000 US Centers for Disease Control and Prevention growth reference (Kuczmarski et al., 2002). Child BMI is classified as underweight (BMI <5th percentile), healthy weight (BMI 5th percentile to <85th percentile), overweight (BMI 85% to <95%), and obesity (BMI ≥95%). Severe obesity is defined as a BMI of 120% or more of the age- and sex-specific 95th percentile or an absolute BMI of 35 kg/m^2 or more, whichever is lower (Kelly et al., 2013).

The US Preventive Services Task Force (USPSTF) (Whitlock, Williams, Gold, Smith, & Shipman, 2005) recommends children ages 6 years and up be screened for obesity at all well-child visits and referred for treatment if their weight trajectories continue to rise despite supportive counseling. Routine monitoring of growth parameters, including BMI, supports active obesity screening in primary and specialty care settings.

Evaluation

The clinical evaluation of overweight/obesity includes a review of systems that covers common medical conditions that may also increase obesity risk, including sleep problems, gastrointestinal symptoms, eating patterns, neurologic disorders that might limit mobility, and symptoms of depression and/or anxiety. The history should include an assessment of the child's growth trajectory and opportunities for physical activity as well as family mealtime routines and foods present in the home. Clinicians should assess the extent to which the child may be consuming large volumes of sugar-sweetened beverages, foods high in fat and/or sugar, and/or low intakes of entire food groups (e.g., vegetables, meat, dairy, grains). Children under the age of 5 years who have severe obesity and characteristics of genetic syndromes (e.g., dysmorphic features) should be referred for further endocrine and/or genetic evaluation (Styne et al., 2017). Behavioral health screens should include anxiety, depression, and bullying. While the American Academy of Pediatrics (AAP) also recommends routine screening for depression in youth ages 12 to 18 years, the presence of obesity may prompt screening at younger ages.

A complete physical exam should be performed, including pulse, blood pressure, and palpation of the thyroid and abdomen, as well as cardiopulmonary examination. Examination of the skin, including infection in intertriginous regions and acanthosis nigricans, is recommended. Examination of the hips and knees should consider orthopedic sequelae of obesity such as slipped capital femoral epiphyses, which may present with symptoms of knee pain (referred pain from the hip). If symptoms are suggestive of hypothyroidism, thyroid-stimulating hormone should be measured. Blood glucose, lipids, and liver enzymes should be measured in all children with obesity (Barlow, 2007; Spear et al., 2007; Styne et al., 2017).

Special Considerations for Children and Youth With Special Health Care Needs

Overweight and obesity are more common in children and youth with autism spectrum disorder (Curtin et al., 2020), attention-deficit/hyperactivity disorder (Cortese & Tessari, 2017), spina bifida (Dosa, Foley, Eckrich, Woodall-Ruff, & Liptak, 2009), depression in females (Sutaria, Devakumar, Yasuda, Das, & Saxena, 2019), and other developmental-behavioral disorders (Halfon, Larson, & Slusser, 2013). Overweight in children and youth with these disorders increases their risk for obesity in adulthood and its associated comorbidities. The increased risk for obesity in these populations is due to multiple factors, some of which relate to the underlying conditions themselves, while some are common to multiple developmental and behavioral disorders (Tables 67.2 and 67.3). For example, children who have physical limitations and limited ambulation will likely have decreased participation in physical activities. Other children with disabilities may lack opportunities for active leisure and sports because they may require accommodations, supervision, and/or assistance to participate. The lack of active leisure opportunity combined with a sedentary lifestyle and increased screen time contributes to obesity. The use of edible primary reinforcers to teach skills may begin in early childhood and may be associated with persistent behavioral patterns and habitual use of food/snacks for calming. Food selectivity, common among children with developmental disabilities, may lead to diets low in fruit and vegetables and high in energy-dense foods. Medications used for challenging behaviors or seizures may predispose to weight gain (Curtin, Jojic, & Bandini, 2014). Sleep disorders may both be worsened by overweight and contribute to overweight as in children without special health care needs. In addition, there are disorder-specific reasons for obesity as a component of several neurobehavioral disorders with onset in childhood.

TABLE 67.2 Examples of Developmental and Behavioral Disorders Causal for Obesity

Disorder	Mechanism
Prader-Willi syndrome	Functional absence of paternally inherited chromosome 15q11–13, lack of satiety Short stature, hypogonadism, mild intellectual disability, skin picking, failure to thrive in infancy, small hands and feet, almond-shaped eyes 1/13,000–15,000 births
Bardet-Biedl syndrome	Autosomal recessive gene that impacts ciliary function, abnormal leptin activity, renal disease, intellectual disability

Despite the recommendations for using BMI to screen for obesity, there can be challenges to obtaining height and weight in children with some developmental disabilities. For example, children with physical disabilities may be unable to stand for a measure of height and weight. Recumbent length can be assessed if the child does not have contractures. If recumbent length is not attainable, arm span, knee height, or tibia length can substitute for height using specific equations (Samson-Fang & Bell, 2013). A wheelchair scale may be needed for some children. Furthermore, the usefulness of BMI in youth with altered body composition is unclear, and in these instances bone density scan measurements or bioelectrical impedance may be more reliable measures of nutritional status (Samson-Fang & Bell, 2013).

A comprehensive set of recommendations on weight management in primary care for children with autism spectrum disorder have been published, which provide suggestions for clinicians working with children and youth and their families, as well as other specialty care providers, schools, and allied health professionals (Curtin et al., 2020).

Parenting Styles and Practices

Parenting style is typically described as fitting in one of four general categories that reflect dimensions of child and parent control and responsiveness (see Chapter 13). An authoritative approach might shape child eating behaviors through structure, support, and reinforcement and is aimed

TABLE 67.3 Examples of Developmental and Behavioral Disorders Associated With Increased Risk for Overweight and Obesity

Disorder	Reasons for Overweight/Obesity
Attention-deficit/hyperactivity disorder	Challenges with participation in active leisure, increased screen time, impulsive eating, less interoceptive awareness
Anxiety	Habitual eating, medication effect (e.g., SSRI)
Autism spectrum disorder	Selective and repetitive eating, limited opportunities for exercise, increased screen time, medication effects (atypical neuroleptic agents)
Depression	Decreased interest in activities, psychomotor slowing, medication effects (e.g., SSRIs)
Motor impairment (muscular dystrophy, myelomeningocele)	Limited opportunities for exercise
Trisomy 21	Hypotonia, hypothyroidism, limited opportunity for active leisure

SSRI, Selective serotonin reuptake inhibitor.

at helping children to make healthy choices. An authoritarian parenting style might try to address child eating behaviors with rules and may use more punitive approaches. An indulgent parenting style may permit children to choose whatever they like to eat without setting limits, and an uninvolved parenting style may provide little monitoring. These latter two parenting styles have been associated with increased rates of obesity (Shloim, Edelson, Martin, & Hetherington, 2015). Parents also influence the child's mealtime and food-related behaviors through practices such as modeling and teaching their children about healthy eating and exercise behaviors, making certain foods available in the home, involving children in food preparation, monitoring or restricting the child's food intake, and using rewards other than food for good behavior (Musher-Eizenman & Holub, 2007; Larsen et al., 2015). Parent practices that are restrictive may be in response to the parent perception of child overweight rather than being a cause of overweight. How caregivers react to and influence child eating behavior is relevant to their role in the interventions used to address obesity (Shloim et al., 2015).

The Role of Pediatric Providers in Weight Management

Weight stigmatization presents significant and harmful risks to individuals with obesity. Some may believe that shame can be a motivating factor to encourage weight loss; however, research has documented an opposite effect. Individuals who experience stigma have been shown to avoid medical care, and paradoxically, gain weight, experience binge eating, and have less engagement in physical activity (Pont, Puhl, Cook, Slusser, & Section on Obesity, & The Obesity Society, 2017). Accordingly, encounters with health care providers must be experienced as supportive and accepting for meaningful change to take place. The AAP has called for physicians to use unbiased and neutral language to ensure that patients do not feel stigmatized during clinical encounters. Neutral terms, such as "weight" and "body mass index" are recommended; "obese," "morbid obesity," and "excessively fat" are to be avoided. Using people-first language (i.e., "patient with obesity") reinforces the notion that obesity is only a medical condition and not a primary descriptor of the individual (Stanford & Kyle, 2018). Clinicians aware of these dynamics approach the matter of the child's weight status with sensitivity and compassion and emphasize healthy lifestyles rather than the child's weight.

Pediatric providers should also gauge the child's and family's willingness and readiness to have discussions related to weight and attainable strategies related to eating and physical activity (see Chapter 91). Motivational interviewing, a technique that focuses on active listening, empathy, and eliciting the patient's own values and goals and capacity for change, has been shown effective for weight management in both adults and children (Gayes & Steele, 2014; vanBuskirk & Wetherell, 2015). The 2007 AAP expert recommendations (Barlow, 2007) contain specific suggestions for communicating with children and families that provide guidance for practitioners, which include ways to approach the issue in a nonjudgmental manner and employing reflective listening techniques with both children and parents to elicit their concerns, beliefs, and values. The USPSTF found that comprehensive obesity treatment was effective and consisted of counseling for healthy diet and physical activity and the use of behavioral management techniques for lifestyle behavior change. The USPSTF also found that frequent and longitudinal care produced the best outcomes. These interventions most commonly entail a multidisciplinary approach, which includes but is not limited to physicians, dieticians, psychologists, and trainers (Barton, 2010). In cases of severe obesity in adolescents bariatric surgery may be warranted, and appropriate referrals for evaluation and intervention should be made.

TAKING A DEVELOPMENTAL APPROACH TO PREVENTION AND TREATMENT

While the evidence for obesity risk factors in the domains of nutrition, physical activity, sleep, and stress does not change, there is a clear difference in how this evidence is translated into treatment across developmental stages from infancy to young adulthood.

Infancy

There is no official definition of obesity in infancy, but infants who have increased pre- or perinatal risk factors for obesity, are crossing weight for length percentiles, and/or are above the 95th percentile in weight for length are at increased risk for later obesity. Fostering healthy nutrition begins with encouraging breastfeeding, breastfeeding continuation, and responsive feeding (Spill et al., 2019). Responsive feeding is the recognition and response of the caregiver to the infant's hunger and satiety cues. Early transition to solid food before 6 months has been linked to later obesity, especially when associated with early formula feeding. Unhealthy food consumption patterns begin early in infancy, and parental role modeling of healthy eating and the creation of healthy home nutritional environments are important strategies for obesity prevention (Birch & Anzman, 2010).

Activity patterns begun in infancy carry through early childhood. The promotion of safe, supervised tummy time with the reduction of excessive time in confining equipment such as car seats, swings, bouncy seats, and strollers promotes not only activity but also motor skill development (Garrett, McElroy, & Staines, 2002). Parents often view television and screen time as educational, even for infants, and are surprised to hear that excessive media use is associated with obesity. Screen time is not recommended for children under 18 to 24 months with the exception of using screen technology (e.g., video chats) with family or family friends (AAP, 2016) (see Chapter 21).

There is an association in early infancy between short sleep duration and increased weight gain (Tikotzky, Har-Toov, Dollberg, Bar-Haim, & Sadeh, 2010). It is important to help parents ensure a safe sleep environment for their infants, keep screens out of the bedroom, and institute bedtime routines (AAP, 2014).

Food insecurity can negatively affect maternal infant feeding styles and contribute to weight gain. Children whose families have access to federal feeding programs (i.e., WIC and SNAP) are less likely to experience food insecurity and have improved weight outcomes (Mabli & Worthington, 2014).

Early Childhood

In early childhood parents and caregivers continue to be important role models for healthy eating at family meals and are instrumental in creating healthy nutritional home environments for children. Specific strategies include reducing or eliminating sugar-sweetened beverages and fast food, serving age-appropriate portions, and offering well-balanced scheduled meals and snacks. Parents may need specific help with picky eating, hunger, and tantrums around food, which may be barriers to establishing healthy feeding patterns.

In general, children under the age of 5 years are failing to meet physical activity guidelines (SHAPE America, 2009) primarily due to lack of time spent in free play and increased screen time (Xu, Wen, Hardy, & Rissel, 2016). Family walks, active games, and outdoor play, as well as family media plans, are all important strategies for improving energy balance at this age.

Short sleep duration in early childhood has been associated with obesity. Late bedtimes, variations in sleep time between weekdays and weekends, and poor sleep quality are all factors that influence sleep duration (Miller, Lumeng, & LeBourgeois, 2015). Bedtime routines, which include no screen time before bedtime and no screens in the bedroom, can help to increase sleep quality and duration.

Negative weight-based stereotypes toward children with overweight emerge as young as the age of 3 years, including weight stigma perpetuated by parents and other family members, teachers, health care professionals, and society at large, including the popular media (Puhl & Heuer, 2009). Parents and caregivers need to be helped to understand the importance of positive parenting on their child's self-esteem and long-term health (Pont et al., 2017).

School Age

Snacking can increase the risk of overweight and abdominal obesity in school-age children and comprises up to 25% of daily energy intake (Roblin, 2007). Parents can be encouraged to offer preplanned and scheduled snacks, composed of healthy foods, and eaten at a table and not in front of a screen. Total physical activity beings to decline in childhood from about the age of 7 years (Farooq et al., 2018), with youth in the most disadvantaged neighborhoods experiencing the biggest declines in physical activity (Clennin et al., 2019). Opportunities for increasing physical activity, including maximizing safe outdoor time and reducing sedentary time, should be identified at home, school, and in the community. Attention to inclusive neighborhood recreational facilities is especially important for children with special health care needs (An et al., 2017).

School-age children need 9 to 12 hours of sleep per night. Adequate sleep contributes to improved attention and behavior, learning and memory, and emotional regulation, in addition to reducing the risk of obesity (Paruthi et al., 2016). Keeping regular nightly sleep routines, including weekends, and turning off screens 30 to 60 minutes before bed with no screens in the bedroom can help improve the amount and quality of a child's sleep.

For children with overweight or obesity, weight stigma is primarily expressed as weight-based victimization, teasing, and bullying (Pont et al., 2017). This can lead to increased vulnerability to depression, anxiety, substance use, low self-esteem, and poor body image (Jensen & Steele, 2009). Pediatric health care providers need to ask about weight bullying, perform a behavioral health screening, and use a patient-centered empowering counseling approach to address the effects of weight bias (Pont et al., 2017).

Adolescence

Adolescents eat more meals away from home, and peer and social pressures often drive their food choices. Stress eating, loss-of-control eating, and binge eating are not infrequent and often include increased consumption of high energy-dense foods (Jääskeläinen et al., 2014). In addition, participation in family meals may decline, removing a protective factor for healthy eating (Neumark-Sztainer, Wall, Story, & Fulkerson, 2004).

Evaluation of adolescents' lifestyle behaviors should include assessing their time spent in sedentary pursuits, which often increase during adolescence and can include screen time, reading, homework, hobbies, and socializing.

Adolescents need 8 to 10 hours of sleep per night. Poor quantity and quality of sleep are linked to obesity and cardiometabolic dysfunction. The combination of evening use of electronic media, required homework, early school start times, and caffeine intake all contribute to poor sleep. Pediatricians should include sleep duration, daytime sleepiness and/or napping, weekend oversleeping, and need for assistance in waking in their sleep histories (Owens, 2014).

Clinicians should screen and counsel for psychosocial stress, depression, and anxiety, which can all contribute to altered eating and activity patterns that result in weight gain.

Young Adulthood

Young adults eat more fast food and drink more sugar-sweetened beverages, snack more, and consume fewer fruits and vegetables than other adult age groups (Allman-Farinelli, Partridge, & Roy, 2016), with the highest risk of weight gain of any age group. Factors that contribute to weight gain include a disinterest in a healthy diet; unhealthy diets of family and friends; social eating of fast food perpetuated by the low cost of unhealthy food and lack of time; and a lack of knowledge, skill, and facility with shopping, planning, and cooking meals. Interest and motivation to improve their health, weight, and self-esteem, getting support and modeling of healthy eating by family and friends, and possessing self-regulation skills all contribute toward healthy eating in young adults (Munt, Partridge, & Allman-Farinelli, 2017).

As in younger children and adolescents, adequate sleep is an important component of maintaining a healthy weight. The use of nonprescription stimulants and cigarette smoking contribute to poor sleep quality in young adults.

Patterns of physical activity and sedentary time vary in young adults; women, Black individuals, parents, and those with overweight engage in less moderate to vigorous activity compared to men, White individuals, those with no children, and those of normal weight. Individuals meeting criteria for overweight and those without children have been shown to have the highest amount of sedentary time. Patterns of high moderate-to-vigorous physical activity alternating with excessive sedentary time are not uncommon.

Understanding the role of cumulative and current stress is important in evaluating obesity risk for young adults. Adverse childhood experiences combined with a lack of protective factors added to current economic stress, educational burden, parenting concerns, and minoritized status can magnify obesity risk from unhealthy nutrition and activity.

CONCLUSION

Weight status and many of the factors that give rise to overweight or obesity over the child and adolescent period can vary and evolve over time. Clinicians who take a developmental perspective in recognizing the role that parents can play in helping to establish eating, activity, and sleep patterns early on, and being able to shift to working with the adolescent or young adult as they become more autonomous in establishing lifestyle patterns for themselves, can help prevent the development of obesity or provide support and guidance to those who have developed overweight/obesity. Having an appreciation for the sociodemographic and psychosocial factors that are associated with weight gain ensures that the clinician takes the whole child into account and can address the causes and consequences of obesity and its sequelae.

REFERENCES

Allman-Farinelli, M., Partridge, S. R., & Roy, R. (2016). Weight-related dietary behaviors in young adults. *Current Obesity Reports*, *5*(1), 23–29. https://doi.org/10.1007/s13679-016-0189-8

American Academy of Pediatrics (AAP). (2014). *Brush, book, bed: How to structure your child's nighttime routine*. https://www.healthychildren.org/English/healthy-living/oral-health/Pages/Brush-Book-Bed.aspx

American Academy of Pediatrics (AAP). (2016). Media and young minds. *Pediatrics*, *138*(5). https://doi.org/10.1542/peds.2016-2591

An, R., Yang, Y., & Li, K. (2017). Residential neighborhood amenities and physical activity among US children with special health care needs. *Maternal and Child Health Journal*, *21*(5), 1026–1036. https://doi.org/10.1007/s10995-016-2198-3

Barlow, S. E. (2007). Expert committee and treatment of child and adolescent overweight and obesity: Expert committee recommendations regarding the prevention. *Pediatrics*, *120*(4), S164.

Barton, M. (2010). Screening for obesity in children and adolescents: US Preventive Services Task Force recommendation statement. *Pediatrics*, *125*(2), 361–367. https://doi.org/10.1542/peds.2009-2037

Baum, C. L., & Ruhm, C. J. (2009). Age, socioeconomic status and obesity growth. *Journal of Health Economics*, *28*(3), 635–648. https://doi.org/10.1016/j.jhealeco.2009.01.004

Birch, L. L., & Anzman, S. L. (2010). Learning to eat in an obesogenic environment: A developmental systems perspective on childhood obesity. *Child Development Perspectives*, *4*(2), 138–143.

Clennin, M. N., Lian, M., Colabianchi, N., Kaczynski, A., Dowda, M., & Pate, R. R. (2019). Associations among neighborhood socioeconomic deprivation, physical activity facilities, and physical activity in youth during the transition from childhood to adolescence. *International Journal of Environmental Research and Public Health*, *16*(19). https://doi.org/10.3390/ijerph16193703

Cortese, S., & Tessari, L. (2017). Attention-deficit/hyperactivity disorder (ADHD) and obesity: Update 2016. *Current Psychiatry Reports*, *19*(1), 4. https://doi.org/10.1007/s11920-017-0754-1

Curtin, C., Hyman, S. L., Boas, D. D., Hassink, S., Broder-Fingert, S., Ptomey, L. T., … Bandini, L. G. (2020). Weight management in primary care for children with autism: Expert recommendations. *Pediatrics*, *145*(1), S126–S139. https://doi.org/10.1542/peds.2019-1895P

Curtin, C., Jojic, M., & Bandini, L. G. (2014). Obesity in children with autism spectrum disorder. *Harvard Review of Psychiatry*, *22*(2), 93–103. https://doi.org/10.1097/hrp.0000000000000031

Dosa, N. P., Foley, J. T., Eckrich, M., Woodall-Ruff, D., & Liptak, G. S. (2009). Obesity across the lifespan among persons with spina bifida. *Disability and Rehabilitation*, *31*(11), 914–920. https://doi.org/10.1080/09638280802356476

Duffey, K. J., & Popkin, B. M. (2013). Causes of increased energy intake among children in the US, 1977–2010. *American Journal of Preventive Medicine*, *44*(2), e1–e8. https://doi.org/10.1016/j.amepre.2012.10.011

Farooq, M. A., Parkinson, K. N., Adamson, A. J., Pearce, M. S., Reilly, J. K., Hughes, A. R., … Reilly, J. J. (2018). Timing of the decline in physical activity in childhood and adolescence: Gateshead Millennium Cohort Study. *British Journal of Sports Medicine*, *52*(15), 1002–1006. https://doi.org/10.1136/bjsports-2016-096933

Friel, C. P., Duran, A. T., Shechter, A., & Diaz, K. M. (2020). US children meeting physical activity, screen time, and sleep guidelines. *American Journal of Preventive Medicine*, *59*(4), 513–521. https://doi.org/10.1016/j.amepre.2020.05.007

Garrett, M., McElroy, A. M., & Staines, A. (2002). Locomotor milestones and babywalkers: Cross sectional study. *BMJ*, *324*(7352), 1494. https://doi.org/10.1136/bmj.324.7352.1494

Gayes, L. A., & Steele, R. G. (2014). A meta-analysis of motivational interviewing interventions for pediatric health behavior change. *Journal of Consulting and Clinical Psychology*, *82*(3), 521.

Halfon, N., Larson, K., & Slusser, W. (2013). Associations between obesity and comorbid mental health, developmental, and physical health conditions in a nationally representative sample of US children aged 10 to 17. *Academic Pediatrics*, *13*(1), 6–13. https://doi.org/10.1016/j.acap.2012.10.007

Jääskeläinen, A., Nevanperä, N., Remes, J., Rahkonen, F., Järvelin, M. R., & Laitinen, J. (2014). Stress-related eating, obesity and associated behavioural traits in adolescents: A prospective population-based cohort study. *BMC Public Health*, *14*, 321. https://doi.org/10.1186/1471-2458-14-321

Jensen, C. D., & Steele, R. G. (2009). Body dissatisfaction, weight criticism, and self-reported physical activity in preadolescent children. *Journal of Pediatric Psychology*, *34*(8), 822–826. https://doi.org/10.1093/jpepsy/jsn131

Kelly, A. S., Barlow, S. E., Rao, G., Inge, T. H., Hayman, L. L., Steinberger, J., … Daniels, S. R. (2013). Severe obesity in children and adolescents: Identification, associated health risks, and treatment approaches: A scientific statement from the American Heart Association. *Circulation*, *128*(15), 1689–1712.

Kuczmarski, R. J., Ogden, C. L., Guo, S. S., Grummer-Strawn, L. M., Flegal, K. M., Mei, Z., … Johnson, C. L. (2002). 2000 CDC growth charts for the United States: Methods and development. *Vital and Health Statistics*, *11*(246), 1.

Kumar, S., & Kelly, A. S. (2017). Review of childhood obesity: From epidemiology, etiology, and comorbidities to clinical assessment and treatment. *Mayo Clinic Proceedings*, *92*(2), 251–265. https://doi.org/10.1016/j.mayocp.2016.09.017

Larqué, E., Labayen, I., Flodmark, C. E., Lissau, I., Czernin, S., Moreno, L. A., … Widhalm, K. (2019). From conception to infancy—Early risk factors for childhood obesity. *Nature Reviews Endocrinology*, *15*(8), 456–478. https://doi.org/10.1038/s41574-019-0219-1

Larsen, J. K., Hermans, R. C., Sleddens, E. F., Engels, R. C., Fisher, J. O., & Kremers, S. P. (2015). How parental dietary behavior and food parenting practices affect children's dietary behavior. Interacting sources of influence? *Appetite*, *89*, 246–257. https://doi.org/10.1016/j.appet.2015.02.012

Mabli, J., & Worthington, J. (2014). Supplemental nutrition assistance program participation and child food security. *Pediatrics*, *133*(4), 610–619. https://doi.org/10.1542/peds.2013-2823

Miller, A. L., Lumeng, J. C., & LeBourgeois, M. K. (2015). Sleep patterns and obesity in childhood. *Current Opinions in Endocrinology and Diabetes Obesity*, *22*(1), 41–47. https://doi.org/10.1097/med.0000000000000125

Munt, A. E., Partridge, S. R., & Allman-Farinelli, M. (2017). The barriers and enablers of healthy eating among young adults: A missing piece of the obesity puzzle: A scoping review. *Obesity Review*, *18*(1), 1–17. https://doi.org/10.1111/obr.12472

Musher-Eizenman, D., & Holub, S. (2007). Comprehensive feeding practices questionnaire: Validation of a new measure of parental feeding practices. *Journal of Pediatric Psychology*, *32*(8), 960–972.

Neumark-Sztainer, D., Wall, M., Story, M., & Fulkerson, J. A. (2004). Are family meal patterns associated with disordered eating behaviors among adolescents? *Journal of Adolescent Health*, *35*(5), 350–359. https://doi.org/10.1016/j.jadohealth.2004.01.004

Ogden, C. L., Fryar, C. D., Martin, C. B., Freedman, D. S., Carroll, M. D., Gu, Q., & Hales, C. M. (2020). Trends in obesity prevalence by race and Hispanic origin—1999–2000 to 2017–2018. *JAMA*, *324*(12), 1208–1210. https://doi.org/10.1001/jama.2020.14590

Owens, J. (2014). Insufficient sleep in adolescents and young adults: An update on causes and consequences. *Pediatrics*, *134*(3), e921–e932. https://doi.org/10.1542/peds.2014-1696

Paruthi, S., Brooks, L. J., D'Ambrosio, C., Hall, W. A., Kotagal, S., Lloyd, R. M., … Wise, M. S. (2016). Consensus statement of the American Academy of Sleep Medicine on the recommended amount of sleep for healthy children: Methodology and discussion. *Journal of Clinical Sleep Medicine*, *12*(11), 1549–1561. https://doi.org/10.5664/jcsm.6288

Pont, S. J., Puhl, R., Cook, S. R., Slusser, W., & Section on Obesity, & The Obesity Society. (2017). Stigma experienced by children and adolescents with obesity. *Pediatrics*, *140*(6). https://doi.org/10.1542/peds.2017-3034

Puhl, R. M., & Heuer, C. A. (2009). The stigma of obesity: A review and update. *Obesity (Silver Spring)*, *17*(5), 941–964. https://doi.org/10.1038/oby.2008.636

Roblin, L. (2007). Childhood obesity: Food, nutrient, and eating-habit trends and influences. *Applied Physiology, Nutrition, and Metabolism*, *32*(4), 635–645. https://doi.org/10.1139/h07-046

Samson-Fang, L., & Bell, K. L. (2013). Assessment of growth and nutrition in children with cerebral palsy. *European Journal of Clinical Nutrition*, *67*(2), S5–S8. https://doi.org/10.1038/ejcn.2013.223

SHAPE America. (2009). *Active start: A statement of physical activity guidelines for children birth-age 5*. Society of Health and Physical Educators.

Shloim, N., Edelson, L. R., Martin, N., & Hetherington, M. M. (2015). Parenting styles, feeding styles, feeding practices, and weight status in 4–12 year-old children: A systematic review of the literature. *Frontiers in Psychology*, *6*, 1849. https://doi.org/10.3389/fpsyg.2015.01849

Spear, B. A., Barlow, S. E., Ervin, C., Ludwig, D. S., Saelens, B. E., Schetzina, K. E., & Taveras, E. M. (2007). Recommendations for treatment of child and adolescent overweight and obesity. *Pediatrics*, *120*(4), S254–S288.

Spill, M. K., Callahan, E. H., Shapiro, M. J., Spahn, J. M., Wong, Y. P., Benjamin-Neelon, S. E., … Casavale, K. O. (2019). Caregiver feeding practices and child weight outcomes: A systematic review. *American Journal of Clinical Nutrition*, *109*(7), S990–S1002. https://doi.org/10.1093/ajcn/nqy276

Stanford, F. C., & Kyle, T. K. (2018). Respectful language and care in childhood obesity. *JAMA Pediatrics*, *172*(11), 1001–1002. https://doi.org/10.1001/jamapediatrics.2018.1912

Styne, D. M., Arslanian, S. A., Connor, E. L., Farooqi, I. S., Murad, M. H., Silverstein, J. H., & Yanovski, J. A. (2017). Pediatric obesity—Assessment, treatment, and prevention: An Endocrine Society Clinical Practice guideline. *The Journal of Clinical Endocrinology & Metabolism*, *102*(3), 709–757.

Sutaria, S., Devakumar, D., Yasuda, S. S., Das, S., & Saxena, S. (2019). Is obesity associated with depression in children? Systematic review and meta-analysis. *Archives of Disease in Childhood*, *104*(1), 64–74. https://doi org/10.1136/archdischild-2017-314608

Tikotzky, L., Har-Toov, J., Dollberg, S., Bar-Haim, Y., & Sadeh, A. (2010). Sleep and physical growth in infants during the first 6 months. *Journal of Sleep Research*, *19*(1 Pt 1), 103–110. https://doi.org/10.1111/j.1365-2869.2009.00772.x

VanBuskirk, K. A., & Wetherell, J. L. (2014). Motivational interviewing with primary care populations: A systematic review and meta-analysis. *Journal of Behavioral Medicine*, *37*(4), 768–780.

Vogelezang, S., Bradfield, J. P., Ahluwalia, T. S., Curtin, J. A., Lakka, T. A., Grarup, N., … Felix, J. F. (2020). Novel loci for childhood body mass index and shared heritability with adult cardiometabolic traits. *PLoS Genetics*, *16*(10), e1008718. https://doi.org/10.1371/journal.pgen.1008718

Whitlock, E. P., Williams, S. B., Gold, R., Smith, P. R., & Shipman, S. A. (2005). Screening and interventions for childhood overweight: A summary of evidence for the US Preventive Services Task Force. *Pediatrics*, *116*(1), e125–e144.

Xu, H., Wen, L. M., Hardy, L. L., & Rissel, C. (2016). A 5-year longitudinal analysis of modifiable predictors for outdoor play and screen-time of 2- to 5-year-olds. *International Journal of Behavioral Nutrition and Physical Activity*, *13*(1), 96. https://doi.org/10.1186/s12966-016-0422-6

Yan, J., Liu, L., Zhu, Y., Huang, G., & Wang, P. P. (2014). The association between breastfeeding and childhood obesity: A meta-analysis. *BMC Public Health*, *14*, 1 7. https://doi.org/10.1186/1471-2458-14-1267

68

Urinary Incontinence and Nocturnal Enuresis

Jaclyn A. Shepard and Sean T. Corbett

For additional material related to the content of this chapter, please see Chapter 88.

> **VIGNETTE**
>
> *Annie is a 7-year-old female with daily symptoms of daytime urinary incontinence, frequency, and urinary urgency, as well as nocturnal enuresis (NE) several nights per week. Constipation symptoms were denied, consistent with the physical exam. An abdominal x-ray as well as a renal and bladder ultrasound were normal. There was no significant postvoid residual on the ultrasound. Given the constellation of symptoms without a defined etiology, a referral to an elimination clinic was initiated. Clinical interview revealed a psychological history significant for chronic worry related to urinary symptoms and in general, which was supported by elevations in the anxiety subscale of a behavioral screening questionnaire. The urology nurse practitioner obtained a uroflow electromyography (EMG) to better understand bladder and pelvic floor function during voiding. Results demonstrated incoordination of the bladder and the sphincter with intermittent sphincter overactivity and a dysfunctional voiding pattern.*

OVERVIEW

Daytime incontinence and NE were traditionally included in a spectrum of disorders known collectively as dysfunctional elimination syndrome. The terminology has evolved into the more descriptive and comprehensive term bladder and bowel dysfunction (BBD), which is comprised of lower urinary tract symptoms (LUTS) and bowel complaints. Common LUTS include dysuria, urgency, urinary frequency, hesitancy, daytime incontinence, enuresis, dribbling, straining, voiding postponement, and urinary retention. The International Children's Continence Society (ICCS) published an updated report on global standardization of pediatric LUT terminology with the goal of enhancing understanding, communication, management, and research across disciplines for providers caring for children and adolescents with various BBD disorders worldwide (Nevéus et al., 2020). Classification of LUTS is based on the relationship to the storage and/or the voiding phases of bladder function. Daytime incontinence and NE are among the storage subgroup and are common LUTS in youth.

According to the traditional classifications of the *Diagnostic and Statistical Manual of Mental Disorders,* fifth edition, and the *International Classification of Diseases and Health-Related Problems,* tenth revision, incontinence is characterized by an involuntary leakage of urine that occurs at least once per month for at least 3 consecutive months in children at least 5 years of age (American Psychiatric Association [APA], 2013; World Health Organization, 1992). It can be subdivided into continuous and intermittent. Continuous incontinence implies constant leakage of urine and is usually the result of congenital anomalies, functional loss, or iatrogenic causes. The focus of this chapter will be on intermittent incontinence, which refers to a distinct leakage of urine at various time points during either the day or night. Daytime incontinence is defined as leakage that occurs intermittently during wake time. Diurnal enuresis is an obsolete term. NE refers to intermittent incontinence encountered only during sleeping periods and is classified as either primary (when nighttime bladder control was never attained) or secondary (reoccurs after at least 6 months of continence) and monosymptomatic or nonmonosymptomatic (Austin et al., 2016). Both daytime incontinence and NE occur commonly in the pediatric population with approximately 10% of 7-year-olds experiencing NE and upward of 6% with daytime incontinence (Maternik, Krzeminska, & Zurowska, 2015; von Gontard & Kuwertz-Bröking, 2019). Children can experience these conditions independently or concurrently and with or without additional LUTS or bowel complaints, such as constipation.

Biobehavioral Framework and Contributing Factors

Pediatric BBD has moved away from psychopathology-driven conceptualizations to a biobehavioral framework given the physiologic and behavioral concomitants of the conditions (Friman, 2019). Consideration of behavioral or psychological factors is essential in the evaluation and management of daytime incontinence and NE, as evidenced by the established efficacy of multicomponent treatment packages (see Shepard, Poler,Jr., & Grabman, 2017 review).

Etiology and Correlates

A complex model of etiology supports the combined role of genetic, neurobiologic, and environmental factors in the development of daytime incontinence and NE. Approximately, 75% of children with NE have a first-degree relative with a history of NE (Friman, 2019), and concordance rates among monozygotic twins are higher than dizygotic twins (von Gontard, 2012). Linkage studies of NE identified several loci on chromosomes 12, 13, and 22 (von Gontard, Schaumburg, Hollmann, Eiberg, & Rittig, 2001), while a positive link to chromosome 17 was identified for daytime incontinence (Eiberg, Shaumburg, Von Gontard, & Rittig, 2001). Neurobiologic mechanisms associated with NE include reduced production of the hormone vasopressin, reduced functional bladder capacity, detrusor overactivity, and impaired arousal (Nevéus, 2017).

The association between NE and sleep is complex. Parents often describe their children as "deep sleepers" who fail to awaken in response to bladder signals, though empirical data are varied. Early polysomnography studies have demonstrated that NE can occur in all stages of sleep, and there is evidence that children with NE may have other sleep-related problems, including more fragmented sleep and higher arousal thresholds than peers without continence difficulties (Ma et al., 2018; Nevéus, Stenberg, Läckgren, Tuvemo, & Hetta, 1999; Wolfish, Pivik, & Busby, 1997). The genetic and neurobiologic risks are modulated by psychosocial factors, particularly for children with secondary enuresis (von Gontard, 2012).

Bowel function is closely related to bladder function and therefore must be part of the evaluation of children presenting with BBD. A thorough medical history and physical exam are vital and often all that is necessary to rule out organic causes of constipation. However, in atypical cases or cases refractory to conventional management additional diagnostic studies may be necessary. Rome III criteria are used to diagnose functional gastrointestinal disorders in children based on symptoms and symptom frequency (Drossman, 2006). The mainstays of therapy are discussed in Chapter 69 and include medications (e.g., maintenance laxation) and behavioral strategies (e.g., toilet sit schedule). Duration of these therapies is vital to the success rates especially when coupled with LUTS. Most children will respond favorably to conventional medical intervention, but patients who continue to struggle with infrequent, painful bowel movements and encopresis despite 6 months of medical intervention may require referral to a pediatric gastroenterologist.

Psychological and behavioral challenges are commonly associated with daytime incontinence and NE, but the relationship is better described as correlational rather than causal. It is estimated that 20% to 40% of youth with daytime incontinence and 20% to 30% of youth with NE meet criteria for a psychiatric disorder (von Gontard et al., 2019), which is consistent with some other chronic medical populations (e.g., pediatric chronic pain [Vinall, Pavlova, Asmundson, Rasic, & Noel, 2016], pediatric epilepsy [LaGrant, Marquis, Berg, & Grinspan, 2020]), but higher than the estimated 10% to 15% prevalence in the general pediatric population (Mellon et al., 2013).

Clinical Disorders

Externalizing Disorders

Externalizing disorders, such as attention-deficit/hyperactivity disorder (ADHD) and oppositional-defiant disorder (ODD), are common in children with daytime urinary incontinence and NE. ADHD is the most widely studied comorbid psychiatric condition in the continence literature (see Chapter 46). Across the NE literature, ADHD prevalence rates are highly variable (9%–53%; von Gontard & Equit, 2015). The highest rates were found in children with monosymptomatic NE (Okur, Ruzgar, Erbey, & Kaya, 2012), though in some cases this may represent selection effects. Despite the larger emphasis on NE in the psychological literature, population studies suggest that school-age children with daytime incontinence are at higher risk of ADHD than those with NE (Joinson, Heron, Emond, & Butler, 2007).

ODD is characterized by a pattern of angry/irritable mood, argumentative/defiant behavior, or vindictiveness (APA, 2013) and has garnered less research than ADHD on the relationship between incontinence and externalizing disorders. However, population study results indicated that nearly 9% of children with NE and approximately 11% of children with daytime urinary incontinence meet criteria for ODD (Joinson, Heron, & von Gontard, 2006). Children with incontinence due to voiding postponement have the highest rate of comorbid behavioral disorders, especially ODD (von Gontard, Niemczyk, Wagner, & Equit, 2016). Overall, children with comorbid externalizing disorders and incontinence exhibit poorer treatment adherence and worse outcomes, identifying this subset as a high-risk group (Niemczyk, Equit, Braun-Bither, Klein, & von Gontard, 2015).

Internalizing Disorders

Children with daytime incontinence and NE experience comorbid internalizing disorders, such as anxiety and depression. Approximately, 11% of children with daytime urinary incontinence and 8% of children with NE exhibit separation anxiety. Prevalence of other comorbid anxiety disorders in NE is similar, including social anxiety (7%), specific phobia (14%), and generalized anxiety (10.5%) (Joinson et al., 2007). The prevalence rate of depression in children with NE is estimated to be 14% (Joinson et al., 2007). Adolescent girls with NE may experience, or at least report, more depressive symptoms than male peers and, when NE persists into late adolescence/early adulthood, adverse psychosocial outcomes may occur (Yeung et al., 2004).

Developmental Disorders

Prevalence rates for daytime incontinence and NE are higher in children with autism spectrum disorder compared to typically developing controls (Niemczyk et al., 2015). In addition, there is evidence that developmental delay identified by 18 months of age leading to later-onset toilet training is associated with daytime incontinence and persistent combined wetting, though not associated with NE alone (Joinson, Grzeda, von Gontard, & Heron, 2019).

Biopsychosocial Factors and Quality of Life

Associations between difficult infant temperament and daytime incontinence during childhood have been established (Joinson, Heron, von Gontard, Butler, Golding, & Emond, 2008; Joinson et al., 2019; Vasconcelos et al., 2017). Compared to healthy peers, children with daytime incontinence also have higher rates of absenteeism and worse academic performance (Filce & LaVergne, 2015). There are associations between urinary incontinence and emotional distress and lower quality of life (QOL) in school-age children, with boys who have combined urinary and fecal incontinence being at greatest risk (Thibodeau, Metcalfe, Koop, & Moore, 2013). Complete remission, as opposed to reduced frequency, of accidents has a greater perceived benefit on QOL for the child (Ikeda et al., 2020). Qualitative data on QOL highlighted practical and emotional social consequences for the child (e.g., inability to play sports or participate in sleepovers due to accidents; embarrassment and anxiety related to stigma; Malhotra et al., 2020), as well as parental frustration about financial cost, increase in laundry, and perceived laziness of the child (Thibodeau et al., 2013). There is emerging evidence that adolescents who experience a delay in bladder control have poorer self-image and more difficulties in peer relationships at school than those who never experienced such delays. Additionally, children with a history of combined daytime incontinence and NE experience more difficulties in peer relationships during adolescence compared to those who experienced either daytime or nighttime accidents alone (Grzeda, Heron, von Gontard, & Joinson, 2017).

EVALUATION

Medical

A central component of evaluation is a thorough history and physical examination, which should include gathering information related to voiding, bowel habits, and dietary factors such as fluid intake (including bladder irritants, Table 68.1) and factors potentially contributing to constipation. Symptoms associated with lower urinary tract dysfunction, including frequency, urgency, voiding symptoms (i.e., hesitance, straining, weak stream, intermittency, and dysuria), and other relevant symptoms of bladder function (i.e., holding maneuvers, sensation of incomplete emptying, urinary retention, postmicturition dribble, various genital/lower urinary track pain) should be assessed (Austin et al., 2016). One should thoroughly assess for constipation by asking about stool frequency, history of large or hard stools, and a history of fecal soiling. The perspectives of the parent/caretaker as well as the child should be assessed as it is not uncommon to have discrepant histories, especially for older children who have more autonomy in managing their bladder and bowel function. Although a thorough history can be time consuming, brevity can limit the effectiveness of the visit and ultimately the management of the patient. Chronic urinary incontinence and the associated physical, practical, and emotional consequences are discouraging and frustrating for families. Therefore ample time with and validation from the provider is a key element in a thorough history. Not only does it foster strong rapport, which in turn facilitates the success of care, but a thorough history at the initial visit may obviate the need for additional testing and examinations.

TABLE 68.1 Common Bladder Irritants

Liquids	Foods
Citrus drinks: orange juice, lemon juice, others	Citrus fruits: oranges, lemons, grapefruit, others
Carbonated drinks: sodas	Sugary foods and candy
Caffeinated drinks: sodas, tea, coffee	Chocolate
Drinks with artificial colors: Hawaiian Punch, Kool-Aid, Hi-C, and others	Melons: watermelon, cantaloupe, and others
Milk and other dairy especially after lunchtime	Ice cream especially after lunchtime

Physical examination should include direct observations of the child specific to apparent holding maneuvers, developmental level, and behavioral issues. The abdominal exam should assess for palpable masses, bladder distention, or stool balls. Evaluation should also include a genital, anal, lower extremity, and lower spine evaluation to assess for abnormalities such as meatal stenosis, anteriorly displaced anus, toe walking, or spinal dysraphism.

Bladder and bowel diaries are invaluable as they relate to diagnosis and management, as an estimated 15% of children will become dry using diaries alone (von Gontard & Kuwertz-Bröking, 2019). For diaries to be most effective, the caregiver/child must adhere to recording symptoms on a daily basis, which can be challenging to maintain. Advancements in technology, including mobile applications, aim to improve adherence through accessibility, ease of use, and engaging, game-like content. There are many such applications currently available that are offered at no cost and are readily accessible (e.g., iUFlow, Pee Tracker, Urination Diary, Gogo Band Parent).

Finally, there are additional tests that can prove helpful in adjunct to evaluation and ultimately management, including urinalysis (infection), renal and bladder ultrasound (kidney and bladder abnormalities), uroflow +/− pelvic floor EMG (dysfunctional voiding), postvoid residual volume measurement, and abdominal x-ray (rectal distention/constipation). Invasive tests such as voiding cystourethrogram/contrast-enhanced voiding ultrasonogram, urodynamics, and spinal magnetic resonance imaging should be reserved for situations in which there is a high index of suspicion for organic uropathies, neurologic issues, or failed initial management (Maternik et al., 2015).

Behavioral

The cooccurrence of psychiatric disorders and developmental disorders with LUTS is described earlier. It is therefore recommended by the ICCS to provide systematic screening for behavioral and psychological symptoms, and to do so as early as possible to initiate timely intervention (Austin et al., 2016). Youth who meet criteria for a psychiatric disorder are at increased risk for nonadherence and worse outcomes if these disorders are not addressed, particularly by adolescence (Vasconcelos et al., 2017).

The increased prevalence of psychological and behavioral correlates in children and adolescents with incontinence underscores the utility of an interprofessional approach to evaluation and management. A pediatric behavioral health provider, such as a clinical psychologist, has extensive training in gathering pertinent behavioral, psychological, and developmental information during a thorough clinical interview. Parent- and self-report questionnaires, including those that are broadband and/or illness/symptom specific (Table 68.2), are often used in adjunct to the initial clinical interview. These measures not only assist with identification of current behavioral, psychological, and developmental concerns, but they also serve to provide quantitative data that can be used

TABLE 68.2 Questionnaires to Assess Lower Urinary Tract Symptoms (LUTS)

Instrument	Purpose	Self-Report (Child Age in Yr)	Parent Report (Child Age in Yr)	Total Items
Dysfunctional Voiding Symptom Score (DVSS)	Identify presence and severity of LUTS	Yes (3–10)	No, but self-report form includes one parent-report item	10
Dysfunctional Voiding and Incontinence Scoring System (Akbal)	Identify presence of LUTS	No	Yes (4–10)	13
Dry Pie	Severity of incontinence	Yes (5–12)	No	1-mo color-coded diary
Incontinence Symptom Index	Identify severity and impairment of urinary incontinence	Yes (11–17)	No	11
International Consultation on Incontinence Questionnaire Pediatric Lower Urinary Tract Symptoms (ICIQ-CLUTS)	Identify presence of LUTS	Yes (10–18)	Yes (5–9)	9—self 9—parent
Urge visual analogue scale	Severity of urgency	Yes (5–12)	No	2 scales

to inform treatment, track outcomes, and identify youth who would benefit from a comprehensive psychological evaluation. In clinical settings brief screening measures are often preferred due to shorter administration and scoring time and overall reduced patient burden. There are several symptom-specific questionnaires available that are used in clinical settings to identify presence and/or severity of LUTS in children (Table 68.2). In addition to symptom severity measures, the Pediatric Urinary Incontinence Quality of Life Score is a cross-cultural, symptom-specific questionnaire that measures the psychosocial and emotional impact of urinary incontinence in children 6 to 17 years of age. It is widely used and has excellent psychometric properties, though clinical cutoff scores have not been published, which may limit its clinical utility (Bower, Sit, Bluyssen, Wong, & Yeung, 2006).

More general, or broadband, questionnaires are helpful in screening for emotional and behavioral problems in children with daytime incontinence and NE. These measures are discussed in more detail in Chapter 82, but may include parent-report questionnaires such as the Child Behavior Checklist (CBCL) or Behavior Assessment System for Children. These measures have strong psychometric properties but are lengthy and may not be feasible to implement in some clinic settings. An alternative parent-report questionnaire is the Short Screening Instrument for Psychological Problems in Enuresis, which was adapted from the CBCL and is widely administered in clinical settings to screen for behavioral and emotional problems in youth with incontinence (Van Hoecke, Baeyens, Vanden Bossche, Hoebeke, & Vande Walle, 2007).

MANAGEMENT

First-Line Interventions

Interventions for daytime incontinence and NE are summarized in Table 68.3. As specified by the ICCS, behavioral or psychiatric comorbidities should be addressed concurrently (Chase, Austin, Hoebeke, McKenna, & International Children's Continence Society, 2010).

Daytime Incontinence

The first-line intervention for daytime incontinence is referred to as urotherapy and involves patient education, lifestyle modifications, skill building, a timed voiding protocol, and constipation management. At the outset of management, families are provided with education about typical bladder function, etiologic factors, and correlates of daytime incontinence, as well as treatment expectations and timelines (Chase et al., 2010). Lifestyle modifications, including adjustments related to adequate fluid intake and reduced bladder irritants (see Table 68.1), are necessary for improvement of LUTS and should be presented in a practical manner (Morgan, Leroy, Corbett, & Shepard, 2019). Skill building helps children learn effective voiding posture and hygiene (e.g., wiping, changing wet clothing). Timed voiding protocols, typically every 2 to 3 hours regardless of sensation to void, are commonly implemented to help set a daily voiding routine. Adjunctive positive reinforcement, typically via sticker charts, a token economy, or a novel potty watch that vibrates to alert the child at set time intervals, may be recommended to address adherence difficulties or to promote developmentally appropriate autonomy and increased self-efficacy. During this protocol, children are taught to double void (e.g., after voiding, return to the toilet a few minutes later to void again) to help fully empty the bladder. Constipation management is also a critical component of first-line treatment and is described in Chapter 69.

Nocturnal Enuresis

In addition to urotherapy, first-line interventions for NE include behavioral treatments using alarm therapy and sometimes medication. Behavioral interventions for NE have been extensively and rigorously studied (Shepard et al., 2017). Alarm therapy uses moisture-sensitive sensors that, upon the start of voiding, sound an alarm to awaken the child (and the caregiver) at the time of the accident, at which point the child then finishes voiding in the toilet. Over time, the child learns through behavioral conditioning to recognize the sensation of a full bladder and awaken to use the bathroom before the alarm sounds.

Alarm therapy has strong evidence of efficacy in the treatment of NE (see Shepard et al., 2017 review). It has demonstrated superiority over stand-alone medication trials and other therapies, qualifying it as an essential component of NE treatment. The course of intervention ranges from 5 to 12 weeks, producing a cure rate of up to 80% and relapse rates as low as 15% (Friman, 2019). Alarm therapy has also demonstrated positive psychological effects for school-age children, particularly improved self-concept, as well as positive parental perception of their children's behavior (Longstaffe, Moffatt, & Whalen, 2000).

Desmopressin (DDAVP) is an antidiuretic hormone that is often included in first-line management of monosymptomatic NE and works primarily by decreasing nocturnal urine production to a level that can be accommodated within the bladder (Nevéus et al., 2020). In the United States DDAVP is typically administered in the evening as 0.2-mg tablets and most often titrated in 0.2 increments to a maximum of 0.6 mg/evening until the desired effect is obtained. It is especially effective for short-term use. Approximately, 30% of children with NE achieve a full response, and 40% achieve a partial response; however, rates of relapse are high with cessation of the medication (Kuwertz-Bröking & von Gontard, 2018). There is a potential additive effect with the combined use of DDAVP and alarm therapy, though the added benefit is observed only while taking the medication and does not affect alarm efficacy long term. DDAVP is generally well tolerated, but rare adverse effects have been reported, including headache, abdominal pain, and emotional disturbances. Water intoxication and hyponatremia are extremely rare but potentially very serious; thus if DDAVP is used for treatment of NE, fluid restriction is important after taking the medication in the evening.

Second-Line Interventions

Daytime Incontinence

At times when urotherapy fails, pharmacologic therapy or a referral for pelvic floor physical therapy (PFPT) may be indicated (Table 68.3). Daytime incontinence is often associated with a variety of LUTS and/or NE, so combination therapy may be required. There are several classes of medications that have been used to address cooccurring symptoms. Anticholinergic (antimuscarinic) medications block

TABLE 68.3 Management of Daytime Incontinence and Nocturnal Enuresis

Daytime Incontinence	Nocturnal Enuresis
First-Line Management — Urotherapy	
• **Standard**	• Standard
Information/demystification, instruction to optimize bladder and bowel function, eating and hydration habits, documentation, and support	Information/demystification, instruction to optimize bladder and bowel function, eating and hydration habits, documentation, and support
• **Specific**	• Specific
Biofeedback, pelvic floor exercises, electrostimulation, cognitive-behavioral therapy, and psychotherapy	Alarm therapy, antidiuretic hormone (DDAVP)
Second-Line Management — Pharmacotherapy	
Anticholinergics	Anticholinergics
Muscarinic receptor agonists or inhibitors of acetylcholine esterase	Tricyclic antidepressants
Alpha-blockers	
Tricyclic antidepressants	
Third-Line Management — Surgical	
1. Intradetrusor or submucosal botulinum toxin injections	2. Removal of tonsils +/– adenoids
Complementary and Alternative Therapies	
1. Acupuncture	
2. Hypnotherapy	

acetylcholine receptors in the detrusor muscle and inhibit overactivity. These medications are not selective and are associated with side effects, which may negatively impact patient adherence (Maternik et al., 2015). Additionally, special consideration needs to be given to constipation prior to initiation of anticholinergic medications. The most commonly used and only US Food and Drug Administration–approved anticholinergic for use in children with overactive bladder is oxybutynin (Maternik et al., 2015). More selective antimuscarinic agents (e.g., propiverine, tolterodine, solifenacin) may demonstrate similar efficacy with less side effects, and thus promote adherence (Maternik et al., 2015). For the underactive bladder, which typically presents with prolonged holding behavior, muscarinic receptor agonists (bethanechol or carabachol) or inhibitors of acetylcholine esterase (distigmine, pyridostigmine, or neostigmine) have been trialed, but data are limited to support their use (Maternik et al., 2015). Alpha-blockers have been used to decrease bladder neck resistance and thus improve bladder emptying, but data remain conflicting (Maternik et al., 2015). Finally, imipramine, a tricyclic antidepressant, has demonstrated efficacy for refractory daytime incontinence in children, but potential side effects warrant caution in its application.

PFPT is a well-established, evidence-based intervention widely used in the management of abdominal and pelvic floor dysfunction. PFPT is comprised of patient education, behavioral strategies, functional exercise training (including effective muscle contraction and increased muscle and body awareness, coordination, and control), biofeedback, and electrotherapy (Ladi-Seyedian, Sharifi-Rad, & Kajbafzadeh, 2019). Early outpatient studies in children with urinary incontinence were promising as evidenced by a significant reduction in episodes of daytime incontinence (Vasconcelos et al., 2006). With advancements in technology, the application of biofeedback as a complementary component to pediatric PFPT has expanded and resulted in consistently positive outcomes (Koenig & McKenna, 2011). In 2010 biofeedback as part of a comprehensive outpatient program was included in the ICCS management guidelines for children with dysfunctional voiding (Chase et al., 2010). Factors impacting the success of biofeedback therapy include patient effort, motivation for treatment, age (>5 years), and treatment delivery by a trained professional in a practical environment (Ladi-Seyedian et al., 2019).

Nocturnal Enuresis

NE can occur independently of other symptoms (monosymptomatic NE) or with LUTS, including daytime incontinence that should be addressed concomitantly. Table 68.3 outlines the pharmacotherapy applicable when first-line interventions, including alarm therapy, fail. Anticholinergic therapy is useful as a second-line antienuretic therapy especially in primary therapy resistant cases in combination with desmopressin and enuresis alarms (Nevéus et al., 2020). Oxybutynin is the most commonly used medication, but the reduced side effect profiles of some of the newer agents offer promise. Finally, imipramine has demonstrated some efficacy by a modest reduction in wetting episodes per week (Caldwell, Deshpande, & Von Gontard, 2013). Its effects are wide ranging and include anticholinergic, antispasmodic, local anesthetic, and central nervous system effects on voiding. Side effects are use limiting, but not prohibitive, especially in therapy-resistant cases. The norepinephrine reuptake inhibitors reboxetine and atomextine are not cardiotoxic, so they may be useful alternatives to imipramine (Kuwertz-Bröking & von Gontard, 2018). For children who continue to be symptomatic after trials of first- and second-line therapies or combinations thereof, another trial of a first-line therapy may be beneficial as the response to treatment may evolve with time. For those who remain resistant, third-line therapies (e.g., complementary, alternative, and surgical options) can be considered (see Table 68.3).

Dry-bed training (DBT) is a multicomponent intervention based on operant conditioning that pairs the urine alarm with other behavioral strategies, including a frequent waking schedule, positive practice (i.e., voiding attempts are made at set intervals regardless of child's urge to urinate), and overcorrection for bedwetting via cleanliness training. It is considered a well-established treatment and has demonstrated a 75% cure rate, which is comparable to that of alarm therapy (Shepard et al., 2017). However, the complexity of the protocol, particularly the first week of intensive hourly waking, may be a less attractive treatment option for families who have not yet tried alarm therapy.

Full-spectrum home training (FSHT) is a multicomponent treatment package that was designed to be less demanding than DBT. FSHT pairs the urine alarm with other behavioral strategies, including retention control with monetary rewards, cleanliness training, self-monitoring and parent monitoring, and graduated overlearning. The inclusion of a relapse prevention component and the removal of rigorous waking schedules are attractive components of this treatment package. FSHT has demonstrated high success rates (84%–89% of youth achieved 14 consecutive dry nights within 6 months) and 12-month relapse rates of 14% to 16%, though it is deemed a probably efficacious intervention due to limited study.

CLINICAL IMPLICATIONS

Interprofessional care teams, often including psychology, pediatric gastroenterology, and pediatric urology, offer the most comprehensive treatment for patients with incontinence. The traditional approach of seeing patients in independent subspecialty clinics over many months and multiple visits can negatively impact patient satisfaction and adherence, as well as risk creating confusion if the providers are not coordinated in their approach. Comprehensive initial visits in an interprofessional clinic may require more upfront costs and investment of time by families and providers, but in turn allow for a coordinated management plan that has the opportunity to improve understanding, adherence, and outcomes. The interprofessional clinic setting also promotes cross-collaboration and education among subspecialists.

Evidence-based interventions for daytime incontinence and NE have behavioral and/or pharmacologic components, therefore treatment success or failure is highly dependent on adherence. For example, alarm therapy, though highly effective, requires a considerable investment from the family system, which may contribute to underutilization, lack of adoption, or discontinued use (Shepard et al., 2017). Parental motivation for treatment is often high at the time they are referred to a specialist, but child investment is variable. A child who is not bothered by persistent incontinence, or who experiences learned helplessness as a result of previous intervention failures, is likely to be apathetic toward treatment. Therefore it is critical that providers help align expectations in treatment by preparing families for the associated demands and to identify and address any current or anticipated barriers. An essential component of this process is to improve self-efficacy by helping children be more active participants in their own care.

Annie, described in the chapter-opening vignette, had a comprehensive evaluation that revealed anxiety and a dysfunctional voiding pattern. Education was provided about bladder function and incontinence and recommended lifestyle modifications (increased water intake, reduced caffeine). Effective voiding posture, a double voiding protocol, and management strategies for NE were discussed. The clinical psychologist provided psychoeducation about the physiologic aspects of anxiety, then modeled and practiced diaphragmatic breathing with the patient. Principles of cognitive-behavioral therapy were also outlined, and an example personalized to the patient was used to demonstrate how anxiety-producing thoughts, paired with the physiologic symptoms of anxiety, reinforce and exacerbate urinary urgency and frequency. Behavior management training, specifically ways to for Annie's parents provide perceived control, were also provided by the psychologist to help manage the patient's anticipatory anxiety. Annie and her parents returned for follow-up 5 months after the initial visit and reported significant improvements after implementing the recommendations. Specifically, Annie experienced complete resolution of daytime incontinence, urgency, and frequency; significant reduction in NE, totaling three episodes over the past 5 months; and reduced anxiety.

FUTURE DIRECTIONS

Technology has advanced patient care in pediatric bladder and bowel disorders. Mobile applications and the integration of child-friendly, interactive, game-like components to existing treatment procedures have demonstrated positive effects. Continuous monitoring devices can be used as a new means of accident prevention overnight (Kwinten et al., 2020). The wireless ultrasonic bladder sensor is designed to be worn on the lower abdomen as it measures nocturnal bladder filling, with the goal of waking the child before the bladder is full. This innovative approach is feasible, offers some advantages over traditional alarm therapy, and has potential for expanding its clinical utility. More recently, heart rate monitors have been used to assess heart rate alterations and their association with NE episodes. Continued efforts to apply novel technology to evaluation and treatment approaches in pediatric BBD disorders will undoubtedly continue to have positive implications for quality of and access to care.

Similarly, there has been an increase in the use of social media platforms to disseminate multimodal information as a means of patient education. This movement stems from patient-reported preferences for using social media to learn about health conditions, and there is evidence that social media use has benefits, such has high impact factor for journals and parental adoption of and preference for this method to learn about children's medical symptoms. Another plausible benefit is helping adolescents, who are deemed higher risk and more likely to have adherence difficulties, to be more active participants in their own care.

REFERENCES

American Psychiatric Association. (2013). *Diagnostic and statistical manual of mental disorders* (5th ed.). Author.

Austin, P., Bauer, S., Bower, W., Chase, J., Franco, I., Hoebeke, P., ... Nevéus, T. (2016). The standardization of terminology of lower urinary tract function in children and adolescents: Update report from the Standardization Committee of the International Children's Continence Society. *Neurourolgy and Urodynamics, 35*, 471–481.

Bower, W. F., Sit, F. K., Bluyssen, N., Wong, E. M., & Yeung, C. K. (2006). PIN-Q: A valid, reliable and reproducible quality-of-life measure in children with bladder dysfunction. *Journal of Pediatric Urology, 2*(3), 185–189.

Caldwell, P. H., Deshpande, A. V., & Von Gontard, A. (2013). Management of nocturnal enuresis. *BMJ (Clinical Research Ed.), 347*, f6259. https://doi.org/10.1136/bmj.f6259

Chase, J., Austin, P., Hoebeke, P., McKenna, P., & International Children's Continence Society. (2010). The management of dysfunctional voiding in children: A report from the Standardisation Committee of the International Children's Continence Society. *Journal of Urology, 183*(4), 1296–1302.

Drossman, D. (2006). Rome III: The new criteria. *Chinese Journal of Digestive Diseases, 7*, 181–185.

Eiberg, H., Shaumburg, H. L., Von Gontard, A., & Rittig, S. (2001). Linkage study of a large Danish 4-generation family with urge incontinence and nocturnal enuresis. *Journal of Urology, 166*(6), 2401–2403.

Filce, H. G., & LaVergne, L. (2015). Absenteeism, educational plans, and anxiety among children with incontinence and their parents. *The Journal of School Health, 85*(4), 241–250.

Friman, P. C. (2019). Incontinence: A biobehavioral perspective. In T. H. Ollendick, S. W. White, & B. A. White (Eds.), *The Oxford handbook of clinical child and adolescent psychology* (pp. 367–381). Oxford University Press.

Grzeda, M. T., Heron, J., von Gontard, A., & Joinson, C. (2017). Effects of urinary incontinence on psychosocial outcomes in adolescence. *European Child and Adolescent Psychiatry, 26*, 649–658.

Ikeda, H., Oyake, C., Oonuki, Y., Fuyama, M., Watanabe, T., Kyoda, T., & Tamura, S. (2020). Complete resolution of urinary incontinence with treatment improved the health-related quality of life of children with functional daytime urinary incontinence: A prospective study. *Health and Quality of Life Outcomes*, *18*(1), 14. https://doi.org/10.1186/s12955-020-1270-2

Joinson, C., Grzeda, M. T., von Gontard, A., & Heron, J. (2019). A prospective cohort study of biopsychosocial factors associated with childhood urinary incontinence. *European Child & Adolescent Psychiatry*, *28*(1), 123–130. https://doi.org/10.1007/s00787-018-1193-1

Joinson, C., Heron, J., Emond, A., & Butler, R. (2007). Psychological problems in children with bedwetting and combined (day and night) wetting: A UK population-based study. *Journal of Pediatric Psychology*, *32*(5), 605–616.

Joinson, C., Heron, J., & von Gontard, A. (2006). Psychological problems in children with daytime wetting. *Pediatrics*, *118*(5), 1985–1993. https://doi.org/10.1542/peds.2006-0894

Joinson, C., Heron, J., von Gontard, A., Butler, U., Golding, J., & Emond, A. (2008). Early childhood risk factors associated with daytime wetting and soiling in school-age children. *Journal of Pediatric Psychology*, *33*(7), 739–750.

Koenig, J. F., & McKenna, P. H. (2011). Biofeedback therapy for dysfunctional voiding in children. *Current Urology Report*, *12*, 144–152.

Kuwertz-Bröking, E., & von Gontard, A. (2018). Clinical management of nocturnal enuresis. *Pediatric Nephrology (Berlin, Germany)*, *33*(7), 1145–1154. https://doi.org/10.1007/s00467-017-3778-1

Kwinten, W., van Leuteren, P. G., van Duren-van Iersel, M., Dik, P., & Jira, P. E. (2020). SENS-U: Continuous home monitoring of natural nocturnal bladder filling in children with nocturnal enuresis—A feasibility study. *Journal of Pediatric Urology*, *16*(2), 196.e1–196.e6.

Ladi-Seyedian, S. S., Sharifi-Rad, L., & Kajbafzadeh, A. M. (2019). Pelvic floor electrical stimulation and muscles training: A combined rehabilitative approach for management of non-neuropathic urinary incontinence in children. *Journal of Pediatric Surgery*, *54*(4), 825–830. https://doi.org/10.1016/j.jpedsurg.2018.06.007

LaGrant, B., Marquis, B. O., Berg, A. T., & Grinspan, Z. M. (2020). Depression and anxiety in children with epilepsy and other chronic health conditions: National estimates of prevalence and risk factors. *Epilepsy & Behavior*, *103*(Pt A), 106828.

Longstaffe, S., Moffatt, M. E., & Whalen, J. C. (2000). Behavioral and self-concept changes after 6 months of enuresis treatment: A randomized, controlled trial. *Pediatrics*, *105*(3), S935–S940.

Ma, J., Li, S., Jiang, F., Jin, X., Zhang, Y., Yan, C., … Li, F. (2018). Relationship between sleep patterns, sleep problems, and childhood enuresis. *Sleep Medicine*, *50*, 14–20.

Malhotra, N. R., Kuhlthau, K. A., Rosoklija, I., Migliozzi, M., Nelson, C. P., & Schaeffer, A. J. (2020). Children's experience with daytime and nighttime urinary incontinence: A qualitative exploration. *Journal of Pediatric Urology*, *16*, 535.e1–535.e8.

Maternik, M., Krzeminska, K., & Zurowska, A. (2015). The management of childhood urinary incontinence. *Pediatric Nephrology*, *30*, 41–50.

Mellon, M. W., Natchev, B. E., Katusic, S. K., Colligan, R. C., Weaver, A. L., Voigt, R. G., & Barbaresi, W. J. (2013). Incidence of enuresis and encopresis among children with attention-deficit/hyperactivity disorder in a population-based birth cohort. *Academy of Pediatrics*, *13*, 322–327.

Morgan, K. E., Leroy, S. V., Corbett, S. T., & Shepard, J. A. (2019). Complementary and integrative management of pediatric lower urinary tract dysfunction implemented within an interprofessional clinic. *Children (Basel, Switzerland)*, *6*(8), 88. https://doi.org/10.3390/children6080088

Nevéus, T. (2017). Pathogenesis of enuresis: Towards a new understanding. *International Journal of Urology*, *24*(3), 174–182.

Nevéus, T., Fonseca, E., Franco, I., Kawauchi, A., Kovacevic, L., Nieuwhof-Leppink, A., … Rittig, S. (2020). Management and treatment of nocturnal enuresis—An updated standardization from the International Children's Continence Society. *Journal of Pediatric Urology*, *16*, 10–19.

Nevéus, T., Stenberg, A., Läckgren, G., Tuvemo, T., & Hetta, J. (1999). Sleep of children with enuresis: A polysomnographic study. *Pediatrics*, *103*, 1193–1197.

Niemczyk, J., Equit, M., Braun-Bither, K., Klein, A. M., & von Gontard, A. (2015). Prevalence of incontinence, attention deficit/hyperactivity disorder and oppositional defiant disorder in preschool children. *European Child & Adolescent Psychiatry*, *24*(7), 837–843. https://doi.org/10.1007/s00787-014-0628-6

Okur, M., Ruzgar, H., Erbey, F., & Kaya, A. (2012). The evaluation of children with monosymptomatic nocturnal enuresis for attention deficit and hyperactivity disorder. *International Journal of Psychiatry in Clinical Practice*, *16*(3), 229–232. https://doi.org/10.3109/13651501.2011.620129

Shepard, J. A., Poler, J. E., Jr., & Grabman, J. H. (2017). Evidence-based psychosocial treatments for pediatric elimination disorders. *Journal of Clinical Child & Adolescent Psychology*, *46*(6), 767–797. https://doi.org/10.1080/15374416.2016.1247356

Thibodeau, B. A., Metcalfe, P., Koop, P., & Moore, K. (2013). Urinary incontinence and quality of life in children. *Journal of Pediatric Urology*, *9*(1), 78–83. https://doi.org/10.1016/j.jpurol.2011.12.005

Van Hoecke, E., Baeyens, D., Vanden Bossche, H., Hoebeke, P., & Vande Walle, J. (2007). Early detection of psychological problems in a population of children with enuresis: Construction and validation of the Short Screening Instrument for Psychological Problems in Enuresis. *Journal of Urology*, *178*(6), 2611–2615. https://doi.org/10.1016/j.juro.2007.08.025

Vasconcelos, M., East, P., Blanco, E., Lukacz, E. S., Caballero, G., Lozoff, B., & Gahagan, S. (2017). Early behavioral risks of childhood and adolescent daytime urinary incontinence and nocturnal enuresis. *Journal of Developmental and Behavioral Pediatrics*, *38*(9), 736–742. https://doi.org/10.1097/DBP.0000000000000516

Vasconcelos, M., Lima, E., Caiafa, L., Noronha, A., Cangussu, R., Gomes, S., … Colozimo, E. (2006). Voiding dysfunction in children. Pelvic-floor exercises or biofeedback therapy: A randomized study. *Pediatric Nephrology (Berlin, Germany)*, *21*(12), 1858–1864. https://doi.org/10.1007/s00467-006-0277-1

Vinall, J., Pavlova, M., Asmundson, G. J., Rasic, N., & Noel, M. (2016). Mental health comorbidities in pediatric chronic pain: A narrative review of epidemiology, models, neurobiological mechanisms and treatment. *Children (Basel, Switzerland)*, *3*(4), 40.

von Gontard, A. (2012). Enuresis. In J. M. Rey (Ed.), *IACAPAP e-textbook of child and adolescent mental health*. International Association for Child and Adolescent Psychiatry and Allied Professions.

von Gontard, A., & Equit, M. (2015). Comorbidity of ADHD and incontinence in children. *European Child & Adolescent Psychiatry*, *24*(2), 127–140. https://doi.org/10.1007/s00787-014-0577-0

von Gontard, A., & Kuwertz-Bröking, E. (2019). The diagnosis and treatment of enuresis and functional daytime urinary incontinence. *Deutsches Arzteblatt international, 116*(16), 279–285.

von Gontard, A., Niemczyk, J., Wagner, C., & Equit, M. (2016). Voiding postponement in children: A systematic review. *European Child and Adolescent Psychiatry, 25*, 809–820.

von Gontard, A., Schaumburg, H., Hollmann, E., Eiberg, H., & Rittig, S. (2001). The genetics of enuresis—A review. *Journal of Urology, 166*, 2438–2443.

von Gontard, A., Vrijens, D., Selai, C., Mosiello, G., Panicker, J., van Koeveringe, G., … Anding, R. (2019). Are psychological comorbidities important in the aetiology of lower urinary tract dysfunction-ICI-RS 2018? *Neurourology and Urodynamics, 38*(5), S8–S17. https://doi.org/10.1002/nau.24016

Wolfish, N. M., Pivik, R. T., & Busby, K. A. (1997). Elevated sleep arousal thresholds in enuretic boys: Clinical implications. *Acta Paediatrica, 86*, 381–384.

World Health Organization. (1992). *ICD-10: International statistical classification of diseases and related health problems*. Author.

Yeung, C. K., Sihoe, J. D. Y., Sit, F. K. Y., Bower, W., Sreedhar, B., & Lau, J. (2004). Characteristics of primary nocturnal enuresis in adults: An epidemiological study. *BJU International, 93*, 341–345.

69

Toileting and Encopresis

Laura Weissman

For additional material related to the content of this chapter, please see Chapters 68 and 93.

> **VIGNETTE**
>
> *Sammy is a 5-year-old boy who presents to clinic because he is frequently stooling in his underwear. He was toilet trained for urine at age 3 without event. He toilet trained for stool later that year but became increasingly resistant to stooling on the toilet after a toilet overflowed in his preschool. Currently he most often stools in his underwear. He does not notify anyone when he needs to stool or has gone. When his parents try to alert him, he denies that he has stooled. He has a full bowel movement every 3 days but has streaks or smears in his underwear in between. There are no concerns about his learning or cognitive functioning but he is described as quite active and impulsive. His parents are worried he is doing this on purpose and seek support.*

SCOPE OF THE PROBLEM

Encopresis (functional fecal incontinence) and toileting failure are common problems in children. The incidence varies with age, but encopresis affects approximately 4% of children ages 4 to 17 (Loening-Baucke, 2007) and is more common in boys than girls. Toileting refusal impacts up to 20% of children during toilet training. Encopresis/functional fecal incontinence can be divided into two categories: retentive (associated with constipation), which includes more than 80% of cases, or nonretentive (not associated with constipation). Although these problems often cause a great deal of stress to children and families, most cases cannot be attributed to an organic illness (with the exception of constipation) and are curable with appropriate and diligent treatment. However, many children with encopresis are also vulnerable to developmental, behavioral, and emotional problems (Joinson et al., 2006). This should be taken into consideration during management, and their functioning should be monitored over time.

BOWEL FUNCTION AND ENCOPRESIS

Normal bowel functioning is shown in Fig. 69.1. A child who is toilet trained or in the process of toilet training has the ability to keep the external sphincter closed until in the appropriate location to defecate. However, if a child develops constipation because of either diet changes, stool withholding, or other factors, stool remains in the rectum and colon. As stool remains there, water is absorbed and it becomes harder and subsequently more difficult to pass. This results in pain with defecation, and more withholding ensues. The rectum dilates as more stool collects. The stretched muscles and nerve fibers do not function appropriately. This means that it is difficult both to control the external anal sphincter and to sense the urge to defecate as the reflex arc becomes less sensitive. When the child squeezes the external anal sphincter to retain stool, some stool may be ejected into the underwear, resulting in staining. Children may also have leakage of wet stool that makes its way past the harder bolus of stool, or they may have complete stool accidents resulting from inability to appropriately control defecation (Fig. 69.2).

TOILET TRAINING

In the United States toilet training typically occurs from 2.5 to 3 years of age, although in other countries it occurs earlier. In the early 20th century a strictly scheduled, parent-centered approach was used for toilet training. Typically, training was initiated before 18 months of age. In the 1940s some pediatricians began advocating for a less rigid approach that emphasized developmental readiness (Brazelton, 1962). Although many different approaches to toilet training exist, the current model endorsed by most experts as well as by the American Academy of Pediatrics is a child-centered process emphasizing developmental readiness as a precursor to toilet training. As part of this approach, three factors must be in place: the developmental and physiologic skills needed for toileting, the ability to understand instruction, and the motivation to perform the task. Children typically reach the developmental milestones needed for toilet training between 18 and 30 months of age (Brazelton et al., 1999). The development of nighttime bowel continence is usually followed by daytime bowel continence, then daytime urine continence, and lastly nighttime urine continence. The readiness skills that a child needs to toilet train include motor, language, and social skills. A child must have the motor skills needed for ambulating, sitting, and assisting with removal of clothing. These skills are usually attained by the age of 18 months. To maintain continence, a child must have voluntary control of the bowels and

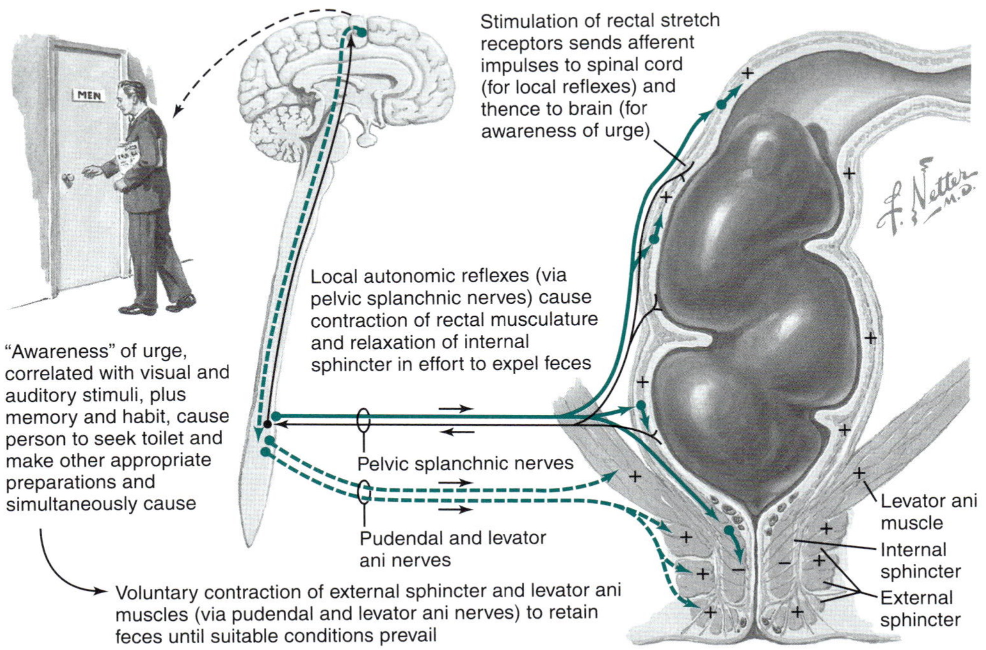

Fig. 69.1 Normal bowel function.

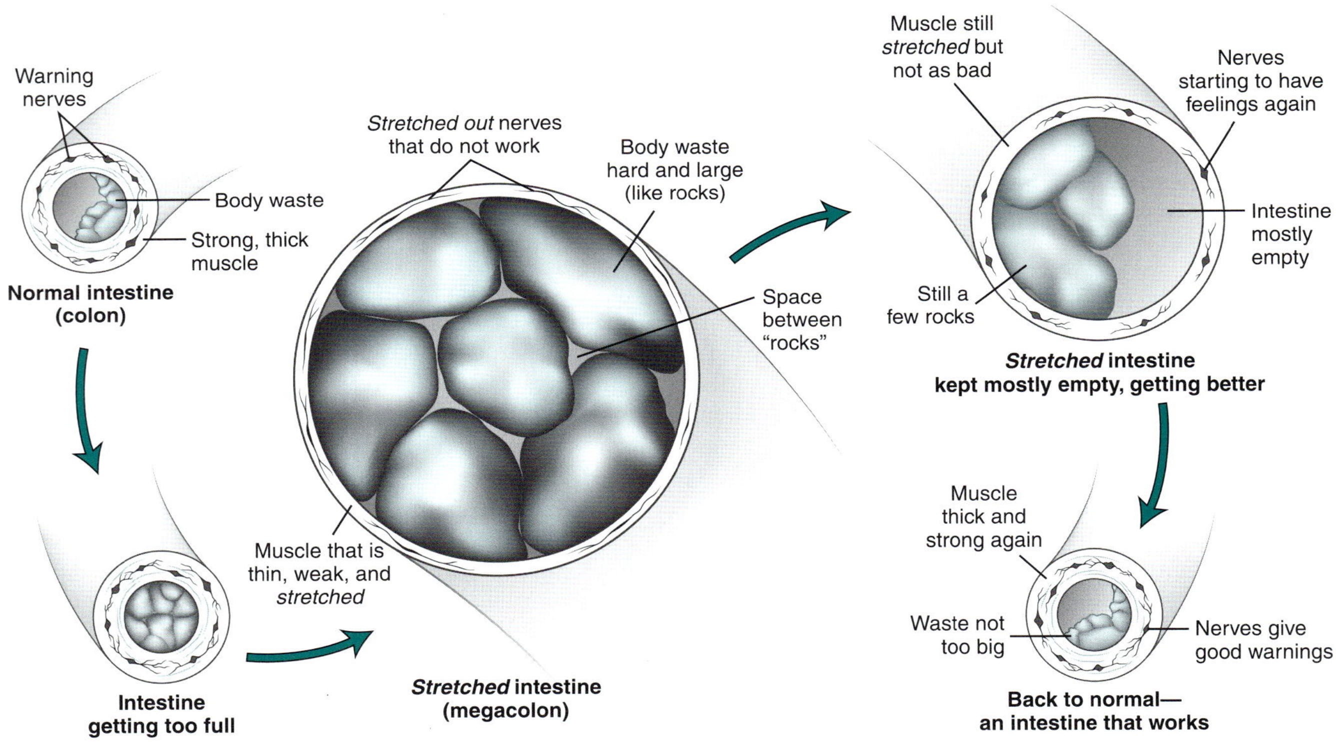

Fig. 69.2 Encopresis. Patient training diagram.

bladder (usually emerging at 9 months, although it must be combined with other described skills for full continence to be achieved) and then be aware of the need to defecate (usually attained at 18 months). The child must have a way of indicating to caregivers the need to use the toilet. Cognitively, the child must understand that certain things go in certain places. Socially, the child needs to recognize the behavior of others and possess the motivation to attain continence.

Once a child has achieved the readiness skills, a step-by-step approach can be used to introduce, model, and facilitate appropriate toileting behavior. A regular discussion in a story format can introduce and normalize toileting behavior for the child. At the same time, the toilet or potty seat can be introduced. This should be a comfortable place to sit, and the child should have a place to rest the feet. In the case of a potty chair this would be the floor; and with a toilet seat, this should be a stool or other support. The child should have time to sit on the potty or toilet either with or without a diaper or pull-up on and with no specific expectation for voiding. As the child becomes comfortable, regular sitting times can be created. During this time there can be books or quiet activities to facilitate and to reinforce sitting. The optimal time for these sittings is approximately 20 to 30 minutes after meals as the gastrocolic reflex increases the urge to defecate. When successful on the toilet or potty, the child should be rewarded with verbal praise or a small token. Over time, a child will learn to request toilet time outside of scheduled sittings. This behavior should also be rewarded. When the child is starting to use the toilet on a regular basis, the diaper or pull-up can be removed and the child can move to underwear.

Children learn how to toilet train at different rates (Blum, Taubman, & Nemeth, 2003). Some children learn quickly in a few days, and others may take a few months. If at any point in time a child is resistant to toileting or demonstrates negative behaviors around toileting, active training should be discontinued temporarily. Research shows that constipation (Blum, Taubman, & Nemeth, 2004; Schonwald, Sherritt, Stadtler, & Bridgemohan, 2004) and difficult temperament traits are associated with challenges in toilet training (Schonwald et al., 2004).

TOILETING REFUSAL/STOOL WITHHOLDING

Toileting refusal or stool withholding presents its own challenges to treatment. This may occur because of physical discomfort, related to constipation or pain, perceived negative experiences in the bathroom, fears, or other reasons. In young children who are resistant to toileting toilet training should be discontinued for a period of months and the child returned to diapers. They should also be assessed for constipation and treated appropriately (Blum, Taubman, & Nemeth, 2004; Tabbers et al., 2014) before continuing with training. For children with toileting refusal who are developing typically and are older than 3 years, management is similar to that for children with encopresis with some modifications. These children often have acquired the basic skills needed for toilet training, but for some other reason, whether it is related to constipation, withholding, temperament, or other conflict or combination, they have been unsuccessful. As with young children, they should be assessed for constipation and treated appropriately (see "Treatment" under Encopresis/Functional Fecal Incontinence, later). They should also be evaluated medically for any contributing organic causes (see Encopresis/Functional Fecal Incontinence for details). The next step of management involves a behaviorally based program to desensitize a child's toileting aversion by decreasing anxiety around toileting. Start with whatever portion of toileting a child is willing to perform. For example, some children will be stooling in a pull-on diaper or underpants at this time. The first goal might be to have them stool in the diaper or underpants in the bathroom or on a specific mat or while sitting on the toilet with the diaper on.. The care provider can use a reward system to encourage completion of the goal. Once the goal is obtained, a new goal is developed using of a stepwise approach that moves the child closer to defecating on the toilet. For example, a child who defecates sitting on the toilet with a diaper on, may next sit on the toilet wearing a diaper in which a hole has been cut to allow the stool to fall into the toilet. The specifics of the plan and the approach depend on where the child starts as well as the temperament of the child. Group toileting programs for children who are late to toilet can be extremely helpful. The peer interaction around the topic can help decrease anxiety for both parents and children.

TOILET TRAINING IN SPECIAL POPULATIONS

Some children have developmental conditions that make toilet training more challenging. For example, children with some chronic illnesses, children in daycare, children with developmental disabilities, and those with neurologic impairment may take longer or need special guidance to master toileting. First, it is important to start out with the same general principles described earlier. If a child has acquired some but not all of the readiness skills described, the strategy for toilet training may be more flexible. For example, a child with developmental delay may have difficulty making the connection between the urge to defecate and the social need to hold. In this case frequent sitting at 1- to 2-hour intervals may be appropriate. Verbal praise for success should continue. Some children will toilet train this way; others may not be able to use the toilet of their own initiation consistently but will stay dry and soil free between sits, thus enabling them to wear underwear. Some children may have difficulty understanding the concepts of being wet and dry, and these may also need to be taught.

Toilet training can be particularly challenging in children with autism spectrum disorder (ASD) because of decreased social and communication skills as well as behavioral rigidity. Children with ASD may be overly sensitive to the sensation of defecating, and they may not know to communicate the urge to void. They are also more prone to anxiety around toileting. It is useful in this case to collaborate with school providers, an ASD consultant or behavioral specialist to design an individualized, structured plan for toilet training. Children with ASD may require a behavioral approach in which training is broken into incremental steps. If the child uses a picture exchange communication system or other communication system (see Chapter 94 and 107), this should be appropriately incorporated into training. This might include the development of a story or picture sequence that demonstrates toileting instruction. If the child suffers from firm stools that might increase resistance to defecation, medications can be used for softening the stools.

In children who have a physical disability, such as spina bifida or cerebral palsy, neurologic factors may make it more difficult or impossible for a child to maintain continence. Although social motivation is likely to be less of a problem, neurologic difficulties present unique challenges, and these children are often at risk for constipation. Stool softening agents such as those described for the treatment of encopresis (later) should be used when needed to make stools soft enough to pass with minimal effort. It is also important to consult the child's specialty providers to determine whether being accident free is an achievable goal. If a child is unable to maintain voluntary continence, timed sittings can help to keep a child dry in between sittings and possibly allow the child to wear underwear, which may be important socially for the child. Catheterization may also be an appropriate option and, in some cases, medically necessary. Try to find out the importance of remaining accident free for the child as this will affect success. If a child does not care about accidents, the child is less likely to be compliant with timed sittings. There are also other medical therapies that may be helpful, such as medications to reduce bladder spasms or to induce longer periods of dryness and surgeries to allow independence with toileting.

ENCOPRESIS/FUNCTIONAL FECAL INCONTINENCE

Overview

Encopresis or functional fecal incontinence is categorized in different ways depending on the classification systems. The *Diagnostic and Statistical Manual of Mental Disorders*, fifth edition, defines encopresis as "the repeated passage of feces into inappropriate places" most commonly underwear (American Psychiatric Association, 2013). Typically this is involuntary, but occasionally it may be intentional. The event must occur at least once a month for at least 3 months, and the chronologic age of the child must be at least 4 years (or for children with developmental delays, a mental age of at least 4 years). The fecal incontinence must not be due exclusively to the direct physiologic effects of a substance (e.g., laxatives) or a general medical condition except through a mechanism involving constipation. The gastroenterology literature often uses the term "functional fecal incontinence" to describe encopresis and divides it into two categories: retentive (associated with constipation) and nonretentive (not associated with constipation). Most commonly, encopresis presents with constipation, but we are beginning to have a better understanding of the nonretentive subtype.

Etiology

Encopresis is a complex disorder likely resulting from physical vulnerability in the context of potentiating environmental and behavioral factors. The primary cause is a physical predisposition to constipation, reduced bowel regularity, and ineffective evacuation. In some cases there may be a history of painful bowel movement with subsequent withholding. Children with attentional deficits, obsessions and compulsions, and oppositional behavior are more prone to encopresis (Joinson et al., 2006). Children with attention deficits may be less attuned to body signals around toileting and may have trouble establishing a regular toilet routine. A large proportion of children seeking treatment of elimination disorders are found to have neurodevelopmental disabilities, including ASD (Peeters, Noens, Philips, Kuppens, & Benninga, 2013). In addition, individuals with challenging or difficult temperament traits may be more prone to encopresis and toileting delays (Schonwald et al., 2004). Certainly environmental factors such as lack of access to the toilet, disorganized home setting, and exposure to trauma or violence can contribute to the development of encopresis. However, a majority of children with encopresis do not have a history of emotional disturbance.

Diagnosis

Diagnosis of encopresis and constipation starts with a thorough history and physical examination. In most cases this is sufficient to identify or rule out any organic disease.

History

Some patients do not present with encopresis until school age, but many have had a history of stool withholding or initial toileting refusal. Some children may have had a history of mild soiling, such as smearing, and are not identified as having encopresis until the condition progresses to more frequent or larger accidents or their soiling affects their functioning with peers or in other settings. In some children with encopresis with or without constipation parents can target a specific illness or other situation that may have immediately preceded withholding behavior, as occurred with Sammy in the chapter-opening vignette.

It is important to evaluate thoroughly for constipation, which might not be apparent to the family. Ask about frequency of symptoms, whether there are entire bowel movement accidents or just staining. Ask about consistency of bowel movements (hard, soft), shape, size, and ease of passage. Some find use of the Bristol Stool Scale (various versions are available online) with caregivers a helpful tool to understand the consistency of stool and how this relates to stool transit time. A child with constipation and encopresis may stool daily but pass only small, hard stools. Ask about times that stool accidents occur. Most children soil between 3 and 7 pm or specifically after or on the way home from school. Soiling at school is usually a marker of a more severe problem. Very rarely do children soil during sleep. Children with significant withholding may soil just as they fall asleep when they finally relax. However, nocturnal soiling can also be a sign of seizures.

Questions about urine accidents (enuresis) are also important. Children with constipation may have enuresis caused by bladder spasms resulting from pressure to the bladder (see Chapter 68). Girls with encopresis are also at risk for urinary tract infections from contamination or poor hygiene. In taking the history ask about any previous interventions tried. Take a diet history and include intolerances or allergies to any foods. Past medical history should review any concerns about growth. Short stature may be a clue to thyroid disease as a cause of constipation. A history of weight loss soon after introduction of solids may be a clue for celiac disease. The neurologic history should include questions about clumsiness or newly acquired lower extremity problems, which might be present in the case of a tethered cord. The gastrointestinal history should also include any history of explosive stools after retention or thin-caliber stools, which may indicate Hirschsprung disease. The family history should include questions about constipation, encopresis, colitis, irritable bowel syndrome, thyroid disease, or similar concerns.

Social history should include screening for history of trauma, ongoing trauma, or other psychosocial stressors that might be contributing to the presentation. Sexual or physical abuse is too important to miss. It is often difficult to ask about these sensitive questions, but they need to be part of the history. The abuse may be from someone other than the parents, so ask about concerns for the child with any other caregivers.

Physical Examination

Clinicians should complete a full physical examination with focus on assessment of the abdomen and genitourinary and neurologic systems. The first part of the examination should include evaluation of the child's overall appearance, including physical habitus and growth parameters, possible dysmorphism, behavior, and social interaction. Abdominal examination may reveal fullness, distention, or a nontender sausage-shaped mass in the lower left quadrant. The absence of this finding does not rule out constipation and may be difficult to appreciate in a child who is overweight or cannot tolerate an abdominal examination. Examine the spine for a sacral dimple, hair, or mass, which might suggest a spinal dysraphism. The neurologic examination needs to be thorough and should include assessment of gait as well as lower extremity reflexes and strength. Increased reflexes or decreased tone could signal a spinal cord abnormality.

Inspect the position of the anus and also look for evidence of soiling. Be alert for any signs of trauma, such as scarring, tears, or reduced rectal tone (see Chapter 15 for further guidance on the evaluation of suspected trauma or abuse). In girls the distance between the posterior fourchette and the anus should be at least one-third the distance between the posterior fourchette and coccyx; in boys the distance between the scrotum and anus should be half the scrotococcygeal distance (Reisner, Sivan, Nitzan, & Merlob, 1984). As part of the comprehensive physical, a digital rectal examination should be performed (Baker et al., 1999); however, this is sometimes difficult or not appropriate during the first visit. In clinical practice it is suggested that a rectal examination be performed during the course of treatment if there is not response to initial management. Increased rectal tone with a history of small-caliber stools and delayed passage of meconium may be a sign of Hirschsprung disease. Decreased rectal tone might be a sign of neurologic concern, such as spinal cord tethering or anomaly, although decreased tone can also be seen with prolonged constipation. Digital rectal examination should also include assessment of the rectal content. A large amount of stool in the rectum has a high positive predictive value for the presence of fecal retention, although absence of stool in the rectum does not rule out fecal retention (Rockney, McQuade, & Days, 1995). Intact neurologic sensation of the anus can be tested by eliciting the anal wink reflex, which involves lightly touching the anus with a cotton swab; this should result in closing of the sphincter. A cremasteric reflex in boys is another way to test lower sacral function; gently stroke the inner thigh and observe for testicular retraction. Table 69.1 lists some of the organic causes of stool withholding and leakage, as well as red flags.

TABLE 69.1 Potential Organic Causes of Constipation or Stool Withholding or Leakage

Disorder or Condition	Historical and Physical Findings
Malformations	
Anal stenosis Partial imperforate anus	Abnormality on inspection and examination of the anus
Neurogenic	
Occult spinal dysraphism Tethered cord Tumor	Increased lower extremity tone Recent onset of symptoms with neurologic signs, back pain, trouble walking up stairs, new-onset incontinence
Endocrine-metabolic	
Multiple endocrine neoplasia III	Variable presentation, including constipation
Thyroid disorder	Constipation, weight gain, decreased energy, cold intolerance
Electrolyte imbalance	Variable presentation, depending on electrolyte affected
Neuromuscular	
Muscular dystrophy	Presents in boys aged 3–5 yr; lower extremity proximal muscle weakness
Hirschsprung disease Cerebral palsy	History of constipation from birth followed by explosive stools; delayed passage of meconium, thin-caliber stools
Medications	Variable presentation, depending on medication
Sexual abuse	Physical signs of trauma or history of abuse (see Chapter 15)
Other celiac	In the case of celiac disease may present as constipation or diarrhea with growth concerns

Laboratory Evaluation and Imaging

In most cases children with encopresis with or without constipation do not require routine laboratory evaluation or imaging. However, if there is clinical suspicion of an organic cause, further investigation is warranted. Laboratory testing might include thyroid function studies and determination of calcium, magnesium, and electrolyte values, depending on history and examination findings. If the history is unclear and physical examination does not confirm constipation, abdominal radiography may be helpful to determine the amount of retained stool (Fig. 69.3). A baseline radiograph can also be useful as a reference to compare to a follow-up after a cleanout is performed. For children who present with urinary incontinence as well as constipation, urinalysis and urine culture may be useful. Constipation can result in pressure on the bladder, and soiling may increase the risk for urinary tract infection, particularly in girls. If a child has

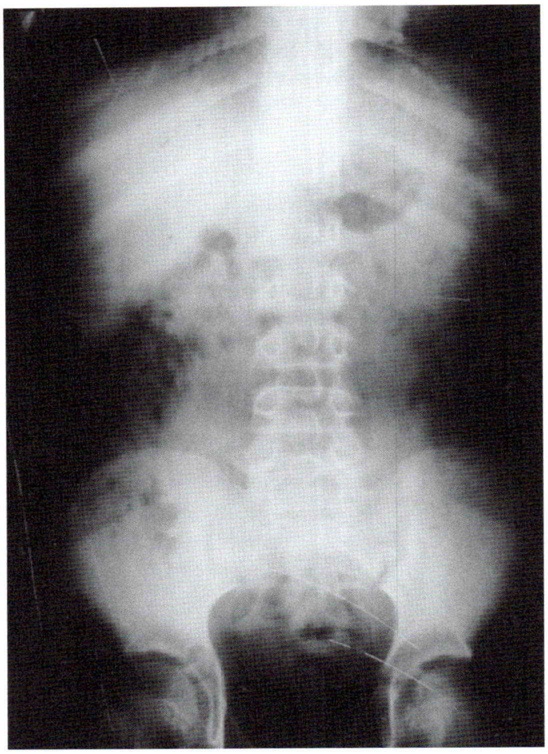

Fig. 69.3 Plain abdominal radiograph.

TABLE 69.2 Sample Treatment Plan for Encopresis

Family education
Clean out
Osmotic laxative with stimulant
or
High-dose PEG with electrolytes
or
In specific circumstances or severe cases:
Day 1: Bisacodyl pill
Day 2: Bisacodyl suppository
Day 3: 1 adult Fleet* enema
(repeat days 1–3 three times for a total of 12 days and then return to office)
Maintenance
Osmotic laxative (i.e., PEG without electrolytes); titrate to maintain soft daily stool and to minimize leakage (see Table 63.3 for other maintenance medications)

PEG, Polyethylene glycol.
*Monobasic sodium phosphate.
Based on a table from Schonwald, A., & Rappaport, L. (2004). Consultation with the specialist. Encopresis: Assessment and management. *Pediatric Reviews, 25,* 278–282.

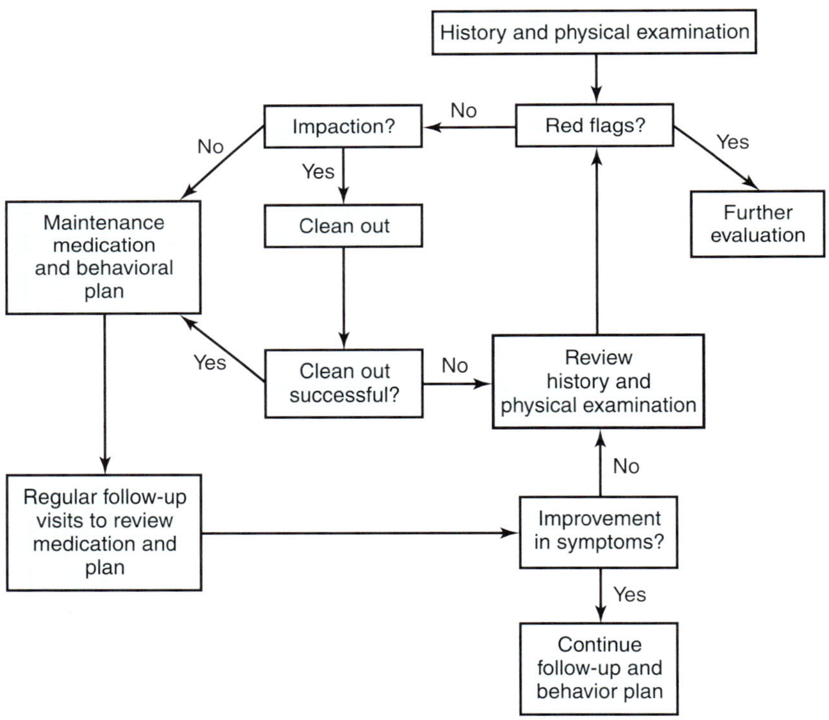

Fig. 69.4 Algorithm for treatment of encopresis.

any lower extremity symptoms, lumbosacral spinal films and lumbosacral magnetic resonance imaging may be useful to rule out a tethered cord or spinal dysraphism. If there is increased rectal tone and a history of inconsistent explosive stools, anal manometry may be useful to evaluate for Hirschsprung disease.

Treatment

Once the diagnosis of encopresis is confirmed by history and physical examination, a multimodal treatment program ensues (Table 69.2; Fig. 69.4). This requires caregiver education regarding encopresis, medical management of the underlying constipation when present, behavioral interventions to encourage the child to use the toilet regularly, followed by a medication maintenance plan once symptoms start to resolve. Encouraging evacuation of stool through regular sitting regimen is essential to success of treatment (Brooks et al., 2000).

Education

Encopresis can be emotionally overwhelming for a child and family. Many families do not understand the underlying pathophysiologic mechanism of this disorder. As a result, by the time most families seek medical attention, the child may have been punished or frequently reprimanded for accidents. The first step in treatment therefore is education to explain the cause and process of encopresis. Explain the cycle of stool retention (see Fig. 69.2) and discuss how physical factors, predisposition to constipation, and in some cases emotional or temperamental traits contribute to encopresis. Let them know that there are many other children with the same problem and that there are many things you and they can do to make things better. Emphasize to the family that this is not the child's fault and explain the relapsing and remitting course of this disorder both before and after treatment. Punitive approaches should be avoided. Although this portion of management may seem intuitive, it is integral to helping a family remain engaged in the treatment program. The family and child may be quite frustrated by this time and have tried other therapies. The use of pictures and handouts can be helpful to moving a family toward understanding.

Cleanout

In children with constipation, intervention includes the cleanout of retained stool and a regimen to maintain regular passage of stool so as not to exacerbate the underlying problem. In most cases, this cleanout can be performed at home. There are many different ways to perform a bowel cleanout. The plan you choose depends on the severity of the constipation and the comfort level of the child and family. Discuss the options with the child and family and consider factors specific to the child, such as maturity, motivation, emotional functioning, and preferred route of administration (Table 69.2 and Table 69.3).

For less severe constipation, a child may benefit from a daily medication to soften the stool, such as an osmotic laxative (polyethylene glycol [PEG] without electrolytes) or lubricant (mineral oil) with or without the addition of a mild to moderate bowel stimulant (senna or bisacodyl tablet) to encourage stool passage until there is cleanout. This less intensive approach is milder and will take longer than an aggressive cleanout.

For severe constipation, a more aggressive cleanout with intensive oral agents over several days or enemas alone or in conjunction with oral cathartics may be useful (see Table 69.2 for regimen). We do not recommend use of enemas in children younger than 5 years or in children with a history of abuse or trauma.

Cleanout can be brief in some children and longer in others. For severe constipation, a child may require reexamination or repeated abdominal radiography to confirm the clearance of stool. Initially, accidents may appear to increase with the introduction of a cleanout regimen. For children who attend school, one option is to use an agent to soften the stool during the week and add a stimulant on the weekends in hopes of decreasing the likelihood of an accident during the school day.

Another option is to use a stronger medication more commonly used in the inpatient settings, such as magnesium citrate or PEG with electrolytes taken by mouth or nasogastric tube.

In a majority of cases, hospitalization or inpatient treatment is never necessary. Aggressive outpatient treatment with a clear treatment plan is typically appropriate. Hospitalization itself can be traumatic and further add to the problem and therefore should be avoided if at all possible. Only severe cases, such as extreme abdominal distress, risk of obstruction, vomiting of feculent material, or extreme parental noncompliance, necessitate hospitalization.

Maintenance

Once cleanout is achieved, or if a child does not require a full cleanout, the next step is maintenance therapy (Table 69.4). Many of the medications used for maintenance are the same as those used for cleanout, such as mineral oil or PEG without electrolytes, but at a lower dose. Other osmotic laxatives, such as lactulose, or stimulants such as senna-based products can also be useful. The goal of maintenance therapy is to encourage regular evacuation of soft bowel movements and to prevent recurrence of constipation.

Often, medications need to be titrated to effect, and the dose may change over time. The choice of medication is often made on the basis of what a child will take on a regular basis. Some children experience gastrointestinal distress with stimulants or strong cathartics. Individuals have varied preferences for pills, liquid preparations, or drinks. PEG without electrolytes is a good choice as it has minimal taste. It can also be safely used for up to 12 months (Loening-Baucke, 2002b). Mineral oil is another option, but the taste and consistency are often more difficult to disguise and is best used when cold and disguised in yogurt or pudding or flavored with chocolate or maple syrups. Prior concerns about the impact of mineral oil on absorption of fat-soluble vitamins are unfounded, and supplementation is not necessary (Sharif, Crushell, O'Driscoll, & Bourke, 2001).

As the constipation resolves, children can be slowly weaned off medications as tolerated. The length of use depends on need as well as on the safety of the medication used. Since it can take the bowels time to recover from prolonged constipation, it is not unusual to require at least 6 months of medications for those with a long history of encopresis. The prolonged use of stimulants and enemas should be avoided because of the side effects and potential for dependence. However, what constitutes prolonged use is difficult to ascertain. To avoid concerns about dependence, stimulants can be used intermittently as described earlier.

Diet

Include a discussion of diet as part of education and maintenance therapy. When possible, parents should encourage high-fiber foods, including fruits, vegetables, and whole

TABLE 69.3 Medications for Cleanout and Maintenance Therapy

Medication	Type of Laxative	Dose	Use	Comments
Polyethylene glycol (PEG) without electrolytes	Osmotic	Cleanout: 1.5g/kg/d divided bid Maintenance: Titrate to effect 1 g/kg/day Typically 8.5–17 g/dose	Cleanout Maintenance Therapy or slower clearout	Taste and texture usually well tolerated Every 17 g needs to be mixed in 8 oz of water or juice
PEG with electrolytes	Osmotic	>6 yr: 25–40 mL/kg/hr PO until clear Maximum: 4 L for children >12 yr	Cleanout	NPO 3–4 hr before ingestion of solution
Lactulose	Osmotic	1–2 g/kg/day qd or bid Maximum: 60 mL/day	Maintenance therapy	
Magnesium hydroxide 400 mg/5mL (milk of magnesia)	Osmotic	2–5 years: 5–15 mL/day qhs or div bid 6–11 years: 15–30 mL/day qhs or div bid ≥12 years: 30–60 mL/day qhs or div bid	Maintenance therapy	Side effects can include cramping, diarrhea, nausea, and vomiting and also fluid and salt losses with prolonged use
Magnesium citrate	Osmotic	2–5 yr: 2–4 mL/kg/day qd or div BID max 60–90 mL/kg 6–12 yr: 100–150 mL PO × 1 or div BID >12 yr: 150–300 mL PO × 1 or div BID	Cleanout	Taste improved when cold and mixed with lemon-lime soda Check drug interactions before prescribing Do not use in patients with poor kidney functioning
Mineral oil	Softener	5–11 yr: 1–3 tsp/day >12 yr: 1–3T/day	Cleanout (use high dose) Maintenance therapy Titrate to effect	May cause leakage of stool and oil Medication best disguised in cold yogurt or pudding Do not use if child is at risk for aspiration Decrease dose if leaking occurs
Docusate sodium	Softener	Given once daily or divided up to 4 times a day <3 yr: 10–40 mg/day 3–6 yr: 20–60 mg/day 6–12 yr: 40–150 mg/day	Maintenance therapy	
Fiber supplement	Bulk-forming agent	Depends on form and brand	Maintenance or As daily supplement for children with low-fiber diets	Many different forms are available, including wafers, powders, tablets, and liquids
Monobasic sodium phosphate enema	Osmotic, enema	1 adult enema (120 mL)	Cleanout	A pediatric enema (65 mL) is often insufficient for treatment of encopretic children Avoid prolonged use Avoid enemas in younger children and children with a history of sexual abuse
Bisacodyl	Stimulant (oral and suppository forms)	<12 yr: 5–10 mg PO/PR qd >12 yr: 5–15 mg PO	Cleanout As described above or during times of relapse	Stronger than a senna product Avoid long-term continuous use as this may lead to dependence
Senna product	Stimulant	15-mg tablets or chocolate squares ½-2 chocolate squares per day ½-2 tablets per day	Cleanout Rescue	Comes in liquid, tablet, or chocolate square Avoid prolonged continuous use as this may lead to dependence

TABLE 69.4 Sample Maintenance Treatment Plan

- Medication for maintenance therapy titrated to effect
- Behavioral plan, including daily sitting with developmentally appropriate reward
- Discussion of diet changes, including increasing fiber and water content
- Encourage increasing activity
- Regular visits with provider to reinforce the plan and continually educate the family

grains as well as fluids. However, diet and fluids alone are not sufficient to treat moderate to severe constipation.

Behavioral Plan

The behavior component of treatment is essential (Brazzelli, Griffiths, Cody, & Tappin, 2011). A child requires a regimen of regular sitting on the toilet for two reasons: first, to encourage the evacuation of stool; second, to help the child become comfortable with using the toilet. Initially, a child may be resistant to sitting on the toilet for many reasons. For one, the child may have developed a fear or aversion to use of the toilet. In addition, the child may have become overwhelmed by the long-standing nature of the problem and be less willing to perform a sitting task. The chronicity and nature of the disorder may have also led to disrupted family dynamics and struggles between parent and child around use of the toilet. However, no matter what the source of the behavior, the plan remains essentially the same.

The behavior plan includes motivating and rewarding a child for sitting on the toilet as opposed to having clean underwear because sitting on the toilet is a behavior the child controls, whereas in children with retentive encopresis, soiling may not be under the child's voluntary control. The best time to sit is 20 to 30 minutes after meals as the gastrocolic reflex encourages defecation; however, it is not necessary to do it at this time only. It may be more convenient for sitting to occur in the morning or directly after school. Depending on age, the child should be encouraged to sit on the toilet one to three times a day for 5 to 10 minutes at a time. The child may have a specific toy, book, electronic device, or desired object during that time. The child is not required to stool but should try if able. There are many different ways to reinforce sitting behaviors. For preschoolers, a sticker chart can be used as a reward, and special toys, devices, or books can be used as reinforcers once a reward goal is achieved. For school-age children, stickers, small sweets, or points to be redeemed for a prize may also be useful, but they can also earn special time, device time, or desired items by sitting. It is important to try to minimize conflict during sitting times. The reward system should be determined collaboratively with the caregiver and child, and the child needs to voice an agreement and understanding. The child then receives a reward for performing the sitting task. If the child does not perform the task, the child should not be punished or reprimanded but gently reminded that if the task is not completed there will be no reward.

Regular scheduled visits with a provider are key to maintaining motivation, to clarify the plan, and to provide encouragement. Often it is easier for a child to perform the task for the provider rather than for a caregiver. If there is a great deal of conflict or resistance, consider eliciting the aid of a psychologist or behavioral specialist. See Chapter 93 for more in-depth discussion of behavioral strategies.

Relapses/Treatment Failure

As described earlier, relapses are common during times of stress. A family should have a plan, which includes medical therapy followed by reinstituting sitting times using reward incentives. In the case of recurrent treatment failure, further workup or specialist intervention might be needed.

Other Therapies

As is common for all children with chronic medical conditions, parents often seek complementary and alternative therapies for their children. The literature is not extensive in regard to complementary and alternative treatments for encopresis. Biofeedback is not routinely recommended and typically only used for those with a specific type of bowel dysfunction in patients amenable to the rigorous treatment protocol.

Outcome

Encopresis tends to be a relapsing and remitting disorder. Most children will improve and many will have resolution of symptoms with treatment. The cure rate is variable but has been reported as 30% to 50% by 1 year and 48% to 75% by 5 years in clinic samples of children with chronic constipation (Loening-Baucke, 2002a). Outcomes vary, depending on the medical complexity of the case as well as other emotional and psychosocial factors involved. The longer the condition is present, the greater the impact on child and family functioning and overall treatment success. It is important therefore to recognize and to treat this disorder as soon as possible. This also includes helping parents anticipate challenges to toilet training.

After further history it is determined that Sammy presents with encopresis/functional retentive fecal incontinence. His parents are provided with information about encopresis and are relieved to find out how common this is and that it is treatable. He is treated with an initial multiday cleanout with PEG without electrolytes with senna and then continues on a maintenance dose of PEG without electrolytes. He is given a behavior plan, which includes a token reward system for sitting on the toilet after meals for 5 minutes three times a day. Over time he starts requesting to use the toilet, and his accidents are less frequent. His token reward plan is modified to take this into account. He is continued on PEG for 6 months and then weaned. His parents are educated around recurrence of accidents around times of stress and successfully manage a mild relapse after a transition in the family.

CONCLUSION

The principles for successful toilet training include recognition of readiness skills and following a stepwise process that recognizes individual developmental, behavioral, and temperamental variation. Management of toilet refusal includes treating constipation, ensuring soft stools, and using a stepwise approach with positive behavioral strategies. Encopresis is common in the pediatric population and is frequently associated with constipation, withholding, and a history of toilet refusal. Encopresis is rarely caused by organic illness, and careful history and physical examination are usually sufficient to rule out organic disease. Successful management of encopresis includes caregiver education, treatment of constipation using a personalized cleanout regimen, use of a structured sitting program with positive behavioral strategies, maintenance medication, a behavioral plan, and a plan for periods of relapse.

REFERENCES

American Psychiatric Association. (2013). *Diagnostic and statistical manual of mental disorders* (5th ed.). Author.

Baker, S. S., Liptak, G. S., Colletti, R. B., Croffie, M., Di Lorenzo, C., Ector, W., & Nurko. S. (1999). A medical position statement of the North American Society for Pediatric Gastroenterology and Nutrition. Constipation in infants and children: Evaluation and treatment. *Journal of Pediatric Gastroenterology and Nutrition*, *29*, 612–626.

Blum, N. J., Taubman, B., & Nemeth, N. (2003). Relationship between age at initiation of toilet training and duration of training: A prospective study. *Pediatrics*, *111*, 810–814.

Blum, N. J., Taubman, B., & Nemeth, N. (2004). During toilet training, constipation occurs before stool toileting refusal. *Pediatrics*, *113*, e520–e522.

Brazelton. T. B. (1962). A child-oriented approach to toilet training. *Pediatrics*, *29*, 121–128.

Brazelton, T. B., Christophersen, E. R., Frauman, A. C., Gorski, P. A., Poole, J. M., Stadtler, A. C., & Wright, C. L. (1999). Instruction, timeliness and medical influences affecting toilet training. *Pediatrics*, *103*, 1353–1358.

Brazzelli, M., Griffiths, P. V., Cody, J. D., & Tappin, D. (2011). Behavioural and cognitive interventions with or without other treatments for the management of faecal incontinence in children. *Cochrane Database of Systematic Reviews*, *12*, CD002240.

Brooks, R. C., Copen, R. M., Cox, D. J., Morris, J., Borowitz, S., & Sutphen, J. (2000). Review of the treatment literature for encopresis, functional constipation, and stool-toileting refusal. *Annals of Behavior Medicne*, *22*, 260–267.

Joinson, C., Heron, J., Butler, U., von Gontard, A., & Avon Longitudinal Study of Parents and Children Study Team. (2006). Avon Longitudinal Study of Parents and Children Study Team: Psychological differences between children with and without soiling problems. *Pediatrics*, *117*, 1575–1584.

Loening-Baucke. V. (2002a). Encopresis. *Current Opinion in Pediatrics*, *14*, 570–575.

Loening-Baucke. V. (2002b). Polyethylene glycol without electrolytes for children with constipation and encopresis. *Journal of Pediatric Gastroenterology and Nutrition*, *34*, 372–377.

Loening-Baucke. V. (2007). Prevalence rates for constipation and faecal and urinary incontinence. *Archives of Disease in Childhood*, *92*(6), 486–489.

Peeters, B., Noens, I., Philips, E. M., Kuppens, S., & Benninga, M. A. (2013). Autism spectrum disorders in children with functional defecation disorders. *Journal of Pediatrics*, *163*(3), 873–878.

Reisner, S. H., Sivan, Y., Nitzan, M., & Merlob, P. (1984). Determination of anterior displacement of the anus in newborn infants and children. *Pediatrics*, *73*, 216.

Rockney, R. M., McQuade, W. H., & Days, A. L. (1995). The plain abdominal radiograph in the management of encopresis. *Archives of Pediatrics and Adolescent Medicine*, *149*, 623.

Schonwald, A., Sherritt, L., Stadtler, A., & Bridgemohan, C. (2004). Factors associated with difficult toilet training. *Pediatrics*, *113*, 1753–1757.

Sharif, F., Crushell, E., O'Driscoll, K., & Bourke, B. (2001). Current topic. Liquid paraffin: A reappraisal of its role in the treatment of constipation. *Archives of Diseases in Childhood*, *85*, 121–124.

Tabbers, M. M., DiLorenzo, C., Berger, M. Y., Faure, C., Langendam, M. W., Nurko, S., … European Society for Pediatric Gastroenterology, Hepatology, and Nutrition, North American Society for Pediatric Gastroenterology, (2014). Evaluation and treatment of functional constipation in infants and children: Evidence-based recommendations from ESPGHAN and NASPGHAN. *Journal of Pediatric Gastroenterology and Nutrition*, *58*(2), 258–274.

70

Sleep and Sleep Disorders in Children

Ronald E. Becker and Judith A. Owens

For additional material related to the content of this chapter, please see Chapters 72, 92, 93, and 98.

VIGNETTES

1. *Andrea is a 15-year-old who states that she "can never get to sleep." She is up for hours after going to bed "waiting to go to sleep." She starts to try to go to bed at 9:30 pm. As she lies in bed, she worries that her sleep problems will affect the next day at school. Once she finally goes to sleep, sometimes as late as 1 am, she stays asleep until morning, but then is very difficult to arouse. She often misses the bus at 6:50 am. She hasn't missed any days of school or been late to school. She sometimes falls asleep during study hall, but not during class. She often participates in after-school activities. She does not nap after school. On weekends she sleeps to 11 am to "catch up."*
2. *Liam is an 8-year-old with autistic disorder and intellectual disability. He is overweight and has been gaining weight. He had a very short sleep duration as a younger child but has seemed to sleep better in the past few years. For the last 6 months Liam has started snoring loudly.*

SLEEP FROM A DEVELOPMENTAL-BEHAVIORAL PERSPECTIVE

The practice of pediatric sleep medicine is closely aligned with that of developmental-behavioral pediatrics. Normal childhood sleep is developmental by its nature, as it changes through the life span. When sleep disorders are present, it is important to consider factors that are intrinsic to the child (health, mental health, and learned experiences) and those that may be extrinsic (sleep environment, family, school and neighborhood/community settings). How well a child sleeps is often inaccurately given moral valence as it may be connected to how "good" the child is perceived to be.

Parent-reported concerns for their children's sleep are common, with as many as 35% expressing concerns in a primary care sample (Byars, Yolton, Rausch, Lanphear, & Beebe, 2012). Children with neurodevelopmental disorders have sleep difficulties reported at a higher rate than the general population. Often they can benefit from standard sleep advice which has been modified to accommodate for their developmental needs related to motor skills, language skills, or anxiety. However, the presence of seizures, the use of neuroactive medications, and higher rates of nocturnal enuresis, sleep apnea, and other medical conditions all disproportionately and negatively impact childhood sleep for children with neurodevelopmental disabilities.

BASIC SLEEP MECHANISMS

The process of falling asleep is regulated by two basic neurologic processes that operate together: The homeostatic process, or sleep drive, refers to the fact that a longer time spent awake will result in increasing sleepiness; endogenous circadian rhythms (biologic clocks) operate independently and influence the timing and duration of daily sleep-wake cycles. Due to the circadian rhythms it can be very challenging for children or adolescents to go to sleep at a time earlier than their body clock may dictate. Sleep patterns are best when both processes are working in concert, and when they are not the result can be unwelcome wakefulness at night or sleep during the day.

The circadian rhythms (which govern many other physiologic systems in addition to sleep-wake cycles) are synchronized to the 24-hour day cycle by environmental cues (zeitgebers), such as timing of meals and other activities. However, the most powerful circadian cue is the light-dark cycle, which exerts a powerful influence on melatonin secretion by the pineal gland, with the timing of morning light being the most important zeitgeber. Thus exposure to morning light is included in the treatment of delayed sleep phase syndrome described later in this chapter.

Sleep is not a uniform process; there are deeper and lighter stages of sleep, with deeper stages of sleep often associated with higher amplitude and slower frequency electroencephalography (EEG) patterns, and so is sometimes referred to as slow-wave sleep. Rapid eye movement (REM) is another sleep stage. REM sleep is associated with voluntary muscle paralysis and a general loss of voluntary muscle tone. It is because loss of tone in the muscles that control the airway that snoring and sleep disorder breathing are more pronounced during this sleep stage. The REM stage is also often most associated with dreaming, although dreams can take place at any stage. Other parasomnias, such as periodic limb movements, are associated with non-REM sleep (slow-wave sleep), and night terrors or sleep walking emerge most often during transitions between deeper and lighter stages of non-REM sleep.

THE SLEEP HISTORY

Screening for sleep problems is important throughout pediatric health care and especially in the care of children with

TABLE 70.1 Elements of the Sleep History

Sleep Schedule
What is the bedtime and lights-out time if different than bedtime?
What is the sleep onset time (may be hard to determine in older children)?
Timing of any wakings during the night and their duration?
What is the morning wake time?
Does schedule vary depending on the day (esp. weekends)?
What are the nap times and nap durations?
What is the daytime schedule (meals, school, other activities)?
Child and Parent Behaviors
What is the child's response to bedtime?
Are parent(s) present for sleep onset?
What are the child behaviors and the parent(s) response during any wakings?
Are the behaviors at night different than during day? Specifically, if there is anxiety at night, is it seen during the day?
How consistent is parent(s) response?
Sleep Environment
Is there a pacifier or other comfort item present?
Does child share the bedroom with siblings or parents?
What kind of bed does the child sleep in (twin bed, bunk or loft, crib [with side rails], bed tent)?
Are there lights on, noise/music/television/other electronic devices playing?
What is the proximity of child's room to parents (same floor of home)?
Social Situation
Who is at home?
Are there any recent changes or stressors?
Are neighbors expressing concern regarding crying infants or toddler?
Medical History
Presence of chronic illness, especially neurologic or respiratory?
Any source of pain?
Medications taken?
Tonsillar enlargement? History of adenotonsillectomy?
Nasal/facial injury?
Family History
Sleep disorders (esp. apnea, sleepwalking, night terrors, leg movements)?
Neurologic disorders?
Other Sleep-Related History
Does the child snore?
Is there sleepwalking, sleep talking, or night terrors?
Enuresis?
Leg movements or discomfort at bedtime?
Evaluate for daytime sleepiness (self, parent, teacher reports)

developmental and behavioral conditions in light of the elevated risk for sleep difficulties in children with these conditions. If a sleep concern is raised, a full sleep history is essential to understanding the problem and developing a treatment plan (Table 70.1). The patient or caregiver should be asked about bedtime, time of sleep onset, timing and duration of any waking in the night, and if any naps are taken. It is important to understand any day-to-day variability in schedule. The history should include questions about snoring or other breathing concerns, excess movements or kicking before bed or during sleep, and any bedwetting or tooth grinding. Behaviors during arousals and the caregiver response to these arousals should be reviewed. Key factors in the sleep environment include whether the bedroom is shared, and the presence of any lights or purposeful sound in the room. Patients of all ages should be asked about the use of devices, including those that may be audio-only. Music that shuts off in the middle of the night can be a potent source of arousal for some children.

It is often helpful to supplement the history with a caregiver-completed sleep log covering 1 to 2 weeks. In this way variability in sleep patterns and average total sleep can be best understood. (Blank log forms are readily available online, including from the American Academy of Sleep Medicine.)

MEASURING SLEEP

Actigraphy

The measurement of sleep continues to be greatly impacted by the emergence of new technologies. This includes a wide range of consumer-facing devices, which are worn on the body, placed on/under a mattress, or even built into an infant's crib, that measure sleep and sleep health to varying degrees of accuracy. It is becoming common for patients and caregivers to employ these devices before seeking clinical care. Most of these devices currently rely primarily on patient movement (actigraphy) as a proxy measure for sleep versus wake and may attempt to report on movement during sleep as a measure of the quality of sleep. However, devices are increasingly collecting data on body temperature and heart rate among other measures, which may improve the accuracy of these devices.

Current clinical/research actigraphy devices also use movement as a measure of sleep versus wake and more often will employ sensors for heart rate, oxygenation, temperature, and ambient light to improve the validity of the sleep measurement. These devices are more likely to have been calibrated against gold standard measures and more often provide the clinician access to the raw data, which allows more clinical correlations and interpretation. However, most of these devices cost far more than the consumer devices and therefore are usually relegated for use in a sleep medicine practice or research program.

Polysomnograms and Multiple Sleep Latency Test

Sleep studies (polysomnograms) are noninvasive, multimodality tests that measure what happens when a patient sleeps. They are best used to diagnose sleep disorders such as sleep apnea, periodic limb movement disorders, and to rule out pathology that may be associated with nocturnal arousal. Overnight polysomnography documents physiologic variables during sleep, including sleep stages and arousals (EEG montage, eye movements, chin muscle tone), cardiorespiratory parameters (airflow, respiratory effort, oxygen saturation, transcutaneous or end-tidal carbon dioxide concentration, and heart rate), and limb movements.

Sleep studies do not typically include a full EEG montage but can also at times identify seizures or seizure-like activity. However, if seizures are highly suspected, overnight EEG is preferred. Sleep studies do not typically answer questions about why an individual may be having trouble falling asleep, and as they are most often one-night studies they do not answer questions about sleep duration. Specialized sleep studies can be extended into the day hours and include the multiple sleep latency test, which involves a series of opportunities to nap, during which patients with excessive daytime sleepiness or narcolepsy (described later) will demonstrate a pathologically shortened sleep onset latency (<5 minutes) and abnormally rapid entry into REM stage sleep during a nap.

Independent of the multiple sleep latency test it can be challenging to identify and quantify daytime sleepiness in children as they often respond to lack of sleep by demonstrating challenges with attention or irritable mood rather than the propensity to fall asleep or nap. The most common survey measure of sleepiness used in adults is the Epworth Sleepiness Scale, and a population-normed modification of this scale for use in pediatrics has recently been published (Maski et. al., 2022).

DEVELOPMENTAL TRAJECTORY OF NORMAL SLEEP

Sleep architecture in neonates and infants is quite different from that in adults, and sleep and sleep-wake patterns begin to resemble those of adults as children mature. There is a dramatic decrease in the proportion of both slow-wave and REM sleep from birth through childhood to adulthood. There is a decrease in the 24-hour total sleep duration from infancy through adolescence, with a more dramatic drop in sleep duration in early childhood followed by a less marked and more gradual continued decrease in nocturnal sleep amounts into late adolescence. Napping is common in infants and toddlers and usually ends before 5 years and becomes virtually impossible for most children until adolescence (Paruthi et al., 2016).

Population studies to develop norms for sleep durations across the age span are challenging to complete and nearly always depend on caregiver report, with the inherent biases of such studies. In addition, these studies typically measure the amount of sleep the child or adolescent achieves rather than the amount needed for optimal functioning, and the prevalence of short sleeping increases dramatically after early adolescence.

Sleep in Newborns

Newborns sleep approximately 16 to 20 hours per day, generally in 1- to 4-hour sleep periods followed by 1- to 2-hour periods awake. Sleep amounts during the day approximately equal the amount of nighttime sleep. Sleep-wake cycles are largely dependent on hunger and satiety; for example, bottle-fed infants generally sleep in longer bouts (3–5 hours) than breastfed infants (2–3 hours). Newborns have two sleep states that are essentially analogous to adult REM and non-REM sleep, active (REMlike; characterized by smiling, grimacing, sucking, and body movements; 50% of sleep) and quiet (non-REMlike), as well as a third indeterminate state.

Sleep in Infants (1–12 months)

Infants generally sleep about 14 to 15 hours per 24 hours at 4 months and 13 to 14 hours total at 6 months; however, there appears to be a very wide intraindividual variation in parent-reported 24-hour sleep duration. Sleep periods last about 3 to 4 hours during the first 3 months and extend to 6 to 8 hours by the age of 4 to 6 months. Most infants between 6 and 12 months of age nap between 2 and 4 hours divided into two naps per day.

Two important sleep-related milestones are normally achieved during the first 6 months of life; these are known as sleep consolidation and sleep regulation. Sleep consolidation is generally described as an infant's ability to sleep for a continuous period that is concentrated during the nocturnal hours, augmented by shorter periods of daytime sleep (naps). Infants develop the ability to consolidate sleep between 6 weeks and 3 months of age, and approximately 70% to 80% of infants achieve sleep consolidation (i.e., "sleeping through the night") by 9 months. Sleep regulation refers to the infant's ability to control internal states of arousal both to fall asleep at bedtime without parental intervention or assistance and to fall back asleep after normal brief arousals during the night. The capacity to self-soothe begins to develop in the first 12 weeks of life and reflects both neurodevelopmental maturation and learning. However, the developmental goal of independent self-soothing in infants at bedtime and after night wakings may not be shared by all cultures and families, and voluntary or lifestyle bed and room sharing of infants and parents is a common and accepted practice in many cultures. Sleep behavior in infancy, in particular, must also be understood in the context of the relationship and interaction between child and caregiver, which has a great impact on the quality and quantity of sleep, as well as of other important factors affecting sleep, such as child temperament, breastfeeding practices, and environmental factors.

Sleep in Toddlers (12–36 months)

Toddlers sleep about 12 hours per 24 hours. Napping can range from 0.5 to 3.5 hours per day. Most toddlers give up a second nap by 18 months. During this stage, both developmental and environmental issues begin to have more of an impact on sleep; examples include an increase in separation anxiety, which may lead to bedtime resistance and problematic night wakings; the development of imagination, which may result in increased nighttime fears; the increased understanding in toddlers of the symbolic meaning of objects, which can lead to increased interest in and reliance on transitional objects to allay normal developmental and separation fears; and an increased drive for autonomy and independence, which may result in increased bedtime resistance. Sleep problems in toddlers are very common, occurring in 25% to 30% of this age group; bedtime resistance is found in 10% to 15% of toddlers, and night wakings in 15% to 20%.

Sleep in Preschoolers (3–5 years)

Preschool-age children typically sleep about 11 to 12 hours per 24 hours; most children give up napping by 5 years, although approximately 25% of children continue to nap occasionally at the age of 5 years. Children in daycare settings will commonly nap at daycare and not at home during this time, which can lead to challenges in establishing a bedtime schedule. Difficulties falling asleep and night wakings (15%–30%), in many cases coexisting in the same child, are still common in this age group. Developmental issues affecting sleep include expanding language and cognitive skills, which may lead to increased bedtime resistance, as children become more articulate about their needs and may engage in more limit testing behavior; developing capacity to delay gratification and to anticipate consequences, which enables preschoolers to respond to positive reinforcement for appropriate bedtime behavior; and increasing interest in developing literacy skills, which reinforces the importance of reading aloud at bedtime as an integral part of the bedtime routine. Bedtime routines and rituals, use of transitional objects, and sleep-wake schedules are all-important sleep-related issues at this developmental stage.

Sleep in Middle Childhood (6–12 years)

Most children this age sleep between 10 and 11 hours a night. Because a high level of physiologic alertness during the day is characteristic of school-age children, the presence of daytime sleepiness in an elementary school–age child is likely to be indicative of significant sleep disruption and fragmentation or insufficient sleep. Middle childhood is also a critical time for the development of healthy sleep habits. Increasing independence from parental supervision and a shift in responsibility for health habits as children approach adolescence may result in less enforcement of appropriate bedtimes and inadequate sleep duration; parents may also be less aware of sleep problems if they do exist, as children this age are less likely to report these to their parents.

Sleep in Adolescents (12–18 years)

Although a number of significant sleep changes occur in adolescence, mostly around circadian cycling, adolescent sleep needs do not appear to differ dramatically from sleep needs of preadolescents, and optimal sleep amounts remain at about 9 to 9.25 hours per night. In adolescence, however, a differential between sleep obtained and that needed very often starts to emerge. A number of studies across different environments and in different cultures have suggested that the average adolescent typically sleeps about 7 hours or less per night and that this accumulating sleep debt may have a significant impact on functioning, performance, and quality of life. Due to biologically mediated changes to the body clock, adolescents are especially at risk for delayed sleep phase syndrome (DSPS) in which they do not feel the need to fall asleep until so late that they do not get adequate sleep before they need to wake up. Regrettably, DSPS can be so common among some cohorts that this negative pattern can be misidentified as "typical teenage sleep."

NEUROBEHAVIORAL AND NEUROCOGNITIVE IMPACT OF INADEQUATE AND DISRUPTED SLEEP IN CHILDREN

There is clear evidence from both laboratory-based studies and clinical observations that insufficient sleep and poor-quality sleep result in daytime sleepiness and behavioral dysregulation, and affect neurocognitive functions, especially attention, working memory, and other executive functions. Insufficient sleep more prominently affects attention and vigilance, whereas fragmented sleep has more impact on mood and mood regulation (increased irritability, decreased positive mood, poor affect modulation).

Behavioral manifestations of sleepiness in children are varied and range from those that are classically sleepy, such as yawning, rubbing eyes, and resting the head on a desk, to externalizing behaviors, such as increased impulsivity, hyperactivity, and aggressiveness, to increased distractibility and off-task behavior. Sleepiness may also result in observable neurocognitive performance deficits, including decreased cognitive flexibility and verbal creativity, poor abstract reasoning, impaired motor skills, decreased attention and vigilance, and memory impairments. Finally, inadequate sleep in children can impact general wellbeing, including cardiac effects, impacts on glucose metabolism, and increased risk for obesity.

Some of the strongest evidence for the negative impact of a sleep disorder is for children with obstructive sleep apnea (OSA). Successful treatment of OSA has been shown in a number of studies to fully or partially reduce associated neurobehavioral and neurocognitive deficits. However, emphasizing the need for timely identification and treatment, there is also evidence that longstanding untreated OSA in children can have lasting impact on cognitive functioning that does not reverse with later treatment (Hunter et al., 2016)

In addition, as parents require adequate sleep for their own functioning, studies have documented the expected secondary effects of children's sleep problems on parents and family functioning. The effects may be particularly prominent on caregivers of children with special health care needs.

GOOD SLEEP HYGEINE

Practices related to sleep that increase the likelihood of an individual falling asleep quickly at bedtime and staying asleep through the night are referred to as good sleep hygiene. These practices can prevent the onset of sleep problems and are typically an important component of intervention for many types of sleep problems. Factors that contribute to good sleep hygiene are shown in Table 70.2.

TABLE 70.2 Sleep Hygiene

Sleep Hygiene for Children	
Sleep schedule	Bedtime and wakeup time should be about the same time every day. There should not be >1 hr difference in bedtime and wakeup time between school nights and nonschool nights.
Bedtime routine	A 20- to 30-min bedtime routine that is the same every night is important in setting the stage for sleep. The routine should include calm activities, such as reading a book or talking about the day, with the last part occurring in the room where the child sleeps.
Bedroom	A child's bedroom should be comfortable, quiet, and dark; a dim nightlight is fine. Children also sleep better in a room that is cool (<75 °F). Avoid using a child's bedroom for time-out or as a punishment. You want your child to think of the bedroom as a good place, not a bad one.
Snack	A light snack (such as milk and cookies) before bed is a good idea. Heavy meals within 1–2 hr of bedtime, however, may interfere with sleep.
Caffeine	Children should avoid caffeinated beverages in general and particularly for at least 3–4 hr before bed. Caffeine can be found in many types of soda, coffee, iced tea, energy and performance drinks, and chocolate.
Evening activities	The hour before bed should be a quiet time. Avoid high-energy activities such as rough play or playing outside, or stimulating activities such as playing computer games.
Television/screens	Keep all screens and devices out of a child's bedroom. Children can easily develop the bad habit of needing the television to fall asleep. It is also much more difficult to control TV viewing if the set is in the bedroom.
Naps	Naps should be geared to a child's age and developmental needs. However, very long naps or too many naps should be avoided, as too much daytime sleep can result in a child's sleeping less at night.
Exercise	Children should spend time outside every day and get daily exercise.
Sleep Hygiene for Adolescents	
Sleep schedule	Wake up and go to bed at about the same time on school nights and nonschool nights. Bedtime and wake time should not differ from one day to the next by more than 1 hr.
Weekends	Do not sleep in on weekends to "catch up" on sleep. This makes it more likely that you will have problems falling asleep at bedtime.
Naps	If you are very sleepy during the day, nap 30–45 min in the early afternoon. Do not nap too long or too late in the afternoon or you will have difficulty falling asleep at bedtime.
Sunlight	Spend time outside every day, especially in the morning, as exposure to sunlight, or bright light, helps keep your body's internal clock on track.
Exercise	Exercise regularly. Exercise may help you fall asleep and sleep more deeply.
Bedroom	Make sure your bedroom is comfortable, quiet, and dark. Make sure that it is also not too warm at night, as sleeping in a room that is >75 °F will make it difficult to sleep.
Bed	Use your bed only for sleeping. Do not study, read, or listen to music on your bed. Keep the electronics (smartphone, computer, television) to a minimum or, better yet, out of the bedroom altogether.

(*Continued*)

TABLE 70.2 Sleep Hygiene—Cont'd

Bedtime	Make the 30–60 min before bedtime a quiet or wind-down time. Relaxing, calm, enjoyable activities such as reading a book and listening to calm music help your body and mind slow down enough to let you get to sleep. Avoid watching television, studying, exercising, or getting involved in energizing activities during the 30 min before bedtime.
Snack	Eat regular meals and do not go to bed hungry. A light snack before bed is a good idea; eating a full meal in the hour before bed is not.
Caffeine	Avoid eating or drinking products containing caffeine in the late afternoon and evening. These include caffeinated sodas, coffee, tea, and chocolate.
Alcohol	Avoid alcohol. Alcohol disrupts sleep and may cause you to awaken throughout the night.
Smoking	Smoking disturbs sleep. Do not smoke at least 1 hr before bed (and preferably, not at all!).
Sleeping pills	Do not use sleeping pills or other over-the-counter sleep aids to help you sleep. These may be dangerous, and the sleep problems often return when you stop the medicine.
Do not drive drowsy	Teenagers are at the highest risk for falling asleep at the wheel, so do not drive when you have not gotten enough sleep.

COMMON SLEEP DISORDERS IN CHILDREN

It can be helpful to characterize sleep disturbances under four basic categories: (1) sleep duration insufficient for sleep need; (2) sleep of sufficient duration, but fragmented or inefficient; (3) circadian rhythm disorders for which sleep is normal in structure but occurring at an undesired time; and (4) disorders of excessive daytime sleepiness (e.g., narcolepsy), which are less common but also possibly underrecognized. For practical purposes, sleep disorders may also be defined as primarily behavioral based versus organic or medical based, although in reality there is much overlap between these categories, and both are influenced by similar psychosocial and physical-environmental factors.

Obstructive Sleep Apnea and Sleep-Disordered Breathing

Sleep-disordered breathing (SDB) in childhood includes a spectrum of disorders that varies in severity, ranging from OSA to primary snoring (defined as snoring without ventilatory abnormalities). The basic pathophysiologic process of OSA involves cessation or restriction of airflow through the nose and mouth during sleep despite respiratory effort and chest wall movement; this disrupts normal ventilation during sleep, resulting in hypoxemia or hypoventilation and a sleep pattern characterized by frequent arousals. Common manifestations of SDB in childhood include loud, nightly snoring; choking or gasping arousals; and increased work of breathing characterized by nocturnal diaphoresis, paradoxical chest and abdominal wall movements, and restless sleep. However, SDB may still be present with less dramatic findings and even manifest primarily with neurobehavioral symptoms, including inattention, hyperactivity, and poor academic functioning. There is growing evidence that children presenting with even mild restriction of respiratory flow at night (upper airway resistance syndrome) may experience some impact on daytime functioning (Smith, Gozal, Hunter, & Kheirandish-Gozal, 2017).

Common risk factors for SDB are those contributing to a reduced upper airway patency and include obstructive features (e.g., adenotonsillar hypertrophy, allergies, reactive airway disease), reduced upper airway size (e.g., obesity, craniofacial syndromes, midfacial hypoplasia, or retrognathia or micrognathia), reduced upper airway tone (e.g., neuromuscular disorders characterized by hypotonia, Down syndrome), as well as genetic factors (family history of SDB) and environmental factors (e.g., secondary smoke exposure).

Specific physical examination findings (growth abnormalities such as obesity or failure to thrive, nasal obstruction with hyponasal speech and adenoidal facies or mouth breathing, or enlarged tonsils) may suggest OSA. However, the presence of large tonsils and adenoids does not necessarily mean the patient has OSA, and in fact there is no constellation of presenting symptoms and physical findings that have reliably been found to differentiate between OSA and primary snoring in the ambulatory setting. Overnight polysomnography remains the gold standard for evaluation and diagnosis of pediatric SDB and would be the recommended evaluation for Liam described in the second opening vignette.

Adenotonsillectomy is generally the first line of treatment for pediatric SDB, although adenotonsillectomy alone may not be curative when other risk factors, such as obesity, are present. Nutrition and exercise counseling should be a routine part of treatment in pediatric SDB in obese children. Positive airway pressure, as either continuous or bilevel positive airway pressure (the most common treatment of OSA in adults), can be an effective and reasonably well-tolerated treatment option for those children and adolescents for whom surgery is not an option or in children who continue to have OSA despite surgery.

Parasomnias

Sleep Terrors, Sleep Walking, and Nightmares

Parasomnias are episodic, often undesirable nocturnal behaviors that typically involve autonomic and skeletal muscle disturbances as well as cognitive disorientation and mental confusion. The most common parasomnias in childhood may be further categorized as those occurring primarily during slow-wave or deep sleep (partial arousal parasomnias), during REM sleep, or at the sleep-wake transition. The partial arousal parasomnias, which include sleepwalking and sleep terrors, typically occur in the first third of the night at the transition out of slow-wave sleep and thus share clinical features of both the awake (ambulation, vocalizations) and the sleeping states (high arousal threshold, unresponsiveness to the environment, amnesia for the event). Sleep terrors are typically differentiated from sleep walking by a very high level of autonomic arousal and behavioral agitation. Both are more common in preschoolers and school-age children and generally, but not always, disappear in adolescence, at least in part because of the relatively higher percentage of slow-wave sleep in younger children and probably also as a corollary of neurodevelopmental maturation. Sleep terrors are considerably less common (1%–3% incidence) than is sleepwalking or sleep talking (40% of the population has had at least one episode). Sleep fragmentation caused by an underlying sleep disorder such as OSA syndrome or behavioral insomnia may increase the frequency of either of these events in a predisposed child. Finally, there appears to be a genetic predisposition for both sleepwalking and night terrors, and it is not uncommon for individuals to have both types of episodes.

In contrast, nightmares, the most common REM-associated parasomnia in childhood, are very common, occur primarily during the last third of the night when REM sleep is most prominent, generally include vivid recall of dream content, and are more likely to be triggered by anxiety or a stressful event. In general, nightmares are fairly easily managed with a combination of behavioral, cognitive, and relaxation strategies. However, very frequent and persistent nightmares in a child warrant further investigation of possible trauma or evaluation for a more global anxiety disorder. Table 70.3 can help clinicians distinguish sleep terrors from nightmares.

Atypical presentations of partial arousal parasomnias are sometimes difficult to distinguish from nocturnal seizures; the index of suspicion for a seizure disorder should be higher in the presence of a previous history of or risk factors for seizures, any unusual or stereotypic movements accompanying the episodes, or postictal phenomena. Subsequent daytime sleepiness is also much more likely with nocturnal seizures. Home videotaping of the episodes may be helpful in making the diagnosis, but overnight polysomnography (with a full EEG seizure montage) may be necessary.

Management of partial arousal parasomnias should first include reassurance and education of the child and family about the benign and self-limited nature of the disorder. Parents may be told that most children stop having sleepwalking episodes or sleep terrors by adolescence. Interim management should include institution of appropriate safety measures, including gates (doorways, top of staircases), locking of outside doors and windows, lighting of hallways, and ensuring safety of the sleeping environment (e.g., reducing clutter on floors), and parent notification measures, such as alarm systems or a bell attached to the bedroom door. Avoidance of possible triggers or exacerbating factors (e.g., sleep deprivation, change in sleeping environment) as well as avoidance of awakening a child during an event should be discussed with parents. In the case of frequent (e.g., nightly) events a technique called scheduled awakenings, which involve having the parent wake the child approximately 15 to 30 minutes before the time of night that the first parasomnia episode typically occurs, can be useful. Pharmacotherapy (with a slow-wave sleep–suppressing drug such as a benzodiazepine or tricyclic antidepressant) should be limited to severe or chronic cases.

Rhythmic Movement Disorders

Rhythmic movement disorders, including body rocking, head rolling, and head banging, are parasomnias that occur largely during sleep-wake transition and are characterized by repetitive, stereotypic movements involving large muscle groups. They are much more common in the first year of life and generally disappear by the age of 4 years, although they may persist into adulthood in rare cases. Although occasionally associated with developmental disorders, most occur in typical children and do not result in physical injury to the child. Treatment is generally parental reassurance and, if appropriate, judicious padding of the sleeping surface.

TABLE 70.3 Factors Distinguishing Sleep Terrors and Nightmares

	Sleep Terrors	Nightmares
Stage of sleep	Partial awakening for slow-wave sleep	Any phase but most commonly rapid eye movement sleep
Child age	2–12 yr most common	Begin in toddler years, occur at any age
Child's appearance	Terrified, panicked, sweating, rapid heart rate and breathing	Fearful
Time since sleep onset	Usually 1–3 hr	Usually> 4 hr
Response to parent entering room	Continue to cry/scream/thrash, do not seem to be awake or know parent is there	Consoled by parent's presence
Recall the next morning	No memory of event unless awakened	Vivid recall of dream
Predisposing factors	Sleep deprivation, illness, stress	Stress, anxiety

Bruxism

Bruxism, or repetitive nocturnal teeth grinding, occurs in as high as 50% of normal infants during eruption of primary dentition, and the incidence of at least occasional episodes approaches 20% in older children. There is some speculation that the underlying pathophysiologic mechanism may be linked to alterations in central nervous system serotonergic and dopaminergic neurotransmission. For this reason, it may be worthwhile to consider the possibility of low body stores of iron as a factor in bruxism as well as for the other movement disorders listed later. At times, bruxism can be triggered by gastroesophageal reflux. Symptomatic treatment (e.g., for temporomandibular joint pain, wearing of teeth surfaces) generally involves the use of occlusal splints, and behavioral treatment (e.g., biofeedback) may also be useful for older children (see Chapter 72 for more information).

Restless Legs Syndrome and Periodic Limb Movement Disorder

Restless legs syndrome and periodic limb movement disorder (RLS/PLMD) are related sleep movement disorders that are frequently overlooked in both adult and pediatric clinical practice. RLS/PLMD is estimated to affect about 10% of adults; increased awareness of the impact on pediatric patients has led to establishing pediatric diagnostic criteria in the last decade and suggests that these difficulties are present in about 1% of the pediatric population (Marcus et al., 2014).

RLS symptoms are typically worse in the evening and are exacerbated by inactivity, leading to significant difficulty in falling asleep. Individuals with RLS describe uncomfortable "creepy-crawly" tingling sensations in the lower extremities rather than pain per se; however, these symptoms are often poorly articulated by the children themselves and may be expressed by parents as "growing pains" or a need to move (Picchietti et al., 2011). RLS is a clinical diagnosis and based on reported symptoms; a sleep study is not helpful in detecting RLS. Periodic limb movements, which often cooccur with RLS (as many as 80% of adults with RLS also have periodic limb movements), are characterized by brief, repetitive, rhythmic jerks primarily of the lower extremities during lighter stages of sleep; these may result in sleep fragmentation related to nocturnal arousals and awakenings. Because they cooccur frequently, a diagnosis of PLMD may help corroborate a diagnosis of RLS and help with management planning.

PLMD is more common among children with attention-deficit/hyperactivity disorder (ADHD) and increasingly recognized in children with autism spectrum disorder (ASD). A strong connection to low body stores of iron has been implicated. Children with developmental disorders may be at risk for iron deficiency due to dietary restriction, or at times due to excessive milk intake (Youssef, Singh, Huntington, Becker, & Kothare, 2013). Anemia is a late sign of iron deficiency, therefore it is recommended that a ferritin level be obtained when these concerns are present. Lab-reported norms for ferritin are typically based on hematologic outcomes, so seeking a ferritin of greater than 50 ng/mL should be the target, and iron supplements should be considered to reach this goal (Gurbani et al., 2019). The diagnosis of PLMD is confirmed with a sleep study, but many would recommend ensuring the ferritin is in the correct range before obtaining a sleep study. When PLMD is present despite appropriate ferritin levels, other treatments can include a variety of agents such as gabapentin, benzodiazepines, and dopaminergic agents.

Narcolepsy

Narcolepsy is a primary disorder of excessive daytime sleepiness that affects approximately 40 per 100,000 people in the United States. Narcolepsy is rarely diagnosed in prepubertal children, but retrospective surveys suggest that it frequently first manifests in late childhood and early adolescence. However, both pediatric and adult patients with narcolepsy often delay seeking medical attention and are frequently mislabeled as having mood disorders, learning problems, and academic failure before the underlying etiology is identified, sometimes as long as several decades later. Most cases are sporadic, but in about 25% of cases there is a family history of narcolepsy; rarely secondary narcolepsy after brain injury or in association with other medical illnesses may occur.

The cardinal and usual initial presenting feature of narcolepsy is repetitive episodes of profound sleepiness that may occur both at rest and during periods of activity (talking, eating). These "sleep attacks" may be very brief (3 seconds or "microsleeps"), resulting primarily in lapses in attention. Children may initially present as being generally tired and prone to napping, although not always in an uncontrolled fashion. Children are less likely to present initially with other features of the so-called narcoleptic tetrad, which essentially represents uncoupling of REM phenomena or the intrusion of REM sleep features (muscle atonia, dream mentation) into wakefulness. In addition to daytime sleepiness, the tetrad includes cataplexy (sudden loss of total body or partial muscle tone, usually in response to an emotional stimulus); hypnagogic (at sleep onset) or hypnopompic (on waking) visual, auditory, or tactile hallucinations; and sleep paralysis (temporary loss of voluntary muscle control) at sleep onset or offset. These symptoms of narcolepsy are also frequently misdiagnosed as part of a psychiatric or neurologic disorder, such as psychosis or a conversion reaction. It is important to note that sleep paralysis can also be present in some adolescents as an isolated symptom and without necessarily implicating a narcolepsy diagnosis.

The pathophysiologic mechanism of narcolepsy is related to alterations in the hypocretin-orexin sleep neuroregulatory system and may have an autoimmune basis. The gold standard for diagnosis is overnight polysomnography followed by a multiple sleep latency test (described earlier). On the multiple sleep latency test, individuals with narcolepsy will demonstrate a pathologically shortened sleep onset latency (<5 minutes) as well as periods of REM sleep occurring immediately after sleep onset. The treatment of narcolepsy generally involves a combination of lifestyle accommodations such as scheduled naps, medications to combat daytime sleepiness (stimulants), and REM sleep suppressants (such as selective serotonin reuptake inhibitors [SSRIs]) to prevent cataleptic attacks.

Behavioral Insomnia of Childhood (Sleep Onset Association and Limit Setting Subtypes)

Insomnia in children and adolescents should be viewed as a constellation of sleep-related symptoms that result from a wide range of possible causes, and not as a diagnosis per se. Practically speaking, the most frequent clinical manifestations of childhood insomnia, particularly in younger children, are bedtime refusal or resistance, delayed sleep onset, and prolonged night wakings requiring parental intervention.

In general, behavioral insomnia of childhood is a disorder of young children (0–5 years) but may persist into middle childhood and beyond. The presenting problem in the sleep onset association subtype of behavioral insomnia is generally one of prolonged night waking resulting in insufficient sleep. In this disorder the young child learns to fall asleep only under certain conditions or in the presence of specific sleep associations, such as being rocked or fed, which are usually readily available at bedtime. During the night, when the child experiences the type of brief arousal that normally occurs at the end of each sleep cycle or awakens for other reasons, the child is not able to get back to sleep (self-soothe) unless those same conditions are available again. As children realize that the rocking or soothing is likely to disappear when they fall asleep, they are also more vigilant at night, which may further increase the likelihood of arousal. The infant then signals the caregiver by crying (or coming into the parents' bedroom if the child is no longer in a crib) until the necessary associations are provided.

The limit setting behavioral insomnia subtype is a disorder most common in children of preschool age and older and is characterized by active resistance, verbal protests, and repeated demands at bedtime ("curtain calls") rather than night wakings. If it is sufficiently prolonged, the sleep onset delay may result in inadequate sleep. This disorder commonly develops from a caregiver's difficulty setting consistent bedtime rules. However, it is important to determine whether the child's resistance at bedtime is due to an underlying problem in falling asleep caused by other factors (e.g., medical conditions such as asthma or medication use, a sleep disorder such as restless legs, or anxiety). It is also important that the parents do not attempt bedtime too far in advance of the child's natural ability to fall asleep and that the expectation for overnight sleep is appropriate to the child's age.

Successful treatment of behavioral insomnia of childhood generally involves a combination of behavioral strategies aimed at eliminating inappropriate sleep onset associations or reducing undesirable bedtime behaviors. Studies indicate that behavioral therapies (discussed further in Chapters 4 and 93) produce reliable and durable changes for both bedtime resistance and night wakings in young children (Gradisar et al., 2016). Most of the interventions described in these studies could be placed into the following categories: extinction and its variants (i.e., unmodified extinction, extinction with parental presence, graduated extinction), positive bedtime routines, scheduled awakenings, bedtime fading with response-cost, positive reinforcement, and parent education/prevention. The introduction of more appropriate sleep associations that will be readily available to the child during the night (transitional objects such as a blanket or toy) in addition to positive reinforcement (e.g., stickers for remaining in bed) is often beneficial. Although these treatments can cause temporary stress due to a changing of rules and expectations, available research is highly reassuring that sleep training does not create any long-term emotional consequences (Price, Wake, Ukoumunne, & Hiscock, 2012).

Problems with limit setting generally respond to some combination of decreased parental attention for bedtime-delaying behavior, establishment of a consistent bedtime routine that does not include stimulating activities such as television viewing, bedtime fading (temporarily setting bedtime to the current sleep onset time and then gradually advancing bedtime earlier), and positive reinforcement (e.g., sticker charts) for appropriate behavior at bedtime.

SLEEP ISSUES IN SPECIAL POPULATIONS

Chronic Health Concerns

Chronic health conditions such as asthma, diabetes, sickle cell disease, and juvenile rheumatoid arthritis in children may predispose children to sleep problems, which in turn are likely to have a further impact on morbidity and quality of life. Additional specific medical conditions that may also have an increased risk of sleep problems include allergies and atopic dermatitis, migraine headaches, seizure disorders, other rheumatologic conditions such as chronic fatigue syndrome and fibromyalgia, and chronic gastrointestinal disorders such as inflammatory bowel disease. More substantial medical challenges can be associated with frequent hospitalization, use of medical technology through the night, or concerns for safety at night that may impact sleep until the underlying disorder is successfully managed.

Anxiety

Symptoms of anxiety are often more pronounced at nighttime. Anxiety at bedtime can present with children who find it difficult to go to sleep on their own, or they may find that anxious thoughts interfere with sleep onset. Children in this situation often benefit from a bedtime that is as late as possible to still accommodate sufficient sleep as this provides less time for ruminating thoughts to take hold. A program of gradual exposure to being alone in the room can also be beneficial. For any children with anxiety that is present both day and night, the best outcomes are achieved when they can engage in a cognitive-behavioral therapy (CBT) approach to their anxiety (see Chapter 98). At times, CBT can be tailored to treatment of insomnia.

Attention-Deficit/Hyperactivity Disorder

Children with ADHD commonly have increased challenge with sleep onset. This is likely a result of the underlying difficulties with impulsivity, hyperactivity, and the ability to settle in for sleep. However, there is also increasing indications that individuals with ADHD have a stronger preponderance to delayed sleep phase, which can persist to adulthood (Yoon,

Jain, & Shapiro, 2012). As noted earlier in this chapter, the symptoms of ADHD can be magnified in the setting of insufficient sleep, which serves to emphasize the importance of maximally supporting a child's sleep needs.

Autism Spectrum Disorder

Although the rate of sleep difficulties is increased in the setting of ASD, most children with ASD are capable of very good sleep. They and their caregivers may need additional support at setting up a bedtime routine that allows the caregivers to be absent at the time of sleep onset. They may also need additional support to minimize the impact of perseverative behaviors at bedtime. A smaller subset of children will have shortened sleep durations or highly fragmented sleep that is not responsive to behavioral or environmental supports. In those cases medication treatment of their sleep disorder should be considered with total sleep durations and daytime performance monitored for improvement.

Specific Genetic Diagnoses

As many genetic syndromes are also associated with global developmental concerns, it is not surprising that most have been associated with sleep disturbances at a higher frequency than the general population. There are specific syndromes of note, and close monitoring of the scientific literature can be helpful when caring for children with known gene differences. For example, Smith-Magenis syndrome can be associated with reversal of intrinsic melatonin cycling, leading to significant sleep schedule disturbance for some. Children with Prader-Willi syndrome may have increased risk of central apnea.

MEDICATIONS FOR SLEEP

There are no US Food and Drug Administration–approved medications for pediatric sleep indications. The potential overuse of medications and/or supplements for pediatric sleep has appropriately been a topic of public concern for some time. As such, a cautious and conservative approach to the use of medications for pediatric sleep is indicated. Medication treatment is usually reserved for treatment of sleep disruption that may be neurologically based (such as high sleep fragmentation or short sleep durations), which is not amenable to a behavioral or schedule-based approach. As such, there can be a rational role for use of medications for sleep indications in specific settings and populations. Treatment may also be considered to address underlying conditions (e.g., anxiety or ADHD) that may impact sleep negatively.

Medications for treatment of sleep difficulties fall into several categories, including prescription and over-the-counter products. It is important for a prescriber to be familiar with mechanisms of action and durations of action for prescribed medications. Some medications are short acting and primarily support sleep onset. These include antihistamines (e.g., diphenhydramine, hydroxyzine) and benzodiazepines/atypical benzodiazepines (e.g., zolpidem). Clonidine is sometimes used in the context of difficulty with sleep onset associated with impulsive or hyperactive nighttime behavior. While this medication can address the underlying behavioral issue, it is very short acting and will sometimes result in rebound arousal in the middle of the night.

Atypical antidepressants such as trazodone and mirtazapine have the dual action of creating initial drowsiness and often supporting sleep maintenance likely through action on both serotonergic and noradrenergic receptors.. Gabapentin has a similar , but less-well-defined, mechanism and can support sleep maintenance . It has been shown to have benefit for children with an autism spectrum disorder (Robinson & Malow, 2013).

Melatonin is currently getting frequent use and is supported by the preponderance of empiric data in the ASD population (Buckley et al., 2020). Short-term safety is well established in those studies, but long-term safety has been less well studied. Most studies show some benefit; although average response yields a modest improvement in sleep durations, some individuals appear to benefit more robustly. Usual dosing would be 1 to 3 mg, typically given 1 to 2 hours before bed. The activity of melatonin is also short, and it does not tend to improve sleep maintenance. Extended-release formulations are a consideration but have not shown much benefit, although few studies have been done.

At times, treatment of daytime drowsiness with stimulant medications can also help reestablish a more regular sleep pattern. This can often be beneficial when daytime napping is interfering with overnight sleep.

SLEEP-RELATED SIDE EFFECTS OF PSYCHOPHARMACOLOGY

Individuals with neurodevelopmental disorders will frequently be prescribed neuroactive medications, and many of these can impact sleep patterns. Proper treatment for a neurodevelopmental disorder frequently results in better sleep, but it is important to recognize the potential for sleep-related side effects. Stimulant medications are well recognized to have the potential to cause or worsen sleep-onset insomnia. This risk is increased when extended-release preparations are used, and usually adjustment of dosing can minimize the sleep impact. Nighttime alpha-adrenergic agents can wear off at night and generate rebound arousal for some children. SSRIs frequently inhibit REM sleep, although this does not usually result in any clinical concern and may be noted mainly on sleep study. However, withdrawal of SSRI can be associated with vivid dreaming or nightmares due to rebound increase in REM stage. Anticonvulsants frequently can cause daytime drowsiness, and some are also associated with overnight sleep fragmentation (perhaps most notably levetiracetam).

CONCLUSION

Sleep problems such as those described for Andrea in the first opening vignette are common in children and adolescents. A thorough history is essential to identifying the factors contributing to the sleep problems. The physical exam and occasionally laboratory testing may be necessary to make a definitive diagnosis. For Andrea, her irregular sleep schedule, catchup sleep on the weekends, trying to go to bed before she is tired, and perhaps anxiety may all be contributing to her sleep problems. Understanding and implementing good sleep hygiene may be sufficient for Andrea and many children with sleep difficulties. In other situations good sleep hygiene may need to be combined with behavioral interventions to improve sleep. Less commonly, pharmacologic interventions will be necessary. For children with OSA surgical intervention may be indicated.

REFERENCES

Buckley, W. A., Hirtz, D., Oskoui, M., Armstrong, M. J., Batra, A., Bridgemohan, C., … Ashwal, S. (2020). Practice guideline: Treatment for insomnia and disrupted sleep behavior in children and adolescents with autism spectrum disorder: Report of the Guideline Development, Dissemination, and Implementation Subcommittee of the American Academy of Neurology. *Neurology*, *94*(9), 392–404. https://doi.org/10.1212/WNL.0000000000009033

Byars, K. C., Yolton, K., Rausch, J., Lanphear, B., & Beebe, D. W. (2012). Prevalence, patterns, and persistence of sleep problems in the first 3 years of life. *Pediatrics*, *129*(2). https://doi.org/10.1542/peds.2011-0372

Gradisar, M., Jackson, K., Spurrier, N. J., Gibson, J., Whitham, J., Williams, A. S., … Kennaway, D. J. (2016). Behavioral interventions for infant sleep problems: A randomized controlled trial. *Pediatrics*, *137*(6). http://www.aappublications.org/news

Gurbani, N., Dye, T. J., Dougherty, K., Jain, S., Horn, P. S., & Simakajornboon, N. (2019). Improvement of parasomnias after treatment of restless leg syndrome/ periodic limb movement disorder in children. *Journal of Clinical Sleep Medicine*, *15*(5), 743–748. https://doi.org/10.5664/jcsm.7766

Hunter, S. J., Gozal, D., Smith, D. L., Philby, M. F., Kaylegian, J., & Kheirandish-Gozal, L. (2016). Effect of sleep-disordered breathing severity on cognitive performance measures in a large community cohort of young school-aged children. *American Journal of Respiratory and Critical Care Medicine*, *194*(6), 739–747. https://doi.org/10.1164/rccm.201510-2099OC

Marcus, C. L., Traylor, J., Gallagher, P. R., Brooks, L. J., Huang, J., Koren, D., … Tapia, I. E. (2014). Prevalence of periodic limb movements during sleep in normal children. *Sleep*, *37*(8), 1349–1352. https://doi.org/10.5665/sleep.3928

Maski, K., Worhach, J., Steinhart, E., Boduch, M., Morse, A., Strunc, M., … Sideridis, G. (2022). Development and validation of the pediatric hypersomnolence survey. *Neurology*. Advance online publication. https://doi.org/10.1212/WNL.0000000000200187

Paruthi, S., Brooks, L. J., D'Ambrosio, C., Hall, W. A., Kotagal, S., Lloyd, R. M., … Wise, M. S. (2016). Recommended amount of sleep for pediatric populations: A consensus statement of the American Academy of Sleep Medicine. *Journal of Clinical Sleep Medicine*, *12*(6), 785–786. https://doi.org/10.5664/jcsm.5866

Picchietti, D. L., Arbuckle, R. A., Abetz, L., Durmer, J. S., Ivanenko, A., Owens, J. A., ... Walters, A. S. (2011). Pediatric restless legs syndrome: Analysis of symptom descriptions and drawings. *Journal of Child Neurology*, *26*(11), 1365–1376. https://doi.org/10.1177/0883073811405852

Price, A. M. H., Wake, M., Ukoumunne, O. C., & Hiscock, H. (2012). Five-year follow-up of harms and benefits of behavioral infant sleep intervention: Randomized trial. *Pediatrics*, *130*(4), 643–651. https://doi.org/10.1542/peds.2011-3467

Robinson, A. A., & Malow, B. A. (2013). Gabapentin shows promise in treating refractory insomnia in children. *Journal of Child Neurology*, *28*(12), 1618–1621. https://doi.org/10.1177/0883073812463069

Smith, D. L., Gozal, D., Hunter, S. J., & Kheirandish-Gozal, L. (2017). Frequency of snoring, rather than apnea–hypopnea index, predicts both cognitive and behavioral problems in young children. *Sleep Medicine*, *34*, 170–178. https://doi.org/10.1016/j.sleep.2017.02.028

Yoon, S. Y. R., Jain, U., & Shapiro, C. (2012). Sleep in attention-deficit/hyperactivity disorder in children and adults: Past, present, and future. *Sleep Medicine Reviews*, *16*(4), 371–388. https://doi.org/10.1016/j.smrv.2011.07.001

Youssef, J., Singh, K., Huntington, N., Becker, R., & Kothare, S. V. (2013). Relationship of serum ferritin levels to sleep fragmentation and periodic limb movements of sleep on polysomnography in autism spectrum disorders. *Pediatric Neurology*, *49*(4), 274–278. https://doi.org/10.1016/j.pediatrneurol.2013.06.012

71

Movement Disorders

Samuel H. Zinner and Jonathan W. Mink

For additional material related to the content of this chapter, please see Chapters 46, 51, and 98.

VIGNETTE

The parent of an 8-year-old mentions concerns about his daughter's "habits." Last year, she began to lick her lips frequently, creating a chapped ring that lasted weeks or more. For several months now, she repeatedly opens her eyes widely, usually while also turning her head away, and often asks "What?" though no one else is speaking to her. She seems to be falling behind in school, particularly with math and reading, and becomes upset when asked to start her homework. She has been viewed as "intense" since she was a toddler and now seems to require rituals especially before going to school, starting homework, and bedtime, counting and then retracing her steps as she heads to her room, repeatedly touching both pages of her workbook until it's "right," and growing very upset if interrupted. As the parent describes these behaviors, the clinician notices the parent blinking repeatedly and intensely.

BACKGROUND

Pediatric movement disorders are common phenomena but often diagnostically challenging. Although symptoms of the most common movement disorders in children (i.e., tics and stereotypies) may be relatively benign and adequately managed in primary care, the differential diagnosis is broad. This requires clinicians to be aware of key features that differentiate benign from more serious conditions, as well as to identify more serious presentations of customarily benign conditions. These latter circumstances are often best managed in coordination with pediatric subspecialist care.

The term movement disorders encompasses a wide range of conditions characterized by distinctive features that emerge from a variety of genetic and acquired causes. Movement disorders are traditionally divided into two broad categories: hyperkinetic, which is common in children, is sometimes referred to as dyskinetic, and is characterized by excessive unintended movements; and hypokinetic, which is rare in children, wherein movements are decreased in amplitude or frequency, and may be accompanied by rigidity.

Despite wide-ranging differences, each of the disorders shares the quality of interference with the initiation or control of normal intended movement, intrusion into voluntary movement patterns, interference with maintained posture, or a combination. Weakness or abnormal muscle tone may accompany but does not cause movement disorders. Similarly, ataxia is traditionally not included as a movement disorder. Clinicians may find it difficult to classify an abnormal movement pattern in part because features overlap across many of these disorders and because their origins can be elusive. To complicate matters, until recently there had been no universally used terminology to categorize abnormal motor patterns in children.

NEUROBIOLOGY/PATHOPHYSIOLOGY

Movement disorders result from biochemical and/or structural abnormalities in circuitry that links cortical and subcortical structures. Most pediatric movement disorders likely arise from dysfunction within the frontal cortex, the basal ganglia, connecting circuits, or a combination. The basal ganglia are thought to play a modulatory role in the control of voluntary movement, perhaps by facilitating desired movements and suppressing competing undesired ones. Cortical input enters the basal ganglia mostly through the striatum. Many neurotransmitter systems come together at this cortical-striatal synapse. It is these systems that serve as the chief targets of neuropharmacologic interventions for basal ganglia–based disorders. Moving beyond this synapse, signals are processed through complex processes of activation and inhibition and then exit the basal ganglia, mostly via the globus pallidus and substantia nigra, providing inhibitory output to the thalamus and brainstem with subsequent modulation of frontal cortical areas.

Each type of movement disorder is phenotypically distinct but shares common circuitry with other movement disorders. The observed clinical differences across various movement disorders arise from differences in anatomic location or neurophysiologic activity in these circuits. The basal ganglia have parallel pathways, which regulate and refine motor actions, but which also influence a variety of nonmotor functions, including emotions, reward-based learning, cognition, and other roles. Indeed, there are few movement disorders that are not accompanied by affective or cognitive symptoms. Differential involvement of these parallel pathways may explain the variability and complexity of nonmotor symptoms described in the chapter.

CLINICAL STARTING POINT

The phenotypic appearance of the abnormal movement(s) and the clinical contexts in which the movements occur are key to determining diagnosis and guiding management.

The movements may not be observed in the clinical setting and may vary across settings or time, so it is helpful to ask the child's caregiver to prepare video recordings. Evaluation begins with characterizing the movements, including symptom onset, pattern, and change over time; whether they are paroxysmal (sudden onset and offset) or continual (repeated) or continuous (without stop); exacerbating or ameliorating influences, including emotional states; the child's awareness or voluntary control of the movements; and presence of associated preceding sensory urge. Evaluation includes a medical history including pre- and perinatal risk factors and development, academic learning, social behaviors, family history (including of similar or related conditions), and a physical examination. The clinician must be alert to deviations from normal timing and patterns of neurodevelopmental skills. Physical examination should include a neurologic assessment with attention to other features and clues such as dysmorphology, involvement of other organ systems, and neurocutaneous lesions. Diagnostic workup, including laboratory and imaging, is sometimes indicated and may require referral to a neurologic or an other relevant subspecialist.

Because movement disorders and the underlying mechanisms are variable, management approaches are specific to the particular movement disorder, the causal disease entity, and the child. Treatment may be supportive, symptomatic, or directed to the disease process itself. Useful management goals include optimizing present and future function and quality of life and reducing pain (Koy et al., 2016).

TIC DISORDERS

Definitions

Tics are common among children, especially among children with other neurodevelopmental disorders, and are commonly overlooked or misdiagnosed. Tics are movements or phonic (often vocal) productions that are sudden, rapid, recurrent, and nonrhythmic. While tics are described as involuntary, most children with tics, particularly as they approach adolescence, can identify an urge preceding some or all tics and can temporarily suppress the tics, albeit at the cost of physical discomfort.

The *Diagnostic and Statistical Manual of Mental Disorders*, fifth edition (*DSM-5*), organizes tic disorders by duration and phenotype. The most common, provisional tic disorder, describes one or more motor and/or vocal tics present for less than 1 year since onset. If tics endure beyond 1 year, often with waxing and waning frequency, the child is diagnosed with a chronic (persistent) motor tic disorder, chronic (persistent) vocal tic disorder (but not both), or Tourette disorder, wherein children have had multiple motor and one or more vocal tics, although not necessarily concurrently. All such tic disorders emerge prior to age 18 years and must not be attributable to the physiologic effects of a substance or another medical condition (American Psychiatric Association, 2013). The delineations between chronic tic disorders (CTDs) and Tourette disorder, and perhaps among all tic disorders, may be artificial; rather, tic disorders may lie along a spectrum of severity. For ease of discussion, tic disorders will be grouped with CTDs.

Tic severity can be considered along objective and subjective dimensions. The Yale Global Tic Severity Scale is the most frequently reported and recommended instrument in clinical investigations and identifies five dimensions of tic severity for both motor and vocal tics (number, frequency, intensity, complexity, and interference), as well as overall subjective functional impairment or distress in psychosocial, family, academic, and work settings (Martino et al., 2017). Table 71.1 identifies common simple and complex motor and phonic tics.

Epidemiology and Natural Course

Tics usually emerge in the first decade of life and most commonly involve muscles in the head, neck, or shoulders. Over time, if persistent, tics may involve more distal muscle groups and may increase in severity, reaching a maximum in the

TABLE 71.1 Tic Classifications

	Simple	Complex
Motor	• Sudden • Brief • "Meaningless" in appearance • Isolated to muscle group • Examples: blinking, eye movements, nose twitching, lip movements, grimacing, opening eyes widely, neck jerks, jaw snaps, gaze shifts, abdominal tensing, extremity clenching or jerking	• Slower and longer • "Purposeful" in appearance • May involve several muscle groups at once or in sequence • May be imitative of movements of self or others • Can involve vulgarity • Examples: head shaking, trunk flexion, stepping, stomping, scratching, gesturing, dystonic expressions or postures, torso twisting
Phonic	• Sudden • "Meaningless" linguistically • Often "allergy"-like • Sometimes voiceless • Examples: grunting, sniffing, throat clearing, coughing, belching, sucking, tongue clicking, hissing, barking, chirping, squealing, whistling	• Often sudden • "Meaningful" linguistic elements • Atypical speech prosody • May be imitative of noises or language of self or others • Can involve vulgarity • Examples: syllables, words, phrases, obscenities, alterations in rate or rhythm or pitch, halting

Adapted from Zinner, S. H., & Mink, J. W. (2010). Movement disorders I: Tics and stereotypies. *Pediatrics in Review, 31*, 223–233 (Table 2).

preteen years followed by a decrease in tic severity during adolescence or early adulthood. However, it is not possible to predict a tic course for any affected individual. Tics often occur in bouts, wax and wane over time (ranging from seconds to years), are highly state dependent (emotion, relaxation, and arousal), and diminish or disappear during sleep. Roughly 20% of children will experience tics at some point in childhood (Scahill et al., 2014), and up to 1% to 3% will have a CTD (Knight et al., 2012). The great majority of children with CTDs have other nontic childhood neurobehavioral disorders. These individuals are at substantial risk for impairment to general health and to social, emotional, academic, and work function. Early identification and coordinated management offer the best advantage to children with CTDs.

Phenomenology

Most children, especially those over age 10 years, can describe a premonitory, unpleasant sensory experience in the muscle groups where tics occur, described as an itch, pressure, tension, or tickle, similar to the sensation that builds around the eye muscles when trying to hold back a blink. This sensory urge is involuntary, while the tic behavior may be performed as a semivoluntary response to the urge, executed with just the right intensity and often with several repetitions, resulting in temporary relief. Drawing this description directly from the child is clinically helpful in distinguishing tics from other causes.

Tics may be strengthened via negative reinforcement (i.e., the sensation serves as an aversive stimulus that drives a behavioral response—the tic—resulting in relief that serves as reinforcement for the tic). While the physiologic mechanisms are not well understood, disinhibition within frontal cortex–basal ganglia systems involving motivation, reward, and patterned learning is involved, likely with dysregulation in dopaminergic pathways, among other neurotransmitter systems, including gamma-aminobutyric acid (GABA), glutamate, and serotonin. Disinhibition appears key in linking tic vulnerability to many of the nontic coexisting phenomena common to CTDs.

Distinctions From Similar Repetitive Behaviors

Clinical context is essential to distinguish tics from other similar repetitive movement patterns. The following neurologic and behavioral patterns are sometimes confused with tics:

1. *Stereotypic movement disorder* (stereotypies) is a common behavior pattern (discussed later).
2. *Habits:* Like tics, habits are repetitive movement patterns often reinforced by environmental antecedents and consequences. Unlike tics, habits may be rhythmic and sustained and do not have a premonitory sensation. They also do not typically change type or anatomic location over time. Examples discussed in Chapter 72 include thumb sucking, nail biting, or skin picking. These behaviors are most common when the child is bored, tired, or anxious.
3. *Somatic cough syndrome (psychogenic) and tic cough (habit):* A cough is a common tic expression that can perplex clinicians and sufferers alike. It has recently been proposed that the term "habit cough" be replaced with "tic cough (habit)" if the behavior has core clinical features of tics, including a premonitory sensation, suppressibility, distractibility, or suggestibility, even in the absence of any other tics. The symptom can be triggered by a preceding respiratory infection, asthma, or an other source, but is maintained beyond the resolution of the trigger. In contrast, "somatic cough syndrome (psychogenic)," which is the proposed new term for psychogenic cough, is a somatic symptom disorder that does not have these tic elements. Organic causes must be ruled out (Vertigan, 2017).
4. *Mannerisms:* Mannerisms are generally stereotyped and sometimes repetitive behaviors infused into intended movements, reactions, or statements. Examples include specific gestures, facial expressions, or vocal inflections. While mannerisms are usually unique to an individual, both children and adults may mimic mannerisms of others as a function of bonding (Chartrand & Lakin, 2013). Mannerisms may serve to convey, accentuate, or hide an intended communication as a means of social connection or of defense. However, among individuals with distorted social communication, including autism, mannerisms may occur more frequently and without clear social purpose.
5. *Compulsions:* Obsessions and compulsions are described more fully in Chapter 51, but a brief discussion is warranted because these behaviors often cooccur with CTDs and likely share genetic and physiologic origins. Like complex tics, compulsions are repetitive behaviors or mental acts that appear purposeful, often in response to an obsession (an unpleasant thought or image) or to meet demands of an idiosyncratic ritual or rule, such as opening and closing a door a number of times until the action feels complete or to ward off a feared but unrelated threat. Among older children and adolescents who do not suffer from cognitive distortion, the behaviors are recognized as illogical. The patterns of some compulsions and some complex motor tics can overlap, so it can be helpful in distinguishing between these by ascertaining the internal experience that precedes and accompanies the behavior; tics will likely have a premonitory sensation that drives the behavior, whereas compulsions may have a preceding image, emotion, or thought that drives the behavior. At times, a distinction cannot be definitively made, for which the term tourettic obsessive-compulsive disorder has been coined (Mansueto & Keuler, 2005).
6. *Seizure:* Complex tics may mimic seizures (particularly absence or focal seizures), with the distinction complicated in particular among children with communication disorders. Urges drive tics, which often can be suppressed, whereas auras (which are focal seizures with maintained awareness) do not drive a voluntary suppression or modify the seizure pattern.

Secondary Tic Disorders

While uncommon, tics may emerge in response to a secondary source, most likely affecting the neural pathways implicated in primary tic disorders. Any such source is an exclusion criterion for a diagnosis of a provisional disorder or

CTD. Identified secondary sources may include autoimmune, neurodegenerative, toxic, drug-induced, neoplastic, and inflammatory processes. Onset of tics in later adolescence or adulthood may be due to a functional neurologic (conversion) disorder in some individuals.

Genetics

The inheritance of tic disorders is poorly understood. Investigation has been complicated by phenotypic heterogeneity, but vulnerability is almost certainly multifactorial and inclusive of genetic, epigenetic, and environmental risk factors. There is no question that tic disorders, tic severity, and common nontic coexisting conditions are heritable. New technologies, including whole exome sequencing and genome-wide association studies, hold promise for large-scale projects to elucidate the underlying pathologic mechanisms and create more safe and effective treatment strategies.

Associated Nontic Neurobehavioral Symptoms

The vast majority of individuals with CTDs have one or more coexisting nontic neurobehavioral conditions, and most of these emerge in childhood (Hirschtritt et al., 2015). Each of these conditions has its own presenting time course distinct from tic emergence and is discussed only briefly as the conditions are described more fully in other chapters.

Attention-Deficit/Hyperactivity Disorder

Attention-deficit/hyperactivity disorder (ADHD; see Chapter 46) is the most common childhood neurodevelopmental disorder and occurs in about half of all children clinically diagnosed with CTDs. Impulsive behaviors, inattention, and distractibility are core features that share disinhibited elements. When coexistent in CTDs, ADHD symptoms typically precede the onset of tics and may impose greater functional and social impairment than do tics. Having ADHD often correlates with additional problems, including psychosocial and emotional, learning, and other behavioral concerns. Management of ADHD usually follows customary ADHD guidelines, and stimulants are generally safe to use with low risk of tic exacerbation (Cohen et al., 2015). Comprehensive clinical practice guidelines are available (Barbaresi et al., 2020).

Anxiety and Mood Disorders

Anxiety disorders (see Chapter 51) frequently cooccur with CTDs, often preceding tic onset. Prevalence estimates range widely from roughly 20% to half or more of children with CTDs, and symptoms can impose substantial functional and qualitative impairment. Anxiety disorders describe disproportionate anticipation of future threat that may have neurologic disinhibition roots and is associated with emotional, physical, and cognitive experiences of fear. Heightened anxiety states can exacerbate tic severity so that optimal tic reduction management, when indicated, targets treatment of coexisting anxiety. Mood disorders (see Chapter 49), including major depression, are also common in children with CTDs, although it is unclear whether these are neurologically related or occur secondary to hardships stemming from tics and other coexisting conditions. Depression is significantly associated with tic severity and presence of other coexisting conditions, including ADHD and anxiety disorders.

Obsessions and Compulsions

Obsessions and compulsions (see Chapter 51) are described earlier and are present in most individuals with CTDs, typically first emerging during adolescence. When the behaviors cause substantial distress, interfere with usual routines, or take an hour or more each day to complete, the term OCD is used. CTDs and OCD are genetically related. When linked to CTDs, obsessions and compulsions usually center on experiences of requiring symmetry or a sense of being just right, such as touching something just so, evening up a stack of paper, counting, and checking and rechecking (see vignette at the beginning of this chapter). When indicated, management may include cognitive and behavioral therapy (see Chapter 98), addressing coexisting anxiety, psychotherapy, and/or psychiatric medications (discussed later).

Academic Difficulties

Tics and the associated neurobehavioral concerns discussed earlier can interfere with academic performance and social participation. Children with CTDs are also at increased risk for learning disabilities (particularly in visual-spatial and visual-motor abilities—see vignette at the beginning of this chapter), organizational challenges, poorer frustration tolerance, medication treatment side effects that impair learning functions, and bullying.

Rage Attacks

Rage attacks are sudden, disinhibited, developmental age-inappropriate episodic anger outbursts in response to trivial provocation or frustration, followed by relief and often regret. These substantially impairing behaviors occur in 20% or more of children with CTDs (Conte et al., 2020).

Autism Spectrum Disorder and Other Social Communication Deficits

Tics coexist with autism spectrum disorder (ASD) or other social communication deficits (see Chapter 41) moderately frequently, ranging from 4.5% to 18% of individuals with CTDs (Eapen et al., 2019). A hallmark of ASD is repetitive behaviors, which often include tics. Shared phenotypic patterns include similar male:female ratio (about 4:1), obsessive-compulsive behaviors, imitative or echoic movements and sounds, and repetitive stereotyped complex behavior patterns. It is not clear to what extent the observation of repetitive behaviors may lead to misdiagnosis with an ASD, so social communication behaviors should be scrutinized if ASD is suspected in a child with a tic disorder.

Sleep Disorders

Difficulties in sleep maintenance and quality, as well as increase in movement-associated arousals and parasomnias, occur in up to half of children with CTDs. Tics tend to diminish but can occur in all stages of sleep and may pose disruption.

Further, medication use, anxiety, and other coexisting conditions can disrupt sleep. Insufficient sleep may influence tic severity during wakefulness (Hibberd et al., 2020).

Evaluation and Management

Families often correctly suspect the diagnosis and seek professional confirmation. Diagnosis may be straightforward, especially when tics are so-called simple. It is important to identify specific concerns from the child and family and any management interests or efforts to date. The clinician should gather a description of current and past tics, ideally including from the individual affected, noting tic onset and course, awareness of any premonitory sensation, degree of suppression control, and relief experienced after tic completion. Some clinicians use a tic severity rating scale, such as the Yale Global Tic Severity Scale, to establish baseline objective and subjective information, to identify more severe tics (e.g., self-injurious and functionally or socially disruptive) that demand heightened attention, and to monitor course or treatment response. All children with tics should also be assessed for presence of the common cooccurring conditions (ADHD, mood disorders, OCD, rage episodes).

Evaluation follows the history and physical examination described earlier, including a family history of tics or obsessions and compulsions (see vignette at the beginning of this chapter). Discreet observation will not necessarily spot tics, which wax and wane and are often suppressed in clinical settings. Attention to common but overlooked or misdiagnosed tics such as sniffing, coughing, and blinking (often presumed as allergic symptoms or as habits), including such behaviors seen in relatives, is useful. Further screening or formal evaluation may be needed when coexisting conditions are suspected.

Generally there is no indication for laboratory workup. Some experts opt for basic measures, including hemogram, renal/hepatic function panel, thyroid panel, ferritin, and urine drug screen for adolescents (Murphy et al., 2013). Brain imaging or electroencephalogram is not routinely indicated. Screening for ADHD and anxiety disorders is recommended. Diagnostic uncertainty or the presence of suspected coexisting conditions may require subspecialty referral.

Prioritize Most Burdensome Symptoms

Optimal management relies on revealing the neurodevelopmental and behavioral range of conditions viewed within the framework of cultural/personal values meaningful to the individual and caregivers. Such values or perspectives may differ within families or between families and educators and/or clinicians. The *DSM-5* diagnostic criteria for tic disorders make no mention of tic severity, and as tics may be quite mild across all severity dimensions, psychoeducation and monitoring, as well as identification and management of tic-modifying factors, often suffice. However, if tic-reduction treatment is desired, realistic goals should be set, aiming to reduce impairment and distress but not tic eradication, and may first target coexisting features that contribute to tic expression such as anxiety or sleep insufficiency.

Psychoeducation

Ascertain the child's and family's current understanding of tics. Doing so sets a framework to build an accurate understanding of tics and coexisting conditions and to help guide the direction and scope of intervention. An aim of psychoeducation is to foster resilience and identity strengths rather than symptoms, alleviate shame, enhance collaboration among all stakeholders (teachers, peers, family), and promote ongoing discussion (Pringsheim et al., 2019b). A healthful lifestyle with adequate sleep and a good diet should be supported; however, to date, no supplementary or elimination dietary interventions are known to impact tics. Families and school personnel can be connected with supporting resources, including the Tourette Association of America (Tourette.org). If active tics limit educational activities such as reading, writing, or speaking, an individualized education plan or Section 504 (of the Rehabilitation Act of 1973) accommodations can provide useful supports (e.g., breaks, preferential seating, a scribe, recorded lessons, separate testing locations; see Chapter 113). Screening for bullying should be specific, as bullying can take many forms and when present, management guidance resources are available (Mingbunjerdsuk & Zinner, 2020).

Useful psychoeducational points may include noting:

1. Tic disorders are neurobiologicallybased and are not deliberate.
2. Tics wax and wane in frequency and intensity, and often occur in bouts.
3. Tics can usually be suppressed to some degree, but at the cost of discomfort and distraction and with possible later rebound of increased tics, which can mislead people to assume tics are deliberate.
4. While tics (when chronic) may persist into adulthood, their severity usually diminishes substantially in late adolescence.
5. Watchful waiting with periodic monitoring is an acceptable management option.

Behavioral Tic Management

Behavioral treatment is particularly suited to motivated individuals whose tics are of moderate severity or whose coexisting conditions have behavioral treatments. The most studied behavioral approach for tic reduction is comprehensive behavioral intervention for tics (CBIT). This approach stems from habit reversal training (HRT), a cognitive and behavioral treatment that disrupts the urge-tic-relief cycle (see Chapter 72). In essence, HRT aims to strengthen the individual's awareness of internal experiences associated with tics (i.e., the sensory urge and emotional states that promote tics) and replace the tic with a competing behavior that is incompatible with performing tics. CBIT adds relaxation training (to reduce internal reinforcers such as stress and anxiety) and functional analysis of before-during-after the tic environmental influences (to reduce external reinforcers that drive and maintain tics, such as avoidance of homework because tics emerge in anticipation).

Tic reduction effectiveness with CBIT among suitable candidates is comparable to that of medication, with goals maintained for at least 6 months or more (McGuire et al., 2014). CBIT is used most reliably in individuals age 9 years and older. Duration of treatment varies depending on tic awareness, motivation, tic severity, and presence of coexisting conditions. The approach can be used with medication, but the effects with combined treatments are unclear. Potential drawbacks include difficulty in access due to paucity of trained providers, poor insurance coverage, and challenges with compliance. Virtual CBIT has preliminary evidence for effectiveness. A self-guided CBIT program (TicHelper.com) has not undergone rigorous scientific investigation.

Exposure with response prevention (ERP) for tics is a lesser studied behavioral approach based on the principle of habituation. ERP relies on suppressing all tics for incrementally increasing durations. The suppression is then paired with exposure (real or imagined) to situations in which tics often occur while mentally focusing on the sensory urges. Head-to-head studies of CBIT and ERP are few but suggest comparable reduction in tic severity.

Medication

No medications eradicate tics. Treatment goals may include reducing the pain, interference, and social costs of tics balanced with acceptable adverse effects. Medication treatment selection is individualized, with determinants that include tic severity and interference, safety considerations, and personal and clinician preferences.

Prescribing decisions are complicated by unclear pathophysiology, phenotypic heterogeneity, coexisting features, and psychosocial variables. Prescribing clinicians should screen patients for use of other prescription or complementary medicines and consider potential drug-drug interactions. Treated patients should be alerted that the waxing and waning pattern will continue during medication use and should not warrant immediate medication adjustment. Ongoing periodic reevaluation is advised.

Currently, there are three US Food and Drug Administration (FDA)–approved medications to treat tics. All three are antipsychotics (haloperidol, pimozide, and aripiprazole). All other medications are prescribed as off-label. Since the physiology is likely very complex structurally and chemically, there are no precise anatomic or neurotransmitter targets. The approved medications target dopamine receptor D2 subtype, following the theory of hyperactive dopaminergic systems. However, new strategies are under investigation.

Experts differ in opinion and practice regarding the sequence in which tic-reduction medications are tried. The following sequence reflects a balance of multiple recently published expert opinions:

1. First tier: Virtually all systematic reviews consider the alpha-2 adrenergic agonists clonidine and guanfacine as first tier. These agents may be especially helpful when treating coexisting ADHD (an indication for which there is FDA approval among some long-acting preparations) with impulsive behaviors, or for sleep initiation. However, these agents are not clearly beneficial in tic reduction in youth without coexisting ADHD (Weisman et al., 2013). The mechanism of action is unknown but may relate to noradrenergic dysregulation in thalamocortical and forebrain networks and that via indirect influences on dopamine systems (Singer, 2013a, 2013b).
2. Second tier: Atypical antipsychotics are second tier. The strongest evidence to date for reducing tic severity is seen with haloperidol, risperidone, and aripiprazole (Pringsheim et al., 2019a), though haloperidol is a typical antipsychotic agent and best considered as third tier, due to heightened risk for extrapyramidal symptoms. Safety and tolerability are not well studied. Adverse effects are variable and may include sedation and somnolence, metabolic disturbances (including weight gain and insulin resistance), prolactin disturbance, gynecomastia, and cardiovascular impact (see Chapter 99). There are specific concerns about coadministration with psychostimulants increasing the risk for arrhythmia, although the evidence is slim.
3. Third tier: Typical (first-generation) antipsychotics, including haloperidol and pimozide, may be quite effective in tic reduction, but the relative increased risk for extrapyramidal symptoms, including dystonia, motor restlessness, rigidity, and tardive dyskinesia, restrict their selection. Nevertheless, risk for extrapyramidal symptoms when prescribed to reduce tics appears quite low (Iasevoli et al., 2020). Topiramate, an anticonvulsant drug, is considered as second tier by some experts, although the evidence of efficacy is not strong at this time. Adverse effects can include somnolence, cognitive interference, and weight loss, but it has a generally more favorable safety and side effect profile than antipsychotics. Other anticonvulsants have not shown adequate evidence of benefit.
4. Botulinum toxin injection: Botox injected into vocal cords for severe vocal tics or localized motor tics results in neuromuscular blocking and may also reduce the premonitory sensation. The therapeutic effect lasts about 3 months. Adverse effects can include weakness and hypophonia.
5. Investigational: Agents and strategies under investigation include vesicular monoamine transporter inhibitors (e.g., tetrabenazine), dopamine D1 receptor antagonism (i.e., ecopipam), and cannabis-based medications.
6. Others: There are multiple case reports and small open-label series describing use and possible response to other agents, including magnesium, pyridoxine, baclofen, levetiracetam, mecamylamine, and others. Because of the normal waxing and waning pattern of tics, open-label series and case reports must be interpreted with caution.

Brain Electrical Stimulation

The mechanisms of potential benefit with targeted electrical brain stimulation are unknown but likely relate to electrical and neurochemical influences on implicated neural circuitry.

Noninvasive. Repetitive transcranial magnetic stimulation (rTMS) induces electrical current in the cortex produced by electromagnetic coils placed over the scalp. rTMS may induce long-term changes to synaptic transmission in cortex-subcortex networks. Evidence of benefit in well-designed trials is lacking (Latorre et al., 2019).

Transcranial direct current stimulation uses direct electric currents applied to the scalp via electrodes and is a fledgling area of active research with limited evidence of benefit in tic treatment (Kleimaker et al., 2020).

Surgical. Deep brain stimulation involves surgical implantation of electrodes into a targeted brain region, usually the internal globus pallidus or in the thalamus. There are very few published pediatric case reports or series treating tics and no pediatric controlled research studies (Coulombe et al., 2019). International guidelines restrict its use to severe and functionally impairing tics after having failed exhaustive behavioral and medical treatment trials and advise consultation with a local ethics committee or institutional review board for use in youth under 18 years of age (Schrock et al., 2015). Short-term improvement is variable. Arguments against its use in youth include the natural course/tendency of tics to improve with maturity, hardware and medical complications, and unknown long-term outcomes.

NONTIC MOVEMENT DISORDERS

Stereotypic Behaviors/Stereotypic Movement Disorder (Primary Motor Stereotypies)

Motor stereotypies are rhythmic and repetitive purposeless behaviors emerging in early childhood. The movements may occur as a primary condition without specific known cause or as a secondary one associated with another neurodevelopmental or genetic condition. Primary and secondary motor stereotypies collectively are classified as stereotypic movement disorder. The diagnostic criteria within the *DSM-5)* for this condition require that the motor behavior interfere with social, academic, or other activities and may result in self-injury. Because many children with primary motor stereotypies do not suffer apparent interference in any of these or other areas, some clinicians may opt to classify the behavior by its more colloquial term, stereotypy.

Examples of stereotypies include bilateral hand flapping, wrist rotations, body rocking, nodding or shaking the head, tongue chewing, lip sucking, or wiggling one's fingers in front of the face. Other behaviors in young children that variably are considered as stereotypies, but other times as habits and therefore can be difficult to classify, include thumb sucking and hair twirling, among others, and may regress or evolve into more mature expressions of stereotypies. The behaviors may also manifest as self-injurious, such as face slapping, eye poking, biting, or head banging, and much less commonly (when associated with some neurodevelopmental or genetic conditions) can be quite severe with resulting bruising, lacerations, retinal detachment, or digital amputation. The behaviors usually endure for stretches of seconds to minutes or longer, are rhythmic and fixed in pattern and body location, and tend not to change in their pattern as the child matures.

While motor stereotypies cooccur in the majority of children with ASD (Chebli et al., 2016), the behavior in these children is not classified as a separate disorder unless the behavior also features self-injury or is sufficiently severe so as to require treatment (American Psychiatric Association, 2013). Stereotypies are common among children with intellectual impairment, particularly when moderate to severe or profound, and especially among such children who are in low-stimulating environments. Other conditions commonly associated with stereotypies include sensory deficits and a variety of neurodevelopmental syndromes, including Lesch-Nyhan (self-biting or mutilation such as fingers), Smith-Magenis ("lick and flip" of fingers, as though flipping pages of a book), Cornelia de Lange (head banging or biting hands), Rett (hand wringing), and intrauterine alcohol exposure. However, it is important to understand that children with primary motor stereotypies may incorrectly be assumed to have a secondary condition, often autism; in fact, the neuropsychological function of most children with primary stereotypies is largely intact (Mahone et al., 2014).

Key Similarities to and Differences From Tics

Qualities of motor stereotypies have some overlap with those of motor tic behaviors, particularly in that the movements of both are common, repetitive, usually relatively benign, precipitated by excitement or stress, reduced by distraction, often have a family history of the movement classification (Harris et al., 2008), and are stereotyped (i.e., the movements are repetitive and purposeless and are viewed by others as a familiar and specific behavior pattern linked to the individual who is affected with the condition). However, in the *DSM-5)*, the term stereotyped was omitted from its description of tic behaviors to avoid confusion with stereotypic movement disorder. It is important to recognize that both tics and motor stereotypies can cooccur within the same individual. Factors distinguishing tics from motor stereotypies are featured in Table 71.2.

Pathophysiology

The pathophysiologic mechanism underlying stereotypies is not understood. Among intellectually low-functioning individuals with substantial communication impairment, the behaviors may provide a ready and routine distraction from boredom or occur as a response to emotional discomfort or physical pain. However, there is increasing evidence to suggest that the movements are physiologically distinct from true voluntary movements, involving separate neurologic pathways within brain cortex, subcortex, and/or cerebellar circuits. Suspected specific neurotransmitter systems at play include dopaminergic, glutamatergic, and/or GABAergic, but strong evidence to date is lacking.

Management

Motor stereotypies generally do not interfere with a child's daily activities. As children mature, the behavior may diminish or resolve, although it may persist at least into adolescence (Oakley et al., 2015). If persistent, the behavior may draw negative attention so that otherwise typically developing children often learn to modify or suppress the behavior. There is emerging evidence that behavioral treatments such as those described for tics earlier and for habits in Chapter 72 may be effective.

TABLE 71.2 Features That Distinguish Tics From Stereotypies

	Tics	Stereotypies
Age at onset	5–7 yr (mean)	<3 yr
Pattern	Variable (wax and wane) and evolve over time	Fixed, patterned, predictable
Movements	Usually emerge in eyes, face, neck, or shoulders May progress over time in distal and peripheral body locations	May emerge in arms/hands, head and neck, body
Noises	Usually emerge as nonlinguistic (e.g., sniffing, throat clearing) Progression over time may mimic language (e.g., words, repetitions)	Nonlinguistic and sustained (e.g., moaning, humming) occurring with movement
Rhythm	Absent	Present
Duration	Brief, rapid (except for dystonic tics)	Continuous, prolonged
Premonitory urge	Present (usually, esp. among older children)	Absent
Precipitant	Excitement, stress, or relaxation	Excitement, stress, states of engrossment, or boredom
Suppression	Voluntary (but with increased inner tension) and usually brief	With distraction, and only rarely with conscious effort
Distraction	Reduces the movement	Instantly stops the movement
Coexisting conditions	Frequent (esp. in chronic tic disorders) including ADHD, obsessions and compulsions, anxiety, and stereotypies	Frequent, including ADHD, obsessions and compulsions, anxiety, and tics
Family history	Often positive (esp. for tics and/or obsessions and compulsions)	Sometimes positive (up to 25%)

ADHD, Attention-deficit/hyperactivity disorder.
Adapted from Singer, H. S., Mink, J. W., Gilbert, D. L, & Jankovic, J. (Eds.). (2016). Motor stereotypies. In *Movement disorders in childhood* (2nd ed., pp. 111–126). Academic Press.

Developmental Coordination Disorder

Developmental coordination disorder (DCD), also referred to as developmental dyspraxia, is a common neurodevelopmental impairment in children and adults emerging early in development. In DCD the acquisition and execution of coordinated motor skills relative to same-age peers is impaired, clumsy, and slow and interferes meaningfully with culturally relevant activities of daily living within family, social, school, or community settings. The etiology is not well understood, and it is not yet clear whether the impairment stems from neuromaturational delay or atypical neurologic networks. Although children with DCD usually have additional neurodevelopmental and/or psychosocial challenges or disorders, the motor skill deficits cannot be better explained by these challenges (American Psychiatric Association, 2013). Approximately 5% to 6% of children are affected with DCD (Blank et al., 2019), with males affected between two and seven times more often than females. While the lifelong trajectory is unclear, some motor differences are likely to persist into adolescence and adulthood.

The impact of DCD is variable and influenced by psychosocial and cultural factors, as well as by coexisting difficulties that may include ADHD (half or more individuals), executive function impairment, emotional difficulties (including anxiety disorders), specific learning disorders, ASD, tremor, and joint hypermobility syndrome; symptoms of these conditions may themselves interfere with motor coordination skills. Among younger children, speech and language delays or disorders frequently occur. Further, it is hypothesized that the nature of the neuromotor control deficits themselves may include impaired automatic internal sensorimotor feedback during movement. Efficient feedback is necessary in visual spatial and temporal cognitive development to allow learning of complex, automatic motor skills. Without this internal feedback, children with DCD may be left to rely more heavily on less precise external observational sources of feedback. Children with DCD are less apt to participate socially and athletically, which may result in isolation, poorer social skills development, and physical inactivity and obesity, compounding potential burden on mental health (Blank et al., 2019).

Evaluation and Comorbidity

Benefit of formal evaluation for DCD among children under 5 years of age is uncertain, as younger children may have typical but delayed motor development ("late bloomers") that will later catch up with peers. Evaluation should be culturally relevant and include a careful gathering of developmental, behavioral, and psychosocial history from parents/caregivers, teachers, and when relevant, from the child as well. Assessment should consider interference with activities of daily living, academic performance, leisure, athletics, and play, and incorporate assessment of both handwriting and keyboarding skills. A neurologic examination and assessment of visual function should be completed. Psychoeducational assessment is often indicated.

Management

Management of DCD should be task and activity oriented and include interventions that are meaningful to the child; be goal oriented and task and context specific; require the child to take an active role; aim to achieve functionality rather than normality, and include active involvement of the parent/caretaker (Blank et al., 2019). Keyboarding skills should be emphasized among children with handwriting impairment. Routine physical exercise that engages the impaired motor coordination skills is also crucial. Coexisting conditions that influence motor performance and adherence to treatment need to be treated effectively.

Chorea

Chorea, derived from Greek to mean "dancing in unison," is a nonrhythmic, nonrepetitive irregular and often continuous dancelike or writhing motion that flows across the body. When of large amplitude, chorea may resemble more flinging movements and be called ballism or ballismus. Chorea is classified as primary (i.e., idiopathic or heredity, and is uncommon in childhood) or secondary (i.e., acquired, and is much more common in childhood). Potential causes are many, including metabolic, infectious, vascular, toxic, autoimmune, or heredodegenerative origins. Most commonly, chorea in children is caused by acute rheumatic fever, referred to as Sydenham chorea, and is believed to occur as an autoimmune antibody response triggered by group A beta-hemolytic streptococcal pharyngitis. Movements may occur anywhere on the body and can include the mouth and tongue. Although symptoms of chorea usually self-resolve, they can be permanent. When symptoms are moderate to severe, chorea can be treated with variable success using neuroleptic agents, antiepileptic drugs, benzodiazepines, tetrabenazine, or alpha-2 adrenergic agonists.

Dystonia

While dystonia is a frequent feature of cerebral palsy (CP), dystonia may also occur in individuals without CP. Dystonia describes abnormal, twisting, repetitive, and patterned motions or atypical sustained postures that result from simultaneous activation of agonist and antagonist muscle groups, particularly during volitional and sometimes highly specific movement. Dystonia may occur focally (such as in torticollis, jaw opening, or in the hands) or with broad generalized body distribution. Dystonia is sometimes accompanied by tremor and may be evoked clinically, such as in having a patient open the mouth or hold the hands outstretched with fingers spread. Dystonia is classified either as acute or chronic. Acute dystonic reactions may be drug induced, as described later, and generally respond to anticholinergic or antihistamine medication and, if ineffective, then to benzodiazepine. Chronic dystonia is further divided in to primary and secondary forms.

Primary forms of chronic dystonia are most often symptomatically isolated without other signs or symptoms except for tremor, tend to have a genetic basis, and are without neuronal degeneration or acquired source. Symptoms typically emerge during adolescence (Fuchs & Ozelius, 2013). Secondary forms of chronic dystonia stem from CP, neuromigrational or other abnormalities of brain development, brain injury, and neurodegenerative diseases. These children may have or develop seizures as well.

Dopa-Responsive Dystonia

This rare genetic form of dystonia typically emerges in the first decade of life (most often in the lower extremities) and over time progressively extends proximally and peripherally by adolescence or adulthood. Symptoms tend to follow a diurnal pattern, with notable improvement in the mornings and then worsening progressively over the course of each day. This form of dystonia is unique in that treatment with levodopa can provide complete symptomatic improvement.

Management

Baclofen may be provided either orally or via surgical intrathecal or intraventricular pump implant. Other medication options include trihexyphenidyl (an anticholinergic agent) and, for focal symptoms, injection of botulinum toxin. Deep brain stimulation is another surgical option among some patients.

Tremor

Tremors are common in children and adults and involve rhythmic oscillation about a joint axis (often in the hands but may involve any voluntary muscle group) with measurable amplitude and frequency. A comprehensive discussion is beyond the scope of this chapter. Briefly tremors are classified into two main groups: primary (or idiopathic) and secondary. Primary tremors in children may emerge as early as infancy, occur usually during voluntary action, and are without associated neurologic features or identifiable causes or abnormal examination findings. Examples include enhanced physiologic tremor (usually occurring with sustained posture with tremor increasing in amplitude during emotional stress, fatigue, or with stimulants such as caffeine or amphetamine) and essential tremor (usually occurring as a posture and action tremor that may worsen as the limb approaches a target [intention tremor]).

In contrast, secondary tremors result from an identifiable cause, such as structural, endocrine, metabolic, degenerative, genetic, toxic, nutritional, or drugs. Tremors can also be part of mixed movement disorders, in which the tremors cooccur with other movement disorders but without being caused by them. The onset and time course of tremors may be acute versus insidious, intermittent versus continuous, and stable versus progressive.

While there are several possible descriptive clinical aspects to the tremorous movements themselves, a useful binary distinction divides tremors into those that occur at rest (rest tremor), which reduce or disappear during action, and tremors that occur during voluntary action (action tremor), which are further subclassified as postural, kinetic (including intention), isometric, and task-specific tremors (Singer et al., 2016c).

Evaluation and Management

In otherwise healthy children, intermittent or persistent tremors should be evaluated to confirm absence of serious and/or treatable sources and to provide reassurance. Evaluation of tremor should include gathering a carefully considered history that also includes developmental, environmental, family, and social information; characterization of the tremor (resting vs. action; laterality; time course; severity); a detailed general and neurologic examination; and reassessment 6 to 12 months later to identify if progressive (for which brain magnetic resonance imaging is usually then appropriate). Medical treatment, if indicated, depends on etiology and is usually guided by a neurologic specialist. Supportive services, including occupational therapy, may be helpful for tremors of functional or psychosocial impact.

Drug-Induced Movement Disorders

Drug-induced movement disorders (DIMD) in children are a relatively common, and commonly overlooked, problem that can emerge from the use of an array of medications, particularly those prescribed to treat social, emotional, and behavioral problems. The movements may take any number of forms, with tremor among the most common, but also rigidity, dystonia, chorea, ataxia, tics, and stereotypies (Singer et al., 2016a). The time course of symptom emergence relative to initiation of medication treatment falls into four groups: acute (immediate or shortly after initiation or dose increase), chronic (early or slowly emerging and lasting weeks or more during treatment), tardive (gradual onset after prolonged treatment), and withdrawal emergent (onset after dose decrease or discontinuation and lasting days or more or until medication is resumed).

The most frequently implicated medications are those with dopamine receptor-blocking activity, in particular the typical and atypical neuroleptics or antipsychotics, but also metoclopramide and prochlorperazine used in the treatment of nausea and vomiting. The benefit of the possibly reduced risk of DIMD in atypical neuroleptics compared to typical ones appears to be offset by rising prescribing, and overprescribing, in children and adolescents for a range of mostly off-label indications, such as aggressive behaviors, correlating with an increasing trend in the frequency of DIMD (Factor et al., 2019). Long-term risk for developing a DIMD with neuroleptic use may be as high as 9.3% (Singer et al., 2016a). Time course for emergence of DIMD with dopamine receptor-blocking drugs may fall into any of the four groups noted earlier, each with a range of potential movement symptoms, including the rare but life-threatening neuroleptic malignant syndrome. In contrast to the fate for many adults, tardive symptoms that emerge in children taking neuroleptics (which are often similar to stereotypies such as lip smacking, chewing, or thrusting of the tongue) may not be permanent. Management may require neurologic and/or psychiatric specialty support and usually includes discontinuation or tapering of the causative drug; it may also include substitution with another medication, supportive care, and, less commonly, use of a medication to counteract the DIMD.

Psychostimulant medications were long thought to cause or exacerbate tic symptoms. However, the evidence is now strong that psychostimulants neither cause nor commonly worsen tic symptoms (Cohen et al., 2015), and they can be used safely in children, including those who have tic disorders. Patients and families should be advised that children with ADHD are at increased risk to develop tics (irrespective of treatment). If tics emerge, management may include psychoeducation and reassurance, dose adjustment, medication substitution, or trial psychostimulant discontinuation and reintroduction.

Selective serotonin reuptake inhibitors (SSRIs) are most commonly used in treating symptoms of mood and anxiety disorders. DIMD may emerge, particularly as myoclonus, akathisia, or tremor. While the risk for a full symptomatic expression of serotonin syndrome (multiple symptoms involving neuromuscular, autonomic, emotional, and cognitive systems) is rare in children, a mild version characterized by hyperreflexia and tremor may emerge, particularly among children treated with multiple medications. Management entails close clinical observation with periodic neurologic examination, stringent documentation of the SSRI association and its symptoms, and for any SSRI-related DIMD possible dose reduction or drug discontinuation.

Other drugs with heightened DIMD potential include a variety of antiseizure medications (particularly phenytoin and carbamazepine, most commonly causing acute ataxia and nystagmus), chemotherapeutic and immunosuppressive agents (varied symptoms), and alcohol and dextromethorphan in cough syrup (ataxia and other symptoms).

Infant/Toddler Specific

Sandifer syndrome, a rare response to gastroesophageal reflux (GER) nearly exclusively in infancy, or less commonly to hiatal hernia, is characterized by brief dystonic hyperextension and arching of the back (opisthotonos) and may include neck turning to the side and stretching of the legs and eye deviation; the infant is usually quiet during the event, which is often confused as seizures. The behavior occurs during wakeful states, usually after feeding. The pathophysiology is unknown but may relate to a vagal reflex or to self-positioning to alleviate GER. Neurologic examination is normal. A pH probe combined with a multichannel intraluminal impedance study to measure bidirectional flow of air, fluid, and solids can be diagnostic (Rosen et al., 2018). The condition usually resolves by age 2 years but can be alleviated with customary GER reduction measures (Mindlina, 2020).

Infantile masturbation, or gratification behavior among infants and toddlers, may appear as unusual postures and movements similar in appearance to dystonia or to seizures. The behavior usually emerges within the first few months of life and may be characterized by stereotyped episodes of staring or having a dazed expression, posturing of the limbs or torso, rubbing the thighs together or rocking the body against an object, facial grimacing, vocalizing (often quiet grunting), and rhythmic pelvic movements. In contrast to behavior during most seizures, the child is responsive throughout the episode and the behavior stops with distraction. Management includes distinguishing sexual behaviors that are frequent, intrusive, or abusive (Kellogg, 2009). Audiovisual recording may be helpful for diagnostic confirmation. Management involves reassurance to caregiver of the harmlessness of the behavior and instructions to calmly redirect the behavior without scolding when it occurs (Yang et al., 2005).

Functional Movement Disorders

Functional movement disorders (FMDs) are characterized by changes in voluntary motor function with clinical findings incompatible with recognized neurologic or medical conditions (American Psychiatric Association, 2013). While common, FMDs in children and teens are sparsely described in the medical literature. The term functional is preferred to other terms, such as psychogenic, as the latter may be offensive or misconstrued to mean the patient is feigning symptoms. The *DSM-5* uses the terms conversion disorder and functional neurologic symptom disorder: with abnormal movement, and this variety in terminology highlights the ambiguity regarding pathophysiology. FMDs occur three to four times more commonly in females than males. Until recently, history of emotional trauma had been assumed for most individuals with FMD, but this assumption is not supported by empirical data and, while many patients with FMD also suffer coexisting mood and anxiety disorders, FMDs are best understood within a combined biologic, psychological, and social framework.

The most common FMDs include tremor, dystonia, and gait disorders; tics and chorea are less common (Schwingenschuh et al., 2008). In contrast to the subset of classical movement disorders in which the movements have a voluntary component, patients with FMD perceive their movements as involuntary (Hallett, 2018).

Common features that can be diagnostically helpful include sudden onset of symptoms often with a precipitating illness or injury, rapid progression unlike the slower course in most movement disorders, pronounced variability in severity and with remissions and recurrences, distractibility, previous or current nonmovement other functional symptoms (including somatization symptoms such as abdominal pain, headache, or fatigue), and history and neurologic examination findings incongruent or inconsistent with classical movement disorders.

Diagnosis relies on positive identification rather than excluding other diagnostic explanations and does not usually require extensive laboratory workup (Edwards & Bhatia, 2012). Management standards are not well established, but treatment generally relies on effective and supportive psychoeducation. Intensive physical therapy and psychotherapy are mainstays in usual treatment. Physical activity and relaxation exercises may be beneficial, and antidepressant medication may be helpful even for patients with no history of mood or anxiety disorders.

CONCLUSION

Pediatric movement disorders are common but can be diagnostically challenging due to complicated overlapping features, elusive origins, developmental and maturational variations, and lack of consistent terminology. Hyperkinetic forms occur much more frequently in pediatric populations than hypokinetic forms. Tic disorders and stereotypies are the most common of the disorders and have both shared and distinctive features. Tic disorders range widely in severity and are often associated with coexisting neurodevelopmental and psychiatric conditions, such as child featured in this chapter's vignette, that may share neuropathologic origins of disinhibition and can contribute to movement severity. Most pediatric movement disorders stem from biochemical and/or structural abnormalities in brain circuitry linking cortical and subcortical structures, particularly the frontal cortex and basal ganglia. Phenotype and clinical context are key to making a correct diagnosis, often assisted by caregiver-prepared video recordings of the movement. Evaluation includes gathering a detailed and targeted medical, developmental, psychosocial, and family history and completing a thorough physical examination, and subspecialty referral may be required. Management is tailored to disorder- and individual-specific elements and may include psychoeducational, lifestyle, behavioral, medicinal, and procedural interventions and monitoring.

REFERENCES

Barbaresi, W. J., Campbell, L., Diekroger, E. A., Froehlich, T. E., Liu, Y. H., O'Malley, E., Pelham, W. E. Jr, Power, T. J., Zinner, S. H., & Chan, E. (2020). Society for Developmental and Behavioral Pediatrics clinical practice guideline for the assessment and treatment of children and adolescents with complex attention-deficit/hyperactivity disorder. *Journal of Developmental and Behavioral Pediatrics*, *41*(2), S35–S57.

Blank, R., Barnett, A. L., Cairney, L., Green, D., Kirby, A., Polatajko, H., Rosenblum, S., Smits-Engelsman, B., Sugden, D., Wilson, P., & Vinçon, S., (2019). International clinical practice recommendations on the definition, diagnosis, assessment, intervention, and psychosocial aspects of developmental coordination disorder. *Developmental Medicine and Child Neurology*, *61*, 242–285.

Chartrand, T. L., & Lakin, J. L. (2013). The antecedents and consequences of human behavioral mimicry. *Annual Review of Psychology*, *64*, 285–308.

Chebli, S. S., Martin, V., & Lanovaz, M. J. (2016). Prevalence of stereotypy in individuals with developmental disabilities: A systematic review. *Review Journal of Autism and Developmental Disorders*, *3*, 107–118.

Cohen, S. C., Mulqueen, J. M., Ferracioli-Oda, E., Stuckelman, Z. D., Coughlin, C. G., Leckman, J. F., & Bloch, M. H.. (2015). Meta-analysis: Risk of tics associated with psychostimulant use in randomized, placebo-controlled trials. *Journal of the American Academy of Child and Adolescent Psychiatry, 54*, 728–736.

Conte, G., Valente, F., Fioriello, F., & Cardona, F. (2020). Rage attacks in Tourette syndrome and chronic tic disorder: A systematic review. *Neuroscience and Biobehavioral Reviews, 119*, 21–36.

Coulombe, M. -A., Elkaim, L. M., Alotaibi, N. M., et al. (2019). Deep brain stimulation for Gilles de la Tourette syndrome in children and youth: A meta-analysis with individual participant data. *Journal of Neurosurgery: Pediatrics, 23*, 236–246.

Eapen, V., McPherson, S., Karlov, L., Nicholls, L., Črnčec, R., & Mulligan, A. (2019). Social communication deficits and restricted repetitive behavior symptoms in Tourette syndrome. *Neuropsychiatric Disease and Treatment, 15*, 2151–2160.

Edwards, M. J., & Bhatia, K. P. (2012). Functional (psychogenic) movement disorders: Merging mind and brain. *Lancet Neurology, 11*, 250–260.

Factor, S. A., Burkhard, P. R., Caroff, S., Friedman, J. H., Marras, C., Tinazzi, M., & Comella, C. L. (2019). Recent developments in drug-induced movement disorders: A mixed picture. *Lancet Neurology, 18*, 880–890.

Fuchs, T., & Ozelius, L. J. (2013). Genetics in dystonia: An update. *Current Neurology and Neuroscience Report, 13*, 410.

Hallett, M. (2018). The most promising advances in our understanding and treatment of functional (psychogenic) movement disorders. *Parkinsonism & Related Disorders, 46*(1), S80–S82.

Harris, K. M., Mahone, E. M., & Singer, H. S. (2008). Nonautistic motor stereotypies: Clinical features and longitudinal follow-up. *Pediatric Neurology, 38*, 267–272.

Hibberd, C., Charman, T., Batoa, R. S., Tekes, S., Hedderly, T., Gringras, P., & Robinson, S. (2020). Sleep difficulties in children with Tourette syndrome and chronic tic disorders: A systematic review of characteristics and associated factors. *Sleep, 43* , zsz308.

Hirschtritt, M. E., Lee, P. C., Pauls, D. L., Dion, Y., Grados, M. A., Illmann, C., King, R. A., Sandor, P., McMahon, W. M., Lyon, G. J., Cath, D. C., Kurlan, R., Robertson, M. M., Osiecki, L., Scharf, J. M., Mathews, C. A., & Tourette Syndrome Association International Consortium for Genetics. (2015). Lifetime prevalence, age of risk, and etiology of comorbid psychiatric disorders in Tourette syndrome. *JAMA Psychiatry, 72*, 325–333.

Iasevoli, F., Barone, A., Buonaguro, E. F., Vellucci, L., & de Bartolomeis, A. (2020). Safety and tolerability of antipsychotic agents in neurodevelopmental disorders: A systematic review. *Expert Opinion on Drug Safety, 19*, 1419–1444.

Kellogg, N. D. (2009). Committee on Child Abuse and Neglect, American Academic of Pediatrics. *Clinical report—The evaluation of sexual behaviors in children. Pediatrics, 124*, 992–998.

Kleimaker, M., Kleimaker, A., Weissbach, A., Colzato, L. S., Beste, C., Bäumer, T., & Münchau, A. (2020). Non-invasive brain stimulation for the treatment of Gilles de la Tourette syndrome. *Frontiers in Neurology, 11*, 592258.

Knight, T., Steeves, T., Day, L., Lowerison, M., Jette, N., & Pringsheim, T. (2012). Prevalence of tic disorders: A systematic review and meta-analysis. *Pediatric Neurology, 47*, 77–90.

Koy, A., Lin, J. P., Sanger, T. D., Marks, W. A., Mink, J. W., & Timmermann, L. (2016). Advances in management of movement disorders in children. *Lancet Neurology, 15*, 719–735.

Latorre, A., Rocchi, L., Berardelli, A., Bhatia, K. P., & Rothwell, J. C. (2019). The use of transcranial magnetic stimulation as a treatment for movement disorders: A critical review. *Movement Disorders, 34*, 769–782.

Mahone, E. M., Ryan, M., Ferenc, L., Morris-Berry, C., & Singer, H. S. (2014). Neuropsychological function in children with primary complex motor stereotypies. *Developmental Medicine and Child Neurology, 56*, 1001–1008.

Mansueto, C. S., & Keuler, D. J. (2005). Tic or compulsion?: It's tourettic OCD. *Behavior Modification, 29*, 784–799.

Martino, D., Pringsheim, T. M., Cavanna, A. E., Colosimo, C., Hartmann, A., Leckman, J. F., Luo, S., Munchau, A., Goetz, C. G., Stebbins, G. T., Martinez-Martin, P., & Members of the MDS Committee on Rating Scales Development. (2017). Systematic review of severity scales and screening instruments for tics: Critique and recommendations. *Movement Disorders, 32*, 467–473.

McGuire, J. F., Piacentini, J., Brennan, E. A., Lewin, A. B., Murphy, T. K., Small, B. J., & Storch, E. A. (2014). A meta-analysis of behavior therapy for Tourette syndrome. *Journal of Psychiatric Research, 50*, 106–112.

Mindlina, I. (2020). Diagnosis and management of Sandifer syndrome in children with intractable neurological symptoms. *European Journal of Pediatrics, 179*, 243–250.

Mingbunjerdsuk, D., & Zinner, S. H. (2020). Coping with tics in school and with peers. *Current Developmental Disorders Reports, 7*, 227–236.

Murphy, T. K., Lewin, A. B., Storch, E. A., & American Academy of Child and Adolescent Psychiatry (AACAP) Committee on Quality Issues (CQI). (2013). Practice parameter for the assessment and treatment of children and adolescents with tic disorders. *Journal of the American Academy of Child and Adolescent Psychiatry, 52*, 1341–1359.

Oakley, C., Mahone, E. M., Morris-Berry, C., Kline, T., & Singer, H. S. (2015). Primary complex motor stereotypies in older children and adolescents: Clinical features and longitudinal follow-up. *Pediatric Neurology, 52*, 398–403.

Pringsheim, T., Holler-Managan, Y., Okun, M. S., Jankovic, J., Piacentini, J., Cavanna, A. E., Martino, D., Müller-Vahl, K., Woods, D. W., Robinson, M., Jarvie, E., Roessner, V., & Oskoui, M. (2019a). Comprehensive systematic review summary: Treatment of tics in people with Tourette syndrome and chronic tic disorders. *Neurology, 92*, 907–915.

Pringsheim, T., Okun, M. S., Muller-Vahl, K., Martino , D., Jankovic, J., Cavanna, A. E., Woods, D. W., Robinson, M., Jarvie, E., Roessner, V., Oskoui, M., Holler-Managan, Y., & Piacentini, J. (2019b). Practice guideline recommendations summary: Treatment of tics in people with Tourette syndrome and chronic tic disorders. *Neurology, 92*, 896–906.

Rosen, R., Vandenplas, Y., Singendonk, M., Cabana, M., DiLorenzo, C., Gottrand, F., Gupta, S., Langendam, M., Staiano, A., Thapar, N., Tipnis, N., & Tabbers, M. (2018). Pediatric gastroesophageal reflux clinical practice guidelines: joint recommendations of the North American Society for Pediatric Gastroenterology, Hepatology, and Nutrition and the European Society for Pediatric Gastroenterology, Hepatology, and Nutrition. *Journal of Pediatric Gastroenterology and Nutrition, 66*, 516–554.

Scahill, L., Specht, M., & Page, C. (2014). The prevalence of tic disorders and clinical characteristics in children. *Journal of Obsessive and Compulsive Related Disorders, 3*, 394–400.

Schrock, L. E., Mink, J. W., Woods, D. W., Porta, M., Servello, D., Visser-Vandewalle, V., Silburn, P. A., Foltynie, T., Walker, H. C., Shahed-Jimenez, J., Savica, R., Klassen, B. T., Machado, A. G., Foote, K. D., Zhang, J. G., Hu, W., Ackermans, L., Temel, Y., Mari, Z., ... Tourette Syndrome Association International Deep Brain Stimulation (DBS) Database and Registry Study Group (2015). Tourette syndrome deep brain stimulation: A review and updated recommendations. *Movement Disorders*, *30*, 448–471.

Schwingenschuh, P., Pont-Sunyer, C., Surtees, R., Edwards, M. J., & Bhatia, K. P. (2008). Psychogenic movement disorders in children: A report of 15 cases and a review of the literature. *Movement Disorders*, *23*, 1882–1888.

Singer, H. S. (2013a). Motor control, habits, complex motor stereotypies, and Tourette syndrome. *Annals of the New York Academy of Sciences*, *1304*, 22–31.

Singer, H. S. (2013b). The neurochemistry of Tourette syndrome. In D. Martino & J. F. Leckman (Eds.), *Tourette syndrome*. Oxford University Press.

Singer, H. S., Mink, J. W., Gilbert, D. L., & Jankovic, J. (Eds.). (2016a). Drug-induced movement disorders in children. In *Movement disorders in childhood* (2nd ed.). Academic Press.

Singer, H. S., Mink, J. W., Gilbert, D. L., & Jankovic, J. (Eds.). (2016b). Motor stereotypies. In *Movement disorders in childhood* (2nd ed.). Academic Press.

Singer, H. S., Mink, J. W., Gilbert, D. L., & Jankovic, J. (Eds.). (2016c). Tremor. In *In Movement disorders in childhood* (2nd ed.). Academic Press.

Vertigan, A. E. (2017). Somatic cough syndrome or psychogenic cough—What is the difference? *Journal of Thoracic Diseases*, *9*, 831–838.

Weisman, H., Qureshi, I. A., Leckman, J. F., Scahill, L., & Bloch, M. H. (2013). Systematic review: Pharmacological treatment of tic disorders—Efficacy of antipsychotic and alpha-2 adrenergic agonist agents. *Neuroscience and Biobehavioral Reviews*, *37*, 1162–1171.

Yang, M. L., Fullwood, E., Goldstein, J., & Mink, J. W. (2005). Masturbation in infancy and early childhood presenting as a movement disorder: 12 cases and a review of the literature. *Pediatrics*, *116*, 1427–1432.

Habit Disorders in Children and Adolescents

Carissa R. Jackel and Nathan J. Blum

For additional material related to the content of this chapter, please see Chapter 71.

VIGNETTE

1. *A 4.5-year-old sucks her thumb at bedtime and while watching television or riding in the car. In the past she sucked her thumb while playing with toys and interacting with other people, but has been sucking only during downtime for about 6 months.*
2. *A 2-year-old bangs his head on his mattress each night as he is falling asleep and during some tantrums. His parents tell him to stop banging and have set up a video camera in the bedroom so they can detect banging more quickly. When he head bangs during a tantrum they hold him to prevent him from hurting himself. On one occasion he hit the corner of a piece of furniture causing a bruise, but in general, the head banging has not caused bruising or swelling. His parents are distressed that the head banging during tantrums seems to be occurring more frequently, when they had been told he would outgrow it.*
3. *A 3-year-old has pulled out the hair on the left lateral side of her scalp and her eyebrows. She tends to pull her hair while sucking her thumb. After pulling out the hair she puts it in her mouth, and her parents report that they have found hair in her stool.*

The three children described in the vignettes are engaged in repeated and rhythmic behaviors that, at least on initial appearance, seem purposeless. These types of behaviors are often referred to as repetitive or stereotypic behavior. Assessment of children with repetitive behaviors is complex because, although this type of behavior is a universal component of typical child development, repetitive behaviors can also occur across a wide spectrum of developmental, emotional, and physical disorders. In addition, the behavior itself may be a concern because it causes tissue damage, is socially undesirable, or causes the individual distress. The cases described represent a range of behaviors. Some are likely to be benign and self-limited, but others might require further assessment and intervention. In this chapter we briefly review the etiology of repetitive behaviors and then discuss their assessment and management.

CLASSIFICATION

Classification of repetitive behaviors or habits is complex as behaviors with a similar appearance may have different causes or significance. Often the habits described in this chapter are referred to as body-focused repetitive behaviors when the behaviors are not associated with functional impairment or distress to the individual and as body-focused repetitive behavior disorders (BFRBD) when associated with impairment, distress, and repeated attempts by the individual to stop the behavior. The *Diagnostic and Statistical Manual of Mental Disorders*, fifth edition (*DSM-5*) (American Psychiatric Association, 2013) classifies some of the behaviors described in this chapter in the section on neurodevelopmental disorders; these include stereotypic movement disorders (SMD; rocking, head banging). The *DSM-5* section on obsessive-compulsive and related disorders (e.g., hair pulling, skin picking) includes a discussion on BFRBD. The primary characteristics that distinguish between SMD and obsessive-compulsive/related disorders are age at onset and the behavior causing distress to the individual. The criteria for SMD include that the onset of the behavior is in the early developmental period (typically <3 years of age) and that the behavior interferes with functioning but does not cause distress to the individual. In contrast, BFRBDs are described as having their onset in adolescence and are associated with distress and repeated attempts to stop the behavior. Repetitive behaviors that occur as part of a general medical or neurologic condition, in response to medications, or as part of a developmental disorder, sensory impairment, or psychiatric disorder are not given a separate diagnosis if the repetitive behaviors that cause dysfunction are thought to be part of the underlying condition. This may occur in autism spectrum disorder, obsessive-compulsive disorder, and body dysmorphic disorder, among other conditions.

ETIOLOGY

Both biologic and environmental factors can be important in causing or maintaining repetitive behaviors. Studies of infants have found that repetitive behaviors are nearly universal phenomena that occur with a distinctive developmental progression. For example, hand sucking occurs in most typically developing infants within 2 hours of birth, object banging and body rocking begin at approximately 6 months of age, and hand clapping begins at 7 to 8 months of age (Kravitz & Boehmm, 1971; Thelen, 1996). The early and nearly universal occurrence of these behaviors and their distinctive developmental progression led to the theory that rhythmic behaviors represent movement patterns encoded in the brain that serve as a transition between uncoordinated movements and more mature goal-directed behaviors (Thelen, 1996). Further facilitating the development of complex behaviors is the brain's ability to create sequences of behavior that link sensory cues with motor behavior without requiring thought. This ability is critical for learning such complex adaptive behaviors as walking or riding a bike, but may also facilitate the development of habits (Leckman & Riddle, 2000). In addition, although habits are often viewed as purposeless, they may serve some adaptive functions such as reducing feelings of anxiety or fear and increasing feelings of security and control.

Pharmacologic, functional neuroimaging, neuroanatomic, and animal studies are beginning to elucidate brain structures and pathways involved in habits, tics, compulsions, and other repetitive behaviors. Much of this research is focused on the cortical-striatal-thalmo-cortical pathways and the dopamine neurotransmitter systems. The striatum is believed to be responsible for habit learning (as opposed to explicit memory based in the hippocampus), and dopamine-containing neurons from the substania nigra modulate the activity of striatal neurons. Activation of striatal dopamine receptors has been demonstrated to produce stereoptypic behaviors in laboratory animals, and some functional neuroimaging studies of individuals with Tourette syndrome suggest that there is increased striatal dopaminergic innervation in this disorder (Albin & Mink, 2006). Furthermore, administration of stimulant medications that increase dopamine levels produces tics or repetitive picking behaviors in some individuals. Environmental factors also influence these behaviors. Repetitive behaviors occur most frequently either during periods of low arousal such as when tired, bored, or distracted by other stimuli (e.g., reading, television) or during periods of high arousal such as when concentrating, angry, or frustrated (Sallustro & Atwell, 1978). Severe sensory deprivation can produce these behaviors in both laboratory animals and humans. The response of parents or others to some repetitive behaviors may serve to reinforce them making it more likely that the behaviors will be maintained over time.

STEREOTYPIC MOVEMENTS

Sucking

Sucking of the hand, fingers, or thumb has been observed *in utero* and is nearly universal in healthy neonates within hours after birth (Kravitz & Boehm, 1971). Nonnutritive sucking occurs in 82% of infants at 5 months of age and 73% of children between 2 and 5 years old (Staufert Gutierrez & Carugno, 2021). Sucking is a biologically driven behavior that develops into a habit in some children. Both genetic and environmental factors contribute to thumb sucking as one twin study found that 58% of monozygotic twins were concordant for frequent thumb sucking as compared to only 33% of dizygotic twins (Ooki, 2005).

Thumb or digit sucking may provide a sense of security to children; soothe them when they are tired, sick, or upset; or provide stimulation to delay the onset of boredom during periods of low stimulation. In some children thumb sucking may occur in response to emotional stress or anxiety, but it has not been found to be consistently associated with specific behavioral or emotional disorders. The habit is usually harmless in infants and young children, but persistence beyond 4 to 6 years of age has been associated with a number of sequelae, especially if it is occurring with high frequency or intensity. In the first vignette the child is over 4 years of age, but the behavior is only occurring during periods of low stimulation and thus is not likely to require treatment. When the behavior is occurring with high intensity and frequency, some of the most frequent sequelae of thumb sucking include dental problems such as an anterior open bite, decreased alveolar bone growth, mucosal trauma, and even altered growth of the facial bones. Thumb or digit sucking is a common cause of paronychia in children, and it may be associated with an increased incidence of accidental ingestion. Deformities of the fingers and thumb may occur. Finally, thumb or digit sucking persisting into the elementary school may have psychological sequelae as the child might be viewed as a less desirable playmate or become insecure due to persistent nagging from parents.

Treatment of thumb sucking is rarely indicated in children younger than age 4 or in older children if it occurs infrequently or only as a temporary response to a stressor. Treatment may be indicated in older children if they are sucking in multiple settings, if it is distressing to them, or if it is causing the complications discussed earlier. A variety of successful treatments for thumb sucking have been described (Table 72.1). If thumb sucking has resulted in significant negative reactions from the parents, a moratorium on parental comments on the thumb sucking should precede any other treatment (see Behavioral Interventions, later). All treatments are most effective when the child is a willing partner in the treatment.

Banging

Rhythmic banging behaviors such as the banging of one's hand or an object against a surface occur commonly in typically developing infants and will not be discussed further.

Head banging is the most dramatic banging behavior and the one that is most likely to elicit concern from parents. Head banging involves the rhythmic hitting of the head against a solid surface, often the crib mattress, but sometimes harder surfaces. It occurs in 5% to 19% of children during the infancy and toddler years. It most often occurs when the child is tired and/or alone, such as during bedtime, but it may also occur as part of a tantrum (Sallustro et al., 1978). Many children who bang their head have had other rhythmic behaviors, often body rocking or head rolling, earlier in infancy. Each episode of head banging usually lasts for less than 15 minutes, but episodes can last for up to a few hours. Although the frequency of head banging declines rapidly after 18 months of age, 1% to 3% of children continue the behavior after 3 years of age, and uncommonly it persists into the elementary school years.

Although most children who bang their head do not have physical illness, in some cases the onset of head banging has been associated with episodes of otitis media and with teething. In these cases head banging is postulated to serve as a pain-relieving function.

TABLE 72.1 Treatments for Thumb or Digit Sucking

Treatment	Description	Efficacy
Psychological interventions/behavioral modifications	Habit reversal Positive reinforcement and negative reinforcement Praise and rewards when not sucking; token rewards Gaining child's cooperation	Significantly more likely to stop sucking than no treatment, in both short and long term Not sufficient data to determine whether one psychological intervention works better than another
Orthodontic appliances	A variety of appliances that must be placed by a dentist, some types of appliances have resulted in injury to the child Appliance interferes with child's placement of the thumb or finger in the mouth	High efficacy when children want to stop sucking, but appliances can be avoided, bent, or broken by children who do not want to cooperate with treatment Efficacious for both short- and long-term cessation of sucking
Barrier techniques	Gloves Bandages Thumb splints	Insufficient data to determine efficacy, but easiest to implement with very low risk
Chemical techniques	Coat thumbnail with aversive taste substance in morning, evening, and if sucking is observed Small rewards offered to child for not sucking during specified intervals	Insufficient data to determine efficacy Aversive taste products are commercially available; typically considered safe
Combination	Psychological intervention and orthodontic appliances Psychological interventions and chemical techniques	

Adapted from Borrie, F. R., Bearn, D. R., Innes, N. P., & Iheozor-Ejiofor, Z. (2015). Interventions for the cessation of non-nutritive sucking habits in children. *The Cochrane Database of Systematic Reviews, 3*, CD008694.

Head banging when a child is relaxed, for example, when falling asleep, is not a sign of a developmental or emotional disorder. In addition, this type of head banging does not cause injuries to the brain, although occasionally it can result in callus formation or abrasions at the site of the banging. Typically developing children who head bang during tantrums do not usually injure themselves, although occasionally they may make a mistake and bang on a surface that is harder or sharper than they expect causing a bruise or laceration, as occurred in the second vignette. The child does not usually bang on this surface a second time. Thus with the exception of children with developmental disabilities (most commonly autism spectrum disorder or severe intellectual disability) or bleeding disorders, head banging does not usually result in significant injury.

Treatment of head banging not associated with risk for serious injury primarily involves reassurance of the parents that head banging alone is not a sign of another disorder and that injury is unlikely. If the child is banging against a hard surface, padding the surface decreases the chance of abrasions or contusions. In most cases parents should be counseled to ignore the behavior while it is occurring. This is especially true for head banging during tantrums, which may be inadvertently reinforced by the parent through holding or comforting the child. Head banging may also be reinforced if it causes a parent to give in to a child's demands in an attempt to stop the head banging. In children with developmental disabilities severe and persistent head banging may place the child at risk for significant intracranial or retinal injury and may necessitate the use of a helmet and pharmacologic treatment in some cases.

Body Rocking

Body rocking occurs in most infants during the first year of life. It usually begins around 6 months of age and has been reported to occur most frequently when infants are listening to music or are alone in their crib. It usually involves a rhythmic forward and backward swaying of the trunk at the hips that occurs in a sitting position but can also occur in the quadruped position. It can be gentle or violent enough to shake or even move a crib. The peak prevalence has been variably reported to be between 6 and 18 months of age, with a rapid decline in the prevalence of the behavior after 18 months of age. Most episodes of uninterrupted body rocking last for less than 15 minutes.

Body rocking persists beyond age 2 years in approximately 3% of typically developing children and its prevalence may increase again at school age. On self-report measures over 20% of adults and college students state that they engage in body rocking. A variety of functions of rocking behaviors have been proposed, including self-stimulation and tension reduction. In children with developmental disorders and children with visual impairments body rocking has been associated with a lack of environmental stimulation, excitement, demands being placed on the child, and eating (Katherine, 2018).

In most cases body rocking does not cause significant functional impairment or stigmatization. However, cases in which rocking occurs throughout most of the day, interfering with functional activities and causing significant impairment or stigmatization, have been described in children and adults. These cases meet criteria for stereotypic movement disorder.

BODY-FOCUSED REPETITIVE BEHAVIORS

Picking

Picking behavior may involve picking the skin or the nose. There has been little systematic study regarding nose picking, although survey studies suggest that over 90% of adolescents and adults report nose picking and 4% to 8% report eating what they picked (Andrade & Srihari, 2001). Young children are often observed to pick their nose in public, whereas older children are more likely to do so when they are alone or when they feel protected from public view. Nose picking may begin in association with rhinorrhea and nasal irritation or itchiness. The most common complication of nose picking is epistaxis. Other complications, such as infections or perforation of the nasal septum, are much less common. When nose picking is associated with allergic symptoms or rhinorrhea resulting from a cold, treatment with antihistamines or decongestants may be helpful.

Individuals may also pick at their skin or at scabs, resulting in excoriations, which at times may become infected. Problematic skin picking has been reported to occur in 2% to 4% of adolescents and adults (Bohne, Keuthen, & Wilhelm, 2005). Skin picking has been described either as a habit occurring during periods of stress and anxiety or as an obsessive-compulsive and related disorder known as excoriation disorder when it is associated with skin lesions, clinically significant distress or impairment in functioning, and repeated attempts to stop the behavior. In some cases skin picking may occur in response to, or be exacerbated by, treatment with stimulant medications. Skin picking occurs relatively commonly in adolescents and adults with Prader-Willi syndrome.

Little systematic information on the treatment of skin or nose picking is available. Emphasizing good hygiene and, with skin picking, blocking access to the picked site until it heals will be sufficient for some children. In more difficult cases behavioral treatment using the habit reversal (HR) procedure (see later) could be attempted. There are reports of improvement in skin picking with treatment using selective serotonin reuptake inhibitors (SSRIs) or N-acetylcysteine, including in children with Prader-Willi syndrome (Bohne et al., 2005; Nwankwo & Jafferany, 2019).

Trichotillomania

Trichotillomania is a disorder characterized by recurrent pulling of one's own hair, resulting in alopecia (Fig. 72.1). Typically, hair is pulled from the scalp, eyebrows, or eyelashes, but hair pulling can involve any site in which hair grows, including axillary and pubic hair. Occasionally hair may be pulled from dolls, pets, or other materials. Many will tickle their lips or nostrils with the hair and some will eat the hair (trichophagia). The *DSM-5* classifies trichotillomania as an obsessive-compulsive and related disorder with a prevalence of 1% to 2%.

The diagnosis of trichotillomania can be difficult. It is not unusual for individuals with trichotillomania to deny hair pulling and to engage in the behavior surreptitiously. Trichotillomania must be distinguished from other causes of

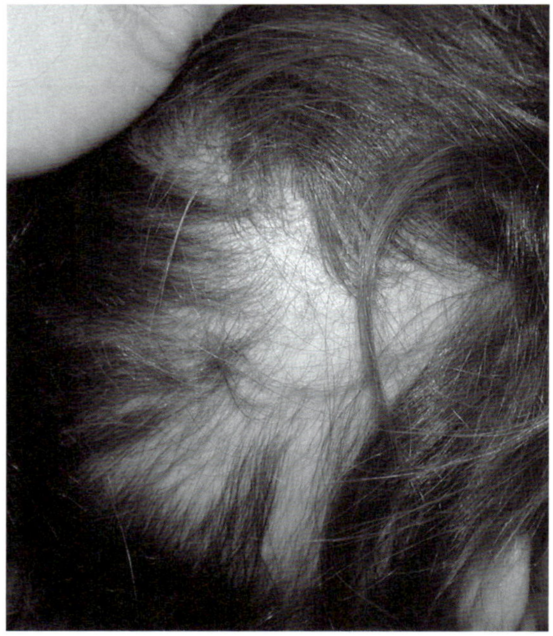

Fig. 72.1 Hair loss due to trichotillomania. Note the nonanatomic distribution of the hair loss and the hairs of multiple different lengths. (Photograph provided courtesy of Dr. Albert Yan.)

alopecia in children, most commonly tinea capitis or alopecia areata. In both trichotillomania and tinea capitis the hair loss is usually patchy, but tinea capitis is usually associated with scaling of the scalp and broken hairs at the scalp. In alopecia areata the hair loss is usually complete in the affected area, whereas in trichotillomania the hair loss is usually incomplete, and hairs of various length are present in the area of alopecia. General thinning of the hair may occur in response to severe stressors, hypothyroidism, hyperthyroidism, and certain medications.

Clinical reports suggest that at least two subtypes of trichotillomania may exist. One form tends to begin in younger children (usually <6 years of age) and is often a habit that is self-limited or effectively treated with behavioral interventions (Woods & Houghton, 2016). In these cases the behavior often occurs in association with thumb sucking and may be most frequent during periods of low stimulation, such as at naptime or bedtime, or may occur when the child is upset. In some cases hair pulling in young children may be associated with anxiety or a developmental disorder. However, trichotillomania that begins in older children and adolescents is more likely to be associated with symptoms of anxiety or depression and is more likely to be chronic (Lewin et al., 2009). Most adults with trichotillomania describe its onset during childhood or adolescence. In all cases the clinician should inquire about trichophagia because treatment is more urgent in children who are eating their hair, to prevent formation of a trichobezoar, which can cause an intestinal obstruction.

A variety of treatments for trichotillomania have been described. In young children who suck their thumb while pulling their hair, treatment of the thumb sucking (see Table 72.1) often stops the hair pulling. This would likely be the approach for the child described in the third vignette, as she sucks her thumb while pulling her hair and is ingesting the hair making it important to stop the hair pulling. For young children who are not sucking their thumb while hair pulling, behavioral treatments (see later) are often effective (Woods & Houghton, 2016). For older children, behavioral treatments using variations of the HR procedure (see later) or HR in combination with cognitive-behavioral therapy are often effective (Woods & Houghton, 2016). Treatment with hypnosis has also been described. There are no US Food and Drug Administration (FDA)–approved medications. SSRIs, clomipramine, and N-acetylcysteine have shown some benefit in adults, but the only randomized clinical trial of a medication, N-acetylcysteine, in children did not show any benefit (Henkel, Jaquez, & Diaz, 2019).

Nail Biting

Nail biting is a common body-focused repetitive behavior in typically developing school-age children, as well as in children with developmental disabilities. It is rare among toddlers, with the incidence increasing to 20% to 33% in 7- to 10-year-olds. The incidence peaks at 45% in adolescents with a subsequent decrease and plateau to 10% in young adulthood (Ellington, 2017). During childhood, the incidence of nail biting is similar in boys and girls but becomes more common in boys during adolescence.

Nail biting has been thought to be an indication of anxiety, but this is not always the case, and boredom and frustration are commonly described reasons among adolescents (Ellington, 2017). Nail biting often runs in families, and children who have parents who were/are nail biters are three times more likely to bite their nails (Bakwin, 1971), even if parents no longer engage in the behavior. This, along with twin studies that show concordance for the habit in monozygotic twins about twice as frequently as dizygotic twins, suggests that there is a genetic component to nail biting (Ooki, 2005).

Nail biting is usually confined to the fingernails, and most individuals bite all 10 nails equally. On occasion, specific fingernails are bitten (or avoided) selectively, and some individuals bite toenails. The bitten nails are short and irregular. Sometimes the skin margins of the nail bed or the cuticle are bitten. This may result in paronychia or, in cases of oral herpes, development of herpetic whitlow on the bitten finger. In severe cases nail biting may cause scarring of the nail bed, bleeding, and damage to the dentition.

When specific stressors related to nail biting can be identified, treatment should be directed at helping the child to cope with these stressors. Behavioral interventions (see later) can be helpful. Good nail hygiene is recommended because the rough nail edges may be irritating and worsen the behavior. In adolescents and adults the HR procedure (see later) can be effective.

BEHAVIORAL TREATMENT OF STEREOTYPIC AND REPETITIVE BEHAVIORS

Behavioral Interventions

Behavioral interventions are typically the initial intervention recommended for stereotypic or repetitive behaviors in young children, if treatment is needed. If the habit has resulted in frequent negative reactions, ridicule, or punishments from the parents, ignoring the behavior to prevent it from being a reliable way to elicit parental attention is often helpful. Typically, this is combined with counseling parents to significantly increase the attention they are providing for appropriate behaviors the child engages in when the habit behavior is not occurring. Procedures that make the habit more difficult to perform or change the sensation elicited by the behavior, such as wearing mittens or short haircuts for children with hair pulling or aversive taste substances for children with thumb sucking, can be effective (Woods & Houghton, 2016). For older children, adolescents, and adults, HR, a multicomponent behavioral intervention, has the best evidence for efficacy (Woods & Houghton, 2016).

Habit Reversal

HR has been demonstrated to be effective for a wide variety of repetitive behaviors, including thumb sucking, nail biting, hair pulling, and tics (Woods & Houghton, 2016). The components of the treatment (Box 72.1) are designed to accomplish four goals: (1) increase the individual's awareness of the habit, (2) teach the individual a competing response to engage

BOX 72.1 Components of Habit Reversal Procedure

I. Increase individual's awareness of habit
   A. Response description—have individual describe behavior to therapist in detail while reenacting the behavior and looking in a mirror.
   B. Response detection—inform individual of each occurrence of the behavior until each occurrence is detected without assistance.
   C. Early warning—have individual practice identifying earliest signs of the target behavior.
   D. Situation awareness—have individual describe all situations in which the target behavior is likely to occur.

II. Teach competing response to habit

The competing response must result in isometric contraction of muscles involved in the habit, be capable of being maintained for 3 min, and be socially inconspicuous and compatible with normal ongoing activities, but incompatible with the habit (e.g., clenching one's fist, grasping and clenching an object). For vocal tics and stuttering, deep relaxed breathing with a slight exhale prior to speech has been used as the competing response

III. Sustain compliance
   A. Habit inconvenience review—have individual review in detail all problems associated with target behavior.
   B. Social support procedure—family members and friends provide high levels of praise when a habit-free period is noted.
   C. Public display—individual demonstrates to others that he or she can control the target behavior in situations where the behavior occurred in the past

IV. Facilitate generalization-symbolic rehearsal procedure

For each situation identified in situation awareness procedure, individual imagines himself or herself beginning the target behavior, but stopping and engaging in the competing response.

in when they feel as if they are about to engage in the habit, (3) help sustain compliance, and (4) facilitate generalization.

Since the original description of HR, modifications of the procedure have also been demonstrated to be effective. Studies that have evaluated components of the original procedure suggest that the training to increase awareness of the habit and the use of the competing response are the most important components of the treatment. The social support procedures may have particular importance in children. Other studies have added components to the HR procedure, including cognitive techniques, progressive muscle relaxation, relaxed breathing, and visual imagery. Recently, digital devices have been developed that can signal the individual when they are starting to engage in the habit behavior. These devices may help with the awareness training component of HR (Henkel et al., 2019). Additional information about behavior management is available in Chapter 93.

OTHER REPETITIVE BEHAVIORS

Bruxism

Bruxism refers to the grinding and clenching of teeth. It is common in both children and adults and may occur during the day (diurnal bruxism) or at night (sleep bruxism). Sleep bruxism is more frequently studied, and in children the incidence has been reported to vary between 6% and 50%, with studies reporting any episodes of bruxism giving higher estimates and those requiring multiple episodes of bruxism (Machado, Dal-Fabbro, Cunali, & Kaizer, 2014).

Investigations of sleep bruxism suggest that the cause is multifactorial. Past theories that focused on dental occlusion problems have been supplanted by the view that a combination of biologic, psychological, and environmental factors interact to cause bruxism. Deficits in dopaminergic transmission, central nervous system maturation, genetic factors, sleep disruptions (including obstructive sleep apnea), stress, anxiety, caffeine, and other medications have all been associated with bruxism, but the relative importance of these factors has not been well delineated (Manfredini et al., 2017). Diurnal bruxism is thought to be related to other oral habits such as nail biting, lip biting, or chewing on objects, as these behaviors tend to occur in similar settings. It is also more common in children with more severe intellectual disability or autism spectrum disorder.

Assessment for sleep bruxism is typically done through history (or questionnaires) and examination of the dentition for tooth wear, but these assessments tend not to correspond well to assessment done by polysomnography, which is considered the gold standard assessment (Castrillon & Exposto, 2018). Electromyographic assessment of the masticatory muscle activity during sleep is being developed as a more objective and accessible assessment.

The most common sign of bruxism is abnormal wearing of the teeth. Hypermobility of the teeth, injury to the periodontium, fractured teeth, and pulpitis may occur, but these are more common in adults than children. Bruxism has also been associated with temporomandibular disorders causing pain and headaches, but the explanation that simple overload of the masticatory muscles is the cause of the pain has not been confirmed (Castrillon & Exposto, 2018).

Treatment of bruxism in children needs to be considered carefully because the bruxism is often transient, and children are less likely to have symptoms than adults. Reassurance is often the only treatment needed. If the child is having significant symptoms, a thorough medical, sleep, and dental evaluation should occur before treatment. If treatment is indicated, the options include interocclusal dental appliances, psychological therapies, pain management strategies, or pharmacologic treatment, but none of these treatments has well established efficacy in children.

Psychological treatments aimed at decreasing stress or teaching the individual to manage stress are helpful in some cases. Nocturnal alarms that arouse the individual during bruxing events have been shown to decrease the frequency and duration of bruxing during treatment, but the gains may not be maintained after treatment. Relaxation training and biofeedback have also been reported to have at least short-term benefit in adults. Exercises, heat applications, ultrasound, and transcutaneous electric stimulation are treatments that may be used to help manage pain. Botulinum toxin injections that decrease the amplitude of the muscle contractions and nonsteroidal antiinflammatory agents may also be helpful for pain management.

Tic Cough (Habit) and Somatic Cough Syndrome (Psychogenic)

These conditions were previously referred to as habit cough and psychogenic cough, respectively, until the American College of Chest Physicians came out with new guidelines in 2015 (Vertigan et al., 2015). They are discussed in more detail in Chapter 71.

Breathholding Spells

Breathholding spells (BHS) are not a habit disorder but are reflexive events in which the child becomes apneic. BHS are divided into three types: cyanotic, pallid, and mixed spells, based on the color of the child's face and lips during the event. Cyanotic spells are the most common and are often precipitated by anger or frustration resulting in crying that may be brief or prolonged and gradually intensifying. The crying stops at end expiration when the child becomes apneic and cyanotic. In some cases the spell resolves at this point as the child takes a deep breath (simple BHS), whereas in other cases the event continues and the child may lose consciousness and have a brief seizure (complex BHS). After the event there may be a period of drowsiness. Pallid spells are similar except that they are more likely to be provoked by pain or fear, and crying prior to the spell may be minimal. The two types of spells may coexist (mixed spells). BHS are reported to occur in 4% to 5% of children. Rarely, they begin in the first month of life, but most frequently begin between 6 and 18 months of age. Approximately, half of children will have resolution of their BHS by 4 years of age, and it would be very unusual for the spells to persist beyond 8 years of age.

The cause of BHS is not completely understood and is likely multifactorial. Autonomic dysregulation, iron deficiency, delayed myelination of the brainstem, child temperament, and parenting factors may all play a role (Leung, Leung, Wong, & Hon, 2019). For cyanotic spells, autonomic dysregulation is thought to lead to inhibition of respiratory effort, and the increased intrathoracic pressure during apnea may lead to a ventilation-perfusion mismatch that cause cyanosis. Pallid spells are related to an overactive vagal response leading to bradycardia or brief asystole. Children with pallid BHS may be at increased risk for having episodes of vasovagal syncope as adolescents or adults. There is a genetic predisposition to BHS with a positive family history found in 20% to 35% of those with BHS (Leung et al., 2019).

The differential diagnosis includes seizures, cardiac arrhythmias, or a brainstem tumor or malformation (e.g., Arnold-Chiari malformation). Anemia may increase the frequency of BHS. BHS have also been reported to occur with increased frequency in children with familial dysautonomia and Rett syndrome, but they would not be the sole manifestation of these disorders. Usually, the history of a provoking event and the presence of color change before the loss of consciousness allow one to distinguish BHS from seizures on clinical grounds, but occasionally an electroencephalogram is helpful. If a child has pallid spells, one should consider obtaining an electrocardiogram or Holter monitor to evaluate for cardiac arrhythmias or conditions associated with arrhythmias.

BHS are frightening to parents. Treatment primarily involves reassurance that the spells will not harm the child and demystification of the events leading to the loss of consciousness. Parents should understand that if the child does lose consciousness, the child will begin breathing at that time. If parents remain fearful of the events they may try to prevent the child from experiencing pain, fear, minor injury, anger, or frustration. In trying to prevent these events the parents may unnecessarily restrict some activities, may have difficulty setting consistent limits, or may provide attention in response to tantrums. In these cases the parents' behavior may reinforce the tantrums, and the child may learn to trigger the BHS during tantrums to get the desired response from the parents.

Iron supplementation has been shown to decrease the frequency of breathholding in children with anemia, but also in children without iron deficiency (Jain, Omanakuttan, Singh, & Jajoo, 2017). A randomized controlled trial found that piracetam, a derivative of gamma-aminobutyric acid that is not FDA approved in the United States, was effective in reducing the frequency of BHS (Sawires & Botrous, 2012). In cases of very frequent and severe (i.e., associated with seizures) pallid BHS treatment with atropine or other anticholinergic medications may be effective (Leung et al., 2019). In very rare cases unresponsive to counseling and pharmacologic treatment, cardiac pacemaker implantation has been used (Sartori et al., 2015).

Rumination

Rumination is characterized by the repetitive regurgitation of food into the mouth followed by rechewing and reswallowing or expulsion. Rumination has been described most frequently in infants and in individuals with developmental disabilities/intellectual disabilities, although recent studies have suggested it more common outside of infancy and in those with average cognitive abilities (Halland, Parthasarathy, Bharucha, & Katzka, 2016; Tack, Blondeau, Boecxstaens, & Rommel, 2011). The differential diagnosis includes gastroesophageal reflux disease (GERD), gastroparesis, achalasia, and eating disorders. Diagnosis can be aided by manometry but is most commonly diagnosed by history using the Rome III criteria (Hyman 2006) (Box 72.2).

Rumination is usually described as effortless regurgitation that occurs 5 to 30 minutes after a meal and persists for about 1 to 2 hours. Abdominal pain has been reported to occur in 40% to 80% of patients, and weight loss, which occurs in 40% to 60%, is especially common in adolescents (Tack et al., 2011). Up to 33% will have other gastrointestinal disorders, including constipation, heartburn, nausea, or diarrhea. Coexisting psychiatric disorders are common, and an underlying eating disorder has been reported in up to 20% (Tack et al., 2011). Complications associated with rumination include weight loss, malnutrition, electrolyte disturbances, halitosis, and dental erosions. A variety of relaxation therapies, such as diaphragmatic breathing, in combination with HR training and cognitive-behavioral therapy have been reported to be effective, although there are refractory cases that can become chronic and difficult to treat and may require intensive interventions such as inpatient treatment.

BOX 72.2 Rome III Definition of Rumination Syndrome in Infants and Adolescents

Infants: Must include all of the following for at least 3 mo:
- Repetitive contractions of the abdominal muscles, diaphragm, and tongue
- Regurgitation of gastric content into the mouth, which is either expectorated or rechewed and reswallowed

Three or more of the following:
- Onset between 3 and 8 mo
- Does not respond to management for gastroesophageal reflux disease or to anticholinergic drugs, hand restraints, formula changes, and gavage or gastrostomy feedings
- Unaccompanied by signs of nausea or distress
- Does not occur during sleep and when infant is interacting with individuals in the environment

Adolescents: Must include all of the following:
- Repeated painless regurgitation and rechewing or expulsion of food that begins soon after ingestion of a meal
- Does not occur during sleep
- Does not respond to standard treatment for gastroesophageal reflux
- No retching
- No evidence of an inflammatory, anatomic, metabolic, or neoplastic process that explains the subject's symptoms

Adapted from Hyman, P. E., Milla, P. J., Benninga, M. A., Davidson, G. P., Fleisher, D. F., & Taminiau, J. (2006). Childhood functional gastrointestinal disorders: Neonate/toddler. *Gastroenterology, 130*(5), 1519–1526.

Infant rumination syndrome (IRS) is associated with severe sensory and emotional deprivation causing failure to thrive and, if untreated, potentially lethal dehydration and malnutrition. IRS has been described in both severely deprived home situations and neonatal intensive care units. In the latter setting efforts to promote parent-infant bonding and make intensive care units more responsive to the needs of infants have made IRS rare.

Rumination has been reported to occur in up to 10% of individuals with severe intellectual disability living in institutions (Fredericks, Carr, & Williams, 1998). These individuals need a thorough evaluation for medical conditions possibly associated with rumination such as GERD, esophagitis, or anatomic defects. The possible role of medications that may alter esophageal function such as antipsychotics and benzodiazepines should be considered. Similar to infants, rumination is thought to begin as a self-stimulatory behavior when it occurs in individuals with intellectual disability. If rumination results in social attention or leads people to avoid asking the individual to engage in tasks, these responses may reinforce the behavior. Increasing overall levels of environmental stimulation and providing reinforcement for alternative behaviors may be effective interventions.

CONCLUSION

A wide variety of repetitive behaviors are common during childhood. Often they are typical variations such as thumb sucking or rocking, requiring only reassurance and counseling of adults not to reinforce the behaviors. However, at times repetitive behaviors may be a sign that a child is experiencing significant distress or the behaviors may occur in conjunction with a significant developmental, behavioral, or emotional disorder. In addition, the repetitive behaviors may become problematic because they cause stigmatization, subjective distress, or tissue damage. Evaluation of all these possibilities is necessary for clinicians to help families develop a plan for effective intervention.

REFERENCES

Albin, R. L., & Mink, J. W. (2006). Recent advances in Tourette syndrome research. *Trends in Neurosciences, 29*(3), 175–182.

American Psychiatric Association. (2013). *Diagnostic and statistical manual of mental disorders* (5th ed.). Author.

Andrade, C., & Srihari, B. S. (2001). A preliminary survey of rhinotillexomania in an adolescent sample. *The Journal of Clinical Psychiatry, 62*(6), 426–431.

Bakwin, H. (1971). Nail-biting in twins. *Development Medicine and Child Neurology, 1971*(13), 304–307.

Bohne, A., Keuthen, N., & Wilhelm, S. (2005). Pathologic hairpulling, skin picking, and nail biting. *Annals of Clinical Psychiatry, 17*(4), 227–232.

Borrie, F. R., Bearn, D. R., Innes, N. P., & Iheozor-Ejiofor, Z. (2015). Interventions for the cessation of non-nutritive sucking habits in children. *The Cochrane Database of Systematic Reviews, 3*, CD008694.

Castrillon, E. E., & Exposto, F. G. (2018). Sleep bruxism and pain. *Dental Clinics of North America, 62*(4), 657–663.

Ellington, E. (2017). Chronic nail biting in youth. *Journal of Psychosocial Nursing and Mental Health Services, 55*(2), 23–26.

Fredericks, D. W., Carr, J. E., & Williams, W. L. (1998). Overview of the treatment of rumination disorder for adults in a residential setting. *Journal of Behavior Therapy and Experimental Psychiatry, 29*(1), 31–40.

Halland, M., Parthasarathy, G., Bharucha, A. E., & Katzka, D. A. (2016). Diaphragmatic breathing for rumination syndrome: Efficacy and mechanisms of action. *Neurogastroenterology and Motility, 28*(3), 384–391.

Henkel, E. D., Jaquez, S. D., & Diaz, L. Z. (2019). Pediatric trichotillomania: Review of management. *Pediatric Dermatology, 36*(6), 803–807.

Hyman, P. E., Milla, P. J., Benninga, M. A., Davidson, G. P., Fleisher, D. F., & Taminiau, J. (2006). Childhood functional gastrointestinal disorders: Neonate/toddler. *Gastroenterology, 130*(5), 1519–1526.

Jain, R., Omanakuttan, D., Singh, A., & Jajoo, M. (2017). Effect of iron supplementation in children with breath holding spells. *Journal of Paediatrics and Child Health, 53*(8), 749–753.

Katherine, M. (2018). Stereotypic movement disorders. *Seminars in Pediatric Neurology, 25*, 19–24.

Kravitz, H., & Boehm, J. J. (1971). Rhythmic habit patterns in infancy: Their sequence, age of onset, and frequency. *Child Development, 42*(2), 399–413.

Leckman, J. F., & Riddle, M. A. (2000). Tourette's syndrome: When habit-forming systems form habits of their own? *Neuron, 28*(2), 349–354.

Leung, A., Leung, A., Wong, A., & Hon, K. L. (2019). Breath-holding spells in pediatrics: A narrative review of the current evidence. *Current Pediatric Reviews, 15*(1), 22–29.

Lewin, A. B., Piacentini, J., Flessner, C. A., Woods, D. W., Franklin, M. E., Keuthen, N. J., & TLC-SAB, (2009). Depression, anxiety, and functional impairment in children with trichotillomania. *Depression and Anxiety, 26*(6), 521–527.

Machado, E., Dal-Fabbro, C., Cunali, P. A., & Kaizer, O. B. (2014). Prevalence of sleep bruxism in children: A systematic review. *Dental Press Journal of Orthodontics, 19*(6), 54–61.

Manfredini, D., Serra-Negra, J., Carboncini, F., & Lobbezoo, F. (2017). Current concepts of bruxism. *The International Journal of Prosthodontics, 30*(5), 437–438.

Nwankwo, C. O., & Jafferany, M. (2019). N-acetylcysteine in psychodermatological disorders. *Dermatologic Therapy, 32*(5), e13073.

Ooki, S. (2005). Genetic and environmental influences on the handedness and footedness in Japanese twin children. *Twin Research and Human Genetics, 8*(6), 649–656.

Sallustro, M. A., & Atwell, C. W. (1978). Body rocking, head banging, and head rolling in normal children. *The Journal of Pediatrics, 93*(4), 704–708.

Sartori, S., Nosadini, M., Leoni, L., de Palma, L., Toldo, I., Milanesi, O., & Suppiej, A. (2015). Pacemaker in complicated and refractory breath-holding spells: When to think about it? *Brain & Development, 37*(1), 2–12.

Sawires, H., & Botrous, O. (2012). Double-blind, placebo-controlled trial on the effect of piracetam on breath-holding spells. *European Journal of Pediatrics, 171*(7), 1063–1067.

Staufert Gutierrez, D., & Carugno, P. (2021). Thumb sucking. In *StatPearls* [Internet]. StatPearls Publishing.

Tack, J., Blondeau, K., Boecxstaens, V., & Rommel, N. (2011). Review article: The pathophysiology, differential diagnosis and management of rumination syndrome. *Alimentary Pharmacology and Therapeutics*, *33*(7), 782–788.

Thelen, E. (1996). Normal infant stereotypes: A dynamic systems approach. In R. L. Sprague & K. M. Newell (Eds.), *Stereotyped movements: Brain and behavior relationships* (pp. 139–164). American Psychological Association.

Vertigan, A. E., Murad, M. H., Pringsheim, T., Feinstein, A., Chang, A. B., Newcombe, P. A., & Irwin, R. S. (2015). Somatic cough syndrome (previously referred to as psychogenic cough) and tic cough (previously referred to as habit cough) in adults and children: CHEST guideline and expert panel report. *Chest*, *148*(1), 24–31.

Woods, D. W., & Houghton, D. C. (2016). Evidence-based psychosocial treatments for pediatric body-focused repetitive behavior disorders. *Journal of Clinical Child and Adolescent Psychology*, *45*(3), 227–240.

73

Sexuality and Its Variations

Laura J. Mintz and Margaret Stager

For additional material related to the content of this chapter, please see Chapters 74, and 75.

VIGNETTES

1. *Ashton is a 10-year-old boy whose parents are concerned about his "feminine tendencies." They explain that from a young age he has enjoyed playing with girls, dancing, playing with dolls, and recently experimenting with makeup. At age ~5 years, they found him playing "doctor" with another boy; no touching was involved with this incident. His parents have noted that his behavior has caused him to be a target for bullies. They ask you if he is transgender or if he is gay, or if there is a way to know if he is gay.*

WE ARE SEXUAL BEINGS FROM BIRTH TO DEATH

In this chapter we discuss typical sexual development over the course of childhood and adolescence, offer common clinical scenarios, and provide guidance for concerns and challenges from patients and families. Understanding sexuality and sexual health is an ongoing dialogue, and definitions are constantly evolving and changing (see Chapter 76).

Research regarding sexuality in children is challenging and fraught with ethical concerns interacting with prevailing cultural values, attitudes, and beliefs; since the work of Floyd Martinson (1973) and others in the 1970s and 1980s, clinicians have understood sexuality as a lifelong experience, beginning prenatally. Instead of an "on" switch beginning in puberty, a more accurate framing situates sexual development as an evolving process of discovery. Sexual development is linked with sexual health, and clinicians have the opportunity to help children and families have positive, open, culturally appropriate, and accepting conversations regarding sexual development. This base of understanding can assist children in building positive self-image and healthy boundaries, which creates a foundation for healthy relationships throughout the life span.

Because of the differences between parental beliefs, popular media, and clinician education, parents often approach clinicians with questions about sexual development. This offers an opportunity to discuss typical childhood sexual development with parents and patients in targeted, supportive, and constructive ways as well as modeling supportive and accepting behavior. Sexual development is linked with gender identity (see Chapter 76).

The World Health Organization (WHO, 2006) offers the following definitions of sexuality and sexual health:

Sexuality is a central aspect of being human throughout life that encompasses sex, gender identities and roles, sexual orientation, eroticism, pleasure, intimacy, and reproduction. Sexuality is experienced and expressed in thoughts, fantasies, desires, beliefs, attitudes, values, behaviors, practices, roles, and relationships. While sexuality can include all of these dimensions, not all of them are always experienced or expressed. Sexuality is influenced by the interaction of biologic, psychological, social, economic, political, cultural, legal, historical, religious, and spiritual factors.

Sexual health is a state of physical, emotional, mental, and social well-being in relation to sexuality; it is not merely the absence of disease, dysfunction, or infirmity. Sexual health requires a positive and respectful approach to sexuality and sexual relationships, as well as the possibility of having pleasurable and safe sexual experiences, free of coercion, discrimination, and violence. For sexual health to be attained and maintained, the sexual rights of all persons must be respected, protected, and fulfilled. These definitions can be used to guide trainees and health care professionals in identifying areas of study and can help caregivers and children think about the interactions between sexuality and sexual health.

TYPICAL SEXUAL DEVELOPMENT BY AGE

Fetal Life and Infancy: A Time of Exploration

In pregnancy a fetus begins to respond to touch from outside the womb and begins to self-explore one's body (including genitals). In infancy this touch and interaction grows, and exploration of the self and the other becomes a critical task. Infants require touch and socialization as an essential component of development, and neglect or discomfort regarding touch has deleterious effects on infant development (Underdown, Barlow, & Stewart-Brown, 2010). The erection and pleasure from genital self-touch is expected in infancy and throughout childhood; parents can be reassured that this is unconcerning.

Toddlerhood: Learning the Self, Learning Others

In the realm of sexuality toddlers display interest in self-touch, which is a frequent cause of parental concern. Clinicians have the opportunity to model nonshaming conversations about self-touch with parents using appropriate and accurate terminology. This is also a time where children learn to distinguish "girl" and "boy" and to learn the accompanying cultural values, attitudes, and beliefs regarding gender roles. Toddlers also enjoy nudity, and parents often are challenged to convey when and where nudity is appropriate. Clinicians should talk with parents about establishing expectations with children for appropriate behavior in ways that toddlers will understand, acknowledging that rules and expectations regarding nudity vary by culture, religion, and context. For toddlers that are or were breastfed, they must learn how to transition from that to other forms of touch. This is occasionally difficult for some children and can result in grabbing the breasts of close family members while they learn and understand the rules of appropriate touch. Toddlers engage in exploration and play with other same-age children. Parents should be guided to encourage these questions from toddlers to create safety and openness in the home regarding sexuality. Clinicians can help parents have these conversations to establish that "private" doesn't mean shameful. The books referenced in the online supplement can help parents to have conversations with their children.

School-Age Children: Healthy Socializing Builds the Framework for Healthy Sexuality

School-age children learn more related to gender roles and expectations and support or sanction of their interests and behavior. Children come to understand the difference between private and public activity and explore their body when alone. This is an important phase for children to understand their own notions of nonsexual and eventually sexual attraction, and many children ask the people in their lives frank questions about sex and sexual activity. Answering openly, honestly, and in a manner that is developmentally appropriate is critical. These conversations help to prevent secrecy regarding sex and to set a groundwork for those conversations moving forward. This helps children to assert boundaries and eventually build sexual relationships that are consensual and helps to prevent unwanted touch, unwanted pregnancy, sexually transmitted infections, and abuse. These conversations can be very challenging, and so clinicians can offer parents resources about this topic (see online supplements).

As school-age children navigate relationships, they also come to understand and enforce norms regarding gender among each other. Many children end up victims of gender-based bullying at this age, particularly those outside of the stereotypical norms of gender. Clinicians should support families to resist bullying (see online supplements). Ashton's parents, in the first vignette, should be encouraged to support their child's interests to further their child's development rather than ignoring it.

As trusted advisors regarding sexual development, clinicians must also explore their own values, attitudes, and beliefs regarding gender roles and sexuality. These personal inventories and practice in neutral conversations are critical elements to ensure that these sensitive conversations are framed in open, inclusive, and nonjudgmental ways. This is difficult across cultural difference; clinicians should learn and understand the values and frameworks regarding sexuality across culture and particularly in populations that they serve. When clinicians encounter their own judgment, it is an important learning experience for them to explore separately from the exam room. Returning to Ashton in the first vignette, this child has shown interest in activities and expressions more stereotypically ascribed to girls, but we challenge you to expand that notion for yourself and for the families you treat. It is our role to support children's development, and encouraging children to explore their interests early on allows them to develop healthy and creative interests as they grow.

Preteens: A Moving Target of Developmental Achievement

Historically, the preteen years have been regarded as a prepubertal time when children are mostly sexually unexperienced and interested in developing their own sexual identity, but pubertal development has shifted to younger ages (Farello, Altieri, Cutini, Pozzobon, & Verrotti, 2019). When this physical development occurs, it can be a cause for concern for preteen children and their families. Menarche and nocturnal arousal and erection can begin at this time as well. Accurate and clear information regarding physical development is critical for young people to come to understand their own body (see online supplements). Reinforcing the message of autonomy, boundaries, and communication with parents and caregivers gives the child the ability to discuss what is happening to them and for adults to appropriately support their children's safety and growth.

The increase in messaging regarding sexuality from online and popular culture, including pornography, has also changed. The Internet can be an excellent source of factually accurate and age-appropriate resources regarding sexuality (see online supplements), but it also contains inaccurate, hypersexualized, and potentially harmful messages regarding sex and sexuality. Given the prevalence of pornographic images, many children encounter them either intentionally or accidentally, and clinicians should ask about this in visits with school-age children and teens (see Chapter 21).

Returning to Ashton, his parents have described typical sexual behavior (self-touch, "playing doctor"), along with gendered behavior that may or may not have anything to do with the child's ultimate understanding of his identity. His parents should be encouraged to address any bullying and to allow him to explore his interests without ascribing gender or sexual identity to them. This allows him to pursue diverse interests without shame or pressure.

Adolescence: Asserting the Self

Adolescence is a time of biologic, social, and emotional growth during which experimentation and exploration of sexual identity, sexual attraction, and romantic relationships may occur. Adolescents begin to experiment with various forms of sexual activity in their personal relationships. Through navigation of these relationships, adolescents begin to formulate and understand their own preferences and desires. Sexual orientation can shift throughout adolescence (and throughout the life span) as people come to understand themselves and their body more clearly. Sexual orientation and gender identity are always intertwined but may be particularly labile at this stage as young people come to understand attraction along with personal identity. Allowing adolescents to continue to define and understand themselves in relation to others can create healthy relationships between adolescents and caregivers to model expectations for safety and acceptance in relationships generally. Clinicians must be clear that gender does not necessarily correlate with anatomy (see Chapter 76), and so it is appropriate to discuss attraction and sexual activity with patients in anatomically specific ways to discuss contraception and sexually transmitted infection prevention as appropriate.

Recent decades have seen expansion of public discourse and conversation regarding the spectrum of sexual orientation. Political and legal achievements by sexual minority persons (legalization of same-sex marriage, increased rights regarding parenting and adoption, etc.) have created an opportunity for young people to openly understand themselves as sexual minorities. A pantheon of ever-evolving terminology exists that sexual minority persons use to describe themselves, and so definitions of sexual orientation will necessarily be incomplete given expanding cultural understanding and practice (see Chapter 76).

VIGNETTES

2. *Mandy is a 14-year-old female assigned child who you are meeting for the first time. In the individual interview Mandy tells you that she is a pansexual and that she is considering if she is nonbinary. She has a girlfriend, and she tells you that her family's religious tradition does not accept members of the LGBTQ+ community. Mandy was caught kissing her girlfriend at religious school, and as such has lost much of her close-knit community "unless I say I am something that I am not." She doesn't want you to talk to her parents because "it's pointless."*

For Mandy, in the second vignette, it is important to consider multiple layers of this patient's disclosure. Firstly, it is appropriate to show appreciation for Mandy's honesty. An important interview technique is to ask which pronouns (she/he/they/etc.) Mandy prefers and whether that should be evident in Mandy's medical record (see Chapter 76). Mandy's sexual risk is unknown until you ask about any specific types of sex engagement. We recommend asking patients about the particular sexual behaviors regarding oral, anal, or vaginal sex, and offering testing, counseling, and treatment options as relevant. Many young women who identify as lesbian, gay, bisexual, or pansexual have sex with people that may result in unintended pregnancy or they may have sex involving sharing of toys that puts them at risk for sexually transmitted infection (Charlton et al., 2018). Discussing the specific sexual acts that a patient is engaging in is essential for appropriate screening, prevention, testing, and treatment.

Many states have legal protections for assessment and treatment of the reproductive and sexual health concerns of adolescents. It is important to understand your state's laws regarding a minor's consent for, and treatment of, reproductive and sexual health (Guttmacher Institute, 2021). Teens often disclose sexual activity and sexual orientation to clinicians without disclosing it to parents, so confidentiality should be discussed with patients. Clinicians should offer to discuss these concerns with patients and families together, and connect patients with appropriate resources, including community resources such as LGBT centers, online groups, or gay-straight alliance (GSA) groups in schools. Clinicians should also be aware of LGBTQ+ affirming therapists, counselors, and/or support groups. It is important for all clinicians to understand their own comfort, values, and competence regarding issues of sexual health and sexuality in adolescents. For adolescents with complex social situations or other developmental differences that providers may be unable to address with cultural competence, it may be appropriate to refer to experienced providers that have board certification and/or special interest or training in adolescent medicine, LGBTQIA+ populations, etc. See Box 73.1 for typical behaviors during developmental stages in youth.

EXPERIENCES IMPACTING/COMPLICATING THE DEVELOPMENT OF SEXUALITY

Initiation of Sexual Activity/Intercourse

The process of sexual initiation is complex and value laden for parents, children, and clinicians. To provide inclusive and nonjudgmental medical care, we must understand our own values and beliefs as related to sex in order to best address the needs of our patients and families. Your feelings and biases about age at sexual debut, sexual activity (and particular sexual activities such as anal sex or same-gender activity), consent, and parental disclosure may affect your ability to interpret a patient's needs as well as parental concerns and legal issues. In the third vignette Jennifer's reluctance to disclose her relationship to her parents may indicate that she understands that her parents may be concerned about her having an older boyfriend or having sexual activity. To respond to this teen, it is appropriate to first affirm her decision to tell you the truth and to discuss issues of consent and mutuality in sexual relationships, pregnancy and sexually transmitted infection prevention, and legal issues that may be involved (varies by location) and to consider sharing this with her parents.

VIGNETTES

3. *Jennifer, a 15-year-old girl, tells you that she has a 17-year-old boyfriend that she hasn't told her family about. They are having oral and vaginal sex without protection. Jennifer has kissed another girl in front of him at his request (which Jennifer felt neutral about), and she tells you that he would like to have anal sex.*

BOX 73.1 Typical Sexual Behaviors in Children and Adolescents

Prenatal/infancy	Self-exploration, including genital (erections), recognition of gendered faces, faces of caregivers, enjoyment of nudity
Toddlers	Discovery and enjoyment of pleasurable self-touch, learning words for genitals, cultural understandings of "girl" and "boy," grabbing breasts of family members, enjoyment of nudity, exploration and play with same-age children
School-age children	Self-touching, moving to private exploration, understanding of privacy and sexual interaction, "doctor" and body-based play with same-age peers
Preteens	Masturbation, exploration of attraction, early puberty causing increased sexualization (apart from the child's internal thoughts)
Adolescents	Masturbation, dating, attraction, sexual experimentation, sexual identity formation

High-Risk Sexual Behavior

Some of the activities described in the third vignette are often framed as high risk, including age discrepancy among partners, sexual activity at 15 years, and anal sex. We caution clinicians against using this term (and these billing diagnoses) because while medical professionals and researchers use this language to describe activities that may put people at statistically higher risk for pregnancy and sexually transmitted infection, patients construe this framing as judgmental and stigmatizing. In internal framing, note writing, and coding we encourage neutral descriptions of sexual activity to give direct and indirect messages to patients and families about sexual health. (See online supplement regarding PrEP and HIV infection for more information.)

Sexual Abuse and Sexual Assault

Both of these topics are discussed in more detail in Chapter 15, and it bears mention to discuss these things in the context of sexual health and sexual identity. Sexual violence does not change sexual orientation; however, an emerging literature suggests that children perceived as sexual and gender minorities (i.e., lesbian, gay, bisexual, or transgender) are at higher risk for targeting by perpetrators of violence (Stephenson et al., 2018), and sexual and gender minorities consistently report higher prevalence of sexual abuse and assault (McCauley, Coulter, Bogen, & Rothman, 2018). Sexuality can be profoundly affected by sexual violence and abuse experiences, thus clinicians should be familiar with appropriate referrals for support regarding sexual violence.

CONCLUSION

Clinicians have an opportunity and obligation to discuss sexual behavior, sexual identity, and sexual practice in age and developmentally appropriate ways with children, preteens, adolescents, and their caregivers. Understanding that both conscious and unconscious biases inform the ways that all people think about sexuality and sexual health are key components of a successful pediatric clinical practice. Clinicians have an important role and opportunity in building long-lasting and robust relationships with caregivers and patients alike in supporting healthy self-esteem, relationships, and sexual health throughout the life span.

REFERENCES

Centers for Disease Control and Prevention. (n.d.). *Terminology: Adolescent and school health*. https://www.cdc.gov/healthyyouth/terminology/sexual-and-gender-identity-terms.htm

Centers for Disease Control and Prevention. (2021). *Sexually transmitted disease surveillance*, 2019. https://www.cdc.gov/std/statistics/2019/default.htm

Charlton, B. M., Roberts, A. L., Rosario, M., Katz-Wise, S. L., Calzo, J. P., Spiegelman, D., & Austin, S. B. (2018). Teen pregnancy risk factors among young women of diverse sexual orientations. *Pediatrics*, *141*(4).

Farello, G., Altieri, C., Cutini, M., Pozzobon, G., & Verrotti, A. (2019). Review of the literature on current changes in the timing of pubertal development and the incomplete forms of early puberty. *Frontiers in Pediatrics*, *7*, 147. https://doi.org/10.3389/fped.2019.00147

Guttmacher Institute. (n.d.). *State policies on later abortions*. https://www.guttmacher.org/united-states/teens/state-policies-teens#

Guttmacher Institute. (2021). *An overview of consent to reproductive health services by young people*. https://www.guttmacher.org/state-policy/explore/overview-minors-consent-law

Martinson, F. M. (1973). *Infant and child sexuality a sociological perspective*. The Book Mark.

McCauley, H. L., Coulter, R. W., Bogen, K. W., & Rothman, E. F. (2018). Sexual assault risk and prevention among sexual and gender minority populations. In: *Sexual assault risk reduction and resistance* (pp. 333–352). Academic Press.

Stephenson, R., Temmerman, M., Blondeel, K., De Vasconcelos, S., García-Moreno, C., & Toskin, I. (2018). Violence motivated by perception of sexual orientation and gender identity: A systematic review. *Bulletin of the World Health Organization* https://doi.org/10.2471/BLT.17.197251

Underdown, A., Barlow, J., & Stewart-Brown, S. (2010). Tactile stimulation in physically healthy infants: Results of a systematic review. *Journal of Reproductive and Infant Psychology*, *28*(1), 11–29. https://doi.org/10.1080/02646830903247209

World Health Organization. (2006). *Defining sexual health* (pp. 1–30). https://www.who.int/reproductivehealth/topics/sexual_health/sh_definitions/en/

74

Sexuality in Children and Youth With Disabilities

Beth Ellen Davis, Susan Hayden Gray, and Jenniffer Herrera

for additional material related to the content of this chapter, please see Chapters 73.and 75

> **VIGNETTE**
>
> *An 11-year-old girl with autism spectrum disorder (ASD) level 3, who is nonverbal and has cooccurring intellectual disability (ID), is transitioning to middle school setting. Parents have questions about their daughter's pubertal changes, hygiene and incontinent care at school, approaching menstruation, need for sexual education, and safety.*

INTRODUCTION

Children who experience physical and developmental disabilities are a growing subset of all children and youth in the United States, comprising between 8% and 10% of the population (Zablotsky, Black, Maenner, Schieve, Danielson, Bitsko, & Boyle, 2019), and more than 10 million children have conditions that moderately or severely affect their daily activities (Hagerman & Houtrow, 2020). Addressing the comprehensive needs of children with disabilities requires an individualized, yet multidimensional approach that ultimately optimizes inclusion and independence, while mitigating isolation and impairment. Even though the physiologic changes of puberty often motivate individuals, parents, teachers, and health clinicians to address sexual health issues (as seen in the chapter-opening vignette), healthy sexuality is a lifelong process and a critical component of each person's sociocultural development and competency, especially for individuals who experience physical or developmental differences (Mona, Cameron, & Clemency Cordes, 2017). In Chapter 73 the foundation was laid for a biopsychosocial approach to sexuality for all children and youth across the life course, to begin to understand the complex nature of healthy sexuality. This chapter is dedicated to encouraging clinician knowledge, skills, and efficacy to move beyond disability toward promotion of healthy sexuality and sexual wellbeing as part of a larger strengths-based comprehensive model of care so as to improve the quality of life for children and youth with disabilities.

Within families, educational systems, communities, cultures, religions, and societies, many barriers to healthy sexuality exist for individuals with disabilities (Roden, Schmidt, & Holland-Hall, 2020). Families and caregivers often see their child with disability as vulnerable, childlike, or asexual and do not acknowledge the child's potential for sociosexual development. While excellent educational resources are available specific to the needs of children with disabilities (Table 74.1) who receive special education through a wide array of eligibility categories (Lipkin, Okamoto, Council on Children with Disabilities, & Council on School Health, 2015), instruction is frequently presented in a circumscribed, inaccessible curriculum (Breuner, Mattson, Committee on Adolescence, & Committee on Psychosocial Aspects of Child and Family Health, 2016). Children with disabilities often need repeated access to inclusive universal design (UD) materials, presented in multiple modalities, to include peer mentoring (Roden et al., 2020).

While primary care clinicians have training in sexual health needs of children, and over a dozen recent clinical reports have been published on sexual health topics in children and youth (Houtrow, Elias, & Davis, 2021), according to individuals and their families, most clinicians do not discuss sexuality in the setting of disability, which results in unmet sexual health education needs (Graham Holmes, Shattuck, Nilssen, Strassberg, & Himle, 2020; Sommarö, Andersson, & Skagerström, 2020). For many clinicians, having an easy-to-remember framework to address multidimensional patient needs in a comprehensive, yet customized way helps to promote regularity in all encounters. The International Classification of Functioning, Disability and Health (ICF) provides a socioecologic framework for all individuals, especially those with disabilities, and connects health, function, and factors related to quality of life (World Health Organization, 2001). A decade ago, a provocative

> *In the patient from the vignette, who is now 11 years of age, were prior opportunities to address sexual health issues possibly missed?*
>
> 1. *As a nonverbal child with ID, how does she communicate "no!" or "wet"? Has communication been optimized? If the child is noncommunicative, then trusted supervision is required in all settings.*
> 2. *The language of growing up and stating the term "briefs" instead of "diapers" by age 5 sends the message to all involved that despite being incontinent, this child is not a baby but a growing, developing sexual being.*
> 3. *Does the school individualized education plan include visual schedules around hygiene care, encourage same-sex caregivers for incontinent care after a certain age, offer appropriate supervised settings for hygiene care? What is the chaperone policy for middle- and high-school students with significant developmental disabilities?*
> 4. *Do family and friends encourage side hugs and high-fives for casual greetings and redirect or reframe inappropriate kissing and touching by the individual?*
> 5. *If child/youth can make choices, setting out choices for clothes or meal preparation and allowing daily opportunities for autonomy are teachable moments.*

TABLE 74.1 Sexual Education Resources for Individuals With Disabilities, Families, Schools, and Clinicians

For Parents, General	
Center for Parent Information and Resources, 2018: www.parentcenterhub.org (also in Spanish)	
Healthybodies.org (Vanderbilt) Boys/Girls: https://www.healthybodies.org/	
Couwenhoven, T. (2015). *Boyfriends & girlfriends: A guide to dating for people with disabilities.* Woodbine House.	
Bright Futures. (2017). *Guidelines for health supervision of infants, children, and adolescents* (4th ed.). https://brightfutures.aap.org/Pages/default.aspx	
Sexuality Resource Center for Parents: Teaching children across the age ranges (0-18): http://www.srcp.org/for_all_parents/development.html	
Raising Special Kids: www.raisingspecialkids.org (also in Spanish)	
Condition-Specific Resources (for Pediatric Clinicians)	
Autism spectrum disorder	www.stwwgepublications.com/pages/publications.html (includes a brochure entitled "Sex Education for Parents of Children With Autism Spectrum Disorders") https://www.autismspeaks.org/docs/family_services_docs/parentworkbook.pdf Kate E. Reynolds to help learn about puberty: "What's Happening to Ellie?" A book about puberty for girls and young women with autism and related conditions. (2015); "What's Happening to Tom?" A book about puberty for boys and young men with autism and related conditions (2015).
Cerebral palsy	Glader, L., & Stevenson, R. (2019). *Children and youth with complex cerebral palsy: Care and management* (chap. 17, 18). Mac Keith Press.
Spina bifida	The Spina Bifida Association: https://www.spinabifidaassociation.org/guidelines/ Centers for Disease Control and Prevention: https://www.cdc.gov/ncbddd/spinabifida/adult.html#sexual-health
Spinal cord injury	Papadakis, J. L., Zebracki, K., Chlan, K. M., & Vogel, L. C. (2017). Sexuality in pediatric spinal cord injury. *Top Spinal Cord Injury Rehabilitation, 23*(1), 42–48. https://doi.org/10.1310/sci2301-42 (there is an excellent table for parents!)
Down syndrome	Chicoine, B., & McGuire, D. (2010). *The guide to good health for teens and adults with Down syndrome.* Woodbine House; (2005). *Teaching children with Down syndrome about their bodies, boundaries, and sexuality: A guide for parents and professionals.* Woodbine House.
Intellectual and developmental disabilities	Brown, F., & Brown, S. (2016). *When young people with intellectual disabilities and autism hit puberty: A parents' Q&A guide to health, sexuality and relationships.* Jessica Kingsley Publishers.
Other	U.S. National Library of Medicine: https://ghr.nlm.nih.gov/condition (an up-to-date genetic review of genetic conditions, easily searchable alphabetically, including rare microdeletions)
For Schools/Educators	
FLASH: Seattle and King County Sexual Health Education Curriculum: https://www.kingcounty.gov/depts/health/locations/family-planning/education/FLASH.aspx	
Advocates for Youth: https://advocatesforyouth.org/wp-content/uploads/storage//advfy/documents/Factsheets/sexual-health-education-for-young-people-with-disabilities-educators.pdf	

Adapted from Houtrow, A., Elias, E., Davis, B. E., & Council on Children With Disabilities. (2021). Promoting healthy sexuality in children and youth with disabilities. *Pediatrics, 148*(1), e2021052043. doi: 10.1542/peds.2021-052043. Epub 2021 Jun 28. PMID: 34183359.

review, titled "The F-Words in Childhood Disability: I swear this is how we should think!" (Rosenbaum & Gorter, 2011), operationalized the ICF framework for child-serving clinicians to approach biopsychosocial factors, including healthy sexuality, at every encounter. The six F-words include function, family, fitness, fun, friends, and future (Fig. 74.1).

GENERAL CONCEPTS WHEN ADDRESSING SEXUALITY NEEDS OF INDIVIDUALS WITH DISABILITIES

It is imperative for children and youth, with and without disabilities, to receive accurate, developmentally appropriate, culturally sensitive sexuality education about safe, healthy, positive attitudes toward themselves, their own body, and others (Bright Futures, 2017) repeatedly, from multiple sources, over time.

Physical Disabilities

Children and youth with physical disabilities are a heterogeneous population, including those with concomitant mental and cognitive impairments, with congenital or acquired conditions, and with gender-specific needs. Compared to the general population, individuals with physical disabilities have significant sexual and reproductive health disparities, unmet sexual education needs, and higher rates of sexual distress (Rowan et al., 2015). Individuals with physical disabilities are as interested in their sexuality, sexual function, and intimacy as their typically developing peers (Eisenburg, Andreski, & Mona, 2015). However, individuals with physical disabilities

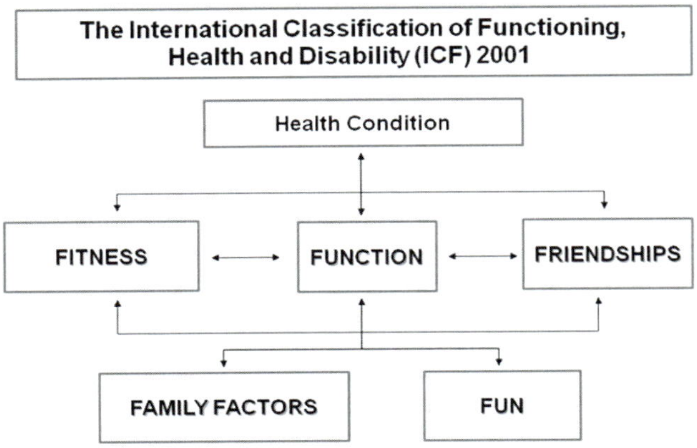

Fig. 74.1 The International Classification of Functioning, Disability and Health framework: The interconnections among elements. (From Rosenbaum, P., & Gorter, J. W. [2012]. The "F-words" in childhood disability: I swear this is how we should think! *Child: Care, Health and Development*, 38[4], 457–463. https://doi.org/10.1111/j.1365-2214.2011.01338.x)

have a much more restricted frame of reference, fewer opportunities to access social activities, and less sexual education than other youth, sometimes merely due to environmental or structural barriers (Welage & Liu, 2011). Individuals with physical disabilities report they are frequently frustrated by adults and health care clinicians who assume coexisting cognitive disability and are treated differently than their cognitively abled peers, feeling disrespected and devalued. As cognitively abled youth, they indicate they want to be provided the same confidential autonomy of other adolescents when discussing sexuality and other sensitive topics, and for others to assume competence first. The needs of children and youth with physical disabilities require an individualized approach to sexual functioning and sexual wellbeing, from biologic (type of disability, medication use), psychological (body image, sexual attraction), educational (appropriate access to resources), and sociocultural (access to relationships) perspectives (Eisenberg, 2015).

Intellectual and Developmental Disabilities

Most individuals with intellectual and developmental disabilities (IDD), especially those with mild IDD and ASD, have typical life spans and mature desires for happiness and wellbeing, including relationships, intimacy, and families. They are interested in their future sociosexual lives, but they lack experiences, volume, and variety of social networks (van Asselt-Goverts, Embregts, Hendriks, Wegman, & Teunisse, 2015) compared to their neurotypical peers. Adults with IDD report sexual experiences but with significantly more unsafe or unintended consequences (Baines, Emerson, Robertson, & Hatton, 2018). At least additive to experiencing a disability itself, people with IDD are also more likely to experience a range of social and material disadvantages (low family socioeconomic position, living in a more deprived area, unmet transportation needs, exposure to violence), which are known across all populations to be associated with risky sexual behaviors and victimization (Baines et al., 2018).

Family and Caregivers

Individuals with disabilities, especially IDD, are much more likely to live with their family well into adulthood and are predominantly cared for by their mother (Braddock, Hemp, Tanis, Wu, & Haffer, 2017). Parents and caregivers are generally uncomfortable talking with their youth about sexual health issues and are much more cautious when it comes to youth with disabilities (Breuner et al., 2016). Parent perspectives around the child's sexuality are often associated with concerns for vulnerability, such as exploitation and victimization, and conversations are often tempered with warnings and negative statements. In one study mothers of youth with ID compared to those without indicated that withholding sexual information was in the best interest of their children, to protect them from possible exploitation, and prioritized their child's protection over less important sexual desires and interest in relationships (Pownall, Jahoda, & Hastings, 2012). Daughters are of great concern to their parents and caregivers, as they try to anticipate hygiene care around menstruation, pregnancy prevention, and the need for personal safety (Holland-Hall & Quint, 2017). At the extreme has been the introduction of a still controversial medical intervention called growth attenuation, which includes parent-directed sterilization and prevention of physiologic puberty in young children with profound ID (see Chapter 111). From an emotional perspective, sexuality, sexual education, and "growing up" sometimes evokes a reexperiencing of grief in parents, when a new chapter of the child's life begins, even years after acceptance of a differently-abled child.

Sexual Education

Many excellent evidence-based sexual education resources are available for individuals with physical disabilities and IDD (and even specific to Down syndrome, spina bifida, spinal cord injury, cerebral palsy, autism, children with ID, among others), their families, their teachers, and health care clinicians (see Table 74.1). Despite available and accessible resources, most individuals with disabilities have significantly unmet sexual health education needs (Graham Holmes et al., 2020; Jahoda & Pownall, 2014). The impact of unmet sexual health education is well described and results in inappropriate or problem behaviors, unprotected sexual activity, increased sexually transmitted infections, inadequate contraception, unintended teen pregnancy, and sexual vulnerability (Baines et al., 2018; Breuner et al., 2016; Roden et al., 2020). Pediatricians can be a source of customized information and recognize they have a role in sex education, but typically they devote little time during a clinical encounter and often wait until it is broached by the patient or parent (Breuner et al., 2016). Thus most adolescents, including teens with disabilities, are obtaining sex education through informal portals such as the Internet or their social networks (Caton & Chapman, 2016; Lindberg, 2016). This is fraught with barriers for individuals with unique physical or medical needs, or who lack literacy skills, or who experience social anxiety.

Contemporary educational literature recommends the use of a UD framework to improve accessibility of learning materials for diverse audiences, especially those with IDD (Roden et al., 2020). Use of clear and defined language, engagement through shared decision making, use of verbal and visual strategies when providing education, and opportunities for questions are successful factors in UD communication. Most sexual education assumes heterotypical relationships and often omits discussions about gender identity, gender diversity, and sexual orientation. For individuals with IDD, who report higher prevalence of gender minority status (George & Stokes, 2018), an open, nonjudgemental approach is needed (Box 74.1).

A lack of information and education on sexuality and disability is felt to be a major contributing factor toward societal stigma attached to the expression of healthy sexuality in individuals with disabilities. Through increased awareness and knowledge across systems of care, societal attitudes and perceptions can change (Sommarö et al., 2020).

Puberty

The onset of puberty often brings anxiety for families of children with physical or developmental disabilities (Gray, S. H., Wylie, M., Christensen, S., Khan, A., Williams, D., & Glader, L., 2021). For parents of girls with physical disabilities, the prospect of menstruation may pose logistical or hygiene challenges, and parents dread dysmenorrhea as another potential source of physical pain for their daughters. For parents of children with IDD, fear of possible sexual misbehavior or abuse is common. The timing of puberty can vary, but most individuals with disabilities have typical pubertal onset and progression (see Chapters 73 and 111). The current American Academy of Pediatrics (AAP) and American College of Obstetricians and Gynecologists (ACOG) guidelines recommend endocrinologic evaluation for girls, including those with disabilities, not having menarche within 3 years after thelarche, and no menses by age 15 (ACOG, 2006). Likewise, precocious puberty usually needs further assessment. Children with some neurodevelopmental disabilities, including cerebral palsy, McCune-Albright syndrome, hydrocephalus, neural tube defects, acquired brain injuries, among others, appear to be at higher risk for precocious puberty.

Human Papillomavirus Vaccination

Sometimes parents of children with disabilities ask to defer vaccination with the human papillomavirus (HPV) vaccine because they assume their children will not be sexually active in the future. The authors strongly recommend routine, on-time immunization for HPV in all children per the AAP/Advisory Committee on Immunization Practices schedule because of the vaccine's efficacy in reducing the incidence of cervical, anal, and penile cancers and because predicting the onset of sexual activity (or sexual abuse) may be difficult if not impossible (Giuliano et al., 2019).

BOX 74.1 Sexual Identity and Orientation Interview—Sample Questions

Many people have a hard time figuring out their sex. Is this something you think about?

1. What sex do you identify with: male (boy), female (girl), transgender, or something else?
2. Who are you attracted to: men, women, both or neither?
3. Are you in a relationship? With whom?

Adapted from Walters, F. P., & Gray, S. H. (2018). Addressing sexual and reproductive health in adolescents and young adults with intellectual and developmental disabilities. *Current Opinions in Pediatrics, 30*(4), 451–458. https://doi.org/10.1097/MOP.0000000000000635

Menstruation and Menstrual Management, Contraception, Pregnancy, Reproductive Care, and Sexually Transmitted Infections

Families of girls with disabilities may have assumptions about how their daughters will deal with menstruation, which are influenced by personal, family, cultural, or religious factors, and so it is worth asking about those before providing anticipatory guidance or advice. Some families of girls with severe disabilities may seek preemptive medical treatment to prevent menses or even request hysterectomy, whereas others may view menstruation as a natural occurrence and something that connects them to their daughters (Gray et al., 2021). Except in unusual circumstances it is often worth taking a watchful waiting approach to the onset of menstruation and being flexible in response to the patient and family's needs (Box 74.2). Numerous recent sources address in detail contraception in this population (Holland-Hall & Quint, 2017;

BOX 74.2 Menstrual Supports and Interventions for Individuals with Intellectual and Developmental Disabilities

- Begin anticipatory guidance about menses at sexual maturity stage 2 or before. Resources range from books (e.g., *The Care and Keeping of You, It's Not the Stork*) to videos and websites (e.g., youngwomenshealth.org, amaze.org).
- Consider consultation with an adolescent specialist or gynecologist prior to menarche if menstrual suppression is desired by family and/or patient.
- Consider a watchful waiting approach at sexual maturity stage 3 with use of washable, absorbent underwear designed for menstrual flow to acclimate girls to wearing menstrual protection.
- Anticipate and make a plan for treatment of dysmenorrhea (e.g., naproxen sodium or ibuprofen in weight-appropriate dosing given at regular intervals for first several days of menses, starting as soon as it is apparent menses are beginning). Nonpharmacologic interventions include heat, TENS unit.
- If menses are interfering with medical treatment of other conditions, hygiene, or quality of life, consider medical intervention with hormonal treatments to make menses lighter, shorter, less painful, or to eliminate menses. Surgical intervention is rarely indicated due to the availability of less invasive/risky medical treatments, and may require a court order.

Adapted from Walters, F. P., & Gray, S. H. (2018). Addressing sexual and reproductive health in adolescents and young adults with intellectual and developmental disabilities. *Current Opinions in Pediatrics, 30*(4), 451–458. https://doi.org/10.1097/MOP.0000000000000635

Walters & Gray, 2018). Additional issues related to menstrual management, contraception, pregnancy, reproductive care, and sexually transmitted infections in individuals with disabilities are covered in Chapters 40, 73, and 111.

> *At age 11, the preteen in the vignette is likely showing signs of puberty, and a careful exam can help project a timeline for preparation and anticipatory guidance. Box 74.2 lists the parent education that this visit affords. Most parents need reassurance that, typically, multiple cycles of menstruation are allowed to occur before suppression is attempted. Conversations about addressing hygiene in middle school can start by asking how this was navigated in elementary school and if any issues had to be resolved. This is often a good time to also discuss opportunities for expanding other social networks such as day or summer camps, where youth with similar conditions attend, usually with a trained 1:1 counselor, medical staff, and extensive supervision.*

SEXUAL ACTIVITY

Just as definitions of disability vary and affect prevalence rates (Hagerman & Houtrow, 2020), defining and describing rates of sexual activity can be challenging. In the United States about 38% of high-school students (age 14–19) reported ever being sexually active, according to the National Youth Risky Behavior Survey from the Centers for Disease Control and Prevention (CDC, 2019). National surveys and self-reports by youth with disabilities support similar rates of sexual motivation and interest to neurotypical peers, but when followed longitudinally over time typically developing young adults become more sexually active and individuals with disabilities do not, especially individuals with more significant physical disability and IDD (Kahn, 2018). The sexual experiences of youth and young adults with disabilities also differ from their typical counterparts with respect to risky behaviors: with evidence of less condom use, less contraception, more sexually transmitted infections, and increased completed pregnancies (Baines et al., 2018).

Adolescents With Intellectual Disabilities

Of the 1% to 2% of the young adult population with ID, the vast majority experience nonsyndromic mild ID, with limited need for social, practical, or conceptual supports. In adulthood similar to their typically developing peers, they are not required to disclose their disability when visiting a medical clinician, and in fact, most health care clinicians are unaware individuals have preexisting IDD (Ames, Massolo, Davignon, Qian, Cerros, & Croen, 2020). If guardianship has not been established, these young adults are expected to and are often capable of addressing their own medical, mental health, and sexuality needs (Bennett, Miller, Stollon, Prasad, & Blum, 2018).

Individuals with disabilities, as they transition to high school and beyond, lose the structure of school- and sports-based social networks, and societal expectations are for youth to initiate and develop their own friendships and relationships. While individuals with disabilities, especially IDD, are interested in sociosexual opportunities, their social networks are considerably smaller than their peers (Caton et al., 2016). For IDD, high interest but low knowledge, along with social naiveté, results in reports of risky behaviors, negative experiences, and vulnerability.

Adolescents With Autism Spectrum Disorders

Navigating the transition to a somewhat spontaneous, social adult world from a supervised, structured school and home setting can be challenging for all adolescents and especially for individuals with ASD (Bennett et al., 2018; Turner, 2017). For individuals with ASD, difficulty with social reciprocity and pragmatic communication directly impact the understanding and development of social relationships, compared with their typical but also cognitively delayed peers (Dewinter, De Graaf, & Begeer, 2017). In a large study youth/adults with ASD did not significantly differ from their neurotypical peers without ASD in their knowledge of sexual language and interest in sexual experiences (Dewinter et al., 2017). However, numerous studies, including self-reports by individuals with ASD, indicate significant unmet needs in sexual awareness and appropriate behavior, including understanding of privacy norms and expectations in social settings (Fernandes, Gillberg, Cederlund, Hagberg, Gillberg, & Billstedt, 2016; Hancock, Stokes, & Mesibov, 2017). Inappropriate sexual behavior may be common, even in individuals with ASD without ID (Fernandes et al., 2016). Additionally, youth with ASD have greater diversity in sexual orientation and gender identity compared with typically developing peers, which brings with it navigation of socially ostracized nonconforming relationships (DeWinter et al., 2017; Hancock et al., 2017). The growing literature about the unique needs of individuals with ASD, separate from other individuals with IDD, create opportunities to customize safety and sex education, understand sexual diversity, prevent problem sexual behaviors, and ensure safety (see Table 74.1) (Hancock et al., 2017).

Adolescents With Spina Bifida or Spinal Cord Injury (Examples of Physical Disability)

Individuals with physical disabilities are similar to their peers in interest, attitudes, and future relationship planning. They are interested in discussing how to manage their physical differences but are unlikely to initiate conversations with their health clinicians (Seburg, McMorris, Garwick, & Scal, 2015). Individuals with spina bifida or spinal cord injury, two specific types of physical disability, experience at least partial lower extremity paralysis, neurogenic bowel and bladder, and loss of nerve signals to their sex organs. The neurologic consequences of spinal cord injury and spina bifida can alter sexual and reproductive experiences and can affect confidence and self-esteem. Women with spinal cord injury or spina bifida tend to have normal fertility and usually require high-risk obstetric care, before and during their pregnancies, and perinatally (Brei & Houtrow, 2017; Rowen, 2015). Men with spina bifida or spinal cord injury tend to have altered fertility and physical activity (Hess & Hough, 2012). People with spina bifida should use nonlatex condoms because of the increased risk of latex allergy in this population. Collaboration with a physical medicine and rehabilitation specialist and/or obstetrics-gynecology specialist helps as transition to adult health care occurs (see Chapters .. and ..).

PROBLEM SEXUAL BEHAVIORS

Taking a dimensional approach to sexual behaviors ranging from typical, to socially inappropriate or problematic, to atypical regardless of situation often helps families of children with IDD, acquired brain injury, or ASD understand behavior according to developmental ability rather than chronologic age. In most settings individuals with physical disabilities without cognitive impairment or social communication deficits are expected to demonstrate sexual behaviors similar to their neurotypical peers.

Problem Sexual Behaviors in Children

Problem sexual behaviors are behaviors that are developmentally inappropriate, intrusive, or abusive (Kellogg, 2009). They can be interpersonal or self-focused and may not be sexually motivated or related to sexual gratification (Mesman, Harper, Edge, Brandt, & Pemberton, 2019). Problem sexual behaviors often persist despite parental attention and supervision and tend to be more preoccupying. It may be difficult to distract a child from the behavior, and children may show feelings of anger, frustration, fear, or anxiety with attempts at redirection. When determining whether a sexual behavior is problematic, one should consider factors that include the type of behavior, frequency, age, environment, and level of imposed harm. There are childhood sexual behaviors that are rare across age ranges and developmental levels and should be a cause for concern (e.g., trying to have sexual intercourse, mouth-to-genital contact, asking others to do sex acts, pretending toys are having sex, and inserting an object or finger into the rectum or vagina). Behaviors that involve children of disparate ages (>4-year age difference) or abilities are also cause for concern, as are those that involve threat, force, or aggression. Behaviors that interfere with social development are considered problematic as well. For example, a child dismissed from a team sport due to inappropriate touching of other players may be displaying a problematic sexual behavior. Problematic sexual behavior among individuals with IDD is common, with an incidence ranging from 15% to 33%. The behaviors are like those in the general population, except that those with IDD tend to be more socially inappropriate than assaultive (Thom, Grudzinskas, & Saleh, 2017). Problematic sexual behavior can range from a child with developmental disability disrobing in public to a youth with ASD asking sexual questions to strangers or sexting (Box 74.3). It can include startling behavior such as frottage and using female family members' undergarments for masturbation and behavior that is illegal (e.g., touching a younger child's genitals or stalking) (Blasingame, 2018). Problematic sexual behavior in this population, and in those with acquired brain injuries and ASD, may be related to poor boundaries/social skills, lack of impulse control, tendency toward repetitive/perseverative behavior, or difficulty understanding abstract concepts such as private versus public or what is hurtful or uncomfortable to others (Blasingame, 2018; Kellogg, 2009) as a result of dysfunction in areas of the brain (including the frontal cortex, amygdala, or temporal lobes) or as a result of their primary condition. In individuals with IDD chronologic age discordant to developmental ability may turn what is normative sexual behavior (for developmental level) into problematic sexual behavior (due to chronologic age). Problematic sexual behavior in individuals with IDD may also stem from a lack of opportunity for social relationships to explore sexuality safely or to learn and practice sociosexual behaviors (Thom et al., 2017).

A biopsychosocial model can guide assessment and treatment of problematic sexual behaviors (Griffiths & Fedoroff, 2014; Miodrag, Richards, Fedoroff, & Watson, 2020). From

BOX 74.3 Problem Sexual Behavior Supports and Resources

Excessive or Public Masturbation

1. Suggested conversation: "Today, we discussed that masturbation is a normal behavior. Excessive and/or inappropriate masturbation is often difficult to control, as it can be a self-reinforcing behavior. We discussed that although inappropriate masturbation, such as public masturbation, may not completely go away, your child can learn to be redirected to perform the behavior in private. The key to approaching this is to ensure that your child both has a personal space and understands the appropriate place for private behaviors. Recommend utilizing a schedule or timer to set boundaries for these behaviors."
2. Specific protocols for minimizing excessive public masturbation include interrupting the behavior, reminding the person of appropriate time and place, redirection, and allowing masturbation in private. Often, working with a behavior therapist who can offer applied behavior analysis is recommended.
3. Resources: Kate, E. Reynolds books: *Things Tom likes: A book about sexuality and masturbation for boys and young men with autism and related conditions* (2015) and *Things Ellie likes: A book about sexuality and masturbation for girls and young women with autism and related conditions* (2015).
4. Inappropriate interactions (stalking), touching, or romantic gestures
   a. Through the Individualized Education Program, request a functional behavior assessment and a behavior intervention plan for positive supports such as social skills group, scripting, video modeling and feedback, self-management, and rule-governed behaviors.
   b. Resource: *Teaching moment: Teaching your kids appropriate and inappropriate touching*: https://www.northshore.org/healthy-you/teaching-your-kids-appropriate-touching/

Adapted from Houtrow, A., Elias, E., Davis, B. E., & Council on Children With Disabilities. (2021). Promoting healthy sexuality in children and youth with disabilities. *Pediatrics, 148*(1), e2021052043. doi: 10.1542/peds.2021-052043. Epub 2021 Jun 28. PMID: 34183359.

a biomedical perspective, knowledge of a syndrome can help explain the nature of a problematic sexual behavior. For instance, individuals with Smith-Magenis syndrome engage in polyembolokoilamania, and skin picking (including rectal picking and digging) is common in Prader-Willi syndrome. Individuals with Williams syndrome are more prone to urinary tract infections, which may present as self-touch as opposed to masturbation, as they may be unable to communicate their symptoms. A person with Tourette syndrome may have a complex tic of a seemingly sexual nature (Griffiths & Fedoroff, 2014). Individuals with ASD have difficulty detecting social cues and may not recognize personal boundaries or that another person does not want to engage in a relationship. Medication side effects should be considered as possible cause of problematic sexual behavior (Griffiths & Fedoroff, 2014; Miodrag et al., 2020). Psychological assessment should include not only assessment of cognitive ability and adaptive functioning but also behavioral assessment, trauma assessment, and assessment of sexual knowledge. All behavior serves a function, and defining the antecedent, the behavior, and the consequences can help identify the function of a specific problem sexual behavior. For instance, a behavioral assessment could help identify whether a child was engaging in a problematic sexual behavior to escape a consequence or to gain attention (Griffiths & Fedoroff, 2014).

Individuals with IDD are more vulnerable to abuse, yet trauma history in this population is rarely addressed (Miodrag et al., 2020). Children with sexual abuse histories have higher rates of problem sexual behavior than children without such a history (Mesman et al., 2019). Assessment of sexual knowledge is important, as a younger developmental versus chronologic age does not mean lack of experience or lack of physical development (Griffiths & Fedoroff, 2014). Behavior may be related to lack of understanding to a certain degree rather than total lack of awareness (Lindsay & Michie, 2013). Finally, social conditions such as living in an environment where sexuality is more open or allows access to sexual material may result in modeling of such behavior (Kellogg, 2009; Mesman et al., 2019). Other socioenvironmental factors that may contribute to problem sexual behaviors are family dysfunction and stress, including poverty, single parenting, domestic violence, parent incarceration, and chronic illness in child or parent (Kellogg, 2009; Lindsay & Michie, 2013; Mesman et al., 2019) as these may inhibit parental guidance and appropriate supervision.

Individuals With Disabilities Are at Risk for Sexual Abuse and Victimization

Individuals with disabilities are almost three times more likely to be sexually abused than peers without disabilities, and risks are even higher for those with IDD and for females. Although studied 30 years ago, it is likely that perpetrators of sexual violence against individuals with disabilities are known to the victim with the majority being in their social network or caregiver role (Crawford-Jakubiak, Alderman, Leventhal, Committee on Child Abuse and Neglect, & Committee on Adolscence, 2017). Individuals with IDD and parents report risk factors that include inadequate awareness of vulnerable social settings, misunderstanding of appropriate relationships and physical contact, desire to conform, and poor knowledge and communication skills to discuss sexual maltreatment (Walters & Gray, 2018).

THE ROLE OF THE DEVELOPMENTAL BEHAVIORAL CLINICIAN

As youth with disabilities, especially IDD, gain increasing agency and control and transition to adulthood, it is critical to better understand the context and outcomes of demands for choice and agency over sexuality and relationships. Often, it is the developmental-behavioral pediatrician (DBP) who is asked by a family about medical prognosis for autonomy and lifetime health-related quality of life. Though no one has a crystal ball, the DBP can share an awareness of the wide intersectional scope of the lives of individuals with disabilities and support their self-awareness and desires around sexuality. Through a longitudinal relationship, the DBP can help reframe sexuality in disability away from the negative for individuals and their families, while addressing safety through education and appropriate supervision. Finally, the DBP can provide a safe space, perhaps not dissimilar to Winnicott's "holding place," (Winnicott, 1971) for youth with disabilities and their families to express their dreams, sexual desires, beliefs, and attitudes as society's understanding moves from sexual marginalization to intersectionality.

Often during a big transition, such as puberty and adolescence, parents "seek permission" to be seen with their youth more often than once a year. Setting up office visits for individuals with disabilities every 6 months as puberty begins (especially for girls) and to establish school and community supports for transition and education is often preferred. There are transition checklists and strategies for individuals with a wide array of disabilities (see Gottransition.gov). As in the vignette, this is a great time to discuss with parents how to build a broader circle of support for their child and encourage them to share their future goals, but also to explore what a happy and meaningful life means through their child's eyes.

REFERENCES

American College of Obstetricians and Gynecologists Committee on Adolescent Health Care. (2006). ACOG Committee Opinion No. 349: Menstruation in girls and adolescents: Using the menstrual cycle as a vital sign. *Obstetrics and Gynecology*, *108*(5), 1323–1328. https://doi.org/10.1097/00006250-200611000-00059

Ames, J. L., Massolo, M. L., Davignon, M. N., Qian, Y., Cerros, H. J., & Croen, L. A. (2020). Transitioning youth with autism spectrum disorders and other special health care needs into adult primary care: A provider survey. *Autism*, 1362361320926318. https://doi.org/10.1177/1362361320926318. Epub ahead of print.

Baines, S., Emerson, E., Robertson, J., & Hatton, C. (2018). Sexual activity and sexual health among young adults with and without mild/moderate intellectual disability. *BMC public health*, *18*(1), 667. https://doi.org/10.1186/s12889-018-5572-9

Bennett, A. E., Miller, J. S., Stollon, N., Prasad, R., & Blum, N. J. (2018). Autism spectrum disorder and transition-aged youth. *Current psychiatry reports, 20*(11), 103. https://doi.org/10.1007/s11920-018-0967-y

Blasingame, G. D. (2018). Risk assessment of adolescents with intellectual disabilities who exhibit sexual behavior problems or sexual offending behavior. *Journal of Child Sexual Abuse, 27*(8), 955–971.

Braddock, D. L., Hemp, R. E., Tanis,E. S., Wu, J., & Haffer, L. (2017). *State of the states in intellectual and developmental disabilities* (11th ed.).

Brei, T., & Houtrow, A. (2017). Spina bifida. *Journal of Pediatric Rehabilitation Medicine, 10*(3–4), 165–166. https://doi.org/10.3233/PRM-170469

Breuner, C. C., Mattson, G., Committee on Adolescence, & Committee on Psychosocial Aspects of Child and Family Health. (2016). Sexuality education for children and adolescents. *Pediatrics, 138*(2), e20161348. https://doi.org/10.1542/peds.2016-1348

Bright Futures. (2017). *Guidelines for health supervision of infants, children, and adolescents* (pp. 217–227, 4th ed.). https://brightfutures.aap.org/Pages/default.aspx

Caton, S., & Chapman, M. (2016). The use of social media and people with intellectual disability: A systematic review and thematic analysis. *Journal of Intellectual Development and Disabilities, 41*(2), 125–139. https://doi.org/10.3109/13668250.2016.1153052

Centers for Disease Control and Prevention. (2019). Youth Risk Behavior Survey data summary and trends report 2009–2019. https://www.cdc.gove/healthyyouth/data/yrbs/pdf

Crawford-Jakubiak, J. E., Alderman, E. M., Leventhal, J. M., Committee on Child Abuse and Neglect, & Committee on Adolscence. (2017). Care of the adolescent after an acute sexual assault. *Pediatrics, 139*(3), e20164243. https://doi.org/10.1542/peds.2016-4243

Dewinter, J., De Graaf, H., & Begeer, S. (2017). Sexual orientation, gender identity, and romantic relationships in adolescents and adults with autism spectrum disorder. *Journal of Autism and Developmental Disorders, 47*(9), 2927–2934. https://doi.org/10.1007/s10803-017-3199-9

Eisenburg, N. W., Andreski, S.-R., & Mona, L. R. (2015). Sexuality and physical disability: A disability-affirmative approach to assessment and intervention within health care. *Current Sexual Health Reports, 7*, 19–29. https://doi.org/10.1007/s11930-014-0037-3

Fernandes, L. C., Gillberg, C. I., Cederlund, M., Hagberg, B., Gillberg, C., & Billstedt, E. (2016). Aspects of sexuality in adolescents and adults diagnosed with autism spectrum disorders in childhood. *Journal of Autism and Developmental Disorders, 46*(9), 3155–3165.

George, R., & Stokes, M. A. (2018). Sexual orientation in autism spectrum disorder. *Autism Research, 11*(1), 133–141. https://doi.org/10.1002/aur.1892

Giuliano, A. R., Joura, E. A., Garland, S. M., Huh, W. K., Iversen, O. -E., Kjaer, S. K., . . . Luxembourg, A. (2019). Nine-valent HPV vaccine efficacy against related diseases and definitive therapy: Comparison with historic placebo population. *Gynecologic Oncology*. https://doi.org/10.1016/j.ygyno.2019.03.253

Graham Holmes, L., Shattuck, P. T., Nilssen, A. R., Strassberg, D. S., & Himle, M. B. (2020). Sexual and reproductive health service utilization and sexuality for teens on the autism spectrum. *Journal of Developmental and Behavioral Pediatrics, 41*(9), 667–679. https://doi.org/10.1097/DBP.0000000000000838

Gray, S. H., Wylie, M., Christensen, S., Khan, A., Williams, D., & Glader, L. (2021). Puberty and menarche in young females with cerebral palsy and intellectual disability: A qualitative study of caregivers' experiences. *Developmental Medicine and Child Neurology, 63*(2), 190–195. https://doi.org/10.1111/dmcn.14698

Griffiths, D. M., & Fedoroff, P. (2014). Persons with intellectual disabilities and problematic sexual behaviors. *Psychiatric Clinics of North America, 37*(2), 195–206.

Hagerman, T. K., & Houtrow, A. J. (2020). Variability in prevalence estimates of disability among children in the National Survey of Children's Health. *JAMA Pediatrics*. https://doi.org/10.1001/jamapediatrics.2020.5073

Hancock, G. I. P., Stokes, M. A., & Mesibov, G. B. (2017). Socio-sexual functioning in autism spectrum disorder: A systematic review and meta-analyses of existing literature. *Autism Research, 10*(11), 1823–1833.

Hess, M. J., & Hough, S. (2012). Impact of spinal cord injury on sexuality: Broad-based clinical practice intervention and practical application. *Journal of Spinal Cord Medicine, 35*(4), 211–218.

Holland-Hall, C., & Quint, E. H. (2017). Sexuality and disability in adolescents. *Pediatric Clinics of North America, 64*(2), 435–449. https://doi.org/10.1016/j.pcl.2016.11.011

Houtrow, A., Elias, E., & Davis, B. E. (2021). Promoting sexuality for children and youth with disabilities. *Pediatrics*. https://doi.org/10.1542/peds.2021-052043

Jahoda, A., & Pownall, J. (2014). Sexual understanding, sources of information and social networks; the reports of young people with intellectual disabilities and their non-disabled peers. *Journal of Intellectual Disabilities Research, 58*(5), 430–441. https://doi.org/10.1111/jir.12040

Kahn, N. F., & Halpern, C. T. (2018). Associations between patterns of sexual initiation, sexual partnering, and sexual health outcomes from adolescence to early adulthood. *Archives of Sexual Behavior, 47*(6), 1791–1810. https://doi.org/10.1007/s10508-018-1176-9

Kellogg, N. D. (2009). Committee on Child Abuse and Neglect Clinical Report—the evaluation of sexual behaviors in children. *Pediatrics, 124*(3), 992–998.

Lindberg, L. D., Maddow-Zimet, I., & Boonstra, H. (2016). Changes in adolescents' receipt of sex education, 2006–2013. *Journal of Adolescent Health, 58*(6), 621–627. https://doi.org/10.1016/j.jadohealth.2016.02.004

Lindsay, W. R., & Michie, A. M. (2013). Individuals with developmental delay and problematic sexual behaviors. *Current psychiatry reports, 15*(4), 350.

Lipkin, P. H., Okamoto, J., Council on Children with Disabilities, & Council on School Health. (2015). The Individuals With Disabilities Education Act (IDEA) for children with special educational needs. *Pediatrics, 136*(6), e1650–e1662. https://doi.org/10.1542/peds.2015-3409

Mesman, G. R., Harper, S. L., Edge, N. A., Brandt, T. W., & Pemberton, J. L. (2019). Problematic sexual behavior in children. *Journal of Pediatric Health Care, 33*(3), 323–331.

Miodrag, N., Richards, D. A., Fedoroff, J. P., & Watson, S. L. (2020). Sex and genes, part 2: A biopsychosocial approach to assess and treat challenging sexual behavior in persons with intellectual disabilities including fragile X syndrome and 22q11.2 deletion syndrome. *Behavioral Sciences & the Law, 38(2)*, 152–172.

Mona, L. R., Cameron, R. P., & Clemency Cordes, C. (2017). Disability culturally competent sexual healthcare. *American Psychology, 72*(9), 1000–1010. https://doi.org/10.1037/amp0000283

Pownall, J. D., Jahoda, A., & Hastings, R. P. (2012). Sexuality and sex education of adolescents with intellectual disability: Mothers' attitudes, experiences, and support needs. *Intellectual and developmental disabilities, 50*(2), 140–154. https://doi.org/10.1352/1934-9556-50.2.140

Roden, R. C., Schmidt, E. K., & Holland-Hall, C. (2020). Sexual health education for adolescents and young adults with intellectual and developmental disabilities: Recommendations for accessible sexual and reproductive health information. *Lancet Child and Adolescent Health, 4*(9), 699–708. https://doi.org/10.1016/S2352-4642(20)30098-5

Rosenbaum, P., & Gorter, J. W. (2012). The "F-words" in childhood disability: I swear this is how we should think! *Child: Care, Health and Development, 38*(4), 457–463. https://doi.org/10.1111/j.1365-2214.2011.01338.x

Rowen, T. S., Stein, S., & Tepper, M. (2015). Sexual health care for people with physical disabilities. *Journal of Sexual Medicine, 12*(3), 584–589. https://doi.org/10.1111/jsm.12810

Seburg, E. M., McMorris, B. J., Garwick, A. W., & Scal, P. B. (2015). Disability and discussions of health-related behaviors between youth and health care providers. *Journal of Adolescent Health, 57*(1), 81–86. https://doi.org/10.1016/j.jadohealth.2015.03.004

Sommarö, S., Andersson, A., & Skagerström, J. (2020). A deviation too many? Healthcare professionals' knowledge and attitudes concerning patients with intellectual disability disrupting norms regarding sexual orientation and/or gender identity. *Journal of Applied Research in Intellectual Disabilities, 33*(6), 1199–1209. https://doi.org/10.1111/jar.12739

Thom, R. P., Grudzinskas, A. J., & Saleh, F. M. (2017). Sexual behavior among persons with cognitive impairments. *Current Psychiatry Reports, 19*(5), 25.

Turner, D., Briken, P., & Schottle, D. (2017). Autism-spectrum disorders in adolescence and adulthood: Focus on sexuality. *Current Opinion in Psychiatry, 30*(6), 409–416.

van Asselt-Goverts, A. E., Embregts, P. J., Hendriks, A. H., Wegman, K. M., & Teunisse, J. P. (2015). Do social networks differ? Comparison of the social networks of people with intellectual disabilities, people with autism spectrum disorders and other people living in the community. *Journal of Autism and Developmental Disorders, 45*(5), 1191–1203. https://doi.org/10.1007/s10803-014-2279-3

Walters, F. P., & Gray, S. H. (2018). Addressing sexual and reproductive health in adolescents and young adults with intellectual and developmental disabilities. *Current Opinion in Pediatrics, 30*(4), 451–458. https://doi.org/10.1097/MOP.0000000000000635

Welage, N., & Liu, K. P. (2011). Wheelchair accessibility of public buildings: A review of the literature. *Disability and Rehabilitation: Assistive Technologies, 6*(1), 1–9. https://doi.org/10.3109/17483107.2010.522680

Winnicott, D. W. (1971). *Playing and reality*. Tavistock Publications.

World Health Organization. (2001). *International classification of functioning, disability and health*. Author.

Zablotsky, B., Black, L. I., Maenner, M. J., Schieve, L. A., Danielson, M. L., Bitsko, R. H., & Boyle, C. A. (2019). Prevalence and trends of developmental disabilities among children in the United States: 2009–2017. *Pediatrics, 144*(4), e20190811. https://doi.org/10.1542/peds.2019-0811

75

Gender and Its Variation in Youth

Claire A. Coyne, Afiya Sajwani, and Diane Chen

For additional material related to the content of this chapter, please see Chapters 9 and 74.

VIGNETTES

1. *Zain is a 6-year-old child designated male at birth. Two years ago, he asked his parents to buy him a skirt following a playdate during which he borrowed his friend's skirt to dress up as Moana, his favorite character. His parents initially discouraged him from wearing skirts in public due to concerns about bullying but noticed increased withdrawal and distress when he was told to change before leaving the house. Now he regularly wears skirts around the house, at school, and in familiar public spaces with his parents. Zain enjoys drawing and painting, playing with Legos, and making jewelry to match his outfits. Zain is often asked if he is a boy or a girl. Sometimes he responds, "I'm a he"; other times, "I'm a girl-boy."*
2. *Josephine or "Joey" is a 10-year-old child designated female at birth. Joey is a "tomboy," gravitating toward playing sports and with trucks and action figures since toddlerhood. In imaginary play, Joey takes on the role of the "father" or "brother," and at school Joey's friends are primarily boys. Parents allow Joey to choose clothing and hairstyles—Joey has not chosen to wear dresses in years and has worn short hair for the last 3 years. Joey is sometimes mistaken for a boy by strangers, which Joey enjoys. Joey has been more withdrawn and tearful over the last 6 months, refusing to go swimming despite this being a favorite summer activity, and choosing to wear baggy sweatshirts despite it being summer. When parents talked to Joey about their concerns, Joey expressed worry and distress about puberty, tearfully telling parents, "I really don't want my chest to get bigger or to get a period because I'm not a girl."*
3. *Xander is a 15-year-old adolescent designated female at birth. Xander recently told parents, "I am not a boy but don't like being a girl" and describes a gender identity of nonbinary. Xander requested parents use they/them/their pronouns and to go by the name Xander rather than the birth name. Xander enjoys marching band, cosplay, and online role-playing games, where they have met transgender and nonbinary peers. Xander identifies as pansexual and has joined the LGBTQ+ group at school. Xander is very distressed by having a monthly menstrual cycle. Xander recently donned a short haircut and asked parents to buy a chest binder. Parents reported that Xander never really cared about clothing in childhood except as related to sensory sensitivities. In middle school, Xander was diagnosed with attention-deficit/hyperactivity disorder and autism spectrum disorder with no intellectual impairment and requires mild supports to manage academic organization. Xander does not feel close to peers at school despite having known them since elementary school. Parents expressed concern that Xander's nonbinary identity may be due to the influence of peers in an online gaming community.*

Gender-diverse identities exist as part of healthy human diversity. Historical research indicates presence of gender diversity in several cultures, including non-Western and precolonial cultures (Hinchy, 2017; M'Baye, 2013). There has been increased visibility of transgender and gender-diverse (TGD) people in popular culture, legal spheres, and research in the last decade, and more people, particularly younger people, are identifying with a gender identity different from their designated sex at birth. Recent studies suggest between 0.004% and 0.6% (Herman, Flores, Brown, Wilson, & Conron, 2017; Meerwijk & Sevelius, 2017) of adults and between 0.7% (Herman et al., 2017) and 2.7% (Rider, McMorris, Gower, Coleman, & Eisenberg, 2018) of high school–age students identify as TGD in the United States.

Health professionals are likely to encounter TGD youth in their clinical practices. Thus it is imperative to have a basic understanding of gender development, the unique barriers TGD youth encounter, and knowledge of available gender-affirming treatment options. This is especially important given the significant physical and mental health disparities (e.g., Day, Fish, Perez-Brumer, Hatzenbuehler, & Russell, 2017) and low rates of health care utilization (Rider et al., 2018) observed in this population. With limited numbers of gender specialists available to support a growing need for gender-affirming care (Korpaisarn & Safer, 2018), pediatricians and other generalist health care clinicians can help bridge this gap by facilitating linkage to care and providing appropriate preventative health care using a gender-affirming approach (Sequeira, Ray, Miller, & Coulter, 2020). Gender-affirmative care embraces gender diversity as normal variations on human diversity and encourages individuals to follow their own path to living authentically without privileging any outcome other than a sense of wholeness and emotional wellbeing (Coyne, Poquiz, Janssen, & Chen, 2020). Pediatric health care settings are key environments in which clinicians can normalize gender diversity with parents and youth, facilitate gender exploration, and promote resilience through gender-affirming practices.

There are many words used to communicate about different aspects of gender diversity (see Table 75.1). Labels for designated sex at birth and gender identity are often incorrectly used interchangeably. A child is usually designated a sex label of male or female at birth based on the appearance of external genitalia. Sometimes a child is designated intersex

TABLE 75.1 Key Terminology

Term	Definition
Cisgender	Describes identifying with the gender corresponding to one's designated sex at birth (e.g., an individual designated female at birth identifying as a woman or designated male at birth identifying as a man).
Designated sex at birth	The sex label that a child is given at birth most often based on the appearance of the external genitalia but also can include hormones and chromosomes. Most people are designated male or female, and this is what is put on their birth certificate. Of note, more US states now allow for a designation of "intersex" on the birth certificate of children born with variations in chromosomes, hormones, or genitalia that do not fit neatly within binary male-female categories.
Gender	The way cultures categorize and assign social norms to groups of people. These groups are often based on designated sex at birth, but understandings of gender vary across time and culture.
Gender-affirming treatment	Medical or surgical treatments that help a person physically change the body to align more closely with a gender identity. Gender-affirming treatments can include puberty blockers, hormones (e.g., estrogen, testosterone), and surgery.
Gender dysphoria	A diagnosis introduced in the DSM-5 to capture clinically significant distress associated with identifying with a gender different from the one corresponding to designated sex at birth. A person might feel uncomfortable with the physical body or with the social roles associated with a perceived gender. The experience of gender dysphoria is highly individual, and not every gender nonconforming person experiences gender dysphoria.
Gender expansive	Describes gender expression or behavior that differs from traditional or cultural norms associated with designated sex at birth. Gender-expansive people may or may not self-identify as transgender.
Gender expression	Cultures often relate physical appearance, clothing choices, accessories, communication patterns, social roles, and behaviors to gender. The way a person uses these gendered items and behaviors is called gender expression. Gender expression is highly individual and may or may not be reflective of a person's other identities.
Gender fluid	Describes a nonbinary gender identity that is dynamic and changing, as opposed to being static. Gender-fluid people can move between genders and may or may not use different gender expressions or pronouns at different times.
Gender identity	A person's innate sense of one's own gender. This can be the same or different from the gender corresponding to the designated sex at birth. A person could feel like a man, woman, nonbinary, agender, etc., regardless of the designated sex at birth.
Nonbinary	Describes identifying outside of the male-female gender binary. Nonbinary can be used as an adjective or an umbrella term encompassing several different gender identities.
Pronouns	Words used to substitute the name of a person. In English language, pronouns are gendered and can be an important part of someone's gender expression. Using the appropriate pronouns for somebody can be a way to affirm the gender identity.
Transgender	Describes not identifying with the gender corresponding to one's designated sex at birth.
Transition	Changes a person makes to one's own appearance, behaviors, or body to affirm the gender identity. There are different types of transitions. A social transition can include changing one's appearance or asking others to use a different name and/or pronouns. A legal transition can include changing one's name and gender marker on government-issued documents such as a birth certificate. A medical transition can include using gender-affirming hormones to induce physical changes that affirm one's gender identity.
Transphobia	On an internalized level, transphobia refers to the shame or discomfort experienced by transgender and gender-diverse (TGD) people as a result of internalizing stigmatizing messaging. On interpersonal and systemic levels, transphobia can refer to the harassment and discrimination of people based on their perceived gender identity. TGD people experience transphobia in different forms, ranging from internalized self-hatred and bullying to discrimination in medical and legal settings.

DSM-5, Diagnostic and Statistical Manual of Mental Disorders, Fifth Edition.

when there is variation in chromosomal, gonadal, or phenotypic sex characteristics (also known as a difference in sex development [DSD]). Gender identity, irrespective of designated sex at birth, refers to a person's innate sense of one's own gender. Gender identities may be broadly categorized under "cisgender" and "transgender" umbrellas. Cisgender refers to a gender identity that aligns with designated sex at birth. Transgender refers to a gender identity that differs from the gender corresponding to one's designated sex at birth. Gender expression is the way a person uses physical appearance, clothing choices, accessories, communication patterns, social roles, and behaviors to communicate gender to others. A person's gender expression may or may not align with designated sex at birth or gender identity. The term *gender minority* describes transgender people, as well as gender-expansive people who do not self-identify as transgender but have gender expression or gender role behaviors that differ from traditional or cultural norms associated with designated sex at birth. Language around gender diversity can evolve, be highly individual, and change depending on the context. Therefore it is important for health care clinicians to use language used by their patients and correct assumptions accordingly. It is also important to note that gender identity, sexual orientation, and gender expression, though interrelated, are different constructs. As an example, Xander, from the third vignette, identifies a gender identity of nonbinary, a sexual orientation of pansexual, and chooses a hairstyle and clothing that reflect an androgynous gender expression.

GENDER DYSPHORIA

Gender dysphoria refers to affective distress due to incongruence between a person's gender identity and the designated sex at birth. The term also reflects the psychiatric diagnosis in the *Diagnostic and Statistical Manual of Mental Disorders*, Fifth Edition (DSM-5) (American Psychiatric Association, 2013), which captures distress and functional impairment associated with gender incongruence. The diagnostic criteria for gender dysphoria differ by developmental stage (Table 75.2).

Notably, there remains significant controversy regarding the inclusion of gender dysphoria as a diagnosis in the DSM-5. Despite DSM moving from a framework of identity-as-pathology (i.e., "gender identity disorder" in earlier

TABLE 75.2 DSM-5 Diagnostic Criteria for Gender Dysphoria

For a diagnosis of gender dysphoria in children, criteria are met if at least two of the following (one of which must be the first criterion) is experienced for at least 6 mo:	
1.	A strong desire to be or insistence that one is of a gender different from the gender associated with one's designated sex at birth.
2.	A strong preference for stereotypically feminine clothing in children designated male at birth. A strong preference for wearing only stereotypically masculine clothing and a strong resistance to wearing stereotypically feminine clothing in children designated female at birth.
3.	A strong preference for cross-gender roles in make-believe play or fantasy play.
4.	A strong preference for toys, games, or activities stereotypically used by the other gender.
5.	A strong preference for playmates of the other gender.
6.	A strong rejection of stereotypically masculine toys, games, and activities and a strong avoidance of rough-and-tumble play in children designated male at birth. A strong rejection of stereotypically feminine toys, games, and activities in children designated female at birth.
7.	A strong dislike of one's sexual anatomy.
8.	A strong desire for the physical sex characteristics that match one's experienced gender.
For diagnosis of Gender Dysphoria in Adolescents and Adults, criteria are met if at least six of the following (one of which must be the first criterion) is experienced for at least 6 mo:	
1.	A marked incongruence between one's experience/expressed gender and primary and/or secondary sex characteristics (or in young adolescents, the anticipated secondary sex characteristics).
2.	A strong desire to be rid of one's primary and/or secondary sex characteristics because of a marked incongruence with one's experienced/expressed gender (or in young adolescents, a desire to prevent the development of anticipated secondary sex characteristics).
3.	A strong desire for the primary and/or secondary sex characteristics of the other gender.
4.	A strong desire to be of a gender different from one's designated sex at birth.
5.	A strong desire to be treated as a gender different from one's designated sex at birth.
6.	A strong conviction that one has the typical feelings and reactions of the other gender (or some alternative gender different from one's designated sex at birth).

DSM-5, Diagnostic and Statistical Manual of Mental Disorders, Fifth Edition.

versions of the DSM) to distress-as-pathology (i.e., "gender dysphoria" in its most recent iteration), some have argued that including gender dysphoria in the DSM at all is antithetical to conceptions of gender diversity as normal variations on human diversity (Davy & Toze, 2018). It is also notable that not all TGD people experience gender dysphoria or meet criteria for it; similarly, not all people who experience gender dysphoria or meet criteria for it identify as TGD. Considering the three vignettes, Joey, in the second vignette, mostly clearly exhibits the level of distress and impairment associated with a diagnosis of gender dysphoria.

GENDER IDENTITY DEVELOPMENT

Gender identity development is a complex process shaped by biological, cognitive, social, and cultural factors. Children and adolescents develop an understanding of their gender identity over time in the context of socialization practices in their family, peer groups, and school settings.

Preschool (Ages 3–5 Years)

By age 3 years, children acquire the concept of gender, can label other people's gender, and reliably identify their own gender (Ruble, Taylor, Cyphers, Greulich, Lurye, & Shrout, 2007). Between ages 3 and 5 years, children develop gender stereotypes and gender-typed preferences, which may include preferences for same-gender peers and clothing and toys marketed for their gender. Transgender children resemble gender-matched cisgender children in their gender-typed preferences and gender expression (Olson & Gülgöz, 2018). Children should feel safe to explore preferences for toys, clothing, and activities. Parents can encourage gender exploration, avoid gendering clothing, toys, and preferences (e.g., "That is a girl toy"), and advocate for their child in settings where other adults and children may need information about and guidance around appropriate responses to gender diversity (e.g., at school, with peers or extended family members). Zain, from the first vignette, describes a gender identity of both "boy" and "girl-boy," and a gender expression that includes preferences for stereotypically feminine clothing (e.g., dresses, movie characters) as well toys and activities that can be categorized as gender neutral (e.g., drawing). Though many children may identify a core, stable gender identity by early childhood, some children like Zain experience their gender in ways that reflect gender fluidity and continue to explore gender as they develop. For parents of children like Zain, health care clinicians can normalize gender fluidity and exploration as part of the process of gender identity development.

Childhood (Ages 6–9 Years)

During childhood, caregivers play a central role in shaping how TGD youth share their gender identity with others and express their gender at home, school, and in public. A child's ability to change pronouns, name, or clothing to match a gender identity is mediated by caregiver acceptance and support. Caregivers' responses can help or hinder how children navigate conversations about gender identity and expression with family members, teachers, and community members. Parents are encouraged to follow their child's lead when exploring the timing and location of changes to names, pronouns, and gender expression. For young children like Zain (see vignette 1) who express clear clothing and toy preferences, we may observe improvement in psychosocial functioning when limits around gender expression are relaxed or removed (e.g., less withdrawn, distressed, and oppositional) (Chen, Hidalgo, & Garofalo, 2017; Durwood, McLaughlin, & Olson, 2017). As part of this process, parents can assess safety in new settings, anticipate potential challenges, and advocate for their children with school staff and family members regarding changes in names, pronouns, or gender expression.

Preteen (Ages 10–12 Years)

Among pediatric patients in gender specialty clinics, most recognized gender identity as different from designated sex at birth in childhood or early adolescence (Kuper, Lindley, & Lopez, 2019). For some children, puberty is an inflection point for gender identity exploration as changes in secondary sex characteristics may elicit significant distress and mark the onset or exacerbation of gender dysphoria. The increased distress and withdrawal described by Joey's parents (see vignette 2) may be associated with the onset of pubertal development and increased anxiety about future development of secondary sex characteristics (e.g., breasts) that are incongruent with Joey's gender identity. Prior to the onset of puberty, declaring a specific gender identity that differs from designated sex at birth or changing chosen name and pronouns may not be necessary or desired for some children. In Joey's case, the positive response to being gendered as a boy and growing discomfort with feminizing pubertal development (e.g., breasts, menstruation) warrant further discussions with Joey, parents, and health care clinicians about gender identity and gender dysphoria. Behavioral health clinicians with experience providing gender-affirmative care can help youth like Joey explore gender and facilitate understanding of the range of social (e.g., changing name and pronouns) and medical (e.g., pubertal suppression) interventions available that may alleviate distress associated with gender dysphoria.

Adolescence (Age 13+ Years)

Adolescence is a critical period for identity development and substantial physical growth that marks transition from childhood to reproductive maturity. Developing secondary sex characteristics may be uniquely distressing for TGD youth as these bodily changes may heighten incongruence between gender and designated sex at birth. Adolescents prioritize relationships with peers during this developmental period and spend less time with parents as part of the process of self-exploration and individuation. For TGD adolescents like Xander (see vignette 3), peer relationships can provide safe spaces to explore gender identity and experiment with social changes in gender expression (e.g., names and pronouns). These relationships may also act as a buffer against conflict with caregivers who are unwilling to support social transition at home or explore options for medical interventions for gender transition.

The process of sharing one's gender minority identity with parents, or "coming out," may be challenging or create disruptions in parent-child relationships (Starks & Millar, 2017). Gender minority youth may resist sharing their gender identity because they fear negative consequences of parental rejection (e.g., emotional distress, financial hardship), and many youth do experience parental rejection, loss of support, or social isolation after coming out (D'Augelli, Grossman, & Starks, 2008). Parental rejection (e.g., trying to change gender identity) during adolescence is associated with poor health outcomes (e.g., substance use, depression, and sexual health risk) in young adulthood (Klein & Golub, 2016). In contrast, family acceptance is associated with positive health outcomes (i.e., self-esteem, general health) in young adulthood (Ryan, Russell, Huebner, Diaz, & Sanchez, 2010).

RISK AND RESILIENCE

TGD youth experience significant physical and mental health disparities compared to their cisgender peers, including higher rates of depression, anxiety, substance use, suicidality, and self-injurious thoughts and behaviors (Reisner et al., 2015). The gender minority stress model (Hendricks & Testa, 2012), adapted from health disparities work in communities of color (Williams, Lavizzo-Mourey, & Warren, 1994), posits that TGD people experience unique stress due to discrimination and stigma associated with their gender minority identity. The interplay between external (discrimination, victimization, rejection, and nonaffirmation) and internal (internalized transphobia, anticipated stigma, concealment of identity) stressors results in poor physical and mental health outcomes. Stigmatizing and discriminatory experiences (e.g., intentional misgendering in nonaffirming school or home environments; lack of access to safe bathrooms) negatively affect mental health and result in internalizing negative beliefs about one's identity, anticipation of future stigma, and pressure to conceal one's identity. Exposure to gender identity–related stressors is linked to major depressive and generalized anxiety disorders (Chodzen, Hidalgo, Chen, & Garofalo, 2019), substance misuse (Day et al., 2017), suicidality and suicide attempts, and school absences and dropout rates (Grossman & D'Augelli, 2007) in TGD children and adolescents.

When working with TGD youth and families, it is important to consider other identity-specific factors and associated experiences of interpersonal and systemic stigma and discrimination. The framework of intersectionality (Crenshaw, 1991) highlights the unique experiences with systemic inequity for TGD people holding multiple marginalized identities along the axes of race, ethnicity, sexual orientation, ability, religiosity/spirituality, and social class. For instance, Black TGD youth disproportionately experience poverty and homelessness (James, Herman, Rankin, Keisling, Mottet, & Anafi, 2016), disparities in educational attainment (Bauermeister, Goldenberg, Connochie, Jadwin-Cakmak, & Stephenson, 2016), and barriers to health care (Goldenberg, Jadwin-Cakmak, Popoff, Reisner, Campbell, & Harper, 2019), which increase health risks. Consequently, clinical care with TGD youth should consider intersecting identities while focusing on reducing external and internal stressors and strengthening resilience factors such as family support, community connectedness, and identity pride (Coyne et al., 2020). With parents and youth, clinicians can highlight the importance of family support (Westwater, Riley, & Peterson, 2019), assertive self-advocacy in school settings (Hillier, Kroehle, Edwards, & Graves, 2020), and connections with supportive communities (Austin, Craig, Navega, & McInroy, 2020) to mitigate the impact of gender minority stressors. For TGD youth holding multiple marginalized identities, clinical interventions should explicitly address the effects of stigma, discrimination, and structural factors along multiple axes of oppression and help youth address experiences with discrimination due to intersecting marginalized identities (Poquiz, Shrodes, Garofalo, Chen, & Coyne, in press). Clinicians should refrain from automatically attributing TGD patients' mental or physical issues to their TGD identity and miss opportunities to provide holistic care (Payton, 2015). Familiarity with gender-inclusive clinical practices can help clinicians to avoid burdening patients with the task of educating their care team about gender diversity in order to access care (James et al., 2016).

GENDER-AFFIRMATIVE INTERVENTIONS

Gender-affirming interventions fall broadly within two categories: social and medical/surgical. Social interventions may include therapeutic support around gender exploration and psychoeducation about gender diversity with parents, extended family, schools, and in other social contexts in which TGD children/adolescents spend time. Gender exploration focuses on supporting youth in better understanding their own experience of gender and determine how they are most comfortable expressing gender in different contexts. Psychoeducation focuses on ways to maximize support and affirmation of gender diversity and minimize stigma in family and social contexts. For some youth, a social gender transition may be indicated to reduce gender dysphoria and facilitate living authentically. Social gender transition can be initiated at any developmental stage and involves changing one's name and/or pronouns and gender expression (i.e., clothing, hairstyle) to more accurately reflect one's gender. Social transitions have a positive impact on mental health in TGD children (Durwood et al., 2017; Olson, Durwood, DeMeules, & McLaughlin, 2016) and adolescents (Russell, Pollitt, Li, & Grossman, 2018).

Gender-affirming medical and surgical interventions for TGD people vary based on an individual's age, developmental stage, and treatment goals and are informed by clinical practice guidelines by the Endocrine Society (Hembree et al., 2017) and the World Professional Association for Transgender Health (Coleman et al., 2012). No medical or surgical interventions are indicated prior to a youth starting puberty. Treatment options are provided in a staged manner to youth, with treatments considered reversible offered first prior to treatments considered partially irreversible or irreversible. For pediatric populations, guidelines recommend a multidisciplinary team approach (including a mental health clinician) to ensure youth and their parents understand the benefits and potential risks or side effects of medical or surgical interventions (Coleman et al., 2012; Hembree et al., 2017).

For TGD youth in early puberty, medications to suppress endogenous sex hormone production may be offered. Gonadotropin-releasing hormone analogs (GnRHa), referred to as puberty blockers, suspend pubertal progression by shutting down the hypothalamic-pituitary-gonadal axis. This prevents gonadal sex hormone production (i.e., testosterone and estrogen). GnRHa are generally considered to be reversible and are intended to provide time for TGD youth to mature and consider fully whether partially irreversible and irreversible medical and/or surgical treatments are aligned with their long-term treatment goals. If GnRHa are discontinued, the hypothalamic-pituitary-gonadal axis will reactivate, and endogenous puberty would progress.

For TGD adolescents in the later stages of puberty or TGD adults, gender-affirming hormones (i.e., testosterone or estrogen) may be prescribed to induce desired secondary sex characteristics (e.g., facial hair and voice deepening mediated by testosterone, breast development mediated by estrogen). Gender-affirming hormone treatment is considered partially irreversible. Some of the physical changes are reversible (e.g., fat distribution), meaning that if hormones are discontinued, physical changes would revert back to pretreatment physicality. Other physical changes, however, are irreversible (e.g., breast development, voice deepening), meaning that if hormones are discontinued, hormone-mediated changes would remain.

Most surgical interventions, which are irreversible, are offered only to TGD adults and may involve removing undesired reproductive organs (e.g., ovaries/uterus, testicles) and/or creating desired genital anatomy (e.g., vaginoplasty, phalloplasty). One notable exception is breast/chest surgery, which may be offered to adolescents desiring these procedures who have parental support and consent (Olson-Kennedy, Warus, Okonta, Belzer, & Clark, 2018).

Additional Considerations in Providing Gender-Affirmative Care

Neurodiversity in Gender-Diverse Youth

The co-occurrence of gender variance and autism spectrum disorder (ASD) among adolescents referred for gender care is well established (e.g., de Vries, Doreleijers, Steensma, & Cohen-Kettenis, 2011); however, more research is needed to characterize the developmental course of gender variance and gender dysphoria among neurodiverse youth (Strang et al., 2018, 2019). Some interpretations of the gender diversity–neurodiversity co-occurrence center on the possibility that neurodiverse youths' propensity for intense restricted interests could predispose them to develop gender dysphoria if the focus of these interests is directed at gender-related behaviors and concepts (VanderLaan et al., 2015). On the other hand, differences in social communication and interpretation among neurodiverse youth may result in their feeling less pressure to adhere to social norms and conform to conventional gender stereotypes compared to neurotypical youth, potentially making it more likely that they will express gender diversity.

Irrespective of etiologic underpinnings of the gender diversity–neurodiversity co-occurrence, awareness of gender identity and gender exploration may emerge later in development for neurodiverse TGD youth due to the impact of neurodiversity-related communication differences on self-advocacy about gender needs, gender exploration, and desired gender transition (Strang et al., 2018). Neurodiverse TGD youth may need multiple opportunities over time to express themselves in gender evaluations and need ASD-related communication accommodations (e.g., visuals) (Strang et al., 2018). Across development, clinicians can initiate conversations with youth and parents about gender diversity to normalize exploration and the common barriers (e.g., concern about harassment) that might prevent youth from feeling comfortable experimenting with gender expression. Creating safe and accepting environments for gender exploration and expression is particularly important to help youth balance concrete experimentation and abstract aspects of gender identity. Due to difficulties with social awareness and executive functioning, neurodiverse TGD youth may experience challenges planning for transition-related care or how to present as their affirmed gender (Strang et al., 2018). A mental health clinician working with Xander (see vignette 3) could foster discussion about gender history, the relationship between gender identity and gender expression, and strategies for exploring how social or medical interventions might alleviate distress. Discussions with Xander's parents can normalize gender expression and help to understand Xander's gender development and gender-related needs.

Nonbinary Presentations and Medical Transition

Nonbinary identities are increasingly common among TGD individuals. Medical clinicians must understand that nonbinary individuals seeking care are not undecided about their gender identity. For nonbinary youth interested in gender-affirming hormone therapy, their specific transition goals may require individually tailored treatment plans (Chen, Edwards-Leeper, Stancin, & Tishelman, 2018). Xander (see vignette 3) is distressed about menstruation and chest development but has not expressed interest in masculine secondary sex characteristics (e.g., deeper voice, body hair). Therefore they may pursue a narrow range of medical interventions (e.g., chest surgery, hormonal management of menstruation) to achieve specific transition goals.

CLINICAL IMPLICATIONS

Pediatric health care clinicians equipped with developmentally appropriate and evidence-based information about gender diversity can create gender-sensitive health care practices that support TGD youth and their parents in settings outside of gender specialty clinics. The treatment needs and goals for TGD youth vary across development and depending on context. Health care provided by gender-affirming clinicians is increasingly politicized in the United States and internationally. Efforts to legislate patient care undermine the capacity for youth and their families who seek effective medical care. Clinicians who understand the developmental course of gender identity exploration and identification, and the range of available supports and interventions (social and medical) can reduce stigma and the impact of gender minority stress in health care settings.

REFERENCES

American Psychiatric Association. (2013). *Diagnostic and statistical manual of mental disorders* (5th ed.). Author.

Austin, A., Craig, S. L., Navega, N., & McInroy, L. B. (2020). It's my safe space: The life-saving role of the internet in the lives of transgender and gender diverse youth. *International Journal of Transgender Health, 21*(1), 33–44.

Bauermeister, J. A., Goldenberg, T., Connochie, D., Jadwin-Cakmak, L., & Stephenson, R. (2016). Psychosocial disparities among racial/ethnic minority transgender young adults and young men who have sex with men living in Detroit. *Transgender Health, 1*(1), 279–290.

Chen, D., Edwards-Leeper, L., Stancin, T., & Tishelman, A. (2018). Advancing the practice of pediatric psychology with transgender youth: State of the science, ongoing controversies, and future directions. *Clinical Practice in Pediatric Psychology, 6*(1), 73–83. https://doi.org/10.1037/cpp0000229.

Chen, D., Hidalgo, M. A., & Garofalo, R. (2017). Parental perceptions of emotional and behavioral difficulties among prepubertal gender-nonconforming children. *Clinical Practice in Pediatric Psychology, 5*(4), 342–352. https://doi.org/10.1037/cpp0000217.

Chodzen, G., Hidalgo, M. A., Chen, D., & Garofalo, R. (2019). Minority stress factors associated with depression and anxiety among transgender and gender-nonconforming youth. *Journal of Adolescent Health, 64*(4), 467–471. https://doi.org/10.1016/j.jadohealth.2018.07.006.

Coleman, E., Bockting, W., Botzer, M., Cohen-Kettenis, P., DeCuypere, G., Feldman, J., … Zucker, K. (2012). Standards of care for the health of transsexual,transgender, and gender-nonconforming people, version 7. *International Journal of Transgenderism, 13*, 165–232.

Coyne, C. A., Poquiz, J. L., Janssen, A., & Chen, D. (2020). Evidence-based psychological practice for transgender and non-binary youth: Defining the need, framework for treatment adaptation, and future directions. *Evidence-based Practice in Child and Adolescent Mental Health, 5*(3), 340–353. https://doi.org/10.1080/23794925.2020.1765433.

Crenshaw, K. (1991). Mapping the margins: Identity politics, intersectionality, and violence against women. *Stanford Law Review, 43*(6), 1241–1299.

D'Augelli, A. R., Grossman, A. H., & Starks, M. T. (2008). Gender atypicality and sexual orientation development among lesbian, gay, and bisexual youth. *Journal of Gay and Lesbian Mental Health, 12*(1-2), 121–143. https://doi.org/10.1300/J529v12n01-08.

Davy, Z., & Toze, M. (2018). What is gender dysphoria? A critical systematic narrative review. *Transgender Health, 3*(1), 159–169. https://doi.org/10.1089/trgh.2018.0014.

Day, J. K., Fish, J. N., Perez-Brumer, A., Hatzenbuehler, M. L., & Russell, S. T. (2017). Transgender youth substance use disparities: Results from a population-based sample. *Journal of Adolescent Health, 61*(6), 729–735.

de Vries, A. L. C., Doreleijers, T. A. H., Steensma, T. D., & Cohen-Kettenis, P. T. (2011). Psychiatric comorbidity in gender dysphoric adolescents. *Journal of Child Psychology and Psychiatry, 52*(11), 1195–1202. https://doi.org/10.1111/j.1469-7610.2011.02426.x.

Durwood, L., McLaughlin, K. A., & Olson, K. R. (2017). Mental health and self-worth in socially transitioned transgender youth. *Journal of the American Academy of Child and Adolescent Psychiatry, 56*(2), 116–123. https://doi.org/10.1016/j.jaac.2016.10.016.

Goldenberg, T., Jadwin-Cakmak, L., Popoff, E., Reisner, S. L., Campbell, B. A., & Harper, G. W. (2019). Stigma, gender affirmation, and primary healthcare use among Black transgender youth. *Journal of Adolescent Health, 65*(4), 483–490.

Grossman, A. H., & D'Augelli, A. R. (2007). Transgender youth and life-threatening behaviors. *Suicide and Life-Threatening Behavior, 37*(5), 527–537. https://doi.org/10.1521/suli.2007.37.5.527.

Hembree, W. C., Cohen-Kettenis, P. T., Gooren, L., Hannema, S. E., Meyer, W. J., Murad, M. H., … T'Sjoen, G. G. (2017). Endocrine treatment of gender-dysphoric/gender-incongruent persons: An Endocrine Society clinical practice guideline. *Journal of Clinical Endocrinology and Metabolism, 102*(11), 3869–3903. https://doi.org/10.1210/jc.2017-01658.

Hendricks, M. L., & Testa, R. J. (2012). A conceptual framework for clinical work with transgender and gender nonconforming clients: An adaptation of the minority stress model. *Professional Psychology: Research and Practice, 43*(5), 460–467. https://doi.org/10.1037/a0029597.

Herman, J. L., Flores, A. R., Brown, T. N., Wilson, B. D., & Conron, K. J. (2017). *Age of individuals who identify as transgender in the United States.* eScholarship. University of California.

Hillier, A., Kroehle, K., Edwards, H., & Graves, G. (2020). Risk, resilience, resistance and situated agency of trans high school students. *Journal of LGBT Youth, 17*(4), 384–407.

Hinchy, J. (2017). The eunuch archive: Colonial records of non-normative gender and sexuality in India. *Culture, Theory and Critique, 58*(2), 127–146.

James, S. E., Herman, J. L., Rankin, S., Keisling, M., Mottet, L., & Anafi, M. A. (2016). The report of the 2015 US Transgender Survey. *National Center for Transgender Equality.*

Klein, A., & Golub, S. A. (2016). Family rejection as a predictor of suicide attempts and substance misuse among transgender and gender nonconforming adults. *LGBT Health, 3*(3), 193–199. https://doi.org/10.1089/lgbt.2015.0111.

Korpaisarn, S., & Safer, J. D. (2018). Gaps in transgender medical education among healthcare providers: A major barrier to care for transgender persons. *Reviews in Endocrine and Metabolic Disorders, 19*(3), 271–275.

Kuper, L. E., Lindley, L., & Lopez, X. (2019). Exploring the gender development histories of children and adolescents presenting for gender affirming medical care. *Clinical Practice in Pediatric Psychology, 7*(3), 217–228. https://doi.org/10.1037/cpp0000290.

M'Baye, B. (2013). The origins of Senegalese homophobia: Discourses on homosexuals and transgender people in colonial and Postcolonial Senegal. *African Studies Review, 56*(2), 109–128. http://www.jstor.org/stable/43904930.

Meerwijk, E. L., & Sevelius, J. M. (2017). Transgender population size in the United States: A meta-regression of population-based probability samples. *American Journal of Public Health, 107*(2), 1–8.

Olson, K. R., & Gülgöz, S. (2018). Early findings from the transyouth project: Gender development in transgender children. *Child Development Perspectives, 12*(2), 93–97. https://doi.org/10.1111/cdep.12268.

Olson, K. R., Durwood, L., DeMeules, M., & McLaughlin, K. A. (2016). Mental health of transgender children who are supported in their identities. *Pediatrics*, *137*(3), e20153223. https://doi.org/10.1542/peds.2015-3223.

Olson-Kennedy, J., Warus, J., Okonta, V., Belzer, M., & Clark, L. F. (2018). Chest reconstruction and chest dysphoria in transmasculine minors and young adults: Comparisons of nonsurgical and postsurgical cohorts. *JAMA Pediatrics* https://doi.org/10.1001/jamapediatrics.2017.5440.

Payton, N. (2015). *Feature: The dangers of trans broken arm syndrome.* Pink News.

Poquiz, J., Shrodes, A., Garofalo, R., Chen, D., & Coyne, C. A. (in press). Supporting pride, activism, resiliency, and community (SPARC): A telemedicine-based group for youth with intersecting gender and racial minority identities. *Transgend Health*.

Reisner, S. L., Vetters, R., Leclerc, M., Zaslow, S., Wolfrum, S., Shumer, D., & Mimiaga, M. J. (2015). Mental health of transgender youth in care at an adolescent urban community health center: A matched retrospective cohort study. *Journal of Adolescent Health*, *56*(3), 274–279. https://doi.org/10.1016/j.jadohealth.2014.10.264.

Rider, G. N., McMorris, B. J., Gower, A. L., Coleman, E., & Eisenberg, M. E. (2018). Health and care utilization of transgender and gender nonconforming youth: A population-based study. *Pediatrics*, *141*(3). https://doi.org/10.1542/peds.2017-1683.

Ruble, D. N., Taylor, L. J., Cyphers, L., Greulich, F. K., Lurye, L. E., & Shrout, P. E. (2007). The role of gender constancy in early gender development. *Child Development*, *78*(4), 1121–1136. https://doi.org/10.1111/j.1467-8624.2007.01056.x.

Russell, S. T., Pollitt, A. M., Li, G., & Grossman, A. H. (2018). Chosen name use is linked to reduced depressive symptoms, suicidal ideation, and suicidal behavior among transgender youth. *Journal of Adolescent Health*, *63*(4), 503–505. https://doi.org/10.1016/j.jadohealth.2018.02.003.

Ryan, C., Russell, S. T., Huebner, D., Diaz, R., & Sanchez, J. (2010). Family acceptance in adolescence and the health of LGBT young adults. *Journal of Child and Adolescent Psychiatric Nursing*, *23*(4), 205–213. https://doi.org/10.1111/j.1744-6171.2010.00246.x.

Sequeira, G. M., Ray, K. N., Miller, E., & Coulter, R. W. (2020). Transgender youth's disclosure of gender identity to providers outside of specialized gender centers. *Journal of Adolescent Health*

Starks, T. J., & Millar, B. M. (2017). Special issues in psychotherapy with sexual minority and transgender and gender nonconforming adolescents: *Handbook of sexual orientation and gender diversity in counseling and psychotherapy* (pp. 239–261). American Psychological Association.

Strang, J. F., Klomp, S. E., Caplan, R., Griffin, A. D., Anthony, L. G., Harris, M. C., … van der Miesen, A. I. R. (2019). Community-based participatory design for research that impacts the lives of transgender and/or gender-diverse autistic and/or neurodiverse people. *Clinical Practice in Pediatric Psychology*, *7*(4), 396–404. https://doi.org/10.1037/cpp0000310.

Strang, J. F., Powers, M. D., Knauss, M., Sibarium, E., Leibowitz, S. F., Kenworthy, L., … Anthony, L. G. (2018). "They thought it was an obsession": Trajectories and perspectives of autistic transgender and gender-diverse adolescents. *Journal of Autism and Developmental Disorders*, *48*(12), 4039–4055. https://doi.org/10.1007/s10803-018-3723-6.

VanderLaan, D. P., Postema, L., Wood, H., Singh, D., Fantus, S., Hyun, J., … Zucker, K. J. (2015). Do children with gender dysphoria have intense/obsessional interests? *Journal of Sex Research*, *52*(2), 213–219. https://doi.org/10.1080/00224499.2013.860073.

Westwater, J. J., Riley, E. A., & Peterson, G. M. (2019). What about the family in youth gender diversity? A literature review. *International Journal of Transgenderism*, *20*(4), 351–370.

Williams, D. R., Lavizzo-Mourey, R., & Warren, R. C. (1994). The concept of race and health status in America. *Public Health Reports*, *109*(1), 26–41.

76

Fundamentals of Developmental, Behavioral, and Psychological Assessment

Melissa Armstrong-Brine, Jessica VanOrmer Simpson, and Terry Stancin

For additional material related to the content of this chapter, please see Chapters 3, 40, 47, 48, 77–90.

VIGNETTE

Abby is an 8-year-old Hispanic female who presents due to concerns for attention-deficit/hyperactivity disorder (ADHD). After a thorough clinical interview with the help of an interpreter, you learn that Abby is one of five children in the home. She has witnessed domestic violence between her parents, which resulted in a 2-month placement in foster care. Her parents are still married, but her father returned to his home country 5 months ago. Abby and her family are primarily Spanish-speaking, although Abby has been enrolled in an English-speaking school since she was 4 years of age. Her mother explains that Abby has been struggling in school academically for several years and has displayed increasing behavioral difficulties over the previous year. Abby is often shy and reserved; her teachers report frequent off-task behaviors, incomplete assignments, and poor retention of academic concepts. Most recently teachers have noted disruptive classroom behaviors (e.g., she makes inappropriate comments in class, gets out of her seat without permission). At home, Abby ignores her mother's directions, refuses to complete homework, and leaves daily tasks incomplete. She has recently begun threatening to run away and makes statements such as, "Why can't I be like other kids?" when confronted with consequences for her misbehavior.

INTRODUCTION TO PSYCHOLOGICAL ASSESSMENT

Psychological assessment frequently combines elements of clinical interviewing, record review, psychological testing, observation, and sound clinical judgment. Together these elements form a picture of the patient in a daily context to formulate a diagnosis, guide treatment recommendations, and, often most importantly, assist others in understanding the patient's behavior in the greater context of the world around them. Psychological assessment is not a static event that occurs over a single session. It is a multifaceted process, distinguished from psychological screening and psychological testing in its breadth, depth, and level of expertise required to do it well. In general, psychological assessment is composed of several stages or steps. It begins with identifying the referral question, then moves to planning the assessment, record review, clinical interview, observation, direct psychological testing, integration of data and conceptualization, and concludes with feedback to family and referral sources, when appropriate. Comprehensive psychological assessment data are most commonly presented to the family and referring clinician in a written report format that includes relevant background information, current concerns and presenting problems, behavioral observations, testing data, a summary of the interpretation, and data-driven recommendations for next steps and treatment.

Screening

Psychological screening refers to the use of measures, usually standardized to some degree, to determine if a condition, trait, or ability is likely to be present in a patient. Screening measures are typically standardized to optimize the rate at which a condition will be identified if it is present. Screening measures require minimal time to administer, score, and interpret, making them ideal to give to a large number of patients in a busy clinic setting. Screening measures can be used to help guide next steps in treatment or to support further evaluation for emotional (e.g., depression, anxiety), cognitive (e.g., intellectual functioning, memory loss), or behavioral (e.g., ADHD, oppositional-defiant disorder, aggressive behaviors) conditions commonly the subject of parental concerns in general and developmental-behavioral pediatric settings. Screening measures should not be utilized as stand-alone measures for purpose of diagnosis because they are intended only to identify patients in need of further evaluation or treatment. Sometimes screening measures can be helpful in tracking treatment outcome by identifying a decrease in the patient's

TABLE 76.1 Psychometric Properties of Screening Measures

Screening Measure Properties

Term	Definition
Specificity	The proportion of people who get a negative result on a screening measure (i.e., the ability of a test to identify people who do not possess the construct/disease) $specifity = \frac{number\ of\ true\ negatives}{number\ of\ true\ negatives + number\ of\ false\ positives}$
Sensitivity	The proportion of people who get a positive result on a screening measure (i.e., how well a test can identify people who possess the construct/disease) $sensitivity = \frac{number\ of\ true\ positives}{number\ of\ true\ positives + number\ of\ false\ negatives}$
Positive predictive value (PPV)	The probability that those who get a positive screening test actually possess the construct/disease (i.e., people who test positive and do have the condition) $PPV = \frac{number\ of\ true\ positives}{number\ of\ true\ positives + number\ of\ false\ positives}$
Negative predictive value (NPV)	The probability that those that get a negative screening test actually do not possess the construct/disease (i.e., people who test negative and don't have the condition) $NPV = \frac{number\ of\ true\ negatives}{number\ of\ true\ negatives + number\ of\ false\ negatives}$

symptoms or documenting that the symptoms no longer reach a level of broad diagnostic significance. Table 76.1 outlines several psychometric aspects of screeners that are important to know (also see Chapter 81).

Psychological Testing

Psychological testing is a lengthier process than screening and includes the use of standardized, norm-referenced measures to identify the level of a patient's emotional, cognitive, or behavioral functioning compared to other individuals with similar characteristics. Psychological testing focuses on the level of a trait, skill, or ability the patient possesses rather than the presence or absence of that trait, skill, or ability. Psychological testing includes administration, scoring, and interpretation of data by a user with knowledge of the measure's psychometric properties and limitations, including the standardization process. The clinician is able to effectively consider patterns of data and not just single scores. Psychological tests are often used in combination as part of the psychological assessment process to identify relationships between abilities, behaviors, and traits and the patient's overall cognitive, behavioral, or emotional presentation. However, neither psychological screening nor psychological testing stand alone to characterize the patient or clarify diagnosis without the personal experience with the patient, context, and clinical judgment inherent in psychological assessment (Srinath, Jacob, Sharma, & Gautam, 2019).

The Purpose of Psychological Assessment

The purpose of a psychological assessment can vary greatly by factors, such as patient presentation, clinical setting, and stage of treatment. However, identifying the purpose of the assessment and the specific referral question(s) guides the evaluation process and sets the stage for effective communication between the clinician, patient, patient's family, and referral source. Common purposes of testing include assisting with diagnostic clarity, objectively measuring personality characteristics or abilities, and guiding treatment planning.

When diagnostic clarification is the purpose of assessment, methods that identify characteristics that support or negate a diagnosis include clinical interview questions, psychological testing, and record review. Assessment methods that distinguish abnormal levels of behaviors, emotions, or cognitive functioning from typical rates are especially useful. For instance, when a diagnostic question of ADHD is the purpose of testing, as for Abby in the chapter-opening vignette, specific questions about ability to follow multistep directions, complete tasks independently, and activity level may be included in the interview; parental report measures of attention and hyperactivity may be completed by parents and teachers; and psychological testing utilizing measures of attentional focus, concentration, processing speed, inhibitory control, and working memory may be administered to the child (Sattler, 2020).

Diagnostic assessment processes (e.g., "Does Abby have ADHD?") can be streamlined to accommodate limited appointment time, provide in-depth information about the patient's specific condition related difficulties, or identify patients appropriate for specific services. However, diagnostically focused assessments may lack breadth, leading to factors contributing to the child's presentation being overlooked or underappreciated and missing other appropriate diagnoses that are impacting the patient's daily functioning.

When psychological assessment is used to objectively measure specific characteristics and/or abilities, the focus is often on using normative data to compare an individual to others of a similar age, sex, or academic standing or to track the individual's progress or decompensation across different time points. While there are a multitude of uses for psychological assessment as an objective measure of personal characteristics, some common reasons include generating a list of diagnostic differentials; determining someone's fit for a particular position, placement, or activity (e.g., return to play after injury, fitness to serve, response to intervention, competency to stand trial); and identifying a baseline of functioning prior to implementation or change in the patient's condition, environment, or treatment (e.g., presurgical evaluation or prior to initiation of chemotherapy; young child with a condition placing him at high risk for neurologic insult such as hemophilia or sickle cell disease). When the purpose of an assessment is to measure a patient's personal characteristics or abilities, the assessment may cover a wide range of domains of functioning, include reporters and observations from different settings, and may seek to find variations in a patient's functioning both compared to normative samples and compared to their own abilities across time. These types of evaluations are often time consuming, but they provide a general overview of the patient's strengths and weakness and are comprehensive in determining factors that may contribute to or exacerbate their condition.

Psychological assessment can also be important as a guide to treatment planning. A combination of diagnostic and objective measurement is often included in assessments when the purpose is treatment planning because recommendations often include both evidence-based, condition-appropriate considerations and factors personal to the patient. Assessment for treatment planning can help to identify treatment goals, including which areas of behavioral, emotional, or cognitive functioning should be targeted in treatment. Psychological assessment can help to elucidate barriers and assets to treatment that can be utilized to guide the selection of one treatment over another or that can be incorporated in treatment to improve outcome. Further, when utilized as a way to track the level of symptoms, functioning, or characteristics over time, assessment can help determine treatment effectiveness and progress over the course of treatment. Particularly in conditions in which treatment is more long term (e.g., trauma, developmental disability) or requires significant medical intervention (e.g., shunt placement, neurosurgery, radiation, chemotherapy), assessment for treatment planning can assist in identifying early cognitive, emotional, and behavioral effects that may not be notable in the daily environment but warrant treatment, as well as symptom resolution or compensation over time so that treatment adjustments can be made accordingly.

Psychological assessment is often an integral aspect of eligibility determination for federal and state programing (e.g., Board of Developmental Disabilities, Social Security Disability Income), treatment access (e.g., organ donation, bariatric surgery), inclusion in research studies (e.g., medication trials, condition-specific treatment programs), and academic supports or services (e.g., special education, SAT/ACT accommodations). In this sense, clinicians become gatekeepers to valuable resources that may or may not be appropriate for the patient and require some formal assessment to make an informed, qualified decision. In these instances, specific guidelines are often determined by the governing organization that identifies a minimum standard for the criteria that must be met to qualify for services and the type of data needed to determine eligibly. Specific interview questions regarding timing (e.g., symptoms appearing prior to a specific age) or the impact of the patient's daily functioning, the psychological tests included in the testing battery, and the data needed to support each type of recommendation (e.g., giving additional time to complete the SAT/ACT) may all be covered in eligibility guidelines. Therefore it is vital that the clinician become familiar with eligibility criteria and guidelines prior to initiating the assessment.

TEST DESIGN AND PSYCHOMETRICS

Measures utilized in psychological assessment can include symptom checklists and informal procedures intended to provide descriptive information on the patient's behavioral, cognitive, and emotional functioning. However, psychological assessment most often includes standardized, norm-referenced measures of functioning that allow the clinician to effectively compare the patient's abilities, skills, and traits to others with similarities in age, educational background, clinical environment, or condition. Standardized, norm-referenced measures have several primary features. First, they are developed and normed under rigorous conditions with large numbers of patients, such as those of clinical trials for medication or devise development. Scores from the normative testing group are subject to statistical analysis allowing for the identification of mean (average) scores and variability in scores across the normative group (e.g., standard deviation). Second, these measures are intended to assess a specific trait or behavior and are not meant to measure other characteristics with any degree of accuracy. Finally, to be accurate, these measures must be administered in the same way, under similar conditions, to patients who have personal traits and backgrounds consistent with those individuals included in the normative sample. Structured administration and scoring procedures are meant to ensure that the measure's statistical properties can be applied appropriately across clinicians and settings. If any of these conditions is unmet, the test cannot be assumed to be a valid or reliable measure on which to base clinical decisions.

It is important to note that standardized measures are not all norm referenced. In a standardized measure, administration and scoring rules are clear and explicit. There may be important environment protocols for testing, such as the elimination of distractions, having a quiet testing environment, and sitting at a table directly across from a patient in a four-legged chair. When a measure has less specific administration and scoring guidelines, the assessment tool is said to be unstandardized. Standardized measures can look at a patient's performance in a valid and reliable manner across time but do not allow a clinician to compare the patient's performance to others unless they have been subject to the normative process. See American Educational Research Association, American Psychological Association, and National Council on Measurement in Education (2014), Frick, Barry, and

Kamphaus (2020), and Sattler (2020) for additional and more detailed information on standardization practices of psychological assessments.

Norm-referenced tests allow for comparison of an individual to other individuals with similar characteristics based on a normative curve, most often the bell curve. This allows the clinician to identify to what extent the patient's ability, characteristic, or behavior falls within normal limits as represented by the middle of the curve or outside of the normal limits as represented by the tails of the curve. Fig. 76.1 illustrates a typical bell curve and the percentage of people who fall within each area of the curve. However, prior to this interpretation, it is important to consider who was included in the normative sample of the test. Many assessment measures include information about the type (e.g., ethnic background, family composition, socioeconomic status) and number of people who were used in the research to establish a measure's accuracy, consistency, and useful. In addition to information included in a testing manual, researchers frequently examine the accuracy and consistency of a measure with underserved or unrepresented populations. Therefore conducting a good literature review can be helpful for patients who may not have been included in the normative sample. Of course, not every ethnicity, sexual orientation, or other areas of diversity are included in a normative sample of a measure, and research may not exist with some diverse populations. The greater the discrepancy between a patient and the norming group in terms of personal characteristics and history, the less valid an assessment tool is for use with patient decisions. Therefore it is up to a clinician to be clear in the interpretation of results or declare that results need to be interpreted with caution. For information on the types of scores made in norm-referenced interpretations see Table 76.2.

Reliability

When selecting tests to include in a psychological assessment it is important to consider the test's reliability. Reliability refers to the degree to which scores from a test are consistent and free from the effects of measurement error. There are a variety of forms of reliability in regard to the psychometric properties of a test (Table 76.3). Choosing the method of estimating a test's reliability depends on the nature of the assessment measure.

One component of a test's reliability is internal consistency. Two main methods for evaluating internal consistency involve administering the test once to a single group of examinees: the split half method and the use of a Cronbach coefficient alpha. The split half reliability method considers whether a test measures a single construct by dividing it into equal halves (e.g., first items vs. last items, odd vs. even numbers) and examining the degree to which results from the halves are correlated. The use of split-half reliability can underestimate a measure's true reliability because as a test length is shortened, reliability correlations tend to decrease. In contrast, a Cronbach coefficient alpha utilizes a special formula to examine the average degree of inter-item consistency. This special formula can be thought of as the average reliability from all possible ways of splitting the test. The use of a Cronbach coefficient alpha is more conservative, considered the lower boundary of a measure's reliability. Cronbach coefficient alpha ranges from 0, meaning there is no reliability, to 1.0, indicating perfect reliability. The general rule of thumb is that a Cronbach coefficient alpha of .80 or above is appropriate for clinical and psychological testing measures with reliability coefficients approaching or above .90

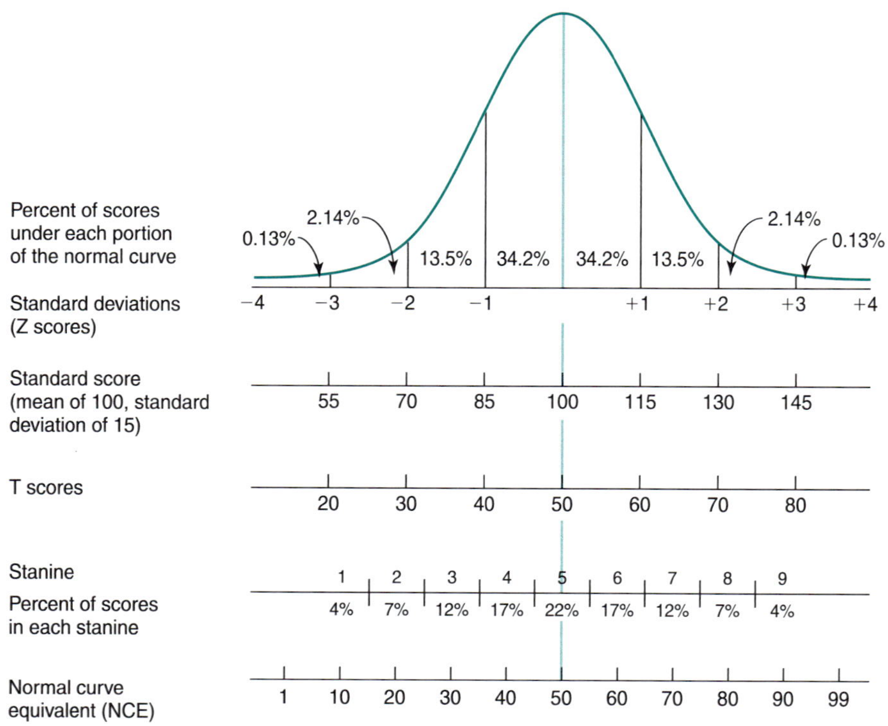

Fig. 76.1 Normal distribution.

TABLE 76.2 Types of Standardized Scores

Types of Scores for Norm-Referenced Interpretation

Type of Score	What It Is	Statistical Formula	Example
Percentile rank (PR)	Percentage of people in the norm sample who achieved lower scores	$PR = \left[\frac{M + (0.5 \times R)}{Y}\right] \times 100$	A percentile rank of 65 indicates that 65% of the norm sample performed lower than the patient
Standard score	Typically has a mean of 100 and a standard deviation of 15	Population mean $\mu = \frac{\sum xi}{N}$ Sample mean $\overline{X} = \frac{\sum xi}{n}$ Population standard deviation $\sigma = \sqrt{\frac{\sum (x-\mu)^2}{N}}$ Sample standard deviation $s = \sqrt{\frac{\sum (x-\overline{x})^2}{n-1}}$	IQ tests often use standard scores; a standard score of 85 indicates a patient performed 1 SD below the norm sample
T-score	A standard score, where the mean is 50 and the standard deviation is 10	$t = \frac{x-\mu}{\sigma/\sqrt{n}}$	On the *BASC-3* a T-score = 75 on the Inattention Scale is 2.5 SD above, indicating clinical significance
Z-score	A standard score where the mean is 0 and a standard deviation is 1	$Z = \frac{x-\mu}{\sigma}$	A Z-Score of 1.5 on a reading accuracy measure indicates patient performed better (i.e., 1.5 SD above the norm sample)
Stanine score	A standard score where the distribution is divided into nine parts; mean is 5 and the standard deviation is 2	N/A	If a patient's stanine score on an inhibition task is 2, the patient is 1.5 SD below the norm sample, which could indicate issues with inhibiting patient's responses

TABLE 76.3 Reliability

Types of Reliability

Term	What It Means	Way To Measure
Internal consistency	Measures whether test items measure the proposed general construct of the test (i.e., does it measure what you want it to?)	Split half method or Cronbach alpha: $\alpha = \left(\frac{K}{K-1}\right)\left(1 - \frac{\sum V_i}{V_T}\right)$
Interrater reliability	Degree of agreement among raters	Percentage agreement Correlation coefficient
Test-retest reliability	Measures test consistency or repeatability of a test (i.e., when a measure is given to the same people twice, are scores similar?)	Correlation coefficient

being excellent (Sattler, 2020). Reliability between .79 and .60 is adequate, but any reliability coefficient below .60 indicates the measure lacks reliability.

Another form of measuring a test's reliability is to examine the interrater reliability. Interrater reliability applies only to assessments that include a subjective scoring component that depends on a rater's judgment, such as a behavioral observation scale or projective personality test. Interrater reliability is calculated using either a correlation coefficient or percent agreement on scores/ratings between two or more raters. The kappa statistic is a type of correlation coefficient used when the scores on a test are on a nominal or ordinal scale of measurement and there are two raters. In contrast, the use of a percent agreement is calculated by dividing the number of items/observations that raters agreed on by the total number of items/observations. Many structured behavioral observation assessments suggest a clinician demonstrate at least 80% interrater reliability prior to administering the test on one's own to ensure they are reliable in administration.

Lastly, the test-retest method of reliability is estimated by administering a test to the same group of examinees on two separate occasions and then correlating the two scores. This correlation coefficient indicates the degree of stability/consistency of a patient's scores over time and is appropriate for tests that assume an attribute is stable over time, unaffected by previous exposure to test items (e.g., cognitive ability). In contrast, it would not be appropriate to use a test-retest reliability correlation coefficient on an assessment of mood due to fluctuations over time, or creativity, which might be affected by having previous exposure to items on the assessment. However, it is important for clinicians to be aware of when a test is appropriate to be readministered, as many have rules on how frequently the same version of a test can be given to a patient. Some assessments have alternative forms available that measure the same areas but contain different test items to avoid the pitfalls of repeat administration.

There are several factors that can impact a measure's reliability (Table 76.4). These factors are important to consider when selecting an assessment measure and when interpreting scores to determine whether the scores are reliable for that particular patient (American Educational Research Association et al., 2014; Sattler, 2020).

TABLE 76.4 Threats to Reliability

Some Threats to Reliability

Threats	How So?
Length of test	When a test is longer in length it helps minimize the effect of measurement error. Therefore, typically the longer the test length, the larger the reliability coefficient.
Range of scores	When norming a test, the degree of similarity between examinees on the attribute being measured affects the reliability. For instance, if all items are really difficult or really easy, all examinees obtain similar scores, thus resulting in a restricted range of scores.
Guessing	As the probability of a patient correctly guessing answers on a measure increases, the reliability of the measure decreases.
Patient/ environmental characteristics	Natural changes in a patient or the environment can impact reliability. These include factors such as the patient's emotional/social functioning and physical health as well as environmental factors that include historic events and changes in societal rules/expectations.
Administration of test	If an examiner does not follow proper protocol for an assessment, administration instructions are poor in quality, or the measure requires subjective scoring, then reliability decreases.

Validity

After establishing a test is reliable, it is vital to ensure an assessment measure has adequate validity for its purpose. A test's validity refers to the degree to a which a test measures what it has been designed to measure (i.e., the accuracy of the test) (Table 76.5).

Construct validity determines the extent to which a test measures a hypothetical trait or abstract characteristic that cannot be directly observed and is inferred by observing its effects. Convergent and divergent validity are used to establish construct validity by comparing a measure's correlations with other measures of similar and dissimilar constructs. When a measure has a high correlation with an assessment tool that measures the same construct or related traits, there is evidence for convergent validity. In contrast, low correlations with tests of unrelated constructs/characteristics provide evidence of divergent validity. For example, a test measuring aggressiveness should have high correlations with other measures of aggressiveness; however, a clinician would want the aggression measure to have lower correlations with measures of assertiveness as these constructs are theoretically different. Face validity is the extent to which a measure appears to cover the purpose of the assessment (i.e., the transparency of a test to the participants). When a test has high face validity it may mean patients are aware of what the test is trying to measure. This feature can sometimes lead patients to change

TABLE 76.5 Summary of Validity

Types of Validity

Term	What It Means
Construct validity	Assesses whether a test measures what it is supposed to. Methods to assess construct validity: • Internal consistency • Factor analysis • Group differences • Convergent and divergent validity
Convergent validity	Measures how much a test is similar to other tests of the same construct
Divergent validity	Measures how much a test is dissimilar to other tests of a different (likely unrelated) construct
Face validity	Degree to which a test is subjectively viewed as covering the concept it is supposed to measure
Predictive validity	Degree to which an assessment tool predicts performance on a criterion/test later on
Concurrent validity	Degree to which an assessment tool predicts performance on an existing measure/ criterion

their responses to either fake bad (i.e., present themselves in a more unfavorable light) or fake good (i.e., present themselves in a more favorable light). However, tests with low face validity may result in a patient being confused why the test is administered or disagreeing with the results.

The extent to which test scores can be used to make conclusions about a patient's performance or status on another measure is known as criterion-related validity. There are two main forms of criterion validity: predictive validity and concurrent validity. Predictive validity refers to an assessment tool's ability to predict a construct, performance, or status in the future. For example, a clinician may want to know whether a patient's performance on an academic test would predict how the patient will perform in school in the upcoming year. Concurrent validity is similar but concerns a measure's ability to predict current status or performance, such as whether an academic test accurately estimates how a patient is performing currently in school.

There are several factors that can impact a measure's validity and the validity of psychological administration of measures, which can influence how measures are interpreted (Table 76.6). For more information on the validity of psychological testing, see American Educational Research Association et al. (2014) and Sattler (2020).

TABLE 76.6 Threats to Validity

Some Threats to Validity

Threats	How So?
Time between testing	Significant time between testing sessions may result in possible changes in the patient due to natural maturation, new symptoms or ailments, or changes in the environment, all of which affect how the patient performs in testing. Practice effects from taking the measure or a similar measure too closely in time also impact validity. Follow an assessment tool's guidelines for when a measure can be readministered.
Lack of representation in norming sample	A patient's personal characteristics such as race, socioeconomic status, language, or education level are considered to determine if the normative data included individuals with similar traits. If the normative group lacks aspects of the patient's diversity, it may be inappropriate to compare the patient to that group.
Biases in test items	Some items may assess skills or knowledge obtained through particular experiences (e.g., formal schooling), which could result in a patient who has not had those experiences performing differently than the normative group.
Criterion contamination	This occurs when a knowledge of how a patient performed on a previous measure or testing affects how they are rated on another measure.
Deviation administration of test	If examiner does not follow proper protocol for an assessment (i.e., improper scoring, distractions in the room, poor instructions), an assessment tool becomes less valid.

Test Construction

Theories and methods of test construction are complex and well outside the scope of this chapter. However, a basic understanding of the theories of test construction is helpful in understanding the ways a test is developed, organized, and found to be reliable and valid. Two theories of test construction are frequently discussed in the research literature and technical manuals of testing measures: classical test theory and item response theory. In applying both theories, questions, items, or tasks are developed, often by a panel of experts, that are thought to measure the construct of interest. A subset of those questions is identified, often through expert consensus, as the best to utilize. That subset is then subject to the normative processes in which hundreds or thousands of individuals answer the questions or complete the tasks. Statistical analyses are utilized to determine the distribution of scores across the sample, reliability, and validity. Readers interested in learning more about test construction should see American Educational Research Association et al. (2014) and Sattler (2020).

Test publishers must update tests regularly due to a variety of threats to reliability and validity that occur over time. Societal changes that impact variables, such as the quality and type of visual stimuli familiar to individuals, specifics of common knowledge, and vernacular (e.g., slang words that may be acceptable responses, phrasing of questions), are considered when updating and renorming a measure. An additional statistical catalyst for updating a test stems from a phenomenon called the Flynn effect, in which average scores on specific performance-based measures, particularly intellectual measures, increase over time. In general, an increase of about 0.3 standard score points occurs each year from the time the test was initially normed. While this change may not seem significant on the surface, it has strong implications for clinical practice particularly when considering high-stakes areas of evaluation, such as diagnosis of intellectual disability for eligibility determination or assessment for competency to stand trial or face maximum penalty in the justice system. Testing experts have suggested that the Flynn effect has been receding over time and is less of an issue today than it was 2 or 3 decades ago. However, recent research has not supported this claim and has confirmed a continued increase of approximately 3 points per decade since 1972 as evidenced by a meta-analysis of 52 well-executed studies (Trahan, Stuebing, Fletcher, & Hiscock, 2014).

For clinical purposes it is important to be aware of the Flynn effect for two reasons. First, a patient's score will likely increase on the same test over time due to a combination of practice effects and the Flynn effect. Second, a score decrease is expected when an individual is given an updated version of a test; the score on the *Wechsler Intelligence Scale for Children, Fifth Edition*, (Wechsler, 2014) will likely be lower than the score on the fourth edition, even if the tests are administered in close temporal proximity to each other. The Flynn effect also supports the need to use only the most recent version of a test for clinical purposes.

COMPETENCIES TO CONDUCT ASSESSMENTS

Competence to conduct psychological assessments requires expertise, clinical skills, and a solid understanding of psychometric statistics, standardization procedures, and interpretation methods. Personal review of testing measures and technical manuals, even when thorough, is only one step in the process of becoming competent in psychological assessment. Coursework in statistics and test development, practice with an already expert testing administrator, and close supervision in the administration of measures and data interpretation are vital aspects of building assessment skills. These training opportunities are key components of all clinical and school psychology training programs and can be sought by long-term consultation with experts in psychological assessment and specific training opportunities through conferences and testing companies. In addition to standard expert training, some assessment measures require specialized training in the form of workshops or long-term supervision. This requirement is most often the case when there are only semistructured administration instructions or there are subjective components of scoring. Examples of measures requiring specialized training are the *Autism Diagnostic Observation Schedule, Second Edition*, and the *Exner System* for the *Rorschach Inkblot Test* (Exner, 1974). Additionally, many experts in psychological assessment find that they need to review each measure to refresh themselves on specific psychometric properties and administration procedures every few years because of natural tendencies to forget details or include more personal approaches to test administration, scoring, and interpretation. The natural loss of detail and gradual introduction of nonstandardized testing practices is referred to as examiner drift and is just one of many common threats to validity and reliability in psychological assessment (American Educational Research Association et al., 2014).

ASSESSMENT PLANNING

An assessment plan is essential to conducting a comprehensive, organized assessment that will answer specific referral questions posed by the family and referring clinician. Once the referral question is clear and confirmed with all parties, the clinician must turn attention to identifying the best process for answering the referral question and generating a hypothesis as to what may be contributing to the aspects of the patient's presentation that are the subject of the referral question. Assessment planning often progresses in phases where details of each aspect of the evaluation are refined as additional information is collected. For instance, the evaluation planned for Abby, in the vignette, who was referred for concerns of attention, might have seemed straightforward until interviews with the family also indicate concerns for trauma and learning problems that must be accommodated in the assessment plan.

SOURCES OF ASSESSMENT DATA

Interview

The clinical interview is the most frequently used evaluation procedure and often the initial step taken when conducting a comprehensive psychological assessment. Thorough clinical interviews are used to obtain historical data on a patient (e.g., presenting concerns, frequency of behaviors, academic information, birth and developmental history), provide the foundation to establish a collaborative relationship with the family, and are useful for case formulation and treatment planning. Clinical interviews may be loosely structured or more standardized and highly structured, requiring the clinician to ask specific questions in certain ways. Loosely structured clinical interviews for child and adolescent assessments may serve as an intake, typically with a parent or guardian of the individual, who can provide the necessary historical background. Depending on the patient's age, a child may also participate during or in parts of the clinical intake interview. Although unstructured interviews provide flexibility during the interview process, they rely heavily on the expertise and knowledge of the clinician who conducts them. Their validity and reliability rely on the skill and accuracy of the clinician to ask appropriate initial and follow-up questions.

In contrast, semistructured and structured interviews have specific questions often with standardized wording, cover specific domains, and follow a standardized format. Several semistructured and structured interviews are designed to assess a broad range of psychological symptoms, such as the *Schedule for Affective Disorders and Schizophrenia for School-Age Children* (*K-SADS*; Ambrosini, 2000). Other structured interviews are used to assess a specific concern or cluster of symptoms, such as the *Autism Diagnostic Interview–Revised* (*ADI-R*; Rutter, LeCouteur, & Lord, 2003). Although semistructured and structured interviews can be beneficial by standardizing the interview process, allowing for reliability among clinicians, they can be time consuming and sometimes constraining on clinicians depending on the degree of structure provided in the interview (see Chapter 77 for more on interviewing).

Observations

Direct behavioral observations of a patient are an important source of assessment data and can be unstructured or structured. Assessment observations can be made during clinic evaluations, while the patient is in the waiting room (e.g., how the child interacts with others in the waiting room), or when the patient is in other natural settings such as at school.

Observations described in a psychological assessment may include effort/motivation, language abilities, attention, social behaviors, thought process, affect/mood, motor control, and behavioral concerns. These observations often help determine if factors such as fatigue or limited compliance may impact the validity of test results.

In contrast, structured observational assessment addresses specific behaviors that are important for diagnosis or treatment monitoring and can be normative or unnormed. Unnormed behavioral observations are typically individually designed to measure specific behaviors or symptoms that are the subject of assessment and often focus on factors such as the circumstances just prior to or after the target behavior, frequency, or duration of the behavior. A functional behavior analysis is an example of an unnormed semistructured observation. Structured normative observations allow a clinician to determine the significance of the child's behavior in comparison to the general or condition-specific population. Norm-referenced observations typically require specific training to learn the assessment procedures and frequently require supervision of administration, scoring, and interpretation to ensure the clinician is providing observation data that are clinically reliable and valid. For example, the *Autism Diagnostic Observational Schedule, Second Edition* (*ADOS-2*; Lord et al., 2012) is a standardized, norm-referenced measure of ASD-related behavior (see Chapter 84 for more on behavioral observations).

Caregiver and Self-Report Measures

Many psychological assessments include measures completed by the patient, parents, teachers, or others who can provide insight into a patient's concerns and inform the case conceptualization. These report measures may entail having the informants rate the frequency of certain behaviors, how true they feel a statement is in relation to the patient, or whether they think a specific statement/behavior/symptom is true or false. Report measures vary on many internal qualities such as reading level, length, informant options, and time reference (e.g., last 6 months, when the child was 4–5 years of age). However, one of the most important factors to consider is the appropriateness of the informant to complete the measure because personal, situational, and measure-specific qualities can impact the validity of the report. For instance, reading level, familiarity with the child, differing demands of environments (e.g., school vs home), and characteristics of the normative sample can all impact the choice of informant (see Frick et al. [2020] and Chapters 81–82 for more on report measures).

Broadband Versus Domain Report Measures

One common distinction made in considering the selection of a report measure lies in the scope of behaviors measured. A broadband report measure evaluates a variety of behaviors (e.g., attention, depression, parenting stress) rather than a specific area, allowing the clinician to consider the breadth of the patient's symptoms and behaviors. Broadband report measures used during psychological assessments include the *Behavior Assessment System for Children, Third Edition* (*BASC-3*; Reynolds & Kamphaus, 2015) and the *Child Behavior Checklist* (*CBCL*; Achenbach & Rescorla, 2001). Broadband measures are often helpful in narrowing the type of symptoms a patient experiences although in a somewhat shallow manner. Domain-specific measures are restricted to specific symptom areas, often those important to determining the type or severity of symptoms related to a condition or area of functioning, for a more in-depth analysis of an area of concern. Domain-specific measures are often very helpful for treatment planning, symptom monitoring, or identification of specific patterns of behavioral concerns. For example, the *Behavior Rating Inventory of Executive Functioning, Second Edition* (*BRIEF-2*; Gioia, Isquith, Guy, & Kenworthy, 2015), is a domain-specific measures that provides a rating for a parents' perceptions of their child's executive functioning at both global and ability-specific levels. However, the limitation of these measures includes their lack of breadth in the range of behaviors they measure. Often many psychological assessments include both a broadband measure and domain-specific measures in particular areas of concern to gain a full picture of the patient's behavioral functioning.

Performance-Based Measures

Clinicians conducting a comprehensive assessment typically include performance-based measures in their testing plan. Performance-based measures, including standardized intelligence and achievement tests, require patients to complete tasks in the assessment environment to determine how they perform in comparison to others (i.e., norm referenced) or in regard to a specific skill (i.e., criterion referenced). Test selection is a nuanced skill as numerous factors must be considered when developing the testing plan, including patient characteristics (e.g., diversity factors, limitations to functioning, attention span), the child's previous testing experience, and expertise of the clinician in accurately administering and scoring particular testing measures.

INTEGRATING INFORMATION

The interpretation and integration of data sources are perhaps the most difficult aspects of the assessment process. To be successful and thorough in data interpretation, well-supervised clinical experience is needed to recognize both common and patient-specific variations in data while integrating that data with patient factors and other sources of information. For the sake of brevity, two specific and basic types of data interpretation will be discussed in this chapter: normative variation and internal variation in performance. It is important to recognize, however, that some higher levels of data interpretation exist, including recognition of disease-specific patterns in data and neuroanatomic correlations of data patterns, and are often included in the work of experts in the fields of neuropsychology and neuroscience (see Sattler [2020] Semrud-Clikeman & Ellison [2009],], and Chapter 87 for further details).

Interpretation of normative variation refers to the process of comparing a patient's scores on norm-referenced measures to those of other individuals of the same age, grade, gender, or some combination of those factors. This level of interpretation allows one to consider absolute or normative strengths and weaknesses of the patient compared to what is considered the standard of ability or skill for the general population (as defined by the normative sample). When a child's scores fall well outside of the average range in a particular area, we can consider that area to be either a cause for concern, as is the case of a very low IQ score suggesting intellectual disability (see Chapter 40), or a factor that may suggest resilience or special ability, as in a superior IQ score, suggesting giftedness (see Chapter 48). These strengths and weaknesses can be integrated with history and context to support specific diagnoses or treatment options.

In contrast, internal variation in performance across or within domains of functioning is used to identify areas where a child shows personal strengths relative to other abilities. Strengths or weaknesses identified in this type of analysis are often called relative due to their relationship to the child's other areas of functioning as opposed to the general population. Internal variability in scores is important to recognize for several reasons. First, variability across or within specific domains, such as attention, can direct the clinician more specifically to the basic skill or ability that requires targeted treatment or can be relied on for compensatory strategies. For instance, a child who has impaired ability in the specific areas of selective attention and attention shifting will likely show improved academic performance if provided a variety of environmental accommodations to support the ability to locate information to which the child needs to attend and strategies to help the child prepare for upcoming transitions. Secondly, internal variation in scores can assist with diagnostic clarification and treatment planning when a child's abilities appear evenly distributed compared to population norms but are variable within the child's overall score profile. For instance, standard scores of 112 and 86 are both within the average range of the normative sample but represent significantly different levels of ability for the child and should be interpreted as such. Finally, internal variation in scores is vital to identifying the validity of cumulative, composite, or index scores. A 70 full-scale IQ in a child who receives a 63 on the verbal comprehension index with a 101 on the visual spatial index should not be considered a valid overall estimate of ability because of the extreme variability in performance. This type of variability often points to a clear deficit associated with a specific condition or indicates that patient (e.g., motivation, alterations in awareness) or environmental (e.g., extraneous noise, administration/scoring error) factors are impacting the test's validity.

One additional consideration when performing a basic interpretation of testing scores lies in the concepts of statistical versus clinical significance. Statistical significance is identified when scores on performance-based tests vary from the normative group, including differences between subtests scores in a particular domain or index score comprising a composite scale. While these types of statistical differences are important to note and explore during interpretation, they may not be cause for concern. Instead, the clinician must consider whether the difference noted is unusual in the population, thus signaling an unusual pattern of ability or skills. As a general rule, a statistical difference is not considered to have clinical significance unless it occurs in less than 10% to 15% of the population (Sattler, 2020). This difference in statistical and clinical significance again highlights the importance of assessing data in the meaningful context of both population norms and patient-specific factors (Frick et al., 2020; Sattler, 2020).

Abby's presentation raises many assessment considerations and challenges, including language, appropriateness of normative data, access to appropriate testing measures, historical events that may confound behavioral reports, informant characteristics, and her ability to maintain attention and compliance in testing. For example, given her bilingual status, which language will be most appropriate for testing? If Spanish is her dominant language, what valid and reliable Spanish language measures are available? Are available measures culturally translated or direct translations of English measure? What is the impact of using an interpreter on the validity and reliability of testing? Are bilingual Latinx children appropriately represented in the normative data? Is there any published research on the performance of children from Latinx backgrounds on the measures to be used? Has Abby received any past testing? If so what measures were utilized? How long ago did testing take place? Will measures of ADHD symptoms be confounded by trauma or anxiety? Does her mother have reading skills at a level that will allow her to reliably respond to parent questionnaires, or will questionnaires need to be presented orally? An assessment plan will need to take all of these challenges into consideration to select appropriate measurement strategies and to synthesize results into recommendations using valid interpretations.

CONCLUSION

Psychological assessment is a complex process that applies clinical knowledge in human development and behavior and patient history with a solid awareness of psychometrics, standardized test administration, and data interpretation to build a complex conceptualization of the patient. To provide effective psychological assessment, a clinician must have specific training and expertise from coursework or test manual review, further refined and developed through guided practice and supervised experience. Psychological assessment has a variety of clinical applications, including diagnostic clarification, treatment planning, and tracking changes in abilities across time for purposes of monitoring outcome or quantifying progression of degenerative conditions. In the following chapters, the reader will find in-depth discussions of many of the components of psychological assessment as well as the types of psychological assessment commonly utilized in the clinical setting.

REFERENCES

Achenbach, T. M., & Rescorla, L. A. (2001). *Manual for the aseba school-age forms and profiles*. University of Vermont, Research Center for Children, Youth, & Families.

Ambrosini, P. J. (2000). Historical development and present status of the schedule for affective disorders and schizophrenia for school-age children (K-SADS). *Journal of the American Academy of Child & Adolescent Psychiatry*, *39*(1), 49–58. https://doi.org/10.1097/00004583-200001000-00016

American Educational Research Association, American Psychological Association, & National Council on Measurement in Education, (2014). *Standards for educational and psychological testing*. Author.

Exner, J. E. (1974). *The Rorschach: A comprehensive system*. Wiley. (vol. 1).

Frick, P. J., Barry, C. T., & Kamphaus, R. W. (2020). *Clinical assessment of child and adolescent personality and behavior* (4th ed.). Springer International Publishing. https://doi.org/10.1007/978-3-030-35695-8

Gioia, G. A., Isquith, P. K., Guy, S. C., & Kenworthy, L. (2015). *Behavior rating inventory of executive function* (2nd ed.). PAR Inc.

Lord, C., Rutter, M., DiLavore, P. C., Risi, S., Gotham, K., & Bishop, S. (2012). *Autism diagnostic observation schedule* (2nd ed.). Western Psychological Services.

Reynolds, C. R., & Kamphaus, R. W. (2015). *Behavior assessment system for children* (3rd ed.). Pearson.

Rutter, M., LeCouteur, A., & Lord, C. (2003). *Autism diagnostic interview-revised manual*. Western Psychological Services.

Sattler, J. M. (2020). *Assessment of children: Cognitive foundations and applications* (6th ed.). Jerome M. Sattler Publisher, Inc.

Semrud-Clikeman, M., & Ellison, P. A. T. (2009). *Child neuropsychology: Assessment and interventions for neurodevelopmental disorders* (2nd ed.). Springer International Publishing. https://doi.org/10.1007/978-0-387-88963-4

Srinath, S., Jacob, P., Sharma, E., & Gautam, A. (2019). Clinical practice guidelines for assessment of children and adolescents. *Indian Journal of Psychiatry*, *61*(2), S158–S175. https://doi.org/10.4103/psychiatry.IndianJPsychiatry_580_18

Trahan, L. H., Stuebing, K. K., Fletcher, J. M., & Hiscock, M. (2014). The Flynn effect: A meta-analysis. *Psychological Bulletin*, *140*(5), 1332.

Wechsler, D. (2014). *Wechsler intelligence scale for children* (5th ed.). Pearson.

77

The Interview in Developmental-Behavioral Pediatrics

John C. Duby, Kelly Blankenship, and Mary Beth DeWitt

For additional material related to the content of this chapter, please see Chapter 91.

VIGNETTE

Jackson is a 27-month-old boy who was referred by his pediatrician due to concerns about delayed language and possible autism spectrum disorder (ASD). Jackson failed the M-CHAT-R at his 24-month visit after his maternal grandparents raised concerns about his development. The clinician looked directly at parents warmly and simply said, "Share with me what brings you in today." His parents recount that he failed the screening test and then quickly add they have heard that boys are frequently late talkers and father did not talk until he was 3. They do not feel there is anything to be concerned about and came today because of the pressure from grandparents. Your observations indicate significant concerns with social interaction, social communication, and restricted and repetitive behaviors consistent with a diagnosis of ASD. The clinician considers how to begin the interview to assure the parents about objectivity and support.

The art of the medical interview is an essential skill for success in the practice of developmental-behavioral pediatrics. Often, an accurate diagnosis becomes evident largely based on the information that is gathered in the interview, which is then augmented by the physical examination and formal developmental and behavioral assessment (Chapters 76, 78, and 90).

Steven Cole and Julian Bird wrote a hallmark text on the medical interview, proposing that the interview has three objectives: (1) developing rapport and responding to patients' emotions; (2) gathering data to understand the patient, including biomedical and psychosocial information; and (3) educating and motivating patients. Further, addressing all aspects of the patient and family as unique, with their own values beliefs, will lead to both better health for the patient and greater satisfaction for the clinician (Cole & Bird, 2014).

INITIATING AND SUPPORTING THE RELATIONSHIP

Clinicians launch their unique role as family health advisors as they begin the initial interview. Our relationship with others is the foundation of all interaction, and in each visit (American Academy of Pediatrics, 2011). The interview is the initial opportunity to build the therapeutic alliance with families we serve and to establish our common goal, to promote optimal growth and development in children (Shah & Ribaudo, 2018). Establishing this alliance is a skill that should be developed, continually evaluated, and maintained. It can and must be taught and facilitated in medical and professional training programs (Levetown, 2008). In fact, it is identified as an art, which requires practice under supervision during its development (Wender, 2009). The clinical-patient relationship and communication is one of the strongest predictors of outcome during a medical visit. Communication skill influences patient disclosure, treatment adherence, and outcomes.

At the heart, the interview requires warmth and trust. As clinicians, we must embrace the alliance and recognize that parents and families are the expert regarding themselves and their children. They, like the family in the vignette, may present with strong emotions, uncertainty, and fear. Clinicians should "walk with" families during these visits, and not lead by a predetermined agenda (Wender, 2009). They should not limit discussion to initial concerns but rather follow the families or patients through their journey. Trainees may be initially preoccupied with the task of obtaining answers to a list of questions and may fail to listen or recognize cues in others (Levetown, 2008). It is critical for clinicians to examine their own biases to ensure that all patients know that they are welcome, that they will be treated with mutual respect, and that high-quality care will be delivered regardless of background using family- and patient-centered care (Trent, Dooley, & Dougé, 2019).

To facilitate a positive relationship, the clinician should, at a basic level, consider the influence of the clinical setting itself, as setting can contribute to comfort and ease. Ideally, the clinician should be seated and aligned with families, not seated behind a desk or computer. Eye contact should be utilized to facilitate the connection. Families should be comfortable, with adequate seating for caregivers and their support, as well as child-sized chairs and friendly activities.

A common but essential tool to develop and maintain the therapeutic alliance is active listening. This skill includes our nonverbal cues of looking and acknowledging through gestures, but also includes open-ended questioning, with reflective and clarifying statements. Barriers to active listening may include time pressures and clinician discomfort with emotional or challenging encounters. Listening is a key component of empathic support. Simple communication skills such as asking questions about psychosocial issues, making supportive statements, and listening attentively will increase disclosure of sensitive information (Wender, 2009). A clinician's expressed interest and support—using open-ended questions such as "How are things going for you as parents?"—can be tremendously valued. Validating stress can open the door for discussion (Duby, 2018; Pickles, Lihn, Boat, & Lannon, 2020). Other examples of open-ended questions to guide conversation include, "What changes have you seen in your child's health/development?" and "What bad, sad, or scary things may have happened to you or your family?" (Duby, 2018).

Barbara Korsch, a respected pioneer in developmental-behavioral pediatrics, guides us to facilitate dialogue and elicit concerns early in the visits as well as to establish parental and child expectations for the visit (Korsch, 2011). Clinicians should guide but not dominate the interaction and should show courtesy and warmth. The child should be incorporated into the interaction. The clinician should be focused when addressing an acute problem and redirect as needed. Following information gathering through shared dialogue, the clinician should counsel and close the visit. One approach is an open to closed "cone" interaction with the gradual narrowing of focus from an initial nondirective approach to a more direct exploration of a specific hypothesis. Other techniques include:

1. Open-ended questions: allowing patients to describe their symptoms using their own vocabulary and personal experiences
2. Facilitation: comments or interviewer behaviors that encourage the patient to continue talking along the same lines (e.g., nodding without interrupting)
3. Summarization: providing an explicit verbal summary of the information gathered so far, which allows the patient to confirm that the physician has understood what has been said, and acts as an opening to further explain the problems and thoughts
4. Surveying problems: briefly scan the full range of a patient's problems, such as by asking, "What else would you like to share?" (Cole & Bird, 2014)

Meeting and Greeting

The first few moments of the interview can set the stage for success or failure. Davies-House and colleagues (2017) investigated how patients want to be greeted by clinicians on a first encounter in the clinical setting. They found that patients preferred to be greeted informally by their first name and didn't mind how the clinician introduced themselves or preferred them to use their first name also. Patients showed a preference to shake hands with their clinician, particularly in older generational cohorts. Most patients believed that it was helpful to know the specific role of the clinician, whether a student, resident, fellow, or attending, and to be provided an explanation of what that meant (Davies-House, Ball, & Balmer, 2017). Many settings have emphasized the importance of making these distinctions by having name badges or color-coded uniforms that clearly identify roles. At the same time, it may be preferable to ask the child and the caregiver how they would like to be addressed and to note and be respectful of their requests.

Expanding on the earlier research, Studer (2003) developed the AIDET mnemonic as a template for improving communication with patients, which has been linked to patient satisfaction. AIDET is widely used in health care settings and enhances clinician and patient satisfaction. The AIDET model provides a framework for initiating every patient interaction. The components are:

Acknowledge: Address each person in the room.
Introduce: Introduce yourself, your role, your specialty, your training.
Duration: Set expectations for the length of the visit.
Explanation: Describe what will happen during the visit
Thank You: Show appreciation for the family's trust.

Agenda Setting

There is often a struggle to be certain that all the family's concerns are heard while effectively managing time. The use of collaborative upfront agenda setting has been shown to identify more concerns early in the visit and result in fewer concerns being raised late in the visit, with no significant difference in visit length. (Brock, Mauksch, Witteborn, Hummel, Nagasawa, and Robins, 2011) found no difference in total concerns addressed, patient or provider satisfaction, or patient trust and functional status when setting a clear agenda at the outset of the visit. Eliciting additional concerns following identification of the chief complaint by asking, "What else is important for us to address today?" can eliminate surprise concerns at the end of the visit and provide an opportunity for the clinician and the family to establish priorities for the visit.

Previous studies have shown that due to feelings of time constraints, the clinician often interrupts the patient during an opening statement. Beckman and Frankel (1984) found that patients were only permitted to complete their opening statement 23% of the time, with the average interruption occurring after just 18 seconds, and that only 2% of those opening statements were subsequently completed. If patients were permitted to complete their opening statements, they only took 2.5 minutes (Beckman & Frankel, 1984). Clinicians should avoid interruption, thus facilitating information gathering and improving satisfaction.

Shah and Ribaudo (2018) identified the SHARE concept as useful when preparing and conducting an interview. Within this framework, components of visits and overall care should strive to be continuous, comprehensive, family centered, coordinated, compassionate, and culturally effective. The SHARE framework identifies the following guidelines:

S: Set the tone by creating a safe holding environment, which provides support to the parent and child and begins to build the therapeutic alliance.

H: Hear parent concerns about health, development, and behavior and how they affect overall family functioning. This may require the use of guided questions.

A: Address specific risk factors and Allow the parent to reflect on how cultural traditions contribute to their expectations of child behavior, health, and development.

R: Reflect with parents on their experience of the child and Reframe in terms of the child's developmental level. Revisit therapeutic goals identified.

E: Empower the parent and child by formulating an action plan to address concerns and goals identified during the visit.

Potential Challenges for Consideration

When working with families, many obstacles can impede the clinician's ability to gather information. There may be language barriers that affect interaction. It is estimated that 25 million Americans speak English "less than very well" and that more than 60 million speak a language other than English at home. Title VI of the Civil Rights Act mandates the use of interpreter services be provided for patients with limited proficiency, and is superior to relying on unstrained staff, family, or friends. Clinicians should remember to address child and family members directly with warmth, using short statements, and allowing for sentence-by-sentence interpretation (Juckett & Unger, 2014).

Social determinants of health have become an increasingly relevant consideration in health care. More than 40% of patients reported that their doctor was unaware of their struggles (Andermann, 2016). Asking about these concerns in a sensitive and culturally appropriate way becomes essential. Behfourez, Drain, and Rhatigan (2014) encouraged clinicians to rethink the social history to include the assessment of broader social factors (Table 77.1).

Access to care for individuals with developmental disabilities is a common concern. Telehealth offers a method to improve access to care by making specialty provider care available in rural, remote, and medically underserved communities (Hooshmand & Foronda, 2018). During the COVID-19 pandemic, it became an almost essential way to provide health care as shelter-in-place mandates quickly spread across the United States. Telehealth has allowed providers to improve access to services that were previously geographically challenging. Underserved and rural areas often benefit from the ability to use telehealth services. In rural areas knowledge and resources regarding ASD is very limited. Telehealth can assist with education of rural community providers, early intervention specialists, education specialists, and families (Goldstein, Klaiman, & Williams, 2017). The use of telehealth may expedite the ability to receive a diagnosis and thus implement early intervention services (Alfuraydan et al., 2020).

A study regarding telemedicine for care of children and adolescents with developmental disabilities found three different factors that parents reported making telemedicine an attractive alternative. These included requiring a travel time of 1 hour for subspeciality care, parent missing work to travel to appointment, and reliance on emergency departments for care or regulation of child's medication (Langkamp, McManus, & Blakemore, 2015).

There have been concerns regarding outcomes and patient satisfaction with telehealth services. Several studies have looked at outcomes and satisfaction levels of telehealth for children with developmental disabilities. Overall,

TABLE 77.1 Social Considerations in the Developmental-Behavioral Pediatric Interview

Social Factor	Screening Strategy	Reference
Health literacy	The Newest Vital Sign	Weiss et al., 2005
Poverty	Do you have difficulty making ends meet at the end of the month?	American Academy of Pediatrics, 2016
Food insecurity	Within the past 12 mo, we worried whether our food would run out before we got money to buy more. Within the past 12 mo, the food we bought just didn't last and we didn't have the money to get more.	Brcic, Eberdt, & Kaczorowski, 2011
Adverse childhood experiences	What bad, sad, or scary things may have happened to you and your family?	Duby, 2018
Impact of racism	Assess for bullying and/or cyberbullying on the basis of race. Assess neighborhood safety, poverty, housing inequity, and academic access. Assess patients who report experiencing racism for mental health conditions, including signs of posttraumatic stress, anxiety, grief, and depressive symptoms, using validated screening tools and a trauma-informed approach to make referrals to mental health services as needed.	Trent et al., 2019

BOX 77.1 Tips for a Successful Virtual Visit—Preparing for Visit

1. Ensure the background being used and clinician's personal appearance are professional.
2. Avoid wearing patterns or stripes as this can be visually confusing to the patient.
3. Natural light sources are often ideal.
4. It is important to have a backup form of communication should there be a technology failure prior to or during the visit.
5. Consider hosting the visit while standing. This can improve the dynamics of the visit and tone of voice.
6. Look in the camera instead of the screen to improve eye contact.
7. Have the patient and family complete screening tools prior to the visit through the patient portal.
8. Train staff to help families connect to the platform if they are having difficulty.

Adapted from AimsCenter. (2020). Telehealth tips for behavioral health. University of Washington. aims.uw.edu/sites/default/files/Telehealth%20Tips%20for%20BH%20Providers_040220%20Final.pdf; Korioth, T. (2021). Pediatric mental health experts share tips to make the most of telehealth visits. *American Academy of Pediatrics News*. https://www.aappublications.org/news/2021/01/15/office-hourstelehealth011521

BOX 77.2 Tips for Successful Virtual Visit—During the Visit

1. Introduce yourself and credentials. Consent procedure should be reviewed discussing risks and benefits of telehealth services. The patient should then verify name and location (important for state licensing and to provide emergency aid if needed during the appointment).
2. Discuss the plan if the service platform is disconnected during the visit. Ask the patient to interrupt you if the patient experiences any technology issues.
3. Setting an agenda can help the patient to know what to expect from the visit, especially if the patient has not used telehealth services in the past.
4. Telehealth visits allow children to be watched in their normal environment. Parents can be coached through interactions by wearing earbuds.
5. During the interaction it can be helpful to be more deliberate and overt in nonverbal responses. It can also be helpful to ask more questions to clarify the meaning attached to facial expressions and/or body language.
6. At the end of the appointment, ask about how the visit could be improved. Set a date and time for the next appointment.
7. If the family does not have the resources needed to conduct a telehealth visit, consider options that might offer bandwidth needed for such services such as schools or libraries.

Adapted from AimsCenter. (2020). Telehealth tips for behavioral health. University of Washington. aims.uw.edu/sites/default/files/Telehealth%20Tips%20for%20BH%20Providers_040220%20Final.pdf; Korioth, T. (2021). Pediatric mental health experts share tips to make the most of telehealth visits. *American Academy of Pediatrics News*. https://www.aappublications.org/news/2021/01/15/office-hourstelehealth011521
(Cowan, Johnson and Close, 2020)

consultations were found to be as effective as in-person visits with high levels of parent satisfaction. One study described children with severe anxiety and autism being more engaged during telepsychiatry visits than during traditional in-person visits (Langkamp et al., 2015). Tips for a successful virtual visit are provided in Boxes 77.1 and 77.2.

Building an Alliance With Children

VIGNETTE CONTINUES

With Jackson and his family, the clinician set up a small table and chairs and a few developmentally appropriate toys. The clinician reflects on the pressure that the parents feel and sets the tone to begin the alliance with, "That must be uncomfortable for you when you have fewer concerns." The clinician then begins to explore with them the developmental milestones and how Jackson interacts with others by using open-ended questions such as "How does Jackson let you know what he needs?" "What does he like to do at home?" and "How does he interact when other children are with him?" Observing repetitive hand flapping, the clinician asks, "Do you see this at home?" or "What do you think he might be trying to tell us with that behavior?"

As clinicians working with children, we must recognize the unique opportunity to build an alliance not only with parents but also with the child. We must recognize developmental aspects as this evolves. In infancy, babies are making sense of their sensory worlds and establishing basic trust in their environment. As caregivers, we should approach our youngest with warmth and soft tone, using gentleness in our voice and touch. This approach can support the development of trust for both the child and parents, and even at the youngest ages we should always narrate what we plan to do with the child. As children develop, toddlers strive for a sense of autonomy, but they also experience basic stranger anxiety and separation issues. To build our alliance we can guide rapport building by allowing some sense of choice and control for little ones and allow some active exploration in the environment. Preschool thought may be characterized by magical thinking and self-focused (egocentric) thought. Children may perceive illness or standard clinical care negatively, perhaps as a punishment for being bad. Clinicians should engage the child and assess for this type of thinking, while reassuring the child that it is not the child's fault. With school age comes advancing verbal and cognitive skills. Children start to be more logical and organized in their thinking. Clinicians should build rapport by asking about interests, friends, and school, and should begin to directly ask about their feelings. As teens, our youth are developing critical behaviors that will carry through their lifetime and are beginning to gain more autonomy from parents. Clinicians should begin to allow time with the parent and with the child separately, and begin to address confidentiality and its limits. Teens can be included in the determination of mutually agreed upon goals for care (Shah & Ribaudo, 2018). Similar tools for

BOX 77.3 Developmental Considerations for Child Interviews

Age	Developmental Stage	Tips
0–3	Symbiotic, separation	Model calm communication for parents of infants Individuation begins to occur; allow closeness with parent Avoid direct, prolonged eye contact Approach the child gently, gradually Use play to capture child's attention Prepare the child for physical contact
3–6	Preschool, age of initiative	Use simple language Encourage child to ask questions Engage child with explanations Some time alone may facilitate relationship
6–12	School age, age of industry	Improved cognitive skills Children like to talk about family, interests Explanation of plans becomes important Spend time alone with child to determine any further concerns
13+	Adolescence, age of identity	Interview adolescent separated from parent to respect growing independence Elicit and address adolescent concerns Emphasize and clarify confidentiality issues Do not pressure the adolescent to talk Address difficult topics (drugs, sex, mental health) in a nonjudgmental manner Always be truthful Acknowledge that the adolescent is responsible for personal health care

Based on From Lui, Y.H and Stein, M.T. (2005). Talking with Children. In Parker, S, and Zuckerman, B. Developmental and behavioral pediatrics: a handbook for primary care. Philadelphia: Lippincott Williams and Wilkins.

the interview, as mentioned earlier, should be considered as we interview children. Use of open-ended questions, pauses, empathy, reflection, and active listening should be used within the context of cultural sensitivity. Consideration should be provided for the child's developmental stage, with guidance and tips listed in Box 77.3.

FAMILY HISTORY

The family history has long been recognized as an opportunity to identify potential genetic risk factors and to assess the potential for family stressors to impact children's development and behavior. Zuckerman and Wong (2019) have suggested that the family history is also an opportunity to disrupt transmission of behavioral health problems. They argue that a family history of at least three generations will assist the clinician in identifying underlying parental concerns and anxiety for themselves and their children. The history should specifically include depression, alcoholism, drug dependency, posttraumatic stress disorder, anxiety, and suicide. Potential follow-up questions for consideration include:

- Because this problem runs in families, do the parents or their siblings have any similar problems? If yes, are they being treated, or do they need support to obtain treatment? If no, are they worried that they may develop some of these problems?
- Do the parents perceive that their own childhood experiences due to the behavioral health problems of their parents currently affect their parenting? Are they, for example, overprotective, overly strict, not emotionally connected, or easily angered? Asking parents such questions provides them with a chance to reflect on the linkage of past and present behaviors.
- Are parents concerned that their children might develop similar or related behavioral health problems, if not imminently, then perhaps in adolescence?
- An extend family history offers a window of opportunity to help parents perceive their children's experience with empathy, recognizing the similarities between their own childhood experiences and their children's. This perspective may also help parents to perceive and reflect on the need, with or without help, to make changes in their parenting to break the chain of intergenerational transmission." (Zuckerman & Wong, 2019)

DISCUSSING DIAGNOSIS AND TREATMENT

After a thorough interview is augmented by the physical examination and developmental-behavioral assessments, a differential diagnosis and treatment plan will be developed. With what has been learned from the clinician's assessment of the family's health literacy, the biologic, genetic, social, and environmental factors that contribute to an accurate understanding of the child's presenting problem should be explained in terms that are easily understood by both parent and child if developmentally appropriate. Often it will be helpful to ask the family for their opinion of what the problem is. The family is often correct, and if so the disposition becomes easier since the clinician can agree with the family's assessment.

VIGNETTE CONTINUES

As in Jackson's case, the family may feel that there is not a problem, that he is just like his father, and that he will be fine if we wait a little longer. This is clearly not fully accurate, in that Jackson exhibits many signs of ASD. It will be important to highlight specific examples of the signs of ASD that were shared in the history and observed during the visit, and again to revisit the fact that these behaviors have been seen at home as well as in the clinical setting. Reviewing the diagnostic criteria in detail may be necessary. Sharing videos of children with similar concerns might be helpful. Offering to arrange a second opinion may be indicated. It will also be beneficial to emphasize the value of early intervention for all developmental concerns, including if he is simply a "late bloomer" like his father. Providing resources on ASD for the family to review and offering to track Jackson's developmental progress with the family may be the best approach. Time and repeated observations can help the family recognize and accept the signs that are supportive of the diagnosis.

The use of Teach Back can be a valuable tool to ensure that the family has understood the diagnosis and next steps (Agency for Healthcare Research and Quality, n.d.). The clinician should start with the most important message. For example:

Jackson fits the picture of a child with ASD.

Then, using plain language, offer two to four key points to support the diagnosis:

You have shared with me that Jackson is not talking like other children his age and that he doesn't seem to try to communicate by pointing. He doesn't respond to his name or look you in the eye. He lines up his cars and gets upset if you move them.

Rephrase the message until there is clear understanding:

Just to be safe, I want to make sure we are on the same page. Can you tell me the signs that I mentioned that make me concerned about autism?

Or: I want to make sure that I explained things clearly. Can you explain to me why I am worried about Jackson having autism?

Always be well prepared for this conversation. Be sure to have all available test results on hand and plan to discuss them in plain language. This should include:

1. Providing a rationale for diagnosis
2. Sharing the possibilities in differential diagnosis and rationale for the conclusion based on history, observations, and test results
3. Discussing co-occurring symptoms and conditions
4. Providing a realistic prognosis
5. Offering recommendations for further evaluation
6. Reviewing intervention options: medical, developmental, rehabilitative, educational, behavioral, recreational, integrative, complementary and alternative, safety
7. Emphasizing the ongoing importance of the primary care medical home
8. Providing resources on diagnosis, treatment, family-to-family support, peer-to-peer support, and sibling support
9. Social prescribing, such as connecting patients with various support resources within and beyond the health system, such as food banks, local women's groups, housing advocacy organizations or employment agencies (Andermann, 2016)

It is important to consider that some families may feel ambivalent or upset to receive a diagnosis. Some families may challenge or even argue the diagnosis with the provider. Motivational interviewing can be a very helpful technique to use in these situations (Desai, 2019). The use of open-ended questions and responding with reflective listening is important. It will help the clinician to be assured they have heard and understood the family's and patient's concerns accurately. It also helps the family to know the clinician is listening and hearing their concerns. Expressing empathy is important as well. It again assures the family that the clinician understands and appreciates what they are thinking and feeling. It can also assure the family that this is a collaboration. Although it will not change the diagnosis, one can assure that the family is understood and working toward a goal with the clinician.

If the family has concerns regarding the diagnosis, it can be helpful to develop discrepancy between the concerns and some symptoms that have been reported. It can be helpful to ask the family open-ended questions about symptoms they are concerned about and review other possible diagnoses. This will help to build discrepancy between other diagnoses and the child's symptoms. If the family continues to exhibit ambivalence with the diagnosis, it can be helpful to roll with resistance at this time. Invite new perspectives and give the family resources on how to find more information. Resistance is often a signal to respond differently. The clinician is there to be collaborative as much as the family chooses (Miller & Rollnick, 2002).

VIGNETTE CONTINUES

With Jackson and his family, it may be helpful to reflect back to the family their concerns. The clinician could say, "I understand there is a family history of speech delay. I also recognize that the behaviors I've observed during the appointment are different than behaviors noted at home." By exhibiting reflective listening at this stage, the family will know their apprehension regarding the observations are understood. It can also be helpful to gain their understanding surrounding symptoms of ASD. The family may have an inaccurate understanding of symptoms causing them to be resistant to acknowledging the validity of the diagnosis. Also, it will be important to understand what having a child with ASD would mean to them. The clinician could say, "Do you know someone with ASD? What symptoms does this person exhibit?" The family may be resistant to the diagnosis because of what they feel this may represent for their own or their child's future. If the family still appears resistant it can be helpful to discuss symptoms they agree are present, such as the speech delay in Jackson's history. They may be willing to initiate speech therapy as a starting point. Families may need time to process the appointment. By using motivational interviewing, it can facilitate engagement while allowing time and space to process the diagnosis.

Shared Decision Making

When considering a plan for intervention, it is important to integrate the concepts of shared decision making into the process. Key features of shared decision making include the following:

1. At least tw parties are involved.
2. Information is exchanged in both directions.
3. All parties are aware of treatment options and what they are.
4. All bring their knowledge and value-related priorities equally into the decision-making process.

Shared decision making is an interactive process in which patients (families and children, especially more cognitively able children) and physicians (and other involved professionals) simultaneously participate in all phases of the decision-making process and together arrive at a treatment plan to be implemented. Offering children information that is appropriate for their developmental age can help their understanding of their condition and treatments, reduce fear, and enhance self-confidence. Together, the clinician and family can consider choices, options, and ultimately decisions (Adams, Levy, & Council on Children With Disabilities, 2017).

Recognizing the Emotional Needs of the Family

Many families with a child with a developmental disability will grieve the loss of their ideal child. For parents with children with developmental disabilities, the gap between the idealized and actual child is generally larger, so the mourning process is more profound. Parents need an opportunity to tell their stories, to have their feelings validated, and to be offered support and community. Discussions about diagnosis and prognosis should be grounded in a hopeful, but realistic view of the future. Parents will often request input on the long-term vision for their child. It is essential to frame that discussion around realistic expectations while emphasizing the child and family's strengths and opportunities for promoting resilience and optimal outcomes. Parents may require support in letting go of what they cannot control while also being provided information on what they can do to help their child (Kennedy, 2015).

It is also important to validate the stress patients and families may be feeling. Begin conversations about emotional health and resilience early, at the time of diagnosis, and address it at most visits. Recognize that parents may have trouble acknowledging their feelings and underreport the extent of their distress. Highlight the importance of self-care for parents (Pickles et al., 2020).

One simple trigger question said with true meaning that can be helpful to open the door for discussion is, "How are you doing?"

MANAGING THE CHALLENGING INTERVIEW

Despite our best efforts to provide optimal care in a collaborative, supportive framework, inevitably some interactions will be challenging for clinicians to navigate. As providers, recognizing the physical or emotional responses triggered in ourselves by challenging patients/families or encounters may allow the provider to effectively partner with instead of confront the patient or family (Lorenzetti, Jacques, Donovan, Cottrell, & Buck, 2013).

Challenges can arise on either side of the therapeutic alliance. Common clinician factors may include negative bias toward specific health conditions, poor communication skills, and situational stressors. Implicit and explicit personally mediated racism is a factor that can affect health care delivery and general health outcomes, and as noted, clinicians need to be aware and examine these biases (Trent et al., 2019). Patient factors may include mental health concerns, multiple and poorly described symptoms, nonadherence to medical assistance, or self-destructive behaviors (Bruener & Moreno, 2011; Lorenzetti et al., 2013). Situational facts include time pressures during visits, patient-staff conflicts, and complex social issues. Recognizing barriers is an important first step in improving health education (Dreger & Tremback, 2002).

The clinician should monitor these factors during the difficult encounter and identify contributing factors. As in all encounters, we should be mindful to use empathic listening and a nonjudgmental caring attitude, but we should also evaluate for underlying patient-state factors that may be influencing the interaction. The clinician should help to identify these factors, discuss these openly, and use patient-centered communication to return to and reach a mutually agreed upon plan.

Korsch (2011) has illustrated several factors that may contribute to the difficult encounter. First, when the clinician-patient relationship may suffer from a mismatch, the clinician should evaluate the communication style. Parents may be overanxious or talk excessively, at which time the clinician can reassure and redirect, providing added structure and boundaries to the session. The clinician should address the problem, utilize and expand the support system, and give it time. For some patients, the clinician may need to schedule more frequent and focused visits, set appropriate boundaries for each visit, and agree on achievable goals (Lorenzetti et al., 2013).

Additionally, Lorenzetti et al. (2013) advised use of a CALMER approach to the difficult encounter by striving to be the catalyst for change, altering thoughts to change feelings, listening and then making a diagnosis, making an agreement, educating, and following up to reach out and discuss feelings.

These more involved visits may be challenging during a busy workday, so clinicians must self-monitor their own frustrations and fatigue and engage in self-care. Strategies to help clinicians identify personal factors that may contribute to a difficult encounter include self-reflection, recognizing biases, and discussions with an experienced colleague or seeking self-support (Lorenzetti et al., 2013).

VIGNETTE CONTINUES

Jackson's parents do not share the concerns of the clinician or his grandparents. Ideally, the clinician should allow for more time with the family or have them return within a week or two to revisit the discussion and provide support. Using empathic listening and a caring attitude, we can illustrate again why we are concerned, and together develop a mutually agreed upon plan for monitoring and intervention. "I understand that you have fewer concerns, but I have heard very few words used during my observations, and Jackson seems content to play alone. We can monitor his development closely, but it would be worthwhile to pursue early intervention programs to allow for specific guidance in facilitating his development and allowing him to interact more consistently with peers. What are your thoughts on that?"

CONCLUSION

The interview is the basis for understanding the biologic, genetic, social, and environmental factors that influence development and behavior. A well-organized interview sets the stage for a successful therapeutic alliance, which will lead to better clinician, patient, and family satisfaction, improved adherence, and long-term outcomes. The experienced clinician will demonstrate warmth and empathy from the moment of meeting and greeting to the shared decision-making process that will lead to agreement on diagnosis and a treatment plan. Motivational interviewing techniques can foster trust, gauge readiness for change, and guide the decision-making process. It is vital that clinician's embrace the use of telehealth technology to enhance access and improve efficiency.

REFERENCES

Adams, R. C., Levy, S. E., & Council on Children With Disabilities, (2017). Shared decision-making and children with disabilities: Pathways to consensus. *Pediatrics, 139*(6), e20170956.

Agency for Healthcare Research and Quality. (n.d.). Teach back quick guide. https://www.ahrq.gov/patientsafety/reports/engage/interventions/teachback.html

AimsCenter. (2020). Telehealth tips for behavioral health. University of Washington. aims.uw.edu/sites/default/files/Telehealth%20Tips%20for%20BH%20Providers_040220%20Final.pdf

Alfuraydan, M., Croxall, J., Hurt, L., Kerr, M., Brophy, S. (2020). Use of telehealth for facilitating the diagnostic assessment of autism spectrum disorder (ASD): A scoping review. *Plos One*, 1–16.

American Academy of Pediatrics Committee on Early Childhood, & Adoption and Dependent Care. (2011). The pediatrician's role in family support and family support programs. *Pediatrics, 128*(6), 1680–1684.

American Academy of Pediatrics Council on Community Pediatrics. (2016). Poverty and child health. *Pediatrics, 137*(4), e20160339. https://doi.org/10.1542/peds.2016-0339.

Andermann, A. (2016). Taking action on the social determinants of health in clinical practice: A framework for health professionals for the CLEAR Collaboration. *CMAJ Podcasts*. https://soundcloud.com/cmajpodcasts/160177-rev.

Beckman, H. B., & Frankel, R. M. (1984). The effect of physician behavior on the collection of data. *Annals of Internal Medicine, 101*(5), 692–696.

Behfourez, H. L., Drain, P. K., & Rhatigan, J. J. (2014). Rethinking the social history. *New England Journal of Medicine, 371*(14), 1277–1279.

Brcic, V., Eberdt, C., & Kaczorowski, J. (2011). Development of a tool to identify poverty in a family practice setting: A pilot study. *International Journal of Family Medicine*, 812. https://doi.org/10.1155/2011/812182.

Brock, D. M., Mauksch, L. B., Witteborn, S., Hummel, J., Nagasawa, P., & Robins, L. S. (2011). Effectiveness of intensive physician training in upfront agenda setting. *Journal of General Internal Medicine, 26*(11), 1317–1323.

Bruener, C. C., & Moreno, A. A. (2011). Approaches to the difficult patient/parent encounter. *Pediatrics, 127*(1), 163–169.

Cole, S. A., & Bird, J. (2014). *The medical interview: The three-function approach* (3rd ed.). Saunders Elsevier.

Cowan, A., Johnson R., Close H. (2020) Telepsychiatry in Psychotherapy Practice. Innov ations in Clinical Neuroscience, 17(4–6), 23–26.

Davies-House, A., Ball, N., & Balmer, C. (2017). Meeting and greeting in the clinical setting—are we doing what patients want? *British Dental Journal, 222*(6), 457–461.

Desai, N. (2019). The role of motivational interviewing in children and adolescents in pediatric care. *Pediatric Annals, 48*(9), e376–e379.

Dreger, V., & Tremback, T. (2002). Optimize patient health by treating literacy and language barriers. *AORN Journal, 75*(2), 280–285, 287, 289–293; quiz 297–300, 303–304.

Duby, J. C. (2018). Social and emotional development. In R. G. Voigt, M. M. Macias, S. M. Myers, & C. D. Tapia (Eds.), *Developmental and behavioral pediatrics* (2nd ed., pp. 223–250). American Academy of Pediatrics.

Goldstein, F. P., Klaiman, C., & Williams, S. (2017). Bridging care gaps: Using tele-health to provide care for people with autism spectrum disorder. *International Journal of Developmental Disabilities, 63*(4), 190–194.

Hooshmand, M., & Foronda, C. (2018). Comparison of telemedicine to traditional face-to-face for children with special needs: A quasiexperimental study. *Telemedicine and e-Health, 24*(6), 433–441.

Juckett, G., & Unger, K. (2014). Appropriate use of medical interpreters. *American Family Physician, 90*(7), 476–480.

Kennedy, D. (2015). Grieving the loss of the ideal child. *MindSpark*. https://mindsparklearning.com/grieving-the-loss-of-the-ideal-child/.

Korioth, T. (2021). Pediatric mental health experts share tips to make the most of telehealth visits. *American Academy of Pediatrics News*. https://www.aappublications.org/news/2021/01/15/officehours telehealth011521.

Korsch, B. (2011). Talking to families. In M. Augustyn, B. Zuckerman, & E. B. Caronna (Eds.), *The Zuckerman handbook of developmental behavioral pediatrics in primary care* (3rd ed., pp. 3–6). Lippincott Williams and Wilkins.

Langkamp, D. L., McManus, M. D., & Blakemore, S. D. (2015). Telemedicine for children with developmental disabilities: A more effective clinical process than office-based care. *Telemedicine and E-Health, 21*(2), 110–114.

Levetown, M. (2008). Communication with children and families: From everyday interactions to skill in conveying distressing information. *Pediatrics, 121*(5), 1441–1460.

Lorenzetti, R. C., Jacques, C. H. M., Donovan, C., Cottrell, C., & Buck, J. (2013). Managing difficult encounters: Understanding physician, patient and situational factors. *American Family Physician, 87*(6), 419–425.

Liu, Y. H., & Stein, M. T. (2019). Talking with children. In M. Augustyn & B. Zuckerman (Eds.), *Parker handbook of developmental and behavioral pediatrics for primary care* (4th ed.). Wolters Kluwer.

Miller, W. R., & Rollnick, S. (2002). *Motivational interviewing* (2nd ed.). Gilford Press.

Pickles, D. M., Lihn, S. L., Boat, T. F., & Lannon, C. (2020). A roadmap to emotional health for children and families with chronic pediatric conditions. *Pediatrics, 145*(2), e20191324.

Shah, P. E., & Ribaudo, J. (2018). Interviewing and counseling children and families. In R. G. Voight, M. M. Macias, S. M. Myers, & C. D. Tapia (Eds.), *Developmental and behavioral pediatrics* (2nd ed., pp. 61–77). American Academy of Pediatrics.

Studer, Q. (2003). *Hardwiring excellence* (pp. 285–292). Fire Starter Publishing.

Trent, M., Dooley, D. G., & Dougé, J. (2019). Section on Adolescent Health, Council on Community Pediatrics, Committee on Adolescence Pediatrics. The impact of racism on child and adolescent health. *Pediatrics*, *144*(2), e20191765.

Weiss, B. D., Mays, M. Z., Martz, W., Castro, K. M., DeWalt, D. A., Pignone, M. P., . . . Hale, F. A. (2005). Quick assessment of literacy in primary care: The newest vital sign. *Annals of Family Medicine*, *3*(6), 514–522.

Wender, E. H. (2009). Interviewing: A critical skill. In W. B. Carey, A. C. Crocker, W. L. Coleman, E. R. Elias, & H. M. Feldman (Eds.), *Developmental-behavioral pediatrics* (4th ed., pp. 747–756). Saunders Elsevier.

Zuckerman, B., & Wong, S. L. (2019). Family history: An opportunity to disrupt transmission of behavioral health problems. *Pediatrics*, *143*(6), e20183383.

78

The Physical Exam: Laying on of Hands...or Not

Jamie T. Rabot, Randall Phelps, and Heidi M. Feldman

For additional material related to the content of this chapter, please see Chapters 76 and 84.

> **VIGNETTE**
>
> ***History:*** *Dylan is a 12-year-old boy with previous diagnoses of attention-deficit/hyperactivity disorder and oppositional-defiant disorder. Multiple medications have been prescribed, with negligible benefits. His mother requests diagnostic reassessment. As you enter, Dylan and his mother are sitting on opposite sides of the room. Dylan responds to your greeting with an angry glare. He answers your introductory questions with only a glower. His mother answers for him. She rapidly enumerates his many challenging behaviors. She awkwardly draws a blank when you ask her to list some strengths. After the history, you ask her to go to the waiting room so you can complete a physical examination.*
>
> ***Physical examination:*** *Alone with Dylan, you struggle to make progress with your usual opening questions. So, you explain that you are going to do a physical examination. You start by first asking to see Dylan's hands. He reluctantly complies, extending his hands. You ask Dylan to squeeze your fingers. Dylan relishes squeezing your fingers a little too hard. You laugh, complimenting his strength, and playfully ask him to stop before he breaks your fingers. You proceed to test strength of his upper extremities. Dylan's expression softens and you reintroduce ice-breaker questions, working toward questions about home life. Dylan soon discloses key details about his mother's excessive drinking and fits of rage.*

Developmental-behavioral diagnosis is primarily based on history. Clinicians in developmental-behavioral medicine, such as psychiatrists and psychologists, may dispense with the physical examination. Certainly, developmental-behavioral diagnoses may often be made on basis of information gleaned from combination of interview, direct observations, questionnaires, and psychological testing. Nevertheless, physical examination serves as a valuable component of the diagnostic workup for three reasons. First, the exam may reveal subtle or previously missed findings that provide the explanation for a developmental disorder. Second, the physical examination offers the clinician an opportunity to model for caregivers approaches that promote calmness and cooperation. Third, the exam offers an opportunity to create an emotional connection with a child. Particularly if the clinician has obtained a long history in which the child was only rarely involved, the physical examination allows the clinician to link back with the child, using a combination of physical and nonphysical means. In the chapter-opening vignette, the exam helped Dylan to relax and thus allowed him to reveal his true feelings. The response of the child to kind and supportive interactions in such cases provides a wealth of information, often as relevant to diagnosis as the physical findings. When done skillfully, the physical exam contributes to the positive relationship among clinicians, parents, and children.

CONDUCTING THE PHYSICAL EXAMINATION

The setting of the physical exam can enhance its utility. The physical examination is often best done after the history, when the information collected during the interview can guide the examination. Moreover, especially if the clinician makes efforts to engage the child in the discussion, the shy or fearful child may have had an adequate chance to warm up or relax.

To establish a positive relationship, the physical exam should begin with conversation with the child. Simple questions, such as the child's favorite foods or the name of the family's pet, serve to demonstrate the supportive nature of the interaction. Repositioning of seating may be helpful to demarcate this actual physical exam from the conversational part of the assessment. Whenever possible, the examiner should be comfortably seated at eye level with the child. The examination should proceed in a systematic and calm manner, allowing the examiner to introduce each part of the examination and to provide reassurance when necessary.

In examining preschoolers, school-age children, and adolescents, we advocate starting with a request to see the patient's hands. The advantage of starting with the hands is that the maneuver is relatively unintimidating. For shy or fearful children, we remain relatively distal, moving closer only as their behavior suggests they are ready. After the children place their hands in ours, we may ask a question about a bracelet, or a scrape, or other distinctive features of the hands. This moment provides an opportunity to assess social and communication skills. We proceed to test upper extremity tone and strength, joint range of motion, dexterity, rapid alternating movements, and right-left discrimination. These tasks are

TABLE 78.2 Nonspecific Dysmorphic Features Associated With Anomalous Brain Development

Body Part	Dysmorphic Features	Pathogenesis/Possible Significance
Cranium	Microcephaly	Reduced brain growth
	Asymmetry	Premature suture fusion, deforming external forces, or abnormal underlying brain growth
Hair	Absent or multiple (>2) parietal whorls	Abnormal brain development between 10 and 16 wk gestation
	"Cowlick," or anterior upsweep of scalp hair	Posterior displacement of junction of parietal and frontal hair streams, resulting from reduced frontal brain development
Eyes	Short palpebral fissures	Deficient frontal brain growth
	Up-slanted palpebral fissures	Relatively deficient frontal brain growth as compared with midface growth
Ears	Low set (below top of helix, below outer canthi)	Delayed morphogenesis, fetal pattern of ear position
	Posterior rotation (axis tilted backward >15 degrees)	Delayed morphogenesis, fetal pattern of posterior ear rotation
Mouth	High arched	Persistent lateral palatal ridges, indicative of oral hypotonia or other oral-motor dysfunction

TABLE 78.3 Miscellaneous Physical Exam Findings of Developmental or Behavioral Significance

Finding	Possible Significance
Tonsillar hypertrophy	Obstructive sleep apnea
Alopecia	Trichotillomania, stereotypies involving scalp
Ecchymoses over soft tissues	Nonaccidental trauma
Bitten nails, cuticles, callouses	Self-mutilation, stereotypies
Characteristic scars	Self-cutting
Discoloration of dorsum of hand, posterior molar acid damage, parotid hyperplasia	Bulimia nervosa

Neurologic Examination

The neurologic examination is a crucial component of the developmental assessment as it may provide evidence for neurologic immaturity or focal neurologic injury. A systematic assessment of the evolution of complex reflexes can indicate neurodevelopmental delay, such as is seen in global developmental delay, or neurodevelopmental deviance, such as is seen in cerebral palsy. A systematic approach, such as has been developed in the Milani-Comparetti Motor Development Screening Test, evaluates the child's posture and tone in different positions, the development of motor skills, the evolution of primitive reflexes, and protective responses to rapid movement (Trembath, Kliewer, & Bruce, 1977).

Careful examination of cranial nerve function may help in elucidating focal lesions. Examples of findings on cranial nerve examination with the corresponding significance are provided in Table 78.4 (Maria, 2005). Clues to developmental diagnoses may be provided by abnormalities of tone, strength, coordination, or deep tendon reflexes. Systematic examination of each of these features should be included in developmental assessments. Table 78.5 summarizes some key findings with their corresponding significance (Maria, 2005).

TABLE 78.4 Significance of Findings on Examination of Cranial Nerves

Finding	Possible Significance
Vertical nystagmus	Brainstem dysfunction
Horizontal or rotary nystagmus	Congenital abnormality, vestibular abnormality, medication side effect
Pupil asymmetry	Intracranial mass effect, midbrain dysfunction, optic nerve abnormality, medication side effect Associated with ptosis and anhydrosis: Horner syndrome (Note: 10% of children have subtle baseline pupil asymmetry.)
Ptosis	Impaired sympathetic innervation, myasthenia gravis, cranial nerve (CN) III dysfunction
Increased width of palpebral fissure	Upper motor neuron dysfunction, CN VII dysfunction
In-turning of eye or impaired abduction	CN VI dysfunction
Positive cover test	Esophoria or exophoria
Upper and lower facial weakness	CN VII dysfunction
Isolated lower facial weakness	Stroke

TABLE 78.5 Key Findings on Neuromuscular Examination and Associated Diagnoses

Key Findings	Possible Significance
Asymmetry of muscle tone, bulk, or range of motion	Cerebral palsy, stroke, peripheral lesion
Weakness Most sensitive: deltoids, wrist extensors, hamstrings, ankle dorsiflexors Least sensitive: handgrip, biceps, quadriceps, gastrocnemius	Neuromuscular disorders
Asymmetry of rapid alternating movements	Dyscoordination, associated with many disorders, including ADHD, ASD
Slowness of attempted rapid pincer movements or toe-tapping	Upper motor neuron dysfunction
Irregularity of attempted rapid pincer movements or toe-tapping	Cerebellar dysfunction
Abnormal finger-nose-finger testing	Tremor, dysmetria, dyscoordination
Decreased deep tendon reflexes	Muscular, peripheral nerve, acute upper motor neuron or cerebellar abnormality
Increased deep tendon reflexes, clonus	Brain or spinal cord lesion, such as cerebral palsy

ADHD, Attention-deficit/hyperactivity disorder; *ASD*, autism spectrum disorder.

WHEN WE ARE UNABLE TO LAY ON HANDS: TELEHEALTH

The COVID-19 pandemic prompted a dramatic and abrupt increase in the use of telehealth. It is highly likely that telehealth will remain a substantial part of our ongoing practice of developmental-behavioral pediatrics. In this section we discuss how we can examine a child when we practice telehealth.

General Principles

Telemedicine is the use of telecommunication technology to exchange medical information and provide clinical care to patients at a distance. Telehealth, which refers to the broader scope of remote health care services, was initially introduced in the 1960s and gained popularity in the 1990s as technological advances increased and associated costs declined (Perednia & Allen, 1995). Initially intended to improve health care delivery for patients in remote settings, telemedicine now has a wide clinical scope with the purpose of providing more convenient, safe, and cost-efficient care. The COVID-19 pandemic catalyzed the rapid adoption of telemedicine. Widespread use was facilitated by lifting regulatory restrictions on the platform used and by insurance companies reassuring reimbursement even for new patient consultations (Hirko & Kerver, 2020).

Advantages of the Telehealth Visit

Telehealth is a cost-effective strategy for increasing access to care for families, especially those who live in rural locations (Soares & Langkamp, 2012). It decreases the nonmedical costs of accessing health care and eliminates common frustrations, such as transportation expense, time in traffic, parking, and navigating a large campus. Prior to the COVID-19 pandemic, data supported a rise in patient satisfaction and a decrease in no-show and short notice cancellation with the use of telemedicine (Joshi, 2014). Advantages of telehealth that are specific for the care of children with neurodevelopmental and behavioral disorders include the ability to see children in their natural environments, including home and school. Telehealth platforms may permit coordination of interdisciplinary teams, regardless of geographic location. An initial telehealth visit can be used to gather initial data or to clarify referral questions for additional subspecialty services that may be needed.

Limitations of the Telehealth Visit

The most obvious limitation in telemedicine, especially for new consultations, is the inability for the clinician to complete all parts of the examination. Thus it is crucial that the clinician determine when a virtual visit is inadequate and have systems in place to expedite an in-person examination visit. The method introduces significant challenges for families with language barriers, lack of access to technology or bandwidth, or knowledge for troubleshooting technological difficulties (Guido-Estrada, 2020). Real-time telemedicine may be difficult with children with developmental disabilities who cannot cooperate with clinicians via remote methods. Asynchronous or store-and-forward telemedicine may offer benefits for children with developmental-behavioral problems due to more flexibility in the timing of data collection for the visit. These include avoiding the need for special equipment or staff during travel, decreasing anxiety for the child and parents, and increasing the likelihood of a successful examination (Langkamp, Mcmanus, & Blakemore, 2015).

Examination in the Telehealth Visit

Like an in-person examination, the telehealth visit offers opportunities to assess a wide array of physical, developmental, and behavioral features and to see a child in interaction with family. The setting is important in telehealth, just as it is in the office.

Patient Privacy and Security

Videoconferencing interactions are generally required to comply with the Health Insurance Portability and Accountability

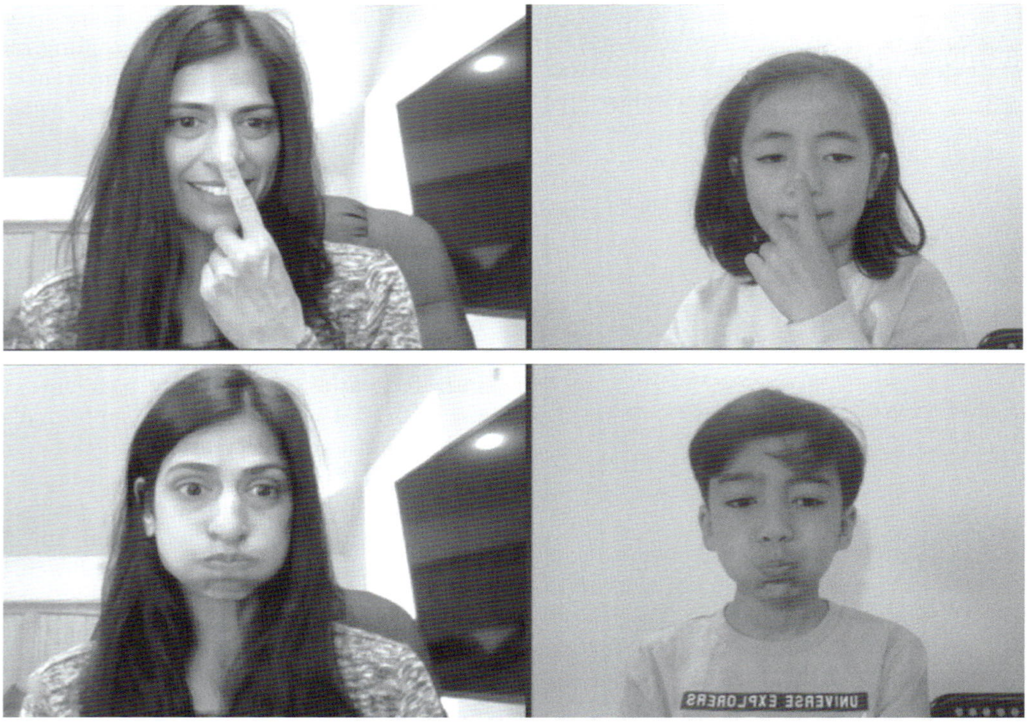

Fig. 78.3 Televisit. Position the camera at a level where it does not cut off the top of the clinician's head. Allow some distance between the camera and clinician to give the impression that the clinician is looking directly at the patient and caregiver. Demonstrate components of virtual neurologic examination and establishing connection with patient virtually.

Act (HIPAA) of 1996. Just as important as HIPAA, pediatric clinicians need to comply with the Children's Online Privacy Protection Act (COPPA, 2013), which assigns parents in control when it comes to collection of personal information from children under 13 years old. Unlike an office visit, it is important to consider the privacy of the family's setting. Ensure that only those individuals who are involved in the visit are present. It is possible to use telehealth to have private conversations with parents while children are not in the same room. Ensure that the child is safe in the home, if the child is not present.

The Clinician's Considerations

The clinician should consider whether the remote connection facilitates interaction and encourages trust. A few tips are as follows (Fig. 78.3): Ensure that the lighting in the room is in front of the clinician, avoid bright lights behind or next to the clinician, allow distance between the camera and clinician to give the impression that the clinician is looking directly at the child and caregiver, look directly into the camera so as to appear to be directly speaking to the patient and caregiver, limit noise, and use a microphone with good sound quality (Northeast Telehealth Resource Center [NTRC], 2020).

The Child and Family Considerations

It is helpful to create instructions for caregivers on how to access the virtual system, including how to get started and how to navigate it. It may be helpful for a medical assistant to check the family in to make sure technology is working well (NTRC, 2020). As with in-person visits, consideration of the child's safety while parents are providing history and during the developmental examination is paramount (Grefe, Hsieh, & Joshi, 2020). To prepare for optimal virtual observations it is helpful to request that the family have materials available at the time of the examination (Table 78.6)

TABLE 78.6 Suggested Items During Virtual Visits to Assist With Behavioral Observation and Neurologic Examination

Child Age	Suggested Toys and Tools
Infant and toddler	Shiny or visually interesting toy Rattle or other noise-making toy Flashlight or other source of light Crayons and paper Soft ball
Preschool and school-age child	Crayons or pen/pencil and paper Favorite books Soft ball, size of tennis ball Cotton swab or soft tool for sensory exam Flashlight or other source of light

The physical (Box 78.1) and neurologic (Box 78.2) examinations can be accomplished via telehealth, using ingenuity and parental engagement. Fig. 78.3 demonstrates how a positive relationship can be established with a child in telehealth,

BOX 78.1 The Virtual Physical Examination

Vital signs and constitutional. Parents can measure height, weight, and head circumference. For the head circumference, ask the parent to measure the head at the largest point on the forehead and around the head just above the ear pinna, using a tape measure. If done during the visit, observe the child for any signs of distress. Make observations of the child's behavior, as in an office visit.

Skin. Request that the parent allow you to examine the entire skin surface and notate any skin lesions. Ask the caregiver to show you the child's back.

Head, eyes, ears, nose, and throat. Observe for signs of facial dysmorphisms. Ask parent to use the video from the camera on the backside of the smartphone to provide a clear view of the oropharynx.

Neck. Instruct the child to look over the right shoulder and then look over the left shoulder. Ask about pain or limitation with motion.

Lungs. Ask patients to deeply inhale and exhale through an open mouth. Listen for coughing or wheezing. Observe for tachypnea and accessory muscle use as signs of impaired respiration.

Heart. Ask the child/caregiver to take the pulse at the wrist. Have them count out the beats they feel. If children have an Apple Watch or similar smartphone technology, including AliveCor from Kardia.10,11, heart rates and electrocardiogram may be displayed via the monitor during the visit or uploaded prior to the visit.

Abdomen. Look for protuberance and scarring. The presence of any feeding tubes (G-tube, J-tube) should be documented as well.

Extremities. Assess for range of motion, signs of deformity, or local inflammation

Adapted from Benziger, Z. (2021). The telehealth ten: A guide for a patient-assisted virtual physical examination. *American Journal of Medicine, 134*(1), 48–51.

BOX 78.2 The Virtual Neurologic Exam

Mental status. Observe level of alertness, awareness, or interaction with the environment. Try to get the child's attention. Observe the interaction with the caregivers, including games such as Peek-a-Boo. Engage in conversation with the child.

Cranial nerves

II, III, IV, VI: Have the caregiver gently hold the child's head, then move a visually interesting toy (or the caregiver's face for infants) in all directions. Observe for nystagmus, disconjugate movements or failure to track and regard. Ask caregivers to dim lights and then shine a light into baby's eyes. Observe for red reflex and subtle nystagmus. Ask parents to cover the child's eyes, one eye at a time while the patient is looking at the camera.

V, VII: Ask the child to open the mouth ("Show me all your teeth!" or "Roar like a lion"). Assess facial symmetry in smiling, chewing, talking.

VIII: Ask about hearing and hearing aids.

IX, X: Assess swallowing.

XI, XII: Observe tongue protrusion at rest and during crying. Assess tongue for fasciculations if close-up is possible.

Motor

Observe the child sitting in the caregiver's lap and while lying on a flat surface, determining whether the infant's posture is normal or is frog-legged vs hyperextended.

Observe movements for symmetry. Ask caregivers to gently pull on each limb and release and observe for normal recoil response.

Motor strength: Ask child to dance like a chicken, get up from the floor, or play Head, Shoulders, Knees, and Toes.

Parents can perform many maneuvers with infants, especially if you model with a doll, such as scarf sign, horizontal and vertical suspension, and weight bearing.

Observe independent sitting, crawling, standing, walking, jumping, running, and hopping (with camera on lower extremities).

Observe reach, grasp, transfer. Observe drawing and writing.

Sensory. Assess vision and hearing during cranial nerve exam. Observe response to touch on different body parts, differentiating left and right, proximal and distal, medial and lateral.

Cerebellar. Observe for tremor or dysmetria with finger-to-nose or reach. Observe gait.

Reflexes. Parents can perform many primitive reflexes with infants, especially if you model with a doll, including rooting, Moro, tonic neck, truncal incurvation, palmar and plantar grasp, and parachute reflex. Deep tendon reflexes are difficult to illicit without a skilled examiner.

Adapted fromGrefe, A., Hsieh, D., Joshi, C., et al. (2020). Pediatric neurological exam via telemedicine. ***Child Neurology Society***, 1e9.

BOX 78.3 Ideal Visits for Telehealth

- Patients who require multiple visits for medication management, including those with attention-deficit/hyperactivity disorder, depression, anxiety disorders
- Behavioral consultations where observations made as well as video recordings done in the child's natural setting may be helpful in diagnosis, including autism assessment
- Visits where treatment plans are often derived from history, including sleep disorders, feeding problems, discipline difficulties, enuresis, and encopresis
- Visits that require split appointments on same-day service (e.g., children with history of trauma, children in split-household families)

similar to what we have described for in-person visits. Box 78.3 lists ideal candidates for telehealth.

CONCLUSION

Physical examination is a valuable feature of the developmental and behavioral evaluation. It may uncover the cause of a developmental or behavioral problem, allowing families to know the reason for the disorder, the prognosis, and the recurrence risk in other family members. Parents can observe approaches to assist their children with developmental and behavioral problems, such as maintaining composure, complying with requests, and responding to positive reinforcement. The laying on of hands, as we saw in the opening vignette with Dylan, facilitates the creation of a relationship between the clinician and the child. When we touch our patients, we make a literal connection that can serve as a warm beginning of a therapeutic alliance. As we expand the use of telehealth evaluations in developmental-behavioral pediatrics, we need to consider substitute strategies for establishing that relationship and alternatives to accomplish our clinical objectives.

REFERENCES

Benziger, Z. (2021). The telehealth ten: A guide for a patient-assisted virtual physical examination. *American Journal of Medicine*, *134*(1), 48–51.

Dixon, S. D., & Stein, M. T. (2006). *Encounters with children: Pediatric behavior and development*. Elsevier Science Health Science.

Grefe, A., Hsieh, D., Joshi, C., et al. (2020). Pediatric neurological exam via telemedicine. *Child Neurology Society*, 1e9.

Guido-Estrada, N. (2020). Embracing telemedicine: The silver lining of a pandemic. *Pediatric Neurology*, *113*, 13–14.

Hirko, K., & Kerver, J. (2020). Telehealth in response to the COVID-19 pandemic: Implications for rural health disparities. *Journal of the American Medical Informatics Association*, *27*(11), 1816–1818.

Holden, E. W., Tarnowski, K. J., & Prinz, R. J. (1983). Reliability of neurological soft signs in children: Re-evaluation of the paness. *Journal of Abnormal Child Psychology*, *10*(12), 163–172.

Jones, K. L. (2006). *Smith's recognizable patterns of human malformation*. Elsevier.

Joshi, C. (2014). Telemedicine in pediatric neurology. *Pediatric Neurology*, *51*, 189–191.

Langkamp, D. A., Mcmanus, M. D., & Blakemore, S. D. (2015). Telemedicine for children with developmental disabilities: A more effective clinical process than office-based care. *Telehealth and e-Health*, 21.

Maria, B. L. (2005). *Current management in child neurology* (3rd ed.). B.C. Decker.

Northeast Telehealth Resource Center. (2020). Tips for professional video conferencing and telepresenting. https://www.netrc.org

Perednia, D. A., & Allen, A. (1995). Telemedicine technology and clinical applications. *JAMA*, *273*(6), 483–488.

Soares, N., & Langkamp, D. (2012). Telehealth in developmental-behavioral pediatrics. *Journal of Developmental and Behavioral Pediatrics*, *33*, 656–665.

Stinnett, T. A., Oehler-Stinnett, J., Fuqua, D. R., & Palmer, L. S. (2002). Examination of the underlying structure of the nepsy: A developmental neuropsychological assessment. *Journal of Psychoeducational Assessment*, *20*(1), 66–82.

Trembath, J. T., Kliewer, D., & Bruce, W. (1977). *The Milani-Comparetti motor development screening test*. University of Nebraska Medical Center. Media Resource Center, C Louis Meyer Children's Rehabilitation Institute.

79

Evaluation of Children Who Are Nonverbal/Minimally Verbal

Casey E. Krueger and Jessica Patel

For additional material related to the content of this chapter, please see Chapters 76 and 84.

VIGNETTE

Isabella is a 4-year 8-month-old girl referred for a neuropsychological evaluation by her neurologist. The purpose of the evaluation is to gain an understanding of her neuropsychological functioning, with an emphasis of nonverbal domains, in order to recommend appropriate school placement for kindergarten and to guide therapeutic treatment recommendations for therapy. She has a history of symptomatic generalized epilepsy and an expressive language delay. Isabella met early developmental milestones on time. She began having seizures around 18 months of age. She continued to make developmental progress in the setting of ongoing seizures in all domains except expressive language. She currently speaks in one- or two-word utterances that are difficult to understand.

Isabella had two seizures in the morning of the evaluation and her mother noted that she is more tired than usual. You observe that Isabella is very friendly, maintains eye contact, and responds appropriately to commands. She points out things that she sees while walking to the evaluation room and asks you to "help" her with the buttons on her raincoat. Isabella becomes frustrated during testing when she does not know the answer. She refuses to complete verbal tasks. She has difficulty maintaining attention and engagement throughout the evaluation and needs praise and rewards after each task.

What are the best methods and tools to evaluate Isabella? Will the evaluation be valid and reliable?

It is common for clinicians in a developmental-behavioral pediatric clinic to see children with limited verbal skills. Of course, this population includes preverbal infants and young children who have not yet learned language and speech. However, preschoolers, school-age children, and adolescents may also be nonverbal or minimally verbal. Clinicians need to understand how to modify their usual approaches to work with this population of children in a competent and effective manner. This chapter will cover the following topics:

- Which children are unable to use verbal language effectively for communication?
- What are specific areas to cover in interview with their families?
- What are critical observations to make of the child during interaction and play?
- How can standardized psychological testing be used effectively in this population?

DEFINING THE POPULATION OF CHILDREN WHO ARE MINIMALLY VERBAL

The terms *nonverbal* and *minimally verbal* are often used to describe children with few to no spoken words or few fixed words or phrases that are used for communication (Kasari, Brady, Lord, & Tager-Flusberg, 2013). In this chapter we use the term *minimally verbal* to describe this population of children. Minimally verbal children may have sensory, neurologic, cognitive, speech, or psychiatric conditions. Table 79.1 summarizes numerous conditions that may lead a child to be minimally verbal.

Unfortunately, many of these children are poorly understood because they are frequently excluded from research studies (Bal, Katz, Bishop, & Krasileva, 2016). Many professionals may assume that the children have autism spectrum disorder (ASD) or are significantly cognitively impaired. However, minimally verbal is not synonymous with intellectually disabled. For example, it is difficult for people with auditory neuropathy to communicate through spoken language because the condition compromises their ability to send speech sounds to the brain for comprehension, but they may have intact cognitive and social function. Landau-Kleffner syndrome is a rare language disorder characterized by the loss of the ability to use or understand language (auditory agnosia) in association with seizures. There may be a complete loss of the ability to speak, while hearing and intelligence are usually preserved (Pearl, Carrazana, & Holmes, 2001). Children with selective mutism, a childhood anxiety disorder characterized by a child's ability to speak only in select social settings, may have an accompanying expressive language disorder; however, this co-occurrence is difficult to assess because of the paucity of language output during evaluations (Wong, 2010). Even when children do function in the range of intellectual disability, being minimally verbal may lead to an underestimate of their cognitive abilities. Children with Down syndrome often have their cognitive skills underestimated in part because their ability to speak is below their receptive language and nonverbal cognitive skills (Hickey, Hickey, & Summar, 2012). Understanding the nuances of these conditions and their impact on a child's overall functioning, including relations to cognition, receptive language, and motor skills, is a critical part of the evaluation process.

TABLE 79.1 **Examples of Children Who May Be Minimally Verbally**

Category	Example	Characteristics
Neurodevelopmental disorder	Autism spectrum disorder (wide variety of skills)	May have severe delays in expressive language and/or language regression
Intellectual disability	Down syndrome	Mild-moderate intellectual disability, better receptive than expressive language, weakness in syntactic processing and verbal working memory, strength in visual-spatial skills
Sensory impairment	Deaf children, auditory neuropathy, progressive hearing loss	May detect some sounds, but have poor speech-perception abilities, difficulty understanding spoken speech
Neurologic disorder	Landau-Kleffner, other seizure disorder, brain injury, tumor	Auditory verbal agnosia (loss of language comprehension) and verbal expression (aphasia)
Motor speech disorder	Severe apraxia	Difficulty coordinating the complex oral movements needed to create sounds into syllables and words, motor speech disorder
Motor disorder	Cerebral palsy and other motor disorders	Verbal dystonia
Psychiatric disorder	Severe trauma, selective mutism	Inability to speak in select settings or at select times

CAREGIVER INTERVIEW

When working with any child or family, the first and most important step in the assessment process is to understand the goals of the current evaluation (Urbina, 2014). This step is generally achieved through a caregiver interview. The interview is the typical strategy for obtaining a complete developmental history, which may be supplemented with a developmental questionnaire (see Chapter 77).

With a minimally verbal child it is particularly important to expand beyond a basic developmental interview to gain information to understand the child's strengths and needs. The history should investigate the child's medical history, including information about any preexisting diagnoses. It is also important to ensure that the child has been evaluated by an audiologist and to understand those findings. In discussing the child's developmental milestones, the history about any regressions that may have occurred and in which domains is also important diagnostically.

While a minimally verbal child may have speech and/or expressive language difficulties, the child may have adequate or strong social communication. The interview should focus on how a child communicates with the family and how, in turn, the family communicates with the child. More specifically, it is important to gain a rich understanding about how the child communicates wants and needs, how the child invites others to interact socially, how the child shares interests with the family, and how the child and family manage joint attention. Children may communicate with gesture, sign, facial expression, exaggerated movements, or stylized actions. Their attempts may be conventional, shared with a large community, or idiosyncratic, shared only with their family or invented by the children. It is important to ask about any use of assistive and augmentative communication strategies (AAC), including picture exchange communication system (PECS), sign language, or electronic devices. Moreover, understanding how and when these are accessed is also critical. Some children use AAC spontaneously with great effect, whereas others may avoid or resist using AAC. For some, AAC is available at school but not at home. It is important to know if the family uses verbal communication, sign, and/or visual supports (pictures, schedules) to communicate with the child and if so how well they work.

Children who are minimally verbal may or may not have delays in their adaptive functioning. It is necessary to ask about their overall daily living skills, communication skills, and adaptive skills. For minimally verbal children, measures of adaptive functioning are of particular importance, as they may help to provide an estimate of their functional ability, particularly when their participation in cognitive evaluations is adversely impacted by their age, ability to participate, or limited verbal production.

Understanding their social skills is also particularly important for not only diagnostic clarification but also for informing treatment recommendations. This domain includes questions surrounding their relationship with their siblings, cousins or close friends, peers at school, their parents, other adults in the community, other professionals who may work with them, and individuals who they do not know well. It is also important to ask about communication used for social purposes, such as requesting, sharing interests, use of gestures, and reciprocal interactions.

CRITICAL OBSERVATIONS TO MAKE OF THE CHILD DURING INTERACTION AND PLAY

It is critical to observe children in their play, interactions with their parents, and interaction with you during the evaluation session. This step is particularly important because minimally verbal children may not be readily assessed with structured instruments. Moreover, children learn language in a social context, making it especially important to examine social behavior. Social skills that are used for communicative purposes can be viewed as foundational prelinguistic skills for all children. Joint engagement serves as a springboard between caregivers and children to promote the development of spoken language. In addition, improving symbolic play has been associated with an increase in expressive language skills for children with autism who are minimally verbal (Chang, Shih, Landa, Kaiser, & Kasari, 2018).

During the observations, noting the level of imitation, joint attention, affect sharing, requesting, and play skills is important as children use these abilities to learn spoken language (Kasari, Gulsrud, Freeman, Paparella, & Hellemann, 2012). Gestural attainment, rate of communication, and parent response contingency were factors found to be significant predictors of language outcomes in young children with developmental disabilities (Brady, Marquis, Fleming, & McLean, 2004). These skills may be observed in toddlers and preschoolers who are predominantly preverbal. Assessing these skills in older minimally verbal children is also important with adaptations, particularly in terms of materials used, to ensure the stimuli are appropriate for the child's developmental age and their interests.

Evaluating for repetitive and atypical behaviors is important. Repetitive speech and repetitive object play, but not repetitive body movements, may differentially predict developmental outcomes, including language (Watt, Wetherby, Barber, & Morgan, 2008). Documentation in this area may include watching how the child interacts with toys and asking simple questions: Does the child always play in the same way with toys? Does the child inspect or spin the toys repetitively? Does the child play with toys appropriately at developmental level?

PSYCHOLOGICAL ASSESSMENT

Deciding on a protocol for evaluating a minimally verbal child is dependent on several factors, including the child's age and presenting concerns. A joint assessment with a speech-language pathologist (SLP) is recommended, if possible (see Chapter 107). A SLP may utilize creative strategies for eliciting communication and interpreting limiting speech output based on observations and/or speech samples. SLPs are in a unique position to plan interventions because of their knowledge and skills in effective communication treatments. Table 79.2 includes information on sample instrument selection depending on age and domain of the child. Please refer to the chapters on neuropsychological (Chapter 87) and cognitive testing (Chapter 85) for detailed information about these domains. As with all assessments, multiple domains are typically assessed.

Nonverbal Cognitive Functioning

Generally speaking, standardized measures of intelligence include measures of both nonverbal and verbal skills; however, children who are minimally verbal would clearly have deficits in their verbal scores. Thus lowered overall cognitive scores could be attributed to a child's language weaknesses rather than a true deficit in overall cognitive abilities.

For children who are nonverbal or minimally verbal, a nonverbal cognitive test provides the best estimate of that child's current cognitive functioning. Alternatively, using a test that offers a nonverbal index can provide estimates of a child's nonverbal functioning (Wechsler, 2012, 2014). Overall, a nonverbal cognitive test provides an estimate of cognitive functioning without the impact of language weaknesses, which is critical for minimally verbal patients.

Selecting a nonverbal cognitive test includes consideration of the child's understanding of language. If the test has verbally presented directions, then the assessment of nonverbal cognition will be confounded by receptive language abilities (DeThorne & Shaffer, 2004). Therefore, if there are also receptive language delays, the child would benefit from a task that has visual, rather than verbal, directions. If the child's receptive language is intact, selecting a test that requires comprehension of verbal instructions may be acceptable. Additional considerations in test selection include if the test is timed or untimed, as untimed tests may provide a better estimate of a child's nonverbal cognitive abilities (Kasari et al., 2013).

Overall, cognitive tests have long been thought to not only provide a snapshot into a child's current abilities but to be predictive of future abilities. In addition, if a cognitive test is appropriately selected, administered, and interpreted in a way that leads to meaningful interventional approaches for a young child, positive changes in the child's academic functioning may occur (Kaufman, Raiford, & Coalson, 2016). Thus ensuring that the test being used for decision making about a child is one that is appropriate for a minimally verbal child is critical to interpretation (see Chapter 76). The Leiter International Performance Scale and the Raven's Colored Progressive Matrices are two of the most widely used tests for an estimate of nonverbal cognitive skills for children with ASD (Kasari et al., 2013). For children with general language weaknesses, the UNIT or TONI-3 are often recommended by language professionals (DeThorne & Shaffer, 2004)

Communication Skills

Language is a complex method of communication (see Chapter 44). Language components include expressive, receptive, articulation, and social language skills, and it is a particularly challenging domain to assess in minimally verbal children.

Receptive language is of particular importance to evaluate with minimally verbal children as this ability is associated with overall level of general intellectual functioning (full-scale IQ) and prognosis (Selassie, Jennische, Kyllerman, Viggedal,

TABLE 79.2 Sample Test Selection by Age and Domain for Minimally Verbal Children

Instrument	Ages	Considerations
Cognitive		
Leiter International Performance Scale, Third Edition (Leiter-3: Roid, Miller, Pomplun, & Koch, 2013)	3–75+ yr	One of the most widely used tests for an estimate of nonverbal cognitive skills for children with autism spectrum disorder (ASD) (Kasari et al., 2013)
Raven's Colored Progressive Matrices (John, 2003)	5+	One of the most widely used tests for an estimate of nonverbal cognitive skills for children with ASD (Kasari et al., 2013)
Test of Nonverbal Intelligence, Fourth Edition (TONI-4; Brown, Sherbenou, & Johnsen, 2010)	6:0–89:11	For children with general language weaknesses, the UNIT or TONI-3 are often recommended by language professionals (DeThorne & Shaffer, 2004)
Universal Nonverbal Intelligence Test 2 (UNIT-2; Bracken & McCallum, 2016)	5–21 yr, 11 mo	For children with general language weaknesses, the UNIT or TONI-3 are often recommended by language professionals (DeThorne & Shaffer, 2004)
Language Skills		
Bayley Scales of Infant and Toddler Development, Fourth Edition (Bayley-4; Bayley & Aylward, 2019)	16 days–42 mo	Includes measures of expressive and receptive language
The MacArthur-Bates Communication Development Inventories (M-CDI; Fenson, Marchman, Thal, Reznick, & Bates, 2006)	8–37 mo	A parent-report inventory of expressive and receptive language
Peabody Picture Vocabulary Test, Fifth Edition (PPVT-5; Dunn, 2019)	2:6–90+ yr	Receptive vocabulary
Preschool Language Scales-5 (PLS-5; Zimmerman, Steiner, & Pond, 2011)	Birth–7:11 yr	Expressive communication and auditory comprehension
Communicative Intent		
Complexity Communication Scale (CCS; Brady et al., 2018)	Infants–adults	Preintentional and intentional expressive communication (joint attention, gestures, language)
Early Social Communication Scales (ESCS; Mundy et al., 2003)	8–30 mo	Nonverbal communication skills

& Hartelius, 2005). Those who are minimally verbal would be expected to show a wide range of skills in this area because they may be extremely delayed or highly advanced.

Children who are minimally verbal may show a variety of expressive and social language responses. Some children may point, gesture, or make word approximations to respond. Other children may use signs or other gestures to indicate a response. Some children may be able to point with a pencil or have a stuffed animal point for them. Use of an AAC device may help children express themselves more fully. Interact with the child first to build rapport and test out communication methods. Note the form and function of words, sounds, and any communication. Also, take note of tone and the use of and responsiveness to nonverbal communication.

While a clinician may use traditional measures of language functioning in children who are minimally verbal and adapt them as needed to incorporate different communication modalities, the standardized scoring methods do not allow adaptation for use with children who communicate using alternative modalities. Thus reporting any adaptations of procedure and how they may have impacted the results is critical.

Behavioral Rating Scales

Children with language disorders have more symptoms of social, emotional, and behavioral problems relative to peers (Norbury, Gooch, & Wray, 2016). Therefore it is important to include measures of emotional and behavioral functioning when evaluating minimally verbally children (Chapter 82). Children with language impairment exhibited lower internalizing scores on the Child Behavior Checklist but higher lethargy and irritability scores on the Aberrant Behavior Checklist compared to verbally fluent children (Fok & Bal, 2019). A limitation of rating scale items is a frequent assumption that expressive language skills are present, which can compromise the validity of the assessment. Examination of individual test items can assist accurate interpretation.

Additional Areas for Consideration

An evaluation of a minimally verbal child may assess academic skills, fine motor or visual-motor concerns, memory skills, or executive functioning tests. Consideration must again be made to allow for nonverbal responses and determining the understanding of verbally presented directions prior to proceeding.

Academics

When evaluating a nonverbal child's academic skills, one may consider a direct observation of a child's academic skills rather than presenting them with a test that may require oral directions or verbal responses. Measures of adaptive functioning (as discussed earlier) may also provide information about a child's academic skills. In addition, children may also be allowed to use assistive technology rather than presenting with verbal responses (Frisby, 2003). The documentation of any modification (e.g., if a child is allowed to respond by writing rather than verbally) is also an important part of the evaluation, as it can give information about how a child may function in an academic environment.

Fine Motor Skills and Visual-Motor Integration

Speech-language impairments have been found to be concordant with fine motor difficulties (Hill, 2001), and children with speech-language impairments have been found to have greater difficulties with visual-motor integration than children without speech-language impairments (Nicola & Watter, 2016). Therefore evaluating these skills and the potential need for occupational therapy or other supportive services is often a necessary part of the evaluation.

Memory

Memory skills are thought to be a critical component of academic performance (Swanson & Alloway, 2012). Working memory indexes are often included as part of the assessment tools discussed earlier; however, additional memory testing may be warranted depending on the diagnostic question. There are a variety of memory tests examining these skills, with some tests offering specific scales for nonverbal (or visual) memory.

CONCLUSION AND CLINICAL IMPLICATIONS

Isabella became frustrated during verbal tasks. The examiner focused on administering tests that did not require a verbal response. Receptive vocabulary, oral comprehension, and nonverbal cognitive functioning were within normal limits. Isabella noticed that things had not gone as planned at the end of the testing session. She told the examiner "sorry" and hugged the examiner. She displayed a high level of empathy and social awareness. A mainstream kindergarten classroom was recommended with push-in supports and increased individualized attention. The evaluation also recommended that Isabella be provided with alternative methods to display her knowledge and communicate. For example, she may demonstrate knowledge via pointing to identify an answer among choices or using an AAC device. Ongoing speech-language therapy was also recommended.

Overall, the evaluation of a minimally verbal child requires sensitivity in terms of ensuring that the evaluation is accurate, reliable, and valid. Minimally verbal children present with a variety of abilities. The assessing clinician should never assume that minimally verbal equates to low abilities. A strength-based approach also emphasizes the child's abilities, skills, and preferences. The psychological or neuropsychological assessment of a minimally verbal child differs from that of a verbal child. Traditional psychological assessment instruments may not be appropriate for the minimally verbal child. Creativity is required to carefully substitute alternative measures or approaches to ensure that the evaluation of the child is as accurate as possible. Additional time may be needed to complete these assessments.

REFERENCES

Bal, V. H., Katz, T., Bishop, S. L., & Krasileva, K. (2016). Understanding definitions of minimally verbal across instruments: Evidence for subgroups within minimally verbal children and adolescents with autism spectrum disorder. *Journal of Child Psychology & Psychiatry*, *57*(12), 1424–1433.

Bayley, N., & Aylward, G. P. (2019). *Bayley scales of infant and toddler development—fourth edition technical manual*. NCS Pearson.

Bracken, B. A., & McCallum, R. S. (2016). *Universal nonverbal intelligence test* (2nd ed.). Pro-Ed.

Brady, N., Marquis, J., Fleming, K., & McLean, L. (2004). Prelinguistic predictors of language growth in children with developmental disabilities. *Journal of Speech, Language, and Hearing Research*, *47*(3), 663–667.

Brady, N. C., Fleming, K., Romine, R. S., Holbrook, A., Muller, K., & Kasari, C. (2018). Concurrent validity and reliability for the communication complexity scale. *American Journal of Speech and Language Pathology*, *27*(1), 237–246.

Brown, L., Sherbenou, S., & Johnsen, K. (2010). *Test of nonverbal intelligence–4 (TONI-4)*. Pro-Ed.

Chang, Y. C., Shih, W., Landa, R., Kaiser, A., & Kasari, C. (2018). Symbolic play in school-aged minimally verbal children with autism spectrum disorder. *Journal of Autism and Developmental Disorders*, *48*(5), 1436–1445. https://doi.org/10.1007/s10803-017-3388-6

Dethorne, L. S., & Schaefer, B. A. (2004). A guide to child nonverbal IQ measures. *American Journal of Speech-Language Pathology*, *13*(4), 275–290.

Dunn. D. M. (2019). *Peabody picture vocabulary test* (5th ed.). NCS Pearson.

Fenson, L., Marchman, V. A., Thal, D. J., Reznick, S., & Bates, E. (2006). *The MacArthur-Bates communicative development inventories: User's guide and technical manual*. Brookes.

Fok, M., & Bal, V. H. (2019). Differences in profiles of emotional behavioral problems across instruments in verbal versus minimally verbal children with autism spectrum disorder. *Autism Research*, *12*(9), 1367–1375.

Frisby. C. L. (2003). Nonverbal assessment of academic achievement with special populations. In R. S. McCallum (Ed.), *Handbook of nonverbal assessment*. Springer.

Hickey, F., Hickey, E., & Summar, K. L. (2012). Medical update for children with Down syndrome for the pediatrician and family practitioner. *Advances in Pediatrics*, *59*(1), 137–157.

Hill. E. L. (2001). Non-specific nature of specific language impairment: A review of the literature with regard to concomitant motor impairments. *International Journal of Language and Communication Disorders*, *36*(2), 149–171.

John. R. J. (2003). Raven progressive matrices. In R. S. McCallum (Ed.), *Handbook of nonverbal assessment*. Springer.

Kasari, C., Brady, N., Lord, C., & Tager-Flusberg, H. (2013). Assessing the minimally verbal school-aged child with autism spectrum disorder. *Autism Research*, *6*(6), 479–493.

Kasari, C., Gulsrud, A., Freeman, S., Paparella, T., & Hellemann, G. (2012). Longitudinal follow-up of children with autism receiving targeted interventions on joint attention and play. *Journal of the American Academy of Child and Adolescent Psychiatry*, *51*(5), 487–495.

Kaufman, A., Raiford, S., & Coalson, D. (2016). *Intelligent testing with the WISC-V*. Wiley.

Mundy, P., Delgado, C., Block, J., Venezia, M., Hogan, A., & Seibert, J. (2003). *Early social communication scales (ESCS)*. University of Miami.

Nicola, K., & Watter, P. (2016). Visual-motor integration performance in children with severe specific language impairment. *Child: Care, Health and Development*, *42*(5), 742–749.

Norbuy, C. F., Gooch, D., Wray, C., Baird, G., Charman, T., Simonoff, E., Vamvakas, G., & Pickles, A. (2016). The impact of nonverbal ability on prevalence and clinical presentation of language disorder: Evidence from a population study. *Journal of Child Psychology & Psychiatry*, *57*(11), 1247–1257.

Pearl, P. L., Carrazana, E. J., & Holmes, G. L. (2001). The Landau-Kleffner syndrome. *Epilepsy Currents*, *1*(2), 39–45.

Roid, G. H., Miller, L. J., Pomplun, M., & Koch, C. (2013). *Leiter international performance scale* (3rd ed.). Stoelting Company.

Selassie, G. R., Jennische, M., Kyllerman, M., Viggedal, G., & Hartelius, L. (2005). Comorbidity in severe developmental language disorders: Neuropediatric and psychological considerations. *Acta Paediatrica*, *94*(4), 471–478.

Swanson, H. L., & Alloway, T. P. (2012). Working memory, learning, and academic achievement. In K. R. Harris, S. Graham, T. C. Urdan, C. B. McCormicktine, G. M. Sinatra, & J. Sweller (Eds.), *APA educational psychology handbook, Vol 1: Theories, constructs, and critical issues* (1st ed.). American Psychological Association.

Urbina. S. (2014). *Essentials of psychological testing*. Wiley.

Watt, N., Wetherby, A. M., Barber, A., & Morgan, L. (2008). Repetitive and stereotyped behaviors in children with autism spectrum disorders in the second year of life. *Journal of Autism and Developmental Disorders*, *38*(8), 1518–1533.

Wechsler. D. (2012). *The Wechsler preschool and primary scale of intelligence* (4th ed.). Pearson Education Incorporated.

Wechsler. D. (2014). *WISC-V: Technical and interpretive manual*. Pearson.

Wong. P. (2010). Selective mutism: A review of etiology, comorbidities, and treatment. *Psychiatry*, *7*(3), 23–31.

Zimmerman, I., Steiner, V., & Pond, R. (2011). *Preschool language scale (PLS-5)*. Pearson Education Incorporated.

80

Assessment of Temperament

Hannah Perrin and Nicole R. Bush

For additional material related to the content of this chapter, please see Chapters 2 and 91.

VIGNETTE

Six-year-old James and his parents present to your office to discuss concerns about James's behavior. James enters the room hesitantly, after significant coaxing from his parents, and avoids eye contact with you, looking down toward the floor. His parents immediately begin talking over one another as they describe that they think something is "wrong" with their son. Ever since the family moved to a new town several months ago, James has become quieter and more withdrawn than usual. His 8-year-old sister loves the new home and has invited new friends from the neighborhood over to play in the backyard. Though his parents have encouraged James to engage with kids at the park or invite children over, James stays close to his parents when meeting new children, declines offers of playdates, and has mostly played alone in his room or with the family's dog, for whom James has always shown a particular fondness. James' parents recall that, since infancy, James has seemed "shy" and hesitant in new experiences, in contrast to his sister, who, like them, is gregarious and willing to try anything.

In the office you have a productive discussion with James' parents regarding their understanding of his temperament, their own temperaments, and how differences between their recall of their own approaches to new situations in their childhood and James' behavior do not necessarily warrant concern. You further discuss how their expectations for James might differ from what they expect for their older daughter, based on each child's individual temperament. You ask James' parents to describe his areas of strength, and they depict a kind, empathetic, sensitive child with a love of music and drawing and a strong affinity for animals. They note that although he had just a few close friends at his prior school, they were positive, stable friendships. You support them in coming to the realization that although he might be "slow to warm up" to the new context, he could flourish in a warm and nurturing environment that encourages and develops his strengths. After discussing ways to scaffold James in connecting with new peers in smaller groups, you encourage them to provide opportunities but be patient as he adjusts to the move and develops friendships at his own pace. You also remind them that supporting James' interests, even in solo or family-based activities, will increase his confidence to take risks in other realms. They resolve to approach James with his temperament in mind going forward.

INTRODUCTION

Temperament constructs have been a part of public discourse for thousands of years. As early as 370 BC, Hippocrates proposed four humors (yellow bile, black bile, blood, and phlegm) corresponded to choleric, melancholic, sanguine, and phlegmatic temperaments, respectively, which he postulated were related to personality and behavior. This construct of temperament has evolved over the years, with several prominent child development researchers developing their own refined definitions of temperament. Within the New York Longitudinal Study launched in 1956 (see for review Hertzig, 2020), Thomas and Chess identified nine traits or dimensions of temperament, including activity level, persistence, distractibility, approach/withdrawal, adaptability, mood, intensity, sensitivity, and regularity, as well as three temperament clusters: difficult, easy, and slow to warm up. Influential theorists advanced this work, creating frameworks that emphasize foundational elements of temperament such as emotion regulation (Goldsmith & Campos, 1982), psychobiological features (Kagan, Reznick, & Snidman, 1987; Rothbart, Derryberry, & Posner, 1994), and the genetic bases of temperament (Buss & Plomin, 1984). Although exact definitions vary depending upon one's preferred framework, current consensus defines temperament as biologically based differences in behavioral and emotional reactivity and regulation that are fairly consistent across contexts or situations. A practical definition is "behavioral style" (Carey, 1998). Although understood to be a set of individual differences that are relatively stable over time, temperament is shaped by environment and experience, with lower stability in infancy and increasing stability in the toddler years (Carey, 1998) that continues into middle childhood.

WHAT DOES TEMPERAMENT PREDICT?

Temperament is considered to be a precursor to personality. It can predict later development of healthy or unhealthy behaviors, lifestyles, and even career choices. For example, researchers surveyed resident and fellow physicians using the temperament and character inventory; the resulting personality profile clusters were strongly associated with physician specialty (although many profiles were found in each specialty, and many specialties were noted in each personality profile cluster) (Sievert et al., 2016). Furthermore, while temperament is distinct from behavioral and emotional adjustment and does not automatically confer a specific disorder to an individual, individuals with certain temperaments can be more prone to certain disorders. For example, James, the 6-year-old child in our vignette, exhibits a high degree of behavioral inhibition, which has been well studied and found to be associated with greater likelihood of developing anxiety than would be expected in children without this temperament trait (Pérez-Edgar & Guyer, 2014). The child who rates high on scales of activity, distractibility, and intensity, and low on persistence, might be more prone to attention-deficit/hyperactivity disorder (ADHD). However, simply having these traits does not confer the diagnosis, which also requires a level of functional impairment that might or might not be present, depending on how well the child's environment is suited to that particular child's needs.

HOW TEMPERAMENT MODIFIES EXPERIENCE OR RESPONSE TO ENVIRONMENT

A child's temperament affects the child, the family, and interactions within the child's larger community across settings and life stages. Differences between a child's temperament and the expectations or behavioral styles of that child's parents, caregivers, or teachers can lead to challenging interactions and affect the child's resulting behavior, or the perception of the child's behavior by others. This goodness of fit between a child and the environment can influence whether an individual's temperament is an asset or a detriment for optimal functioning for that child and the system within which the child is embedded (Chess & Thomas, 1999). Indeed, individual differences in temperament are understood to confer variation in sensitivity to environment, termed differential susceptibility or biological sensitivity to context (Ellis, Boyce, Belsky, Bakermans-Kranenburg, & van Ijzendoorn, 2011) (see Chapter 2). While these concepts simplify a fairly complex understanding of variations in temperament, they are supported by a growing body of evidence (Bush & Boyce, 2016) and have wide appeal with practitioners and parents. Within this framework, individuals with less sensitive temperament are thought to be fairly impervious to influences from the social environment, whereas those with more sensitive temperament are thought to be at greater risk for behavioral and emotional problems when reared in adverse environments, while demonstrating superior outcomes in enriched environments that optimize opportunities for thriving. Such a framework can be helpful to parents by highlighting that their "sensitive" child, whom they see as struggling in certain contexts, may actually outperform peers in social competence, wellbeing, and academic outcomes when exposed to warm, nurturing environments. In contrast, the highly active and impulsive child, who may present challenges in highly structured, sedate settings, could thrive in environments that support energetic individuals with quick decision making. Additionally, although some temperaments place children at greater risk for developing problems when faced with stressors and adversities (such as adverse childhood experiences [see Chapter 15]), the very features that may confer risk for trauma may also make those children more responsive to positive parenting or therapeutic intervention (Boyce, 2016).

Culture plays an important role in social attitudes about individual difference characteristics, particularly for children. These culture-specific attitudes shape evaluations of children's behavioral displays, adults' responses to them, and the impact the characteristics will have across settings and development for child functioning (Chen, 2018). Given cultural influences, and recent evidence for race-based disparities in child diagnoses related to behavior (Kang & Harvey, 2020), it is important to consider our own biases as clinicians when assessing and providing feedback to families (Schnierle, Christian-Brathwaite, & Louisias, 2019).

ASSESSMENT OF TEMPERAMENT

Temperament is a helpful construct for both families and professionals to comprehend when considering a child's response to a certain stimulus or situation. It is important to support parents' understanding that there is a wide range of so-called normal when it comes to child temperament, and that qualities they see in their child as abnormal might not be cause for alarm. In fact, two parents of the same child might disagree on perceptions of their child, based on their own temperament, experiences, or culture. Or, as in the case of James, having a sibling with a contrasting temperament can influence how a parent sees the child. In this case James' exuberant sister draws a sharp contrast with James' temperament and more closely resembles their parents' own qualities, leading to potential bias against James' behavioral style.

The American Academy of Pediatrics (AAP) and *Bright Futures* recommend that pediatricians discuss temperament with families in routine well-child care, beginning in infancy (AAP, 2007). Several tools have been developed to assist with temperament assessment, including observational measures that can be conducted by a trained professional, and parent/caregiver questionnaires. However, many of these tools were developed for research purposes and are not feasible in day-to-day clinical encounters. Additionally, there is substantial concern about the validity of parent-rated temperament questionnaires (Gagne, Van Hulle, Aksan, Essex, & Goldsmith, 2011), in part due to the long-standing evidence for poor correspondence between parent ratings and single-visit observations conducted by professionals (Planalp, Van Hulle, Gagne, & Goldsmith, 2017).

A few high-quality, structured task-based observational rating scales are available and in common use. The Neonatal Behavioral Assessment Scale (NBAS) (Brazelton & Nugent, 2011) is used for infants beginning a few hours after birth (for infants at least 35 weeks of gestational age) until 2 months of age (or older if developmentally delayed) and measures 28 neurobehavioral items. Developed as a briefer tool, the Newborn Behavioral Observations (NBO) System (Nugent, Keefer, Minear, Johnson, & Blanchard, 2007) is based on the NBAS, measures 18 neurobehavioral items, and can be administered postnatally to infants at least 36 weeks of gestational age until 3 months postterm. Use of both instruments in clinical contexts may improve outcomes for caregivers and their infants (Barlow, Herath, Bartram Torrance, Bennett, & Wei, 2018). The Lab-TAB instruments (for a review, see Goldsmith & Rothbart [1991]; for a recent empirical example, see Planalp et al. [2017]) measure temperament in a laboratory setting beginning at 6 months of age and extending through middle childhood. In addition to standardized tasks, clinicians can also make informal observations, with the clinic providing an excellent stimulus to ascertain children's responses to challenges, such as meeting unfamiliar staff, being expected to wait for appointments, and inoculation or other potentially stressful procedures.

Numerous parent-rated questionnaires for various stages of development spanning from early infancy through middle childhood are used to assess temperament, most notably those developed by teams led by Rothbart (Rothbart, 1981; Rothbart, Ahadi, Hershey, & Fisher, 2001) and Carey (Carey & McDevitt, 1978; Fullard, McDevitt, & Carey, 1984; Hegvik, McDevitt, & Carey, 1982; McDevitt & Carey, 1978; Medoff-Cooper, Carey, & McDevitt, 1993). In addition, some medical practices and other organizations have created their own tools, such as the Infant Toddler Temperament Tool (IT^3), an online survey for parents and caregivers (Center for Early Childhood Mental Health Consultation, 2021). Collectively, parent-rated tools provide helpful information on caregiver perceptions of their child's behavioral and emotional style and how it might be impacting the child's and the family's functioning. Because of the concern regarding validity of parent-rated temperament questionnaires, experts typically advocate for a combination of parent-rated questionnaires and observation tools. However, this combination is time intensive and generally not feasible for many clinicians. If parent ratings are used as the primary tool, research finds that questionnaires that are specific and ask about concrete behaviors (rather than general feelings), such as the Children's Behavior Questionnaire (Rothbart et al., 2001), tend to be less susceptible to parent biases (Gagne et al., 2011). Other respondents, such as teachers or childcare providers, can also supply the clinician with their observations in home and school settings using standardized questionnaires, which ascertain children's temperament across settings and perceiving adults.

HOW AND WHEN TO INTERVENE

Carey (1998) argued that pediatric clinicians can play an essential role in teaching parents about their children's temperaments—that they are real, important for both the parent and child, and best managed by accommodation. Educating parents/caregivers and teachers about child temperament allows caregivers to reflect on their own biases and adjust their expectations. This education is especially important when there is significant dissonance between the child's temperament and the caregivers' expectations and when caregivers are attempting to force children to behave in ways that are counter to their natural temperament. Educating and empowering caregivers can support them in interpreting differences in a holistic or positive light and help them to adapt the environment to suit the needs of the child and optimize positive functioning. For example, children with an inhibited, fearful temperament might struggle in a chaotic home or classroom environment, but those same children may thrive in an environment with clear expectations and strong adherence to routines. Children with deep-seated empathy might experience great distress if frequently exposed to sad events, such as news stories of mass casualties, but that temperamental quality might also facilitate success in mentoring younger peers or new classmates. Exuberant, impulsive children are likely to benefit from support with transitions, consistent expectations, and consequences around behavior; they are likely to require opportunities to release energy in settings where they are perceived positively, such as frequent body movement breaks, dance, or sports. Such adaptations of the environment may prevent significant interpersonal challenges with peers and adults, benefitting both the children and those in their social system. With a comprehensive understanding of a child's temperament, caregivers can include preventative measures in the home or school setting, such as regular mindfulness activities for children who are high in affective arousal or who struggle with behavioral or emotional self-regulation, movement breaks for children with high activity

BOX 80.1 Interventions

The pediatrician can suggest the following interventions, which may help, but should keep the focus on helping the child to make difficult transitions in ways best suited to the child's particular temperamental profile.

- Validate the parents' feelings of stress, inadequacy, or even anger at the baby or each other. By listening well and acknowledging such emotions, the pediatrician gets useful information about interactions at home.
- Ask routinely about sources of support as well as stressors. With a better knowledge base, the pediatrician can help absolve the parents of some of the inevitable self-blame and can help focus the discussion on interactions between baby and caregivers and between the caregivers themselves, rather than on "what's wrong with the baby."
- Teach parents how to be aware of their baby's temperament and what it means.
- Encourage parents to see the child's distress as reflecting a difficulty adapting to environmental change, so it will be easier to guide their attempts to comfort the child.
- Teach parents methods to calm their baby based on the child's temperament. Many children do better if left alone for a short while than they do when bombarded with further stimulation as the parents attempt to comfort them. Swaddling, quiet rocking, and calm, gentle handling can also be effective and are more likely to occur when parents understand the nature of the infant's state of arousal.
- Lastly, make parents aware that their child's temperament also affects their sleeping and feeding patterns. If caregivers can come to see the child's waking as related to daytime activity levels and not necessarily to unsatisfied hunger, their responses can be more adaptive and appropriate.

levels, or enhanced preparation warnings about and tolerance during transitions between activities for children who struggle to shift attention or are highly sensitive to change. Parents are thereby adjusting the environment to encourage and optimize for the child's particular strengths (Box 80.1).

CONCLUSION

Temperament is an important and often underutilized construct to explain differences among children's personalities and behaviors. Temperament is distinct from qualities that indicate clinical disorders and should be interpreted in context. Multiple tools have been developed to assess temperament, although reports are susceptible to bias by the rater, and observational ratings are often not feasible to administer in clinical encounters, limiting their use. Educating parents, teachers, and other caregivers about temperament can help to normalize healthy variability in individual differences in reactivity and regulation, support identification of ways to adjust expectations or modify environments to suit a child's needs, result in a happier and healthier home and school experience, and optimize child functioning.

REFERENCES

American Academy of Pediatrics. (2007). *Bright futures* (3rd ed., p. 369).

Barlow, J., Herath, N., Bartram Torrance, C., Bennett, C., & Wei, Y. (2018). The Neonatal Behavioral Assessment Scale (NBAS) and Newborn Behavioral Observations (NBO) system for supporting caregivers and improving outcomes in caregivers and their infants. *Cochrane Database of Systematic Reviews*, 3. https://doi.org/10.1002/14651858.CD011754.pub2

Boyce, W. T. (2016). Differential susceptibility of the developing brain to contextual adversity and stress. *Neuropsychopharmacology*, *41*(1), 142–162. https://doi.org/10.1038/npp.2015.294

Brazelton, T. B., & Nugent, J. K. (2011). *The Neonatal Behavioral Assessment Scale*. Mac Keith Press.

Bush, N. R., & Boyce, W. T. (2016). Differential sensitivity to context: Implications for developmental psychopathology. In D. Cicchetti (Ed.), *Developmental psychopathology* (pp. 107–137). John Wiley and Sons, Inc.

Buss, A. H., & Plomin, R. (1984). *Temperament: Early developing personality traits*. Erlbaum.

Carey, W. B. (1998). Teaching parents about infant temperament. *Pediatrics*, *102*(E1), S1311.

Carey, W. B., & McDevitt, S. C. (1978). Revision of the infant temperament questionnaire. *Pediatrics*, *61*(5), 735–739.

Center for Early Childhood Mental Health Consultation. (2021). *Infant Toddler Temperament Tool (IT3)*. https://www.ecmhc.org/temperament/index.html

Chen, X. (2018). Culture, temperament, and social and psychological adjustment. *Developmental Review*, *50*, 42–53. https://doi.org/10.1016/j.dr.2018.03.004

Chess, S., & Thomas, A. (1999). *Goodness of fit: Clinical applications from infancy through adult life*. Bruner/Mazel.

Ellis, B. J., Boyce, W. T., Belsky, J., Bakermans-Kranenburg, M. J., & van Ijzendoorn, M. H. (2011). Differential susceptibility to the environment: An evolutionary-neurodevelopmental theory. *Development and Psychopathology*, *23*(1), 7–28. https://doi.org/10.1017/S0954579410000611

Fullard, W., McDevitt, S. C., & Carey, W. B. (1984). Assessing temperament in one- to three-year-old children. *Journal of Pediatric Psychology*, *9*(2), 205–217. https://doi.org/10.1093/jpepsy/9.2.205

Gagne, J. R., Van Hulle, C. A., Aksan, N., Essex, M. J., & Goldsmith, H. H. (2011). Deriving childhood temperament measures from emotion-eliciting behavioral episodes: Scale construction and initial validation. *Psychological Assessment*, *23*(2), 337–353. https://doi.org/10.1037/a0021746

Goldsmith, H. H., & Campos, J. J. (1982). Toward a theory of infant temperament. In R. N. Emde & R. J. Harmon (Eds.), *The development of attachment and affiliative systems* (pp. 161–193). Springer.

Goldsmith, H. H., & Rothbart, M. K. (1991). Contemporary instruments for assessing early temperament by questionnaire and in the laboratory. In J. Strelau & A. Angleitner (Eds.), *Explorations in temperament. Perspectives on individual differences*. Springer.

Hegvik, R. L., McDevitt, S. C., & Carey, W. B. (1982). The middle childhood temperament questionnaire. *Journal of Developmental & Behavioral Pediatrics*, *3*(4).

Hertzig, M. E. (2020). New York Longitudinal Study (NYLS). In V. Zeigler-Hill & T. K. Shackelford (Eds.), *Encyclopedia of personality and individual differences* (pp. 3236–3239). Springer International Publishing.

Kagan, J., Reznick, J. S., & Snidman, N. (1987). The physiology and psychology of behavioral inhibition in young children. *Child Development*, *58*, 1459–1473.

Kang, S., & Harvey, E. A. (2020). Racial differences between black parents' and white teachers' perceptions of attention-deficit/hyperactivity disorder behavior. *Journal of Abnormal Child Psychology*, *48*(5), 661–672. https://doi.org/10.1007/s10802-019-00600-y

McDevitt, S., & Carey, W. (1978). The measurement of temperament in 3 and 7 year-old children. *Journal of Child Psychiatry & Psychology*, *19*, 245–253.

Medoff-Cooper, B., Carey, W. B., & McDevitt, S. (1993). The early infancy temperament questionnaire. *Journal of Developmental & Behavioral Pediatrics*, *14*(4), 230–235.

Nugent, J. K., Keefer, C. H., Minear, S., Johnson, L. C., & Blanchard, Y. (2007). *Understanding newborn behavior and early relationships: The Newborn Behavioral Observations (NBO) system handbook*. Paul H Brookes Publishing.

Pérez-Edgar, K. E., & Guyer, A. E. (2014). Behavioral inhibition: Temperament or prodrome? *Current Behavioral Neuroscience Reports*, *1*(3), 182–190. https://doi.org/10.1007/s40473-014-0019-9

Planalp, E. M., Van Hulle, C., Gagne, J. R., & Goldsmith, H. H. (2017). The infant version of the Laboratory Temperament Assessment Battery (Lab-TAB): Measurement properties and implications for concepts of temperament. *Frontiers in Psychology*, *8*(846). https://doi.org/10.3389/fpsyg.2017.00846

Rothbart, M. K. (1981). Measurement of temperament in infancy. *Child Development*, *52*, 569–578.

Rothbart, M. K., Ahadi, S. A., Hershey, K. L., & Fisher, P. (2001). Investigations of temperament at three to seven years: The children's behavior questionnaire. *Child Development*, *72*(5), 1394–1408.

Rothbart, M. K., Derryberry, D., & Posner, M. I. (1994). A psychobiological approach to the development of temperament. In J. E. Bates & T. D. Wachs (Eds.), *Temperament: Individual differences at the interface of biology and behavior* (pp. 83–116). American Psychological Association.

Schnierle, J., Christian-Brathwaite, N., & Louisias, M. (2019). Implicit bias: What every pediatrician should know about the effect of bias on health and future directions. *Current Problems in Pediatric and Adolescent Health Care*, *49*(2), 34–44. https://doi.org/10.1016/j.cppeds.2019.01.003

Sievert, M., Zwir, I., Cloninger, K. M., Lester, N., Rozsa, S., & Cloninger, C. R. (2016). The influence of temperament and character profiles on specialty choice and well-being in medical residents. *Peer Journal*, *4*, e2319–e2319. https://doi.org/10.7717/peerj.2319

81

Developmental Surveillance and Screening

Benjamin W. Sanders, Brittany S. Bassitt,
Luis A. Rivas Vazquez, and Katharine E. Zuckerman

For additional material related to the content of this chapter, please see Chapters 5, 6, and 76.

VIGNETTE

An 18-month-old boy, previously born at 34 weeks of gestation, presents for his well-child check. His mother completed a developmental screening tool at the beginning of today's visit. Developmental surveillance at his 15-month visit revealed a mild fine motor delay. At that time, the clinician gave his mother an activity handout to promote his fine motor development. Today, he has persistent fine motor delay despite working through the activity sheet. The mother also expresses concern about language delay, as the patient only says three words. The screening tool reveals that he does not scribble while holding a crayon, he does not feed himself with a spoon, and he is unable to successfully stack two blocks. His physical exam is unremarkable, his immunizations are current for age, and he has no other medical problems. An autism screening questionnaire is also completed without any concerning findings. The clinician refers the patient to early intervention (EI) and audiology and recommends follow-up in 1 month to monitor his progress and consider referral to a developmental specialist.

BACKGROUND

A large body of evidence supports the effectiveness of EI programs and early childhood special education (ECSE) in promoting optimal outcomes for children with developmental delays and risks. Early identification of disability risk is key, as infancy marks a critical period of high neuroplasticity and in which benefits of treatment far outweigh societal costs. Developmental screening using a validated tool, together with developmental surveillance, improves detection of developmental delays and disabilities.

Definitions and Chapter Scope

The 2020 American Academy of Pediatrics (AAP) clinical report on developmental surveillance and screening defines developmental screening as "the use of standardized tools to identify and refine" a child's risk for developmental delay that has not been previously identified (Lipkin & Macias, 2020). Developmental surveillance is a "flexible, longitudinal, continuous, and cumulative process in which knowledgeable health care professionals identify children who may have developmental problems." The components of surveillance include eliciting and attending to the parents' concerns about their child's development; obtaining, documenting, and maintaining a developmental history; making accurate and informed observations of the child; identifying risks and protective factors; and maintaining an accurate record of the process and findings. In the 2020 AAP clinical report additional emphasis was placed on a sixth component: sharing and obtaining opinions and findings with other professionals, such as child-care providers, home visitors, preschool teachers, and developmental therapists, especially when concerns arise (Lipkin & Macias, 2020). While surveillance is conducted at every well-child visit, screening consists of an objective, standardized tool completed at a set point in time. Both surveillance and screening allow the clinician access to valuable information regarding development to improve detection of delays (AAP Committee on Children with Disabilities, 2001).

Developmental screening should be distinguished from other types of developmental assessment in early childhood. General developmental screening traditionally assesses a child's progress in domains of communication, gross motor, fine motor, and adaptive/problem-solving skills, usually in the first 5 years of life. Autism spectrum disorder (ASD) screening is now an important part of health care screening, given the importance of identifying the condition early. Social-emotional screening is also recommended by the AAP. Lastly, since social adversity in a child's life affects long-term development, screening for social risk factors and offering corresponding resources to interested families may prove beneficial. For purposes of this chapter in informing clinical practice, we focus on screening children in the domains of general development and ASD, with brief mention of social-emotional screening.

Developmental screening occurs in many early childhood settings, including primary health care, subspecialty and multidisciplinary clinics, EI and ECSE, and early educational settings such as Head Start. We focus here on primary care as a model since child health care settings have near-universal access to children with regular visits under age 5 years. Surveillance and screening guidelines for primary care are also well established, and the literature offers insights into key principles that apply to early detection of developmental delays and linkage to services in other settings.

Child Find and the Child Abuse Prevention and Treatment Act

EI and ECSE—the public programs providing developmental services to at-risk children—are specified by Parts B and C of the Individuals with Disabilities Education Act (IDEA) and are described in more detail in Chapters 103, 104, and 113. The Child Find component of IDEA Part B mandates that states must identify and evaluate "all children with disabilities residing in the State" and "determine which children are currently receiving needed special education" (IDEA Part B, 34 CFR §300.111[a][1]). Part C obligates participating states to do the same for "all infants and toddlers with disabilities" (IDEA Part C, 34 CFR §303.302[b]). States must also make the public aware of these services through "all primary referral sources (especially hospitals and physicians)" (34 CFR §303.301) and provide for prompt referral by these sources to IDEA services (34 CFR §303.303). Child Find's emphasis on early identification and timely linkage to services creates opportunities for collaboration between health care clinicians and their state's EI and ECSE programs.

The Child Abuse Prevention and Treatment Act (CAPTA, PL 93-247) mandates additional referrals to EI and ECSE for children "involved in a substantiated case of child abuse or neglect" (CAPTA §106[b][2][A][xxi]). It includes infants affected by parental substance abuse and was designed to address the frequent cooccurrence of child maltreatment and developmental disabilities.

Clinician Screening Rates

Pediatric clinician adoption of developmental screening has gradually increased since its formal recommendation by the AAP in 2001. Only 21% of pediatricians reported screening for development using a validated tool in 2002, with improvement to 63% in 2016 (Lipkin et al., 2020). Parent surveys corroborate this trend (Hirai, Kogan, Kandasamy, Reuland, & Bethell, 2018). This increase has been driven by endorsement by professional organizations, Medicaid reimbursement, and adoption as national care quality metrics. Barriers to developmental screening are discussed later.

IDENTIFYING CHILDREN AT RISK FOR DELAYS AND DISABILITIES

In its third revision the AAP 2020 clinical report on general developmental screening reaffirms its prior recommendation that the pediatric clinician perform developmental surveillance at every well-child visit and screening at 9, 18, and 30 months for children without identified developmental problems or risks (Fig. 81.1) (Lipkin & Macias, 2020). Formal developmental screening at these intervals increases clinical detection of developmental concerns at key early ages where many signs are just beginning to appear. If developmental concerns arise outside of these screening visits, screening tools should be employed; however, screening is not recommended for every well-child visit unless clinical concerns arise. In contrast, developmental surveillance should be integrated with developmental screening in a seamless overall process that facilitates early detection and linking to services. The 2020 clinical report also adds detail to its clinical algorithm and puts increased emphasis on assessing children for school readiness at 4 to 5 years old (see Chapter 83).

Autism Screening

ASD is especially responsive to treatment early in its course, and thus screening in primary care is of high importance. The 2020 AAP clinical report on ASD reaffirmed the prior recommendation for routine ASD screening at 18 and 24 month well visits with a standardized tool (Hyman, Levy, & Myers, 2020) and referral of children with positive screening results to specialty services. Eighteen and 24 months of age were chosen as key times for ASD screening due to the rapid growth of language and social communication skills between the ages of 1 and 2 years. Delays in language and social development—and definitely regressions—by this age should alert clinicians to a possible autism concern.

Social-Emotional Screening

Social-emotional development in early childhood is important and closely related to other developmental domains (Adams & Tapia, 2013). The AAP Bright Futures Recommendations for Preventive Pediatric Health Care (AAP Committee on

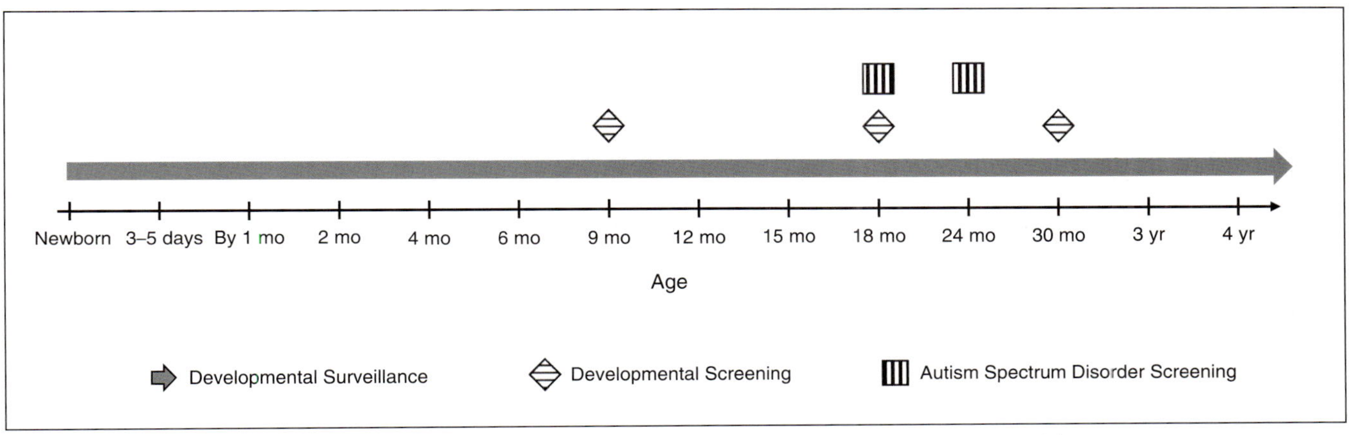

Fig. 81.1 Periodicity diagram. Screening for developmental delays and autism spectrum disorder at well-child visits.

Practice & Ambulatory Medicine, Bright Futures Periodicity Schedule Workgroup, 2021) recommends a behavioral assessment at each well-child visit throughout childhood. The 2015 AAP clinical report on social-emotional screening offers guidance to screen "with standardized, well-validated measures beginning in infancy" with proper preparations to address identified needs (Weitzman & Wegner, 2015). Clinicians should do this "at regular intervals" they determine to be appropriate for their practice. Table 81.1 lists validated screening tools for children starting in infancy.

TABLE 81.1 Commonly Used Parent-Completed Tools for Developmental Screening

Screening Tool	Suggested Ideal Uses; Age Range	No. of Items	Parent Completion Time	Validation Quality	Language Availability[a]	Cost	Literacy Level
General Developmental Screening							
Ages and Stages Questionnaire (ASQ-3)	Development; 1–66 mo	30	10–15 min	Sens: 86% Spec: 85%	English, Spanish, French, Korean …	Purchase	Grades 4–6
Parents' Evaluation of Developmental Status (PEDS)	Development; 0–8 yr	10	2 min	Sens: 86% Spec: 83%	English, Spanish, Chinese, Vietnamese …	Purchase	Grade 5
Parents' Evaluation of Developmental Status—Developmental Milestones (PEDS-DM)	Development; 0–11 yr	6–8	5 min	Sens: 83% Spec: 84%	English, Spanish, Chinese, Arabic …	Purchase	Grades 3–4
Survey of Wellbeing of Young Children (SWYC)	Development, social-emotional development, autism, maternal depression, social determinants of health; 1–66 mo	10–17	10 min	Sens: 76% (milestones); 75%–94% (POSI[b]); >70% (PPSC[c]) Spec: 77% (milestones); 41%–48% (POSI); >70% (PPSC)	English, Spanish, Vietnamese, Arabic, Haitian-Creole …	Free	Grade 6
Autism Screening							
Modified Checklist for Autism in Toddlers (M-CHAT-R/F)	Autism screening; 16–30 mo	20	5–10 min	Sens: 91% Spec: 95%	English, Spanish, Vietnamese, Arabic, French …	Free	Grade 5
Social Communication Questionnaire	Autism screening; 4 yr	40	10 min	Sens: 85% Spec: 75%	English, Spanish, Korean, Russian, German …	Purchase	Grade 6
Parent's Observations of Social Interactions (POSI)[d]	Autism screening; 16–35 mo	7	5 min	Sens: 75%–94% Spec: 41%–48%	English, Spanish Vietnamese, Arabic …	Free	Grade 5
Screening Tool for Autism in Toddlers & Young Children (STAT)	Level 2 autism screening; 24–35 mo	12	20–30 min[e]	Sens: 83% Spec: 86%	English	Purchase	[e]
Rapid Interactive Screening Test for Autism in Toddlers	Level 2 autism screening; 18–36 mo	9	5–10 min[e]	Sens: 100% Spec: 84%	English	Purchase	[e]

TABLE 81.1 **Commonly Used Parent-Completed Tools for Developmental Screening—cont'd**

Screening Tool	Suggested Ideal Uses; Age Range	No. of Items	Parent Completion Time	Validation Quality	Language Availability[a]	Cost	Literacy Level
Social-Emotional Screening							
Ages and Stages Questionnaire: Social Emotional 2 (ASQ: SE)	Social-emotional; 1–72 mo	19–33	10–15 min	By age and disability Sens: 78% Spec: 95%	English, Spanish	Purchase	Grades 4–5
Pediatric Symptom Checklist (PSC) 17b and 35b	Social emotional; 4–16 yr, ≥11 yr	17, 35	<5 min, <5 min	Compared to CGAS in middle and low income: Sens: 95% and 88% Spec: 68% and 100%	English, Spanish, Chinese, Filipino …	Free	Grades 5–6
Strength and Difficulties Questionnaire (SDQ)	Social emotional; 4–17 yr; also 3–4 yr version; youth self-report 11–16 yr	25; 22 items for 3–4 yr	5–10 min	Sens: 63%–94% Spec: 88%–98%	English, Spanish, Chinese, Tagalog …	Permission	Grade 6
SWYC: Baby Pediatric Symptom Checklist (Baby PSC)	Social emotional; 1–18 mo	12	~5 min	Correlation with ASQ-SE 0.61, 0.70	See SWYC above	Free	Grade 6
SWYC: Preschool Pediatric Symptom Checklist (Preschool PSC)	Social emotional; 18–65 mo	18	~5 min	Correlation with ASQ-SE 0.88, 0.89	See SWYC above	Free	Grade 6

ASQ-3: https://agesandstages.com/wp-content/uploads/2015/03/DOHVE-ASQ-3-and-ASQ-SE-Issue-Brief_Cleared.pdf
PEDS: https://pedstest.com/AboutOurTools/LearnAboutPEDS/IntroductionToPEDS.html
SWYC: https://www.tuftschildrenshospital.org/The-Survey-of-Wellbeing-of-Young-Children/Parts-of-the-SWYC
M-CHAT: https://m-chat.org/en-us/page/learn-about-m-chat/about-us
SCQ: https://www.wpspublish.com/scq-social-communication-questionnaire
POSI: https://www.tuftschildrenshospital.org/The-Survey-of-Wellbeing-of-Young-Children/Parts-of-the-SWYC/POSI
ASQ-SE: https://agesandstages.com/products-pricing/asqse-2/
PSC: https://www.massgeneral.org/psychiatry/treatments-and-services/pediatric-symptom-checklist/
SDQ: https://www.sdqinfo.org
[a]More languages and information available at the above links. Availability of a tool in multiple languages does not correlate to validation of the tool in such languages.
[b]POSI: Parent's Observations of Social Interactions
[c]PPSC: Preschool Pediatric Symptom Checklist
[d]The POSI (Autism), the Baby PSC and the Preschool PSC (both Social Emotional) are all separable components of the Survey of Wellbeing of Young Children (SWYC).
[e]Test is administered by trained professionals.
Adapted from Lipkin, P. H., & Macias, M. M. (2020). Promoting optimal development: Identifying infants and young children with developmental disorders through developmental surveillance and screening. *Pediatrics, 145*(1), e20193449. https://doi.org/10.1542/peds.2019-3449

Surveillance and Screening Must Be Family Centered

Identifying children at risk for delays and disabilities must be family centered. Developmental care is a dynamic, cooperative activity between parents and clinicians. Social stigma, mistrust based on a history of racial or cultural mistreatment, beliefs about mental health and development, and many other factors shape a family's approach to their child's development. Clinicians should elicit parents' level of concern and state of readiness about their child's development, and this should guide the clinician's approach to care. Conversations about a child's development can and should span multiple visits as parents often shift their perspectives incrementally. Likewise, the clinician's level of concern should influence the conversation. Ultimately, the family will decide what to do for their child, and the clinician's opportunity to positively influence a child's health emerges from respect and understanding shared between them and the family.

Beyond the United States

In some settings outside of the jurisdiction of IDEA Part C universal screening may not have the same utility when treatment resources are limited. The World Health Organization (WHO) recommends family-centered longitudinal developmental surveillance ("monitoring") and reserves screening tools for when warranted by clinical concerns (WHO, 2020). Marlow, Servili, and Tomlinson (2019) reviewed screening tools for use in developing countries in their 2019 paper.

VALIDATION AND EVIDENCE FOR SCREENING

Validation

Validation tests a tool to establish that it does what it is intended to do. Validation often involves comparison of a tool against another known tool or a full diagnostic evaluation (proxies for the elusive gold standard) in a representative sample of a population. Among other benefits, developmental screening tools balance clinicians' relative specificity with more sensitivity—the ability to detect milder delays often missed by clinical skills alone.

Validation may evaluate any combination of a tool's predictive power (criterion validity, including sensitivity and specificity), harmony with its theoretical basis (construct validity), or adequate coverage of the topic being measured (content validity). Validation also requires establishing a tool's reliability, or consistency of results across time, people, and circumstances. Sensitivity and specificity above 70% is considered adequate due to the difficulty in creating a parental report tool that is reliable, valid, and short enough for use in clinical settings.

Establishing a tool's generalizability (external validity) is a judgment call on the extent to which the tool's validation results may be applied to another population. Screening tools lose validity when used in dissimilar populations, other ages of children, or with modified or absent questions. Translations into other languages—a common practice born out of necessity—seemingly allow broader access to the tool, but unless separately validated they are not in themselves truly validated tools.

Evidence for Screening

Developmental screening has been shown to be effective in identifying children with developmental delays in a number of validation trials (Brothers, Glascoe, & Robertshaw, 2008; Sheldrick & Perrin, 2013; Squires, Bricker, & Potter, 1997). Use of a validated tool increases sensitivity in detecting developmental delays, especially in cognitive and behavioral areas of development. Guevara et al. (2013) in a large randomized trial demonstrated that children who received formal screening were identified with delays more often, were referred more often, and were found eligible for EI services more often than children receiving surveillance alone. Evidence correlating screening with improved developmental outcomes is more sparse. In a systematic review of evidence for screening for speech-language delays by the US Preventive Services Task Force (USPSTF) a majority of studies correlate screening with improved outcomes in speech and language, although study designs were too heterogeneous to permit metaanalysis (Wallace et al., 2015).

Likewise for ASD, symptoms can be reliably identified before 30 months of age, and ASD often responds very well to EI. Surveillance alone is inadequate, since social and emotional symptoms are more difficult to recognize clinically, they may not present during a visit, and parents are less likely to volunteer their concerns about them (Hyman et al., 2020). The USPSTF, in a systematic review of evidence for ASD screening, found insufficient evidence to recommend screening. They cited a lack of specificity of current tools and an absence of evidence linking screening directly with developmental outcomes (Siu & Force, 2016). The AAP and others continue to recommend screening for ASDs given that an outcomes study would be an enormous undertaking and difficult to justify given early treatment is effective, most children with ASD are identified years after toddlerhood and in the meantime large racial and income disparities permeate ASD identification and treatment (Hyman et al., 2020).

IMPLEMENTATION OF DEVELOPMENTAL SCREENING IN CLINICAL SETTINGS

Studies demonstrating the feasibility of routine developmental screening describe the importance of an established office workflow with clear staff roles, choosing appropriate screening tools, maximizing the function of the electronic health record (EHR), reimbursement, and monitoring screening rates as a part of ongoing quality improvement (King et al., 2010; Schonwald, Huntington, Chan, Risko, & Bridgemohan, 2009; Silver et al., 2017). Readers may consider consulting resources listed in Further Reading at the end of this chapter.

Components of an Effective Implementation

To begin, determine the specific needs and capacities of clinic staff and patients. Anticipate barriers to success, and seek buy-in from everyone involved in the process, including families, nursing, and front desk staff. Identify one or more champions of surveillance and screening in the office. Choose a tool of the appropriate length and language, while considering other factors such as EHR integration.

Your team can then establish a preliminary and imperfect workflow that describes who will do what, when, and where from previsit through to referral results and follow-up (Silver et al., 2017). Plan to accommodate families with Limited English Proficiency (see Gerdes & Yun [2015] in Further Reading), and remember that some parents will not be sufficiently literate to read the screening tool questions. Consider how secondary screening, such as the follow-up questions of the Modified Checklist for Autism in Toddlers–Revised with Follow-up (M-CHAT-R/F), will be conducted. Check with payers to identify their criteria for reimbursement using the Current Procedural Terminology (CPT) code 96110, including the modifier code 59 to allow its use twice at the 18-month visit when screening for both ASD and general development. Identify follow-up resources and make a plan to follow up positive screens to make sure families access care. Ensure someone has responsibility for each workflow task identified.

Next, to pilot the plan, structure an iterative approach to refine the screening process using quality improvement techniques such as plan-do-study-act (see Autism Toolkit in Further Reading). Make sure to solicit feedback from multiple viewpoints; this will be more efficient in the end and it will reinforce investment of team members. After implementation, work on reducing barriers to billing for the service and optimizing the EHR to support surveillance and screening. With an eye to long-term sustainability, find ways to support the designated developmental champion and consider adding developmental screening rates as a measure in the clinic's ongoing quality monitoring. Getting everyone involved and starting small are keys to success, because while they may seem inefficient at first, these approaches germinate resiliency and team capacity later on.

Common Implementation Challenges

Clinicians consistently name time as a principal barrier to conducting developmental screening. This has improved over time with payer reimbursement and use of newer brief tools. Of note, Schonwald and colleagues (2009) found screening with a validated tool made developmental care more efficient, as it helped identify parent concerns prior to the visit and helped structure the clinician-parent conversation.

A related challenge comes when parents do not complete the screening tool before the visit, which delays scoring and interpretation. Patient portals or mailed screening tools can facilitate completion before visits. However, this may capture at most 10% of eligible families and use rates are associated with racial, income, and other inequities (El-Toukhy, Méndez, Collins, & Pérez-Stable, 2020).

Reliably distributing screening tools to the correct children at the correct visits can be difficult, especially without automated age-based notifications in the EHR (King et al., 2010). Many clinics review charts before visits and note in the electronic record that developmental screening is indicated. Less reliable is for staff to determine eligibility at the visit check-in. If the EHR does not provide age-based reminders, clinic staff may agree on a reliable location in the patient record to store typed notes and even manually add flags to alert the next user that a screening is due.

Securing buy-in on the part of all clinicians can be challenging. Many clinicians feel that screening tools offer little assistance to their own clinical abilities. While the evidence suggests otherwise, this perception may be based on the observation that screening tools are often less specific than clinician judgment (Sheldrick, Merchant, & Perrin, 2011). Screening tools contribute needed sensitivity for milder but important cases that are otherwise missed. Early and consistent engagement of each clinician is key to managing this challenge. See the Results section later in this chapter for discussion of integrating clinical judgment with screening results. Staff turnover is another challenge to successful implementation and underscores the importance of early project buy-in across clinic roles.

Copyrights ensure many screening tools come with a cost, and may even prevent their incorporation into the EHR. Publishers may grant permission for local use of a screening tool in the EHR if it can be modified locally. In addition, some copyrights are less restrictive than others, so if a particular screening tool is preferred, reach out to their publisher to discuss details.

Developmental Care and the Electronic Health Record

Make use of existing functions, regardless of the level of an EHR's pediatric sophistication. Alerts to distribute a screening tool may be configured to trigger automatically in some cases. Store longitudinal developmental data in the same location for every patient, such as the comments section of a chronic condition on the problem list. Discuss with technical support how to make billing for the screening as easy as possible. Parents completing screening tools on a tablet can help address some of the challenges listed earlier. As mentioned, asking parents to fill out developmental screening tools on the patient portal before the visit may be insufficient to equitably improve screening rates.

Special Populations and Circumstances

Screening for general developmental status is appropriate upon return to primary care after an extended hospitalization or stay in a subacute care facility. Premature infant development in typical clinical practice is evaluated adjusting for prematurity until 24 months of age. However, keep in mind that measurable effects of prematurity on development extend throughout childhood.

Children with mild delays who are already enrolled in EI also benefit from developmental screening, so that the clinician may track progress and identify additional issues that need evaluation. Children with moderate or severe developmental disabilities present unique considerations. Most screening tool validation studies exclude children with identified developmental disabilities, and so use of tools in this context lies outside the validation studies. Some tools, such as the Parents Evaluation of Developmental Status (PEDS), may be better suited in this context since they focus on parental concern rather than on specific milestones. Many experienced clinicians choose surveillance to track progress over time in this scenario.

Children in foster care have a higher risk of developmental delays from congenital, environmental, and psychosocial causes (Adams & Tapia, 2013). We recommend screening children in foster care for developmental and ASD risk outside of the recommended routine visits due to this elevated risk, especially when historical data are lacking due to instability of their medical home. Although these children are often referred prior to presenting to clinic, clinicians should nevertheless assess the child's development and refer to EI or ECSE if indicated.

Children growing up in multilingual households deserve careful consideration. A multilingual environment alone does not increase a child's risk of communication disorders, but early on children learning more than one language may score lower on standardized screening tools that are validated among children only learning one language. More important is offering a screening tool to the child's caregiver in the native language whenever possible to improve the chances of accurate reporting (see Gerdes & Yun [2015] in Further Reading). However, as noted earlier, translation does not guarantee validation in the target language.

RESULTS

Interpretation of Results

The clinician should interpret the results of a developmental screening tool rapidly and give an impression to the family during the same clinical encounter. Clinicians should score the tool according to the tool developer's algorithm, and minimize rewording of questions or discounting of answers due to social or cultural considerations, since doing so may insert bias. Multiple studies show that clinicians often do not take action based on a positive screening test result, which may cause concerning delays in care. A unilateral wait-and-see approach by the clinician—especially when presented with parental concern about a child's development—is inappropriate and does a disservice to the child and family. As a result, clinicians should consider carefully if they plan to *not* refer a child with a positive test result. Clearly, there are some situations in which a child with a positive screening result should not be referred for services (for instance, a child who is already enrolled in services, or a child with prematurity who is developing typically for corrected gestational age). However, overall, clinicians should err on the side of referral when they are uncertain.

Clinicians should remind families that screening does not produce a diagnosis. Screening permits early identification of developmental delay, which is a common pathway for many causes for clinicians to consider; a more specific medical diagnosis may not be established until after treatment has begun. For instance, a child with an isolated communication delay might indicate an expressive language disorder, an early indication of ASD, or a hearing impairment. Asking follow-up questions about parents' observations and concerns will help inform next steps.

Borderline Results

Many developmental screening tools are more sensitive and specific at the extremes of the score range than near the cutoff (Sheldrick et al., 2019b), therefore shared decision making may be needed for children with borderline scores. The decision whether to seek additional services as a result of a positive screening test may depend on parent preferences, specific concerns, and service availability, among other factors (Sheldrick et al., 2019a). It is also important to consider that while developmental delays in early childhood generally are predictive of academic and social risks as children age, the specific pattern of developmental delays in any particular child has limited predictive value. For a child with borderline scores, it may be acceptable to offer opportunities for developmental promotion (e.g., through the Centers for Disease Control and Prevention's Learn the Signs. Act Early. resources or Vroom, see Further Reading) and rescreen the child at the next visit. Inserting a reminder in the EHR to rescreen at the next visit may be helpful.

Communicating Results and Forming a Plan

When communicating screening test results to a family, it is important to consider the family's state of knowledge and concern. For instance, many parents have never heard the word *autism*, or they may know very little about the condition (Zuckerman, Chavez, Regalado Murillo, Lindly, & Reeder, 2018). Parents also may not share clinicians' concerns about the child's development and/or behavior, may experience stigma related to developmental conditions, or may have inaccurate views about developmental services (for instance, confusing them with child protective services [Jimenez, Barg, Guevara, Gerdes, & Fiks, 2012], or expecting that they are expensive). As a result, it is useful to frame the discussion in terms of opportunities for support rather than deficits and prognoses. A discussion of developmental screening also provides an opportunity for shared decision making in that clinicians can help prioritize those skills and services that parents perceive as most valuable. After a plan is made, documenting the delay and the plan in the EHR is essential so that it can be readdressed at the next visit.

REFERRAL

Children who have a positive result on a general developmental screener should be referred to their local EI or ECSE agency. Though services are often available elsewhere, EI has a federal mandate to evaluate and treat children within 45 days of referral, and thus is often the fastest route to services. Children with receptive or expressive language delays should also be referred for an audiology evaluation. If children have delays in multiple areas, have a profound delay in any area, or have other indications of a developmental syndrome on history or physical exam, they should also be referred to a developmental specialist.

Children who have a positive result on an autism screener should additionally be referred for autism evaluation. Relying on EI to perform an autism evaluation, or waiting to engage EI until after an autism evaluation, is not recommended as it may lead to delays in diagnosis and treatment.

AFTER REFERRAL

Loss to follow-up after referring a child to EI/ECSE is a common problem, with anywhere from one-third to two-thirds of referred children never completing their eligibility determinations (Atkins, Dolata, Blasco, Saxton, & Duvall, 2020; McManus et al., 2020). Communication barriers play a role, and many families express low acceptability for the entry process and receiving services (Jimenez et al., 2012). Families of racial minorities and families with low income are especially at risk for not engaging in services (McManus et al., 2020). For these reasons, it is important to define a follow-up process within the office workflow. Having a health care professional send a referral directly instead of only giving parents a phone number to call has been associated with an almost threefold higher likelihood of success (Jimenez et al., 2014). Referral navigators can be effective but expensive (Conroy et al., 2018). Tracking referrals proactively can be effective, but studies done in the pre-EHR era have found this very time consuming (King et al., 2010). Here we encourage clinicians to consider use of their EHR's referral function or the registry function if present. Regardless, we recommend clinicians habitually discuss the outcome of EI/ECSE referrals with their patient families at their next clinic visit by asking about the child's progress and the caregiver's satisfaction with it. In addition, placing a developmental concern on the problem list of a child's medical record enables its future consideration, such as when assessing their school readiness.

FURTHER READING

AAP Autism Toolkit. https://toolkits.solutions.aap.org/autism/home

AAP. *Developmental surveillance. What, why and how* [Video]. YouTube. https://youtu.be/sceYLUHhgnU

AAP. *Screening/testing coding fact sheet*. https://www.aap.org/en-us/Documents/coding_factsheet_developmental-screeningtestingandEmotionalBehvioraassessment.pdf

Alabama Child Health Improvement Alliance and the University of Alabama. *Tools for developmental screening* [Video]. YouTube. https://www.youtube.com/watch?v=hlqgVrHIogw

Bricker, D., Macy, M., Squires, J., & Marks, K. (2013). *Developmental screening in your community: An integrated approach for connecting children with services*. Paul H. Brookes Publishing.

CDC Learn the Signs. Act Early. & AAP. (2017). *Don't just wait & see change package*. https://downloads.aap.org/DOCHW/Developmental_Surveillance_Screening_P2_Change_Package_FINAL.pdf

CDC Learn the Signs. Act Early. *With Milestone Tracker app*. https://www.cdc.gov/ncbddd/actearly/index.html

Gerdes, M., & Yun, K. (2015). *Translating standardized pediatric questionnaires: A simple tool for providers*. https://policylab.chop.edu/sites/default/files/pdf/publications/Translating_Standardized_Pediatric_Questionnaires.pdf

Glascoe, F. P. (2013). *Identifying and addressing developmental-behavioral problems: A practical guide for medical and non-medical professionals, trainees, researchers and advocates*. PEDStest.com, LLC.

Help Me Grow National Center, including links to local programs. https://helpmegrownational.org/

Screening Technical Assistance & Resource (STAR) Center—Developmental Screening. https://www.aap.org/en-us/advocacy-and-policy/aap-health-initiatives/Screening/Pages/Early-Childhood-Development.aspx

Vroom. *Bezos Family Foundation mobile app*. https://www.vroom.org/

REFERENCES

Adams, R. C., & Tapia, C. (2013). Early intervention, IDEA Part C services, and the medical home: Collaboration for best practice and best outcomes. *Pediatrics*, *132*(4), e1073–e1088. https://doi.org/10.1542/peds.2013-2305. Reaffirmed 2017. https://doi.org/10.1542/peds.2017-0649

American Academy of Pediatrics Committee on Children With Disabilities. (2001). Developmental surveillance and screening of infants and young children. *Pediatrics*, *108*(1), 192–195. https://doi.org/10.1542/peds.108.1.192

American Academy of Pediatrics Committee on Practice and Ambulatory Medicine, Bright Futures Periodicity Schedule Workgroup. (2021). 2021 recommendations for preventive pediatric health care. *Pediatrics*, *147*(3) https://doi.org/10.1542/peds.2020-049776

Atkins, K. L., Dolata, J. K., Blasco, P. M., Saxton, S. N., & Duvall, S. W. (2020). Early intervention referral outcomes for children at increased risk of experiencing developmental delays. *Maternal and Child Health Journal*, *24*(2), 204–212. https://doi.org/10.1007/s10995-019-02830-4

Brothers, K. B., Glascoe, F. P., & Robertshaw, N. S. (2008). PEDS: Developmental milestones—An accurate brief tool for surveillance and screening. *Clinical Pediatrics*, *47*(3), 271–279. https://doi.org/10.1177/0009922807309419

Conroy, K., Rea, C., Kovacikova, G. I., Sprecher, E., Reisinger, E., Durant, H., … Toomey, S. L. (2018). Ensuring timely connection to early intervention for young children with developmental delays. *Pediatrics*, *142*(1), e20174017. https://doi.org/10.1542/peds.2017-4017

El-Toukhy, S., Méndez, A., Collins, S., & Pérez-Stable, E. J. (2020). Barriers to patient portal access and use: Evidence from the Health Information National Trends Survey. *Journal of the American Board of Family Medicine*, *33*(6), 953–968. https://doi.org/10.3122/jabfm.2020.06.190402

Guevara, P. J., Gerdes, M., Localio, R., Huang, V. Y., Pinto-Martin, J., Minkovitz, S. C., … Pati, S. (2013). Effectiveness of developmental screening in an urban setting. *Pediatrics*, *131*(1), 30–37. https://doi.org/10.1542/peds.2012-0765

Hirai, A. H., Kogan, M. D., Kandasamy, V., Reuland, C., & Bethell, C. (2018). Prevalence and variation of developmental screening and surveillance in early childhood. *JAMA Pediatrics* https://doi.org/10.1001/jamapediatrics.2018.1524

Hyman, S. L., Levy, S. E., & Myers, S. M. (2020). Identification, evaluation, and management of children with autism spectrum disorder. *Pediatrics*, *145*(1), e20193447. https://doi.org/10.1542/peds.2019-3447

Jimenez, E. M., Barg, K. F., Guevara, P. J., Gerdes, M., & Fiks, G. A. (2012). Barriers to evaluation for early intervention services: Parent and early intervention employee perspectives. *Academic Pediatrics*, *12*(6), 551–557. https://doi.org/10.1016/j.acap.2012.08.006

Jimenez, E. M., Fiks, G. A., Shah, R. L., Gerdes, M., Ni, Y. A., Pati, S., & Guevara, P. J. (2014). Factors associated with early intervention referral and evaluation: A mixed methods analysis. *Academic Pediatrics*, *14*(3), 315–323. https://doi.org/10.1016/j.acap.2014.01.007

King, M. T., Tandon, D. S., Macias, M. M., Healy, A. J., Duncan, M. P., Swigonski, L. N., … Lipkin, H. P. (2010). Implementing developmental screening and referrals: Lessons learned from a national project. *Pediatrics*, *125*(2), 350–360. https://doi.org/10.1542/peds.2009-0388

Lipkin, P. H., & Macias, M. M. (2020). Promoting optimal development: Identifying infants and young children with developmental disorders through developmental surveillance and screening. *Pediatrics*, *145*(1), e20193449. https://doi.org/10.1542/peds.2019-3449

Lipkin, P. H., Macias, M. M., Baer Chen, B., Coury, D., Gottschlich, E. A., Hyman, S. L., ... Levy, S. E. (2020). Trends in pediatricians' developmental screening: 2002–2016. *Pediatrics*, *145*(4). https://doi.org/10.1542/peds.2019-0851

Marlow, M., Servili, C., & Tomlinson, M. (2019, February). A review of screening tools for the identification of autism spectrum disorders and developmental delay in infants and young children: Recommendations for use in low- and middle-income countries. *Autism Research*, *12*(2), 176–199. https://doi.org/10.1002/aur.2033

McManus, B. M., Richardson, Z., Schenkman, M., Murphy, N. J., Everhart, R. M., Hambidge, S., & Morrato, E. (2020). Child characteristics and early intervention referral and receipt of services: A retrospective cohort study. *BMC Pediatrics*, *20*(1), 84. https://doi.org/10.1186/s12887-020-1965-x

Schonwald, A., Huntington, N., Chan, E., Risko, W., & Bridgemohan, C. (2009). Routine developmental screening implemented in urban primary care settings: More evidence of feasibility and effectiveness. *Pediatrics*, *123*(2), 660–668. https://doi.org/10.1542/peds.2007-2798

Sheldrick, R. C., Frenette, E., Vera, J. D., Mackie, T. I., Martinez-Pedraza, F., Hoch, N., ... Carter, A. S. (2019a). What drives detection and diagnosis of autism spectrum disorder? Looking under the hood of a multi-stage screening process in early intervention. *Journal of Autism and Developmental Disorders*. https://doi.org/10.1007/s10803-019-03913-5

Sheldrick, C. R., & Perrin, C. E. (2013). Evidence-based milestones for surveillance of cognitive, language, and motor development. *Academic Pediatrics*, *13*(6), 577–586. https://doi.org/10.1016/j.acap.2013.07.001

Sheldrick, R. C., Schlichting, L. E., Berger, B., Clyne, A., Ni, P., Perrin, E. C., & Vivier, P. M. (2019b). Establishing new norms for developmental milestones. *Pediatrics*, *144*(6), e20190374. https://doi.org/10.1542/peds.2019-0374

Sheldrick, R. C., Merchant, S., & Perrin, E. C. (2011). Identification of developmental-behavioral problems in primary care: A systematic review. *Pediatrics*, *128*(2), 356–363. https://doi.org/10.1542/peds.2010-3261

Silver, R. B., Newland, R. P., Hartz, K., Jandasek, B., Godoy, L., Lingras, K. A., ... Seifer, R. (2017). Integrating early childhood screening in pediatrics: A longitudinal qualitative study of barriers and facilitators. *Clinical Practice in Pediatric Psychology*, *5*(4), 426–440. https://doi.org/10.1037/cpp0000214

Siu, A. L., & US Preventive Services Task Force, (2016). Screening for autism spectrum disorder in young children: USPSTF recommendation statement. *The Journal of the American Medical Association*, *315*(7), 691–696. https://doi.org/10.1001/jama.2016.0018

Squires, J., Bricker, D., & Potter, L. (1997). Revision of a parent-completed developmental screening tool: Ages and stages questionnaires. *Journal of Pediatric Psychology*, *22*(3), 313–328. https://doi.org/10.1093/jpepsy/22.3.313

Wallace, F. I., Berkman, D. N., Watson, R. L., Coyne-Beasley, T., Wood, T. C., Cullen, K., & Lohr, N. K. (2015). Screening for speech and language delay in children 5 years old and younger: A systematic review. *Pediatrics*, *136*(2), e448–e462. https://doi.org/10.1542/peds.2014-3889

Weitzman, C., & Wegner, L. (2015). Promoting optimal development: Screening for behavioral and emotional problems. *Pediatrics*, *135*(2), 384–395. https://doi.org/10.1542/peds.2014-3716

World Health Organization. (2020). Monitoring children's development in the primary care services: Moving from a focus on child deficits to family-centred participatory support. *Report of a virtual technical meeting*, 9–10. June 2020. https://apps.who.int/iris/rest/bitstreams/1310553/retrieve

Zuckerman, K. E., Chavez, A. E., Regalado Murillo, C., Lindly, O. J., & Reeder, J. A. (2018). Disparities in familiarity with developmental disabilities among low-income parents. *Academic Pediatrics*, *18*(8), 944–951. https://doi.org/10.1016/j.acap.2018.06.011

82

Evaluation of Emotion and Behavior

Laura A. Shaffer and R. Emily Gonzalez

For additional material related to the content of this chapter, please see Chapter 76.

VIGNETTE

Four-year-old Anthony Diaz is the eldest of three children born in Guatemala to predominantly Spanish-speaking parents. Anthony's family immigrated to the United States when he was 3 years old, and he was separated from his parents for approximately 6 months in the process. Upon reunification with his parents, Anthony had lost previously acquired language milestones, regressed with toilet training, had diminished appetite, and experienced frequent nightmares. In his initial evaluation the pediatric clinician noted delays in fine and gross motor skills as well as in speech and language development. Anthony's emotional and behavioral presentation was most notable for restricted affect, anxiety, avoidant eye contact, and an exaggerated startle response. His parents share that he cries when taken to preschool and spends most of his day sitting by himself, quiet and apparently overwhelmed. Parents are ambivalent about seeking care for Anthony, sharing concerns about their inability to afford medical care and worries about being reported to authorities for their son's developmental delays. Parents believe that Anthony's symptoms will improve with time for adjustment and decreased stress.

Growing numbers of children and adolescents are experiencing emotion and behavior concerns and are more likely to present initially in pediatric settings than in specialty mental health settings. Current estimates of US children diagnosed with a mental disorder consistently fall in the range of 13% to 20%. Among children living below 100% of the poverty level, 22% had a mental, behavioral, or developmental disorder (Cree et al., 2018). Even greater numbers of children have subthreshold symptoms and would benefit from intervention to prevent worsening (Stiffler & Dever, 2015). Early identification and treatment can make a difference in the lives of children with emotion and behavior concerns and their families.

The most commonly diagnosed mental disorders in children in the United States are attention-deficit/hyperactivity disorder (ADHD) (9.4%), behavior problems (7.4%), anxiety (7.1%), and depression (3.2%) (Danielson, Bitsko, Ghandour, Holbrook, & Blumberg, 2018; Ghandour et al., 2019). Emotion and behavior concerns are even more prevalent in children with neurodevelopmental disorders (ND) and developmental disabilities (DD) (Lai et al., 2019). Nearly two out of five youth with autism spectrum disorder (ASD) have clinically elevated levels of anxiety (van Steensel, Bögels, & Perrin, 2011). Children with chronic health conditions are twice as likely as children without to have cooccurring mental health or substance abuse disorders (Perrin, Asarnow, Stancin, Melek, & Fritz, 2019). Thus pediatric settings are crucial arenas for routine assessment of emotion and behavior.

Emotion and behavior concerns often are missed in pediatric settings (Maruish, 2018). A review by the American Academy of Pediatrics Task Force on Mental Health (AAP-TFM, 2019) found that less than one in three children with mental health problems are identified in primary care. Clinicians' ability to correctly identify children with behavioral health concerns based on clinical judgment alone was quite low with sensitivities ranging from 14% to 54% (Sheldrick, Merchant, & Perrin, 2011). Detection of behavioral health concerns is even more problematic for children of different racial and ethnic groups (Liang, Matheson, & Douglas, 2016).

Routine assessment in pediatric settings has the potential to mitigate these oversights and disparities. Pediatric clinicians are optimally positioned to screen, diagnose when able, and know when to refer for more extensive evaluation. More systematic evaluation of emotion and behavior problems enables clinicians to make appropriate recommendations and referrals as well as provide resources as a bridge to evidence-based treatment and track symptoms over time. Emotion and behavior assessment also supports more value-based health care payment models.

ASSESSMENT METHODS

The American Psychological Association (APA, 2020) defines assessment as "complex activity integrating knowledge, clinical judgement, reliable collateral information, and psychometric constructs with expertise in an area of professional practice or application" (p. 5). This typically involves synthesis of information from multiple sources or reporters and multiple methods. No single instrument is diagnostic. The assessment of emotion and behavior in pediatrics generally follows a progression from global screening to broadband assessment to symptom-specific or narrowband assessment to formal diagnostic assessment (Stiffler & Dever, 2015). More in-depth discussions of global screening and diagnostic assessment through psychological testing are provided in Chapters 76 and 81, respectively. Broadband and narrowband assessment measures are described further here. Specific examples of these measures identified by experts in the field (AAP-TFM, 2019; Andrews, Cho, Tugendrajch, Marriott, & Hawley, 2020; Holmbeck et al., 2008) are detailed in Tables 82.1 and 82.2. Included instruments generally have suitable reliability and validity with general populations. The majority of emotion and behavior assessment measures for children have not yet been well researched for populations with neurodevelopmental differences, and few studies have established reliability and validity with translated measures. Users should review information provided in the technical manuals for the instruments to fully inform selection, administration, scoring, and interpretation.

Broadband Measures

Broadband measures identify general maladjustment as well as possible arrays of symptom severity for specific disorders (Stiffler & Denver, 2015). They contain more items, take longer to complete, and are more complicated to score and interpret than screening measures. Because of their greater complexity, broadband measures tend to be proprietary, requiring certain professional credentials and fees to use. Broadband assessments of emotion and behavior can take the form of omnibus rating scales, structured interviews, or projective tests.

Omnibus Rating Scales

Omnibus rating scales (see Table 82.1) typically consist of broad composite internalizing and externalizing symptom scores in addition to more specific scales related to different symptom and adaptive function clusters that are derived from norm-based scoring. Most are available in parent, teacher, and youth self-report forms. Self-report inventories have been shown to be less valid for children younger than 8 to 9 years old but can still be informative regarding children's perceptions of their functioning (Frick, Barry, & Kamphaus, 2020). Though lengthier than global screeners, omnibus rating scales are still time efficient and facilitate multiinformant assessment (Frick et al., 2020). They also tend to have national normative samples, increasing their utility by facilitating comparisons of individual youth to their age- and gender-matched peers instead of simply using symptom counts to determine clinical cutoffs. Furthermore, omnibus rating scales have much more extensive data demonstrating reliability and validity and thus are considered by many to be the gold standard to which other measures are compared. These advantages lend to their suitability for use in pediatric settings.

Structured Diagnostic Interviews

Structured diagnostic interviews typically consist of a standardized set of questions organized by the *Diagnostic and Statistical Manual of Mental Disorders*, fifth edition (*DSM-5*) (American Psychiatric Association, 2013) diagnosis and can be used to assess disruptive behavior disorders, affective disorders, and anxiety disorders in children and adolescents in addition to screening for schizophrenia. Most interviews take anywhere from 30 minutes to 2 hours to complete and have parallel child and parent versions to promote multiinformant assessment. Interviews allow for gathering information about the parameters of a child's behaviors and symptoms such as onset, duration, and temporal sequencing that is not obtained from rating scales (Frick et al., 2020). However, structured diagnostic interviews are time intensive and dependent on *DSM-5* criteria, which makes them less useful for assessing behaviors that do not closely align with these criteria and for making norm-referenced interpretations (Frick et al., 2020). These disadvantages make interviews less practical for use in pediatric settings outside the context of fuller psychological assessment.

Projective Techniques

Projective techniques require test takers to respond to unstructured or ambiguous stimuli and include methods such as drawings (e.g., Draw a Person and Kinetic Family Drawing), incomplete sentences, apperception or storytelling tasks (e.g., Roberts Apperception Technique for Children), and inkblot tests (e.g., Rorschach). These tests are rooted in psychodynamic theory and are based on the projective hypothesis that stimuli that allow for a variety of interpretations encourage revelation of information respondents otherwise would not share in response to direct questioning. There are two approaches to the interpretation of projectives: Psychometric and clinical (Frick et al., 2020). The psychometric approach allows for the comparison of a child's score to a normative group and requires the maintenance of rigorous standardization in administration and scoring as well as acceptance of limited data. The clinical approach affords greater flexibility in administration and scoring but is more susceptible to idiosyncratic influences as a result. Use of projective techniques is controversial because of the debate over these disparate approaches. Accordingly, their use in child and adolescent assessment has been declining in the United States.

Narrowband Measures

As their name implies, narrowband measures gather more domain-specific information regarding children's emotional and behavioral functioning. Narrowband assessment methods include rating scales, structured interviews, and clinician observer-based measures. Most of these measures are faster to administer because they are briefer and more focused than broadband measures. Rating scales are available in multiple informant versions and are designed to assess a particular domain of functioning such as anxiety, depression, or executive functions (see examples in Table 82.2). Use of structured interviews to assess targeted emotion or behavior concerns typically involves administering a domain-specific section of a full diagnostic interview. (Observational assessments are discussed in Chapter 84.) In addition to allowing for the collection of more detailed information about specific domains from multiple informants, many narrowband measures, particularly rating scales, are well validated and normed, are easily administered and scored, capture low-frequency behaviors, and allow for more specific monitoring of treatment progress. One potential drawback to narrowband measures is they do not allow for the assessment of behavior or emotion concerns

TABLE 82.1 Broadband Rating Scales of Emotion and Behavior in Children and Adolescents

Instrument	Domains Assessed	Number of Items and Respondents	Age Group	Administration Time	Technical Notes	Cultural/ Linguistic Considerations	Availability
Achenbach System of Empirically Based Assessment (ASEBA)	Yields overall scores for internalizing, externalizing, and total problems Has specific syndrome and *DSM*-oriented scales	100–113 items Parent report: Child Behavior Checklist (CBCL/1.5–5yr and CBCL/ 6–18yr) Teacher Report Form (C-TRF & TRF) Youth Self-Report (YSR) (11–18yr)	1.5–18yr	15–20min	Differentiates between children referred and not referred for mental health disorders Children with DD had higher total problems scores on the CBCL than children with ASD and mental health concerns	Norms available for a number of countries including the US >110 translations	Proprietary
Behavior Assessment System for Children, Third Edition (BASC-3)	Yields scores for externalizing problems, internalizing problems, behavioral symptoms index, adaptive skills, 7 content scales, 4 clinical indexes, 5 executive functioning indexes, and a validity index	105–192 items Parent Report (PRS-P, PRS-C, PRS-A) Teacher Report (TRS-P, TRS-C, TRS-A) Self-Report (SRP-C, SRP-A, SRP-COL)	2–21yr	10–30min	Clinical norms available, norms for students diagnosed with ADHD; profile analyses presented for children identified with a diagnosis of ADHD, ASD, emotional/ behavioral disturbances, hearing impairment, specific LD, or speech/language disorder; PRS recommended for use in youth with long-term physical problems	Translation: Spanish	Proprietary
Infant-Toddler Social Emotional Assessment (ITSEA)	Problem total, competence total, externalizing, internalizing, dysregulation, competence, maladaptive item cluster, social relatedness cluster, atypical item cluster	170 items Parent/caregiver and childcare provider report, can be completed as interviews	1–3yr	20–30min	Low test-retest reliability; lack of empirical support for reliability and validity of childcare provider form	Translation: Spanish	Proprietary

ADHD, Attention-deficit/hyperactivity disorder; *ASD*, autism spectrum disorder; *DD*, developmental disabilities; *DSM, Diagnostic and Statistical Manual of Mental Disorders*; *LD*, learning disabilities.

Note: Most information obtained from the *Mental Measurements Yearbook* and Publisher's websites. Additional citations for articles reviewed to evaluate each tool's psychometric properties are available from the corresponding author on request.

TABLE 82.2 **Narrowband Assessment Measures of Emotion and Behavior in Children and Adolescents**

Instrument	Domains Assessed	Number of Items and Respondents	Age Group	Administration Time	Technical Notes	Cultural/Linguistic Considerations	Availability
Children's Depression Inventory (CDI, 2003 Update)	Depression (negative mood, interpersonal problems, ineffectiveness, anhedonia, and negative self-esteem)	27 items, youth 17 items, parent 12 items, teacher	7–17 yr	10 min	Manual states the validity of using the CDI in cross-cultural applications has not been established, as diagnostic classifications and symptoms vary from culture to culture	Translation: Spanish	Proprietary
Center for Epidemiological Studies Depression Scale for Children (CES-DC)	Depression (mood, somatic complaints, and interpersonal problems)	20 items, youth	6–17 yr	10 min	Measure is adapted from the adult CES-D. Several psychometric validity studies have been published for different ethnic cultures in the adult population Modified version may not differentiate well between depressed and nondepressed adolescents	Translations: Chinese, French, German, Italian, Japanese, Korean, Russian, & Spanish	Freely accessible
Patient Health Questionnaire for Adolescents	Anxiety, eating problems, mood problems, and substance abuse	83 items, youth	13–18 yr	3–10 min		11 translations including Spanish	Freely accessible
Beck Depression Inventory-II (1996 revision of the BDI)	Depression	21 items, youth	14+ yr	5–10 min	Discriminates between adolescents who do and do not meet *DSM* criteria for a major depressive disorder. The normative sample is predominantly White (91%); more research is needed on the use of the BDI-II with diverse groups of adolescents	Cross-cultural validation of psychometric properties in several countries, different populations. Translations: Arabic, Chinese, Farsi, German, Japanese, Norwegian, Spanish, Swedish, & Turkish	Proprietary
Parent Version-Young Mania Rating Scale (P-YMRS)	Mania, hypomania, and functional interference	11 items, parent	5–17 yr	5–10 min	Discriminates bipolar mood disorder vs. unipolar disorder, disruptive behavior disorder, and other diagnoses	Translation: Spanish	Freely accessible
Ask Suicide-Screening Questions (ASQ) Toolkit	Suicidal ideation	4+ items, youth	8+ yr	<5 min		13 translations including Spanish	Freely accessible

Suicidal Ideation Questionnaire (SIQ) and Suicidal Ideation Questionnaire, Jr. (SIQ-J)	Suicidal ideation	SIQ: 30 items, grades 10–12 SIQ-J: 15 items, grades 7–9	12+ yr	10 min	Good psychometric properties (including sensitivity, predictive validity) with diverse normative groups (clinical, nonclinical, different cultural backgrounds). Strong favorability as the screening tool to use with youth compared to other measures	Translation: French	Proprietary
GAD-7	Generalized anxiety	7 items, youth	13+ yr	5 min		Translations: Arabic, Bengali, French, German, Greek, Hebrew, Hindi, Spanish, Turkish, & Urdu	Freely accessible
Screen for Child Anxiety-Related Emotional Disorders (SCARED)	Panic/somatic, generalized anxiety, separation anxiety, social phobia, and school phobia	41- and 66-item versions Parent report Youth self-report	8–18 yr	10 min		Cross-cultural validation of psychometric properties in several countries. 13 translations including Spanish	Freely accessible
Spence Children's Anxiety Scale	Social phobia, panic disorder, agoraphobia, generalized anxiety disorder, obsessive-compulsive disorder, separation anxiety disorder, specific phobias/ fear of physical injury	38 items, parent report 44 items, child report 3–5 items, preschool version	8–15 yr	10 min	Limited normative information for preschool version No US data available	Cross-cultural validation; Translations: Arabic, Bengali, French, German, Greek, Hebrew, Hindi, Spanish, Turkish, & Urdu	Freely accessible
Multidimensional Anxiety Scale for Children, Second Edition (MASC-2)	Separation anxiety/ phobias, generalized anxiety disorder, social anxiety, obsessions and compulsions, physical symptoms, harm avoidance, anxiety	50 items, youth self-report 50 items, parent report	8–19 yr	15 min	Limited normative information for different ethnic/racial groups	Translations: Chinese, Dutch, Icelandic, Swedish, & Taiwanese	Proprietary

(*Continued*)

TABLE 82.2 Narrowband Assessment Measures of Emotion and Behavior in Children and Adolescents—Cont'd

Instrument	Domains Assessed	Number of Items and Respondents	Age Group	Administration Time	Technical Notes	Cultural/Linguistic Considerations	Availability
Children's Yale-Brown Obsessive Compulsive Scale	Severity, functional interference of obsessive-compulsive disorder symptoms	70 questions, semistructured interview	6–17 yr	15–25 min	The modified scale 2 (CYBOCS-PDD) contains only the five compulsion severity items (range 0–20) and has shown excellent reliability (ICC = 0.97) and internal consistency (alpha = 0.85)	14 translations including Spanish	Freely accessible
NICHQ Vanderbilt Scales	Inattention, disruptive behavior, anxiety, depression; home and school functional interference (interpersonal relationships, academic)	55 items, parent/teacher 43 items, parent follow-up 26 items, teacher follow-up	6–12 yr	10 min		Translations: Spanish	Freely accessible
Trauma Symptom Checklist for Children (TSCC), Adolescent Self-Report (TSCC-A), and Young Children (TSCY)	Anxiety, depression, anger/aggression, posttraumatic stress intrusion, posttraumatic stress avoidance, posttraumatic stress arousal, posttraumatic stress total, dissociation, sexual concerns	54 items, child 44 items, adolescent (44-item TSCC-A does not include sexual concern items) TSYC: 90 items, parent report	8–16 yr	15–20 min	Psychometrics supported by multisite sample of children exposed to multiple forms of trauma Limited normative information for translated versions	Translations for TSCC, TSCC-A: Chinese, Dutch, French, Japanese, Latvian, Slovenian, Spanish, & Swedish Translations for TSYC: Spanish & Swedish	Proprietary
UCLA Posttraumatic Stress Disorder Reaction Index (PTSD RI), Revised for *DSM-5* (2013)	Exposure to traumatic experiences and impact of traumatic events	20 items, child 21 items, parent 22 items, youth	7–12 yr (child, parent) 13+ yr (youth)	15–20 min		Cross-cultural validation in 11 countries of a 4-factor structure aligning with *DSM-V* criterion; 10 different translations	Proprietary
Child and Adolescent Trauma Screen (CATS)	Trauma screen Functional impairment	3–6 items, parent version 7–17 items, youth self-report	3–17 yr	10 min	Limited normative information for 3–6 version Satisfactory psychometric properties across international samples for youth version	Cross-cultural validation studies (Germany, Norway) Translations: German, Norwegian, & Spanish	Freely accessible

DSM-5, Diagnostic and Statistical Manual of Mental Disorders, fifth edition.

Note: Most information obtained from the *Mental Measurements Yearbook* and Publisher's websites. Additional citations for articles reviewed to evaluate each tool's psychometric properties are available from the corresponding author on request.

beyond the scope of the particular measure. Some argue that this could be significantly limiting given the high cooccurrence of psychiatric disorders and symptom profiles and call for a more globally focused evaluative process (Derogatis, 2017; Stiffler & Dever, 2015).

IMPLEMENTATION OF EMOTION AND BEHAVIOR ASSESSMENTS IN CLINICAL SETTINGS

Emotion and behavior assessment requires careful planning. There are several resources available to provide guidance for assessment program implementation (Maruish, 2018) and to guide pediatric clinicians in assessment with ethnically and culturally diverse families (Cora-Bramble & Schaefer, 2011; Godoy & Carter, 2013; Kohn-Wood & Hooper, 2014). Psychologists often are integral to the establishment of effective emotion and behavior assessment programs because of their strong training in foundations of assessment. Psychologists are well positioned to assist in selecting appropriate measures, establishing protocols for office procedures, training in administration and scoring of instruments, and formulating clinical decision-making protocols (Ward-Zimmerman & Berlinsky, 2018). The development of the assessment workflow needs to incorporate a number of factors, including instrument selection, procurement, administration, scoring, and interpretation as well as how results will be communicated to families.

Instrument Selection

Selecting an assessment instrument calls for careful consideration on a number of fronts, including relevancy, technical properties, and feasibility for families and clinical practices. A summary of general considerations compiled by Maruish (2018) is presented in Table 82.3. It is helpful to select measures that allow for collection of information from multiple informants such as caregivers, teachers, and youth themselves to provide a fuller picture of the child's functioning across settings and as perceived by different key individuals. Ideally, assessment of emotion and behavior problems in youth with ND/DD would entail the use of instruments with norms and demonstrated psychometric integrity specific to this population, but the reality is that much of this work has yet to be done. Recommended technical criteria for assessment instruments are that they be tested against a gold standard for assessing the target problem in the population of interest and have adequate validity (e.g., Chronbach alpha > 0.80) and reliability (e.g., interrater reliability > 0.4) (Thabrew, McDowell, Given, & Murren, 2017). In a review of 44 instruments to assess emotion and behavior problems in youth with long-term physical concerns none met all of the technical criteria to qualify as an ideal instrument and most had demonstrated psychometric integrity only with the general population (Thabrew et al., 2017). Thus clinicians must select from measures developed for the general population.

Access/Purchasing Requirements

Central to the establishment of assessment procedures is the premise that clinicians should use only those tests for which they have the appropriate training and expertise. Some instruments are available for public use, whereas others require permission and proof of credentials that meet the educational and training qualifications required by the publisher. Purchase privileges are tiered such that a bachelor's degree is often sufficient for obtaining and administering certain screening measures, and the use of more comprehensive assessment tools requires a master's or doctoral degree in specified fields with training in the ethical administration, scoring, and interpretation of clinical assessments related to the intended use of the instruments.

Administration of Measures

Emotion and behavior rating scales have several options for how and by whom they can be administered. These measures may be sent to families and teachers electronically or by mail prior to visits, provided by frontdesk staff and self-administered in the waiting room, administered by support staff with appropriate training, or administered by clinicians as part of the visit. Instruments can be paper-pencil, electronic, or orally administered using interactive voice-response technology. Electronic administrations may facilitate identification of concerns that otherwise might have been underidentified due to greater ease in accessing other language versions and adolescents' tendency to disclose more emotion and behavior concerns on electronic platforms than in interviews or on paper (AAP-TFM, 2019). Nonproprietary instruments can be integrated into the electronic health record (EHR) to be pulled into the patient encounter at the time of the visit. Many propriety measures can be administered on publishers' web-based platforms, a number of which have options to interface with the EHR. Optimizing use of the EHR to make results rapidly available in addition to embedded decision support and referral tools can increase clinical utility.

Scoring and Interpretation

Established tools for emotion and behavior assessment are accompanied by guidelines for scoring and interpretation. Rating scales can be scored by trained staff members with consultation from clinicians when questions arise such as how to handle missing data. Shorter measures can be scored quickly by hand, and longer measures typically have electronic scoring systems available. Staff can then enter the scores into the EHR to be reviewed and interpreted by the pediatric clinician. Ethical and meaningful interpretation is more complex than simply comparing the results to cutoff scores for the normative sample. The clinician must also consider contextual factors such as how a child's ND/DD and ethnicity, culture, and language might impact scores and resemblance to the reference group. Valid interpretation to inform clinical decision making about diagnosis and recommendations typically requires additional information gathered through pertinent follow-up questions or additional measures.

Valid interpretation of assessment findings also includes the synthesis of data from multiple informants across different settings. Interpretation of convergent findings is straightforward. More commonly, clinicians are faced with interpreting discrepant findings across informants. Correlations between different sources tend to be low to moderate, ranging from 0.20 to 0.60 with higher levels of correspondence occurring when informants complete reports about concerns that they both have relatively greater opportunities to observe (e.g., externalizing behaviors vs. internalized emotions) or observe within the same context (e.g., parents in the same household vs. parent-teacher) (De Los Reyes et al., 2015). There are numerous reasons informant discrepancies may arise, including characteristics of the raters themselves, varying demands and behaviors across settings, and differing opportunities for informants to observe behaviors (De Los Reyes, 2013; Frick et al., 2020). Key to interpreting and synthesizing discrepant findings is explaining the discrepancies and any methodologic confounds (De Los Reyes, 2013; Frick et al., 2020). Understanding why certain concerns are noted by certain reporters in certain settings allows for a more individualized, context-specific approach that better reflects youths' functioning. Collateral information such as that from other raters or observations in clinic can be useful in testing hypotheses about reasons for discrepancies and help clarify situational and observer differences (De Los Reyes, 2013). Repeated measurements over time can also be informative and clarifying when there are discrepant reports across informants (Frick et al., 2020).

Providing Feedback

For assessment to be clinically meaningful there must be feedback to the family that includes interpretation of the findings and recommendations for next steps. Feedback may occur in oral and written forms. Regardless of the method, findings should be communicated clearly and in a culturally sensitive manner. It is also important to discuss implications of findings and formulate recommendations in the context of a child's ND/DD.

TABLE 82.3 General Considerations for Selecting Assessment Instruments for Emotion and Behavior

Instrument Feature	Important Considerations
Relevancy to the intended purpose of the assessment	• Is appropriate for measuring the targeted domain(s) in the targeted population(s)
Source of information	• Was developed to obtain information from the desired source of information (e.g., obtaining patient information from a parent using an instrument developed for administration to parents)
Instrument content	• Has no irrelevant, inappropriate, or offensive item content
Psychometric integrity	• Meets generally accepted standards for validity and reliability • Has demonstrated responsiveness (for individual data) and/or sensitivity (for group data) to changes in patient status
Availability of relevant normative data	• Has norms that are appropriate for the targeted population
Comprehensibility of results	• Results can be easily understood by the clinician, patient, family members, and other relevant stakeholders
Actionable information	• Provides the clinician with information that can be used to improve services to the patient
Assessment across the continuum of care	• Is appropriate for use with patients receiving care at any level of service (e.g., inpatient, outpatient, partial hospitalization)
Ease of use	• Is easy to administer, score, interpret, and provide feedback
Clinical utility	• Provides information that cannot be obtained any other way • Yields classification accuracy that is better than other measures of the same construct • Is cost effective and easy to use
Brevity	• Is considered short from the patient's perspective
Reading level	• Requires no higher than an eighth-grade reading level, with sixth grade or lower preferable • Or, can be administered via another mode that does not require reading (e.g., audiotape, interactive voice response) and yields comparable results
Cost	• Inexpensive to use for multiple administrations to a single patient
Overall practicality and feasibility	• Given all considerations, is practical for use in the intended setting, with the intended population, for the intended purpose(s)
Translated and adapted versions	• Was developed according to commonly accepted procedures and guidelines • Has met psychometric and other standards for equivalency with the original version of the instrument

Maruish (2013). Outcome assesment in health settings. In K.F. Geisinger. *APA handbook of testing and assesment in clinical and counseling psychology* (pp. 303–321). Washington, DC: American Psychological Association.

Financial Considerations

Emotion and behavior assessment carries costs for both health care professionals and families. Whereas there are many free instruments available, some require a fee for use. Other assessment costs include personnel time for training, administration, and scoring; instrument and data storage; and communicating assessment results to families and referring clinicians, schools, or other third parties. Many of these costs can be recuperated by coding and billing for emotion and behavior assessments as a separate current procedural terminology (CPT) code, but families are asked to cost-share when fees are not covered by their insurance. Creating an implementation plan that includes workflow for coding and billing helps optimize coverage and reduce costs for families.

Securing Data

Pediatric clinicians using emotion and behavior assessment tools are responsible for maintaining the security of the content and results of these measures. Copyrighted materials such as the instruments, specific items, administration manuals, and scoring guides should be kept separate from patient records. Web-based scoring platforms linked to many copyrighted assessment measures provide encrypted scoring and password protection to facilitate security of the measures and patient information. Within patient health records, standard practices such as EHR encryption, password protection, and signed consent for records release secure the results.

CULTURAL AND LANGUAGE CONSIDERATIONS

Clinicians should be sensitive to diverse cultural, ethnic, and religious backgrounds when they assess children's emotion and behavior. Whereas little has been done to examine the intersectionality of ethnic minority and disability status in assessment, there is growing evidence that instruments to assess youth emotion and behavior may be biased or lack cultural equivalence (Bevan, Liu, Wallis, & Pinto-Martin, 2020; Caballero et al., 2017; Liang et al., 2016). The majority of normative samples for most standardized instruments are for a White population, complicating instrument selection and interpretation of scores for children from different racial and ethnic groups. Furthermore, adaptation of tests for persons of another culture and language too often refers only to translation of test items with little concern for the integrity of meaning, context of items, and appropriate standardization (Dubay & Watson, 2019). Whereas many measures have been translated into languages other than English, there is little research on the conceptual and psychometric equivalence across different language versions and different cultural groups (Dubay & Watson, 2019). The absence of this information further complicates decision making about validity. Many commonly used emotion and behavior assessment measures are less accurate in detecting symptoms in minority groups (Council of National Psychological Associations for the Advancement of Ethnic Minority Interests, 2016) and youth with long-term physical conditions and DD (Thabrew et al., 2017). In the case of Anthony, in the chapter-opening vignette, the clinician must take into consideration that available behavioral Spanish-language assessment instruments function differently because of both language and culture and thus likely are not as psychometrically valid as English versions used in the general population (Bevan et al., 2020).

CLINICAL IMPLICATIONS

Assessment of emotion and behavior in pediatric settings is an integral tool for treatment planning, treatment monitoring, and outcomes. Wider use of culturally sensitive assessment with multiple methods and collateral informants stands to improve identification of concerns among youth with ND/DD who are typically at greater risk for emotion and behavior problems. It is important to keep in mind that instruments are not diagnostic on their own, but they do provide useful information concerning the need for more in-depth assessment and intervention. This connection to services is essential to optimizing the value of assessment. Thus in addition to clear protocols for implementation, pediatric clinicians must establish channels to refer for further evaluation and treatment when indicated by the assessment. Unfortunately, this can be a challenge due to the shortage of pediatric behavioral health clinicians in the United States, especially those trained to work with ND/DD populations, and other barriers including lack of culturally responsive services and social stigma. Including psychologists on the integrated health team helps to reduce some of these barriers in addition to developing sound assessment practices.

Anthony's case illustrates the complexity and potential benefits of assessment despite limitations in the field related to specific use of assessment tools with ND/DD and ethnic minority populations. To conduct a culturally sensitive assessment, the clinician would need to be proficient in Spanish or use a trained interpreter to conduct the interview, assessment, and feedback; select measures that are appropriately translated and culturally validated; and seek consultation from the literature or a colleague familiar with the assessment of ethnic minority children and the important sociocultural variables specific to the assessment of Latinx children. A good starting point for standardized assessment with Anthony would be a broadband measure such as the Child Behavior Checklist that is available in Spanish and has been demonstrated to have adequate validity with Latinx populations (Gross et al., 2006; Sivan, Ridge, Gross, Richardson, & Cowell, 2008). When interpreting the findings and formulating recommendations, the clinician would need to take into account cultural variations in conceptualization of behavioral difficulties and recommendations. Critical aspects of feedback to Anthony's parents in addition to identification of specific emotion and behavior concerns would be education about the benefits of intervention, resources for culturally appropriate referrals to address Anthony's developmental delays, and discussing their fears and concerns about cost and external authorities.

REFERENCES

American Academy of Pediatrics, Task Force on Mental Health. (2019). *Addressing mental health concerns in primary care: A clinician's toolkit*. Author.

American Psychiatric Association. (2013). *Diagnostic and statistical manual of mental disorders* (5th ed.). Author.

American Psychological Association, APA Task Force on Psychological Assessment and Evaluation Guidelines. (2020). *APA guidelines for psychological assessment and evaluation*. https://www.apa.org/about/policy/guidelines-psychological-assessment-evaluation.pdf

Andrews, J. H., Cho, E., Tugendrajch, S. K., Marriott, B. R., & Hawley, K. M. (2020). Evidence-based assessment tools for common mental health problems: A practical guide for school settings. *Children & Schools*, *42*(1), 41–52. https://doi.org/10.1093/cs/cdz024

Bevan, S. L., Liu, J., Wallis, K. E., & Pinto-Martin, J. A. (2020). Screening instruments for developmental and behavioral concerns in pediatric Hispanic populations in the United States: A systematic literature review. *Journal of Developmental & Behavioral Pediatrics*, *41*(1), 71–80. https://doi.org/10.1097/DBP.0000000000000724

Caballero, T. M., Ross DeCamp, L., Platt, R. E., Shah, H., Johnson, S. B., Sibinga, E. M. S., & Polk, S. (2017). Addressing the mental health needs of Latino children in immigrant families. *Clinical Pediatrics*, *56*(7), 648–658. https://doi.org/10.1177/0009922816679509

Cora-Bramble, D., & Schaefer, D. M. (2011). *Culturally effective care toolkit*. American Academy of Pediatrics. www.aap.org/en-us/professional-resources/practice-support/Patient-Management/Pages/Culturally-Effective-Care-Toolkit.aspx

Council of National Psychological Associations for the Advancement of Ethnic Minority Interests. (2016). *Testing and assessment with persons & communities of color*. American Psychological Association. https://www.apa.org/pi/oema

Cree, R. A., Bitsko, R. H., Robinson, L. R., Holbrook, J. R., Danielson, M. L., Smith, D. S., & Peacock, G. (2018). Health care, family, and community factors associated with mental, behavioral, and developmental disorders and poverty among children aged 2–8 years—United States, 2016. *Morbidity and Mortality Weekly Report*, *67*(5), 1377–1383. https://doi.org/10.15585/mmwr.mm6750a1

Danielson, M. L., Bitsko, R. H., Ghandour, R. M., Holbrook, J. R., & Blumberg, S. J. (2018). Prevalence of parent-reported ADHD diagnosis and associated treatment among US children and adolescents, 2016. *Journal of Clinical Child and Adolescent Psychology,*, *47*(2), 199–212. https://doi.org/10.1080/15374416.2017.1417860

De Los Reyes, A. (2013). Strategic objectives for improving understanding of informant discrepancies in developmental psychopathology research. *Development and Psychopathology*, *25*, 669–682. https://doi.org/10.1017/S0954579413000096

De Los Reyes, A., Augenstein, T. M., Wang, M., Thomas, S. A., Drabick, D., Burgers, D. E., & Rabinowitz, J. (2015). The validity of the multi-informant approach to assessing child and adolescent mental health. *Psychological Bulletin*, *141*(4), 858–900. https://doi.org/10.1037/a0038498

Derogatis, L. R. (2017). Screening for psychiatric disorders in primary care settings. In M. E. Maruish (Ed.), *Handbook of psychological assessment in primary care settings* (2nd ed., pp. 167–192). Taylor & Francis.

Dubay, M., & Watson, L. R. (2019). Translation and cultural adaptation of parent-report developmental assessments: Improving rigor in methodology. *Research in Autism Spectrum Disorders*, *62*, 55–65. https://doi.org/10.1016/j.rasd.2019.02.005

Frick, P. J., Barry, C. T., & Kamphaus, R. W. (2020). *Clinical assessment of child and adolescent personality and behavior* (4th ed.). Springer. https://doi.org/10.1007/978-3-030-35695-8

Ghandour, R. M., Sherman, L. J., Vladutiu, C. J., Ali, M. M., Lynch, S. E., Bitsko, R. H., & Blumberg, S. J. (2019). Prevalence and treatment of depression, anxiety, and conduct problems in US children. *The Journal of Pediatrics*, *206*, 256–267. https://doi.org/10.1016/j.jpeds.2018.09.021

Godoy, L., & Carter, A. S. (2013). Identifying and addressing mental health risks and problems in primary care pediatric settings: A model to promote developmental and cultural competence. *American Journal of Orthopsychiatry*, *83*(1), 73–88. https://doi.org/10.1111/ajop.12005

Gross, D., Fogg, L., Young, M., Ridge, A., Cowell, J. M., Richardson, R., & Sivan, A. (2006). The equivalence of the Child Behavior Checklist/1 1/2-5 across parent race/ethnicity, income level, and language. *Psychological Assessment*, *18*(3), 313–323. https://doi.org/10.1037/1040-3590.18.3.313

Holmbeck, G., Welborn Thill, A., Bachanas, P., Garber, J., Bearman Miller, K., . . . Zukerman, J. (2008). Evidence-based assessment in pediatric psychology: Measures of psychosocial adjustment and psychopathology. *Journal of Pediatric Psychology*, *33*(9), 958–980. https://doi.org/10.1093/jpepsy/jsm059

Kohn-Wood, L. P., & Hooper, L. M. (2014). Cultural competency, culturally tailored care, and the primary care setting: Possible solutions to reduce racial/ethnic disparities in mental health care. *Journal of Mental Health Counseling*, *36*(2), 173–188. https://doi.org/10.17744/mehc.36.2.d73h217l81tg6uv3

Lai, M. C., Kassee, C., Besney, R., Bonato, S., Hull, L., Mandy, W., & Ameis, S. H. (2019). Prevalence of co-occurring mental health diagnoses in the autism population: A systematic review and meta-analysis. *Lancet Psychiatry*, *6*(10), 819–829. https://doi.org/10.1016/S2215-0366(19)30289-5

Liang, J., Matheson, B. E., & Douglas, J. M. (2016). Mental health diagnostic considerations in racial/ethnic minority youth. *Journal of Child and Family Studies*, *25*(6), 1926–1940. https://doi.org/10.1007/s10826-015-0351-z

Maruish, M. E. (2013). Outcome assesment in health settings. In K. F. Geisinger (Ed.), *APA handbook of testing and assessment in clinical and counseling psychology*. (pp. 303–321). American Psychological Association.

Maruish, M. E. (2018). *Handbook of pediatric psychological screening and assessment in primary care*. Routledge.

Perrin, J. M., Asarnow, J. R., Stancin, T., Melek, S. P., & Fritz, G. K. (2019). Mental health conditions and health care payments for children with chronic medical conditions. *Academic Pediatrics*, *19*(1), 44–50. https://doi.org/10.1016/j.acap.2018.10.001

Sheldrick, R. C., Merchant, S., & Perrin, E. C. (2011). Identification of developmental behavioral problems in primary care: A systematic review. *Pediatrics*, *128*, 356–363. https://doi.org/10.1542/peds.2010-3261

Sivan, A. B., Ridge, A., Gross, D., Richardson, R., & Cowell, J. (2008). Analysis of two measures of child behavior problems by African American, Latino, and non-Hispanic Caucasian parents of young children: A focus group study. *Journal of Pediatric Nursing*, *23*(1), 20–27. https://doi.org/10.1016/j.pedn.2007.07.005

Stiffler, M. C., & Dever, B. V. (2015). *Contemporary issues in psychological assessment. Mental health screening at school:*

Instrumentation, implementation, and critical issues. Springer International Publishing. https://doi.org/10.1007/978-3-319-19171-3

Thabrew, H., McDowell, H., Given, K., & Murren, K. (2017). Systematic review of screening instruments for psychosocial problems in children and adolescents with long-term physical conditions. *Global Pediatric Health*, *4*, 1–25. https://doi.org/10.1177/2333794X17690314

van Steensel, F. J., Bögels, S. M., & Perrin, S. (2011). Anxiety disorders in children and adolescents with autistic spectrum disorders: A meta-analysis. *Clinical Child and Family Psychology Review*, *14*(3), 302–317. https://doi.org/10.1007/s10567-011-0097-0

Ward-Zimmerman, B., & Berlinsky, E. B. (2018). Psychologists' facilitation of behavioral health screening in pediatric primary care: Rationale and practicalities. In M. E. Maruish (Ed.), *Handbook of pediatric psychological screening and assessment in primary care* (pp. 93–115). Routledge.

83

Evaluation of School Readiness: Beyond ABCs

Jaime W. Peterson, Doris Valenzuela-Araujo, Kylie M. L. Seeley, and Shelly Reggiani

For additional material related to the content of this chapter, please see Chapters 7, 18, 86, and 113.

VIGNETTE

What could an ideal evaluation of school readiness look like?

A Ready Child in a Ready Clinic: Mia frequented the clinic since she was an infant and looked forward to the new book she received at each visit. Her mother felt comfortable asking questions about Mia's health and development. The staff was welcoming, respected their culture, and communicated with them in their preferred language. The clinic decor, the picture books and toys for children, and the magazines and pamphlets positively reflected many races and cultures. On this occasion with the clinician, Mia looked with curiosity at the pictures on the table in front of her and proudly answered many questions about the pictures.

A Ready School: Mia was very excited to start kindergarten. Her pre-K program, located near the school site, partnered with the school for open houses for incoming kindergarteners. The school staff created a welcoming environment for children and families, communicating with families in their preferred language, establishing bidirectional communication pathways, embedding multicultural approaches to the open house events, and honoring the home cultures and customs of the incoming families. Centering on families, their cultural asset and wellness, was a cornerstone of the school's approach to education.

A Ready Family: The kindergarten teachers, in partnership with Mia's pre-K staff, visited Mia and her family at their home as part of an intentional transition to kindergarten. They learned about Mia's home culture, her strengths and interests, and formed a relationship of trust with the family. During the home visits, the pre-K staff and kindergarten teachers spoke Mia's home language and demonstrated cultural respect. Mia's family felt comfortable answering their questions and asking their own.

A Ready Community: Mia's elementary school partnered with culturally specific, local organizations that provide families with after-school care, health care, housing, parenting support, and nutritional resources. Families see these partner organizations, who are frequently at school events, as an integral part of the school community. Families coming into the school can access flyers printed in their home language with images of children and families who reflect themselves and their community.

INTRODUCTION

As you can see, school readiness goes far beyond an evaluation of the child's mastery of preacademic skills to a broad consideration of the child, school, family, and community. In this chapter we will review the evolution of the concept of school readiness and the importance of school readiness to child health and academic performance. We will explore facets of kindergarten readiness rooted in a family's cultural strength that expand beyond traditional monocultural or English language–dominant approaches. Finally, we will explore the role of clinicians and pediatric health systems in assessing and promoting school readiness.

WHAT IS SCHOOL READINESS?

School readiness was traditionally defined as a measure of a child's academic proficiency at kindergarten entry. Furthermore, until recently, the emphasis was only on the child's preacademic skills, such as reading, mathematics, and writing. Even in the evaluation of the children, we have broadened our view. Currently, we consider school readiness skills in terms of five developmental domains: cognitive, language and communication, physical, social-emotional, and self-help approaches to learning skills (Box 83.1). Using this expanded definition, clinicians play a vital role in evaluating school readiness by assessing and monitoring these skills across development and providing child- and family-specific supports (Hagan & Duncan, 2017).

The expanded definition of school readiness still has two fundamental constraints: (1) the expectation of readiness falls on the child and (2) the expected skills are based on dominant culture and are not culturally responsive. In the United States the dominant culture is defined as that of people who are White and of European descent whose norms, traditions, beliefs, and systems of functioning are recognized and generally unquestioned by the vast majority of institutions in the country, including schools (Gulati-Partee & Potapchuk, 2014).

Current conceptualizations of school readiness, from early childhood education (ECE) and public health, are broader than the original definition and are more culturally responsive. School readiness is viewed beyond that of the child and includes the readiness of families, communities, and schools (Administration for Children and Families, 2015; Institute of Education Sciences, 2018). The United Nations International Children's Emergency Fund (UNICEF) outlines the three dimensions of school readiness as "ready children," "ready

BOX 83.1 Child School Readiness Skills by Developmental Domain[a]

1. **Cognitive:** Abilities for learning such as memory and attention to learn sound-letter associations, spatial relations, and number concepts (expected at entry)
2. **Physical:** Child health and nutrition, gross and fine motor skills, perception, vision, and hearing
3. **Language development:** Language and speech sufficient for communication and learning and literacy
4. **Social-emotional development:** Emotional health, ability to form relationships with adults and children, ability to separate from family and caregivers
5. **Approaches to learning:** Self-regulation (behavior and emotions to follow class rules and successful group participation) and executive functioning (impulse control and focus, initiative, and curiosity)

[a]*Cultural considerations:* Family norms for behavior, communication, and self-expression are rooted in one's culture and may differ from those of others, both within and outside of a same racial group. From Hagan, J. F., & Duncan, P. M. (Eds.). (2017). *Bright futures: Guidelines for health supervision of infants, children, and adolescents* (4th ed.). American Academy of Pediatrics.

schools," and "ready families" (UNICEF, 2012). The National Association for the Education of Young Children (2009) states "children are not innately ready or not ready for school: their skills and development are strongly influenced by their families and through their interactions with other people and environments before coming to school." The Institute of Education Sciences' (2018) comprehensive approach for school readiness (Box 83.2) is a model for pediatrics to move beyond the "ready child" and toward the shared understanding that "a ready child results from a ready family, school and community." The chapter-opening vignette captured this broad conceptualization:

A ready child has the skills, knowledge, and attitudes necessary for success in primary school, later learning, and life. Physical, cognitive, language, social, and emotional development are essential ingredients of school readiness.

A ready family supports the child's learning by preparing for kindergarten by reading daily with the child, engaging the child in conversation and activities where the child practices listening and speaking, and maintains a positive home-to-school connection.

A ready "school" or "learning environment" is prepared to deliver evidence-based instruction; hire and continually train knowledgeable teachers, principals, and staff; and be culturally responsive of all its students.

A ready community ensures access to health care, provides quality childcare and early education, and invests in resources for families such as health care, safe housing, access to healthy and affordable food, and transportation.

BOX 83.2 A Comprehensive Definition of School Readiness: A Ready Child, a Ready Family, a Ready School, and a Ready Community

School readiness is about children, families, early environments, schools, and communities. Children are not innately "ready" or "not ready" for school. Their skills and development are strongly influenced by their families and through their interactions with other people and environments before coming to school.[a] School readiness refers not only to ready children, but to ready communities, families, and schools:

A *ready child* has the skills, knowledge, and attitudes necessary for success in primary school, later learning, and life.[b,c]

Strong physical, cognitive, language, social, and emotional development; has been well cared for physically, interacts socially with others, has a positive self-perception, can understand the emotions of others, and can interpret and express feelings; and approaches learning with enthusiasm and curiosity, has developed language and listening skills, and has cognition skills and general knowledge; and is prepared to learn successfully in school.

A *ready family* is ready for the child to start school, supports the child's learning by preparing for kindergarten, reads daily with the child, and maintains a positive home-to-school connection.[d]

Supports child in learning and through transition to kindergarten in the preferred language; reads to the child daily and engages in conversation and activities where the child practices listening and speaking; and continues to engage in the child's learning through the school years.

A *ready school* is ready to receive kindergarten students when it is prepared to deliver evidence-based instruction, hire and continually train knowledgeable teachers and principals, and be culturally responsive of all its students.[a,c,d]

Uses curriculum in kindergarten and the early grades that builds on prior learning; takes into account individual differences in language, culture, and prior experience; and employs teachers who reflect the cultural and linguistic diversity of the students who know how to teach young children and have the resources to do so.

A *ready community* is ready to support its children when it ensures access to health care, provides quality childcare and early education, and invests in resources for families.[a,c,d]

Helps ensure that children have access to health care, immunizations, and nutrition; helps ensure that families have access to quality early childcare and education; and invests in resources and activities that support families and promote school readiness such as nurse home visiting programs, community programs, high-quality and affordable preschools, safe housing, libraries, and parks.

[a]National Assocation for the Education of Young Children (2009)
[b]Administration for Children and Families (2015)
[c]Maxwell and Clifford (2004)
[d]Institute of Education Sciences (2018)

WHY SHOULD WE EVALUATE SCHOOL READINESS IN A CHILD?

Children who enter kindergarten with the skills, knowledge, and attitudes to meet its academic, social, and emotional demands are more likely to succeed academically throughout their school years and be healthy into their adult life (Peterson, Loeb, & Chamberlain, 2018). Entering school behind developmentally increases the likelihood children will struggle academically, drop out of school, engage in high-risk behaviors such as substance use, or be arrested (Fitzpatrick, Boers, & Pagani, 2020; Yoshikawa, 1995). By contrast, entering school on target developmentally decreases the likelihood children will repeat grades and increases chances that they will achieve higher graduation rates and better adult health outcomes (Duncan et al., 2007). Higher math skills at school entry are associated with later achievement (Duncan et al., 2007), less anxiety, more physical activity, and a healthier weight (Fitzpatrick et al., 2020). Higher reading abilities are associated with increased school connection and academic engagement (Fitzpatrick et al., 2020). Strong social-emotional skills are associated with emotional self-regulation for learning and academic achievement (Duncan et al., 2007). Children who start ready across multiple domains see a lasting impact on academic achievement, health, and economic prospects later in life (Campbell et al., 2014; Magnuson & Duncan, 2016; Yoshikawa, 1995).

In the United States many children, especially those living in poverty, who are often children of color, enter kindergarten behind their more affluent White peers and struggle to catch up; this difference is called the school readiness gap (Garcia & Weiss, 2017; Lee & Burkham, 2002; Reardon & Portilla, 2016). The initial gap is important because children who start behind tend to stay behind, contributing to later academic achievement gaps in math and early reading between Black and White students, Hispanic and White students, and low- and high-income students (Bassok, Fitzpatrick, Greenberg, & Loeb, 2016; National Center for Education Statistics, 2011; Reardon & Portilla, 2016; Vanneman, Hamilton, Anderson, & Rahman, 2009). It is important to recognize that the child's limitation in school readiness skills may be the result of long-standing environmental conditions, including inequality, systemic racism, and institutional and societal practices. These forces perpetuate the cycle of poverty and limit access to comprehensive early childhood experiences that promote child-level skills in school readiness: high-quality preschool programs, libraries, safe spaces for play, books in the home, and role models with experience in the education system (Trent, Dooley, & Dougé, 2019).

HOW SHOULD WE ASSESS SCHOOL READINESS IN A CHILD?

Use of Culturally Responsive Assessment Tools

Traditional school-based kindergarten readiness assessments measure a child in relationship to an educational standard of what a typical child should know and be able to do at the time of the assessment. It is important for practitioners and educators alike to note that such assessments, when normed on native English-speaking, middle- to upper-class children who had access to prekindergarten programs, take for granted the inherent privileges and advantages this population has at the start of school. Practitioners and educators must consider if the school readiness tool being used assesses for skills and traits that determine school readiness based on a standard exhibited by those in the dominant culture (Gulati-Partee & Potapchuk, 2014) and if the level of readiness assessed can be attributed solely to a child's racial, cultural, socioeconomic, and linguistic group membership. School readiness assessments that are culturally responsive honor a child's race and ethnic heritage as assets to the child's identity (Box 83.3). As such, the validity and reliability of assessments are ensured when the assessment has been created for and normed on a cross section of children by race, home language, culture, socioeconomic status, gender, and family makeup.

School readiness and early childhood assessments, when intentionally developed to be culturally responsive, can inform clinicians about early childhood milestones and can contribute to the preparedness of school systems to welcome

BOX 83.3 Factors to Consider When Designing Culturally Responsive School Readiness Assessments

- **Designed for and normed** on a cross section of children by **race, home language, culture, socioeconomic status, gender, and family makeup.**
  - Take into account the cultural norms, assets, and capabilities of children across races and cultures.
  - Mitigate the risk of misunderstanding and misinterpreting cultural expressions and ways of being as not on track or at risk.
  - Take into account the behavioral and social norms of races and cultures vs. the standard set by a single culture way of being.
- Administered in **the home language** of the child, ideally by a person familiar to the child, who understands the **home culture** of the child, and whom the child trusts.
  - Consider if the assessment is a direct translation from English, which may retain the frame of the dominant culture or if it was created in the language the child speaks, accounting for cultural expression, norms, and nuances of the child.
  - Note the cultural frame from which the assessment was designed.
- Scored appropriately if the child is **a dual language learner** (is learning ≥2 languages).
  - Children who are **dual language learners** develop receptive and expressive language at different ways and rates than monolingual children (Sousa, 2010).
- Administered with the assistance of a bilingual **cultural broker** who can help the child access an assessment given in English or by a practitioner who is not from the same racial or cultural group as the child.
  - A **cultural broker** is someone who has the lived experience with the cultural group who speaks the same home language as the child. The person has a strong understanding of the cultural norms of the family and their context as members of a culturally specific group within the community.
- Designed to be **strengths based.**
  - **Strength-based approaches** acknowledge and honor what the child has accomplished vs. focusing primarily on what the child is missing. These assessments allow practitioners to see and respond to a child's social-emotional awareness, sense of self, relationships with others, and development of personal and academic skills through an asset-based vs. a deficit-based lens.

and serve their youngest and potentially most vulnerable learners. Assessments results should be used to develop culturally responsive approaches to the kindergarten curriculum and experience. Culturally responsive approaches described by Ladson-Billings (1995) support children in framing their own thinking; honor and build on their cultural interests, heritage, and strengths; and examine curriculum from multiple viewpoints while creating a safe and inclusive environment where children can critically think and solve problems.

Assessing School Readiness in Pediatrics

The trusted relationship between families and pediatric primary care clinicians offers an important opportunity to screen, assess, monitor, and promote school readiness of children. The goals of universal developmental screening, outlined by the American Academy of Pediatrics and Bright Futures (Hagan & Duncan, 2017) are early detection of delays, referral for diagnosis, and connection to community-based services as soon as possible to maximize each child's learning potential (see Chapter 81). Assessing school readiness is distinct from universal developmental screening: It aims to measure a child's school readiness abilities to guide parents as they prepare their child for school during the preschool years and to prepare schools for the children they will need to educate. At present, a single, comprehensive assessment tool that is culturally sensitive and available in multiple languages does not yet exist. Given the broad definition of child school readiness domains, a single measure may not be possible. A host of tools (screeners and assessments) are currently used in practice, from informal methods to more complex measures. A combination of measures is likely required to assess all five school readiness domains.

HOW SHOULD WE INTERPRET SCHOOL READINESS ASSESSMENTS?

In the past school readiness assessments have been used inappropriately to make a diagnosis or to delay school entry (American Academy of Pediatrics, 1995). Once a culturally responsive, validated tool has been selected, the purpose of a school readiness assessment session should be a shared, collaborative experience with a strengths-based approach rather than a judgment of a "ready" or "unready" child. The assessment should be administered by a clinician who can act as a cultural broker. The results should be used to start a conversation about the individual child's strengths and areas for growth in the context of the family and home environments. Open-ended questions allow for exploration of parent perspectives:

What are your concerns or curiosities about your child starting school?

What surprised you about the assessment we did with your child?

Are there areas on the assessment you would like to practice with your child? Which ones do you feel unsure about or less confident? We can use this time to practice together.

How frequently in your child's day do you, or another caregiver, practice with your child? For example, read books or tell stories? Practice counting, shapes, or colors? Talk to your child about feelings and ideas?

What types of opportunities does your child have for cooperative play with other children or time to practice sharing or taking turns? How frequently are you, or another caregiver or family member, able to access books in your home language with your child or engage in play?

What types of barriers have you encountered when accessing programs like preschool, the library, or early intervention? Are you worried about using any of these programs? What other resources or tools do you wish you could access for your child?

Would you like to learn about community programs to help your child continue to grow in these areas?

A clinician can tailor support by sharing school readiness knowledge and may offer (1) a safe place to practice behaviors, such as how to do shared reading (regardless of literacy level); (2) access to books, such as through Reach Out and Read (ROAR); and/or (3) connection to early childhood resources, such as through parenting groups, childcare, libraries, and preschools. For instance, a first-time parent may not understand how comparing sizes or sorting objects is helpful for learning math; a parent with limited literacy may need reassurance that describing the pictures in the story is as valuable for promoting reading and language skills in their child as reading the text verbatim; or a parent new to the United States may need guidance to successfully navigate the nuances of ECE programs, including eligibility or enrollment processes. These conversations are ongoing and should be revisited during subsequent well-child checks to monitor progress or identify new barriers. Efforts in primary care to use local school readiness data to tailor clinic interventions is an emerging area of interest.

NEW MODELS FOR ASSESSING SCHOOL READINESS IN ACTION

Three examples show how communities, schools, and health systems are trying to move beyond "the ready child" and incorporate the role of the family, schools, and communities to assess and address school readiness, as reflected in the opening vignette. Two are bold, progressive efforts within Medicaid systems to break down system silos and change care delivery. First, the All:Ready Network of cross-sector organizations rethinks how systems work to promote the readiness of families, communities, and learning environments (All:Ready, 2020; Figs. 83.1). Second, the New York Advanced Primary Care Model restructures the New York Medicaid system to support the holistic needs of families and children to promote school readiness and health (New York's First 1,000 Days Initiative, 2018; see Fig. 83.2). The third is UNICEF's international framework for assessment, monitoring, and evaluating the readiness of children, schools, and families for school (Fig. 83.3). These models highlight how pediatric systems can assess and support school readiness to ultimately improve the overall health and success of all children.

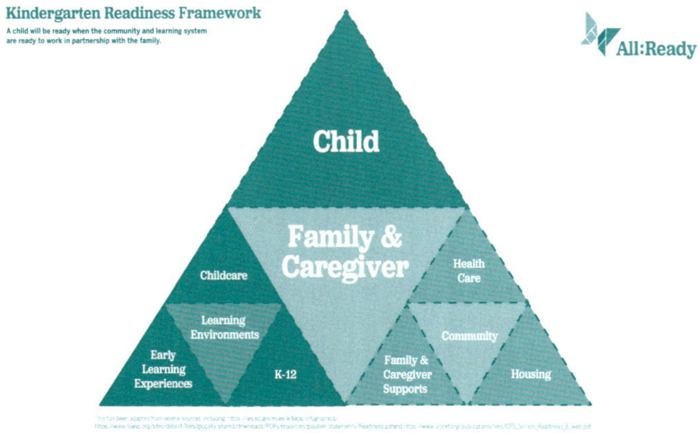

Fig. 83.1 Spotlight 1: All:Ready (Oregon). In 2017 Health Share of Oregon approved a strategic investment in All:Ready, a regional school readiness network. Health Share unites over 60 organizations from different sectors (health, education, community, and family supports) to address the gap between health and education outcomes in our children ages 0 to 5 years. Using collaborative decision making and an antiracism framework, All:Ready is committed to redesigning how systems work together so that race, class, and disability are no longer predictors of school readiness. To redesign systems, this framework shifts the responsibility off the child and on to the system by asking:

As a caregiver and family: Does a family share stories or read to their children daily? Are we reducing disparities in infant mortality and low birthweight?

As a community: Are we ensuring that children have access to affordable, safe, and stable housing? Are all children accessing well-child checks, immunizations, and preventive dental visits?

As a learning environment: In what ways do we value parents as their child's first teacher and consider individual differences in language, culture, prior experience, and family educational values, goals, and preferences? Is childcare affordable for all families?

CLINICAL IMPLICATIONS

Children who enter school "ready" to learn are likely to experience good health and educational success. The school readiness gap impacts many children, especially children living in poverty and children of color, due to multiple interacting environmental forces, including ongoing systemic racism and oppression. Pediatric clinicians are trusted partners in the health and education of children and can guide families on the school readiness journey. Clinicians have a responsibility to work collectively with families and caregivers, learning environments from ECE to K-12, and community partners to ensure all sectors are "ready" to support children.

Clinicians support school readiness by building trusted relationships with families, celebrating strengths of the children, and identifying areas for growth in school readiness domains. The assessment includes the readiness of the family, discussing the importance of school readiness and encouraging preschool; and understanding the community's local resources (e.g., Head Start, preschools, libraries, home visiting programs) to tailor recommendations for each family (Williams & Lerner, 2019). To the extent possible, clinics should include staff and providers that reflect the linguistic, cultural, and racial diversity of the community. Additionally, clinics should consider investment in a range of early interventions to promote school readiness, such as ROAR, parenting groups, community resource navigators, math/literacy texting programs, and individual coaching sessions (Cates, Weisleder, & Mendelsohn, 2016; Peterson, Huffman, & Bruce, 2020; York, Loeb, & Doss, 2019). Health systems need to work with learning systems, families, and communities to decrease barriers to access, utilization, and

New York State Model of Advanced Primary Care for Children

Well Child Visits→		
Bright Futures scope and schedule - including all EPSDT required services	Care Coordination/Case Management→	
Screening - services tailored to need (no one size fits all care)	All Pediatric Practices include care coordination	Family Support Services→
Disparities in needs and outcones addressed	Tired with more intensive services for higher complexity (based on risk stratification-guided by screening)	Child/Family support programs integrated into practice (e.g. Reach Out and Read, Healthy Steps)
2 Generation approach to anticipatory guidance, parent education - focused on social emotional support	Care Coordination requires Pediatric specific skills (Early Childhood needs, Education system needs, etc)	Integrated Behavioral Health in Primay Care Setting
Family engagement - culturally competent and trauma informed are prioritized	2 Generation approach	Referrals to and integration with other services (e.g. child care, early intervention, home visiting, peer supprt, early childhood mental health)
Primary Care augmentations following BF recommendations (e.g Reach Out and Reach)		2 Generation approach
IT supported pre and Post visit engagement		
Good access to care		

Fig. 83.2 Spotlight 2: First 1,000 Days on Medicaid (New York). In 2017 New York Medicaid recognized that the earliest years of life greatly influenced long-term health and wellbeing. Over 200 stakeholders from education, child development, child welfare, pediatrics, public health, and mental health came together to develop evidence-based recommendations for how New York State Medicaid could improve outcomes for the youngest New Yorkers, age 0 to 3 years. The 10 recommendations included funding for mental health consultations, implementing statewide home visits and *kindergarten readiness assessments, promoting early literacy*, providing peer *family navigators* and dyadic therapy, *development of a cross-sector referral system*, creation of a Preventive Pediatric Care Clinical Advisory Group, and expanding the Centering Pregnancy model. (From New York's First 1,000 Days Initiative, 2018.) *Italics highlight examples of clinically embedded SR screening and individualized supports.*

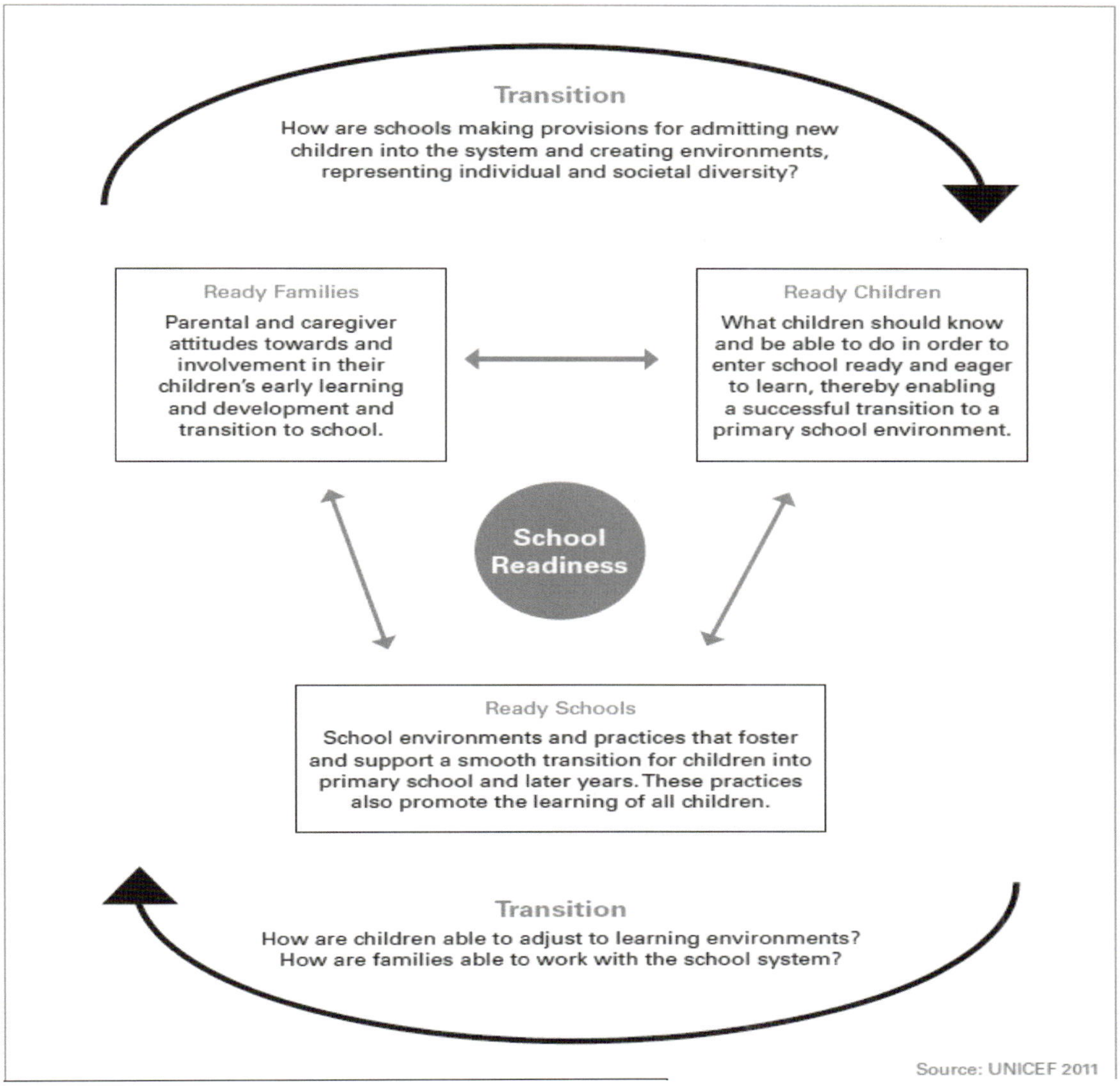

Fig. 83.3 Spotlight 3: UNICEF School Readiness Framework (2012). UNICEF's child-friendly schools provides a conceptual framework for the assessment, monitoring, and evaluation of three key components of school readiness: children's readiness for school, schools' readiness for children, and families' readiness for school. Key factors to selecting measures include the purpose of the assessment, whether the instrument measures school readiness or delay in development, and cultural relevance. Notably, the readiness of a child's community is not part of the UNICEF framework although it is an integral component of child development.

acceptability of school readiness resources and services across the early learning landscape; share data across sectors to understand school readiness on a population level; and consider school readiness as a health outcome for various interventions. Finally, clinicians have a responsibility to advocate for evidence-based policies and programs shown to improve school readiness (i.e., poverty reduction and access to high-quality ECE).

REFERENCES

Administration for Children and Families. (2015). *The head start early learning outcomes framework: Ages birth to five (HSELOF)*. Department of Health and Human Services.

All:Ready. (2020). *Health Share of Oregon*. https://www.healthshareoregon.org/allready

American Academy of Pediatrics Committee on School Health and Committee on Early Childhood, & Adoption and Dependent Care. (1995). The inappropriate use of school "readiness" tests. *Pediatrics*, *95*(3), 437–438.

Bassok, D., Fitzpatrick, M., Greenberg, E., & Loeb, S. (2016). Within- and between-sector quality differences in early childhood education and care. *Child Development*, *87*(5), 1627–1645. https://doi.org/10.1111/cdev.12551

Campbell, F., Conti, G., Heckman, J. J., Moon, S. H., Pinto, R., Pungello, E., & Pan, Y. (2014). Early childhood investments substantially boost adult health. *Science*, *343*(6178), 1478–1485. https://doi.org/10.1126/science.1248429

Cates, C. B., Weisleder, A., & Mendelsohn, A. L. (2016). Mitigating the effects of family poverty on early child development through parenting interventions in primary care. *Academic Pediatrics*, *16*(3), S112–S120. https://doi.org/10.1016/j.acap.2015.12.015

Duncan, G. J., Dowsett, C. J., Claessens, A., Magnuson, K., Huston, A. C., Klebanov, P., & Brooks-Gunn, J. (2007). School readiness and later achievement. *Developmental Psychology*, *43*(6), 1428.

Fitzpatrick, C., Boers, E., & Pagani, L. S. (2020). Kindergarten readiness, later health, and social costs. *Pediatrics*, *146*(6). https://doi.org/10.1542/peds.2020-0978

Garcia, E., & Weiss, E. (2017). *Education inequalities at the school starting gate: Gaps, trends, and strategies to address them.* Economic Policy Institute. https://www.epi.org/publication/education-inequalities-at-the-school-starting-gate/

Gulati-Partee, G., & Potapchuk, M. (2014). Paying attention to white culture and privilege: A missing link to advancing racial equity. *The Foundation Review*, *6*(1), 4.

Hagan, J. F., & Duncan P. M. (Eds.). (2017). *Bright futures: Guidelines for health supervision of infants, children, and adolescents* (4th ed.). American Academy of Pediatrics.

High, P. C., American Academy of Pediatrics Committee on Early Childhood, Adoption, Dependent Care, & Council on School Health. (2008). School readiness. *Pediatrics*, *121*(4), e1008–e1015. https://doi.org/10.1542/peds.2008-0079

Institute of Education Sciences. (2018). *Preparing a school ready child.* https://ies.ed.gov/ncee/edlabs/infographics/pdf/REL_SE_preparing_a_school_ready_child.pdf;https://ies.ed.gov/ncee/edlabs/infographics/pdf/REL_SE_The_Ready_School_The_Ready_Community.pdf

Ladson-Billings, G. (1995). But that's just good teaching! The case for culturally relevant pedagogy. *Theory into Practice*, *34*(3), 159–165.

Lee, V. E., & Burkham, D. (2002). *Inequality at the starting gate: Social background differences in achievement as children begin kindergarten.* Economic Policy Institute.

Magnuson, K., & Duncan, G. J. (2016). Can early childhood interventions decrease inequality of economic opportunity? *Russell Sage Foundation Journal of the Social Sciences*, *2*(2), 123–141.

Maxwell, K. L., & Clifford, R. M. (2004). *School readiness assessment. Young children.* Research in Review. https://www.calstatela.edu/sites/default/files/groups/Anna%20Bing%20Arnold%20Children's%20Center/Docs/naeyc_school_readiness_article.pdf

National Association for the Education of Young Children. (2009). *School readiness position statement.* https://www.naeyc.org/sites/default/files/globally-shared/downloads/PDFs/resources/position-statements/Readiness.pdf

National Center for Education Statistics. (2011). *The nation's report card: Mathematics and reading 2011 (NCES).* Author. 2012–458.

New York's First 1,000 Days Initiative. (2018). Schuyler Center for Analysis and Advocacy. http://www.scaany.org/wp-content/uploads/2018/02/1st1K_Budget_overview_02-18.pdf

Peterson, J. W., Huffman, L. C., Bruce, J., Prata, N., Harley, K. G., & Chamberlain, L. J. (2020). A clinic-based school readiness coaching intervention for low-income Latino children: An intervention study. *Clinical Pediatrics (Philadelphia)* https://doi.org/10.1177/0009922820941230

Peterson, J. W., Loeb, S., & Chamberlain, L. J. (2018). The intersection of health and education to address school readiness of all children. *Pediatrics*, *142*(5). https://doi.org/10.1542/peds.2018-1126

Reardon, S. F., & Portilla, X. A. (2016). Recent trends in income, racial, and ethnic school readiness gaps at kindergarten entry. *AERA Open*, *2*(3), 2332858416657343.

Sousa, D. A. (2010). *How the ELL brain learns.* Corwin Press.

Trent, M., Dooley, D. G., & Dougé, J. (2019). The impact of racism on child and adolescent health. *Pediatrics*, *144*, 2.

UNICEF. (2012). *School readiness: A conceptual framework.* https://www.unicef.org/publications/files/CFS_School_Readiness_E_web.pdf

Vanneman, A., Hamilton, L., Anderson, J. B., & Rahman, T. (2009). *Achievement gaps: How Black and White students in public schools perform in mathematics and reading on the National Assessment of Educational Progress. Statistical Analysis Report.* National Center for Education Statistics. NCES 2009-455.

Williams, P. G., & Lerner, M. A. (2019). School readiness. *Pediatrics*, *144*(2), e20191766.

York, B. N., Loeb, S., & Doss, C. (2019). One step at a time: The effects of an early literacy text-messaging program for parents of preschoolers. *Journal of Human Resources*, *54*(3), 537–566. https://www.muse.jhu.edu/article/729993

Yoshikawa, H. (1995). Long-term effects of early childhood programs on social outcomes and delinquency. *The Future of Children*, *5*(3), 51–75. http://www.ncbi.nlm.nih.gov/pubmed/8835514

Observational Assessment in Developmental-Behavioral Pediatrics

Jordan Ezell Klein and Laura Arnstein Carpenter

For additional material related to the content of this chapter, please see Chapters 41, 76, and 79.

VIGNETTE

Janelle is a 9-year-old girl with a history of moderate intellectual disability and autism spectrum disorder (ASD). She can use some short phrases, although much of her speech is repetitive and nonfunctional. For the past 2 years she has engaged in self-injurious hand biting that has left a large callous on her hand. This behavior happens only at school. Her teacher reports that Janelle bites her hand when she is overstimulated, and that redirecting Janelle to the classroom sensory corner when she is upset almost always stops this behavior. A behavioral consultant comes into the classroom to collect antecedent-behavior-consequence (ABC) data (see Fig. 84.1 later). Because the behavior is occurring frequently, only a few days of data collection are needed. The data show that Janelle is redirected to the sensory corner about 50% of the time and that hand biting is ignored or not noticed the rest of the time. The consultant concludes that the behavior serves an escape/avoidance function for Janelle and is her way of communicating, "I don't want to do this." About 50% of the time, she is redirected to the sensory corner and thus successfully escapes/avoids nondesired tasks. The consultant designs an intervention to teach Janelle to use index cards to request a break from demands (see Fig. 84.2 later). Other components of the intervention include daily scheduled noncontingent access to the sensory corner, temporarily decreasing the frequency and difficulty of demands, and using a picture schedule to link nonpreferred and preferred activities (e.g., "first worksheets, then swings").

INTRODUCTION

Observational assessment in developmental and behavioral pediatrics is a powerful tool that is used to provide objective information about behavior. Observational assessments involve the systematic recording of information about a child's behavior either within the natural environment (e.g., the home, the classroom) or during a structured assessment session. For example, if a child is having difficulty sleeping, a clinician may ask parents to systematically record information regarding what time they try to put the child to bed, how they put the child to bed, what time the child actually falls asleep, and each time the child wakes up after falling asleep and what happens during these wakeful periods. After 1 week of recording this information, the provider will have baseline information regarding the number of hours the child is sleeping as well as information about where to intervene in the child's sleep. Objective observational data may reveal highly specific information that could not be obtained through parent interview or a standard rating scale. For example, recording systematic information about a child's sleep may reveal that parents are trying to put the child to bed much later than they realized or that sleep problems only occur on nights after the child has taken a late nap. Thus observational assessments are often used in situations in which standard behavioral recommendations are not having the desired impact or in which briefer parent/teacher rating scales have not provided enough detailed information to formulate or evaluate an intervention.

One of the most commonly used applications of observational assessments is in obtaining baseline information about a behavior prior to intervention and then systematically evaluating the response to an intervention. For example, if a child is prescribed a new medication aimed at improving attention, the teacher may be asked to record the proportion of time the child sits in the assigned spot during circle time each morning in the weeks before and after starting the medication. Systematic recording of data can be particularly useful in determining whether a behavior is changing in subtle ways that may not be obvious to a casual observer. For example, a parent may report that a child "doesn't seem to care" when losing a privilege following an aggressive episode. However, a review of data on aggression can help to objectively determine whether these events are changing in frequency or intensity over time.

Although observational assessments typically take more time and effort than traditional behavior checklists and caregiver/teacher interviews (see Chapter), they can also add vital important information to the diagnostic assessment process. Observational assessments may be helpful in supplementing parent/teacher-reported measures to provide a more comprehensive diagnostic evaluation that includes multiple pieces of information. For example, observational assessment is often included in diagnostic evaluations of behaviorally defined disorders such as ASD and attention-deficit/hyperactivity disorder (ADHD). For these disorders, parent/teacher interviews and checklists are often combined with structured behavioral assessment performed by the clinician to arrive at an accurate diagnosis. Observational assessments may be particularly helpful in classifying behaviors that may have diagnostic overlap. For instance, social avoidance and difficulty initiating conversations are behaviors, consistent with both anxiety and ASD. Thus without direct observation of the behaviors, it is difficult to discern if the child has anxiety, ASD, or both disorders.

Although observational assessment can be an incredibly powerful tool, it is important to be aware of some of the possible sources of error associated with this approach (Kantowitz, Roediger, & Elmes, 2009). First, people will sometimes change their behavior when they know they are being observed, a phenomenon sometimes called the Hawthorne effect. For example, if an observer comes into a classroom to take data on a child's disruptive behavior, that child may engage in more or less disruptive behavior than typical due to the presence of a second adult in the classroom. This effect can be minimized by collecting observations over a longer period of time (e.g., 1 week vs. 1 day). Second, the observer's expectations or beliefs may incur differential attention to information that confirms these beliefs, and the observer may disregard information that is not consistent with the expectations. This is known as the observer-expectancy effect. For example, if a clinician has been told that a child has ADHD, the clinician may pay special attention to behaviors consistent with this diagnosis. This effect can be minimized by providing clear and objective definitions for the behaviors being observed and by collecting this information in an objective manner. For example, the clinician may record percent of time in seat versus out of seat for a child being evaluated for possible hyperactivity. Observer expectations and beliefs can also directly impact children's behavior. For example, parents who expect that their child will comply with a direction may give subtle cues that increase the chance of compliance, and the reverse may also be true. This source of error can be minimized through the use of an impartial observer when collecting observational assessment information.

OBSERVATIONAL ASSESSMENT METHODS

In the context of observational assessments behavior is defined as the interplay between an individual and the environment that can be objectively observed and reliably measured (Cooper, Heron, & Heward, 2007; Umbreit, Ferro, Liaupsin, & Lane, 2007). Importantly, behavior is not the absence of another behavior. For instance, "not throwing toys" is not a measurable behavior, whereas "using toys appropriately" is an observable and measurable behavior (Heron, Cooper, & Heward, 2015). Internalized behavior and motives are also not observable behaviors and are usually captured most accurately through other means (i.e., self-report measures, clinical interviews). Lastly, in behavioral observations the goal is observation rather than interpretation. The observer is not trying to determine if an individual hit a classmate because of anger or meanness, but to document that the behavior occurred regardless of function (motive). The recorded information can later be interpreted to determine the function of the behavior.

Identifying and describing a target behavior is the first step in observational assessments. A clear, concrete definition of the target behavior increases the consistency and reliability of the behavior observations. Ideally, when describing a target behavior, it should pass the stranger test, whereby a stranger could identify and observe the child's target behavior solely on the description (Howell, Hosp, & Kurns, 2008). For instance, a target behavior of "attitude problem" is vague and could be interpreted differently by different observers (e.g., talking back to a parent when given a task, rolling eyes). This target behavior would not pass the stranger test because it needs to be defined in specific, measurable terms. On the other hand, "arguing when given an instruction" is more specific, and the likelihood of a stranger identifying that behavior as the same behavior the observer is targeting is high. Clearly describing the targeted behavior in measurable terms is the first step in objectively and reliably defining child behavior.

After a target behavior has been clearly identified and described, the observer can begin systematically tracking the child's behavior. Behavioral observations are an objective way to track behavior patterns, and in some cases to determine the function of a child's behavior. Through systemized behavior tracking, the examiner is able to quantify observed behaviors. There are four main methods for tracking and quantifying child behavior: time sampling, event sampling, duration sampling, and latency sampling (Table 84.1). Aligning the tracking method to the observation question will ensure that the most useful data for quantifying the target behavior are collected.

Time Sampling

Time sampling provides an estimate of the average percentage of time that a behavior occurred during the observation. There are several approaches to time sampling, including partial interval recording, whole interval recording, and momentary time sampling. In partial interval recording the observer simply checks a box to indicate whether or not the behavior occurred at any time during each interval. For example, if a classroom day is divided into seven periods, then at the end of each period, the observer simply checks off whether or not the target occurred at any point during the period behavior (e.g., whether the child got out of the chair without permission). In whole interval recording at the end of each period the observer checks off whether the behavior occurred continuously for the entire period (e.g., whether the child stayed in the chair without getting up for the entire interval). Finally, in momentary time sampling the observer checks off whether the behavior was occurring at one specific time point out of each of the seven periods (whether or not the child was in the chair at one specific predetermined instance).

Event Sampling

Event sampling involves recording the exact number of times that a behavior occurs during a set time interval. Short, discrete behaviors (e.g., a neck tic, yelling out in class) lend themselves

TABLE 84.1 Definitions and Applications of Various Observational Assessment Methods

Question	Sampling Method	Definition	Ideal Use	Example
Approximately how much time of the observed time does the behavior occur?	Time sampling	The percentage of time the behavior occurs during predetermined observation periods	Best for behaviors that occur so frequently that counting the exact amount would be difficult Efficient because the child does not need to be observed continuously	Jimmy worked on his worksheet during 5 of the 10 predetermined observations (50% of the time).
How often does the behavior occur?	Event sampling	Number of times a behavior occurs during an observation period	Best for discrete behaviors in a short period of time Can be counted or tallied	Neveah poked her classmate 5 times from 10:00 a.m. to 10:15 a.m.
How long does the behavior occur or last?	Duration	Percent or average amount of time that a behavior occurs during observation period	Best for behaviors that last more than a few seconds or that have varying length Can use a stopwatch or timer to measure amount	Alyssa spent 25% of math class in her seat (15 out of 60 min).
How long does it take for the behavior to occur?	Latency	The amount of time it takes for an individual to perform the target behavior	Best for behaviors with a clear beginning and for building new behaviors	Rashawn took 10 min to sit in his seat after the bell rang.

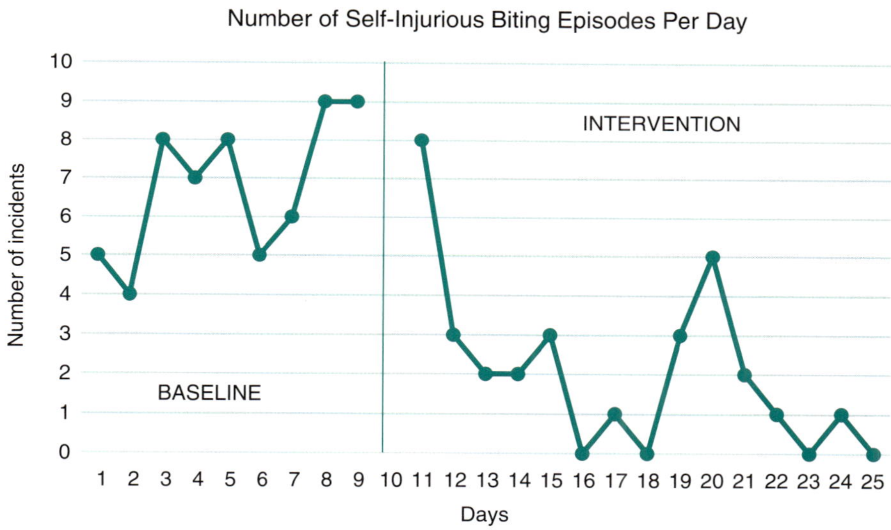

Fig. 84.1 Response to intervention for Janelle (chapter vignette).

to event sampling. The chapter vignette involves tracking of self-injurious biting using event sampling (see Fig. 84.1 later).

Duration Sampling

Duration sampling involves using a timer to determine how long a behavior occurs during a specified interval. Behaviors that last a variable amount of time (e.g., staying in one's chair when expected to do so) may be best quantified through duration sampling.

Latency Sampling

Latency sampling involves calculating the amount of time it takes for an individual to perform a target behavior. For example, a stopwatch can be started once an instruction is given and stopped once the instruction is followed, to determine the latency to comply with the instruction. Latency sampling is often used when building new behaviors (e.g., how long it takes a child to get ready for school after waking up in the morning).

FUNCTIONAL BEHAVIOR ASSESSMENT

Once a child's behavior has been clearly defined and then quantified through tracking, the observer can then analyze the surrounding events to create hypotheses about what may be increasing or decreasing the likelihood of the behavior. A core tenet of behaviorism is that behavior serves a function. In other words children communicate through their behavior, and understanding the function of problem behaviors is essential for designing effective and meaningful interventions. The primary functions of child behavior fall into four categories: escape, avoidance, attention, gaining access to tangibles, and/or self-stimulation. The same behavior may serve different functions for people or even in the same person at different times. For example, one child who cries loudly may be communicating that he needs attention, while another child who cries loudly may be communicating that a task is too hard and that she needs help. Clearly different interventions are needed to decrease loud crying for these two children.

Functional behavior assessment (FBA) is a key component of the applied behavior analysis treatment approach for children with autism and other neurodevelopmental disorders. FBA is the process of gathering and analyzing information about a behavior to determine its function (Hanley, Iwata, & McCord, 2003). The FBA may include interviews with patients with disabilities and their caregivers, record reviews, and systematic direct observation. One type of observational assessment commonly used in this process is collection of antecedent-behavior-consequences of the target behavior (Fig. 84.2):

1. Antecedent. The antecedent (A) to a behavior is the context, event, or stimulus that precedes the presence of the target behavior. In the chapter-opening vignette task demands precede Janelle's self-injurious biting, making task demands the antecedent.
2. Behavior. The target behavior (B) is the clearly defined behavior of interest that is specific and observable. The target behavior is the behavior that is recorded during the observational assessment. For Janelle, the target behavior is self-injurious hand biting. Thus we have established the antecedent as demands and the behavior as biting.
3. Consequence. The final step is to understand the consequence (C) or the event or reaction that occurs directly after or in response to the target behavior. The consequence can help determine if the behavior is being reinforced, which leads to a maintenance or increase of the behavior (Christ, 2008). For Janelle, she is removed to a sensory corner about 50% of the time after biting her hand.

ABC data, interviews, record reviews, and other relevant information can be used to develop hypotheses regarding the relationship between the behavior and the environment. Making an incorrect assumption about why a child is displaying the target behavior can lead to an inappropriate and ineffective response. For instance, when a child hits her seatmate during math, she may be moved to time-out as a consequence, or her teacher may decide to sit next to her to better control her behavior. Moving her to time-out may inadvertently reward escape-motivated behavior by allowing her to skip her math work, even if it is just for a short period of time. On the other hand, having her teacher sit next to her may inadvertently reward attention-seeking behavior, even when the attention is negative. Without knowing the function of the hitting behavior, we risk implementing consequences that may be ineffective or may even cause the behavior to occur more frequently.

The FBA is a systemized process of compiling information and data about a target behavior to form evidence-based hypotheses about the function of the behavior (Alberto & Troutman, 2009; Scott, Anderson, & Spaulding, 2008). From the ABC data, the observer is able to determine what

Date & Time	Antecedent (What happened right before the behavior?)	Behavior (What did the behavior look like and how long did it last?)	Consequence (What happened immediately after the behavior?)	Possible Function
3/1 at 1:49	asked to pack up backpack	bit hand hard for 30 seconds and screamed	ignored (teacher helping another child)	demand avoidance
3/2 at 9:15	asked to sit in chair to do worksheets	bit hand and slapped at wall	directed to sensory corner	demand avoidance
3/2 at 11:15	sorting papers	sat on ground, screamed, bit hand	directed to sensory corner	escape
3/2 at 12:03	asked to clean up from lunch	bit hand and cried loudly	direction given again, more firmly	demand avoidance
(continue for several days)				

Fig. 84.2 ABC data sample for Janelle (chapter vignette). To draw accurate conclusions, ABC data may need to be collected over several days or longer depending on the frequency of the behavior.

situations (antecedents) may trigger the behavior and what consequences may maintain the behavior. In some cases it may also be necessary to collect information on other events that may make the behavior more or less likely, such as time of day, hunger, sleep, illness, and other factors (setting events). Using the ABCs, the observer is able to determine what situations (antecedents) and actions (consequences) reinforce or increase the target behavior (Kerr & Nelson, 2010). This information is then used to determine the function or the goal of the behavior.

Collecting ABC data and completing the FBA is not only important for systematically developing hypotheses about why the behavior is occurring but also helps develop an appropriate and effective intervention. For instance, if the function of a behavior is attention, then attention may be withheld until the positive behavior is shown. So, a student who receives attention when he leaves his seat is instead ignored until he returns to his seat, where he will receive positive attention. Thus attention is now used to positively reinforce the goal behavior and not the problem behavior. Some children may need to be explicitly taught an alternative way to seek attention, such as raising their hand in class or quietly and gently placing a hand on a parent's arm. Teachers and caregivers may also need to be reminded to pay attention to positive attention-seeking behavior (The IRIS Center for Training Enhancements, 2009).

Importantly using the FBA approach to inform interventions tends to lead to a focus on developing prosocial behaviors and adaptive skills rather than on punishing undesired behaviors. Understanding why a behavior occurs allows for an intervention that addresses the function or goal underlying problem behavior, which leads to long-term, positive change in the child's behavior (Ingram, Lewis-Palmer, & Sugai, 2005). In the vignette for this chapter an intervention was designed for Janelle based on the escape/avoidance function determined from the ABC data. The intervention included use of an index card to request a break, along with some additional classroom modifications. A graph of the number of self-injurious biting episodes per day (i.e., event sampling) shows that this behavior decreased dramatically after the implementation of this intervention (Fig. 84.1).

PUBLISHED INSTRUMENTS FOR OBSERVATIONAL ASSESSMENT

Thus far the observational assessment methods described involve collecting information that is personalized and specific to one child. However, there are also several commercially available tools that can be used to collect observational information for behavioral challenges and for symptoms of ASD.

Behavior

The Behavior Assessment System for Children, Third Edition (BASC-3) and Achenbach (CBCL) checklists include comprehensive parent/teacher/self-report rating scales and are described in detail in Chapter. In addition to checklists, both of these systems also include behavioral observational measures. The BASC-3 Student Observation System (SOS) can be used for any school-age child. It is completed by a teacher or other observer in the classroom and uses momentary time sampling during 3-second intervals spaced 30 seconds apart over a 15-minute period to quantify both adaptive (e.g., positive peer interactions) and maladaptive (e.g., inappropriate vocalizations) behaviors. The SOS does not include normative data. The Achenbach Direct Observation Form (DOF) is intended to be used with children 6 to 11 years of age in any group setting. The observer scores on-task behavior in 1-minute intervals for 10 minutes, and then rates 88 problem items related to domains such as attention, oppositional behavior, and social withdrawal. The DOF includes normative data, and local comparisons can be made by observing and scoring a comparison child.

Autism Spectrum Disorder

Standardized observational assessments are particularly useful for disorders with subjective behavioral diagnostic criteria such as ASD. These assessments can help to objectively quantify subjective diagnostic criteria (e.g., reduced use of eye contact, lack of social reciprocity). The Autism Diagnostic Observation Schedule, Second Edition (ADOS-2; Lord et al., 2012) is the most well-researched observational assessment for ASD. The ADOS-2 is a semistructured, observational measure designed to assess symptoms consistent with ASD in individuals 12 months and older. The ADOS-2 has five modules to choose from based on the child's language level and age. Each module contains a series of structured tasks designed to elicit social communication and other behaviors. Throughout the administration, the examiner tracks the quantity and quality of social behaviors such as eye contact, requesting, sharing enjoyment, and interactive play, as well as communicative behaviors such as conversation and gestures. Additionally, during the observation the examiner notes the presence of any restrictive or repetitive behaviors such as stereotyped speech, sensory interests, repetitive play, or unusual motor movements. The semistructured format creates space for the examiner to probe for specific behaviors both directly in tasks and throughout the entire assessment. For instance, in determining whether the child responds to her name, the examiner follows structured prompts to directly elicit the child's attention in response to hearing her name. Other behaviors such as eye contact and social approaches are observed throughout the entire observation. Once the 30- to 60-minute face-to-face assessment section is completed, the examiner scores approximately 35 clearly defined items related to ASD. These scores are used to calculate an overall score that reflects whether or not the child's behaviors during the ADOS-2 fall in the autism spectrum range. Importantly, this tool is just one part of a comprehensive assessment, and the final diagnosis is based on expert clinical judgment.

The ADOS-2 allows direct observation of behaviors consistent with ASD by a trained clinician. Without direct observation by clinicians, diagnosing ASD requires parents and teachers to report the diagnostic nuances that distinguish ASD from other overlapping symptoms. For instance, children with anxiety and children with ASD may both present with social avoidance, poor eye contact, and sensory avoidance with a child with ASD, which may present similarly in screening measures. Clinical observation aids in distinguishing the source of the observed behavior. The use of observational assessments such as ADOS-2 has been shown to distinguish cooccurring and overlapping disorders such as intellectual disabilities (Thurm, Farmer, Salzman, Lord, & Bishop, 2019). Through the use of observational measures, a trained clinician is able to better assess for differential diagnoses that a questionnaire might be unable to detect.

As noted in the introduction, one disadvantage to behavioral observations is the subjectivity and potential bias that comes with each observer. Thus standardization of observations is important for consistent scoring across clinicians. The ADOS-2 has an extensive training process for clinicians to become either clinically reliable or research-reliable administrators of the measure. Even with extensive training, the standard for reliability of observational measures such as the ADOS-2 is around 80% accuracy. Although the ADOS-2 is considered the gold standard for an ASD measure, diagnostic sensitivity is highest when multiple sources of information are used together (Brian, Zwaigenbaum, & Ip, 2019; Kim & Lord, 2012).

CLINICAL IMPLICATIONS

Observational assessments give clinicians the power to more accurately assess and understand challenging or maladaptive behaviors. Behavioral observations can elicit and support evidence-based hypotheses of subjective impressions of problem behavior. Clinicians often have to determine the function of a behavior based on parent or teacher report, as they are not usually present during times when problem behavior occurs, such as a tantrum at bedtime or when recess is ending. Thus utilizing a structured system for describing observed behaviors provides clinicians with the information necessary to determine the function of a behavior and therefore develop the most appropriate behavioral intervention.

Importantly, the results of observational assessments are often meaningful for the consumer as well as the clinician. Caregivers may be motivated by data that show slow but steady improvements in response to intervention that may not be obvious based on general recall. Patients themselves may also be motivated when they are able to view objective data showing their progress (e.g., serial pictures of improving eyebrow growth in response to trichotillomania treatment). Some clinicians have even used diagnostic observation measures (e.g., ADOS-2) to develop operational definitions of behaviors that link directly to intervention goals, making goals more personally meaningful (Guercio & Hahs, 2015).

Overall, observational assessments are excellent tools that can provide rich insight into the nuances of child behavior. In addition to providing evidence-based and meaningful data, many of the methods described in this chapter are free and readily accessible. The minimal number of materials required for tracking child behavior and completing ABCs and FBAs reduces the barriers for clinicians to assess and intervene with problem behavior. Accessibility is essential for schools and families that may lack resources because of funding or location. Additionally, technology has become integrated into many of these methods and measures to improve efficiency and to allow for remote collection of data.

REFERENCES

Alberto, P. A., & Troutman, A. C. (2009). *Applied behavior analysis for teachers* (8th ed.). Pearson Education, Inc.

Brian, J. A., Zwaigenbaum, L., & Ip, A. (2019). Standards of diagnostic assessment for autism spectrum disorder. *Paediatrics and Child Health (Canada)*, *24*(7), 444–451. https://doi.org/10.1093/pch/pxz117

Christ, T. (2008). Best practices in problem analysis. In A. Thomas & J. Grimes (Eds.), *Best practices in school psychology* (pp. 159–176). National Association of School Psychologists.

Cooper, J. O., Heron, T. E., & Heward, W. L. (2007). *Applied behavior analysis* (2nd ed.). Prentice Hall.

Guercio, J. M., & Hahs, A. D. (2015). Applied behavior analysis and the Autism Diagnostic Observation Schedule (ADOS): A symbiotic relationship for advancements in services for individuals with autism spectrum disorders (ASDs). *Behavior Analysis in Practice*, *8*(1), 62–65.

Hanley, G. P., Iwata, B. A., & McCord, B. E. (2003). Functional analysis of problem behavior: A review. *Journal of Applied Behavior Analysis*, *36*, 147–185. https://doi.org/10.1901/jaba.2003.36-147

Heron, T., Cooper, J., & Heward, W. (2015). Applied behavior analysis. In E. Neukrug (Ed.), *The Sage encyclopedia of theory in counseling and psychotherapy* (pp. 51–55). Sage Publications, Inc. https://doi.org/10.4135/9781483346502.n25

Howell, K. W., Hosp, J. L., & Kurns, S. (2008). Best practices in curriculum-based evaluation. In A. Thomas & J. Grimes (Eds.), *Best practices in school psychology* (pp. 349–362). National Association of School Psychologists.

Ingram, K., Lewis-Palmer, T., & Sugai, G. (2005). Function-based intervention planning: Comparing the effectiveness of FBA function-based and non-function-based intervention plans. *Journal of Positive Behavior Interventions*, *7*, 224–236.

Kantowitz, B., Roediger, H. L., & Elmes, D. G. (2009). *Experimental psychology* (10th ed.). Cengage Learning.

Kerr, M. M., & Nelson, C. M. (2010). *Strategies for addressing behavior problems in the classroom* (6th ed.). Pearson.

Kim, S. H., & Lord, C. (2012). Combining information from multiple sources for the diagnosis of autism spectrum disorders for toddlers and young preschoolers from 12 to 47 months of age. *Journal of Child Psychology and Psychiatry*, *53*(2), 143–151.

Lord, C., Rutter, M., DiLavore, P., Risi, S., Gotham, K., & Bishop, S. (2012). *Autism Diagnostic Observation Schedule–2nd edition (ADOS-2)*. Western Psychological Services.

Scott, T. M., Anderson, C. M., & Spaulding, S. A. (2008). Strategies for developing and carrying out functional assessment and behavior intervention planning. *Preventing School Failure*, *52*(3), 39–49.

The IRIS Center for Training Enhancements. (2009). *Functional behavioral assessment: Identifying the reasons for problem behavior and developing a behavior plan*. http://iris.peabody.vanderbilt.edu/fba/chalcycle.htm

Thurm, A., Farmer, C., Salzman, E., Lord, C., & Bishop, S. (2019). State of the field: Differentiating intellectual disability from autism spectrum disorder. *Frontiers in Psychiatry*. https://doi.org/10.3389/fpsyt.2019.00526

Umbreit, J., Ferro, J., Liaupsin, C. J., & Lane, K. L. (2007). *Functional behavior assessment and function-based intervention: An effective practical approach*. Prentice Hall.

85

Developmental, Cognitive, and Intelligence Testing

Stephanie K. Takamatsu, Eleanore M. Hall, and Allison G. Dempsey

For additional material related to the content of this chapter, please see Chapters 76, 79, and 81.

VIGNETTE

Nathan is a 4-year, 9-month-old White male with a prenatal diagnosis of 22q deletion syndrome (also known as DiGeorge syndrome). He lives with both his parents and is an only child. English is the primary language spoken in the home. Nathan was referred to a developmental-behavioral pediatrician (DBP) for evaluation due to his genetic diagnosis and its known developmental and behavioral comorbidities, specifically delays in language, social, and cognitive development. His medical history is significant for a cardiac anomaly, feeding difficulties, and growth delay, as well as delayed developmental milestones and sleep disturbances. Prolonged hospital stays were common in his first year of life due to cardiac surgery and medical complications. Because of his medical challenges and health care needs, he has not been enrolled in any formal childcare or preschool setting. Nathan receives private therapy services, including physical therapy for gross motor delays and occupational therapy for feeding challenges. His parents' current concerns are that he speaks single words and has a few two-word phrases and has difficulty following and attending to commands. On meeting Nathan, the clinician also noted significant behavioral signs of anxiety. The DBP is aware of possible comorbidities that could explain delays and also considers the prolonged early hospital stays and reduced opportunities for social engagement with peers. Suspecting that Nathan may be exhibiting some learning challenges, the physician administers the Kaufman Brief Intelligence Test, Second Edition (KBIT-2), which is a brief cognitive assessment that measures verbal and nonverbal ability among individuals 4 years and older (Kaufman & Kaufman, 2004). The standard scores produced were over 1 standard deviation below the mean, and the DBP decided to refer the child for psychological testing to (1) determine current developmental level, (2) determine whether delays are consistent with a neurodevelopmental comorbidity, and (3) generate specific recommendations for intervention.

This chapter promotes interdisciplinary collaboration by helping medical clinicians to understand the history of intellectual and developmental testing, and when, how, and why psychological testing can support patient care. It will provide a broad overview of the differences between intellectual and developmental testing, the historical context in which they were developed, and the current limitations to test administration and interpretation. The chapter will detail the psychologist's approach to testing, including instrument selection, methodology, score interpretation, consideration of scores in diagnostic decision making, and treatment planning (see Chapter 76 for more background related to psychological assessment).

HISTORY OF INTELLECTUAL AND DEVELOPMENTAL TESTING

History of Intellectual Testing

Intelligence testing emerged in the early 20th century, when the Binet-Simon Intelligence Scale was developed for the purposes of evaluating schoolchildren. As described by Kranzler, Benson, & Floyd, (2016), significant changes in the United States at the turn of the 20th century, including compulsory schooling, created both a surge in school attendance and a need to efficiently evaluate students' ability levels to place them on "tracks" based on their perceived abilities. Intelligence tests were thus used to determine educational tracks into which students could be placed. Educational tracks based on intelligence testing were eliminated during the civil rights movement amidst concerns and legal battles over the impact of race, ethnicity, and socioeconomic status (SES) on test scores (with minoritized groups and students from low-SES backgrounds disproportionately placed in lower tracks).

In the 1970s new legislation emerged that changed the function of intelligence testing in children. Under the Individuals with Disabilities in Education Act (IDEA; Public Law 94-142), first published in 1975 and originally called the Education of All Handicapped Children Act, intelligence testing was now used to identify children in need of additional school services. This new approach to intelligence testing aimed to provide "free and appropriate education" to all children, at school age and beyond (Kranzler et al., 2016).

History of Theories of Intelligence

Although early tests sought to determine intellectual level or mental age, future iterations measured results through an intelligence quotient (IQ; i.e., a standardized number that describes a person's developmental skill level in comparison to chronologic age). The Cattell-Horn-Carroll (CHC) theory of cognitive abilities offers the most widespread theory of intelligence (Flanagan & Dixon, 2014; McGrew & Flanagan, 1998). This model conceptualizes intelligence as consisting of various hierarchically arranged cognitive abilities. At the highest level is the most general factor of intelligence: *g*. The second level down contains numerous broad cognitive abilities, such as fluid reasoning *(Gf)*, comprehension-knowledge *(Gc)*, short-term memory *(Gsm)*, long-term storage and retrieval *(Glr)*, and visual processing *(Gv)*. The bottom tier contains more than 80 narrow cognitive abilities. The CHC theory provides common language and theoretical ground for test developers and providers (Kranzler et al., 2016). Indeed, most contemporary intelligence tests are based on this theory.

History of Developmental Testing

Although intellectual and cognitive abilities are considered relatively stable traits, they are not considered to be measurable and/or stable until early school age, or approximately 7 years due to rapid development in the cortex and prefrontal cortex in early childhood (Schneider, Niklas, & Schmiedeler, 2014). Thus developmental testing was created to monitor early childhood precursors to the formation of intellectual skills (language, motor movements, early cognitive skills).

The first standardized developmental assessments emerged in the latter half of the 20th century, when the Head Start movement began in the United States, and there was a need to monitor progress in early childhood. The Denver Developmental Screening Test was developed in 1967 and was the first developmental screening tool to identify young children (<6 years of age) who were at risk for developmental delays. With the inclusion of early childhood populations in IDEA legislation in 1986, developmental testing became increasingly widespread.

In recent decades a growing recognition of the importance of early intervention led pediatricians, educators, and developmental specialists to call for routine monitoring of development through standard screening to identify children in need of further testing and intervention. In 2001 the American Academy of Pediatrics (AAP, 2001) recommended universal developmental screening for all children in pediatric practices. They refined these guidelines in 2006, calling for standardized screening in pediatric primary care with validated developmental screening tools when parents or health care clinicians noted concern at their 9-, 18-, and 30-month well-child visits (American Academy of Pediatrics, 2006). The AAP also called for ongoing surveillance at every preventive visit as well as autism-specific screening at 18 and 24 months of age.

USES AND LIMITATIONS OF TESTING

Uses of Developmental Versus Intellectual Testing

Clinicians must determine whether developmental or intellectual testing is most appropriate for a given child. Developmental testing is most appropriate for infants and toddlers and is used to monitor development in children born at risk for developmental delays, to determine eligibility for early intervention services, and to aid in diagnostic decision-making and treatment planning. Developmental testing does not equate to a child's IQ, and developmental test scores are typically not strong predictors of future performance (Månsson, Stjernqvist, Serenius, Ådén, & Källén, 2019).

Intellectual or cognitive testing is typically completed with children at school age (≥5–6 years) and adults. The tests are used to assess an individual's strengths and weaknesses across cognitive domains (e.g., verbal comprehension, visual-spatial, fluid reasoning processing speed, and attention and memory), to determine whether cognitive impairments are present, and to indicate a potential need for additional services and supports. Although intellectual testing is appropriate to use with young children, results from those under the age of 7 years should be interpreted as representing the child's skills at a particular point in time because intellectual abilities are not yet considered stable at these ages.

Limitations of Testing

Environmental Influence on Intelligence Scores

Intelligence has been shown to be a product of both heredity and environmental factors. Many researchers have examined the impact of environmental influences on intelligence and suggest that differences in intellectual abilities sometimes observed among minoritized youth and their White counterparts are a product of unequal access to resources and opportunities. This discrepancy was underscored by research at the turn of the 21st century, which showed that increased educational opportunities for children of low SES led to significant, lasting gains in IQ (Wahlsten, 1997). However, it is also important to note that increased access to resources and affluent school districts alone does not automatically close the testing gap, as placing minoritized youth in predominately White or affluent districts can lead to emotional distress and feelings of isolation for the child. Thus intellectual tests can reflect societal disadvantage rather than a person's true abilities.

Cultural and Linguistic Influence on Test Scores

Culture and language must be considered in determining the appropriateness of developmental, cognitive, and intelligence tests for any given child (American Educational Research Association, 2014). Although tests such as the Weschler Intelligence Scales for Children (WISC-V) have been updated to reduce cultural bias (e.g., amended informational questions and updated images), a child's primary language, acculturation status, and time spent in the United States all have the potential to significantly influence performance on assessment measures (as summarized by Ortiz, Piazza, Ochoa, & Dynda, 2018). For example, if a child is bilingual, the clinician must consider the amount of academic instruction the child has received in the native language. A child's ability to carry on a conversation in English is not an appropriate measure of proficiency; the demands on an English-speaker-normed test may exceed the child's capacity.

Psychological tests are largely validated on native English speakers who are of White ethnicity (e.g., WISC-V; Wechsler, 2014b). The WISC-V Spanish was adapted using a sample of bilingual, primarily Spanish-speaking children in the United States, with the process being overseen by a panel of bilingual psychologists (Muñoz, Weiss, & Prifitera, 2019). However, the size of the WISC-V Spanish test's normative sample (N = 220; Wechsler, 2014a) falls below the minimum size recommended by the International Test Commission Guidelines and is 10 times smaller than that of the traditional WISC-V. To address the lack of empirical support for standardized testing in culturally and linguistically diverse populations, the following are needed to improve validity: (1) testing in an examinee's native language, (2) modifying or adapting subtests with high linguistic or cultural loading, and (3) administering nonverbal tests or a combination thereof (Ortiz et al., 2018).

REASONS FOR REFERRING FOR DEVELOPMENTAL, INTELLECTUAL, OR COGNITIVE TESTING

DBPs who work with patients like Nathan, from the chapter-opening vignette, who have conditions with known comorbidities of developmental delays and learning difficulties, may engage in closer monitoring of the child and plan to refer for testing at specific timepoints in development, thus ensuring that the child receives continued supports. Physicians should consider several factors when referring a child for testing, including age of the child, domains of concern, and reason for testing (e.g., differential diagnosis, eligibility determination, treatment planning). Once a referral for testing is deemed appropriate, the physician must determine how to connect the child and family and how to communicate with the clinician about the reason for the referral. Referral decisions and clinician-to-clinician communication vary according to the availability of integrated behavioral health care in a pediatric practice. These are briefly described next.

Integrated Behavioral Health Models

Integrated behavioral health models are increasingly common in primary and specialty pediatric practices associated with larger medical centers. They are especially common in clinics for children with medical conditions that place them at high risk for developmental and/or learning and behavioral difficulties, such as in neonatal follow-up clinics, DBP practices, cardiac follow-up clinics, and clinics for those with specific genetic variations. In an integrated behavioral health care model psychologists or other behavioral health clinicians are regular members of the care team. In some specialty care clinics developmental and intellectual testing at established timepoints in development may be part of routine care in the clinic.

In an integrated model the clinician may verbally communicate with the testing clinician about the concerns that necessitate the testing referral. The physician and the behavioral health clinician may then collaborate in writing a report, making diagnostic decisions, and treatment planning. As the testing may take place in the same setting as the medical practice, there are often reduced barriers to receiving testing, including reduced stigma for receiving behavioral health services, greater ease of scheduling, and improved communication among the clinicians.

Referral Model

In settings in which clinicians who can complete testing and interpretation are not integrated into the practice a consultation model may be used. In this model of care the physician may need to make a more formalized, written referral, and the family will then need to arrange scheduling through the separate clinic. Once testing is completed and the clinician in the outside clinic/setting writes the report, the physician must then receive and review the report (either directly from the clinician or from the parents of the child) and then use the report to aid in decision making related to care for the child.

Physicians may refer to clinicians in various settings for testing, including early intervention, schools, specialized pediatric and/or behavioral care settings (e.g., psychology or neuropsychology clinics), or other outpatient centers. Each setting has its own goal and area of specialty that will guide the test selection and recommendations. Limitations of this type of model relate to the goals and processes of the referral setting. Thus reason for testing should guide the decision regarding the appropriate setting to refer the child.

Referrals to Early Intervention

If a physician refers a young child to early intervention services, testing will be completed to determine eligibility. For those who meet criteria, appropriate early intervention services are determined and an individualized family service plan for special education preschool programming is developed. Testing will not be used for diagnosis or treatment planning outside of services available through early intervention. That is, early intervention testing does not provide diagnoses, such as autism spectrum disorder or global developmental delay; formal diagnosis of these conditions may be needed for insurance to cover more intensive services, such as applied behavior analysis or intensive physical or feeding therapies. Lastly, given the predetermined cutoff for service eligibility, some children with delays may not meet criteria for early intervention and will need to seek services elsewhere.

Referrals for Testing in Public Schools

As another example, testing completed in schools for children at school age will not be used for diagnostic decision making and will instead focus on eligibility determination for special education services. A physician does not make a direct referral for testing and may instead recommend that a family who has concerns about their child's learning approach the school to ask for an evaluation to determine eligibility for services. The primary goal of testing in an academic setting is to assess a child's current educational performance and how a disability or learning delay impacts the child's participation and success in the general academic curriculum. The evaluation results are used to determine eligibility for in-school services via an individualized education plan. The two criteria for eligibility include (1) whether a student meets the educational determination of a disability (based on 13 categories of disability), and (2) the child's need for special education services to function in school. Since both criteria are necessary, a child may present with a disability but be ineligible for services if the symptoms are not interfering with learning (see Chapter 86 for more on educational assessment).

Referrals to Psychology Practices

Referrals to specialty care practices for psychological testing may be necessary when a child of any age demonstrates a complex symptom presentation that requires rule-out of several diagnoses or symptom etiologies. Given the complexity of such cases, formal testing for various conditions, such as intellectual disability or autism spectrum disorder, is often needed. Specialty care testing is also especially important for children with medical complexities, like Nathan in the case vignette, who have medical complications that can affect development and cognitive functioning (see Chapter 87 for more on neuropsychological testing).

Framing Referral Questions

Regardless of referral model (to integrated behavioral health or external referrals), the physician must carefully consider the reason for referring a child for testing and appropriately frame the referral question. The inclusion of more detail in a referral question increases the likelihood that the results of the testing will be of benefit to the referring physician and family. A detailed referral may also assist clinicians in making a case for preauthorization for testing from insurance companies. The following information should be included in a referral question, unless a different format is requested by the clinic: (1) brief summary of child and relevant medical details (including sleep, feeding, medical diagnoses), (2) any past interventions and/or medications to treat presenting issues, (3) complicating factors such as medical conditions (e.g., vision/hearing/motor difficulties) or social/developmental/home factors (e.g., parents going through divorce, recent relocation), (4) possible rule-out diagnoses and/or explanations for behaviors, and (5) specific questions (e.g., What is the appropriate diagnosis? What treatment does this child need?).

In the case of Nathan the DBP could frame the referral as follows: Referring this 4-year, 9-month-old White male with DiGeorge syndrome and significant cardiac complications for developmental and psychological testing. He has a history of feeding difficulties and motor delays and is currently receiving occupational and physical therapy. Child displays sleep problems and delayed language milestones. I also observed some anxiety in the office. He speaks in single words and two-word phrases, and parents have concerns about his attending to and following directions. He has been in and out of the hospital in his first year and has no childcare or school experience. No hearing or vision concerns. Referral questions are (1) Does he meet criteria for diagnosis of language or developmental delay or other disorder? (2) What (nonpharmacologic) services does he need for anxiety, sleep, and social development? (3) Does he need additional or more intensive developmental therapies?

TESTING PROCESS AND INTERPRETATION

For the remainder of this chapter we will be discussing the process that the testing clinician (referred to as psychologist hereafter) completes once a child has been referred for testing. We primarily focus on the process within health care settings, though many aspects of test selection and interpretation may be similar for early intervention and school settings.

Record Review, Clinical Interview, and Rating Scales

Once a psychologist receives the referral for testing, the first step in the testing process is to obtain and review detailed information about the child's background, including medical and school records, previous testing reports, and social, family, and developmental history. The psychologist then gathers additional information through a clinical interview with the parents/caregivers and occasionally with other adults familiar with the child (e.g., teachers, home care nurses). The psychologist will also typically ask parents and teachers to provide additional information about the child's social-emotional functioning, behaviors, and adaptive skills using standardized rating scales. This information is used to further refine testing questions and identify factors that need to be considered in selecting a test battery (see Chapter 82 for more on evaluation of emotions and behavior).

Test Selection

Psychologists have a wide range of psychological tests available for assessment (Tables 85.1 and 85.2), with certain intellectual and developmental tests being commonly used across evaluations. However, test selection is an idiographic, evolving process based on each child's presentation, with psychologists taking the individuals' physical, linguistic, developmental, and cultural context into account in building, reevaluating, and amending the test battery. For example, limitations in expressive or receptive language and/or speech production may interfere with the validity of certain measures that have complex verbal instructions or require verbal process.

There has also been consideration of the role telehealth can play in testing and when it is and is not appropriate. For many families, testing can present significant financial challenges, including the need to take off a full day of work and obtain childcare, purchase gas to travel to the appointment, and the emotional stress related to traveling with children long distances. While there are options for conducting both developmental and intellectual/cognitive testing through telehealth, research is continuing to be conducted to assess the effectiveness of these approaches.

Referring back to the case of Nathan, the psychologist, prior to meeting with Nathan and his family, first considers the referral question. A review of medical records and previous testing evaluations from his occupational and physical therapists confirms that Nathan does not have any notable impairments in hearing or vision that would interfere with standardized administration of any tests.

Because Nathan is out of the age range of the Bayley-4 (norms stop at 42 months), a developmental assessment, the psychologist determined that an intellectual/cognitive test for young children would be more appropriate. Given the referral question about diagnosis of develop-

mental delays, the psychologist selected to administer tests that would assist with ruling out the following diagnoses: Global developmental delay, attention-deficit/hyperactivity disorder, and generalized anxiety disorder (or other form of anxiety disorder). The following test battery is developed: The Wechsler Preschool & Primary Scale of Intelligence, Fourth Edition (WIPPSI-IV) to assess cognitive skills, and two parent report measures—the Adaptive Behavior Assessment System, Third Edition (ABAS-3) to assess daily living skills and the Child Behavior Checklist (CBCL) for ages 1.5 to 5 years to assess anxiety and behaviors.

Test Administration

Throughout testing, psychologists also take note of each child's unique presentation and record these in the report as behavioral observations. Standardization of the testing environment and procedures can reveal notable behaviors, mood, or thought content that contribute to the psychologist's understanding of the child and what tests might be relevant. When conducting developmental testing, the following is typically noted in behavioral observations: (1) who was present; (2) any concerns (or lack thereof) related to vision, hearing, motor weaknesses; (3) presence/absence of any atypical behaviors or social skills; (4) child's energy level/fatigue

TABLE 85.1 Most Commonly Used Intellectual/Cognitive Tests for Children

Test Name	Age Range (Y:M)	Year Edition Published	Domains Assessed
Differential Ability Scales, Second Edition (DAS-II)	2:6–17:11	2007	Verbal, nonverbal reasoning, spatial,
Kaufman Assessment Battery for Children, Second Edition Normative Update (KABC-II NU)	3:0–18:11	2018	Simultaneous, sequential, planning, learning, knowledge
Reynolds Intellectual Assessment Scales, Second Edition (RIAS-2)	3:0–94:11	2015	Verbal, nonverbal, composite memory, speeded processing, composite intelligence
Stanford-Binet Intelligence Scales, Fifth Edition (SB-5)	2:0–85+	2003	Fluid reasoning, knowledge, quantitative, visual-spatial, working memory
Wechsler Intelligence Scale for Children (WISC-V)	6:0–16:11	2014	Verbal comprehension, visual spatial, working memory, fluid reasoning, processing speed
Wechsler Preschool and Primary Scale of Intelligence (WPPSI-IV)	2:6–7:7	2012	Verbal comprehension, visual spatial, working memory (fluid reasoning, processing speed for 4:0–7:7)
Woodcock-Johnson IV Tests of Cognitive Abilities (WJ IV COG)	2:0+	2014	Comprehension-knowledge, fluid reasoning, short-term working memory, cognitive processing speed, auditory processing, long-term retrieval, visual processing

Note: Nonverbal tests, which are covered in another chapter, are not included in this table.

TABLE 85.2 Most Commonly Used Developmental Tests

Test Name	Age Range (Y:M)	Year Edition Published	Domains Assessed via Direct Assessment	Domains Assessed via Parent Report (Interview or Questionnaire)
Battelle Developmental Inventory, Third Edition (BDI-3)	0:0–7:11	2020	Cognitive, communication, motor	Social-emotional, adaptive
Bayley Scales of Infant and Toddler Development (Bayley-4)	16 days–3:6	2019	Cognitive, language, motor	Social-emotional, adaptive
Developmental Assessment of Young Children, Second Edition (DAYC-2)	0:0–5:11	2012	Cognition, communication, physical development	Social-emotional, adaptive
Developmental Profile, Third Edition (DP-3)	0:0–12:11	2007	n/a	Adaptive behavior, cognition, social-emotional development, physical development, communication
Mullen Scales of Early Learning (Mullen)	0:0–5:8	1995	Visual reception, language, motor	n/a

and attentiveness to tasks; and (5) presence or absence of any disruptive behaviors. When conducting intellectual or cognitive testing, the following is typically noted in behavioral observations: (1) interest, engagement, motivation; (2) any concerns (or lack thereof) related to vision, hearing, language processing or production, and/or motor weaknesses; and (3) presence/absence of any atypical or disruptive behaviors or social skills concerns. For both types of testing, the behavioral observations should include an assessment whether the results of testing should be considered valid and/or interpreted with caution and a reason for this conclusion.

In first meeting Nathan the psychologist noted he presented with anxious behaviors (e.g., limited eye contact, limited verbal responses, and he stayed close to his parents). Given Nathan's initial presentation, his history of frequent medical appointments, and that he has rarely been asked to separate from a parent, the psychologist decided that one parent would stay in the room with Nathan, while the other sat in the waiting room to limit distractions. The psychologist also spent additional time with Nathan at the beginning of session building rapport, and although Nathan was observed to check in with eye contact frequently with his father, Nathan's motivation and comfort increased over time. During the evaluation, Nathan was observed to have significant difficulty remaining in his seat and focused on the task at hand. He also appeared to have difficulty related to low muscle tone (e.g., appeared to have difficulty remaining in an upright posture). Modification to standardized testing was determined to be necessary as the results would not be an accurate measurement of his skills since he was not attending to the tasks and appeared to physically fatigue as testing continued. Nathan benefitted from use of a more supportive chair, reminders of appropriate behaviors, labeled praise, and a visual schedule that limited language demands, and helped him understand expectations and when a task would be over. While the modification helped Nathan regulate his behaviors, he continued to show difficulties attending. Thus the results of this assessment were considered an underestimate of his true abilities and should be interpreted with caution.

Interpretation of Testing Scores

Skilled psychologists take all steps possible to set up the testing environment to allow for a valid assessment of a child's developmental, intellectual, or cognitive functioning. However, as described in previous sections, multiple factors can influence testing results. Thus the first step in test interpretation is to identify and consider all factors that influenced a child's performance on the day of the assessment.

If the psychologist believes the scores can be considered a valid reflection of a child's abilities, the next step is to examine the standardized scores to make interpretations about a child's functioning. Scores are typically interpreted from broad to specific. That is, typically psychologists look at the global level (i.e., general ability), to the domain level (e.g., verbal processing, working memory), to the most specific, individual subtest levels. On the global level, the summary/full-scale IQ score (i.e., *g*) is often the first score to be interpreted because it is the best predictor of achievement and performance. It is a summary score derived from all subtests administered; however, this summary score is not always interpretable, particularly when there is a significant difference in scores between domains.

Domain scores represent specific groups of skills, such as verbal processing and working memory (representative of the individual CHC factors) and are typically derived from scores on two to three subtests. Differences across domain scores are used to derive conclusions about a child's cognitive strengths and weaknesses and to identify areas of needed support in various settings. Similar to global scores, domain scores are sometimes uninterpretable due to drastic variations in scores on individual subtests that comprise them, thus requiring interpretation of scores on an individual subtest level. For example, a child may perform in the borderline range on the domain of working memory; however, if we look at individual subtest scores, the child performed in the average range on a processing speed task requiring brief scanning of visual stimuli and decision making about the stimuli, marking the answer with a slash or dot; in contrast, the child scored in the impaired range on a task requiring quick copying of visual stimuli. In this case the psychologist might hypothesize that the child has a challenge with fine motor skills rather than working memory and will then look for similar patterns on subtests requiring similar skills. Large differences in domain and/or subtest scores (i.e., splintered skill sets) are often seen among children diagnosed with neurologic injuries or genetic conditions.

Reporting Scores and Interpretations

The psychologist reports and interprets the results of testing, integrated with information obtained from record review, clinical interviews, and ratings scales. In addition to these written portions, a report typically also includes one or more tables that summarize testing data in the form of standardized scores. We highly recommend that readers look to the report's conclusion or summary section to understand results and diagnosis, not simply to the report's tables, as multiple factors described earlier go into the interpretation of scores.

Looking back at our case vignette, Nathan showed a varied cognitive profile on the WIPPSI-IV (Table 85.3). Use of the summary score/full-scale IQ is inappropriate and would not be representative of his actual abilities because there is a significant discrepancy between his index scores. Instead, looking at each of his index (domain) scores separately provides a more accurate understanding of his cognitive abilities. For instance, his performance on the verbal comprehension index suggests that his verbal skills are delayed compared to same-age peers. The visual spatial index score and fluid reasoning index (scores) indicated that these domains of cognitive functioning are relative strengths for Nathan compared to his performance across other indices. This also suggests that he has near- or age-

TABLE 85.3 Testing Results for Nathan (Clinical Vignette) on the Wechsler Preschool and Primary Scale of Intelligence

Domain Score	Composite Standard Score	Qualitative Description
Verbal comprehension (VCI)	76	Borderline
Visual spatial (VSI)	86	Low average
Fluid reasoning (FRI)	92	Average
Working memory (WMI)	75	Borderline
Processing speed (PSI)	69	Extremely low

Note: VCI is a measure of verbal reasoning and comprehension; VSI is a measure of ability to attend, organize visual details and understand part-whole relationships; FRI is a measure of fluid and inductive reasoning skills; WMI is a measure of visual and visual-spatial working memory; and PSI is a measure of one's ability to quickly and correctly scan and sequence visual information.

appropriate skills in his ability to organize visual information (e.g., putting together puzzles and recreating designs) and to use logic to solve problems (e.g., completing patterns). His lower scores on both the working memory index (WMI) and processing speed index (PSI) suggest difficulties in his executive functioning skills.

Using Testing for Diagnostic Decision Making

Psychological testing often culminates in a diagnosis. For clinicians, the universal language of a diagnosis facilitates efficient, interdisciplinary conceptualization of a child's presentation. For families, a diagnosis may serve as a roadmap through which caregivers can better understand and help their child. At times, the results of an evaluation may indicate that a diagnosis is not warranted. Data may show conflicting or ambiguous results. For example, a child's behaviors and functioning may be explained by multiple factors that cannot be isolated (e.g., traumatic history, mood concerns) rather than a reflection of developmental, intellectual, or cognitive abilities. A diagnosis may be deferred until further clarification is possible. Alternatively, children may not meet criteria for a diagnosis at the time of an evaluation due to subthreshold symptoms/scores, though may still benefit from recommendations based on results.

Results from cognitive/intellectual testing revealed that Nathan's verbal cognitive abilities are delayed, and his nonverbal cognitive abilities are closely comparable to that of his same-age peers. Given this profile, the psychologist ruled out a global developmental delay or concerns for an intellectual disability. Nathan does meet criteria for a developmental coordination disorder, indicating difficulties with coordination and motor skills. Although his language is delayed, the psychologist did not provide a formal diagnosis because formal testing was not completed and it was recommended that Nathan receive a comprehensive speech and language evaluation to assess his current skills and needs for additional intervention services.

Other diagnoses that were considered included generalized anxiety disorder (or another anxiety disorder) and attention-deficit/hyperactivity disorder. Behavioral observations, parent report, and cognitive/intellectual testing support difficulties with anxiety and his executive functioning skills. However, significant consideration was given to Nathan's history of frequent medical stays, language delays, and lack of exposure to other children and a structured preschool setting. It is possible that his anxiety symptoms may decrease with exposure to other children and continued improvement in his communication skills. In addition, a diagnosis of attention-deficit/hyperactivity disorder requires that symptoms be present across at least two environments because behaviors in settings can differ significantly. Thus Nathan was not provided with either diagnosis at this time, but the psychologist noted that these behaviors should be monitored.

Providing Feedback and Recommendations

The feedback session that follows the evaluation is one of the most important components of the psychological assessment process. It is at this appointment that families learn the psychologist's conceptualization of their child's presentation, begin to make sense of symptoms or behaviors, and learn what steps they can take to best help their child. Caregivers may experience a range of emotions at feedback sessions, ranging from grief over a diagnosis to relief at learning answers to long-held questions. A family's cultural background may also inform their perspective on a diagnosis, their conceptualization of behavior, and the level of stigma around certain services. In some cases these views may reduce the likelihood that a family will accept the results of an evaluation and pursue the psychologist's recommendations.

The psychologist approaches the feedback session—as well as the entire evaluation process—with this in mind. Psychologists are trained to reflect and validate caregivers' experiences, use language the family uses, align with their goals, and approach the assessment as a collaborative partnership. While the testing psychologist is an expert in evaluation, the caregiver is an expert on the child. Such a stance increases the likelihood that families will place trust in their clinician at the feedback session. Recommendations can provide caregivers, educators, and professionals with appropriate next steps and a better understanding of the child's unique strengths and areas of difficulty, as well as how to tailor strategies to help the child engage and perform best. The length and specificity of the recommendations section are subject to differences in resources between settings and geographic areas.

In the case of Nathan his psychologist provided recommendations that helped his parents and future teachers to best support him based on his individual profile. For example, the psychologist noted that Nathan's nonverbal cognitive abilities are an area of strength compared to his verbal abilities and he will need significant modifications (e.g., limited language demands, as he may struggle to find words to communicate his needs and meaning; include multimodal forms of teaching to increase his comprehension of material) for him to showcase his skills.

Nathan's profile also suggests that he will benefit from behavioral supports (e.g., increased time on tasks, more frequent feedback, visual schedules, increased positive reinforcement for desired behaviors, starting out with easier problems first to build confidence). Sleep concerns were also noted in the referral question, which was assessed in this evaluation through clinical interview. Behavioral sleep strategies were discussed in the feedback, and it was recommended that the referring DBP consider ordering a sleep test, due to parents' concerns of snoring. Nathan will need to be reevaluated once he enters a structured preschool setting. This would be a core component of the psychologist's recommendations, as a reevaluation would allow for analysis if his anxiety symptoms have decreased, and of his behavior across settings, thus confirming or refuting a potential attention-deficit/hyperactivity disorder. Repeated intellectual/cognitive testing would also allow for comparison of his scores over time, assess progress, and gain a sense of his developmental trajectory. This could be completed via repeated testing with the psychologist, or potentially, ongoing monitoring using the KBIT-2 or similar measure by the DBP.

CONCLUSION

Developmental and intellectual/cognitive testing is an important service that guides diagnostic decision making, treatment planning, and progress monitoring for children seen in DBP practice. This chapter provided an overview of when physicians should consider referrals for testing and how to use evaluation results to guide their clinical decisions. Understanding of the uses and limitations of tests and framing appropriate referral questions are critical to DBP practice. By having a foundational understanding in the different referral options and what an evaluation entails, a physician can better ensure a family is directed to the appropriate setting, saving the family both resources and time. Physicians can also educate families on their options and provide guidance on what they can expect. This can be a critical step to help prevent feelings of frustration and confusion and to help families better prepare for the upcoming evaluation. Specifically, having this early discussion can help families use the time while they wait for the evaluation to formulate their own questions and concerns, and notice new or ongoing behaviors with potentially a different lens. This in turn can help them feel they are active participants and have an important role in the evaluation.

As the case vignette represents, significant time and consideration is taken in understanding the broad contexts that can influence a child's symptom presentation and testing performance. It is essential that a clinician not only can administer a standardized test but can synthesize all relevant data and use the information to advocate for the necessary resources and interventions. A well-written referral question can help guide the evaluation process and facilitate interprofessional collaboration and care.

REFERENCES

American Academy of Pediatrics, & Committee on Children With Disabilities. (2001). Developmental surveillance and screening of infants and young children. *Pediatrics*, *108*, 192–195. https://doi.org/10.1542/peds.108.1.192

American Academy of Pediatrics, Council on Children With Disabilities, Section on Developmental Behavioral Pediatrics, & Bright Futures Steering Committee and Medical Home Initiatives for Children With Special Needs Project Advisory Committee. (2006). Identifying infants and young children with developmental disorders in the medical home: An algorithm for developmental surveillance and screening. *Pediatrics*, *118*, 405–420. https://doi.org/10.1542/peds.2006-1231

American Educational Research Association (AERA), American Psychological Association, & National Council on Measurement in Education. (2014). *Standards for educational and psychological testing*. AERA.

Flanagan, D. P., & Dixon, S. G. (Ed.) (2014). The Cattell-Horn-Carroll theory of cognitive abilities. In *Encyclopedia of special education: A reference for the education of children, adolescents, and adults disabilities and other exceptional individual* (4th ed.). John Wiley & Sons, Inc. https://doi.org/10.1002/9781118660584.ese0431

Horn, J. L., & Cattell, R. B. (1966). Refinement and test of the theory of fluid and crystallized general intelligences. *Journal of Educational Psychology*, *57*(5), 253–270. https://doi.org/10.1037/h0023816

Kaufman, A. S., & Kaufman, N. L. (2004). *Kaufman brief intelligence test* (2nd ed.). (KBIT-2). American Guidance Service.

Kranzler, J. H., Benson, N., & Floyd, R. G. (2016). Intellectual assessment of children and youth in the United States of America: Past, present, and future. *International Journal of School & Educational Psychology*, *4*(4), 276–282. https://doi.org/10.1080/21683603.2016.1166759

Månsson, J., Stjernqvist, K., Serenius, F., Ådén, U., & Källén, K. (2019). Agreement between Bayley-III measurements and WISC-IV measurements in typically developing children. *Journal of Psychoeducational Assessment*, *37*(5), 603–616. https://doi.org/10.1177/0734282918781431

McGrew, K. S., & Flanagan, D. P. (1998). *The intelligence test desk reference (ITDR): Gf-Gc cross-battery assessment*. Allyn & Bacon.

Muñoz, M., Weiss, L., & Prifitera, A. (2019). *Testing Hispanics with WISC-V and WISC-V Spanish: WISC-V: Clinical use and interpretation* (pp. 197–221) (2nd ed.). Elsevier.

Ortiz, S. O., Piazza, N., Ochoa, S. H., & Dynda, A. M. (2018). Testing with culturally and linguistically diverse populations: New directions in fairness and validity. In D. P. Flanagan & E. M. McDonough (Eds.), *Contemporary intellectual assessment: Theories, tests, and issues* (4th ed.). Guilford Press.

Schneider, W., Niklas, F., & Schmiedeler, S. (2014). Intellectual development from early childhood to early adulthood: The impact of early IQ differences on stability and change over time. *Learning and Individual Differences*, *32*, 156–162. https://doi.org/10.1016/j.lindif.2014.02.001

Wahlsten, D. (1997). The malleability of intelligence is not constrained by heritability. In B. Devlin, S. E. Fienberg, D. P. Resnick, & K. Roeder (Eds.), *Intelligence, genes, and success: Scientists respond to the bell curve* (pp. 71–87). Springer.

Wechsler, D. (2014a). *WISC-V administration and scoring manual* (5th ed.). Pearson.

Wechsler, D. (2014b). *WISC-V technical and interpretive manual.* PsychCorp.

86

Educational Testing and Evaluation of Academic Performance

Sara Kupzyk, Brenda Bassingthwaite, and Tina Scott-Mordhorst

For additional material related to the content of this chapter, please see Chapters 18, 83, and 104.

VIGNETTES

1. *Clara is a 2-year-old White female who lives with her biological parents with noticeable repetitive behaviors and limited social skills. Her parents describe that she is doing superb with academic tasks such as identification of shapes and letters; she sometimes "gets stuck" on things like singing the same song and repeating phrases; and she gets cranky if her routine is not followed. You conduct a screening for autism spectrum disorder (ASD) and refer the family for comprehensive evaluation. The evaluation confirms that she has ASD. The family is referred to early intervention services and to the local Child Find System in the state to determine if she qualifies for educational services. A release form is signed to share information between the clinic (e.g., evaluation, health status, diagnosis) and the school (e.g., evaluation conducted, educational verification, plans). After the educational evaluation is completed, the school multidisciplinary team (which includes the parents) meets to review the information and determines that Clara meets the educational verification criteria for ASD. An individualized family service plan (IFSP) is developed, and Clara begins early intervention services.*
2. *Marco is a 16-year-old Black male in ninth grade who receives medication management for attention-deficit/hyperactivity disorder (ADHD)–predominantly inattentive type. He completes a depression screener at the beginning of the appointment that indicates he is experiencing a significant number of depressive symptoms. Marco wants to discontinue medication because he does not feel like it is helping anymore. He is also thinking about dropping out of school. He used to like school for the social aspect, but he ended up in a class this year that has a lot of reading, he can't keep up, and his girlfriend made fun of him for being a slow reader. His father is getting calls about how poorly Marco is doing and legal ramifications related to truancy and feels that the school is not helping Marco as they should be, especially since he has always had an individualized education plan (IEP). When asked about the educational verification and services and goals outlined on his IEP, his father states that he went to the last meeting, but he did not know what was in the IEP but signed it in agreement because he did not know what to say. Medication and psychology services are discussed, and a release of information is obtained for communication with the school. The clinic social worker connects Marco and his father with the parent resource center for support and helps the family generate questions to discuss with the school to improve their understanding of Marco's learning needs and plan and his rights related to special education services. The father arranges a follow-up meeting with the IEP team at the school to update the plan with new information and revise the goals and services he receives to increase school success.*

IMPORTANCE OF UNDERSTANDING EDUCATIONAL TESTING AND EVALUATION

Medical school teaches students anatomy, physiology, diseases, and treatments. Over the last several years, they have added interpersonal skill building into the curriculum. What medical students are not taught well is how to work with institutions outside of the hospital or medical setting, particularly schools. Schools operate on their own set of laws, jargon, and boundaries, which pose potential barriers to collaboration. Despite the challenges of these two institutions working together, collaboration needs to happen for children and adolescents to have academic success and social-emotional health. Clinicians who work with children and adolescents are confronted with questions and concerns about a child's education, often when a family is in crisis. Information in these situations typically comes from a distraught, confused parent, guardian, advocate, or primary caregiver (we will use the term *parent* throughout to refer to these roles). The chapter-opening vignettes highlight the importance of learning about how educational systems work in order to help families navigate the medical and educational systems in a more coordinated manner.

POLICIES RELATED TO EDUCATIONAL TESTING AND EVALUATION

Standardized testing of students began in the mid-19th century as a means to decide how to place students, allocate resources, hold schools accountable, and influence teaching and learning standards (US Congress, 1992). Development of standardized intelligence and achievement tests and technology that allowed for multiple choice scanning and scoring formats made it easier to test students in larger groups (US Congress, 1992). Today, states are required to conduct annual testing for accountability and school improvement practices.

Unfortunately, the educational system and testing are not always equitable, culturally sensitive, and free of bias, particularly for students of underrepresented populations. While laws (e.g., 1896 *Plessy v. Ferguson*; 1954 *Brown v. Board of Education*; and 1967 *Hobson v. Hansen*) have helped to integrate schools and have limited the use of tests that were standardized on White, middle-class populations, there continue to be racial disparities in educational programs and disciplinary practices that school systems need to address (e.g., Cruz, Firestone, & Rodle, 2021). Children with disabilities also have faced a challenging history in education. Through the 1970s, children with significant disabilities were kept home or institutionalized because they were deemed "uneducable." Children with less severe disabilities were expected to learn in the same manner as their peers, with no additional supports. Events such as these have contributed to mistrust in education and ongoing disproportionality. As a result, laws aimed at increasing access to appropriate education and the expectation for success for all students have been passed (Table 86.1) (see Chapter 104 for related information on special education and inclusion). Although access has improved, some families continue to have mistrust, and having a trusted clinician supporting a collaborative relationship can be pivotal to increasing trust between families and educators.

Testing and Laws Focused on Equal Opportunity

The National Assessment of Educational Proficiency test was initiated in 1969 to measure what students in the United States know and can do in different subjects (reading, math, science). The test is taken by a representative sample of students in grades 4, 8, and 12. Reports are made available to the public and can be obtained based on demographic variables, including gender, age, and disability status (National Center for Education Statistics, 2020). No Child Left Behind (NCLB), in 2002, increased focus on accountability and measurement of achievement, with the goal of closing disparities in performance across

TABLE 86.1 Laws and Policies Related to Educational Assessment

Year	Law/Policy	Goal/Purpose
1965	Elementary and Secondary Education Act (ESEA)	Civil rights law aimed at improving the quality of education by providing grants and funding for districts serving low-income students, books, special education centers, and state educational agencies
1973	Section 504 of the Rehabilitation Act	Protects the rights of individuals who have a disability that limits one or more major life activities; schools provide accommodations or modifications to enable the student an equal opportunity to participate in academic and extracurricular activities
1975	Education for All Handicapped Children Act	Provided the right to free and appropriate public education (FAPE) in the least restrictive environment (LRE) for children ages 3–21 yr
1986	Education for All Handicapped Children Act	Outlines the special education process for children with disabilities ages birth–3 yr
1990	IDEA	Amended the Education for All Handicapped Children Act; outlines responsibilities for identification, assessment (multidisciplinary), and educational programming for students with disabilities; describes that parents should be included throughout the process
1994	Goals 2000: Education America Act	Defined national education goals and framework for meeting the goals; provided funding to states to create and implement improvement plans aimed at improving student achievement
1997	IDEA Amendments	Included functional behavior assessment to inform behavior plans
2002	No Child Left Behind Act (NCLB; previously ESEA)	Placed focus on accountability for and measures to close the achievement gap; included requirements for testing, meeting yearly goals, and penalties for not making sufficient progress
2004	IDEA Amendments	Added procedural safeguards related to change of placement, manifestation determinations, and timelines for related appeals and hearings; included "scientifically based" instructional practices and use of a process to determine if a student responds to scientific, research-based intervention as part of the evaluation procedures for a specific learning disability (SLD).
2005	Title I of ESEA	Provides funding to schools that include a high percentage of students from low-income families to support academic programming
2015	Every Student Succeeds Act (ESSA; previously ESEA/No Child Left Behind [NCLB])	Affords more flexibility to schools than NCLB. Requires states to develop a plan that includes (1) specific academic standards, (2) administration of annual tests to determine if students are meeting the standards (an alternative test for students with significant cognitive disabilities), (3) an accountability system, and (4) process for identifying schools in need of additional support and improvement

demographics. In 2015 NCLB was replaced by Every Student Succeeds Act (ESSA), which requires states to develop plans related to annual tests, accountability, and a process for providing supports to schools in need of improvement. The common elements across these laws are the recognition of the need to improve the quality of instruction and student outcomes regardless of students' background (e.g., race, culture, income).

While testing can be helpful for monitoring progress, determining if achievement gaps are closing, and improving educational outcomes, there are limitations and problems with current testing approaches. High-stakes decisions about a student (e.g., graduation, admission, educational placement) or school (e.g., sanctions, effectiveness of instruction) should not be based on one assessment. Use of one measure contradicts the American Psychological Association (APA, 2020) guidelines for assessment that recommend use of multiple sources, especially for young children. In response to concern with use of a single measure for decision making, fewer states now require exit exams (Gewertz, 2019), and some universities no longer require students to submit ACT or SAT scores with their application (Tugend, 2019).

Furthermore, the standardized tests cover a narrow range of content that is typically assessed using multiple-choice and short-answer questions. The tests rarely measure more in-depth understanding of content, critical thinking, or problem-solving skills. The content varies across states, as do proficiency standards and expected yearly progress, with some states setting more stringent expectations than others, making it difficult to compare progress from state to state. Fairness in use of testing continues to be a concern despite efforts to remove bias (González Canché, 2019). There should be careful consideration of the potential impact of cultural biases and attitudes when conducting assessments (APA, 2020). Finally, testing takes significant time and can increase stress and related problems (e.g., anxiety, depression, decreased motivations) for teachers and students (Fullerton, 2020). Lastly, the tests do not inform instruction. They are designed as summative measures providing only information about the student's overall performance.

The Department of Education (2015) encouraged Congress to address these concerns in the Elementary and Secondary Education Act (ESEA) by placing a cap on the amount of time students spend taking standardized tests, improving information to parents about assessments given, requiring use of multiple measures to examine student progress, increasing investments in innovative assessment, decreasing redundancy, and improving the quality of assessments. Overall, it was recommended that tests given to students should be worth taking in that they are aligned with what is being taught, engage critical thinking skills, and provide information to guide instruction.

Laws Focused on Students With Disabilities

In 1973 Section 504 of the Rehabilitation Act outlined protections for individuals with disabilities that limit one or more major life activities (e.g., epilepsy, ADHD, asthma, anxiety), including access to modifications (e.g., extra time for assignments, administration of medication, modification of physical activities) to enable students to have an opportunity to participate in academic and extracurricular activities. In 1975 the Education for All Handicapped Children Act was passed, giving all children ages 3 through 21 (later referred to as Part B) the right to a free and appropriate education in the least restrictive environment. In 1986 the law added the requirement to identify and provide services to children with disabilities from birth through age 3 (Part C). In 1990 the law was renamed the Individuals with Disabilities Education Act (IDEA). IDEA outlined the responsibilities for identification, assessment (Box 86.1 lists the 13 disability categories), educational programming, and transition planning. In 2004 additional procedural safeguards, timelines, the use of scientifically based instructional practices, and use of a process to determine response to instruction were added (see A Multitiered System of Support, later).

BOX 86.1 IDEA Disability Categories

Autism	Multiple disabilities
Deafness	Orthopedic impairment
Deaf-blindness	Other health impairment
Developmental delay	Specific learning disability
Emotional disturbance	Speech or language impairment
Hearing impairment	Traumatic brain injury
Intellectual disability	Visual impairment, including blindness

IDEA, Individuals with Disabilities Education Act.

TYPES OF ASSESSMENTS

Educational laws have consistently included reference to using methodologically sound assessments to identify a student's need and eligibility for different types of educational services (e.g., academic, behavioral, speech and language, gifted). In school-based assessment an evaluation team may work together to identify specific assessment questions prior to engaging in the assessment process. Questions may be asked about the student's cognitive functioning and performance in academic, social-emotional behavior, language, and motor skills.

Norm-Referenced Assessments

Norm-referenced assessments are scaled based on a normative sample (Table 86.2). These assessments can be evaluations of developmental progress in all areas of functioning. The student's results are compared to a norming sample of same-age and sometimes same-gender peers. Results indicate where the student's performance falls within the norming sample.

Criterion-Referenced Assessments

Criterion-referenced assessments indicate whether a student has met a preestablished criterion (see Table 86.2). Sometimes educational teams will ask questions about whether a student has mastered instructional content or prerequisite skills needed for a new content area. When students have not met a criterion, an intervention can be planned to develop the skills they are lacking. It is important to keep in mind that with both types of assessment, the educational team should focus on identifying

TABLE 86.2 Types of Assessments

Assessment	Definition	Interpretation
Norm referenced	An assessment that is standardized using a normative group.	Performance is scored by comparing the individual score to that of the norming group. Examples of common normative groups include age range, grade level, and gender. Individual results may be shared using a percentile ranking or a discussion of whether the individual is below, within, or above the average range within the normative group.
Criterion referenced	An assessment that is standardized based on meeting specific criterion that usually indicates mastery of content.	Performance is scored by comparing the individual's score to a predefined criterion. Examples of criterion-referenced tests include academic assessments that evaluate whether an individual demonstrates appropriate knowledge and skills on the assessment. Individual results are shared often using an accuracy measure (e.g., percentage correct) that is compared to the criterion. Results are discussed in terms of whether the individual successfully met criterion or not.
Curriculum-based measurement	An assessment method in which materials from the curriculum are used to determine an individual's mastery of content areas (e.g., reading, writing, mathematics).	Performance is scored by comparing an individual's score to a predefined criterion that is measured by accuracy and fluency. Assessments are typically short in duration (between 1 and 5 min). Examples include a reading fluency probe in which the student reads a passage aloud for 1 min and the correct words per minute are graphed. These assessments can be administered weekly so that educators can evaluate the student's progress in the evaluated academic area.
Portfolios	An assessment method in which work products that the individual has completed are reviewed to demonstrate progress in skills over a period of time.	This is the most subjective of all the assessment measures. The sampling of types of work products varies across subjects and across teachers. There are no specified criteria for what should be included or how to score the work products. Typically, the collection of work products shows a progression in the skills that are trying to be measured. An example includes reviewing drawings and handwriting samples across time to see if fine motor and visual perceptual skills are improving.

the educational supports needed to address the student's needs as identified by the assessment. Sometimes the educational supports are a part of the special education system, but sometimes the school team may be intervening with general education supports. By understanding the discrepancy the student has from the normative standard, educators know how much "catching up" the student may need to do, which may help identify how intensive the intervention needs to be. By understanding criterion skills that are lacking, the educational team knows where the focus of intervention needs to be.

While we highlighted the use of norm-referenced and criterion-referenced assessments in determining deficits students may have, they are also used to identify strengths in some students. It is common to use these assessments to determine if students should receive talented and gifted programming or extended learning plans or be accelerated into a higher grade level for an academic area in which they are especially talented.

Curriculum-Based Evaluation

One common type of educational assessment that incorporates both norm-referenced measures and criterion-referenced measures is curriculum-based evaluation (CBE). CBE is "any set of measurement procedures that use direct observation and recording of a student's performance in a local curriculum as a basis for gathering information to make instructional decisions" (Deno, 1987, in Shinn, 1989, p. 62). Curriculum-based measurement (CBM) is a type of CBE that allows educators to assess and monitor progress a student is making within a district's curriculum (see Table 86.2). CBM uses curriculum materials to measure constructs such as reading, writing, and math. These assessments can be scored by either looking at a norming sample or specific criterion.

Portfolio Assessments

Portfolio assessment is a fourth type of assessment used in schools. Portfolios are a combination of work samples or products that the student has completed across a period of time. The purpose is to look at the changes in these products over time. Portfolio assessments are more subjective because there may not be an objective standard for scoring the work samples. Portfolio assessments serve a variety of purposes. Portfolios may be used for all students within a grade to demonstrate their growth in a skill area over time. Educators may discuss these portfolios with parents during conferences and point out the areas of growth they observe. Portfolios may also be used for students with significant intellectual disabilities who are benefiting from an alternate curriculum rather than the general education curriculum.

A MULTITIERED SYSTEM OF SUPPORT: A FRAMEWORK FOR ASSESSMENT AND INTERVENTION

Overview of MTSS

When educational systems became accessible to all students, there began an interest in developing a system that effectively met the needs of all students. Traditional models of support focused on assessing a student's eligibility for more intensive services (i.e., discrepancy model for special education). When a student did not qualify for services, there were few alternatives available to support the student's success. This system left some students falling through cracks because they needed more support than what the general education environment provided, but they were not eligible to receive the accommodations and instructional supports that students entitled to special education received (Fuchs & Fuchs, 2006).

As it became evident that this model was not effective for all learners, tiered models of support focusing on academic and behavioral needs began to be discussed. The MTSS framework has been discussed actively in educational research and practice since the 1980s. The MTSS framework assists educators in considering levels of supports that are targeted to meet student needs (Reschly & Bergstrom, 2009). Currently, most MTSS models discuss a three-tiered system that includes universal (tier 1), targeted (tier 2), and intensive (tier 3) supports. These tiers are typically aligned with different educational interventions that are delivered in the general education classroom (tier 1), supplemental instruction along with general education instruction in a general education classroom (tier 2), and long-term interventions that involve special education (Reschly, 2014).

A successful MTTS school meets the needs of all students by supporting them with the differing levels (or intensity) of instruction and intervention across the three tiers. The process for supporting students includes (1) using evidence-based instruction and interventions that are matched to the student's needs, (2) conducting universal screening and frequent progress monitoring, (3) making data-based decisions by reviewing progress monitoring data and other data regularly, and (4) having levels of intervention that vary to match the needs of the student (Leonard, Coyne, Oldham, Burns, & Gillis, 2019; Reschly, 2014). This framework is used to address academic (e.g., Coyne, Oldham, Leonard, Burns, & Gage, 2016; Reschly, 2014) and social-emotional behavioral health needs (e.g., Sugai & Horner, 2006; Weist et al., 2018). The student's needed level of support is identified through district-wide assessments (e.g., screening measures), individual assessments of areas of concerns, and measuring the student's response to intervention. When an MTSS framework is implemented with high fidelity, students with and at risk for disabilities can demonstrate accelerated achievement (Coyne et al., 2018). Table 86.3 provides purposes of educational testing across the tiers and common school-based assessments administered in groups or individually. For additional information about social-emotional behavioral health needs within an MTSS framework, see Wood and McDaniel (2020) and Briesch, Nissen, Long, & Chafouleas, (2020).

Universal (Tier 1)

School systems operating within an MTSS identify assessments and interventions that are used across the three tiers to provide support to students. Tier 1 is defined as the universal tier because instruction and supports are available to all students. Academic curricula within tier 1 create the foundation for the system and are considered general education. It is designed to help prevent concerns by using curricula that are evidence based and demonstrated to be effective in teaching skills. Schools with a strong tier 1 often find that 80% to 85% of the students are successful given these universal supports (Reschly, 2014).

Educational policies enacted within the past 20 years have had a growing impact on the use of assessments at tier 1. Schools are mandated to publish outcomes of the district-wide assessments that specify the percentage of students meeting proficiency standards. This information can be used in some states to withhold funding or support parents who want their child to go to a school that has a higher number of students meeting proficiency standards. An important aspect of operating within an MTSS framework is identifying screening measures to determine whether a student is being successful with the instruction and supports provided to the student. At the universal level, all students will participate in screening assessments that help to identify their progress. The type of screening assessment given often varies by age. For example, in the early elementary school grades it may be more common for school teams to use CBM to evaluate developing reading, math, and writing skills. During mid to late elementary school, it becomes more common for school districts to use group-administered norm-referenced tests to measure academic skills in general (e.g., reading comprehension) or core content knowledge (e.g., science, history). These assessment results help to identify how effective the chosen curricula are for the students within the district (see Table 86.3 for examples of assessments).

An outcome of the assessments that are administered within tier 1 is to identify students who may be at risk for learning concerns. It is common for a teacher to consider the results of the assessment in conjunction with other records of the student (e.g., progress on daily work). If a student does not perform within the desired range of the assessment, it would be common for a discussion to occur between the teacher and the student's parents about whether more assessment or targeted supports are needed for the student. There may be factors that influenced the student's performance on the test (e.g., test anxiety, bad day) that may make the screening less valid. Parents should always be encouraged to talk with school personnel when they have concerns about their

TABLE 86.3 Purposes of Assessment and Commonly Used Educational Assessment Instruments

Universal: Tier 1

Purposes of Assessment

Measuring program effectiveness/accountability
Identifying students at risk for learning or social-emotional behavioral concerns using screening tools

Type of Test	Skills Assessed	Examples of Common Tests
Group achievement	Reading and language skills (e.g., word analysis, reading comprehension, spelling, grammar, language expression); mathematics skills (e.g., computation, reasoning, problem solving); science; social studies	American College Test California Achievement Test Comprehensive Test of Basic Skills Iowa Assessments Metropolitan Achievement Test, Eighth Edition Stanford Achievement Test, Tenth Edition Test of General Education Development Scholastic Aptitude Test
Individual benchmark assessments	Fluency of skills (e.g., reading, writing, math computation; math application); reading comprehension; fluency of prereading skills	Curriculum-based measurement (reading, math, and written language); dynamic indicators of basic early literacy skills; informal reading inventories

Targeted: Tier 2 or Intensive: Tier 3

Purposes of Assessment

Monitoring progress with targeted interventions
Making eligibility decisions
Informing individualized interventions

Type of Test	Skills Assessed	Examples of Common Tests
Individual achievement	Reading and language skills (e.g., letter and word recognitions, phonemic awareness, reading comprehension, verbal reasoning); mathematics skills (e.g., computation, problem solving, mathematical reasoning)	Diagnostic Achievement Battery-3 Kaufman Test of Educational Achievement–3 Peabody Individual Achievement Test–Revised Scholastic Achievement Test for Adults Wechsler Individual Achievement Test, Third Edition Wide Range Achievement Test, Fifth Edition Woodcock-Johnson Tests of Achievement, Fourth Edition
Reading assessment	Letter identification and recognition; phonetics; sound blending; sight word recognition and identification; oral reading accuracy and fluency; oral reading comprehension; silent reading comprehension; vocabulary; spelling	Dynamic Indicators of Basic Early Literacy Skills Formal Reading Inventory Gates-MacGinitie Reading Tests, Fourth Edition Gates-McKillop-Horowilz Reading Diagnostic Test, Second Edition Nelson-Denny Reading Tests Tests of Reading Comprehension, Fourth Edition Test of Early Reading Ability, Fourth Edition
Writing, spelling, and language	Listening comprehension; story retelling; following directions; sentence repetition; sentence formation; sentence completion; grammar; composition; writing fluency	Clinical Evaluation of Language Fundamentals, Fifth Edition Oral and Written Language Scales, Second Edition Test of Early Written Language, Third Edition Test of Written Expression Test of Written Spelling
Mathematics	Numeration; rational numbers; addition; subtraction; multiplication; division; measurement; time; money; geometry; estimation; interpretation of data; problem solving; applications; vocabulary	KeyMath Diagnostic Assessment, Third Edition Sequential Assessment of Mathematics Inventories Stanford Diagnostic Mathematics Test, Fourth Edition Test of Early Mathematics Ability, Third Edition Test of Mathematics Ability, Third Edition

Adapted from Reed, M. S. (2009). Educational assessment. In W. B. Carey, A. C. Crocker, W. L. Coleman, E. R. Elias, & H. M. Feldman (Eds.), *Developmental-behavioral pediatrics* (4th ed., pp. 811–827). Saunders Elsevier.

child's academic development. The meeting may include only the general education teacher, but it could also include other teachers, the principal, or guidance counselor, depending on the concerns of the parent (Table 86.4).

Targeted (Tier 2)

Tier 2 of an MTSS framework includes targeted assessments and interventions for students who are not meeting academic benchmarks. It is expected that between 15% and 20% of all students will need targeted interventions through tier 2 supports (Hoover, 2011). The need for these targeted assessments and interventions can be identified by the universal screenings, parent concerns, and/or nonschool professionals (e.g., medical clinician, mental health clinician). Depending on the types of concerns, a meeting may be held to discuss whether additional assessment is needed to identify an appropriate intervention. Some school districts will have a team of staff members that comprise a tier 2 team, which may be referred to as a student assistance team, building assistance team, or problem-solving team. The team may include other teachers within the school building, the principal or assistant principal, the school counselor, and personnel who have specialized training in the area of concern (see Table 86.4).

The team will identify whether additional assessment is needed to make decisions about intervention. When an academic assessment is conducted at this tier, it will likely be done within a one-to-one setting focused on the area of concern. The purpose of the assessment is to identify what types of interventions are more likely to help the student become successful in the area of concern. CBM is often used because the measures are brief, provide a snapshot of student skills in a particular area, and can be used to monitor progress.

Tier 2 interventions supplement the instruction that is provided in tier 1 (Hoover, 2011). If there is a concern in the area of reading, for example, the student receives reading instruction through the general education curriculum and participates in an intervention. It is common that interventions are administered through the student's general education teacher, a specialist (e.g., reading specialist/interventionist; behavior specialist/interventionist), guidance counselor, or special education teacher (Hoover, 2011). When the intervention is designed, the team identifies the instructional intensity of the intervention, a goal for the student to achieve, and a means of monitoring the student's progress. Instructional intensity includes consideration of the instructional minutes, instructional frequency, and instructional duration (Mellard, McKnight, & Jordan, 2010). These interventions may take several months, depending on the length of the curriculum and the frequency of intervention sessions. Interventions targeting a specific strategy to use may be shorter in duration.

TABLE 86.4 Potential Educational Team Members

Team Members	Description of Role
Parents/legal guardians	Provide insight into their child and are critical when making decisions about intervention
Student	Shares needs, contributes to setting goals, and provides feedback on programming
Principal/administrator	Manages the organization and climate (safety, wellbeing) of the school, serves as an instructional leader, supports program accountability
Classroom teacher	Provides group and differentiated instruction; shares information about the student's current abilities and potential barriers to learning
School counselor	Provides social-emotional classroom lessons, short-term counseling to individual students, and referrals for long-term supports
Additional Team Members at the Targeted/Intensive Tiers	**Description of Role**
Special education teacher	Ensures the needs of the student with disabilities are being met and that accommodations are being implemented
Paraeducator/educational assistant	Provides daily behavioral and instructional support to students with disabilities
School psychologist	Consults with teachers, families, and other support staff; conducts assessments to inform programs; provides direct support and interventions for mental health, learning, and behavior
Physical therapist	Provides intervention and strategies to improve movement, reduce or manage pain, and prevent disability
Occupational therapist	Uses therapeutic techniques to rehabilitate, improve, or maintain student's ability to perform everyday activities
Speech-language pathologist	Provides intervention and strategies to improve student's speech sounds, language, literacy, social communication, voice, fluency, cognitive-communication, and feeding and swallowing
Applied behavior analyst	Conducts behavioral assessments, designs interventions to improve adaptive behaviors and decrease maladaptive behaviors, provides training and coaching support

Research has shown variability in instructional intensity across school systems (Mellard et al., 2010).

Identifying a goal for the intervention and a means to monitor the student's progress toward that goal are also discussed when the intervention is designed. Intervention goals should be specific, measurable, achievable, realistic, and timely. Because the student was already identified as at risk, the team is encouraged to closely monitor the student's progress so that if the intervention is not successful, the team can talk about additional steps they can take to support the student. Best practice is that progress monitoring would occur frequently enough so that the team can review the data within a short amount of time and see whether the student is making progress. Simmons et al. (2002) recommend that progress monitoring occur as frequently as every 2 to 4 weeks depending on the intensity of the instruction (i.e., the more intensive the instruction, the more frequently progress should be measured). There are a variety of measures that can be used to monitor the student's academic progress throughout the intervention. CBM is often used with a focus on fluency (e.g., words read per minute, math facts completed per minute) and accuracy of skills (e.g., words read correctly, percentage correct) in the areas of concern. If a curriculum is being used for the intervention, there will likely be some assessment tools included for the team to review.

Sometimes it can feel to the teacher and the parents that tier 2 is a hoop to go through before the student can be evaluated for special education services. There are situations when the concern is so great for the student that the team may decide to conduct an evaluation for special education services while they are providing the targeted intervention. However, in many cases the targeted intervention can be successful and no further assessment or intervention is needed.

Intensive (Tier 3)

Although tier 3 within MTSS may include continued intensive services without special education supports, when a disability is suspected, a multidisciplinary evaluation should be conducted to determine if the child meets criteria for special education services (IDEA) or a 504 Plan. Fig. 86.1 outlines the process for special education evaluation and intervention. If parent(s) consent to the evaluation, it is conducted by a multidisciplinary team (MDT) (see Table 86.4). Individual team makeup will vary depending on the concerns presented.

An evaluation must be completed in all areas of suspected disability (e.g., intellectual/cognitive, academic achievement, speech, physical, occupational skills, behavior). Furthermore, the evaluation must be conducted in the student's native language or mode of communication and include more than one procedure/assessment to determine the student's educational needs. For students suspected of having a specific learning disability, a severe discrepancy between intellectual ability and achievement has historically been used for verification. Due to significant concerns with the use of such a model (see Fuches & Young, 2006), IDEA was amended in 2004 to no longer require the use of the severe discrepancy model and made it permissible for schools to use a "process that determines if the child responds to scientific, research-based intervention as part of the evaluation procedures" (IDEA, 2004). This approach to identification of specific learning disabilities

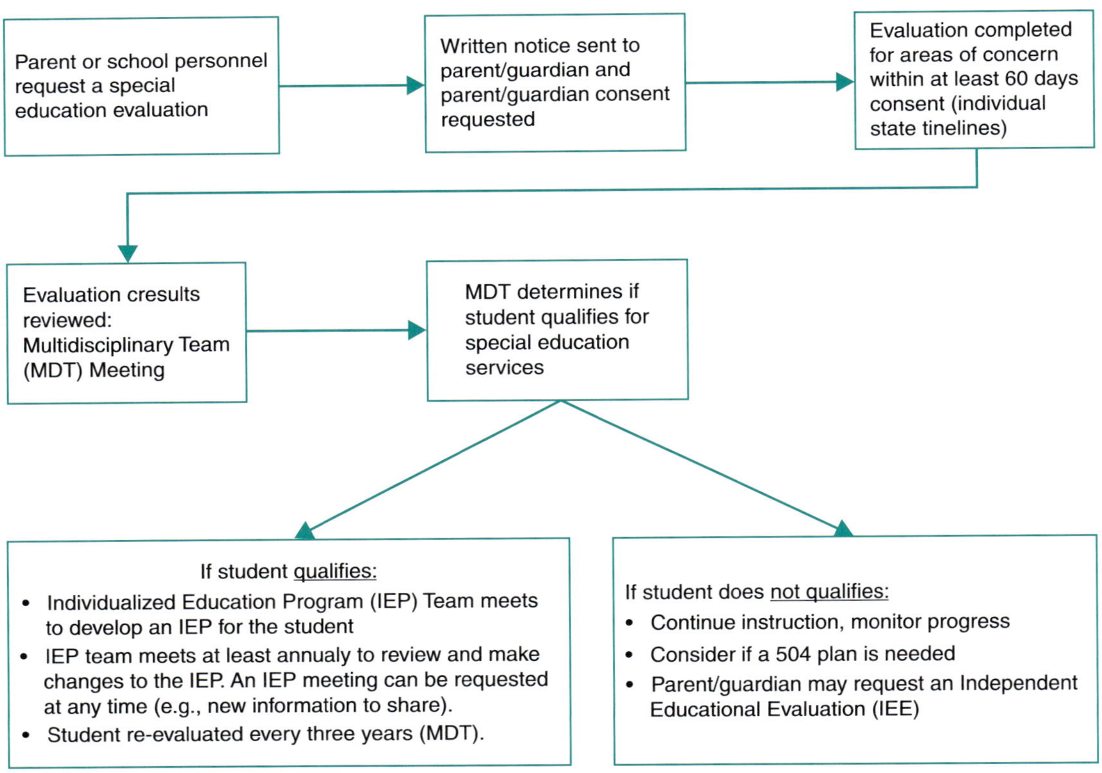

Fig. 86.1 Navigating the special education evaluation and intervention process.

is commonly referred to as response to intervention. Within this process, a student is provided scientific, research-based intervention to increase the team's confidence that the student's low performance in a specific area is not due to poor instruction and to evaluate interventions appropriate to meet the student's needs. If the student does not show positive response to the intervention or the intervention cannot be maintained with general education supports, the team can consider that information when determining eligibility. Table 86.3 includes common assessments that may be conducted as part of the evaluation process for learning concerns.

If the MDT determines the student meets disability verification criteria (see Box 86.1), an IFSP (ages birth–3 years) or IEP (ages 3–21 years) is developed. If the student attends a private or home school, the student may be able to receive special education services through the public school system, but this varies by state. The plan is implemented and reviewed at least annually, but it can be modified sooner if changes are indicated. Progress toward the annual goals is monitored and parents are notified of progress. Students receiving special education services are reevaluated every 3 years to determine if the student continues to meet the verification criteria or if services should be discontinued. If the student does not meet criteria as a child with a disability under IDEA, the team may consider if a 504 Plan is indicated. If parents disagree with the results of the evaluation, they can request an independent educational evaluation (IEE) to be conducted at the school's expense. The results of an IEE are shared with the MDT who review the results and recommendations to consider if the student meets the verification criteria. If needed, parents may seek mediation, file a state complaint, or file a due process complaint to aid in resolving disagreements.

TABLE 86.5 Clinical Actions and Recommendations for Pediatricians

Diagnosis and Monitoring
• Medical evaluation and diagnosis
• Questions to ask parent or adolescent:
  • How is your child doing in school?
  • Has your child been evaluated for special education?
  • Does your child have an IFSP or IEP?
  • Do you have any questions about the school verification or IFSP/IEP?
  • Do you feel like your child is getting all of the services needed as part of the IFSP/IEP?

Referring for Services and Sharing Information
• Obtain relevant release of information
• Share impact of medical diagnosis and medication on education
  • Early childhood: refer to local Child Find System
  • School age: provide documentation or letter describing diagnosis and potential educational impacts
    a. May indicate potential need for a special education services or a 504 Plan
• Referrals may also be made for private services such as physical, occupational, or speech therapy, psychology
• Help families advocate for their child's needs
• Facilitate understanding of medical diagnosis
• Reinforce the importance of parents in the process
• Help parents compose questions to ask clinicians to better understand the services and how they can support their child's development

Providing Resources • Compile list of local clinicians and support groups • Compile list of quality websites (e.g., parent information from Department of Education, Office of Special Education Programs) • Connect with state parent resource center (Center for Parent Information and Resources: https://www.parentcenterhub.org/)

IEP, Individualized education plan; *IFSP,* individualized family service plan.

Physician Contributions Across the Tiers and Overcoming Barriers to Coordination

Physicians have many roles and responsibilities while treating children and adolescents, including history taking, completing physical exams, and diagnosing and treating patients. These are well acknowledged, but physicians are also advocates. They are in a unique position to support students across the continuum of medicine, education, and other systems. It is especially important for children with disabilities and complex medical conditions to have an established medical home and coordinated care (see care mapping, Boston Children's Hospital, 2021; Antonelli & Lind, 2012). Table 86.5 lists actions clinicians can take to bridge the gap between the clinic and school. To facilitate this valuable role, many primary care offices have psychologists, social workers, and care coordinators embedded in their clinics.

When children/adolescents are given a diagnosis or treatment plan by a physician that may impact their education, it can be shared with schools after appropriate consent has been obtained. Examples of relevant information to communicate include hearing or vision problems, ADHD, ASD, traumatic brain injury, learning disabilities, chronic illness, depression, and anxiety. It is important to note that school teams must consider diagnoses and information from clinicians or other outside evaluators, but they do not have to use it in their educational plan for the student. However, sharing the information may spur educational evaluation and inform individualized special education plans or 504 Plans. Similarly, information from a school evaluation can provide valuable information to inform medical diagnosis. For example, a clinician should consider if symptoms of ADHD are due to ADHD or a specific learning disability (e.g., more hyperactive during specific instruction due to academic difficulties).

Navigating the medical and educational systems can be daunting and at times perplexing to families. To aid families, physicians can first help parents to understand their child's medical diagnosis and how a medical diagnosis differs from an educational verification. Medical diagnoses are based on criteria outlined in the *International Classification of Diseases.* To receive an educational verification, the child must meet the criteria outlined in IDEA/related state regulations. It is possible for a child to meet educational verification criteria but not medical criteria and vice versa because the criteria differ. For example, a child may be given a medical diagnosis of ASD, but the school team determines that the diagnosis does not impact their education and therefore special education is not warranted. Parents may also present at the pediatrician's office thinking their child has been given the diagnosis of ASD because the child is getting services at school. When appropriate, it is beneficial for children to receive a medical diagnosis and educational verification because it increases access to services. Educational verification provides access to individualized, special education services. A medical diagnosis of a disability may provide access to a 504 Plan, disability services or waivers, therapies, etc. Should developmental-behavioral clinicians be advocates? They are advocates by the nature of their training and profession. This is particularly true of primary care and developmental-behavioral clinicians who are in the unique position of knowing families in a very intimate way and can support their patients and families by working closely with school professionals.

In Clara and Marco's cases the medical team was instrumental in conducting evaluation, monitoring progress, providing referrals to appropriate resources, and advocating to meet the child's needs. Through these efforts and ongoing communication and collaboration, there is a higher likelihood of positive outcomes for all parties involved.

REFERENCES

American Psychological Association, APA Task Force on Psychological Assessment and Evaluation Guidelines. (2020). *APA guidelines for psychological assessment and evaluation.* https://www.apa.org/about/policy/guidelines-psychological-assessment-evaluation.pdf

Antonelli, R., & Lind, C. (2012). Care mapping: An innovative tool and process to support family-centered, comprehensive care coordination. Poster session presented at the annual Primary Care Innovation Conference of the Harvard Medical School Primary Care Center, Boston, MA.

Boston Children's Hospital. (2021). *Organizing care and relationships for families: Care map.* https://www.childrenshospital.org/integrated-care-program/care-mapping

Briesch, A. M., Nissen, K., Long, S., & Chafouleas, S. M. (2020). A review of state-level procedural guidance for implementing Multitiered Systems of Support for Behavior (MTSS-B). *Journal of Positive Behavior Interventions, 22*(3), 131–144. https://doi.org/10.1177/1098300719884707

Coyne, M. D., Oldham, A., Dougherty, S. M., Leonard, K., Koriakin, T., Gage, N. A., Burns, D., & Gillis, M. (2018). Evaluating the effects of supplemental reading intervention within an MTSS or RTI reading reform initiative using a regression discontinuity design. *Exceptional Children, 84*(4), 350–367.

Coyne, M. D., Oldham, A., Leonard, K., Burns, D., & Gage, N. (2016). Delving into the details: Implementing multitiered K–3 reading supports in high-priority schools. In B. Foorman (Ed.), Challenges to implementing effective reading intervention in schools. *New Directions for Child and Adolescent. Development, 154*, 67–85.

Cruz, R. A., Firestone, A. R., & Rodle, J. E. (2021). Disproportionality: Reduction in exclusionary school discipline: A best-evidence synthesis. *Review of educational research, 91*(3), 397–431. https://doi.org/10.3102/0034654321995255

Deno, S. L. (1987). Curriculum-based measurement. *Teaching Exceptional Children, 20*(1), 40–42. https://doi10.1177/004005998702000109

Fuchs, D., & Fuchs, L. S. (2006). Introduction to response to intervention: What, why, and how valid is it? *Reading Research Quarterly, 41*(1), 93–99.

Fuches, D., & Young, C. (2006). On the irrelevance of intelligence in predicting responsiveness to reading instruction. *Exceptional Child, 73*, 8–30.

Fullerton, S. G. (2020). Examining the impact of high-stakes testing accountability evaluation on subject-area teachers serving grades 3 to 8 in Pennsylvania. *In Dissertation Abstracts International Section A: Humanities and Social Science, 18*, 12-A.

Gewertz, C. (2019). What tests does each state require? *Education Week.* https://www.edweek.org/teaching-learning/what-tests-does-each-state-require

González Canché, M. (2019). Repurposing standardized testing for educational equity: Can geographical bias and adversity scores expand true college access? *Policy Insights from the Behavioral and Brain Sciences, 6*(2), 225–235.

Hoover, J. J. (2011). Making informed instructional adjustments in RTI models: Essentials for practitioners. *Intervention in School and Clinic, 47*(2), 82–90.

Leonard, K. M., Coyne, M. D., Oldham, A. C., Burns, D., & Gillis, M. B. (2019). Implementing MTSS in beginning reading: Tools and systems to support schools and teachers. *Learning Disabilities Research & Practice, 34*(2), 110–117. https://doi.org/10.1111/ldrp.12192

Mellard, D., McKnight, M., & Jordan, J. (2010). RTI tier structures and instructional intensity. *Learning Disabilities Research & Practice, 25*(4), 217–225.

National Center for Education Statistics. (2020). *About NAEP: A common measure of student achievement.* https://nces.ed.gov/nationsreportcard/about/

Reed, M. S. (2009). Educational assessment. In W. B. Carey, A. C. Crocker, W. L. Coleman, E. R. Elias, & H. M. Feldman (Eds.), *Developmental-behavioral pediatrics* (4th ed., pp. 811–827). Saunders Elsevier.

Reschly, D. J. (2014). Response to intervention and the identification of specific learning disabilities. *Topics in Language Disorders, 34*(1), 39–58. https://doi.org/10.1097/TLD.0000000000000003

Reschly, D. J., & Bergstrom, M. K. (2009). Response to intervention. In T. B. Gutkin & C. R. Reynolds (Eds.), *The handbook of school psychology* (4th ed., pp. 434–460). Wiley.

Shinn, M. R. (1989). *Curriculum-based measurement: Assessing special children.* The Guildford Press.

Simmons, D. C., Kame'enui, E. J., Good, R. H., Harn, B. A., Cole, C., & Brawn, D. (2002). Building, implementing, and sustaining a beginning reading improvement model: Lessons learned school by school. In M. R. Shinn, H. M. Walker, & G. Stoner (Eds.), *Interventions for academic and behavior problems II: Preventative and remedial approaches.* NASP Publications.

Sugai, G., & Horner, R. R. (2006). A promising approach for expanding and sustaining school-wide positive behavior support. *School Psychology Review*, *35*(2), 245–259. https://doi.org/10.1080/02796015.2006.12087989

Tugend, A. (2019). *Questioning their fairness, a record number of colleges stop requiring the SAT and ACT*. Hechinger Report. https://hechingerreport.org/questioning-their-fairness-a-record-number-of-colleges-stop-requiring-the-sat-and-act/

US Congress, Office of Technology Assessment. (1992). *Testing in American schools: Asking the right questions (OTA-SET-519)*. US Government Printing Office. https://www.princeton.edu/~ota/disk1/1992/9236/9236.PDF

US Department of Education. (2015). *Fact sheet: Testing action plan*. https://www.ed.gov/news/press-releases/fact-sheet-testing-action-plan

Weist, M. D., Eber, L., Horner, R., Splett, J., Putnam, R., Barrett, S., Perales, K., Fairchild., A., & Hoover, S. (2018). Improving multitiered systems of support for students with "internalizing" emotional/behavioral problems. *Journal of Positive Behavior Interventions*, *20*(3), 172–184. https://doi.org/10.1177/1098300717753832

Wood, B. J., & McDaniel, T. (2020). A preliminary investigation of universal mental health screening practices in schools. *Children and Youth Services Review*, *112* https://doi.org/10.1016/j.childyouth.2020.104943

87

Neuropsychology in Developmental-Behavioral Pediatrics Practice

Melissa Armstrong-Brine and Leslie Speer

For additional material related to the content of this chapter, please see Chapters 76, and 85.

VIGNETTE

Heather, a 7-year-old, White female, was referred for a neuropsychological evaluation due to concerns regarding increasing difficulties with academic learning, memory, fine motor skills, and reduced emotional control. A clinical interview and review of records indicate that Heather has spina bifida with hydrocephalus and had a shunt revision 3 years prior. Parents, teachers, and medical team question if symptoms indicate the presence of a learning disability, intellectual disability, or possibly symptoms of anxiety. There is also concern symptoms may be early signs of a shunt malfunction.

DEFINING NEUROPSYCHOLOGY

Neuropsychology is a specialized branch of clinical psychology that focuses on brain-behavior relationships through the detailed analysis of behavior, emotional functioning, and cognitive abilities. Neuropsychology combines tenants from neurology, neuropsychiatry, neurochemistry, and neuropharmacology as well as clinical psychology to seek a comprehensive understanding of the impact of central nervous system (CNS) dysfunctions on an individual's overall functioning. Neuropsychologists utilize a combination of mental status and neurobehavioral evaluation, direct observation, collateral source report, and standardized normative measures to identify patterns of cognitive, emotional, and behavioral characteristics that correspond with anomalies in the CNS.

The field of neuropsychology, while rooted in theories and practices dating to ancient Greek and Egyptian times, is relatively new as a designated discipline of psychology. Important modern neuropsychological principles and knowledge can be traced to the 1800s with finding such as Broca and Wernicke's linking specific areas of brain injury to distinct patterns of language impairment and pivotal theories of brain organization purposed by neurologists, particularly Luria. However, the modern practice of neuropsychology was not truly introduced until the mid-1900s when physicians such as Reitan and Halstead began to utilize behavioral performance to characterize and localize neurologic impairment through notable changes in overt functioning of patients on motor, cognitive, and physical evaluation. Pediatric neuropsychology, which includes a focus on the changes in functioning incurred when a developing CNS experiences disruption, did not emerge until the latter half of the 1900s and remains an evolving field that some may say is still in the infancy period. For a detailed account of the history of neuropsychology, please see Vallar and Caputi (2020).

WHO IS A NEUROPSYCHOLOGIST?

Neuropsychologists are doctoral level psychologists, often in the areas of clinical or school psychology, who have specific training in assessment, intervention, and research related to the connection between the brain and behavior, cognition, and emotional functioning. Aspirational training guidelines for neuropsychologists are outlined in a document developed in 1997 by a joint task force composed of experts from the Division of Clinical Neuropsychology (Division 40) of the American Psychological Association and the International Neuropsychological Society. Because the conference for this task force was hosted by the University of Houston, the guidelines are referred to colloquially as the "Houston Guidelines." Under the Houston Guidelines, a neuropsychologist is defined as "a professional psychologist trained in the science of brain-behavior relationships. The clinical neuropsychologist specializes in the application of assessment and intervention principles based on the scientific study of human behavior across the lifespan as it relates to normal and abnormal functioning of the central nervous system" (Hannay et al., 1998).

The Houston Guidelines outline training expectations at the three primary stages of training in professional psychology (e.g., doctoral training, clinical internship, and fellowship). In addition to core coursework in general psychology and clinical psychology, the Houston Guidelines set forth expectations for course work and clinical experience in areas of functional neuroanatomy, neuroimaging and other neurodiagnostic techniques, neurochemistry, neurologic conditions, nonneurologic conditions that can impact the CNS, neuropsychological research, and specialized neuropsychological assessment and intervention techniques. Although 1 year of postdoctoral fellowship training is often expected for clinical psychologists, the Houston Guidelines indicate that advanced fellowship training equivalent to 2 years of full-time experience should be required for neuropsychologists prior to eligibility for board certification. While not required to practice, neuropsychologists are often board certified by one of three organizations, including the American Board of Clinical Psychology of the American Board of Professional Psychology (ABPP-CN), the American Board of Professional Neuropsychology (ABPN), or the American Academy of Pediatric Neuropsychology (ABPdN). ABPP-CN is likely the most widely recognized and rigorous professional boarding agency for neuropsychology and within the last decade devised procedures for specialized certification in child neuropsychology, which are completed in addition to standard ABPP-CN certification procedures.

NEUROPSYCHOLOGICAL EVALUATION DIFFERS FROM PSYCHOLOGICAL EVALUATION

Like psychological or psychoeducational assessment, neuropsychological evaluation has a variety of purposes, including diagnostic clarification, treatment planning, and determining eligibility for specific status or services (e.g., competence to stand trial, disability eligibility). While neuropsychological evaluation often includes elements of both psychological and psychoeducational evaluation, neuropsychological evaluation has two main differences from psychological and psychoeducational assessment. First, neuropsychological evaluation takes a deep look at behavior and cognition in a wider range and more discrete level of ability not addressed in psychological or psychoeducational evaluation. On the basic level, neuropsychological evaluation includes consideration of areas of cognitive functioning, such as memory and executive functioning not commonly included in other types of psychological evaluation. At a more significant level, neuropsychological evaluation includes a more refined look at domains of cognitive and behavioral functioning by dissecting broad areas of ability into specific components that allow for a greater specificity in the type or "localization" of neurologic disturbance. Second, neuropsychological evaluation takes evaluation a step further to correlate the patient's behavioral, cognitive, and emotional presentation with known or suspected underlying neurologic compromise (e.g., "axonal injury"; diffuse brain differences related to fetal alcohol exposure) likely impacting the patient. See Chapter 76 for more on psychological assessment.

WHEN TO REFER FOR A NEUROPSYCHOLOGICAL EVALUATION

A variety of concerns can prompt a referral for a neuropsychological evaluation. Neuropsychological evaluations are often utilized to obtain a baseline of an individual's abilities, acquire general levels of functioning and an overall learning profile, as well as provide diagnostic clarity. A neuropsychological evaluation can also provide insight into an individual's response to treatment (e.g., medication, therapy, academic intervention). Following an injury, neuropsychological evaluations are often used to assess the impact of the injury on development and cognitive functions. When a medical condition is thought to impact certain aspects of development or functioning, a neuropsychological evaluation is often initiated to capture an initial baseline of functioning when the condition is first identified, and then additional evaluations are conducted to measure subsequent impact over time. The overall goal of a neuropsychological evaluation is to assist patients, families, and professionals with understanding current needs, facilitating treatment planning, and monitoring progress and response to treatment over time.

It is common for neuropsychological reevaluations to be conducted. These reevaluations can be initiated for a variety of reasons, and the intervals at which they are scheduled varies. The interval between evaluations is typically based on initial referral concern and the individual's condition. With treatment monitoring, the testing protocol generally consists of brief, targeted assessments, done at shorter intervals, based on the expected action of the prescribed medication or therapy. When providing ongoing evaluation of medical and psychiatric conditions, which are thought to impact development and functioning, repeated assessments are conducted throughout adolescence and young adulthood, often every 3 years. The interval between evaluations, however, can be adjusted as needed depending on the course of treatment and response to intervention (Bernstein, 2009).

NEUROPSYCHOLOGY IN PRACTICE

Neuropsychologists practice in a range of settings, including hospitals, rehabilitation centers, developmental-behavioral pediatric clinics, jails, schools, and private practice. They participate in clinical care, research, and administrative roles to contribute to the overall health and wellness of children and adults with a range of neurologic, psychiatric, and educational conditions. Neuropsychologists combine perspectives from medicine (biologic basis of behavior), psychiatry (behavioral criteria for disorder-specific conditions as outlined in the *Diagnostic and Statistical Manual of Mental Disorders*, fifth edition [American Psychiatric Association, 2013]), neuropsychology (brain-behavior relationships), and education (variations in learning ability and academic skills when typical exposure to learning has been provided) (Bernstein et al., 2009).

Neuropsychologists collect data on patients by reviewing medical, educational, and other relevant records, conducting a clinical interview with the patient and a collateral source (e.g., parent/guardian, caregiver, case manager), behavioral observations of the patient, and standardized, norm-referenced measures of cognitive functioning.

Neuropsychological testing batteries vary in scope, organization, and content across providers. While traditional neuropsychological evaluation often assesses a wide range of domains over a full day or two of testing, more recently many neuropsychologists have moved to time-limited assessment batteries that target specific behaviors, abilities, and skills known to be commonly impacted by the area neuroanatomic difference in the brain, medical condition, and/or reported concern. Focused batteries have come into common practice largely due to reimbursement limitations, difficulties many patients have in attending to and maintaining effort in long testing sessions, and long waiting lists as the number of patients needing neuropsychological evaluation has grown faster than the number of neuropsychologists in practice. Further, some neuropsychologists utilize a fixed battery of testing in which they administer a relatively stable list of tests to all patients, while others, particularly when using a focused approach to neuropsychology, use a flexible battery where they tailor testing to the patient's specific condition, concerns, or reason for assessment. Both flexible and fixed testing batteries have pros and cons. Most notably flexible batteries allow the neuropsychologist to explore specific areas of concern in depth but may result in the neuropsychologists overlooking areas of difficulty not commonly associated with the patient's condition or outside of the patient's awareness. In contrast, comprehensive and fixed batteries may provide more breadth in the skills, abilities, and behaviors assessed, but they may lack depth in analyzing areas of specific difficulty or concern for the patient. Fixed batteries are also highly useful in research by allowing for comparison of patients with a variety of conditions or presentations across domains of functioning.

Perhaps most notably, compared to other forms of psychological or educational evaluation, neuropsychologists consider large domains of cognitive and behavioral functioning and higher-order skills commonly viewed as solitary constructs in the general population as composed of a set of more specific abilities that interact or build on one another. Because of the focus on brain-behavior relationships, neuropsychologists are acutely aware that neurologic substrates of large domains of ability such as language, attention, or memory are often not localized to one specific region of neuroanatomy but instead arise from a complex web of neural connections and neurochemical communications that encompass many different areas of the CNS. Through this awareness, neuropsychologists consider broad areas of subjective concern but then break those areas down to the substrate abilities and skills often associated with defined areas of CNS neuroanatomy. Thus through a process of deductive reasoning or examination of associative ability, they can identify specific areas of cognitive difficulty that can be utilized to support a fine-grained treatment plan and guide pharmacologic or behavioral interventions with a fair level of biologic and behavioral detail to target the patient's specific needs.

As mentioned previously and in Chapter 76, neuropsychologists have extensive training and years of supervised practice to develop the clinical and technical expertise needed to effectively administer and interpret data from standardized cognitive and psychological measures within a framework of brain-behavior relationships. Their knowledge is also vital to developing an assessment plan that will provide enough data to competently answer the referral questions and sufficiently explore the presenting concerns. Table 87.1 outlines common cognitive domains covered in a neuropsychological evaluation and lists some, certainly not all, of the common associated abilities within those domains. To visually illustrate this approach to refined understanding of a patient's abilities, Fig. 87.1 depicts the substrates commonly assessed as they combine to comprise the large concept of "attention"—one of the domains of considerable importance in most neuropsychological assessments. To effectively measure these nuances of attention, the neuropsychologist may use parent and teacher report measures to look for daily behavioral signs of inattention, hyperactivity, and emotional functioning to help discern the etiology and specific pattern of attention difficulties experienced by the patient. Additional evaluation components may include observation of behaviors associated with distractibility and limited inhibitory control, performance-based paper-pencil tasks looking at visual attention, working memory, and processing speed, and computerized measures of vigilance, divided attention and response speed, to clarify the patient's specific attentional difficulties and build a case for support services and accommodations personalized for the patient. For additional information on neuropsychological domains and methods, please see Chapters 76, 82, 84, 85, and 88, and Ida Sue Baron's book *Neuropsychological Evaluation of the Child*, second edition (2018).

CODING AND BILLING FOR NEUROPSYCHOLOGICAL SERVICES

A thorough understanding of neuropsychology billing is well outside the scope of this chapter. That said, an informed provider who refers patients for neuropsychological evaluation may wish to understand the general procedures included in billing so that they can educate their patients as needed. Under a fee-for-service payment model there are a variety of services that are provided and billed throughout the course of a neuropsychological evaluation. These services include aspects of the evaluation conducted while the patient is present such as the clinical interview, test administration, and provision of feedback. However, sometimes surprisingly to patients, billing also incorporates professional services that are completed outside of patient facing time such as scoring of testing, integration of a variety of patient data (e.g., record review of medical chart and previous evaluations, consultation with other treating providers), report writing, and interpretation. These services are typically documented based on time spent delivering the service with the exception of two commonly used time-based billing codes used for the clinical interview and administration of a single automated instrument via electronic platform with automated results.

NEUROPSYCHOLOGICAL REPORT

The primary work product of neuropsychologists includes a written report that documents data collected from a number

TABLE 87.1 **Domains of Functioning Commonly Assessed in Neuropsychology**

Domain	Common Subdomains	Description	Example Measures
Intelligence	Please see Chapter 85 of this text.	The general mental ability to learn from, adapt, and respond to one's environment and experiences	*Wechsler Intelligence Scale for Children*, Fifth Edition *Kaufman Assessment Battery for Children*, Second Edition *Leiter International Performance Scales*, Third Edition *Stanford-Binet Intelligence Scale*, Fifth Edition
Academic Achievement	Please see Chapter 85 of this text.	Level at which one has reached age- or grade-based expectations for learning academic skills and information	*Wechsler Individual Achievement Test*, Fourth Edition *Woodcock Johnson, Test of Achievement*, Fourth Edition *Wide Range Achievement Test*, Fifth Edition
Memory		The encoding, storage, and retrieval of information through a complex neural process	*Wide Range Assessment of Memory and Learning*, Third Edition *Children's Memory Scale* *Test of Memory and Learning*, Second Edition
	Short-term or immediate memory	Registration of information perceived from the environment and ability to maintain that information in conscious awareness (Baron, 2018)	
	Long-term memory	Ability to consolidate and store information for hours, days, months, or years	
	Recognition memory	Ability to accurately identify previously encountered information from a particular source vs. novel information or information from another source	
	Prospective memory	Often referred to as "remembering to remember"; requires one to have an intention to act and use environmental cues (e.g., time of day, specific event) to prompt one to act	
Executive Functioning	Overall		*NEPSY-2* *Delis Kaplan Executive Functioning System* *Behavior Rating Inventory of Executive Functioning*, Third Edition Subtests of IQ, memory, and executive functioning measures such as Digit Span; Spatial Span; Arithmetic Tower of London; Stroop Color-Word Test; Subtests of NEPSY-2 such as Inhibition and Response Set
	Working memory	Brief (a few seconds) memory system where information can be processed and manipulated	
	Planning/ organizing	Thinking ahead to select the best process to achieve a goal; preparing thoughts, action, or materials to complete a task	
	Inhibition	Ability to ignore distractions, resist temptations, and avoid a common or learned response to provide a competing, accurate, or functional response	
	Mental flexibility	Ability to think about something in more than one way and identify similarities and difference between objects or concepts	
	Initiation/ self-monitoring	Ability to initiate and keep track of one's progress on daily tasks	

TABLE 87.1 Domains of Functioning Commonly Assessed in Neuropsychology—cont'd

Domain	Common Subdomains	Description	Example Measures
Attention			*Test Everyday Attention for Children*, Second Edition *NEPSY-2* *Test of Variables of Attention* *Conner's Continuous Performance Test*, Third Edition *Dichotic Listening Tasks*
	Focused attention	Ability to perceive and respond to a stimulus over time when monitoring information	
	Selective attention	An element of focused attention involving selecting one target stimulus from a large array of stimuli	
	Sustained attention	Maintaining attention across time or repetition for the purpose of conscious task completion	
	Attention control/ shifting	Ability to move one's focused attention between competing demands or one task demand to another; involves both removing attention from one stimulus then selecting and attending to another stimuli in a seamless manner	
	Divided attention	Being able to attend to two stimuli at one time for the purpose of multitasking or purposeful activity (e.g., listening to a lecture while typing notes)	
Language			*Clinical Evaluation of Language Fundamentals*, Third Edition *Preschool Language Scale*, Fifth Edition *Peabody Picture Vocabulary Test*, Fourth Edition *Expressive Vocabulary Test*, Fourth Edition
	Receptive language	Ability to process and understand spoken language	
	Expressive language	Ability to generate purposeful speech with appropriate grammar, syntax, and vocabulary	
	Verbal fluency	Level of effort required to produce words that fit a specific request, such as words that begin with a specific letter	
Sensory/motor		Using sensory information to produce a response; requires intact basic sensory reception	*Wide Range Assessment of Visual Motor Abilities*, Second Edition *Finger Tapping Test* *Grooved Pegboard* *Beery-Buktenica Test of Visual Motor Integration*
	Fine motor dexterity	Ability to manipulate small objects effectively and efficiently	
	Fine motor speed	How quickly one can use movement of muscles involved in fine motor tasks	
	Visual-motor integration	Coordination of visual information with a motor output	
Visual-spatial		Ability to perceive, analyze, and understand visual information for the purpose understanding orientation in space or identify objects	*Rey-Osterrieth Complex Figure (Copy)* *Judgment of Line Orientation* *Hooper Visual Organization Test* *Block Design Subtests*
Validity		Measure of how appropriate the patient's effort is during the course of testing	*Test of Memory Malingering* *Word Memory Test* *Rey 15-Item Visual Memory Test*

The list of references for tests outlined in this table are available in the online supplement.

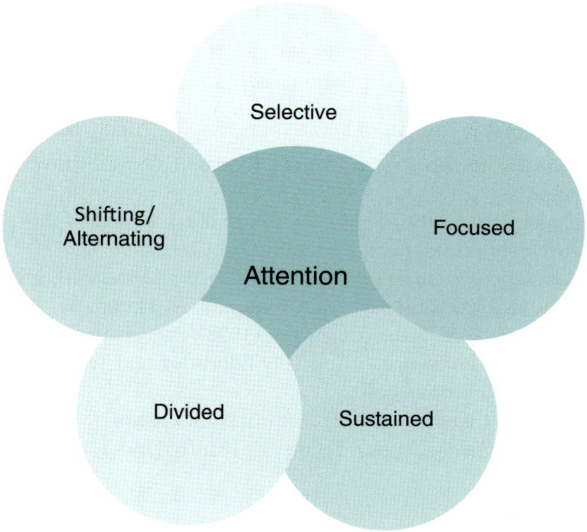

Fig. 87.1 Subdomains of attention.

of subjective and objective sources, a conceptualization of the relationship between the pattern of data and the patient's biological and behavioral presentation, a medical or psychological diagnosis appropriate for the patient's presentation, and recommendations to guide treatment planning or further diagnostic investigation. Neuropsychological reports range significantly in structure and length. Some neuropsychological reports are comprised of a three-page letter to the referral source outlining the significant findings of testing and recommendations with little reference to general patient history or specific testing scores. Other reports are 20- to 25-page documents providing a comprehensive psychosocial history, detailed analysis of each score by testing measure, a finely detailed summary of conceptualization based on all data collected, and specific, targeted recommendations that include refined goals for intervention and identified referral sources the clinician feels will best meet the patient's remediation and personal needs. Box 87.1 outlines the common sections of a neuropsychological report although, again, it is important to note there is some variability in the specific format and content of neuropsychological reports.

Heather's neuropsychologist is aware of several common cognitive findings in children with spina bifida and hydrocephalus, including significant visual-spatial difficulties compared to verbal difficulties, memory problems, and compromised visual-motor coordination and dexterity. While spina bifida is also commonly associated with executive functioning difficulties, Heather's young age makes many measures of executive functioning inappropriate; however, measures of verbal and design fluency and inhibition may be included in testing to assess these abilities. Heather's neuropsychologist will also review medical records to determine the type of her spina bifida, the location of her spinal anomaly, and specific characteristics of her hydrocephalus and shunt (e.g., intercranial pressure history, exact location of placement) to refine the neuropsychological testing plan based on the literature on neuropsychological functioning in spina bifida. Specific motor limitations will be considered and addressed in the testing plan. Given concerns for anxiety, the neuropsychologist will include parent and teacher report measures of anxiety in the test plan. Finally, given possible shunt malfunction, the neuropsychologist will compare previous neuropsychological testing conducted shortly after Heather's shunt placement to her current performance to assess for changes that may suggest decompensation due to shunt malfunction.

BOX 87.1 Sections Contained in a Neuropsychological Report

Reason for Referral

- Identifies basic demographic information, referral source, and basic intentions of the evaluation.

Background History

- Includes information pertinent to understanding the patient's social, educational, medical, family, cultural, and behavioral/emotional history that are important for context, but may not be directly related to the current concerns.

Results

- Text and tables outline specific scores and ranges for measures. Often includes patterns of performance with reference to unusual differences both within patient scores and as compared to normative data.

Diagnosis

- *Diagnostic Statistical Manual of Mental Disorders*, Fitth edition and/or *ICD-10* diagnosis.

History of Presenting Problems

- Reviews behavioral, emotional, cognitive factors involved in the current concerns with attention to specific medical, psychosocial, or historical details that may contribute.

Review of Records/Previous Testing

- Discusses general details of important medical, educational, other historical records while attributing information to the original source. Often includes review of medical tests and specific educational evaluations.

Summary/Interpretation

- Text and tables outline specific scores and ranges for measures. Often includes patterns of performance with reference to unusual differences both within patient scores and as compared to normative data.

Recommendations

- Identifies referrals, supports, treatments, and resources appropriate for the patient based on the conceptualization presented in the summary/interpretation section.

CONCLUSION

Neuropsychology utilizes a combination of norm-referenced, standardized measures of cognition and behavior, known medical facts, and subjective observation and clinical judgment. Neuropsychologists possess training in both general clinical psychology and neuroanatomic and neurochemical substrates of psychiatric, neurologic, behavioral, and educational conditions. They work in a range of occupational settings and because of the nuances of functioning examined by neuropsychologists and the comprehensive nature of the evaluation process, neuropsychological evaluations can be time consuming and effortful for patients. However, the effort required for neuropsychological evaluations is generally outweighed by the detailed analysis of the patient's presentation as it relates to CNS involvement and specific treatment recommendations provided in the neuropsychological report.

REFERENCES

American Psychiatric Association. (2013). *Diagnostic and statistical manual of mental disorders* (5th ed.). Author.

Baron, I. S. (2018). *Neuropsychological evaluation of the child: Domains, methods, & case studies* (2nd ed.). Oxford University Press.

Bernstein, J. H. (2009). Neuropsychological assessment of the developing child. In H. Feldman (Ed.), *Developmental-behavioral pediatrics* (4th ed., pp. 828–835). Saunders-Elsevier.

Hannay, H. J., Bieliauskas, L. A., Crosson, B. A., Hammeke, T. A., Hamsher, K. S., & de Koffler, S. P. (1998). Proceeding of The Houston Conference on Specialty Education and Training in Clinical Neuropsychology.

Vallar, G., & Caputi, N. (2020). *The history of human neuropsychology*. https://doi.org/10.1016/B978-0-12-809324-5.23914-X

88

Evaluation of Adaptive Functioning

Micah O. Mazurek, Sophie Brunt, and Erica Fornaris Rouch

For additional material related to the content of this chapter, please see Chapter 76.

VIGNETTE

Timothy is an 8-year-old boy who is socially motivated but struggles with communication, academic skills, behavioral regulation, and self-care. As a toddler, Timothy was diagnosed with mild cerebral palsy and global developmental delay due to motor and language delays. He was later diagnosed with a language disorder and attention-deficit/hyperactivity disorder (ADHD). Timothy has lived with a foster family for the past 2.5 years. He was removed from his biological parents' care due to unsanitary living conditions and parental drug use and violence at home. He spends about half his school day in a special education resource classroom and the rest in the general education classroom. His teachers describe him as a happy child, but his performance is about two grade levels below academic expectations and he often appears distracted or confused in the classroom. Timothy also has challenges with conversational skills and answering questions. He wears pull-ups for toileting, struggles with understanding safety conventions, and often plays with younger children instead of same-aged peers. His foster parents reported that he has thrived in their care and that his behavior has improved dramatically. However, he still has trouble regulating his emotions, and his frustration can quickly escalate to anger and aggressive kicking or hitting.

INTRODUCTION

The concept of adaptive functioning refers to a person's ability to meet expectations for age-appropriate personal and social responsibilities in everyday life. Difficulties with adaptive functioning have significant implications for daily life and independence across the life span. As such, assessment of adaptive functioning should be an integral component of developmental assessment, diagnosis, and treatment planning. Characterizing adaptive functioning is essential for classification and diagnosis of neurodevelopmental disorders, and it is necessary for determining the amount and type of support needed for optimizing independence and quality of life. There are key conceptual frameworks that inform the understanding and assessment of adaptive behavior, as well as its subsequent application to diagnosis, eligibility, and intervention planning. This chapter will provide an overview of these constructs and the various purposes of adaptive behavior assessment and common assessment approaches and tools.

ADAPTIVE BEHAVIOR DEFINITIONS AND FRAMEWORKS

Long before the development of formal intelligence tests, the ability to use everyday skills and adjust to environmental demands has been an indicator of general intelligence. By the same token, deficits in everyday adaptive functioning have been central to the overall conceptualization of intellectual disability (see for review, Oakland & Daley, 2013). However, following the advent of standardized tests of intelligence in the early 1900s, the diagnostic criteria for intellectual disability focused largely on intelligence test scores alone rather than everyday functioning (see for review, Tassé et al., 2012). It was not until the late 1950s that associated impairment in adaptive behavior was formally included in the operational definition of intellectual disability by the American Association on Mental Deficiency (AAMR, now the American Association on Intellectual and Developmental Disabilities [AAIDD]) (Heber, 1959). The AAIDD (2010) continues to be a leading authority on the conceptualization and assessment of adaptive behavior, which it currently defines as "the collection of conceptual, social, and practical skills that have been learned and performed by people in their everyday lives" (p. 43).

Adaptive functioning is defined by cultural and social norms, and expectations for independence and responsibility increase across the life span. As such, adaptive behavior is best understood from within an ecologic framework, with consideration of an individual's developmental, environmental, and cultural contexts. In general, however, adaptive behavior can be conceptualized as comprising three primary domains: *practical*, *conceptual*, and *social*. Practical skills refer to performance of daily living and self-care activities (hygiene, dressing, safety, etc.). Conceptual skills include communication, functional academic skills, and planning and self-direction. Skills within the social domain include interpersonal skills, social-emotional competence, and social responsibility (AAIDD, 2010; Tassé et al., 2012; Thompson, McGrew, & Bruininks, 1999). It is important to note that the concept of adaptive behavior refers to typical *performance* of these skills, not just ability. Overall, these skills are important for day-to-day functioning across settings (from home to community) and activities (from personal interactions to

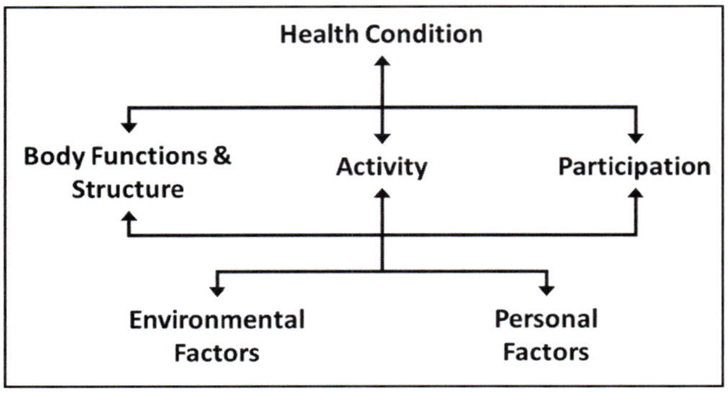

Fig. 88.1 International Classification of Functioning, Disability and Health (ICF) biopsychosocial model.

work or academic tasks). Adaptive behavior is a fundamental aspect of functioning across the life span, making it an important consideration for overall developmental assessment.

At the broadest level, the construct of disability itself is closely related to adaptive functioning. The World Health Organization (WHO) developed a standard framework for conceptualizing disability and functioning, the *International Classification of Functioning, Disability and Health* (ICF). This model was first proposed in 1980 and has undergone an ongoing process of refinement (WHO, 1980, 2001, 2007). The ICF is part of a larger body of international standards for classification of health and health conditions. While the *International Classification of Diseases* (ICD) provides an etiologic framework for diagnostic classification (WHO, 1993), the ICF is designed to provide a complementary framework for characterizing an individual's overall health and health-related functioning. The ICF framework is based on the biopsychosocial model (Engel, 1977), which views health and disability as products of dynamic interconnections among biologic, psychological, and sociocultural factors (Borrell-Carrió, Suchman, & Epstein, 2004) (Fig. 88.1). This framework depicts the interaction between health conditions and contextual factors, as well as different aspects of functioning and disability. Within this model, impairments can be experienced at the physical level (problems or limitations in bodily function), at the activity level (difficulties engaging or executing activities), or at the participation level (problems in everyday situations).

Overall, the activities and participation components of the ICF framework are directly relevant to the concept of adaptive behavior as they capture aspects of day-to-day individual and social functioning. Specifically, ICF classifies activities and participation across nine domains: (1) learning and applying new knowledge, (2) general tasks and demands, (3) communication, (4) mobility, (5) self-care, (6) domestic life, (7) interpersonal interactions and relationships, (8) major life areas, and (9) community, social, and civic life. Within each domain, the magnitude of the problem (ranging from 0 = no problem to 4 = complete problem) is captured, as well as both capacity and performance. Capacity refers to the individual's ability to execute the task or action, while performance refers to the degree to which the individual actually engages in the task or activity. In contrast to an assessment tool or diagnostic system, the ICF framework is intended to provide a common coding and classification system across systems and users for documenting aspects of health and functioning (WHO, 2001). The results of adaptive functioning evaluations may be particularly useful in informing classification and coding across ICF domains (WHO, 2013).

PURPOSE OF ADAPTIVE BEHAVIOR ASSESSMENT

Assessment of adaptive behavior is critical for diagnosis, eligibility determination, treatment planning, and progress monitoring for children with or at risk for developmental disorders. Ultimately, the overall purpose of adaptive assessment is to inform the selection of supports and services that will meet the unique needs of each individual. As such, it is important to identify both strengths and challenges, and to understand them within the context of the individual's age, family, culture, and community.

Regarding diagnostic determination, impairment in adaptive functioning is an essential component of the diagnostic criteria for intellectual disability across classification systems. For example, *ICD-11* defines intellectual disability as being "characterised by significantly below average intellectual functioning and adaptive behaviour" (WHO, in press). The AAIDD criteria for intellectual disability also require "significant limitations both in both intellectual functioning and in adaptive behavior as expressed in conceptual, social, and practical adaptive skills" (AAIDD, 2010). Similarly, the *Diagnostic and Statistical Manual of Mental Disorders,* fifth edition (*DSM-5*; American Psychiatric Association [APA], 2013) diagnostic criteria for intellectual disability require concurrent impairment in intellectual functioning and adaptive behavior. Criterion B requires evidence of "deficits in adaptive functioning that result in failure to meet developmental and sociocultural standards for personal independence and social responsibility" (APA, 2013).

Adaptive assessment results are also important for eligibility determination for special education services and many other community-based programs and services. The Individuals with Disabilities Education Improvement Act of 2004 (IDEA, 2004) governs the provision of early intervention, special education, and related services for infants, toddlers, and youth with disabilities in the United States, and it includes specific mention of adaptive functioning. IDEA specifies that infants, toddlers, and young children (ages 3–9 years) may be found eligible for early intervention and/or special education services if they are experiencing developmental delays in one or more areas: cognitive development, physical development, communication development, social or emotional development, and adaptive development.

Beyond diagnosis and classification, assessment of adaptive functioning is important for individualized intervention planning, progress monitoring, and outcome assessment (Harman, Smith-Bonahue, & Oakland, 2010). Understanding how a child is functioning in daily life is critical for characterizing overall development, identifying strengths and weaknesses, and determining specific treatment strategies and needs for support. Effective intervention planning should prioritize the skills needed to achieve age-appropriate independence in daily tasks, and it should take into account the individual's family and environmental context to maximize relevance, consistency, and impact of intervention strategies (Harrison & Oakland, 2015; Saulnier & Klaiman, 2018). Early intervention can be helpful in promoting improvement in overall adaptive functioning for children with a range of developmental disabilities (Ahn & Hwang, 2018; Rogers & Vismara, 2008; Sandbank et al., 2020; Woodman, Demers, Crossman, Warfield, & Hauser-Cram, 2018). Ultimately, improvements in adaptive skills are among the most meaningful intervention outcomes because of their importance for independent living, particularly among individuals with developmental disabilities.

ASSESSMENT OF ADAPTIVE FUNCTIONING

Assessment of adaptive functioning should ideally include a comprehensive norm-referenced measure of adaptive behavior, along with supplemental information gained from interviews, observations, and other sources of information. National and international guidelines emphasize the importance of standardized measures, in addition to clinical evaluation, when assessing adaptive functioning (AAIDD, 2010; APA, 2013; WHO, in press). In fact, both *ICD-11* and AAIDD diagnostic criteria for intellectual disability require specific evidence of adaptive functioning at two or more standard deviations below the mean on standardized measures that are normed on the general population (AAIDD, 2010; WHO, in press).

While direct observation of skill performance in natural environments can be informative, this is not generally feasible within the context of a clinical assessment. Thus collecting information from respondents who can report on an individual's daily performance across home, school, and community settings is often the most efficient way to gather ecologically valid information. In general, gathering information from multiple informants (such as parents and teachers) is useful for understanding an individual's functioning across settings (Floyd et al., 2015). Informal clinical interviews may also yield additional information about factors that differentially affect a child's performance of skills in certain social situations or environmental settings. However, these methods should be considered supplemental to the use of standardized norm-referenced assessments.

There are a number of standardized assessment tools that can be useful in evaluating adaptive behavior. The most widely used comprehensive measures of adaptive functioning are the Vineland Adaptive Behavior Scales, Third Edition (Sparrow, Cicchetti, & Saulnier, 2016), Adaptive Behavior Assessment System, Third Edition (ABAS-3) (Harrison & Oakland, 2015), and Scales of Independent Behavior–Revised (SIB-R) (Bruininks, Woodcock, Weatherman, & Hill, 1996). These tools are similar in that they are standardized, norm-based instruments that provide scores for an individual's functioning across domains relative to same-aged peers. They also demonstrate solid psychometric properties (Floyd et al., 2015) and rely on information provided by caregivers, teachers, or others with sufficient knowledge of an individual's functioning in everyday environments. The properties of these measures are illustrated in Table 88.1, and they are described in more detail in the sections that follow.

TABLE 88.1 Standardized Norm-Referenced Adaptive Behavior Measures

Instrument	Age Range	Respondent	Format	Time to Administer	Scores/Domains
Vineland-3	Birth–90 yr (varies by form)	Parent/caregiver or teacher	Interview or rating scale completed by parent/caregiver or teacher (available in paper or electronic formats)	10–40 min	Standardized adaptive behavior composite score *Core domain scores:* 1. Communication 2. Daily Living Skills 3. Socialization *Optional domains:* • Motor skills • Maladaptive behaviors
ABAS-3	Birth–89 yr (varies by form)	Parent/caregiver, teacher, or self (for adults)	Rating scale completed by parent/caregiver or teacher; self-rating option for adults (available in paper or electronic format)	15–20 min	Standardized general adaptive composite score *Core domain scores:* 1. Conceptual 2. Social 3. Practical
SIB-R	3 mo–80 yr (varies by form)	Parent/caregiver	Structured interview or rating scale completed by parent/caregiver (paper format only)	Full scale form: 1. 45–60 min Short form and early development form: 1. 15–20 min	Standardized broad independence score *Domain scores:* 1. Motor skills 2. Social interaction and communication 3. Personal living 4. Community living

ABAS-3, Adaptive Behavior Assessment System, Third Edition; *SIB-R*, Scales of Independent Behavior–Revised; *Vineland-3*, Vineland Adaptive Behavior Scales, Third Edition.

Vineland Adaptive Behavior Scales, Third Edition (Vineland 3)

The Vineland-3 is a comprehensive, standardized, norm-referenced measure of adaptive behavior for individuals across the life span (birth–90 years). It is available in three formats: interview, parent/caregiver, and teacher forms (Sparrow et al., 2016). The interview form is a semistructured, open-ended interview designed to be administered verbally to a parent or caregiver who is knowledgeable about the child's everyday adaptive behavior at home. The parent/caregiver form is a rating form designed to be completed by a caregiver directly who is familiar with the child's functioning, and the teacher form is designed to be completed by someone who is familiar with the child's functioning in a school/preschool/daycare setting. The parent/caregiver and teacher forms are available in a paper version or online for administration via computer, tablet, or smartphone, and the interview version is available in a paper version or online for administration via computer or tablet.

Each version is available in a comprehensive form, which includes more items in greater detail, and a domain-level version, which is briefer and contains fewer items. Both forms include three core domains, which make up the adaptive behavior composite (ABC): communication, daily living skills, and socialization. The comprehensive form also offers subdomain scores for each domain. The communication domain includes receptive, expressive, and written subdomains; the daily living domain includes personal, domestic, and community subdomains; and the socialization domain includes interpersonal relationships, play and leisure, and coping subdomains. The motor skills and maladaptive behavior domains are optional for both forms. The comprehensive form offers subdomain scores within the motor domain (fine and gross subdomains) and the maladaptive behavior domain (internalizing, externalizing, and critical items subdomains).

Test items pertain to how often an individual engages in a certain behavior independently without help, prompting, or reminders. All items use a three-point Likert-type response format with scores 0 (never), 1 (sometimes), and 2 (usually or often). If administering the comprehensive form, a ceiling is reached on a subdomain after four consecutive scores of 0, and the interviewer can proceed to the next subdomain. The Vineland can be scored manually or online using the Q-Global platform. Both the comprehensive and domain-level versions provide an ABC standard score, as well as a standard score for each domain. The comprehensive form also includes v-scale scores for each subdomain ($M = 15$; $SD = 3$), which are summed to calculate the domain scores.

All three formats have generally good-to-excellent internal consistency and test-retest reliability for individual domains and the ABC, with very few falling in the fair range. In addition, test-retest reliability between the electronic and paper versions of each form was excellent, and thus formats should be considered comparable. Interrater reliability ranged from good to excellent on the interview and parent/caregiver forms, but it fell in the poor-to-fair range for a few subdomains on the teacher form. The Vineland-3 has well-established construct and content validity, and it is highly correlated with other measures of adaptive functioning (e.g., ABAS-3) (Sparrow et al., 2016).

Adaptive Behavior Assessment System, Third Edition

The ABAS-3 is another comprehensive norm-referenced measure of adaptive functioning that measures an individual's ability to complete daily living skills independently (Harrison & Oakland, 2015). It is available in five different forms: parent/primary caregiver form (ages 0–5 years), parent form (ages 5–21 years), teacher/daycare provider form (ages 2–5 years), teacher form (ages 5–21 years), and an adult form (ages 16–89). The adult form may be administered as a self-report or be completed by a parent, family member, counselor, or someone else who is familiar with the individual's everyday skills and behaviors. The test can be administered on paper or online using the WPS Online Evaluation System.

The ABAS-3 assesses adaptive behavior across three main adaptive functioning domains: conceptual, social, and practical, which correspond to the adaptive functioning domains considered within both *DSM-5* and AAIDD criteria for intellectual disability (AAIDD, 2010; APA, 2013). The three ABAS-3 domains comprise the general adaptive composite (GAC), and scores are provided for specific adaptive skill subdomains within each domain. The conceptual domain includes communication, functional academics, and self-direction subdomains; the social domain includes leisure and social subdomains; and the practical domain includes community use, home or school living, health and safety, self-care, and work subdomains. A motor subdomain is included for young children and is supplemental for older individuals. Test items pertain to how often the individual is able to perform the skill or behavior when needed, and responses are recorded on a 4-point rating scale: 0 = Is not able, 1 = Never (or almost never when needed), 2 = Sometimes when needed, and 3 = Always (or almost always when needed).

Each domain and the GAC produce a standard score ($M = 100$; $SD = 15$), confidence interval, and percentile rank. Each of the adaptive skill subdomains produces scaled scores ($M = 10$; $SD = 3$), and age equivalents may be calculated. In addition, each score corresponds to a descriptive category: extremely low, low, below average, average, above average, high. The ABAS-3 GAC has been shown to have good-to-excellent internal consistency and test-retest reliability, and well-established concurrent validity correlating highly with the Vineland-2 (Harrison & Oakland, 2015).

Scales of Independent Behavior–Revised

The SIB-R is a comprehensive standardized assessment system that measures an individual's adaptive and maladaptive behaviors across settings (Bruininks et al., 1996). It is available in three forms: the full scale form (for ages 3 months–80 years), short form (containing a subset of 40 items from the full form), and early development form (for ages 3 months–8 years). It may be administered either as an interview or as a checklist.

The SIB-R includes an adaptive behavior section and a problem behavior section. The adaptive behavior items pertain to how often an individual engages in a behavior independently, on a 4-point scale: 0 = Never or rarely (even if asked), 1 = Does, but not well (or about one-fourth of the time, may need to be asked), 2 = Does fairly well (or about three-fourths of the time, may need to be asked), 3 = Does very well (always or almost always without being asked). Adaptive behavior subscales include motor skills, social interaction and communication skills, personal living skills, and community living skills. The problem behavior section includes internalized, externalized, and asocial subscales, and items are rated on frequency (0–5) and severity (0–4) of the behavior.

The adaptive behavior section of all formats produces a general broad independence standard score, and the full scale form additionally includes individual domain standard scores for each of the four domains ($M = 100$; $SD = 15$), as well as percentile ranks and age equivalents. The early development and short form versions do not provide domain scores. In addition, a support scale score can be calculated from the adaptive behavior and problem behavior scores. This score indicates how much support the individual may need in certain areas. For all forms, internal consistency ranged from fair to excellent, and test-retest reliability ranged from good to excellent for each domain score as well as the broad independence score. Validity has been established by numerous studies (Bruininks et al., 1996); however, it should be noted that the SIB-R has not been revised in over 20 years, so the normative data need to be updated.

Timothy's foster parents shared concerns with his developmental-behavioral pediatrician that Timothy was not being provided enough academic support at school. Given his long-standing challenges with learning and self-care, this raised concerns about a possible intellectual disability (ID). The possibility of ID had been raised during a school evaluation several years prior, but it was deemed difficult to disentangle from Timothy's unstable home environment, ADHD, and behavioral challenges. Given the need for diagnostic clarity, his developmental-behavioral pediatrician referred Timothy for a comprehensive interdisciplinary evaluation.

To assess Timothy's intellectual functioning and current language abilities, the interdisciplinary assessment team administered standardized cognitive and speech-language assessments. Assessing his adaptive skills was also important to understand his current day-to-day functioning and assess for the possibility of intellectual disability. Timothy's foster mother and teacher completed adaptive behavior scales to enable the team to assess his functioning across the home and school settings. They also completed standardized rating scales to provide information about his social, emotional, and behavioral functioning and symptoms across settings. A thorough parent interview and record review was also important for understanding the role of Timothy's home environment and early experiences in his development.

Based on the assessment results, Timothy was found to have many social-emotional strengths, including social motivation, an interest in helping others, and a generally cheerful and friendly demeanor. However, Timothy's intellectual functioning was found to be well below expectations for his age. On the Differential Ability Scales, Second Edition (DAS-II), he obtained standard scores in the very low range (standard scores of [SS] ≤70) in multiple areas of cognition, including verbal (SS = 58), nonverbal (SS = 62), and spatial (SS = 63) reasoning. On a language assessment with the Clinical Evaluation of Language Fundamentals, Fifth Edition (CELF-5), Timothy's performance was within the very low range across expressive language (SS = 59) and receptive language (SS = 70). Based on parent report on the Vineland Adaptive Behavior Scales, Third Edition (VABS-3), Timothy's communication (SS = 40), socialization (SS = 48), and daily living skills (SS = 44) were in the low range and significantly below expectations compared to same-aged peers. His teacher also reported adaptive skills challenges across communication (SS = 50), socialization (SS = 58), and daily living skills (SS = 49). Lastly, in completing the Behavior Assessment System for Children, Third Edition (BASC-3) both his foster mother and teacher indicated that Timothy had clinically significant challenges with hyperactivity, inattention, and conduct problems.

Overall, measures of Timothy's language, cognitive, and adaptive skills functioning clustered in the same range, well below age expectations. Interview and medical records revealed that these challenges had been present throughout Timothy's early developmental period and had persisted in recent years despite a stable home and behavioral improvement. Based on his significant weaknesses in intellectual functioning and deficits in adaptive functioning across conceptual, social, and practical skills, Timothy met criteria for a diagnosis of ID. His adaptive functioning deficits, including challenges with self-care, safety awareness, and socialization and communication, appeared directly related to his underlying level of cognitive functioning. Timothy's language delays were conceptualized as part of his intellectual disability, so a diagnosis of language disorder was not warranted. Timothy continued to meet criteria for an ADHD diagnosis due to ongoing difficulties with attention and hyperactive behavior that were above and beyond what is expected in the context of ID.

Key recommendations offered to Timothy's caregivers included increasing individualized instruction in school, speech-language services for functional communication and pragmatic language, and parent resources for managing challenging behavior. Specific recommendations to target adaptive functioning were also made, including explicitly teaching daily living skills (e.g., toileting, understanding safety, cleaning up after himself) and functional academic skills (e.g., counting, writing his name) across home and school settings. Timothy's foster parents and teachers were encouraged to use visual supports and repetition to help teach Timothy the steps involved in daily living tasks and steps for coping with frustration.

CONCLUSION

Evaluation of adaptive functioning should be an essential element of developmental assessment, particularly for individuals with or at risk for developmental delays or disabilities.

Overall, a comprehensive multiinformant approach is recommended, including the use of standardized, norm-referenced measures of adaptive behavior. Accurate assessment of an individual's level of adaptive behavior as compared to same-aged peers is important for diagnostic assessment, classification of functioning, and eligibility determination. Ultimately, adaptive behavior assessments should directly inform the interventions and services that promote improve overall functioning and quality of life.

REFERENCES

Ahn, S., & Hwang, S. (2018). Cognitive rehabilitation of adaptive behavior in children with neurodevelopmental disorders: A meta-analysis. *Occupational Therapy International.*

American Association on Intellectual and Developmental Disabilities. (2010). *Intellectual disability definition, classification, and systems of supports* (11th ed.). American Association on Intellectual and Developmental Disabilities.

American Psychiatric Association. (2013). *Diagnostic and statistical manual of mental disorders* (5th ed.). Author.

Borrell-Carrió, F., Suchman, A. L., & Epstein, R. M. (2004). The biopsychosocial model 25 years later: Principles, practice, and scientific inquiry. *The Annals of Family Medicine, 2*(6), 576–582.

Bruininks, R. H., Woodcock, R. W., Weatherman, R. F., & Hill, B. K. (1996). *Scales of independent behavior-revised. SIB-R.* Riverside Publishing.

Engel, G. L. (1977). The need for a new medical model: A challenge for biomedicine. *Science, 196*(4286), 129–136.

Floyd, R. G., Shands, E. I., Alfonso, V. C., Phillips, J. F., Autry, B. K., Mosteller, J. A., . . . Irby, S. (2015). A systematic review and psychometric evaluation of adaptive behavior scales and recommendations for practice. *Journal of Applied School Psychology, 31*(1), 83–113.

Harman, J. L., Smith-Bonahue, T. M., & Oakland, T. (2010). Assessment of adaptive behavior development in young children. In E. Mpofu & T. Oakland (Eds.), *Rehabilitation and health assessment: Applying ICF guidelines* (pp. 333–352). Springer Publishing Company.

Harrison, P. L., & Oakland, T. (2015). *Adaptive behavior assessment system—Third edition (ABAS-3): Manual.* Western Psychological Services.

Heber, R. (1959). A manual on terminology and classification in mental retardation. *American Journal of Mental Deficiency.*

Individuals with Disabilities Education Improvement Act of 2004. Public Law 108–446. U.S. Code. 20 2004. § 1400 et seq.

Oakland, T., & Daley, M. (2013). Adaptive behavior: Its history, concepts, assessment, and applications. In K. F. Geisinger, B. A. Bracken, J. F. Carlson, J.-I. C. Hansen, N. R. Kuncel, S. P. Reise, & M. C. Rodriguez (Eds.), *APA handbook of testing and assessment in psychology, vol. 3. Testing and assessment in school psychology and education* (pp. 183–212). American Psychological Association.

Rogers, S. J., & Vismara, L. A. (2008). Evidence-based comprehensive treatments for early autism. *Journal of Clinical Child & Adolescent Psychology, 37*(1), 8–38.

Sandbank, M., Bottema-Beutel, K., Crowley, S., Cassidy, M., Dunham, K., Feldman, J. I., . . . Mahbub, P. (2020). Project AIM: Autism intervention meta-analysis for studies of young children. *Psychological Bulletin, 146*(1), 1.

Saulnier, C. A., & Klaiman, C. (2018). *Essentials of adaptive behavior assessment of neurodevelopmental disorders.* John Wiley & Sons.

Sparrow, S., Cicchetti, D., & Saulnier, C. (2016). *Vineland adaptive Behavior Scales* (3rd Ed.). Pearson.

Tassé, M. J., Schalock, R. L., Balboni, G., Bersani, H., Jr, Borthwick-Duffy, S. A., Spreat, S., . . . Zhang, D. (2012). The construct of adaptive behavior: Its conceptualization, measurement, and use in the field of intellectual disability. *American Journal on Intellectual and Developmental Disabilities, 117*(4), 291–303.

Thompson, J., McGrew, K., & Bruininks, R. (1999). Adaptive and maladaptive behavior: Functional and structural characteristics. *Adaptive Behavior and Its Measurement: Implications for the Field of Mental Retardation*, 15–42.

Woodman, A. C., Demers, L., Crossman, M. K., Warfield, M. E., & Hauser-Cram, P. (2018). Part C early intervention dosage and growth in adaptive skills from early childhood through adolescence. *Early Childhood Research Quarterly, 43*, 73–82.

World Health Organization. (in press). *ICD-11 for mortality and morbidity statistics.*

World Health Organization. (1980). *The international classification of impairment, disability and handicap.* Author.

World Health Organization. (1993). *International statistical classification of diseases and related health problems* (10th ed.). Author.

World Health Organization. (2001). *International classification of functioning, disability and health.* Author.

World Health Organization. (2007). *International classification of functioning, disability and health: children & youth version.* Author.

World Health Organization. (2013). *How to use the icf: a practical manual for using the international classification of functioning, disability and health (ICF).* Author.

89

Assessments of the Central Nervous System

Fiona M. Baumer and Emily M. Spelbrink

For additional material related to the content of this chapter, please see Chapters 29, 30, and 31.

VIGNETTE

A full-term neonate is transferred to the neonatal intensive care unit due to a concerning exam in the delivery room. He is nondysmorphic but has poor cry, minimal reactivity, and low tone. There were no complications with the pregnancy or delivery. Blood gas is normal. Head ultrasound (HUS) is unrevealing of bleed or significant malformation. On the first day of life, he develops episodic, nonsuppressible jerking of the right arm. Electroencephalography (EEG) shows decreased amplitude and frequent sharp waves over the left hemisphere and then confirms seizures starting in the central region of the left hemisphere. Seizures cease after phenobarbital. Magnetic resonance imaging (MRI) with vascular imaging demonstrates a left hemispheric stroke due to left middle cerebral artery occlusion (Fig. 89.1, row 1).

When assessing a child with a neurologic or developmental complaint, such as the child in the vignette, clinicians are tasked with determining the etiology, appropriate treatment, and prognosis. A growing number of tests that measure central nervous system structure and function are available to complement the history and physical exam (Table 89.1). Advances in neuroimaging allow us to visualize the brain and spinal cord at increasingly nuanced levels. Meanwhile, well-established techniques, such as EEG, are more readily available than in the past. This chapter reviews the mechanisms, advantages, limitations, and indications for the diagnostic studies most commonly used in assessment of the central nervous system, focusing on how to target these studies to clinical questions and interpret their results. Special attention is given to MRI and EEG. An overview of advanced techniques reserved for subspecialty care or research is provided in Table 89.2.

STRUCTURAL ASSESSMENT OF THE CENTRAL NERVOUS SYSTEM

Neuroimaging is one of the most efficient tools for diagnosing the etiology of developmental disability, particularly when combined with a strong clinical hypothesis. Imaging has the highest diagnostic yield in children with acute neurologic deficits (Moeschler et al., 2014) and can be particularly helpful in infants or young children who do not demonstrate the same localizing exam findings as older children and adults (Tsze & Valente, 2011). Current neuroimaging techniques are used to: (1) identify, characterize, and time existing brain abnormalities (see Chapter 29); (2) monitor the progression of evolving disease processes; and (3) visualize the effects of disease on brain function in real time. Discovery of imaging biomarkers of neurodevelopmental diseases is also ongoing.

BRAIN IMAGING

Head Ultrasound

Mechanism, Advantages, and Limitations

HUS is a portable, painless, and rapid test that uses sound waves to visualize the brain. Due to its portability, HUS can easily be obtained serially, even in critically ill children. It is restricted to infants for whom the anterior fontanelle is sufficiently open (usually <5 months of age). Classic sonography through the anterior fontanelle provides only a limited view of the posterior fossa, so posterior fontanelle sonography has been increasingly incorporated into the exam. HUS requires a trained technologist and a physician well versed in its interpretation (Orman et al., 2015).

Indications

- HUS screening for intraventricular hemorrhage (IVH) is routine care for premature infants under 30 weeks of gestational age and for older infants with clinical concern (Hand, Shellhaas, & Milla, 2020). HUS can monitor progression of hemorrhage and ventriculomegaly to determine if surgical intervention is required (see Chapter 34).
- Neonates with suspected hypoxic ischemic injury, as in the vignette, undergo HUS before therapeutic hypothermia to evaluate for IVH. HUS of severe or remote hypoxic ischemic injury may reveal cerebral edema or cystic changes. However, the sensitivity of HUS for hypoxic ischemic injury is low and thus MRI is used to assess fully the extent of the injury.
- In the outpatient setting HUS is used to evaluate cases of macro- and microcephaly and to assess infants for ventriculomegaly, fluid collections, and major brain malformations.

Computed Tomography

Mechanism, Advantages, and Limitations

Computed tomography (CT) is a rapid test that uses radiation to visualize intracranial structures. CT is sensitive to

Magnetic Resonance Imaging and Magnetic Resonance Spectroscopy

Mechanism, Advantages, and Limitations

MRI is a versatile imaging technique that provides insight into normal anatomy, macrostructural and microstructural pathology, and even molecular abnormalities. MRI aligns protons in water molecules using a strong magnetic field and then disrupts this alignment with specific radiofrequency pulses. Images are created by measuring the frequencies emitted during the "relaxation" of these protons back to their baseline state. Different images highlight distinct tissue properties: these are referred to as MRI sequences. MRI can visualize the fetal brain as early as 16 weeks of gestation, though level of anatomic detail improves as myelination matures (Barkovich & Barkovich, 2019). MRI use is limited by higher cost, availability, longer scan duration, and need for patient stillness. MRI can be combined with IV gadolinium contrast to assess vascular or inflammatory processes, but careful consideration is required with children due to risk of deposition of gadolinium in various organ systems (Ho, Campeau, Ngo, Udayasankar, & Welker, 2017).

Indications

- MRI is used to assess for structural changes (e.g., in children with global developmental delay/intellectual disability; see Chapter 40) or evaluate focal neurologic findings (e.g., early hand preference). T1-weighted MRI sequences are sensitive to gray matter and typically characterize anatomy, while T2-weighted images are sensitive to water content/edema and typically characterize pathology. MRIs can highlight macrostructural changes such as alterations in brain size (e.g., megal/microencephaly), pathologic formation of the cortex (e.g., lissencephaly, polymicrogyria), or absence/abnormality of typical structures (e.g., agenesis of the corpus callosum, vermian hypoplasia). MRI can also detect microstructural changes such as gray matter heterotopias and focal cortical dysplasias. Such findings, along with clues that can be visualized outside of the central nervous system (e.g., optic nerve hypoplasia), often make a diagnosis or direct further workup (Ho et al., 2017).
- MRI is indicated in children with acute/subacute neurologic changes, symptoms of elevated intracranial pressure, or developmental regression to assess for new or progressive lesions. T2-weighted and fluid-attenuated inversion recovery (FLAIR) sequences are sensitive to edema and other pathology. These images are particularly useful in detecting processes of at least several hours duration, such as white matter injury from acute disseminated encephalomyelitis. Diffusion-weighted imaging (DWI) assesses water movement and can detect injuries occurring only minutes before. DWI is critical to assess for ischemic stroke or hypoxic ischemic injury. In the clinical vignette DWI showed the left hemispheric stroke that caused the infant's seizures and encephalopathy (Ho et al., 2017).
- MRI can be used to estimate when in development an injury occurred. Specific pathologies are seen after injury during specific developmental windows. For example, transmantle schizencephaly suggests an insult in the second trimester (Barkovich, Guerrini, Kuzniecky, Jackson, & Dobyns, 2012). Comparing DWI, T1, and T2 images can determine if an injury is acute, subacute, or remote, as the appearance of injured tissue changes predictably with time. More immediately, MRI with gadolinium contrast can assess whether an inflammatory process is active or quiescent (e.g., in multiple sclerosis), as only active lesions show contrast enhancement (Ho et al., 2017).
- Serial MRIs of progressive neurologic disorders determine if and when to proceed with intervention, such as surgery for low-grade tumors or ventriculomegaly.
- Magnetic resonance spectroscopy (MRS) can be combined with structural imaging to assess chemical composition of the brain. MRS estimates relative concentrations of more than 20 metabolites, including: (1) N-acetylaspartate (NAA), a neuronal marker that decreases in neurodegenerative disorders and is increased in Canavan disease; (2) creatine (Cr), a marker of cellular metabolism; (3), choline (Cho), a marker of cell membrane integrity that rises with cell destruction such as in high-grade tumors; and (4) lactate (Lac), a marker of anaerobic metabolism that is elevated in ischemic injury and some metabolic/mitochondrial disorders. MRS is not a part of standard MRI protocols and must be ordered separately; it can add up to 30 minutes of additional scanner time (Vigneron, 2006).

Considerations When Ordering MRI

A variety of other MRI sequences exist to address specific clinical indications. For example, various sequences exist to assess for blood, while others look at the cranial nerves. More detailed imaging can be directed to areas of specific concern (e.g., thin sections of the temporal lobes in epilepsy patients). Therefore providing a detailed clinical history and speaking with the radiologist about specific concerns prior to MRI may enhance the yield and safety of the study (Ho et al., 2017).

Spinal Imaging

Mechanism, Advantages, and Limitations

The spinal cord, nerve roots, and vertebrae can be imaged with many of the previously described techniques, with many of the same advantages and limitations.

Indications

- Spinal ultrasound or MRI can evaluate sacral dimples, hemangiomas, or hair tufts over the spine to assess for spina bifida occulta or tethered cord.
- Spinal imaging is indicated when neurologic or developmental symptoms localize specifically to the spine (e.g., motor delays confined to the lower extremities with concomitant bowel or bladder dysfunction). Acute neurologic symptoms that localize to the spine, such as sudden onset of flaccid paralysis to an extremity, also require urgent spinal imaging (Rossi, Martinetti, Morana, Severino, & Tortora, 2016; Roth et al., 2016).
- Spinal imaging should be considered in addition to brain imaging whenever there is concern for a process that can affect the entire central nervous system (e.g., tumors,

inflammatory or autoimmune disorders, infections, and metabolic/genetic degenerative disorders) (Rossi et al., 2016).

- Surveillance imaging may be required for conditions associated with vertebral or cord abnormalities (e.g., to monitor for atlantoaxial instability in trisomy 21 or syringomyelia in Chiari malformation) (Rossi et al., 2016).

Considerations When Ordering Spinal Imaging

CT of the spine is fast but involves radiation. CT should be used when there is concern for acute injury that might require emergent surgical intervention. MRI is higher resolution and preferable for subacute or chronic processes (Rossi et al., 2016). Another consideration is that the spinal cord and vertebral levels are not equivalent, and imaging studies are often based on vertebral level. For example, to assess for cord lesions at L1 or below, order both thoracic and lumbar spine sequences.

VASCULAR IMAGING

Vascular imaging is obtained when there is concern for pathology specific to arterial or venous structures. Contrast agents and/or specific imaging sequences can enhance visualization of these vessels. Common indications for vascular imaging include concern for congenital vascular malformations, increased intracranial pressure (suggestive of dural venous sinus thrombosis or intracranial hemorrhage), stroke or transient ischemic attack, vessel dissection or trauma, vessel inflammation, and surgical planning. In the vignette the left middle cerebral artery etiology of the stroke was detected by vascular imaging. Vascular imaging characterizes the diameter, patency, and anatomy of large arteries and veins and is less sensitive for visualizing arterioles, venioles, and capillaries. However, with appropriate radiologic guidance, even small aneurysms and subtle arteriopathies may be visualized.

Direct Angiography

Mechanism, Advantages, and Limitations

Direct angiography is an invasive technique in which a catheter is advanced from a large peripheral vessel (e.g., femoral artery) to the vessel of interest (e.g., the carotid artery). Contrast is then injected as serial x-rays are taken. While considered the gold standard, direct angiography has largely been replaced by other modalities given that it carries a risk of significant complications (e.g., contrast-related bronchospasm, hemorrhage, arterial dissection) near 3% (Barkovich & Barkovich, 2019).

Indications

Direct angiography is still used in children when noninvasive angiographic techniques do not obtain adequate images or during endovascular intervention (Barkovich & Barkovich, 2019).

Computed Tomography Angiography/Venography

Mechanism, Advantages, and Limitations

In CT angiography (CTA) and CT venography (CTV) a single bolus of IV contrast dye is injected. Timed CT is used to gather images first of the arterial and then of the venous systems. As with all CT imaging, CTA/CTV has the drawback of exposing the patient to radiation. However, it provides higher resolution images of the vessels than those obtained with MRI (Kamalian et al., 2016).

Indications

CTA/CTV is indicated for children when urgent vascular imaging is needed and MRI is not available. Additionally, it is standard of care for most vascular malformations, particularly those requiring intervention. CTA is also better at assessing interaction between vasculature and bony structures (e.g., in bow hunter syndrome, where bony impingement causes transient ischemia).

Magnetic Resonance Angiography/Venography

Mechanism, Advantages, and Limitations

Various MRI techniques to image vessels exist (Kuo, Nagpal, Ghoshhajra, & Hedgire, 2019). The main noncontrast method, referred to as time of flight (TOF) imaging, uses radiofrequency pulses to saturate proton spin of the brain tissue; subsequent movement of blood thus makes vessels stand out from the brain parenchyma. TOF has the advantages of not requiring radiation or contrast, but the images can be of poor quality. Higher-resolution vascular images can be obtained with the addition of gadolinium contrast. With stronger magnets, small branch vessels may be better visualized by MR angiography (MRA) than on CTA (Yoon, McNally, Taussky, & Park, 2016).

Indications

MRA/MR venography (MRV) is the preferred vascular imaging modality for children. It is often used to evaluate congenital vascular anomalies (e.g., Sturge-Weber syndrome, vein of Galen malformation) and acquired or evolving vascular lesions (e.g., acute stroke, arteriopathies such as moyamoya).

Considerations When Ordering MRA/MRV

It is advantageous to consult with a neuroradiologist before ordering MRV imaging to ensure that the most appropriate sequences are obtained.

> **VIGNETTE CONTINUED**
>
> *The infant's seizures stop. He is discharged home off of phenobarbital. As he grows, he shows early lefthand preference at 6 months and develops a more notable right hemiparesis. With developmental services, he meets milestones and has average scores on cognitive testing. At age 7 years, he develops seizures of right-body jerking occurring several times per week, which cannot be controlled by medications. His neurologist recommends epilepsy surgery. EEG shows left hemispheric seizures, and magnetoencephalogram (MEG) identifies an onset directly anterior to the stroke bed. The family worries that surgery will worsen his hemiparesis or affect language, but functional MRI shows that right-hand motor and language function are supported by the right hemisphere.*

FUNCTIONAL ASSESSMENT OF THE CENTRAL NERVOUS SYSTEM

Human behavior is governed not only by the structural connections but also by the functional interactions between neurons and brain regions. Neurophysiologic techniques that directly measure electrical and magnetic cortical activity and functional imaging techniques that infer brain activity by measuring hemodynamic changes are both important for central nervous system assessment.

NEUROPHYSIOLOGIC STUDIES

Electroencephalogram

Mechanism, Advantages, and Limitations

EEG (Fig. 89.2) measures electrical activity generated by the cortex providing real-time information on the order of milliseconds. EEG does not measure action potentials from individual neurons but rather current flow at the synapses, which is generated by the summed activity of thousands of neurons. Therefore the signal at each EEG electrode represents activity from at least 6 cm^2 of underlying cortex. Due to this, a major limitation of EEG is that it lacks spatial specificity and provides only a broad sense of what brain regions are affected. EEG predominantly records activity from cortical pyramidal cells, which are close to the surface and organized such that their activity travels to the scalp. Activity from deeper brain structures (e.g., the brainstem, thalamus, and hippocampus) influence EEG indirectly by their interactions with pyramidal cells (Holmes & Khazipov, 2007).

Indications

- EEG is indicated if patients have behavioral events concerning for seizures. If the spell occurs during the EEG recording, a definitive diagnosis of seizure can often be confirmed or excluded. Even if the spell is not captured, identification of EEG abnormalities associated with epilepsy (spike-wave/epileptiform discharges) can aid in clinical decision making. Generalized discharges appear in both hemispheres synchronously, whereas focal discharges present in only one region at a time (Hirsch et al., 2021). The pattern of

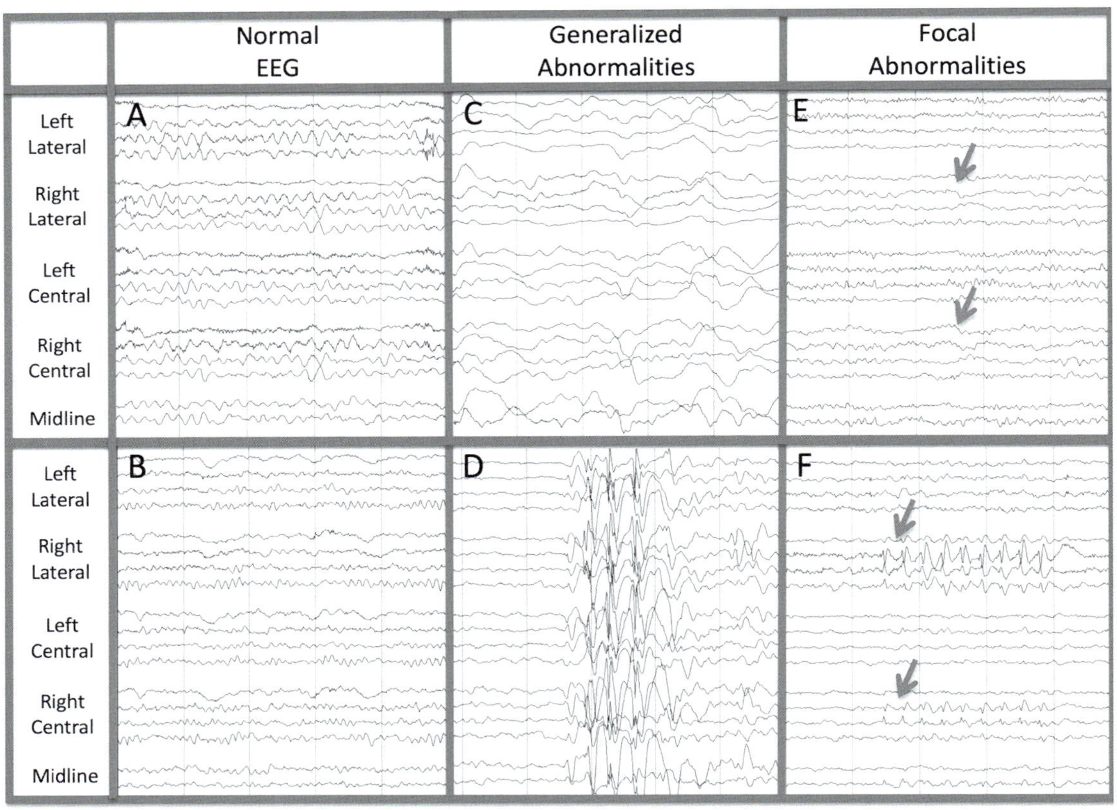

Fig. 89.2 Electroencephalogram assessment of brain function. Bipolar longitudinal montage, sensitivity 10 to 15 μV/mm; *green lines* = 1 second. The first column demonstrates evolution of the normal awake background with age; background rhythms increase in frequency over childhood, as illustrated by the change between age 11 months (A) and 7 years (B). The normal background consists of continuous activity that is symmetric in amplitude and synchronous in timing between the left and right hemispheric electrodes. The second column illustrates generalized abnormalities, including generalized slowing of background rhythms (C) and generalized spike waves occurring at three times per second (D), both of which are seen in the left and right hemispheric electrodes simultaneously. This pattern of generalized spike waves is typical to absence epilepsy. The third column shows focal abnormalities. The *arrow* highlights slowing specific to the right lateral (temporal) electrodes (E); such slowing often warrants neuroimaging to assess for a focal lesion. Focal right hemispheric spikes (F) are more prominent in the right lateral (specifically temporal) than the right central electrodes. In the correct clinical context such focal centrotemporal spikes suggest childhood epilepsy with centrotemporal spikes (benign rolandic epilepsy).

epileptiform discharges in conjunction with the clinical history are often adequate to diagnose specific pediatric epilepsy syndromes. For example, generalized spike waves are a feature of multiple pediatric epilepsy syndromes, but their speed and appearance differ between common disorders such as childhood absence epilepsy and severe conditions such as Lennox-Gastaut syndrome. The distribution of epileptiform discharges across the scalp and relation to behavioral state can also be telling. For example, focal centrotemporal discharges that increase during sleep suggest childhood epilepsy with centrotemporal spikes (formerly benign rolandic epilepsy) (Kim, Korff, Kim, & Nordli, 2015).

- EEGs are indicated in the setting of developmental plateau or regression, even without suspected seizures, to assess for an epileptic encephalopathy. Epileptic encephalopathies are a group of conditions in which abnormal EEG activity itself contributes to developmental difficulties. For example, children with neonatal brain injury can develop continuous spike-wave activity during sleep associated with profound language or behavioral regression, even without any seizures. For these children, cognitive problems do not improve unless the EEG abnormalities are treated (Auvin, Cilio, & Vezzani, 2016).
- EEG also assesses background brain activity, though it is rarely ordered explicitly for this purpose. The EEG background should be continuous, synchronous and symmetric between hemispheres, and organized (with characteristic rhythms seen in different electrodes). Lack of continuity indicates significant cortical dysfunction, which may be reversible (e.g., when due to a metabolic disturbance) or irreversible (e.g., after hypoxic ischemic injury). Amplitude asymmetry between hemispheres suggests a unilateral intra- (e.g., stroke) or extracranial (e.g., subdural hemorrhage) abnormality. In the vignette the EEG asymmetry was consistent with the stroke. Asynchrony in timing of activity between hemispheres, particularly after age 2 years, raises the question of callosal abnormalities (Lynn, Buchanan, Fenichel, & Freemon, 1980). Poorly organized activity indicates an encephalopathic state, though not a specific etiology. In disorders such as infantile spasms normalizing the background activity is an important aim of treatment. Background activity should have an appropriate mix of frequencies for the child's age. Generalized slowing seen in both hemispheres simultaneously indicates global cerebral dysfunction and can be due to acute illness or chronic developmental or genetic disorders. Focal slowing, in contrast, raises concern for structural lesions and is generally an indication for neuroimaging (St. Louis et al., 2016).
- EEG monitoring is increasingly part of standard care for children in intensive care units. Children with or at risk for acute brain injury often have seizures visible to EEG but without obvious clinical manifestations, variably termed subclinical, nonconvulsive, or electrographic-only seizures (Herman et al., 2015). Neonates undergoing therapeutic hypothermia for hypoxic ischemic injury are routinely monitored as 50% to 60% experience electrographic-only seizures after birth (Glass et al., 2014). Older children are often monitored when mental status is altered in the setting of injury, such as hemorrhage, traumatic brain injury, central nervous system infection, ischemic stroke, hypoxic-ischemic injury after cardiac or respiratory arrest, or recent neurosurgery. Similarly, EEG monitoring should be considered in those with fluctuating mental status without a clear etiology or children undergoing medical paralysis (e.g., extracorporeal membrane oxygenation). Monitoring is also indicated for children who do not recover their baseline mentation after clinical seizures stop, as they are at high risk for subclinical seizures or subclinical status epilepticus (Herman et al., 2015).

Considerations When Ordering EEG

Several factors determine the most appropriate choice of EEG. When a child first presents with an event concerning for a seizure, a routine 30- to 60-minute EEG screening for epileptiform discharges may be adequate to guide treatment. The sensitivity of routine EEGs for capturing epileptiform abnormalities is 30% to 70% (Baldin, Hauser, Buchhalter, Hesdorffer, & Ottman, 2014), though it improves if the child sleeps (Baldin, Hauser, Buchhalter, Hesdorffer, & Ottman, 2017). Longer EEG recordings are often necessary when it is critical to confirm if specific events are seizures. For example, 15% to 20% of children with autism spectrum disorder have epileptiform abnormalities without seizures (Capal et al., 2018), and thus if the question is whether movements are seizures versus stereotypy, capturing an event may be necessary to clarify. Prolonged EEGs can often be arranged in both the inpatient and outpatient setting. Inpatient EEGs with video tend to be more sensitive and specific, especially for brief or subtle spells, while outpatient studies may be more practical for families and capture the child in the home environment.

Magnetoencephalogram

Mechanism, Advantages, and Limitations

Magnetoencephalogram (MEG) measures brain activity by recording the magnetic field induced by cortical current flow. MEG has several advantages when compared to EEG. First, magnetic fields are less prone to distortion as they pass through the dura, scalp, and skull. Second, MEG is better able to detect signals generated by cortex folded within sulci, which represents a substantial amount of the cortical surface. Finally, because it uses many sensors, MEG can localize the origin of brain activity with millimeter precision while simultaneously providing high temporal specificity. The clinical application of MEG is more limited than EEG, however, as it requires expensive and highly specialized equipment as well as computationally complex postcollection analysis.

Indications

As seen in the vignette, MEG is primarily used to localize the seizure onset zone or to identify eloquent cortex (areas necessary for functions such as movement or language) in patients with epilepsy. The research applications of MEG to study functional brain connectivity are also growing (Proudfoot, Woolrich, Nobre, & Turner, 2014).

Functional MRI

Mechanism, Advantages, and Limitations

Functional MRI (fMRI) uses changes in blood oxygenation levels to determine function of specific brain regions. When neuronal activity increases, an initial decline in oxygen is followed by a rebound increase in blood flow; blood oxygen level–dependent (BOLD) fMRI measures this sudden increase in oxygenation. fMRI has high spatial sensitivity, localizing brain activity even from deep structures, often within 1 cm. In contrast to EEG and MEG, fMRI has limited temporal specificity as it infers activity based on hemodynamic changes that occur in the order of seconds (Chen & Glover, 2015).

Indications

Clinically, fMRI is used to identify regions of eloquent cortex prior to neurosurgery in order to define borders for resection and to predict postsurgical deficits. fMRI is frequently used before tumor resection or epilepsy surgery as both conditions often cause anatomic remapping of important functions. This can be particularly true in pediatric patients, like the patient in the vignette who showed atypical language lateralization to the right hemisphere. Most clinical fMRI studies are task based, comparing BOLD signal during specific tasks with that seen in the resting state. Such studies are time intensive and require patient cooperation, and thus may be of limited utility in children or individuals with developmental disorders. Resting-state fMRI measures spontaneous fluctuations in BOLD signal while the patient is at rest. Brain regions demonstrating correlated BOLD changes are considered part of a functional network, such as the attention or sensorimotor network. To date, resting-state fMRI has largely been confined to research, but there is growing interest in its clinical applications because it gathers information on multiple brain regions simultaneously and can be performed even with sedation (Silva, See, Essayed, Golby, & Tie, 2018).

DIRECT ASSESSMENT OF THE CENTRAL NERVOUS SYSTEM

Sampling of tissue or fluid from the central nervous system can provide direct measurements of brain health. We limit our discussion here only to lumbar puncture (LP), but brain biopsies or surgical pathology specimens can also shed insight into neurologic or developmental problems.

Lumbar Puncture

Mechanism, Advantages, and Limitations

In an LP a needle is inserted into the thecal space to remove cerebrospinal fluid (CSF) for analysis. LP is a common procedure performed in a wide variety of circumstances by a breadth of practitioners. It requires a sterile field and relatively still patient. Absolute contraindications include active bleeding or local skin infection, low platelets or coagulopathy, noncommunicating hydrocephalus, and impending brain herniation, which can be precipitated by CSF removal. Common adverse events include site pain, nerve root discomfort, or positional low-pressure headache following the procedure (Costerus, Brouwer, & van de Beek, 2018).

Indications

- LPs can diagnose pathology that affects the cellular or molecular composition of the CSF, including infectious, inflammatory, autoimmune, and oncologic processes.
- LP is more sensitive for detecting subarachnoid hemorrhage than imaging and should be considered if clinical suspicion is high and imaging is negative or ambiguous.
- LP can be used to assess for elevated intracranial pressure or to therapeutically relieve pressure.
- Various chemotherapies and gene therapies for oncologic and neurodegenerative processes may be administered into the thecal space via LP.
- CSF studies allow disease-specific biochemical testing for many developmental disorders; details of these studies can be found in Chapters 24, 30, and 36.

CONCLUSION

This chapter provides a brief overview of imaging and neurophysiologic techniques currently available to assess the central nervous system. Despite major technological advances, the history and physical exam remain the cornerstone of patient assessment and should direct choice and interpretation of ancillary studies. When in doubt, discussing the patient with the radiologist and clinical neurophysiologist ahead of time may aid you in ordering the most appropriate tests and allow them to incorporate advanced techniques directed at your specific clinical question. When working with children or patients with developmental disabilities, it is important to consider the feasibility of completing a study and to be particularly judicious when ordering tests that require sedation, radiation, and/or contrast.

REFERENCES

Auvin, S., Cilio, M. R., & Vezzani, A. (2016). Current understanding and neurobiology of epileptic encephalopathies. *Neurobiology of Disease*, *92*(Pt A), 72–89. https://doi.org/10.1016/j.nbd.2016.03.007

Baldin, E., Hauser, W. A., Buchhalter, J. R., Hesdorffer, D. C., & Ottman, R. (2014). Yield of epileptiform electroencephalogram abnormalities in incident unprovoked seizures: A population-based study. *Epilepsia*, *55*(9), 1389–1398. https://doi.org/10.1111/epi.12720

Baldin, E., Hauser, W. A., Buchhalter, J. R., Hesdorffer, D. C., & Ottman, R. (2017). Utility of EEG activation procedures in epilepsy: A population-based study. *Journal of Clinical Neurophysiology*, *34*(6), 512–519. https://doi.org/10.1097/WNP.0000000000000371

Barkovich, M. J., & Barkovich, A. J. (2019). MR imaging of normal brain development. *Neuroimaging Clinics of North America*, *29*(3), 325–337. https://doi.org/10.1016/j.nic.2019.03.007

Barkovich, A. J., Guerrini, R., Kuzniecky, R. I., Jackson, G. D., & Dobyns, W. B. (2012). A developmental and genetic classification for malformations of cortical development: Update 2012. *Brain, 135*(5), 1348–1369. https://doi.org/10.1093/brain/aws019

Capal, J. K., Carosella, C., Corbin, E., Horn, P. S., Caine, R., & Manning-Courtney, P. (2018). EEG endophenotypes in autism spectrum disorder. *Epilepsy and Behavior, 88*, 341–348. https://doi.org/10.1016/j.yebeh.2018.09.036

Chen, J. E., & Glover, G. H. (2015). Functional magnetic resonance imaging methods. *Neuropsychology Review, 25*(3), 289–313. https://doi.org/10.1007/s11065-015-9294-9

Costerus, J. M., Brouwer, M. C., & van de Beek, D. (2018). Technological advances and changing indications for lumbar puncture in neurological disorders. *The Lancet Neurology, 17*(3), 268–278. https://doi.org/10.1016/S1474-4422(18)30033-4

Duncan, J. S., Winston, G. P., Koepp, M. J., & Ourselin, S. (2016). Brain imaging in the assessment for epilepsy surgery. *The Lancet Neurology, 15*(4), 420–433. https://doi.org/10.1016/S1474-4422(15)00383-X

Glass, H. C., Wusthoff, C. J., Shellhaas, R. A., Tsuchida, T. N., Bonifacio, S. L., Cordeiro, M., … Chang, T. (2014). Risk factors for EEG seizures in neonates treated with hypothermia: A multicenter cohort study. *Neurology, 82*(14), 1239–1244. https://doi.org/10.1212/WNL.0000000000000282

Hand, I. L., Shellhaas, R. A., & Milla, S. S. (2020). Routine neuroimaging of the preterm brain. *Pediatrics, 146*(5). https://doi.org/10.1542/peds.2020-029082

Herman, S. T., Abend, N. S., Bleck, T. P., Chapman, K. E., Drislane, F. W., Emerson, R. G., … Hirsch, L. J. (2015). Consensus statement on continuous EEG in critically ill adults and children, part I: Indications. *Journal of Clinical Neurophysiology, 32*(2), 87–95. https://doi.org/10.1097/WNP.0000000000000166

Hirsch, L. J., Fong, M. W. K., Leitinger, M., LaRoche, S. M., Beniczky, S., Abend, N. S., … Gaspard, N. (2021). American Clinical Neurophysiology Society's standardized critical care EEG terminology: 2021 version. *Journal of Clinical Neurophysiology, 38*(1), 1–29. https://doi.org/10.1097/WNP.0000000000000806

Ho, M. L., Campeau, N. G., Ngo, T. D., Udayasankar, U. K., & Welker, K. M. (2017). Pediatric brain MRI part 1: Basic techniques. *Pediatric Radiology, 47*(5), 534–543. https://doi.org/10.1007/s00247-016-3776-7

Holmes, G. L., & Khazipov, R. (2007). Basic neurophysiology and the cortical basis of EEG. In A. S. Blum & S. B. Rutkove (Eds.), *The clinical neurophysiology primer* (pp. 19–33). Humana Press. https://doi.org/10.1007/978-1-59745-271-7_2

Kamalian, S., Lev, M. H., & Gupta, R. (2016). Computed tomography imaging and angiography—Principles. *Handbook of Clinical Neurology, 135*, 3–20. https://doi.org/10.1016/B978-0-444-53485-9.00001-5

Kim, S. H., Korff, C. M., Kim, A. J., & Nordli, D. R. (2015). A practical, simple, and useful method of categorizing interictal EEG features in children. *Neurology, 85*(5), 471–478. https://doi.org/10.1212/WNL.0000000000001805

Kuo, A. H., Nagpal, P., Ghoshhajra, B. B., & Hedgire, S. S. (2019). Vascular magnetic resonance angiography techniques. *Cardiovascular Diagnosis and Therapy, 9*(1), S28–S36. https://doi.org/10.21037/cdt.2019.06.07

Lynn, R. B., Buchanan, D. C., Fenichel, G. M., & Freemon, F. R. (1980). Agenesis of the corpus callosum. *Archives of Neurology, 37*(7), 444–445. https://doi.org/10.1001/archneur.1980.00500560074011

Mehyar, L. S., Abu-Arja, M. H., Stanek, J. R., Elbeshlawi, I., & AbdelBaki, M. S. (2019). The risk of developing secondary central nervous system tumors after diagnostic irradiation from computed tomography in pediatrics: A literature review. *Pediatric Neurology, 98*, 18–24. https://doi.org/10.1016/j.pediatrneurol.2019.03.028

Moeschler, J. B., Shevell, M., Saul, R. A., Chen, E., Freedenberg, D. L., Hamid, R., … Tarini, B. A. (2014). Comprehensive evaluation of the child with intellectual disability or global developmental delays. *Pediatrics, 134*(3), e903–e918. https://doi.org/10.1542/peds.2014-1839

Orman, G., Benson, J. E., Kweldam, C. F., Bosemani, T., Tekes, A., de Jong, M. R., … Huisman, T. A. G. M. (2015). Neonatal head ultrasonography today: A powerful imaging tool!. *Journal of Neuroimaging, 25*(1), 31–55. https://doi.org/10.1111/jon.12108

Proudfoot, M., Woolrich, M. W., Nobre, A. C., & Turner, M. R. (2014). Magnetoencephalography. *Practical Neurology, 14*(5), 336–343. https://doi.org/10.1136/practneurol-2013-000768

Rossi, A., Martinetti, C., Morana, G., Severino, M., & Tortora, D. (2016). Diagnostic approach to pediatric spine disorders. *Magnetic Resonance Imaging Clinics of North America, 24*(3), 621–644. https://doi.org/10.1016/j.mric.2016.04.001

Roth, C. J., Angevine, P. D., Aulino, J. M., Berger, K. L., Choudhri, A. F., Fries, I. B., … Bykowski, J. (2016). ACR appropriateness criteria myelopathy. *Journal of the American College of Radiology, 13*(1), 38–44. https://doi.org/10.1016/j.jacr.2015.10.004

Silva, M. A., See, A. P., Essayed, W. I., Golby, A. J., & Tie, Y. (2018). Challenges and techniques for presurgical brain mapping with functional MRI. *NeuroImage: Clinical, 17*, 794–803. https://doi.org/10.1016/j.nicl.2017.12.008

St. Louis, E., Frey, L., Britton, J., Hopp, J., Korb, P., Koubeissi, M., … Pestana-Knight, E. (2016). *Electroencephalography (EEG): An introductory text and atlas of normal and abnormal findings in adults, children, and infants*. American Epilepsy Society. https://doi.org/10.5698/978-0-9979756-0-4

Tsze, D. S., & Valente, J. H. (2011). Pediatric stroke: A review. *Emergency Medicine International, 2011*, 1–10. https://doi.org/10.1155/2011/734506

Vigneron, D. B. (2006). Magnetic resonance spectroscopic imaging of human brain development. *Neuroimaging Clinics of North America, 16*(1), 75–85. https://doi.org/10.1016/j.nic.2005.11.008.

Yoon, N. K., McNally, S., Taussky, P., & Park, M. S. (2016). Imaging of cerebral aneurysms: A clinical perspective. *Neurovascular Imaging, 2*(1), 6. https://doi.org/10.1186/s40809-016-0016-3

90

Integration of Data Sources and Uncertainty

Alison Schonwald and Bridget Kiley

For additional material related to the content of this chapter, please see Chapter 76.

VIGNETTE

Parker is an 8-year-old with worsening moodiness. Early friendships have not been sustained, and classroom behavior is disruptive. In school Parker is always moving, calls out answers, and can talk incessantly. In addition, at home Parker screams and cries when told to stop playing a videogame or stop an activity to come to a meal. An initial evaluation diagnosed autism spectrum disorder (ASD) with generalized anxiety disorder, but a subsequent evaluation by a different professional resulted in an attention-deficit/hyperactivity disorder (ADHD) diagnosis. School testing identifies average scores on cognitive and academic testing. Parker's family is left confused and unsure of the next steps.

Care of youth with developmental and behavioral (DB) needs often includes ambiguity. Ambiguity is defined as "a state of being doubtful; uncertain; inexplicable; capable of being understood in two or more possible senses or ways" (*Merriam-Webster*, n.d.). Most DB diagnoses are inexact, with definitions that have varied over time. The nonlinear journey of diagnosis and treatment is impacted by a range of constantly changing influences. Managing ambiguity becomes a frequently used skill for practitioners in the DB field. This chapter explores the factors that contribute to the ambiguity intrinsic to DB care, concluding with guidance in supporting families managing uncertainty.

FACTORS CONTRIBUTING TO UNCERTAINTY IN DIAGNOSIS AND CARE

Developmental Changes

Primary to the diagnostic uncertainty faced in DB pediatric care is that children are in a never-ending state of development. The constant state of change for children is unmistakable across every realm: physical, cognitive, language, motor, social, and emotional domains. In early childhood progress across stages is often drastic and uneven, forward and backward, faster and then slower. Typical developmental trajectories vary with genetic predisposition, temperament, resources, and adversities that children may face.

One area of growth may accentuate the slower pace of another. For example, some children have strong language skills, generating complex sentences with impressive vocabulary; this may not translate into a similarly sophisticated appreciation of emotional nuance. Alternatively, weak language skills may result in underestimation of learner's potential, as many areas of nonverbal reasoning capacity are less evident.

Developmental assessment seeks to quantify the child's skills in comparison to expectations for age. However, these assessments do not necessarily indicate true capacity or future potential. Developmental assessment of infants and toddlers fails to fully predict later performance on intelligence testing in typically developing children, perhaps as some intelligence facets are not yet developed (McCall & Carriger, 1993). For example, one study of 162 children assessed at 2.5 years with the Bayley Scales of Infant and Toddler Development III, compared to Wechsler Intelligence Scale for Children, Fourth Edition scales at 6.5 years of age, showed only weak positive correlations between most scores (Månsson et al., 2019). By 11 years of age, individual IQ score correlates well over time (Deary & Brett, 2015). Thus even when evaluation includes use of standardized measures, results from early childhood testing may change considerably on reassessment. Standardized measures reflect where a child performs, within a normal distribution, in the moment of time the testing takes place. We cannot be certain precisely how the behaviors and skills reported or demonstrated will change over time in the course of development.

Defining Normal

Diagnosing symptoms and skills as outside the range of normal, thus warranting a DB diagnosis, requires an established definition of normal. A larger question becomes, "What is normal?" A child is not a number or a score, although scores provide specific and useful information. Furthermore, most clinical encounters lack the luxury of direct testing with standardized tools, limiting access to standardized norms. Ambiguity in DB care is heightened by the difficulties we have in precisely defining normal.

In the field of child development screening and surveillance are recommended to identify DB concerns as discussed in Chapters 81 and 82. Each screen is scored to identify a risk for clinical findings with a recommendation for next steps, often including referral for further evaluation. Screening tools should also be used when clinical concerns arise, and clinicians are expected to provide developmental surveillance at all visits (Weitzman et al., 2015).

But what exactly does this mean? Whether clinicians provide surveillance with observation, interview, physical exam, and/or standardized surveys, questions arise.

- Exactly how late can a milestone be reached and still be within the normal range?
- How low is "low tone"?
- What if one parent observes a skill, but the other does not?
- How often does a skill have to be displayed to indicate mastery?
- What if a skill is observed in some settings and not in others?

Surveillance is fraught with uncertainty. While use of screening tools improves rates of identifying children at risk for developmental concerns (Schonwald, Huntington, Chan, Risko, & Bridgemohan, 2009), results are meant to be interpreted by the clinician. The ambiguity that infuses surveillance similarly impacts screening.

Parent Perspectives

Ambiguity in care is also fueled by varied perspectives held by clinicians and parents. Regardless of clinicians' experience and skill, parents are experts on their child's behavior. At times, perspectives conflict, resulting in multiple interpretations of a child's skills or behaviors.

Parents as experts on their child's behavior is a central principle of the Touchpoints model. Touchpoint principles highlight the importance of both the clinician-parent relationship and the parent-child relationship. These concepts are embedded in the tenet that child development comes in bursts and regressions (Brazelton & Sparrow, 2007). In acknowledging parents as the experts on their children, clinicians are faced with reconciling differences that may arise in regard to a child's profile.

Why are parental perspectives sometimes at odds with those of the clinician?

- Parents can educate themselves via extensive resources available on the Internet, where a great deal of accurate information is available for the layperson. For example, the Centers for Disease Control and Prevention website (CDC, 2020) includes checklists, photos, and a tracker for developmental milestones from birth to age 5 years, freely available through its Learn the Signs Campaign. Similarly, the American Academy of Pediatrics (healthychildren.org) provides lists of age-based developmental expectations paired with advice about developmental promotion (American Academy of Pediatrics, n.d.). Parents may find these resources appealing, but they still need support in understanding why early identification is important and what to do next. Those providing primary care to children and teens are left to respond to the information parents bring (Raspa et al., 2015).
- Parents may experience their children through an emotional lens. Children with secure attachment, for example, may feel socially connected to parents, when in fact social communication skills are confused with emotional reciprocity. Psychological defense mechanisms may protect parents from full recognition of a child's deficits, so "putting a positive spin" on delays can shield a parent from painful awareness.
- Parents are often familiar with the idea that "we shouldn't compare" one child with another, and so they may also intentionally discount differences observed when comparing their child to same-aged peers.
- Parents also have their own experiences (trauma, difficulties in school, ruptured relationships) that impact how they perceive their child's behaviors. When a child displays behavior reminiscent of a parent's own past, the parent may misattribute the underlying cause to one that aligns with the parent's personal experience. While in some scenarios a parent who lived similar challenges can profoundly understand a child's situation, in other scenarios parents project their own histories as inaccurate interpretations of the child's behavior.
- Vulnerable child syndrome is a specific framework that helps us understand why some parents perceive concerns disproportionate to those concerns held by a clinician. When vulnerable child syndrome occurs, a child is viewed by parents as being at higher risk for problems than current health indicates, often after the child suffered a serious or life-threatening event (Schmitz, 2019). This evolves into a maladaptive family dynamic that can present with exaggerated reporting of a child's signs and symptoms, leaving the health care clinicians to disentangle contradictory information.
- Culture-informed parent perspectives on child development also vary widely and may result in disparate reports between parents and clinicians. We all are influenced by the history, customs, language, and religion inherent to surrounding communities and institutions. Within a culture and ethnicity, great heterogeneity exists, while patterns of parent-child interaction between groups are nonetheless present (Kuchirko & Tamis-LeMonda, 2019). For example, in traditional Chinese culture, a child making eye contact with an adult may be considered rude and arrogant; in Chinese culture pointing with one's index finger is not practiced. Caretakers may not endorse concerns about these developmental skills, while clinicians might find these as concerning for ASD (Zhang, Wheeler, & Richey, 2006). In some cultures,disability may be considered punishment for sins or caused by evil spirits, resulting in stigma and family reluctance to report on or agree with developmental concerns (Bhayana & Bhayana, 2018). How clinicians and caretakers view and describe child development can subsequently clash.
- A final consideration is where a parent might be in one's "journey." We have considered that parents may come to the clinical scenario with their own histories, facts, and cultural perspectives; sometimes parents are simply moving through well-documented stages in processing their child's DB needs: they may be at a stage mismatched with the clinician's view and approach. In one study of parents of children diagnosed with ASD three periods emerged in the parental experience, termed their diagnostic odyssey:

(1) making sense of the child's developmental differences, (2) navigating the diagnosis, and (3) finally connecting to services (Lappé et al., 2018). In moving through the diagnostic odyssey a parent may still be making sense of the child's profile and not ready to proceed toward treatment, despite clinical recommendations.

Caregivers may experience grief when facing a child's diagnosis, perhaps grieving the loss of the imagined or expected future. They may pass through various levels of denial, anger, bargaining, depression, and acceptance (Kübler-Ross & Kessler, 2005), sometimes in a nonlinear fashion. The timeline of the process is as individual as the person experiencing it. Denial is an effective defense mechanism, allowing us to protect ourselves from information too painful to integrate immediately. We may feel anger and express it toward our child, care providers, or partner. Bargaining reflects an effort to gain control of outcomes, while depression may include feeling stuck in sadness and feelings of loss. In finally finding acceptance, we tackle realities of a diagnosis.

Partnering with parents means working to understand their perspective rather than focusing solely on resolving ambiguity.

Scientific Advances

With scientific advances comes the expansion of research-based understandings of diseases and disorders. Diagnostic frameworks, labels, and subsequent treatments shift as the field grows in understanding diagnostic and treatment options. Again, ambiguity ensues; new and different ways of making sense of a clinical scenario permeate thinking, obviating previous conceptions.

Attention-Deficit/Hyperactivity Disorder

Eloquently described by Lange, Reichl, Lange, Tucha, and Tucha (2010), overactive and inattentive children have had a variety of labels since the 1700s. Sir George Frederic Still, the so-named father of British pediatrics, described children with "an abnormal degree of passionateness" and "wanton mischievousness" with "exaggeration of excitability" in the early 1900s. In the same era early brain damage (e.g., from perinatal anoxia) with subsequent behavior or learning problems was described. After an encephalitis epidemic (1917–1918), surviving children often had a so-called postencephalitic behavior disorder. Described as hyperactive, distractible, and unmanageable in school, their hyperkinesis led children to continually touch, take, and destroy. In the 1960s minimal brain dysfunction was proposed as the most appropriate term by the Oxford International Study Group of Child Neurology. Referring to those with near average to above intelligence, symptoms of affected children included poor attention, impulse, or motor function.

Recognizing that many children with this symptom constellation had no brain damage, and that hyperactivity was the most marked symptom, the term hyperkinetic impulse disorder emerged. The term hyperkinetic reaction of childhood appeared in the 1968 *Diagnostic and Statistical Manual of Mental Disorders* (American Psychiatric Association [APA], 1968), second edition (*DSM-II*), defined by only two descriptive sentences. In the *DSM-III* (1980) three symptoms (hyperactivity, impulsivity, inattention) with numerical cutoffs were offered, and the disorder was renamed attention-deficit disorder (ADD) with or without hyperactivity (Lange et al., 2010). In 1987 the revised *DSM-III-R* renamed the disorder ADHD (APA, 1987), which continued in the *DSM-IV* (1994) and *DSM-5* (APA, 2013). Yet parents still frequently refer to ADD when hyperactivity is absent, confused why clinicians diagnose ADHD.

Autism Spectrum Disorder

In the 1960s childhood autism was misattributed to a cold and distant ("refrigerator") mother causing socially unavailable children (Mandy & Lai, 2016). We now know that 74% to 93% of risk for autism is heritable (Tick, Bolton, Happé, Rutter, & Rijsdijk, 2016). Previously a rare and strictly defined profile, ASD is now understood to be heterogeneous and common (Lord, Elsabbagh, Baird, & Veenstra-Vanderweele, 2018). As is the case with ADHD, diagnostic options for autism diagnoses evolved over time.

Autism first appeared in the *DSM-III*, defined by essential features occurring within the first 30 months of age (APA, 1980). Criteria were broadened in the 1987 revised *DSM-III-R*, when pervasive developmental disorder–not otherwise specified (PDD-NOS) was added to describe those more mildly affected.

By 1994, the *DSM-IV* presented more of a spectrum concept, including five conditions: autism, PDD-NOS, Asperger disorder, childhood disintegrative disorder, and Rett disorder (APA, 1994). These subtypes were then eliminated in the 2013 *DSM-5*, as research found the previous subtypes were not reliably confirmed across clinicians or time (Lord et al., 2006, 2012). With only ASD as a diagnostic option, the model of a spectrum was consolidated. Rett disorder was removed, as its genetic etiology was confirmed in 1998 (Sirianni, Naidu, Pereira, Pillotto, & Hoffman, 1998). Childhood disintegrative disorder was also removed, as advancements in testing led to more specific etiologic explanations (Lord & Bishop, 2015).

Similar changes in the name for what we now call intellectual disability are discussed in Chapter 1.

Early Childhood Adversity

The vicious cycles of chronic disease and poverty were long attributed to inherited risk for medical and mental health disease, along with the absence of models of healthy behaviors and lack of opportunity for change. The National Research Council (NRC) and the Institute of Medicine (IOM) released *From Neurons to Neighborhoods: The Science of Early Childhood Development* (Shonkoff, Phillips, & National Research Council U.S., 2000), highlighting the science and advances in the understanding of childhood development. We now know that chronic and toxic stress experienced by young children interrupts the development of many body systems (including neurologic, cardiovascular, and immunologic), impacting health outcomes (see Chapter 15; Shonkoff et al. 2012). Thus the model of intervention shifts dramatically to addressing social determinants of health.

For many DB disorders, names and explanations have varied over time. As the constant change in child development creates a foundation of uncertainty in DB care, the regular change in names and explanations of DB diagnoses creates another layer of ambiguity. Sometimes abrupt and other times subtle, these transformations require agility in thinking about affected children. Clinical care takes on an element of ambiguity, requiring clinicians and families to embrace the inexactness of the field and to consider the various stressors and factors that contribute to child development.

Variations Across Disciplines

Several clinicians may be involved in the diagnosis and care of youth with DB needs. Some children are cared for by a primary care provider only, others may have a larger team of specialists (Table 90.1). Training for each discipline varies, with regional and programmatic differences within each discipline. The focus of a clinical visit may vary from one specialist to another. Finally, it is important to note that clinicians generally confirm only those diagnoses within their own specialty area.

Consider the child in the vignette: A psychologist diagnoses ASD with generalized anxiety disorder, another specialist diagnoses ADHD, and school testing identifies average range cognitive and academic function. The psychologist may utilize direct assessment of attention, mood, social communication, repetitive behaviors, and perseverative interests, along with standardized surveys completed by caregivers and teachers. In contrast, a neurologist, primary care provider, or developmental pediatrician may review previous testing, examine and interact with the child, and review history with parents. School testing may focus on discrete cognitive and academic skills, and performance in the classroom setting.

Understandably confusing to a family, each diagnosis might nonetheless have both value and validity. Ideally, each clinician explains their specific role in caring for the child. Rather than presenting the parent with conflicting diagnostic perspectives, clinicians should speak to treatment goals complementary to those addressed by others. For example, for the child in our vignette, the following plan might be appropriate:

- The psychologist recommends in-school and at-home therapies to address the social communication and cognitive rigidities of ASD, provides parental psychoeducation, and provides cognitive-behavioral therapy to address generalized anxiety disorder.
- The physician recommends in-school and at-home supports to accommodate for ADHD as it impacts learning and adaptive function, and provides psychopharmacology.
- The school implements accommodations to promote attention, provides counseling to complement therapy for anxiety, and provides direct social skills instruction

Returning to the definition of ambiguity as a state of being doubtful, uncertain, inexplicable, and capable of being understood in two or more possible senses or ways, we see that the inconsistent terminology across disciplines can create doubt and uncertainty in the diagnosis. However, we also see opportunities to align perspectives as complementary in addressing a child wholistically.

TABLE 90.1 Professionals Involved in Diagnosis and Management of Developmental-Behavioral Pediatric Conditions

• Audiologist	• Physiatrist
• Behavior Therapist	• Physical Therapist
• Board-Certified Behavior Analyst	• Physician Assistant
• Developmental Behavioral Pediatrician	• Psychiatric and Mental Health Clinical Nurse Specialist
• Guidance Counselor	• Psychiatrist
• Licensed Mental Health Counselor	• Psychologist
	• School Psychologist
• Neurologist	• Speech and Language Pathologist
• Nurse Practitioner	
• Occupational Therapist	• Social Worker

METHODS FOR APPROACHING AMBIGUITY IN CARE

Data Gathering

Children's behavior can fluctuate from one setting to another, challenged by varying demands and supported by different relationships. Regardless of a clinician's discipline, gathering information from a range of sources can illuminate the picture of a child's profile. Given the abundance of ambiguity in developmental-behavioral pediatric (DBP) care, information from multiple sources can clarify the specific strengths and difficulties a child displays in multiple situations, in comparison to other same-age peers. Questionnaires can be broad or narrow. They may be repeated over time to monitor change. Importantly, validated questionnaires are interpreted in various ways, such as:

- Level of risk for the diagnosis of a disorder
- Presence of adequate symptoms to meet diagnostic criteria
- Indication of need for further evaluation
- Increased specificity of the nature of the concern

Surveys are often given to caregivers and teachers, self-reports are often given to older children and adolescents. It is particularly important that more than one individual completes a survey to understand function across contexts.

Data gathering through validated surveys can bring clarity:

1. How much do these behaviors interfere in school?
2. Are symptoms improving or worsening?
3. Which area of concern is most problematic?

However, no single score or survey suffices to make a diagnosis. For example, every symptom of ADHD can be endorsed for a child suffering from severe anxiety. Likewise, social skills deficits can come from ADHD and not ASD. Gathering data rounds out the picture of the whole child, reflecting how the child or teen functions within the everyday world.

Uncertainty Management Theory

Arising from ambiguous, complicated, unpredictable, and vague situations, uncertainty emerges when probability is anything more than 0% or less than 100%. Uncertainty can be frustrating, interfering with decision making and planning, generating anxiety and unrest. However, uncertainty can also allow for optimism and hope. For a single person and situation, uncertainty can be both positive and negative simultaneously. The ambiguity and impact of uncertainty incorporates the variability of the affected person's experiences and interpretations, emotions, behavioral and psychological responses. We explored why ambiguity infuses DB care, and now grapple with how to face this ambiguity.

According to uncertainty management theory (UMT), managing uncertainty requires considering the multiple layers of context, their interconnectedness, and the time frames in which they occur (Brashers, 2001). Uncertainty is rife in medical decision making, particularly in relation to children with DB disorders; UMT is a particularly well-suited approach to the uncertainty common in DBP care (Table 90.2).

As clinicians, we engage in uncertainty management through communication with families. Communication is a reciprocal and multilayered process. For example, parents told of a new diagnosis of dyslexia for their child may ask, "Will he always have dyslexia?" "Will he be able to go to college?" and "Did I not read to him enough as a baby?"

On the surface, these questions are unanswerable. But what are families really saying? Likely, families are saying, "I just want the best for him" and "Will he be okay?"

Meeting families "where they are" means that clinicians must recognize the needs of families to do the following:

1. Manage information, sometimes conflicting, unexpected, and complicated
2. Learn to live with chronic uncertainty
3. Maintain hope at the same time

TABLE 90.2 Implication of Uncertainty Management Theory In Developmental-Behavioral Pediatric Practice

1. Appreciate the role of uncertainty for parents, which may both provoke anxiety and maintain hope
2. Understand that information seeking and avoidance may be in service to managing emotions stemming from uncertainty
3. Recognize that each person's experiences, interpretations, and emotions impact how they face uncertainty and ambiguity
4. Optimize communication, which requires listening for the unspoken questions and concerns, or "reading between the lines"
5. Intentionally create a "fair interpersonal process" for trusting clinician-patient relationships to develop

In replying, we can provide manageable, clear information in a supportive and hopeful manner: "Several reading programs have been shown to be very effective in treating dyslexia. Let's work hard to get that started for him."

In some cases clinicians find that incorrect information is used by families to help reduce their uncertainty. For example, families of children with ASD may believe the disproved role of vaccines as causative. Similarly, parents often describe difficult births as a presumed explanation for a child's otherwise unexplained disabilities. Information seeking often reflects an understandable desire to mitigate uncertainty. On the other hand, families may avoid, consciously or unconsciously, information seeking sometimes to maintain or increase uncertainty and thus allow for more hope and optimism (Rains & Tukachinsky, 2015). UMT is therefore a helpful framework that unpacks the process through which individuals encounter and manage health-related uncertainty (Brashers, 2001). As clinicians working with families and patients affected by DB disorders, UMT can inform a supportive and collaborative approach.

Both collaboration and perception of fair treatment are important in the development of a trusting clinical relationship. In the world of organizational psychology the experience of a fair interpersonal process has positive effects on a multitude of workplace functions. Van den Bos & Lind (2002) suggest that "the key function of fairness is that it provides people with a way to cope with uncertainties." We can apply this concept to the clinical relationship in health care; when both clinician and patient feel a "fair interpersonal process" is unfolding, uncertainty is reduced. The experience of personal attention, the receipt of direct, honest, and manageable explanations of decisions, and the sense that there is an investment in overall time and attention contribute to the development of trusting relationships. In DB care, where so much is ambiguous, connections that are collaborative and trusting can bolster a family's ability to manage chronic uncertainty.

Shared Decision Making

Shared decision making (SDM) is a process in which clinicians and patients work together to make decisions and select tests, treatments, and care plans based on clinical evidence that balances risks and expected outcomes with patient preferences, goals, and values (as discussed further in Chapter 77) (Wyatt et al., 2015). SDM plays a central role when facing uncertainty in clinical care as it creates a structure through which clinicians and families navigate uncertainty in care. Practical suggestions for SDM implementation are included in Table 90.3.

Opel (2018) proposes a four-step framework that distinguishes when SDM should be physician guided (when one option is more favorable in benefit/burden ratio) versus parent guided (when no option is more favorable). A continuum of roles played then reflects the degree to which each option is preference sensitive. Given the importance of quality communication in SDM, the role of cultural humility in SDM is accentuated (Derrington, Paquette, & Johnson, 2018).

TABLE 90.3 Stepwise Approach to Shared Decision Making in Pediatrics

- Ask (Who should hear this? What type of information would be helpful?)
- Tell (clear statements about new information, expecting an emotional response)
- Second ask (What questions do you have? Should we talk more now?)
- More than one acceptable option (state this explicitly)
- Describe different paths (different options with benefits and risks)
- Elicit concerns or questions
- Elicit values (What does this new information mean to you? What are you hoping for? What are you worried about?)
- Determine how much pediatrician input is desired in decision making
- Make a recommendation if appropriate and ask for a decision
- Make plans for follow-up

Adapted from Walter, J. K., Hwang, J., & Fiks, A. G. (2018). Pragmatic strategies for shared decision-making. *Pediatrics, 142*(3), S157–S162.

SDM therefore can weave together the many contributors to ambiguity in DB care, and then utilize data gathering and UMT when faced with uncertainty. While asking for and listening to caregiver questions, a trusting and fair relationship is forged. Explicit statements about data gathered, new information and diagnostic considerations, various (sometimes conflicting) perspectives, and intervention options all become part of a conversation, wherein a family's emotional process, values, and priorities emerge. Responsive, dynamic care then unfolds.

CONCLUSION

Care of youth with DB needs often includes ambiguity. Managing that ambiguity is a necessary skill for practitioners in the field. Understanding and effectively implementing strategies based on UMT and SDM may allow clinicians to more effectively provide clinical care in the face of uncertainty.

REFERENCES

American Academy of Pediatrics. (n.d.). *Ages & stages.* healthychildren.org. https://www.healthychildren.org/English/ages-stages/Pages/default.aspx

American Psychiatric Association. (1968). *Diagnostic and Statistical Manual of Mental Disorders* (2nd ed.). Author.

American Psychiatric Association. (1980). *Diagnostic and Statistical Manual of Mental Disorders* (3rd ed.). Author.

American Psychiatric Association. (1987). *Diagnostic and Statistical Manual of Mental Disorders* (3rd ed.). Author. rev.

American Psychiatric Association. (2013). *Diagnostic and Statistical Manual of Mental Disorders* (5th ed.). Author.

Bhayana, A., & Bhayana, B. (2018). Approach to developmental disabilities in newcomer families. *Canadian Family Physician (Medecin de Famille Canadien), 64*(8), 567–573.

Brashers, D. (2001). Communication and uncertainty management. *Journal of Communication, 51*, 477–497.

Brazelton, T. B., & Sparrow, J. (2007). *The touchpoints model of development.* Brazelton Touchpoints Center. http://www.brazeltontouchpoints.org/wp-content/uploads/2011/09/Touchpoints_Model_of_Development_Aug_2007.pdf

Centers for Disease Control and Prevention. (2020). *Child development basics.* https://www.cdc.gov/ncbddd/childdevelopment/facts.html

Deary, I. J., & Brett, C. E. (2015). Predicting and retrodicting intelligence between childhood and old age in the 6-day sample of the Scottish Mental Survey 1947. *Intelligence, 50*, 1–9.

Derrington, S. F., Paquette, E., & Johnson, K. A. (2018). Cross-cultural interactions and shared decision-making. *Pediatrics, 142*(3), S187–S192.

Kübler-Ross, E., & Kessler, D. (2005). *On grief and grieving: Finding the meaning of grief through the five stages of loss.* Scribner.

Kuchirko, Y. A., & Tamis-LeMonda, C. S. (2019). The cultural context of infant development: Variability, specificity, and universality. *Advances in Child Development and Behavior, 57*, 27–63.

Lange, K. W., Reichl, S., Lange, K. M., Tucha, L., & Tucha, O. (2010). The history of attention deficit hyperactivity disorder. *Attention Deficit and Hyperactivity Disorders, 2*(4), 241–255.

Lappé, M., Lau, L., Dudovitz, R. N., Nelson, B. B., Karp, E. A., & Kuo, A. A. (2018). The diagnostic odyssey of autism spectrum disorder. *Pediatrics, 141*(4), S272–S279.

Lord, C., & Bishop, S. L. (2015). Recent advances in autism research as reflected in DSM-5 criteria for autism spectrum disorder. *Annual Review of Clinical Psychology, 11*, 53–70.

Lord, C., Elsabbagh, M., Baird, G., & Veenstra-Vanderweele, J. (2018). Autism spectrum disorder. *Lancet (London, England), 392*(10146), 508–520.

Lord, C., Petkova, E., Hus, V., Gan, W., Lu, F., Martin, D. M., … Risi, S. (2012). A multisite study of the clinical diagnosis of different autism spectrum disorders. *Archives of General Psychiatry, 69*(3), 306–313.

Lord, C., Risi, S., DiLavore, P. S., Shulman, C., Thurm, A., & Pickles, A. (2006). Autism from 2 to 9 years of age. *Archives of General Psychiatry, 63*(6), 694–701.

Mandy, W., & Lai, M. C. (2016). Annual research review: The role of the environment in the developmental psychopathology of autism spectrum condition. *Journal of Child Psychology and Psychiatry, and Allied Disciplines, 57*(3), 271–292.

Månsson, J., Stjernqvist, K., Serenius, F., Ådén, U., & Källén, K. (2019). Agreement between Bayley-III measurements and WISC-IV measurements in typically developing children. *Journal of Psychoeducational Assessment, 37*(5), 603–616.

McCall, R., & Carriger, M. (1993). A meta-analysis of infant habituation and recognition memory performance as predictors of later IQ. *Child Development, 64*(1), 57–79.

Merriam-Webster. (n.d.). *Ambiguous.* https://www.merriam-webster.com/dictionary/ambiguous

Opel, D. J. (2018). A 4-step framework for shared decision-making in pediatrics. *Pediatrics, 142*(3), S149–S156.

Rains, S. A., & Tukachinsky, R. H. (2015). An examination of the relationships among uncertainty, appraisal, and information-seeking behavior proposed in uncertainty management theory. *Health Communication, 30*, 339–349.

Raspa, M., Levis, D. M., Kish-Doto, J., Wallace, I., Rice, C., Barger, B., Green, K. K., & Wolf, R. B. (2015). Examining parents' experiences and information needs regarding early identification of developmental delays: Qualitative research to inform a public health campaign. *Journal of Developmental and Behavioral Pediatrics: JDBP*, *36*(8), 575–585.

Schmitz, K. (2019). Vulnerable child syndrome. *Pediatrics in Review*, *40*(6), 313–315.

Schonwald, A., Huntington, N., Chan, E., Risko, W., & Bridgemohan, C. (2009). Routine developmental screening implemented in urban primary care settings: More evidence of feasibility and effectiveness. *Pediatrics*, *123*(2), 660–668.

Shonkoff, J. P., Garner, A. S., Committee on Psychosocial Aspects of Child and Family Health. Committee on Early Childhood, Adoption, Dependent Care, & Section on Developmental and Behavioral Pediatrics. (2012). The lifelong effects of early childhood adversity and toxic stress. *Pediatrics*, *129*(1), e232–e246.

Shonkoff, J. P., Phillips, D. A., & National Research Council (U.S.), (2000). *From Neurons to Neighborhoods: The Science of Early Child Development*. National Academy Press.

Sirianni, N., Naidu, S., Pereira, J., Pillotto, R. F., & Hoffman, E. P. (1998). Rett syndrome: Confirmation of X-linked dominant inheritance, and localization of the gene to Xq28. *American Journal of Human Genetics*, *63*(5), 1552–1558.

Tick, B., Bolton, P., Happé, F., Rutter, M., & Rijsdijk, F. (2016). Heritability of autism spectrum disorders: A meta-analysis of twin studies. *Journal of Child Psychology and Psychiatry, and Allied Disciplines*, *57*(5), 585–595.

van den Bos, K., & Lind, E. A. (2002). Uncertainty management by means of fairness judgments. In M. P. (2002). Zanna (Ed.), *Advances in experimental social psychology* (vol. 34, pp. 1–60). Academic Press.

Walter, J. K., Hwang, J., & Fiks, A. G. (2018). Pragmatic strategies for shared decision-making. *Pediatrics*, *142*(3), S157–S162..

Weitzman, C., Wegner, L., Section on Developmental and Behavioral Pediatrics, Committee on Psychosocial Aspects of Child and Family Health, Council on Early Childhood, Society for Developmental and Behavioral Pediatrics, & American Academy of Pediatrics. (2015). Promoting optimal development: Screening for behavioral and emotional problems. *Pediatrics*, *135*(2), 384–395.

Wyatt, K. D., List, B., Brinkman, W. B., Prutsky Lopez, G., Asi, N., Erwin, P., Wang, Z., Domecq Garces, J. P., Montori, V. M., & LeBlanc, A. (2015). Shared decision making in pediatrics: A systematic review and meta-analysis. *Academic Pediatrics*, *15*(6), 573–583.

Zhang, J., Wheeler, J. J., & Richey, D. (2006). Cultural validity in assessment instruments for children with autism from a Chinese cultural perspective. *International Journal of Special Education*, *21*, 109–114.

91

Counseling and Readiness to Change

Rebecca A. Baum and Cody A. Hostutler

For additional material related to the content of this chapter, please see Chapters 92, 93, 98, and 101.

VIGNETTE

Dr. Caplan meets with the mother of Jon, a 3-year-old boy recently diagnosed with autism spectrum disorder (level 3) with accompanying intellectual disability. The diagnosis came as a surprise to his mother, Ms. Rivers, who is overwhelmed by her son's behavior. Applied behavioral analysis (ABA) was recommended, but Ms. Rivers has not yet called to begin the referral process. Jon's family has been under a lot of stress lately. Jon's father left, and Ms. Rivers recently lost her job. She wants what's best for Jon, but she feels it might be easier if she just stayed home with Jon rather than pursuing ABA.

BACKGROUND: WHY READINESS TO CHANGE MATTERS

For many clinicians, years are spent learning about evidence-based practice and the *what* behind the information we share with our patients and families. Relatively little time, in comparison, is spent on the *how,* meaning the way in which we share information. Both aspects of communication are important, but how information is communicated is especially important when the clinical concern involves some type of behavior change. Specific communication strategies, traditionally considered part of mental health practice, can potentially lead to better outcomes for patients and clinicians alike. These communication strategies represent a paradigm shift from the traditional, physician-centric model of "doctor knows best." The purpose of this chapter is to support both trainees and seasoned practitioners in the implementation of evidence-based practices that promote effective counseling and behavior change.

Dr. Caplan decides to tell Ms. Rivers about the evidence behind ABA to convince her to follow through with the ABA referral. He tells her that 40 hours/week is best, but that it's okay if they only do 25 hours/week. Ms. Rivers listens quietly and nods along, feeling guilty that she's having thoughts that this all seems too hard. She decides to stay home with Jon to avoid what seems like a complicated process yet feels bad about her choice. She doesn't schedule a follow-up visit with Dr. Caplan because she doesn't want to have to tell him about her choice.

The Transtheoretical Model

Decades ago, Prochaska and colleagues aimed to better understand how behavior change occurs. Their efforts evolved into the transtheoretical model (TTM), which captures the key elements of behavior change that transcend individual evidence-based practices (EBP; Prochaska & DiClemente, 1983). The TTM describes that change occurs across a continuum and that clinicians can help to support an individual's progress along that continuum. Moreover, research involving the TTM suggests that advice or recommendations are more likely to be followed when tailored to where the patient is on this continuum of change (Miller, 2016). Not surprisingly, patients who are "farther along" on this continuum tend to have better outcomes (Krebs, Norcross, Nicholson, & Prochaska, 2018). The TTM has been widely studied in clinical scenarios where behavior change is a necessary part of treatment (e.g., addiction, smoking cessation, obesity) (Krebs et al., 2018).

Stages of Change

As described by Prochaska, the change continuum begins at the precontemplative stage, where individuals feel that they "don't have a problem" and are content with the status quo. Individuals in the precontemplative stage who present for care may have been coerced or encouraged by external forces (e.g., the court system, referring provider, or school) rather than being internally motivated to seek care. In the contemplative stage the individual may recognize the problem but not yet feel that it is significant enough for behavior change to occur, or that behavior change is too much effort. Individuals in the preparation stage are feeling more ready to make a change, but they have not yet taken the necessary steps for change to occur; or, they may be willing to take small steps but not larger ones that may be needed for effective change to occur. In the action stage individuals are ready to make the changes necessary to modify their behavior or environment for effective change to occur. The maintenance phase refers to

TABLE 91.1 Description of the Stages of Change

Stage of Change	Description	Sample Language	Goal
Precontemplative	Problem is not yet realized; may be coerced into care	*My child doesn't have autism ... he's just a little shy.*	Increase awareness of need to change
Contemplative	Problem is recognized, but the cost of change may be too great	*I know my child has autism, but he'll probably talk when he's ready.*	Resolving ambivalence by increasing motivation and confidence in ability to change
Preparation	Individual has the intent to change but is interested mainly in small steps	*I'll start looking into ABA when I have time to see who takes our insurance.*	Work collaboratively to select appropriate goals and change strategies
Action	Individual has the intent to change and is ready to take the steps necessary	*I'm going to change my work schedule around so that we can get in 20 hours/week*	Help support consistent implementation of change strategies and monitoring of progress
Maintenance	Behavior change has occurred and change has been effective; some effort is needed to maintain gains	*We're making great progress! I just need to check in with the ABA team lead every 2 weeks to make sure we're on track*	Generalizing change strategies to anticipate future barriers and prevent relapse
Relapse	Recurrence of previous interfering behaviors	*We got off track over summer vacation. I guess it's not surprising since we were out of our routine. Back to visual schedules!*	Cope with relapse, understand it as an expected part of the change process, and resume effective change strategies

the period when effective change has occurred but ongoing attention is needed to prevent relapse or maintain the gains that occurred. Because behavior change can be hard, patients should also be counseled about how to manage the relapse stage, when previously managed behaviors recur. Prochaska's stages of change are summarized in Table 91.1.

Stages of Change and Clinical Practice

The TTM has special meaning when applied to the pediatric population. When considering behavior change in the pediatric population, clinicians may be working with parents, family members, or the children themselves. Studies in the adolescent population suggest that the TTM can be useful when considering health behavior change, such as condom use, substance use, and obesity (Crossman, 2016; Redding et al., 2014; Serafini, Shipley, & Stewart, 2016). Studies in teens with disabilities are sparse. A certain developmental level is necessary to fully engage in the stage of change process, and, similar to other aspects of health care for individuals with disabilities, the discussion should be tailored to their developmental level. Nonetheless, the TTM likely has applications when working with older children/teens, including those with disabilities, and their parents when behavior change is necessary.

Applying the TTM benefits both patients and families and also clinicians. Studies suggest that the TTM contributes to patient satisfaction and likely improves outcomes. It has been suggested that the TTM can also improve provider satisfaction and possibly reduce burnout (Pollak et al., 2016; Shute, 2019), although further study is needed.

Limitations of the Transtheoretical Model

While there are many benefits to assessing and linking counseling to a patient's readiness to change, it is not without limitations. First, clinicians may not be able to wait for readiness when urgent or safety challenges are present. For example, crisis interventions may need to be put in place prior to a patient being ready to change if there is a clear and imminent risk of harm to self or others. Second, a degree of cognitive ability and clarity is required to work through stages of change, and it may be particularly difficult to experience success when mental status is altered. Third, stages of change are not perfectly sequential, and moving from precontemplation to action is typically not accomplished within the course of a single office visit. Office visits may not occur frequently enough to maintain momentum or sustain changes in motivation. Fourth, there are sometimes barriers that exist outside the direct reach of the individual clinician or medical team (e.g., poverty, systemic racism). Despite these limitations, use of readiness to change informed approaches to counseling can save time, reduce patient and provider frustration, and strengthen the clinician-patient relationship even when immediate behavior change is out of reach.

APPLICATION TO CLINICAL PRACTICE

The TTM tells us that good advice that is poorly timed is likely not to be followed. So how can a busy clinician best tailor evidence-informed counseling to each individual patient and family? The next section provides guidance for putting the TTM into practice.

Assessing Readiness to Change

Formal measures have been developed to assess where the patient/family is in the change process. These measures may be more applicable for research or mental health clinicians and more difficult to use in a busy medical practice. Instead, the patient/family's language can help us understand where they are in the change process (see Table 91.1). A parent may appear resistant to change or content with how things are (e.g., "I got spanked when I was little, and that's how I'm raising my kids when they act out" [precontemplative]). We may hear change talk (e.g., "I'd really like to stop spanking, but I've tried everything and nothing else seems to work" [contemplative] or "I've signed up for parenting classes, and his father and I are talking about other types of parenting strategies" [preparation]). These statements invite additional discussion to clarify the individual's intent to change and steps taken so the clinician can best support the change process. Other strategies include asking patients/families about a timeline for change. Are they willing to change within 1 month, within 6 months, or more than 6 months? Those who are not willing to change within 6 months are likely to be precontemplators; contemplators are willing to change within 6 months, preparers within 1 month, and those who are already changing their behavior are in the action phase.

Jon's mother may be at the contemplative stage: She recognizes that Jon has autism and that he needs treatment, but navigating the complex process of ABA seems too daunting with all of the other things she's juggling. She may not be ready to hear about the potential complexities of establishing an ABA program. She may even be at the precontemplative stage and questioning the diagnosis of autism. If she does not agree, Dr. Caplan may need to start there before launching into a discussion about ABA. Clarifying her stage of change can help Dr. Caplan know how to move forward.

Another helpful tool in determining a person's readiness for change is a change ruler. A change ruler helps to measure patients' readiness to change by having them report on a 0–10 scale how important it is for them to make a change and how confident they feel that they can make a change. Asking these two questions can help clinicians understand what is driving each patient's stage of change. For example, two patients may both be resistant to change; however, one might find change important (8 out of 10), but has limited confidence in the ability to change (2 out of 10); the other might not believe the change to be a priority (3 out of 10), but feels confident about making the change if that is desired (8 out of 10). While both of these patients are reluctant to change, their reasoning is quite different and requires different therapeutic approaches. It is a much better use of time to talk about the *why* for the patient high in confidence, but low in importance and the *how* for the patient low in confidence.

While it is tempting to immediately ask patients low on the readiness scale why their score is not higher or what can be done to increase the score, it is important to first ask why it is greater than 0 or a number lower than the number they give you. This provides an opportunity to elicit change talk rather than reasons why change is hard. Only once you have elicited change talk does one move forward with asking what would have to happen to increase the score.

Facilitating Readiness to Change

Inherent in the TTM is the implication that the clinician's approach changes to accommodate patients and their readiness to change. Many clinicians make the mistake of assuming that if a patient or family comes to an appointment, then the patient/family is ready to make a change. That is, they assume that the patient/family is in the action phase and ready to proceed with advice and recommendations accordingly. Instead, the clinician's role may well be to identify where the patient/family is on the change continuum and aim to support the move from one stage to the next. Specific strategies can be helpful in this regard. Consciousness raising can be helpful in moving a patient or family from the precontemplative to contemplative stage. With this strategy, patients/families begin to increase their awareness of the problem and the advantages associated with change. Dramatic relief involves coming to terms with the challenges associated with the status quo. As individuals move toward contemplation and preparation, they begin to evaluate themselves through the process of self-reevaluation, finally realizing that they have the power to change their behavior, a process termed self-realization. Change is sustained during the action phase through reinforcement, and new, replacement behaviors are learned, a process called counterconditioning. Once effective change has occurred, stimulus control helps the individual maintain positive change by learning to manage triggers that may lead to relapse. Fig. 91.1 summarizes strategies that can help facilitate movement along the change continuum.

Motivational Interviewing

While the TTM provides a useful framework for understanding the stages and process of change, techniques from motivational interviewing (MI) (Miller & Rollnick, 2012) can provide specific strategies to facilitate behavior change. MI is a collaborative, patient-centered counseling approach to help patients explore and resolve ambivalence about

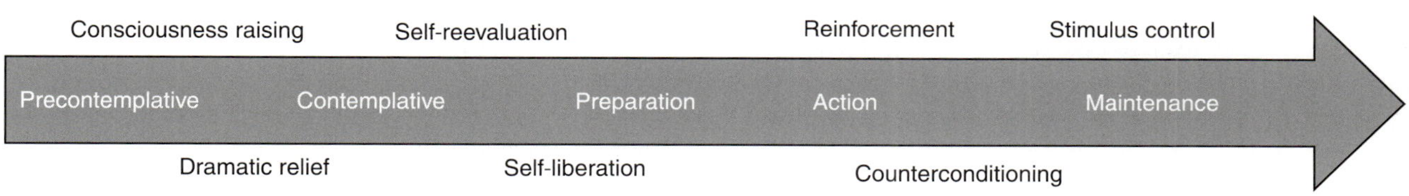

Fig. 91.1 Strategies to facilitate movement along the change continuum.

making change. The overarching approach, or spirit, of MI focuses on collaboration, evocation, and patient autonomy. In addition to understanding specific MI tools, embracing the overarching spirit of MI is important, as it is best understood as a style of communicating rather than a checklist or protocol of questions. Implementing both specific MI tools in the context of this overall spirit of collaboration and autonomy will help clinicians best apply these communication strategies flexibly across a variety of situations. Table 91.2 illustrates how this approach differs from traditional medical practice.

Guiding Principles

Four guiding principles—resisting the righting reflex, understanding patient motivations, listening to the patient, and empowering the patient—can help clinicians stay true to the spirit of MI. The righting reflex refers to the tendency to tell patients what to do. It may feel earned from years of school or an inherent part of the patient/provider hierarchy, but it can reduce patient autonomy and marginalize patients' preferences and opinions. Instead, clinicians are encouraged to elicit and attempt to understand their patients' desire to change and to maintain the status quo. This involves actively listening to what patients say, including their nonverbal communication, specific wording, and what they chose to share or not share. Ultimately it is the patient's decision to make a change. For example, rather than stating the health benefits of stopping smoking to encourage a patient to quit, a better approach may be to understand the patient's motivation, barriers, and previous attempts. The guidance can then be framed in that context: "It sounds like you've tried to quit smoking before, and you're really motivated to try again. Would it be okay if we talked about some strategies that have been helpful for some of my other patients?" The spirit of MI is built upon the foundational belief that the clinician's role is to help support behavior change by empowering patients to make changes that are meaningful to them.

OARS (Open-Ended Questions, Affirmations, Reflective Listening, Summary Statements)

The OARS acronym (open-ended questions, affirmations, reflective listening, summary statements) illustrates specific tools that can be used when talking with families that are consistent with the overall spirit of MI.

Strategic use of open-ended questions can help obtain information that is more accurate and complete. For example, asking, "You haven't been having any sad feelings lately, have you?" is not likely going to elicit the same information as "How have you been feeling lately?" Further, closed questions (e.g., yes or no) lead to a forced choice, and when patients and families are ambivalent about change, a closed question may force them into a no and miss opportunities to elicit, explore, and build upon any ambivalence that may be present. For example, if Dr. Caplan asks Ms. Rivers whether she is willing to start ABA therapy and she is having reservations, she

TABLE 91.2 Comparing Aspects of the Spirit of Motivational Interviewing With Traditional Medical Care

	Motivational Interviewing	Traditional Medical Care
Sample language	**Collaboration** Assumes provider needs to partner with patient to understand and build a patient's own desire to change. *Let's figure out together how we can find a therapist who will work well with you and your child.*	**Righting Reflex** Assumes a patient's perspective is impaired and needs corrected and persuaded. *You need to start counseling to work on your parenting skills for your child to get better.*
Sample language	**Evocation** Providers seek to activate patients' own motivation for change by eliciting their own reasons for change. The provider then links the behavior change to things the patients care about. *What would it take for you to consider starting a medication for ADHD? I'm wondering about how things might go at your job if you keep having to pick him up from school?*	**Education** Patient is presumed to lack the insight, education, or skills needed to make a change, and the provider needs to tell the patient what to do. *Your child will keep getting in trouble at school unless you start him on medication. Research has shown us that stimulant medications are the most effective treatment.*
Sample language	**Patient Autonomy** Assumes that behavior change is ultimately up to the patient and has right and freedom not to change. *It sounds like you have some concerns about starting a stimulant medication. Would it be okay if we talk about the pros and cons of this type of medication, then see if we can make a decision about what's best?*	**Provider Authority** Assumes that the provider is the expert, and that patients need to adhere to providers recommendations. *There are other ADHD medications besides stimulants, but they aren't as effective. I know you've heard about side effects from these medications, but they're still the most effective. That's what I recommend.*

will likely answer "no," whereas asking for her thoughts on ABA therapy will allow her to discuss the ambivalence she is experiencing.

Affirmations are statements that recognize the patient/family strengths and link them to values or behaviors that lead to the desired change, no matter how big or small. To be effective, affirmations should be genuine and congruent with the patient's actual behavior. A useful equation for effective affirmations is: You + Behavior = Positive trait or Sign of motivation. It is best to start affirmations with "You ..." rather than "I ..." as it focuses more on the behavior, values, and desire to change within the patient rather than being more about the clinician's approval. For example, instead of Dr. Caplan telling Ms. Rivers, "I appreciate you coming to this appointment to discuss treatment options," it would be more effective for him to say, "You coming to this appointment shows how much you care about getting Jon the help he needs."

Reflective listening serves two primary purposes: (1) checking to make sure your understanding is accurate and (2) demonstrating to the patient and family that you heard and understood them. Reflections can also help highlight ambivalence, elicit further change talk, and help to prevent time-consuming and unhelpful cycles of communication where the clinician repeatedly provides education to convince the family of something, while the family continues to repeat their concern in response without moving forward. There are many types of reflections, some being simple and others complex (Table 91.3).

Summary statements can be helpful at the start of a visit, reviewing previous visits and establishing consensus; to end a visit, reviewing shared goals and next steps; and to transition the conversation, reviewing agreed-upon reasons for change. It is helpful to begin by indicating you are using a summary and to check to make sure the patient agrees with your summary: "To summarize our last visit ... is that right?"; "Let me see if I understand so far ..."; "So, what I've heard from you is ..., have I missed anything?" Like reflections, summaries can be simple and restate the primary themes, or they can be complex by drawing pieces of the current and previous conversations together to move the conversation forward or to emphasize ambivalence or desire for change. Summaries can also serve as a gentle way to mark the end of a listening period and on to the next task.

Change Talk

To help facilitate behavior change, clinicians can use specific questions that help to elicit a patient's motivation for change. Through active listening, clinicians will also be able to hear certain language from their patients that can be amplified to help move them along the change continuum. Table 91.4 summarizes the DARN-CAT mnemonic to help clinicians remember the various aspects of change talk: desire, ability, reason, need, commitment, action, and taking steps. In traditional medical care we often assume that desire to change is all that is needed. In fact, it is farther down the change continuum. For example, ability to change is more urgent than desire and demonstrates higher-level commitment to change than desire alone. Matching change talk to stages of change and providing advice accordingly provides the best opportunity for success for patients and clinicians alike.

TABLE 91.3 Types of Reflections

Simple Reflections: Simple reflections add little meaning or emphasis to the original statement		
	Description	**Sample Language**
Repeat	Simply restates	Patient: "I think I want to start taking my medication again." Clinician: "You think you want to start taking your medication again."
Rephrase		Patient: "I think I want to start taking my medication again." Clinician: "You're thinking it might be helpful to start taking your medication again."
Complex Reflections: Complex reflections extend the meaning or elicit change talk		
Reframing	Offering a new interpretation	Patient: "I've tried counseling a hundred times before and it never works." Clinician: "You have made so many attempts, it sounds like getting better is really important to you and you haven't found the therapist or type of therapy that works for you yet."
Double sided	Reflects both sides of a patient's ambivalence	"*On one hand*, you would like to start occupational therapy; *on the other hand*, you worry about finding the time for it."
Amplified	Exaggeratedly reflecting what the patient says to elicit the other side	Grandmother: "No one at the school cares about my grandson." Clinician: "It sounds like every single person at the school is hoping that your grandson fails." Grandmother: "Well, I don't think they want him to fail, especially not his special education teacher, but I think they are just too busy to do what is right."

TABLE 91.4 **DARN-CAT Mnemonic for Change Talk**

	Language to Elicit Change Talk (Clinician)	Change Talk (Patient/Family)
Desire	*Why do you want to make this change?*	*I want to …* *I wish that …* *It would be nice if …*
Ability	*How might you be able to do it?*	*I can …* *I could …* *I am able to …*
Reason	*What is one good reason to make a change?*	*If I __, then __.*
Need	*What do you need to make this change?*	*I'll need to do __ to make it happen.*
Commitment	*What do you intend to do?*	*I'm planning to ...*
Action	*What are you ready to do?*	*I'm in the process of ...*
Taking Steps	*What have you done?*	*I've already ...*

Dr. Caplan decides to explore Ms. Rivers ambivalence about ABA by asking open-ended questions while also listening for change talk. Dr. Caplan learns that Ms. Rivers wants to do what's best for Jon, but she's worried that she won't be able to navigate the insurance issues surrounding ABA. She wants to spend time with him and worries that 25 hours/week would not give her much time with Jon. She does not want to let him down, and she also has a lot on her plate. Dr. Caplan uses a double-sided reflection to highlight the ambivalence:

Dr. Caplan: On one hand, you're worried that setting up ABA seems like a complex process and that it may take valuable time away from you and Jon; on the other hand, it seems like you want to do what is best for Jon and realize there might be some benefits to starting ABA. Do I have that right?

Ms. Rivers: Yes, that's right.

Dr. Caplan: I have an idea that might help us get the best of both worlds. Would you be interested in connecting with our family navigator? She's been through the process, and she can talk with you about what it was like and how she balanced finding time with her child while getting him involved in ABA.

Ms. Rivers: It would really help to hear from another parent. I'd really like that—it would make me feel like I'm making an informed decision.

Dr. Caplan: Great! I'll get that set up, and then maybe we can check in again after your conversation.

PUTTING IT ALL TOGETHER

For busy clinicians, time is an often-cited barrier to effective communication. The TTM and MI can be used successfully in a busy practice with just a few modifications in the way clinicians take a history, ask questions, and provide advice. The following framework can be used as a reminder to implement strategies that encompass the *how* of facilitating behavior change:

1. Engage: use open-ended questions, affirmations, reflective listening, and summary statements
2. Focus: help set the agenda for the visit by incorporating what's important to the patient/family
3. Evoke: reinforce change talk and amplify the case for change
4. Plan: focus on how to make change happen

Learning and successfully implementing these techniques takes training and practice. Resources are available to support both trainees and seasoned professionals in learning these skills. Brief videos on MI in pediatric practice are available at https://www.aap.org/en-us/advocacy-and-policy/aap-health-initiatives/Mental-Health/Pages/motivational-interviewing.aspx. Courses of varying lengths are available at the Motivational Interviewing Network of Trainers, https://motivationalinterviewing.org/, and both informal and formal training can be accessed through a variety of resources. Graduate medical education programs are beginning to incorporate TTM and MI as a component of evidence-based practice, but an increased emphasis on training, practice opportunities, and ongoing feedback is likely needed to ensure competence (Hauer, Carney, Chang, & Satterfield, 2012; Pollak et al., 2015).

REFERENCES

Crossman, J. M. (2016). Planning, practising and prioritising wellness through an integrative behaviour change plan. *Health Education Journal*, *75*(7), 823–832. https://doi.org/10.1177/0017896916629171

Hauer, K. E., Carney, P. A., Chang, A., & Satterfield, J. (2012). Behavior change counseling curricula for medical trainees: A systematic review. *Academic Medicine*, *87*(7), 956–968. https://doi.org/10.1097/ACM.0b013e31825837be

Howard, K. R. (2007). Childhood overweight: Parental perceptions and readiness for change. *The Journal of School Nursing*, *23*(2), 73–79. https://doi.org/10.1177/10598405070230020301

Krebs, P., Norcross, J. C., Nicholson, J. M., & Prochaska, J. O. (2018). Stages of change and psychotherapy outcomes: A review and meta-analysis. *Journal of Clinical Psychology*, *74*(11), 1964–1979. https://doi.org/10.1002/jclp.22683

Miller, K. L. (2016). Patient centered care: A path to better health outcomes through engagement and activation. *NeuroRehabilitation*, *39*(4), 465–470. https://doi.org/10.3233/nre-161378

Miller, W. R., & Rollnick, S. (2012). *Motivational interviewing: Helping people change*. Guilford Press.

Pollak, P. I., Nagy, P., Bigger, J., Bilheimer, A., Lyna, P., Gao, X., … Armstrong, S. (2016). Effect of teaching motivational interviewing via communication coaching on clinician and patient satisfaction in primary care and pediatric obesity-focused offices. *Patient Education and Counseling*, *99*(2), 300–303. https://doi.org/10.1016/j.pec.2015.08.013

Prochaska, J., & DiClemente, C. (1983). Stages and processes of self-change in smoking: Towards an integrative model of change. *Journal of Consulting and Clinical Psychology*, *5*, 390–395.

Redding, C. A., Prochaska, J. O., Armstrong, K., Rossi, J. S., Hoeppner, B. B., Sun, X., … Velicer, W. F. (2014). Randomized trial outcomes of a TTM-tailored condom use and smoking intervention in urban adolescent females. *Health Education Research*, *30*(1), 162–178. https://doi.org/10.1093/her/cyu015

Serafini, K., Shipley, L., & Stewart, D. G. (2016). Motivation and substance use outcomes among adolescents in a school-based intervention. *Addictive Behaviors*, *53*, 74–79. https://doi.org/10.1016/j.addbeh.2015.10.004

Shute, D. (2019). Motivational interviewing: Benefits and advice for busy physicians. *Contemporary OB/GYN*, *64*(10), 38–40.

92

Common Factors and Lifestyle Interventions

Jeremy Kruger and Larry Wissow

For additional material related to the content of this chapter, please see Chapters 35, 67, 70, and 91.

VIGNETTE

Nick is a 10-year-old boy with difficult-to-control asthma and significant anxiety around bedtime as a result of some past asthma exacerbations at night, who is seen with his single mother. His mother reports that Nick has had more breakthrough episodes and some nighttime awakenings that are hard to distinguish between either respiratory issues or anxiety. Nick has started asking his mother to wait for him to fall asleep in case he stops breathing, and she has resisted his request to sleep in her room. Nick has stopped participating in soccer due to fear of having a major asthma attack and dying; instead, he is spending more time alone in his room playing video games. In response to an inquiry about other family stressors, his mother reports that her elderly father had a stroke. Though he is now recovering, she has had to split her care-taking time between her child and her parents.

Children frequently need care for long-standing behavioral, emotional, and medical problems with indeterminant or multifactorial causes. In this situation treatment may need to target mechanisms that are believed to mediate symptoms across a range of potential diagnoses. In this chapter we discuss two clusters of these treatments, one based on psychotherapeutic interactions and one based on lifestyle factors.

COMMON FACTOR SKILLS DERIVED FROM PSYCHOTHERAPY

The term 'common factors' refers to the finding that certain approaches influencing outcomes are included across psychotherapies (Karver, Handelsman, Fields, & Bickman, 2005), suggesting that they provide a foundation for therapeutic relationships. The common factors include the development of a positive bond between the patient and provider, agreement on the goals and methods of care, and patient perceptions that the provider is genuine, empathetic, and providing hope. Variation in use of common factors contributes more to outcomes than do differences between therapies or therapists' adherence to a particular protocol (Laska, Gurman, & Wampold, 2014). Common factors also play a role in pharmacotherapy outcomes (De Nadai et al., 2017).

The interactional style involved in common factors overlaps with the style of motivational interviewing (see Chapter 91) and other approaches to individuals struggling with complex decisions (Miller & Rollnick, 1992). The style addresses situations with strong emotional overlays where ambivalence, demoralization, and anger can create barriers to collaboration. Providers create a setting where family concerns can be expressed, where families take the lead in developing goals and the strategies to attain them, and where information offered corresponds to families' expressed needs.

In the following paragraphs we divide common factor-related skills into four groups corresponding to four goals for individual visits and longitudinal relationships.

Identifying Treatment Goals

Clinicians must first communicate an understanding of the patient or parent(s) concerns. Patient/parent(s) will feel reassured that their problems have been accurately described, "make sense to someone else," and can be helped in some way. Opportunity is given to disclose a full range of concerns, including safety issues. In the process the clinician and patient/parent come to agreement on the most important concerns, allowing the clinician to offer the most specific and credible advice.

Essential Skills

- Use open-ended questions, ask about psychosocial issues even for established patients, and ask "anything else" before settling on an agenda for the visit.
- Actively involve all parties to the visit; ensure that all get a chance to contribute to agenda setting.
- Tactfully redirect conversation, if it rambles, through summarizing, making lists, and asking for priorities.
- Reframe or normalize the story so that it fits with a helpful and hopeful paradigm with a direct relationship to a possible treatment plan.

Reducing Patient and Parent Levels of Distress and Conflict (At Least Temporarily)

Families frequently express negative emotions during the visit. Managing these feelings is important in building the therapeutic relationship.

Essential Skills

- Use turn taking.
- Reinterpret negative feelings as concern, offering empathy for people who are angry or hurt.

- Ask speakers to rephrase statements that propose negative generalizations or attribute behavior to negative traits about the patient or family member.
- Promptly address "ruptures" in the relationship with the patient/parent: Apologize for miscues and restate commitment to alliance.

Immediate Relief

When families come for complex problems, considerable time can be spent gathering diagnostic information and ordering evaluations whose results will not be known for some time. Families should be able to leave each visit with at least one thing that they can do to improve the problem even if only in a small way or for the short term. Initial suggestions often include interventions that are likely to be helpful across many different eventual diagnoses (e.g., managing a parenting issue or conflict; improving sleep, activity, or diet). They may also include more condition-specific advice such as development of a behavior plan, counseling, referral, medication, or developing an emergency or crisis intervention plan. Ideally, they directly address the family's priority issue and involve a tactic that the family has identified as likely to succeed.

Essential Skills

- Manage requests for advice in a way that takes into account the patient's and parent's stage of willingness to take action (see Chapter 91), concerns about barriers, and attitudes toward particular actions. Elicit patient/parent's ideas about actions and present lists of options incorporating patient/parent's ideas rather than a single standardized "prescription."
- *If advice is not requested overtly by patient/parent*, ask for permission to give it (e.g., "Is it okay to discuss how your divorce may be impacting your child's behavior?").
- *If patient/parent feel unsure or hopeless that actions can help*: Quantify confidence that action can be taken. Ask what would improve hope even just a bit. When possible, point out past successes, and collaboratively think about the circumstances in which they occurred and how they might be replicated. Identify exceptions to the problem when things did work out. Make vague goals into specific goals that can measured and achieved in small steps.
- *If patient/parent is ambivalent or rejecting of advice*: "Roll with resistance" rather than confronting or avoiding it. Ask patient/parent to clarify the importance of the problem and ask what would increase importance. Explore pros and cons of action. Ask for permission to give more information or advice, and solicit their reaction to what you have said. Elicit larger goals and ask tactfully how current behavior fits with goals.

Agreement on Next Steps

By the end of the visit, the goal is for the patient/parent and clinician to agree on steps that will be taken to develop a differential diagnosis and longer-term treatment plan (repeat visit, results of referral, etc.) if that becomes necessary.

Essential Skills

- Work to clearly understand treatment goals from the patient/parent perspective. How will you track attainment of those goals?
- Explore barriers to any plans (logistic, financial, cultural, linguistic, or concerns from others in the family). What assistance might the family need to be able to move on to these next steps?
- Assure continuity and means of contact. How can the family get back in touch with you or your office/clinic to troubleshoot advice or in a crisis?
- To the extent possible, pledge your ongoing partnership as treatment goes on.

Using Common Factor Skills in Developing Collaborations That Support Families

In addition to working with families, clinicians often need to work effectively with other providers and agencies to create individualized systems of care. Principles from the common factor skills can aid in developing these systems, too. Both medical home standards and guidelines for integrated care emphasize processes required to achieve integration and coordination among collaborating providers, including creating registries, tracking referrals, and developing mechanisms for communication of patient information (http://uwaims.org; http://integrationacademy.ahrq.gov/atlas/frameworkIBHC). However, while setting up structures and processes are important, relationships are most critical to successful collaborative patient care. For example, a state program designed to support primary care providers' ability to help families with children's mental health concerns developed a telephone "warm line" that primary care providers called for assistance. One of the factors that promoted primary care providers' willingness to call was face-to-face training from child mental health specialists. Familiarity with the specialists overcame primary care providers' fears that they would appear uninformed or unskilled (Gadomski et al., 2014).

LIFESTYLE FACTORS RELATED TO MENTAL HEALTH

While psychotherapy and/or medication typically form the backbone of mental health treatment, lifestyle affects primary, secondary, and tertiary prevention of mental health problems. Interventions that increase physical activity and improve sleep and diet can influence development, treatment, and prognosis. Similar to the common factor interviewing techniques, these interventions are often effective across multiple diagnoses and thus may be appropriate recommendations for initial intervention even if the diagnosis is uncertain. Evidence for the benefit of each of these types of lifestyle changes is detailed in this section.

Physical Activity

The US Department of Health and Human Services (DHHS; 2018) advises children and adolescents between ages 6 and 17 years to engage in at least 60 minutes of physical activity per day, mostly of moderate to vigorous aerobic intensity, with at least 3 days per week involving muscle/bone-strengthening activity. Sedentary behavior in youth is associated with increased mood problems and lower psychological wellbeing (e.g., life satisfaction and happiness; Rodriguez-Ayllon et al., 2019). While the exact amount of physical activity needed to confer mental health benefits is unclear, most recommendations suggest at least 45 minutes daily, including 3 to 5 days of moderate to vigorous aerobic activity. Unfortunately, among US high school students, only 20% meet these guidelines (Hosker, Elkins, & Potter, 2019).

The relationship between physical activity and mental health can be understood through neurobiologic and psychological lenses. Exercise increases levels of brain-derived neurotrophic factor (BDNF), a neurotrophin thought to enhance neuroplasticity, neural connectivity, and angiogenesis, in turn playing important roles in cognition, learning, and memory (de Azevedo et al., 2020) while reducing depression and anxiety (Martinowich, Manji, & Lu, 2007). Physical activity can further modulate dopamine, serotonin, norepinephrine, endorphins, endocannabinoids, inflammatory and oxidative stress, and the hypothalamic-pituitary-adrenal axis. Psychologically, exercise can serve to improve self-concept, autonomy, mastery, resilience, and distress tolerance (Hosker et al., 2019; Rodriguez-Ayllon et al., 2019).

Setting habits and expectations toward more active lifestyles while young can increase likelihood of active lifestyles later in life. However, broad recommendations to increase physical activity are unlikely to yield much behavioral change. Supervised exercise interventions provide more step-by-step guidance, accountability, and potentially social interactions. They can also be helpful for children with atypical development or physical disabilities, who are more likely to be inactive and may need the added support of a physical activity professional. Sports participation, particularly team sports, is associated with improved mental health and may be preferable for many youth over nonsport exercise (Hosker et al., 2019). Sports offer opportunities for pleasure, social connectedness, and self-discipline. On a systems level, incorporating regular physical activity into existing community institutions such as school settings and after-school programs may confer the greatest benefit to the larger population (Firth, Solmi, et al., 2020).

Mood and Anxiety Problems

Across age, gender, and geographic regions around the world, physical activity has been shown to be protective against depression (Schuch et al., 2018). Similarly, exercise can attenuate symptoms of anxiety in children and adolescents, particularly social anxiety. Among adolescents and young adults, higher levels of activity are associated with lower odds of hopelessness, suicidal ideation, suicide attempts, and nonsuicidal self-injury (Boone & Brausch, 2016; Hosker et al., 2019). Physical activity moderates the relationship between depressive symptoms and self-harming behaviors, though less so for those who are primarily motivated to exercise for appearance or weight concerns. Furthermore, obesity can have a significant negative impact on mood and self-image (see Chapter 67). While many of these findings relate to longer-term outcomes of exercise, intense exercise is one of many skills taught in dialectical-behavioral therapy to manage acute moments of distress and in turn reduce self-destructive behaviors (Linehan, 2015). The European Psychiatric Association and the Royal Australian and New Zealand College of Psychiatrists recommend exercise as a first-line treatment for depression, one to implement even before pharmacotherapy or psychotherapy (Firth et al., 2020b). As symptoms of depression and anxiety frequently include fatigue, avoidance, and social isolation, sedentary behavior often predominates, so influencing behavioral change can be challenging yet paramount in breaking the cycle.

Attention and Behavior Problems

In general, exercise is associated with cognitive and academic benefits, including improved learning, memory, attention, and processing speed, as well as greater school achievement and fewer disruptive behaviors in the classroom (Hosker et al., 2019; Khalife et al., 2014). In children with attention-deficit/hyperactivity disorder (ADHD), a single bout of physical activity can modulate attention, vigilance, and impulsivity. Longer-term benefits include those on core ADHD symptoms, executive functioning, and social-emotional functioning. In studies of exercise interventions for children with ADHD those that were sports based had the lowest dropout rates, suggesting that perhaps sports were more engaging to sustain attention and motivation (Vancampfort et al., 2016).

Neurodevelopmental Disorders

Children with autism spectrum disorder (ASD) and other neurodevelopmental disabilities on average engage in less physical activity than neurotypical youth (Srinivasan, Pescatello, & Bhat, 2014), yet they stand to benefit from physical activity across multiple domains. In addition to improvements in physical health such as decreased risk for obesity, exercise in youths with ASD can improve hyperactivity, disruptive behaviors, aggressive or self-injurious behaviors, stereotypies, sleep, academic performance, interpersonal relations, and gross motor coordination. Collaboration with any involved family, caregivers, special educators, and physical and occupational therapists can serve to maximize uptake of physical activity with associated long-term benefits.

Psychosis and Substance Use Problems

Adolescents who exercise more tend to have lower levels of alcohol, marijuana, and cigarette use (Hosker et al., 2019). Less data exist to show the influence of physical activity on psychotic disorders, particularly in youths, though some studies suggest that increased physical activity reduces risk of incident psychosis (Firth et al., 2020b). Adolescents who develop a psychotic illness tend to exhibit less physical activity and poorer cardiorespiratory fitness. Moreover, second-generation antipsychotics are known to increase risk of adiposity and insulin resistance, thereby emphasizing exercise as a necessity to maintain physical health.

TABLE 92.1 Examples of Aerobic, Muscle-, and Bone-Strengthening Physical Activities for Children and Adolescents

Type of Physical Activity	Preschool-Age Children	School-Age Children	Adolescents
Moderate-intensity aerobic	• Games such as tag or follow the leader • Playing on a playground • Tricycle or bicycle riding • Walking, running, skipping, jumping, dancing • Swimming • Playing games that require catching, throwing, and kicking • Gymnastics or tumbling	• Brisk walking • Bicycle riding • Active recreation, such as hiking, riding a scooter without a motor, swimming • Playing games that require catching and throwing, such as baseball and softball	• Brisk walking • Bicycle riding • Active recreation, such as kayaking, hiking, swimming • Playing games that require catching and throwing, such as baseball and softball • House and yard work, such as sweeping or pushing a lawn mower • Some videogames that include continuous movement
Vigorous-intensity aerobic	• Games such as tag or follow the leader • Playing on a playground • Tricycle or bicycle riding • Walking, running, skipping, jumping, dancing • Swimming • Playing games that require catching, throwing, and kicking • Gymnastics or tumbling	• Running • Bicycle riding • Active games involving running and chasing, such as tag or flag football • Jumping rope • Cross-country skiing • Sports such as soccer, basketball, swimming, tennis • Martial arts • Vigorous dancing	• Running • Bicycle riding • Active games involving running and chasing, such as flag football • Jumping rope • Cross-country skiing • Sports such as soccer, basketball, swimming, tennis • Martial arts • Vigorous dancing
Muscle strengthening	• Games such as tug of war • Climbing on playground equipment • Gymnastics	• Games such as tug of war • Resistance exercises using body weight or resistance bands • Rope or tree climbing • Climbing on playground equipment • Some forms of yoga	• Games such as tug of war • Resistance exercises using body weight, resistance bands, weight machines, handheld weights • Some forms of yoga
Bone strengthening	• Hopping, skipping, jumping • Jumping rope • Running • Gymnastics	• Hopping, skipping, jumping • Jumping rope • Running • Sports that involve jumping or rapid change in direction	• Jumping rope • Running • Sports that involve jumping or rapid change in direction

From US Department of Health & Human Services. (2018). *Physical activity guidelines for Americans* (2nd ed.). https://health.gov/sites/default/files/2019-09/Physical_Activity_Guidelines_2nd_edition.pdf

Assessment

In any child, particularly those at higher risk of mental health problems, clinicians should first review with the patient/parent the type, frequency, duration, and intensity of physical activity in which the child is already engaging. Assessing their preferred modes of physical activity, preferences for independent activities versus those with peers, and any obstacles that are interfering with activity can be informative. In particular, competing activities such as screen time, social barriers, logistical barriers (e.g., environmental, transportation, time limitations), or medical/physical disabilities are vital to bring forward. Conversely, any concerns that an individual may be exercising too much, as may be seen in eating disorders, should give the clinician pause in recommending a vigorous exercise regimen.

Recommendations

Recommendations should start according to the child's activity preferences and abilities to maximize long-term adherence—generally speaking, those activities that the child finds most enjoyable are most likely to be continued. The amount of activity should typically start low and go slow in increasing duration, frequency, and intensity. Starting with easily achievable goals (e.g., walking for a few minutes) that are mutually agreed upon by the patient may make uptake more likely. Providers should advise replacement of sedentary activities (e.g., screen time) for physical activities with peers or family whenever possible (Hosker et al., 2019). Table 92.1 provides a menu of activities to consider by age group.

TABLE 92.2 Duration of Sleep Needed by Age Group

Age	Sleep Duration in Hours
4–12 mo	12–16 (including naps)
1–2 yr	11–14 (including naps)
3–5 yr	10–13 (including naps)
6–12 yr	9–12
13–18 yr	8–10

Based on Paruthi, S., Brooks, L. J., D'Ambrosio, C., Hall, W. A., Kotagal, S., Lloyd, R. M., Malow, B. A., Maski, K., Nichols, C., Quan, S. F., Rosen, C. L., Troester, M. M., & Wise, M. S. (2016). Recommended amount of sleep for pediatric populations: A consensus statement of the American Academy of Sleep Medicine. *Journal of Clinical Sleep Medicine, 12*(6), 785–786. https://doi.org/10.5664/jcsm.5866

Sleep

The causes, assessment, and recommendations for sleep problems are discussed in detail in Chapter 70 and are thus discussed only briefly here. The American Academy of Sleep Medicine (Paruthi et al., 2016) recommendations for amount of sleep for each age group are shown in Table 92.2. An estimated 60% of middle school students and 70% to 75% of high school students get less sleep than clinically advised. Contributing factors to inadequate sleep are multifactorial, including screen use, caffeine intake, academic and extracurricular demands, early school start times, and social engagements (Owens et al., 2014). Many psychiatric disorders themselves can impair sleep, including depression, anxiety, bipolar disorder, ADHD, and neurodevelopmental disorders. Confounding medical conditions, neurologic sleep disorders, substance use, and medication side effects can also play a role.

Insufficient sleep is linked to a number of physical problems across the life span, including hypertension, obesity, diabetes, and risk of accidents and injuries. From a neuropsychiatric standpoint, sleep deficiency can contribute to problems in attention, behavior, and learning, as well as depression, suicidal ideation, suicide attempts, and self-harm (Paruthi et al., 2016). Sleep and psychiatric symptoms often have a bidirectional relationship, where many disorders can underlie sleep problems, while sleep problems can exacerbate mental health problems.

Improving sleep has been shown to help with mood, attention, behavior, learning, memory, academic performance, emotion regulation, self-esteem, self-acceptance, optimism, quality of life, and mental and physical wellness (Firth et al., 2020b; Hosker et al., 2019; Paruthi et al., 2016). The Canadian 24-Hour Movement Guidelines for Children and Youth (age 5–17 years) advise sleep durations consistent with Table 92.2, in combination with 60+ minutes of physical activity and less than 2 hours of screen time. Youths who adhered to all three of these domains had improved mental health outcomes, particularly in depression and anxiety, with a possible incremental dose effect for each of the three (Sampasa-Kanyinga et al., 2020). Thus while physical activity is strongly tied with mental health outcomes as previously described, there seems to be an additive benefit with adequate sleep.

Diet/Nutrition

The majority of Americans do not follow a healthy diet pattern, and 41% of children and adolescents in the United States are overweight or obese (US Department of Agriculture [USDA] & DHHS, 2020). With increasing trends toward obesity across the Western world, there has been an increased focus on how dietary patterns can affect physical and mental health throughout the life span (see Chapter 67).

Mood and Anxiety Problems

Several studies have demonstrated correlation between unhealthy diet in childhood and adolescence with poorer mental health, as well as some weaker evidence that healthy diet is associated with better mental health, especially regarding depression and anxiety (Khalid, Williams, & Reynolds, 2016; O'Neil et al., 2014;). The definition of "healthy" varies but generally emphasizes intake of high-nutrient foods such as fruits, vegetables, and fish, while limiting foods high in saturated fat, refined carbohydrates/sugar, processed foods, and sweetened beverages. Patterns of food variety, adequacy, moderation, and balance, as well as regularity of meal consumption may also be considered when judging healthy versus unhealthy. In some adult-based literature some specific dietary patterns, including a Mediterranean-style diet, a low-inflammatory index diet, low glycemic index, or one rich in omega-3 fatty acids and other polyunsaturated fatty acids, confer a reduced risk of depression. Likewise, higher consumption of sugar-sweetened beverages is associated with greater risk of depression (Firth et al., 2020a, 2020b).

Proposed explanations to link diet and mental health are broad (Firth et al., 2020a; O'Neil et al., 2014): (1) The placebo effect may apply, as how one sees the quality of their diet may have an influence on their mood and mental wellbeing, and similarly, guilt about eating patterns can negatively impact one's mental state. (2) Reverse causation is possible—that is, those with internalizing symptoms may eat more poorly as a form of self-medication or stress relief with comfort foods, or may put less care into what they eat or don't eat. Indeed, a core symptom of depression is change in appetite and eating patterns, and classically the atypical variant of depression features craving of simple carbohydrates along with hypersomnia. (3) With increased consumption of carbohydrates, the body's compensatory response to lower plasma glucose (e.g., insulin release) may then overshoot and influence a stress response involving an increase in cortisol, adrenaline, growth hormone, and glucagon that all may influence anxiety and irritability. (4) Nutritional deficiencies may influence mental illnesses, particularly folate, zinc, magnesium, and omega-3 fatty acids, though targeted supplementation has not yielded consistently positive results in prevention or treatment of mental illness. (5) In animal models high-fat, high-refined sugar diet is associated with a reduction in BDNF, neuronal plasticity, and learning (Molteni, Barnard, Ying, Roberts, & Gómez-Pinilla, 2002), in contrast to the enhancing effects of physical activity on these systems as described earlier. (6) Dietary-induced inflammation may contribute to depression, and similarly the microbiome may serve as a mediator to this process. This is an emerging field, and translational clinical outcomes remain limited (Firth et al., 2020a; O'Neil et al., 2014). (7) Socioeconomic factors likely serve as a strong mediator between diet and mental health, where financial, geographic, educational, and time barriers to maintaining a healthy diet can disproportionally affect those with mental illness, and socioeconomic stressors can directly impact mental health.

Attention and Hyperactivity Problems

A large-scale cross-sectional study in Germany (van Egmond-Fröhlich, Weghuber, & de Zwaan, 2012) demonstrated significant associations between ADHD symptoms and low dietary quality and high caloric intake, particularly in girls. Specific dietary interventions have been examined, with limited positive outcomes. Although some studies suggest that children with ADHD may benefit from some types of elimination diets (Firth, Solmi, et al., 2020; Pelsser, Frankena, Toorman, & Rodrigues Pereira, 2017), there is not currently sufficient evidence to recommend dietary intervention to treat ADHD.

Neurodevelopmental Disabilities

Children with ASD and other neurodevelopmental disorders frequently demonstrate food selectivity, with strong preferences for some foods and aversions to others, and many may not take in adequate nutritional requirements. The microbiome and nutrition-related factors are speculated to play a role in some autistic symptoms. Gluten-free/casein-free diets, ketogenic diets, and use of pre- and probiotics have shown inconsistent results in their effect on ASD symptoms, and these studies tend to lack methodologic strength. Thus there is not sufficient evidence to recommend these interventions (Peretti et al., 2019). Likewise, the data around specific nutritional deficiencies' influence on behavioral symptoms remains equivocal. Children with ASD are at higher risk of iron deficiency, which influences motor, behavioral, and cognitive development. Routine screening of iron levels in individuals with ASD may be beneficial. Overall, dietary and nutritional interventions for children with neurodevelopmental disorders do not have a strong evidence base beyond typical recommendations for a healthy diet.

Assessment

In evaluating dietary patterns clinicians should ask children and caregivers what, with whom, when, where, and why children are eating, as shown in Table 92.3.

Recommendations

The USDA and DHHS outline specific dietary guidelines discussed in Chapter 35. In practice, clinicians should shift the focus from "what not to eat" to "what to eat," to gradually promote healthful choices and not prompt undereating. As children and adolescents face increased energy and growth requirements compared to adults, calorie restriction and intermittent fasting are not advised. Caution should also be lent toward those at risk of eating disorders, and for anyone

TABLE 92.3 Questions for Evaluation of Dietary Patterns

What	Types and variety of foods/beverages (e.g., nutrient-dense foods vs. calorically dense, processed or fast foods, and those high in sugar, sodium, and saturated fats), food aversions/pickiness, and any vitamins/supplements
With whom	How often children are eating with family/caregivers vs. alone? What are the dietary patterns of family members?
When	Number of meals and snacks per day. Do they eat breakfast? Timing of meals in the day/night.
Where	Is there a safe, comfortable, and consistent dining place? How often do they eat in vs. go out? Are there screens or other distractors present?
Why	Eating for nourishment, satiate hunger or cravings, enjoyment, comfort, and/or management of emotion, stress, or boredom

Adapted from Hosker, D. K., Elkins, R. M., & Potter, M. P. (2019). Promoting mental health and wellness in youth through physical activity, nutrition, and sleep. *Child and Adolescent Psychiatric Clinics of North America, 28*(2), 171–193. https://doi.org/10.1016/j.chc.2018.11.010

the focus should be on promoting health rather than specifically modulating weight or appearance.

For picky eaters, offering a choice between different healthy options and in small portions to start may facilitate added dietary balance over time. Aiming for deliberate meal and snack times can serve to regulate food volume and quality, as well as more evenly serving energy needs. In particular, eating breakfast has been shown to improve psychosocial and academic functioning. Furthermore, clinicians should promote mindful eating and limiting eating in distracting spaces such as in front of screens or schoolwork; families should plan for at least five meals per week together while trying to make for enjoyable experiences at the table or gathering space. Parental eating patterns tend to influence children's eating patterns, and striving for healthy living can be a family endeavor (Hosker et al., 2019).

CONCLUSION

The initial evaluation of children with behavioral or emotional symptoms may occur in primary care, developmental-behavioral, or psychiatry practices. Sometimes the initial diagnosis will not be clear and will require additional testing, referral, or time to make the diagnosis. In other cases the family may not be ready for such evaluation and treatment. Interventions derived from common factors in therapy and lifestyle changes may be important initial therapeutic approaches that may improve many behavioral and emotional symptoms, build the therapeutic alliance, and increase the likelihood of successful intervention.

For Nick, described in the opening vignette, an intervention plan was developed that involved problem solving around medication administration and bedtime routines, safely reincorporating physical activity based on Nick's preferences, and reassuring Nick about his and his grandfather's health.

REFERENCES

Boone, S. D., & Brausch, A. M. (2016). Physical activity, exercise motivations, depression, and nonsuicidal self-injury in youth. *Suicide and Life-Threatening Behavior*, *46*(5), 625–633. https://doi.org/10.1111/sltb.12240

de Azevedo, K. P. M. D., de Oliveira, V. H., Medeiros, G. C. B. S. D., Mata, D. N. D. S., García, D. N., Martínez, D. G., … Piuvezam, G. (2020). The effects of exercise on BDNF levels in adolescents: A systematic review with meta-analysis. *International Journal of Environmental Research and Public Health*, *17*(17), 6056. https://doi.org/10.3390/ijerph17176056

De Nadai, A. S., Karver, M. S., Murphy, T. K., Cavitt, M. A., Alvaro, J. L., Bengtson, M., … Storch, E. A. (2017). Common factors in pediatric psychiatry: A review of essential and adjunctive mechanisms of treatment outcome. *Journal of Child and Adolescent Psychopharmacology*, *27*(1), 10–18. https://doi.org/10.1089/cap.2015.0263

Firth, J., Gangwisch, J. E., Borsini, A., Wootton, R. E., & Mayer, E. A. (2020a). Food and mood: How do diet and nutrition affect mental wellbeing? *BMJ*, m2382. https://doi.org/10.1136/bmj.m2382

Firth, J., Solmi, M., Wootton, R. E., Vancampfort, D., Schuch, F. B., Hoare, E., … Stubbs, B. (2020b). A meta-review of "lifestyle psychiatry": The role of exercise, smoking, diet and sleep in the prevention and treatment of mental disorders. *World Psychiatry*, *19*(3), 360–380. https://doi.org/10.1002/wps.20773

Gadomski, A. M., Wissow, L. S., Palinkas, L., Hoagwood, K. E., Daly, J. M., & Kaye, D. L. (2014). Encouraging and sustaining integration of child mental health into primary care: Interviews with primary care providers participating in Project TEACH (CAPES and CAP PC) in NY. *General Hospital Psychiatry*, *36*(6), 555–562. https://doi.org/10.1016/j.genhosppsych.2014.05.013

Hosker, D. K., Elkins, R. M., & Potter, M. P. (2019). Promoting mental health and wellness in youth through physical activity, nutrition, and sleep. *Child and Adolescent Psychiatric Clinics of North America*, *28*(2), 171–193. https://doi.org/10.1016/j.chc.2018.11.010

Karver, M. S., Handelsman, J. B., Fields, S., & Bickman, L. (2005). A theoretical model of common process factors in youth and family therapy. *Mental Health Services Research*, *7*(1), 35–51. https://doi.org/10.1007/s11020-005-1964-4

Khalid, S., Williams, C. M., & Reynolds, S. A. (2016). Is there an association between diet and depression in children and adolescents? A systematic review. *British Journal of Nutrition*, *116*(12), 2097–2108. https://doi.org/10.1017/s0007114516004359

Khalife, N., Kantomaa, M., Glover, V., Tammelin, T., Laitinen, J., Ebeling, H., … Rodriguez, A. (2014). Childhood attention-deficit/hyperactivity disorder symptoms are risk factors for obesity and physical inactivity in adolescence. *Journal of the American Academy of Child & Adolescent Psychiatry*, *53*(4), 425–436. https://doi.org/10.1016/j.jaac.2014.01.009

Laska, K. M., Gurman, A. S., & Wampold, B. E. (2014). Expanding the lens of evidence-based practice in psychotherapy: A common factors perspective. *Psychotherapy*, *51*(4), 467–481. https://doi.org/10.1037/a0034332

Linehan, M. M. (2015). *DBT skills training manual* (2nd ed.). The Guilford Press.

Martinowich, K., Manji, H., & Lu, B. (2007). New insights into BDNF function in depression and anxiety. *Nature Neuroscience*, *10*(9), 1089–1093. https://doi.org/10.1038/nn1971

Miller, W. R., & Rollnick, S. (1992). *Motivational interviewing: Preparing people to change addictive behavior*. The Guilford Press.

Molteni, R., Barnard, R., Ying, Z., Roberts, C., & Gómez-Pinilla, F. (2002). A high-fat, refined sugar diet reduces hippocampal brain-derived neurotrophic factor, neuronal plasticity, and learning. *Neuroscience*, *112*(4), 803–814. https://doi.org/10.1016/s0306-4522(02)00123-9

O'Neil, A., Quirk, S. E., Housden, S., Brennan, S. L., Williams, L. J., Pasco, J. A., … Jacka, F. N. (2014). Relationship between diet and mental health in children and adolescents: A systematic review. *American Journal of Public Health*, *104*(10), e31–e42. https://doi.org/10.2105/ajph.2014.302110

Owens, J. Adolescent Sleep Working Group, Committee on Adolescence, Au, R., Carskadon, M., Millman, R., . . . O'Brien, R. F. (2014). Insufficient sleep in adolescents and young adults: An update on causes and consequences. *Pediatrics*, *134*(3), e921–e932. https://doi.org/10.1542/peds.2014-1696

Paruthi, S., Brooks, L. J., D'Ambrosio, C., Hall, W. A., Kotagal, S., Lloyd, R. M., … Wise, M. S. (2016). Recommended amount of sleep for pediatric populations: A consensus statement of the American Academy of Sleep Medicine. *Journal of Clinical Sleep Medicine*, *12*(6), 785–786. https://doi.org/10.5664/jcsm.5866

Pelsser, L. M., Frankena, K., Toorman, J., & Rodrigues Pereira, R. (2017). Diet and ADHD, reviewing the evidence: A systematic review of meta-analyses of double-blind placebo-controlled trials evaluating the efficacy of diet interventions on the behavior of children with ADHD. *PLoS One*, *12*(1), e0169277. https://doi.org/10.1371/journal.pone.0169277

Peretti, S., Mariano, M., Mazzocchetti, C., Mazza, M., Pino, M. C., Verrotti Di Pianella, A., & Valenti, M. (2019). Diet: The keystone of autism spectrum disorder? *Nutritional Neuroscience*, *22*(12), 825–839. https://doi.org/10.1080/1028415x.2018.1464819

Rodriguez-Ayllon, M., Cadenas-Sánchez, C., Estévez-López, F., Muñoz, N. E., Mora-Gonzalez, J., Migueles, J. H., … Esteban-Cornejo, I. (2019). Role of physical activity and sedentary behavior in the mental health of preschoolers, children and adolescents: A systematic review and meta-analysis. *Sports Medicine*, *49*(9), 1383–1410. https://doi.org/10.1007/s40279-019-01099-5

Sampasa-Kanyinga, H., Colman, I., Goldfield, G. S., Janssen, I., Wang, J., Podinic, I., … Chaput, J. P. (2020). Combinations of physical activity, sedentary time, and sleep duration and their associations with depressive symptoms and other mental health problems in children and adolescents: A systematic review. *International Journal of Behavioral Nutrition and Physical Activity*, *17*(1). https://doi.org/10.1186/s12966-020-00976-x

Schuch, F. B., Vancampfort, D., Firth, J., Rosenbaum, S., Ward, P. B., Silva, E. S., … Stubbs, B. (2018). Physical activity and incident depression: A meta-analysis of prospective cohort studies. *American Journal of Psychiatry*, *175*(7), 631–648. https://doi.org/10.1176/appi.ajp.2018.17111194

Srinivasan, S. M., Pescatello, L. S., & Bhat, A. N. (2014). Current perspectives on physical activity and exercise recommendations for children and adolescents with autism spectrum disorders. *Physical Therapy*, *94*(6), 875–889. https://doi.org/10.2522/ptj.20130157

US Department of Agriculture, and US Department of Health and Human Services. (2020). *Dietary guidelines for Americans, 2020–2025.* https://www.dietaryguidelines.gov/sites/default/files/2021-03/Dietary_Guidelines_for_Americans-2020-2025.pdf

US Department of Health & Human Services. (2018). *Physical activity guidelines for Americans* (2nd ed.). https://health.gov/sites/default/files/2019-09/Physical_Activity_Guidelines_2nd_edition.pdf

van Egmond-Fröhlich, A. W. A., Weghuber, D., & de Zwaan, M. (2012). Association of symptoms of attention-deficit/hyperactivity disorder with physical activity, media time, and food intake in children and adolescents. *PLoS One*, *7*(11), e49781. https://doi.org/10.1371/journal.pone.0049781

Vancampfort, D., Firth, J., Schuch, F. B., Rosenbaum, S., Probst, M., Ward, P. B., … Stubbs, B. (2016). Dropout from physical activity interventions in children and adolescents with attention deficit hyperactivity disorder: A systematic review and meta-analysis. *Mental Health and Physical Activity*, *11*, 46–52. https://doi.org/10.1016/j.mhpa.2016.09.002.

93

Behavioral Parent Training and Consultation

Cy Nadler and Nathan J. Blum

For additional material related to the content of this chapter, please see Chapters 4, 46, 94, and 98.

VIGNETTE

Tom is a 5-year-old boy whose parents are concerned about his demanding, defiant, and sometimes aggressive behavior. He dawdles each morning, and it can take 45 minutes to get him dressed because he frequently changes his mind about what clothes he wants to wear. His parents have to yell or threaten to get him to "finally finish getting dressed." When he is happy, he is smiling and exuberant. However, he can have severe tantrums in response to even mild frustrations such as running out of his favorite cereal. Sometimes he screams and cries for so long that he is red in the face and drenched in sweat. Explaining to him that they are going to be late, yelling, threatening, and ignoring him do not consistently work and on a few occasions one of his parents had to go to the store to get the cereal he wanted to get him to calm down. Tom has been late for school and his parents have been late for work. In the evenings he fights with his younger sister, resists getting ready for bed, and gets up repeatedly to ask for another story or a drink. When the parents say "no" he will cry and scream, sometimes waking his sister. His kindergarten teacher reports similar tantrums and noncompliance, as well as occasional aggression toward peers. However, the teacher also notes that Tom has a few good friends and is able to do the activities that she expects kindergarten students to do.

Behavior problems in childhood, such as the noncompliance, aggression, and negative emotional episodes described in the vignette, are among the most common topics discussed by parents and caregivers at primary care visits and represent some of the most frequent reasons for referral to developmental-behavioral and mental health care (Rushton, Bruckman, & Kelleher, 2002). These behaviors are also common during development for virtually all children; this means that parents may struggle to identify when and where to seek outside assistance, and the popular self-help literature and the Internet are teeming with advice that is often not informed by the robust intervention research that has been done.

The ubiquity of child behavior problems makes familiarity with evidence-based parenting strategies critical for medical, mental health, and allied professionals who encounter pediatric populations. An estimated 7.4% of youth between 3 and 17 years of age have a diagnosed externalizing (disruptive) behavioral disorder such as oppositional defiant disorder, conduct disorder, or attention-deficit/hyperactivity disorder (ADHD) (Ghandour et al., 2019), with much higher rates observed among youth with developmental disabilities and/or other mental health diagnoses. While sometimes identified or reported at higher rates among males, oppositional defiant disorder lifetime prevalence rates for males and females are not significantly different (Nock, Kazdin, Hiripi, & Kessler, 2007). Diagnostic criteria emphasize a developmental onset for each of the specific externalizing conditions, along with two distinct and well-replicated trajectories. The subset of youth who manifest clinically significant behavior problems in preschool and/or early grade school, sometimes referred to as early starters, are more likely to experience higher degrees of chronicity and severity (including increased rates of persistent callous-unemotional and antisocial traits), while those whose symptoms emerge after age 10 (late starters) tend to have less severe behavioral presentations (e.g., curfew violations, adolescent drug use) that are more likely to remit in adulthood, though they may have higher rates of other mental health problems.

Known genetic contributors to the development of externalizing behavior disorders are beyond the scope of this chapter, but theoretically and empirically identified influences from the social environment directly inform the evidence-based interventions described in the chapter. Specifically, behavioral frameworks highlight the reasons why children misbehave (the functions of their behavior; see Chapter 4), and how child behaviors such as aggression interact with and influence the behaviors of parents, teachers, siblings, and peers (Patterson, 1982). For instance, if a child screams and hits his mother when she tries to take his tablet away and this aggression results in more tablet time, the child's aggression has been positively reinforced with access to the tablet; simultaneously, the mother's acquiescence (i.e., leaving the child alone for a few more minutes) has been negatively reinforced by the avoidance of further screaming and aggression. Conceptually, this creates a reinforcement trap for both the child and parent, such that they are both more likely to engage in these same behaviors when conflicts arise in the future. The same trap exists when parents inadvertently discover that their own hostile strategies (yelling and scolding, spanking, etc.) are intermittently successful at interrupting the child's behaviors, such that the parent's use of negative emotional strategies are reinforced when the child stops misbehaving and the child learns to briefly discontinue the problem behavior in the presence of the parent's heightened emotionality. This potentially self-perpetuating interaction pattern is termed the coercive cycle and is heavily influenced by social learning theories (see Chapter 4). This same foundation suggests that parent modeling of hostile behaviors such as yelling, physical aggression, and relational aggression also have the further potential to inspire and shape the child's repertoire for coercive behaviors.

The chronic occurrence of negative (coercive) interaction patterns (regardless of what biologic, environmental, and social factors occasioned their occurrence) leads to clinically significant disruptive and aggressive behaviors. Not surprisingly, these externalizing behavior problems also place children at increased risk for a wide range of negative outcomes both during childhood and later in adulthood, including higher rates of other mental health conditions, substance abuse, academic/vocational, and even legal and health problems (Erskine et al., 2016). Very fortunately, the consistent interruption of coercive processes along with targeted modeling, prompting, and reinforcement of prosocial behaviors can alter a child's trajectory over time, especially when intervention is initiated early. The parent-mediated approaches for young children discussed in this chapter are specifically intended both to decrease proximal behavior problems and mitigate the risk for distal negative outcomes.

EVIDENCE-BASED PARENT TRAINING PACKAGES

The coalescence of behavioral and social learning theory frameworks with the attachment literature in the 1960s and 1970s, and specifically the work of psychologist Constance Hanf (and her trainees), led directly to the development of multiple manualized and evidence-based parent training packages (Kaehler, Jacobs, & Jones, 2016). Table 93.1 presents a summary of the primary packages and how they are delivered.

Parent-Child Interaction Therapy

Parent-Child Interaction Therapy (PCIT) (McNeil & Hembree-Kigin, 2010), like several other programs, employs a two-stage model inspired by Hanf's original work. First, the therapist coaches the parent on skills that enhance their ability to deliver positive reinforcement in a child-led play context (child-directed interaction) that is explicitly similar to traditional play therapy, with the key difference being that (outside of therapist demonstrations) the parent is the child's play partner. Therapists typically employ a "bug in the ear" communication system to deliver feedback and guidance to the parent in real time from behind a one-way window. The second phase (parent-directed interaction) employs therapist modeling and parent coaching approaches to teach the delivery of effective instructions, use of warnings, and implementation of timeout to respond to noncompliance (see later for discussion of these strategies). Typically, PCIT lasts at least 12 sessions, but formal PCIT relies on objective mastery criteria to determine when parents are ready to finish each phase. The efficacy of PCIT is well established, and employing mastery criteria leads to more robust decreases in externalizing behavior problems (Thomas, Abell, Webb, Avdagic, & Zimmer-Gembeck, 2017).

Incredible Years

Incredible Years (IY) (Webster-Stratton & Bywater, 2019) encompasses a suite of aligned curricula to support parents of children from infancy through middle childhood. IY programs are group based (serving 8–12 families at a time), relying heavily on the use of brief video vignettes to demonstrate parenting strategies and stimulate discussion among participants and facilitators. Like PCIT, the IY preschool basic program content begins with teaching child-directed play and using positive reinforcement strategies, progressing to topics such as giving instructions and implementing timeout; IY also explicitly addresses topics that include how parents can encourage social-emotional development, school readiness, and successful daily routines; use incentives to shape behavior; and combine these strategies to address a range of parents' individual concerns. Group discussions are intended to be collaborative among the parents (rather than the facilitators in an expert role). IY has been investigated in several randomized controlled trials and has perhaps the most robust replication support of the various parent training packages (Furlong et al., 2012).

TABLE 93.1 Evidence-Based Behavioral Parent Training Packages

Program	Age Range (yr)	Primary Format	Approx. Number of Sessions	Session Length (min)	Live Coaching?	Video Models?
Parent-Child Interaction Therapy (PCIT)	2–7	Single family	12–16	60	Yes	
Incredible Years (IY; Basic)	3–6	Group of parents	18–20	120		Yes
Triple P (Standard)	0–12	Single family	8–12	60	Yes	
Helping the Noncompliant Child	3–8	Single family	8–10	75–90	Yes	
Defiant Child	2–12	Single family	10	60	Yes	
Community Parent Education Program (COPE)	3–12	Group of parents	10	120		Yes
Parent Management Training–Oregon Model (PMTO)	4–12	Single family	15–25	60	Yes	

Triple P Positive Parenting Program

Triple P (Sanders, Kirby, Tellegen, & Day, 2014) is a multi-tiered framework aimed at mitigating negative outcomes associated with behavioral, emotional, and developmental problems in childhood. Levels of intervention span from low-intensity universal prevention through media to high-intensity intervention for individual families, with Standard Triple P being the moderate-intensity level most analogous to the other parent training packages. Not unlike PCIT, Standard Triple P uses a behavioral skills training format where the therapist models and then coaches the parent on implementing a series of child management strategies that are tailored to the child's age, including facilitating positive relationships via child-led interactions, delivery of positive reinforcement (including attention/praise and tokens), teaching and encouraging appropriate behavior, delivering instructions effectively, and responding to problem behaviors using strategies such as planned ignoring and timeout. Well over a hundred studies of various permutations of Triple P have been published, showing strong evidence for parent skill development as well as child behavior change (Sanders et al., 2014).

Helping the Noncompliant Child and Defiant Children

Helping the Noncompliant Child (HNC; McMahon, Long, & Forehand, 2011) and Defiant Children (DC; Barkley, 2013) share many similarities in terms of content and format to PCIT, including the use of live therapist coaching on how to provide contingent reinforcement for appropriate behaviors and to actively ignore minor misbehaviors, as well as how to deliver effective commands and consequences. DC also incorporates some additional guidance on school-based challenges often associated with ADHD. While fewer large-scale trials have investigated HNC and DC compared to other programs, consistent evidence across smaller studies (along with the programs' similarity to packages such as PCIT) provide them with a solid evidence base.

Community Parent Education Program

Community Parent Education Program (COPE; Cunningham, 2006) is a group-based program, supporting up to 25 to 30 parents at a time to maximize access to care. Similar to IY, COPE relies on video examples, role plays, and group-based problem solving to maintain engagement and ensure tailored guidance is offered to each family. The problem-solving mnemonic PASTE (*p*ick one solvable problem, *a*nalyze advantages and disadvantages of possible solutions, *s*elect the best option, *t*ry it, and *e*valuate the outcome) is used as a framework for approaching child behavior problems, introducing concepts such as attention and rewards, planned ignoring, managing transitions, instructions and warnings, and timeout. The program has been subject to limited rigorous investigation as a stand-alone program (Furlong et al., 2012).

Parent Management Training–Oregon Model

The Parent Management Training–Oregon Model (PMTO; Forgatch & Patterson, 2010) is the applied extension of the research that originally advanced coercion theory. A significant emphasis is placed on interrupting patterns of negative parent-child interaction that may perpetuate coercive processes by fostering positive interactions and relationships, implementing predictable discipline strategies, increasing parental monitoring (to reduce opportunities for covert problem behaviors), and improving the parent's ability to problem-solve situations in real time. Of note, children are not present during these sessions; live coaching is exclusively during role plays with the therapist. Phone check-ins are used to provide feedback and support between sessions as parents begin implementing the skills with their children in the home setting. PMTO (including numerous international adaptations) has been subjected to a number of rigorous trials, with strong evidence for both proximal improvements in child behavior and longitudinal maintenance of gains.

BEHAVIORAL COUNSELING DURING MEDICAL CARE

Initiating Counseling

Clinicians providing care to children with developmental or behavioral challenges commonly see parents seeking recommendations about managing their child's challenging behaviors. As a medical clinician, one of the first considerations is whether to provide the recommendations in the context of the child's medical visit or refer for family behavioral counseling or one of the evidence-based parent training programs described earlier. Multiple clinician, family, and practice setting factors will contribute to this decision.

At the time parents seek advice from a professional about their child's behavior they have likely already experienced significant worry about the behavior and often feel frustrated by multiple previous unsuccessful attempts to manage the behavior. Parents who may feel overwhelmed and in need of extra support from family and friends commonly feel blamed by these individuals for their child's behavior and, in the worst cases, become increasingly isolated. Parents may need significant support from the clinician and need to feel that the clinician understands the magnitude of the challenges and is optimistic that they can help (see Chapter 91). Parents often need to know that the clinician does not blame them for their child's behavior. Instead, the clinician and parents need to identify the characteristics of the child, environment, and adult expectations that are making it challenging for the child to behave appropriately. Through this process the adults can come to better understand the child's behavior and think about how they may need to modify the environment, support the child, or respond differently to child behaviors to increase the likelihood of the child meeting expectations for appropriate behavior.

Assessment of Child Characteristics

Developmental Stages

There are a number of child characteristics that can increase the likelihood that a child will engage in behaviors that adults find challenging, including progression through developmental stages. Psychosocial development during the toddler and preschool years requires improving self-regulation, increasing independence, and increasing social reciprocity with peers (see Chapters 7). As children learn these skills, there can be challenges, and parents may be concerned about acting-out behaviors, defiant behaviors, emotional sensitivity, or conflicts with peers. Adolescence is another developmental stage associated with an increased frequency of challenging behaviors as adolescents seek to establish their own identity while learning about sexual behaviors, negotiating drug and alcohol use, and often taking on the increased responsibilities associated with operating a motor vehicle or employment (see Chapters 8–10). This may lead to parental concerns about risky behaviors, arguments, and defiance.

Temperament

Temperament refers to a child's behavioral style and is discussed further in Chapter 80. Although the dimensions of temperament are the subject of some debate, children who tend to be inflexible, intense in their reaction to stimuli, have a more negative mood, and/or are irregular in sleep and eating patterns are often more challenging for parents. Other temperament characteristics may also be a concern to parents particularly when there is a mismatch between the child's characteristics and the expectations of caretakers (Carey, 1990). For example, a child with a high activity level may not be viewed as challenging by parents who are also very active, but might be seen as problematic by parents with a more sedate lifestyle. Tom, described in the chapter-opening vignette, seems somewhat inflexible and can be intense when he is happy but also when he is upset, which may contribute to his difficult behaviors.

Developmental Delays and Disabilities

Developmental delay and intellectual disability are associated with an increased risk of challenging behaviors (see Chapter 40). Failure to complete a task due to a skill deficit may be misinterpreted as defiance or resistance. This may be particularly likely when a child has delays in one stream of development but not others. For example, young children with strong language skills but weak fine motor skills may be seen as defiant or resistant when they have trouble completing written assignments if their weak fine motor and writing skills are not recognized.

Communication delays as occur in language disorders and autism spectrum disorders among other disabilities are often associated with challenging or disruptive behaviors. As noted earlier in this chapter, disruptive behaviors often serve a communicative function. For example, tantrums can be very effective ways for children to get caretakers' attention, escape from task demands, or sometimes to get caretakers to give the child something the child wants. In children with limited ability to communicate their wants and needs using language disruptive behaviors may be the most effective strategy to communicate these wants or needs.

Selecting the Behavior to Change

If one is going to provide behavioral recommendations to the caretakers, it is important to discuss with the adults and child (if developmentally appropriate) what behavior to work on changing. Some of the factors to consider are included in Table 93.2. The most important factors to consider in selecting the behavior are that it is important to all the adults involved in the situation, is important for child functioning, and that it is one that you are fairly certain the child can be successful in accomplishing when motivated. Generally, behavioral plans that target increasing appropriate behavior are more effective than ones that focus on decreasing inappropriate behavior. One also wants to define the behavior in such a way that any involved adult and the child will know when the behavior has occurred. Defining the behavior in a general way, such as telling the truth, could be problematic as frequently the adult may not know when it is happening and when it is not happening. If one is not sure that the child can accomplish the full task, breaking the task down into smaller units or shorter periods of time can increase the likelihood that the child will be successful. The clinician should also consider other factors related to the child or environment that might impact the likelihood of success. For example, a child may be very likely to be successful with a behavior when rested and well fed but may be unsuccessful when tired or hungry. Other stressors such as a chaotic, noisy environment may also make some behaviors more challenging for a child.

TABLE 93.2 Questions to Consider in Selecting the Behavior to Change
Is the behavior important to all the adults in the situation?
Is the behavior important to child functioning?
Can you define the behavior you want the child to do?
Can you know when the behavior occurred?
Is the behavior within the child's skills and capacity?
Does the behavior occur at a time the child is likely to be successful?

Parents often identify many specific child problem behaviors that they would like to change. Alternatively, they may nominate a general goal (e.g., listening to parents) that encompasses a large variety of behaviors occurring in many different settings. Selecting multiple behaviors or these types of general behaviors to change is problematic as successfully implementing the plan requires significant adult effort in monitoring the child's behavior and consistently responding to different behaviors. It is often hard for parents or other caretakers to sustain the effort and monitoring needed to successfully implement the plan across multiple behaviors or setting. This leads to inconsistent implementation of the plan and failure to promote the desired behavior. Potentially even more problematic, the inconsistent implementation often serves to intermittently reinforce inappropriate behavior. As described in Chapter 4, intermittent reinforcement is one of the most successful ways to maintain a behavior and thus may make it harder to decrease inappropriate behavior in the future.

Elements of Evidence-Based Parent Training Programs

The evidence-based parent training programs described at the beginning of this chapter are packages of behavioral interventions that have strong evidence for helping manage problematic child behavior. The premise of these programs is that the likelihood of a specific behavior occurring is influenced by what happens prior to the behavior (antecedents) and what happens after the behavior (consequences; see Chapter 4). Although there are some differences in the programs, there are also many elements that are common across these programs (Chorpita & Daleiden, 2009; Kaehler et al., 2016). These common elements are likely the factors most associated with the success of the programs and thus are strategies to consider when providing behavioral recommendation to a child's parents.

Modifying the Environment

Modifying the environment can be one of the most effective ways to decrease problem behaviors. Clinicians commonly recommend these approaches when they encourage childproofing the home for toddlers or not having tempting high-calorie foods in the home if a child repeatedly tries to sneak access to them. A child who is easily distracted during homework may be provided a quiet workplace. As these examples demonstrate, a large number of potential environmental modifications may encourage appropriate behaviors. It is always worth considering if there are environmental modifications that can help with a problem behavior as once the environmental modification is made, these interventions require little ongoing effort. In contrast, most of the recommendations related to changing the consequences of behavior require significant adult effort, monitoring, and often adapting the intervention to maintain effectiveness.

Effective Instructions

Giving effective instructions is an important skill. The first consideration is whether the instruction is important enough to adults that they are willing to praise compliance or manage noncompliance. Often adults give instructions that are not that important to them and then ignore noncompliance so that children learn that they do not have to follow adult instructions. If adults give an instruction, they should ensure that they have the child's attention by making eye contact or touching them to gain the child's attention prior to giving the instructions. Instructions should be given in a calm but firm tone specifying what the adult wants the child to do, as opposed to telling the child what not to do. A single simple instruction is more likely to result in compliance than a complex or multistep instruction. Instructions should not be worded as a question unless the child has a choice.

If the child does not comply with the instruction, then adults need to be prepared to manage the noncompliance. If the behavior is dangerous to the child or others an immediate consequence should be implemented (see Punishment, later), but in other situations it is appropriate to give the child a single warning as an if-then statement such as "If you don't (instruction), then (consequence)."

Modeling Appropriate Behavior

Modeling appropriate behavior is important as children often imitate the adults. If the adults often lose control, scream, curse, or engage in other behaviors they find inappropriate in children, then the clinician will need to help parents learn alternative strategies (including self-management) that do not emotionally or physically escalate the situation. It is often helpful to encourage adults to think of themselves as a coach trying to teach new skills. Typically, adults will understand that yelling, screaming, or cursing at children would not be an effective way to teach them a new skill and that calmly giving instructions and using strategies such as encouraging small improvements is more likely to be effective. If caretakers are using corporal punishment, the discussion of the need to model appropriate behavior may help to discourage the use of these strategies. A child who gets hit by an adult who is upset may think it is okay to hit when upset, too.

Increasing Praise

Increasing praise for appropriate behavior is one of the most common components of parent training programs for young children. Adult attention is typically a powerful motivator for young children's behavior. When coercive parent-child interactions have developed, it is often true that child misbehavior is producing parental attention more frequently than appropriate child behavior. Increasing praise and attention for appropriate behavior is an important first step toward beginning to decrease the coercive interactions and teach the child that appropriate behavior will result in adult attention. The child-directed interaction described for PCIT (see earlier) may be valuable in demonstrating to parents the absence of problem behaviors when they provide undivided attention and place no demands on the child for a few minutes. Often parents need instruction on how to do this as they may not realize they are placing subtle demands on the child during play by making suggestions, attempting to teach or quiz the child, or asking leading questions such as "Do you want to build a castle?" One strategy to avoid this is to encourage parents to observe and describe their child's play and praise the child for good ideas with comments such as "You are driving the train along the track" or "That is nice sharing your toy with me." Parents can also be encouraged to frequently notice appropriate behaviors. This is often described as "catching the child being good" and involves praising the child as the child engages in routine appropriate behaviors that previously were not acknowledged.

Differential Attention or Reinforcement

Differential attention or differential reinforcement goes beyond increasing praise for appropriate behavior to strategically using adult attention (or other reinforcers) to encourage appropriate behavior and discourage inappropriate behavior. Often it may be helpful to give caretakers a goal of providing attention four to five times more often for appropriate behavior than for inappropriate behavior. Typically to reach this goal, caretakers will have to ignore many of the problem behaviors they have been attending to in the past. Clinicians counseling parents to use this strategy need to warn parents about the extinction burst discussed in Chapter 4. In this situation when the parents stop providing attention for problem behaviors that have resulted in adult attention in the past, there may be an initial increase in these inappropriate behaviors as the child tries to use the coercive strategies that worked in the past to get adult attention (Lehrman & Iwata, 1996). It is only after the child consistently experiences that coercive strategies are far less effective than appropriate behaviors that adults will start to see a decrease in the inappropriate behaviors.

Reward Systems

Reward systems or token economies are incorporated into many behavioral plans to reinforce specific target behaviors. As described in Table 93.2, it is important to select a limited number of target behaviors that one thinks the child can successfully accomplish. If the child is not frequently earning the reward, the reward system is not likely to be very motivating to the child and it is likely to fail. When using a reward system to teach or encourage a behavior that has not been occurring frequently, the reward system will be most effective if the child earns the reward each time the child exhibits the behavior (a continuous, fixed ratio schedule; see Chapter 4). Once a behavior is well established, parents can shift to an intermittent reinforcement schedule to maintain the behavior over time.

There are many types of rewards that can be offered (Table 93.3). One may need to change the rewards relatively frequently to maintain the child's interest in the reward system. Time-based rewards are important to consider as they are easy to make incremental such that the child can earn progressively more time with improving performance. When children want larger tangible rewards, they may earn tokens or points toward the award. For younger children who may not understand tokens or points, a picture of the item can be cut into a few puzzle pieces and they can earn puzzle pieces toward the desired reward.

Sometimes caretakers will resist using reward systems stating that they do not think they should have to "bribe" children to get them to behave. Clinicians must be able to help families distinguish between using positive rewards and bribes. With positive rewards, the reward is generally agreed upon in advance and used to recognize the child's effort in doing something that is difficult for the child. By definition, bribes are things given to an individual to encourage misbehavior. In the course of parenting this may occur when the adult offers a "reward" because the child is misbehaving. For example, if a child is refusing to come into the house and the adult says, "I will let you play your videogames if you come in now," this is a bribe because the adult was not going to let the child play the videogame until the child resisted coming into the house. Thus the reward of playing the videogame is reinforcing the child's resistance to come into the house and is a bribe that will likely increase the frequency of the child resisting coming into the house in the future. Using rewards is often an effective way to teach children to engage in desired behaviors. Bribes should be discouraged as they may discontinue inappropriate behavior in the moment but increase the likelihood that inappropriate behaviors will continue to occur in the future.

Many families seeking professional support will have tried reward systems unsuccessfully. Usually, this is either because (1) the task or behavior required is not clear or too difficult for the child or (2) the reward is not functioning as a reinforcer (i.e., it is not valued enough by the child to effect behavior).

TABLE 93.3 Sample of Rewards for Children

Time-Based Rewards

- Time playing a child-chosen game with parent
- Time doing a child-chosen activity with parent
- Time or number of books parent reads to child at bedtime
- Time playing outside or at a playground
- Time on electronic games

Nontime-Based Rewards

- Adult praise and/or attention
- Special activity the child wants to do
- Playdate with a friend
- Stickers
- Toy or treat the child wants
- Grab bag or spin the wheel that selects special toy, treat, or activity
- Connect the dots to earn special toy, treat, or activity
- Puzzle pieces to earn a toy, treat, or activity (see text for further explanation)
- Tokens or points that can be exchanged for privileges, toys, treats, or activities

TABLE 93.4 Factors to Consider When a Reward System Is Not Working

Task or Behavior Is Not Clear or Too difficult

- Is the task or desired behavior clearly defined in a way the child understands?
- Does the task require too many steps?
- Is the change in behavior or skill requested too large?
- Is the child making an effort to change behavior that is not being recognized?
- Are other stressors, fatigue, or hunger interfering with child's ability to comply?

The Reward Is Not Reinforcing

- Has the child lost interest in a reward that was initially reinforcing?
- Does the child have other ways to get the reward other than the target behavior?
- Is the child infrequently earning the reward?
- Is there a long time between the behavior and the reward?
- Is the reward being used as a bribe?
- Are problem behaviors being intermittently reinforced?

More specific factors to consider in each of these domains are shown in Table 93.4.

Punishment

Punishment may be included in behavior management plans, but punishment should not be the only component of a plan. Punishment may help to teach a child what an adult does not want the child to do, but it does not teach the child what the child should do instead. The most commonly recommended punishment strategies are timeout from positive reinforcement (e.g., timeout) and loss of privileges or response-cost systems. Consistent with evidence that corporal punishment is unnecessary, often ineffective, and can be harmful, spanking or other forms of corporal punishment are not recommended (Sege, Siegel, & Council on Child Abuse and Neglect, & Committee on Psychosocial Aspects of Child and Family Health, 2018).

Timeout involves briefly removing the child from the opportunity to obtain positive reinforcement such as adult attention or participating in fun activities typically by sitting on a chair, step, or some other location. Timeout is most effective when children have been getting a high level of attention, praise, and other forms of positive reinforcement as this increases the contrast between time in and timeout. Although recommendations for the duration of timeout vary between different parenting programs, there is general agreement that the child should demonstrate at least a brief period of being in control and regulated prior to being released from timeout (Kaehler et al., 2016); this "calm criterion" prevents children from being inadvertently reinforced with escape following yelling and other misbehavior during the timeout. A base duration of not longer than 1 minute for each year of the child's age is a reasonable guide, with diminishing returns for school-age children after 5 to 10 minutes. If a child does not stay in a timeout chair, then the child may be sent to one's room (as long as the room does not have a television, videogames, or a lot of the child's other favorite activities available) or the child may lose privileges (see later) (Everett, Hupp, & Olmi, 2010).

If a child loses privileges it should be for a brief period. This could involve loss of a story at bedtime, loss of access to electronic games for the remainder of the day, or in older children grounding where they are not allowed to do things with friends for a short period. If a token economy is implemented, a response-cost system can be added in which there are certain behaviors for which the child loses tokens or points. However, if children are losing more points than they are earning or losing a privilege for an extended period, then the behavior management plan is unlikely to be effective. In these situations the child is not earning the reward or accessing the privilege and thus the reward or privilege loses its reinforcing value. One alternative to time-based grounding that can avoid the prolonged loss of privileges is "job grounding" in which the child is grounded or not allowed access to a favorite activity until completing an extra (brief) chore. In all of these situations it is important for the adults to specify the consequences for specific behaviors prior to the behaviors occurring and not implement punishments based primarily on their level of frustration at the time of the behavior.

In approaching Tom's case we have already identified some temperament characteristic that may contribute to the challenging behaviors, including his inflexibility. Tom also receives a lot of parental attention by escalating his emotional responses. Often during daily routines, appropriate behaviors that a child like Tom engages in, do not result in attention. Tom's parents might be counseled to strategically (i.e., differentially) provide less attention in response to tantrums and more attention to his appropriate behaviors. The clinician will need to prepare the parents for the fact that Tom will have some severe tantrums, both because of his temperament and his learning history.

The clinician and parents will need to decide on what behavior they want to prioritize to change. The morning routine and bedtime routine might both be logical options, but Tom is tired at bedtime and if the behavior plan results in a tantrum, he may wake his sister making it more challenging for his parents to ignore tantrums. Thus working with the parents on the morning routine might be more likely to be successful. Perhaps modifying an antecedent by having Tom select the clothes the night before would be helpful. A time-based reward system could be implemented for completing the morning routine that is taking 45 minutes currently. If Tom has the ability to independently put on the clothes laid out the night before, the parents could set a timer for 45 minutes as soon as Tom starts getting ready and expect Tom to dress independently. With any remaining time once Tom is dressed, the parent could agree to play Tom's favorite game with him. This system has a built-in response-cost system as any delaying Tom does in getting ready in the morning means less time to play his favorite game with his parents. As Tom and his parents begin having more positive interactions, counseling could address the bedtime routine and his noncompliance with timeout.

EXTENSIONS TO IMPROVE ACCESS, ENGAGEMENT, AND OUTCOMES

Concurrent with efforts over the last several decades to refine and validate the parent training packages described earlier, considerable attention has also been directed to extending these models beyond typically developing preschool children with externalizing behavior problems, tailoring the delivery of care to meet the needs of specific populations, and considering strategies to more effectively and efficiently disseminate the strategies embedded in these models.

Parent training for youth with cooccurring developmental/cognitive differences and mental health challenges is an area of notable growth. For children with autism, PCIT (with and without alterations), as well as tailored versions of other programs that include a suite of extensions (e.g., Stepping Stones Triple P, Incredible Years Autism & Language Delays) are all available and show promise, though research supporting use for children with disabilities lags behind the evidence in typically developing children (Postorino et al., 2017). RUBI (Research Units in Behavioral Intervention; Bearss et al., 2015) was specifically constructed to integrate traditional parent training strategies with behavior analytic approaches with a well-established efficacy for youth with autism and other developmental differences (see Chapter 94). Parent training approaches have even been successfully applied for youth with brain injuries (Wade et al., 2017) and internalizing disorders (Carpenter, Puliafico, Kurtz, Pincus, & Comer, 2014).

Mode and intensity of delivery has also become an important area for expansion. Programs that originated as single-family models have been adapted for group delivery, and Triple P's lower intensity universal prevention level reaches the entire continent of Australia. A two-session group adaptations of PCIT called the Child-Adult Relationship Enhancement (CARE) workshops is becoming increasingly popular as a psychoeducational offering (Gurwitch et al., 2016). While there is no shortage of parent self-help content in popular books and online that is not studied, at least one widely available parenting book, *1-2-3 Magic* (as well as a DVD adaptation), shows at least preliminary evidence for reducing child behavior problems without any therapist involvement (Porzig-Drummond, Stevenson, & Stevenson, 2015).

Even prior to the COVID-19 pandemic, telehealth-based adaptations of parent training models had been of great interest. Some programs already relied on "bug in the ear" coaching where the therapist is not present in the room, and others were designed to be delivered without the child present; in both cases the logistics of virtual delivery are quite reasonable. While more research is needed on how telehealth delivery performs (for child outcomes, parent satisfaction and access), available data suggest that virtual delivery yields the same degree of improvement for behavior problems as in-person intervention (Florean, Dobrean, Păsărelu, Georgescu, & Milea, 2020).

Despite the availability of many evidence-based programs, parents face many barriers in identifying and accessing effective sources of support. Primary care clinicians are ideally positioned to provide anticipatory guidance regarding behavior issues, especially in very young children who respond quickly enough to planned ignoring and positive reinforcement that the techniques can be demonstrated during a brief encounter. Increasingly, primary care offices are embedding behavioral health professionals to facilitate "warm hand-offs," and these models (including brief consultation, as well as the delivery of full parent training packages in the primary care setting) appear successful at meeting families where they are to address externalizing behavior and other mental health concerns (Asarnow, Rozenman, Wiblin, & Zeltzerf, 2015). Like primary care–based interventions, models designed to be embedded in community settings such as schools minimize the new people and places that a family must connect with to access parenting guidance. Schools will sometimes offer the psychoeducational as well as group-based programs described earlier, but several behaviorally oriented approaches designed specifically for use in school settings have demonstrated strong effects in terms of short- and long-term child outcomes. The Family Check Up (FCU; Shaw & Shelleby, 2014) is modeled as much after evidence-based intervention for adult substance abuse as it is the literature on child behavior management. FCU integrates motivational interviewing techniques to engage parents in collaboration around their child's behavior problems, followed by a 12-session structured intervention inspired by PMTO; families are then invited to annual checkups where their progress is monitored and the parents are supported in the ongoing use of the key strategies. FCU has focused specifically on reaching families who are at the highest risk for poverty and other known risk factors for child externalizing problems as well as negative adult outcomes, with strong evidence for delivery in primary care and through Women, Infants, and Children Nutritional Supplement (WIC) programs in addition to schools. There is an additional dose-response relationship showing that the effects of the program increase as a function of the number of annual behavioral check-ups attended by families (Asarnow et al., 2015), underscoring the value of longitudinal contact with families even after the completion of a parent training package.

Despite the generally robust research supporting the parent training approaches described here, the age ranges for the traditional packages taper off as children reach the teen years. Multisystemic Therapy (MST; Van der Stouwe, Asscher, Stams, Deković, & van der Laan, 2014) is the most well-established model for mitigating significant challenges in adolescence, sometimes serving as a therapeutic alternative to psychiatric hospitalization or even incarceration when the chronicity as well as intensity of behavior problems have progressed. MST integrates behavioral parent training strategies with cognitive-behavioral therapy (see Chapter 98), components of other family therapy models focused on conflict reduction (see Chapter 97), and elements of other intensive and wraparound outpatient models for managing psychiatric conditions (borderline personality disorder, schizophrenia, etc.). Controlled studies of MST show small but significant effects on youth delinquency and youth psychopathology, but less consistent impacts on a range of other important youth and family outcomes (Van der Stouwe et al., 2014). At a population level, prevention and early intervention approaches remain the best option for improving the long-term trajectories of youth with externalizing behavior disorders.

Parent engagement in the coaching process, whether a family is participating in a brief CARE workshop or a multi-year FCU program, is arguably the most modifiable factor that prevents children from benefiting in evidence-based programs. The reality is that an estimated 25% of families referred to behavioral parent training programs never actually attend; worse yet, an additional 26% drop out prior to completing the program (Chacko et al., 2016). Data are mixed regarding whether family-level variables such as socioeconomic status, parent mental health, and the severity of the child's behavior problems impact the likelihood of a family completing a behavioral parent training program, but it is reasonable to assume that these variables (among other sociodemographic considerations) impact the likelihood of being included in such research. Evidence-based strategies to boost parent engagement (including strategies specifically for fathers) are available, but they remain chronically underutilized in clinical practice in part because the traditional programs do not explicitly embed them. The FCU data provide strong evidence that meaningful individualization at the family level can significantly improve long-term engagement and outcomes for children, including for those who are most underserved by our health and mental health systems (McCabe, Yeh, & Zerr, 2020).

CONCLUSION

Parents have sought (and offered) advice on how to manage behavior problems in childhood for far longer than behavioral scientists have formally studied these questions. That said, the core concepts described here are supported by a robust evidence base. Guiding parents to use praise to encourage appropriate behaviors, avoid inadvertently encouraging problem behaviors through their reactions, and employ predictable family routines and consequences that diffuse negative interactions is an incredibly rewarding clinical experience that pediatric clinicians of all disciplines can enjoy, especially when aware of the wide range of resources available to guide their work. Every practice region will have variation in terms of what services are available, and clinicians are encouraged to familiarize themselves with options ranging from evidence-based self-help all the way through intensive services to help families access the appropriate level of support. Moreover, clinicians are urged to consider the directions in which parenting supports have evolved and stay abreast of developments that continue to reduce the barriers for marginalized families to access high-quality and timely guidance tailored to their needs. Good therapists have always individualized interventions (even manualized ones) for their patients, and the growing evidence for adaptations and embedded engagement efforts will only enhance our ability to both personalize care and improve child and family outcomes.

REFERENCES

Asarnow, J. R., Rozenman, M., Wiblin, J., & Zeltzer, L. (2015). Integrated medical-behavioral care compared with usual primary care for child and adolescent behavioral health: A meta-analysis. *JAMA Pediatrics*, *169*(10), 929–937.

Barkley, R. A. (2013). *Defiant children: A clinician's manual for assessment and parent training* (3rd ed.). Guilford Press.

Bearss, K., Johnson, C., Smith, T., Lecavalier, L., Swiezy, N., Aman, M., McAdam, D. B., Butter, E., Stillitano, C., Minshawi, N., Sukhodolsky, D. G., Mruzek, D. W., Turner, K., Neal, T., Hallett, V., Mulick, J. A., Green, B., Handen, B., Deng, Y., ... Scahill, L. (2015). Effect of parent training vs parent education on behavioral problems in children with autism spectrum disorder: A randomized clinical trial. *JAMA*, *313*(15), 1524–1533.

Carey, W. B. (1990). Temperament risk factors in children: A conference report. *Journal of Developmental and Behavioral Pediatrics*, *11*, 28–34.

Carpenter, A. L., Puliafico, A. C., Kurtz, S. M., Pincus, D. B., & Comer, J. S. (2014). Extending parent–child interaction therapy for early childhood internalizing problems: New advances for an overlooked population. *Clinical Child and Family Psychology Review*, *17*(4), 340–356.

Chacko, A., Jensen, S. A., Lowry, L. S., Cornwell, M., Chimklis, A., Chan, E., & Pulgarin, B. (2016). Engagement in behavioral parent training: Review of the literature and implications for practice. *Clinical Child and Family Psychology Review*, *19*(3), 204–215.

Chorpita, B. F., & Daleiden, E. L. (2009). Mapping evidence-based treatments for children and adolescents: Application of the distillation and matching model to 615 treatments from 322 randomized trials. *Journal of Consulting and Clinical Psychology*, *77*(3), 566–579.

Cunningham, C. E. (2006). COPE: Large-group, community-based, family-centered parent training. In R. A. Barkley (Ed.), *Attention-deficit hyperactivity disorder: A handbook for diagnosis and treatment* (pp. 480–498). Guilford Press.

Erskine, H. E., Norman, R. E., Ferrari, A. J., Chan, G. C., Copeland, W. E., Whiteford, H. A., & Scott, J. G. (2016). Long-term outcomes of attention-deficit/hyperactivity disorder and conduct disorder: A systematic review and meta-analysis. *Journal of the American Academy of Child & Adolescent Psychiatry*, *55*(10), 841–850.

Everett, G. E., Hupp, S. D., & Olmi, D. J. (2010). Time-out with parents: A descriptive analysis of 30 years of research. *Education and Treatment of Children*, *33*, 235–259.

Florean, I. S., Dobrean, A., Păsărelu, C. R., Georgescu, R. D., & Milea, I. (2020). The efficacy of internet-based parenting programs for children and adolescents with behavior problems: A meta-analysis of randomized clinical trials. *Clinical Child and Family Psychology Review*, *23*(4), 510–528.

Forgatch, M. S., & Patterson, G. R. (2010). Parent management training—Oregon model: An intervention for antisocial behavior in children and adolescents. In J. R. Weisz & A. E. Kazdin (Eds.), *Evidence-based psychotherapies for children and adolescents* (pp. 159–177). The Guilford Press.

Furlong, M., McGilloway, S., Bywater, T., Hutchings, J., Smith, S. M., & Donnelly, M. (2012). Behavioural and cognitive-behavioural group based parenting programmes for early-onset conduct problems in children aged 3 to 12 years. *Cochrane Database of Systematic Reviews*, *2*, CD008225. https://doi.org/10.1002/14651858.CD008225.pub2

Ghandour, R. M., Sherman, L. J., Vladutiu, C. J., Ali, M. M., Lynch, S. E., Bitsko, R. H., & Blumberg, S. J. (2019). Prevalence and treatment of depression, anxiety, and conduct problems in US children. *Journal of Pediatrics*, *206*, 256–267.

Gurwitch, R. H., Messer, E. P., Masse, J., Olafson, E., Boat, B. W., & Putnam, F. W. (2016). Child–Adult Relationship Enhancement (CARE): An evidence-informed program for children with a history of trauma and other behavioral challenges. *Child Abuse & Neglect*, *53*, 138–145.

Kaehler, L. A., Jacobs, M., & Jones, D. J. (2016). Distilling common history and practice elements to inform dissemination: Hanf-model BPT programs as an example. *Clinical Child and Family Psychology Review*, *19*(3), 236–258.

Lehrman, D. C., & Iwata, B. A. (1996). Developing a technology for the use of operant extinction in clinical settings: An examination of basic and applied research. *Journal of Applied Behavior Analysis, 29*, 345–382.

McCabe, K. M., Yeh, M., & Zerr, A. A. (2020). Personalizing behavioral parent training interventions to improve treatment engagement and outcomes for culturally diverse families. *Psychology Research and Behavior Management, 13*, 41.

McMahon, R. J., Long, N., & Forehand, R. L. (2011). Parent training for the treatment of oppositional behavior in young children: Helping the noncompliant child. In *Clinical handbook of assessing and treating conduct problems in youth* (pp. 163–191). Springer.

McNeil, C. B., & Hembree-Kigin, T. L. (2010). *Parent child interaction therapy*. Springer Publishing Company.

Nock, M. K., Kazdin, A. E., Hiripi, E., & Kessler, R. C. (2007). Lifetime prevalence, correlates, and persistence of oppositional defiant disorder: Results from the National Comorbidity Survey Replication. *Journal of Child Psychology and Psychiatry, 48*(7), 703–713.

Patterson, G. R. (1982). *A social learning approach to family intervention: Vol. 3. Coercive family process*. Castalia.

Porzig-Drummond, R., Stevenson, R. J., & Stevenson, C. (2015). Preliminary evaluation of a self-directed video-based 1-2-3 Magic parenting program: A randomized controlled trial. *Behaviour Research and Therapy, 66*, 32–42.

Postorino, V., Sharp, W. G., McCracken, C. E., Bearss, K., Burrell, T. L., Evans, A. N., & Scahill, L. (2017). A systematic review and meta-analysis of parent training for disruptive behavior in children with autism spectrum disorder. *Clinical Child and Family Psychology Review, 20*(4), 391–402.

Rushton, J., Bruckman, D., & Kelleher, K. (2002). Primary care referral of children with psychosocial problems. *Archives of Pediatrics & Adolescent Medicine, 156*(6), 592–598.

Sanders, M. R., Kirby, J. N., Tellegen, C. L., & Day, J. J. (2014). The triple P positive parenting program: A systematic review and meta-analysis of a multi-level system of parenting support. *Clinical Psychology Review, 34*(4), 337–357.

Sege, R. D., Siegel, B. S., & Council on Child Abuse and Neglect, & Committee on Psychosocial Aspects of Child and Family Health. (2018). Effective discipline to raise healthy children. *Pediatrics, 142*(6), 12.

Shaw, D. S., & Shelleby, E. C. (2014). Early-starting conduct problems: Intersection of conduct problems and poverty. *Annual Review of Clinical Psychology, 10*, 503–528.

Thomas, R., Abell, B., Webb, H. J., Avdagic, E., & Zimmer-Gembeck, M. J. (2017). Parent-child interaction therapy: A meta-analysis. *Pediatrics, 140*(3).

Van der Stouwe, T., Asscher, J. J., Stams, G. J. J., Deković, M., & van der Laan, P. H. (2014). The effectiveness of Multisystemic Therapy (MST): A meta-analysis. *Clinical Psychology Review, 34*(6), 468–481.

Wade, S. L., Cassedy, A. E., Shultz, E. L., Zang, H., Zhang, N., Kirkwood, M. W., & Taylor, H. G. (2017). Randomized clinical trial of online parent training for behavior problems after early brain injury. *Journal of the American Academy of Child & Adolescent Psychiatry, 56*(11), 930–939.

Webster-Stratton, C., & Bywater, T. (2019). The Incredible Years® series: An internationally evidenced multimodal approach to enhancing child outcomes. In B. H. Fiese, M. Celano, K. Deater-Deckard, E. N. Jouriles, & M. A. Whisman (Eds.), *APA handbooks in psychology. APA handbook of contemporary family psychology: Family therapy and training* (pp. 343–359). American Psychological Association.

94

Applied Behavior Analysis for Autism Spectrum Disorder

Amanda E. Bennett and Lauren B. Fishbein

For additional material related to the content of this chapter, please see Chapters 4, 41, and 93.

VIGNETTE

Johnny is a 3-year-old male who was recently diagnosed with autism spectrum disorder (ASD). His language skills, adaptive skills, and cognitive functioning are in the low to very low range. His speech is echolalic, and he does not respond to his name. Johnny has some difficulties expressing his wants and needs and engages in head banging and aggression. His parents report these behaviors occur at seemingly random times, and traditional discipline strategies have not worked.

After receiving his diagnosis, Johnny was enrolled in a center-based applied behavior analysis (ABA) program for 40 hours per week. He showed improvement in his cognitive skills, self-help skills, and communication skills. His head banging and aggression decreased from multiple times a day to a few times per month. Johnny's parents learned that the function of Johnny's behavior was to get items he wanted such as preferred toys and snacks. Johnny has made meaningful improvements such as mastering toilet training, improving self-feeding, and increasing his communication through a combination of speech and use of visual supports.

A few years later, Johnny is in third grade, he is in a mainstream classroom with an individualized education plan, and is performing at the same level as his typically developing peers in many domains. He has started to demonstrate increased anxiety and still struggles to have reciprocal conversation and make friends. His parents are seeking out effective interventions to address social-emotional concerns.

*This chapter will include both person-first ("a person with autism") and identity-first ("an autistic person") language to respect differing perspectives on how to address this population (Haller, 2016).

INTRODUCTION TO AUTISM SPECTRUM DISORDER

ASD is a neurodevelopmental disorder comprised of deficits in social communication skills and presence of repetitive, restricted, stereotypical, and/or sensory-focused behaviors or interests, as discussed in Chapter 41 and listed in the *Diagnostic and Statistical Manual of Mental Disorders*, fifth edition (*DSM-5*; American Psychiatric Association, 2013). In addition, many autistic individuals have cooccurring symptoms or disorders, including intellectual disability, attention-deficit/hyperactivity disorder (ADHD), anxiety, irritability, sleep disturbances, seizures, and gastrointestinal problems (Kuhlthau, McDonnell, Coury, Payakachat, & Macklin, 2018). These cooccurring symptoms can impact developmental progress and community participation (Joshi et al., 2013).

HISTORY OF AUTISM TREATMENT APPROACHES

Applied behavior analysis (ABA) became increasingly accepted during the deinstitutionalization movement of the 1960s and 1970s as behavioral science demonstrated efficacy in producing clinically meaningful outcomes such as increases in prosocial behaviors, adaptive skills, and communication for individuals with autism as well as individuals with intellectual disability (Fishbein, Rouse, Minshawi, & Fodstad, 2017). Prior to identifying ABA as a way to decrease problem behaviors and build skills, treatment for ASD relied on psychodynamic theory that autism was caused by "refrigerator mothers" who were characterized as cold and uncaring. This left little hope for families of children with ASD (Lovaas, 1979). Treatments for children with autism shifted away from psychodynamic approaches as behavioral studies demonstrated that analyzing and manipulating variables within an individual's environment decreased problem behaviors and increased skill development across various domains of functioning (Lovaas, 1987).

ABA is based on Skinner's theory of behaviorism and the experimental analysis of behavior (Cooper, Heron, & Heward, 2007). As described in Chapter 4 this theory proposes that causes of behavior can be found within the environment. Thus within a given context behaviors are strengthened (i.e., reinforced) or reduced (i.e., extinguished) depending on whether the behavior is followed by a favorable or unfavorable outcome (Roane, Fisher, & Carr, 2016). Therefore by examining the antecedents and consequences of a specific target behavior, these factors could be manipulated to bring about behavior change (Roane et al., 2016). In the case of Johnny, in the chapter-opening vignette, his aggressive behavior was maintained by the fact that he got items he wanted after engaging in the behavior. Using behavioral theory terminology, his behavior was reinforced by providing access to tangible items.

PRINCIPLES OF APPLIED BEHAVIOR ANALYSIS

ABA therapy focuses on the systematic evaluation of the frequency of specific behaviors and using this data to develop interventions that change behaviors and/or enhance skill development through principles of reinforcement and punishment. In the context of behavioral theory reinforcement is considered to occur when the frequency of a given target behavior is increased, whereas punishment occurs when the frequency of a given target behavior is decreased. Behavior analysis is a science that involves studying how to alter the environment so that appropriate behaviors are more likely to occur while inappropriate behaviors will be less likely to occur (Cooper et al., 2007). Strategies used in ABA programs include but are not limited to rewarding behaviors to increase the likelihood they will happen again (i.e., reinforcement), reinforcing successive approximations of a behavior (i.e., shaping), gradually decreasing the amount of prompting provided when teaching a skill (i.e., fading), breaking down tasks into individual parts (i.e., chaining), removing reinforcement to decrease a behavior (i.e., extinction and punishment), demonstrating how to complete a task (i.e., modeling), and providing varying levels of assistance to teach the correct response (i.e., prompting) (Cooper et al., 2007).

There are several important elements of ABA that were initially described by Baer, Wolf, & Risley, (1968) and continue to guide ABA programming. First, behavioral procedures must be applied in nature. This dictates that behaviors that are selected for change should be used to improve a person's life to a socially significant degree. Second, the interventions must be behavioral such that the behaviors targeted for change are clearly defined, focusing on specific behaviors that can be reliably measured. The analytic component requires that the functional relation between the reinforcers (or punishers) and the behavior can be demonstrated by reliable changes in the behavior that are objectively measured. The technological element of ABA indicates that the behavior change procedures are clearly identified and described such that anyone reading them should be able to apply the techniques and replicate the same results. The effective component requires that improvements are sufficient for the intervention to make a socially significant impact on the individual's life. Finally, generality indicates that improvements are generalizable by demonstrating that behavior change lasts over time and across multiple environments beyond the original intervention setting (Baer et al., 1968; Cooper et al., 2007).

ABA AS AN EVIDENCE-BASED INTERVENTION FOR ASD

Behavioral treatments have been applied to build complex behaviors such as language or academic skills and to decrease behavioral excesses such as self-stimulatory behavior and aggression, but it was largely the work of Ivar Lovaas that began in the 1970s that demonstrated the effectiveness of ABA for young children with autism. His interventions differed from previous studies in that the interventions were provided across settings and across different people to help maintain and generalize gains. His landmark study (Lovaas, 1987) reported that young children (age <40–46 months) who received 40 hours per week of ABA demonstrated dramatic improvements when compared to a group that received 10 hours or less of one-to-one treatment per week. Both groups received treatment for 2 or more years and outcomes were assessed between ages 6 and 7 years. Children in the group receiving up to 40 hours per week of ABA therapy 5 to 7 days per week gained an average of 30 IQ points more than the comparison group, and these improvements remained stable over time. Of children in the experimental group, 47% achieved average cognitive functioning and were in a mainstream educational placement compared to 2% of children in the comparison group. Not only was this study important in demonstrating that early intervention can have a significant impact on a child's intellectual functioning, but it was also noted that treatment gains were easy to detect, objectively measure, and socially significant (e.g., educational placement as an outcome variable) (Lovaas, 1987). These types of intensive ABA-based intervention are now often referred to as early intensive behavioral intervention (EIBI).

Lovaas's model focused on both enhancing skill development and reducing problem behavior and relied heavily on a specific teaching approach called discrete trial training (DTT), which includes repetitive practice with immediate feedback that is either corrective or reinforced through praise or the delivery of a preferred reinforcer (e.g., toy, edible) (Roane et al., 2021). For example, when teaching a child to respond to his name, the provider calls the child's name and then provides immediate feedback. This is practiced in a repetitive fashion for a specified number of trials. At each trial, if the child exhibits the correct response (i.e., making eye contact/turning to look toward the person), he is given reinforcement (e.g., "good job looking!" and/or an edible treat). If the child does not respond by looking or turning, he is given corrective feedback and the process is repeated until all trials have been completed. Responses on each trial are recorded as correct or incorrect, and data are analyzed to determine if the child is making improvements. If the child meets mastery criteria (e.g., 85% correct across 2 consecutive weeks), he will move on to the next step of the specified program, or the goal is considered mastered and the focus becomes maintenance and generalization. Once the child is responding in a one-on-one setting, he will move on to practicing this goal in a group setting. If the child does not demonstrate improvements based on objective analysis of data, the team reevaluates the teaching procedures to ensure effectiveness. For example, the targeted skill may need to be changed, the teaching approach may need to be modified, or the reward may need to be changed to enhance motivation. It is important to ensure that when starting a new goal, the child will have a chance at some level of success so that he learns the contingency (relationship) between the correct response and the positive consequence that immediately follows (Cooper et al., 2007; Roane et al., 2016).

Replication studies have further supported the evidence base for the use of EIBI for young children with ASD. For example, Eldevik et al. (2009) found that EIBI is effective for improving adaptive and cognitive skills. Smith and Iadarola (2015) reviewed research on ABA treatments in children 5 years and younger, for two types of ABA, EIBI delivered one-on-one and teacher implemented ABA, both of which were found to have strong empirical support. Additionally, the National Standards Report (National Autism Center, 2009) found 11 evidence-based treatments for ASD, all of which had a behavioral component.

Limitations of the ABA literature for ASD intervention include a small number of randomized controlled trials (RCTs) compared to the large number of studies utilizing within-subject research designs. Additionally, there needs to be more research on a wider variety of target behaviors across individuals with differing presentations of ASD and across development, as much of the literature is focused on young children with communication and cognitive delays.

ABA FOR CHALLENGING BEHAVIOR

ABA researchers have demonstrated that using an experimental procedure the function of a particular problem behavior can be identified (Iwata, Dorsey, Slifer, Bauman, & Richman, 1994). Behaviorism posits that all behaviors serve one of four functions, and that problem behaviors persist because they serve a function that has been reinforced. These four functions include attention (social positive reinforcement), escape/avoidance (negative reinforcement), tangible (positive reinforcement), and automatic (nonsocial positive or negative reinforcement). An experimental functional analysis (EFA) includes a series of experimental manipulations of the environment to determine the factors reinforcing the behavior. The different conditions typically include access to attention, access to tangible items, escape from a demand, and a control condition in which the child is provided attention, preferred tangible items, and no demands are placed on the child. Using a visual analysis (Fig. 94.1), the function of the behavior can be identified and used to inform treatment planning (Cooper et al., 2007; Iwata et al., 1994; Tarbox et al., 2009). The results in the figure show that the target behavior of head banging occurred at increased frequency when the behavior resulted in attention and when it resulted in escape/avoidance.

When results from an EFA demonstrate an automatic function (similar rates of the problem behavior across all conditions, including the control condition), medical reasons contributing to the behavior should be considered. For example, a child with an ear infection or a toothache may start hitting herself in the head, suggesting the behavior is maintained by automatic negative reinforcement (i.e., relieves the pain momentarily).

There have been variations developed on this procedure, such as brief functional analyses, but the principles and basic framework have remained the same (Tarbox et al., 2009). In addition to an EFA already described, two additional methods of identifying the function of a behavior include indirect

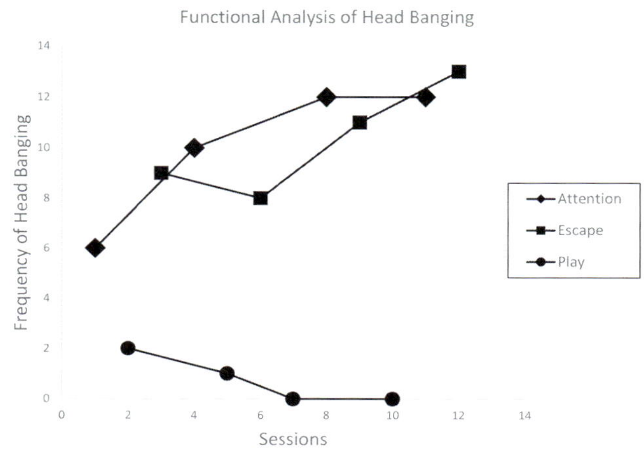

Fig. 94.1 Experimental functional analysis results.

and descriptive assessments. There are important differences across these types of assessments in terms of the reliability of the results they produce and the ease of implementation and data collection. Indirect assessments can include rating scales that have been empirically developed and validated. Assessments such as the Questions About Behavioral Functioning (QABF; Paclawskyj, Matson, Rush, Smalls, & Vollmer, 2000) or the Functional Assessment Screening Tool (FAST; Iwata & DeLeon, 2005) are examples of rating scales that can be completed quickly to identify a hypothesized function.

Descriptive assessments are often completed in an ABC format, in which the *a*ntecedents, *b*ehavior, and *c*onsequences are observed in a child's natural environment. Descriptive assessments can be helpful in classroom and home settings and are often used in outpatient behavioral parent training to help inform the development of function-based behavioral interventions. This requires careful observation, as the observer must notice the target behavior, immediately record what happened right before (antecedent), and then what happened following the behavior (consequence) (Table 94.1). The advantage of an EFA is that it allows for more control over the environment and produces more reliable results. However, EFAs are cumbersome to design and implement, are time

TABLE 94.1 Example of Descriptive Assessment

ABC Data Sheet		**Target Behavior: Physical Aggression**	
Date and time	**Antecedent** (What happened right before the behavior occurred?)	**Behavior** (Describe the behavior, hitting, kicking, throwing)	**Consequence** (What happened immediately after? How did you respond?)
1/1/21 at 12:05pm	*Went to turn the TV off before lunch*	*Threw the remote and hit me in the head*	*Told him "That's not nice, you hurt me"*

intensive, and require advanced training and additional staffing resources. Thus they tend to be used in highly controlled settings, such as inpatient or residential behavioral settings, where there is adequate staffing, time, safety resources, training, and data collection methods that will allow for each condition of the EFA to be conducted across multiple trials and across several days. Both direct and indirect functional assessments have been found to produce conclusive results, but descriptive assessments often do not (Tarbox et al., 2009).

Functional assessments are important as the results are used to develop function-based interventions, which allow a person to learn new ways to meet the same function as the unwanted behavior being engaged in. Within ABA the goal is to teach a skill that the individual can use to achieve the same outcome so that they no longer need to engage in the problem behavior to get the need met. For example, for the child whose data are shown in Fig. 94.1, the fact that head banging occurred at increased frequency when it resulted in attention and when it resulted in escape/avoidance might lead to the development of an intervention that teaches the child alternative ways to request attention or to request not to do a task. Further, if one does not identify the proper function of a behavior, inadvertent reinforcement of the unwanted behaviors may occur (Tarbox et al., 2009). For example, if a child is engaging in tantrums when presented with an assignment, and the function is assumed to be escape from demands, the teacher may repeat the demand or provide corrective feedback under the assumption that letting him out of his work would further reinforce the tantrum. However, if the results from a functional analysis find the tantrums serve an attention-seeking function, the verbal feedback from the teacher could inadvertently reinforce the behavior by providing a verbal response and attention in the form of corrective feedback. In contrast, if the function had been accurately identified, the teacher would have likely used planned ignoring and differential attention, in which the teacher ignores the tantrum and reinforces the child for getting attention in an alternative, more adaptive way (e.g., raising his hand, or saying "excuse me" and then immediately receiving attention from his teacher).

Identifying the function of a problem behavior has become a standard practice under the Individuals with Disabilities Education Act (IDEA) (Tarbox et al., 2009). The results are used to develop a behavior intervention plan based on teaching the student to engage in alternative behaviors to meet that same function. Using functional communication training could be included in the child's behavior intervention plan, whereby the child is given a way to ask for what is wanted, and upon exhibiting the appropriate behavior the child is then reinforced with receiving whatever is requested (e.g., a drink, help, or a break).

QUALIFICATIONS OF ABA PROVIDERS

When looking for appropriate ABA providers, it is important to find practitioners who are certified by the Behavior Analysis Certification Board (BACB). Practitioners may have a degree in the field of ABA or in related fields such as speech therapy, psychology, or occupational therapy (Roane et al., 2016). To become certified, individuals must complete the BACB educational and supervisory requirements to sit for the certification exam to become either a Board Certified Behavior Analyst (BCBA) or a Board Certified Associate Behavior Analyst (BCaBA) (Behavior Analyst Certification Board Handbook, 2020; Cooper et al., 2007). The former requires the person have a graduate level degree in ABA or a related field, while the latter requires a bachelor's degree. Additionally, Registered Behavior Technicians (RBTs) are paraprofessionals typically with high school degrees. Both BCaBAs and RBTs practice under the supervision of a BCBA. The BACB has a specific code of ethics for behavior analysts that was developed and is followed through the Association for Behavior Analysis International (Roane et al., 2016).

Other considerations for identifying quality providers include programs that provide parent training and input. Parents and families are important for ensuring skill generalization to the home and the community and to ensure focus on producing socially meaningful change for the autistic individual and/or family. Families should also seek out behavioral therapy providers that have a well-developed, explicit, and individualized learning plan, a BCBA supervising direct care providers, and a systematic way of reviewing data and making data-based decisions about programming changes and needs. Families should expect to receive progress reports and be informed on their child's progress on goals in all domains of focus (e.g., adaptive, preacademic, social, communication, and motor skills).

VARIATIONS IN ABA THERAPY FOR ASD

Dosage (Hours of Therapy)

While Lovaas advocated for EIBI to be delivered on an intensive basis (e.g., up to 40 hours/week), in practice, children under 5 years are recommended to receive EIBI for a minimum of 25 hours per week, especially when focusing on basic developmental skills such as joint attention and imitation. As kids get older, the number of hours tends to be reduced. For example, a child may receive 15 hours to target more complex social behaviors such as perspective taking and emotion recognition (Roane et al., 2016).

Variations on ABA Modalities

Over the past few decades, evidence-based ABA interventions have included numerous variations of the principles with varying levels of evidence supporting their use. Early models of ABA are often referred to as EIBI based on Lovaas's original description, with the majority of EIBI interventions using the DTT approach described earlier. DTT trials have demonstrated effectiveness in teaching a number of specific skills, and the traditional DTT model remains a well-established intervention for children with ASD (Smith & Iadarola, 2015). However, variations of ABA (Table 94.2) that utilize a more naturalistic approach to teach specific skills, such as pivotal response training (PRT), natural environment training,

TABLE 94.2 Features and Evidence for Different Applied Behavioral Analysis (ABA) Modalities

ABA Modality	Features	Clinical Implications
Discrete Trial Teaching (DTT)	Distraction-free setting with one-on-one instruction Five unique steps: 1. Cue: brief, clear instruction or question 2. Prompt: hand-over-hand or modeling by teacher, gradually faded with success 3. Responses: correct/incorrect; may accept approximations initially with gradual fading of prompts 4. Consequences: positive reinforcement or removal of attention/"no" response 5. Intertrial intervals: pause 1–5 sec between consequence and next cue Recommended strategy for very specific skill development and/or academic skills Mimics antecedent-behavior-consequence (ABC) contingency model	*Clinical delivery:* 1. Registered Behavior Technician (RBT) supervised by Board Certified Behavior Analyst (BCBA) or BCBA *Limitations:* 1. Risk for potential implementation errors: a. Inadequate reinforcement for correct responses b. Poorly timed trials c. Unnecessarily harsh consequences for incorrect responses d. Limited variability of stimuli/exercises Concerns for controlled/scripted nature of training resulting in poor generalization of skills Relies heavily on trainer-initiated activities
Pivotal Response Training (PRT)	Naturalistic language training strategy Implemented in naturalistic, play-based context Utilizes reinforcement for communication attempts and therapist modeling through play Emphasizes "pivotal" areas/skills: 1. Motivation to interact with others 2. Self-management 3. Self-initiation 4. Responsiveness to multiple cues 5. Includes parent training component and parents actively carry out interventions	*Clinical delivery:* Psychologists, speech-language pathologists, or special education teachers *Limitations:* Outcomes impacted by other factors: • Child's age • Severity of autism symptoms • Child's language proficiency • Parental stress • Treatment fidelity Variability in intervention components Limited research on outcome predictors, comparisons with control groups, and components that constitute a PRT intervention model Variability in implementation impacted by trainer background, attitudes toward people with disabilities, and child-trainer relationship
Natural Environment Training (NET)	Utilizes rewards to establish behaviors based on spontaneity Emphasizes rewarding requests ("mands") in the natural setting Typically embedded into child's typical daily environment Capitalizes on ability to identify and use child's preferred motivators	*Clinical delivery:* same as for DTT *Limitations:* May be limited by child's interests, making it difficult to expand teaching opportunities No specific script or curriculum
Verbal Behavior Therapy	Classifies language components based on function: 1. Mand = request 2. Tact = comment to share experience or draw attention 3. Intraverbal = word used to respond to a question 4. Echoic = repeated ("echoed") word Combines DTT with naturalistic strategies to promote use of language with respect to social events that precede and follow communication events Emphasizes "errorless learning" through a series of prompts to emphasize correct use of language Verbal Behavior Milestones Assessment and Placement Program (VB-MAPP) is an assessment tool, curriculum guide, and skill tracking system based on the verbal behavior therapy approach (Fig. 94.2)	*Clinical delivery:* Psychologist, BCBA, special education teacher, speech language pathologists *Limitations:* Limited research on impact on adaptive or functional skills

TABLE 94.2 Features and Evidence for Different Applied Behavioral Analysis (ABA) Modalities—Cont'd

ABA Modality	Features	Clinical Implications
Picture Exchange Communication System (PECS) (Fig. 94.3)	https://pecsusa.com/pecs/ Combines DTT with naturalistic strategies Emphasizes requesting specific activities/items by handing pictures cards to others Common choice for nonverbal individuals	*Clinical delivery:* Speech-language pathologists Others who have completed PECS training *Limitations:* Benefits not consistently sustained after intervention Individuals with milder symptoms of ASD had greater improvements than those with more severe symptoms
Early Start Denver Model (ESDM)	https://www.esdm.co/ Developmentally informed curriculum addressing all developmental domains Core teaching strategies focus on: 1. Interpersonal exchange and positive affect 2. Shared engagement with real-life materials and activities 3. Adult responsivity and sensitivity to child cues 4. Focus on verbal and nonverbal communication Combines individualized therapist-driven interventions with parent training for every day using during routine activities (feeding, dressing, bathing, etc.)	*Clinical delivery:* Therapists who meet the following criteria: • Work with young children with ASD • Educational degree and professional license to practice independently • Part of interdisciplinary team • Completion of introductory and advanced ESDM workshops and certification supervision procedures *Limitations:* Intensive model (frequent individualized therapist-led sessions over 2 yr) has strongest evidence for impacting child behaviors Specific training protocol for ESDM therapists to become certified in ESDM
Treatment and Education of Autistic and Related Communication–Handicapped Children (TEACCH) (Fig. 94.4)	https://teacch.com/ Emphasizes close working relationship between practitioners and parents Adapt intervention to individualized characteristics of the patient Curriculum goals based on baseline standardized test results Structured teaching protocol includes organizing environment and activities to optimize learning and avoid frustration Arrange activities in a predictable fashion (visual schedules) Organize materials and tasks to minimize reliance on adult directions/prompts Targets activities of daily living, communication, social skills, executive function, attention, and engagement	*Clinical delivery:* Professional certification program through University of North Carolina *Limitations:* Expensive and intensive training required

verbal behavior therapy, and picture exchange communication system, have demonstrated improved communication and cognitive performance in smaller samples (Delprato, 2001; Lima et al., 2018; Peterson, 2004; Roane et al., 2016; Stock, Mirenda, & Smith, 2013).

Another emerging modality, the Early Start Denver Model (ESDM), combines ABA principles with a focus on developmental milestones specifically emphasizing imitation, verbal and nonverbal communication, social and emotional sharing, and play (Roane et al., 2016). The model often utilizes an interdisciplinary team to deliver the intervention with improvements in developmental growth for toddlers when the intervention was delivered intensively and directly by therapists. However, when parents were trained to implement ESDM in follow-up studies, outcomes were not different from comparison treatments (Roane et al., 2016).

A final program, Treatment and Education of Autistic and Related Communication–Handicapped Children (TEACCH), emphasizes structure and predictability in the classroom or center-based program to increase functional skills and minimize frustration and distractions. Moderate to large gains have been reported in social behaviors and reduction of maladaptive behaviors (Virues-Ortega, Julio, & Pastor-Barriuso, 2013), and a preliminary trial of a parent-mediated TEACCH intervention revealed similar benefits on social communication skills (Turner-Brown, Hume, Boyd, & Kainz, 2019).

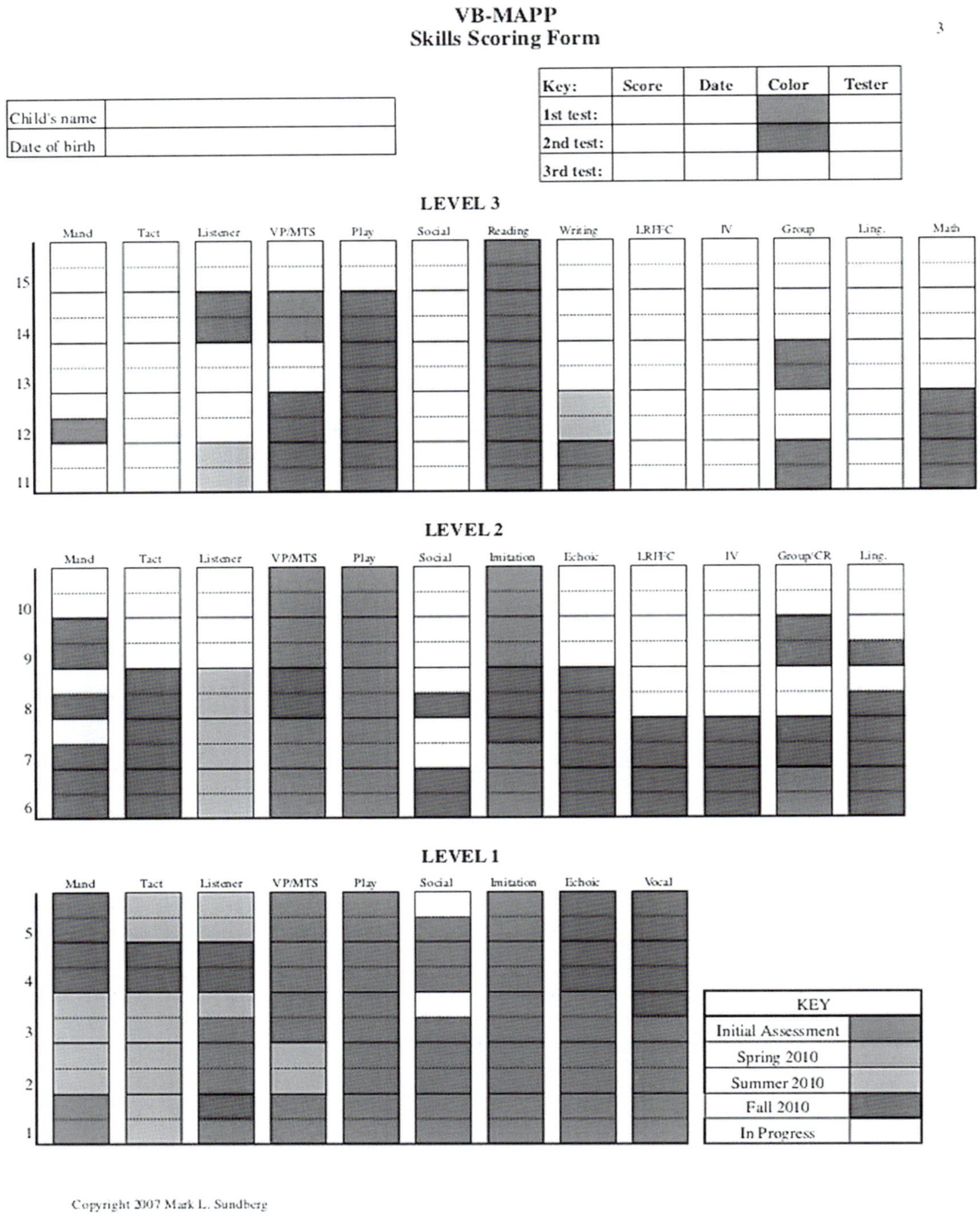

Fig. 94.2 Example of VB-MAPP. With kind permission from Mark Sundberg.

Table 94.2 includes descriptions of the differentiating features and clinical delivery requirements for the ABA modalities included in the majority of autism-specific treatment plans.

Home-Based Versus Center-Based Approaches

The many studies of the various models of ABA therapy have delivered interventions in a range of settings, including clinical center-based intervention programs, special education classrooms, mainstream classrooms, institutions, medical settings, and homes. Potential benefits of center-based instruction include opportunities to deliver interventions with same-age peers for modeling and practicing of skills, increased frequency of one-on-one therapist-driven interventions, and an environment specifically designed to support an ABA-based intervention. Home-based interventions, however, offer opportunity for the child to learn and practice skills in the child's natural

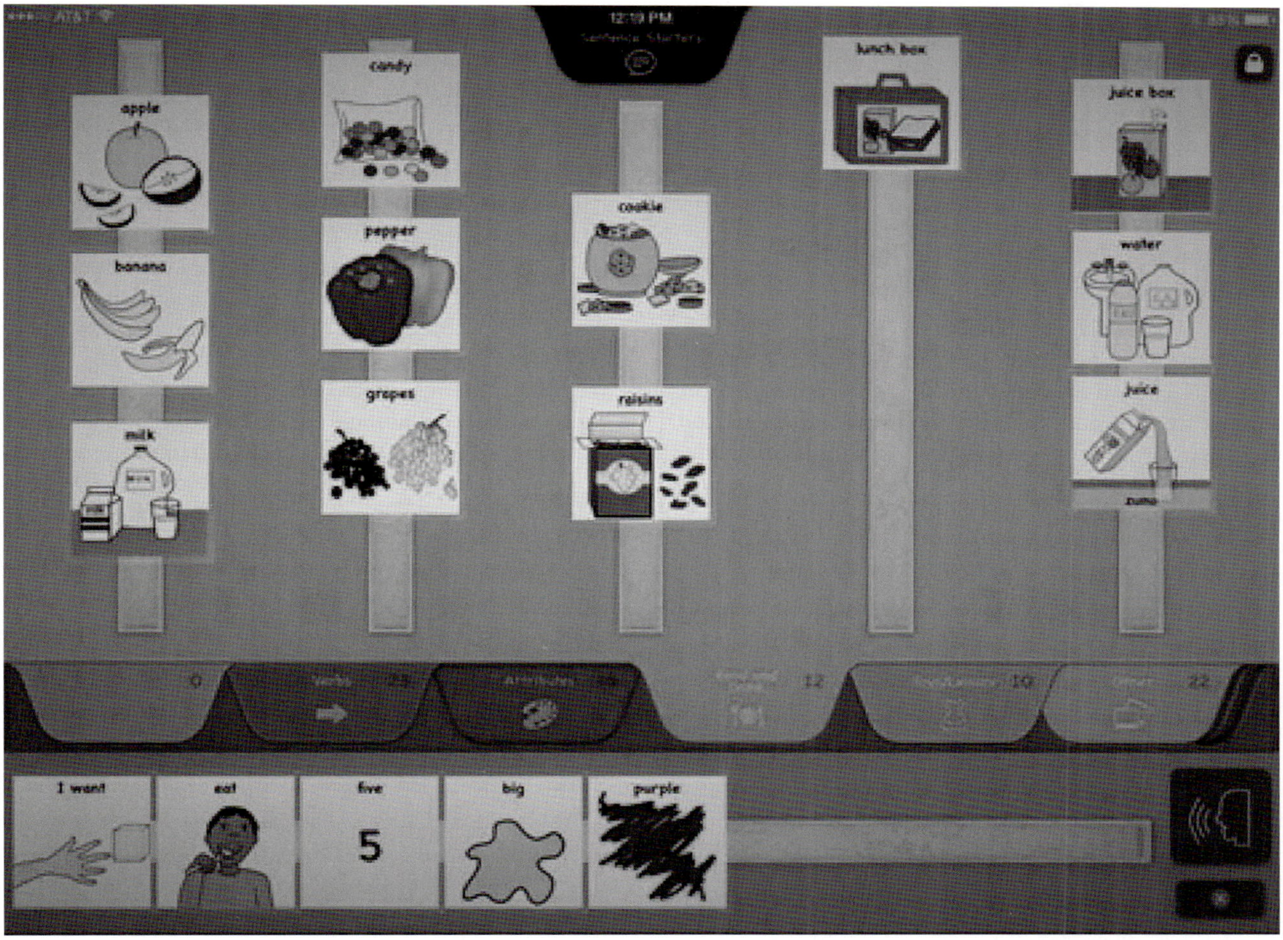

Fig. 94.3 Example of Picture Exchange Communication System (PECS) board. (From https://i.ytimg.com/vi/9wRykZKrl7I/maxresdefault.jpg)

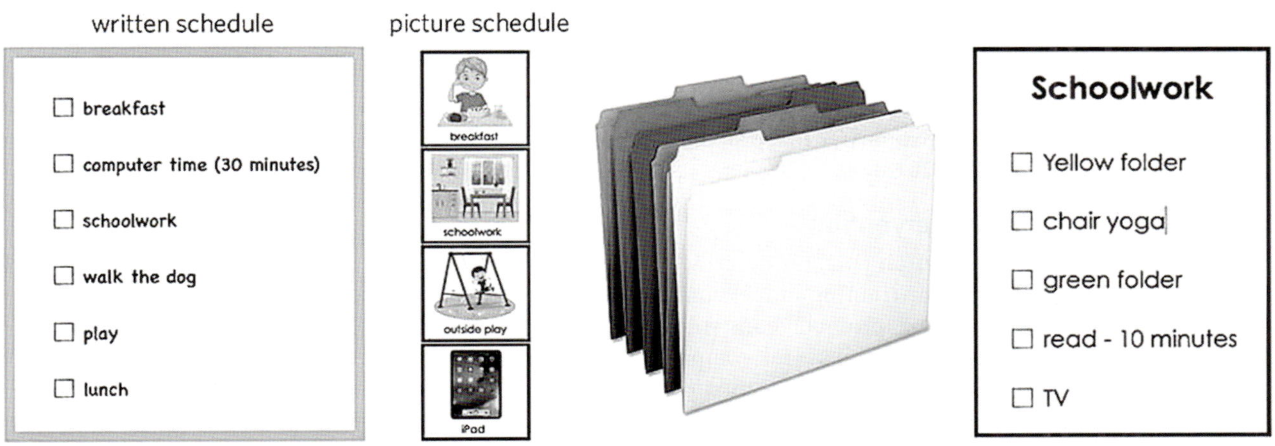

Fig. 94.4 Sample of Treatment and Education of Autistic and Related Communication–Handicapped Children (TEACCH) materials. University of North Carolina TEACCH® Autism Program.

environment, potentially leading to improved generalization of newly acquired skills with family and others in the child's community. In spite of the potential impact of setting on outcomes, few studies have specifically evaluated the setting of intervention when reporting outcomes after ABA-based interventions. One retrospective study comparing center-based interventions and home-based interventions in a sample of children 3 to 12 years old with ASD demonstrated significantly greater mastery of skills per hour of center-based intervention compared to home-based intervention (Dixon et al., 2016).

OTHER BEHAVIORAL MODELS

While ABA-based interventions have the strongest evidence supporting their use for autistic people, other behavioral models offer alternative approaches to the traditional ABA methods for addressing social communication deficits and behavior challenges associated with ASD.

Developmental, Individual Difference, Relationship-Based/Floortime Play

Developmental, Individual Difference, Relationship-based (DIR), often called floortime play, consists of encouraging spontaneous and structured or unstructured play sessions to promote relationship building, two-way communication, social engagement, complex thinking, and problem solving (Greenspan & Wieder, 1999; Rojas-Torres, Alonso-Esteban, & Alcantud-Marín, 2020). Several small trials or single-subject case reports have highlighted improvements in child behavior, family interactions, and ASD symptoms. A pilot RCT of adding DIR-based floortime play to conventional intervention for preschool children with ASD found that those receiving DIR-based floortime play demonstrated greater improvements in ASD symptoms and improved emotional development. A 1-year follow-up study demonstrated continued improvements in symptoms as well as family relationships (Rojas-Torres et al., 2020). Other studies utilizing DIR-based floortime play principles have demonstrated improvements in functional development, parent-child interactions, overall symptom severity, and improved ability of parents to read and respond to their child's social demands (Rojas-Torres et al., 2020). However, there have been concerns with experimental design and validity of the outcomes measures used in the treatment trials. Many of the measures were created specifically to assess effects of DIR/floortime and not standardized. Other concerns about the intervention include the lack of structure resulting in increased frustration for the child, limited ability to reinforce specific skills through repetition, and the possibility of reinforcing nonfunctional or inappropriate play skills (Ross, Harrison, & Zane, 2018).

Relationship Development Intervention

Relationship development intervention (RDI) is described as a cognitive-developmental parent-training model comprising an intensive parent-training protocol consisting of 6 days of trainings on theory, principles, and components of RDI as well as weekly or biweekly consultation meetings with an RDI consultant and 6-month intensive reevaluation of skills (Gutstein, Burgess, & Montfort, 2007). Through participation in the RDI program, parents learn how to perceive and scaffold learning opportunities for the autistic child to respond in flexible and thoughtful ways to novel and increasingly unpredictable settings. One published study includes a chart review of 16 children age 20 to 96 months with ASD and reported reduced ASD symptoms and increased mainstream educational placement in children receiving the RDI intervention. However, limitations of the study include lack of a control group and small sample size (Gutstein et al., 2007).

Behavior Therapy and Modified Cognitive-Behavioral Therapy

The application of behavioral interventions to treat common challenges for autistic individuals is increasingly frequent. Given the heterogeneity of ASD presentations, there is a need for more research on the efficacy of modified behavioral and cognitive-behavioral interventions (Roane et al., 2016), but a metaanalysis focused on these behavioral interventions for adolescents and adults with autism is promising as it found medium to strong effect sizes addressing areas of academic skills, phobias, vocational skills, challenging behaviors, and daily living skills (Roth, Gillis, & DiGennaro Reed, 2014).

Children with ASD also may present with high levels of comorbid psychopathology (Vasa et al., 2014). Some research has shifted to focusing on how to treat these co-occurring problems through adaptations of more transitional ABA approaches. There is support for the use of modified cognitive-behavioral therapy (M-CBT) to address concerns, including anxiety, depression, and social skills. CBT is focused on helping the patient identify unhelpful thought patterns that may be impacting the individual's emotions and behaviors and challenging those unhelpful thoughts to shift the way the individual thinks about a problem (see Chapter 98). The theory is that by changing thoughts, this will change emotions related to those thoughts, as well as the behaviors an individual engages in. Similarly, by changing behaviors, this can help shift thinking styles and emotions. Oftentimes in CBT, a patient starts to identify unhelpful thoughts and then practices applying the use of positive self-talk and coping skills to reduce negative emotions. For anxiety, this typically includes the use of exposure therapy; for autistic individuals, it includes providing differential reinforcement for facing fears. Behavioral interventions have been used to address fears and phobias such as medical and dental phobias and M-CBT has demonstrated efficacy for reducing anxiety in individuals with high functioning autism, as defined by average IQ and language skills (Sukhodolsky, Bloch, Panza, & Reichow, 2013).

Behavioral parent training has been an additional approach to helping parents address challenging behaviors in children with ASD. In a RCT comparing medication and combination of medication plus parent training the combination group was superior to medication alone for reducing challenging behaviors such as aggression, tantrums, and self-injury (Aman et al., 2009). Additionally, in one of the largest RCTs of behavior intervention for ASD parent behavior training was found to be significantly more effective at reducing disruptive behaviors as compared to parent education (Bearss et al., 2015). Results from these studies underscore the importance of parent implementation of behavioral strategies to reduce challenging behaviors and facilitate generalization of treatment gains from the treatment setting into the home setting.

CONCLUSION

ABA therapy may vary greatly in the specific methodologies but has generally good evidence supporting its use to increase skill development and reduce problematic behaviors. Much of the research on ABA for children with ASD is based on lower functioning individuals who present with cognitive and communication delays. With increased awareness of ASD, however, there has been increased heterogeneity that will require ongoing empirical investigation regarding which specific treatments work best for various presenting problems and levels of functioning (Roane et al., 2016). Clinicians treating autistic individuals should familiarize themselves with local providers and agencies that provide ABA interventions, including their experience with specific methodologies and/or treatment goals and what documentation may be required for a client to qualify for services.

REFERENCES

Aman, M. G., McDougle, C. J., Scahill, L., Handen, B., Arnold, L. E., Johnson, C., … Research Units on Pediatric Psychopharmacology Autism Network. (2009). Medication and parent training in children with pervasive developmental disorders and serious behavior problems: Results from a randomized clinical trial. *Journal of the American Academy of Child and Adolescent Psychiatry*, *48*(12), 1143–1154. https://doi.org/10.1097/CHI.0b013e3181bfd669

American Psychiatric Association. (2013). Autism spectrum disorder. *Diagnostic and statistical manual of mental disorders* (5th ed.). https://doi.org/10.1176/appi.books.9780890425596

Baer, D. M., Wolf, M. M., & Risley, T. R. (1968). Some concurrent dimensions of applied behavior analysis. *Journal of Applied Behavior Analysis*, *1*, 91–97.

Bearss, K., Johnson, C., Smith, T., Lecavalier, L., Swiezy, N., Aman, M., … Scahill, L. (2015). Effect of parent training vs parent education on behavioral problems in children with autism spectrum disorder: A randomized clinical trial. *JAMA*, *313*(15), 1524–1533. https://doi.org/10.1001/jama.2015.3150

Behavior Analyst Certification Board. (2020). *Behavior Analyst Certification Board handbook*. https://www.bacb.com/wp-content/uploads/2020/11//BCBAHandbook_210513.pdf

Cooper, J. O., Heron, T. E., & Heward, W. L. (2007). *Applied behavior analysis* (2nd ed.). Pearson Education Inc.

Delprato, D. (2001). Comparisons of discrete-trail and normalized behavioral language interventions for young children with autism. *Journal of Autism & Developmental Disorders*, *31*(3), 315–325.

Dixon, D. R., Burns, C. O., Granpeesheh, D., Amarasinghe, R., Powell, A., & Linstead, E. (2016). A program evaluation of home and center-based treatment for autism spectrum disorder. *Behavior Analysis in Practice*, *10*(3), 307–312. https://doi.org/10.1007/s40617-016-0155-7

Eldevik, S., Hastings, R. P., Hughes, J. C., Jahr, E., Eikeseth, S., & Cross, S. (2009). Meta-analysis of early intensive behavioral intervention for children with autism. *Journal of Clinical Child and Adolescent Psychology: The Official Journal for the Society of Clinical Child and Adolescent Psychology, American Psychological Association, Division 53*, *38*(3), 439–450. https://doi.org/10.1080/15374410902851739

Fishbein, L., Rouse, M. L., Minshawi, N., & Fodstad, J. C. (2017). Historical development of treatment. In J. L. Matson (Ed.), *Handbook of treatments for autism spectrum disorders*. Springer.

Greenspan, S. I., & Wieder, S. (1999). A functional developmental approach to autism spectrum disorders. *Journal of the Association for Persons with Severe Handicaps*, *24*(3), 147–161. https://doi.org/10.2511/rpsd.24.3.147

Gutstein, S. E., Burgess, A. F., & Montfort, K. (2007). Evaluation of the relationship development intervention program. *Autism*, *11*(5), 397–411. https://doi.org/10.1177/1362361307079603

Haller, B. (2016). *Journalists should learn to carefully traverse a variety of disability terminology* [online commentary]. (2016). National Center on Disability and Journalism. https://ncdj.org/2016/01/journalists-should-learn-to-carefully-traverse-a-variety-of-disability-terminology/

Hardan, A. Y., Gengoux, G. W., Berquist, K. L., Libove, R. A., Ardel, C. M., Phillips, J., … Minjarez, M. B. (2015). A randomized controlled trial of Pivotal Response Treatment Group for parents of children with autism. *Journal of Child Psychology and Psychiatry*, *56*(8), 884–892. https://doi.org/10.1111/jcpp.12354

Iwata, B., & DeLeon, I. (2005). *The functional analysis screening tool*. The Florida Center on Self Injury, University of Florida.

Iwata, B. A., Dorsey, M. F., Slifer, K. J., Bauman, K. E., & Richman, G. S. (1994). Toward a functional analysis of self-injury. *Journal of Applied Behavior Analysis*, *27*, 197–209.

Joshi, G., Wozniak, J., Petty, C., Martelon, M. K., Fried, R., Bolfek, A., … Biederman, J. (2013). Psychiatric comorbidity and functioning in a clinically referred population of adults with autism spectrum disorders: A comparative study. *Journal of Autism and Developmental Disorders*, *43*, 1314–1325. https://doi.org/10.1007/s10803-012-1679-5

Kuhlthau, K. A., McDonnell, E., Coury, D. L., Payakachat, N., & Macklin, E. (2018). Associations of quality of life with health-related characteristics among children with autism. *Autism*, *22*(7), 804–813. https://doi.org/10.1177/1362361317704420

Lima Antão, J., Oliveira, A., Almeida Barbosa, R. T., Crocetta, T. B., Guarnieri, R., Arab, C., … Abreu, L. C. (2018). Instruments for augmentative and alternative communication for children with autism spectrum disorder: A systematic review. *Clinics (Sao Paulo, Brazil)*, *73*, e497. https://doi.org/10.6061/clinics/2017/e497

Lovaas, O. I. (1979). Contrasting illness and behavioral models for the treatment of autistic children: A historical perspective. *Journal of Autism and Developmental Disorders*, *9*, 315–323. https://doi.org/10.1007/BF01531442

Lovaas, O. I. (1987). Behavioral treatment and normal educational and intellectual functioning in young autistic children. *Journal of Consulting and Clinical Psychology*, *55*, 3–9.

National Autism Center. (2009). *National standards report: National Standards Project—addressing the need for evidence-based practice guidelines for autism spectrum disorders*. Author.

Paclawskyj, T. R., Matson, J. L., Rush, K. S., Smalls, Y., & Vollmer, T. R. (2000). Questions about behavioral function (QABF): A behavioral checklist for functional assessment of aberrant behavior. *Research in Developmental Disabilities*, *21*(3), 223–229. https://doi.org/10.1016/S0891-4222(00)00036-6

Peterson, P. (2004). Naturalistic language teaching procedures for children at risk for language delay. *Behavior Analyst Today*, *5*(4), 404–424.

Roane, H. S., Fisher, W. W., & Carr, J. E. (2016). Applied behavior analysis as a treatment for autism spectrum disorder. *Journal of Pediatrics*, *175*, 27–32.

Rojas-Torres, L. P., Alonso-Esteban, Y., & Alcantud-Marín, F. (2020). Early intervention with parents of children with autism spectrum disorders: A review of programs. *Children (Basel, Switzerland)*, *7*(12), 294. https://doi.org/10.3390/children7120294

Ross, R. K., Harrison, K. L., & Zane, T. (2018). Focus on science: Is there science behind that?: Autism and treatment with DIR/floor time. *Science in Autism Treatment*, *15*(1), 20–24.

Roth, M. E., Gillis, J. M., & DiGennaro Reed, F. (2014). A meta-analysis of behavioral interventions for adolescents and adults with autism spectrum disorders. *Journal of Behavioral Education*, *23*, 258–286.

Smith, T., & Iadarola, S. (2015). Evidence base update for autism spectrum disorder. *Journal of Clinical Child and Adolescent Psychology: The Official Journal for the Society of Clinical Child and Adolescent Psychology, American Psychological Association, Division 53*, *44*(6), 897–922. https://doi.org/10.1080/15374416.2015.1077448

Stock, R., Mirenda, P., & Smith, I. (2013). Comparison of community-based verbal behavior and pivotal response treatment programs for young children with autism spectrum disorder. *Research in Autism Spectrum Disorders*, *7*, 1168–1181.

Sukhodolsky, D. G., Bloch, M. H., Panza, K. E., & Reichow, B. (2013). Cognitive-behavioral therapy for anxiety in children with high-functioning autism: a meta-analysis. *Pediatrics*, *132*(5), e1341–e1350. https://doi.org/10.1542/peds.2013-1193

Tarbox, J., Wile, A. E., Najdowski, A. C., Findel-Pyles, R. S., Balasanyan, S., Caveney, A. , … Tia, B. (2009). Comparing indirect, descriptive, and experimental functional assessments of challenging behavior in children with autism. *Journal of Developmental and Physical Disabilities*, *21*, 493–514.

Turner-Brown, L., Hume, K., Boyd, B. A., & Kainz, K. (2019). Preliminary efficacy of family implemented TEACCH for toddlers: Effects on parents and their toddlers with autism spectrum disorder. *Journal of Autism and Developmental Disorders*, *49*(7), 2685–2698. https://doi.org/10.1007/s10803-016-2812-7

Vasa, R. A., Carroll, L. M., Nozzolillo, A. A., Mahajan, R., Mazurek, M. O., Bennett, A. E., … Bernal, M. P. (2014). A systematic review of treatments for anxiety in youth with autism spectrum disorders. *Journal of Autism and Developmental Disorders*, *44*(12), 3215–3229. https://doi.org/10.1007/s10803-014-2184-9

Virues-Ortega, J., Julio, F. M., & Pastor-Barriuso, R. (2013). The TEACCH program for children and adults with autism: A meta-analysis of intervention studies. *Clinical Psychology Review*, *33*(8), 940–953. https://doi.org/10.1016/j.cpr.2013.07.005

95

Crisis Management in Developmental-Behavioral Pediatrics

Brittany R. Myers and Raman Marwaha

For additional material related to the content of this chapter, please see Chapter 15.

VIGNETTE

A 13-year-old male with mild intellectual disability and learning difficulties presents in clinic for assessment. Parents report that he has always had angry outbursts, but in the last year he seems increasingly irritable and aggressive at home. When you meet with him alone, he may describe any of the following crises: Suicidality, aggression, homicidaity, anxiety, abuse or neglect, psychotic symptoms, intoxication, or a caregiver mental health crisis.

INTRODUCTION

The potential crises mentioned in the chapter-opening vignette are not uncommon in developmental-behavioral pediatrics. In clinical practice we often work with children with significant behavioral and emotional concerns, and we work with families that are often under a high degree of stress. Sometimes patients and their families present to us already in crisis. Other times, we discover a crisis during a routine assessment and then must handle that crisis while managing a busy clinic.

This chapter offers general guidelines for managing different types of crises that may present in pediatric clinical practice across multiple settings (e.g., ambulatory setting, inpatient, emergency department). Other chapters will include more in-depth review of pertinent theories and literature on many of the topics. This chapter focuses on practical management of various acute crises presenting in developmental-behavioral pediatric practice settings. Every patient and crisis are unique and will require consideration of multiple factors, including the patient's current presentation, social and family context, culture, sources of support and protective factors, available resources, legal and ethical guidelines, and clinician comfort. This chapter does not present "right answers" for how to handle every crisis but rather aims to give clinicians a framework to guide conceptualization and decision making during a crisis, which should then be clinically tailored to each individual patient's needs. Throughout this chapter, we refer back to the vignette, each time changing some details to illustrate how the same patient may present with different crises that need to be addressed differently.

SUICIDALITY AND SELF-HARM

Suicide is currently the second leading cause of death in adolescents and young adults from 10 to 34 years of age (Hedegaard, Curtin, & Warner, 2020), and suicide rates continue to increase annually (Hedegaard, Curtin, & Warner, 2018). Suicidal ideation is most commonly associated with depression, but children and adolescents may experience suicidal ideation in many other circumstances, for example, when they are feeling very anxious or frustrated, when they have experienced trauma, when they are being bullied, when they are having school or relationship difficulties, or when they are adjusting to life changes. Chapters 49 and 50 cover mood disorders and suicidality in more detail. This chapter focuses on assessing acute suicidality.

Our 13-year-old male (from the vignette) with mild intellectual disability and learning difficulties presents in clinic for aggressive behavior. When parents leave the room, he shares that he often wishes he weren't alive, and sometimes he cuts himself.

Assessment

When assessing mood concerns and suicidality, it is important to speak with adolescent patients alone. Younger children may feel more at ease with parents in the room, so it may be helpful to offer young patients both choices and use clinical judgment to decide who should be present. When meeting with minor patients alone, the clinician should always first review together the rules around teen privacy and limits to confidentiality. Both the patient and the caregivers should understand in advance that the clinician may break patient confidentiality to share with caregivers any concerns for safety, including self-harm, harm to others, and in some cases concerns for abuse. Laying down these ground rules before assessing the patient alone provides transparency and helps to preserve the clinician's relationship and trust with the teen.

When assessing suicidality with the teen alone, the clinician should first build rapport and learn about the patient's interests, strengths, and support network. The clinician should then assess the history of mood concerns and both past and recent suicidal ideation, including onset, frequency,

TABLE 95.1 Considerations for Management of Suicide/Homicide Risk by Risk Level, Including Possible Levels of Care and Safety Plan

Type of Risk	Level of Risk	Possible Level of Care	Elements of Safety Plan
Suicidal ideation	High/ imminent	• Inpatient psychiatric hospitalization • Emergency department	• Do not leave patient unsupervised • Sweep environment to remove dangerous objects • Transfer to higher level of care
	Moderate	• Intensive outpatient • Partial hospitalization • Outpatient therapy • Psychiatry	• Identify warning signs • Coping skills, including behavioral and social distractions • Names of supportive adults to help manage future crises • Remove access to lethal means of harm: guns, pills, sharps, and other dangerous objects • Increased parental monitoring • Give crisis numbers
	Low	• Outpatient therapy • Psychiatry	
Homicidal ideation	High/ imminent	• Inpatient psychiatric hospitalization • Emergency department	• Do not leave patient unsupervised • Sweep environment to remove dangerous objects • Transfer to higher level of care • Consider duty to warn/protect
	Moderate	• Intensive outpatient • Partial hospitalization • Wrap-around services • Outpatient therapy • Psychiatry	• Inform caregivers • Identify warning signs • Coping skills, including relaxation techniques, distraction • Names of supportive adults to help manage future crises • Remove access to lethal means of harm: guns, pills, sharps, and other dangerous objects • Increased parental monitoring • Give crisis numbers • Consider duty to warn/protect
	Low	• Outpatient therapy • Psychiatry	

duration, and nature of suicidal thoughts. Is the patient having passive thoughts like "I wish I had never been born," or active thoughts like "I want to kill myself"? The clinician should next assess any previous suicidal behaviors or attempts and then assess current thoughts, plans, and intent. While having a suicide plan places teens at higher risk for suicidal behavior, some adolescents who do not endorse a plan for suicide may still have considered possible methods or may act impulsively in a moment of distress, placing them at risk. When assessing suicidal behaviors, the clinician should differentiate between suicide attempts and nonsuicidal self-injury such as cutting or burning oneself. This distinction is important because previous suicide attempts increase risk of future attempts. The clinician should also consider the lethality of previous attempts and the patient's access to lethal objects.

Intervention

Once it has been established that a patient is at risk for suicidality, the patient should not be left alone, and efforts should be made to ensure the safety of the clinical environment by removing any potentially dangerous objects. These steps will look different depending on the setting, and institutions often have specific safety protocols around suicidality. Based on the patient's current suicidality, risk, and protective factors, the clinician then must determine patient disposition and link the patient to the appropriate level of care. If the patient does not appear to be at imminent risk for self-harm, the clinician can work with the family to create a safety plan with close follow-up. If the patient appears to be at imminent risk of harming themself, the clinician should facilitate transfer to a higher level of care. When determining disposition, the clinician should also consider the patient's sources of support and whether the patient and family appear able to follow a safety plan (Table 95.1).

VIOLENT OUTBURST AND AGGRESSION

Another crisis that commonly arises in developmental-behavioral pediatrics is aggression or agitation.

Let us return to our 13-year-old patient in the vignette: When you interview him alone, he becomes angry and starts to break and throw things in the office.

Assessment

Before acting, the clinician should first form a working conceptualization of the problem at hand. Aggressive outbursts in children and adolescents can arise for many reasons, and it is helpful to have ideas of what is triggering the behavior to guide the clinician's response. It is important first to consider the child's age and developmental level. Children may become agitated when they do not have the language abilities to express themselves verbally or when there are developmental delays or sensory sensitivities. Children may become aggressive when they are frustrated, tired, frightened, or in pain. Aggression can also be a sign of an underlying mood, anxiety, or attention concern or trauma. In assessing aggression one should consider the patient's history of previous violence with weapons or access to weapons as this increases the potential risk of harm to self or others. See Chapter 55 for discussion of disruptive behaviors and aggression.

Intervention

In responding to aggressive behavior in a clinical setting safety of all parties is the highest priority. Clinicians should never put themselves in harm's way and should also prioritize the safety of the patient, the patient's family, and other patients and staff in the clinic. As the child starts to become agitated, there may be ways for the clinician to defuse the situation before behavior escalates. If the patient is agitated during a medical procedure, it may be helpful to give the patient a break, avoid further triggers, distract the patient, or give the patient some choices. Once a patient is agitated, clinicians should strive to remain calm, lower the volume of their voice, and speak to the patient in a nonthreatening manner.

When dealing with aggressive behaviors in children, one should always use the least restrictive means possible to manage the situation safely: The clinician should attempt to ensure that there are no dangerous objects (e.g., sharps, blunt objects) in the room, or attempt to move the patient to a safer space to calm down if safe to do so. If the patient is a threat to clinicians, staff, or other patients, the clinician should follow organizational guidelines for violent patients; this may include using a panic button, calling police, calling the appropriate code, or use of restraint or seclusion. Clinicians should be aware that police involvement and/or use of restraint in some cases may further escalate a situation or further traumatize a patient, particularly given the context of widespread incidences of police brutality in communities of color and systemic racism both in the justice system and in medicine. Clinicians should reflect on their own biases when making decisions to use more restrictive measures. Studies of clinician bias have found that clinicians were more likely to use restraint when patients were Black, younger, male, uninsured, homeless, or were diagnosed with psychotic disorders, bipolar disorders, posttraumatic stress disorder, or substance use disorders (Schnitzer et al., 2020).

Once the patient is calm, the clinician next should determine the patient's disposition and appropriate discharge plan. If the patient remains a risk to themself or others, the clinician can facilitate transfer to the emergency room or a higher level of care. If the clinician and caregivers feel that the patient is safe for discharge home, the clinician can go over a safety plan and consider appropriate referrals for the family (e.g., outpatient therapy, intensive outpatient, wrap-around services). See Table 95.1 for more information on safety planning.

Restraint and Seclusion

The term *restraint* refers to any method, device, or material that reduces a patient's freedom of movement or manages a patient's behavior that is not a standard of treatment for the patient's condition (Condition of participation: Patient's rights, 2019). Restraint may only be used when a patient presents an imminent risk to themself or others and other less restrictive measures to manage the behavior have failed. Restraint can mean physical restraint (i.e., use of physical methods to restrain) or chemical restraint (i.e., use of medications to restrain). The use of chemical restraint is preferable to physical restraint due to increased risk of injury when using physical restraint. Table 95.2 lists medications that can be used for aggression in children (Pappadopulos et al., 2003). Seclusion refers to the involuntary confinement of a patient away from others when they are severely violent or at imminent danger to themselves.

There are very specific guidelines for use of restraint and seclusion, including in what circumstances restraint may be used, who has authority to order restraints, how staff must be trained, how long patients can be kept in restraints, how often they must be reassessed, and how use of restraint must be documented. Clinicians using restraint or seclusion should be aware of state, local, and institutional policies and professional guidelines around restraint.

THREATS OF HARM TO OTHERS

Sometimes patients present to clinic with homicidal ideation, or thoughts of harming others.

> *Returning to our 13-year-old patient: This time, in the visit parents express concerns that he has been increasingly aggressive toward siblings. The patient discloses that he sometimes has thoughts of killing his sister, and once a few months ago he went and got a knife and considered stabbing her but did not.*

Assessment

To determine appropriate next steps, the clinician first needs to know more about the history and onset of homicidal ideation, precipitating events and triggers, frequency, and duration of homicidal thoughts, and whether homicidal thoughts are currently happening. If the patient is not currently endorsing homicidal thoughts, it is important to know when the most recent thoughts occurred, and clinicians should further evaluate the nature of the homicidal thoughts. As in suicidal thoughts, homicidal or aggressive thoughts can be passive (e.g., "I wish that person would die") or more active (e.g., "I want to kill that person") and can vary in specificity, plan, intent, lethality, and access to means.

Intervention

The appropriate level of intervention depends on the results of the abovementioned assessment. As with suicidal thoughts, if a patient appears to be an imminent risk of harm to others, the clinician should recommend a higher level of care such as inpatient psychiatric hospitalization. The clinician must also consider whether there is sufficient concern to trigger a duty to warn any identifiable potential victims or duty to protect others. If the clinician feels that the patient is safe to be discharged home with caregivers, the clinician should first engage in safety planning with the family (see Table 95.1). If a patient is having thoughts of harming or killing others,

TABLE 95.2 **Medication Considerations for Crisis Management in Children**

Name	Dosage/Route	Route	Indication
Atypical Antipsychotic			
Aripiprazole	2.5–30 mg/daily	PO	Schizophrenia, bipolar mania
Risperidone	0.25–6 mg/daily; q6	PO, PO disintegrating tablet, IM, IV	Aggression associated with autism, disruptive behavior disorder[a]
Quetiapine	12.5–600 mg/daily	PO	Schizophrenia, bipolar mania
Olanzapine	2.5–20 mg/daily; q6	PO, sublingual tablet, IM, IV	Disruptive behavior disorder[a]
Paliperidone	3–12 mg/daily	PO	Schizophrenia, disruptive behavior disorder[a]
Lurasidone	20–80 mg/daily	PO	Schizophrenia, bipolar depression
Typical Antipsychotic			
Haloperidol	0.5–30 mg/daily; q6	PO, IM, IV	Schizophrenia, bipolar mania[a] Disruptive behavior disorder[a]
Mood Stabilizer			
Lithium	300–1200 mg/daily (therapeutic range: 0.8–1.2 mEq/L)	PO	Bipolar mania, aggression[a]
Valproic acid	15–20 mg/kg/day In two to three daily doses (therapeutic range: 85–110 mcg/mL)	PO, liquid	
Benzodiazepines			
Lorazepam	0.25–6 mg/daily; q6	PO, IM, IV	Aggression,[a,b] panic attack,[a,b] Anxiety[a,b]
Clonazepam	0.25–2 mg/daily in divided doses	PO	Panic attack,[a,b] anxiety[a,b]
Antihistamine			
Diphenhydramine	12.5–50 mg each dose; q6	PO, IM, IV	Agitation[a,c]
SSRIs			
Sertraline	12.5–200 mg daily	PO	Panic disorder, generalized anxiety disorder
Paroxetine	10–50 mg daily	PO	Panic disorder, generalized anxiety disorder Social anxiety disorder

[a]Off label.
[b]Use with caution as can cause paradoxic disinhibition, sedation and has addiction potential when used long term.
[c]Use with caution as can cause paradoxic disinhibition.
IM, Intramuscular; *IV*, intravenous; *PO*, per oral; *q6*, can be given every 6 hr for aggression; *SSRIs*, selective serotonin reuptake inhibitors.

it is imperative to ensure that there is no access to firearms, sharps/knives, or other objects that could potentially be used as a lethal weapon when homicidal thoughts arise. If parents feel confident in their ability to monitor the patient and keep the patient safe from hurting themself and others with the safety plan in place, the patient may be discharged home with a safety plan, outpatient referrals, and close follow-up.

Duty to Warn and Duty to Protect

Depending on the nature of the homicidal threat or plan, its specificity, and the degree of potential danger to other identifiable individuals, the clinician may be obligated to break confidentiality to carry out our duty to warn or protect. In the seminal *Tarasoff v. Regents of the University of California* (1976) case the California Supreme Court ruled that when a therapist determines "that his patient presents a serious danger of violence to another, he incurs an obligation to use reasonable care to protect the intended victim …" The ruling further specified that depending on the nature of the threat, the clinician may be obligated to warn the intended victim, notify police, or take "whatever other steps are reasonably necessary" to protect the intended victim. Since this decision, there have been several other court cases and laws further clarifying this matter, but guidelines and expectations on this vary from state to state, so it is important to be familiar with the relevant state laws for specific guidance about when clinicians must report a potential threat, and to whom. Clinicians are encouraged to consult with colleagues and legal counsel as needed if faced with this decision.

CONCERNS FOR ANXIETY OR PANIC

The prevalence of anxiety disorders in children has increased significantly over the last 10 years (Ghandour et al., 2019). Currently, 1 in 10 children from age 12 to 17 years suffers from significant anxiety (Ghandour et al., 2019). See Chapter 51 for further discussion of childhood anxiety. This section will focus on addressing acute anxiety during a visit.

Let us refer again to our hypothetical vignette: In the visit parents state that the patient has been experiencing chest pain, shortness of breath, shaking, sweating, and dizziness. When discussing this, the patient becomes anxious and begins to shake, cry, and hyperventilate.

Assessment

In this scenario the clinician should strive to be a calming and reassuring presence for the patient. Before attempting to assess the patient's anxiety, the clinician will likely first have to take a step back and help the patient to calm down (e.g., using deep breathing, mindfulness grounding techniques, or by discussing the patient's interests). Caregivers can also be significant sources of support in these moments. Once the patient seems calmer, the clinician should assess history and nature of current symptoms, including symptom onset, frequency, duration, triggers, and precipitating events. Anxiety in some situations may be developmentally appropriate and should be differentiated from clinical anxiety. For example, toddlers commonly develop separation anxiety and anxiety with strangers, and many children commonly fear darkness or monsters.

Given that many anxiety symptoms overlap with other medical conditions, it is important to rule out organic concerns such as hyperthyroidism, asthma, lead intoxication, caffeine intoxication, pheochromocytoma, arrhythmias, and seizures. The clinician should also consider any recent changes to medications and consider ordering additional testing such as bloodwork, electrocardiogram, electroencephalogram, and other scans as indicated.

Intervention

When other diagnoses have been ruled out and the clinician feels confident that the patient is presenting with anxiety or panic, the clinician has an opportunity to educate the patient and family about physiologic symptoms of anxiety and the link between thoughts, feelings, and bodily symptoms. It may be helpful to provide specific psychoeducation on panic attacks: panic attacks can arise when individuals experience physiologic arousal (either related to anxiety or for other organic reasons) and they make a catastrophic interpretation of bodily symptoms (e.g., "I must be dying!"). Catastrophic thinking further amplifies physiologic arousal, which further increases catastrophic thinking, and so on. The clinician can help to break this cycle by reassuring the patient and demonstrating relaxation strategies. Once the patient is calm, the clinician may consider appropriate referrals or medications (see Table 95.2).

CONCERNS FOR DISCLOSURE OF ABUSE, NEGLECT, SEXUAL ASSAULT, OR DOMESTIC VIOLENCE

Estimated prevalence of child abuse, neglect, and exposure to violence varies. Analysis of national data from Child Protective Services indicates that an estimated 9.2 children per 1000 were victims of abuse and neglect in 2018 (US Department of Health & Human Services, 2018). However, self-report surveys with children suggest that rates are much higher than are reported to Child Protective Services; one national survey found that 15% of children reported experiencing physical, emotional, or sexual abuse (Finkelhor, Turner, Shattuck, & Hamby, 2015). Pediatric health professionals serve an important role in identifying and reporting abuse and neglect. Children have long-standing relationships with their primary care providers, and pediatric visits often give children the opportunity to speak with a trusted adult confidentially. Pediatricians also may identify possible signs of abuse during physical exam or when discussing parenting strategies.

Returning to our vignette: In the visit the patient privately shares that when he is in trouble his father punches him. He shows you a bruise on his chest from a recent argument.

Assessment

As in previous scenarios, the clinician should first review rules around adolescent confidentiality and limits to confidentiality, as well as rules around mandated reporting. All medical and behavioral health clinicians are mandated to report concerns for abuse or neglect to local Child Protective Services. After a disclosure of potential abuse, the clinician should thank the patient for disclosing, and should strive to create a safe, supportive, and nonjudgmental space for the patient. Then, the clinician should gather more information about the possible abuse by calmly asking open-ended and nonleading questions. Medical clinicians should also document signs of potential abuse notable upon physical exam. Throughout the information-gathering process, the clinician should strive to avoid retraumatization by only asking the patient to recount the details of the traumatic event that are necessary to assess current safety and to possibly make a mandated report. The clinician should empower the patient by being transparent, giving the patient choices where possible, and asking for consent before touching the patient, particularly during sensitive portions of the exam.

Intervention

Following assessment, the clinician should avoid victim-blaming or lecturing, particularly when the trauma took place in the context of some risky behavior (e.g., while patient was out at a party, using substances, sneaking out). Depending on the nature of the trauma, the medical clinician may also need to order additional testing to further assess the extent of injuries and, if relevant, possible sexually transmitted infections or pregnancy.

Next, the clinician will need to decide whether the concerns mandate a report to local Child Protective Services and whether it is appropriate to share that plan with the family. When making the decision around what information to share with the family, it is important to consider what information was shared with the clinician, by whom, and in what context. When parents or caregivers disclose concerning parenting behaviors or events that trigger the mandated reporting, the clinician can consider informing the family that they will be making a report; this transparency can help to maintain trust between the clinician and the family. However, when the child discloses potential abuse by a caregiver during a confidential session, the clinician should always consider the patient's current safety, the safety of other children in the home, and risk of caregiver retaliation against the child when deciding whether to discuss reporting with the family in advance. The clinician should consider the severity of allegations and whether the child is safe to return home with the caregiver following the visit.

If the clinician must disclose allegations of abuse with caregivers that the teen shared privately (e.g., allegations of abuse perpetrated by a third party), the clinician should give the teen choices about how the information is shared (e.g., whether the teen wants to be present, who should lead the discussion), and should ally with the patient in helping to manage caregivers' emotional reactions in the room, particularly victim-blaming by the parent. This is especially critical because studies indicate that loved ones' reactions to survivors' first disclosure of abuse predict the course of mental health outcomes (Dworkin, Brill, & Ullman, 2019). See Chapters 15 and 56 for discussions on trauma and stress disorders.

This discussion should serve as a guide outlining various factors that clinicians may take into consideration when managing disclosures of trauma or abuse, but each case should be treated individually, considering details of the allegations, patient and family factors, applicable state laws, ethical and professional guidelines, and institutional policies. Once patient safety and reporting issues have been managed, the clinician may consider appropriate referrals.

ACUTE PRESENTATION OF CONCERNS FOR PSYCHOSIS

Psychotic-like experiences such as hallucinations and delusion exist on a continuum, and recent studies suggest that prevalence rates for psychotic-like experiences in the general population are between 5% and 8% (Van Os, Linscott, Myin-Germeys, Delespaul, & Krabbendam, 2009), but prevalence rates for psychotic disorders such as schizophrenia are estimated as falling around 0.05% (Kessler et al., 2005). In children prevalence rates of subclinical psychotic-like experiences may be as high as 17% (Kelleher et al., 2012), and while some of these children may go on to develop a psychotic disorder in adulthood, the majority do not (Van Os et al., 2009). Typical onset of schizophrenia is in late adolescence or early adulthood; childhood onset of schizophrenia is extremely rare. Psychotic symptoms can also present across other affective and developmental disorders in children. Chapter 52 discusses schizophrenia and thought disorders in more detail. This chapter will focus on acute management of concerns for psychosis in children.

When revisiting our vignette, in today's visit, the patient shares that he has been hearing voices whispering to him and he sometimes sees dark figures at night.

Assessment

Appropriate treatment planning first depends on a quality assessment of the patient's symptoms. The clinician should be aware of the age of the child and level of development and language abilities. The clinician should gather history of these symptoms, including content and nature of symptoms (e.g., auditory, visual, delusions), frequency, onset, duration, triggers, and contexts in which symptoms occur. The clinician should ask about precipitating events, including stressors, illnesses, injuries, and changes in medications. The clinician should also note how caregivers react to possible hallucinations and whether parental responses or attention could be maintaining these symptoms. The clinician should also assess other emotional or behavioral symptoms, as well as family history of similar concerns.

If the patient is presenting with auditory or visual hallucinations, the clinician should interview the child using open-ended and nonleading questions. Are voices speaking in the patient's own voice or a voice recognizable to the patient? Are voices distressing to the patient? Are voices commanding or encouraging any dangerous behaviors? Can the patient distinguish these voices from reality? The clinician should also make detailed observations of the patient's behavior and appearance, such as changes to the patient's thought processes, agitation, or changes in personal hygiene. In addition to positive symptoms such as hallucinations or delusions, patients with psychotic disorders may exhibit negative symptoms such as blunted affect, poverty of speech, reduction of motivation and activity, withdrawal, and anhedonia.

Using this information, the clinician can start to form a working conceptualization of the presenting concerns and can consider possible rule-outs. Young children and children with developmental delays may have difficulties differentiating between voices and their internal monologues or may appear to others as if they are talking to themselves. Children who are anxious or who have sleep problems may report seeing shadows or monsters at nighttime. Intrusive or obsessive thoughts can sometimes be mistaken for psychotic symptoms. Children who have experienced trauma of grief may experience flashbacks or see visions of departed loved ones. Seeing spirits or figures can also be grounded in cultural norms and beliefs.

The clinician should also consider common medical rule-out diagnoses such as ingestion of toxins, medication interactions or side effects, delirium, seizure, brain tumor, Wilson disease, porphyria, endocrine and electrolyte disorders, substance use, and sleep disorders. Visual hallucinations in children, specifically, are more commonly organic in nature. The clinician may need to order additional testing, such as bloodwork for signs of infection, thyroid function, and other endocrine abnormalities, urine sample for tox screen, magnetic resonance imaging, electroencephalogram, or sleep study.

Intervention

The provider should next determine the appropriate level of care. If the patient does appear to be experiencing acute psychotic symptoms, the clinician should decide if the patient needs to be transferred to an inpatient medical or psychiatric unit to stabilize and further assess symptoms. If the patient does not appear to be at acute risk to oneself or others but is experiencing psychotic symptoms, the clinician may consider starting a medication. (Table 95.2 provides information about medications that can be used for psychotic symptoms.) The clinician may also consider referrals to outpatient psychology or psychiatry, as well as referrals to other services such as neurology, ophthalmology, audiology, endocrinology, or sleep specialists. Upon discharge, the clinician should encourage close monitoring of the patient, remove access to lethal means of self-harm, and give emergency resources. If the symptoms do not appear to be causing distress or danger or appear developmentally appropriate, the clinician may choose to simply provide education and continue to monitor.

POTENTIALLY INTOXICATED CHILD OR CAREGIVER

Alcohol and other substance use are very common in adolescence. By 12th grade, 40% of high school students reported using alcohol in the past month, 28% reported using marijuana in the past month, 14% had tried prescription drugs, and 17% had tried other substances such as cocaine, heroin, ecstasy, or hallucinogens (Underwood et al., 2020). Chapter 53 discusses substance use in more detail, but this section will focus on managing intoxication acutely.

> *Returning to the vignette: In this visit when you speak with the patient alone, you notice that he is slurring his speech, is dysregulated, and appears to be intoxicated.*

Assessment

As in the other crises discussed, assessment should focus first on issues of patient safety—in this case concern for possible overdose. The clinician can make behavioral observations, noting, for example, whether the patient is able to speak coherently or is disoriented, inattentive, irritable, or agitated. Acute mental status change in a pediatric patient has a wide differential diagnosis, including central nervous system infections, tumor, seizures, endocrine abnormalities, and electrolyte imbalance, apart from toxic ingestion. If the patient reports having recently used substances, the clinician should gather information about what substances the patient has been using, when the substance was last used, and in what quantities.

Intervention

If the clinician is concerned about a possible overdose, the focus should be on immediate stabilization of the patient's airway, breathing, and circulation. Once the patient is stable, then further workup can be done, including urine toxicology, complete blood count, basic metabolic panel, and blood alcohol level. If the patient is stable and coherent, the clinician can also try to gather more information about the patient's frequency of use, what substances the patient is using, and in what contexts. The clinician may also screen for other risky behaviors. It is important to find out from the patient whether parents are aware of the substance use, and the clinician should be knowledgeable of relevant legal/ethical guidelines around adolescent confidentiality when considering disclosing substance use to parents. Many states have laws that allow teens to seek confidential substance use treatment without parents' knowledge. If the patient appears to be at imminent risk of harm or appears to have overdosed as a suicide attempt, the clinician should connect to a higher level of care. If the patient appears safe to discharge home, the clinician can consider appropriate outpatient referrals.

CAREGIVER MENTAL HEALTH CRISIS

Although developmental behavioral clinicians typically work primarily with children, this work frequently involves close collaboration and collateral work with parents and caregivers. Sometimes during visits, parents may share personal challenges or details of their own mental health concerns. This can sometimes place developmental-behavioral clinicians in the position of managing and stabilizing parental mental health crises.

> *So, let us review our vignette: In the visit the patient's mother shares she is very depressed and sometimes cannot get out of bed to care for the kids or take them to school.*

Assessment

As in our previous examples, the next steps to managing this crisis depend on a quality assessment of the presenting concerns. The provider should be mindful of parents' privacy by speaking to the parent alone when asking about their mental health and should ask permission to document in the parent's own medical record instead of the child's if possible. The provider should assess presenting concerns using a supportive and nonjudgmental tone with particular focus on symptoms that could threaten the safety of the parent or children (i.e., parental suicidality, homicidality, abuse or neglect, substance use, domestic violence, psychosis).

Intervention

If there are no acute safety concerns, then the intervention focuses on providing emotional support and validation to the parent and helping the parent to connect to adult mental health treatment. If parent mental health concerns present acute safety concerns to the parent or child, the clinician can involve other services such as social work, psychology, psychiatry, or Child Protective Services, and/or transport to a local emergency room.

CONCLUSION

Given their focus on working with children with behavioral and developmental concerns, clinicians in developmental-behavioral pediatrics often find themselves working with families in distress or even crisis. In general, when faced with an acute crisis, clinicians should first focus on addressing immediate safety concerns to the patient, staff, and others and should then focus on stabilization, triage, and linking to appropriate services. The types of crises discussed in this chapter are often a product of complex, long-standing behavioral health concerns or family stressors, so the goal in these moments is not to resolve all concerns but to manage the family's acute needs. It is important to remember that you are never alone in managing a crisis; clinicians should mobilize available team members in a crisis, including front desk staff, nurses, other physicians, and interdisciplinary team members. Where possible, it can be helpful to take a break to consult with colleagues to discuss potential treatment plans and available resources. Clinicians should also always be aware of relevant legal and ethical guidelines, state laws, and institutional policies that can help to guide decision making. Finally, clinicians should make a conscious effort to slow down and remain calm during a crisis; crises are stressful for clinicians, too. After managing a crisis, clinicians should pause to take care of themselves by engaging in relaxing activities and connecting with loved ones.

REFERENCES

Condition of participation: Patient's rights, 42 C.F.R. § 482.13 (2019).

Dworkin, E. R., Brill, C. D., & Ullman, S. E. (2019). Social reactions to disclosure of interpersonal violence and psychopathology: A systematic review and meta-analysis. *Clinical Psychology Review*, *72*, 101750.

Finkelhor, D., Turner, H. A., Shattuck, A., & Hamby, S. L. (2015). Prevalence of childhood exposure to violence, crime, and abuse: Results from the national survey of children's exposure to violence. *JAMA Pediatrics*, *169*(8), 746–754.

Ghandour, R. M., Sherman, L. J., Vladutiu, C. J., Ali, M. M., Lynch, S. E., Bitsko, R. H., & Blumberg, S. J. (2019). Prevalence and treatment of depression, anxiety, and conduct problems in US children. *Journal of Pediatrics*, *206*, 256–267.

Hedegaard, H., Curtin, S. C., & Warner, M. (2018). *Suicide rates in the United States continue to increase*. US Department of Health and Human Services, Centers for Disease Control and Prevention, National Center for Health Statistics.

Hedegaard, H., Curtin, S. C., & Warner, M. (2020). Increase in suicide mortality in the United States, 1999–2018. *NCHS Data Brief*, *362*, 1–8.

Kelleher, I., Connor, D., Clarke, M. C., Devlin, N., Harley, M., & Cannon, M. (2012). Prevalence of psychotic symptoms in childhood and adolescence: A systematic review and meta-analysis of population-based studies. *Psychological Medicine*, *9*, 1–7.

Kessler, R. C., Birnbaum, H., Demler, O., Falloon, I. R., Gagnon, E., Guyer, M., Howes, M. J., Kendler, K. S., Shi, L., Walters, E., & Wu, E. Q. (2005). The prevalence and correlates of nonaffective psychosis in the National Comorbidity Survey Replication (NCS-R). *Biological Psychiatry*, *58*(8), 668–676.

Pappadopulos, E., Macintyre Ii, J. C., Crismon, M. L., Findling, R. L., Malone, R. P., Derivan, A., Schooler, N., Sikich, L., Greenhill, L., Schur, S. B., Felton, C. J., Kranzler, H., Rube, D. M., Sverd, J., Finnerty, M., Ketner, S., Siennick, S. E., & Jensen, P. S. (2003). Treatment recommendations for the use of antipsychotics for aggressive youth (TRAAY). Part II. *Journal of the American Academy of Child & Adolescent Psychiatry*, *42*(2), 145–161.

Schnitzer, K., Merideth, F., Macias-Konstantopoulos, W., Hayden, D., Shtasel, D., & Bird, S. (2020). Disparities in care: The role of race on the utilization of physical restraints in the emergency setting. *Academic Emergency Medicine*, *27*(10), 943–950.

Tarasoff v. Regents of the University of California (Supreme Court of California June 1, 1976).

Underwood, J. M., Brener, N., Thornton, J., Harris, W. A., Bryan, L. N., Shanklin, S. L., Deputy, N., Roberts, A. M., Queen, B., Chyen, D., Whittle, L., Lim, C., Yamakawa, Y., Leon-Nguyen, M., Kilmer, G., Smith-Grant, J., Demissie, Z., Everrett Jones, S., Clayton, H., & Dittus, P. (2020). *Youth risk behavior surveillance—United States, 2019*. Centers for Disease Control and Prevention.

US Department of Health & Human Services, Administration on Children, Youth and Families, Children's Bureau. (2018). *Child maltreatment* (pp. 1–274). Author.

Van Os, J., Linscott, R. J., Myin-Germeys, I., Delespaul, P., & Krabbendam, L. J. P. M. (2009). A systematic review and meta-analysis of the psychosis continuum: Evidence for a psychosis proneness-persistence-impairment model of psychotic disorder. *Psychological Medicine*, *39*(2), 179.

Individual Therapy for Children and Adolescents: Play Therapy and Interpersonal Therapy as Developmentally Centered Relational Change Modalities

Karla K. Fehr, Abby Hughes-Scalise, Bethany Leraas, and Kristen Boog

For additional material related to the content of this chapter, please see Chapter 15.

VIGNETTE

Anika is a 15-year-old teenager with a 5-year-old sister, Grace. Anika and Grace are currently living with their father full time and have had minimal contact with their mother since their parents' recent separation. Anika's father is worried about how the separation is affecting both of his daughters. He has noticed that Anika has been more withdrawn and tearful. She has also "stopped caring" about school and is at risk of failing two of her courses, a stark contrast from her honor roll performance in previous semesters. Grace is having difficulty falling asleep independently. She refuses to go to bed until her father lays down with her, becomes "panicked" if her father is not there when she wakes, and is receiving insufficient sleep. The children's father is seeking suggestions for what to do to help his daughters.

EFFECTIVENESS OF THERAPY WITH CHILDREN AND ADOLESCENTS

Psychotherapy can be defined as an intervention "intended to alleviate psychological distress, reduce maladaptive behavior, or enhance adaptive behavior through counseling, structured or unstructured interaction, a training program, or a predetermined treatment plan" (Weisz et al., 1995, p. 452). Within this broad definition, psychotherapy can be practiced from a variety of theoretical orientations, including psychodynamic, client-centered, cognitive, behavioral, and family systems perspectives. Psychotherapy is a first-line treatment for many emotional and behavioral disorders of childhood and has been demonstrated to be a helpful augment to psychiatric medication (March et al., 2004; The MTA Cooperative Group, 1999; Walkup et al., 2008).

While child psychotherapy has been practiced for decades, research into its effectiveness is a relatively recent endeavor. In the late 1980s and 1990s four influential meta-analyses were published demonstrating positive effects of child psychotherapy with mean effect sizes ranging from moderate to large (Casey & Berman, 1985; Kazdin et al., 1990; Weisz et al., 1987, 1995). Since the publication of these seminal articles, much work has been done in the area of treatment outcome research, although recent results are generally consistent with earlier studies. Weisz et al. (2017) conducted an updated metaanalysis of randomized treatment trials and yielded a mean posttreatment effect size of 0.46 indicating a moderate effect of psychotherapy. The mean effect size for follow-up studies (mean: 44.26 weeks posttreatment) was 0.36, providing evidence for moderate long-term effects of psychotherapy. The authors attributed the lower effect sizes found in this metaanalysis compared to those previously conducted to methodologic advances in effect size calculation that are now considered standard in metaanalyses (Weisz et al., 2017). Treatment effects were generally larger for anxiety compared to externalizing problems and depression and for individuals with only one problem type compared to individuals with comorbid difficulties. Treatment type was not a significant moderator of treatment effects, and there was no evidence of differential treatment effects based on age or ethnicity. Taken together, evidence suggests that child psychotherapy is moderately effective at improving psychosocial functioning regardless of treatment approach, presenting concern, or patient characteristics, and these effects are maintained over time.

While metaanalytic evidence supports positive effects of child psychotherapy, a substantial amount of variance is not accounted for by specific treatment approaches. Thus researchers have examined the interpersonal and process-related factors that could also contribute to therapeutic change. These variables, often referred to as common factors, include the therapeutic alliance, client expectations for change, and therapist characteristics. While first developed in the context of adult psychotherapy, models of common factors have been developed for youth psychotherapy. The therapeutic alliance has received the greatest attention in the literature and refers to the relationship between the therapist and client and agreement on the tasks and goals of therapy. A recent metaanalysis found a positive moderate effect of child-therapist alliance on therapy outcomes (Karver et al., 2018). The effect of the parent-therapist alliance on treatment outcomes was of similar magnitude. A strong alliance with parents may contribute to better child outcomes through greater treatment adherence, attendance, and generalization of skills outside of sessions. In fact, research has demonstrated that parent involvement in therapy is associated with better outcomes compared to child-only interventions.

The contribution of client and parent expectations to youth psychotherapy outcomes has also been examined. Expectations refer to the degree that the client believes therapy is inherently helpful, can explain the source of distress or problem behavior, and will be beneficial to them personally. In a recent study positive expectations for treatment held by youth were associated with greater compliance and mastery of exposure exercises in treatment for anxiety (Wu et al., 2020). While these positive youth expectations were not directly related to symptom change, they were predictive of greater treatment compliance that in turn predicted greater symptom reduction. A similar pattern was found for parental expectations highlighting the importance of understanding parent expectations for treatment as well (Wu et al., 2020). Higher treatment expectations have been associated with greater symptom reduction across presentations, including among youth with depression and obsessive-compulsive disorder.

Characteristics of the therapist, including interpersonal skills, empathy, and effective implementation of treatment strategies, also contribute to treatment outcomes. Therapist relationship variables (e.g., being perceived as too directive, controlling, or confrontational) were moderate predictors of premature termination and were more predictive than pretreatment child or parent variables (de Haan et al., 2013). Taken together, the literature on common factors suggests that process variables are as important as the specific treatment approach in optimizing outcomes in child psychotherapy. These relational components of psychotherapy are central to interpersonal, supportive, and play-based treatment approaches.

The children's father raises concerns with Dr. Phelps, the children's primary care physician. Dr. Phelps is wondering whether Anika is struggling with adjustment-related stress or clinically significant depressive symptoms. Grace presents as temperamentally anxious in session, and Dr. Phelps is considering the possibility of separation anxiety brought on by the parents' separation. As Dr. Phelps works in an interdisciplinary care setting, he recommends that the family meet with one of the behavioral health specialists in clinic. Dr. Phelps briefly explains the integrated behavioral health model of their clinic and provides psychoeducation on how behavioral health services can help assess mood, anxiety, and adjustment concerns and identify appropriate treatment options, if applicable. The family agrees to meet with the clinic's behavioral health specialist, Maria.

INTEGRATED BEHAVIORAL HEALTH

While the research is clear that therapy is effective for children and adolescents, access to services and other barriers prevent many children and adolescents from getting the mental health services they need. Unfortunately, only about 21% of children with clinically significant mental health concerns receive treatment (Kataoka et al., 2002). Some of the barriers to obtaining care for patients and families include limited access to services, mental health–related stigma, and logistical challenges (e.g., long waitlists, lack of insurance coverage, transportation). If evidence-based treatments are not provided, limited changes in mental health functioning are likely to be obtained, which may result in resistance to finding another clinician in addition to not addressing the child's needs. Integrated behavioral health (IBH) increases access to services by integrating a behavioral health clinician in the medical care setting. The IBH arrangement can range from colocation of services (i.e., the mental health clinician collaborates with medical clinicians in the medical office to coordinate care but maintains own treatment plans and schedule) to truly integrated services (i.e., the mental and medical clinician provide care together with an integrated treatment plan, joint appointments, and shared electronic health record; Stancin & Perrin, 2014).

The IBH clinician may provide a range of therapeutic services, depending on the practice goals and needs. IBH clinicians may conduct brief, evidence-based treatments for a wide range of mental health (e.g., anxiety, depression, disruptive behavior) and behavioral health (e.g., sleep, toileting) concerns. They may provide consultations to families to answer questions about development, conduct brief assessments to assist with diagnostic clarity and treatment planning, provide preventive intervention to improve child outcomes when early risk factors are indicated, or coordinate care across agencies (e.g., coordinating with the school to ensure appropriate 504 Plan accommodations are put in place for a child newly diagnosed with attention-deficit/hyperactivity disorder [ADHD]). Warm handoffs allow the behavioral health clinician to conduct a consultation while the patient is present for the medical appointment, resulting in increased integration of services as well as being able to address behavioral health needs immediately when identified. The IBH clinician is also a resource for the medical team providing consultation or training on behavioral health topics. Curbside consultations provide the medical clinician with informal behavioral health consultation regarding how the medical clinician may be able to manage the behavioral health concern even without the IBH clinician directly assessing the patient. The IBH clinician can also assist at a systems level with developmental and psychosocial screening and prevention of and early intervention for developmental, behavioral, and psychosocial symptoms throughout childhood.

IBH benefits the patients, medical clinicians, and behavioral health clinicians. First, IBH in the pediatric setting has been shown to improve behavioral health outcomes as compared to treatment as usual (Asarnow et al., 2015). Integrated care results in more comprehensive care for families, and the ability to easily collaborate and coordinate care is a benefit to medical and behavioral health clinicians resulting in more comprehensive care. Second, contact with an IBH clinician increases follow-through with referrals for mental health treatment. Parents in rural locations report a greater willingness to seek services in a primary care office compared to other locations where mental health services are typically obtained such as community mental health clinics or schools

(Fehr et al., 2020). Furthermore, parents in urban and rural locations indicate a desire to obtain behavioral health information as part of their typical medical care (Leraas et al., 2020; Riley et al., 2019). Third, IBH has the potential to result in more efficiency for the medical clinician. In the primary care setting pediatricians spend almost double the amount of time in visits addressing behavioral health concerns as compared to medical concerns only. Integration of behavioral health services also provides benefits at the systems level. Having an IBH clinician onsite can increase medical clinicians' comfort with managing less severe mental health concerns, thus increasing the behavioral health services available to patients across the practice. Integration of behavioral health also reduces utilization of psychiatric crisis services such as emergency department visits.

Dr. Phelps brings Maria to Anika and Grace's clinic room and introduces her to the family with a "warm handoff." Maria directs a few additional questions to Anika, Grace, and her father related to the daughters' symptom onset and severity. Grace's father shares that while Grace has always been "a little on the anxious side," her current difficulties related to sleep initiation and separation anxiety at bedtime only surfaced following her mother's move from the family home. Anika reports that while she currently feels "probably the worst" she's ever felt, depression symptoms have been present since she started high school. She voiced feeling overwhelmed with the idea of "being an adult soon" and that this has been even harder with her mom out of the house ("I feel like all of a sudden I have to act really grown up, and I don't feel up for it").

THERAPEUTIC STRATEGIES FOR MEDICAL CLINICIANS AND SUPPORTIVE THERAPY

Mental health clinicians integrate supportive strategies into treatment to assist in building rapport with and providing emotional support to patients and families. Rasmussen and Kealy (2020) define supportive psychotherapy as "talking therapy that aims to support client's adaptive functioning through non-interpretive interventions" (p. 282). In addition to integrating supportive techniques into another treatment approach, supportive therapy can be helpful for patients experiencing stressors (e.g., divorce, loss) but who are otherwise well adjusted. Further, it has been suggested that supportive therapy may be indicated for individuals with chronic medical conditions who may not need intense directive treatment. In cases where patients decline directive treatment that is recommended supportive therapy may temporarily support them until they are ready to initiate directive treatment. When patients would benefit from more directive approaches, such as those that teach skills (e.g., cognitive coping), supportive therapy would not be the treatment of choice and a referral to the appropriate type of behavioral health treatment would be recommended.

The unstructured nature and goals of alleviating distress and disability makes supportive psychotherapy techniques ideally suited for the doctor-patient relationship. There are several supportive psychotherapy techniques that therapists use as part of their treatments that medical clinicians can also implement in their practice, including reflective listening, empathic summaries, reassurance, praise, and encouragement. Reflective listening skills are those where the clinician repeats back the patient's statements to indicate that the clinician has been attentive to the patient. Empathic summaries are when the clinician summarizes the patient's statements in an understanding and emotionally sensitive way. Praise, reassurance, and encouragement can be used to encourage adaptive behaviors (e.g., physical activity, adherence) and validate struggles the patient may be experiencing. See Chapters 91, 97, 98, 101, and 102 for additional discussion regarding therapeutic strategies.

Supportive therapy techniques are likely to be particularly helpful to medical clinicians when discussing sensitive topics, including assessing mental health needs and making referrals. For example, reflective listening and empathic summaries may be helpful in supporting an assessment of mental health symptoms (or following up on positive screening results if utilized within the medical practice). Validation, praise, and reassurance are important once mental health symptoms are disclosed. For example, a medical clinician may validate an adolescent who discloses a depressed mood, praise the client for sharing concerns, and reassure the client that depression is not uncommon in adolescence and there are effective ways to help teenagers learn to cope with and improve these feelings. It is important that children, adolescents, and their families feel that their concerns are heard and taken seriously as well as feel hopeful about the potential benefits that therapy can provide. As noted, expectations about the benefits of therapy are related to outcomes. An IBH clinician can also assist in discussing and facilitating a referral to a community mental health clinician if more intensive or consistent services are needed than can be provided within the integrated care model.

Maria validates Anika, Grace, and their father's willingness to discuss the family's current difficulties. She empathically summarizes the family's struggles and reinforces the need to seek further therapeutic intervention. She provides psychoeducation about the therapy process and in this context reassures the family that things can get better with professional support. Maria shares her perception that the current difficulties experienced by both daughters are connected to changes in core family relationships. In addition, these changes are happening at crucial developmental stages for both daughters: for Grace, the transition to elementary school, and for Anika, during adolescence. As such, Maria suggests that developmentally informed relational approaches to therapy would most effectively address Anika's and Grace's symptoms. Specifically, she refers Anika to a therapist trained in interpersonal therapy and Grace to a psychologist with experience working with young children with anxiety and sleep difficulties from a play-based perspective.

THERAPEUTIC APPROACHES: THE THERAPEUTIC RELATIONSHIP AS THE VEHICLE OF CHANGE

Behavioral and cognitive-behavioral therapy (CBT) approaches are considered first-line treatments for addressing child and adolescent mental health concerns in the context of individual therapy. CBT and other empirically supported treatments are reviewed more extensively in Chapter 98, and it is important to acknowledge empirical support for the effectiveness of these approaches. CBT and behavioral therapy have proven effective at symptom reduction across a wide variety of youth mental health concerns, including ADHD and disruptive behavior, depression, anxiety, and insomnia.

These skills-oriented treatments, however, are not always effective, and significant rates of dropout remain a barrier to symptom improvement. A metaanalysis of treatment dropout in child and adolescent treatment demonstrated a mean dropout rate of 28.4% to 50% (de Haan et al., 2013). This indicates that even in the context of rigorous empirical examinations of therapy, one-quarter to one-half of children receiving this treatment drop out before treatment is complete.

Even when clients stay in skills-based treatments, not everyone responds positively. Anxiety disorders, arguably the class of disorders that responds most consistently and effectively to CBT, still post a nonresponse to treatment rate ranging from 15% to 50%. Many factors have been identified as possible explanations for poor treatment response in CBT, including low adherence by the therapist and client/family, low client motivation, higher symptom severity, the presence of comorbidity, and poor therapeutic alliance. Familial factors, including parenting stress and maternal mental health, and logistical barriers (e.g., lack of childcare, transportation, wait time) are common reasons for poor treatment engagement in behavioral therapy for young children with disruptive behavior. In addition, skills-based approaches that rely heavily on language and client insight into thoughts and behaviors may not be developmentally appropriate for young children.

The therapeutic relationship has consistently been recognized as having a critical role in psychotherapy for youth. Relational approaches have long understood the therapeutic relationship in the context of attachment theory. With this understanding comes an acknowledgment that much of what we learn from our early attachment relationships is not expressed in words. Memories, feelings, and physiologic responses often exist outside of conscious/verbal awareness, and yet they have an enormous impact on the therapy relationship and the therapeutic process.

Thus alternate therapeutic approaches, including play therapy, and interpersonal approaches may be beneficial as an adjunct to empirically supported treatments or if the empirically supported treatment is not working. In addition, there may be clinical indicators (e.g., presenting concern, client demographics, parent-child relationship, client insight) that suggest a developmentally informed therapeutic approach emphasizing relationships, such as play therapy or interpersonal therapy, may be useful as a primary approach to treatment.

Relational Approaches

Relational approaches in psychotherapy offer a potential alternative to skills-based approaches and are often informed by attachment theory. This theory asserts that in early development an individual learns about the world through interactions with caregivers, or attachment figures. The quality of these attachment relationships impacts a person's perception of whether the world is a safe, predictable place and whether the person can depend on others in times of distress. Attachment relationships also strongly influence how a person regulates one's own emotions in times of uncertainty and confusion.

In adolescence the definition of attachment figure expands. Adolescents begin to form meaningful, intimate attachments with not only their caregivers but also romantic partners, close friends, and other individuals outside of their immediate family. Adolescents approach these relationships through the lens of their own attachment style. Attachment style is organized along two primary dimensions: attachment avoidance and attachment anxiety. Attachment avoidance captures the level to which an individual relies on attachment figures for regulating emotional distress, while attachment anxiety captures the level of an individual's tolerance for perceived threats to interpersonal security. Youth high in attachment anxiety and/or attachment avoidance are conceptualized as having an insecure attachment style. Insecure attachment styles have been associated with higher levels of psychopathology. Within this framework of attachment theory, relational therapy approaches use the therapeutic relationship as well as the here-and-now experiences of the client to process past relational issues (including insecure attachment), identify relational patterns and internal models of the self and the other, and generate adaptive alternatives. Many therapy modalities incorporate elements of a relational approach as well as an attachment-based focus. Two such therapy approaches, play therapy and interpersonal therapy, are discussed next.

Play Therapy

Play is a developmentally appropriate and enjoyable medium that can be used to engage young children. Play-based therapy approaches are typically considered for children ages 4 to 10 (Russ, 2004). Play is incorporated into a variety of theoretical orientations, including psychodynamic, client centered, and cognitive behavioral. Depending on theoretical orientation, the therapist may be directive or nondirective. In a directive approach (e.g., cognitive behavioral) the therapist is involved in the play and provides structure to elicit specific play themes or opportunities (e.g., a story about a boy who is afraid of the dark, having a doll practice a specific coping strategy). In a nondirective approach (e.g., psychodynamic, client centered) the therapist observes and comments on the child's play while following the child's lead.

The specific ways in which play is utilized and the treatment goals of the play reflect the theoretical orientation of the treatment approach. For example, in psychodynamic therapy, play is seen as an approach to gain insight into children's mental health and assist the child in working through and mastering the conflicts they are experiencing (Russ, 2004). Through play, the child is able to process conflicts and feelings in a safe way and ultimately gain mastery of the situation or emotion. In client-centered play therapy, the therapeutic relationship is used to express acceptance of the child and assist the child in developing confidence in one's own abilities (Landreth, 2012). This is conveyed by the therapist observing, accepting, and commenting on the child's play. In cognitive-behavioral play therapy specific scenarios are presented allowing the child the opportunity to gain exposure to anxiety-provoking scenarios as well as identify and practice coping skills (Knell, 2016). In addition to exposure to the anxiety-inducing scenarios, coping strategies are directly taught and practiced through the play.

Across theoretical orientations, Russ (2004) identified four ways in which pretend play can result in therapeutic change. First, as children use pretend play naturally to express their emotions, play in therapy can be used for the child to communicate feelings and thoughts they are otherwise not able to state directly. Second, the therapist's empathic and attentive response to the child contributes to the child feeling understood and development of the therapeutic relationship. A third mechanism is by helping the child gain insight or work through conflicts. Fourth, play allows distance from reality letting the child practice behaviors, ideas, and interpersonal interactions and explore alternate outcomes of situations.

Empirical Support

Pretend play relates to positive psychosocial outcomes such as coping, problem solving, and wellbeing (Russ, 2004). In addition, pretend play intervention can improve outcomes relevant to therapy goals (e.g., increased emotional understanding). Regarding outcomes of play therapy, a 2005 metaanalysis of the effect of play therapy found that almost 80% of the research conducted examined outcomes associated with play therapy from a client-centered approach (Bratton et al., 2005). The results of this metaanalysis and another specifically examining the effect of client-centered play therapy (Lin & Bratton, 2015) indicated overall moderate to large treatment effect sizes. Larger effect sizes were obtained when including only children younger than 7 years of age as compared to children above the age of 7 (Lin & Bratton, 2015). Furthermore, the mean effect size for treatment was larger when examining outcomes of global behavior problems, caregiver-child relationship stress, and improvements in self-efficacy as compared to externalizing behavior problems (Lin & Bratton, 2015).

Support for cognitive-behavioral play therapy has been demonstrated in case studies of children ages 3 to 8 years with presenting concerns of anxiety, stressful or traumatic life experiences, and encopresis (Knell, 2016). Brief, standardized treatment approaches based on cognitive-behavioral play therapy principles have also been examined for reducing school anxiety (Pearson, 2008), improving behavioral sleep difficulties (Fehr et al., 2016), and improving adjustment in siblings of children diagnosed with cancer (Fehr et al., 2017). Cognitive-behavioral play therapy can also be used in combination with empirically supported parent-focused behavioral or cognitive-behavioral treatment. Thus cognitive-behavioral play therapy may be appropriate for very young children presenting with concerns of anxiety, coping with stressors, school adjustment, or behavioral sleep difficulties, especially when used as an adjunct to parent-focused treatment.

The literature suggests that child-centered play therapy is likely most useful for children under the age of 7 years and with presenting problems such as parent-child relationship stressors or concerns about the development of self-efficacy. Individual factors that impact whether and how play is incorporated include the child's ability to engage in play, developmental level, age, and ability to verbalize (Russ, 2004). For example, for children who struggle to engage in pretend or those who can already discuss the presenting problems directly, play therapy may not provide an additive benefit to empirically supported treatment. Play therapy is not recommended for the treatment of ADHD (Koocher et al., 2015) and should not be considered a first-line treatment for other behavioral disorders, given the empirical support for well-established behavioral approaches, especially when presenting concerns are behavioral and seem related to ineffective or negative parenting strategies (Knell, 2016). Play-based approaches (e.g., cognitive-behavioral play therapy) may be considered when they can provide a child-focused component to complement empirically supported treatment. For example, inclusion of a child-focused treatment component teaching cognitive-behavioral coping strategies through play to address the child's distress at bedtime may be a useful adjunct to empirically supported behavioral treatment of bedtime resistance in young children (Fehr et al., 2016).

Given the presence of comorbid anxiety and bedtime resistance, Grace begins working with Dr. Kaul, a psychologist with experience in pediatric behavioral sleep medicine. Dr. Kaul begins teaching Grace's father empirically supported behavioral strategies to address her bedtime resistance. However, Grace's father reports concern regarding the behavioral strategies (i.e., setting limits at bedtime) adding to the distress she is experiencing related to her mother's departure. Knowing that anxiety and sleep difficulties are frequently comorbid, including in preschool-age children, and that there are common elements in cognitive-behavioral treatment for sleep difficulties and anxiety (Fehr et al., 2020), Dr. Kaul decides to incorporate a child-focused treatment component focused on coping skills to complement behavioral strategies and address Grace's separation anxiety. This play-based approach also provides Grace with a venue to explore and process her feelings and fears related to her parents' separation, mother's absence, and the change in the parenting structure. Dr. Kaul spends time each session providing cognitive-behavioral play therapy to Grace and parent management to her father. After three sessions, Grace's anxiety at bedtime has subsided, and Grace's father reports a willingness to engage with the behav-

ioral strategies he previously felt she was not prepared to cope with. In addition, he notes significant improvements in her daily sleep duration and daytime mood. Dr. Kaul plans to continue to provide support through play to allow Grace to explore her thoughts and feelings about relationships within the family while Grace's father implements the remaining behavioral sleep strategies, but the family agrees that significant improvements have been made both in Grace's sleep habits and anxiety.

Incorporating Play Therapeutically

The play therapy literature referenced earlier focuses on the use of pretend play as the agent of change. However, play may also be utilized within treatment to achieve another goal. In fact, most therapy approaches that include very young children in the treatment process do incorporate play to some degree. While this may be done therapeutically, the term play therapy is typically reserved for situations in which the hypothesized mechanism of change occurs through the play itself. For example, engaging a child in play or a game in order to build rapport or using play to facilitate communication or assist the child in understanding information (e.g., using dolls to show how a medical procedure will be completed) alone may not be considered play therapy. A variety of empirically supported treatments utilize play as a modality to achieve the treatment goal. In parent-child interaction therapy (PCIT) a well-established treatment for disruptive behaviors, parents learn to use specific behavioral strategies while playing with their child. Although the parent plays with their child in a therapeutic manner, the proposed mechanism of change is the improved parental management skills and parent-child relationship. See Russ and Niec (2011) for empirically supported treatment approaches that incorporate play-based strategies.

Pretend play strategies may be particularly helpful to integrate as part of a medical clinician's repertoire (Fehr, 2020). In addition to the benefit of playful interactions on building rapport, formal or informal observations of a child's pretend play can provide insight into a child's functioning and developmental level. Related areas of functioning such as social interactions (e.g., observing the manner in which children request their parent become involved in their play) or the parent-child relationship (e.g., assessing positive affect and mutual enjoyment during joint parent-child play) can also be assessed by observing the child's play with parents or the medical staff. Pretend play may also be used as a modality to facilitate communication with a child during a medical visit. For example, a clinician may provide education to ease anxiety about how a medical procedure will be completed by demonstrating on a teddy bear prior to performing the procedure on the child. A clinician could also engage in a play narrative with a shy child by using a stuffed animal or puppet (including the child's stuffed animal) to talk with the child. Finally, there is a significant research base demonstrating that engaging in pretend play reduces stress and increases coping in children, including in medical and dental settings (see Moore & Russ, 2006, for review). Thus offering an opportunity to engage in pretend play during stressful situations, which could include being in the doctor's office and getting vaccinations or having other medical procedures, may reduce stress during the medical appointment. Clinicians who wish to encourage play should provide play materials that include structured and unstructured toys (Russ, 2004). Unstructured toys should be provided that encourage emotional expression (e.g., aggressive types of animals) and imagination (e.g., blocks, other undefined objects that can be used for multiple purposes). Stuffed or plastic animals, a set of family dolls and dollhouse, and realistic toys that can be used for medical play are helpful to provide along with materials such as paper and crayons and playdoh. Medical clinicians can also encourage parents to engage with their children in pretend play and reinforce the use of pretend play as a positive coping strategy for children (Moore & Russ, 2006).

Individual Therapy Modalities for Adolescents

When considering best practice for therapy with adolescents, it is essential to understand normative adolescent development. While cognitive skills–based approaches have been adapted for adolescents and to address familial or relationship issues in this developmental stage, relational functioning is not a primary component in the work. This is at odds with the notion that a core developmental task in adolescence is the process of navigating increasingly nuanced interpersonal relationships. Adolescents are experiencing tension related to conflicting goals of (1) increasing their autonomy from their family unit while also (2) developing increased intimacy and meaningful connection in relationships outside of their primary caregivers. Peers in particular have a strong impact on the adolescent's well-being and identity development. In this social-developmental context adolescents are also navigating increased interpersonal conflict.

For youth specifically, factors such as low parent involvement and insecure caregiver attachment have been shown to predict treatment nonresponse in skills-based treatments. Given that an adolescent's interpersonal context impacts their treatment response, and the fact that social relationships are a central task in adolescent development, alternative therapeutic approaches are needed that more directly acknowledge and integrate interpersonal functioning into the therapeutic process.

Interpersonal Therapy

Interpersonal therapy for adolescents (IPT-A; Jacobson et al., 2017) is used primarily to treat adolescent depression and is considered a well-established treatment for this disorder (Weersing et al., 2017). It has also been adapted to treat depression in the context of comorbid anxiety, specific learning disorders, and/or ADHD. IPT-A intentionally conceptualizes depression from an attachment lens and stresses that symptoms of depression cannot be divorced from an adolescent's interpersonal context. IPT-A further asserts that, while the etiology of adolescent depression is multifactorial, the onset and course of depression are strongly linked to the adolescent's significant interpersonal relationships (Jacobson et al., 2017).

The goal of IPT-A is to decrease depressive symptoms by holding the therapist-client relationship as a model for healthy attachment. The therapist then uses this relationship as a vehicle to promote healthy attachments with other individuals in the adolescent's life. In a traditional outpatient course of IPT-A treatment is divided into three phases, each centered on distinct clinical foci (Jacobson et al., 2017). The first phase lasts one to three sessions and focuses on (1) building a strong therapeutic alliance and (2) identifying a problem area to focus on in the second phase of treatment. IPT-A identifies four potential interpersonal problem areas: grief surrounding the loss of an important relationship, difficulties with role transition into adolescence, conflict around expectations in an important relationship (role dispute), and interpersonal issues due to a social skills deficit.

Once a problem area has been identified, the middle phase of IPT-A starts by educating the adolescent on the connection between the interpersonal struggles and depression symptoms. Over time, the therapist introduces communication, problem solving, and affective awareness skills to address the adolescent's core problem area. Typically these skills are learned and practiced in six to eight sessions in the context of one important relationship outside of the therapy context (e.g., a caregiver, friend, romantic partner). The termination phase (the final one to three sessions of treatment) consists of reviewing symptom improvement and encouraging independent and generalized use of learned skills (Jacobson et al., 2017).

Empirical Support

A recent metaanalysis that investigated the impact of IPT-A on depression in adolescents demonstrated improved depressive symptoms across all 10 studies included (Mychailyszyn & Elson, 2018). IPT-A was also found to be significantly more effective than control/placebo groups across studies. Notably, IPT-A has demonstrated a positive impact on attachment style (Gunlicks-Stoessel et al., 2019). In a study of 40 adolescents who received a 16-week randomized controlled trial of IPT-A adolescents who showed a decrease in depressive symptoms over the course of treatment also showed significant decreases in attachment anxiety and attachment avoidance. The research literature on IPT-A demonstrates that an interpersonal approach can be effectively used to treat one of the most debilitating and prevalent disorders in the adolescent population (Jacobson et al., 2017).

Anika meets with an IPT therapist, Laurel. During the initial treatment phase, Laurel identifies difficulties with role transition into adolescence as Anika's core problem area, though she also acknowledges Anika's feelings of grief over how her relationship with her mother has changed since her mother moved out of the family home. In the middle phase of treatment Laurel and Anika focus on improving her communication with her father around her difficulties, as well as increasing her affective awareness around negative emotional states. She is able to acknowledge that her feelings of grief toward her mother actually reflect her insecurity about transitioning to the increased independence of adolescence. Engaging in problem solving when negative affect or interpersonal difficulties arise allows Anika to effectively approach, rather than avoid, the responsibilities of adolescence. Over the course of treatment, both Anika and her father report improvements in their relationship, and Anika reports feeling more confident about the tasks ahead of her as she continues to move toward young adulthood.

Therapeutic Relationship to Process Adolescents' Experiences

The developmental stage of adolescence leaves our adolescent clients particularly vulnerable to experiencing tension between what they feel and what they can express. For adolescents struggling significantly with this discrepancy (such as adolescents with a history of trauma or adolescents who present with somatic disorders), traditional talk therapy can feel overwhelming and frustrating (Ogden & Goldstein, 2017). A therapy process focused almost exclusively on language often results in these adolescents feeling as though they are failing therapy. In turn, therapists working with these adolescents may feel as though the adolescent is not really trying or is holding something back intentionally, rather than conceptualizing this presentation as a disconnect between what the mind can say and what the body is trying to express.

When these situations arise, it can be helpful to integrate interventions focused specifically on increasing the adolescent's understanding of the mind-body connection within the context of the therapeutic relationship. This work ranges from noticing and exploring patterns of physiologic response when sensitive topics are broached in session, to using grounding strategies during session as a somatic resource of self-regulation when processing trauma, to incorporating mindfulness-based strategies using biofeedback as a way for clients to understand how their physiologic arousal can impact their mood and psychosocial functioning (Ogden & Goldstein, 2017).

CONCLUSION

Therapy for children and adolescents is effective at improving outcomes across theoretical orientation. Although the strength of the empirical support for specific theoretical orientations varies based on presenting problems (as described across chapters in this volume), consideration of developmental and relational factors is also important when determining the most appropriate treatment referral for youth. Knowledge of the empirical evidence for diverse symptom presentations and supportive therapy strategies may assist medical clinicians in making effective referrals. In addition, medical clinicians can assist families in determining whether treatment being obtained is indicated for their presenting concerns and when developmentally focused relational approaches are likely to be beneficial. IBH can also assist with connecting families with effective treatment approaches.

REFERENCES

Asarnow, J. R., Rozenman, M., Wiblin, J., & Zeltzer, L. (2015). Integrated medical-behavioral care compared with usual primary care for child and adolescent behavioral health: A meta-analysis. *JAMA Pediatrics*, *169*(10), 929–937.

Bratton, S., Ray, D., Rhine, T., & Jones, L. (2005). The efficacy of play therapy with children: A meta-analytic review of treatment outcomes. *Professional Psychology: Research and Practice*, *36*(4), 376–390.

Casey, R. J., & Berman, J. S. (1985). The outcome of psychotherapy with children. *Psychological Bulletin*, *98*, 388–400.

de Haan, A. M., Boon, A. E., de Jong, J. T. V. M., Hoeve, M., & Vermeiren, R. J. M. (2013). A meta-analytic review on treatment dropout in child and adolescent outpatient mental health care. *Clinical Psychology Review*, *33*, 698–711.

Fehr, K. (2020). Assessment of play processes. In M. Clark (Chair) (Ed.), *Come play with us! Teaching the art of play for developmental promotion, evaluation, and community engagement in the face of a pandemic*. Workshop presented at the annual meeting of the Society for Developmental & Behavioral Pediatrics.

Fehr, K., Chambers, D., & Ramasami, J. (2021). The impact of anxiety on behavioral sleep difficulties and treatment in young children: A review of the literature. *Journal of Clinical Psychology in Medical Settings* , *28*(1), 102–112..

Fehr, K., Leraas, B., & Littles, M. (2020). Integrated behavioral health in rural pediatric primary care: Behavioral and mental health needs, barriers, and parent preferences. *Journal of Pediatric Psychology*, *45*(8), 910–920.

Fehr, K., Russ, S., Anderson, J., Leigh Josie, K., & Cousino, M. (2017). Application of a cognitive-behavioral play intervention to pediatric populations: A pilot study for siblings of children diagnosed with cancer. In C. Sieberg (Chair) (Ed.), *Behavioral interventions for pediatric health conditions: Results from prospective studies*. Symposium presented at the annual meeting of the Association for Behavioral and Cognitive Therapies.

Fehr, K., Russ, S., & Ievers-Landis, C. (2016). Treatment of sleep problems in young children: A case series report of a cognitive-behavioral play intervention. *Clinical Practice in Pediatric Psychology*, *4*(3), 306–317.

Gunlicks-Stoessel, M., Westervelt, A., Reigstad, K., Mufson, L., & Lee, S. (2019). The role of attachment style in interpersonal psychotherapy for depressed adolescents. *Psychotherapy Research*, *29*(1), 78–85.

Jacobson, C. M., Mufson, L. H., & Young, J. F. (2017). Treating adolescent depression using interpersonal psychotherapy. In J. R. Weisz & A. E. Kazdin (Eds.), *Evidence-based psychotherapies for children and adolescents* (3rd ed., pp. 66–82). The Guilford Press.

Karver, M. S., De Nadai, A. S., Monahan, M., & Shirk, S. R. (2018). Meta-analysis of the prospective relation between alliance and outcome in child and adolescent psychotherapy. *Psychotherapy*, *55*(4), 341–355.

Kataoka, S. H., Zhang, L., & Wells, K. B. (2002). Unmet need for mental health care among U.S. children: Variation by ethnicity and insurance status. *The American Journal of Psychiatry*, *159*(9), 1548–1555.

Kazdin, A. E., Bass, D., Ayers, W. A., & Rodgers, A. (1990). Empirical and clinical focus of child and adolescent psychotherapy research. *Journal of Consulting and Clinical Psychology*, *58*(6), 729–740.

Knell, S. (2016). Cognitive-behavioral play therapy. In K. O'Connor, C. Schaefer, & L. Braverman (Eds.), *Handbook of play therapy* (2nd ed., pp. 119–133). Wiley.

Koocher, G., McMann, M., Stout, A., & Norcross, J. (2015). Discredited assessment and treatment methods used with children and adolescents: A Delphi poll. *Journal of Clinical Child & Adolescent Psychology*, *44*(5), 722–729.

Landreth, G. (2012). *Play therapy: The art of relationship* (3rd ed.). Routledge/Taylor & Francis Group.

Leraas, B. C., Ramasami, J., & Fehr, K. K. (2020). *Parent preferences for behavioral health information in rural pediatric primary care.* [Poster presentation]. Society of Pediatric Psychology Annual Conference, Virtual.

Lin, Y., & Bratton, S. (2015). A meta-analytic review of child-centered play therapy approaches. *Journal of Counseling & Development*, *93*, 45–58.

March, J., Silva, S., Petrycki, S., Curry, J., Wells, K., Fairbank, J., … Treatment for Adolescents with Depression Study (TADS) Team (2004). Fluoxetine, cognitive-behavioral therapy, and their combination for adolescents with depression: Treatment for adolescents with depression study (TADS) randomized controlled trial. *Journal of the American Medical Association*, *292*(7), 807–820.

Moore, M., & Russ, S. (2006). Pretend play as a resource for children: Implications for pediatricians and health professionals. *Journal of Developmental & Behavioral Pediatrics*, *27*(3), 237–248.

Mychailyszyn, M. P., & Elson, D. M. (2018). Working through the blues: A meta-analysis on Interpersonal Psychotherapy for depressed adolescents (IPT-A). *Children & Youth Services Review*, *87*, 123–129.

Ogden, P., & Goldstein, B. (2017). Embedded relational mindfulness (ERM)© in child and adolescent treatment: A sensorimotor psychotherapy perspective. *European Journal of Trauma & Dissociation*, *1*(3), 171–176.

Pearson, B. (2008). Effects of a cognitive behavioral play intervention on children's hope and school adjustment. *Dissertation Abstracts International*, *69*(6).

Rasmussen, B., & Kealy, D. (2020). Reflections on supportive psychotherapy in the 21st century. *Journal of Social Work Practice*, *34*(3), 281–295.

Riley, A., Walker, B., Wilson, A., Hall, T., Stormshak, E., & Cohen, D. (2019). Parents' consumer preferences for early childhood behavioral intervention in primary care. *Journal of Developmental & Behavioral Pediatrics*, *40*, 669–678.

Russ, S. (2004). *Play in child development and psychotherapy: Toward empirically supported practice*. Erlbaum Associate Publishers.

Russ, S., & Niec, L. (Eds.). (2011). *Play in clinical practice: Evidence-based approaches*. Guilford Publications.

Stancin, T., & Perrin, E. (2014). Psychologists and pediatricians: Opportunities for collaboration in primary care. *American Psychologist*, *69*(4), 332–343.

The MTA Cooperative Group. (1999). A 14-month randomized clinical trial of treatment strategies for attention-deficit/hyperactivity disorder. *Archives of General Psychiatry*, *56*(12), 1073–1086.

Walkup, J. T., Albano, A. M., Piacentini, J., Birmaher, B., Compton, S. N., Sherrill, J. T., … Kendall, P. C. (2008). Cognitive behavioral therapy, sertraline, or a combination in childhood anxiety. *The New England Journal of Medicine*, *359*(26), 2753–2766.

Weersing, V. R., Jeffreys, M., Schwartz, K. T. G., & Bolano, C. (2017). Evidence-base update of psychosocial treatments for child and adolescent depression. *Journal of Clinical Child & Adolescent Psychology*, *46*(1), 11–43.

Weisz, J. R., Kuppens, S., Ng, M. Y., Eckshtain, D., Ugueto, A. M., Vaughn-Coaxum, R., … Fordwood, S. R. (2017). What five decades of research tells us about the effects of youth psychological therapy: A multilevel meta-analysis and implications for science and practice. *American Psychologist*, *72*(2), 79–117.

Weisz, J. R., Weiss, B., Alicke, M. D., & Klotz, M. L. (1987). Effectiveness of psychotherapy with children and adolescents: A meta-analysis for clinicians. *Journal of Consulting and Clinical Psychology*, *55*(4), 542–549.

Weisz, J. R., Weiss, B., Han, S. S., Granger, D. A., & Morton, T. (1995). Effects of psychotherapy with children and adolescents revisited: A meta-analysis of treatment outcome studies. *Psychological Bulletin*, *117*(3), 450–468.

Wu, M. S., Caporino, N. E., Peris, T. S., Perez, J., Thamrin, H., Albano, A. M., Kendall, P. C., Walkup, J. T., Birmaher, B., Compton, S. N., & Piacentini, J. (2020). The impact of treatment expectations on exposure process and treatment outcome in childhood anxiety disorders. *Journal of Abnormal Child Psychology*, *48*, 79–89.

97

Family Systems Therapy and Its Importance in Developmental-Behavioral Pediatrics

Robyn Mehlenbeck and Paige J. Trojanowski

For additional material related to the content of this chapter, please see Chapters 12 and 13.

> **VIGNETTE**
>
> *Maggie is a 13-year-old cisgender female who has depression and is on the autism spectrum with mild social impairments. She has become more isolated than usual, her grades are dropping, and her mother finds her crying in her room several times per week. Her mother identifies as Latina, and Maggie and her mother live with Maggie's maternal grandparents, her younger brother, and younger sister. Her father identifies as White but is not part of her life.*

An immediate thought when we say "family therapy" is that there is a problem with the family we are seeing. This can be due to divorce, disconnect between children and parents, extended family dysfunction, among other things. Moreover, anyone who treats children recognizes that children do not function independently. Rather, they function as part of a system—the immediate system is the family with whom they live. The larger system includes school, extended family, peers, government, religious systems, etc. By the end of this chapter, our hope is that you think of family therapy as a means of improving a child's functioning by helping the system—not because that system is necessarily broken, but rather that the system has the strengths to help the child.

WHAT IS FAMILY THERAPY?

Family therapy is where the family is the unit of concern and intervention involves the family and its relationships. There is a long history of different types of family therapy (Cottrell & Boston, 2002), and while many professionals working in pediatrics recognize the importance of involving the family, there is minimal research to determine the efficacy of different types of family therapy. A recent reference, *The Handbook of Systemic Family Therapy*, describes the research to date on family systems treatment for a variety of childhood concerns, including chronic health conditions, mental health issues, and neurodevelopmental issues, and is an excellent reference (Wampler & McWey, 2020). Family systems is based on Bowen's theory of families, and a brief description of this can be found at https://www.thebowencenter.org/core-concepts-diagrams.

We would be remiss if we did not acknowledge the important contributions of developmental-behavioral pediatricians William Coleman and William Cohen in this discussion of family therapy. The reader is referred to *Developmental and Behavioral Pediatrics*, fourth edition, for additional historical detail, as well as key strategies to implement family systems interviewing and intervention (Carey, Crocker, Coleman, Elias, & Feldman, 2009).

Defining the Family

To identify who should be involved in family therapy, we first must define the family. Maggie, from the chapter-opening vignette, may identify her family as the people she lives with (i.e., her mother and siblings only) or include her father, though not physically present, in her definition of her family. Family therapy should consider who has the most direct influence in her system. In this case it would be helpful to include her maternal grandparents in any family therapy, as they clearly have influence in her day-to-day life. Sometimes siblings should be involved as they contribute to the family system (and sometimes give you the most honest look at the full system).

Why Family Systems?

A family system is defined as a collection of individuals in a relationship with one another such that if any single individual changes significantly then all others change. For example, a young child with autism becomes the focus of his mother's attention, to the exclusion of the marital relationship. Would that child do better if his parent's marital relationship was stronger? A child with type 1 diabetes may have a parent who is so anxious about her medical state that she is restricted from playdates. Imagine the stress in the family when her siblings are permitted to go on playdates but she is not. In both cases helping the family system make some changes will benefit the child tremendously. In Maggie's case we can argue that if some of the relationships in her family system change, it will influence both her depression and her overall functioning.

EVIDENCE FOR FAMILY SYSTEMS INTERVENTIONS

Pediatric Psychology

Changes in the family system are inevitable when a child is diagnosed with a chronic illness or a neurodevelopmental disorder. The pediatric psychology literature suggests that significant family reorganization and changes in child expectations can occur in response to disease onset (Rolland, 2019;

Weihs & Reiss, 2000). These adjustments change over time as adolescents mature, but they can lead to conflict or misunderstandings among family members at multiple levels. Siblings of a chronically ill child may be at higher risk of psychological health/adjustment problems compared to children without siblings with chronic illness (Sharpe & Rossiter, 2002); however, more research is needed to understand sibling coping as well as their role in helping the affected child to cope. Interventions with a family systems approach involve more than one member of the family and may include psychoeducation, disease training, skill building , clarification of expectations and roles, goal setting, and disease management routines (Kazak, Rourke, & Crump, 2003). They may also include more foundational family interventions (e.g., relationship skills, collaborative problem solving, communication). Although research supporting family systems continues to be minimal, there is good evidence for some family interventions in pediatric psychology in the areas of type 1 diabetes and obesity, as two examples (Wysocki et al., 2006).

A well-supported family program is the Behavioral Family Systems Therapy for Diabetes (BFSTD; Wysocki et al., 2006). It combines problem-solving training ("problem definition, generation of solutions, group decision making, planning, implementation and monitoring of the selected solution, and renegotiation or refinement of ineffective solutions"), communication training ("instructions, feedback, modeling, and rehearsal targeting common parent–adolescent communication errors"), cognitive restructuring ("targeted family members' irrational beliefs, attitudes, and attributions about one another's behavior that could impede effective parent–adolescent communication"), and functional-structural family therapy ("targeted anomalous family systemic characteristics [e.g., weak parental coalitions and cross-generational coalitions] that could impede effective problem solving and communication") (Wysocki et al., 2006).

A metaanalysis of 20 studies with largely White samples examined the Comprehensive Behavioral Family Lifestyle Interventions for obesity, reporting a small but significant effect for family interventions on dietary intake, physical activity, and behavior strategies to reduce weight in adolescents (Janicke et al., 2014). Interventions relied on family-based change and parent modeling of behavior as critical agents of change. Skelton and colleagues (2012) and Pratt and Skelton (2018) also provide evidence for family systems intervention with weight management. Consistent with family systems theory, they argue that families strive for equilibrium within and outside the family system, which can make behavioral changes difficult if there is not a full family change. Thus for interventions to be successful, you must understand the relationships among family members to best assess the ability to make behavior changes, including targeting individuals who have more power, such as caregivers or parents, of the family system to increase likelihood of change. For example, it is important to fully understand family routines and rituals to ensure ability to change behaviors during obesity interventions (e.g., family mealtime, dietary restrictions, dietary

BOX 97.1 Overview of Select Techniques Emphasized in Family Therapy

Technique/Skill	Description
Circular questions	Asking another family member to comment on the behavior, opinion, or reaction of another family member (e.g., "How would your mom say that things have been going over the past week?" or "How do you think your son feels when you ——?"). Therapists may elicit responses from each family member for the same question. These questions help each family member to take new perspectives and reinforces talking to each other.
Family communication	Provide family with guidelines for positive communication (e.g., having discussion when both parties are calm, showing empathy, not bringing up past faults, tone of voice, active listening). Use guidelines during communication role plays and during sessions to build family's ability to communicate effectively and without argument. Provide feedback and observations of family communication style throughout sessions as needed.
Family problem solving	Systematic method of problem solving, involving the whole family in generating potential options, evaluating options, and selecting the course of action. Therapist works with the entire family to help them work through the following steps: • Identify/select the problem • Generate options from: make a list of a wide range of options from doing nothing to things requiring larger-scale change • Rate the likelihood of success with each option (thinking about the advantages and disadvantages of each option) • Help family to select the best option • Evaluate success of chosen option
Family connectedness and strengths	Help the family to recognize their strengths as a family and to validate their experience of negative emotions and conflict during times of stress. Explain that positive family interactions need to outnumber negative family interactions to maintain positive family relations. Therapist may ask family members to share what they appreciate about the other family members and explore each family member's role in maintaining a positive environment.

BOX 97.2 Linear Versus Circular Questions

Linear Question	Circular Question
1. Tell me what brought you in today?	1. Why did your mother decide to bring you in today?
2. What are you most upset about?	2. Which parent understands most what upsets you?
3. When did you last cut yourself?	3. Do your parents know when you last cut yourself?
4. Have you ever experienced physical abuse?	4. Do your parents worry that you have ever been abused?
5. Does your mom understand you?	5. Who understands you the best?

patterns), and these patterns might be distinct in different families, particularly when culture and background are taken into consideration. The reader is referred to Pratt and Skelton (2018) for an excellent flow chart, including both assessment for family intervention for weight management and an outline of a family systems theory informed approach (i.e., focusing on strengths of the family, rules, structure, relationships and communication affecting weight management, reorganization of families around healthy behaviors) versus more traditional behavioral intervention (e.g., focusing on goal setting, problem solving, monitoring) (Pratt & Skelton, 2018).

Children With Autism Spectrum Disorder and Other Neurodevelopmental Difficulties

Although evidence-based treatments for autism spectrum disorder (ASD) are almost entirely behavioral or cognitive-behavioral in nature (i.e., behavior management, parent training, language training, modeling, social skills, using stories to teach skills) (Chorpita et al., 2011; Flessner & Piacentini, 2017), some research indicates that a family-centered approach may be helpful (Gabovitch & Curtin, 2009). For example, families with a child with ASD report significant family stress associated with caring for a child with ASD, which impacts family functioning. In addition, the reciprocal influences between an individual with ASD and other family members (e.g., lack of spontaneity, daily routines, emotion management, help with tasks of daily living) can result in greater family conflict and poor psychosocial health of family members (Cridland, Jones, Magee, & Caputi, 2014). Importantly, effects on the family unit can also be positive, such as improved communication, patience, and empathy (Cridland et al., 2014). Other data suggest that severe family stress in these families may be particularly related to lack of coparent support and ability to socialize, both of which may be addressed through a family systems approach (Sim et al., 2018). Improving caregiver communication, supportiveness, and division of responsibility may improve overall family functioning and protect against the development of negative outcomes in families with a child with ASD.

Despite family therapy/family systems therapy in ASD not being studied widely, many evidence-based behavioral interventions do have a family-centered approach, relying on the family to determine goals, values, and concerns and encouraging the family to be actively involved in the intervention implementation, and a family-centered approach is strongly recommended in the Missouri Autism Consensus Statement in their *Guide to Evidence-based Interventions* (2012). Family dynamics, cultural considerations, resources, and educational background are all considered in the implementation of behavioral, skill-based interventions.

WHAT IS INVOLVED IN FAMILY SYSTEMS THERAPY?

Returning to Maggie, the family decided that her mother and grandparents should be involved in treatment to start, especially as Maggie's mother worked several jobs and Maggie spent a lot of time with her grandparents. Maggie's mother and grandparents were initially leery of participating as they were worried that they would be blamed for Maggie's problems, and they felt that the doctors needed to "fix" Maggie. Treatment started with explaining how important they were to helping Maggie feel better and that they were the experts on their daughter/granddaughter. Clinicians discussed the family strengths and how each member's strengths had contributed to good family functioning in the past. Maggie's grandparents mentioned that they were religious, and that they did not think Maggie prayed enough. If she went to church more with them, she would meet other teens her age, and could attend the youth group. Psychoeducation was provided regarding depression, and the concepts of cognitive-behavioral therapy were included in the family session, as cognitive-behavioral and behavioral interventions, when they are indicated, are often part of family intervention as well. Maggie agreed to attend church with her grandparents over the next week, and her grandparents stated that they would "make sure" Maggie talked to some other teens. We know that behavioral activation is a key part of treating depression. In Maggie's case capitalizing on the family's frequent visits to church helped get her out of the house.

This is an example of a first-order change in family systems; it addresses the initial problem (staying isolated, likely contributing to her depression), but it is very linear in intent. First-order change is defined as an action that is increased or decreased to obtain changes but occurs within the existing system. It often occurs at the individual level. Getting out of the house might help Maggie feel better initially, but this does not address the second-order systems changes needed to maintain improvement. Second-order systems changes are those that rewrite systems rules and relationships. In the next session, this might be addressed by discussing how Maggie's mother and grandparents work together to address Maggie's ASD and subsequent social difficulties. This might lead to helping Maggie identify when she feels most confident in social interactions, with both mother and grandparents acknowledging how they protect Maggie from social interactions given their assumption that she is "not good at them."

This portion of treatment for Maggie exemplifies a few core assumptions that are present in any family systems intervention. First, the focus is on family strengths and how the family is key to helping their child. This is often a shift from focusing on the so-called problem child. Second, the family is the source of healing, not blame. In psychology there is a history of blaming parents (particularly mothers) for children's problems. Family systems approaches take the opposite tack, assuming blame is not helpful. Rather, the focus is on identifying ways to reorganize the family to promote healthy behaviors and functioning. Doing so also allows the clinician to work within the family's belief system with increased cultural sensitivity.

The third assumption is that family systems are reality based, in that the child lives at home with the family. Most therapists will see a child/family once a week for 50 minutes. This is an artificial setting, and changes will not be maintained if they are not enacted and supported in their real life. Finally, family systems treatment utilizes the therapist as a coach, not the expert. This is very different from a typical medical model where a patient comes to ask for advice or direction to address a specific issue. Rather, our goal is to help caregivers feel empowered to take care of their children, and caregivers are truly the experts on their children. This can be difficult for both providers and families alike, but if we help families make significant second-order changes within their belief system, knowing their children best, the changes are likely to last.

In addition to these base assumptions, there are several additional key factors to consider when implementing family systems therapy. Pratt and Skelton (2018) summarize the key tenets succinctly:

> *Families determine membership; subsystems exist, such as parent-child, spouse, and sibling relationships; families strive to maintain equilibrium; resources are needed for adaptation and change; existence of family rules; and likely the most important tenet describing behaviors, first- and second-order change. First-order change is how a family receives input from their surrounding environment. Second-order changes require the reorganization of rules and routines to make lasting first-order changes and changes to the overall family environment. (p. 621)*

Family systems therapy is a way of thinking and approaching concerns, and it changes the focus of the intervention to the system. However, as demonstrated in Maggie's case, it does not preclude other interventions from being implemented, including behavioral or cognitive-behavioral interventions (both strongly evidence-based interventions for children with ADHD, disruptive behavior, anxiety, and depression). In fact, family systems work can enhance this work by helping the family learn and reinforce skills with their children. Many child therapists include family therapy sessions while treatment for this very reason.

It should be noted that there are exceptions to when family systems therapy is indicated. One of the prime exceptions is in cases of child abuse. A child should never be required to stay in a room or work directly with a family member who was/is abusive without significant trauma work first. Even then, it needs to be carefully determined if family systems therapy is an appropriate follow-up intervention. The priority is always to protect the child.

Key Techniques for Systems Interventions

Interventive Interviewing

Interventive interviewing is a technique that uses questions as intervention (Box 97.1). Thus even your initial evaluation is considered an intervention. Clinicians' questions help the family recognize patterns and start to identify where changes need to be made from the beginning. For example, during intake, you are observing that a 9-year-old boy is sitting in his mother's lap. You ask about other times when the child is asked to engage with new people and how both mother and child respond. These questions will target not only whether the child can separate from mom, but also how mother reacts to encourage or discourage healthy separation (Tomm, 1987, 1988). Using questions as intervention may be a mind shift for the provider, as we typically think about assessment, treatment plan, and intervention separately.

Circular Questions Versus Linear Questions

One way to engage in interventive interviewing is the use of circular questions (Box 97.2). Circular questions ask not only about content, but also about the relationship between two or more members of the family system. This type of question also encourages a patient or caregiver to think through a different perspective. For example, if you ask a question such as "What is your mother most concerned about today?" the child is likely to look at mother to try to guess what she is thinking. Or, if the child knows exactly what mother is concerned about, you have just gained additional information about their communication. If the child guesses wrong, the benefit here is the chance to prompt the child and mother to talk about the concerns, modeling healthy communication between them and reinforcing their relationship.

During assessment, we are taught to ask linear questions to gather content. For example, "What is your primary concern? Does your child make eye contact when you play together?" This is an excellent way to gather content about the concerns, but it does not maximize your ability to gather information and insert some intervention from the beginning, as we are not trained to think like this. Depending on the age of the child, you might ask the caregiver, "What does your child think your main concern is?" or ask the child, "Does your mother realize how hard it is for you to make eye contact when you play together?" Having two to three circular questions prepared in advance will help you use them in your initial interview. This way, you have some benefit of this technique without struggling to focus on it during your face-to-face time.

BOX 97.3 Family Communication Strategies

Steps Toward Positive Communication

Timing Is Key

Find a time when both people are ready to talk.
Avoid times when people are tired/upset/etc.
Take a break if the conversation starts to get too heated.

Stick to the Facts; Stick to the Present

Be specific—don't beat around the bush.
Don't dig up the past.
Avoid judgment and name-calling.
Use a clear, calm, and sincere voice.

Give to Get

Start with a statement that shows you care about the other person's feelings or perspective.
- Teen example: I know you've been worried about me lately. Is that true? I also want to be able to spend time with my friends.
- Parent example: I've noticed you've been really angry lately about the rules. Is that right? I want to be sure you're safe.

Use Active Listening

Look at the person with calm neutral face.
Stay focused on the other person and don't get distracted by surroundings.
- Nod head and say "Uh-huh."
- Ask questions.
- Repeat back what you have heard, not just the facts but the feelings, too.

BOX 97.4 Improving Family Activities

Tips for Improving Family Activities

Be present in the moment and pay full attention to the activity. Do not text, check e-mail, get on the phone, or engage in other distracting behaviors.
This allows for:
- More positive interactions
- Understanding of what is going on with one another
- A foundation for working together

Share what you like about the activity and what the other person is doing.
- "I really enjoy it when ______."
- "Thanks for ______."

Do not criticize or reprimand one another.
Ignore minor misbehaviors.
Defer all problems to a later time.
Avoid controversial subjects.
Have fun just being together.
Practice good communication and listening skills.

Specific Family Communication Strategies

Family systems therapy often includes some basic family communication strategies. As you work with a family, patterns often emerge that are hard to shake. Different subgroups within the family often have different patterns of communication. Helping each member of the system review and implement some basic communication strategies can improve family relationships. Boxes 97.3 and 97.4 illustrate several specific strategies that can be helpful as you work with families and are adapted from the *Core Competency Manual* developed by Esposito-Smythers, Spirito, Kahler, Hunt, & Monti, (2011). These include active listening, staying with the present issue (i.e., not bringing up past events), being aware of timing of serious discussions, and intentionally noticing positive interactions.

HOW DO I HELP FAMILIES, WITH AND WITHOUT FAMILY THERAPY?

Thinking About Your Client and Family

Including a family systems approach is helpful to case conceptualization, and it is especially useful to highlight with trainees. Thinking from a systems perspective helps curb bias and promotes understanding of systemic/structural/policy level factors that can influence child health beyond personal/individual factors and behavior choices. This practice takes time and an intentional focus on identifying changes that will benefit the child. Many practitioners are used to first-order changes and can help a parent focus on providing healthier foods in the house (if worried about obesity, for example), or in Maggie's case, working on getting her out of the house more. However, thinking through the family system will help practitioners consider second-order changes. For Maggie, this might include helping her advocate for herself, altering the relationships between the caregivers in the home, and helping them view Maggie differently.

Using Brief Face-to-Face Time to Maximize Content and Reinforce Relationship

Family systems interventions start in your office or exam room. How you ask the questions and assess the family functioning sets the tone for your visit, as well as allows you an opportunity to get additional information that you would not get by deeming the visit "assessment only." Any interaction with a child or family is an intervention. Taking this perspective will help you be a better practitioner and will help the family function better. Start by asking one to two circular questions in your intake and see what happens (see Box 97.2). Did you get more information than if you asked one of the direct questions? Did the family connect with each other, even a little bit, in your office?

Assessing Need for Family Therapy

A family systems approach addresses how a family understands, labels, and talks about the presenting problems, pediatric illness, disability, or disorder. Key themes in family systems therapy that should be assessed include family boundaries (i.e., Is there an enmeshed family dynamic? Is a key member of the system disengaged?), family roles (negotiator, helper, trouble-maker, organizer, etc.), family rules (both spoken or unspoken), family climate (emotional and physical), and family equilibrium (stability, consistency, customs, routines, or lack thereof) (Christian, 2006). Family systems therapy is recommended when there is conflict, unhealthy dynamics in the family, relationships that are being minimized or neglected, or when a family gets into a pattern that is hard to break (e.g., a parent's only interaction with the child is around the child's diabetes and blood sugars). There may be other times where you can make a difference by identifying the family strengths and common goals (most families truly want the best for their children!) and utilizing this to encourage family systems therapy.

Referring for Treatment

Not all family therapy is the same, so it is important to identify therapists who are familiar with systems treatment, work with multiple members of a family, and are accessible. When referring for family therapy, be sure to talk with the family about how family therapy can help them, focusing on their strengths. It is critical to ensure that families do not feel blamed for the issues, rather that they are key to helping their child. If you connect with colleagues in the community, and can facilitate a warm handoff, that is also going to help with the transition to treatment and increase follow-through on the part of the family.

Fortunately, Maggie's mother and grandparents did commit to family systems therapy. One of the key factors that had not been addressed was the absence of her father, and her family's unwillingness to discuss him at all. This was a result of cultural factors as well as shame. Maggie ended up feeling the effects of his absence without understanding why or where it came from. Maggie's ASD diagnosis "confirmed" for grandparents that their daughter was "being punished" for her actions. During family systems treatment, these issues were able to be addressed, and Maggie's grandparents came to see the effect they had on their granddaughter, even as they were most upset at their daughter. Maggie's depression improved, and she was increasingly willing to practice social interactions at church, which increased her confidence in herself. While this may have happened with typical behavioral treatments (social skills groups, individual CBT for depression), family systems addressed the underlying issue that allowed for significant family changes, improving Maggie's life.

CONCLUSION

Children live with their families, and the family has a significant effect on a child's functioning. This is true whether a child has an illness, a developmental disorder, or is developing typically as expected. The benefits of family systems approaches are treating a child by highlighting their unique family strengths, helping the family make changes to spoken and unspoken rules and structure, and helping the family maintain any changes that they make. Focusing on the family unit also helps destigmatize the child and improves the wellbeing of everyone in the family. By working within the family's belief system, their culture and background, you can share your knowledge and help the family incorporate it in a way that makes sense to them. Families who understand the role of the system also incorporate behavioral interventions better and make sustained changes.

REFERENCES

Carey, W. B., Crocker, A. C., Coleman, W. L., Elias, E. R., & Feldman, H. M. (2009). *Developmental behavioral pediatrics* (4th ed.). Elsevier.

Chorpita, B. F., Daleiden, E. L., Ebesutani, C., Young, J., Becker, K. D., Nakamura, B. J., ... Starace, N. (2011). Evidence-based treatments for children and adolescents: An updated review of indicators of efficacy and effectiveness. *Clinical Psychology: Science and Practice*, *18*(2), 154–172. https://doi.org/10.1111/j.1468-2850.2011.01247.x

Christian, L. G. (2006). Understanding families: Applying family systems theory to early childhood practice. *Young Children*, *61*(1), 12–20.

Cottrell, D., & Boston, P. (2002). Practitioner review: The effectiveness of systemic family therapy for children and adolescents. *Journal of Child Psychology and Psychiatry*, *43*(5), 573–586. https://doi.org/10.1111/1469-7610.00047

Cridland, E. K., Jones, S. C., Magee, C. A., & Caputi, P. (2014). Family-focused autism spectrum disorder research: A review of the utility of family systems approaches. *Autism*, *18*(3), 213–222. https://doi.org/10.1177/1362361312472261

Esposito-Smythers, C., Spirito, A., Kahler, C. W., Hunt, J., & Monti, P. (2011). Treatment of co-occurring substance abuse and suicidality among adolescents: A randomized trial. *Journal of Consulting and Clinical Psychology*, *79*(6), 728–739. https://doi.org/10.1037/a0026074

Flessner, C. A., & Piacentini, J. C. (2017). *Clinical handbook of psychological disorders in children and adolescents: A step-by-step treatment manual.* Guilford Publications.

Gabovitch, E. M., & Curtin, C. (2009). Family-centered care for children with autism spectrum disorders: A review. *Marriage & Family Review*, *45*(5), 469–498. https://doi.org/10.1080/01494920903050755

Janicke, D. M., Steele, R. G., Gayes, L. A., Lim, C. S., Clifford, L. M., Schneider, E. M., ... Westen, S. (2014). Systematic review and meta-analysis of comprehensive behavioral family lifestyle interventions addressing pediatric obesity. *Journal of Pediatric Psychology*, *39*(8), 809–825. https://doi.org/10.1093/jpepsy/jsu023

Kazak, A. E., Rourke, M. T., & Crump, T. A. (2003). Families and other systems in pediatric psychology. *In Handbook of pediatric psychology* (pp. 159–175) (3rd ed.). The Guilford Press.

Missouri Autism Guidelines Initiative. (2012). *Autism spectrum disorders: Guide to evidence-based interventions.* https://autismguidelines.dmh.mo.gov/

Pratt, K. J., & Skelton, J. A. (2018). Family functioning and childhood obesity treatment: A family systems theory-informed approach. *Academic Pediatrics*, *18*(6), 620–627. https://doi.org/10.1016/j.acap.2018.04.001

Rolland, J. S. (2019). Families, health, and illness. *In Handbook of health social work* (pp. 331–357). John Wiley & Sons, Ltd. https://doi.org/10.1002/9781119420743.ch15

Sharpe, D., & Rossiter, L. (2002). Siblings of children with a chronic illness: A meta-analysis. *Journal of Pediatric Psychology*, *27*(8), 699–710. https://doi.org/10.1093/jpepsy/27.8.699

Sim, A., Vaz, S., Cordier, R., Joosten, A., Parsons, D., Smith, C., & Falkmer, T. (2018). Factors associated with stress in families of children with autism spectrum disorder. *Developmental neurorehabilitation*, *21*(3), 155–165. https://doi.org/10.1080/17518423.2017.1326185

Skelton, J. A., Buehler, C., Irby, M. B., & Grzywacz, J. G. (2012). Where are family theories in family-based obesity treatment? Conceptualizing the study of families in pediatric weight management. *International Journal of Obesity*, *36*(7), 891–900. https://doi.org/10.1038/ijo.2012.56

Tomm, K. (1987). Interventive interviewing: Part II. Reflexive questioning as a means to enable self-healing. *Family Process*, *26*(2), 167–183. https://doi.org/10.1111/j.1545-5300.1987.00167.x

Tomm, K. (1988). Interventive interviewing: Part III. Intending to ask lineal, circular, strategic, or reflexive questions? *Family Process*, *27*(1), 1–15. https://doi.org/10.1111/j.1545-5300.1988.00001.x

Wampler, K., & McWey, L. (2020). Systemic family therapy with children and adolescents. *In The handbook of systemic family therapy* (Vol. 2). Amazon.com: Books. 9781119702184 Books.

Weihs, K., & Reiss, D. (2000). Family reorganization in response to cancer: A developmental perspective: *Cancer and the family* (2nd ed.). John Wiley & Sons Ltd.

Wysocki, T., Harris, M. A., Buckloh, L. M., Mertlich, D., Lochrie, A. S., Taylor, A., … White, N. H. (2006). Effects of behavioral family systems therapy for diabetes on adolescents' family relationships, treatment adherence, and metabolic control. *Journal of Pediatric Psychology*, *31*(9), 928–938. https://doi.org/10.1093/jpepsy/jsj098

98

Cognitive-Behavioral Therapy in Developmental-Behavioral Pediatrics

Megan E. Tudor, Shereen J. Cohen, Breanna M. Winder-Patel, and Kathleen Angkustsiri

For additional material related to the content of this chapter, please see Chapters 49, and 51.

VIGNETTE 1

Raquel is a 9-year-old girl with a history of vocal and motor tics, aggressive tantrums, and general anxiety. Cognitive-behavioral therapy (CBT) was implemented wherein Raquel collaborated with her therapist on setting personal goals and creating individualized weekly plans for changing both her behavior and thinking patterns. Treatment consisted first of psychoeducation about tics wherein Raquel was surprised to learn that it was possible to change them, previously believing that they were entirely out of her control. She monitored her vocal tics (throat clearing) and motor tics (nose scrunching) daily while learning to identify the urges she felt in her body (bottom of throat and tip of nose). Raquel began practicing a "competing response" for her tics, such as swallowing, while earning small rewards for her daily practice. To externalize her anxiety and anger symptoms, Raquel created original characters to represent her anger and anxiety (the "Angry Rabbit" and "Silly Worry Brain"). She learned to identify early warning signs, in contrast to her previous belief that her emotions were all there or not there. She actively participated in cognitive restructuring wherein she challenged her anxious thoughts, such as "If I can't do this perfectly then I shouldn't do it at all," to "Everyone makes mistakes sometimes, it's part of learning." Raquel and her mother agreed upon a daily behavior plan to practice new responses to anger (e.g., communicating, drawing in a quiet part of the house) and anxiety (e.g., trying small new activities every day, practicing making mistakes as a family). Raquel's mother consistently applied positive praise and small rewards for target behaviors, while using planned ignoring to cease attention for outbursts. Over 12 sessions, Raquel experienced marked reduction in all symptom categories. A more complete account of this case is published elsewhere (Tudor, Bertschinger, Piasecka, & Sukhodolsky, 2018).

COGNITIVE-BEHAVIORAL THERAPY

CBT is one of the most widely studied psychotherapy intervention models with adaptations for an immense number of disorders in children, adolescents, and adults alike. CBT for youth and adolescents has met the growing need for evidence-based practice (EBP; or empirically supported treatment [EST]) within health care at large, with a wealth of supported CBT models for an array of common childhood psychological disorders (Box 98.1) (APA Presidential Task Force, 2006). CBT, with its emphasis on actively changing maladaptive behavioral and thinking patterns, is now accepted as the gold standard intervention for children and adolescents. CBT may be a particularly appropriate intervention for this age group given its history of modularity of treatment components, focus on short-term treatment, ease of modification or individualization, and overall transdiagnostic emphasis (Friedberg et al., 2014). CBT for youth has proven increasingly popular not only among dedicated clinics but also in schools and medical care settings (see Box 98.1).

A Brief History of CBT

In the 1950s empirical studies demonstrated that the prevailing psychotherapeutic treatments of the time appeared to be no more effective than no treatment at all, indicating a need for novel, improved interventions. By this time, Pavlov and Watson had conducted extensive research on classical conditioning, including the automatic behavioral responses related to hunger and fear. Subsequently, Skinner and others built upon these concepts through the study of operant conditioning (described in further detail later). This foundation of behavioral learning principles would prove revolutionary in the field of psychotherapy. Behavioral therapy initially emerged as a treatment for children with severe behavior problems and, eventually, became integrated with the concepts of social learning theory and cognitive processing work, resulting in the basis of CBT that is pervasive across the field of clinical psychology today (Benjamin et al., 2011).

The B in CBT—Behavior

Behavioral learning is essential to the philosophy, principles, and subsequent strategies of CBT. CBT therapists work from the core belief that all beings engage in behavior that results in a preferred outcome and avoid engaging in behaviors that result in a negative outcome (Fig. 98.1). Thus behavior is a series of actions that have been reinforced because a positive outcome has occurred. As examples, a child who receives access to watching a favorite TV show every night after washing dishes becomes more likely to wash dishes. Or a child who earns a "chore pass" wherein she can forego doing a chore if she receives an A on her spelling test becomes more likely

BOX 98.1 Psychological Disorders Treated With Cognitive-Behavioral Therapy

	Children/Adolescents	Adult
Established EBP	Anxiety Disruptive behavior (ODD/CD) OCD PTSD Schizophrenia/psychosis Self-injurious thoughts/behaviors Substance abuse	Anorexia ADHD Binge eating disorder Bulimia Chronic headache Chronic pain Depression Generalized anxiety disorder Schizophrenia Insomnia Irritable bowel syndrome OCD Panic disorder Social anxiety PTSD
Emerging as EBP	Anorexia Bulimia Trichotillomania Excoriation Depression Anger problems	Gambling addiction Substance use disorder

ADHD, Attention-deficit/hyperactivity disorder; *CD*, Conduct disorder; *EBP*, evidence-based practice; *OCD*, obsessive-compulsive disorder; *ODD*, Oppositional-defiant disorder; *PTSD*, posttraumatic stress disorder.

	Behavior Increases	Behavior Decreases
Stimuli Added	Positive Reinforcement	Positive Punishment
Stimuli Removed	Negative Reinforcement	Negative Punishment

Fig. 98.1 Basic behavioral learning principles.

to study for her test. Consistently, behavior is expected to decrease when a negative outcome occurs or a positive experience is removed. To illustrate, a child who is made to do the boring and unpleasant task of cleaning out underneath the kitchen sink in response to hitting his sister becomes less likely to hit his sister in the future. Similarly, a teenager whose highly desirable cell phone is removed for 2 hours when she cusses in front of her mother is likely to show a decrease in her cussing behavior. Additionally, the concept of extinction is relevant to CBT in that long-standing behaviors that have been maintained through a history of responses are then extinguished by removing these previously predictable reinforcements. For example, a small child reliably receives a new toy or treat when he cries while grocery shopping; his parent's response has served to stop his crying and his parent's embarrassment but, in the context of treatment, will be extinguished by removing reinforcement and eventually decreasing inappropriate behavior. These tenets appear deceptively simple yet often reflect a complex and multilayered conceptualization that integrates individual motivators, cultural differences, consistency of approaches, and calibrations of reward/punishment ratios, to name a few.

Overall, CBT recruits behavioral learning principles with the assumption that behavior can be changed (e.g., more or less likely to occur) with appropriately tailored responses from individuals or the environment around them, thus leading to a vast array of strategies and behavioral concepts that are integrated into CBT based on particular behavioral goals.

Examples of Behavioral Strategies

A central tenet of CBT for youth is that it can be presented modularly and flexibly, rather than a one-size-fits-all approach, even for manualized programs (e.g., Kendall et al., 2008). This conceptualization renders CBT attractive for treating youth across many diagnostic categories and age groups. Some behavioral strategies practiced within CBT may be especially common and critical to treatment success (Box 98.2). Behavioral strategies used in CBT are apparent descendants of earlier, traditional behavioral therapies (e.g., applied behavior analysis). For youth, typically practiced strategies may include exposure for anxiety, behavioral activation for depression, or parent management training for disruptive behavior and, in many cases, may integrate an array of behavioral strategies to simultaneously target various behavioral goals. Altogether these common strategies aim to provide children with new behavioral experiences and therefore new opportunities to be reinforced.

BOX 98.2 Selected Behavioral Strategies in Cognitive-Behavioral Therapy

Behavioral Strategy	Description
Role playing/behavioral rehearsal	Children act out specific, new behaviors as a form of practice in a safe environment. For example, an anxious child role playing asking a sales clerk a question with the trusted therapist in advance of an in vivo exposure. For young children, this process may also occur in the context of play, drawing, or performance.
Behavioral activation	Changes to daily routine or activities to provide youth opportunities for pleasure or reinforcement.
Reward programs/token economy	Use of specific positive reinforcement planning for in-session behavior and out-of-session behavior that will be met with agreed upon rewards and/or points or tokens that can be exchanged for rewards. Consists of various specifics, including clear definition of desired behavior, type of rewards, time of delivery, ratio of behavior to reward, constant reevaluation of effectiveness, etc.
Shaping	As per child's overall temperament and preferences, delivering verbal or physical positive feedback for small steps toward desired behavior.
Modeling	As completed by therapist and/or parents, acting out and narrating particular sequences of desired behavior to serve as a template for behavior in child.
Exposure	Gradually exposing children to previously feared or anxiety-inducing stimuli or situations at a rate that allows child to gain a new experience and positive association (e.g., mastery) over time.
Parent management training	Training parents in various behavioral techniques to elicit desired behaviors over time, including use of effective demands/requests, time warnings, planned ignoring, time-out, praise, special parent-child time, etc., with an emphasis on positive reinforcement over punishment strategies

The C in CBT—Cognitive

The cognitive aspects of CBT are founded upon the theory that humans make errors in their thinking, sometimes called cognitive distortions (Beck et al., 1979) (Box 98.3). Thoughts influence emotions and behaviors, and therefore by altering thoughts, one can alter mood or behavioral choices. Thus by examining maladaptive thoughts, challenging them, and coming to a different conclusion, children, adolescents, and adults can reduce the experience of negative emotions (e.g., depression or anxiety). Cognitive therapy is most often paired with behavioral intervention, especially for children and adolescents, to learn experientially how cognitions can impact emotions and ultimately actions and outcomes (see Box 98.3).

Examples of Cognitive Strategies

A common early step in any CBT treatment is psychoeducation. Psychoeducation is the process of providing information about the child's diagnosis and symptoms, as well as the theoretical underpinnings of CBT. For example, one may provide statistics on how common a disorder is, common features of the disorder, and how the child (and parent) can expect changes to occur. Therapists explain the connection between thoughts, feelings, and actions to help the client and parents understand the function of all future CBT strategies.

Another staple of cognitive therapy and CBT is cognitive restructuring, consisting of the patient identifying and challenging maladaptive thoughts (described in further detail later). This process may consist of multiple steps but can be expanded or simplified depending on the age and cognitive ability of the client. For example, prior to about age 7 years, a typically developing child may not be able to engage in metacognition or self-thought.

Let us consider, for example, a teenager who is walking down the hallway in school. This teen passes a friend, and the friend does not say hello. This teen might jump to the conclusion that her friend doesn't like her anymore, which taps into her core belief that she is in fact entirely unlikable, and she spends her lunchbreak alone in the bathroom for the remainder of the week. This teenager shares this with her therapist, who will now try to restructure the client's thoughts, including identifying the thought, labeling the negative emotions associated with the thought, examining the evidence for and against the thought, and, ultimately, considering more realistic or adaptive interpretations of

BOX 98.3 Common Cognitive Distortions

Cognitive Distortion	Description
All-or-nothing thinking	Placing experiences in one of two opposite categories (e.g., flawless or defective, immaculate or filthy, saint or sinner, good or bad)
Overgeneralizing	Drawing sweeping inferences (e.g., "I can't control my temper") from a single instance
Jumping to conclusions	Focusing on one aspect of a situation in deciding how to understand it (e.g., "the reason I haven't gotten my test grade yet is because I failed it")
Mind reading	Believing one knows what another person is thinking, with very little evidence
Fortune telling	Believing one knows what the future holds, while ignoring other possibilities
Emotional reasoning	Believing that something must be true, because it feels like it is true
Inappropriate blaming	Using hindsight to determine what one "should have done," even if one could not have known the best thing to do at the time; ignoring mitigating factors; or ignoring the roles played by others in determining a negative outcome

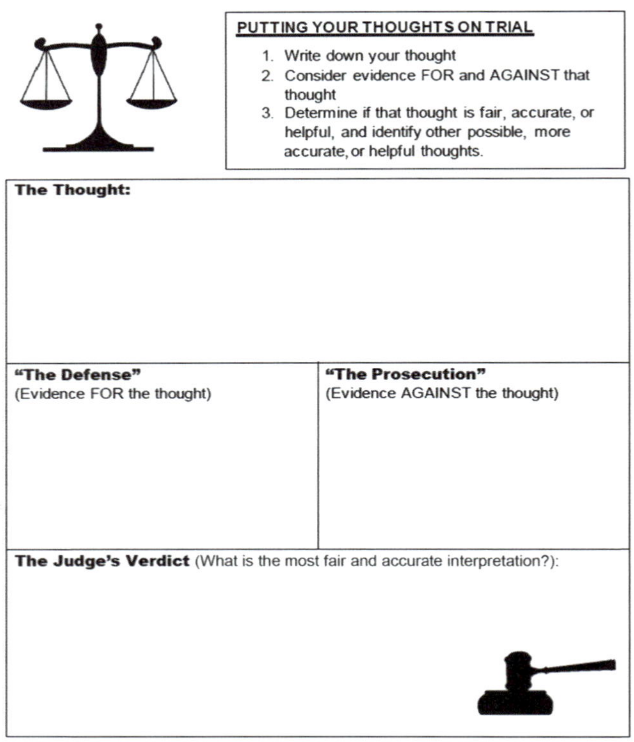
PUTTING YOUR THOUGHTS ON TRIAL

1. Write down your thought
2. Consider evidence FOR and AGAINST that thought
3. Determine if that thought is fair, accurate, or helpful, and identify other possible, more accurate, or helpful thoughts.

The Thought:

"The Defense" (Evidence FOR the thought)

"The Prosecution" (Evidence AGAINST the thought)

The Judge's Verdict (What is the most fair and accurate interpretation?):

Fig. 98.2 Sample cognitive restructuring worksheet.

the event (e.g., her friend had a big test that day and was stressed). For younger children, this process may often integrate illustrations, games, or other forms of visuals to organize the thought process. For adolescents, similar developmentally appropriate metaphors, such as "putting a thought on trial" may be integrated (Fig. 98.2).

It can also be helpful to engage the child in analyzing the cause and effects of the behavior (i.e., chain analysis). Returning to the previous example, the teenager could learn that the anxiety trigger that led her to thinking no one likes her and feeling anxious also led her to further self-isolation. Helping the teen see that her behavioral response moves her further from the goal of being liked and accepted by others can be a helpful cognitive strategy.

Cognitive work in CBT may take other directions that reflect particular psychopathology. For example, hypothesis testing is often central to treating youth with anxiety or obsessive-compulsive disorder (OCD). For example, "I believe that if I walk by a dog it will attack me" is identified, examined, and eventually tested through actual exposure to feared stimuli to determine if the thought is true or false. Various developmentally appropriate metaphors, such as becoming "detectives" or "scientists," may motivate youth challenging these thoughts. Further, in some cases, simply identifying an opposite thought and asking the child to recite this as a mantra of sorts can be sufficient for emotional and behavioral change. For example, if a child frequently has the thought, "I can't do it," then practicing the new phrase, "I can do it," can be effective at reducing maladaptive thoughts.

For younger children, it may also be helpful to externalize the maladaptive thoughts by assigning them a character and/or a name. Recalling Raquel's "Angry Rabbit" and "Silly Worry Brain" from the first vignette, these are examples of a child externalizing distressing thoughts and feelings. These strategies make the maladaptive thoughts more concrete for children and allows for concepts such as "fighting back" or "talking back," which may be especially engaging. As another example, an 11-year-old girl presenting with anxiety named her self-deprecating thoughts "Oogie," who says things like "You can't do this" or "You're weak." She then named the voice of her inner cheerleader "Boogie," who says things like "Yes you can!"

Relaxation-Based Strategies

Controversy exists around the necessity or utility of integrating relaxation-based strategies into CBT for youth, especially as a possible distractor from the inherent experience of anxiety during exposures (e.g., Benito et al., 2020). Nevertheless, a number of relaxation-based strategies can and frequently are included in youth treatment. Diaphragmatic breathing, sometimes called belly breathing, is a strategy used for reducing feelings of anxiety by activating the parasympathetic nervous system, which in turn suppresses the sympathetic nervous system, reducing overall physiologic arousal. When teaching this strategy to children, it can often be helpful for therapists to engage more fun and imaginative strategies. For example, to illustrate making the stomach move up and down, one can have the child lie down and place a stuffed animal on the stomach. Another strategy is asking the child to pretend to smell a flower, and then to slowly blow out a birthday candle or blow a big bubble. Similarly, progressive muscle relaxation is another strategy shown to help reduce physiologic arousal (anxiety, anger, etc.). Typically, one begins by tensing and tightening the muscles in the feet for a few (5–6) seconds, then releasing the tension. The child may be asked to pretend to squeeze lemons into lemonade. To achieve a more individualized, engaging experience, therapists may refer to preferred characters to reflect different forms of the body (e.g., Elastigirl from *The Incredibles*).

Typical Format of CBT

Children and adolescents referred to CBT may encounter a wide range of experiences in terms of session format and duration of treatment. In the context of research studies CBT is often delivered across 12 to 16 weekly sessions, typically 45 to 60 minutes in duration. Overall, a commonality across CBT is an emphasis on an active treatment approach with out-of-session practice, sometimes called homework or assignments, which is intended to enhance skill development daily between sessions. Ultimately, CBT is designed to encourage independence and, as such, CBT therapists typically aim for length of treatment to be as brief as possible with a focus on maintenance and ongoing progress that may be achieved by the patient (and often the patient's family) after sessions end; occasional booster sessions are often encouraged.

Individual and Group Models

CBT for youth is offered in individual and group formats. As the demand for mental health services rises, group-based CBT has proven a popular and effective treatment option. As an example, Wergeland and colleagues (2014) conducted a study comparing individual and group CBT for youth with anxiety disorders and found both treatment modalities to be more effective than no treatment and equally effective at the end of treatment and at 1-year follow-up. Similarly, researchers have found group CBT to be an effective treatment for youth with social anxiety, depression, and OCD (e.g., Keles & Idsoe, 2018).

In both individual and group-based interventions it is not only valuable but even necessary to involve parents and families in treatment to support the child in applying the skills learned in therapy across more settings and situations. Many studies have found added benefit to including parents and families in CBT; indeed, given the importance of out-of-session practice, parent involvement is considered integral to CBT effectiveness.

An Important Note About Appropriate Training in CBT

Due to the predominance of CBT among psychological clinics and practitioners, including for youth, it is sometimes erroneously assumed that CBT can be easily adopted and effectively administered. This ideal seems to be further perpetuated by the easily accessible CBT manuals available on the Internet. This is a tempting notion, but it is simply is not the case. CBT is a specialized treatment that first necessitates strong foundational therapeutic skills and then requires in-depth training, supervision, and continued education. Such a wealth of experience is consistent with doctoral-level psychologists who typically receive years of graduate and postdoctoral training learning to effectively administer CBT and conducting related research. It is therefore not surprising that attempts at providing brief training to other professionals, such as physicians, have shown rather mixed results (Dorflinger et al., 2016). Despite the apparent present-day pervasiveness of CBT for youth, the mental health needs of youth far exceed treatment availability. A dire need for more dissemination of CBT and training of appropriate professionals continues to exist.

Appropriateness of CBT Referral

There are several aspects to consider in determining the appropriateness of CBT referral that go beyond clinical diagnosis. Firstly, a referring clinician must consider if the child is experiencing excessive, impairing psychological symptoms versus a realistic problem that needs to be solved. An example often seen in anxiety clinics is a child referred for anxiety related to academics or bullying. In such cases the family would be better served in advocating for educational supports. Additionally, given the active nature of CBT, families (including parents) must be prepared to put in effort toward the treatment goals on a daily basis. While parent motivation is a necessity for effective CBT, children's initial apprehension or refusal is not necessarily a deterrent to treatment readiness and may often be inherent to their symptom profile (e.g., anxiety, irritability, oppositionality). Skilled therapists are typically aware of these obstacles and will work to build rapport. However, if a child recurrently and totally refuses treatment after various appropriate efforts, it is possible that the child is not yet ready for this particularly demanding treatment modality; in such instances other approaches (e.g., medication management) may be appropriate (discussed further later). Such a pattern may result in a therapist shifting to parent-focused sessions and education. Lastly, the cognitive skills in traditional CBT include some level of cognitive ability, including expressive and receptive language, short- and long-term memory, and causal reasoning. While CBT was previously assumed a poor fit for youth with intellectual impairments, more recent research has examined modifications to CBT for these youth with promising results (Hronis et al., 2017).

Common Applications of CBT in Children and Adolescence

Anxiety

Childhood anxiety and fear is normative during particular developmental windows, including separating from parents in toddlers, nervousness about their dark bedroom at night in young children, and concern about social evaluation in adolescence. Normative anxiety and fear are helpful for children and adolescents to learn about the world around them. However, when anxiety reaches a degree that significantly impairs daily life, including school, friendships, and family functioning, it is considered a disorder that warrants specialized treatment. Anxiety disorders, including separation anxiety, social phobia, specific phobia, and generalized anxiety disorder, are the most common psychological diagnoses among children aged 3 to 17 years with 7.4% of children meeting criteria for an anxiety disorder (Ghandour et al., 2018) (see Chapter 51).

Gradual exposure. A major component of CBT for anxiety is gradual exposure, which consists of facing the anxiety-inducing stimuli or situation in small steps over time. The exposure process targets the anxiety-relief loop that occurs when a child recurrently avoids the feared object or situation. Avoidance gives initial relief and illusion of safety; however, the next time the child encounters the feared object or situation, the child will feel anxious again, thus perpetuating the cycle. The evidence is robust for the use of gradual exposure for youth anxiety disorders (Higa-McMillan et al., 2016). Exposure therapy typically includes psychoeducation about anxiety and the fear-avoidance loop, followed by development of a fear hierarchy or fear ladder that will guide step-by-step exposures in order of least difficult to most difficult with the child's collaboration. Coping thoughts are taught to challenge long-held fearful thoughts, and reinforcement programming is applied to encourage the child to face the fear (i.e., rewards for completing exposure activities). CBT for anxiety in youth is focused around building the child's confidence and praising mastery of previously avoided stimuli, which relies heavily on parents consistently encouraging brave behavior and reducing their own accommodation of fear avoidance. To illustrate, a 7-year-old child with a significant fear of dogs, which is limiting a family's ability to go to others' homes, the park, or school events, would ultimately participate in gradual exposure to dog-related stimuli (e.g., stuffed animal dogs, photos of dogs, recordings of dogs) and eventually interacting with actual dogs and going to areas where dogs may be present. With practice of brave mantras and use of appropriately motivating rewards by therapist and parents, the child would learn to make more positive associations with dogs and establish a newfound ability to face the fear. Another relevant anxiety treatment vignette is presented later in this chapter (see CBT for Youth With Neurodevelopmental Differences).

Obsessive-Compulsive and Related Disorders

OCD is defined by the presence of both obsessions and compulsions. Obsessions are distressing thoughts, urges, or images that are met with attempts to ignore, suppress, or neutralize distress through carrying out compulsive behavior. These compulsions can be repetitive acts (e.g., washing, checking) or thoughts (e.g., praying, repeating verbal rituals) that impair and impede daily functioning. It may be easier to identify compulsions in children than obsessions because children may not be able to verbalize or explain the obsessions driving their compulsions. Common themes of obsessions and compulsions relate to cleanliness, symmetry, taboo thoughts/urges, and fear of causing harm. For example, a fear of one's house catching on fire may result in repetitive checking of appliances, outlets, and things around the home.

A number of other disorders that may be categorized as body-focused repetitive behaviors (BFRBs) in the literature are discussed in Chapters 51, 71, and 72. These include trichotillomania, which is characterized by compulsive hair pulling, and excoriation, which is characterized by compulsive and recurrent skin picking. Both disorders are further defined by recurrent attempts to stop or reduce the impulsive behavior, causing clinically significant distress and/or impairment in functioning. These disorders may commonly cooccur with attention-deficit/hyperactivity disorder (ADHD) and anxiety (e.g., Lochner et al., 2019).

Exposure and Response Prevention and Habit Reversal Training

One specific intervention model found to be effective in treating OCD and related disorders is exposure and response prevention. Similar to CBT for anxiety, youth with OCD participate in gradual exposure to fear-stimuli. Unique to OCD treatment is the focus on resisting the strong urge to engage in the compulsive behavior. Youth with contamination-related obsessions (e.g., intrusive thoughts that they have caught AIDS whenever they ride public transportation followed by showering for 4 hours) might begin by refraining from washing their hands after standing near a subway entrance, ultimately leading up to riding a subway without bathing for an entire day. Consistent with CBT for anxiety (described earlier), children and adolescents learn about their symptom patterns, new adaptive and realistic ways of challenging irrational thoughts, and are encouraged to take pride in their mastery of new skills.

Habit reversal training/therapy is generally used to treat BFRBs as well as tic disorders. Tic disorders, such as Tourette disorder, have also been successfully treated using comprehensive behavioral interventions for tics. There is significant overlap between these interventions, and as such, core components of both of these interventions will be discussed simultaneously. As with most CBT programs, these interventions begin with psychoeducation. The clinician will next focus on awareness training, helping patients identify the physical and emotional sensations of the premonitory urge to tic or engage in the compulsive behavior. Patients are also asked to self-monitor, logging how many times within a certain time frame (e.g., 30 minutes) they engage in the behavior they are trying to reduce, in addition to the situations or settings in which the behavior is most likely to occur. Data collection is followed by identifying opportunities for response blocking (e.g., wearing a hat during long car rides to impede hair pulling) and/or the creation of a competing response to the undesired behavior. A good competing response is a behavior that is incompatible with the tic or compulsive behavior, which can be performed continuously for 1 minute and is less noticeable or aversive than the tic or compulsive behavior. For example, a patient with a vocal tic might press the lips together and take slow deep breaths when the premonitory urge to vocalize is experienced. Similarly, a patient with trichotillomania or excoriation may be prompted to sit on the hands or play with a fidget toy whenever the urge arises, with a corresponding reward program to reinforce engagement in the practice of these new adaptive behaviors (see Chapters 71 and 72 on related disorders).

VIGNETTE 2

Adrienne was a 12-year-old White female who presented at a community clinic with the primary complaint that she could not stop pulling out her hair (to the extent that her eyebrows were nearly gone). Adrienne was diagnosed with trichotillomania and identified her patterns of hair-pulling behavior, which was largely limited to times during which she was engaged in homework. Adrienne elected to wear gloves when completing her homework. This physically prevented her from engaging in hair pulling while she was wearing the gloves, leading to eventual extinction of the behavior. She was also taught to use diaphragmatic breathing to manage anxiety during homework time. Adrienne was also asked to record each day how many hairs she had pulled. Each week, she set a goal (e.g., <10/week), and if she met that goal she could reward herself with a predetermined reinforcer (e.g., purchasing a new desired song on iTunes). With parental support, Adrienne met treatment goals after two therapy sessions. Skills generalized to resisting pulling even without gloves, and her eyebrows eventually grew back over subsequent weeks.

Depression

Depression in youth occurs at a rate of 2.8% in childhood and nearly doubles in adolescence to 5.6% (Costello et al., 2006). Depression in youth can present with unique challenges to identification, given the differing presentations that can occur across the life span. Irritability may present as the predominant symptom in younger children in contrast to the more commonly expected presentation of depressed mood that may emerge later in adolescence (American Psychiatric Association, 2013). Depression also poses a singular risk in its association with suicidality and suicide, which is currently the second leading cause of death among adolescents in the United States (American Academy of Child and Adolescent Psychiatry, 2018; see also Chapters 49 and 50 for more on mood disorders and suicide).

CBT for depression. CBT for depression in youth demonstrates an emerging evidence base, especially for mild cases (Oud et al., 2019). According to research evidence thus far, effectiveness of CBT for depression may rely on specific treatment components, such as behavioral activation, cognitive restructuring, and significant involvement of parents in treatment. Behavioral activation techniques (as noted previously) focus on disrupting children's preexisting patterns of behavior. In the context of depression youth typically become withdrawn and expectant of negative experiences. This withdrawal serves only to reinforce the youth's negative self-schemas and lackluster experiences. Behavioral activation encourages gradual introduction of other routines that require youth to venture out and make themselves available to new, more reinforcing experiences (e.g., go to the store and pick out a preferred cereal, go to an extracurricular club and possibly of find a like-minded peer).

Similarly, cognitive restructuring related to depression in youth relates to challenging the deeply ingrained negative views of oneself, their future, and the world around them. Such thought patterns are associated with an external locus of control comprised of beliefs that youth have no control over their experiences but rather they are mere helpless recipients of the injustices of the world around them. CBT emphasizes new thought patterns that focus on their sense of efficacy in their experiences and awareness of evidence that contradicts negative schemas (e.g., "My classmate asking me to be a project partner does not fit with my belief that everyone thinks I am dumb").

Despite some emerging promising evidence for this treatment, ongoing research is needed to discern the exact levels of depression severity, depression types, and various other mediating or moderating factors related to the complex picture of depression in youth (e.g., family relational factors, situational factors) that may contribute to the efficacy of CBT for depression in youth (Oar et al., 2017).

VIGNETTE 3

Vasiliy is a 16-year-old man who identifies as queer. He has had muscular dystrophy with some signs of onset since childhood (e.g., weakening facial and left arm muscles). Vasiliy's prognosis was much like others in his family who had lost most muscle control by middle age. He described feeling tormented by thoughts of his future as wheelchair bound, especially given that skateboarding was his primary passion in life. Vasiliy fell into social withdrawal, declining academic performance, and only variably attending to basic daily self-care, with recurrent thoughts of "It doesn't matter, I'm going to lose everything." Vasiliy was initially reserved and flippant during therapy sessions, which were arranged by his mother, but he slowly warmed up to the therapist's humor, rolling with resistance, and other attempts at alliance building (e.g., formulating personal goals as opposed to mother's goals). While appealing to Vasiliy's sardonic humor, the therapist guided him to identify that his recurrent thoughts were maintaining his depressed mood. He practiced new realistic variations, such as "I'm going to lose some of my physical abilities decades from now" and "Muscular dystrophy will not stop what I do today." He gradually began to visit the skatepark again and experience pleasure as he had in the past.

CBT for Youth With Neurodevelopmental Differences

Youth with neurodevelopmental differences, such as autism spectrum disorder (ASD), ADHD, or intellectual disability (ID), are at significantly heightened risk for mental health conditions, such as anxiety disorders, in comparison to their typically developing peers (e.g., van Steensel et al., 2011), and a growing body of research supports the effectiveness of CBT for these populations (e.g., Kester & Lucyshyn, 2018). Diagnostic overshadowing often results in mental health conditions going overlooked when a more salient condition, such as ASD, is present (Mason & Scior, 2004). This occurs, in part, due to the challenges of assessing for mental health symptoms in the context of limited language and/or cognitive functioning. These obstacles may become especially problematic given that screening measures were designed and standardized for typically developing children (Kerns et al., 2020).

Recent research also suggests that distinct presentations of clinical phenomena may exist among youth with neurodevelopmental differences that are not captured by traditional *Diagnostic and Statistical Manual of Mental Disorders* diagnoses, such as unique presentations of anxiety (Table 98.1) (American Psychiatric Association, 2013). Fortunately, a growing body of research aims to increase accurate assessment of anxiety in youth with neurodevelopmental disorders (e.g., Scahill et al., 2019).

Common Modifications to CBT for Neurodiverse Youth

CBT may be most effective for youth with neurodevelopmental differences when thoughtful modifications are applied (Beidas et al., 2010). These modifications may vary depending on the child's level of cognitive functioning, including language ability, cognitive ability, and executive functioning skills. Common modifications may include adjusting the content to make it more concrete with visual tools, reducing abstract language, involving parents in many or all aspects of treatment if necessary, and incorporating the child's special interests to enhance motivation. Beidas and colleagues (2010) further describe ways to provide "flexibility within fidelity" by structuring the session with breaks and point systems, delivering the therapy in a way that is as interactive as possible (e.g., throwing a ball back and forth while conversing) and making the therapy room distraction free. Indeed, CBT for youth with ASD or ID may often primarily emphasize the "B" principles and strategies rather than the "C" components of CBT. Rather than adapting traditional CBT, some programs have been designed specifically for youth with ASD (e.g., Reaven et al., 2012; Wood et al., 2009). Overall, efforts to disseminate CBT to individuals with ASD and to train more professionals to deliver this much-needed treatment remain increasingly important in the field of clinical psychology.

In Combination With Pharmacologic Intervention

Medication management may be an efficacious addition to CBT for some youth. CBT is considered first-line treatment for mild-moderate anxiety (Walter et al., 2020; Wang et al., 2017a, 2017b) and depression in children and adolescents (Cheung et al., 2018). For moderate-severe anxiety in children ages 6 and older, a multimodal approach, including medication and psychotherapy, is recommended by the American Academy of Child and Adolescent Psychiatry, and combination therapy is more effective than either modality alone. Medications, particularly selective serotonin reuptake inhibitors (SSRIs), may be considered alone if psychotherapy is unavailable or for severe symptoms when individuals are unlikely to benefit from CBT until symptoms are stabilized. SSRIs may be as effective as CBT alone (Wang et al., 2017a, 2017b), but evidence suggests that combined therapy may be best, and there are more side effects with SSRI therapy than CBT (see Chapter 99).

VIGNETTE 4

Nico is a 10-year-old with a previous diagnosis of ASD with an IQ of 79. He was worrying throughout the day indicated by many "what if" thoughts (e.g., "What if I fall off a building?" "What if I'm late?" "What if my parents are upset with me?") that interfered to such a degree that his parents opted for homeschooling. In addition to generalized anxiety, Nico was also anxious about specific sounds such as the microwave beeping or cell phone rings. His face would get flushed, he would ask many questions about the sounds, cry, and try to avoid them even before they occurred. Lastly, Nico experienced excessive anxiety about potential changes in his routine or novelty, such as his mother going a new way in the car or a new topic introduced at school. His parents put in significant effort to prime or prepare him for upcoming changes and, even with the preparation, he was anxious and asked for reassurance often.

The Coping Cat CBT program (Kendall & Hedtke, 2006) was used to target Nico's anxiety with modifications for ASD. In therapy Nico was taught to view himself as Iron Man and his anxiety as the Mandarin (archenemy of Iron Man). Once Nico learned to identify how he felt in his body when he was anxious and his thoughts related to anxiety, he learned to "fight back" against it. Strategies included problem solving, looking for proof of anxious thoughts, and "channeling" Iron Man against the Mandarin if there was no proof of his fears. A fear ladder was constructed related to specific sounds with a coping thought during exposures, such as: "Eh, it is just a sound. Maybe my mom's hands are full, and I can help her out." The same exposure procedure applied to Nico's fears of change (e.g., doing a different therapy session format, parents going a different way in the car). Nico's preferred coping thought was, "I get used to it after a bit of time and my anxiety goes down," which was consistent with his experience during exposures. Nico was reinforced instantly for exposure practice, in the form of telling his psychologist about superheroes and supervillains. Nico's autism symptoms were observed as a meaningful component of treatment planning and contributed to a longer than average course of treatment (e.g., 35 sessions) but not a barrier to treatment or ultimate success. Posttreatment, all of Nico's anxieties and related impairment had significantly reduced.

TABLE 98.1 Distinct Anxiety Types Associated With Autism

Anxiety Disorder	Description	Example(s)
Uncommon phobia	Similar to specific phobia but with distinct and unusual content	Fears of black toilets, cartoon eyeballs, hearing "wooing"
Special interest fear	Excessive anxiety related to a restricted or repetitive interest	Excessive worry about loss of or access to Lego, missing the garbage truck in the morning
Other social fear	Social confusion fears	Avoidance of others without traditional symptom of fear of negative evaluation
Fear of change	Anxious anticipation of and distress following changes in routine, environment, etc.	Worry about changes in routine or about overall novelty, such as teacher getting haircut, deviation from daily routine

There are only a few pharmaceutic clinical trials focused on pediatric anxiety and depression. However, there is considerable evidence for the effectiveness and safety of SSRIs (Walter et al., 2020). Only three SSRI medications (sertraline, fluoxetine, and fluvoxamine) have US Food and Drug Administration (FDA) approval for OCD but not other forms of anxiety. The only medication that carries an FDA indication for non-OCD anxiety is duloxetine, a serotonin and norepinephrine reuptake inhibitor (SNRI), for generalized anxiety disorder in children ages 7 and older. However, the evidence for SSRIs is stronger than that for SNRIs (Walter et al., 2020), with SSRIs recommended for initial use in treating anxiety. SNRIs can be considered if SSRIs have been ineffective. For depression, only fluoxetine (>8 years) and escitalopram (>12 years) have FDA approval for children and adolescents, although randomized clinical trials support the use of other SSRIs.

Parental resistance to the use of psychiatric medication include concern for side effects of SSRIs, particularly suicidal ideation, which warrants close monitoring. It can be helpful to review safety data with families, including counseling that 4 to 6 weeks may be necessary to observe therapeutic effects, and to provide evidence that combined treatment may be most effective as compared to CBT alone. Children may experience gastrointestinal symptoms or behavioral activation consisting of motor or mental restlessness, insomnia, irritability, or disinhibition. SSRIs can interact with other medications and can cause serious symptoms (serotonin syndrome) that require immediate medical attention. SNRIs have similar side effects as SSRIs, with additional concern for hypertension or other cardiovascular effects. There is insufficient evidence for the use of benzodiazepines or tricyclic antidepressants (Wang et al., 2017a, 2017b).

VIGNETTE 5

Blake was an 11-year-old multiracial male. At the time of referral, Blake was in foster care with a significant history of trauma and ADHD. He had recently been placed in a new, third foster home with three of his siblings. Blake had begun exhibiting severe aggressive emotional outbursts, which seemed to be escalating in severity. Blake's clinician began CBT, including identifying emotions and thoughts, and building relaxation and coping skills. Unfortunately, Blake's ADHD was interfering with his ability to remain focused in therapy and gain skills being targeted. Additionally, the physiologic arousal he experienced when faced with any trauma trigger was severe to such a degree that he was unable to access any of the skills he was learning in CBT. Subsequently, Blake was referred for a psychiatric consult and was prescribed clonidine to help manage his physiologic arousal. His aggressive outbursts quickly diminished in both frequency and severity, with significantly improved engagement in therapy, and led to success that was unlikely to have been achieved without concurrent medication management.

New Waves of CBT

In recent decades new treatments that have emerged that have expanded from CBT (the purported "first" wave of therapy being behavioral and "second" being cognitive techniques) with an emphasis on novel strategies toward changing not only patients' behaviors and the thoughts but the contexts and functions that they may take. Various forms of treatment have emerged, though dialectical behavior therapy (DBT) and acceptance and commitment therapy (ACT) have undoubtedly gained the most traction in the field at large, with an evidence base that remains in progress (Öst, 2008). These treatments are closely aligned with tenants of mindfulness and, while ongoing research is warranted (especially for child and adolescent treatments), their rising popularity and possible effectiveness in treating a range of clinical profiles is worthy of review.

Dialectical Behavior Therapy

DBT was founded as a treatment for chronically suicidal individuals and evolved into specialized treatment for youth and adults with borderline personality disorder (Linehan, 2015). Evidence continually emerges to suggest that DBT may also be effective in treating an array of symptoms related to the general area of emotion dysregulation (Dimeff & Koerner, 2007), a trait which arguably underlies all psychological diagnoses.

DBT is unique in both its progression of treatment and therapist role. Stages of treatment evolve from stabilization and decreasing threatening or harmful behavior, to building skills of both emotion regulation and interpersonal

VIGNETTE 6

Brenda is a 16-year-old Latina diagnosed with social anxiety disorder. She is on her high school track team, where she is occasionally expected to lead warm-up and stretching exercises, an activity she dreads. She expressed extreme fear of being called on or raising her hand during class, stating she's afraid of saying something "stupid," despite being a straight A student. Brenda's therapist first applied a traditional CBT framework; however, her willingness to engage in exposure was hindered by her anxiety, including crying at the thought of calling even one of her own family members. From an ACT perspective, Brenda was struggling with experiential avoidance and cognitive fusion. Brenda was guided through mindfulness meditations with a focus on physical sensations, emotions, and thoughts. She and her therapist identified the following top five values: (1) family, (2) physical health, (3) friendship, (4) humor, and (5) adventure. By acting in line with her values (e.g., reaching out to family and friends), Brenda was able to build a broader behavioral repertoire and extinguish fear responses. By learning to accept her thoughts and feelings rather than fight with or avoid them, Brenda is able to learn experientially that it's her reactions to her own thoughts and feelings that prevent her from living in line with her core values.

effectiveness, to achieving a sense of long-term stable happiness that does not rely on chaotic, reactive sense of self or interactions with others. Therapists practicing DBT must strike a fine balance of acceptance with rapid change and independence (hence the dialectical nature of the therapy). DBT emotion regulation skill building is deeply rooted in the practice of mindfulness (e.g., acceptance of experiences) to dislodge maladaptive black-and-white thinking. DBT is often intensive and may include multiple simultaneous therapy formats (e.g., individual, group, emergency therapeutic services), though it has been adapted to more traditional models of therapy delivery.

DBT has been initially examined for youth, especially adolescents, for a myriad of clinical presentations, including mood disorders, eating disorders, nonsuicidal self-injury, and trichotillomania, among others (MacPherson et al., 2013). Overall, much more extensive research is needed to establish DBT as an EST, particularly in regard to different age groups and clinical presentations. Furthermore, comparative studies between DBT and more traditional CBT will serve to best inform treatment in years ahead.

Acceptance and Commitment Therapy

Like CBT, ACT is, at its core, founded upon the foundational behavioral principles of classical and operant conditioning. Unlike CBT, which emphasizes examining evidence for and against one's thoughts, ACT emphasizes the impact of one's thoughts on behavior, as well as how that behavior aligns or fails to align with personal values. The underlying principle of ACT is that people experience cognitive fusion, which refers to the rigid fusing of thoughts with self or thoughts with reality. Thus ACT aims to defuse cognitions with a variety of thought experiments, metaphors, and behavioral strategies that ultimately support acceptance rather than avoidance of experiences. ACT relies heavily on the concept of mindfulness and the related practice of meditation, encouraging clients to notice any thoughts, emotions, urges, or physical sensations without judging, avoiding, fighting with, or pushing away. The objective truth is not the goal in ACT but rather the workability of the response to one's own internal processes.

As a relatively newer treatment modality, ACT for children and adolescents remains minimally studied. Halliburton and Cooper (2015) reported that evidence appears to support the efficacy of ACT for teens with OCD, depression, anorexia, disruptive behavior, chronic pain, posttraumatic stress disorder, and even the emotional and behavioral sequelae of ASD. Some evidence also suggests that ACT may be effective for children with anxiety (Hancock et al., 2018). At this time, ACT appears to be a promising treatment for youth, but further research is necessary.

CONCLUSION

CBT for children and adolescents is now supported by several decades of research. CBT's central targets of changing thought and behavioral patterns may be appropriate for youth with a range of clinical presentations. The future of CBT and its descendants, DBT and ACT, requires further investigation and training to ensure best applications for special groups and dissemination to the many youth who may benefit.

REFERENCES

American Academy of Child and Adolescent Psychiatry. (2018). *Suicide in children and teens*. www.AACAP.org

American Psychiatric Association. (2013). *Diagnostic and statistical manual of mental disorders* (5th ed.). Author.

APA Presidential Task Force on Evidence-Based Practice. (2006). Evidence-based practice in psychology. *American Psychologist, 61*, 271–285.

Beck, A. T. (1993). Cognitive therapy past, present, & future. *Journal of Consulting and Clinical Psychology, 61*(2), 194–198.

Beck, A. T., Rush, A. J., Shaw, B. F., & Emery, G. (1979). *Cognitive therapy of depression: A treatment manual. Guilford* Press.

Beidas, R. S., Benjamin, C. L., Puleo, C. M., Edmunds, J. M., & Kendall, P. C. (2010). Flexible applications of the coping cat program for anxious youth. *Cognitive and Behavioral Practice, 17*, 142–153.

Benito, K. G., Machan, J., Freeman, J. B., Garcia, A. M., Walther, M., Frank, H., ... Franklin, M. E. (2020). Therapist behavior during exposure tasks predict habituation and clinical outcome in three randomized controlled trials for pediatric OCD. *Behavior Therapy.*

Benjamin, C. L., Puleo, C. M., Settipani, C. A., Brodman, D. M., Edmunds, J. M., Cummings, C. M., & Kendall, P. C. (2011). History of cognitive-behavioral therapy (CBT) in youth. *Child and Adolescent Psychiatric Clinics of North America, 20*(2), 179–189.

Costello, E. J., Erkanli, A., & Angold, A. (2006). Is there an epidemic of child or adolescent depression? *The Journal of Child Psychology and Psychiatry, 47*, 1263–1271.

Dimeff, L. A., & Koerner, K. (Eds.). (2007). *Dialectical behavior therapy in clinical practice: Applications across disorders and settings*. Guilford Press.

Dorflinger, L. M., Fortin, A. H., & Foran-Tuller, K. A. (2016). Training primary care physicians in cognitive behavioral therapy: A review of the literature. *Patient Education and Counseling, 99*(8), 1285–1292.

Friedberg, R. D., Hoyman, L. C., Behar, S., Tabbarah, S., Pacholec, N. M., Keller, M., & Thordarson, M. A. (2014). We've come a long way, baby! Evolution and revolution in CBT in youth. *Journal of Rational-Emotive & Cognitive-Behavior Therapy, 32*, 4–14.

Ghandour, R. M., Sherman, L. J., Vladutiu, C. J., Ali, M. M., Lynch, S. E., Bitsko, R. H., & Blumberg, S. J. (2018). Prevalence and treatment of depression, anxiety, and conduct problems in US children. *The Journal of Pediatrics, 206*, 256–267.

Halliburton, A. E., & Cooper, L. D. (2015). Applications and adaptations of Acceptance and Commitment Therapy (ACT) for adolescents. *Journal of Contextual Behavioral Science, 4*(1), 1–11.

Hancock, K. M., Swain, J., Hainsworth, C. J., Dixon, A. L., Koo, S., & Munro, K. (2018). Acceptance and commitment therapy versus cognitive behavior therapy for children with anxiety: Outcomes of a randomized controlled trial. *Journal of Clinical Child and Adolescent Psychology, 47*(2), 296–311.

Higa-McMillan, C. K., Francis, S. E., Rith-Najarian, L., & Chorpita, B. F. (2016). Evidence base update: 50 years of research on treatment for child and adolescent anxiety. *Journal of Clinical Child & Adolescent Psychology, 45*(2), 91–113.

Hronis, A., Roberts, L., & Kneebone, I. I. (2017). A review of cognitive impairments in children with intellectual disabilities: Implications for cognitive behaviour therapy. *British Journal of Clinical Psychology, 56*(2), 189–207.

Keles S., & Idsoe T. (2018). A meta-analysis of group Cognitive Behavioral Therapy (CBT) interventions for adolescents with depression. *Journal of Adolescence, 67*, 129–139.

Kendall, P. C., Gosch, E., Furr, J. M., & Sood, E. (2008). Flexibility within fidelity. *Journal of the American Academy of Child & Adolescent Psychiatry, 47*, 987–993.

Kendall, P. C., & Hedtke, K. (2006). *Cognitive-behavioral therapy for anxious children: Therapist manual* (3rd ed.). Workbook.

Kerns, C. M., Winder-Patel, B., Iosif, A. M., Nordahl, C. W., Heath, B., Solomon, M., & Amaral, D. G. (2020). Clinically significant anxiety in children with autism spectrum disorder and varied intellectual functioning. *Journal of Clinical Child & Adolescent Psychology*, 1–16.

Kester, K. R., & Lucyshyn, J. M. (2018). Cognitive behavior therapy to treat anxiety among children with autism spectrum disorders: A systematic review. *Research in Autism Spectrum Disorders, 52*, 37–50.

Linehan, M. M. (2015). *DBT skills training manual*. Guilford Press.

Lochner, C., Keuthen, N. J., Curley, E. E., Tung, E. S., Redden, S. A., Ricketts, E. J., Bauer, C. C., Woods, D. W., Grant, J. E., & Stein, D. J. (2019). Comorbidity in trichotillomania (hair-pulling disorder): A cluster analytical approach. *Brain and Behavior, 9*(12), e01456.

MacPherson, H. A., Cheavens, J. S., & Fristad, M. A. (2013). Dialectical behavior therapy for adolescents: Theory, treatment adaptations, and empirical outcomes. *Clinical Child and Family Psychology Review, 16*(1), 59–80.

Mason, J., & Scior, K. (2004). "Diagnostic overshadowing" amongst clinicians working with people with intellectual disabilities in the UK. *Journal of Applied Research in Intellectual Disabilities, 17*(2), 85–90.

Oar, E. L., Johnco, C., & Ollendick, T. (2017). Cognitive behavioral therapy for anxiety and depression in children and adolescents. *Psychiatric Clinics of North America, 40*, 661–674.

Öst, L. (2008). Efficacy of the third wave of behavioral therapies: A systematic review and meta-analysis. *Behaviour Research and Therapy, 46*(3), 296–321.

Oud, M., de Winter, L., Vermeulen-Smit, E., Bodden, D., Nauta, M., Stone, L., van den Heuvel, M., Taher, R. A., de Graaf, I., Kendall, T., Engels, R., & Stikkelbroek, Y. (2019). Effectiveness of CBT for children and adolescents with depression: A systematic review and meta-aggression analysis. *European Psychiatry, 57*, 33–45.

Reaven, J., Blakeley-Smith, A., Culhane-Shelburne, K., & Hepburn, S. (2012). Group cognitive behavior therapy for children with high-functioning autism spectrum disorders and anxiety: A randomized trial. *Journal of Child Psychology and Psychiatry, 53*(4), 410–419.

Scahill, L., Lecavalier, L., Schultz, R. T., Evans, A. N., Maddox, B., Pritchett, J., … Edwards, M. C. (2019). Development of the parent-rated anxiety scale for youth with autism spectrum disorder. *Journal of the American Academy of Child & Adolescent Psychiatry, 58*(9), 887–896.

Tudor, M. E., Bertschinger, E., Piasecka, J., & Sukhodolsky, D. G. (2018). Cognitive behavioral therapy for anger and aggression in a child with Tourette's syndrome. *Clinical Case Studies, 17*, 220–232.

van Steensel, F. J. A., Bögels, S. M., & Perrin, S. (2011). Anxiety disorders in children and adolescents with autistic spectrum disorders: A meta-analysis. *Clinical Child and Family Psychology Review, 14*(3), 302–317.

Walter, H. J., Bukstein, O. G., Abright, A. R., Keable, H., Ramtekkar, U., Ripperger-Suhler, J., & Rockhill, C. (2020). Clinical practice guideline for the assessment and treatment of children and adolescents with anxiety disorders. *Journal of the American Academy of Child & Adolescent Psychiatry, 59*(10), 1107–1124.

Wang, Z., Whiteside, S. P., Sim, L., Farah, W., Morrow, A. S., Alsawas, M., Barrionuevo, P., Tello, M., Asi, N., Beuschel, B., Daraz, L., Almasri, J., Zaiem, F., Larrea-Mantilla, L., Ponce, O. J., LeBlanc, A., Prokop, L. J., & Murad, M. H. (2017a). Comparative effectiveness and safety of cognitive behavioral therapy and pharmacotherapy for childhood anxiety disorders: A systematic review and meta-analysis. *JAMA Pediatrics, 171*(11), 1049–1056.

Wang, Z., Whiteside, S., Sim, L., Farah, W., Morrow, A., Alsawas, M., Moreno, P. B., Tello, M., Asi, N., Beuschel, B., Daraz, L., Almasri, J., Zaiem, F., Gunjal, S., Mantilla, L. L., Ponte, O. P., LeBlanc, A., Prokop, L. J., & Murad, M. H. (2017b). *Anxiety in children*. Comparative Effectiveness Review 192. (Prepared by the Mayo Clinic Evidence-based Practice Center under Contract No. 290-2015-00013-I.) AHRQ Publication No. 17-EHC023-EF. Agency for Healthcare Research and Quality.

Wergeland, G. J., Fjermestad, K. W., Marin, C. E., Haugland, B. S., Bjaastad, J. F., Oeding, K., Bjelland, I., Silverman, W. K., Ost, L. G., Havik, O. E., & Heiervang, E. R. (2014). An effectiveness study of individual vs. group cognitive behavioral therapy for anxiety disorders in youth. *Behaviour Research and Therapy, 57*, 1–12.

Wood, J. J., Drahota, A., Sze, K., Har, K., Chiu, A., & Langer, D. A. (2009). Cognitive behavioral therapy for anxiety in children with autism spectrum disorders: A randomized, controlled trial. *Journal of Child Psychology and Psychiatry, 50*(3), 224–234.

99

Psychopharmacology

DePorres Cormier II and Alison Schonwald

For additional material related to the content of this chapter, please see Chapters 41, 46, 71, and 93.

> **VIGNETTE 1**
>
> *Alex is a 12-year-old with attention-deficit/hyperactivity disorder (ADHD) and long-standing inattention and fidgetiness. Trials of stimulants between 8 and 10 years of age were not tolerated due to weight loss and insomnia. With the increased challenge of middle school, Alex's grades are dropping. Work is not completed, directions are not followed, and test performance is inconsistent. While parents attempt to support executive function needs, they question whether a different medication may be helpful.*

Clinical care for developmental-behavioral conditions includes thoughtful use of psychopharmacology. Aimed at optimizing the life course of affected children and adolescents, medication-related decisions are complex. This chapter provides an overview of medications commonly used to improve function by reducing impairing inattention, hyperactivity, impulsivity, anxiety, depression, irritability, and aggression in youth. Practical guidance provided includes dosing, monitoring, and side effect profiles. The common developmental-behavioral pediatrics uses of the medications approved by the US Food and Drug Administration (FDA) are discussed, as are common unapproved or off-label uses. Balancing the risks and benefits of medications is emphasized.

STIMULANTS

Alex, from the chapter-opening vignette, has already been tried on stimulant medication. In addition to the assessment for ADHD (see Chapter 46), the following assessments related to use of stimulants should have been completed prior to starting these medications:

1. Medical history, including history of syncope, shortness of breath, chest pain, or other cardiovascular symptoms
2. Family history of cardiac disease, sudden unexplained death before 40 years of age, inherited rhythm disturbance
3. Social history, including risk assessment for substance misuse and diversion
4. Comprehensive physical examination, including weight, height, heart rate, and blood pressure

Stimulant medications are the first-line treatment of ADHD symptoms for school-age children and adolescents. Used for more than half a century, extensive literature and experience support the efficacy and safety of stimulant medications. These medications include those based on methylphenidate or amphetamine, each now available in various preparations with a range of doses, delivery systems, and flavors (Table 99.1).

Mechanism of Action

While the exact mechanisms of action of stimulants are unknown, both methylphenidate- and amphetamine-based preparations affect ADHD symptoms primarily by impacting dopamine. Methylphenidate promotes release of stored dopamine from presynaptic vesicles and inhibits the reuptake of dopamine from the synaptic cleft in a dose-dependent fashion. Amphetamines cause release of newly synthesized dopamine. Dopamine serves as an inhibitory neurotransmitter, concentrated in the basal ganglia and frontal cortex. Brain circuits that connect the frontal cortex with the basal ganglia play a central role in attention, organization and planning, functions deficient in those with ADHD (see Chapter 46).

Methylphenidate is a racemic mix of d- and l-threo enantiomers. The d-threo enantiomer of methylphenidate is more pharmacologically active than the l-threo enantiomer, leading to the development of the dexmethylphenidate formulations. Dextroamphetamine exerts more central nervous system stimulation than levoamphetamine, although both isomers are effective in treating ADHD (Heal, Smith, Gosden, & Nutt, 2013). Mixed amphetamine salts are a 3:1 mixture of d-amphetamine:l-amphetamine. The amphetamine prodrug, lisdexamfetamine dimesylate, has a lysine bound to an amphetamine, which is then metabolized by red blood cells via enzymatic hydrolysis (Heal et al., 2013). Both noradrenaline and serotonin systems may also be impacted by stimulant medications but are less central to the treatment of ADHD symptoms.

Efficacy

Several metaanalyses and literature reviews confirm the efficacy of stimulant medication in treating the core symptoms of ADHD (Chang et al., 2019). Amphetamine- and methylphenidate-based medications are more effective than atomoxetine and alpha-2 adrenergic agonists. The best results are generally found when using stimulant medication together with behavioral treatment. Secondary impacts of stimulant treatment include reduced risk of injury, reduced rate of motor vehicle accidents, improved academic performance, reduced short-term rate of criminality, and reduced rates of substance abuse (Keilow et al., 2018).

TABLE 99.1 Stimulant Medications Used to Treat Attention-Deficit/Hyperactivity Disorder

Generic Name	Medication Class	Brand Name	Starting Dose	Max Dose
Methylphenidate (immediate release)	Methylphenidate based	Ritalin	5 mg BID	60 mg/day
Methylphenidate (extended release)	Methylphenidate based	Metadate CD, Ritalin LA	10–20 mg	60 mg
Methylphenidate (evening dose)	Methylphenidate based	Jornay PM	20 mg	100 mg
Methylphenidate OROS	Methylphenidate based	Concerta	18 mg	54–72 mg
Methylphenidate (patch)	Methylphenidate based	Daytrana	10 mg	30 mg
Dex-methylphenidate (immediate release)	Methylphenidate based	Focalin	2.5 mg BID	20 mg
Dex-methylphenidate (extended release)	Methylphenidate based	Focalin XR	5 mg	30 mg
Mixed amphetamine salts (immediate release)	Amphetamine based	Adderall	2.5–5 mg/day	40 mg/day
Mixed amphetamine salts (extended release)	Amphetamine based	Adderall XR	5–10 mg	30 mg
Dextroamphetamine	Amphetamine based	Dexedrine	2.5–5 mg	40 mg/day
Lisdexamfetamine	Amphetamine based	Vyvanse	10 mg	70 mg

Side Effects

The best dose of a stimulant medication for an individual will balance efficacy with tolerability. Reported rates of side effects may be underestimated, as study participants may drop out in response to those side effects. Nonharmful side effects are reported in more than half of users of methylphenidate, most commonly appetite suppression and headache. Amphetamine-based preparations have greater rates of side effects, including appetite suppression and weight loss, insomnia, nausea, vomiting, and increased blood pressure and heart rate (Heal et al., 2013), and emotional lability.

Blood pressure and heart rate increases are small. For example, a 2017 systematic review of 14 clinical trials calculates (small) statistically significant changes caused by amphetamine-based medication on diastolic pressure and heart rate; methylphenidates did not cause statistically significant changes. Small prepost effects on systolic blood pressure are seen in use of both medications (Hennissen et al., 2017). In fact, some but not all metaanalyses find the changes to be clinically insignificant (Liang et al., 2018). While no significant increase in risk of serious cardiovascular events occurs in the typical population of children and teens treated with stimulants, before starting stimulant medication patients must be screened for family history of cardiac disease, exercise-induced syncope, shortness of breath, or other cardiovascular disease (Clavenna & Bonati, 2017). Those with underlying cardiac disease may be at increased risk for sudden death, resulting in the FDA black box warning for stimulants (Thomas, Stansifer, & Findling, 2011). Stimulant medications are not associated with significant changes on electrocardiography (ECG), including on the QT interval (Cortese et al., 2013).

Growth may be delayed, but treatment cessation may normalize growth, and studies suggest only modest ultimate impact on weight and height (MTA Cooperative Group, 2004). High-dose dextroamphetamine may worsen tics, but methylphenidate does not worsen tics in most people (Osland, Steeves, & Pringsheim, 2018).

Approved Indications

Numerous preparations of methylphenidate- and amphetamine-based medications are FDA approved to treat ADHD. Most approval begins at 6 years of age, though Dexedrine and mixed amphetamine salts are approved down to age 3 years. However, this is related to criteria in place at the time of amphetamine approval, as methylphenidate is more extensively studied in younger children. In addition to ADHD, several preparations are FDA approved to treat narcolepsy.

Off-Label Uses

Use of stimulants to treat symptoms of oppositional defiant disorder and other disruptive behavior disorders is supported by some evidence (Golubchik & Weizman, 2018). The side effect of appetite suppression has led to efforts to use stimulants to treat obesity in specific populations with limited benefit. Due to the noradrenergic effects of methylphenidate, it is sometimes used to augment depression treatment in adults (Trenque, Herlem, Abou Taam, & Drame, 2014). Both stimulants are used in selected older adults to improve alertness and cognitive performance.

Dosing

Medication initiation begins at the lowest dose available, with incremental increases, approximately every week, until target symptoms are adequately improved with minimal or tolerable medication side effects. Maximum dose guidelines are generally guided by FDA labeling, yet higher doses are sometimes required to reach optimal clinical impact.

Monitoring

Monitoring of ADHD symptoms using a standardized checklist along with a physical exam, including heart rate, blood pressure, weight, and height, should occur at least every 6 months, with symptom checklist done more frequently after dose or medication changes. Baseline and follow-up ECG are not indicated unless history and exam suggest otherwise (Thomas et al., 2011).

Interactions

Methylphenidate is metabolized in the liver but not by the cytochrome p450 isoenzymes, preventing interactions with the many psychoactive medications metabolized through the p450 system. However, interactions can occur with medications that cause increased heart rate, blood pressure, or other cardiovascular changes (changes that could be exacerbated by stimulants). Amphetamines have similar interactions. In addition, they are metabolized via oxidation and deamination, possibly involving 2YP2D6, and thus potentially interact with medications that inhibit this isoenzyme (and thus increase the amphetamine level).

Clinical Pearls

Stimulant management requires a careful balance of impact to target symptoms with minimization of adverse effects. Considerations to guide clinical practice in optimizing this balance include the following:

- Appetite: Stimulants should generally be taken in the morning after a hearty breakfast. Lunch may include only low-volume, high-protein options. Children often eat a larger dinner or more evening snacks to compensate for reduced daytime intake.
- Sleep: Giving the medication as early as possible in the morning can minimize impact on sleep onset. Sleep hygiene (see Chapter 70) takes on increased importance when medication-induced insomnia occurs.
- Rebound: Some children experience irritability during the period of time when stimulants wear off. Adding a lower dose of short-acting medication before the wear-off period can reduce the irritability. Alternately, managing the wear-off period with low-demand, low-stress activities can allow this challenging period to pass without incident.

The choice of which stimulant to initiate for ADHD treatment depends on several factors: (1) duration of action desired, (2) formulation (whether or not the child can swallow a pill), and (3) insurance coverage.

Long-acting formulations may differ pharmacokinetically. Serum concentration may slowly rise and then fall (as in Adderall XR and OROS preparation of methylphenidate) or may have biphasic peaks. Biphasic release may be comparable at each point (Ritalin LA and Focalin XR) or one peak might be higher than the other (Metadate CD). These variations can be used to customize medication choice.

ALPHA-2 ADRENERGIC AGONISTS

Clonidine and guanfacine, each in short- and long-acting forms, are used to treat ADHD symptoms (Table 99.2). The long-acting forms of both medications are FDA approved as monotherapy and adjunctive treatment for ADHD. They are considered second-line treatments for ADHD.

Mechanism of Action

The exact mechanism of action of guanfacine and clonidine is not fully understood. They are thought to treat ADHD symptoms by imitating noradrenaline effects on alpha-2 adrenoceptors, which are highly concentrated in the prefrontal cortex (Martinez-Raga, Knecht, Szerman, & Martinez, 2013). Clonidine binds alpha-2A, B, and C receptor subtypes, while guanfacine is more selective to alpha-2A. Clonidine is more sedating, likely due to its impact on alpha-2C receptors in the locus coeruleus associated with hypotensive and sedative actions (Naguy, 2016).

Efficacy

Both short- and long-acting formulations of guanfacine and clonidine are effective in reducing symptoms of ADHD, when used as monotherapy and adjunctive therapy (Huss, Dirks, Gu, Robertson, Newcorn, & Ramos-Quiroga, 2018). They may work synergistically with stimulants.

Side Effects

Both guanfacine and clonidine can cause common, dose-related, and often quickly self-resolving side effects, including somnolence, dizziness, fatigue, and headache. Small decreases in heart rate and blood pressure can result from treatment with guanfacine- or clonidine-based medications, used alone or as adjuncts to stimulant treatment. There are no statistically significant changes in QTc interval; risk for serious cardiovascular adverse events is low when used at appropriate doses, but these medications can cause orthostatic hypotension, hypotension, and rarely syncope (Huss

TABLE 99.2 Nonstimulant Medications Used to Treat Attention-Deficit/Hyperactivity Disorder

Generic Name	Medication Class	Brand Name	Starting Dose	Max Dose
Guanfacine (immediate release)	Alpha-adrenergic	Tenex	0.5–1 mg	3 mg/day
Guanfacine (extended release)	Alpha-adrenergic	Intuniv	1 mg	7 mg
Clonidine (immediate release)	Alpha-adrenergic	Catapres	0.05–0.1 mg	0.3 mg/day
Clonidine (extended release)	Alpha-adrenergic	Kapvay	0.1 mg	0.4 mg
Clonidine transdermal patch	Alpha-adrenergic	Catapres TTS	0.1 mg	0.3 mg
Atomoxetine	Noradrenaline reuptake inhibitor	Strattera	0.5 mg/kg 40 mg if >70 kg	1.4 mg/kg 100 mg if >70 kg

et al., 2018; Martinez-Raga et al., 2013). In overdoses they can cause significant bradycardia.

Guanfacine tends to be less sedating and less potent in lowering blood pressure when compared to clonidine (Martinez-Raga et al., 2013). Rebound hypertension can occur with abrupt cessation; medications should be weaned instead.

Approved Indications

Guanfacine ER and clonidine ER are both FDA approved as monotherapy and adjunctive therapy to treat ADHD. In their short-acting forms both are approved as centrally acting antihypertensives.

Off-Label Uses

Guanfacine XR can be used to treat oppositional defiant disorder symptoms in children with cooccurring ADHD, as well as reduce tics (see Chapter 71) and ADHD symptoms when cooccurring (Osland et al., 2018). When used for children with autism spectrum disorder (ASD) and ADHD, reduction in oppositional behavior and repetitive behaviors has been demonstrated (Politte et al., 2018). Clonidine is often used to treat insomnia associated with ADHD and stimulant medication or other neurodevelopmental disorders. Clonidine-based medications are often used in opiate detoxification and posttraumatic stress disorder. It can also be used for neuroleptic-induced akathisia.

Dosing

Clonidine is available and used for ADHD as oral short-acting tablets (given three to four times daily) and as a long-acting tablet (given twice daily) (see Table 99.2), and as a transdermal patch delivering a consistent dose across the day for 7 days. For each formulation, the medication is often started once daily at a low dose to minimize sedation, and the dose is increased weekly to effect as tolerated. Clinicians treating children often start at fractions of the available doses (e.g., at 0.025 mg) of clonidine once or twice daily.

Short-acting guanfacine is usually dosed twice daily. Similar to use of clonidine, clinicians treating children often start with once daily dosing and may use fractions of the available doses (e.g., at 0.25 mg) once or twice daily, increasing weekly to effect as tolerated. Guanfacine XR can be given in the morning or the evening. Some initiate treatment with bedtime dosing to prevent daytime sedation, moving the dose to the morning after several days. Originally approved at 1 to 4 mg per dose, additional evidence expanded the range of efficacy and safety of guanfacine extended release to up to 7 mg per dose (0.12 mg/kg), which may be necessary for adolescents (Huss et al., 2018). When switching between short- and long-acting medications one cannot simply use the same dose. Due to different pharmacokinetic profiles one should titrate the new medication as described earlier.

Monitoring

Monitoring should include baseline history (including cardiac- specific history), physical exam, heart rate, blood pressure, weight, height, and standardized symptom checklist. Every 6 months, the clinician should obtain a repeat height, weight, heart rate, and blood pressure, as well as symptom checklists. Baseline and follow-up ECG are not indicated unless history and exam suggest otherwise (Thomas et al., 2011).

Interactions

Guanfacine is mainly metabolized by CYP3A4, so its dose may need to be increased up to twofold if adding a potent CYP3A4 inducer (such as phenobarbital or rifampin). Adding a potent inhibitor (such as ketoconazole, erythromycin, or fluconazole) calls for halving the guanfacine dose (Schoretsanitis, de Leon, Eap, Kane, & Paulzen, 2019). Clonidine is a CYP2D6 substrate (Schoretsanitis et al, 2019). No serious cardiovascular adverse events are reported when combining either clonidine- or guanfacine-based medication with psychostimulants (Martinez-Raga et al., 2013).

Clinical Pearls

Children and teens with ADHD who cannot tolerate an increase in stimulant due to concerns with poor appetite, insomnia, or anxiety may benefit from adjunctive treatment with a long-acting alpha agonist.

Long-acting clonidine can be particularly helpful in children whose sleep problems involve both long latency and night waking. Both long-acting formulations require pill swallowing.

ATOMOXETINE

Atomoxetine is a second-line treatment for ADHD as a monotherapy and can be used as adjunctive therapy (see Table 99.2).

Mechanism of Action

Atomoxetine is a highly selective noradrenaline reuptake inhibitor that was originally developed as a potential antidepressant but never approved for that indication (Scott, Ripperger-Suhler, Rajab, & Kjar, 2010). By blocking noradrenaline reuptake and increasing the levels of this neurotransmitter at the synapse, atomoxetine impacts the functions of the prefrontal cortex related to ADHD symptoms. It was the first nonstimulant medication FDA approved (in 2002) to treat ADHD (Martinez-Raga et al., 2013).

Efficacy

Atomoxetine reduces ADHD symptoms on parent and teacher rating scales (Waxmonsky et al., 2010). Both stimulant and guanfacine ER monotherapy treatments result in a larger reduction of ADHD symptoms compared to atomoxetine (Joseph et al., 2017). Parents particularly have observed greater improvements when atomoxetine is combined with behavior therapy (Waxmonsky et al., 2010).

Side Effects

Atomoxetine is generally well tolerated and often chosen when stimulants are not tolerated. Adverse effects usually occur early in treatment and include dry mouth, nausea, constipation, decreased appetite, dizziness, sweating, dysuria, sexual problems, and insomnia (Martinez-Raga et al., 2013). Symptoms typically self-resolve. Increases in heart rate and blood pressure are generally clinically insignificant (Martinez-Raga et al., 2013). Atomoxetine potentially exacerbates tics in those with ADHD (Yang, Li, Gao, & Zhao, 2017). As is the case with selective serotonin reuptake inhibitors (SSRIs), there is an increased rate of suicidal thinking in those taking atomoxetine (Fedder et al., 2020). Atomoxetine should be used with care in those with hepatic impairment; if used, dosing should be adjusted and careful monitoring should occur (Fedder et al., 2020).

Approved Indications

Atomoxetine is approved to treat ADHD in children over 6 years, adolescents, and adults. Atomoxetine is a second-line medication for most with ADHD, and it may be first-line treatment for those with cooccurring substance abuse as it does not have abuse potential.

Off-Label Uses

While not robust, the literature suggests atomoxetine may reduce oppositional defiant behaviors. The literature is mixed as to whether atomoxetine improves anxiety and/or depression cooccurring with ADHD. The presence of anxiety or depression does not correlate with response to atomoxetine in children treated for ADHD (Scott et al., 2010).

Dosing

Atomoxetine dosing is weight based. Children start at 0.5 mg/kg/day with increases every 2 to 3 weeks to effect or a maximum of 1.4 mg/kg/day. It can be given once daily or divided into two doses. Capsules should be taken whole and not opened. Atomoxetine can be discontinued abruptly without a taper (Fedder et al., 2020).

Monitoring

Monitoring should include baseline history (including cardiac specific history), physical exam, heart rate, blood pressure, weight, height, and standardized symptom checklist. Every 6 months, repeat height, weight, heart rate, and blood pressure, as well as symptom checklists. Baseline and follow-up ECG are not indicated unless history and exam suggest otherwise. Liver damage is rare; routine liver function testing is not indicated. Sexual dysfunction is a potential side effect and should be monitored in adolescents and young adults.

> **VIGNETTE 2**
>
> *A 13-year-old boy with a history of well-controlled ADHD presents with an 8-week history of depressed mood on most days. Upon further questioning, he endorses that he has been spending less time with his friends and has become less interested in his community basketball team, which he previously enjoyed. His parents state he is "sad and just kind of out of it" most days and just "lies around" during the weekends. His academic performance, which had previously been stellar, has slipped considerably. He does not have any suicidal ideation and there is no prior history of suicide attempts. You diagnose major depressive disorder (MDD) and recommend cognitive-behavioral therapy. His family has many questions regarding possible medication use, including side effects.*

Interactions

Primarily metabolized by CYP2D6, atomoxetine carries a risk of many drug-drug interactions. Further, its metabolism can vary from person to person due to genetic polymorphism across races and ethnicities.

Clinical Pearls

There is no abuse potential for atomoxetine. Thus it may be considered for those with risk for abuse or diversion of stimulant medication.

Unlike stimulants, atomoxetine may take many weeks for full therapeutic effects (Fedder et al., 2020).

SELECTIVE SEROTONIN REUPTAKE INHIBITORS

Mechanism of Action

SSRIs are a class of medications commonly used in both pediatric and adult populations for the treatment of anxiety and mood disorders. Information about commonly used SSRIs is in Table 99.3. Serotonin is a neurotransmitter associated with a variety of human responses, such as mood, reward, memory, attention, and appetite. SSRIs work by selectively blocking serotonin uptake through inhibition of ATPase. This inhibition increases the length of time serotonin can act in the postsynaptic binding sites. This inhibition alone, however, does not fully account for SSRIs' therapeutic benefit. Full therapeutic effect, which often takes weeks after initiation of an SSRI, is likely due to additional downstream effects of serotonin reuptake inhibition. This includes an increase in production of brain natriuretic peptide and modification to the serotonin receptor (Krishnan & Nestler, 2008).

While SSRIs, as their name implies, selectively bind to serotonin receptors, this selectivity is not absolute. Some SSRIs also partially inhibit other neurotransmitters. Specifically, paroxetine partially inhibits the reuptake of norepinephrine, as does sertraline with dopamine. Additionally, paroxetine also exhibits some anticholinergic activity (Schatzberg & DeBattista, 2019).

Efficacy

Multiple studies have demonstrated the effectiveness of SSRIs in the treatment of pediatric anxiety disorders (Locher et al., 2017). This effectiveness appears to be enhanced when combined with cognitive-behavioral therapy, as demonstrated in the Child/Adolescent Anxiety Multimodal Study (Piacentini et al., 2014).

Side Effects

In general, SSRIs are well tolerated. The most common side effects include gastrointestinal symptoms such as nausea,

TABLE 99.3 Medications Used to Treat Depressive and Anxiety Disorders

Generic Name	Medication Class	Brand Name	On-Label Uses	Off-Label Uses	Starting Dose	Max Dose
Fluoxetine	SSRI	Prozac	MDD 8–18 yr OCD 7–17 yr	Migraines GAD	10 mg	60 mg
Sertraline	SSRI	Zoloft	OCD 6–17 yr	GAD Separation anxiety	25 mg	200 mg
Citalopram	SSRI	Celexa	None in pediatrics	MDD	10 mg	40 mg
Escitalopram	SSRI	Lexapro	MDD 12–17 yr	MDD GAD	5 mg	20 mg
Fluvoxamine	SSRI	Luvox	OCD 8–17 yr	GAD	25 mg	200 mg (ages 8–11 yr) 300 mg (ages 12–18 yr)
Paroxetine	SSRI	Paxil	None in pediatrics	MDD	10 mg	60 mg
Duloxetine	SNRI	Cymbalta	GAD 7–17 yr		40 mg	120 mg
Venlafaxine	SNRI	Effexor	None in pediatrics	Social anxiety MDD GAD	37.5 mg	225 mg
Imipramine	Tricyclic antidepressant	Trofanil	None in pediatrics	Enuresis	10 mg	75 mg
Bupropion	Aminoketone antidepressant	Wellbutrin	None in pediatrics	MDD ADHD	100 mg	300 mg

GAD, Generalized anxiety disorder; *MDD*, major depressive disorder; *OCD*, obsessive-compulsive disorder; *SNRI*, selective norepinephrine reuptake inhibitor; *SSRI*, selective serotonin reuptake inhibitor. Of the SNRIs, only duloxetine and venlafaxine are shown due to limited pediatric data in other SNRIs.

vomiting, diarrhea, and cramping. The gastrointestinal symptoms are due to the presence of gut-lined serotonin receptors. These symptoms usually resolve in 2 to 4 weeks. Slow titration of the medication may help with symptoms. Another potential side effect of SSRIs, particularly paroxetine, is sedation. This can be mitigated by taking the dose at night (Schatzberg & DeBattista, 2019). An additional side effect, particularly in prepubescent children, is behavioral activation. This is characterized by the onset of hyperactivity, restlessness, and irritability. It is usually managed by either lowering the dose of the SSRI, discontinuing, or changing to a different medication (Luft, Lamy, DelBello, McNamara, & Strawn, 2018).

When SSRIs are abruptly stopped or decreased, a collection of symptoms known as discontinuation syndrome can emerge, predominantly characterized by fatigue, dizziness, lightheadedness, drowsiness, and nausea. In adults onset of discontinuation syndrome typically occurs within 1 to 3 days of abrupt cessation or significant dose decrease and can last for 2 weeks. Management typically involves either symptomatic treatment or, if possible, restarting the SSRI with a more gradual taper. While there are limited data in children, evidence in adults indicates that the likelihood of developing a discontinuation syndrome after the abrupt cessation of an SSRI is inversely proportional to the SSRI's half-life. As such, individuals taking SSRIs with a longer half-life, such as fluoxetine, are less likely to develop a discontinuation syndrome than those taking other SSRIs such as sertraline and paroxetine.

In 2004 the FDA issued a black box warning for SSRIs due to concern for an increase in suicidal thoughts and behavior. This was based on a metaanalysis of 24 short-term clinical trials (up to 4 months) with over 4400 pediatric participants. The rate of suicidal thoughts and behavior was 4% in participants taking SSRIs compared to 2% in participants taking placebo. No suicides were completed in this analysis (FDA, 2018). The FDA recommends: "All patients being treated with antidepressants for any indication should be monitored appropriately and observed closely for clinical worsening, suicidality, and unusual changes in behavior, especially during the initial few months of a course of drug therapy, or at times of dose changes, either increases or decreases" (Eli Lilly, 2017).

Another potentially serious adverse effect is serotonin syndrome, which is classically characterized by a triad of mental status changes, autonomic hyperactivity, and neuromuscular abnormalities. Its presentation is variable, and early symptoms may be overlooked. Mild cases of serotonin syndrome can present with tachycardia, diaphoresis, and mydriasis. In moderate cases patients' additional symptoms may include hypertension and hyperthermia. More severe cases can be associated with delirium, hypertonicity, and shock. Serotonin syndrome is caused by excess serotonin. In the context of SSRIs and similar medications serotonin syndrome can be caused by inadvertent or intentional administration of either multiple serotonergic medications or a single serotonergic medication at a high dose. Additionally, serotonin syndrome can be caused by a combination of a serotonergic drug such as an SSRI and a drug that inhibits CYP2D6 metabolism. As such, clinicians must remain cognizant of all a patient's prescriptions and over-the-counter medications. Examples of medications used in mood and anxiety disorders whose combinations can precipitate serotonin syndrome include SSRIs, tricyclic antidepressants (TCAs), and monoamine oxidase inhibitors. Other medications that can precipitate serotonin syndrome include opiate analgesics, antibiotics, and antiemetics. Serotonin syndrome is a clinical diagnosis. Mild cases are managed supportively, with more severe cases requiring inpatient care and the administration of serotonin antagonists (Boyer & Shannon, 2005).

Approved Indications

Some SSRIs have received approval through the FDA for the treatment of MDD and obsessive-compulsive disorder (OCD) in childhood (see Table 99.3).

Off-Label Uses

Despite lacking FDA approval there is evidence to support the use of most SSRIs in the treatment of MDD and OCD, as well as the use of SSRIs in other anxiety and mood disorders. Examples of off-label use of SSRIs include fluvoxamine for the use of generalized anxiety disorder and fluoxetine for migraines. Additionally, there are small, randomized controlled trials favoring the use of fluoxetine and fluvoxamine for repetitive behaviors in ASD.

Dosing

After an informed discussion of benefits, side effects, and alternatives, dosing of an SSRI should start at the lowest dose possible. For young children and those with developmental disorders, a starting dose below the dose given in Table 99.3 may be recommended. Dose increases should be slow, with increases occurring every 2 to 3 weeks along with close monitoring of effectiveness and adverse effects. Some patience is warranted when treating with SSRIs, as the full therapeutic effect can often take 12 weeks to emerge.

Monitoring

Laboratory monitoring for SSRIs is generally not warranted. Symptom checklists should be conducted at follow-up visits, as well as questions regarding suicidal ideation, particularly during medication initiation and dose increases.

Interactions

SSRIs undergo hepatic metabolism largely via the CYP450 isoenzymes. Half-lives for SSRIs can vary considerably. The half-lives of fluvoxamine and paroxetine range from 15 to 20 hours, whereas sertraline has a half-life of approximately 25 hours. Escitalopram and citalopram's half-lives range from 32 to 35 hours. Fluoxetine has the longest half-life of the SSRIs at approximately 72 hours. Additionally, fluoxetine and sertraline produce active metabolites, which can extend their functional half-lives. Fluoxetine produces norfluoxetine, which has an additional half-life of 7 to 14 days, whereas sertraline produces N-desmethylsertarline, which has a half-life of 2 to 3 days (Schatzberg & DeBattista, 2019).

Many SSRIs, particularly fluoxetine, are simultaneously substrates and inhibitors of the CYP2D6 enzyme. Thus concentrations of other medications that utilize CYP2D6 for metabolism may be increased with concomitant administration of an SSRI. Examples of medications that utilize CYP2D6 include risperidone, TCA, oxycodone, and clonidine (Mayo Clinical Labs, 2014).

Clinical Pearls

Set expectations so that youth and their families are prepared for the extended time SSRIs may take to reach clinical efficacy. Prepare families for the black box warning of suicidality so that they don't first learn of it from the package insert. Typically dosed once daily, move the dose to bedtime if sedation occurs, or to the morning if insomnia occurs.

SEROTONIN-NOREPINEPHRINE REUPTAKE INHIBITORS

Mechanism of Action

Serotonin-norepinephrine reuptake inhibitors (SNRIs) are a class of medications that, like SSRIs, are often used in the treatment of anxiety and mood disorders. Examples of these medications are included in Table 99.3. SNRIs act by inhibiting the reuptake of both serotonin and norepinephrine, increasing the level of these neurotransmitters at the synapse. The degree of norepinephrine transporter inhibition varies between different SNRIs, with duloxetine demonstrating strong inhibition effects and venlafaxine exhibiting comparably mild inhibitory effects (Nelson & Baker, 2019).

Efficacy

Multiple metaanalyses have demonstrated the effectiveness of SNRIs in the treatment of pediatric anxiety. A 2017 meta-analysis found that SNRIs are effective in pediatric depressive and anxiety disorders, though with a smaller effect size than SSRIs (Locher et al., 2017).

Side Effects

Common side effects from SNRIs are similar to those from SSRIs, including gastrointestinal symptoms. Additionally, use of SNRIs may lead to increases in blood pressure and heart rate, likely due to their effects on norepinephrine (Nelson & Baker, 2019). Most increases are modest, ranging to 2 to 7 mmHg and 1 to 4 beats per minute. Hypertension due to SNRIs often resolves by decreasing the dose. When prescribing SNRIs, blood pressure and heart rate should be obtained before initiation and monitored at subsequent follow-up visits. Liver toxicity, defined as elevations in amino transaminases, has been seen with duloxetine. As with SSRIs, there is a risk of serotonin syndrome when SNRIs are administered concomitantly or within close temporal proximity to other serotonergic drugs. SNRIs can also precipitate a discontinuation syndrome similar to that seen with SSRIs if the dose is quickly reduced or discontinued.

Approved Indications

Currently, only duloxetine has FDA approval for pediatric use in the treatment of generalized anxiety disorder in ages 7 to 17 years.

Off-Label Uses

Off-label uses of SNRIs that have been described in the literature include anxiety disorders, depressive disorders, chronic pain syndromes, and headaches (Urits et al., 2019). The evidence for some of these indications in the pediatric population is sparse.

Dosing

As with SSRIs, prescribing SNRIs in pediatrics should start with a discussion of expected benefits, potential side effects, and alternative interventions. Dosing, particularly in children with developmental disorders, should begin at the lowest dose, with slow incremental increases.

Monitoring

No laboratory monitoring is indicated for SNRIs, though blood pressure should be monitored. Additionally, children on duloxetine should be monitored for clinical signs of liver toxicity.

Interactions

Of the commonly used SNRIs, only duloxetine is a potent inhibitor of CYP450 isoenzymes. Just as with SSRIs that are inhibitors of CYP450, concentrations of other medications that utilize CYP450 for metabolism, such as risperidone, TCA, oxycodone, and clonidine, may be increased with concomitant administration of duloxetine. Half-lives of SNRIs are similar and range from 9 to 12 hours (Mayo Clinical Labs, 2014).

TRICYCLIC ANTIDEPRESSANTS

Tricyclic antidepressants (TCAs) work by inhibiting the reuptake of norepinephrine and serotonin, though they also exhibit anticholinergic and antihistamine activity. Examples of these medications include amitriptyline, imipramine, and desipramine. Prior to the widespread use of SSRIs, TCAs were commonly used for the treatment of depressive and anxiety disorders. The side effect profile of TCAs, particularly compared with SSRIs, have limited their current use in pediatrics. Serious side effects of TCAs include prolonged QT interval, decreased seizure threshold, sedation from antihistamine activity, and confusion or delirium due to anticholinergic activity. Additionally, overdoses of TCAs can be fatal. Given this side effect profile, clinicians prescribing TCAs in children should be aware of any relevant cardiac or seizure history and should consider alternative medication options if warranted. There is some evidence supporting the use of TCAs such as imipramine in the treatment of nocturnal enuresis (see Table 99.3), with results suggesting similar efficacy to desmopressin (Caldwell, Sureshkumar, & Wong, 2016).

BUPROPION

Bupropion is an aminoketone antidepressant, structurally different from SSRIs, SNRIs, and TCAs. It is occasionally used as an off-label treatment of MDD and ADHD, particularly when first-line medications for these disorders, such as SSRIs and stimulants, are ineffective (see Table 99.3). In its sustained release formulation (Zyban), bupropion is approved for smoking cessation treatment in adults. Efficacy at treating ADHD is less than that of stimulants and atomoxetine (Stuhec, Munda, Svab, & Locatelli, 2015). Bupropion acts by inhibiting the presynaptic reuptake of dopamine and norepinephrine. Side effects of bupropion include hypertension, weight loss, and lowering of the seizure threshold. As such, bupropion is contraindicated in individuals with epilepsy, anorexia nervosa, or bulimia and should be used cautiously in individuals with cardiovascular conditions (GlaxoSmithKline, 2017).

Clinical Pearls

Given the efficacy and tolerability of SSRIs, other medication classes are used far less often for anxiety and depression and related symptoms in children and adolescents. However, an alternative medication may be ideal for select patients who either do not respond to or tolerate SSRIs. A working knowledge of SNRIs and bupropion expands the range of therapeutic interventions accessible to affected youth.

VIGNETTE 3

Violet is a 15-year-old with ASD and intellectual disability, moderate in severity. She functions at a 5-year-old level. A generally happy youngster, Violet has had considerable mood swings for the past 3 years. She becomes aggressive and self-injurious daily. Her family and school provide the maximum of behavioral therapy they can access, but her behavior can be unsafe to herself and to others.

ANTIEPILEPTICS

Mechanism of Action

Many brain targets have been proposed for mood stabilizers. The underlying pathology of bipolar disorder remains poorly understood but is thought to reflect an imbalance of neurotransmission, with excess dopamine and glutamate transmission but reduced cholinergic muscarinic transmission. Valproate increases gamma-aminobutyric acid (GABA) concentration in the brain. Carbamazepine inhibits high-frequency firing of sodium channels to treat seizures but also serves as an antagonist of adenosine receptors, involved in modulation of neurotransmitter release (Weisler, 2006). Topiramate has many mechanisms that potentially explain its mood-stabilizing capacity in adults: it blocks sodium and calcium channels, inhibits the excitatory glutamate pathway, and enhances the inhibitory effect of GABA. Lamotrigine also blocks sodium channels, inhibits calcium channels, and inhibits glutamate release (Findling, 2015).

Efficacy

Valproate and carbamazepine demonstrate effectiveness in treating mania and mixed episodes of bipolar disorder in children and adolescents. Limited data support the efficacy of lamotrigine in treating older adolescents with bipolar disorder (Findling, 2015).

Side Effects

Side effects of valproate include weight gain, nausea, sedation, and tremor. Less common but significant are pancreatitis, thrombocytopenia, alopecia, and hepatic failure. Female patients should be monitored for signs of polycystic ovary syndrome. Side effects of topiramate are anorexia, weight loss, and sedation. Carbamazepine can cause hematologic side effects such as agranulocytosis and aplastic anemia, as well as additional side effects of hepatotoxicity, hyponatremia, and dermatologic reactions. Lamotrigine can cause dermatologic reactions such as Stevens-Johnson syndrome and toxic epidermal necrolysis, for which children under 16 years are at greater risk than are adults.

Approved Indications

Valproate is approved as monotherapy and adjunctive therapy for complex partial seizures in children as young as 10 years. Topiramate is used as monotherapy for partial-onset or primary generalized tonic-clonic seizures in children as young as 2 years of age and as adjunctive therapy for partial-onset seizures or primary generalized tonic-clonic seizures associated with Lennox-Gastaut syndrome in children as young as 2 years. Carbamazepine is used as monotherapy for partial, generalized, and tonic-clonic seizures in children, including those under 6 years of age. Lamotrigine is used as adjunctive therapy for children aged 2 and older with partial-onset seizures, primary generalized tonic-clonic seizures, and generalized seizures due to Lennox-Gastaut syndrome. It is also used as monotherapy in patients 16 and older with partial-onset seizures converting from other specific treatments.

Off-Label Uses

Antiepileptics are sometimes used off-label in the treatment of bipolar disorder. Valproate, for example, along with lithium and atypical antipsychotics, remains a primary treatment for early-onset bipolar disorder. Best outcomes result from combination treatments, such as an antiepileptic or lithium plus an antipsychotic (Pavuluri et al., 2004). As is the case for valproate, carbamazepine data come mostly from adult populations; it may be effective for juveniles insufficiently responsive to lithium. Lamotrigine, approved for acute mania and maintenance treatment of bipolar disorder in adults, is also sometimes used for juvenile bipolar disorder (Pavuluri et al., 2009). It is a first-line treatment for depression in adults with bipolar disorder and may also be useful in the pediatric population, both for bipolar and unipolar depression. Neither gabapentin nor topiramate has been found to be helpful in treating adult bipolar disorder. Topiramate is sometimes used to counteract weight gain from psychoactive medications, though data supporting its efficacy are lacking.

Several initial studies demonstrate potential utility of antiepileptic medication to treat problematic symptoms associated with ASD. For example, topiramate may reduce irritability, stereotypic behavior, and hyperactivity when used as an adjunct to risperidone (Rezaei et al., 2010). Valproate may also reduce irritability in children and adolescents with ASD. Atypical antipsychotics are used more commonly, however, due to the better risk/benefit ratio, ease of management (i.e., no need to check for therapeutic levels), and more extensive evidence supporting efficacy.

Dosing

Dosing of these medications generally follows guidelines for their use as antiepileptics.

Monitoring

Before any antiepileptic is started, females of child-bearing age should undergo pregnancy testing with advice about potential teratogenic effects of these medications. Valproate and carbamazepine serum levels are monitored.

Interactions

Carbamazepine is metabolized in the p450 isoenzyme system (CYP3A4) and therefore interacts with many similarly metabolized medications, including oral contraceptives. Likewise, topiramate is a mild CYP2C19 inhibitor and CYP3A4 inducer. Valproate is a weak inhibitor of CYP2C9 enzyme activity and may interact with other medications that interact with CYP2C9 substrates (Gunes et al., 2007). Strong or moderate inducers of CYP3A4 may enhance metabolism of lamotrigine. Clinicians should be cautious about coadministration of lamotrigine with valproate, which may increase risk of severe and possibly life-threatening rash.

Clinical Pearls

Clinicians should monitor behavioral changes in children and teens with developmental disabilities when first treated for seizure disorders. Antiepileptics often interact with other psychoactive medications.

ATYPICAL ANTIPSYCHOTICS

Use of antipsychotic medications began in the 1950s. The addition of atypical antipsychotics with similar efficacy yet lowered side effect risk occurred in the 1990s. This group of

TABLE 99.4 Side Effects of Commonly Used Atypical Antipsychotics

Side effects	Aripiprazole	Clozapine	Olanzapine	Quetiapine	Risperidone	Ziprasidone
Anticholinergic	0	+++	++	0/+	0	0
EPS	++	0	0/+	0	+	0
Neutropenia	0/+	++	0/+	0/+	0/+	+
Diabetes mellitus	0/+	+++	+++	++	+	0/+
↑ Lipid	0/+	+++	+++	++	+	0/+
↑ Prolactin	0/-	0	+	0	++	+
↑ QTc	0/+	+	0/+	+	+	+++
Sedation	0/+	+++	++	+++	+	0/+
↑ Weight	+	+++	+++	++	++	+

EPS, Extrapyramidal side effects. Range reduced (–) → most increased (+++)

TABLE 99.5 Prescribing Guide for Commonly Used Atypical Antipsychotics

Generic Name	Aripiprazole	Olanzapine	Quetiapine	Risperidone	Ziprasidone
Brand name	Abilify	Zyprexa	Seroquel	Risperdal	Geodon
Starting dose mg/day	2 mg	2.5 mg	50 mg	0.25 mg	20 mg divided BID
Max dose mg/day	20–30 mg	10 mg	800 mg	6 mg	160 mg divided BID
Interactions with cytochrome P450 system	CYP2D6 CYP3A4	CYP2D6 CYP1A4	CYP3A4	CYP2D6	CYP3A4
Indication for irritability in autism spectrum disorder	X			X	No pediatric indications
Indication for pediatric or adolescent bipolar	X	X	X	X	
Indication for pediatric or adolescent schizophrenia	X	X	X	X	
Indication for Tourette disorder	X				
Lowest age of approval in years	6	9	10	5	

medications is therefore also referred to as second-generation antipsychotics. Clozapine was the first available atypical antipsychotic but has no pediatric indications and a particularly high risk of side effects; it is rarely used in children, limited to treatment-resistant conditions.

Several atypical antipsychotics are currently available in the United States and Canada. Some of the more commonly used atypical antipsychotics are shown in Tables 99.4 and 99.5. More recently developed atypical antipsychotics include paliperidone, asenapine, iloperidone, and cariprazine. A growing body of literature supports the efficacy of these more recently developed antipsychotics, but the discussion in this chapter will focus on those that have more research and clinical experience for treatment of children and adolescents. Several additional atypical antipsychotics are used around the world.

Mechanism of Action

The method in which atypical antipsychotic medications address a range of developmental and mental health symptoms is not fully understood. All atypical antipsychotics block dopamine (D2) receptors and serotonin (5HT2A) receptors while agonizing 5HT1A receptors.

Efficacy

Risperidone reduces irritability, aggression, tantrums, and self-injury associated with ASD. Greater magnitude of effect is observed in those with more severe behaviors at baseline (Levine et al., 2016). Aripiprazole reduces irritability and aggression associated with ASD (Devane et al., 2019).

Current research suggests that risperidone and aripiprazole are broadly equivalent in efficacy (DeVane et al., 2019). Further, emerging evidence confirms clinical experience that both medications reduce ADHD symptoms in those with ASD (Lamberti et al., 2016).

Risperidone and aripiprazole are both effective in treating acute mania and mixed episodes in youth with bipolar I disorder (Findling et al., 2013). The combination of olanzapine and fluoxetine treats bipolar depression, though weight gain and triglycerides should be monitored closely. Quetiapine effectively treats mania in youth with bipolar I but not depression. Ziprasidone may also effectively treat bipolar mania in pediatric patients (Findling et al., 2013).

Both positive and negative symptoms of schizophrenia in youth respond to treatment with risperidone. Aripiprazole is generally well tolerated and effective in treating and maintaining youth with schizophrenia (Pagsberg et al., 2017). Studies indicate efficacy of olanzapine and quetiapine as well (Pagsberg et al., 2017).

Antipsychotics may be useful for tics (see Chapter 71).

Side Effects

The risk of the assorted side effects (discussed later) varies substantially across the different commonly used atypical antipsychotics (see Table 99.4). Younger age tends to increase risk for side effects, while prior exposure to atypical antipsychotics seems somewhat protective. Increased risk of side effects is conferred with polypharmacy. One meta-analysis of children and adolescents with ASD treated with atypical antipsychotics found central nervous system adverse events (increased appetite, sedation, headache) most common, followed by endocrine disorders (weight gain, elevated prolactin) and gastrointestinal disorders (Alfageh et al., 2019) (see Table 99.4).

Adults are at increased risk of type 2 diabetes mellitus with atypical antipsychotic use, as are youth. Adverse changes in glucose metabolism are most strongly linked to olanzapine. Overall, the risk of diabetes is increased two to three times with antipsychotic treatment (Galling et al., 2016).

Prolactin is increased transiently with risperidone treatment, which can lead to galactorrhea and gynecomastia, though it rarely results in discontinuation (McKinney & Renk, 2011). Risk of elevated prolactin varies across antipsychotics (see Table 99.4).

Extrapyramidal side effects (EPSs) are drug-induced movement disorders caused by dopamine-receptor blockers. The spectrum of EPS includes relatively acute symptoms of dystonia, akathisia, and parkinsonism (tremor, rigidity, slowed truncal/extremity motor function), along with more chronic tardive dyskinesia (see Chapter 71) and tardive akathisia. Withdrawal dyskinesia can occur with abrupt cessation of medication.

Olanzapine results in greater weight gain compared to other atypical antipsychotics. Enuresis is reported for youth taking risperidone, in addition to increased appetite and weight gain. Aripiprazole is associated with weight gain, somnolence, and vomiting. Weight gain is most likely in younger patients with higher baseline weight Z score. Sedation was more likely in those who are antipsychotic naïve (Mankoski et al., 2013). Neuroleptic malignant syndrome (NMS) is rare but potentially fatal (McKinney & Renk, 2011). Symptoms start with mental status change, followed by muscle rigidity, dystonia, fever, elevated creatinine phosphokinase and white blood cells, increased respiratory rate and heart rate, hyperthermia, and profuse diaphoresis. When NMS is suspected, the causative agent should be discontinued, with referral to a hospital for supportive care and close monitoring.

Approved Indications

Risperidone and aripiprazole are both FDA approved for the treatment of irritability associated with ASD in children age 5 and over, and 6 and over, respectively (see Table 99.5).

Asenapine, aripiprazole, olanzapine, quetiapine, and risperidone are FDA approved as monotherapy treatment for manic or mixed episodes for children and teens with bipolar I disorder, who are 9 to 10 years and older (olanzapine approval starts at 13 years old). Olanzapine and lurasidone are also approved for depressive episodes associated with bipolar I when combined with fluoxetine in children and adolescents as young as 10 years. Quetiapine is approved for acute treatment of manic episodes in youth 10 to 17 years with bipolar 1 disorder, both as monotherapy and adjunct to lithium or valproate. Aripiprazole is also FDA approved for acute and maintenance treatment of manic and mixed episodes in children 10 to 17 years with bipolar disorder. Risperidone is similarly approved for treatment of bipolar mania in children and adolescents 10 to 17 years old.

Aripiprazole, olanzapine, lurasidone, quetiapine, and risperidone are approved for treatment of schizophrenia for 13- to 17-year-olds, and paliperidone is approved for children 12 years and over.

Aripiprazole is approved for treatment of Tourette disorder in children and teens 6 to 18 years.

Off-Label Uses

Atypical antipsychotics along with valproate and lithium remain a primary treatment for early-onset bipolar disorder, although only olanzapine is FDA approved for treatment of this disorder. Best outcomes result from combination treatments: antiepileptic or lithium + antipsychotic (Pavuluri et al., 2004). Clozapine may be beneficial, but its side effect profile limits its use (Thomas et al., 2011).

Oppositional defiant disorder and conduct disorder are among the most common diagnoses linked to antipsychotic use in children and adolescents. Evidence supports variable efficacy of risperidone, possibly by reducing anxiety, and with small to medium effect sizes (Jahangard et al., 2017).

Dosing

For treating bipolar disorder, aripiprazole should be started at 2 mg/day for 2 days, then titrated to 5 mg/day for 2 days, and then increased to a target dose 10 mg/day. Further increases in dose may be made in 5-mg increments on a weekly basis to a maximum 30 mg. With risperidone, dosing should start at 0.5 mg/day, with an increase of 0.5 to 1 mg at an interval of greater than 2 weeks, to a target dose 0.5 to 6 mg/day.

When treating behavioral symptoms associated with ASD, aripiprazole should be started at 2 mg/day, then titrated weekly by up to 5 mg/week, with a target dose of 10 to 15 mg/day (see Table 99.5). With risperidone, dosing should start at 0.25 mg/day for children under 20 kg and 0.5 mg/day for 20 kg and above. Increase by 0.25 to 0.5 mg every 2 weeks or more, to a target dose of 0.5 to 3 mg/day. With both these medications, clinicians often start younger children at lower doses and increase more slowly.

When treating Tourette disorder, aripiprazole is dosed at 2 mg/day, titrating to 5 mg/day, with a target dose of 10 mg/day by day 8. The dose can be increased up to 20 mg/day.

Monitoring

Before starting any atypical antipsychotic medication, review personal and family history of obesity, diabetes, elevated lipids, high blood pressure, or cardiovascular disease; document baseline weight, height, body mass index, blood pressure, lipid profile, and fasting glucose or hemoglobin A1c. Weight should be checked at 4, 8, and 12 weeks after starting and then every 3 months. Baseline ECG and prolactin are often advised, given risks of QTc changes and hyperprolactinemia with some antipsychotics. However, conventional doses of risperidone do not appear to lengthen the QTc interval in children and teens (Vo et al., 2016). EPS should be monitored regularly (e.g., using the Abnormal Involuntary Movement Scale).

Interactions

Atypical antipsychotics have numerous potential interactions due to metabolism via the cytochrome p450 system (see Table 99.5).

Clinical Pearls

Starting at a low dose and slowly increasing the dose is particularly important when using atypical antipsychotics, as most side effects are dose dependent. Updating a patient's medication list at each visit is particularly important, given the many medication interactions possible with these medications.

MISCELLANEOUS MEDICATIONS

Numerous medications have been purported to treat symptoms associated with child and adolescent developmental and mental health disorders. Selected medications are reviewed briefly in this section.

Lithium

Mechanism of Action

The method through which lithium exerts its mood-stabilizing effects is not fully understood. Both neuroprotective and neuroproliferative effects have been demonstrated, along with modulation of neurotransmitters (including dopamine, glutamate, and GABA).

Efficacy

Lithium is not well studied in children or teens, but it is used to treat bipolar disorder (Duffy & Grof, 2018). Most evidence relates to the manic and mixed phases of illness, most commonly observed in affected youth. Higher response rates and lower relapse rates may result when combined with antipsychotic medication (Stepanova & Findling, 2017). Lithium is considered the mainstay of bipolar maintenance in adults.

Side Effects

Lithium is generally well tolerated. Early indications of lithium toxicity include ataxia, dysarthria, and reduced motor coordination. Levels well above the therapeutic window can result in seizures, coma, and death. Dehydration should be avoided as it can lead to lithium toxicity. Mild to moderate side effects include headache and nausea/vomiting, sedation, diarrhea, polyuria and polydipsia, acne, and weight gain. Long-term treatment can cause nephrogenic diabetes insipidus (Thomas et al., 2011).

Approved Indications

Lithium is approved to treat acute mania and mixed episodes, and for maintenance therapy, for children as young as 7 years of age with bipolar disorder.

Off-Label Uses

Lithium is sometimes used in severely depressed and high-risk teens inadequately treated with antidepressants or with considerable suicide risk (West-Ward Pharmaceuticals, 2018).

Dosing

Lithium dosing should start at 20 mg/kg/day or 900 mg/day divided into two to three daily doses, whichever is lower. It should be increased toward therapeutic range according to response and side effects. Weight-based dosing is another option (<30 kg start at 300 mg twice daily; >30 kg start at 300 mg three times daily). Increases should occur by 300 mg every 4 to 5 days until therapeutic response is achieved or blood level reaches 1.2 mEq/L.

Monitoring

Baseline labs include serum electrolytes, renal function, thyroid function, and blood counts. Renal function should be reassessed every 2 to 3 months in the first 6 months of treatment and then every 6 months. Thyroid function should be monitored every 6 months. Baseline pregnancy test in females should be confirmed before lithium is initiated due to potential cardiac malformations such as Ebstein anomaly. Baseline ECG is also recommended, given the risk for lithium-induced cardiac side effects in those with preexisting cardiac disease (Thomas et al., 2011). Lithium levels should be monitored, with a target blood level of 0.6 to 1.2 mEq/L. After a therapeutic level is achieved on a stable dose for 3 months, levels should continue to be checked every 3 months (Thomas et al., 2011).

Interactions

Lithium is not metabolized, but its narrow therapeutic range requires careful consideration of any coadministered medications that might impact its serum level (e.g., thiazide diuretics may increase the concentration of lithium, while osmotic diuretics can decrease its concentration). Most relevant for children and adolescents is the interaction between lithium and nonsteroidal antiinflammatory medication, which can decrease renal clearance and potentiate toxicity by increasing lithium concentration (Finley, 2016).

Amantadine and Memantine

Mechanism of Action

Both amantadine and memantine are thought to impact neurologic symptoms via their roles as NMDA receptor antagonists, thus impacting glutamatergic neurotransmission.

Efficacy

Research on the use of amantadine and memantine to impact the behavior of children and teens with ASD is variable but suggests they may have a role as augmentation to risperidone (King et al., 2001).

Side Effects

Both amantadine and memantine are well tolerated with mild side effect profiles, although amantadine may cause sedation (King et al., 2001).

Approved Indications

Amantadine is approved as prophylaxis and treatment for influenza A virus. Memantine is approved to treat mild to moderate dementia of Alzheimer type.

Off-Label Uses

In the pediatric population amantadine has been used to treat fatigue associated with multiple sclerosis as well as traumatic brain injury. It is also used as adjunctive treatment for aggressive behavior in hospitalized children and teens (McGrane, Loveland, & Zaluski, 2016).

Dosing

Memantine dosing is weight based, ranging from 3 mg/day for those under 20 kg to 15 to 20 mg/day for those over 60 kg. Amantadine is dosed differently across studies (e.g., in one study dosing was 100 mg/day for those <30 kg and 150 mg/day for those >30 kg, divided into two doses). A second study dosed 5 mg/kg/day twice per day (King et al., 2001).

Monitoring

No laboratory monitoring is indicated for these medications.

Interactions

Both medications can have anticholinergic-like side effects, which can be increased by other medications with anticholinergic properties.

Clinical Pearls

Given the lack of robust evidence supporting their use, neither amantadine nor memantine is a mainstream choice to treat children and teens with ASD and/or aggression. However, their benign side effect profiles make them appealing adjuncts to treatment.

N-Acetylcysteine

Mechanism of Action

The mechanism of action of N-acetylcysteine (NAC) is not fully understood and may be related to its antiglutaminergic and antioxidant properties.

Efficacy

Data on the efficacy of NAC is limited and mixed, with some research indicating improvement of irritability, hyperactivity, and compliance of children 4 to 12 years with ASD. NAC is used to augment treatment with risperidone (Ghanizadeh & Moghimi-Sarani, 2013).

Side Effects

NAC is well tolerated with rare severe side effects.

Approved Indications

NAC is approved as an antidote for acetaminophen overdose to prevent or minimize hepatic injury.

Off-Label Uses

Use of NAC to address behavior of children with ASD is off-label.

Dosing

In studies of NAC given to children with ASD doses vary. In one participants were given 1200 mg/day divided into two doses (Ghanizadeh & Moghimi-Sarani, 2013). In a second participants under 20 kg were given 200 mg/dose three times per day, and those over 20 kg received 300 mg three times per day (Nikoo, Radnia, Farokhnia, Mohammadi, & Akhondzadeh, 2015).

Monitoring

No laboratory monitoring is indicated.

Clinical Pearls

As the efficacy of NAC is not well proven, its use is limited to occasions when evidence-based interventions fail or have intolerable side effects.

Naltrexone

Mechanism of Action

An opioid antagonist, naltrexone is posited to address symptoms associated with ASD via its role in blocking the action of naturally occurring opioid peptides and brain serotonin (Roy, Roy, Deb, Unwin, & Roy, 2015).

Efficacy

There is limited and mixed data regarding use of naltrexone for youth with ASD. A review of 10 studies, mostly using a randomized controlled crossover design, including 155 children with ASD, determined that 77% showed improvement in irritability and hyperactivity with naltrexone treatment (Roy et al., 2015). It has also been used to treat self-injurious behavior.

Side Effects

Naltrexone is generally well tolerated with adverse effects that include weight loss and sedation.

Approved Indications

Indications are for treatment of alcohol dependence and for blockade of effects of exogenously administered opioids.

Off-Label Uses

Naltrexone has been used for hyperactivity, irritability, and self-injury associated with ASD or intellectual disability.

Dosing

Previous studies of naltrexone for youth with ASD generally include doses ranging from 0.5 to 1.5 mg/kg.

Monitoring

No laboratory monitoring is indicated.

Interactions

Naltrexone may interact with other opioid-containing medications, such as cough and cold remedies, antidiarrhea medication, and opioid analgesics.

Clinical Pearls

Like amantadine and memantine, the mild side effect profile of naltrexone makes it an appealing option for treatment-resistant children and adolescents, despite the lack of robust evidence supporting its use.

POLYPHARMACY

Polypharmacy is often used in children with developmental disorders, with one study estimating that approximately 35% of children with ASD were taking two or more psychotropic medications. Polypharmacy appears to be more common in older children and those with multiple developmental and behavioral disorders (Spencer et al., 2013). Given the limited data on the safety and efficacy of polypharmacy in children with developmental and behavioral disorders, additional attention must be taken in these scenarios to ensure a child's medication regimen balances meeting their behavioral needs while minimizing side effects and adverse medication interactions. A review of all a child's medications should be performed at every visit to ensure accuracy of the medication list, assess for the potential for medication interactions, and determine the necessity of each medication in addressing its specific target symptoms.

CONCLUSION

Use of pharmacotherapy is often a helpful treatment component for impairing symptoms of many developmental and behavioral health conditions in children and adolescents. Medication can be appropriate and impactful across a broad age span and for a spectrum of symptoms, as illustrated in the vignettes above. However, every medication brings a set of risks carefully balanced with benefits. Safe and optimal care requires clinicians to update themselves regularly regarding this frequently expanding field.

REFERENCES

Alfageh, B. H., Wang, Z., Mongkhon, P., Besag, F. M. C., Alhawassi, T. M., Brauer, R., & Wong, I. C. K. (2019). Safety and tolerability of antipsychotic medication in individuals with autism spectrum disorder: A systematic review and meta-analysis. *Paediatric Drugs*, *21*(3), 153–167.

Boyer, E., & Shannon, M. (2005). Current concepts: The serotonin syndrome. *New England Journal of Medicine*, *352*(11), 1112–1120.

Caldwell, P., Sureshkumar, P., & Wong, W. (2016). Tricyclic and related drugs for nocturnal enuresis in children. *Cochrane Database of Systemic Reviews*, *1*. https://doi.org/10.1002/141651858.CD002117.pub2

Chang, Z., Ghirardi, L., Quinn, P. D., Asherson, P., D'Onofrio, B. M., & Larsson, H. (2019). Risks and benefits of attention-deficit/hyperactivity disorder medication on behavioral and neuropsychiatric outcomes: A qualitative review of pharmacoepidemiology studies using linked prescription databases. *Biological Psychiatry*, *86*(5), 335–343.

Clavenna, A., & Bonati, M. (2017). Pediatric pharmacoepidemiology—A Safety and effectiveness of medicines for ADHD. *Expert Opinion on Drug Safety*, *16*(12), 1335–1345.

Cortese, S., Holtmann, M., Banaschewski, T., Buitelaar, J., Coghill, D., Danckaerts, M., … Sergeant, J. (2013). European ADHD Guidelines Group. Practitioner review: Current best practice in the management of adverse events during treatment with ADHD medications in children and adolescents. *Journal of Child Psychology and Psychiatry*, *54*(3), 227–246.

DeVane, C. L., Charles, J. M., Abramson, R. K., Williams, J. E., Carpenter, L. A., Raven, S., … Bragg, J. E., Jr (2019). Pharmacotherapy of autism spectrum disorder: Results from the randomized BAART clinical trial. *Pharmacotherapy*, *39*(6), 626–635.

Duffy, A., & Grof, P. (2018). Lithium treatment in children and adolescents. *Pharmacopsychiatry*, *51*(5), 189–193.

Eli Lilly. (2017). *Prozac (fluoxetine) [package insert]*. US Food and Drug Administration. https://www.accessdata.fda.gov/drugsatfda_docs/label/2017/018936s108lbl.pdf

`Fedder, D., Patel, H., & Saadabadi, A. (2020). *Atomoxetine*. StatPearls Publishing.

Findling, R. L., Cavuş, I., Pappadopulos, E., Vanderburg, D. G., Schwartz, J. H., Gundapaneni, B. K., & DelBello, M. P. (2013). Efficacy, long-term safety, and tolerability of ziprasidone in children and adolescents with bipolar disorder. *Journal of Child and Adolescent Psychopharmacology*, *23*(8), 545–557.

Finley, P. R. (2016). Drug interactions with lithium: An update. *Clinical Pharmacokinetics*, *55*(8), 925–941.

Food and Drug Administration. (2018). *Suicidality in children and adolescents being treated with antidepressant medications*. https://www.fda.gov/drugs/postmarket-drug-safety-information-patients-and-providers/suicidality-children-and-adolescents-being-treated-antidepressant-medications

Galling, B., Roldán, A., Nielsen, R. E., Nielsen, J., Gerhard, T., Carbon, M., Stubbs, B., Vancampfort, D., De Hert, M., Olfson, M., Kahl, K. G., Martin, A., Guo, J. J., Lane, H. Y., Sung, F. C., Liao, C. H., Arango, C., & Correll, C. U. (2016). Type 2 diabetes mellitus in youth exposed to antipsychotics: A systematic review and meta-analysis. *JAMA Psychiatry*, *73*(3), 247–259. Erratum in: *JAMA Psychiatry, 73*(4), 412.

Ghanizadeh, A., & Moghimi-Sarani, E. (2013). A randomized double blind placebo controlled clinical trial of N-acetylcysteine added to risperidone for treating autistic disorders. *BMC Psychiatry*, *13*, 196.

GlaxoSmithKline. (2017). *Wellbutrin (bupropion) [package insert]*. US Food and Drug Administration. https://www.accessdata.fda.gov/drugsatfda_docs/label/2017/018644s052lbl.pdf

Golubchik, P., & Weizman, A. (2018). The effect of methylphenidate treatment on suspiciousness in children with ADHD alone or comorbid with ODD. *International Journal of Psychiatry in Clinical Practice*, *22*(2), 109–114.

Gunes, A., Bilir, E., Zengil, H., Babaoglu, M. O., Bozkurt, A., & Yasar, U. (2007). Inhibitory effect of valproic acid on cytochrome P450 2C9 activity in epilepsy patients. *Basic & Clinical Pharmacology & Toxicology*, *100*(6), 383–386.

Heal, D. J., Smith, S. L., Gosden, J., & Nutt, D. J. (2013). Amphetamine, past and present—A pharmacological and clinical perspective. *Journal of Psychopharmacology (Oxford, England)*, *27*(6), 479–496.

Hennissen, L., Bakker, M. J., Banaschewski, T., Carucci, S., Coghill, D., Danckaerts, M., Dittmann, R. W., Hollis, C., Kovshoff, H., McCarthy, S., Nagy, P., Sonuga-Barke, E., Wong, I. C., Zuddas, A., Rosenthal, E., Buitelaar, J. K., & ADDUCE Consortium, (2017). Cardiovascular effects of stimulant and non-stimulant medication for children and adolescents with ADHD: A systematic review and meta-analysis of trials of methylphenidate, amphetamines and atomoxetine. *CNS Drugs*, *31*(3), 199–215.

Huss, M., Dirks, B., Gu, J., Robertson, B., Newcorn, J. H., & Ramos-Quiroga, J. A. (2018). Long-term safety and efficacy of guanfacine extended release in children and adolescents with ADHD. *European Child and Adolescent Psychiatry*, *27*(10), 1283–1294.

Jahangard, L., Akbarian, S., Haghighi, M., Ahmadpanah, M., Keshavarzi, A., Bajoghli, H., Brand, S. (2017). Children with ADHD and symptoms of oppositional defiant disorder improved in behavior when treated with methylphenidate and adjuvant risperidone, though weight gain was also observed—Results from a randomized, double-blind, placebo-controlled clinical trial. *Psychiatry Research*, *251*, 182–191.

Joseph, A., Ayyagari, R., Xie, M., Cai, S., Xie, J., Huss, M., & Sikirica, V. (2017). Comparative efficacy and safety of attention-deficit/hyperactivity disorder pharmacotherapies, including guanfacine extended release: A mixed treatment comparison. *European Child & Adolescent Psychiatry*, *26*(8), 875–897.

Keilow, M., Holm, A., & Fallesen, P. (2018). Medical treatment of attention deficit/hyperactivity disorder (ADHD) and children's academic performance. *PloS One*, *13*(11), e0207905.

King, B. H., Wright, D. M., Handen, B. L., Sikich, L., Zimmerman, A. W., McMahon, W., … Cook, E. H., Jr. (2001). Double-blind, placebo-controlled study of amantadine hydrochloride in the treatment of children with autistic disorder. *Journal of the American Academy of Child and Adolescent Psychiatry*, *40*(6), 658–665.

Krishnan, V., & Nestler, E. (2008). The molecular neurobiology of depression. *Nature*, *455*(7215), 894–902.

Lamberti, M., Siracusano, R., Italiano, D., Alosi, N., Cucinotta, F., Di Rosa, G., … Gagliano, A. (2016). Head-to-head comparison of aripiprazole and risperidone in the treatment of ADHD symptoms in children with autistic spectrum disorder and ADHD: A pilot, open-label, randomized controlled study. *Paediatric Drugs*, *18*(4), 319–329.

Levine, S. Z., Kodesh, A., Goldberg, Y., Reichenberg, A., Furukawa, T. A., Kolevzon, A., & Leucht, S. (2016). Initial severity and efficacy of risperidone in autism: Results from the RUPP trial. *European Psychiatry: The Journal of the Association of European Psychiatrists*, *32*, 16–20.

Liang, E. F., Lim, S. Z., Tam, W. W., Ho, C. S., Zhang, M. W., McIntyre, R. S., & Ho, R. C. (2018). The effect of methylphenidate and atomoxetine on heart rate and systolic blood pressure in young people and adults with attention-deficit hyperactivity disorder (ADHD): Systematic review, meta-analysis, and meta-regression. *International Journal of Environmental Research and Public Health*, *15*(8), 1789.

Locher, C., Koechlin, H., Zion, S. R., Werner, C., Pine, D. S., Kirsch, I., ... Kossowsky, J. (2017). Efficacy and safety of selective serotonin reuptake inhibitors, serotonin-norepinephrine reuptake inhibitors, and placebo for common psychiatric disorders among children and adolescents: A systematic review and meta-analysis. *JAMA Psychiatry*, *74*(10), 1011–1020.

Luft, M., Lamy, M., DelBello, M., McNamara, R., & Strawn, J. (2018). Antidepressant-induced activation in children and adolescents: Risk, recognition and management. *Current Problems in Pediatric and Adolescent Health Care*, *48*(2), 50–62.

Mankoski, R., Stockton, G., Manos, G., Marler, S., McQuade, R., Forbes, R. A., & Marcus, R. (2013). Aripiprazole treatment of irritability associated with autistic disorder and the relationship between prior antipsychotic exposure, adverse events, and weight change. *Journal of Child and Adolescent Psychopharmacology*, *23*(8), 572–576.

Martinez-Raga, J., Knecht, C., Szerman, N., & Martinez, M. I. (2013). Risk of serious cardiovascular problems with medications for attention-deficit hyperactivity disorder. *CNS Drugs*, *27*(1), 15–30.

Mayo Clinical Labs. (2014). *Cytochrome P450 2D6 known drug interaction chart*. https://www.mayocliniclabs.com/it-mmfiles/Cytochrome_P450_2D6_Known_Drug_Interaction_Chart.pdf

McGrane, I. R., Loveland, J. G., & Zaluski, H. J. (2016). Adjunctive amantadine treatment for aggressive behavior in children: A series of eight cases. *Journal of Child and Adolescent Psychopharmacology*, *26*(10), 935–938.

McKinney, C., & Renk, K. (2011). Atypical antipsychotic medications in the management of disruptive behaviors in children: Safety guidelines and recommendations. *Clinical Psychology Review*, *31*(3), 465–471.

MTA Cooperative Group. (2004). National Institute of Mental Health multimodal treatment study of ADHD follow-up: Changes in effectiveness and growth after the end of treatment. *Pediatrics*, *113*(4), 762–769.

Naguy, A. (2016). Clonidine use in psychiatry: Panacea or panache. *Pharmacology*, *98*(1–2), 87–92.

Nelson, S., & Baker, M. (2019). Antidepressant medications. In R. Bowers, J. Jackson, & C. Wetson (Eds.), *Green's child and adolescent clinical psychopharmacology* (6th ed.). Wolters Kluwer. https://doi.org/10.1176/appi.books.9781615372997.AS03

Nikoo, M., Radnia, H., Farokhnia, M., Mohammadi, M. R., & Akhondzadeh, S. (2015). N-acetylcysteine as an adjunctive therapy to risperidone for treatment of irritability in autism: A randomized, double-blind, placebo-controlled clinical trial of efficacy and safety. *Clinical Neuropharmacology, 38*(1), 11–17.

Osland, S. T., Steeves, T. D., & Pringsheim, T. (2018). Pharmacological treatment for attention deficit hyperactivity disorder (ADHD) in children with comorbid tic disorders. *Cochrane Database of Systematic Reviews, 26*, 6.

Pagsberg, A. K., Jeppesen, P., Klauber, D. G., Jensen, K. G., Rudå, D., Stentebjerg-Olesen, M., … Fink-Jensen, A. (2017). Quetiapine extended release versus aripiprazole in children and adolescents with first-episode psychosis: The multicentre, double-blind, randomised tolerability and efficacy of antipsychotics (TEA) trial. *The Lancet Psychiatry, 4*(8), 605–618.

Pavuluri, M. N., Henry, D. B., Carbray, J. A., Sampson, G., Naylor, M. W., & Janicak, P. G. (2004). Open-label prospective trial of risperidone in combination with lithium or divalproex sodium in pediatric mania. *Journal of Affective Disorders, 82*(1), S103–S111.

Pavuluri, M. N., Henry, D. B., Moss, M., Mohammed, T., Carbray, J. A., & Sweeney, J. A. (2009). Effectiveness of lamotrigine in maintaining symptom control in pediatric bipolar disorder. *Journal of Child and Adolescent Psychopharmacology, 19*(1), 75–82.

Piacentini, J., Bennett, S., Compton, S. N., Kendall, P. C., Birmaher, B., Albano, A. M., ... Walkup, J. (2014). 24- and 36-week outcomes for the Child/Adolescent Anxiety Multimodal Study (CAMS). *Journal of the American Academy of Child and Adolescent Psychiatry, 53*(3), 297–310.

Politte, L. C., Scahill, L., Figueroa, J., McCracken, J. T., King, B., & McDougle, C. J. (2018). A randomized, placebo-controlled trial of extended-release guanfacine in children with autism spectrum disorder and ADHD symptoms: An analysis of secondary outcome measures. *Neuropsychopharmacology, 43*(8), 1772–1778.

Rezaei, V., Mohammadi, M. R., Ghanizadeh, A., Sahraian, A., Tabrizi, M., Rezazadeh, S. A., & Akhondzadeh, S. (2010). Double-blind, placebo-controlled trial of risperidone plus topiramate in children with autistic disorder. *Progress in Neuro-Psychopharmacology & Biological Psychiatry, 34*(7), 1269–1272.

Roy, A., Roy, M., Deb, S., Unwin, G., & Roy, A. (2015). Are opioid antagonists effective in attenuating the core symptoms of autism spectrum conditions in children: A systematic review. *Journal of Intellectual Disability Research: JIDR, 59*(4), 293–306.

Schatzberg, A., & DeBattista, C. (2019). Antidepressants: *Schatzberg's manual of clinical psychopharmacology* (9th ed.). American Psychiatric Association Publishing. https://doi-org.ezp.slu.edu/10.1176/appi.books.9781615372997.AS03

Schoretsanitis, G., de Leon, J., Eap, C. B., Kane, J. M., & Paulzen, M. (2019). Clinically significant drug-drug interactions with agents for attention-deficit/hyperactivity disorder. *CNS Drugs, 33*(12), 1201–1222.

Scott, N. G., Ripperger-Suhler, J., Rajab, M. H., & Kjar, D. (2010). Factors associated with atomoxetine efficacy for treatment of attention-deficit/hyperactivity disorder in children and adolescents. *Journal of Child and Adolescent Psychopharmacology, 20*(3), 197–203.

Spencer, D., Marshall, J., Post, B., Kulakodlu, M., Newschaffer, C., Dennen, T., ... Jain, A. (2013). Psychotropic medication use and polypharmacy in children with autism spectrum disorders. *Pediatrics, 132*(5), 833–840.

Stepanova, E., & Findling, R. L. (2017). Psychopharmacology of bipolar disorders in children and adolescents. *Pediatric Clinics of North America, 64*(6), 1209–1222.

Stuhec, M., Munda, B., Svab, V., & Locatelli, I. (2015). Comparative efficacy and acceptability of atomoxetine, lisdexamfetamine, bupropion and methylphenidate in treatment of attention deficit hyperactivity disorder in children and adolescents: A meta-analysis with focus on bupropion. *Journal of Affective Disorders, 1*(178), 149–159.

Thomas, T., Stansifer, L., & Findling, R. L. (2011). Psychopharmacology of pediatric bipolar disorders in children and adolescents. *Pediatric Clinics of North America, 58*(1). 173–xii.

Trenque, T., Herlem, E., Abou Taam, M., & Drame, M. (2014). Methylphenidate off-label use and safety. *SpringerPlus, 3*, 286.

Urits, I., Peck, J., Orhurhu, M. S., Wolf, J., Patel, R., Orhurhu, V., ... Viswanath, O. (2019). Off-label antidepressant use for treatment and management of chronic pain: Evolving understanding and comprehensive review. *Current Pain and Headache Reports, 23*(9), 66.

Vo, L. C., Snyder, C., McCracken, C., McDougle, C. J., McCracken, J. T., Aman, M. G., … Scahill, L. (2016). No apparent cardiac conduction effects of acute treatment with risperidone in children with autism spectrum disorder. *Journal of Child and Adolescent Psychopharmacology, 26*(10), 900–908.

Waxmonsky, J. G., Waschbusch, D. A., Pelham, W. E., Draganac-Cardona, L., Rotella, B., & Ryan, L. (2010). Effects of atomoxetine with and without behavior therapy on the school and home functioning of children with attention-deficit/hyperactivity disorder. *The Journal of Clinical Psychiatry, 71*(11), 1535–1551.

Weisler, R. H. (2006). Carbamazepine extended-release capsules in bipolar disorder. *Neuropsychiatric Disease and Treatment, 2*(1), 3–11.

West-Ward Pharmaceuticals. (2018). *Lithium [package insert]*. US Food and Drug Administration. https://www.accessdata.fda.gov/drugsatfda_docs/label/2018/017812s033,018421s032,018558s027lbl.pdf

Yang, R., Li, R., Gao, W., & Zhao, Z. (2017). Tic symptoms induced by atomoxetine in treatment of ADHD: A case report and literature review. *Journal of Developmental and Behavioral Pediatrics: JDBP, 38*(2), 151–154.

100

Hypnosis, Biofeedback, and Meditation

Howard Hall, Fatima Malik, and Suzanne Rusnak

For additional material related to the content of this chapter, please see Chapters 64, 91, and 98.

> **VIGNETTE 1**
>
> *Robert, a 3-year-old, falls down some stairs splitting his lip and knocking a tooth into his maxillary bone. He is bleeding profusely and screaming with both pain and fright. His parents run to him with fear on their face asking if he is alright. They yell for a neighbor to bring a towel and ice. They comment to each other that they can't believe how much he is bleeding and stating he is going to need stitches. He is rushed to the emergency room where they are told their child will need about 10 stitches.*

INTRODUCTION

Self-regulation refers to the process of gaining awareness of the mind-body connection, in order for the individual to develop some measure of control over selected psychological or physiologic processes. Self-regulation empowers the child to learn how to self-manage stress and discomfort (e.g., by controlling autonomic arousal associated with anxiety-provoking situations). Self-regulation or mind-body skill training aims to cultivate empowering emotional states and self-control via self-directed therapeutic affirmations and suggestions.

There are a variety of strategies used to teach self-regulation in the health care setting (Table 100.1). These approaches may be a primary treatment in some cases and in others may help manage pain, anxiety, or other symptoms associated with a condition (Table 100.2). In this chapter we will focus on three approaches: self-hypnosis, biofeedback, and meditation.

These interventions differ in their approach to teaching self-regulation but also have important similarities. One unifying aspect of almost all forms of therapy is the use of language. To begin this chapter, we will introduce the concepts of therapeutic language and integrative therapeutic breath control. Clinicians who do not teach hypnosis, biofeedback, or meditation can use these approaches to help children manage fear, pain, and anxiety that commonly occur in all health care settings.

THERAPEUTIC LANGUAGE

Critical to self-regulation interventions is the therapeutic use of language and invitation. Therapeutic conversations are affirmative rather than dismissive, emphasize strengths over weaknesses, and are consistent with the patient's experiences and background. When working with children, language can highlight that children view the world differently than adults. Children are curious, seeking to understand the world around them. They may be open to suggestions about how to understand the world.

The first vignette describes a common occurrence for parents and children, but a parent (who also happened to be trained in hypnosis) provides an instructive case on how one might use therapeutic language as opposed to the more common approach taken by the parents in the vignette. As Robert paused for breath from screaming, his parent told him quickly, simply, sympathetically, and emphatically, "That hurts, awful Robert. That hurts terrible." Thus Robert knew that his parents understood and agreed with him and his current situation. Then they told Robert, "And it will keep right on hurting" articulating Robert's own fear and judgment. After he took his next breath, they told him, "And you really wish it would stop hurting." The following suggestion was offered: "Maybe it will stop hurting in a little while, in just a minute or two." The parent emphasized that the child's blood was strong and red and the bleeding and swelling were the "right" response for his body.

The need for stitches was discussed in a way to avoid a negative reaction. This was done by stating regretfully that, while he would have to have stitches in his lip, it was doubtful if he would have as many stitches in his lip as he could count. In fact, it looked as if he would not even have 10 stitches, and Robert could count to 20. Regret was expressed he could not have 17 stitches, like one of his friends, but comfort was offered in the statement that he would have more stitches than a couple sibling. In this way Robert was enabled to face the question of stitches without fear or anxiety but with hope of high accomplishment (Erickson, 1958).

Learning the therapeutic language of hypnosis equips a clinician to incorporate it in other self-regulation modalities such as biofeedback and meditation, as well as in everyday pediatrics (Sugarman, 2006). For example, if a child has a tic cough (see Chapter 71), it is important for the clinician to

TABLE 100.1 Self-Regulation Approaches

1. Mindfulness Meditation	Cultivating of non-judgmental awareness and attention mind through observing inner thoughts, emotions, and sensations
2. Yoga	An ancient science and philosophy of the mind, body, and soul that includes movement, posture, and the breathing techniques
3. Hypnotherapy	An altered state of awareness usually involving relaxation during which the individuals experience high suggestibility
4. Biofeedback	The use of electronic or electromagnetic instruments to measure and feed back physiologic processes, which then can be altered by the individual in the desired direction
5. Positive self-talk	Use of positive self-talk as in cognitive behavioral therapy (see Chapter 98)
6. Progressive muscle relaxation	Alternately tightening and then relaxing specific muscle groups throughout the body
7. Diaphragmatic breathing	Developing an effortless, slow, and deep rhythmic breathing pattern usually in the range of 5–7 breaths/min
8. Self-monitoring	Keep an accurate record of mind, body, and symptom change over time
9. Mind-body education	Explaining in a developmentally appropriate manner how body systems work, to provide a logical understanding of optimal health. In addition, it is important to explore how changes in thinking cause changes in physiologic processes and vice versa
10. Autogenics	Employing self-administered, repetitive suggestions involving sensations of warmth, heaviness, and relaxations throughout the body

Gertz, D. S., & Culbert, T. (2009). Pediatric self-regulation. In *Developmental-behavioral pediatrics* (pp. 911–922 [table 91-1]). WB Saunders.

TABLE 100.2 Applications of Hypnotherapy, Meditation, and Biofeedback

Applications of Hypnotherapy	
Habit problems	Thumb sucking Biting Hair pulling Enuresis Speech and voice Intractable cough Habitual drug abuse Tics and tremors
Behavioral problems	Anger Adjustment disorder Self-regulation Adjustment to counseling
Developmental disorders	Pediatric learning problems Performance and attention problems
Psychophysiologic problems (augmentative treatment)	Asthma Tourette syndrome Irritable bowel syndrome Warts Medical procedures and examinations Seizures
Pain	Acute Chronic (recurrent/constant)
Psychological disorders	Generalized anxiety disorder Social anxiety Performance anxiety Posttraumatic stress disorder Obsessive-compulsive disorder Phobia Insomnia Conversion reactions Depression
Chronic illness (augmentative treatment)	Asthma Cancer Hemophilia Juvenile rheumatoid arthritis Transplant Inflammatory bowel disease
Applications of Meditation	
Global functioning	Emotional regulation Increases compassion for self and others Enhanced attention Improved performance
Psychological	Anxiety Depression Stress

TABLE 100.2 Applications of Hypnotherapy, Meditation, and Biofeedback—cont'd

Physiologic	Hypertension Immune function Pain
Applications of Biofeedback	
Acute and chronic pain	Pediatric burn patients Rheumatoid arthritis Migraine headaches Tension-type headaches Pain related to cancer
Autonomic dysfunction	Hypertension Reynold disease Reflex sympathetic dystrophy
Biobehavioral disorders	Enuresis Encopresis
Movement and posture disorders	Gait training Cerebral palsy Torticollis
Developmental disorders	Attention-deficit/hyperactivity disorder Autism

consider how language may influence the child's symptoms. If parents focus on the cough or model how the child coughs, the child will often start coughing. Instead, the clinician would focus on the child's strengths, and not the child's problems. This is discussed further in the next vignette.

DIAPHRAGMATIC BREATHING

VIGNETTE 2

Sarah, an 8-year-old female, presented with a disruptive, harsh, barking cough that was interfering in classroom and social settings. A thorough medical evaluation was negative. At the initial consultation, the therapist let the parents know that they would not talk about the cough habit in front of the child, nor were they permitted to bring up this subject. During the initial visit, the therapist learned that Sarah was keenly interested in sports. The use self-regulation approaches in sports psychology programs was discussed, and Sarah was taught diaphragmatic breathing. The cough was never mentioned, and Sarah never coughed during the visit. As she was walking out of the room, Sarah stopped and asked, "What about my cough?" The therapist answered: "Oh! That's just a habit." The parents became plural experts on not focusing on her cough habit and on providing a lot of attention to nonhabit behaviors. Over time Sarah learned biofeedback and hypnosis for sports, and the cough became rare.

Similar to the use of therapeutic language, breath control/focus is used in almost all the self-regulation techniques and in everyday clinical settings. Diaphragmatic breathing technique is known as belly breathing because fully contracting the diaphragm causes the abdomen to expand while the chest remains relatively still. It can be easily taught and has been shown to help individuals relax, lower heart rate and blood pressure, decrease pain, and improve athletic performance (Giardino et al., 2004; Lin et al., 2012; Siepmann et al., 2008). Younger children or those who find it difficult can focus on blowing bubbles or balloons with some of the same effects.

This approach can be introduced by focusing on extending the out-breathing, which triggers the natural response of in-breath. The child is asked to allow the breath to come in through the nose and to place one hand on the abdomen and purse the lips for an extended out-breath. The child spends the bulk of the time blowing out rather than breathing in. It can be helpful to describe this as blowing out slowly through a straw to encourage a very long extended out-breath with pursed lips. While doing this, the child can imagine breathing out warm, happy feelings from the heart.

HYPNOTHERAPY

VIGNETTE 3

Carl, a 13-year-old male diagnosed with dysautonomia and postural tachycardia syndrome (POTS), developed taste aversion to even bland foods such as boiled rice or cow's milk. Anything he ate made him nauseous. He was referred for comanagement to the hypnotherapy clinic. Conversational hypnotic induction was used. The story of wild rats and how they learn to avoid developing taste aversion in garbage-laden areas was presented in a manner to evoke curiosity (Liu, 2011). How interesting was it that the wild rats could avoid getting sick from toxic food in garbage dumps by nibbling a little and walking away, instead of eating large servings? Similarly, Carl was encouraged to make almond milk smoothies with different fruits and vegetables each time (to vary the taste so as to avoid the conditioned taste aversions). He also sipped the drinks slowly and did not drink it all down in one swallow, just like the rats that would nibble the new foods.

Principles and Procedures

Hypnosis is focused awareness of consciousness, like zooming in to the scene with a camera lens and then observing the details. This heightened awareness, informally known as the trance state, makes the mind more receptive to suggestions. This therapeutic tool has been of interest to Western medicine since at least the early 18th century (Kohen & Olness, 2012). In hypnotherapy a hypnotic state is induced by increasing focus on calming and comforting imagery/ideas. The therapist utilizes the child's internal resources and interests to create a mental imagery and induce relaxation. The goal is to achieve a healthy altered state of consciousness (i.e., modified sensations and perceptions) in which the child is more susceptible to suggestions. In this state of high susceptibility to suggestions mastery-oriented suggestions are given for

TABLE 100.3 Steps of Hypnotherapy

Interview	Discussion about what is "hypnosis" and how and why we will utilize it in treatment. Understanding child's developmental level, likes/interests, hopes and motivations and also aligning/understanding the goal of the parent, the therapist, and the child.
Induction techniques	Visual (multisensory), imagery (e.g., favorite place), ideomotor technique (e.g., magnet fingers), storytelling technique, progressive relaxation techniques, eye fixation techniques, distraction and utilization techniques.
Invitation	Inviting to use the induction techniques to create dissociation and focused attention.
Intensification	Enhancing the experience of the hypnotic state of narrowed focus by combining it with another complimenting technique (e.g., using magnet fingers [ideomotor induction] for invitation and combining it with visual [multisensory] experience for intensification).
Suggestions	Specific, personalized goal-oriented therapeutic suggestions made in hypnotic language that are ego-strengthening in this state of hypnosis.
Anchoring	Posthypnotic suggestions that encourage the person to take control and increase the expectancy of making the therapeutic change. It allows the person to access this self-hypnosis experience regularly and whenever needed.
Realerting	This can be more or less structured, depending on the client's age and preference (e.g., "When you are done, you are done.").
Debriefing	Discussion about the experience and what was it like for the patient.

the individual's therapeutic goal. Hypnotherapy has specific techniques that cannot be learned without proper training. The specific steps of hypnotherapy have been summarized in Table 100.3. Diaphragmatic breathing can be incorporated as a means of intensification.

The goal of hypnotherapy is to instill self-mastery or a skill set of interpersonal communication to facilitate a therapeutic change in maladaptive psychophysiologic reflexes. Hypnotherapy allows the utilization of inner control on healing. It also enables a patient to be more consciously engaged with other treatment modalities. In the last 2 centuries there has been an influx of research and work on the development of this tool and its utilization in children.

Core features of hypnosis may vary with the child's developmental stage. In the early childhood years the approach does not look like conventional methods, but moments of intense focus/relaxation are picked up by a trained therapist who will embed suggestions during a playful conversation. Children naturally go in and out of trance state/imaginative absorption and may or may not close their eyes during a formal therapy session. For adolescents, hypnotherapy will be similar to the adult experience, but it is important to understand the technique may require some modification based on the developmental/emotional/behavioral state of the child. The interview before therapy is to understand the developmental stage and interests of the child and align the goals of the parent, patient, and therapist. Once the technique is chosen, the therapy process is focused to increase inner absorption to enhance self-mastery and create a therapeutic change. It is important that when creating the change, the clinician be mindful of the patient's personal goals and provide clear choices and suggestions for the patient.

In clinical settings children can enter natural trance states (e.g., when presenting in pain or when they are afraid or preoccupied by the lights and gadgets in the examination room). Thus a clinician should be mindful of such moments and be careful in the use of language. Even when unintentional, negative or misunderstood suggestions in such states can be accepted as true (Kohen & Olness, 2012). However, positive suggestions can create the shift toward a therapeutic goal, behavioral modification, and self-control. By mastering language use as suggested earlier, principles of hypnotherapy can be applied to regular clinical/hospital practice even when not using formal hypnotherapy (Kaiser et al., 2018).

Applications of Hypnosis

Hypnotherapy can be a component of treatment of several conditions such as pain, habit problems, psychophysiologic and psychological disorders (see Table 100.2) (Kohen & Olness, 2012). In some cases the hypnotherapy may be the primary treatment modality, but in many of the conditions it will be a supplement to other treatment modalities that may allow decreasing the dose or frequency of medications or other treatments. There is a dearth of large-scale randomized controlled trials to guide clinicians in determining what conditions or patients are most likely to respond to this intervention.

Carl, described in the third vignette, had improvement in his taste aversion with hypnosis. As his taste aversion improved, the therapist began working with him on controlling his autonomic symptoms using biofeedback.

BIOFEEDBACK

VIGNETTE 4

A 12-year-old girl, Julia, diagnosed with Raynaud syndrome, was referred by her rheumatologist. When exposed to cold, even holding a cold drink, her hands turn white and her fingers get numb. When her fingers warm up, they turn red and tingle.

Principles and Procedures

Biofeedback is defined as "a process that enables an individual to learn how to change physiological activity for the purposes of improving health and performance" (Schwartz, 2010). Precise electronic and electromechanical instruments measure physiologic activity such as brain waves, heart rate, breathing, muscle activity, and skin temperature. These instruments can rapidly and accurately feed back this information to the user (e.g., in visual, auditory, kinesthetic, or multimedia format). The individual learns to use this information and control these physiologic reactions/processes by changing behavior, thoughts, and emotions. Thus biofeedback allows an immediate and objective observation of this mind-body interaction (Schwartz & Andrasik, 2017). Over time these changes can endure without continued use of an instrument.

Biofeedback has many similarities to hypnotherapy. As the instrument provides the patient physiologic information, the therapist uses hypnotic suggestions to encourage the patient to create the change in the therapeutic direction. The therapist intensifies this experience with ego-strengthening phrases (i.e., phrases that encourage feelings of personal adequacy and vitality). As the positive results are observed by both the clinician and the patient, the therapist uses future-oriented empowering suggestions (posthypnotic) for continued practice to sustain this change (Kaiser et al., 2018).

Biofeedback equipment is widely available, simple to use, and can be fairly inexpensive. Examples range from simple devices that monitor color variation with skin temperature changes, to more complex computerized software and applications; it is now even available in videogame format. Newer technologies monitor heart rate variability with relaxation and increasingly provide child-friendly feedback formats.

Applications of Biofeedback

Biofeedback alone and integrated with other interventions has evidence in the successful management of various clinical disorders such as acute and chronic pain, including pain associated with migraine headaches (Olness et al., 1987), tension-type headaches (Labbé & Ward, 1990), or rheumatoid arthritis (Lavigne et al., 1992). Electromyography (EMG) biofeedback, urodynamics, and anorectal manometry have been utilized for biobehavioral disorders such as fecal incontinence (Olmsted et al., 1980) and enuresis (Kjølseth et al., 1994). Biofeedback in the form of electrodermal activity or finger temperature has been described for the management of autonomic dysfunction in conditions that include Raynaud disease (Rose & Carlson, 1987), hypertension (Ewart et al., 1987), and reflex sympathetic dystrophy (Barowsky et al., 1987). Surface EMG biofeedback has evidence for neuromuscular retraining such as gait training in children with cerebral palsy (Flodmark, 1986) and spasmodic torticollis (Jahanshahi et al., 1991). There is conflicting literature on neurofeedback treatment for attention-deficit/hyperactivity disorder (Fox et al., 2005) and executive functions in autism spectrum disorders (Kouijzer et al., 2009).

For Julia, described in the fourth vignette, after the history and rapport building, biofeedback principles were explained to her and her parents. A thermometer with a cord and a temperature probe was prescribed (cost <$12). The probe was taped on her nondominant hand to get a baseline temp. Then, Julia was invited to allow her hand temperature to increase (if she got too competitive with attempting to change the temperature, the temperature went down). As she relaxed, the finger temperature went up by 4°F. She was excited to practice this more at home, and on follow-up she reported a marked decrease in symptoms.

MEDITATION

Principles and Procedures

One form of meditation that has been used in medical settings is mindfulness. Kabat-Zinn (2003), creator of Mindfulness-Based Stress Reduction (MBSR), describes mindfulness as a way of paying attention to the present moment, on purpose, and nonjudgmentally. Formal and informal practices are used to train the mind and body in this increased awareness and higher quality of attention. The results are a better understanding of our experience—emotional, mental, and physical—from moment to moment and the freedom to consciously choose responses to those experiences. The position is one of nonjudgmental witnessing that allows for less reactivity and more intentionality. Practitioners gain a greater understanding of the mind-body connection and how to use this connection in an integrated way to recognize what is happening in any given moment and in choosing helpful versus unhelpful responses. In this way attentional control, cognitive control, emotion regulation, and self-related processes are positively impacted.

Mindfulness practices include formal meditation, as well as more informal practices that can be done periodically throughout the day, or as needed. In meditation children can be taught to focus their attention on an anchor (i.e., the breath, sensations, or sounds), noticing thoughts as they arise and choosing to return the attention to the anchor rather than getting caught in the content of the thoughts. They might also practice a more open, or choiceless awareness in which there is an open monitoring of experience. The children notice stimuli as they arise and pass through their field of awareness without needing to react. The length of these practices depends on the developmental age of the child, but the practices can be done daily. This way of meditating strengthens children's attentional control and their ability to notice the activities of the mind and body without being reactive to them. They can begin to see the temporary nature of experience.

In informal practice children learn to bring mindful attention to an activity they are doing by attending to sensory experiences involved in things such as washing hands, walking, or eating. This allows for present moment awareness and brings the attention out of the cognitive realm where stressful, fearful thoughts can negatively impact health and coping. Children can also learn to attend to their breath at any moment—again, taking the awareness out of the cognitive and into the present. They can learn to breathe in deeply and exhale slowly, as well, stimulating the parasympathetic nervous system, and feeling the sensations of the breath in the body.

There are a wide variety of sources for training in teaching mindfulness. The most codified and researched program for adults is MBSR. There is an outgrowth of MBSR that is designed specifically for teens (MBSR-T). In addition, there are several well-respected programs designed to train individuals in teaching mindfulness in school settings. The Mindful School programs have shown efficacy in benefitting both teacher and students to stay grounded, decrease stress, and regain focus (Smith et al., 2012). Similarly, Learning to BREATH curriculum, a mindfulness-based program for middle and high school students, has been shown to increase emotional regulation, attention, and performance (Broderick, 2013; Metz et al., 2013). These methods can be adapted to meet the needs of a more specialized setting, such as in pediatrics.

In terms of psychological treatment there have been several therapeutic interventions developed that are informed by mindfulness. Mindfulness-based cognitive therapy (MBCT), dialectical behavior therapy (DBT), and acceptance and commitment therapy are all treatment modalities that rely heavily on principles and practices of mindfulness. Each of these interventions has been adapted for use with children.

Applications of Mindfulness Meditation

There is a growing body of research in mindfulness meditation for children that indicates that, when taught by a trained instructor or practitioner, it can be helpful for anxiety, depression, stress, hypertension, pain, focusing, and attention issues. Mindfulness meditation has also been shown to be well tolerated and often enjoyed by participants.

The overall health benefits of mindfulness practice in adults have been well demonstrated (Grossman et al., 2004; Sedlmeier et al., 2012), including the pioneering work on MBSR (Chiesa & Serretti, 2009). Neurobiologic research has indicated the positive influence of mindfulness training on immune function and overall brain function (Davidson et al., 2003). Similarly, there is evidence supporting a variety of positive outcomes of mindfulness in management of anxiety (Hoge et al., 2013), improved levels of performance on attentional tasks (Jha et al., 2007), increased empathy (Shapiro et al., 2007), emotion regulation (Desbordes et al., 2012), and reduced physical symptoms and stress (Grossman et al., 2004). A comparatively smaller number of studies involving mindfulness and pediatric populations have indicated similarly meaningful relationships between mindfulness and levels of attention (Napoli et al., 2005), stress and anxiety (Semple et al., 2005), blood pressure (Brown-Wright et al., 2011), pain (Semple et al., 2018), and global functioning with regard to emotional regulation and management of emotional reactivity (Kallapiran et al., 2015; Oberle & Schonert-Reichl, 2017).

TABLE 100.4 Training in Self-Regulation Techniques

Certification Courses for Hypnotherapy *For Children:*
• **The National Pediatric Hypnosis Training Institute (NPHTI)** (www.nphti.org) provides pediatric-specific hypnosis skills training workshop [20+ hr] where experiential learning is strongly emphasized.
For Adults:
• **The American Society of Clinical Hypnosis (ASCH)** (founded by Milton H. Erickson, MD in 1957) offers certificate courses and networking opportunities.
Certification Courses for Biofeedback **Biofeedback Certification International Alliance (BCIA)** accredits didactic programs and is recognized as the certification body for the practice of biofeedback by the following organizations: • Association for Applied Psychophysiology and Biofeedback (AAPB) • Biofeedback Federation of Europe (BFE) • International Society for Neurofeedback and Research (ISNR)
Certification Courses Offered by BCIA for health care professionals: • Biofeedback (BCB) • Neurofeedback (BCN) • Pelvic Muscle Dysfunction Biofeedback (BCB-PMD) • Heart Rate Variability Biofeedback (BCB-HRV or BCN-HRV)
Stens offers professional biofeedback practice training with its online Professional Biofeedback Certification Program (https://www.stens-biofeedback.com/biofeedback-course).
The International Society for Neuroregulation & Research (ISNR) (https://isnr.org) supports education and excellence in neurotherapy, neurofeedback training, and neurofeedback research.
Certification Courses for Meditation/Mindfulness-Based Therapies Mindfulness-Based Stress Reduction. (MBSR) (https://www.brown.edu/public-health/mindfulness/classes). MBSR-T (https://www.stressedteens.com/training-for-professionals). MBCT (Mindfulness-based Cognitive Therapy https://www.mbct.com). Learning to BREATHE (https://learning2breathe.org). MBCT-C (https://www.cebc4cw.org/program/mindfulness-based-cognitive-therapy-for-children-mbct-c/detailed).

SUMMARY

Improving self-regulation in children can occur through multiple modalities. Strategies utilizing language and breathing are applicable to almost all pediatric health care providers to help children with fear, anxiety, or pain. Strategies such as hypnosis, biofeedback, or meditation combine language and breathing with other therapeutic approaches and may be effective as the primary treatment or to augment treatment response for a wide variety of conditions seen in pediatrics. Table 100.4 provides resources for clinicians interested in training in these techniques.

REFERENCES

Barowsky, E. I., Zweig, J. B., & Moskowitz, J. (1987). Thermal biofeedback in the treatment of symptoms associated with reflex sympathetic dystrophy. *Journal of Child Neurology*, *2*(3), 229–232.

Broderick, P. C. (2013). *Learning to breathe: A mindfulness curriculum for adolescents to cultivate emotion regulation, attention, and performance*. New Harbinger Publications.

Brown-Wright, L., Gregoski, M., Barnes, V., & Treiber, F. (2011). Impact of stress reduction interventions on hostility and ambulatory systolic blood pressure in African American adolescents. *The Journal of Black Psychology*, *37*, 210–233. https://doi.org/10.1177/0095798410380203

Chiesa, A., & Serretti, A. (2009). Mindfulness-based stress reduction for stress management in healthy people: A review and meta-analysis. *The Journal of Alternative and Complementary Medicine*, *15*(5), 593–600.

Davidson, R. J., Kabat-Zinn, J., Schumacher, J., Rosenkranz, M., Muller, D., Santorelli, S. F., … Sheridan, J. F. (2003). Alterations in brain and immune function produced by mindfulness meditation. *Psychosomatic Medicine*, *65*(4), 564–570.

Desbordes, G., Negi, L. T., Pace, T. W., Wallace, B. A., Raison, C. L., & Schwartz, E. L. (2012). Effects of mindful-attention and compassion meditation training on amygdala response to emotional stimuli in an ordinary, non-meditative state. *Frontiers in Human Neuroscience*, *6*, 1–15.

Erickson, M. H. (1958). Pediatric hypnotherapy. *American Journal of Clinical Hypnosis*, *1*(1), 25–29. https://doi.org/10.1080/00029157.1958.10401769

Ewart, C. K., Harris, W. L., Iwata, M. M., Coates, T. J., Bullock, R., & Simon, B. (1987). Feasibility and effectiveness of school-based relaxation in lowering blood pressure. *Health Psychology*, *6*(5), 399.

Flodmark, A. (1986). Augmented auditory feedback as an aid in gait training of the cerebral-palsied child. *Developmental Medicine & Child Neurology*, *28*(2), 147–155.

Fox, D. J., Tharp, D. F., & Fox, L. C. (2005). Neurofeedback: An alternative and efficacious treatment for attention deficit hyperactivity disorder. *Applied Psychophysiology and Biofeedback*, *30*(4), 365–373.

Giardino, N. D., Chan, L., & Borson, S. (2004). Combined heart rate variability and pulse oximetry biofeedback for chronic obstructive pulmonary disease: Preliminary findings. *Applied Psychophysiology and Biofeedback*, *29*(2), 121–133.

Grossman, P., Niemann, L., Schmidt, S., & Walach, H. (2004). Mindfulness-based stress reduction and health benefits: A meta-analysis. *Journal of Psychosomatic Research*, *57*(1), 35–43.

Hoge, E. A., Bui, E., Marques, L., Metcalf, C. A., Morris, L. K., Robinaugh, D. J., … Simon, N. M. (2013). Randomized controlled trial of mindfulness meditation for generalized anxiety disorder: Effects on anxiety and stress reactivity. *The Journal of Clinical Psychiatry*, *74*(8), 786–792.

Jahanshahi, M., Sartory, G., & Marsden, C. D. (1991). EMG biofeedback treatment of torticollis: A controlled outcome study. *Biofeedback and Self-Regulation*, *16*(4), 413–448.

Jha, A. P., Krompinger, J., & Baime, M. J. (2007). Mindfulness training modifies subsystems of attention. *Cognitive, Affective, & Behavioral Neuroscience*, *7*(2), 109–119.

Kabat-Zinn, J. (2003). Mindfulness-based interventions in context: Past, present, and future. *Clinical Psychology: Science and Practice*, *10*(2), 144–156.

Kaiser, P., Kohen, D. P., Brown, M. L., Kajander, R. L., & Barnes, A. J. (2018). Integrating pediatric hypnosis with complementary modalities: Clinical perspectives on personalized treatment. *Children*, *5*(8), 108.

Kallapiran, K., Koo, S., Kirubakaran, R., & Hancock, K. (2015). Effectiveness of mindfulness in improving mental health symptoms of children and adolescents: A meta-analysis. *Child and Adolescent Mental Health*, *20*(4), 182–194.

Kjølseth, D., Madsen, B., Knudsen, L. M., Peter Nørgaard, J., & Christian Djurhuus, J. (1994). Biofeedback treatment of children and adults with idiopathic detrusor instability. *Scandinavian Journal of Urology and Nephrology*, *28*(3), 243–247.

Kohen, D. P., & Olness, K. (2012). *Hypnosis and hypnotherapy with children*. Routledge.

Kouijzer, M. E., de Moor, J. M., Gerrits, B. J., Congedo, M., & van Schie, H. T. (2009). Neurofeedback improves executive functioning in children with autism spectrum disorders. *Research in Autism Spectrum Disorders*, *3*(1), 145–162.

Labbé, E. E., & Ward, C. H. (1990). Electromyographic biofeedback with mental imagery and home practice in the treatment of children with muscle-contraction headache. *Journal of Developmental and Behavioral Pediatrics*, *11*(2), 65–68.

Lavigne, J. V., Ross, C. K., Berry, S. L., Hayford, J. R., & Pachman, L. M. (1992). Evaluation of a psychological treatment package for treating pain in juvenile rheumatoid arthritis. *Arthritis & Rheumatism: Official Journal of the American College of Rheumatology*, *5*(2), 101–110.

Lin, G., Xiang, Q., Fu, X., Wang, S., Wang, S., Chen, S., … Wang, T. (2012). Heart rate variability biofeedback decreases blood pressure in prehypertensive subjects by improving autonomic function and baroreflex. *The Journal of Alternative and Complementary Medicine*, *18*(2), 143–152.

Liu, C. (2011). The Garcia effect: A tailored taste for survival. *Berkeley Scientific Journal*, *16*, 1.

Metz, S. M., Frank, J. L., Reibel, D., Cantrell, T., Sanders, R., & Broderick, P. C. (2013). The effectiveness of the learning to BREATHE program on adolescent emotion regulation. *Research in Human Development*, *10*(3), 252–272.

Napoli, M., Krech, P. R., & Holley, L. C. (2005). Mindfulness training for elementary school students: The attention academy. *Journal of Applied School Psychology*, *21*(1), 99–125.

Oberle, E., & Schonert-Reichl, K. A. (2017). Social and emotional learning: Recent research and practical strategies for promoting children's social and emotional competence in schools. In J. L. Matson (Ed.), *Handbook of social behavior and skills in children* (pp. 175–197). Springer International Publishing. https://doi.org/10.1007/978-3-319-64592-6-11

Olmsted, R. W., Olness, K., McParland, F. A., & Piper, J. (1980). Biofeedback: A new modality in the management of children with fecal soiling. *The Journal of Pediatrics*, *96*(3), 505–509.

Olness, K., MacDonald, J. T., & Uden, D. L. (1987). Comparison of self-hypnosis and propranolol in the treatment of juvenile classic migraine. *Pediatrics*, *79*(4), 593–597.

Rose, G. D., & Carlson, J. G. (1987). The behavioral treatment of Raynaud's disease: A review. *Biofeedback and Self-Regulation*, *12*(4), 257–272.

Schwartz, M. S. (2010). A new improved universally accepted official definition of biofeedback: Where did it come from? Why? Who did it? Who is it for? What's next? *Biofeedback*, *38*(3), 88–90. https://doi.org/10.5298/1081-5937-38.3.88

Schwartz, M. S., & Andrasik, F. (2017). *Biofeedback: A practitioner's guide*. Guilford Publications.

Sedlmeier, P., Eberth, J., Schwarz, M., Zimmermann, D., Haarig, F., Jaeger, S., & Kunze, S. (2012). The psychological effects of meditation: A meta-analysis. *Psychological Bulletin, 138*(6), 1139.

Semple, R. J., Reid, E. F., & Miller, L. (2005). Treating anxiety with mindfulness: An open trial of mindfulness training for anxious children. *Journal of Cognitive Psychotherapy, 19*(4), 379–392.

Shapiro, S. L., Brown, K. W., & Biegel, G. M. (2007). Teaching self-care to caregivers: Effects of mindfulness-based stress reduction on the mental health of therapists in training. *Training and Education in Professional Psychology, 1*(2), 105.

Siepmann, M., Aykac, V., Unterdörfer, J., Petrowski, K., & Mueck-Weymann, M. (2008). A pilot study on the effects of heart rate variability biofeedback in patients with depression and in healthy subjects. *Applied Psychophysiology and Biofeedback, 33*(4), 195–201.

Smith, A., Guzman-Alvarez, A., Westover, T., Keller, S., & Fuller, S. (2012). *Mindful schools program evaluation.* University of California–Davis Center for Education and Evaluation Services.

Sugarman, L. I. (2006). *Hypnosis in pediatric practice: Imaginative medicine in action [video documentary DVD and learning guide booklet].* Crown House Publishing.

Growth Mindset as a Brief Intervention: Research to Practice

Irene M. Loe, Kara K. Wright, and Claudia M. Mueller

For additional material related to the content of this chapter, please see Chapters 8, 9, and 18.

VIGNETTES

Toddler. *Diego and his parents present for his 3-year-old well-child visit. His mother notes he is even more "head strong" now than he was during his "terrible twos." He is an increasingly picky eater and refuses anything green. She stops offering a food if Diego rejects it more than once. He is "very stubborn and strong willed." How can the clinician counsel Diego's mother?*

Elementary school student. *Evelyn, a second grader, is seen for her 8-year-old well visit. Her dad is worried that she is reluctant to read books that are a "reach" for her, preferring to reread the ones she has already mastered. The teacher indicates she is making progress but sees the same reluctance to pick up a challenging book. Evelyn says she's worried about not reading well and prefers the books she's already good at reading so "I won't make any mistakes." How can the clinician reframe the situation to encourage both Evelyn and her dad?*

Preteen. *Ahmed, a fifth grader, had enjoyed participating in his local recreation center soccer league for 3 years. When asked about soccer at his well visit, he says, "It's not much fun this year." In private his mother says he seems frustrated by the higher level of competition. He likes practice and playing with his friends, but he commented that he's no longer the "best one on the team." What can Ahmed's parents say to help him reduce his frustration?*

Middle school student. *In the summer between seventh and eighth grade Chanel's mother calls the clinic to share her concerns about bullying that took place last year. She hopes Chanel gets off to a better start this year and is concerned that she may avoid participating in activities at school out of fear of bullying, despite the school's support. Chanel has three good friends and has not had difficulties in the past navigating social situations. What advice would help Chanel?*

High school student. *Alex is a high school sophomore with diabetes and attention-deficit/hyperactivity disorder (ADHD). He doesn't like to check his blood sugar at school and frequently forgets to take his stimulant medication. He says it doesn't make much difference since he "was born this way." What can a clinician do to increase his adherence?*

College student. *Gabriella is in her first semester at a 4-year university. Her parents immigrated to the United States, and she is the first person in her family to attend college. Gabriella feels overwhelmed by her course load and out of place as no other graduates from her high school enrolled at the same university. She heard of a campus group for first-generation students but hasn't found time to attend any of their meetings. What counseling or resources might be helpful for Gabriella?*

WHAT IS GROWTH MINDSET?

A mindset can be defined as an established set of attitudes and, within the study of psychology, is identified as a powerful influence on human behavior. A significant body of work, most notably by Carol Dweck and her associates (Dweck, 2006;Dweck & Yeager, 2019), demonstrates that when individuals hold a mindset about the characteristics of a personal attribute, their attitudes, goals, and behaviors may be altered according to this belief. These "implicit" beliefs are based on assumptions that people make about the malleability of personal attributes and exist on a continuum. At one end, "fixed" mindset reflects the idea that a particular attribute or ability is set and unchangeable. At the other end, a "growth" mindset reflects the belief that this same attribute is malleable and subject to change and development.

Individuals' mindsets may be categorized by responses to simple statements about attribute malleability. Consider the statement, "You can learn new things, but you can't really change your basic intelligence." If you agree, you are showing a fixed mindset regarding intelligence; if you disagree, you are showing a growth mindset. The opposing views yield differing psychological frameworks, including judgments, goals, and responses to setbacks. A fixed mindset leads individuals to see failures in any arena as evidence of stable, low ability; a growth mindset does not carry the same negative judgment. Furthermore, mindsets have been linked to differing goals: Fixed mindset results in a "performance" goal, which emphasizes the appearance of high ability and avoidance of failure; growth mindset is associated with a "mastery" goal, which focuses on learning, even if it involves temporary setbacks. Finally, mindsets can result in contrasting responses to challenge. A growth mindset is linked to challenge-seeking behaviors and resilience after failure; a fixed mindset is associated with giving up and avoidance of challenge. Interestingly, these two mindsets are independent of actual ability; even students of high capability in math, for example, can have a fixed mindset of their skill, which leads them to respond negatively to challenge or failure.

How mindsets develop for individuals remains an area of active study. What is clear is that mindsets can be created or modified through feedback. Mueller and Dweck (1998) demonstrated that praise to fifth-grade students after an academic setback determined their enjoyment, persistence, and ultimate performance on subsequent school tasks. Praise of effort resulted in a growth mindset and adaptive responses to challenge. Praise for ability or "smartness" resulted in a fixed mindset and poor postfailure responses. In other words praise for effort teaches individuals that success results from hard work, which gives them a goal to strive for even amid a challenge or poor outcome. Praise for ability, on the other hand, sends the message that success is primarily a consequence of innate skill without an obvious avenue for development in the face of failure (Table 101.1).

The concept of a growth mindset has proven a fruitful way to improve resilience and achievement within academic settings. Mindset theory has been expanding and applied to other domains of life, such as social and interpersonal interactions (Yeager et al., 2013, 2014) and to health beliefs and behaviors (Mueller et al., 2017). In all these areas growth mindset has been linked to more adaptive outcomes than has fixed mindset. Importantly, individuals do not necessarily hold a fixed or a growth mindset across all domains of life. Their mindsets appear to be specific to each area; the same individual might endorse a growth view of intelligence and a fixed view of sports ability.

TABLE 101.1 Clinical Indicators of Mindset

Indicator	Growth Mindset	Fixed Mindset
What does the individual think it takes to succeed?	Effort, practice, hard work	Intelligence, talent, innate ability
What is the individual's typical response to new challenges?	Yes, please	No, thank you
How does the individual respond to setbacks?	The individual looks for new approaches and strategies.	The individual blames others, becomes defensive, or gives up.
What might you see if the individual experiences failure?	The individual tries again with a new approach.	The individual lies about performance, makes excuses.
What might you expect if you know the test is very difficult?	Sustained effort at studying	Cheating, procrastination

Adapted from Dweck, C. S., & Master, A. (2009). Self-concept. In: *Developmental-behavioral pediatrics* (4th ed.). Elsevier.

WHY IS GROWTH MINDSET IMPORTANT?

Interventions designed to promote a growth mindset in students by emphasizing the malleability of the mind (e.g., "the brain is a muscle that gets stronger through hard work") initially demonstrated practical improvements in challenge seeking, persistence, and grades for students from junior high school to college (Blackwell et al., 2007; Yeager et al., 2019). Growth mindset now holds promise as a brief intervention in many areas. Recent interventions have targeted multiple domains in various age groups. We want to demonstrate how growth mindset can improve functional outcomes in three different domains: (1) academic skills, (2) social skills and interpersonal relationships, and (3) health.

Academic Skills

Academic Achievement

The associations of growth mindset to positive academic behaviors, such as challenge seeking and persistence, and outcomes in terms of academic achievement have been well studied. Exciting progress has also been made with interventions promoting growth mindset in students from junior high school to college (Aronson et al., 2002; Blackwell et al., 2007; Yeager et al., 2019). An early study by Blackwell and colleagues followed seventh graders longitudinally across 2 years, measuring their mindset of intelligence and achievement-related beliefs on entry and academic achievement in math as they progressed (Blackwell et al., 2007). They found that students with growth mindset had stronger learning goals and viewed learning as motivating; they were more likely to believe hard work was necessary and effective for achievement compared to students with fixed mindset. Students with growth mindset were also less likely to attribute failure to lack of ability and were more likely to endorse increased effort or a change in strategy compared to those with fixed mindset. Evaluation of math growth trajectories showed that baseline scores were not different for students with fixed versus growth mindset but pulled apart over the 2 years. Students with growth mindset outperformed those with fixed mindset, controlling for prior achievement. Motivational patterns mediated this effect—students with growth mindset had positive motivational beliefs, which were related to increasing grades (Blackwell et al., 2007).

A subsequent growth mindset intervention study was conducted with different junior high students who were diverse in terms of racial/ethnic background and lower socioeconomic status than in the prior study (Blackwell et al., 2007). The intervention focused on the malleability of intelligence by (1) emphasizing that learning changes the brain by forming new connections and (2) putting students in charge of this process. Materials were presented in workshop format with trained workshop leaders and included readings with analogies (e.g., the brain is a muscle that gets stronger with effort or practice) and examples (e.g., babies become smarter as they learn), activities, and discussions. The control group received similarly structured workshops but without analogies and examples of how intelligence is malleable. The intervention group changed their theory of intelligence, with more students endorsing growth rather than fixed mindset postintervention, compared to the control group (Blackwell et al., 2007). Teachers cited a larger proportion of students in the intervention group as showing positive change in motivation. The intervention reduced the typical downward trajectory of math growth typically seen at the transition to junior high. The benefits of the intervention were greatest for students in the intervention group who endorsed fixed mindset at baseline; students in the control group with fixed mindset at baseline had math scores that continued to decline (Blackwell et al., 2007).

Several randomized trials have now been conducted with thousands of students to assess online growth mindset interventions (Paunesku et al., 2015; Yeager et al., 2016). Such studies have found that mindsets and academic outcomes can change under certain conditions (Dweck & Yeager, 2019). An elegant study took the intervention to scale—providing a short (<1 hour) online intervention in a nationally representative sample of US high schools (Yeager et al., 2019). The study had several strengths, including scalability with no training of teachers, an effectiveness trial in a population-generalizable sample, and adherence to a comprehensive preregistered analysis plan. Postintervention, in the targeted lower-achieving adolescents, fixed mindset was reduced relative to the control condition. In addition, lower-achieving adolescents in the intervention group earned higher GPAs in math, science, social studies, and English/language arts at the end of ninth grade compared to the control group (Yeager et al., 2019). A model analyzing poor performance rates estimated that the intervention would prevent 5.3% of 1.5 million US students from being "off track" for graduation, a relative risk reduction of 11% (Yeager et al., 2019). Additionally, the intervention led to increased overall enrollment in advanced mathematics courses; the effects were stronger for the highest achieving 25% of schools compared to the lower 75% of schools (Yeager et al., 2019). The intervention produced a greater difference in end-of-year GPAs relative to the control group when the behavioral norm surrounding students was supportive of a growth mindset belief system (i.e., peers sought out academic challenges) (Yeager et al., 2019). Given the heterogeneity in school environments, this finding was an important initial step in understanding school environments that support growth mindset.

Attrition or Dropout

The transition to community college or university is highly stressful and can result in dropout. Studies of mindset at this stage began as in-person interventions and have since been adapted as online, scalable "light touch" interventions (Yeager et al., 2016). In studies of this transition the interventions often integrate growth mindset and social belonging. Social belonging interventions stem from observations that negative stereotypes threaten people's social standing. Belonging interventions convey that (1) challenges to belonging are normal in an academic transition for all students, and (2) a sense of belonging can increase over time (Walton & Yeager, 2020). Such approaches counteract the common conclusion drawn by underrepresented minorities and/or first-generation students in college who think, "People like me don't belong here" (Walton & Yeager, 2020). A belonging mindset communicates that "people like you belong in your school or in a given academic field" (Rattan et al., 2015). In three double-blind experiments researchers administered a lay theory intervention—that is, an approach that helps college students "understand that challenges in the transition to college are common and improvable; thus, that early struggles need not portend a permanent lack of belonging or potential" (Yeager et al., 2016). The lay theory intervention had positive impacts; it raised first-year full-time college enrollment among students from socially and economically disadvantaged backgrounds and it raised disadvantaged students' cumulative first-year GPA (Yeager et al., 2016). Follow-up surveys found other intervention-related benefits, including improved overall college experience, greater use of student support services, larger friendship networks, and more mentor relationships. Another randomized study of incoming first-year students at a large public university found that a growth mindset intervention significantly improved GPA for Latinx students by about 0.4 point, or a 72% reduction in the GPA gap between White and Latinx students (Broda et al., 2018). These findings at the postsecondary level hold promise for reducing achievement gaps and attrition for disadvantaged students.

Reading

A large-scale, randomized field trial in Denmark evaluated a reading intervention with a growth mindset approach (Andersen & Nielsen, 2016). Seventy-two classrooms with almost 1600 second graders were randomized to treatment or control groups. The treatment targeted parents' growth mindsets, mastery-oriented interactions between parents and child, and parental praise for child effort rather than performance and results. Parents in the treatment group received a booklet and access to an online video. The materials gave examples of how parents could use a mastery-oriented approach when reading with their child and encouraged parents to praise the child's effort rather than performance. Families received three books and information on how to find reading materials in the community. The control group received "treatment as usual." Treatment improved both language and text comprehension, as well as decoding, after 3 and 7 months. Expressive skills measured on a writing test also improved. Compared to the control group, 2 months of additional gain in reading score was seen in the treatment group after 2 months; this decreased to 1 month of gain by

7 months. These effects were not driven by children with high socioeconomic status and applied to children of immigrants and children with lower maternal education (Andersen & Nielsen, 2016). The effects were larger for parents identified with fixed mindset preintervention. The results from this low-cost, scalable intervention suggest that such approaches are feasible and warrant additional study.

Language

In a study of 10-month-old infants a "Pointing to Success" intervention that targeted the pointing gestures of parents was combined with a growth mindset approach to increase parents' and infants' use of pointing and child vocabulary growth (Rowe & Leech, 2019). Parents in the intervention group received a brief training program, emphasizing the malleability of children's language development and parents' role in shaping that development. The teaching was coupled with a 5-minute video on the importance of pointing and repeated growth mindset messaging, a set of developmentally appropriate toys, and weekly text messages between 10 and 12 months that reminded parents to play 15 minutes/day and reinforced the message about pointing. Parents in the control group received the same toys and were told to play with their child but did not receive the pointing or growth mindset information. By 12 months of age, the intervention group had increased their pointing more than the control, and children also increased their gesture use with parents, but there was no effect on child vocabulary (Rowe & Leech, 2019). The effect of the intervention was stronger for parents with fixed mindset at baseline—their children had increased vocabulary growth from 10 to 18 months of age. The addition of growth mindset messaging to a parent intervention boosted positive results, especially for those at higher risk on the basis of fixed mindset at baseline.

Social/Interpersonal Skills

Social

The social domain is another area in which mindset theory has been examined. One fundamental question is whether people look at other people through a fixed or growth mindset frame. In this case the mindset dimension went from fixed ("the kind of person someone is, is something very basic about the person and cannot be changed much") to growth ("everyone, no matter who they are, can significantly change their basic characteristics") (Dweck & Yeager, 2019). Compared to those with growth mindset, people who believed in fixed traits inferred traits more quickly from behavior, invested those traits with more predictive power, and made stronger predictions about what a person might do in the future based on that trait. Judgments arising from mindset applied not only to individuals but also to groups with a role in stereotyping. A fixed mindset was associated with greater attention to information that supported or was consistent with stereotypes than to information that contradicted the stereotype (Dweck & Yeager, 2019). Fixed versus growth mindset was also assessed in relation to prejudice; fixed mindset states "people have a certain amount of prejudice and they can't really change that," whereas growth mindset states "no matter who people are, they can always become a lot less prejudiced" (Dweck & Yeager, 2019). Individuals who believed prejudice was fixed were more worried about discovering prejudice in themselves or appearing prejudiced to others; this belief was separate from individuals' level of implicit or explicit prejudice. These individuals had less interest in diversity-related activities, interracial interactions, and increased symptoms of anxiety during interracial interactions. The findings suggest that education about diversity should identify prejudice and simultaneously emphasize the malleability of prejudicial attitudes and the need for supporting intergroup interactions.

Bullying

In applying mindset theory to personality Yeager and colleagues (2011) examined fixed versus growth mindset in relation to personality characteristics, applying them to both self-views (i.e., fixed self-view of "maybe I'm not a likable person") and views of others (i.e., fixed view of others—people with aggressive behavior are "fundamentally bad people"). Moving into interventions, strategies were applied though in-person workshops to see if a change in personality mindsets in high school students led to reductions in aggressive behavior (Yeager et al., 2013). Students received a growth mindset message of "people's behaviors often come from thoughts and feelings, which live in the brain, and can be changed" (Yeager et al., 2013, 2014). For the intervention group, aggression measured through a behavioral paradigm was reduced 1 month later; students also wrote an increased number of prosocial notes to students, indicating greater empathy; and teacher-rated student conduct was also improved at year end (Yeager et al., 2013).

In applying the fixed versus growth mindset theory to social adversity studies found associations between a fixed mindset of personality and more negative immediate reactions to social adversity in adolescents starting high school (Yeager et al., 2014). By the end of the school year, fixed mindset was associated with greater stress, poorer health, and lower grades (Yeager et al., 2014). In a series of two related studies in high school students with differing demographics, including socioeconomic status, a brief intervention emphasizing malleability of personality resulted in less negative reactions to an immediate experience with social adversity (e.g., exclusion by peers in an online computer game), lower overall stress and physical illness, and better academic performance over the year in the intervention compared to control group (Yeager et al., 2014). The paradigm has been extended into the areas of stress and depression, both highly prevalent in adolescent life (Dweck & Yeager, 2019).

International Relations

Halperin and colleagues examined the effects of teaching growth mindset about groups to Israelis and Palestinians

(Dweck & Yeager, 2019). In this scenario the emphasis was placed on the potential for groups to change—that is, groups do not have a fixed, inherent nature to be evil or violent; rather, they have the potential for change and growth. The other group was not named in the teaching to decrease resistance to the proposed teaching. The growth mindset groups showed more positive attitudes toward the other party and greater willingness to consider concessions for the sake of peace compared to the control groups (Dweck & Yeager, 2019).

Health

Mindsets play an important role in how individuals respond within the domain of health. Mindsets of health can be viewed on a continuum of malleability from fixed to growth (Mueller et al., 2017). Individuals with a fixed mindset see health as a stable quantity that is not easily changeable. Unsurprisingly, they tend to place emphasis on the genetic origin of illness (John-Henderson et al., 2021). Individuals with a growth mindset of health view health as a fluid quality that can be increased through effort. Consequently, they place greater value on the behavioral components of disease than on genes.

Health mindsets affect motivation, effort, and engagement in health behaviors. Induction of a growth mindset about body weight was associated with a positive change in dietary choices in a laboratory setting (Ehrlinger et al., 2017). In a sample of American Indian college students a growth health mindset was associated with lower body mass index, which was partly accounted for by higher levels of physical activity (John-Henderson et al., 2020). In healthy adolescents a growth mindset was associated with less negative interpretations of illness severity and more optimistic judgments of recovery from illness than was a fixed mindset of health (John-Henderson et al., 2021).

A growth mindset of health is beneficial for individuals facing health challenges. A growth mindset was associated with lower blood sugar levels and better glucose monitoring for young adolescents with diabetes (John-Henderson et al., 2021). For individuals working on weight control, a growth mindset of health was associated with better dietary success (Burnette, 2010). Smokers with a growth mindset of health have demonstrated decreases in smoking (Thai et al., 2020). Scoliosis patients with growth mindsets report higher quality of life assessments (Joseph et al., 2020). A growth mindset has been linked to improved pain perception and analgesic use after surgical interventions in children and adolescents (Sujka et al., 2018).

We suggest that mindsets may shape individuals' views of the implications of illness or injury for overall health. Taken together, the findings have important consequences for clinicians, caregivers, and patients themselves. An awareness of how their patients view health, as fixed or malleable, might change how clinicians introduce new diagnoses or how they motivate patients to follow medical instructions. Current studies on mindset interventions in the context of health conditions such as obesity and diabetes are underway (Robinson et al., 2013).

HOW DO WE PROMOTE GROWTH MINDSET IN PEDIATRICS?

It remains unclear how best to promote growth mindset in young children. Studies show that the nature of parent and teacher mindsets do not automatically correlate with children/students' mindsets (Gunderson et al., 2013; Haimovitz & Dweck, 2017; Park et al., 2016). Teacher behaviors that emphasize understanding, the process of learning, and process praise are predictive of student growth mindset rather than teachers' mindsets (Park et al., 2016). Parents' beliefs about what will motivate children are more important than parent mindset (Haimovitz & Dweck, 2017). Parents' beliefs about failure as motivating (i.e., experiencing failure enhances performance and productivity) as opposed to failure as demotivating (i.e., experiencing failure hurts learning and growth) were associated with different parental practices. Parents who viewed failure as enhancing had children who saw their parents as more focused on learning and improving, and less focused on having them prove their ability through school performance. These parents discussed what children could learn from the experience, how they could study mistakes to improve, and how they might ask for help.

Parent approaches and behaviors can motivate children and promote growth mindset. Children as young as kindergarten age are sensitive to the effects of person and process praise. During a role-playing procedure, kindergarteners received person praise ("You're really good at this") or process praise ("You must have tried really hard"). After receiving praise, the children role-played two setback experiences and were reassessed. Children receiving person praise were more likely to endorse a fixed mindset and showed less resilient responding, whereas children receiving process praise were more likely to endorse growth mindset, show higher persistence and more positive self-assessments (Dweck & Yeager, 2019). Recent work in home environments examined parents' chronic use of person or process praise with toddlers (Gunderson et al., 2013). The use of process praise from 14 to 38 months predicted children's growth mindset and challenge-seeking at age 7 to 8 years, although the use of person praise in the toddler years did not subsequently predict fixed mindset (Gunderson et al., 2013). Measures of academic achievement 1 to 2 years later found an indirect relationship in which growth mindset in second to third grade related to process praise as toddlers was predictive of math and reading comprehension in fourth grade (Gunderson et al., 2018). Another study of parents of 8- to 10-year-olds tracked parents' use of person or process praise (Pomerantz & Kempner, 2013). In contrast, the use of more frequent person praise predicted children's fixed mindset, above and beyond their earlier mindset. These findings suggest that parenting behaviors and practices can have longstanding effects on children's mindsets (Table 101.2).

TABLE 101.2 Differentiation of Process Praise and Person Praise

Process Praise	Person Praise
Appreciation of effort	Appreciation of talent
Understanding what the child did to achieve success	Attributing success to a child's innate abilities
Clarity on why a performance was noteworthy	General praise of the performance and child

Reprinted from Dweck, C. S., & Master, A. (2009). Self-concept. In: *Developmental-behavioral pediatrics* (4th ed.). Elsevier.

***Toddler**. In Diego's case having a strong-willed temperament and picky eating are not uncommon in toddler/preschool years. Coupling a growth mindset approach with the usual pediatric advice about offering a variety of foods on multiple occasions and in different ways provides a way to introduce the growth mindset concept to the family. Encouraging growth mindset in parents themselves may help them feel less frustrated and give them an opportunity to begin using process rather than person praise with their young son.*

***Elementary school student**. Evelyn, the second grader who is worried about not reading well and making mistakes, is showing signs of fixed mindset. Even if her father has a growth mindset, he can be encouraged to model the idea that challenges and mistakes are opportunities for learning. He can help her think about different strategies when she makes mistakes. Process praise can switch the emphasis to the process of learning in order to grow and strengthen her reading.*

***Preteen**. Ahmed, the fifth grader who is no longer the best soccer player on the team, is withdrawing from play. His parents can encourage Ahmed to focus on effort and practice and not be afraid of losing a goal or game. A mistake or loss can be viewed as a challenge and an opportunity to learn and grow.*

***Middle school student**. Chanel was bullied in the past and has transitioned to a new school year. It's important to find out what strategies she used to deal with bullying and explore how she views the bullies and herself. She can be taught to consider why the bully might be behaving that way, that people can change, and that her situation will likely improve with time as people change.*

***High school student**. Alex, the sophomore with diabetes and ADHD, has had trouble with monitoring his glucose and medication adherence. The pediatrician tells him about growth mindset as it applies to health—that these conditions are not solely determined by his genes and that health is malleable. His actions can have a significant effect in preventing poor outcomes related to both diabetes and ADHD.*

***College student**. Gabriella, the freshman Latina student, is having a difficult transition to college. She should be encouraged to join the campus group for first-generation students and seek counseling from college advisors. It's important for her to hear that the transition to college is difficult for many students, is likely to improve, and is not predictive of later success. A trusted mentor could also reinforce that she belongs in the university setting and that early setbacks do not mean she is unqualified but, instead, are opportunities to learn and improve.*

TABLE 101.3 Recommendations

Praise and Criticism
- Praise effort and improvement, not ability.
- Do not praise easy successes.
- Give honest, constructive critiques.

Convey That
- Abilities can be developed.
- Effort and learning make the brain grow stronger.
- Success is about progress, not easy perfection.

Show Children That
- Challenges are fun.
- Mistakes are interesting and helpful.

Reprinted from Dweck, C. S., & Master, A. (2009). Self-concept. In: *Developmental-behavioral pediatrics* (4th ed.). Elsevier.

WHAT ARE THE CAVEATS FOR IMPLEMENTING GROWTH MINDSET?

While evidence of the beneficial effects from promoting growth mindset is strong, there are caveats. Contexts are important. Linking process to an outcome, such as learning, can promote growth mindset. However, praising effort that has not been effective may be problematic—it may imply acceptance that children cannot learn and that they are receiving effort praise in consolation. For example, if a child with unidentified dyslexia puts forth consistent effort toward reading but isn't making progress, praise for the effort may sound hollow and undermine the child's effort. In this case the child needs a new approach and may need to seek help rather than continuing unfruitful efforts with the same strategy. Emphasizing effort or hard work may also be ineffective when it does not seem genuine or appears controlling or manipulative (Haimovitz & Dweck, 2017) (Table 101.3).

The term *false growth mindset* refers to a misunderstanding or oversimplification of the core message. Telling children to try hard may not be sufficient to foster a growth mindset. In classrooms the emphasis on effort should be coupled with offering other supports, such as good strategies, mentorship, connections, and access to resources (Dweck & Yeager, 2019). Some educators either provide information on growth mindset without any follow-up or resources to support students, or treat all children the same, leaving struggling students to feel "blamed" (i.e., due to lack of or not enough effort) or advanced students to remain unchallenged. Many unanswered questions include how to provide better support to parents and educators and how to create growth mindset cultures in homes and classrooms. Improved understanding of the use of process praise and what behaviors are motivating in the context of failures or success will be helpful in providing specific guidance.

HOW CAN WE APPLY MINDSET TO PUBLIC EDUCATION AND PUBLIC HEALTH?

Many of the interventions reviewed in this chapter have evolved to brief, online light touch interventions that are scalable. While the effect sizes on GPA (0.1–0.2 points) and other outcomes are small, when taken to scale these findings can have significant impact at a broader population level (Dweck & Yeager, 2019; Yeager et al., 2019). Such findings have policy implications for the education and health sectors.

In education several California school districts have adopted growth mindset as a core social-emotional learning competency. Analysis of a longitudinal dataset of 221,840 fourth- through seventh-grade students in California school districts found that growth compared to fixed mindset corresponded to increased average annual growth of .07 and .05 standard deviations in English and math, respectively, or an equivalent of 48 and 35 additional days of learning (Claro & Loeb, 2019). Education policymakers may be able to leverage evidence-based mindset interventions to reduce racial, gender, and social class achievement gaps (Rattan et al., 2015). Recommendations include federal funding and programs to implement existing mindset interventions and develop new ones, offering validated training to teachers, and establishing academic mindsets as a priority by the Department of Education, among others (Rattan et al., 2015).

In the area of health pediatric clinicians can empower parents and patients by counseling on growth mindset as it applies to health. A teen with diabetes can be taught that outcomes related to diabetes are not solely determined by her genes—her actions and behaviors with more frequent glucose monitoring and adherence to diet, medication, and exercise recommendations can have a significant impact on her long-term health. Such counseling could apply to other chronic illness for which there is decreased adherence during adolescence, such as ADHD. Parents can also be taught about growth mindset and encouraged to apply growth mindset principles to their parenting. Understanding the differences between process and person praise, modeling how to handle setbacks or mistakes, and conveying challenges and mistakes as opportunities for learning are strategies parents can use to provide a strong foundation for developing a growth mindset in children. Future research should continue to focus on how parents, in addition to teachers, can best foster growth mindsets.

CONCLUSION

Mindset is an example of a brief intervention with powerful and long-term effects. Clinicians should consider how to integrate mindset messages in their work. Similarly, education and public health interventions may benefit from inclusion of growth mindset messages. However, brief interventions are unlikely to solve severe or persistent problems and represent but one approach in a diverse armamentarium.

REFERENCES

Andersen, S. C., & Nielsen, H. S. (2016). Reading intervention with a growth mindset approach improves children's skills. *Proceedings of the National Academy of Sciences of the United States of America*, *113*(43), 12111–12113.

Aronson, J., Fried, C. B., & Good, C. (2002). Reducing the effects of stereotype threat on African American college students by shaping theories of intelligence. *Journal of Experimental Social Psychology*, *38*(2), 113–125. https://doi.org/10.1006/jesp.2001.1491

Blackwell, L. S., Trzesniewski, K. H., & Dweck, C. S. (2007). Implicit theories of intelligence predict achievement across an adolescent transition: A longitudinal study and an intervention. *Child Development*, *78*(1), 246–263.

Broda, M., Yun, J., Schneider, B., Yeager, D. S., Walton, G. M., & Diemer, M. (2018). Reducing inequality in academic success for incoming college students: A randomized trial of growth mindset and belonging interventions. *Journal of Research on Educational Effectiveness*, *11*(3), 317–338. https://doi.org/10.1080/19345747.2018.1429037

Burnette, J. L. (2010). Implicit theories of body weight: Entity beliefs can weigh you down. *Personality and Social Psychology Bulletin*, *36*(3), 410–422. https://doi.org/10.1177/0146167209359768

Claro, S., & Loeb, S. (2019). *Students with growth mindset learn more in school: Evidence from California's CORE school districts* [working paper]. https://files.eric.ed.gov/fulltext/ED600488.pdf

Dweck, C. S. (2006). *Mindset: The new psychology of success*. Random House.

Dweck, C. S., & Yeager, D. S. (2019). Mindsets: A view from two eras. *Perspectives on Psychological Science: A Journal of the Association for Psychological Science*, *14*(3), 481–496. https://doi.org/10.1177/1745691618804166

Ehrlinger, J., Burnette, J. L., Park, J., Harrold, M. L., & Orvidas, K. (2017). Incremental theories of weight and healthy eating behavior. *Journal of Applied Social Psychology*, *47*(6), 320–330. https://doi.org/10.1111/jasp.12439

Gunderson, E. A., Gripshover, S. J., Romero, C., Dweck, C. S., Goldin-Meadow, S., & Levine, S. C. (2013). Parent praise to 1- to 3-year-olds predicts children's motivational frameworks 5 years later. *Child Development*, *84*(5), 1526–1541.

Gunderson, E. A., Sorhagen, N. S., Gripshover, S. J., Dweck, C. S., Goldin-Meadow, S., & Levine, S. C. (2018). Parent praise to toddlers predicts fourth grade academic achievement via children's incremental mindsets. *Developmental Psychology*, *54*(3), 397–409. https://doi.org/10.1037/dev0000444

Haimovitz, K., & Dweck, C. S. (2017). The origins of children's growth and fixed mindsets: New research and a new proposal. *Child Development*, *88*(6), 1849–1859.

John-Henderson, N. A., Tintzman, C. S., Counts, C. J., & Mueller, C. M. (2020). Health mindsets as a predictor of physical activity and body mass index in American Indian college students. *Journal of Health Psychology*, *26*(12). https://doi.org/10.1177/1359105319901284

John-Henderson, N., Wright, R., Fotuhi, O., Zuckerman, B., Nally, L., & Mueller, C. M. (2021). The influence of health mindset on perceptions of illness and behaviors among adolescents. *International Journal of Behavioral Medicine*. https://doi.org/10.1007/s12529-021-09972-2

Joseph, G. P., Segovia, N. A., Wright, R. C., Mueller, C., & Tileston, K. R. (2020). Mindset correlates with health-related quality of life assessment in patients with adolescent idiopathic scoliosis. *Spine Deformity*. https://doi.org/10.1007/s43390-020-00243-w

Mueller, C. M., & Dweck, C. S. (1998). Praise for intelligence can undermine children's motivation and performance. *Journal of Personality & Social Psychology*, *75*(1), 33–52.

Mueller, C., Rowe, M. L., & Zuckerman, B. (2017). Mindset matters for parents and adolescents. *JAMA Pediatrics*, *171*(5), 415–416. https://doi.org/10.1001/jamapediatrics.2016.5160

Park, D., Gunderson, E. A., Tsukayama, E., Levine, S. C., & Beilock, S. L. (2016). Young children's motivational frameworks and math achievement: Relation to teacher-reported instructional practices, but not teacher theory of intelligence. *Journal of Educational Psychology*, *108*(3), 300–313. https://doi.org/10.1037/edu0000064

Paunesku, D., Walton, G. M., Romero, C., Smith, E. N., Yeager, D. S., & Dweck, C. S. (2015). Mind-set interventions are a scalable treatment for academic underachievement. *Psychological Science*, *26*(6), 784–793. https://doi.org/10.1177/0956797615571017

Pomerantz, E. M., & Kempner, S. G. (2013). Mothers' daily person and process praise: Implications for children's theory of intelligence and motivation. *Developmental Psychology*, *49*(11), 2040–2046. https://doi.org/10.1037/a0031840

Rattan, A., Savani, K., Chugh, D., & Dweck, C. S. (2015). Leveraging mindsets to promote academic achievement: Policy recommendations. *Perspectives on Psychological Science: A Journal of the Association for Psychological Science*, *10*(6), 721–726.

Robinson, T. N., Matheson, D., Desai, M., Wilson, D. M., Weintraub, D. L., Haskell, W. L., McClain, A., McClure, S., Banda, A. J., Sanders, L. M., Haydel, K. F., & Killen, J. D. (2013). Family, community and clinic collaboration to treat overweight and obese children: Stanford GOALS—A randomized controlled trial of a three-year, multi-component, multi-level, multi-setting intervention. *Contemporary Clinical Trials*, *36*(2), 421–435. https://doi.org/10.1016/j.cct.2013.09.001

Rowe, M. L., & Leech, K. A. (2019). A parent intervention with a growth mindset approach improves children's early gesture and vocabulary development. *Developmental Science*, *22*(4), e12792. https://doi.org/10.1111/desc.12792

Sujka, J., St., Peter, S., & Mueller, C. M. (2018). Do health beliefs affect pain perception after pectus excavatum repair? *Pediatric Surgery International*, *34*(12), 1363–1367. https://doi.org/10.1007/s00383-018-4354-x

Thai, C. L., Rice, E. L., Taber, J. M., Kaufman, A. R., & Klein, W. M. P. (2020). Implicit theories of smoking and association with interest in quitting among current smokers. *Journal of Behavioral Medicine*, *43*(4), 544–552. https://doi.org/10.1007/s10865-019-00058-9

Walton, M. & Yeager, D. S. (2020). Seed and soil: Psychological affordances in contexts help to explain where wise interventions succeed or fail. *Current Directions in Psychological Science*, *29*(3), 219–226. https://doi.org/http://dx.doi.org/10.1177/0963721420904453

Yeager, D. S., Hanselman, P., Walton, G. M., Murray, J. S., Crosnoe, R., Muller, C., Tipton, E., Schneider, B., Hulleman, C. S., Hinojosa, C. P., Paunesku, D., Romero, C., Flint, K., Roberts, A., Trott, J., Iachan, R., Buontempo, J., Yang, S. M., Carvalho, C. M., Dweck, C. S. (2019). A national experiment reveals where a growth mindset improves achievement. *Nature*, *573*(7774), 364–369. https://doi.org/10.1038/s41586-019-1466-y

Yeager, D. S., Johnson, R., Spitzer, B. J., Trzesniewski, K. H., Powers, J., & Dweck, C. S. (2014). The far-reaching effects of believing people can change: implicit theories of personality shape stress, health, and achievement during adolescence. *Journal of Personality & Social Psychology*, *106*(6), 867–884. https://doi.org/10.1037/a0036335

Yeager, D. S., Trzesniewski, K. H., & Dweck, C. S. (2013). An implicit theories of personality intervention reduces adolescent aggression in response to victimization and exclusion. *Child Development*, *84*(3), 970–988. https://doi.org/10.1111/cdev.12003

Yeager, D. S., Trzesniewski, K. H., Tirri, K., Nokelainen, P., & Dweck, C. S. (2011). Adolescents' implicit theories predict desire for vengeance after peer conflicts: Correlational and experimental evidence. *Developmental Psychology*, *47*(4), 1090–1107. https://doi.org/10.1037/a0023769

Yeager, D. S., Walton, G. M., Brady, S. T., Akcinar, E. N., Paunesku, D., Keane, L., Kamentz, D., Ritter, G., Duckworth, A. L., Urstein, R., Gomez, E. M., Markus, H. R., Cohen, G. L., & Dweck, C. S. (2016). Teaching a lay theory before college narrows achievement gaps at scale. *Proceedings of the National Academy of Sciences of the United States of America*, *113*(24), e3341–e3348. https://doi.org/10.1073/pnas.1524360113.

102

Treatment of Developmental, Behavioral, and Mental Health Conditions via Technology

Philip B. Cawkwell, Bayan Jalalizadeh, Eric McDonald, and John E. Leikauf

For additional material related to the content of this chapter, please see Chapter 46.

VIGNETTE

Emma, mother to Jeremy (age 12) and Ella (age 8), is preparing for a follow-up visit with the children's behavioral health clinician. Despite living 200 miles from the medical center, she has been able to access care directly in her home, via a telehealth application. In anticipation of the visit she has filled out psychometric evaluation forms for both children, which have been automatically scored and uploaded for the clinician to assess. She checks that Jeremy's smart watch has also uploaded his recent sleep log and activity tracker for review. Jeremy may have a mood disorder and has completed digital cognitive-behavioral exercises and biofeedback sessions; the clinician will review the daily mood and symptom ratings that have been provided via smartphone to determine the next steps. Ella was recently diagnosed with attention-deficit/hyperactivity disorder (ADHD), inattentive presentation. She has been playing a videogame designed to improve her focus; data from her recent sessions have been sent to the clinician. She has also been using a (VR) virtual reality device to overcome her phobia of public speaking. The clinician logs in and congratulates the family on their adherence to these digital treatments.

INTRODUCTION

Although this futuristic scenario may seem implausible, all the technologies discussed in the opening vignette are in various stages of development, from early research studies to recent US Food and Drug Administration (FDA; 2019a, 2019b) approvals. The World Health Organization (2007) defines health technology as the "application of organized knowledge and skills in the form of devices, medicines, vaccines, procedures and systems developed to solve a health problem and improve quality of lives." Technology in health care is rapidly evolving. The potential is vast. In this chapter we will consider a diverse array of applications of technology for treatment of behavioral and developmental health conditions, including telehealth, phone and app-based treatments, wearable devices, VR, videogames, and procedural technologies.

TELEHEALTH

The Centers for Medicare & Medicaid Services defines telehealth as two-way, real-time, audio and visual interaction between a patient and a clinician at a distant location (American Academy of Child and Adolescent Psychiatry [AACAP], 2021a). First developed by the National Aeronautics and Space Administration in the 1970s for use during space travel, telehealth had, until recently, been seen largely as a way to reach remote or otherwise underserved communities, particularly with specialty care such as pediatric mental and behavioral health services that are in limited supply (AACAP, 2021a; Soares & Langkamp, 2012). Significant advantages include time and travel saved, ease of assembling multiple participants from the patient's life and/or clinical teams, insight into a patient's living conditions, and potentially greater comfort on the part of some patients.

Telehealth services remained in limited use until the COVID-19 pandemic. In March and April 2020 many outpatient health care clinicians rapidly switched to full-time or nearly full-time telehealth practices. Among privately insured individual medical visits, the proportion of telehealth claims increased 86-fold in April 2020 compared with April 2019 (Herzer & Pronovost, 2021). Factors that enabled such a rapid change in clinical practice included widespread availability of broadband Internet access, devices allowing synchronous two-way audio-video communication, software enabling secure or encrypted audio and video communication appropriate for patient confidentiality and Health Insurance Portability and Accountability Act compliance, and the willingness of both payers and regulators to facilitate remote visits (Zulman & Verghese, 2021). These experiences will undoubtedly have a transformational effect on service delivery in the years to come. It remains to be seen exactly when families, clinicians, and payers choose telehealth when it again becomes discretional.

Prepandemic evidence regarding telehealth visits for mental health generally supports feasibility and acceptance across a variety of studied clinical encounter types, with more limited evidence for clinical effectiveness and cost savings (Bashshur et al., 2016). Herzer and Pronovost (2021) have recommended considering the following principles in evaluating the value and quality of telehealth in the future relative to in-person clinical care: safe and effective, efficient and timely, patient centered, and equitable. Professional organizations, including the AACAP (2021a) and the American Academy of Pediatrics (AAP, 2021), have provided useful online guides that include primers on the use of telehealth. These guides are becoming increasingly nuanced and updated as experience grows. Of particular interest to readers of this volume may be sources such as guidelines for interviews of youth with neurodevelopmental disorders (AACAP, 2021b). However, best practices for many scenarios still have yet to be determined.

Despite the recent success in rolling out telehealth rapidly on a massive scale, several challenges remain. Telehealth visits can address specific disparities in health care access related to the dimensions of time and space. Fundamentally, telehealth does not increase the number of health care clinicians; subspecialists will likely remain undersupplied, thus limiting access. Access to the physical equipment and the skills to effectively communicate with digital technology are unevenly distributed throughout the population, including among health care clinicians. We can anticipate residency programs increasing formal standards for training in telehealth modalities appropriate to different specialties and significant need for continuing medical education modules in this area, but these processes will take time (Accreditation Council for Graduate Medical Education, 2020). It is also likely that new and unforeseen demands will be placed on clinicians, such as increased patient load, ergonomic challenges, and the phenomenon of Zoom fatigue (Bailenson, 2021), the experience that interactions via videoconference are significantly more tiring than in-person interactions. For patient skills, extensive formal training in the technology used by health care networks seems likely to be limited. Similarly, while it is not hard to envision scenarios in which giving a mobile device to a patient may be worth the cost from a system point of view, it is questionable whether this cost will be borne by health care payers. The Federal Communications Commission (2021) estimates that 14.5 million Americans do not have access to broadband service where they live and that approximately 100 million Americans still do not subscribe to broadband Internet service. Will these services eventually be seen as a necessary part of health care? If so, who will be seen as rightfully paying for them?

PHONE- AND APPLICATION-BASED TREATMENTS

As smartphones and mobile devices equipped with Internet access and sensors have proliferated, so too have efforts to create programs, or applications (apps), or "software functions" under current FDA terminology, that assist in clinical care. Health-related apps are available to the almost 4 billion smartphone users worldwide (Statista, 2022). Through the last 2 decades, innovation was happening very quickly in this space, though health care has traditionally been slower than other sectors of the economy to adopt new technologies due largely to concerns about safety and efficacy and rigors of the regulatory process.

The FDA regulates software functions using the same risk-based framework as it uses for other medical devices. Smartphones and tablets themselves are not considered medical devices and are not regulated by the FDA. However, historically, the FDA has regulated "software as a medical device" in which software was generally attached or complementary to the function of hardware, such as within a magnetic resonance imaging scanner or an electrocardiogram, and with slower update cycles. Such devices classified as moderate (class II) or high risk (class III) continue to require significant premarket review (Shuren et al., 2018). The FDA released guidance in 2013, updated in 2015 and 2019, clarifying its current position that many software functions do not carry the same level of risk and so will not be subject to FDA review; the hope is that this new process facilitates innovation and access. It was also recognized that many software functions exist cross-platform and are updated weekly based on rapid feedback from user interactions; it would be impractical to submit each software update for each platform separately to regulatory review, and many such updates have little impact on risk level to users (FDA, 2019a)

Software functions that generally do not qualify as a device and thus do not need regulatory review include those that (1) help patients self-manage a condition without providing specific treatment suggestions, (2) automate simple tasks for health care clinicians, or (3) facilitate communication with health care clinics. The FDA also clarified that it intends to exercise discretion in enforcing regulation of software functions that may qualify as a device but pose low risk. Many of these are in the behavioral health space, including functions that help maintain coping skills, provide motivational reminders, provide location information via Global Positioning System related to health conditions (e.g., preidentified high-risk areas for persons with substance use disorders), and enhance motivation for exercise through videogames (FDA, 2019b).

Clinicians prefer recommending treatments, including software, that have been shown to work in randomized, controlled, clinical trials (RCTs). A recent estimate found that only about 2% of mobile health apps had been evaluated in published articles, the vast majority for adults (Martínez-Pérez et al., 2015). Another recent metaanalysis found 37 studies evaluating mobile health apps for youth (Fedele, 2017), most targeting behavior change for chronic disease, with a modest effect size overall ($d = 0.22$). Specific complicating issues arise in the conduct and evaluation of studies of mobile apps that may limit the number of studies performed relative to the number of apps available. Automated mobile consent processes, which are commonly used in studies of apps for adults and necessary for scale, are not always possible for enrolling persons under age 18, particularly for youth with developmental and behavioral challenges. It is not clear how to evaluate the efficacy of "blinding" in placebo or sham conditions or the practicality of evaluating a continually evolving software function within a controlled trial. Technology companies with popular products (e.g., Amazon, Facebook, Google) continuously randomize users to different experimental conditions without the consent or knowledge of the user as they test new features and modifications to software.

Experimentation on users without their knowledge or consent is not the culture or practice in health care; informed consent is a bedrock principle of research on clinical interventions. Finally, privacy concerns are significant. The mobile devices are not regulated as medical devices and yet many apps along with the operating systems themselves collect very large amounts of data from users. Therefore some loss of privacy is inherent in use of the devices, even if the software function of interest is low or minimal risk. In the absence of high-quality evidence for the efficacy of most mobile health apps the American Psychiatric Association has offered a comprehensive model online at psychiatry.org for evaluating mobile health tools in clinical practice.

WEARABLE DEVICES

Worn devices, ranging from wristbands and smart watches to shirts with embedded textile sensors, are being developed and actively studied for their potential to promote early intervention, monitor physiologic data, improve adherence and efficacy, and develop new treatment modalities. Their functional features typically involve accelerometers and actigraphy, light and audio sensors, eye tracking, electrode systems, and interactive displays. Many wearable electronic devices provide monitoring and feedback to users; preliminary findings show that feedback systems are more likely to be used if the user interface is perceived as accessible and the feedback provided is objective and transparent (Choo et al., 2017).

In the monitoring of symptoms and signs wearable devices can measure movement, light, vital signs, heart rate variability, respiration activity, and unobtrusive passive analytics. Some devices, for example, combine measured physical data along with multiple-daily cognitive tasks and brief mood assessments to follow severity of specific psychiatric diagnoses (Cormack et al., 2019).

Another potential use of wearable technologies is for medication adherence monitoring. As one example, patients can take ingestible digital tablets along with their prescribed medication to track frequency of medication ingestion and vital signs (Kane et al., 2013). As another example, a piezoelectric necklace was developed, which can distinguish among medicine swallows and other movements of the neck and mouth; these data can be coupled with smart pill bottle technologies to determine frequency of medicine use (Kalantarian et al., 2016).

Wearable devices can also be used for immediate feedback during therapeutic processes. For example, small audio recording devices placed in the pocket of clothing can quantify a child's communicative interactions and environmental audio data and interface with smartphone applications to display prompts or visual rewards to assist children undergoing speech and language therapy practice in the home environment (Choo et al., 2017).

An increasing number of wearable devices seek to facilitate treatment of psychiatric and developmental disorders by means of biofeedback. These are being studied for various modalities of biofeedback, including heart rate and heart rate variability, electromyography, electrodermal activity, skin temperature, respiratory feedback of end-tidal carbon dioxide, and electroencephalography (EEG) (Hunkin et al., 2019). However, high-quality research on the efficacy of biofeedback in the treatment of pediatric psychiatric and developmental disorders is thus far lacking.

Visual stimuli and feedback can be utilized by wearable glasses technologies for a variety of purposes, including improvement in socialization in children with autism spectrum disorder (Voss et al., 2019). However, data are still sparse regarding the broad applicability and effectiveness of wearable visual technologies for the treatment of psychiatric and developmental disorders.

VIRTUAL REALITY

While VR in its earliest forms has existed since the 1960s, it is just now becoming affordable and available to the average consumer. Within medicine, research is underway on the potential uses of VR, understanding factors that improve effectiveness, and VR's applications for treatment. VR has shown promise in the treatment of anxiety disorders, such as through repeated exposure, and prevention of pain, such as through distraction.

The goal of VR is to immerse the user into a computer-generated world, which substitutes for the real world to create the sensation of being in an interactive, life-sized environment. Two factors comprise the VR's sense of presence (i.e., its immersiveness) for the user: place illusion (PI) and plausibility illusion (Psi) (Slater, 2009). PI refers to the ability of VR to create the sense of "being there" by matching the contingencies of the brain's sense of head rotation, movement, leaning, or other positional data with what is visually being seen. The closer the match, the better the PI. Psi refers to how the virtual environment reacts to the user and to itself. The better the physics of a ball flying through the air in the VR match what is experienced in reality, the better the Psi. If a computer-generated human reacts to the user entering its surrounding space (i.e., making eye contact briefly or keeping appropriate physical distance), the better the Psi for the user.

Given that VR's usefulness in treatment, particularly for anxiety, hinges on its ability to create mock exposures to life-like situations, the better the PI and Psi, and thus the VR's presence, the more effective treatment it will be. Exposures via VR prove particularly advantageous when compared to in vivo in situations that (1) may be dangerous (e.g., a venomous spider), (2) are difficult to access repeatedly (e.g., an operating room), and (3) may be enhanced with real-time coaching and feedback from a therapist. Additionally, VR environments may be tightly controlled to allow for specific gradation in the intensity and duration of the exposure. One RCT provided a preoperative VR of the operating theater as intervention to children scheduled for elective surgery ($n = 69$) resulting in lower Yale Preoperative Anxiety Scale scores as well as better marks on the Induction Compliance Checklist and the

Procedural Behavior Rating Scale (Ryu et al., 2017). A similar RCT showed diminished preoperative anxiety with a preoperative VR intervention (Eijlers et al., 2019).

VR has also been studied as an intervention for pain in multiple settings, including oncologic care and venous access. Used as distraction during the painful procedures, it was found to be significantly more effective in reducing pain and anxiety than care as usual in a metaanalysis. While it was "difficult to differentiate between the added value of VR over other forms of distraction (e.g. watching television)," VR creates a significantly more immersive experience than other forms of distraction, which may result in more pain reduction as it limits attention available for pain perception (Eijlers et al., 2019).

Limitations of the current literature on VR is that it is centered around support for novel uses for VR rather than methodologically rigorous evaluations of efficacy. Furthermore, many studies thus far have relied on self-report (Eijlers et al., 2019). Ultimately there is clear theoretical plausibility for VR's effectiveness in treatment and prevention of anxiety and pain, which has so far been corroborated by preliminary studies and therefore warrants further, more rigorous study.

VIDEOGAMES

Videogames have continually increased in popularity, dating back to the 1970s with the introduction of games such as *Pong* and *Space Invaders*, initially played in arcades. In 2020 three in four households have at least one person who plays videogames (Entertainment Software Association, 2020). Negative impacts of videogame playing, such as the potential for addiction, have long been the focus of medical research. Recently, however, the concept of videogames as a treatment tool has been given serious focus. In June 2020 the FDA granted clearance to the first prescription treatment delivered via videogame, *EndeavorRx*.

EndeavorRx is a videogame played on a cell phone or tablet, where children navigate a character through a course while collecting targets and avoiding obstacles. The device makers describe it as a "digital therapeutic ... designed to improve attention and related cognitive control processes by training interferences management." A randomized, double-blind trial of 348 patients aged 8 to 12 years with ADHD found that 4 weeks of this intervention resulted in significant improvement on the Test of Variables of Attention (TOVA—a computer-based continuous performance test) compared to the placebo (a videogame that targeted cognitive domains not associated with ADHD) (Kollins et al., 2020).

In the mental health sphere several RCTs have been conducted looking at therapeutic videogames for anxiety reduction in teens (Barnes & Prescott, 2018). *MindLight* is a game where players are taught cognitive-behavioral therapy techniques and use a glowing light on their head (which reacts to EEG activity) to navigate through the virtual world. *Dojo* is a game in which players are taught coping skills by the "dojo master," including deep breathing, after which the player undertakes tasks. Both games have shown potential to decrease anxiety symptoms, although questions around adaptability, feasibility, duration of effect, and comparison to gold standard treatment remain unanswered. Limitations and concerns about utilizing videogames for mental health treatment must be considered. As of now, few studies have compared videogames to a psychotherapeutic gold standard, many do not contain a robust control group, longitudinal studies are lacking, and the sample sizes in a majority of these studies are quite limited.

PROCEDURAL TECHNOLOGIC INTERVENTION

ADHD is a high-prevalence neurodevelopmental disorder that warrants the attention of clinicians for early intervention to mitigate risk of complications later in life (see Chapter 46). Currently, stimulant medications, the first-line treatment, come with several adverse effects, such as for irritability, sleep disturbances, decreased appetite, and growth suppression. Other avenues may allow treatment without adverse effects. Two promising noninvasive procedures with minimal risk include trigeminal nerve stimulant (TNS) and EEG neurofeedback (NF) (McGough et al., 2019).

The rationale for TNS is that the trigeminal nerve has connections with the locus coeruleus, reticular activating system, and solitary tract, and that these brain regions are involved in a variety of cognitive functions, including maintenance of attention. TNS has been shown on positron emission tomography to activate multiple brain regions, including the anterior cingulate cortex and the parietotemporal cortex, which have been associated with ADHD and executive functioning (McGough et al., 2019). TNS is minimally invasive; it consists of a device with small wires that run to an adhesive electrode worn across the forehead over the V1 branch of the trigeminal nerve, which emits a low-level current while the child is asleep (McGough et al., 2019). As of 2020, two studies by McGough and colleagues, including an open trial and a sham-controlled double blind study, have shown promise for the effectiveness of TNS in treatment of ADHD symptoms. In the pilot study TNS was well accepted by the patients and their families and was not associated with any clinically meaningful side effects or adverse events. The first RCT demonstrated efficacy of TNS over a sham treatment. The Monarch external TNS system was the first device approved by the FDA for treatment of ADHD. These studies are yet to be replicated to solidify its role as a regular treatment.

NF is a promising nonpharmacologic intervention for ADHD. It works through improvement of self-regulation of brain activity through a brain-computer interface. NF possibly relies on procedural learning, which may result in longer clinical benefits than traditional treatment (Van Doren et al., 2019). NF protocols have yet to be standardized; most studies have not been adequately blinded. These features limit the evidence for efficacy, despite several RCTs and metaanalyses (Van Doren et al., 2019). NF, as of this writing, shows promise for sustained clinical benefit without continued NF training at 2- to 12-month followup.

CONCLUSIONS AND LIMITATIONS TO TREATMENT WITH TECHNOLOGY

The potential clinical use of new technologies, particularly those that leverage recent advances in consumer communication and information technology, for the management of psychiatric, neurological, and developmental disorders is exciting. Many of the technological advances we saw in the opening vignette regarding Jeremy and Ella have arrived, such as telehealth visits and electronic psychometric evaluations. Wearable devices and therapeutic videogames are being actively tested in high-quality randomized clinical trials. These approaches may substantially alter clinical practice in the near future. However, several limitations must be considered. First, development of such technologies is still in the early stages. Most technologic treatments have few, if any, ratings of efficacy or effectiveness from clinical trials. Many have not yet been directly compared against current gold standard treatments (Miralles et al., 2020). While measurements of physiologic signs by wearable devices are beginning to show promise, there appear to be significant differences across individual studies at this time.

Second, even with the previously discussed relaxation of regulation of mobile apps, the process for development and approval of medical technologies is still adapting to new technologies and will need to continue to evolve. There will almost certainly be lags as the regulatory process catches up. In addition to the challenges outlined earlier with mobile apps, emerging artificial intelligence technologies are widely expected to proliferate throughout decision making in clinical medicine. The current regulatory approach does not properly account for fundamental issues, including sources of bias and the need to evaluate on prospective data that are inherent in machine learning and artificial intelligence algorithms (Wu et al., 2021).

Third, these technologies allow various third parties to interact with individuals' personal health information, including app developers, live mediators, and Internet carriers. These third parties do not have the same ethical and legal responsibilities as health care professionals when managing personal health information (Martínez-Pérez et al., 2015). It is important to determine who owns the users' data, who may access such data, in what contexts they may do so, and whether any single party bears the responsibility for the well-being or harm of the patients when using particular technologies. When data are collected on large scales, risks include the introduction of measurement bias, population bias, and selection bias. Missing data due to user adherence or unforeseen errors need to be considered to avoid incorrect data interpretation and ineffective treatment recommendations (Hicks et al., 2019). These issues will only increase in importance with the wide proliferation of artificial intelligence algorithms.

Fourth, a technology, mobile application, or device is unlikely to be utilized if there is poor perceived user experience, high perceived complexity, specific knowledge needed for use, an inability to offer services in the needed languages, or a lack of a culturally informed approach (Baldwin et al., 2017). Limitations in cost, device availability, and Internet access can also inadvertently prevent specific populations from receiving such technologic interventions, significantly impacting the feasibility of these tools and introducing the ethical challenge of just and equitable provision of care (Aamir et al., 2018).

The rapid advances in technology in recent decades push our field to adapt our clinical, regulatory, and research practice. If we can keep up, tools like telehealth, virtual reality, and mobile device monitoring of symptoms may in the near future, seem as routine to patients like Jeremy and Ella as the stethoscope and x-ray do to patients and clinicians today.

REFERENCES

Aamir, J., Ali, S. M., Kamel Boulos, M. N., Anjum, N., & Ishaq, M. (2018). Enablers and inhibitors: A review of the situation regarding mHealth adoption in low- and middle-income countries. *Health Policy and Technology*, *7*(1), 88–97. https://doi.org/10.1016/j.hlpt.2017.11.005

Accreditation Council for Graduate Medical Education. (2020). *ACGME response to COVID-19: Clarification regarding telemedicine and ACGME surveys*. https://acgme.org/Newsroom/Blog/Details/ArticleID/10125/ACGME-Response-to-COVID-19-Clarification-regarding-Telemedicine-and-ACGME-Surveys

American Academy of Child and Adolescent Psychiatry. (2021a). *Telepsychiatry*. https://www.aacap.org/telepsychiatry

American Academy of Child and Adolescent Psychiatry. (2021b). *Tips for clinicians treating patients diagnosed with neurodevelopmental disorders via telepsychiatry*. https://www.aacap.org/App_Themes/AACAP/Docs/clinical_practice_center/business_of_practice/Telepsych/NDD_Tip_Sheet_Clinician_Version.pdf

American Academy of Pediatrics. (2021). *Telehealth support*. https://www.aap.org/en-us/professional-resources/practice-transformation/telehealth/Pages/What-is-Telehealth.aspx

Bailenson, J. N. (2021). Nonverbal overload: A theoretical argument for the causes of zoom fatigue. *Technology, Mind, and Behavior*, *2*(1). https://doi.org/10.1037/tmb0000030

Baldwin, J. L., Singh, H., Sittig, D. F., & Giardina, T. D. (2017). Patient portals and health apps: Pitfalls, promises, and what one might learn from the other. *Healthcare*, *5*(3), 81–85. https://doi.org/10.1016/j.hjdsi.2016.08.004

Barnes, S., & Prescott, J. (2018). Empirical evidence for the outcomes of therapeutic video games for adolescents with anxiety disorders: Systematic review. *JMIR Serious Games*, *6*(1), e3. https://doi.org/10.2196/games.9530

Bashshur, R. L., Shannon, G. W., Bashshur, N., & Yellowlees, P. M. (2016). The empirical evidence for telemedicine interventions in mental disorders. *Telemedicine Journal and E-Health*, *22*(2), 87–113. https://doi.org/10.1089/tmj.2015.0206

Choo, D., Dettman, S., Dowell, R., & Cowan, R. (2017). Talking to toddlers: Drawing on mothers' perceptions of using wearable and mobile technology in the home. *Studies in Health Technology and Informatics*, *239*, 21–27.

Cormack, F., McCue, M., Taptiklis, N., Skirrow, C., Glazer, E., Panagopoulos, E., ... Barnett, J. H. (2019). Wearable technology for high-frequency cognitive and mood assessment in major depressive disorder: Longitudinal observational study. *JMIR Mental Health*, *6*(11), e12814. https://doi.org/10.2196/12814

Eijlers, R., Utens, E., Staals, L. M., de Nijs, P. F. A., Berghmans, J. M., Wijnen, R. M. H., ... Legerstee, J. S. (2019). Systematic review and meta-analysis of virtual reality in pediatrics: Effects on pain and anxiety. *Anesthesia and Analgesia*, *129*(5), 1344–1353. https://doi.org/10.1213/ane.0000000000004165

Entertainment Software Association. (2020). *2020 essential facts about the video game industry*. https://www.theesa.com/wp-content/uploads/2020/07/Final-Edited-2020-ESA_Essential_facts.pdf

Fedele, D. A., Cushing, C. C., Fritz, A., Amaro, C. M., & Ortega, A. (2017). Mobile health interventions for improving health outcomes in youth: A meta-analysis. *JAMA Pediatrics*, 171(5), 461–469.

Federal Communications *Commission*. (2021). *Annual broadband deployment report*.

Herzer, K. R., & Pronovost, P. J. (2021). Ensuring quality in the era of virtual care. *JAMA*, *325*(5), 429–430. https://doi.org/10.1001/jama.2020.24955

Hicks, J. L., Althoff, T., Sosic, R., Kuhar, P., Bostjancic, B., King, A. C., … Delp, S. L. (2019). Best practices for analyzing large-scale health data from wearables and smartphone apps. *NPJ Digital Medicine*, *2*, 45. https://doi.org/10.1038/s41746-019-0121-1

Hunkin, H., King, D. L., & Zajac, I. T. (2019). Wearable devices as adjuncts in the treatment of anxiety-related symptoms: A narrative review of five device modalities and implications for clinical practice. *Clinical Psychology: Science and Practice*, *26*(3), e12290.

Kalantarian, H., Motamed, B., Alshurafa, N., & Sarrafzadeh, M. (2016). A wearable sensor system for medication adherence prediction. *Artificial Intelligence in Medicine*, *69*, 43–52. https://doi.org/10.1016/j.artmed.2016.03.004

Kane, J. M., Perlis, R. H., DiCarlo, L. A., Au-Yeung, K., Duong, J., & Petrides, G. (2013). First experience with a wireless system incorporating physiologic assessments and direct confirmation of digital tablet ingestions in ambulatory patients with schizophrenia or bipolar disorder. *Journal of Clinical Psychiatry*, *74*(6), e533–e540. https://doi.org/10.4088/JCP.12m08222

Kollins, S. H., DeLoss, D. J., Cañadas, E., Lutz, J., Findling, R. L., Keefe, R. S. E., … Faraone, S. V. (2020). A novel digital intervention for actively reducing severity of paediatric ADHD (STARS-ADHD): A randomised controlled trial. *The Lancet Digital Health*, *2*(4), e168–e178. https://doi.org/10.1016/S2589-7500(20)30017-0

Martínez-Pérez, B., de la Torre-Díez, I., & López-Coronado, M. (2015). Privacy and security in mobile health apps: A review and recommendations. *Journal of Medical Systems*, *39*(1), 181. https://doi.org/10.1007/s10916-014-0181-3

McGough, J. J., Sturm, A., Cowen, J., Tung, K., Salgari, G. C., Leuchter, A. F., … Loo, S. K. (2019). Double-blind, sham-controlled, pilot study of trigeminal nerve stimulation for attention-deficit/hyperactivity disorder. *Journal of the American Academy of Child and Adolescent Psychiatry*, *58*(4), 403–411. https://doi.org/10.1016/j.jaac.2018.11.013. e403.

Miralles, I., Granell, C., Díaz-Sanahuja, L., Van Woensel, W., Bretón-López, J., Mira, A., … Casteleyn, S. (2020). Smartphone apps for the treatment of mental disorders: Systematic review. *JMIR mHealth and uHealth*, *8*(4), e14897. https://doi.org/10.2196/14897

Ryu, J. H., Park, S. J., Park, J. W., Kim, J. W., Yoo, H. J., Kim, T. W., … Han, S. H. (2017). Randomized clinical trial of immersive virtual reality tour of the operating theatre in children before anaesthesia. *British Journal of Surgery*, *104*(12), 1628–1633. https://doi.org/10.1002/bjs.10684

Shuren, J., Patel, B., & Gottlieb, S. (2018). FDA regulation of mobile medical apps. *JAMA*, *320*(4), 337–338. https://doi.org/10.1001/jama.2018.8832

Slater, M. (2009). Place illusion and plausibility can lead to realistic behaviour in immersive virtual environments. *Philosophical Transactions of the Royal Society of London B Biological Sciences*, *364*(1535), 3549–3557. https://doi.org/10.1098/rstb.2009.0138

Soares, N. S., & Langkamp, D. L. (2012). Telehealth in developmental-behavioral pediatrics. *Journal of Developmental and Behavioral Pediatrics*, *33*(8), 656–665. https://doi.org/10.1097/DBP.0b013e3182690741

Statista. (2022). *Number of smartphone users worldwide from 2016 to 2023*. https://www.statista.com/statistics/330695/number-of-smartphone-users-worldwide/

US Food and Drug Administration. (2019a). *Device software functions including mobile medical applications*. https://www.fda.gov/medical-devices/digital-health-center-excellence/device-software-functions-including-mobile-medical-applications

US Food and Drug Administration. (2019b). *Examples of software functions for which the FDA will exercise enforcement discretion*. https://www.fda.gov/medical-devices/device-software-functions-including-mobile-medical-applications/examples-software-functions-which-fda-will-exercise-enforcement-discretion

Van Doren, J., Arns, M., Heinrich, H., Vollebregt, M. A., Strehl, U., & Loo, S. K. (2019). Sustained effects of neurofeedback in ADHD: A systematic review and meta-analysis. *European Child and Adolescent Psychiatry*, *28*(3), 293–305. https://doi.org/10.1007/s00787-018-1121-4

Voss, C., Schwartz, J., Daniels, J., Kline, A., Haber, N., Washington, P., … Wall, D. P. (2019). Effect of wearable digital intervention for improving socialization in children with autism spectrum disorder: A randomized clinical trial. *JAMA Pediatrics*, *173*(5), 446–454. https://doi.org/10.1001/jamapediatrics.2019.0285

World Health Organization. (2007). *Health technology assessment*. https://www.who.int/health-technology-assessment/about/healthtechnology/en/

Wu, E., Wu, K., Daneshjou, R., Ouyang, D., Ho, D. E., & Zou, J. (2021). How medical AI devices are evaluated: Limitations and recommendations from an analysis of FDA approvals. *Nature Medicine*, *27*(4), 582–584. https://doi.org/10.1038/s41591-021-01312-x

Zulman, D. M., & Verghese, A. (2021). Virtual care, telemedicine visits, and real connection in the era of COVID-19: Unforeseen opportunity in the face of adversity. *JAMA*, *325*(5), 437–438. https://doi.org/10.1001/jama.2020.27304

103

Early Intervention

Dawn M. Magnusson and Mary A. Khetani

For additional material related to the content of this chapter, please see Chapters 6, 7, 81, 104, and 113.

VIGNETTES

1. *Elijah is 18 months old and has a 25% delay in his communication skills. He points to objects and people but does not say any words. Elijah is an only child, and his primary caregiver is a former preschool teacher who stays home with him. He began receiving early intervention services 3 months ago, and his individualized family service plan (IFSP) includes one 60-minute speech therapy session per month at home. During these visits, Elijah's caregiver and therapist discuss and practice ways they can encourage Elijah's expressive communication and manage their evening routines more smoothly.*
2. *Jade is 18 months old and has a 25% delay in her gross motor skills. Although she is walking independently, she easily loses her balance and prefers crawling up/down stairs. Jade is the youngest of four children whose caregivers work full time. She began receiving early intervention services 3 months ago, and her IFSP includes weekly 30-minute physical therapy sessions at a large, center-based childcare program. During these sessions, Jade's therapist facilitates her participation in center-based activities (e.g., outdoor play, exploration) to encourage her gross motor development. Before leaving, the therapist reviews strategies with Jade's teacher, and leaves a note for Jade's caregivers summarizing the visit.*

WHAT IS EARLY INTERVENTION?

Early intervention is often used to describe various community-based services and supports available to young children and their families. Here, we refer to early intervention (EI) as the federal grant program, under Part C of the Individuals with Disabilities Education Act (IDEA), that supports states in operating a comprehensive system of services and supports for infants and toddlers with or at risk for developmental disabilities, ages birth through 2 years. An infant or toddler with developmental disability refers to a child under the age of 3 years who needs EI services for one of two reasons: (1) The child is experiencing a developmental delay in physical, cognitive, communication, social-emotional, or adaptive development (based on scores from standardized diagnostic assessments), or (2) the child has a diagnosed condition that has a high probability of resulting in developmental delay (US Code of Federal Regulations, 2022). EI services reflect the therapeutic supports required to meet the needs of infants and toddlers and their families (Box 103.1 lists examples of EI service personnel). To the extent possible, EI services are provided in the child's natural environments, those settings considered typical for infants or toddlers without disabilities (e.g., home, daycare, park).

A BRIEF HISTORY OF PART C EARLY INTERVENTION

The actions of families and advocacy groups in the 1950s and 1960s laid the foundation for increased protections and educational opportunities for children with disabilities. Prior to this time, many individuals with disabilities lived in restrictive state institutions where families had little opportunity to inform care decisions. On November 29, 1975, President Ford signed into law the Education of All Handicapped Children Act (EHA; Public Law [P.L.] 94-142), guaranteeing access to "a free appropriate public education in the least restrictive environment to every child [aged 5 to 18 years] with a disability," while also protecting the rights of children with disabilities and their families. This landmark legislation mandated that children receive family-informed individualized education plans (IEPs) and that services occur in the least restrictive environment.

As part of its reauthorization in 1986 (P.L. 99-457), EHA was amended to address the developmental needs of infants and toddlers with developmental delay. The first 3 years of life represent a sensitive period in early brain development; the brain grows to approximately 80% of its full size, and more than 1 million new neural connections are formed every second. After a period of rapid proliferation, connections are refined through a process known as pruning to improve efficiency. As the maturing brain becomes more specialized and proficient, it is less able to reorganize and adapt to novel stimuli. Recognizing these first 3 years of life as critical to a child's future health and development, Congress acknowledged "an urgent and substantial need" to optimize the development of infants and toddlers, enhance the capacity of families to meet their children's needs, and reduce future costs to the educational system.

The 1990 reauthorization (P.L. 110-476) changed the law's name from EHA to the Individuals with Disabilities Education Act, or IDEA. Under Part C of IDEA, the federal government provides financial assistance to states to (1) develop and

BOX 103.1 Examples of Early Intervention Service Personnel

Audiologist	Family therapist	Nurse	Occupational therapist
Pediatrician/primary care	Physical therapist	Psychologist	Registered dietician
Social worker	Special educator	Speech and language pathologist	Vision specialist

implement a statewide, comprehensive EI system for infants and toddlers with disabilities and their families; (2) facilitate payment of EI services from federal, state, local, and private sources; (3) enhance state capacity to provide high-quality EI services to infants and toddlers with disabilities and their families; (4) enhance the capacity of state and local agencies to identify, evaluate, and meet the needs of all children, especially low-income, Black, Indigenous and other racially minoritized children, and children in foster care; and (5) encourage states to expand opportunities for infants and toddlers at risk of experiencing developmental delay. The 1997 reauthorization encouraged states to formally monitor children at risk for developmental delay, while the 2004 reauthorization granted states permission to allow families to continue EI services beyond the child's third birthday and up to their entry into kindergarten. (See Chapter 113 for additional information on IDEA.)

FEDERAL REQUIREMENTS AND STATE IMPLEMENTATION

Federal Requirements

According to US Federal Code, statewide EI systems must include specific components to qualify for and maintain federal assistance (§303.110). Key among them are:

- Policies and procedures to ensure that EI services are available to all infants and toddlers with disabilities and their families
- An interagency coordinating council that supports implementation of the Part C program
- A single line of responsibility in the form of a lead agency that administers programs and activities funded under Part C, IDEA
- A rigorous definition of "developmental delay" used by the state to appropriately identify infants and toddlers with disabilities
- A comprehensive child find system responsible for identifying infants and toddlers with disabilities and connecting them to EI services
- Timely, comprehensive, and multidisciplinary evaluations that reflect families' concerns, priorities, and resources
- IFSPs
- Policies and procedures to ensure receipt of services in the natural environment
- Central directories of EI services, resources, and experts

State Implementation

Beyond these federal requirements, states are afforded notable discretion in designating a lead agency, defining eligibility criteria, and funding EI services. US states and territories are required to designate a lead agency to oversee the administration and coordination of EI services. In addition to overseeing all child find activities, these agencies are additionally responsible for conducting needs assessments, raising public awareness regarding EI, disseminating state and federal legislative updates, and allocating funds. The majority of lead agencies are housed within Departments of Education (n = 15) or Departments of Health (n = 12) (Early Childhood Technical Assistance [ECTA] Center, 2020a). The remaining agencies (n = 17) are housed within a variety of departments, including Developmental Services, Health and Human Services, and Public Health. Little is known about the relationship between lead agency and Part C EI characteristics or outcomes. Twardzik, MacDonald, & Dixon-Ibarra, (2017) examined the relationship between lead agency and Part C EI enrollment and found the odds of enrolling in Part C EI to be higher when the state lead agency was health versus education, controlling for state-level eligibility criteria, population size, and screening rates. Given that pediatric clinicians account for the majority of referrals to Part C EI, health agencies may be better equipped to coordinate referrals within the same department. By comparison, lead agencies housed within departments of education may experience challenges coordinating across multiple systems (Twardzik et al., 2017). It is worth noting that children and families frequently enroll in multiple, simultaneous programs managed across numerous departments. Each program gathers relevant data on participating children and families; most states lack the political and technical infrastructure needed to support data integration and information sharing across programs and state agencies. The Early Childhood Data Collaborative was established to support states in developing integrated data systems across early childhood programs and may serve as a useful resource for states as they seek to improve interagency coordination (IDEA Early Childhood Data Systems, 2021).

Federal regulations mandate that Part C EI services be available to all infants and toddlers with disabilities and their families. Recall that an infant or toddler with a disability is any child under the age of 3 years who needs EI services because of developmental delay or a diagnosed condition that has a high probability of resulting in developmental delay (§303.21). There is no singular set of federal criteria to define developmental delay, forcing states to establish their own and select which diagnoses have a high probability of delay. In addition, states may choose to include children at risk for experiencing developmental delay as the result of documented biologic, social, or environmental factors. There are 26 definitions of developmental delay used by states to establish EI eligibility criteria (ECTA Center, 2020b). Twenty-three states use percent delay criteria ([1 − observed age/chronologic age] × 100), 17 use some combination of percent delay and standard deviation criteria, and 16 use standard deviation criteria. The most common definition for developmental delay (used by 8 states) is 2 standard deviations (SD) below the mean in one or more developmental areas or 1.5 SDs below the mean in two or more developmental areas. It is important to recognize that Elijah and Jade, from the vignettes, would likely not qualify for EI services in many states and territories.

Estimates of the percentage of infants and toddlers likely eligible for Part C EI, based on varying state definitions of developmental delay, range from 2% to 78% (Rosenberg, Robinson, Shaw, & Ellison, 2013). In contrast, the proportion of infants and toddlers enrolled in Part C EI ranges from 0.9% to 10.1%. (US Department of Education, 2020). States using the broadest eligibility criteria make more children candidates for Part C EI than systems can currently handle. Complicating the issue is the impression that children with mild delays are more often enrolled in Part C EI, while infants and toddlers with more significant delays go unserved (Tang, Feldman, Huffman, Kagawa, & Gould, 2012). Among a national cohort of infants or toddlers with disabilities, children living in states with broad eligibility criteria were more likely to participate in EI compared to children living in states with narrow eligibility criteria. While this finding is perhaps intuitive, evidence suggests Part C EI eligibility policy does not affect children equally. For example, in states with narrow versus broad eligibility criteria children experiencing poverty are less likely than those with relative socioeconomic advantage to participate in EI services (McManus, McCormick, Acevedo-Garcia, Ganz, & Hauser-Cram, 2009), while children with significant delays are less likely than children with mild delays to participate in EI services (McManus & Rosenberg, 2012). One might expect that infants and toddlers with disabilities could get their developmental needs met outside of the EI system (e.g., outpatient physical, occupational, or speech therapy clinic). However, findings suggest children living in states with narrow Part C EI eligibility were less likely to have their developmental needs met than children living in states with broad eligibility criteria (Magnusson & McManus, 2017). Taken together, these findings suggest eligibility criteria may reflect the robustness of state early childhood systems to care for infants and toddlers with disabilities more broadly. Little is known about states' selection of EI eligibility criteria; gaining insight to the rationale underlying these criteria may inform the development of more uniform, evidence-based standards, thereby allowing more accurate comparisons of child find efforts between states.

Finally, as alluded to earlier, the federal government provides financial assistance to states to implement comprehensive EI systems for infants and toddlers with disabilities and their families. And while all states currently receive funding under IDEA Part C, many use additional public or private funding sources such as Medicaid, Child Care and Development Block Grants, Temporary Assistance for Needy Families, Early Head Start, and Maternal and Child Health (MCH) Title V. Some state programs calculate and collect sliding monthly fees based on family size and income, although in many states EI services are provided at no additional cost to the family. Little is known about the relationship between state-level funding mechanisms, Part C EI characteristics, and outcomes.

CORE PRINCIPLES

In addition to the federal requirements described previously, key principles guide delivery of EI services in natural environments. The Office of Special Education Programs (OSEP) convened a national workgroup that established several consensus-based principles supported by research from child development, family systems, and human ecology. Several professional organizations subsequently adopted the guiding principles put forth by OSEP, illuminating the alignment of Part C EI best practices within existing professional scopes of practice and codes of ethics (Whipple, 2014). The following section highlights three of these key principles.

Family-Centered Care

Family-centered care is positively associated with improved service access, service efficiency, communication, and care satisfaction (Kuhlthau et al., 2011). Moreover, the MCH Bureau endorses family-centered care as an integral component of effective early childhood systems. Family-centered care reflects a number of core characteristics identified by various national groups, including Family Voices, MCH Bureau, American Academy of Pediatrics (AAP), and Institute for Patient- and Family-Centered Care. Those characteristics put forth by the AAP (Institute for Patient- and Family-Centered Care, 2012) include:

- Respect for cultural differences
- Flexibility
- Information sharing
- Partnership and collaboration
- Strengths-based conversations

Routine-Based Learning in Natural Environments

To the extent possible, EI services must be provided in children's natural environments, those places where children and families spend their time. This emphasis on natural environments is about much more than the location of services (Jennings, Hanline, & Woods, 2012). First, it affords EI professionals valuable opportunities to understand children's daily routines and work alongside family members to integrate developmental interventions within the context of regularly occurring activities. Second, infants and toddlers learn best within the context of daily routines. Embedding interventions within children's daily routines affords children the opportunity to practice functional skills that contribute in meaningful ways to their overall developmental progression and participate fully in their role as a child and member of the family. Third, in addition to being functional, daily routines are predictable and occur multiple times throughout the day, providing children with numerous opportunities to practice new skills. Finally, evidence suggests that routine-based EI services provided in children's natural environments more effectively promote children's development than traditional, biomedical interventions provided in clinical settings while strengthening the ability of caregivers to meet children's needs within the context of naturally occurring, daily activities.

Primary Coaching

The Division of Early Childhood identified primary coaching as an evidence-based strategy to be used by EI providers to engage families as decision makers and promote caregiver-implemented interventions (Lorio, Romano, Woods, & Brown, 2020). Adult learning theory posits that adults learn best when they are able to build upon existing knowledge, integrating new information and skills into an existing framework. Kemp and Turnbull (2014) described a continuum of coaching practices in EI. On one end of the continuum, the provider is viewed as the "expert," directing intervention choices and teaching caregivers how to implement select interventions. On the other (and arguably preferred) end of the continuum, providers and caregivers work collaboratively to identify goals, priorities, and support needs (Kemp & Turnbull, 2014). In building capacity the focus shifts to strengthening caregivers' confidence and competence in supporting their children. Coaching strategies used to support caregiver-implemented interventions reflect family-centered principles and include joint planning, information sharing, direct teaching, demonstration, practice, feedback, problem solving, and reflection (Lorio et al., 2020).

EVIDENCE SUPPORTING PART C EARLY INTERVENTION

Part C EI is charged with enhancing local and state capacity to identify, evaluate, and meet the needs of children, especially Black, Indigenous and other racially minoritized children, and children with limited financial resources living in urban or rural areas. Given the public funds tied to Part C EI systems, calls for evidence regarding program implementation and effectiveness are justifiable. This section summarizes the evidence supporting EI, drawing attention to the challenges and opportunities in conducting process and outcome evaluations of Part C programs.

Process Evaluation

The following section summarizes key Part C process indicators published annually by the ETCA Center (2020a; US Department of Education, 2020).

Child Find

Child Find for Children Birth to Three (indicator C6) is the percent of infants and toddlers birth to 3 years of age with IFSPs in place. States are evaluated based on their performance relative to the national average (mean), despite significant state-level variations in EI eligibility criteria. In fiscal year 2018 an average of 3.48% of infants and toddlers had IFSPs in place (range: 0.9%–10.1%). This estimate has steadily increased since FY 2013 when 3% of infants and toddlers had IFSPs in place. Of interest is the fact that the range has also grown during this time, from 1.2% to 7.9% in 2013 to 0.9% to 10.1% in 2018.

Setting

Setting (indicator C2) is the percent of infants and toddlers with IFSPs who primarily receive EI services in natural environments. Indicator C2 is a compliance indicator with a target of 100%. Setting determination is based on information provided in each child's IFSP. In FY 2018 98% of EI services were provided in natural environments (range across states: 83%–100%). This estimate has remained relatively constant since FY 2013, while the range has diminished, from 74% to 100% in FY 2013 to 83% to 100% in FY 2018).

Timeliness

Timeliness (indicator C7 [i.e., adherence to Part C's 45-day timeline]) is the percent of EI-eligible infants and toddlers with IFSPs for whom an evaluation and initial IFSP meeting were conducted within Part C's 45-day timeline. Indicator C7 is a compliance indicator with a target of 100%. Determinations of timeliness are gathered from each state's data system and/or local monitoring practices, including onsite verification visits and chart reviews. In FY 2018 96% of initial IFSP meetings were deemed "timely" (range: 68%–100%). This estimate has remained relatively constant since FY 2013, while the range has fluctuated over this same time period.

Service Use

While not a formal indicator of compliance, service use is typically captured in the EI service record and has been used to examine the care experience. Service use is typically captured in terms of quantity (amount, duration, intensity) and quality (e.g., family centeredness). When these data are paired with child and family demographic and outcomes data, there has been opportunity to build new evidence of social disparities in EI service use (McManus et al., 2020; Richardson et al., 2019) and associations between EI service use and child and family outcomes (Khetani et al., 2020).

Outcome Evaluation

As described previously, Part C EI seeks to enhance the development of infants and toddlers with disabilities and increase the capacity of families to meet children's needs. The following section summarizes key Part C outcome indicators published annually by ECTA (2020a; US Department of Education, 2020) as well as germane literature examining EI effectiveness in advancing child and family outcomes.

Infant and Toddler Outcomes

Infant and Toddler Outcomes (indicator C3) reflect the percent of infants and toddlers with IFSPs who demonstrate improved (1) social-emotional skills, (2) use of knowledge and skills, and (3) use of appropriate behaviors to meet their needs. The majority of states and jurisdictions (40/56) use the Child Outcomes Summary (COS) process to measure and report child outcomes. Table 103.1 summarizes indicator C3 for FY 2018.

TABLE 103.1 Indicator C3 (Infant and Toddler Outcomes) for Fiscal Year 2018

Indicator Component	Percent of Children Who Substantially Increased Their Skills by the Time They Turned 3 Yr or Exited the Program: Mean (Range)	Percent of Children Who Were Functioning Within Age Expectations by the Time They Turned 3 Yr or Exited the Program: Mean (Range)
A: Social-emotional	66% (30%–90%)	56% (18%–84%)
B: Knowledge and skills	72% (34%–92%)	47% (14%–83%)
C: Behaviors	74% (50%–93%)	58% (17%–92%)

A number of historical and contemporary studies have additionally explored the effectiveness of Part C EI in enhancing child outcomes. These studies are divided into two phases based on their timing relative to the passage of P.L. 99-457. First-generation studies, defined as those conducted before the passage of P.L. 99-457, allowed more rigorous evaluations of EI services vis-à-vis randomized controlled trials. It is worth noting that, in addition to employing randomization strategies, many first-generation studies were based on programs with considerable resources and highly trained staff to ensure fidelity to the intervention protocol. In contrast, second-generation studies of EI programs operating under Part C, IDEA face two fundamental methodologic challenges. First, Part C EI services are mandated for all eligible children, making randomization unethical and a violation of federal law. Second, Part C programs serve a much more diverse population of children and families than those included in many first-generation studies. As a result, there is no uniformly defined intervention with set services, frequencies, or intensities across treatment groups. Despite these limitations, a number of second-generation studies have applied innovative research methods to administrative data to assess the effect of EI services on the developmental and functional outcomes of young children. Like their predecessors, these contemporary health services studies found clinically and statistically meaningful associations between EI service use and functional outcomes across three outcome indicators: social-emotional skills (Richardson et al., 2020),) cognition (Litt, Glymour, Hauser-Cram, Hehir, & McCormick, 2018), and adaptive behaviors (McManus, Richardson, Schenkman, Murphy, & Morrato, 2019). Developmental and intervention science suggests the benefits to children's development are the direct result of enhancing developmental influences on children's outcomes (e.g., child-caregiver interactions, routine- and family-based experiences) (Guralnick, 2011).

Future research will likely center around two key areas. First, the general population of infants and toddlers with disabilities is largely heterogenous with varying etiologies, developmental trajectories, and contextual factors. Thus intervention studies will require well-defined subgroups of children and families, unambiguous intervention strategies, and distinct child and family outcomes (Guralnick, 2017). Second, as we alluded to earlier, little is known about the influence of program- and systems-level variations on child and family outcomes. Additional research is needed to explore the influence of relevant program- and systems-level factors on child and family outcomes.

Family Outcomes

Family Outcomes (indicator 4) reflect the percent of families who report that EI services have helped the family to (1) know their rights, (2) effectively communicate their child's needs, and (3) access desired services, programs, and activities to help their child develop and learn. Despite a general consensus that it is important to evaluate family outcomes, it has historically been challenging to establish standards for assessing these outcomes (Bailey et al., 2006). States have multiple options for the measures they use to collect family outcomes data. The most commonly used options are the Family Outcomes Survey (FOS; Bailey et al., 2011) and the National Center for Special Education Accountability Monitoring Survey (NCSEAM; National Center for Special Education Accountability Monitoring, 2005). States may tailor survey content (e.g., modifying words and phrases, adding supplemental items) and administration (e.g., timing of survey release to families) as needed. Table 103.2 summarizes indicator C4 for FY 2018.

Relatively few studies have examined the effectiveness of Part C EI in enhancing family outcomes. Families who receive EI services are generally satisfied and perceive positive benefits (Hebbeler et al., 2007). Bailey et al. (2006) found that most caregivers participating in EI felt competent to care for and advocate for their children's needs. Many families struggle, however, when it comes to participating in community-based activities and managing their children's behavior in these situations (Khetani, Cohn, Orsmond, Law, & Coster, 2013). Future studies on EI service use and family outcomes would benefit from the use of family-reported outcome measures that yield a more comprehensive profile of the young child's community participation. Recent efforts to implement participation assessments in EI are underway (Albrecht et al., 2020) and may hold promise for strengthening family-provider relationships while enabling a more robust evaluation of EI services and family outcomes.

TABLE 103.2 Indicator C4 (Family Outcomes) for Fiscal Year 2018

Indicator Component	Mean (Range)
A: Know their rights	91% (64%–100%)
B: Effectively communicate their children's needs	91% (65%–100%)
C: Help their children develop and learn	93% (73%–100%)

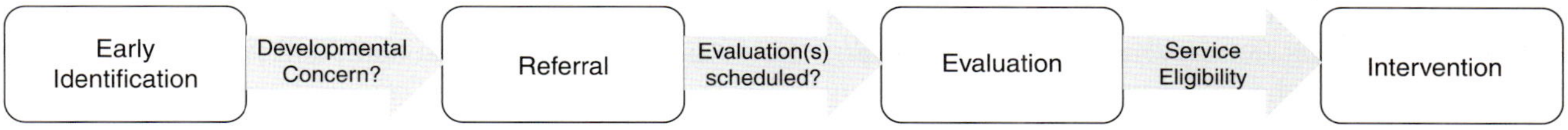

Fig. 103.1 Key steps in the early identification to intervention pathway for infants and toddlers experiencing developmental disabilities.

EARLY IDENTIFICATION TO INTERVENTION PATHWAY

Fig. 103.1 illustrates key steps in the early identification to intervention pathway for infants and toddlers experiencing developmental disabilities: early identification, referral, evaluation, and intervention. Decisions along this pathway are informed by a multitude of clinic-level factors, including resource availability, existing decision support, staffing cohesion, time, and reimbursement, and by provider-level factors such as beliefs regarding referral requirements and EI effectiveness. They also are informed by a host of child- and family-level factors, including caregiver knowledge and beliefs, family values and priorities, community networks, and various social and financial stressors (Jimenez, Barg, Guevara, Gerdes, & Fiks, 2012; Jimenez et al., 2014; Magnusson, Minkovitz, Kuhlthau, Caballero, & Mistry, 2017). Efforts to improve early identification and intervention for infants and toddlers with developmental delay have focused on enhancing organizational processes and changing provider behaviors. Relatively little attention has been paid to understanding caregiver beliefs, values, and priorities along this pathway (Harkness & Super, 2020). For many families, especially underserved families, evidence-based developmental screening guidelines and EI service recommendations presented during the well-child visit use concepts and language that lack cultural relevance and meaning (Magnusson et al., 2017; Zuckerman, Chavez, Regalado Murillo, Lindly, & Reeder, 2018). As a result, many caregivers feel disengaged from the decision-making process while others fee ambivalent toward or overwhelmed by service options.

We begin to see early identification and intervention disparities attenuated when caregivers feel as though they are partners in the decision-making process (Magnusson & Mistry, 2017). Regrettably, some Black, Indigenous and other racially minoritized caregivers report going along with referral and service recommendations, not because they value those decisions but because they feel it is important to "do whatever the doctor says" out of guilt or fear (Magnusson et al., 2017). Others are unaware that a referral has been made or do not understand the rationale behind the referral (Jimenez et al., 2012). Such ambivalence can make families more vulnerable to practical obstacles (e.g., scheduling evaluations and treatment sessions). For those children and families with significant needs (e.g., developmental, social, financial), it can be difficult if not impossible to identify core issues and prioritize potential solutions (Magnusson et al., 2017). Thus pediatric clinicians play a critical role in supporting the early identification to intervention pathway, serving as the central gateway to Part C EI and other developmental services. They are well positioned to work alongside caregivers to address concerns, inform the evaluation, interpret results, coordinate services, and monitor the child's progress (AAP Committee on Children with Disabilities, 2001). The following section takes a closer look at each step of the pathway and suggests actions pediatric clinicians can take to support families along the way. As you work through each step, compare and contrast the experiences of Elijah, Jade, and their families, from the vignettes. How might your care differ in these two scenarios?

Early Identification

Every EI program funded under Part C IDEA must include a comprehensive child find system that ensures rigorous standards for appropriately identifying infants and toddlers with disabilities for EI services (§303.302). Pediatric clinicians play an important role in identifying children at risk for developmental delay. Please refer to Chapter 81 for a more comprehensive examination of the pediatric clinician's role in screening for developmental delay, communicating results in a culturally responsive manner, and forming a shared action plan.

Referral

The majority of referrals to Part C EI originate in pediatric primary care, though anyone familiar with a child's development can submit a referral (§303.303). Thus it is critical for primary care clinicians to remain informed about current EI policies to ensure children and families are well supported throughout the process (Rose, Herzig, & Hussey-Gardner, 2014). The decision to initiate a referral represents an important opportunity to talk with families about developmental milestones, understand their beliefs and expectations, and elicit their priorities and preferences (Adams et al., 2013). It also represents an opportunity to learn about those formal and informal supports that guide decisions. Many caregivers seek the support of family members and peer support groups to further navigate complex health and EI service systems (AAP Committee on Children with Disabilities, 1999). Family Voices is just one example of a nationwide network of families that can assist caregivers and providers throughout the early identification to intervention pathway.

Evaluation

Each state's lead agency must ensure that children under the age of 3 years who are referred to Part C EI receive a timely, comprehensive, and multidisciplinary evaluation. The evaluation refers to the process used by a multidisciplinary team to determine a child's initial and continuing eligibility under Part C, IDEA (§303.321). A child's medical record may be used to establish eligibility (without conducting a formal evaluation of the child) if those records indicate the child has a diagnosed condition with a high probability of developmental delay (as defined by each state). The evaluation additionally involves interviewing the child's caregivers, administering a validated assessment tool(s), and gathering information from family members, other caregivers, social workers, and medical providers to understand the full scope of the child's unique strengths and needs. A family-directed assessment further helps identify the family's resources, priorities, and concerns and the supports and services required to enhance the family's capacity to meet the child's needs. In supporting the evaluation process the pediatric clinician is encouraged to:

1. Learn their state's EI eligibility criteria
2. Guide families through the evaluation process and acquaint them with their state's eligibility criteria
3. Inform the multidisciplinary evaluation by providing relevant medical information and/or diagnoses
4. Seek feedback from the evaluation team regarding the child's eligibility
5. Interpret and discuss evaluation results with child's family
6. Notify families of their rights. If, based on the evaluation, the lead agency determines a child is not eligible for services, the lead agency must provide the primary caregiver with written notice, and include in the notice information about the family's right to dispute the eligibility determination through various resolution mechanisms under Part C EI (303.430).

Intervention

An IFSP is created for each EI-eligible child by a multidisciplinary team that includes the child's primary caregivers as formal members of that team (§303.430). This plan summarizes the child's health and developmental status; describes the family's resources, concerns, and priorities; outlines measurable and time-bound outcomes for the child and family; and lists all EI services required to meet the unique needs of the child and family. In addition to describing the frequency and length of service sessions, the plan describes where these services will take place. The IFSP must be reviewed at least every 6 months to determine (1) the degree to which progress is being made and (2) whether modifications are required. The annual meeting includes a formal reevaluation of the child's development to further inform goals and services. Through their role in the pediatric medical home, clinicians are encouraged to support the provision of EI services through the following activities:

- Review the IFSP and provide input regarding proposed health-related services to ensure these services are appropriate and comprehensive.
- Coordinate all primary and subspecialty care for those children with complex medical needs.
- Communicate all relevant medical information to members of the multidisciplinary team.
- Be aware of potential costs to the family.
- Maintain an updated list of local and regional resources available within your state and your local Part C program.
- Talk with caregivers about service options and models. Caregivers (and providers) can become confused when an infant is dually served by professionals within a biomedical model and professionals within a family-centered model (i.e., pediatric medical home and Part C EI). Unless these services (and related models) are carefully explained and closely coordinated, caregivers (and providers) can develop mistrust of one professional or the other.
- Work alongside caregivers to monitor their child's progress.
- Avail themselves to Part C EI programs as a means of fostering colearning and strengthening referral networks.
- Serve as knowledgeable, thoughtful advocates for Part C EI and other early childhood programs.
- Explore opportunities to participate on state, regional, or national councils/boards tasked with oversight of early childhood programs.

EI CHALLENGES AND INNOVATIONS

National estimates suggest between 15% and 25% of infants and toddlers experience developmental delay, while 3.48% use EI services, suggesting delays are underidentified and/or services are underutilized. If we look more closely at each step along the early identification to intervention pathway (see Fig. 103.1), we see that a significant number of children are lost along the way. Compounding this issue is the fact that Black, Indigenous and other racially minoritized children are least likely to have their delays identified (Magnusson, Palta, McManus, Benedict, & Durkin, 2016) and to use EI services (McManus et al., 2020). Socioeconomic status also is associated with disparities in early identification and intervention. Children with developmental delay who experience poverty (Magnusson et al., 2016) or whose parents have limited formal education or English proficiency (Knuti Rodrigues, Hambidge, Dickinson, Richardson, & Davidson, 2016) are less likely to have their delays identified and to use EI than children with relative socioeconomic advantage. Table 103.3 highlights national initiatives underway to support children, families, and health professionals along the early identification to intervention pathway.

CONCLUSION

EI services, authorized under Part C IDEA, are intended for all infants and toddlers experiencing developmental disabilities. In addition to the federal requirements guiding EI programs under Part C, there exist a number of key principles that further inform EI service delivery in natural environments, including family-centered care, routine-based learning, and primary coaching. States are afforded notable discretion in developing core program elements, including designating a lead agency, establishing eligibility criteria, and funding state programs. If we look more closely at each step of the early identification to intervention pathway, we see that many children and families are lost along the way. Pediatric clinicians play a central role in supporting children and families along this pathway. The provision of services within the pediatric medical home lays a strong foundation for the provision of family-centered, culturally responsive care. In addition, assorted programs exist to support children, families, and health professionals along the early identification to intervention pathway.

TABLE 103.3 National Initiatives to Support the Early Identification to Intervention Pathway

Name	Description
2-1-1	A national telephone access number to state and county call centers that connect individuals and families to local health and human services.
Assuring Better Child Health and Development (ABCD)	ABCD is funded by the Commonwealth Fund and administered by the National Academy for State Health Policy to assist states in improving the delivery of early child development services for low-income children and their families by strengthening primary health care services and systems that support the healthy development of children ages 0–3 yr.
Birth to Five: Watch Me Thrive	A coordinated federal effort to encourage healthy child development, universal developmental and behavioral screening for children, and support for the families and providers who care for them.
Center for Early Childhood Data Systems (DaSy)	The DaSy Center is a national technical assistance center that works with states to support IDEA early intervention and early childhood special education state programs in building high-quality data systems and using data to improve results for young children with disabilities and their families.
Healthy Steps	An evidence-based pediatric primary care program that promotes the health, well-being, and school readiness of babies and toddlers, with an emphasis on families living in low-income communities.
Learn the Signs. Act Early.	A program of the US Department of Health and Human Services, Centers for Disease Control and Prevention that encourages parents of children ages birth to 5 yr and their providers to learn the signs of health development, monitor every child's development, and act early on possible concerns.

REFERENCES

Adams, R. C., Tapia, C., Murphy, N. A., Norwood, K. W., Burke, R. T., Friedman, S. L., … Mucha, S. (2013). Early intervention, IDEA part C services, and the medical home: Collaboration for best practice and best outcomes. *Pediatrics, 132*(4), e1073–e1088. https://doi.org/10.1542/peds.2013-2305

Albrecht, E. C., Kaelin, V. C., Rigau, B. L., Dooling-Litfin, J. K., Scully, E. A., Murphy, N. J., … Sciarcon, L. (2020). Pilot implementation of an electronic patient-reported outcome measure for planning and monitoring participation-focused care in early intervention. *BMC Medical Informatics and Decision Making, 20*(1). https://doi.org/10.1186/s12911-020-01189-9

American Academy of Pediatrics Committee on Children with Disabilities. (1999). The pediatrician's role in development and implementation of an Individual Education Plan (IEP) and/or an Individual Family Service Plan (IFSP). *Pediatrics, 104*(1 I), 124–127. https://doi.org/10.1542/peds.104.1.124

American Academy of Pediatrics Committee on Children with Disabilities. (2001). Developmental surveillance and screening of infants and young children. *Pediatrics, 108*(1), 192–196. https://doi.org/10.1542/peds.108.1.192

Bailey, D. B., Hebbeler, K., Spiker, D., Scarborough, A., Mallik, S., & Nelson, L. (2006). Thirty-six-month outcomes for families of children who have disabilities and participated in early intervention. *Pediatrics, 116*(6), 1346–1352. https://doi.org/10.1542/peds.2004-1239

Bailey, D. B., Raspa, M., Olmsted, M. G., Novak, S. P., Sam, A. M., Humphreys, B. P., … Guillen, C. (2011). Development and psychometric validation of the Family Outcomes Survey-Revised. *Journal of Early Intervention, 33*(1), 6–23. https://doi.org/10.1177/1053815111399441

Early Childhood Technical Assistance Center. (2020a). *Part C lead agencies*. https://ectacenter.org/partc/ptclead.asp

Early Childhood Technical Assistance Center. (2020b). *State and jurisdictional eligibility definitions for infants and toddlers with disabilities under IDEA part C*. https://ectacenter.org/topics/earlyid/state-info.asp?sid=DC

Electronic Code of Federal Regulations. (2022). *Title 34 Subtitle B Chapter III Part §303.21—early intervention program for infants and toddlers with disabilities*. https://www.ecfr.gov/cgi-bin/text-idx?SID=18eacf51596c8ed46f64c374ed8f7fd7&mc=true&node=pt34.2.303&rgn=div5#_top

Guralnick, M. J. (2011). Why early intervention works: A systems perspective. *Infants and Young Children, 24*(1), 6–28. https://doi.org/10.1097/IYC.0b013e3182002cfe

Guralnick, M. J. (2017). Early intervention for children with intellectual disabilities: An update. *Journal of Applied Research in Intellectual Disabilities, 30*(2), 211–229. https://doi.org/10.1111/jar.12233

Harkness, S., & Super, C. M. (2020). Culture and human development: Where did it go? and where is it going? *New Directions for Child and Adolescent Development, 2020*(173), 101–119. https://doi.org/10.1002/cad.20378

Hebbeler, K., Spiker, D., Bailey, D., Scarborough, A. A., Mallik, S., Simeonsson, R. J., … Nelson, L. (2007). *Early intervention for infants and toddlers with disabilities and their families: Participants, services, and outcomes*. https://www.researchconnections.org/childcare/resources/13407

Institute for Patient- and Family-Centered Care. (2012). Patient- and family-centered care and the pediatrician's role. *Pediatrics, 129*(2), 394–404. https://doi.org/10.1542/peds.2011-3084

Jennings, D., Hanline, M. F., & Woods, J. (2012). Using routines-based interventions in early childhood special education. *Dimensions of Early Childhood, 40*(2), 13–23. https://www.wvsha.org/wp-content/uploads/events-manager-uploads/session-handouts/HandoutPreschoolLanguage2.pdf

Jimenez, M. E., Barg, F. K., Guevara, J. P., Gerdes, M., & Fiks, A. G. (2012). Barriers to evaluation for early intervention services: Parent and early intervention employee perspectives. *Academic Pediatrics, 12*(6), 551–557. https://doi.org/10.1016/j.acap.2012.08.006

Jimenez, M. E., Fiks, A. G., Shah, L. R., Gerdes, M., Ni, A. Y., Pati, S., & Guevara, J. P. (2014). Factors associated with early intervention referral and evaluation: A mixed methods analysis. *Academic Pediatrics*, *14*(3), 315–323. https://doi.org/10.1016/j.acap.2014.01.007

Kemp, P., & Turnbull, A. P. (2014). Coaching with parents in early intervention: An interdisciplinary research synthesis. *Infants and Young Children*, *27*(4), 305–324. https://doi.org/10.1097/IYC.0000000000000018

Khetani, M. A., Cohn, E. S., Orsmond, G. I., Law, M. C., & Coster, W. J. (2013). Parent perspectives of participation in home and community activities when receiving part C early intervention services. *Topics in Early Childhood Special Education*, *32*(4), 234–245. https://doi.org/10.1177/0271121411418004

Khetani, M. A., McManus, B. M., Albrecht, E. C., Kaelin, V. C., Dooling-Litfin, J. K., & Scully, E. A. (2020). Early intervention service intensity and young children's home participation. *BMC Pediatrics*, *20*(1). https://doi.org/10.1186/s12887-020-02182-x

Knuti Rodrigues, K., Hambidge, S. J., Dickinson, M., Richardson, D. B., & Davidson, A. J. (2016). Developmental screening disparities for languages other than English and Spanish. *Academic Pediatrics*, *16*(7), 653–659. https://doi.org/10.1016/j.acap.2015.12.007

Kuhlthau, K. A., Bloom, S., Van Cleave, J., Knapp, A. A., Romm, D., Klatka, K., … Perrin, J. M. (2011). Evidence for family-centered care for children with special health care needs: A systematic review. *Academic Pediatrics*, *11*(2), 136–143. https://doi.org/10.1016/j.acap.2010.12.014

Litt, J. S., Glymour, M. M., Hauser-Cram, P., Hehir, T., & McCormick, M. C. (2018). Early intervention services improve school-age functional outcome among neonatal intensive care unit graduates. *Academic Pediatrics*, *18*(4), 468–474. https://doi.org/10.1016/j.acap.2017.07.011

Lorio, C. M., Romano, M., Woods, J. J., & Brown, J. (2020). A review of problem solving and reflection as caregiver coaching strategies in early intervention. *Infants and Young Children*, *33*(1), 35–70. https://doi.org/10.1097/IYC.0000000000000156

Magnusson, D. M., & McManus, B. (2017). State-level disparities in caregiver-reported unmet therapy need among infants and toddlers with developmental delay in the United States. *Physical Therapy Journal of Policy, Advocacy, and Leaderhip*, *17*(1), 3–13.

Magnusson, D. M., & Mistry, K. B. (2017). Racial and ethnic disparities in unmet need for pediatric therapy services: The role of family-centered care. *Academic Pediatrics*, *17*(1), 27–33. https://doi.org/10.1016/j.acap.2016.06.010

Magnusson, D. M., Minkovitz, C. S., Kuhlthau, K. A., Caballero, T. M., & Mistry, K. B. (2017). Beliefs regarding development and early intervention among low-income African American and Hispanic mothers. *Pediatrics*, *140*(5). https://doi.org/10.1542/peds.2017-2059

Magnusson, D. M., Palta, M., McManus, B., Benedict, R. E., & Durkin, M. S. (2016). Capturing unmet therapy need among young children with developmental delay using national survey data. *Academic Pediatrics*, *16*(2), 145–153. https://doi.org/10.1016/j.acap.2015.05.003

McManus, B., McCormick, M. C., Acevedo-Garcia, D., Ganz, M., & Hauser-Cram, P. (2009). The effect of state early intervention eligibility policy on participation among a cohort of young CSHCN. *Pediatrics*, *124*(S4). https://doi.org/10.1542/peds.2009-1255G

McManus, B. M., Richardson, Z., Schenkman, M., Murphy, N. J., Everhart, R. M., Hambidge, S., & Morrato, E. (2020). Child characteristics and early intervention referral and receipt of services: A retrospective cohort study. *BMC Pediatrics*, *20*(1), 84. https://doi.org/10.1186/s12887-020-1965-x

McManus, B. M., Richardson, Z., Schenkman, M., Murphy, N., & Morrato, E. H. (2019). Timing and intensity of early intervention service use and outcomes among a safety-net population of children. *JAMA Network Open*, *2*(1), e187529. https://doi.org/10.1001/jamanetworkopen.2018.7529

McManus, B. M., & Rosenberg, S. A. (2012). Does the persistence of development delay predict receipt of early intervention services? *Academic Pediatrics*, *12*(6), 546–550. https://doi.org/10.1016/j.acap.2012.07.003

National Center for Special Education Accountability Monitoring. (2005). *Family survey—early intervention*. https://ectacenter.org/~pdfs/calls/2017/2005_NCSEAM_Survey_Sample.pdf

Richardson, Z. S., Khetani, M. A., Scully, E., Dooling-Litfin, J., Murphy, N. J., & McManus, B. M. (2019). Social and functional characteristics of receipt and service use intensity of core early intervention services. *Academic Pediatrics*, *19*(7), 722–732. https://doi.org/10.1016/j.acap.2019.02.004

Richardson, Z. S., Scully, E. A., Dooling-Litfin, J. K., Murphy, N. J., Rigau, B., Khetani, M. A., & McManus, B. M. (2020). Early intervention service intensity and change in children's functional capabilities. *Archives of Physical Medicine and Rehabilitation*, *101*(5), 815–821. https://doi.org/10.1016/j.apmr.2019.10.188

Rose, L., Herzig, L. D., & Hussey-Gardner, B. (2014). Early intervention and the role of pediatricians. *Pediatrics in Review*, *35*(1). https://doi.org/10.1542/pir.35-1-e1

Rosenberg, S. A., Robinson, C. C., Shaw, E. F., & Ellison, M. C. (2013). Part C early intervention for infants and toddlers: Percentage eligible versus served. *Pediatrics*, *131*(1), 38–46. https://doi.org/10.1542/peds.2012-1662

Tang, B. G., Feldman, H. M., Huffman, L. C., Kagawa, K. J., & Gould, J. B. (2012). Missed opportunities in the referral of high-risk infants to early intervention. *Pediatrics*, *129*(6), 1027–1034. https://doi.org/10.1542/peds.2011-2720

The Center for IDEA Early Childhood Data Systems. (2021). *DaSy Center*. https://dasycenter.org/

Twardzik, E., MacDonald, M., & Dixon-Ibarra, A. (2017). The relationship between state lead agency and enrollment into early intervention services. *Journal of Early Intervention*, *39*(3), 253–263. https://doi.org/10.1177/1053815117708999

US Department of Education. (2020). *2020 Part C SPP/APR indicator analysis*. https://sites.ed.gov/idea/files/PartC-IndicatorAnalysis-FFY2018.pdf

Whipple, W. (2014). *Key principles of early intervention and effective practices: A crosswalk with statements from discipline specific literature*. https://ectacenter.org/~pdfs/topics/eiservices/KeyPrinciplesMatrix_01_30_15.pdf

Zuckerman, K. E., Chavez, A. E., Regalado Murillo, C., Lindly, O. J., & Reeder, J. A. (2018). Disparities in familiarity with developmental disabilities among low-income parents. *Academic Pediatrics*, *18*(8), 944–951. https://doi.org/10.1016/j.acap.2018.06.011

104

Special Education Services

Nathaniel S. Beers and Cara Coleman

For additional material related to the content of this chapter, please see Chapters 18, 81, 86, 103, 105, and 113.

VIGNETTES

1. *Courtney is a 4-year-old with complex medical and developmental needs. She has spastic quadriplegia as well as significant cognitive impairment. She has a g-tube and tracheostomy and uses a wheelchair for mobility. Prior to school, she was enrolled in early intervention, where she received physical and occupational therapy and speech-language services. She requires g-tube feeds in addition to medication administration and intermittent suctioning during the school day. She has some vocalizations for communication. The age equivalent on her most recent developmental assessment was 1 year 6 months.*

   Courtney transitioned from early intervention to school-based special education services after turning 3 years old. She is currently in an inclusion prekindergarten class. She receives special education instruction inside the classroom. She receives speech and occupational therapy inside the classroom and is pulled out for individual therapy. She receives physical therapy outside of the classroom. She has a nurse assigned to her for her intermittent suctioning and g-tube feeds.

2. *Shawn is a 14-year-old Black teen who has entered middle school (seventh grade) with a diagnosis of attention-deficit/hyperactivity disorder (ADHD) and a history of behavior issues and suspensions. Shawn has a love of airplanes, draws them all the time, and dreams of flying someday. Shawn had a 504 plan throughout elementary school that focused on accommodations such as behavioral strategies (e.g., home/school communication system and behavior contracts), environmental strategies in classroom (e.g., seating and separate space), and accommodation of assignments and evaluation methods (e.g., reduced amount of homework and testing in segments). Shawn was recently suspended for kicking his desk when a classmate took his drawing notebook. It is his second suspension in two-quarters of middle school, and because the desk hit a classmate there has been discussion of involving the school resource officer, a law enforcement officer responsible for school safety and crime prevention. Shawn's middle school math and English teachers note that he is in fact bright, but assessments indicate that he is two grade levels behind in both subjects. The teachers have asked for a formal assessment for autism spectrum disorder (ASD), specifically noting that Shawn struggles to put his feelings into words, appears to have little social awareness, becomes easily overwhelmed in group settings, and turns to drawing airplanes when he has difficulty understanding or focusing on the classroom activity.*

   Shawn had numerous discipline issues in elementary school, and the school record indicates that they were "all related to his ADHD diagnosis and inability to listen to and respect adults." The family moved from out of state last year because his father is in the military. Both parents indicate that since Shawn was young, they noted their concerns to the pediatrician, but he was not referred for evaluation. When he entered kindergarten and began to have behavior issues, the pediatrician diagnosed him with ADHD and prescribed Ritalin. The pediatrician wrote a letter regarding the diagnosis to share in developing the 504 plan. Since then, Shawn has cycled through a number of medications for ADHD and has tried out medication for anxiety and depression as well. Shawn's history of engaging with peers, such as challenges eating lunch in the cafeteria, asking to go to the library for airplane books at recess, or difficulty during PE class or any group activities, were often treated as discipline issues, not as instructive for additional evaluation.

OVERVIEW OF THE INDIVIDUALS WITH DISABILITIES EDUCATION ACT

Special education plays a major role in the health and development of children and adolescents with over 7.5 million individuals served by state and local governments as well as community organizations. Additionally, over 1 million students enrolled in school are receiving services due to eligibility through Section 504 of the Rehabilitation Act. This chapter will help clinicians understand the system of special education and how clinicians can partner to support patients and families access special education services.

History of IDEA

Special education as we currently know it is not a new service provided in schools. Individuals with Disabilities Education Act (IDEA) (P.L. 94-142) was first passed in 1975 and was most recently reauthorized in 2015 (see Chapter 113). IDEA put in place the mandate for a free and appropriate public education (FAPE) for all students ages 3 to 21 years old in the least restrictive environment (LRE). Since the original law passed, it has been updated to ensure access to general education curriculum, services for infants and toddlers (birth to 5 years old), and planning for transition to school services and then to adulthood. In recent years there has been a focus on ensuring the achievement of students with disabilities is being adequately monitored to ensure ongoing academic progress. There have also been additions to increase student and parent engagement by providing more procedural safeguards while trying to reduce the administrative burdens for schools.

Special education in the public nomenclature often includes services covered by several other federal laws. Section 504 of the Rehabilitation Act of 1973 (n.d.) is designed to prohibit discrimination against those with disabilities in programs receiving federal funding. This requires meeting needs of students with disabilities as adequately as students without disabilities and is overseen by the US Department of Education. Similarly, individuals with disabilities also receive additional antidiscrimination protections from Americans with Disabilities Act (ADA) of 1990 (n.d.). The ADA requires the provision of "reasonable accommodations" and provides support for students who are at schools, camps, little leagues, and other programs not receiving federal funds to ensure adequate access to school and the broader community. The ADA is also critical in helping ensure individuals with disabilities can be part of the community by ensuring resources are in place to make the community accessible. Finally, the No Child Left Behind Act, the current version of which is Every Student Succeeds Act (n.d.; ESEA), created a requirement for highly qualified teachers and evidence-based interventions, which has been mirrored in subsequent reauthorizations of IDEA.

IDEA Versus 504

In their simplest forms IDEA provides the structure for special education and related services (occupational, physical, speech, and behavioral therapies) to be in place for individuals with disabilities, and Section 504 focuses on the accommodations needed to access school for those not qualifying for special education services. Each of these laws specify criteria for eligibility, evaluations, processes, and services that are compared in Table 104.1.

TABLE 104.1 Overview of IDEA Versus Section 504

	IDEA	Section 504
Overview	A federal education law to provide special education and related services to children with disabilities; applies to state and local educational agencies	A federal civil rights law to prevent discrimination on the basis of disability; applies to educational and noneducational programs and activities that receive or benefit from federal assistance at the state and local levels; provides and guarantees access to education
Eligibility	Children are determined through evaluation to be eligible for services; specific categories of disability are defined; disability must affect the child's educational performance	Broadly define eligibility for any person with a physical or mental impairment limiting one or more life activities, having a record of such impairment, or regarded as having an impairment; includes children who need specialized instruction as well as those who do not (e.g., children with asthma, temporary disabilities)
Funding	Federal funding assists states in meeting the mandate; state and local funding is also applied in the implementation of the law	No federal funding is provided; funding is under state and local jurisdiction
Evaluation	Requires a comprehensive evaluation by a multidisciplinary team, including the collection of information from a variety of sources; requires parents to provide written consent; reevaluation required every 3 yr	Requires the compilation of information from a variety of sources; does not require testing; requires parents to be notified; reevaluation required periodically
Free appropriate public education	Requires an IEP that is appropriate to the child's unique educational needs and designed to help the child receive educational benefit; provided at no cost to parents	Requires a plan that identifies accommodations to permit equal access to education and its benefits compared with nondisabled peers; provided at no cost to parents
Placement	Requires placement be made by a knowledgeable team made up of specific types of personnel; requires parents to be a part of the decision-making process	Requires placement to be determined by a knowledgeable committee but does not prescribe membership; parents are not required to be on the committee; placement is usually in regular education
Procedural safeguards and due process	Requires and describes specific procedures for written consent, impartial hearings, pendency; requires notice to parents before a change in placement; enforced by the US Department of Education, Office of Special Education	Requires procedural safeguards for notice, access to records, and impartial hearings; local education agencies may develop their own or adopt IDEA procedural safeguards; does not require parent notice before a change in placement but does require notice; enforced in schools by US Department of Education, Office of Civil Rights

IDEA, Individuals with Disabilities Education Act; *IEP*, individualized education plan.
Data from Council for Exceptional Children, 2002; Henderson, 2007; Rosenfeld, 2006.

EQUITY IN SPECIAL EDUCATION

Within special education there are longstanding inequities related to identification, quality of services, and outcomes. The disparities in special education lead to late diagnoses in some areas and overidentification in others, lead to inadequate services for some students and overly restrictive placements for others, and contribute in the long term to increased levels of behavioral interventions, including restraints and suspensions. Since 1997, IDEA has required states to monitor for racial and ethnic disparities.

Data has shown overidentification of Black and Indigenous students, with Black students 40% and Indigenous students 70% more likely to be identified as disabled. There is variability within types of disabilities. For emotional and intellectual disabilities, Black students are twice as likely to be classified. However, compared to White peers, Black children are likely to be diagnosed a year later with ASD. Black and Asian students are also significantly more likely to be in a more restrictive placement than White students (Harper, 2017).

This overidentification creates additional inequities when looking at behavioral management in schools. Students with disabilities are suspended at over twice the rate of nondisabled students. These out-of-school suspensions are associated with high rates of dropout but also higher rates of school-related arrests, seclusion placements, and restraints for students with disabilities compared to their peers. The inequitable application of discipline is even more stark for Black and Brown students with disabilities with nearly 50% of special education students incarcerated being Black despite making up less than 20% of the overall special education population (Disability Rights Education and Defense Fund, n.d.).

PARTNERING WITH CHILDREN AND ADOLESCENTS AND THEIR FAMILIES

Pediatric clinicians can play a very important role in the special education process by partnering with patients and their families. The process as outlined in the next sections of this chapter can be complex and daunting for even the most knowledgeable. It is critical to empower patients and their families with information as well as the understanding that they are the expert on what their child needs or what their own needs are.

Clinicians can play an important role in early detection of developmental and behavioral concerns. The American Academy of Pediatrics (AAP) strongly recommends regular developmental and behavioral screenings throughout childhood (AAP Bright Futures, 2021) to help identify children with developmental and behavioral concerns earlier and with greater accuracy. The frequency and types of screenings recommended can be found on the AAP Periodicity Schedule. The screenings will help identify children and adolescents in need of additional evaluations (see Chapter 81).

While anyone involved with the child can make a referral for special education assessment, pediatric clinicians can help support their patients and families by making a referral when a concern is identified during a visit. Many clinicians use a templated letter to clearly put the school system on notice for the need to move forward with a more formal assessment for special education concerns. Clinicians can also participate as part of the team meetings. Historically, these were not reimbursable by insurance companies, but there are new billing codes that would allow the time to be billed either by a physician (CPT code 99367) or by a nonphysician health care professional (CPT code 99368). In addition, telehealth codes afford a new opportunity for supporting families in this type of meeting.

Just as in clinical practice, the importance of documentation in the special education process is paramount. From the referral through transition to adult services, pediatric clinicians should partner with patients and families to maintain a record of communication with the school system as well as progress once deemed eligible for special education services. These records will help the family monitor the process and assist in accountability.

Patients and families are inundated with formal evaluations and documents as part of the special education process. Many of these evaluations and reports use very technical language. While clinicians are rarely education experts, they can play an important role in helping families understand the evaluations as well as the types of services and interventions recommended. As with any complex process, the jargon used by experts can create impediments for patients and families to engage on equal footing. This is where clinicians can help empower patients and families by interpreting the jargon. Furthermore, helping families to embrace their role as expert on their child also involves encouraging them to value their own observations and experiences as crucial to understanding evaluations and advancing educational strategies.

Patients and their families are the experts in their care. Frequently in the medical and educational worlds, they are marginalized by experts. Clinicians can play an important role in arming them with documentation (referrals and letters) as well as language to empower them. Simply reminding the patient and family that they know their needs best and that they are an equal partner in the process can dramatically change the outcomes. Additionally, ensuring that families are connected to organizations specializing in special education such as Parent Training and Information Centers (www.parentcenterhub.org) or to their school district's parent center can help families become well versed in special education law, process, and advocacy.

The individualized education plan (IEP) process, unfortunately, can often involve conflict arising from differing opinions as to goals, services, and supports. Access to services and supports can be contentious, especially when budgets are tight, supply is limited, and understanding of needs is not shared. A collaborative approach to the function of an IEP is a key strategy for unification. For example, a variety of team members working on drafts of goals or other aspects of an IEP ahead of the actual meeting will focus on developing the best goal for a child and filling in supports and services to respond to what was built. Clinicians can support families by acknowledging the possibility of conflict and encouraging collaborative planning in creative, flexible, and responsive ways for each individual child.

During the eligibility process as well as throughout the special education process, clinicians can play a critical role in supporting families in monitoring their child's status. It is important for families to bring documents from the special education process to visits, including evaluations, IEPs, and quarterly and annual monitoring reports, which give patients and families an opportunity to ask questions about parts they do not understand. It provides clinicians a chance to review progress made as well as to ensure understanding by the patients and families. Periodic monitoring also carves out time to discuss whether the IEP continues to meet a child's needs and begin to create or plan new ideas for goals. All of this will help empower patients and families during the process.

It is impossible to acknowledge the need to partner with patients and families without addressing the needs that have been created in a distant-learning or virtual-learning environment as witnessed during the COVID-19 pandemic. Children with disabilities were dramatically impacted by the lack of access to in-person instruction. Patients and families have known about the challenges in maintaining services and progress during school breaks, and the regulations around the extended school year (ESY) were meant to address some of those issues. However, ESY programs were built on providing in-person instruction and services. Without that option, patients and families were left advocating for services in a virtual space with limits to what was possible. There are several principles to keep in mind in supporting families during this type of experience, whether during a pandemic or an individual illness.

1. The special education process affords patients and families significant flexibility to work with schools to define the goals and instruction based on the needs of the student.
2. The IEP is not a static document but can be changed as the student and the environment change.
3. Patients and families need to be empowered to prioritize goals based on their current needs. Clinicians and educators can often get focused on their goals for the patient or student instead of allowing the voice of the patient/student and family to be heard.

THE SPECIAL EDUCATION PROCESS

The process by which children with disabilities access special education and related services is delineated through a combination of federal and state laws and regulations. The federal laws, such as IDEA and Section 504 of the Rehabilitation Act, lay out what all states must do to meet the needs of children with disabilities. However, these laws also leave room for states to interpret rules and pass their own laws as to application. As such, there may be variation between states, as well as between types of programs and school districts within states. Notably, state laws cannot contradict federal laws, nor can they provide less than the federal requirements; but state laws can offer additional protections. Broadly, the special education process consists of the following major steps: identification, assessment and eligibility, development of IEP, implementation, and evaluation (Office of Special Education and Rehabilitative Services, 2000).

The process portion of this chapter has been written in a specific format. Each aspect of the process begins with an overview that identifies and describes the law and the process, and is followed by a section highlighting ways the clinician and family can partner relative to each aspect of the process, as represented through the vignettes of Courtney and Shawn described at the beginning of the chapter. At times the language and information (e.g., requirement of written notice or timeline) may appear formal; however, both ensure that the clinician learns the jargon that families and school districts will be using.

Identification

Identification Process Overview

Child Find. Child Find is a legal requirement of IDEA (34 CFR sec. 300.111). Specifically, Child Find requires school districts to have a process to identify and evaluate children who may need special education and related services (e.g., counseling, speech therapy). Children birth to age 21 years are covered under the mandate, including those who may be homeschooled, homeless, in foster care, or in private school, and infants or toddlers who may need early intervention. Information about Child Find is typically shared with the public through outreach efforts such as media campaigns, social media, handouts, posts in public places, and school or health fairs. The information attempts to raise awareness about disabilities, possible supports, and contact information for follow-up.

Anyone can refer a child to Child Find, including families, clinicians, and teachers, by requesting an evaluation verbally or in writing. Schools are not required to respond to every request for evaluation, especially if there is no reason (i.e., evidence) to suspect a child has a disability that requires services and supports. However, under IDEA, if a school knows or has reason to suspect a child has a disability, then they must evaluate the child (34 CFR §300.111[c]). Notably, the Child Find mandate does not require a child to have a specific disability diagnosis to evaluate or receive special education services to be evaluated, nor does the school have to determine disability diagnosis prior to providing services. Families may pursue a due process hearing if they disagree with a denial to evaluate. At that hearing, families, clinicians, professionals, and teachers may share their child's story with an independent hearing officer and present evidence, such as evaluation results or samples of their child's work. If Child Find determines an evaluation is needed, families must provide consent to do so. Once consent to evaluate is given, school districts must complete the evaluation within 60 calendar days. This timeline is important to monitor to ensure that a child does not fall further behind simply awaiting evaluation and to open up access to due process review.

Response to intervention. Most school years begin with teachers assessing the reading, writing, and math skills of all students in their class. These assessments often reveal multiple students struggling for a variety of reasons (e.g., English as a second language, frequent absences, inadequate teaching, or undiagnosed disability), and therefore allow the teacher and school to begin to monitor the progress of students and develop interventions. The goal of response to intervention (RTI) is for the school to intervene before a child falls behind, as noted by the RTI Action Network (www.rtinetwork.org). RTI is not a specific program or type of teaching. Instead, RTI is a proactive approach. RTI specifically represents a move from a reactive model to one that emphasizes early research-based interventions to assess a student's skills and use the data to develop targeted research or evidence-based interventions.

There is no one way to provide interventions. RTI is often set up as a multitiered system of supports. The first tier involves the use of interventions as part of classroom-wide instruction. Within the classroom setting, a teacher can break students into small groups focused on different skills or learning styles, often called differentiated instruction. If progress monitoring (recorded and reported through regular assessments) reveals a child has not made adequate progress, a school may offer the next level of RTI through small group instruction for more targeted support. Note that this is provided in addition to, not as replacement for, regular classroom instruction, often given during enrichment or specials, such as art or physical education. The third tier involves intensive intervention through one-on-one instruction daily in small groups or individual lessons. Children can receive both RTI and special education services. RTI recognizes children who are at risk of falling behind, and many are referred for evaluation for eligibility for special education services, but one does not automatically lead to the other.

***Shawn:** Some may wonder how a young man has reached middle school approximately two grade levels behind in math and English despite receiving RTI and a 504 plan. Although Shawn received a variety of levels of RTI instruction in both of the elementary schools he attended, it appears as though progress within that type of instruction, and/or referral for evaluation, may have been hindered by misdiagnosis of ADHD and a superficial focus on behavior, which were viewed as oppositional defiance, rather than potential signs of ASD. It is important for clinicians to keep in mind the equity issues discussed earlier in this chapter, which helps explain what has happened to Shawn and informs what needs to happen moving forward. Additionally, the effects of inequities and Shawn's experience thus far with diagnosis and education may negatively affect the family's trust in the school and health care systems. Cognizance of this reality for the family could help the clinician foster a relationship based in trust and honesty.*

Assessment and Eligibility

Process Overview

Initial evaluation must be provided at no cost to the family and conducted by qualified professionals. Schools must evaluate a child in all areas related to the suspected disability and must employ a variety of tools and strategies to assess and collect information about the child's functioning, development, and academics. Schools cannot use a single assessment as the sole criteria for eligibility. Furthermore, screening by a teacher or educational diagnostician to determine instructional strategies (e.g., RTI) does not constitute evaluation. However, information from clinicians, families, therapists, or other relevant professionals can inform the evaluation process. To ensure equity and accurate assessment, IDEA requires that the school assess the child in the language and form most likely to yield accurate information about the child's abilities.

Once evaluation and assessment are completed and results are compiled in a written report, a team of qualified professionals and the family determine whether the child has a qualifying disability and identify the educational needs of the child. Copies of the evaluation report and documentation of eligibility must be provided to the family. Obtaining and maintaining copies of such reports is important for families and providers alike as the information from the evaluation is to be used in determining the contents of the child's IEP, and how to help the child make progress in the general education curriculum. If families and/or providers disagree with the evaluation results (e.g., disagree with disability classification) or eligibility determination, families can obtain an evaluation from an expert from the private sector, at the school's expense.

***Shawn:** Shawn's teachers have referred him for evaluation for ASD based on their observations and data teaching him in the first 2 quarters of middle school. Families with children who have been struggling to get the right supports, services, and diagnosis for their child may look forward to a new evaluation, but at the same time they may feel distrust and wariness. Shawn's clinician connected the family with the Parent Training Information Center (www.parentcenterhub.org) to ensure that they understand the IEP process and are empowered to partner and advocate within it. His clinician participated in the evaluation process by jointly reviewing and discussing the results. Moving the conversation from evaluation to action for Shawn comes next in the process.*

DEVELOPMENT OF THE IEP OR 504 PLAN

Overview of the IEP Development Process

The Team and the Meeting

An IEP meeting must be convened within 30 calendar days of a child's determination of eligibility for special education (34 CFR §322, §323, §501). The school and family must agree on when and where to hold the IEP meeting. Families must be provided 10 days written notice (unless they consent to a meeting with <10 days notice) of the IEP meeting, its purpose, time, location, attendees, and that they may invite others who have knowledge of their child. IEP meetings do not require in-person attendance; agreement as to alternate means of participation, such as by phone or video, can be reached (34 CFR §300.321). Absence of an IEP team member may be excused if the member's service is not being discussed or modified in the meeting or if the member submits information in writing and the school and family provide written consent. An IEP does not need to be completed in one meeting; however, consent of the family to the IEP is required prior to implementation of special education services.

IDEA outlines that, at a minimum, an IEP team consists of the child's family, a general education teacher, a special education teacher, a school administrator, evaluation personnel, and anyone else who the family and school district think appropriate to attend (34 CFR §300.321). Note that some members may play more than one role on the IEP team, and therefore the team does not necessarily consist of one member per role. Additional team members could include interpreters, supports for the family (friend, attorney, advocate, etc.), clinicians (e.g., pediatrician, specialist, home health nurse), therapists, transition specialists, or tutors. IDEA also encourages that children attend their own IEP meetings. A child's attendance at an IEP meeting can make the process come alive, adults can learn things about the child they did not previously know, and requests or suggestions from a child can carry significant weight. The role that a child plays as part of an IEP team can vary depending on age and comfort level, and it can expand and adjust over time. Involvement in IEP development for a child may make the program more meaningful and enable development of social and self-advocacy skills that are important for life and especially important as a child with a disability transitions to adulthood.

Courtney: *While Courtney and her family have been through the IFSP for early intervention and have an IEP in place, they still feel intimidated by the many experts at the table during the IEP development process. The IFSP process for early intervention services is designed to take a holistic view of the child and family needs. This differs from the IEP process that focuses solely on the child and mostly on the child's educational needs. The IEP development process can be overwhelming for many families, even those with prior experience navigating early intervention or special education services. Clinicians can support families by reminding them they are the expert on their child. If they are feeling overwhelmed, they can invite other family members to be part of the team meetings. Clinicians can also support the family by participating in the IEP meetings. Clinicians can join the meeting virtually or in person, as well as submit a letter or statement for the IEP record. Clinicians can support families by thinking through who might be able to join or what information may be helpful to the IEP team and meeting. Another strategy many expert parents recommend is to ensure the child is able to be in the room or is visually represented with a picture. This can help the team remain focused on the child.*

Shawn: *While Shawn and his family have gone through the process of developing a 504 plan, there are differences with the development of an IEP. The focus will move from accommodations in response to an ADHD diagnosis, to the development of goals and identification of special education supports and related services with the new diagnostic data. Inquiring as to Shawn's interest in joining the meeting is prudent given he is 14 years old and the need to begin transition planning. Additionally, joining the IEP process at the level Shawn is comfortable may offer him a chance to partner positively with adults and to develop social skills.*

Developing the IEP, Goals, Services, and Accommodations

Simply stated, the IEP process is a way to talk about a child's needs and to create a plan to meet those needs. It is a process with formal and legal requirements, but equally important are the more informal collaborative aspects of the process that take place over time and with a variety of the IEP team members. An IEP is a legally binding contract, and therefore it can be a powerful tool for ensuring that a child's educational needs related to the disability are met. It is also important to view an IEP as a fluid instrument or tool that can be reviewed and revised at any time to ensure that it continues to meet a child's needs. While strict timelines and requirements are in place to ensure minimum protections are afforded (such as a review once a year), nothing prevents a child, family, provider, or school from working to ensure more. To ensure that this IEP contract is enforceable and carried out as written, the IEP team must work to ensure that all aspects of supports and services are written within the IEP document.

The form of an IEP may vary between states or school districts, and of course each plan will vary as it is developed to meet each child's unique needs. However, IDEA requires that each IEP must include a statement of the child's present levels of performance; annual goals; measurement, special education, related services, and supplementary aids and services; modifications to state or district-wide assessments; transition goals and services (by age 16); dates when services will begin and end; amount of services, including how often and where they will take place; and age of majority statements (between ages 18 and 21) (34 CFR §300.310).

Present Levels

The foundation of an IEP begins with, and is anchored in, the present levels of academic achievement and functional performance (PLAFP, or present levels) that give rise to the goals of the program. Therefore it is critical to be thorough in this section and ensure time is taken to gather and provide input. Notably, the present levels statement does not solely include information about academic performance but also how a child functions in routine activities of daily living. Present levels should cover all areas of development in which the child may need support, with particular focus on how a child's disability affects the ability to learn and do things similar to children without disabilities. Content for the present levels may be drawn from observations, tests, evaluations, and assessments provided by any of the IEP team members and should reflect the strengths and interests of the child, as well concerns. Families and clinicians can request to review and contribute to the writing of present levels. Once agreed upon by the IEP team, the present levels become an important part of not just the IEP but also the child's permanent school record.

Goals

Using a detailed and in-depth present-level statement as the foundation, the IEP team can build goals targeting a wide range of skills, such as academic, developmental, functional, basic, social, or emotional, to meet the needs of a child and help the child become independent, communicate with others, and interact with others. IDEA requires that annual IEP goals be measurable and "include both academic and functional goals designed to meet the needs arising from the child's disability to enable the child to be involved in and make progress in the general education curriculum, and meet each of the child's other educational needs that result from the disability" (§300.320[a][2][i][A][B]). Goals can be developed collaboratively prior to the actual IEP meeting and should be created using the SMART (specific, measurable, action oriented, realistic, and time limited) framework. Additionally, goals should answer who, what, how, where, and when to be carried out as written (Rebhorn, 2017).

As stated earlier in this chapter, IDEA requires that children with disabilities be educated with their peers without disabilities to the maximum extent appropriate for each child (34 CFR §300.114). Multiple disabilities do not necessarily mean that a child should be removed from the general education class (34 CFR §300.116[e]). An explanation of removal from the general education setting must be written in the IEP. Services and supports can be included in the IEP as part of a FAPE to assist a child with disabilities to succeed in the general education setting and achieve the IEP goals. Supplementary supports and services can include special education, related services, supplementary aids and services, accommodations and modifications, and program modifications or supports for school staff (34 CFR §300.320, 39, 34, 105, 42). These supports and services are designed according to a child's unique strengths, abilities, and needs, thus illustrating the power of an IEP with truly individualized educational programs. For example, an IEP can include assistance with speaking or moving using speech-language pathology or physical therapy as so-called related services. Accommodations and modifications can involve seating a child in the front row and presenting tests orally and without time limits. Medical and health care needed by a child to participate in one's education are accommodations. There is no need to develop a 504 plan for health care needs and an IEP separately. These "health care plans" can be included in the IEP to implement and enforce.

Courtney: *Courtney has both medical and educational needs. The IEP should reflect the service hours and location of both areas as well as the related goals. As Courtney develops, the staffing and goals need to adjust as well. For children with medical needs like Courtney, schools may have difficulty understanding the diagnoses as well as the actual medical needs. Right now, Courtney requires an assigned nurse for her medical needs and may need physician orders to be able to receive these depending on the jurisdiction. Clinicians may not be experts on educational goals, but reviewing goals with parents and concerns they have can be an important support provided to families.*

Shawn: *To ensure strong partnership in the development of an IEP for Shawn there must be engagement in contributing to and reviewing of the draft IEP documents and goals prior to the IEP meeting. Efforts to discuss and contribute to drafts of any aspect of an IEP prior to the meeting are helpful in ensuring all IEP team members, including parents, are part of the process. The focus must be on Shawn's unique needs, not past missteps, nor actual or perceived limitations in services. Families and clinicians can be involved with the development of the present levels, contributing concrete observations of his skills, activities of daily living, routines, and needs that were not fully captured with the previous information. For example, clinicians and families can partner to write a paragraph that includes observations regarding the effect of the move and middle school transition on Shawn's ability to socialize and focus, describe helpful community activities in which he is involved, and document clinical medical efforts to support Shawn's diagnoses. In terms of SMART IEP goal development, clinician contributions to the present levels can directly lead into supportive discussions with the family or direct involvement with the creative development of goals, as well as suggestions for special education and related services. For example, a clinician can lend one's medical knowledge about ASD diagnosis to the discussion of how to write a goal that uses Shawn's love of airplanes to help him with a goal focused on helping him improve his ability to infer information from text and elaborate his thoughts in writing.*

Transition

Throughout the special education process there are multiple transitions that a child and family will experience. This is above and beyond the annual transition of class or grade or the significant transitions of actual schools. Each of the transitions discussed in this section brings a new set of terms and challenges for the family to navigate.

Part C to Part B

Early intervention services are found within Part C of IDEA, and therefore can often be referred to as Part C services (See Chapter 103). Transition to preschool is a huge step for any child, especially for those with disabilities. There are so many aspects of this transition, notably the program model shifts from family-centered services to child-centered education programs. Family involvement, including as decision makers, is mandatory in early intervention. Whereas, in Part B programs the school assumes educational responsibility. As with any transition, time, planning, and communication are critical. Families can visit possible preschool classrooms. Part C encourages families to step into the role of advocate of their child, becoming familiar with system, services, and their rights. Shifting that role from Part C to Part B is natural but will take time, encouragement, and partnership. This transition is recommended to occur over 6 months, but can take longer if needed.

Adolescence to Adulthood

As to transition into adulthood, IDEA specifically states:

> **Transition Services**. *(b)eginning not later than the first IEP to be in effect when the child turns 16, or younger if determined appropriate by the IEP team, and updated annually, thereafter, the IEP must include (1) Appropriate measurable postsecondary goals based upon age appropriate transition assessments related to training, education, employment, and, where appropriate, independent living skills; and (2) The transition services (including courses of study) needed to assist the child in reaching those goals (34 CFR §300.43).*

IDEA clearly requires that an IEP with measurable postsecondary goals, linked to specific transition services to achieve those goals, be in effect when the child turns 16 years old. This requires planning prior to implementation at age 16. Transition services refers to a "coordinated set of activities" for a child with disabilities tied directly back to the findings of Congress in IDEA "our national policy of ensuring equality of opportunity, full participation, independent living, economic self-sufficiency for individuals with disabilities" (20 U.S.C. 1400[c][1]). Transition services are unique to the skills, interests, and needs of each youth, but all focus on the future. As such, IDEA requires that schools invite youth with disabilities to attend IEP meetings or ensure their interests and preferences are expressed and considered in some way, where postsecondary goals and transition services are discussed (34 CFR §300.43[a][1]). Transition services require extensive planning over years as the youth nears age 16 and beyond. Requirements for review continue. See Chapter 105 for additional information on the transition to adulthood.

> ***Shawn:*** *Although Shawn is 14 years old, given the challenges he has had thus far in obtaining the right services to support his educational and medical needs, beginning transition discussions now is critical so that he does not fall even further behind. Additionally, empowering youth like Shawn to become involved in his own care and advocacy can help him to overcome some of the trauma he may have experienced, as well as develop important social and life skills. Clinicians can support Shawn to become involved in his care, education, and future planning by encouraging his involvement, discussing review of evaluations and/or drafts of IEP goals, and assisting him to prepare for the IEP meetings. Critical to clinician efforts to support youth is a people-first/family-centered approach that begins with speaking directly with Shawn and asking him questions.*

Alternative Placements

School districts must offer a continuum of alternative placements for children with disabilities. The LRE is considered to be the regular education classroom in the child's neighborhood school. If the IEP team determines that the child's needs cannot be met in that setting with supplemental aids and services, alternative placements may be offered, such as a special education class, a general education class, or placement in a special education school, home, hospital, residential placement, or some other setting as determined by the team (34 CFR §300.116). If a district is unable to meet the needs of a child, it may contract with other agencies or districts or make any other arrangement consistent with IDEA so that the child's needs are met. Alternative placements must be provided at no cost to the family.

Implementation of IEP

Once developed, an IEP cannot be implemented without the consent of families. Families can sign immediately or ask for time to consider the entire IEP as written. However, it is important to keep track of effective or annual review dates. Families can consent to only certain aspects of an IEP (i.e., by signing and adding written statement as to disagreement) or disagree in entirety. If disagreement does arise, the IEP team should attempt to discuss, problem solve, and reach resolution. If agreement cannot be reached, families may request mediation or a due process hearing to resolve the conflict or file a complaint with the state Department of Education (34 CFR §300.153, 507, 508, 510, 511). While alternate resolution is being pursued, the child can continue receiving services under the current IEP not under dispute (34 CFR §300.300).

Quarterly Reporting

IDEA requires that an IEP contain a statement as to how families will be regularly informed of a child's progress and whether that progress is sufficient to enable the child to achieve (34 CFR §300.320). Families must be informed at least as often as children without disabilities, therefore the minimum is quarterly reporting such as with report cards. The IEP team will determine how and when "periodic report" will be given and will include in writing as part of the IEP.

IEP Review and Revision

The IEP team must convene at least once a year to review a child's educational progress, the program, and plan for the next year. The review must take place prior to the annual review date.

Although IDEA requires only an annual review, a review of the IEP and its goals may occur at any time (34 CFR §300.320). This annual review is a minimum requirement of review, not a maximum. Families, teachers, or other IEP team members may request a "review and revision" of an IEP at any time if they feel that the program or a specific service or goal is not meeting a child's needs. Indeed, review and revision can be used by the IEP as a strategy to ensure that IEP goals or a specific goal or service meets a child's educational needs after a quarter or two of implementation of the goal, rather than waiting an entire year for such discussions. Additionally, any changes made to an IEP (e.g., an adjustment in amount of a service or where it is to be provided) require an IEP meeting. The school and families can also agree to develop a written document modifying or amending an IEP instead of convening an IEP meeting.

Triennial Reevaluation or Three-Year Review

IDEA requires that schools reevaluate a child receiving special education services every 3 years (34 CFR §300.303). Reevaluation can, however, occur more frequently or not at all if the school and family agree otherwise and do so in writing. Reevaluation is not simply additional testing, but rather involves a complete look at a child's needs, whether educational needs have changed, and determine if a child still qualifies for special education services.

> ***Shawn:*** *Shawn's family may be concerned that waiting an entire year between IEP meetings may contribute to falling further behind. As noted earlier, the review regulations lay out the minimum that is required. Clinicians can support a family by emphasizing this point and encouraging a request for review and revision of a goal if it requires modification to meet a child's needs, as well as offering medical advice and observations to the review and revision. Similarly, families such as Shawn's fear reevaluation because of past negative experiences, fear of losing services, and fear of losing access. Clinicians can support families through this process by being available to discuss concerns, review evaluation results, and map the results to necessary supports and services for an IEP.*

Developing a 504 Plan

As noted earlier in this chapter, Section 504 of the Rehabilitation Act is a different law than IDEA with different eligibility requirements, protections, and enforceability mechanisms. However, the process for development should essentially mirror that of an IEP with the convening of a team, a meeting, a written plan, and a binding legal document complete with accommodations, supports, and services crafted to meet the unique needs of, and prevent discrimination against, a child with a disability. Similarly, the team will focus on collecting data, developing a SMART plan, specifying everything in writing, and designing a plan for each child's unique needs. Therefore the earlier guidance for the IEP process and for partnership is relevant and informative for clinicians working on a 504 plan with families.

> ***Courtney:*** *Courtney has an IEP and thus is not eligible for a 504 plan. If she did not have educational needs, she could be eligible for a 504 plan to ensure she had the needed health services to ensure access school. Clinicians can play an important role in helping communicate the medical needs of a child in school.*

RESOURCES

Readers are encouraged to learn more about special education through the following resources.

A Guide to the Individualized Education Program: https://www2.ed.gov/parents/needs/speced/iepguide/iepguide.pdf

Transition from Part C to Preschool: https://ectacenter.org/topics/transition/transition.asp

A Transition Guide to Postsecondary Education and Employment for Students and Youth With Disabilities: https://www2.ed.gov/about/offices/list/osers/transition/products/postsecondary-transition-guide-august-2020.pdf

Protecting Students With Disabilities: https://www2.ed.gov/about/offices/list/ocr/504faq.html

REFERENCES

American Academy of Pediatrics. (2021). *AAP Bright Futures periodicity schedule*. https://downloads.aap.org/AAP/PDF/periodicity_schedule.pdf

Americans With Disabilities Act of 1990, as amended. (n.d.). https://www.ada.gov/pubs/adastatute08.pdf

Code of Federal Regulations. (2022). *Title 34, Subtitle B, Chapter 3, Sec 300*. https://www.ecfr.gov/cgi-bin/text-idx?tpl=/ecfrbrowse/Title34/34cfr300_main_02.tpl

Council for Exceptional Children. (2022). *Understanding the differences between IDEA and Section 504*. http://www.ldonline.org/article/6086

Disability Rights Education and Defense Fund. (n.d.). *School to prison pipeline*. https://dredf.org/legal-advocacy/school-to-prison-pipeline/

Every Child Succeed Acts. (n.d.). https://www.ed.gov/essa?src=rn

Harper, K. (2017). *Five things to know about racial and ethnic disparities in special education*. Child Trends. https://www.childtrends.org/publications/5-things-to-know-about-racial-and-ethnic-disparities-in-special-education

Henderson, K. (2007). *Overview of ADA, IDEA, and Section 504*. http://www.kidsource.com/kidsource/content3/ada.idea.html

Rebhorn, T. (2017). *Developing your child's IEP*. Center for Parent Information and Resources. https://www.parentcenterhub.org/pa12/#ref21

Rosenfeld, S. J. (2006). *Section 504 and IDEA: Basic similarities and differences*. http:www.wrightslaw.com/advoc/articles/504_IDEA_Rosenfeld.html

Section 504 of the *Rehabilitation Act of 1973*, as amended, 29 U.S.C. 794. (n.d.). https://www.govinfo.gov/content/pkg/USCODE-2010-title29/pdf/USCODE-2010-title29-chap16-subchapV-sec794.pdf

US Department of Education/Office of Special Education and Rehabilitative Services. (2000). *A guide to the individualized education program*. https://www2.ed.gov/parents/needs/speced/iepguide/iepguide.pdf

105

Transition to Adulthood for Young Adults With Intellectual and Developmental Disabilities

Judy Lu Kim and Albert Hergenroeder

VIGNETTE

Maria is a 20-year-old female with spastic quadriplegic cerebral palsy, mild intellectual disability, and seizure disorder who has received primary and specialty care at the local children's hospital system since infancy. Maria's pediatrician has been caring for her since birth and usually sees Maria three to four times a year for well-child visits and acute visits. Maria also sees a physical medicine and rehabilitation specialist, neurologist, and orthopedist twice a year at the multidisciplinary cerebral palsy clinic affiliated with the children's hospital. At Maria's last visit, her pediatrician recommended that she transfer care to an adult primary care provider by the time she turns 21. Maria's mother, who is a single parent and works full time, has become increasingly anxious about Maria's future. Maria will age out of the public school system in several months, and plans thereafter are not yet determined. Additionally, Maria has become increasingly irritable and defiant over the past year, causing additional stress in their household. Maria has expressed to her teachers that she feels "tired of it all." Maria's mother feels helpless and unsure of how to navigate the future.

INTRODUCTION

A development disability is a lifelong condition that is present before age 22, results in impairment in physical and/or cognitive functioning, and causes substantial limitations in major life activities (The Developmental Disabilities Assistance and Bill of Rights Act of 2000, n.d.). Intellectual disability is a type of developmental disability that is characterized by significant limitations in both intellectual functioning and adaptive behavioral and occurs before age 18 (American Association on Intellectual and Developmental Disability [AAIDD], n.d.). People with intellectual/developmental disabilities (IDD) have experienced increasing life expectancy in recent decades, and increasing numbers of adolescents with IDD are transitioning into adulthood (Lauer & McCallion, 2015).

For most adolescents and young adults (AYA), the transition into adulthood is complex and multifaceted, involving issues such as emerging independence, autonomous decision making, and sexuality, as well as changes in health care, education, employment, and housing. For AYA with IDD, the transition into adulthood can be even more challenging, given their unique health care and adaptive needs. Like Maria, described in the vignette, many AYA with IDD have spent substantial time in the pediatric health care setting, and the thought of transitioning to another provider can be daunting. Therefore AYA with IDD require intentional planning and support for the transition into adulthood. The goal of this chapter is to provide guidance for pediatric health care providers on how to work with AYA with IDD, as well as their families and health care team members, as they transition from pediatric to adult-based health care.

TRANSITION TO ADULT-BASED HEALTH CARE

Health Care Transition Overview

Priority and Goals of Health Care Transition for AYA With IDD

Advances in health care, nutrition, and medication have resulted in increasing life expectancy of individuals with IDD in recent decades (Lauer & McCallion, 2015). As a result, increasing numbers of AYA with IDD are entering adulthood each year. Additionally, the prevalence of any developmental disability among children and youth ages 3 to 17 in the United States has increased significantly from 16.2% between 2009 and 2011 to 17.8% between 2015 and 2017 (Zablotsky et al., 2019). According to the 2016 National Survey of Children's Health, approximately 5 million adolescents between ages 12 and 17 in the United States have special health care needs, yet only 17% received transition-planning support (Lebrun-Harris et al., 2018).

A well-accepted definition of transition from pediatric to adult-based care was introduced by the Society for Adolescent Medicine in 1993, which defines transition as "the purposeful, planned movement of AYA with chronic physical and medical conditions from child-centered to adult-oriented health care systems" (Blum et al., 1993). While this transition occurs for all AYA, it is particularly complex and challenging for many AYA with IDD given their complex health care and adaptive needs. The goal of health care transition (HCT) for young adults with special health care needs was outlined in a consensus statement from the American Academy of Pediatrics (AAP), American Board of Family Medicine (ABFM), and American College of Physicians (ACP) and is threefold: to maximize lifelong potential, to ensure high-quality and developmentally appropriate health care services, and to continue services without interruption during the transition from adolescence to adulthood (AAP et al., 2002). Achievement of this goal requires intentional planning and collaboration between AYA, their families, health care providers, and other service providers.

Challenges to Health Care Transition for AYA With IDD

AYA with IDD face challenges to HCT on multiple levels. These challenges may be at the level of the individual or family, health care provider, health care system, or insurance/ health care funding. Examples are provided in Table 105.1, and more detailed information on barriers to transition is described in the AAP's 2018 Clinical Report on Supporting the Health Care Transition From Adolescence to Adulthood in the Medical Home (White, Cooley, Transitions Clinical Report Authoring Group; American Academy of Pediatrics; American Academy of Family Physicians; American College of Physicians, 2018). For example, the barrier most widely reported by young adults with special health care needs and their parents/caregivers is the difficulty of losing longstanding relationships with pediatric providers. Adult and pediatric health care providers also report several barriers to transition, including lack of coordination and communication between practices. Pediatric providers have reported not knowing adult providers who are knowledgeable and willing to care for individuals with IDD. Adult providers have reported need for more training in chronic conditions of childhood and better handoff of information from pediatric providers (Gray et al., 2018). Lastly, significant changes in health insurance eligibility and benefits at age 18 put individuals with IDD at risk for loss of services or fragmented care if they are not adequately prepared (Sufian, Passamano, & Sopchak, 2018). Insurance coverage options are reviewed in greater detail later in this chapter.

TABLE 105.1 Challenges to Health Care Transition for Adolescents and Young Adults (AYA) With Intellectual/Developmental Disabilities (IDD)

Factor	Examples
Patient and family factors	Compared to peers with no IDD, AYA with IDD have greater medical complexity, including: • Increased medical comorbidities (Lunsky, 2019) • Increased medication use, polypharmacy (Lee, 2020) • Increased utilization of health care services (e.g., hospitalization, private duty nursing, therapies) (Kim, Stevens, Carbone, & Jones, 2020) • Need for support and adaptive modifications for activities of daily living, communication, mobility, decision making, and learning Attitudinal barriers (White et al., 2018): • Resistance to losing longstanding relationships with pediatric providers • Fear of leaving pediatric health care setting • Perceived low quality of care in adult setting Socioeconomic factors affecting ability to navigate or access care (e.g., language barrier, loss of insurance) (White et al., 2018) Lack of patient/family understanding of health conditions, poor adherence to care, lack of self-advocacy skills (White et al., 2018) Unrealistic patient/family expectations regarding care coordination support, provider time/attention, and access to services (White et al., 2018)
Health care provider factors	Pediatric provider not aware of adult providers knowledgeable and experienced in caring for individuals with IDD (White et al., 2018) Pediatric providers' perceived low quality of care in adult setting Pediatric provider resistance to letting go of longstanding relationship with patient Limited time to discuss transition by pediatric provider Pediatric provider's limited understanding of transition support needs of AYA with IDD Lack of communication and handoff between pediatric and adult health care provider Adult providers' lack of experience and training on IDD associated conditions (Gray et al., 2018) Adult providers' inexperience in providing developmentally appropriate care
Health care system factors	Lack of coordination and communication between pediatric and adult health care systems (Davies, Rennick, & Majnemer, 2011) Differences between pediatric and adult-based approach to health care: • Family-focused vs. individual-focused care • Limited multidisciplinary services in adult setting • Limited care coordination in adult setting • Limited resources for adults with IDD in the adult setting
Insurance/ funding factors	Potential loss of insurance due changes in eligibility criteria at age 18 yr Limited services covered by public insurance for adults Limited providers in network with public insurance for adults

Morbidity and Mortality Associated With Poor Health Care Transition

Morbidity and mortality increase in the posttransition period if HCT planning, transfer, and arrival in the adult health care system is not successful. Complications increase as the complexity of an individual's condition increases, and those with disabilities affecting cognition and mental health tend to have poorer transition experiences (Bloom et al., 2012). Inadequate transition support for AYA with complex chronic disease is associated with delayed or forgone care, decline in health status, and increased hospitalization rate (Dunbar et al., 2019). For example, surgery and hospitalization rates were higher in a group of patients with inflammatory bowel disease who had not gone through a transition program compared to those who did (Cole, Ashok, Razack, Azaz, & Sebastian, 2015). Similarly, patients with congenital heart disease who did not participate in a HCT program had longer time to first adult appointment and deterioration in functional status across the transition to adult-based care compared to patients who participated in a formal HCT program (Hergenroeder et al., 2018).

Differences Between Pediatric- and Adult-Based Approach to Care

Pediatric providers should educate and prepare patients and families for differences in approach to care and availability of services in the pediatric and adult health care settings.

Pediatric Versus Adult Provider Approach to Care

Because of the key roles that parents play as caregivers and primary decision makers for their children, pediatric providers often provide care that is family focused with high parental engagement. On the other hand, adult providers are often more patient focused and assume an individual's independent decision-making capacity. Additionally, pediatric providers are often more attuned to providing care that is developmentally appropriate for an individual, regardless of age. In contrast, adult providers are more accustomed to providing age-appropriate care and may struggle with adapting delivery of care and communication in a way that is developmentally appropriate. Pediatric providers should prepare AYA with IDD for engaging with adult health care providers. Ideas include:

Allow the young adult with IDD to participate in clinic visits as much as possible. If appropriate, allow for independent portion of visits.

Educate the young adult on how to describe the medical condition(s).

Optimize the young adult's self-management skills as developmentally appropriate.

Include information regarding adaptive function (e.g., communication, self-direction, decision-making support) in health records or medical summary that will be handed off to receiving adult providers.

Care Coordination and Service Availability

In the pediatric setting care for patients with IDD is often delivered in integrated, multidisciplinary teams, and care coordination is more readily available to help patients navigate care and access services. In the adult setting, however, patients and families often must assume a greater role in navigating and coordinating care, which may be spread across various providers in different practice settings (Okumura, Harris, & Kleinhenz, 2018). Those who are unprepared for navigating care independently are at risk for fragmented care, loss of services, and overall poor transition experience. In preparation for changes in delivery and coordination of care pediatric providers can educate the AYA with IDD and/or their parents/caregivers on how to:

Appropriately and independently access care (e.g., how to contact health care providers for routine appointments and acute concerns, request medications, contact support services regarding therapy or equipment needs)

Create a list of members of the individual's health care team, their roles and responsibilities, and contact information

Create a care notebook, which should include medical history and health care team members' information (see Table 105.3 [later] for sample templates).

There are also significant differences in availability of services in the pediatric and adult health care setting. For example, insurances often cover long-term therapies for pediatric patients to optimize function in the developmental period. For adults, however, many insurances will cover only short-term therapies to address acute changes in function or symptoms. Similarly, individuals who receive private duty nursing services at home often experience a reduction or loss of insurance coverage for nursing services upon reaching adulthood. For many individuals with IDD, the loss or reduction of private duty nursing is a major disruption that may impair a parent's ability to work out of the home or affect the quality of care the individual receives in absence of a trained nurse. In addition, services such as sedation for anxiety-provoking procedures and child life specialist support are more readily available in the pediatric setting. Adults with IDD may have difficulty accessing sedation for procedures that are usually completed in the general population without sedation, such as lab draws, dental exam, gynecologic exams, or imaging studies. As a result, necessary procedures may be forcibly completed, delayed, or foregone. In preparation for potential loss of services pediatric providers can:

Educate patients and families on the potential loss of services (such as nursing and therapies), and assess the young adult and/or caregivers' ability to continue necessary care independently.

Utilize behavioral therapy services early in the developmental period to facilitate desensitization for procedures that could potentially be completed without sedation in the future. For example, desensitization interventions have been shown to be effective in helping children with autism spectrum disorder successfully accept a dental exam seated in a dental chair in absence of oral sedation or protective stabilization (Yost, Nelson, Sheller, McKinney, Tressel et al., 2019).

Try forms of sedation that may be more easily accessible in the adult setting, such as oral anxiolytics (e.g., benzodiazepines).

Decision-Making Support

In the pediatric setting parents are often the primary decision makers and care providers. Upon reaching the age of majority, individuals cross the threshold into adulthood and assume the legal rights and responsibilities as independent decision makers. In most states this occurs at age 18 but can be up to age 21. This transition in decision-making responsibility can be particularly challenging for individuals with IDD and their families, as parents are often accustomed to making decisions on behalf of their child with IDD, even through adolescence and adulthood. If appropriate, individuals with IDD should receive preparation, support, and opportunity for independent decision making over the course of their lifetime. Some adults with IDD, however, may need lifelong support for decision making, and several legal options are available. In general, an individual's role in decision making should be maximized, and thus the least restrictive form of support should be pursued. Options for decision-making support are summarized in Table 105.2. More detailed information regarding self-determination and decision-making support can be found in Chapter 117.

When deciding on which form of decision-making support is most appropriate, it is important to remember that an individual's physical function and verbal communication skills might not correlate with intellectual function. For example, someone like Maria, described in the vignette, may have significant physical limitations but still have capacity to be an autonomous decision maker. Neurocognitive evaluation by a psychologist may be helpful in situations where the most appropriate type of decision-making support is unclear. Additionally, even if guardianship is appropriate, health care providers and guardians should still aim for an individual's input and assent to care. Lastly, when handing off care to receiving adult providers, the pediatric provider should include within a medical summary or transfer letter information regarding the individual's decision-making capacity, level of intellectual functioning, and preferences for communication to help guide interactions with new providers.

Evidence and Framework for Transitioning to Adult-Based Care

Evidence Base for Transition Planning Practices

In a scoping review of research on transition in young adults with chronic conditions Acuña Mora et al. (2019) reported a dramatic increase in the number of peer-reviewed articles on HCT, from six papers published between 1989 and 1994 to 196 published in 2015 alone. The authors reported strong theoretic groundwork regarding the need for policies that facilitate successful HCT. The evidence base for best practices, however, is not well established (Acuña Mora et al., 2019). Additionally,

TABLE 105.2 Decision-Making Support Options

Option (From Most to Least Restrictive)	Legal Decision Maker	Description	Requirements
Guardianship	Guardian	Designation of guardianship indicates the transfer of decision-making rights from an individual to a guardian (e.g., parent, relative, or court-appointed guardian). Total guardianship allows a guardian to make all decisions. Partial guardianship allows an individual to retain decision-making rights in designated domains.	Guardianship is appropriate for individuals who do not have capacity to make decisions. A physician who is familiar with the individual is usually involved in assessing capacity. The guardianship process goes through the court system and can be costly (due to attorney and court fees) and time intensive.
Supported decision making (SDM)	Individual retains legal decision making right.	SDM is an alternative to guardianship that allows an individual to designate a supporter(s) to assist with making decisions, but the individual retains decision-making rights.	States vary in their approach to SDM. In most states the SDM agreement is a legal document signed by the individual, supporter, and witness(es) or public notary.
Medical power of attorney (MPOA)	Individual retains decision-making rights until deemed incapacitated. Thereafter the designated agent assumes decision-making rights.	MPOA is a type of advance directive in which an individual appoints someone (an agent) to make decisions on one's behalf in the event that the individual is no longer able to make decisions.	At the time of designation of MPOA, an individual must be competent to voluntarily designate an agent. The rules and requirements for MPOA vary by state. In most states the MPOA is a legal document signed by the individual, agent, and witness(es) or public notary.

much of the available research and evidence is regarding populations with homogeneous diagnoses. A systematic review of HCT practice service models by Betz, O'Kane, Nehring, & Lobo. (2016) found that most studies included in the review focused on populations with single chronic conditions of childhood, such as type 1 diabetes, sickle cell disease, organ transplant, juvenile idiopathic arthritis, cystic fibrosis, inflammatory bowel disease, and human immunodeficiency virus. The literature on transition programs for these populations shows promising results for improving transition by having the AYA meet with their adult provider before the transfer to adult care. Similar to the findings of Acuña Mora et al., however, there was not sufficient empirical data to ascribe improved outcome to a specific intervention or model of care to support HCT (Betz et al., 2016). Additionally, diagnostically heterogeneous and complex populations, such as those with IDD, likely need a different approach to transition planning than populations with homogeneous diagnoses. Therefore while there is widespread agreement that AYA with IDD have unique health and adaptive needs that warrant tailored transition planning support, how this transition support should be delivered is not well established.

Framework for Health Care Transition

Although clinical practices vary in their delivery of transition support, there are shared elements among HCT programs. Got Transition, a program of the National Alliance to Advance Adolescent Health, outlines six core elements of HCT (GotTransition.org, n.d.) that are considered basic components of a HCT program (Fig. 105.1). Clinicians and practices may vary in how they implement these elements, and this approach to HCT planning does not require implementation of all these elements nor implementation in a linear fashion. Some practices may choose to implement a few elements while others may implement all elements. The gottransition.org website contains various tools and resources for how these elements can be implemented in various clinical settings.

In general, HCT planning is a three-stage process that involves (1) transition preparation, (2) transfer to adult care, and (3) integration into adult care (Berens, Blazo, & Peacock, 2020). The six core elements are included within each of these three steps. The first stage, transition preparation, includes core elements 1 through 4 (transition policy, tracking and monitoring, transition readiness assessment, and transition planning) and is typically initiated in the pediatric setting at the onset of adolescence. Although transition policy is the first core element of HCT planning, in the authors' experience large practices may have difficulty reaching consensus on specific elements of a HCT policy, such as expected age of transfer or criteria for transfer. Even if details of a transition policy cannot be agreed upon, a practice can still address other elements of transition preparation. If a policy is developed, however, it should be discussed with AYA with IDD and their families well in advance of transfer, as the increased complexity of individuals with IDD may require more time and preparation for transition. Transition preparation also typically involves development of self-management skills. AYA with IDD, however, may vary in their capacity for independence. For individuals who have lifelong dependence on caregivers, pediatric providers should assess the primary caregivers' understanding of the individual's health conditions and provide education for skills needed for daily care (e.g., catheterization, gastrostomy change, tracheostomy care). In preparation of eventual transfer the pediatric provider should work with young adults and their families to create a medical summary that includes the following (Betz, 2018): diagnosis and date of confirmation, condition severity, comorbidities, previous surgeries, previous significant hospitalizations, medications, daily treatments required for management of chronic conditions (e.g., catheterizations, airway clearance regimen), adaptive equipment, special diets, allergies, and name and contact information of health care team members. Table 105.3 provides examples of medical summary templates.

Stage 2, transfer to adult care, usually occurs between ages 18 and 21 and involves the actual transfer of care to adult providers. This may be a multistep process that occurs over a period of months to years as individuals may choose to first transfer to adult primary care and then gradually transfer to adult specialty care. Especially for AYA with IDD who may have complicated medical or behavioral histories, the transfer process should include written or verbal handoff from pediatric to adult providers. Sample transfer checklists can be found at GotTransition.org and https://ddprimarycare.surreyplace.ca/wp-content/uploads/2019/09/2.5-TAY-Transition-Transfer-Tool.pdf. At minimum, the transfer packet should include an updated medical summary for receiving adult providers. Practices should also establish processes to ensure transfer completion, as patients may experience unexpected delay or barriers to establishing care with adult providers

Lastly, integration into adult care (stage 3) involves an ongoing effort to integrate into the adult health care setting and adjust to changes in services and resources. This often requires collaboration and communication between the adult and pediatric health care team, social workers,

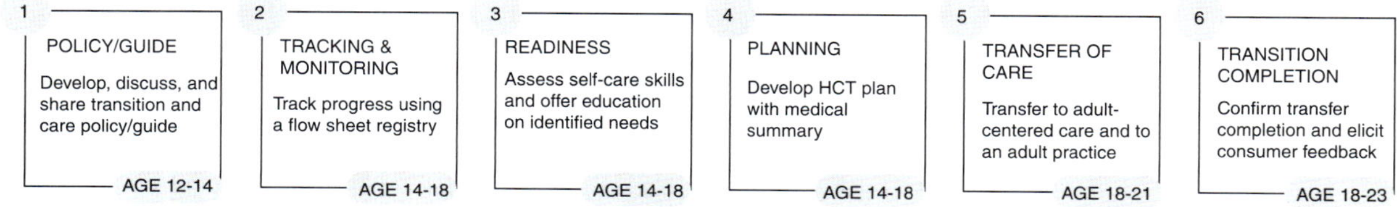

Fig. 105.1 Six core elements. (Copyright © 2020 GotTransition®. Non-commercial use is permitted, but requires attribution to Got Transition for any use, copy or adaptation. https://www.gottransition.org/six-core-elements/)

TABLE 105.3 Examples of Medical Summaries

Got Transition	**Sample Medical Summary and Emergency Care Plan** https://www.gottransition.org/6ce/?leaving-medical-summary-emergency-plan
American College of Physicians	**Pediatric to Adult Care Transitions Toolkit** https://www.acponline.org/clinical-information/high-value-care/resources-for-clinicians/pediatric-to-adult-care-transitions-initiative/condition-specific-tools
Sick Kids Good 2 Go Transition Program	**My Health Passport** https://wapps.sickkids.ca/myhealthpassport/
American Academy of Pediatrics	**Building Your Care Notebook** https://medicalhomeinfo.aap.org/tools-resources/Pages/For-Families.aspx
Medical Home Portal	**Care Notebook** https://www.medicalhomeportal.org/living-with-child/after-a-diagnosis-or-problem-is-identified/caring-for-children-with-special-health-care-needs/managing-and-coordinating-care/care-notebook
Epic UserWeb Community Library	**Transition of Care Portable Medical Summary in Epic UserWeb Community Library**

and care coordinators from insurance and community programs to ensure that the young adult has access to necessary specialists, insurance resources, and community support services. Especially for individuals with IDD, integration into adult care may take years or continue throughout one's lifetime.

Insurance Coverage Changes and Options in Adulthood

The transition to adulthood also includes substantial changes to health insurance that require advance preparation to ensure continued coverage into adulthood. For example, Supplemental Security Income (SSI) is a public program that provides monthly cash benefit and Medicaid coverage for individuals who meet low-income and medical eligibility requirements, and eligibility criteria changes at age 18. Individuals who received SSI benefits as a minor will have to meet new adult medical eligibility criteria at age 18, and some individuals may be at risk for losing SSI benefits and Medicaid insurance if they do not meet the often more stringent adult eligibility criteria. On the other hand, individuals who did not previously qualify for SSI benefits as a minor due to parental income may be eligible for SSI when they turn 18 as only the individual's income is considered. Review for medical eligibility is completed by the Social Security Administration (SSA) and is based on review of medical records. Therefore pediatric providers should be diligent to document individuals' functional and cognitive limitations and whether they preclude engagement in full-time employment.

Young adults with IDD have several options for health insurance (Table 105.4). Pediatric providers should discuss upcoming insurance changes at least 3 months prior to the young adult's 18th birthday to ensure continued coverage and make referrals for social work assistance if needed (Sufian et al., 2018).

Pediatric providers should also prepare young adults for changes in insurance benefits, particularly after transitioning from pediatric to adult Medicaid programs (typically at age 21). Many individuals experience reduction or discontinuation of long-term therapies, private duty nursing, and coverage of certain durable medical equipment (DME). Therefore prior to the transition to adult Medicaid programs, pediatric providers should ensure that DME is updated and fully functional and that individuals or caregivers are skilled to provide care previously provided by private duty nurses or therapists.

Medicaid waiver programs are important sources of coverage for medical care and services not covered by insurance. For many adults with IDD, waivers help cover private duty nursing services, respite care, medical equipment, and long-term therapies. Waiver programs and eligibility criteria vary by state, but in most states individuals with significant disease burden or adaptive and supportive needs qualify for a waiver waitlist. Wait times, however, vary significantly by state and can range from months to over 10 years long. Information regarding Medicaid waiver programs can be found on each state's health or social services department website.

PSYCHOSOCIAL ISSUES DURING TRANSITION INTO ADULTHOOD

In addition to changes in health care, the period of transition to adulthood is accompanied by substantial changes in psychosocial domains, including education and employment, sexuality, mental health, and housing. While it is beyond the scope of this chapter to explore each of these domains in detail, some of these issues are discussed in greater depth in other chapters (see Chapters 75, and 111). The following section provides pediatric providers with a general overview of emerging issues and resources available for young adults with IDD.

Postsecondary Opportunities

For many young adults, graduation from high school is an exciting experience and a gateway to new opportunities. For some AYA with IDD and their families, however, life after graduation may be fraught with uncertainty, fear, and loss—loss of a daily routine, educational engagement, support services, and socialization with peers (McKenzie, Ouellette-Kuntz, Blinkhorn, & Démoré, 2017). Before young adults

TABLE 105.4 Options for Health Insurance for Adults With Intellectual/Developmental Disabilities (IDD)

Option	Description
Medicaid public insurance	Medicaid eligibility varies by state. If living in a state with expanded Medicaid coverage, an individual may qualify for Medicaid as an adult with low income. If living in a state that did not expand Medicaid coverage, then the individual will have to meet low-income and medical eligibility requirements.
Medicare public insurance	Social Security Disability Insurance (SSDI) is a federal program that provides monthly cash benefits and Medicare coverage, regardless of one's assets. An adult with IDD may qualify for Medicare in two primary ways: (1) Disabled Adult Child Program: adults with disabilities may be eligible for SSDI and Medicare if their parent becomes eligible for Medicare; (2) Disability Insurance: individuals who previously worked may be eligible for SSDI if they experience a change in health status that prevents them from continued employment.
Parental private insurance plan	Under the Affordable Care Act, young adults can stay on parental health insurance plan until age 26. Some employer-sponsored insurance plans will allow adult dependents with disabilities to stay on their parent's insurance plan after age 26. Parents should talk to their insurance plan or employer regarding this option before their child turns 26. Documentation of the dependent's disabilities by a physician may be required.
Employer-sponsored private insurance	Some adults with IDD are able to sustain employment. If so, they should be encouraged to seek employment that provides health insurance benefits.
Health Insurance Marketplace	The health insurance marketplace is a government-operated forum that offers health insurance plans for purchase. Marketplace insurance plans are subsidized for individuals and based on income. Since the Affordable Care Act, individuals with IDD can no longer be denied coverage based on their preexisting conditions.
COBRA coverage	The Consolidated Omnibus Budget Reconciliation Act (COBRA) allows for continuation of health insurance for a limited period after a qualifying event (e.g., death of policyholder, termination or layoff).

with IDD age out of the school system (typically at age 21 or 22), pediatric providers should discuss options for continued education or programs to help maximize lifelong potential. Social workers and the school system can also help identify opportunities after graduation, as all students receiving special education must have a transition plan as part of their individualized education plan (IEP). Common postsecondary opportunities include:

Postsecondary education. Some individuals may seek college or university education. For these individuals, pediatric providers should ensure these young adults can independently manage their medical conditions and access adult health care providers, especially if they move out of the home. Young adults should reach out to their institution's office for students with disabilities to access accommodations and services necessary for their educational and experiential success. Many postsecondary educational programs are also expanding services for students with intellectual disabilities. More information on postsecondary educational opportunities can be found at www.thinkcollege.net and www.aucd.org.

Employment. Some individuals with IDD start vocational training in the school system as early as middle school, and vocational skills and job training are the focus of many "18+" programs in school. Individuals who desire to transition from the school system to the workforce can seek further vocational training and employment support through their state's workforce agency or disability program, Medicaid waiver program, or other community programs that provide supported employment for individuals with IDD. Individuals who have Medicaid and are employed should be aware of income limits associated with Medicaid eligibility. More information about employment can be found at https://choosework.ssa.gov/index.html and https://askearn.org/.

Day habilitation program. Day habs are community-based programs that provide opportunities for individuals with IDD to continue to develop vocational, social, and life skills. Some programs also include sheltered workshops to provide supervised employment. Day hab is usually paid by Medicaid waiver programs or out of pocket.

Adult daycare. Adult daycare centers provide care and supervision for adults with disabilities who need assistance with daily activities and/or supervision. These centers may allow family members to continue working out of the home and provide respite for caregivers. Adult daycare is covered by many states' Medicaid plans.

Sexuality

During adolescence and into adulthood, young adults with IDD may experience changes in sexual development and start asking questions or develop an interest in sexuality, sexual behaviors, body image, gender identity, or special relationships. Pediatric providers and caregivers should be prepared to educate and answer questions related to sexuality and respect the inherent sexual rights that individuals with IDD possess (AAIDD, 2008). Given the higher rate of sexual abuse among individuals with disabilities compared to those without disabilities (Office of Justice Programs, 2017), it is particularly important that pediatric providers and caregivers provide developmentally appropriate education regarding names of body parts, sexual development, appropriate sexual behaviors, privacy, safety, and consent. Pediatric providers should encourage parents and caregivers to be the primary teachers of sexual education for their child in a way that is developmentally appropriate and aligned with the family's values, culture, and beliefs. Sexual education resources geared toward individuals with IDD can be found at https://www.respectability.org/resources/sexual-education-resources/. The National Council on Independent Living (https://ncil.org/sex-ed-for-individuals-with-i-dd/) also has video-based sexual education resources designed for individuals with IDD.

Mental Health

AYA with IDD have reported high rates of mental health conditions such as anxiety, depression, and obsessive-compulsive disorder during the period of transition into adulthood, between ages 14 and 22 (Schwartz et al., 2020). Cooccurring mental health conditions can negatively impact quality of life, physical health, relationships, and educational and social participation. Unfortunately, only 1 in 10 children and adolescents with mental health conditions receive specialized mental health care (Munir, 2016). Individuals with IDD face even greater barriers to accessing adequate mental health supports due to underrecognition of mental health conditions, lack of professionals trained to care for individuals with IDD, and inaccessibility of services due to services designed for neurotypical individuals or due to lack of transportation (Schwartz et al., 2020). When caring for AYA with IDD, pediatric providers should screen for changes in mood or behavior, which may at times be based on caregiver report. If changes are identified, the provider should evaluate for underlying medical causes (e.g., headache, dental pain, musculoskeletal pain, infection), environmental causes (e.g., change in routine, new caregiver, inadequate communication, or lack of activities), or mental health condition. Pediatric providers should be wary of diagnostic overshadowing, the false attribution of changes in behavior or mood to the individual's IDD without consideration for possible underlying physical or mental health issues. Pediatric providers should not delay referral to mental health providers such as psychiatrists or therapists if additional expertise is needed for diagnosis or treatment of mental health conditions

Housing Options

As individuals with IDD witness siblings and peers move out of their families' homes, some may explore options for housing that provide greater independence. For some individuals, this may mean moving to a part of their family's home that provides greater privacy when desired. For others, this may mean moving into a group home with supervision, living with roommates, or living independently. The National Council on Independent Living (ncil.org) provides national and local resources on independent living for people with disabilities. Medicaid waiver programs and community programs for individuals with IDD can also provide guidance and support for individuals exploring housing options.

Over the course of 9 months, Maria's pediatrician worked with Maria, her mom, and her pediatric specialists to identify an adult primary care provider, neurologist, and physical medicine specialist that are in network with Maria's current and future insurance and that care for other young adults with cerebral palsy. An adult orthopedist was not necessary at the time of transfer as Maria had no anticipated need for surgery. With the guidance of her pediatrician, Maria and her mom created a care notebook, including a medical summary and supported decision-making agreement to give to her new adult providers. Maria has a Medicaid waiver, and she and her mom were encouraged to speak with their waiver case manager regarding options for postsecondary programs in their area. This would provide Maria the opportunity for continued socialization with peers and allow her mom to continue working. After obtaining further history from Maria and ruling out new underlying medical issues, the pediatrician recommended starting a selective serotonin reuptake inhibitor (SSRI) medication and referral to a counselor for treatment of depression, likely triggered by loss of friends who have already graduated from high school. Both Maria and her mother reported notable improvement in mood and behavior after 4 months. Although Maria's future remains unknown, she and her mother now face the upcoming transitions with greater preparation, anticipation, and hope.

REFERENCES

Acuña Mora, M., Saarijärvi, M., Moons, P., Sparud-Lundin, C., Bratt, E. L., & Goossens, E. (2019). The scope of research on transfer and transition in young persons with chronic conditions. *The Journal of Adolescent Health: Official Publication of the Society for Adolescent Medicine, 65*(5), 581–589. https://doi.org/10.1016/j.jadohealth.2019.07.014

American Academy of Pediatrics. (2002). A consensus statement on health care transitions for young adults with special health care needs American Academy of Family Physicians, & American College of Physicians-American Society of Internal Medicine. *Pediatrics, 110*(6 Pt 2), 1304–1306.

American Association on Intellectual and Developmental Disability. (n.d.). *Defining criteria for intellectual disability*. https://www.aaidd.org/intellectual-disability/definition

American Association on Intellectual and Developmental Disability. (2008). *Joint position statement of AAIDD and The Arc on Sexuality*. https://www.aaidd.org/news-policy/policy/position-statements/sexuality

Berens, J., Blazo, M., & Peacock, C. (2020). Transitioning to adult care. In S. U. Dhar, S. C. Nagamani, & T. N. Eble (Eds.), *Handbook of clinical adult genetics and genomics: A practice-based approach* (pp. 59–69). Elsevier.

Betz, C. (2018). Different healthcare transition models. In A. C. Hergenroeder & C. M. Wiemann (Eds.), *Health care transition: Building a program for adolescents and young adults with chronic illness and disability* (pp. 363–377). Springer.

Betz, C. L., O'Kane, L. S., Nehring, W. M., & Lobo, M. L. (2016). Systematic review: Health care transition practice service models. *Nursing Outlook, 64*(3), 229–243. https://doi.org/10.1016/j.outlook.2015.12.011

Bloom, S. R., Kuhlthau, K., Van Cleave, J., Knapp, A. A., Newacheck, P., & Perrin, J. M. (2012). Health care transition for youth with special health care needs. *The Journal of Adolescent Health: Official Publication of the Society for Adolescent Medicine, 51*(3), 213–219. https://doi.org/10.1016/j.jadohealth.2012.01.007

Blum, R. W., Garell, D., Hodgman, C. H., Jorissen, T. W., Okinow, N. A., Orr, D. P., & Slap, G. B. (1993). Transition from child-centered to adult health-care systems for adolescents with chronic conditions. A position paper of the Society for Adolescent Medicine. *The Journal of Adolescent Health: Official Publication of the Society for Adolescent Medicine, 14*(7), 570–576. https://doi.org/10.1016/1054-139x(93)90143-d

Cole, R., Ashok, D., Razack, A., Azaz, A., & Sebastian, S. (2015). Evaluation of outcomes in adolescent inflammatory bowel disease patients following transfer from pediatric to adult health care services: Case for transition. *The Journal of Adolescent Health: Official Publication of the Society for Adolescent Medicine, 57*(2), 212–217. https://doi.org/10.1016/j.jadohealth.2015.04.012

Davies, H., Rennick, J., & Majnemer, A. (2011). Transition from pediatric to adult health care for young adults with neurological disorders: Parental perspectives. *Canadian Journal of Neuroscience Nursing, 33*(2), 32–39.

Dunbar, P., Hall, M., Gay, J. C., Hoover, C., Markham, J. L., Bettenhausen, J. L., … Berry, J. G. (2019). Hospital readmission of adolescents and young adults with complex chronic disease. *JAMA Network Open, 2*(7), e197613. https://doi.org/10.1001/jamanetworkopen.2019.7613

GotTransition.org. (n.d.). *Got transition*. GotTransition.org. https://www.gottransition.org/

Gray, W. N., Schaefer, M. R., Resmini-Rawlinson, A., & Wagoner, S. T. (2018). Barriers to transition from pediatric to adult care: A systematic review. *Journal of Pediatric Psychology, 43*(5), 488–502. https://doi.org/10.1093/jpepsy/jsx142

Hergenroeder, A. C., Moodie, D. S., Penny, D. J., Wiemann, C. M., Sanchez-Fournier, B., Moore, L. K., & Head, J. (2018). Functional classification of heart failure before and after implementing a health care transition program for youth and young adults transferring from a pediatric to an adult congenital heart disease clinics. *Congenital Heart Disease, 13*(4), 548–553. https://doi.org/10.1111/chd.12604

Kim, J., Stevens, P., Carbone, P. S., & Jones, K. B. (2020). Health care use and spending of pediatric patients with an intellectual or developmental disability. *Medical Care, 58*(5), 468–473. https://doi.org/10.1097/MLR.0000000000001293

Lauer, E., & McCallion, P. (2015). Mortality of people with intellectual and developmental disabilities from select US state disability service systems and medical claims data. *Journal of Applied Research in Intellectual Disabilities: JARID, 28*(5), 394–405. https://doi.org/10.1111/jar.12191

Lebrun-Harris, L. A., McManus, M. A., Ilango, S. M., Cyr, M., McLellan, S. B., Mann, M. Y., & White, P. H. (2018). Transition planning among US youth with and without special health care needs. *Pediatrics, 142*(4), e20180194. https://doi.org/10.1542/peds.2018-0194

Lee, I. (2020). Pharmacist interventions for persons with intellectual disabilities: A scoping review. *Research in Social and Administrative Pharmacy.* https://doi.org/10.1016/j.sapharm.2020.03.009

Lunsky, D. (2019). High health care costs among adults with intellectual and developmental disabilities: A population-based study: High health care costs. *Journal of Intellectual Disability Research, 63*(2), 124–137. https://doi.org/10.1111/jir.12554

McKenzie, K., Ouellette-Kuntz, H., Blinkhorn, A., & Démoré, A. (2017). Out of school and into distress: Families of young adults with intellectual and developmental disabilities in transition. *Journal of Applied Research in Intellectual Disabilities: JARID, 30*(4), 774–781. https://doi.org/10.1111/jar.12264

Munir, K. M. (2016). The co-occurrence of mental disorders in children and adolescents with intellectual disability/intellectual developmental disorder. *Current Opinion in Psychiatry, 29*(2), 95–102. https://doi.org/10.1097/YCO.0000000000000236

Office of Justice Programs. (2017). *Crime against persons with disabilities, 2009-2015.* Statistical Tables.

Okumura, M. J., Harris, I. S., & Kleinhenz, M. (2018). Understanding the pediatric and adult healthcare system: Adapting to change. In A. C. Hergenroeder & C. M. Wiemann (Eds.), *Health care transition: Building a program for adolescents and young adults with chronic illness and disability* (pp. 75–83). Springer.

Schwartz, A. E., Young Adult Mental Health/Peer Mentoring Research Team, Kramer, J. M., Rogers, E. S., McDonald, K. E., & Cohn, E. S. (2020). Stakeholder-driven approach to developing a peer-mentoring intervention for young adults with intellectual/developmental disabilities and co-occurring mental health conditions. *Journal of Applied Research in Intellectual Disabilities: JARID, 33*(5), 992–1004. https://doi.org/10.1111/jar.12721

Sufian, B., Passamano, J., & Sopchak, A. (2018). Healthcare insurance changes as youth become young adults. In A. C. Hergenroeder & C. M. Wiemann (Eds.), *Health care transition: building a program for adolescents and young adults with chronic illness and disability* (pp. 75–83). Springer.

The Developmental Disabilities Assistance and Bill of Rights Act of 2000 [Public Law 106-402, 106th Congress]. (n.d.). https://www.in.gov/gpcpd/board-and-staff/join-the-board/federal-definition-of-developmental-disabilities/#:~:text=The%20Developmental%20Disabilities%20Assistance%20and,of%20mental%20and%20physical%20impairments

White, P. H., Cooley, W. C; Transitions Clinical Report Authoring Group; American Academy of Pediatrics; American Academy of Family Physicians; American College of Physicians. (2018). Supporting the health care transition from adolescence to adulthood in the medical home. *Pediatrics, 142*(5), e20182587. https://doi.org/10.1542/peds.2018-3610

Yost, Q., Nelson, T., Sheller, B., McKinney, C. M., Tressel, W., & Chim, A. N. (2019). Children with autism spectrum disorder are able to maintain dental skills: A two-year case review of desensitization treatment. *Pediatric Dentistry, 41*(5), 397–403.

Zablotsky, B., Black, L. I., Maenner, M. J., Schieve, L. A., Danielson, M. L., Bitsko, R. H., … Boyle, C. A. (2019). Prevalence and trends of developmental disabilities among children in the United States: 2009–2017. *Pediatrics, 144*(4), e20190811. https://doi.org/10.1542/peds.2019-0811

Rehabilitation Services: Occupational Therapy and Physical Therapy

M. Kathleen Kelly and Meg Stanger

For additional material related to the content of this chapter, please see Chapters 29, 30, and 31.

VIGNETTE

Max was referred to the physical therapist (PT) at 14 weeks of age for torticollis. The PT conducted a detailed examination of neck strength and range of motion (ROM) in the context of a standardized neuromotor assessment. The PT noted the child was pale and had a decreased activity level for his age. His mother reported that he chokes or coughs during feeds, but said the pediatrician thought he likely had reflux. After this initial visit, the PT reached out to Max's pediatrician to discuss these red flags, and a plan was developed to monitor these concerns and initiate a referral to an occupational therapist (OT) for the feeding difficulties.

At the follow-up visit 2 weeks later, his head tilt remained unchanged despite the family reliably doing the prescribed home program, and swallowing difficulties were worse. Max's color was dusky, he was irritable, difficult to console, and had an episode of retching without emesis. Concerned that this presentation was not consistent with torticollis or typical reflux, the PT contacted his pediatrician immediately. Max was diagnosed with a medullary astrocytoma requiring urgent surgical resection and resulting in left hemiplegia. He endured multiple courses of chemotherapy over the next few years.

The OT and PT were integral members of Max's medical, rehabilitation, and educational team over the next 5+ years. They provided evidence-based interventions to address his functional limitations and participation restrictions. Outcome measures were used to monitor the impact of chemotherapy on his developing neurologic, musculoskeletal, and cardiopulmonary systems and to track his progress in rehabilitation. When Max was transitioning to school, they worked closely with his teachers and other related service providers to ensure continuity of care and goals.

In partnership with Max's family child- and family-centered care plans were implemented that evolved with his changing medical and developmental status.

According to the World Health Organization (WHO, 2020) rehabilitation is defined as "a set of interventions designed to optimize functioning and reduce disability in individuals with health conditions in interaction with their environment."

*The authors would like to acknowledge Kimberly Kubistek, OTD, OTR/L, Coordinator of Occupational Therapy Services—UPMC Children's Hospital of Pittsburgh for contribution to the case vignette and chapter review.

The essence of rehabilitation is a person-centered approach to optimizing function and meaningful participation. The space of rehabilitation can be occupied by several professionals depending on the context, but mostly includes physical medicine and rehabilitation physicians, OT, PT, speech-language pathologists, orthotists and prosthetists, assistive technology professionals, rehabilitation-related counselors, and behavioral health professionals. With the advances in medicine, science, and technology, the prevalence of children living with developmental differences and complex health care conditions has increased (see Chapter 1). As a result, care needs shift from life saving to life optimizing. This shift requires intentional focus on the provision of supports and services to enhance the child's quality of life. It is in this context that OT and PT play a critical role on the child's medical, rehabilitation, and/or educational team with their collective expertise in identifying and managing the cognitive, physical, sensory, and social-emotional impairments that limit meaningful participation in everyday life.

This chapter provides the reader with an appreciation of how these professions have evolved and their contribution to contemporary pediatric rehabilitation, especially for children who have neurodevelopmental and behavioral challenges. The case of Max, in the vignette, illustrates the depth and scope of knowledge and practice that OT and PT offer to the health care and/or educational teams serving these children and families. Later in the chapter we will discuss the discipline-specific approach to addressing the complexity of issues that unfolded over the first few years of Max's life.

HISTORICAL PERSPECTIVE AND EVOLUTION OF THE PROFESSIONS

The OT and PT professions share a rich history in their evolution and formation of professional identities (Tables 106.1 and 106.2). Both formally emerged in the United States during the early part of the 20th century at a time when the practice of medicine was well established. Although young in comparison, these professions have undergone significant changes during their 100+-year histories and now join medicine as highly respected and vibrant health care professions. For both, World War I was a significant factor in their formative years, although historical accounts note that each has roots preceding the start of the war. In 1917 a physical reconstruction program was created to model what had been in place in

TABLE 106.1 Evolution of the Occupational Therapy (OT) Profession

1917	First meeting of the National Society for the Promotion of Occupational Therapy
1921	Name changed to the American Occupational Therapy Association (AOTA)
1931	First BS program established at Milwaukee-Downer College
1994	Accreditation Council for OT Education (ACOTE) founded and recognized by the US Department of Education
1999	ACOTE establishes postbaccalaureate entry for OT
2017	100-year anniversary of OT profession
2019	Official policy from AOTA: entry-level education for OT is at the master's *or* doctoral level
2021	First offering of board-certified specialist exam in pediatrics (previous specialty certification was peer-review of a professional portfolio)

Adapted from American Occupational Therapy Association. (2017). http://www.otcentennial.org/events/1920

TABLE 106.2 Evolution of the Physical Therapy (PT) Profession

1921	First meeting of the American Women's Physical Therapeutic Association (AWPTA)
1927	First BS program established at New York University
1947	Name changed to the American Physical Therapy Association (APTA)
1960	First 2-year graduate program established at Western Reserve University (now Case Western)
1978	Commission on Accreditation of PT Education (CAPTE) was founded and recognized as the sole entity to grant accreditation status to entry-level PT education programs
1980	Resolution to raise the minimum entry-level education to a postbaccalaureate degree by 1991
1986	First cohort of board-certified clinical specialists in pediatric PT
1993	First Doctor of Physical Therapy (DPT) program established at Creighton University
2000	Clinical residency and fellowship programs approved for credentialing
2021	100-year anniversary of PT profession

Adapted from American Physical Therapy Association. (2021). https://centennial.apta.org/home/timeline/

the European countries already at war. These programs were "directed toward the restoration of the wounded solder to military duty as soon as possible, or if that was not feasible, to return him to civilian life in physical condition which would enable him to o function in the highest degree possible consistent with his injury" (US Army Medical Department, 2009a).

In August 1917 the Surgeon General's Office established the Division of Special Hospitals and Physical Reconstruction: "Physical reconstruction was defined as maximum mental and physical restoration of the individual achieved by the use of medicine and surgery, supplemented by physical therapy, occupational therapy or curative workshop activities, education, recreation, and vocational training." At that time, the scope of physical therapy "consisted of hydrotherapy, electrotherapy, and mechanotherapy, active exercise, indoor and outdoor games, and massage." The function of the OT reconstruction aides was "to teach crafts on the wards to patients who had impaired motor function or who were neurotic or mentally disoriented. Gradually, the occupational therapy aides also assumed responsibility for curative workshop activities in the treatment of ambulatory patients, taking over this function from enlisted personnel and male civilian instructors who had been concerned with vocational training but not medical treatment." Applicants to the reconstruction program came from several places, including the National Society for the Promotion of Occupational Therapy (US Army Medical Department, 2009b).

In addition to the impact of the war, the polio epidemic influenced the growth of the rehabilitation professions. For the PT profession, much of their professional identity and knowledge base was gained from extensive work with infants, children, and adults who were infected with the poliovirus. Many of the interventions directed at improving muscle strength and flexibility are still being used in PT practice today (Neumann, 2004).

As the polio epidemic was coming to an end in the 1960s, civil rights and social equality movements were beginning. The stigma of disability was lessening, and there was a "reawakening of hope and possibilities" for individuals with disabilities (Minnesota Council on Developmental Disabilities, 2021). The Education for All Handicapped Act (EHA) was passed in 1975, signifying an end to children with disabilities being excluded from public education (see Chapter 113). Over the next two decades the law was reauthorized and eventually became known as Individuals with Disabilities Education Act (IDEA) and included supports and services to children (and their families) from birth to 21 years of age. This law created many new opportunities for OT and PT and promoted expansion of practice in pediatric settings beyond hospitals or medical systems.

CONTEMPORARY PRACTICE

By the start of the 21st century, OT and PT were solidly established as respected health care professions. Over time, each had undergone substantial academic transformations with an intention to shift to science-driven and evidence-based professions. As the knowledge base of each profession grew, so did the need to keep up with rapid advances in science, technology, and the changing landscape of health care delivery. Additionally, the expanded roles of OT and PT (and other related service providers) in the school system created the need for new graduates to practice at a more sophisticated level than existed in the past and with more autonomy than their predecessors had. From a practical standpoint, it was also becoming difficult to fit didactic and clinical curricula into the structure of a 4-year degree. As a result, both professions eventually shifted to graduate-level training. Currently, for PT, the entry-level degree is the professional doctorate (DPT degree); for OT, the entry-level degree can be a master's (MOT degree) or a professional doctorate (OTD degree). Additionally, there are opportunities for pediatric specialization through board certification (OT and PT) and residency and fellowship training programs (PT).

Pediatric content is a required part of the educational curricula in OT and PT programs, thus graduates are prepared to work in a variety of settings with patients/clients across the life span. Pediatric therapy practitioners typically work in acute care pediatric hospitals, outpatient clinics, early intervention agencies, or in schools. Within these settings, OT and PT professionals each bring a unique perspective to the care and management of children with a variety of neurodevelopmental and behavioral challenges. OT also has expertise in providing mental health services for children; as such, they may provide mental health services in settings such as community mental health treatment clinics, therapeutic day schools, and shelters (American Occupational Therapy Association, 2021b).

SCOPE OF PRACTICE

OT and PT can evaluate and diagnose within their respective scopes of practice, but most often they work with a referral source to collaborate on the child's plan of care. These highly trained professionals contribute to the comprehensive and holistic assessment of children across the spectrum of development, health, and function. Although different with respect to their philosophical foundations, each shares an embrace of child- and family-centered care, culturally sensitive practices, and an evidence-based approach to clinical decision making (see Chapter 1). In addition, both professional bodies use the International Classification of Function, Disability, and Health—Children and Youth version (ICF-CY) (WHO, 2007) as a conceptual framework to guide practice, research, and education. While it is beyond the scope of this chapter to provide an in-depth perspective, we will briefly describe each profession's scope of practice as it relates to pediatric care.

Occupational Therapy

Occupational therapy practitioners work with children, youth, and their families, caregivers, and teachers to promote active participation in activities or occupations that are meaningful to them (American Occupational Therapy Association, 2021).

OT are unique in their therapeutic use of occupations to promote health, wellbeing, and participation. As such, the defining principle of the OT profession is the meaningful participation in one's occupation. The OT Practice Framework defines nine specific categories of occupations (Table 106.3). In the context of pediatric practice participation in these occupations can include play and creative learning, academic skills, life skills, sleep, and social interactions. Utilizing the ICF-CY, pediatric OT have expertise in assessing these occupation areas as they inform the child's developmental and/or functional status. Assessment tools include standardized measures; performance-, functional, and/or play-based measures; and clinical expertise. Broadly speaking, OT practitioners focus on the quality and rate of fine motor skill development, oral-motor skills, visual-motor coordination, cognitive development, sensory processing and integration, motor planning, age-appropriate activities of daily living, social and emotional skills, positive mental health, and adaptive equipment needs. Therapeutic interventions are targeted toward facilitation of skill acquisition or teaching compensatory/adaptive skills, with a focus on embedding these skills within the child's natural routines and contexts (American Occupational Therapy Association, 2021a; Laverdure & Beisbier, 2020).

Pediatric physical therapy aims to optimize movement for lifelong meaningful participation of all children (APTA Academy of Pediatric Physical Therapy, 2021).

Physical Therapy

PT practitioners can best be described as movement specialists and as such are skilled in identifying and managing impairments that impact movement, motor development, and/or motor control. PT combine their expertise in movement science with a strong understanding of the contributions from the neurologic, musculoskeletal, cardiopulmonary, and integumentary systems to functional movement. Pediatric PT utilize a wide variety of tests and measures to capture the ICF-CY constructs of body structure/function, activity and participation, and contextual factors. As part of their examination and evaluation process, the PT may also identify when the child is at risk for some type of movement dysfunction, thus their scope of practice also includes a role in primary and secondary prevention. Within and beyond the medical setting, PT are also well equipped to design and implement strategies aimed at promotion of health, wellness, and fitness especially for children with chronic health and developmental impairments. In this context, pediatric PT work with the child and family to identify opportunities for participation in activities that promote lifelong fitness.

Pediatric PT work with children who have a wide range of conditions and abilities that impact, or have the potential to impact movement, motor skill acquisition or motor control. They use the history, examination, and evaluation findings to develop an individualized plan of care in partnership with the family and other members of the child's care team (medical or educational). At the core of PT practice is a focus on functional movement and mobility that is age and/or context appropriate. PT interventions are directed at facilitation of motor skill acquisition or retraining, muscle strengthening and flexibility, balance and postural control, motor control strategies, cardiorespiratory endurance, pain management, integumentary integrity, orthotic and prosthetic training, serial casting and splinting, and adaptive and durable medical equipment needs.

We chose Max's case to illustrate the breadth and depth of clinical decision-making skills that pediatric OT and PT practitioners bring to the care of children with complex health care and developmental needs. Max was first seen in PT for routine management of torticollis, a common and treatable condition that is usually responsive to PT interventions. His PT noted several red flags during the initial evaluation and quickly recognized that his failure to improve was inconsistent with the expected trajectory of a torticollis diagnosis. He was ultimately seen by a neurologist who diagnosed him with a brain tumor, a medullary astrocytoma. Following surgical resection of the tumor Max's condition evolved over time and required skillful management of his changing status from a neurodevelopmental and functional perspective. Table 106.4 outlines the issues that this child faced in infancy, toddler/preschool years, and early school age, aligned with the array of assessments that the OT and PT might use to evaluate and monitor these issues, and their respective approaches to treatment.

Max is representative of the many children that OT and PT professionals care for in a variety of practice settings. His treatment spanned several years and required episodes of intensive intervention to align with the family's goals and concerns and fit in with their time constraints; many times, these factors meant prioritizing one therapy over another. During each episode of care, it was critical to provide Max with evidence-based interventions; it was equally important to incorporate a shared decision-making approach with him and his family, his medical team, and the education professionals.

TABLE 106.3 Occupations as Defined by the Occupational Therapy (OT) Practice Framework

Occupations are "the everyday activities that people do as individuals, in families, and with communities to occupy time and bring meaning and purpose to life. Occupations include things people need to, want to and are expected to do."

Definition	Examples
Activities of daily living (ADLs): self-care activities that are completed on a routine basis	Bathing/personal hygiene Dressing Eating and swallowing; feeding Functional mobility
Instrumental activities of daily living (IADLs): activities to support daily life within home and community	Care of pets Communication management
Health management: activities related to developing, managing, and maintaining health and wellness routines ... to support participation in other occupations	Social-emotional health promotion Physical activity Personal care device management
Rest and sleep: activities related to obtaining restorative rest and sleep to support healthy, active engagement in other occupations	Rest Sleep preparation and sleep participation
Education: activities needed for learning and participating in the educational environment	Formal and informal educational participation
Work: labor or exertion related to the development, production, delivery, or management of objects or services; benefits may be financial or nonfinancial	Employment interests and pursuits Volunteer exploration and participation
Play: activities that are intrinsically motivated, internally controlled, and freely chosen ... play is a complex and multidimensional phenomenon that is shaped by sociocultural factors	Play exploration and participation
Leisure: nonobligatory activity that is intrinsically motivated and engaged in during discretionary time	Leisure exploration and participation
Social participation: activities that involve social interaction with others, including family, friends, peers, and community members, and that support social interdependence	Ability to exhibit behaviors that are expected during family, friendship, and peer group participation

Adapted from American Occupational Therapy Association. (2020). Occupational therapy practice framework: Domain and process (4th ed.). *American Journal of Occupational Therapy, 74*(S2). https://doi.org/10.5014/ajot.2020.74S2001

CLINICAL IMPLICATIONS

OT and PT each bring a unique and holistic perspective to the management of children with complex health and developmental needs. They have expertise in understanding the anatomic, physiologic, and psychosocial impact of illness, injury, disease, or developmental differences on a child's function. OT support a child's ability to participate and engage in meaningful roles through the therapeutic use of occupations; PT support a child's ability to engage and participate by focusing on optimizing movement and the physiologic systems that support movement. By incorporating relevant, child-focused, and child-initiated goals these rehabilitation professionals create opportunities for children to thrive.

TABLE 106.4 Highlights of Max's Occupational Therapy (OT) and Physical Therapy (PT) Interventions From Infancy to Early School Age

	Focus of Episode of Care	Assessment Measures and Approaches	Interventions
		INFANCY	
OT	Feeding difficulties Left upper extremity (UE) weakness and decreased bimanual UE play	Oral motor assessments Peabody Developmental Motor Scales (PDMS-2)	Parent training for safe feeding (e.g., pacing, tongue lateralization) Constraint-induced movement therapy (CIMT): alternating with episodes of bimanual skills
PT	Positional head tilt Delayed and asymmetric motor skills Limited endurance during motor activities	Neck range of motion (ROM) (active/passive) PDMS-2 Monitor physiologic responses and breathing pattern Screen/monitor neurologic function to assess chemo toxicity*	Therapeutic exercise to increase neck ROM (active/passive) Facilitate developmental motor skills Graded age-appropriate motor activities
		TODDLER/PRESCHOOL	
OT	Difficulty chewing and swallowing (worked with speech-language pathologist) Fine motor weakness UE movement impairments on left side Difficulty with dressing	Behavior Assessment Scale of Oral Function in Feeding (BASOFF) Oral Motor Assessment Scale (OMAS) Assisting Hand Assessment (AHA) Pediatric Evaluation of Disability Index (PEDI): fine motor subtests	Oral-motor skill activities CIMT: as above Fine motor skills: hand strengthening, activities of daily living (ADL) for feeding, beginning dressing, and prewriting skills
PT	Frequent falls (due to decreased balance and left-sided weakness) Impaired postural control and ataxia Difficulty with running, jumping, riding tricycle, climbing (could not play with peers) Endurance limitations	PDMS-2 Dynamometry; MMT PEDI: gross motor subtests OMNI Rating of Perceived Exertion (RPE)	Dynamic balance and transitional activities Strengthening exercises: sit to stand, squats, calf raises, core strengthening Aerobic activities incorporating peer play skills: jumping, running, ball skills
		EARLY SCHOOL AGE	
OT	ADL difficulties in school: cutting his food, carrying his tray, dressing Difficulty with bimanual activities Visual-motor and perceptual motor impairments (e.g., difficulty writing; tracing letters/numbers)	PEDI: fine motor subtests AHA Beery Visual Motor Integration	Fine motor skills focused on independent dressing, writing, cutting, etc. Hand strengthening exercises Bimanual activities focused on dressing (buttons and zippers); meals; carrying lunch tray, etc. Compensatory strategies for independence with ADL (e.g., tying shoes)
PT	Endurance limitations Functional mobility limitations when speed is required Difficulty participating in age-appropriate play and recreation with siblings and peers	OMNI RPE 6-Minute Walk Test Bruininks-Oseretsky Test of Motor Proficiency (BOT-2) Test of Gross Motor Development-2 Pediatric Balance Scale	Aerobic training incorporating age-appropriate activities Core stabilization activities Coordination activities and high-level gross motor skills (emphasizing eye-hand coordination)

*Parent education for carryover at home was provided throughout episodes of care.

REFERENCES

American Occupational Therapy Association. (2017). http://www.otcentennial.org/events/1920

American Occupational Therapy Association. (2020). Occupational therapy practice framework: Domain and process (4th ed.). *American Journal of Occupational Therapy*, *74*(S2). https://doi.org/10.5014/ajot.2020.74S2001.

American Occupational Therapy Association. (2021a). *Learn about occupational therapy for children and youth*. https://www.aota.org/about-occupational-therapy/patients-clients/childrenandyouth.aspx

American Occupational Therapy Association. (2021b). *Mental health in children and youth: The benefit and role of occupational therapy*. https://www.aota.org/About-Occupational-Therapy/Professionals/MH/children-youth-mental-health.aspx

American Physical Therapy Association. (2021). https://centennial.apta.org/home/timeline/

APTA Academy of Pediatric Physical Therapy. (2021). https://pediatricapta.org/about-pediatric-physical-therapy/APTA-academy-pediatric-physical-therapy.cfm

Laverdure, P., & Beisbier, S. (2020). Occupation- and activity-based interventions to improve performance of activities of daily living, play, and leisure for children and youth ages 5 to 21: A systematic review. *American Journal of Occupational Therapy*, *75*(1). https://doi.org/10.5014/ajot.2021.039560

Minnesota Council on Developmental Disabilities. (2021). *Parallels in time: A history of developmental disabilities*. https://mn.gov/mnddc/parallels/five/5a/1.html

Neumann, D. (2004). Polio: Its impact on the people of the United States and the emerging profession of physical therapy. *Journal of Orthopedic & Sports Physical Therapy*, *34*(8), 479–492.

US Army Medical Department. (2009a). *Physical therapists before World War II*. https://history.amedd.army.mil/corps/medical_spec/chapterIII.html

US Army Medical Department. (2009b). *Occupational therapists before World War II*. https://history.amedd.army.mil/corps/medical_spec/chapteriv.html

World Health Organization. (2007). *International classification of functioning, disability and health—children and youth version*. https://apps.who.int/iris/bitstream/handle/10665/43737/9789241547321_eng.pdf;sequence=1

World Health Organization. (2020). *Rehabilitation*. https://www.who.int/news-room/fact-sheets/detail/rehabilitation

107

Speech-Language Pathology for Developmental-Behavioral Disorders

Cheryl Messick

For additional material related to the content of this chapter, please see Chapter 44.

VIGNETTE

The primary care clinician referred Isabella for a speech-language evaluation through the early intervention program when she turned 18 months of age. Her mother was concerned because she was behind in communication compared to her older brother. She had not yet acquired any real words, despite meeting all other major developmental milestones at the appropriate ages. Isabella's father was bilingual (Spanish and English) and the mother spoke English, the primary language used in the home. When Isabella's paternal grandmother visited from Mexico each summer, Spanish was spoken in the home. Isabella's mother had not graduated from high school; her father had completed 2 years of community college.

The speech-language evaluation revealed that Isabella's receptive language skills were mildly delayed in English and very delayed in Spanish. Her expressive language skills were moderately and severely delayed in English and Spanish, respectively. An analysis of Isabella's speech sound skills revealed that she primarily vocalized using vowels and occasionally produced the consonants /m, b, d/. She showed strengths in social communication skills, using nonverbal means, such as facial expression and gestures, to communicate. She was found eligible for early intervention services that were then provided in the home. The therapist focused on training the parents to model words and sentences. The therapist also encouraged Isabella to play with sounds and to speak. Isabella made progress in producing more consonants, acquiring words, and she began to use a few two-word phrases. At 33 months, anticipating the end of early intervention services, her parents discontinued speech-language services.

At 4 years of age, Isabella was enrolled in preschool. The teacher suggested that a speech-language screening be completed because it was difficult to understand the child. Based on positive screening results, a full speech-language evaluation was completed. The evaluation revealed that Isabella's speech was unintelligible 65% of the time and was very delayed in producing consonants correctly. Receptive and expressive language skills were moderately delayed. Isabella was enrolled in speech-language services, provided two times per week at her preschool program. The goals focused on improving speech intelligibility, developing age-appropriate expressive vocabulary, and expanding the length and complexity of sentences. Treatment also addressed preliteracy skills such as identifying letters, creating rhyming chains (e.g., cat, mat, bat), and blending sounds together to make words (e.g., b. a. t, that says bat).

Isabella continued to have speech-language services when she enrolled in elementary school. At 7 years of age, learning support services were added, due to concerns about reading, writing, and spelling skills. Isabella continued to have speech-language services with the focus on building vocabulary, morphology, and grammar skills important to academic learning.

INTRODUCTION TO SPEECH-LANGUAGE PATHOLOGY

Speech-language pathologists (SLPs) are "experts in communication" (American Speech-Language-Hearing Association, n.d.), whose work focuses on preventing, assessing, diagnosing, and treating speech, language, and swallowing disorders. They work directly with individuals and consider the impact of communication disorders on individuals, families, and the social context. At a basic level, communication skills may affect one's ability to participate in interactions with others and to convey thoughts, ideas, and needs. A child's communication skills influence their ability to make friends, to learn in school, and to engage in activities for fun and enjoyment (e.g., playing with peers, pursuing interests/hobbies, and participating in group activities). The ability to communicate effectively through speaking and writing impacts the vocational and career pathways available to a young adult (Catts, Fey, Tomblin, & Zhang, 2002; Johnson, Beitchman, & Brownlie, 2010; Rudolph, 2017). In the long run, communication skills contribute significantly to the goal of living an independent life (Young et al., 2002). Communication skills, when they are impaired, can have a broad and significant impact on life and career pathways.

SLPs provide services across the life span, from birth through geriatrics, addressing varied types of communication. SLPs provide evidence-based practice and collaborate with team members through the lens of family- and patient-centered care (see Chapter 1). They advocate for the rights and needs of individual patients to secure services and to optimize communication skills. They are often referred to in the lay community as speech-language therapists, or speech therapists. In this chapter we focus on SLPs who specialize in children.

The requirements to practice as an SLP include a master's or doctoral degree in speech-language pathology from a program that is accredited by the Council for Academic Accreditation in Audiology and Speech-Language Pathology (CAA). The SLP curriculum addresses knowledge and skills across nine communication disorder areas: articulation, fluency, voice and resonance, receptive and expressive language, swallowing, augmentative and alternative communication, impact of hearing on speech/language, cognitive aspects of communication, and social aspects of communication. Understanding the differentiating characteristics and underlying etiologies of each disorder area serves as the foundation for developing clinical skills to prevent, assess, and provide treatment. SLP graduate education focuses on the development of professional competencies, such as communication, interprofessional teaming, clinical reasoning, and cultural competence to work with diverse populations. SLP students participate in clinical rotations with adult and children in varied types of settings. Following graduation, SLPs complete a mentored clinical fellowship (CF) for 36 weeks before becoming fully certified and licensed with a Clinical Competence in Speech-Language Pathology (CCC-SLP).

SETTINGS AND TEAM MEMBERS

Like other rehabilitation disciplines (see Chapter 106), SLPs are employed in a variety of setting types. The setting in which an SLP works influences the types of services provided and the team members with whom they collaborate. Broadly speaking, SLPs work in medical, community, and educational settings. Telehealth services are becoming a common format for speech-language services offered within medical and community settings.

Pediatric SLPs employed in medical settings may provide inpatient services to children receiving acute care and intensive rehabilitation. In acute care assessment and diagnosis services are often the primary focus. For example, referrals to an SLP may request an assessment of swallowing abilities to determine risk for aspirating food/liquids into the lungs. Acute care services also may address augmentative/alternative communication strategies to optimize functional communication of the child who is in the medical setting. In inpatient rehabilitation, assessment, diagnosis, and intensive treatment are often aimed at optimizing the child's current communication skills while rebuilding any skills that had been lost. SLPs collaborate with occupational therapists (OT) and physical therapists (PT) (see Chapter 106) and other members of the medical team. In preparation for discharge the entire team works with the family to plan the transition to home- and community-based services.

Medical outpatient services are often provided by SLPs within specialized interdisciplinary clinics, such as cleft palate/craniofacial clinics, neonatal intensive care unit follow-up clinic, autism centers, and aerodigestive disorder programs. The team members include the range of professionals engaged with the child and family, including the pediatrician and specialists (e.g., neurology, nutrition, and genetic counseling), as well as rehabilitation team members (e.g., audiology, OT, PT, and social work). The electronic record system provides team members with current documentation of the range of services provided across the medical system. Outpatient speech-language services may also be offered in community settings, such as not-for-profit clinics and private practice offices. Some community-based agencies focus exclusively on speech-language services, while others provide interdisciplinary care.

The majority of pediatric SLPs (53%) work for educational agencies, which provide speech-language services free of charge to children who qualify by meeting eligibility criteria, established through federal and state laws for individuals from birth through 21 years of age (see Chapters 103, 104, and 113) (American Speech-Language-Hearing Association, n.d.). Services through state-funded early intervention begin with Birth-to-Three programming, which is provided in the young child's natural environment, typically the home or a daycare facility (see Chapter 103). Services focus on training parents/caretakers to promote the development of early communication skills. For children in the 3- to 5-year age range, services typically take place in the least restrictive educational environment (see Chapter 113), a classroom or program that includes children who are nondisabled. These services often take place in preschool and daycare settings and target communication skills to prepare children for kindergarten. School-age services are provided through school districts, beginning in kindergarten and extending through 21 years of age for children with significant special needs. The educational team includes teachers (regular and special education), learning support staff (e.g., resource teacher, vocational trainer), psychologists, SLPs, OT, PT, and other specialists, depending on the child's needs (e.g., visually impaired support, teacher of the hearing impaired, adaptive physical education).

As seen in the vignette, at 18 months of age, Isabella's services were provided as home-based early intervention. At the age of 4 years, Isabella's communication skills were reevaluated and she received speech-language services in the preschool setting. When Isabella began kindergarten, speech-language services were transitioned to the elementary school. Across childhood, children with significant speech-language deficits transition to new service agencies and providers multiple times. SLPs and the other team members play a critical role in helping families to anticipate, plan for, and make successful transitions.

ASSESSMENT METHODS

Identification of Children at Risk for Language Disorders

It is challenging to predict which children with early delays in communication will have ongoing language disorders (see Chapter 44). Some children identified as having deficits as toddlers show normal communication skills by preschool or early school age, while others have long-term language deficits. Recent systematic review and metaanalysis studies provide guidance to facilitate early referral and identification of children at risk for long-term language disorders (Fisher, 2017; Rudolph, 2017). Expressive language milestones in two areas have been used as red flags for referral to speech-language services: delayed acquisition of words and the absence of two-word phrases at 24 months. Deficits in language comprehension have also been found to be a strong predictor of long-term expressive language difficulties (Fisher, 2017). Additionally, four case history factors can serve to differentiate toddlers at risk for long-term language disorders: maternal education, birth order, child's biologic sex, and the 5-minute Apgar score (Table 107.1). Each of these case history factors is as predictive as communication milestone delays to identify children at risk for long-term language deficits.

Examination of the profile for Isabella shows that as early as 18 months, there were factors indicating that she was at risk for long-term communication deficits. She was behind in word acquisition and her mother did not graduate from high school. Her exposure to two languages, Spanish and English, did not place her at enhanced risk for language disorders (see Chapter 44).

Assessment of Speech and Language/Swallowing

When a child is referred for an assessment of communication skills, the initial focus is guided by the specific reason for the referral, the symptoms observed, and the background information obtained from case history and thorough caretaker interview. The child's speech-language skills are addressed in terms of five broad components of language: phonology, semantics, syntax, morphology, and pragmatics. Understanding of language (receptive language) and production of language is considered independent of one another. Each of the areas is addressed in a speech-language evaluation with some components being screened and others assessed in depth depending on the child's presenting symptoms and the reasons for referral (Table 107.2).

A thorough evaluation includes measures using norm-referenced tools, interview assessments, and observational methods (see Chapter 79). The norm-referenced tools allow comparison of the child's abilities to that of peers and determine the extent and severity of the deficits. Interview assessments provide detailed information from the parent/caretaker/teacher on the child's typical behaviors. Observational measures allow in-depth analysis of speech-language skills, which are key to developing treatment plans. (Table 107.2 provides a summary of assessment tools that were appropriate for use with Isabella at different ages.)

Assessment of Swallowing

Swallowing disorders are part of an SLP's scope of practice. For swallowing and feeding concerns, SLPs and/or OTs may be involved, depending on individual areas of expertise and training as well as institutional practice. SLPs have in-depth knowledge of the anatomic structures and physiologic processes involved both in articulating sounds and masticating/swallowing food. The assessment of swallowing conducted by SLPs includes behavioral observations of a child eating/drinking and instrumental assessment using radiography, referred to as a cookie swallow test or a modified barium swallow (MBS) study. The MBS is designed to determine whether the child is at risk for aspirating food/liquids into the lungs. Treatment recommendations include guidance on recommended textures, thickness, and/or consistency of foods/liquids to prevent aspiration and recommendations to the medical team and family regarding nonoral feeding. Guidance on posture and positioning to facilitate safe swallowing may also be addressed. SLPs typically do not implement treatment focused on expanding the range of food types/textures a child is willing to eat or focusing on sensory issues such as decreasing a child's sensitivity to touch around the mouth area. Those areas of concern are typically addressed by OTs.

TABLE 107.1 Factors Associated With Risk of Long-Term Speech-Language Disorder

Areas to Consider	Risk Factoris
Expressive communication symptoms	• Late talker: delayed acquisition of words (Reilly et al., 2010) • Lack of word combinations at 24 mo (Rudolph & Leonard, 2016)
Receptive communication	• Language comprehension deficits (Fisher, 2017)
Case history factors (Rudolph, 2017)	• Maternal education: did not graduate from high school • Biologic sex: male • Scored very low on 5-minute Apgar • Birth order: later born

SERVICE DELIVERY MODELS USED IN TREATMENT

Across a child's course of speech-language services, different models of service delivery will be implemented. At a broad level, services may be provided directly by the SLP or indirectly by training others to implement the communication treatment program. For example, the home-based services provided for Isabella by the Birth-to-Three SLP focused specifically on teaching the parents to implement strategies to promote the development of language skills. A successful parent training program can provide a child with frequent practice and reinforcement of target behaviors on a daily basis. In the indirect model the SLP plays a crucial role in designing the intervention, training others to implement the program, tracking progress, and modifying the goals and methods when needed.

TABLE 107.2 Assessment Tools Used to Measure Isabella's Communication Skills

Age	Area of Language Assessed	Type of Assessment	Specific Tools That Can Be Used
18 mo	Auditory comprehension and expressive communication	Norm referenced	*Preschool Language Scales-5 (PLS-5)*
	Language comprehension Language expression	Parent interview tool (norm referenced)	*Receptive-Expressive Emergent Language-4 (REEL-4)*
	Word/sentence use and understanding	Parent inventory (norm referenced)	*MacArthur-Bates Communication Development Inventory (CDI)*
	Analysis of speech sounds, word approximations, and pragmatic behaviors	Observations	Spontaneous speech-language sample in real time or analysis of videotape
4 yr	Receptive and expressive language Language content Language structure Core language score	Norm referenced	Subtests and Total score of the *Clinical Evaluation of Language Fundamentals, Preschool-3 (CELF-P3)*
	Articulation inventoryPhonologic processesSounds in words and sentences	Norm referenced	*Clinical Assessment of Articulation and Phonology-2 (CAAP-2)*
	Analysis of speech and language in conversation	Observation	Spontaneous speech-language sample
	Description of spontaneous play behaviors	Observation	*Westby Symbolic Play Scale*
	Print knowledge Definitional vocabulary Phonologic awareness	Norm referenced	*Test of Preschool Early Literacy (TOPEL)*
7 yr	Listening comprehension Oral expression Written expression	Norm referenced	*Oral & Written Language Scales–II (OWLS II)*
	Associations Synonyms Semantic absurdities Antonyms Definitions Flexible word use	Norm referenced	*The WORD Test-3 (Elementary)*
	Language strategies Logic Experiences	Norm referenced	*Test of Problem Solving-3 Elementary (TOPS-3E)*

Direct services often include one-on-one treatment, which would be the typical format used in outpatient settings. The SLP works directly with the child to facilitate the development of target behaviors and practice to use the behavior consistently. This format of service delivery is particularly important when a new skill, approach, or goal is being focused on (Case-Smith & Holland, 2009; Nippold, 2012). Direct services are one model of service delivery used in school settings and are often referred to as pull-out treatment, as the child is removed or pulled out of the classroom and taken to another room to work on speech-language goals. In the schools 18% of services include individual treatment sessions, and 73% of services are group-based pull-out sessions.

Isabella's preschool services might include individual treatment to improve the intelligibility of her speech and work on early literacy concepts, while the language goals are approached through group-based treatment providing opportunities for peer modeling and carryover of goals to conversation with classmates. At the age of 7 years, Isabella's speech-language services would incorporate a collaborative model with the classroom teacher, reading specialists, SLP, and parents working together to promote Isabella's academic learning. Speech-language services would target content important for classroom learning using a group treatment model to teach vocabulary and oral language skills for upcoming units in science class (e.g., synonyms and antonyms).

In terms of treatment effectiveness for children with long-term language deficits it is important to initiate speech-language services as soon as possible. The intervention design should incorporate active attention and participation by the child and should be based on evidence-based practice implemented in a culturally responsive manner. To maximize progress, SLPs must provide clear feedback as well as reinforcement and acknowledgment of the progress being made. Once communication behaviors are developed, it is critical to create opportunities to extend use of the behaviors in varied activities and settings (Gillam & Loeb, 2010).

TREATMENT EFFECTIVENESS

Many studies have documented that therapies within the scope of SLP practice are effective at improving communication in children. Sufficient research has been completed that the results can be summarized in systematic reviews and metaanalyses. A landmark metaanalysis reviewed the results of treatment studies of children with primary speech-language disorders (Law, Garrett, & Nye, 2004) and concluded that speech-language therapy is likely to be effective for children with phonologic and expressive vocabulary difficulties. The evidence was mixed concerning the effectiveness of treatment for children with receptive language and expressive syntactic difficulties. Interestingly, the effects were comparable whether the intervention was delivered by trained parents or by clinicians. Duration of intervention greater than 8 weeks was associated with better outcomes than shorter durations. Since then, a scoping review evaluated treatments for receptive language skills, or oral comprehension, and found that regardless of the approach—modifying the environment, targeting the child's language, or targeting the child's language processing—the results of the intervention were positive (Tarvainen et al., 2020). Another metaanalysis found the evidence suggested that recasting, the practice of repeating and expanding what a child says, has large effect sizes on grammatic skills. This method is easy for parents to learn and integrate into their communication with their children. Metaanalyses also found large positive effect sizes on behavioral interventions for stuttering.

Speech-language interventions are also effective for speech-language difficulties that occur as part of other conditions. A metaanalysis of parent-implemented language interventions found a positive impact on receptive and expressive skills in children with intellectual disability (Roberts & Kaiser, 2011). A metaanalysis of intensive multidisciplinary intervention for pediatric feeding disorders was conducted. SLPs were among the core disciplines overseeing care. The results showed that overall effect size for patients successfully weaning from tube to oral feeding was substantial (Sharp, Volkert, Scahill, McCracken, & McElhanon, 2017). Interventions that taught morphology to children had positive effects on phonologic awareness and reading comprehension as well as morphology awareness and vocabulary (Goodwin & Ahn, 2010). Finally, early speech-language interventions for young children with autism found that early and combined therapist-parent intervention yielded greater change in terms of spoken language than usual treatments (Hampton & Kaiser, 2016).

SUMMARY

SLPs are master's or doctoral prepared professionals who may practice independently or as part of an interdisciplinary team in medical, rehabilitative, and educational settings. They use a wide range of assessment strategies and service delivery models. The publication of systematic reviews and metaanalyses inform practicing SLPs about the effectiveness of approaches for populations that are treated in developmental-behavioral pediatric practices.

REFERENCES

American Speech-Language-Hearing Association. (n.d.). *Employment settings for SLPs*. https://www.asha.org/Students/Employment-Settings-for-SLPs

American Speech-Language-Hearing Association. (n.d.). *Who are speech-language pathologists and what do they do?* https://www.asha.org/public/who-are-speech-language-pathologists/

Brandel, J., & Loeb, D. F. (2011). Program intensity and service delivery models in the schools: SLP survey results. *Language Speech and Hearing in the Schools*, *42*(4), 461–490.

Case-Smith, J., & Holland, T. (2009). Making decisions about service delivery in early childhood programs. *Language Speech and Hearing in the Schools*, *40*, 416–423.

Catts, H. W., Fey, M. E., Tomblin, J. B., & Zhang, X. (2002). A longitudinal investigation of reading outcomes in children with language impairments. *Journal of Speech, Language & Hearing Research*, *45*, 1142–1157. https://doi.org/10.1044/1092-4388(2002/093)

Fisher, E. L. (2017). A systematic review and meta-analysis of predictors of expressive-language outcomes among late talkers. *Journal of Speech Language & Hearing Research*, *60*, 2935–2948. https://doi.org/10.1044/2017_JSLHR-L-16-0310

Gillam, R., & Loeb, D. F. (2010). Principles for school-age language intervention: Insights from a randomized controlled trial. *The ASHA Leader.*

Goodwin, A. P., & Ahn, S. (2010). A meta-analysis of morphological interventions: Effects on literacy achievement of children with literacy difficulties. *Annals of Dyslexia*, *60*(2), 183–208.

Hampton, L. H., & Kaiser, A. (2016). Intervention effects on spoken-language outcomes for children with autism: A systematic review and meta-analysis. *Journal of Intellectual Disability Research*, *60*(5), 444–463.

Johnson, C. J., Beitchman, J. H., & Brownlie, E. B. (2010). Twenty-year follow-up of children with and without speech-language impairments: Family, educational, occupational, and quality of life outcomes. *American Journal of Speech-Language Pathology*, *19*, 51–65. https://doi.org/10.1044/1058-0360(2009/08-0083

Law, J., Garrett, Z., & Nye, C. (2004). The efficacy of treatment for children with developmental speech and language delay/disorder.

Nippold, M. (2012). Different service delivery models for different communication disorders. *Language Speech Hearing in the Schools*, *43*(2), 117–120.

Reilly, S., Wake, M., Obioha, C. U., Bavin, E., Prior, M., Cini, E., ... Bretherton, L. (2010). Predicting language outcomes at 4 years of age: Findings from early language in Victoria study. *Pediatrics*, *126*(6), e1530–e31537. https://doi.org/10.1542/peds.2010-0254

Roberts, M. Y., & Kaiser, A. P. (2011). The effectiveness of parent-implemented language interventions: A meta-analysis. *American Journal of Speech-Language Pathology*, *20*(3), 180–199.

Rudolph, J. M. (2017). Case history risk factors for specific language impairment: A systematic review and meta-analysis. *American Journal of Speech-Language Pathology*, *26*, 991–1010. https://doi.org/10.1044/2016_AJSLP-15-0181

Rudolph, J. M., & Leonard, L. B. (2016). Early language milestones and specific language impairment. *Journal of Early Intervention, 38*, 41–58. https://doi.org/10.1177/1053815116633861

Schooling, T., Venediktov, R., & Leech, H. (2010). *Evidence-based systematic review: Effects of service delivery on the speech and language skills of children from birth to 5 years of age.* National Center for Evidence-Based Practice in Communication Disorders, ASHA.

Sharp, W. G., Volkert, V. M., Scahill, L., McCracken, C. E., & McElhanon, B. (2017). A systematic review and meta-analysis of intensive multidisciplinary intervention for pediatric feeding disorders: How standard is the standard of care?. *The Journal of Pediatrics, 181*, 116–124.

Tarvainen, S., Stolt, S., & Launonen, K. (2020). Oral language comprehension interventions in 1–8-year-old children with language disorders or difficulties: A systematic scoping review. *Autism & Developmental Language Impairments, 5*, 2396941520946999.

Young, A. R., Beitchman, J. H., Johnson, C., Douglas, L., Atkinson, L., Escobar, M., & Wilson, B. (2002). Young adult academic outcomes in a longitudinal sample of early identified language impaired and control children. *Journal of Child Psychology and Psychiatry, 43*, 635–645. https://doi.org/10.1111/1469-7610.00052

108

Art and Music Therapy

Colleen Kahn and Catherine Crouse

For additional material related to the content of this chapter, please see Chapters 96 and 97.

> **VIGNETTE 1**
>
> *Isabella is a shy, soft-spoken 12-year-old girl. She lives with her parents and two younger sisters. Isabella is mature, competent, thoughtful, and responsible. She often takes on a motherly role as her mother works two full-time jobs. Isabella first started having pain in her leg during a junior high physical education class. Although she felt intimidated, Isabella summoned the courage to tell her teacher about the pain in her leg while running. The physical education teacher, Mr. Morris, ignored her, adding, "You're lazy, run faster and catch up with your classmates." After school, she told her mother about the pain. Exhausted, her mother said, "It's fine, you're fine, the pain will go away." For the next few weeks the pain persisted, and participating in physical education became traumatic. Isabella's mother then scheduled an appointment with a pediatrician, who, after a quick question-and-answer session, assessed that Isabella was experiencing growing pains. Isabella's pain persisted 2 excruciating months until one day she could not walk in physical education. She was transferred from school to the nearest children's hospital. After numerous invasive tests and scans, Isabella and her family received the diagnosis of acute lymphocytic leukemia (ALL). Isabella was in for a long road of chemotherapy, radiation, and possibly stem cell transplant. She would be in and out of the hospital for the next several years.*

INTRODUCTION

According to the National Coalition of Creative Arts Therapies Association, Inc. (n.d.), "Creative Arts Therapists are human service professionals who use arts-based interventions and creative processes for the purpose of ameliorating disability and illness and optimizing health and wellness." Creative arts therapies include art, dance, drama, music, and poetry. Each discipline has a professional association that defines guidelines for training, requirements for becoming credentialed, standards, and the scope of practice (National Coalition of Creative Arts Therapies Associations, Inc., n.d.). Creative arts therapists provide support in several settings, including schools, psychiatric care, medical care, and communities. Art and music therapists commonly work in pediatric health care. Each modality is readily adapted to meet the needs of children receiving medical treatment and their families. This chapter will focus on art therapy and music therapy.

ART THERAPY

History

Art therapy has become an essential mental health profession since its inception in the 1940s. Psychiatrists pioneered the use of creativity in healing and treatment (Cohen, 2017). In the United Kingdom Adrian Hill coined the term art therapy for applying image-making in therapeutic practices. Hill discovered medicinal benefits that a person can gain through painting or drawing while in a recovery process. Art therapy can engross a patient's mind, which can assist the patient in building a strong defense against the illness (King, 2016). In the United States Margaret Naumburg was the first psychotherapist to use art therapy both to diagnose and treat mental health conditions. She directly influenced the introduction of a graduate-level program at New York University. Naumburg utilized art to assist a patient through interpersonal conflicts (Junge, 2010). Art was exclusively interpreted by the patient, rather than the therapist. These two approaches are embedded in modern-day art therapy.

Definition

The American Art Therapy Association (AATA) defines art therapy as an integrative mental health and human services profession that enriches the lives of individuals, families, and communities through active artmaking, creative process, applied psychological theory, and human experience within a psychotherapeutic relationship (American Art Therapy Association, n.d.b). Art therapists are clinicians who work with people of all ages across a broad spectrum of practice. Guided by ethical standards and a defined scope of practice, their education and supervised training prepares them for culturally proficient work with diverse populations in a variety of settings. Honoring individuals' values and beliefs, art therapists work with people who are challenged with medical and mental health problems and with individuals seeking emotional, creative, and spiritual growth.

Art Therapy Credentials

To become an art therapist, a master's degree in the field of art therapy or a postprofessional certification in art therapy is required. Postgraduate credentials, Registered Art Therapist (ATR) or Board-Certified Art Therapist (ATR-BC), are conferred by the Art Therapy Credentials Board (ATCB).

Applicants' educational and training background must meet stringent criteria for credentialing. In several states licensure is required. All these requirements serve to protect the public and ensure that only those who are fully qualified to practice the specialized profession of art therapy are recognizable by the use of the title.

Art Therapy Assessments

Art therapy assessments are used to determine a client's level of functioning, set goals and formulate treatment objectives, assess strengths, gain understanding of a client's presenting problems, plan treatment, and evaluate progress (American Art Therapy Association, n.d.a). The evaluation of instrument validity and reliability is imperative in this field, as it is with psychological assessments (see Chapter 76). Art therapy assessments include Cognitive Art Therapy Assessment (CATA), House-Tree-Person (HTP), Kinetic Family Drawing (KFD), and Person Picking and Apple from a Tree (PPAT). Fig. 108.1 shows a child's PPAT production (Betts & Groth-Marnat, 2014).

Art Therapy in Medical and Pediatric Settings

In medical art therapy it is critical to establish rapport between patient and therapist. A working alliance with patients and families using appropriate process skills, such as active listening, reflective empathy, and installation of hope, is proportionately important (Case & Dalley, 2006). In the case of Isabella, in the vignette, an art therapist would explore and help her to process fears and feelings associated with her diagnosis. An art therapist can gain insight into hidden emotions through directives drawings. The "tip of the iceberg" art directive is based on the analogy of the tip of the iceberg: What you see on the surface is not the whole. Isabella's drawing can be seen in Fig. 108.2. Above the water are the words resilient, brave, strong, and independent. Isabella is struggling to verbalize the inhibited emotions—the words written below the surface, including alone, tired, unheard, hurt, scared, powerless, weak, annoyed, and feeling not good enough. Isabella drew a cancerous shark, lurking underneath the water and a killer whale identified as Mr. Morris, her physical education teacher. Isabella was able to express herself clearly without using words, demonstrating the power of art therapy.

Another simple yet powerful art therapy directive is "what's in your heart." Fig. 108.3 shows the creation of a 10-year-old girl with anxiety and depressive symptoms. This child reported feeling "fine" most of the time and, when pressed

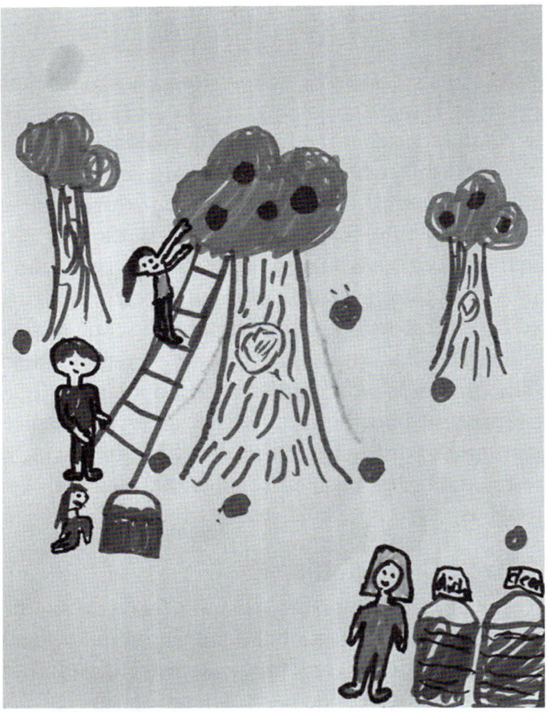

Fig. 108.1 An example of a child's production for the Person Picking and Apple from a Tree (PPAT) directive.

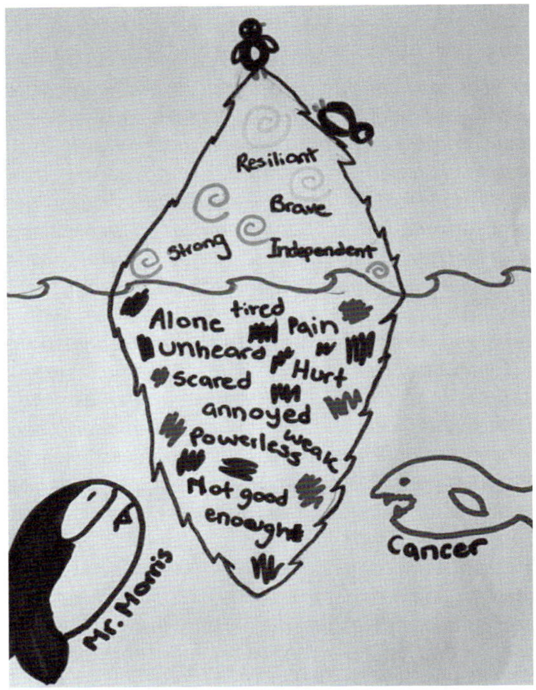

Fig. 108.2 An example of the "tip of the iceberg" art directive, produced by a child who appeared to manage a serious medical condition well and who had many strong feelings beneath the surface.

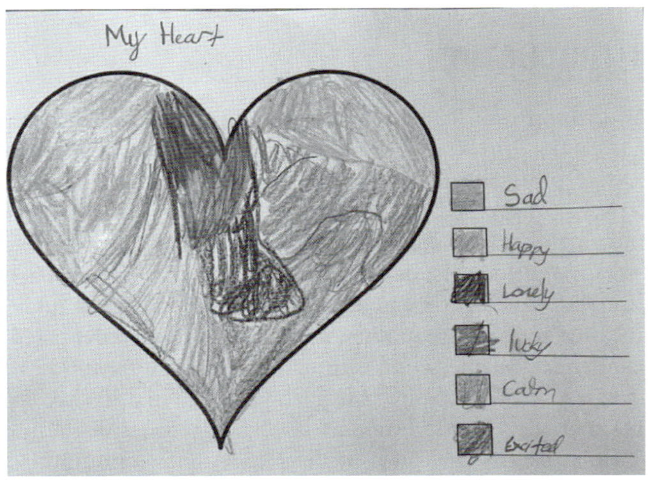

Fig. 108.3 A production in relation to the "what's in your heart" directive in which the child estimated the proportion of different emotions felt during a medical illness.

verbally about her feelings, disclosed "Nothing, I'm fine." When asked to draw what is in her heart, additional feelings emerged. Art therapy allows pediatric patients to draw upon emotions in a developmentally appropriate way Horovitz & Eksten, 2009. This child, like Isabella, was able to express emotions without saying words.

Art therapy can be particularly useful with children who have experienced trauma due to its ability to circumvent language barriers. Malchiodi (2011), an innovator in medical art therapy, asserts that art therapy is especially appropriate for children and adolescents because many prefer to express their experiences nonverbally. Art allows children to explore memories and emotions subtly and symbolically (Malchiodi, 2008).

Research on Art Therapy, Brain Functions, and Stress Measures

Research in art therapy is emerging. For example, Kaimal, Ray, & Muniz, (2017) measured blood flow to the prefrontal cortex as participants completed three art activities. All three visual self-expression tasks activated the medial prefrontal cortex, indicating that artmaking activated reward centers (Kaimal et al., 2017). Thus engaging in visual expression resulted in what is typically perceived as a pleasurable experience. Kaimal et al. (2016) tested cortisol levels, a stress hormone, in 39 individuals making art. The results showed that 45 minutes of creating art in a studio setting with an art therapist significant lowered cortisol levels (Kaimal et al., 2016). Art therapy research has also demonstrated art therapy can help individuals to manage anxiety, depression, grief, stress, pain, irritability, and anger, and improve communication in children and adolescents with trauma or medical conditions (Cohen-Yatziv & Regev, 2019).

VIGNETTE 2

Asher was born prematurely, at 27 weeks of gestational age (GA), admitted to the neonatal intensive care unit (NICU), diagnosed with respiratory distress syndrome, and intubated. His care team noted he was extremely sensitive to stimulation. When Asher reached 28 weeks GA and remained intubated, the team recommended that he receive music therapy support. The music therapist implemented the passive music listening protocol to reduce stress, improve vital signs, and promote tolerance to stimulation. The music therapist observed Asher closely for signs of overstimulation and stopped the intervention when he was unable to tolerate the stimulation. The music therapist then began to work closely with Asher's caregivers, providing education on appropriate uses of music with premature infants and helping parents identify their baby's cues to promote bonding and attachment. At 33 weeks GA, the music therapist trained his caregivers on the Multimodal Neurologic Enhancement (MNE) protocol to help reduce the child's hyperresponsiveness. They learned to provide auditory stimulation via humming and singing, vestibular stimulation via rocking, and tactile stimulation via touch. At 34 weeks GA, when Asher was extubated, he showed signs of oral aversion due to prolonged intubation. The music therapist used the Pacifier Activated Lullaby device (PAL) at bedside, a device that provides contingent music, based on Asher's ability to suck, swallow, and breathe. The PAL promoted positive oral experiences; helped him to coordinate the suck, swallow, and breathe reflex; and prepared him for the transition to oral feeding.

MUSIC THERAPY

Definition

The American Music Therapy Association (AMTA) defines music therapy as "the clinical and evidence-based use of music interventions to accomplish individualized goals within a therapeutic relationship by a credentialed professional who has completed an approved music therapy program" (AMTA, n.d.). The profession uses music to address physical, emotional, cognitive, behavioral, and social needs of an individual within a therapeutic relationship.

Music Therapy Credentials

Music therapists at the bachelor level receive training in musical foundations, clinical foundations, and music therapy foundations in accordance with the AMTA (2013) Professional Competencies. Graduate and doctoral degrees include advanced clinical practice, such as music in counseling, medical music therapy, behavioral health counseling, and research. Once educational requirements are completed, music therapists complete a 1200-hour internship under the supervision of an experienced Board-Certified Musical Therapist (MT-BC), which focuses on clinical training. Certification through the Certification Board of Music Therapists (CBMT) requires education, clinical training, and an examination; the MT-BC remains certified for 5 years (CBMT, 2020). Clinicians must practice within the CBMT Code of Professional Practice and recertify at the end of the 5-year cycle (CBMT, 2011). Music therapy recertification encourages therapists to engage in continuing education, pursue professional development, and participate in professional service opportunities.

Music Therapy Treatment Process

Music therapy services begin with a referral from a member of the interdisciplinary team (Hanser, 2000). The music therapist conducts an initial session to establish therapeutic rapport with the patient. A comprehensive assessment leads to setting goals and objectives and creating an individualized treatment plan. Ongoing assessment is crucial to the therapeutic process, allowing the therapist to adjust the treatment plan, as needed, to meet patients where they are. If the clinician assesses that music therapy services are no longer indicated, the clinician is responsible for terminating services (Hanser, 2018).

Music therapists address therapeutic needs in developmental, rehabilitative, habilitative, medical, mental health, preventive, wellness care, or educational areas (AMTA, 2015). According to the AMTA Scope of Music Therapy Practice (2015), "music therapy interventions may include music improvisation, receptive music listening, song writing, lyric discussion, music and imagery, singing, music performance, learning through music, music combined with other arts, music-assisted relaxation, music-based patient education, electronic music technology, adapted music intervention, and movement to music."

Research on Music Therapy and Brain Function

"Brain research involving music has shown that music has a distinct influence on the brain by stimulating physiologically complex cognitive, affective, and sensorimotor processes" (Thaut & Hoemberg, 2016, p. 1). Fig. 108.4 summarizes the impact of music on areas of the brain. Music elements include pitch or melody, timbre, rhythm or tempo, duration, and dynamics, each of which may impact neural structures.

Research shows that music promotes and enhances neuroplasticity. Music increases dopamine, promotes neural synchrony, and provides clear signals in the brain (Stegemoller, 2014). A music therapist may utilize music in the health care setting to decrease perceptions of pain, encourage mood elevation, or promote a more relaxed state when a person is experiencing anxiety. In a rehabilitation context music therapists utilize music to encourage new neural connections following an injury, stimulate speech, and promote movement.

Music Therapy in Pediatric Medical Care

"Pediatric medical music therapy is the use of music and the therapeutic relationship to promote healthy coping and safeguard the child's psychosocial wellbeing during inpatient and

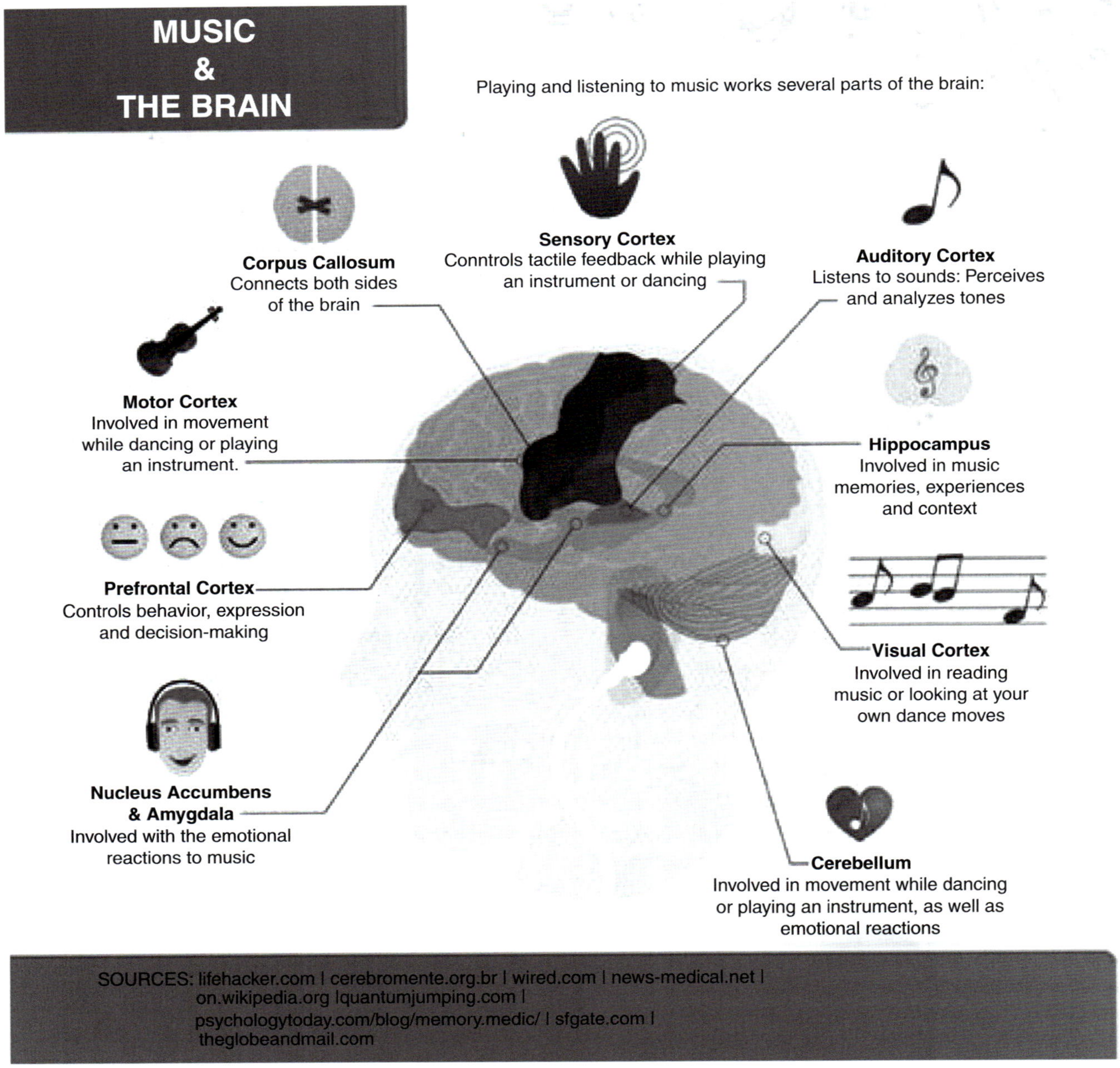

Fig. 108.4 A schematic rendering of brain regions that may be affected during music therapy.

outpatient treatment" (Ghetti, 2011). Music therapists working in the medical setting provide support to patients and families throughout their hospitalization or care. Therapists may facilitate soothing music to promote relaxation and decrease nausea during a patient's treatment, allowing the patient to experience music passively. Additionally, therapists may engage a patient in active music making, including play and exploration, to help normalize the hospital environment and promote development.

Common music therapy interventions utilized in the medical setting include active music making, therapeutic singing, movement to music, songwriting, music technology, music-assisted relaxation, and family-centered music. A meta-analysis (Standley & Whipple, 2003) indicates that medical treatments supported by music therapy are tolerated significantly better than those without music. Music therapists support procedures and treatments, such as lumbar punctures, intravenous line starts or removals, chest tube removals, dressing changes, respiratory treatments, and lab draws. Knott et al. (2020) collected data from music therapists practicing in the pediatric medical setting and Table 108.1 details units and populations served.According to research, music therapy reduces pain, anxiety, and behavioral distress in patients and helps caregivers and nurses feel more relaxed (Whitehead-Pleaux, Zebrowski, Baryza, & Sheridan, 2007). Patients who received music therapy services during their hospital stay had a higher overall satisfaction rating than patients who did not receive music therapy (Yinger & Standley, 2011). Walworth (2005) demonstrated how music therapy can reduce hospital costs through decreased need for sedation, shorter procedure times, and less staff required to support the procedures.

Music therapy is also an effective way to support patients and families during the dying process (see Chapter 11). Music therapists often cotreat with members of the interdisciplinary team, such as child life, chaplaincy, or rehab services, when goals and objectives established by each discipline align. The music therapists may offer music-assisted reminisce, songwriting, heartbeat recordings, and live, preferred music during withdrawal of care.

Music Therapy in the NICU

As in the second vignette, music therapists support premature infants in the NICU. Positive outcomes, such as shortened length of stay, improved oxygenation saturation levels, improved stimulation tolerance, reduction in stress behaviors, enhanced bonding, and improved interactions, make music a beneficial addition in the treatment of fragile infants who are developing outside of the womb (Gooding, 2010). Understanding the auditory and neurologic development of premature infants is crucial for music therapists to provide safe and effective music therapy interventions in the NICU (Standley & Walworth, 2010).

CONCLUSION

Art therapy and music therapy both allow nonverbal modes of expression. Creative art therapies have many functions for children and adolescents with developmental-behavioral conditions. These therapies are likely to improve mental, physical, and emotional wellness and to reduce pain, stress, and anxiety. They provide children and families with opportunities to experience autonomy and control within circumstances that may otherwise offer minimal control. They may

TABLE 108.1 Units and Populations Served by Music Therapists

Units and Populations Served

Question	No. of Responses	Sum Responses	%
Units served	115		
Pediatric intensive care		83	72.2
Medical		81	70.4
Hematology/oncology		74	64.3
Neonatal intensive care		68	59.1
Surgical		58	50.4
Rehabilitation		54	47.0
Cardiac intensive care		53	46.1
Outpatient		46	40.0
Other		30	26.1
Emergency		11	9.6
Radiology		9	7.8
Laboratory (procedural/ testing)		8	7.0
Populations served	115		
Medically complex/ multiple disabilities		95	82.6
Mechanically ventilated		91	79.1
Hematology/oncology		87	75.7
Brain injuries		87	75.7
Chronic conditions		85	73.9
Trauma		78	67.8
Premature infants		73	63.5
Bone marrow/stem cell transplant		58	50.4
Mental health		52	45.2
Organ transplant		48	41.7
Burn care		47	40.9
Other		14	12.2

Note. Other units reported included Outpatient Clinics, Behavioral Health, and Psychiatry. Other populations reported included Neurologic, Eating disorder, Orthopedic, Palliative Care, Spinal cord and injury,and Dialysis.

From Knott, D., Biard, M., Nelson, K. E., Epstein, S., Robb, S. L., & Ghetti, C. M. (2020). A survey of music therapists working in pediatric medical settings in the United States. *Journal of Music Therapy, 57*(1), 34–65. https://doi.org/10.1093/jmt/thz019

expose thoughts and feelings that are difficult for children to verbalize and may allow caregivers, therapists, and the care team to offer support and comfort that is equally difficult to verbalize. They encourage the expression of emotions. Art and music therapists are educated, trained, and board certified. Yet no previous experience with art or music is necessary for individual children and their families to benefit from these modalities. Burgeoning research in these fields confirms their central role in the patient and family experience, making them conducive to integrated care plans that seek to treat serious conditions and to enhance mental health and vitality.

REFERENCES

American Art Therapy Association. (n.d.a). *Art therapy assesments bibliography*. https://arttherapy.org/research/

American Art Therapy Association. (n.d.b). *Definition of profession*. https://www.arttherapy.org/upload/2017_DefinitionofProfession.pdf

American Music Therapy Association. (n.d.c). *What is music therapy?* https://www.musictherapy.org/about/musictherapy/

American Music Therapy Association. (2013). *Professional competencies*. https://www.musictherapy.org/about/competencies/

American Music Therapy Association. (2013). *Scope of music therapy practice*. https://www.musictherapy.org/about/scope_of_music_therapy_practice/

Betts, D. J., & Groth-Marnat, G. (2014). The intersection of art therapy and psychological assessment: Unified approaches to the use of drawings and artistic processes. In L. Handler & A. Thomas (Eds.), *Figure drawings in assessment and psychotherapy: Research and application* (pp. 268–285). Routledge.

Case, C., & Dalley, T. (2006). *The handbook of art therapy* (2nd ed.). Routledge.

Certification Board for Music Therapists. (2011). *CBMT code of professional practice*. http://www.cbmt.org/wp-content/uploads/2020/10/CBMT-CoPP-0920-40339-V2.pdf

Certification Board for Music Therapists. (2020). *CBMT board certification exam*. https://www.cbmt.org/candidates/examination/

Cohen, R. (2017). *Outsider art and art therapy: Shared histories, current issues, and future identities*. Jessica Kingsley Publishers.

Cohen-Yatziv, L., & Regev, D. (2019). The effectiveness and contribution of art therapy work with children in 2018—What progress has been made so far? A systematic review. *International Journal of Art Therapy*, *24*, 100–112. https://doi.org/10.1080/17454832.2019.1574845

Ghetti, C. M. (2011). Active music engagement with emotional-approach coping to improve well-being in liver and kidney transplant recipients. *Journal of Music Therapy*, *48*(4), 463–485. https://doi.org/10.1093/jmt/48.4.463

Gooding, L. F. (2010). Using music therapy protocols in the treatment of premature infants: An introduction to current practices. *The Arts in Psychotherapy*, *37*(3), 211–214. https://doi.org/10.1016/j.aip.2010.04.003

Hanser, S. B. (2000). *The new music therapist's handbook* (2nd ed.). Berklee Press.

Hanser, S. B. (2018). *The new music therapist's handbook* (3rd ed.). Berklee Press.

Horovitz, E. G., & Eksten, S. L. (2009). *The art therapists' primer: A clinical guide to writing assessments, diagnosis, and treatment*. Charles C Thomas.

Junge, M. B. (2010). *The modern history of art therapy in the United States*. Charles C Thomas. https://search-ebscohost.com.laneproxy.stanford.edu/login.aspx?direct=true&db=nlebk&AN=389214&site=ehost-live

Kaimal, G., Ayaz, H., Herres, J., Dieterich-Hartwell, R., Makwana, B., Kaiser, D. H., & Nasser, J. A. (2017). Functional near-infrared spectroscopy assessment of reward perception based on visual self-expression: Coloring, doodling, and free drawing. *The Arts in Psychotherapy*, *55*, 85–92.

Kaimal, G., Ray, K., & Muniz, J. (2016). Reduction of cortisol levels and participants' responses following art making. *Art Therapy: Journal of the American Art Therapy Association, 33*(2), 74–80.

King, J. L. (2016). *Art therapy, trauma, and neuroscience: Theoretical and practical perspectives*. Routledge: Taylor & Francis Group.

Knott, D., Biard, M., Nelson, K. E., Epstein, S., Robb, S. L., & Ghetti, C. M. (2020). A survey of music therapists working in pediatric medical settings in the United States. *Journal of Music Therapy*, *57*(1), 34–65. https://doi.org/10.1093/jmt/thz019

Malchiodi, C. A. (2008). A group art and play therapy program for children from violent homes. In C. A. Malchiodi (Ed.), *Creative interventions with traumatized children* (pp. 247–263). Guilford Press.

Malchiodi, C. A. (2011). *Handbook of art therapy* (2nd ed.). Guilford Press.

National Coalition of Creative Arts Therapies Associations, Inc. (n.d.). *About NCCATA*. https://www.nccata.org/aboutnccata

Standley, J. M., & Walworth, D. (2010). *Music therapy with premature infants: Research and developmental interventions* (2nd ed.). American Music Therapy Association.

Standley, J. M., & Whipple, J. (2003). Music therapy with pediatric patients: A meta-analysis: *In Music therapy in pediatric healthcare: Research and best practice* (pp. 1–18). American Music Therapy Association, Inc.

Stegemoller, E. L. (2014). Exploring a neuroplasticity model of music therapy. *Journal of Music Therapy*, *51*(3), 211–227. https://doi.org/10.1093/jmt/thu023

Thaut, M. H., & Hoemberg, V. (2016). *Handbook of neurologic music therapy*. Oxford University Press.

Walworth, D. D. (2005). Procedural-support music therapy in the healthcare setting: A cost-effectiveness analysis. *Journal of Pediatric Nursing*, *20*(4), 276–284. https://doi.org/10.1016/j.pedn.2005.02.016

Whitehead-Pleaux, A. M., Zebrowski, N., Baryza, M. J., & Sheridan, R. L. (2007). Exploring the effects of music therapy on pediatric pain: Phase 1. *Journal of Music Therapy*, *44*(3), 217–241. https://doi.org/10.1093/jmt/44.3.217

Yinger, O. S., & Standley, J. M. (2011). The effects of medical music therapy on patient satisfaction: As measured by the Press Ganey Inpatient Survey. *Music Therapy Perspectives*, *29*(2), 149–156. https://doi.org/10.1093/mtp/29.2.149.

109

Integrative Medicine for Disorders of Development and Behavior

Ann Ming Yeh, Rachel Lee Gilgoff, and Jenna Arruda

For additional material related to the content of this chapter, please see Chapters 41, 46, 70, and 100.

VIGNETTE

Sam is a 6-year-old who has moderate to severe autism, sleep difficulty, and constipation. His current obsession, investigating trash, is interfering with social relationships. After his parents made dietary changes for him, eliminating gluten and casein and increasing fruits and vegetables, they saw a reduction in hyperactivity and improved sleep. With this improvement, Sam's family sought integrative medical care to discuss the addition of supplements and hyperbaric oxygen therapy to his program, as recommended by a friend. Developmental history was significant for happy infant who was always sensitive to loud noise and who slept poorly. The child showed severe regression between 18 and 24 months of age. On physical exam, Sam was nonverbal, averted gaze to eye contact, engaged in self-stimulating behavior, and made repeated attempts to check the office trash can. The integrative medicine clinician reviewed the evidence for various treatments and encouraged shared decision-making. His parents decided to start methylated vitamin B12 treatment and not pursue hyperbaric oxygen treatments. They realized that they were not practicing good sleep hygiene with their son. Two weeks later, Sam's mother messaged the clinic to share news of a "language explosion." At 3 months follow-up visit his mother reported that he met the whole year's individualized education plan (IEP) goals within 3 months. Sam verbally signaled his need for the restroom and parroted "hello" to the examiner with maternal prompting.

INTRODUCTION

Definitions

Integrative medicine is care that brings conventional and complementary approaches together in a holistic, coordinated way to emphasize a patient- and family-focused approach to all aspects of wellness (including physical, emotional, social, and community aspects). Integrative medicine treats the whole child rather than a single organ system. Complementary medicine was a term used historically to indicate nonmainstream practices in parallel with, but not coordinated with, conventional medicine. Alternative medicine was a term used historically to refer to nonmainstream practices instead of conventional medicine. However, integrative medicine aims to apply evidence-based modalities (or where evidence is lacking, evidence-informed modalities) in conjunction with conventional medicine in an organized and directed manner. In this chapter, we begin with a general introduction to the use of integrative medicine. We then focus on two conditions of major importance in developmental-behavioral pediatrics: autism spectrum disorders (ASD), as with Sam in the vignette, and attention-deficit/hyperactivity disorder (ADHD). We discuss symptoms, possible mechanisms of those symptoms, and integrative treatments that could be used to address those symptoms. We then turn to controversial topics in integrative medicine.

High Prevalence of Integrative Medicine Use

The American Academy of Pediatrics (AAP) 2017 Position Statement on integrative medicine reported that 1 in every 10 children had used complementary therapy in the last year and more than 50% of children with chronic illness used at least one form of complementary therapy (McClafferty et al., 2017). Children with neurodevelopmental disorders may use integrative approaches even more frequently. Parents often seek alternative approaches because of dissatisfaction with conventional medical therapies and persistent disruptive behavior. However, they often do not report use of complementary and alternative medicine to their primary care clinician. Common modalities include supplements (e.g., multivitamins, methyl B12 injections), dietary changes (e.g., gluten-free and casein-free [GFCF] diet), and mind-body interventions (e.g., meditation, yoga, breathing exercises, and progressive muscles relaxation). Interestingly, the modalities parents choose are not necessarily the most efficacious among the diverse alternative and complementary interventions that have been studied. It behooves clinicians to inquire about alternative and integrative treatments and to become familiar with common interventions to guide patients and families in their safe use. Integrative modalities are listed in Table 109.1.

Principles of Integrative Medical Care

Identifying the patient's health goals and values allows for selection of therapies that are consistent with the family's beliefs and scientific evidence.

- **Safety first**. While some integrative therapies may not always have clear efficacy, only treatments generally accepted as safe should be utilized. Response to an intervention should be closely monitored and, like conventional

TABLE 109.1 Modalities of Integrative Medical Care

Dietary supplements	A dietary supplement is any product designed to supplement the diet that includes an amino acid, vitamin, mineral, herb, or botanical (DSHEA, 1994). Dietary supplements are notoriously underregulated compared with pharmaceuticals. Therefore, it is important to help patients verify quality products.
Mind-body	Mind-body interventions are practices that utilize mental focus, breathing techniques, and at times body movements, to help connect the body and the mind. Mind-body techniques activate the body's automatic relaxation response and reduce the harmful effects of stress. Examples include biofeedback, breathing techniques, meditation, mindfulness, and manipulative and movement-based therapies such as yoga and martial arts.
Physical environment	Our physical environment impacts our health, metabolically and psychologically. This category includes the physical space we move about and environmental exposures (such as air pollution, pesticides, and other toxins).
Nutrition	A healthy, well-balanced diet and good eating habits play a significant role in a child's growth, development, and gastrointestinal health. Recent research on the gut microbiome indicates that nutrition may have further implications on the immune system, mood, and behavior.
Relationships	Relationships and relational health are an important part of any child's life and particularly important for a child with developmental or behavioral problems who may struggle to initiate or maintain relationships. Community involvement and caregiver support are included here.
Sleep	Quality sleep is important for attention, behavior, learning, and memory. Children with problems of development and behavior are at risk of sleep onset difficulty, dysregulated sleep cycles, and sleep inefficiency.
Physical activity	Regular exercise helps children build and maintain strong bones and muscles and encourages positive mood, healthy growth, and restful nighttime sleep.

therapies, discontinued if there is no clear therapeutic effect. Fig. 109.1 is a useful guideline for evaluating any treatment. The amount and quality of data on the treatment informs decision making. Fig. 109.2 shows the framework from the AAP for classifying evidence and recommendations used in this chapter. In the case of supplements, Table 109.2 has resources for verifying supplement quality.

- **Less is more**. A stepwise approach to any new intervention is important so clinicians and patients know what had an effect. Symptom logs may help inform this decision.
- **Let the child guide**. Listening to the child and the child's response to a given intervention will often guide next steps. While conventional medicine loves protocols, integrative medicine offers a personalized approach. Motivational interviewing techniques may be especially helpful, not only to identify children's own goals for their health but also to create a partnership between the family and the clinician to assess readiness for change.
- **Therapeutic language**. Integrative modalities do not propose to cure any particular condition. The expectations of treatment effects should be clearly set between the family, patient, and clinicians. Further, the language used to explain a diagnosis, treatment, or intervention can have a significant impact on the patient's potential for wellness (see discussion on hypnosis in Chapter 100). Harnessing the power of expectation using therapeutic language can be therapy in itself.

AUTISM SPECTRUM DISORDER AND INTEGRATIVE MEDICINE

The genetics, epigenetics, and individual physiology of autism may vary greatly among individuals (see Chapter 41). Integrative medicine supports a genetically influenced, environmentally impacted systemic model of autism. As opposed to a genetic, brain-based paradigm, this model better explains the commonalities in nonneurologic symptoms (in particular, gastrointestinal, metabolic, and immune symptoms) experienced in greater frequency by children with autism than by children in the general population. To date there are no approved medical therapies that target core symptoms of ASD. Thus clinicians may consider integrative approaches that target observed commonalities, which in turn could alter brain function and, in some children, reduce the core symptoms of autism.

We will highlight these systemic differences, or susceptibilities, and provide suggestions for intervention. (Table 109.3, in the online supplement, summarizes a comprehensive review of integrative approaches to ASD. References for the articles in that table also are in the online supplement.) The text in the following sections highlights selected recommended therapies (see the online supplement for references in the table).

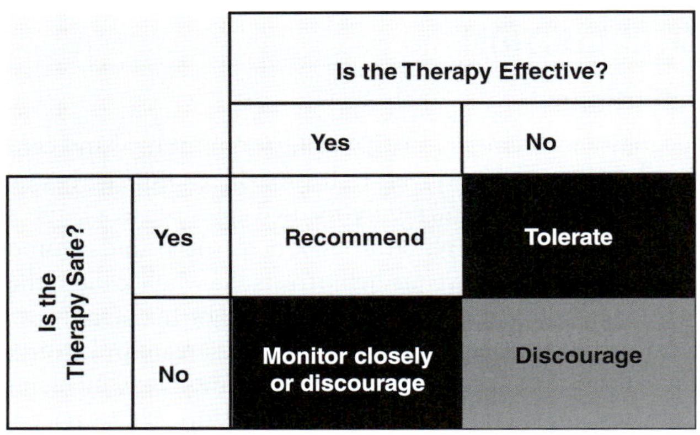

Fig. 109.1 Guide to treatment recommendations. (From Kemper, K. J., & Cohen, M. [2004].)

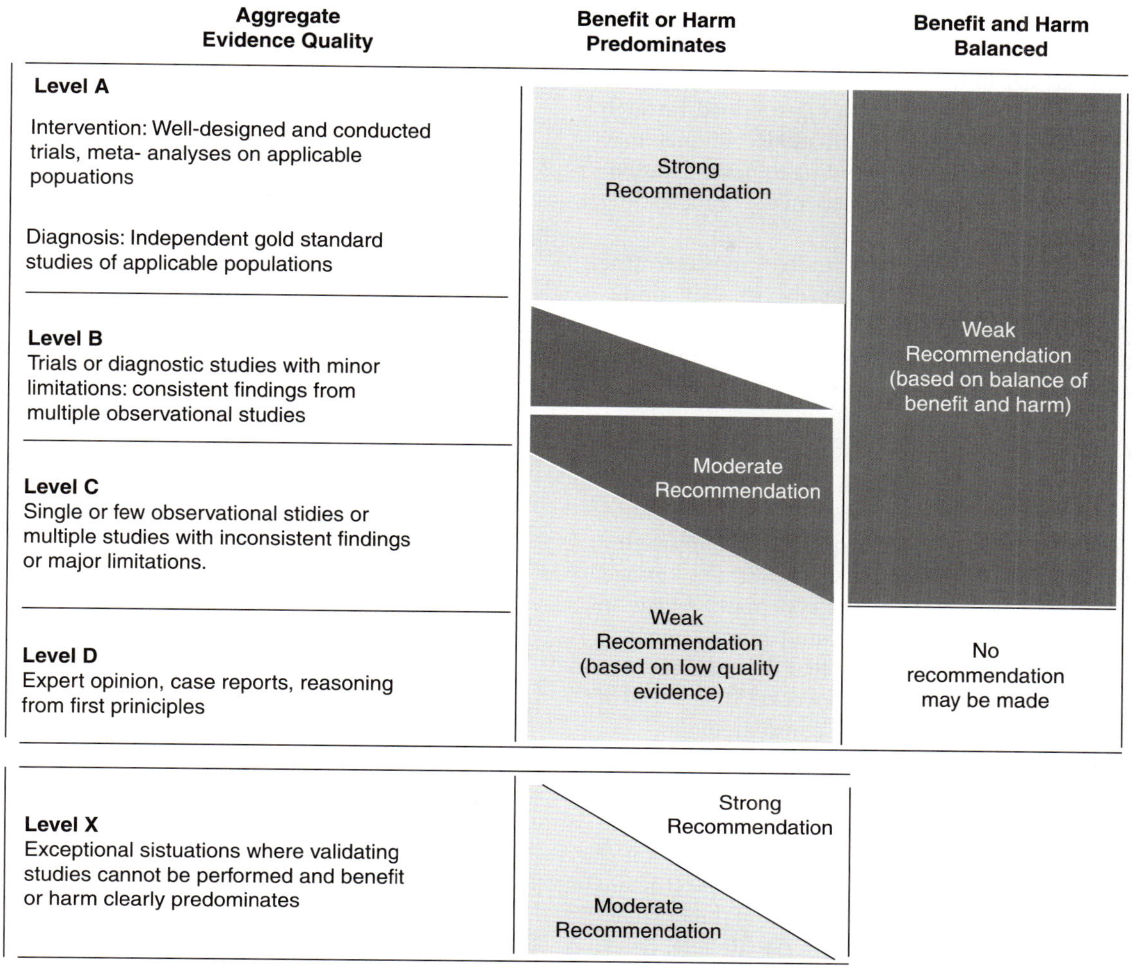

Fig. 109.2 Evidence grading system from the American Academy of Pediatrics. (Steering Committee on Quality Improvement and Management, 2004).)

TABLE 109.2 Resources to Assess Supplement Quality

Resource	Website	Notes
Natural Medicine Database	Naturalmedicines.therapeuticresearch.com	Database on supplements and herbal medicines with monographs and an herb-herb and herb-medication checker
Consumer Labs	Consumerlabs.com	Private company that publishes test results on health, wellness, and nutrition products.
Certification:		
National Sanitation Foundation (NSF)	Nsf.org	Organization that provides onsite inspections of manufacturing facilities and retesting of products to meet standards to maintain certification
US Pharmacopeia (USP)	Usp.org	Organization that designates USP verified mark if a product meets testing and evaluation criteria
Good Manufacturing Practices (GMP)	Fda.gov	System established by the US Food and Drug Administration for ensuring products are consistently produced and controlled according to quality standards

It is important to recognize that each of these treatments may be suitable for a subset of children with ASD. In some cases, we have indications of patients who may respond positively. However, because we do not necessarily have biomarkers for treatment, we often begin with safe approaches for which recommendations rise to level B or C and for which recommendations are classified as moderate (see Fig. 109.2).

Gastrointestinal Disturbances

Gastrointestinal dysfunction and nutritional deficiencies are common comorbidities in ASD. Several pathways have been proposed that support integrative treatments. The first posits that ASD is associated with impaired intestinal permeability and an altered microbiome. Multiple studies have shown altered composition of the fecal microbiota and metabolic products of the gut microbiome in ASD. The theory is that increased epithelial and mucosal permeability provides a mechanism for passage of food-derived peptides through the intestinal mucosa, creating a higher antigenic load through the gastrointestinal tract. Immune cells and cytokines may then cross the blood-brain barrier, binding to brain endothelial cells and inducing immune responses in the brain leading to behavioral disruption.

Many interventions have been studied to determine if gastrointestinal and nutritional approaches can modulate core symptoms of ASD (see Table 109.3 in the online supplements). Following are three safe strategies with weak recommendation.

Probiotics

Probiotics can influence microbiota composition, intestinal barrier function, and alter mucosal immune response. Existing research has been of variable quality and consistency, making determination of appropriate species, strains, dosage, and duration murky. The most recent systematic review in 2019 (Liu, Wan, Huang et al, 2019) found improvement in ASD behaviors in high-quality studies that offered treatment with *Lactobacillus plantarum* for 3 to 4 weeks. Thus a trial of probiotic for children with ASD can be considered.

Prebiotics

Prebiotics are nondigestible compounds that, through breakdown by gut microorganisms, modulate the composition of the gut microbiome. Prebiotics such as inulin-type fructans can be consumed to increase the number of bifidobacteria and butyrate-producing colonic bacteria (Rivière, Selak, Lantin, Leroy, & De Vuyst, 2016). Practically speaking, prebiotic supplementation is achieved by increasing high prebiotic foods such as onions, garlic, asparagus, bananas, artichokes, apples, cocoa, or oats to the diet. For more selective eaters, adding tasteless inulin powder (commonly sourced from chicory root) to a beverage is practical.

Gluten-Free and Casein-Free (GFCF) Diet

Intestinal permeability may improve in patients with autism on a GFCF diet. Some children with ASD may demonstrate increased immune reactivity to gluten by mechanism distinct from celiac disease which has been interpreted as increased intestinal permeability or heightened immunologic reactivity in these patients (Lau et al., 2013). An alternative theory, the opioid excess theory, suggests that metabolism of gluten and casein results in production of peptides with an opioid activity that enter the bloodstream when gut permeability is high, bind to opioid receptors, and affect central nervous system processes causing both gastrointestinal side effects and behavioral problems (Ly, Bottelier, Hoekstra, Arias Vasquez, Buitelaar, & Rommelse, 2017). A multiyear, randomized controlled trial (RCT) of 72 Danish children concluded the GFCF diet may have positive developmental outcomes for selected children (Whiteley et al., 2010); however, other clinical trial data found no symptom changes in patients following a GFCF diet.

Impaired Metabolism

Children with ASD have been reported to have increased incidence of mitochondrial dysfunction, notably impaired methylation capacity, abnormal folate metabolism, and increased incidence of and susceptibility to oxidative stress (Manivasagam et al., 2020). A subset of patients may have mitochondrial autism, hallmarked by multiorgan system disease and regression (Weissman et al., 2008). Neuroinflammation, glial activation, and cytokine release are likely involved.

Methylated Vitamin B12

Methylcobalamin is a cofactor for methylation, which can be impaired in patients with autism. In children with autism, additional methylcobalamin may be beneficial even if patients do not have B12 deficiency. Subcutaneous administration of methylcobalamin is preferred to oral or sublingual administration because it allows for steady rather than pulsatile release. The data classify methylcobalamin as level B evidence and moderate recommendation. Therefore we often recommend a trial of subcutaneous methylated B12 prescribed by a trained clinician.

Folinic Acid

A double-blinded, placebo-controlled trial of 48 children with ASD found statistically significant and clinically meaningful effect of d,l-leucovorin on primary outcome measure of verbal communication (Frye et al., 2018). Presence of folate receptor alpha autoantibody may predict treatment response to folinic acid. Based on the data, a trial of folinic acid is reasonable to determine response.

Minimize Oxidative Stress

Children with autism have been considered to have increased susceptibility to oxidative stress compared to children in the general population. Practical strategies to reduce oxidate stress and environmental exposures in all children include avoidance of air pollution (including tobacco exposure), avoidance of ultraviolet radiation, regular exercise, and an antioxidant-rich diet.

Immune Dysregulation

Gene-environment interactions may lead to a dysfunctional immune response in some patients with autism. One proposed mechanism suggests there is antigen trafficking of environmental triggers through an impaired intestinal barrier and subsequent passage of the antigen/immune-activated complexes through a permissive blood-brain barrier (Fiorentino et al., 2016). Immunocytochemical studies of cerebrospinal fluid in patients with ASD have demonstrated an active neuroinflammatory process and microglial cell activation in the cortex, white matter, and cerebellum, suggestive of a chronic inflammatory process (Vargas, Nascimbene, Krishnan, Zimmerman, & Pardo, 2005). Children with autism are more likely to have food allergy, respiratory allergy, and skin allergy, suggestive of inflammation.

Vitamin D3

Vitamin D is a neuroactive steroid that affects brain development and function, gene regulation, neurotransmission, and plays a role in myelination. A meta-analysis found that children with ASD have lower vitamin D levels than peers (Wang et al., 2016). Vitamin D supplementation is safe and well tolerated, and because children in general are often deficient, checking a serum level and supplementing to normalization is recommended and in line with pediatric clinical guidelines.

Omega-3

Omega-3 long-chain polyunsaturated fatty acids (LCPUFA) hold an essential role in neurotransmitter and glutamatergic signaling and both have immunomodulatory, antiinflammatory, and antioxidant properties. Omega-3 supplementation can be recommended for ASD symptom management.

Lifestyle Factors

Quality sleep, well-balanced nutrition, regular physical activity, and mind-body practices each have important regulatory, mood, and antiinflammatory benefits for the body (see Chapter 92). Lifestyle interventions should be included in the care plan for children with autism.

Aberrant Neurobiology

Children with autism exhibit functional and structural neurologic connectivity differences when compared with peers. Functional MRI (fMRI) studies of visual, auditory, and tactile processing as well as social stimuli in autistic patients show differences in cortical activation patterns compared with typically developing peers (Baum, Stevenson, & Wallace, 2015). Neurohormonal impairments, including the production and cycling of hormones such as melatonin, oxytocin, and vasopressin, are also suspected to contribute to autistic symptoms, including deficits in social function, communication, and sleep physiology. A history of sleep difficulty, as in the vignette, is common in children with ASD. Integrative therapies targeted at these aberrations can be considered.

Sensory Integration Therapy

Sensory integration therapies (SIT) include vestibular and proprioceptive functions to improve balance, coordination, and sensorimotor function. While individualization is clinically useful, it makes the larger rigorous study of the modalities' effectiveness very challenging. A systematic review of three eligible studies of SIT based on Ayres Sensory Integration therapy found it to be an evidenced-based practice by Council for Exceptional Children standards (Schoen et al., 2019).

Oxytocin

Oxytocin modulates neural activity in response to social and emotional processing. Clinical trial evidence for oxytocin's impact on social function has been mixed. However, the most recent study of intranasal oxytocin in pediatrics found a clinically and statistically relevant improvement in social abilities when data were stratified by pretreatment oxytocin level, which previous studies had not accounted for (Parker et al., 2017). A trial of intranasal oxytocin is reasonable, and patient selection may be augmented by measurement of pretreatment neuropeptide levels.

Acupuncture

Acupuncture increases brain levels of arginine-vasopressin and oxytocin, both involved in modulation of social behavior (Zhang et al., 2012). Transcutaneous electrical acupoint stimulation (TEAS) shows promise in treating core symptoms of ASD. In a single-blind, controlled study of patients with autism undergoing TEAS 30 minutes daily, 5 days per week over 12 weeks, researchers found statistically significant improvements in control of emotional response, fear or anxiety, intellective relations, and general impressions on rating scales (Zhang et al., 2012). Treated participants also demonstrated an increase in the varieties of accepted food after TEAS treatment. Results are more favorable when acupuncture is provided in tandem with standard-of-care rehabilitative therapies than when it is in isolation. We think that acupressure, TEAS, or acupuncture could be considered in children with ASD who can access and tolerate the procedures.

Sleep Therapies

As with any child who has sleep difficulty, children with autism may benefit from improvements in sleep hygiene and from behavioral approaches. Melatonin (see Chapter 70) can be utilized safely and may decrease sleep latency but may not impact total sleep time. In children with high-functioning autism, consideration should be given to cognitive-behavioral therapy for insomnia (CBT-I). CBT-I has demonstrated feasibility and safety to help sleep cycle regulation in pediatric ASD.

CONCLUSIONS

The heterogeneity of symptoms in ASD predicts that no single treatment will benefit every affected child. Parents are eager to try integrative methods and many are safe, accessible, and may provide benefit in some children. Close guidance and monitoring by a clinician is important.

ATTENTION-DEFICIT/HYPERACTIVITY DISORDER AND INTEGRATIVE MEDICINE

As with ASD, the range of clinical manifestations in ADHD likely reflects several different pathways as well as moderating and mediating factors in symptom expression (see Chapter 46). Genetics, prenatal or perinatal stress, prenatal and postnatal toxin and drug exposures, pregnancy and birth complications, brain injury, polychlorinated biphenyls, nutritional status, and psychosocial adversity (including high levels of family conflict, institutional deprivation, and adverse childhood experiences) have all been associated with ADHD symptoms. These factors, in turn, may alter the balance of hormones and neurotransmitters, cause neuroinflammation, and/or lead to deficits in neural activity and dysregulated brain circuitry. There are no current guidelines to identify and treat the specific underlying pathophysiology on an individual basis for children and adolescents with ADHD. Integrative medicine offers interventions that can be used to support traditional approaches, reduce medication dosing, and provide an alternative for families reluctant to start medications. (Table 109.4, in the online supplement, includes a comprehensive list of treatments that have been tried for ADHD. The references for those articles are also online.) Here we will focus on nutrition and mind-body approaches as particularly relevant.

Nutrition

Children with ADHD are more likely to have unhealthy diets, including low vegetable intake and high amounts of sugar, fat, and nutrient-poor foods, compared with peers (see Chapter 35). Animal studies have shown that the Western diet (high in saturated fats, refined carbohydrates, and processed foods) is associated with altered brain function; this raises concerns for links to altered human neurodevelopment, cognitive function, and ADHD. Thus improving the diet as well as adding supplements may improve ADHD symptoms.

Supplements

Omega-3 Fatty Acids

Studies have found that children and adolescents with ADHD are more likely than normal controls to be deficient in omega-3 fatty acids. Systematic reviews and meta-analyses, while noting study quality issues, have reported a small but significant effect of omega-3 fatty acid supplementation improving ADHD symptoms (Bloch & Qawasmi, 2011). Improved effects were seen with supplements with higher doses of eicosapentaenoic acid (EPA) than docosahexaenoic acid (DHA). Overall, given that omega-3 supplementation is generally well tolerated with minimal safety risks, omega-3 supplementation, particularly with higher ratio of EPA to DHA, total 1 to 2 g, may be helpful for children with ADHD.

Iron

Low ferritin levels may impact catecholamine production, and children with ADHD have been found to have lower brain iron concentrations than healthy controls. While systematic reviews have shown mixed results, some meta-analyses have found significantly lower ferritin levels in children with ADHD than healthy controls but no difference in serum iron levels between groups (Tseng et al., 2018). In a small, double-blinded RCT children (aged 5–8 years) with ADHD, low serum ferritin levels (<30 ng/mL), and without anemia received 80 mg/day of ferrous sulfate (n = 18) or placebo (n = 5) for 12 weeks. Iron supplementation improved both ferritin levels (29.1 +/− 17.6 ng/mL to 55.7 +/− 20.4 ng/mL) and ADHD symptoms on questionnaires (Konofal et al., 2008). We recommend checking serum ferritin levels in children with ADHD and offering iron supplementation for low serum ferritin levels even in the absence of anemia.

Mind-Body

For children with ADHD who may have altered neurobiology and dysregulated brain circuitry, traditional behavioral approaches may cause increased frustration and worsening symptoms. Mind-body interventions such as neurofeedback, cognitive training, mindfulness, meditation, and experiencing nature offer alternative approaches to restore healthy neurobiology, teach self-regulation skills, and promote relaxation and holistic healing.

Neurofeedback

Neurofeedback is an electroencephalography-based form of biofeedback in which children watch gamelike visuals on a screen and are rewarded when their brain produces the desired brain wave patterns (see Chapter 102). Neurofeedback may particularly support and strengthen underlying neural networks that are involved in attention and self-regulation. While meta-analyses and systematic reviews have found conflicting results, neurofeedback shows significant promise in providing lasting improvements in attention and hyperactivity (Arns et al., 2020). Studies have also identified neurofeedback to have an additive effect to traditional therapy and may allow for decreased medication dosages. Overall, there is a large body of literature that suggests that neurofeedback is safe and may be helpful for some children and adolescents with ADHD.

Mindfulness/Meditation

Like neurofeedback there are conflicting results among meta-analyses citing concerns with the quality of studies and risk for bias. However, studies of well-developed mindfulness-based intervention programs such as mindfulness-based stress reduction, mindfulness-based cognitive-behavioral therapy, mindful awareness programs, and mindfulness-based family intervention as well as yoga have reported positive effect sizes for inattention and hyperactivity symptoms (Cairncross & Miller, 2020; Chimiklis et al., 2018; Xue, Zhang, & Huang, 2019). While more research is needed, mindfulness practices are very safe and can be routinely recommended to patients with ADHD.

Nature

A small study of 17 children with ADHD found their concentration improved after a 20-minute walk in a park with effect sizes similar to methylphenidate (Taylor & Kuo, 2009). In general, exposure to nature has been shown to increase cognitive function, attention, physical activity, resilience, sleep, family functioning, and attachment, as well as decrease frustration and screen time (Kuo, 2015). Clinicians should consider encouraging all children and families, particularly children with ADHD, to get outside and experience nature.

CONCLUSION

As with ASD, no single treatment will benefit every affected child. Overall, a healthy antiinflammatory or Mediterranean diet, omega-3 fatty acid supplementation, mindfulness practices, and time in nature could be recommended to all patients with ADHD. Consider checking labs for ferritin, zinc, vitamin

D, and magnesium and treating if low (see Table 109.4 in the online supplement). Neurofeedback and cognitive training (see Table 109.4 online) are safe and may be helpful but can be expensive as they are not routinely covered by insurance. (Additional interventions are reviewed online in Table 109.4.)

CONTROVERSIAL TREATMENTS IN INTEGRATIVE MEDICINE

Medical Marijuana

Marijuana (also known as cannabis) is derived from the plant *Cannabis sativa*. Several jurisdictions in the United States have legalized marijuanna for recreational and/or medicinal use. In children with behavior and developmental diagnoses, however, there is a paucity of robust research on cannabis-derived products in ASD and ADHD. Significant safety concerns exist regarding recreational cannabis use in the developing child and adolescent brain, including cannabis use disorder, cannabis withdrawal syndrome, cannabis allergy, cannabis hyperemesis syndrome, and vaping-induced lung injury. Additional cautions of using medical marijuana include drug interactions, where cannabidiol (CBD) is a potent inhibitor of cytochrome P450 enzymes. Further, the lack of manufacturing standards and oversight can provide a challenge for clinicians looking to recommend a reputable product with accurate dosing that is free of contamination.

In ASD treatment, a recent systemic review by Fusar-Poli et al. (2020) of 10 studies (8 trials and 2 abstracts) indicated that cannabinoids showed promise in treating certain ASD-associated symptoms such as "improved behavioral problems, hyperactivity, sleep disorders, ... and reduced the number of prescribed medications and significantly reduced the frequency of seizures in patients with comorbid epilepsy." Cannabinoids had unclear effects on ASD core symptoms because several studies analyzed did not report on core symptom outcome measures. As of this publication there are four ongoing trials of cannabinoids for ASD patients registered at clinicaltrials.gov, and therefore additional results of prospective double-blinded trials are needed to support these early findings before drawing strong conclusions.

Given the concerns about safety and regulatory issues, cannabis products cannot be safely recommended across the board for all patients seen in developmental-behavioral pediatric practices. Yet, some research suggests that despite the known issues with cannabis, in a subset of highly selected patients with ASD refractory to other conventional treatments, CBD with no or low levels of tetrahydrocannabinol may be considered as a last-line therapy if there is a clear and understood discussion about the risks and the benefits (Bostwick, 2012).

Chelation Therapy

Chelation therapy is a chemical process in which patients use chelation agents such as ethylenediaminetetraacetic acid or dimercaptosuccinic acid to remove heavy metals or toxins from the body. Although the US Food and Drug Administration has only approved chelation therapy for patients with known and proven lead poisoning, others have explored it for neurodevelopmental disorders such as autism. The premise for this treatment is the hypothesis that children with ASD have heavy metal accumulation, and these heavy metals interfere with developmental processes. However, there is poor clinical evidence that chelation therapy is effective. Further, chelation therapy has serious risks, including renal injury, hypocalcemia, arrhythmia, hypertension, headache, hypoglycemia, thrombophlebitis, and death (Brown, Willis, Omalu, & Leiker, 2006). The routine use of chelation therapy for children with ASD is not proven to be efficacious, is not safe, and is not recommended.

Hyperbaric Oxygen Therapy (HBOT)

HBOT is a treatment in which a patient is within an oxygen chamber and the atmospheric pressure is slowly increased to well above sea level (up to 1.3 atm). The physiologic premise for using HBOT is to increase the partial pressure of oxygen to deliver more oxygen to hypoperfused cerebral tissues in autistic children and improve neuroinflammation through antiinflammatory mechanisms. Only one RCT of 60 children age 2 to 7 years found improved symptom scores in patients randomized to receive 40 1-hour sessions at 1.3 atm (24% oxygen) compared with placebo (chamber at atmospheric pressure and ambient air) (Rossignol et al., 2009). Other RCTs have not replicated these results. Regarding safety, some studies report adverse effects of tympanic membrane rupture due to barotrauma, and nonverbal children may not be able to express discomfort. Further, the time and cost of HBOT treatments are significant: up to $150 per 1-hour session with some families pursuing a course of 10, 40, or up to 120 sessions. Given the significant cost and time investment, the lack of robust evidence for efficacy and potential harm, HBOT is not recommended for treatment of ASD.

Sam, in the vignette, had a favorable response to his parents' initiation of an elimination diet. His parents were very interested in supplements given his poor progress with educational interventions. They liked the rationale and data for methyl B12 and were willing to administer the subcutaneous injections. The integrative clinician steered them away from HBOT for reasons discussed in the chapter. They recognized that they had not instituted a reliable bedtime routine and were willing to try it. They were pleased with the results of these treatments. If Sam's symptoms continue to improve, lifestyle interventions might be more feasible than they had been thus far. Ongoing monitoring is critical.

CONCLUSION

Integrative medicine is frequently pursued by families for various behavior and development conditions. These modalities may play an increasing role as we learn about the underlying mechanisms. Individualization will be important as many of the mechanisms and proposed treatments seem to affect only subsets of the population.

REFERENCES

Arns, M., Clark, C. R., Trullinger, M., deBeus, R., Mack, M., & Aniftos, M. (2020). Neurofeedback and Attention-Deficit/Hyperactivity-Disorder (ADHD) in children: Rating the evidence and proposed guidelines. *Applied Psychophysiology and Biofeedback*, *45*(2), 39–48. https://doi.org/10.1007/s10484-020-09455-2

Baum, S. H., Stevenson, R. A., & Wallace, M. T. (2015). Behavioral, perceptual, and neural alterations in sensory and multisensory function in autism spectrum disorder. *Progress in Neurobiology*, *134*, 140–160. https://doi.org/10.1016/j.pneurobio.2015.09.007

Bloch, M. H., & Qawasmi, A. (2011). Omega-3 fatty acid supplementation for the treatment of children with attention-deficit/hyperactivity disorder symptomatology: Systematic review and meta-analysis. *Journal of the American Academy of Child and Adolescent Psychiatry*, *50*(10), 991–1000. https://doi.org/10.1016/j.jaac.2011.06.008

Bostwick, J. M. (2012). Blurred boundaries: The therapeutics and politics of medical marijuana. *Mayo Clinic Proceedings*, *87*(2), 172–186. https://doi.org/10.1016/j.mayocp.2011.10.003

Brown, M. J., Willis, T., Omalu, B., & Leiker, R. (2006). Deaths resulting from hypocalcemia after administration of edetate disodium: 2003-2005. *Pediatrics*, *118*(2), e534–536. https://doi.org/10.1542/peds.2006-0858

Cairncross, M., & Miller, C. J. (2020). The effectiveness of mindfulness-based therapies for ADHD: a meta-analytic review. *Journal of Attention Disorders*, *24*(5), 627–643

Chimiklis, A. L., Dahl, V., Spears, A. P., Goss, K., Fogarty, K., & Chacko, A. (2018). Yoga, mindfulness, and meditation interventions for youth with ADHD: Systematic review and meta-analysis. *Journal of Child and Family Studies*, *27*(10), 3155–3168

Fiorentino, M., Sapone, A., Senger, S., Camhi, S. S., Kadzielski, S. M., Buie, T. M., Kelly, D. L., Cascella, N., & Fasano, A. (2016). Blood–brain barrier and intestinal epithelial barrier alterations in autism spectrum disorders. *Molecular Autism*, *7* https://doi.org/10.1186/s13229-016-0110-z

Frye, R. E., Sequeira, J. M., Quadros, E. V., James, S. J., & Rossignol, D. A. (2013). Cerebral folate receptor autoantibodies in autism spectrum disorder. *Molecular Psychiatry*, *18*(3), 369–381. https://doi.org/10.1038/mp.2011.175

Fusar-Poli, L., Cavone, V., Tinacci, S., Concas, I., Petralia, A., Signorelli, M. S., Díaz-Caneja, C. M., & Aguglia, E. (2020). Cannabinoids for people with ASD: A systematic review of published and ongoing studies. *Brain Sciences*, *10*(9). https://doi.org/10.3390/brainsci10090572

Kemper, K. J., & Cohen, M. (2004). Ethics meet complementary and alternative medicine: New light on old principles. *Contemporary Pediatrics*, *21*(3), 61–68

Konofal, E., Lecendreux, M., Deron, J., Marchand, M., Cortese, S., Zaïm, M., Mouren, M. C., & Arnulf, I. (2008). Effects of iron supplementation on attention deficit hyperactivity disorder in children. *Pediatric Neurology*, *38*(1), 20–26. https://doi.org/10.1016/j.pediatrneurol.2007.08.014

Kuo, M. (2015). How might contact with nature promote human health? Promising mechanisms and a possible central pathway. *Frontiers in Psychology*, *6*, 1093. https://doi.org/10.3389/fpsyg.2015.01093

Lau, N. M., Green, P. H. R., Taylor, A. K., Hellberg, D., Ajamian, M., Tan, C. Z., Kosofsky, B. E., Higgins, J. J., Rajadhyaksha, A. M., & Alaedini, A. (2013). Markers of celiac disease and gluten sensitivity in children with autism. *PLOS ONE*, *8*(6), e66155. https://doi.org/10.1371/journal.pone.0066155

Liu, J., Wan, G. -B., Huang, M. -S., Agyapong, G., Zou, T., Zhang, X. -Y., Liu, Y. -W., Song, Y. -Q., Tsai, Y. -C., & Kong, X. -J. (2019). Probiotic therapy for treating behavioral and gastrointestinal symptoms in autism spectrum disorder: A systematic review of clinical trials. *Current Medical Science*, *39*(2), 173–184. https://doi.org/10.1007/s11596-019-2016-4

Ly, V., Bottelier, M., Hoekstra, P. J., Arias Vasquez, A., Buitelaar, J. K., & Rommelse, N. N. (2017). Elimination diets' efficacy and mechanisms in attention deficit hyperactivity disorder and autism spectrum disorder. *European Child & Adolescent Psychiatry*, *26*(9), 1067–1079. https://doi.org/10.1007/s00787-017-0959-1

Manivasagam, T., Arunadevi, S., Essa, M. M., SaravanaBabu, C., Borah, A., Thenmozhi, A. J., & Qoronfleh, M. W. (2020). Role of Oxidative Stress and Antioxidants in Autism. In M. M. Essa & M. W. Qoronfleh (Eds.), *Personalized Food Intervention and Therapy for Autism Spectrum Disorder Management* (pp. 193–206). Springer International Publishing. https://doi.org/10.1007/978-3-030-30402-7_7

McClafferty, H., Vohra, S., Bailey, M., Brown, M., Esparham, A., Gerstbacher, D., Golianu, B., Niemi, A. -K., Sibinga, E., Weydert, J., Yeh, A. M., & Medicine, S. on I. (2017). Pediatric Integrative Medicine. *Pediatrics*, *140*(3), e20171961. https://doi.org/10.1542/peds.2017-1961

Rivière, A., Selak, M., Lantin, D., Leroy, F., & De Vuyst, L. (2016). Bifidobacteria and Butyrate-Producing Colon Bacteria: Importance and Strategies for Their Stimulation in the Human Gut. *Frontiers in Microbiology*, *7*, 979. https://doi.org/10.3389/fmicb.2016.00979

Rossignol, D. A., Rossignol, L. W., Smith, S., Schneider, C., Logerquist, S., Usman, A., Neubrander, J., Madren, E. M., Hintz, G., Grushkin, B., & Mumper, E. A. (2009). Hyperbaric treatment for children with autism: A multicenter, randomized, double-blind, controlled trial. *BMC Pediatrics*, *9*, 21. https://doi.org/10.1186/1471-2431-9-21

Schoen, S. A., Lane, S. J., Mailloux, Z., May-Benson, T., Parham, L. D., Roley, S. S., & Schaaf, R. C. (2019). A systematic review of ayres sensory integration intervention for children with autism. *Autism Research*, *12*(1), 6–19. https://doi.org/10.1002/aur.2046

Steering Committee on Quality Improvement and Management. (2004). Classifying Recommendations for Clinical Practice Guidelines. *Pediatrics, 114*(3), 874-877.

Taylor, A. F., & Kuo, F. E. (2009). Children with attention deficits concentrate better after walk in the park. *Journal of Attention Disorders*, *12*(5), 402–409. https://doi.org/10.1177/1087054708323000

Tseng, P. -T., Cheng, Y. -S., Yen, C. -F., Chen, Y. -W., Stubbs, B., Whiteley, P., Carvalho, A. F., Li, D. -J., Chen, T. -Y., Yang, W. -C., Tang, C. -H., Chu, C. -S., Yang, W. -C., Liang, H. -Y., Wu, C. -K., & Lin, P. -Y. (2018a). Peripheral iron levels in children with attention-deficit hyperactivity disorder: A systematic review and meta-analysis. *Scientific Reports*, *8*(1), 788. https://doi.org/10.1038/s41598-017-19096-x

Vargas, D. L., Nascimbene, C., Krishnan, C., Zimmerman, A. W., & Pardo, C. A. (2005). Neuroglial activation and neuroinflammation in the brain of patients with autism. *Annals of Neurology*, *57*(1), 67–81. https://doi.org/10.1002/ana.20315

Weissman, J. R., Kelley, R. I., Bauman, M. L., Cohen, B. H., Murray, K. F., Mitchell, R. L., Kern, R. L., & Natowicz, M. R. (2008). Mitochondrial Disease in Autism Spectrum Disorder Patients:

A Cohort Analysis. *PLoS ONE*, *3*(11). https://doi.org/10.1371/journal.pone.0003815

Whiteley, P., Haracopos, D., Knivsberg, A. -M., Reichelt, K. L., Parlar, S., Jacobsen, J., Seim, A., Pedersen, L., Schondel, M., & Shattock, P. (2010). The ScanBrit randomised, controlled, single-blind study of a gluten- and casein-free dietary intervention for children with autism spectrum disorders. *Nutritional Neuroscience*, *13*(2), 87–100. https://doi.org/10.1179/147683010X12611460763922

Xue, J., Zhang, Y., & Huang, Y. (2019). A meta-analytic investigation of the impact of mindfulness-based interventions on ADHD symptoms. *Medicine*, *98*(23). https://doi.org/10.1097/MD.0000000000015957

Zhang, R., Jia, M. -X., Zhang, J. -S., Xu, X. -J., Shou, X. -J., Zhang, X. -T., Li, L., Li, N., Han, S. -P., & Han, J. -S. (2012). Transcutaneous electrical acupoint stimulation in children with autism and its impact on plasma levels of arginine-vasopressin and oxytocin: A prospective single-blinded controlled study. *Research in Developmental Disabilities*, *33*(4), 1136–1146. https://doi.org/10.1016/j.ridd.2012.02.001

Community-Based Interventions

Lisa Ramirez and Katie Davis

For additional material related to the content of this chapter, please see Chapters 15 and 20.

VIGNETTE

In one midwestern state suicide has overtaken accidental death/injuries as the leading cause of death in children ages 10 to 14 (Ohio Department of Health, 2019). Several school districts within the county have reached out to local pediatricians and mental health professionals asking for support in recognizing and addressing a recent increase in suicidal statements, gestures, and deaths. A needs assessment highlighted several challenges and opportunities within these districts. One of the biggest barriers identified involves the stigma surrounding mental health concerns, leaving many caregivers hesitant to disclose that their child is in distress and schools unaware that their students need and/or are receiving mental health services. Access to mental health services, due to insurance barriers, long wait lists, and confusion about roles of various mental health professionals, was another significant issue. Interestingly, the needs assessment also revealed that many of the high school students reported general education around mental health as their most significant unmet need. These school systems recognize that they need assistance in addressing mental health gaps, but they are unsure of how to engage their partners, and what level of support would be appropriate. Several of these school districts are in underresourced neighborhoods that have a complicated history with many of the medical systems in the area, and there is often skepticism in accepting services from medical and mental health organizations. This scenario highlights an opportunity for professional intervention in a specific school community, and introduces several challenges encountered when exploring community partnerships and community-based interventions.

INTRODUCTION

Community-based interventions are programs that are delivered in a community context (loosely defined within this chapter as a group of people with some characteristics in common, including geographic area, age, and cultural identities) and are intended to meet an identified need (Jason, Glantsman, O'Brien, & Ramian, 2019). There are wide ranges of specific targets and intentions behind community-based interventions, which could vary based on the level of intervention intended and community of interest. Often, community-based interventions imply that the curriculum/intervention/efforts are delivered in a setting outside of the traditional medical/mental health setting. While there are a multitude of examples of community interventions, this chapter will focus on a general overview of community-based interventions, discuss important considerations, highlight two specific examples, and provide resources for additional information.

WHAT IS COMMUNITY-BASED INTERVENTION?

In traditional models mental health systems tend to respond to patients and families once problems arise, including once a diagnosable mental health problem has been recognized, or once a patient or family has concerns about functioning. Conversely, pediatric health clinicians generally spend a lot of time on prevention. They see children and families regularly and provide guidance on how to promote healthy development, and they screen for developmental problems. Clinicians are also ready to address problems that arise (e.g., in sick visits and while staffing inpatient floors). In this sense preventing problems and reacting to presenting problems are opposite ends of the intervention continuum, but much of the connection and intervention happens in their own institutions, organizations, or systems, not out in the community.

Conversely, many community interventions follow a public health model, which tends to focus on environmental and social determinants of health and mental health outcomes. As we continue to understand the vast influence various systems and environmental factors have on the wellbeing of children and their families, community interventions offer rich opportunities to improve health and wellness and to address complex problems.

Community-based interventions can be categorized and conceptualized in a variety of ways. One approach is to begin by considering community as (1) the setting for the intervention, (2) the overall target of the intervention, (3) a collection of internal resources, and/or (4) the agent itself (McLeroy, Norton, Kegler, Burdine, & Sumaya, 2003). Jason et al. (2019) stressed the importance of differentiating community-based interventions as either professionally led or grassroots, the latter of which implies collaboration between community members and their professional partners. As implied by the name, grassroots initiatives focus on understanding the ecology of the community and adapting interventions based on the feedback and needs of the community members. As those invested in creating behavior change understand, using individual and community assets to encourage sustainable change is preferred; however, not all communities are ready or able to act as their own change agents.

Complex Problems

Health professionals are often tasked with addressing complex problems—medical, behavioral, or developmental in nature—yet are limited by system factors (e.g., resources are accessible and can be modified). One of the most attractive parts of community-based interventions is that it allows access to patients and their families, in their home environment, often where they are engaged or experiencing the identified challenges. This allows access to multiple systems where complex problems are often entangled. For context, only 20% of an individual's health outcomes are determined by the medical care they receive; the remaining 80% of outcomes are determined by environment and social determinants of health (Manatt & Phillips, 2019). Professionals interested in patients' and families' health need to consider more factors than what can be addressed in the proverbial office.

Clinicians within a medical system serve as experts on child and adolescent health to support youth and their families. Their expertise also lends well to serving as partners in community-based interventions. Clinicians are in a unique position to be able to gauge and understand the root or cause of the identified problem and intervene in a broader way—both directly and/or to empower a community to improve certain outcomes (McLeroy et al., 2003). There are challenges associated with community collaborations. Before jumping prematurely into creating community-based interventions, there are several considerations, including identifying the actual (unmet) need, resources available to address the (unmet) need, and identifying expertise/ability/willingness to create the intervention (Lopez, 2016).

CONSIDERATIONS IN COMMUNITY-BASED INTERVENTIONS

Inherently, delivering services in a community implies that collaboration must occur, at minimum, between the entity delivering the intervention and the community setting in which the services are being delivered. However, there are often multiple layers of systems (e.g., caregivers, transportation entities, community advocates, schools, and legal partners) that can be critical when working with children and families. In this section we will highlight important considerations for these important collaborations.

Cultural Humility and Sociocultural Implications

Culture has many definitions/applications in these contexts and it is important to consider the culture of the community (demographic, religious, political, openness to collaboration, etc.) and the relative culture of the service provider. Lack of consideration and awareness of cultural mismatches/challenges can greatly diminish the effectiveness of the intervention if we make cultural missteps. One example is the difference between the medical culture and culture of a (hypothetical) community center. For those of us that operate in medical systems, the medical culture can be hierarchic in nature, with clear expectations of roles and responsibilities, and an emphasis on health literacy. Communities may place more of an emphasis on relationships and connection than on expertise and hierarchy. Additionally, while medical culture values privacy, many communities rely on a network of support and services. Leaders in a community may not understand—and even misinterpret—why the medical professionals may be uncomfortable discussing individuals involved in the interventions (e.g., ethical standards related to communications related to patient care), which may set the stage for distrust and disruptions in communication and the larger relationship. Appreciation of these differences in cultures can be critical in setting up partnerships in a meaningful way that will feel respectful and beneficial to all parties involved.

We would be remiss to discuss cultural humility without discussing two important topics: trauma-informed care and systemic racism. Although the concept of trauma-informed care may not be new, the framework has gained more traction in pediatric health care settings, at least in part due to the increased awareness of the impact of adverse childhood experiences (ACEs) on children. Beyond the individual impact of trauma and ACEs, trauma-informed care provides explicit concepts to practice and can be a critical framework when partnering with communities. The six core tenets of trauma-informed care are (1) safety, (2) trustworthiness and transparency, (3) peer support, (4) collaboration and mutuality, (5) empowerment and choice, and (6) cultural, historical, and gender issues (Centers for Disease Control and Prevention [CDC], 2020). As alluded to in the vignette at the opening of the chapter, there is often an inherent distrust between communities and medical/mental health systems due to historical traumas perpetrated by those in positions of privilege. Trauma-informed care can be an important practice in regaining trust in communities that have historically been exploited (see Chapter 15 for more information on trauma-informed care).

Systemic racism, often used interchangeably with structural racism, refers to the tendency of policies, practices, and attitudes to systemically reinforce inequities between racial groups (Aspen Institute, n.d.). Since 2019 various local and state leaders declared racism a public health crisis or emergency. Public health and medical organizations also joined in raising their voices and sharing of research to demonstrate the implications systemic racism has on an individual's health and outcomes. Awareness and acknowledgment of systemic racism aids in shifting discriminatory norms and allowing health and community partners to have honest and transparent communication around barriers that may hinder engagement, recruitment, equitable recruitment in outcome evaluation, and many other areas critical to understanding the true impact of these interventions (see Chapter 20).

Ethical Standards

Ethical considerations are critical in community-based intervention initiatives. Each partner has particular ethical standards. In medical systems the Health Insurance Portability and Accountability Act (US Department of Health and Human Services, 2003) guides our standards for communicating and handling patient information. However, schools and other educational entities are informed by the Family Educational Rights and Privacy Act (US Department of Education, 2020), whose standards and thresholds vary from medical standards. Also, health policies or law may enable youth to access prevention services legally as a mature minor (many states afford this right for sexual health and mental health services), yet lack of funding or processes to support policies inhibits access to care. In the interest of effective and meaningful communication discussions around ethical standards should be an early consideration when exploring collaborative partnerships.

With regard to ethical considerations, youth are often amenable to prevention initiatives, unlike adult populations, when interventions tend to be reactive in nature. However, youth also introduce issues of assent and parental consent, developmental considerations, caregiver influence, and substantial environmental influences (e.g., school/education, peers). Youth are considered vulnerable populations by many regulatory authorities, and higher standards may apply to community-based initiatives focused on youth and families.

Sustainability

The content of community-based interventions is often not reimbursable or billable within the medical system (insurance, Medicaid, Medicare), and ensuring sustainable funding for these programs can be difficult. Community-based interventions are frequently supported by grants or philanthropic sources, which can be beneficial when exploring the feasibility of the intervention. However, there is a need to balance determining feasibility with finding ways to establish sustainability so that intervention initiatives do not become a series of inconsistent pilots, which can inadvertently damage long-term trust between health entities and communities. Examples of means for sustainability include partnering with managed care organizations to fund prevention work that decreases long-term health costs; aligning with local/state/federal funding streams that focus on specific outcomes targeted by intervention programming; finding local philanthropic partners that are interested in similar initiatives; and identifying possible billable services related to your intervention programming, which is often more realistic in level 2 and 3 programming (which we will cover in tiered preventions).

Fortunately, many community-based interventions can result in long-term cost savings, which is often a benefit of prevention initiatives. Some examples include the Communities Putting Prevention to Work intervention (prevention initiatives focused on obesity, tobacco use, and secondhand smoke), which the CDC estimated would save $5.96 billion (about $18 per person in the United States) by 2020 (CDC, 2013). The Sycamore Institute (Melton, 2019) reports that unaddressed ACEs cost the state $5 billion annually in health and missed work expenditures, which implies that community-based interventions to screen, identify, and address ACEs may save at least a portion of the billions they are losing. While systems may not be reimbursed for the direct services provided by the community-based initiatives, the long-term and/or downstream savings may be enough to convince an organization that community interventions are a worthwhile investment. In alignment with these thoughts it is essential to explore advocacy and policy changes that support long-term prevention funding that results in additional cost savings. Cost savings are not only financial: if funders and policymakers identify multiple returns on investment, such as increased graduation rate or decrease in juvenile recidivism, they also will see cost savings in both the medical and social arenas.

Tiered Response to Intervention

In traditional medical and mental health models interventions can be conceptualized as occurring across a continuum of response to the identified target need or outcome. One common framework is the three-tiered level of prevention/intervention that is often used in educational and public health settings. The first tier of the framework is often referred to as primary prevention and focuses on preventing a particular outcome. Primary intervention is also known as universal intervention because the prevention efforts are universally available to a wider population. Public health may consider primary prevention to focus on health promotion and promoting protective factors before disease occurs (CDC, n.d.; MacArthur, n.d.), and educational settings may identify primary interventions as those geared toward all students to promote academic success (Center on PBIS, n.d.).

The second tier focuses on screening individuals to identify those at risk for a particular problem or outcome. These secondary prevention/intervention services are delivered to a targeted group of individuals that have been identified as needing a targeted, often small group intervention to prevent further progression of the disease, deficit, or problem (CDC, n.d.; Center on PBIS, n.d.; MacArthur, n.d.). Examples of secondary interventions may include services for students who have been flagged for elevated levels of depression/anxiety symptoms, children identified as having reading problems, and regular sexual health testing in teens who are sexually active.

The third tier is referred to as tertiary intervention/prevention and focuses on managing active disease, or providing intensive, individualized educational services or mental health treatment. Tertiary interventions may include drug and alcohol treatment for adolescents who have addiction issues, individualized education plans in school settings, and medication for medical diagnoses (CDC, n.d.; Center on PBIS, n.d.; MacArthur, n.d.).

Evidence Base

The emphasis on evidence-based practice is inherent in medical and mental health training. Clinicians are often accustomed to delivering evidence-based services in controlled settings and ways (e.g., medical office, prescribed course of treatment), but community interventions introduce factors that are not often considered or easily controlled (e.g., built environment, motivation to engage, accessibility and relevance). Demonstrating effectiveness in a medical office, clinic, or setting does not mean that it will generalize to a community-based implementation. Additionally, conducting evaluations of community-based interventions can be more challenging than standard evaluations, and it may be 2 years or more before it is possible to begin to measure the effects of the programs (CDC, 2013). Furthermore, unlike direct interventions to reduce active and measurable problem/outcomes (e.g., lowering blood pressure or A1c or weight), community-based interventions are often undertaken to ameliorate, reduce, or altogether prevent specific outcomes, which can take months, years, or decades to understand the impact of the programming. Consider prevention of lead exposure: early childhood intervention initiatives and other long-term health interventions require years to gather and analyze relevant outcomes.

As mentioned earlier in the chapter, having the participation of community members in the design and implementation of the community intervention is a valuable step that can address collaboration, cultural considerations, and other challenges. For this reason, community-based participatory action research continues to increase in use and popularity. Additionally, many challenges faced by professionals are also familiar to community members who are actively engaged in their own strategies for addressing these issues. Joining forces can add professional input and resources, while capitalizing on strategies that may be more effective in attracting and engaging desired/targeted community members.

Health System as a Partner for Communities

Medical/health care delivery/mental health systems have the potential to be valuable partners within the community. Often, health systems have established relationships with schools, community organizations, neighborhoods, libraries, recreation centers, and other partners. If we are cognizant about nurturing relationships and building trust, it will be less cumbersome when approaching community partners for conversations about collaborations to address a widespread problem/challenge. Subject matter experts (SME; e.g., physicians, psychologists, nurses, social workers) may serve a critical role in ensuring evidence-based, or as close to evidence-based as possible, theory/curriculum/interventions are central to community-based initiatives. SMEs are obviously well suited for professionally led initiatives and can be invaluable to grassroots efforts if they attend to the components of successful community-based participatory collaborations.

Health systems may also be able to provide valuable resources within the partnership. Many clinicians work in environments where resources are more readily available than in the communities with which they are partnering. Examples of valuable resources may include access to physical health care, care coordinators, physical space, medical equipment, research, supplies, and administrative infrastructure.

COMMUNITY-BASED INTERVENTION IN ACTION

There are a multitude of successful community-based initiatives that range from universal to individualized in nature, within a variety of targeted communities. There are resources available in which established community-based interventions are listed. One such resource is a compendium of proven community-based prevention initiatives (New York Academy of Medicine, 2013), which includes programs focused on preventing asthma, injury and violence, and tobacco and alcohol use. Although this chapter does not provide the space to review existing community-based interventions in depth, we will discuss two specific areas of community-based interventions: suicide and bullying.

Suicide

This chapter opened by highlighting in the vignette the increase of suicide rates in the youth population in one Midwestern state. This data trend is unfortunately matched across the United States, with suicide being the second leading cause of death for 10- to 24-year-olds (National Institute of Mental Health, 2021). Research has demonstrated that fixed risk factors include but are not limited to family history of suicide, previous suicide attempt, personal mental health problems that predispose to suicide, and social and environmental risk factors that include bullying, impaired child-parent relationships, school difficulties, or stressful life experiences (Shain, 2016). Individual protective factors can include relationships with peers, family, school, or religion that may mitigate risk factors of suicide (Shain, 2016).

A systematic review (Zalsman et al., 2016) of suicide prevention strategies noted that school-based suicide awareness programs have been shown to reduce suicide attempts and suicidal ideations. Signs of Suicide (SOS; Mindwise Innovations, 2021) is one school-based intervention used in middle and high schools and is recognized in the Substance Abuse and Mental Health Services Administration (SAMHSA) Evidence-Based Practice Resource Center (pre-2015) (Suicide Prevention Resource Center, 2016). SOS is a tier 1 prevention program developed by mental health professionals in collaboration with school communities. It has separate curricula for each grade band, and the curricula have demonstrated a decrease in self-reported suicide attempts and increased knowledge of mental health issues related to suicide among students (Aseltine et al., 2007). SOS is typically offered with in-person or virtual sessions and provides training and support materials for school staff and families. Students report having increased knowledge about suicide, feeling more comfortable asking for help, and believing stigma around mental health is reduced within the school climate. The program has been delivered across the United States to a diverse group of students and demonstrates effectiveness across gender and race (Mindwise Innovations, 2021).

Notably, despite the increase in general suicide prevention research, there continues to be limited research in low- to middle-income countries and among youth with high suicide risk factors. Additionally, most of the research in this area has evaluated adult interventions that were modified for youth, as there are few interventions that have been created for youth (Robinson et al., 2018).

As was highlighted in the opening vignette, youth suicide is a serious and complex problem that has demonstrated benefit from community-based interventions, yet many of the issues highlighted in the considerations section apply to suicide interventions. Different geographic regions and cultures have differing views on the appropriateness of discussions around suicide. Logically, sustainability in a program targeting suicide and suicide prevention among youth is an important consideration, and school communities would be upset if a successful program were to be removed from their community due to lack of available funding.

Bullying

Like suicide trends, the prevalence of bullying victimization rates in children is on the rise in the United States (Patchin, 2019). Bully victimization in childhood can increase risk for negative physical and mental health problems across the life span and can ultimately impact financial and educational attainment (Wolke et al., 2013). The need for effective and efficacious prevention programs related to bullying is well documented, and bullying prevention programs are effective at reducing perpetration and victimization by up to 20% (Gaffney, Ttofi, & Farrington, 2019).

Vreeman and Carroll's (2007) systematic review of research on school-based bullying prevention programming highlighted the inherent value of implementing whole-school interventions that spark wide-reaching cultural change across systems (e.g., students, teachers, administrators) instead of classroom curriculum or small group–based programming aimed only at shifting individual/student behaviors.

Importantly, Olweus and Limber's (2010) experiences implementing the Olweus Bullying Prevention Program across US schools emphasized how critical the school communities were to the success of the program. Despite general success of the program in decreasing rates of bully victimization and antisocial behaviors in the intervention schools, the readiness and attitudes of the broader school community—including school staff and student caregivers, and ranging from insufficient time to implement proper training to disbelief that bullying was a problem impacting their community—directly affected program fidelity and sustainability. The authors highlighted that piecemeal and/or short-term solutions do not produce the cultural changes needed to decrease bullying behavior. In this case the more engaged and collaborative the community partner was, the stronger (in direct and long-term impacts) the positive effects. This reinforces the ethical consideration that providing the curriculum, or content, to the community partner may not be enough to address the identified problem if the community is not fully engaged with the efforts. This also highlights the need for community stakeholders (in this case the school) to be involved in the planning process to identify barriers for implementation and program delivery that stem from internal and/or community sociocultural norms or biases.

ADDITIONAL RESOURCES

Thus far, this chapter has covered broad theory and considerations in community-based interventions, as well as provided a few examples of actual interventions. However, this last section provides resource recommendations for planning and engaging in community-based interventions.

Programming Framework

SAMHSA's (2019) prevention guidebook provides a comprehensive manual covering five critical steps for successful implementation of prevention initiatives: assessment, capacity, planning, implementation, and evaluation. The manual also discusses sustainability, cultural competence, evaluation strategies, and reporting outcomes.

The Center for Community Health and Development's (n.d.) *Community Toolbox* provides a free, online, practical toolbox for individuals and organizations interested in becoming involved in community-based initiatives, and the toolbox provides step-by-step instructions for addressing many of the issues we have highlighted in this chapter.

Community-Based Participatory Research

As mentioned earlier in the chapter, a key factor to successful community-based interventions is including patients/community members in the process from the planning stages. The foundations of community-based participatory research (CBPR) are well-established fundamentals that can aid in establishing a solid foundation in community collaborations. PolicyLink and the UC Berkeley School of Public Health have created a report on CBPR that provides background and strategies for meaningful relationships (Minkler, Garcia, Rubin, & Wallerstein, 2012). Similarly, the previously mentioned *Community Toolbox* (Center for Community Health and Development, n.d.) has devoted an entire section to CBPR.

Data Sets

Clinicians assess patients based on both objective and subjective data to provide recommendations and care. When partnering with the community, a population-level approach may be needed for analysis. A variety of data sets on child health exist to both assess and improve health outcomes. We refer you to Appendix A of *Children's Health, The Nation's Wealth: Assessing and Improving Child Health* (Ettinger, 2004), a comprehensive list of existing data sets to use within your collaborative needs assessments. This table provides information about existing data sets, categorized by age of the participants, the periodicity (e.g., single data point, longitudinal) of the data collection, and the geographic detail (local, state, national, international), and includes direct links to the specific data sets.

One example of a frequently referenced data set in community-based interventions in the CDC's (2017) Youth Risk Behavior Surveillance System (YRBSS). The YRBSS was created to monitor risky health behaviors in teenagers across the United States, including unintentional injuries and violence, drug and alcohol use, dietary behaviors and physical activity, and some mood and mental health areas. The YRBSS data set can be examined at local, state, and national level. The data are commonly used to identify high-risk behaviors that may benefit from community-based interventions, including to educate and raise awareness of youth high-risk behaviors to parents, schools, youth-based community organizations, and health care institutions.

CONCLUSION

As illustrated in the opening vignette and highlighted throughout the chapter, communities often struggle with health—including medical and mental health—challenges that lend themselves to community-based intervention. Clinicians are uniquely suited to collaborate with community partners to establish meaningful interventions. These collaborations may be preventive in nature or targeted in addressing chronic and/or severe problems. We have highlighted important considerations in community-based work, described several programs, and directed the reader toward further resources for learning about and engaging in community-based interventions. We hope to have left you with a sense of the value our profession can provide in collaborative, community-based partnerships and have encouraged you to consider providing your professional expertise to communities in your area.

REFERENCES

Aseltine, R. H., James, A., Schilling, E. A., et al. (2007). Evaluating the SOS suicide prevention program: A replication and extension. *BMC Public Health, 7*, 161. https://doi.org/10.1186/1471-2458-7-161

Aspen Institute, Roundtable for Community Change. (n.d.). *Glossary for understanding the dismantling structural racism/promoting racial equity analysis*. aspeninstitute.org. https://www.aspeninstitute.org/wp-content/uploads/files/content/docs/rcc/RCC-Structural-Racism-Glossary.pdf

Center for Community Health and Development. (n.d.). *Table of contents. Community tool box*. https://ctb.ku.edu/en/table-of-contents

Center on PBIS. (n.d.). *Tiered framework*. PBIS.org. https://www.pbis.org/pbis/tiered-framework

Centers for Disease Control and Prevention. (n.d.). *Prevention*. https://www.cdc.gov/pictureofamerica/pdfs/Picture_of_America_Prevention.pdf

Centers for Disease Control and Prevention. (2013). *Brief executive summary, community based interventions, 2010–2013*. National Center for Chronic Disease Prevention and Health Promotion, Division of Community Health. https://www.cdc.gov/nccdphp/dch/programs/communitiesputtingpreventiontowork/pdf/community-based-interventions-executive-brief-update.pdf

Centers for Disease Control and Prevention. (2017). *Youth risk behavior survey*. https://www.cdc.gov/healthyyouth/data/yrbs/

Centers for Disease Control and Prevention. (2020). *Infographic: 6 guiding principles to a trauma-informed approach*. https://www.cdc.gov/cpr/infographics/6_principles_trauma_info.htm

Ettinger, A. S. (2004). Appendix A: Datasets for measuring children's health and influences on children's health: *Children's health, the nation's wealth: Assessing and improving child health*. National Academies Press.

Gaffney, H., Ttofi, M. M., & Farrington, D. P. (2019). Evaluating the effectiveness of school-bullying prevention programs: An updated meta-analytical review. *Aggression and Violent Behavior, 45*, 111–133.

Jason, L. A., Glantsman, O., O'Brien, J. F., & Ramian, K. N. (2019). Introduction to the field of community psychology. In *Introduction to community psychology*. Pressbooks.

Lopez, C. (2016). *Analyzing community problems and designing and adapting community interventions. Center for Community Health and Development*. University of Kansas.

Macarthur, S. (n.d). *Preventative health care and public health*. MPH Online. https://www.mphonline.org/preventative-care-guide/

Manatt, P., & Phillips, L. L. C. (2019). *Medicaid's role in addressing social determinants of health*. RWJF.org. https://www.rwjf.org/en/library/research/2019/02/medicaid-s-role-in-addressing-social-determinants-of-health.html

McLeroy, K. R., Norton, B. L., Kegler, M. C., Burdine, J. N., & Sumaya, C. V. (2003). Community-based interventions. *American Journal of Public Health, 93*(4), 529–533.

Melton, C. (2019). *The economic cost of ACEs in Tennessee medical costs and worker absenteeism from health issues attributed to adverse childhood experiences*. The Sycamore Institute. https://www.sycamoreinstitutetn.org/economic-cost-adverse-childhood-experiences/.

Mindwise Innovations. (2021). *Suicide prevention*. https://www.mindwise.org/suicide-prevention/

Minkler, M., Garcia, A. P., Rubin, V., & Wallerstein, N. (2012). *Community-based participatory research: A strategy for building healthy communities and promoting health through policy change*. PolicyLink.

National Institute of Mental Health. (2021). *Statistics: Suicide*. https://www.nimh.nih.gov/health/statistics/suicide.shtml

New York Academy of Medicine. (2013). *A compendium of proven community-based prevention programs*. https://citeseerx.ist.psu.edu/viewdoc/download?doi=10.1.1.591.4666&rep=rep1&type=pdf

Ohio Department of Health. (2019). Suicide deaths increased by 45% among all Ohioans and by 56% among youth ages 10–24 from 2007–2018. https://odh.ohio.gov/wps/wcm/connect/gov/b9f06188-5026-4695-ae03-06226dc49f22/ODH+News+Release+--+Ohio+Suicide+Demographics++Trends+Report.pdf?MOD=AJPERES&CONVERT_TO=url&CACHEID=ROOTWORKSPACE.Z18_M1HGGIK0N0JO00QO9DDDDM3000-b9f06188-5026-4695-ae03-06226dc49f22-mVCCixj

Olweus, D., & Limber, S. P. (2010). Bullying in school: Evaluation and dissemination of the Olweus Bullying Prevention Program. *American Journal of Orthopsychiatry, 80*(1), 124.

Patchin, J. W. (2019). *School bullying rates increase by 35% from 2016 to 2019*. Cyberbullying Research Center. https://cyberbullying.org/school-bullying-rates-increase-by-35-from-2016-to-2019

Robinson, J., Bailey, E., Witt, K., Stefanac, N., Milner, A., Currier, D., … Hetrick, S. (2018). What works in youth suicide prevention? A systematic review and meta-analysis. *EClinicalMedicine, 4*, 52–91.

Shain, B. (2016). Suicide and suicide attempts in adolescents. *Pediatrics, 138*(1).

Substance Abuse and Mental Health Services Administration. (2019). *A guide to SAMHSA's strategic prevention framework*. https://www.samhsa.gov/sites/default/files/20190620-samhsa-strategic-prevention-framework-guide.pdf

Suicide Prevention Resource Center. (2016). *SOS sings of suicide middle school and high school prevention program*. sprc.org https://sprc.org/resources-programs/sos-signs-suicide

US Department of Education. (2020). *Family Educational Rights and Privacy Act (FERPA)*. https://www2.ed.gov/policy/gen/guid/fpco/ferpa/index.html

US Department of Health and Human Services. (2003). *OCR privacy brief: Summary of the HIPAA privacy rule*. https://www.hhs.gov/sites/default/files/privacysummary.pdf

Vreeman, R. C., & Carroll, A. E. (2007). A systematic review of school-based interventions to prevent bullying. *Archives of Pediatrics & Adolescent Medicine*, *161*(1), 78–88.

Wolke, D., Copeland, W. E., Angold, A., & Costello, E. J. (2013). Impact of bullying in childhood on adult health, wealth, crime, and social outcomes. *Psychological Science*, *24*(10), 1958–1970.

Zalsman, G., Hawton, K., Wasserman, D., van Heeringen, K., Arensman, E., Sarchiapone, M., … Zohar, J. (2016). Suicide prevention strategies revisited: 10-year systematic review. *The Lancet Psychiatry*, *3*(7), 646–659.

Endocrine and Gynecologic Management of Children With Severe Disabilities

Shanlee Davis and Eliza Buyers

For additional material related to the content of this chapter, please see Chapter 74.

> **VIGNETTE**
>
> *EM is a 9-year-old female with optic nerve hypoplasia sequence, epilepsy, and profound intellectual and physical disabilities resulting in immobility and need for full support of all activities of daily living. She was diagnosed with growth hormone (GH) deficiency and hypothyroidism in infancy and has been on levothyroxine 50 mcg daily, but parents elected not to treat with GH. There is increasing distress about how EM's parents will be able to safely care for her as she grows. Her mom is her primary caregiver and transfers are already very difficult; despite precautions, a recent fall resulted in a femur fracture. EM's parents are interested in learning if growth attenuation is an option. They are also anxious about upcoming pubertal changes, specifically menstrual periods, which will add an additional hygiene burden and may worsen her seizures. She already sees many pediatric subspecialists but does not see endocrinology or gynecology.*

This clinical vignette presents numerous endocrine- and gynecologic-related concerns that are common in children with severe disabilities, including fragility fractures, central hormone deficiencies, growth attenuation, and menstrual suppression. These topics and more will be discussed in this chapter with a focus on recognizing when consultation with endocrine and/or gynecology specialist is warranted.

ENDOCRINE MANAGEMENT OF CHILDREN WITH DEVELOPMENTAL DISABILITIES

Bone Density and Preventing Fragility Fractures

Clinical Presentation of Osteoporosis and Fragility Fractures in Children With Developmental Disabilities

Children with severe developmental disabilities have numerous risk factors for low bone mineral density and subsequently risk for fractures (Table 111.1). Although estimates vary in this heterogenous group of conditions, a systematic review found that 12% to 23% of children with severe cerebral palsy suffer one or more fractures, with an annual incidence of 4% (Mergler et al., 2009). Unlike children without disabilities who commonly fracture their upper extremities, the majority of fractures in nonambulatory children with disabilities are in the lower extremities. Further, fractures often occur with minimal trauma and may even go unrecognized if the child cannot communicate location of pain. Therefore clinicians must astutely consider an occult fracture when a child presents with irritability, feeding intolerance, and other unrelated symptoms.

The Role of Imaging to Screen for Fracture Risk

The role of dual x-ray absorptiometry (DXA) in children with severe developmental disabilities and immobility is unclear. While some clinical care guidelines recommend use of DXA as a screening tool, there are limited data on how to interpret results and how these results inform management. Most nonambulatory children will have low bone mineral density; however, low bone mineral density alone in absence of a fracture history is not diagnostic of osteoporosis in youth, and this finding would not necessarily have clinical implications. DXA can be useful in the setting of a fracture history that is unclear, as well as in monitoring the effect of treatment. It is worth noting that hardware implants, hip dysplasia, neuromuscular scoliosis, contractures, and short stature can all present logistical challenges for both lumbar spine and distal femur DXA assessments. If DXA is performed, lateral distal femur or whole body are preferred. As research and clinical care evolve, there may be a more defined role for DXA to quantify risk for fractures in children with developmental disabilities, but at this time, imaging should be considered on a case-by-case basis. Peripheral quantitative computed tomography of the distal skeleton, such as the tibia, may prove to be more useful for risk stratification in this population; however, this is not yet clinically available at most centers.

Management of Low Bone Mineral Density and Osteoporosis

The primary management for addressing bone health in children with severe developmental disabilities is prevention by reducing the modifiable risk factors (see Table 111.1) (Ozel et al., 2016). Most of these risk factors are present early in life and therefore contribute to reduced bone mineral accrual throughout childhood and adolescence. In addition, minimizing fall risk, including seizure control and equipment for transfers, is important to prevent fractures. If osteoporosis is present and the risk for future fractures is deemed to be high, bisphosphonate treatment can be considered (Fehlings et al., 2012). Bisphosphonates inhibit bone turnover resulting in increased

TABLE 111.1 Risk Factors Threatening Bone Health in Children With Severe Developmental Disabilities and Clinical Considerations for Minimizing These Risks

Risk Factor	Clinical Monitoring/Risk Reduction
Minimal/no weight bearing	Physical therapy; consider weight-bearing physical activity (although there is minimal supporting evidence)
Hypotonia or dystonia	Physical therapy
Feeding difficulties, malnutrition, gastrostomy	Optimizing nutrition to avoid over- or underfeeding; ensure appropriate micronutrient intake (Jesus & Stevenson, 2020)
Medication side effects Antiepileptic drugs Glucocorticoids Loop diuretics Proton pump inhibitors	Minimize polypharmacy when possible; attempt to reduce glucocorticoid dosing
Vitamin and mineral deficiencies Vitamin D deficiency Calcium	Dietician involvement to ensure the recommended daily intake of calcium and vitamin D are being met; measure serum 25-hydroxy-vitamin D and replace if low; consider 25 mcg vitamin D for all
Hormone deficiencies Growth hormone deficiency Sex steroid deficiencies	If appropriate for the clinical context, assess for hormone deficiencies and replace if present
Primary or secondary metabolic bone disorder	If low bone mineral density is present, assess serum calcium, phosphate, magnesium, parathyroid hormone, creatinine, and alkaline phosphatase as well as urinary calcium, phosphate, and creatinine

bone mass and presumably decreased fracture risk. However, there is limited research on long-term safety of bisphosphonates in pediatrics outside of the osteogenesis imperfecta population.

In our clinical vignette EM has had one known long bone fracture in addition to multiple risk factors for low bone mineral density. Assessing for modifiable risk factors contributing to poor bone health is indicated, including measuring blood and urine biomarkers, encouraging weight-bearing physical activity, eliminating bone-toxic medications if possible, and considering replacing GH. If there is a history of more than one long bone fracture, DXA would be useful to quantify bone density to make the diagnosis of osteoporosis and consider whether she is a possible candidate for bisphosphonate treatment.

General Screening and Management Considerations of Endocrine Conditions for Children With Complex Medical Conditions

Hypopituitarism

Overview of the hypothalamic-pituitary-organ axes. Insults to the central nervous system and genetic disorders can be accompanied by disturbances of the hypothalamic-pituitary axis (Table 111.2; Fig. 111.1). The anterior pituitary gland secretes hormones that regulate linear growth (GH), the thyroid gland (thyroid-stimulating hormone [TSH]), the adrenal cortex (adrenocorticotropic hormone [ACTH]), and the gonads (follicle-stimulating hormone and luteinizing hormone). For all of these axes, the end-organ hormone provides negative feedback at both the level of the hypothalamus and the pituitary to ensure hormonal homeostasis. Congenital or acquired dysfunction of the hypothalamic-pituitary system can result in some or all of these axes being affected.

Vasopressin, or antidiuretic hormone (ADH), is secreted by the posterior pituitary gland to maintain volume and salt homeostasis. Vasopressin acts on receptors in the renal collecting duct to increase renal reabsorption of water. Children with pituitary dysfunction can secrete too little ADH (diabetes insipidus), too much ADH (syndrome of inappropriate ADH [SIADH]), or a combination of both, depending on the clinical scenario.

Symptoms of hypopituitarism. In the newborn period hypopituitarism will often present with hypoglycemia from deficiency of ACTH and/or GH. Central hypothyroidism may be identified on newborn screening if a primary thyroxine screen is used; however, this can be missed if a primary TSH screen is used, as in many states. The absence of these early manifestations does not rule out hypothalamic-pituitary dysfunction, however. Additionally, pituitary deficiencies can develop long after the initial insult. Referral to endocrinology for assessment of pituitary function is indicated in numerous clinical scenarios (Box 111.1).

Screening for pituitary dysfunction. The best screening for GH deficiency is with measurement of serum insulin-like growth factor 1 (IGF-1), which is a product of the liver that can be measured at any time and does not depend on the pulsatile nature of GH. Random serum GH is almost never useful. A low IGF-1 alone is not sufficient to diagnose GH deficiency, however, particularly in young children or children who are underweight. Screening for central hypothyroidism should include free thyroxine (T4), as TSH is often inappropriately

TABLE 111.2 **Pituitary Hormone Deficiencies**

Pituitary Hormone	End Organ or Gland	End Hormone	Symptoms of Deficiency	Treatment
Adrenocorticotropic hormone	Adrenal cortex	Cortisol; androgens	Hypoglycemia, hypotension, fatigue, prolonged illnesses	Hydrocortisone
Thyroid stimulating hormone	Thyroid gland	Thyroxine	Poor growth, fatigue, constipation, dry skin	Levothyroxine
Luteinizing hormone, follicle-stimulating hormone	Gonads	Estradiol, progesterone; testosterone, inhibin B	Delayed puberty; amenorrhea (Calcaterra et al., 2019)	Estradiol, progesterone; testosterone
Growth hormone	Bone, soft tissues	–	Poor linear growth; hypoglycemia	Somatropin (GH)
Antidiuretic hormone	Kidney	–	Polyuria, polydipsia, hypernatremia	Desmopressin; chlorothiazide

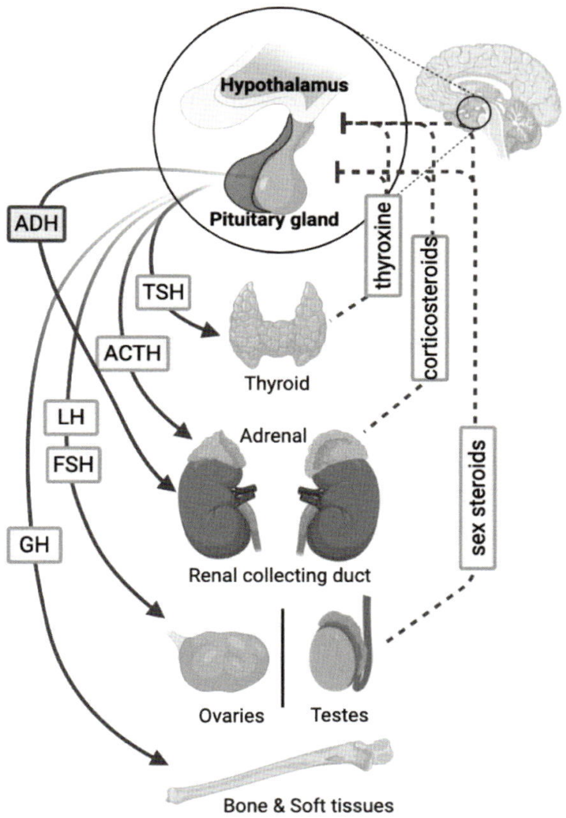

Fig. 111.1 Primary organs and hormones involved in the hypothalamic-pituitary axes. The anterior *(blue)* and posterior *(pink)* pituitary gland secretes hormones into the systemic circulation in response to signals from the hypothalamus. Each of these hormones acts on the specific target glands/organs pictured. In many cases these target glands then secrete hormones that have physiologic actions throughout the body as well as provide negative feedback to the hypothalamus and pituitary gland. *ACTH*, Adrenocorticotropic hormone; *ADH*, antidiuretic hormone; *FSH*, follicle-stimulating hormone; *GH*, growth hormone; *LH*, luteinizing hormone; *TSH*, thyroid-stimulating hormone. **The color figure is available in the Online version.*

BOX 111.1 **Indications for Endocrine Referral for Evaluation of Pituitary Function**

- Radiologic evidence of an abnormal pituitary gland or features of optic nerve hypoplasia sequence
- Poor growth velocity or height percentile >2 SD below mid-parental height percentile in absence of a genetic condition associated with short stature
- Hypoglycemia
- No breast development by age 13 or testicular enlargement by age 14
- Primary or secondary amenorrhea
- Increased thirst and/or urination after diabetes mellitus is ruled out
- Hyper- or hyponatremia
- Recurrent hypotensive illnesses; "crashing" quickly when ill

normal in central hypothyroidism. Evaluation of the adrenal and gonadal axes is more complex and should be undertaken by an endocrinologist in most situations. If diabetes insipidus and/or SIADH is expected, first-morning fasting serum and urine sodium and osmolality can be obtained, but additional evaluation will likely be required for a definitive diagnosis.

Management of pituitary disorders. In most cases treatment of pituitary deficiencies involves replacing the end-organ hormone. Although all pituitary hormones play important roles in growth, health, and development, deficiency of ACTH resulting in adrenal insufficiency is the most serious of these and can be life threatening if not diagnosed and treated appropriately. Depending on the clinical situation, children with central adrenal insufficiency may or may not need daily (maintenance) corticosteroids, usually given as oral hydrocortisone in doses of 5 to 8 mg/m^2/day. All children with central adrenal insufficiency require stress dose steroids in the setting of illness (e.g., fever, vomiting, diarrhea), significant injury (e.g., fracture, motor vehicle accident), and procedures requiring general anesthesia. Stress dose hydrocortisone dosing is 30 to 50 mg/m^2/day. Children should have both enteral and parenteral hydrocortisone as well as an action plan on how and when to administer stress dose steroids.

Central hypothyroidism is treated with oral levothyroxine titrated to maintain free T4 in the normal range. Hypogonadotropic hypogonadism is treated with gradually increasing doses of sex steroids (testosterone or estradiol) to induce secondary sex characteristics at a normal pubertal age. Most often this is via injections of testosterone for males and transdermal estradiol patch for females, although other formulations are available. Sex steroid replacement is continued after puberty is complete to maintain systemic health benefits, particularly bone health.

GH deficiency is treated with daily subcutaneous injections of GH. The primary goal of treatment is to normalize linear growth velocity and ultimately adult height, which may not be an appropriate goal for some children with severe developmental disabilities who depend on others for transfers and care. GH plays a role in body composition and bone health as well, and although these outcomes have not been assessed in clinical trials, lower dosing may be used if height is not the primary goal. Aside from the rare case of GH deficiency causing hypoglycemia, GH treatment is optional, and the risks and benefits should be weighed on an individual basis.

Management of diabetes insipidus can be the most challenging of all the pituitary disorders, particularly for children who do not have an intact thirst mechanism or cannot communicate their thirst. Desmopressin is synthetic ADH that acts on the vasopressin receptors in the kidney, resulting in water retention. The most serious side effect is the potential for severe hyponatremia if there is too much fluid intake while desmopressin is active. In children who have a liquid diet (formula, breastmilk) chlorothiazide may be preferred to reduce the risk of hyponatremia from inadvertently consuming too much fluid due to hunger rather than thirst.

In our clinical vignette EM has a diagnosis of both central hypothyroidism and GH deficiency, but GH deficiency was not treated because height was not a priority for this patient. It may, however, be a modifiable risk factor contributing to her low bone mineral density, and a low dose of GH could be considered. Although she is stable on thyroid hormone replacement, ongoing endocrine care is warranted to ensure appropriate dose titration as she grows and monitoring for the development of other pituitary deficiencies over time.

Precocious Puberty

The hypothalamic-pituitary-gonadal (HPG) axis is inactive until the onset of puberty, typically starting at 8 to 12 years of age for girls and 9 to 13 years of age for boys. If secondary sex characteristics present prior to age 8 for girls or 9 for boys, this is premature (or precocious) puberty. Central precocious puberty can be diagnosed if breast development or testicular enlargement is caused by activation of the HPG axis. Central precocious puberty is more common in children with abnormalities of the central nervous system, likely secondary to a loss of inhibitory signals that are usually present during childhood. Left untreated, central precocious puberty will result in earlier fusion of the growth plates and shorter adult height (Bruzzi et al., 2017). Treatment of central precocious puberty is achieved with a gonadotropin releasing hormone agonist, either via injection or subcutaneous implant. Shared decision making should be used when determining whether to pursue treatment for central precocious puberty in children with severe developmental disabilities. Whether or not treatment is pursued, a brain magnetic resonance imaging to evaluate for new central nervous system pathology (e.g., tumor) as well as assessment of pituitary function are often indicated.

Sometimes puberty signs occur in absence of activation of the HPG axis, called peripheral precocious puberty. In most cases peripheral precocity is benign and self-limited, but pathologic processes should be considered and ruled out. Anecdotally, early pubic hair development frequently occurs in children with severe neurodevelopmental disabilities. This usually reflects production of androgens from early activation of the adrenal glands (adrenarche) for reasons not fully understood. If premature adrenarche is isolated and is not associated with other pubertal signs, increased growth velocity, or advanced bone age, then observation is usually appropriate.

Concerns for Abnormal Growth

Challenges with measuring height. Linear growth in children is one of the most sensitive markers of overall health. Accurate height measurement is essential for evaluating growth velocity as well as calculating body mass index and surface area that are used to assess nutritional status and dose certain medications. However, obtaining accurate and reliable height measurements in children with developmental disabilities has many logistical challenges. The gold standard for height measurement is a wall-mounted Harpenden stadiometer, but this requires the child to be able to stand independently. Even if the child physically can stand, behavior or physical conditions such as scoliosis, contractures, and long bone deformities can lead to inaccurate height interpretations. There have been multiple methods proposed to measure height in nonambulatory children, including recumbent stadiometers, summation of segmental measurements, calculations based on lengths of particular body segments (i.e., tibial length), surrogate measurements such as arm span, and proprietary devices. Unfortunately, these methods require specialized equipment and/or training that is often not an investment primary care practices are willing to make, and as an unfortunate result, height is frequently not documented for nonambulatory children. Furthermore, these methods have wide limits of agreement with standing height in even typical children, so interpretation on standard growth charts should be cautioned. Nevertheless, accurate height measurement remains a crucial vital sign. Providers caring for children with developmental disabilities should prioritize standardization of height assessments in their practices by using consistent techniques and repeat measurements to improve accuracy. The method used should be documented in the child's medical record to appropriately interpret measurements over time.

BOX 111.2 Growth Charts for Specific Conditions

Turner syndrome
Down syndrome
Russell-Silver syndrome
Cornelia de Lange syndrome
Rubinstein-Taybi syndrome
Prader-Willi syndrome
Williams syndrome
22q11 deletion syndrome
Marfan syndrome
Achondroplasia
Quadriplegic cerebral palsy

Interpretation of height and linear growth. Height should be plotted on the appropriate sex-specific growth curve. For children with a known genetic condition associated with an alternative growth pattern, height can also be plotted on their condition-specific growth curve, if available (Magic Foundation (n.d.); Box 111.2); however, these growth charts are often developed from small sample sizes and do not necessarily reflect optimal growth in these conditions.

Interpreting whether growth is indicative of a pathologic etiology involves much more than a single height measurement. Growth velocity, or the change in height over a period of time, should be assessed (prepubertal children should grow 5–8 cm/yr). If biological parents' heights are available, midparental height should be calculated. Attention should also be paid to weight, head circumference, proportions, and body symmetry.

Evaluation of abnormal growth. Children with unexplained abnormal growth should be evaluated to rule out pathologic causes, even if the family would not be interested in treating the height itself. Concerning growth patterns warranting evaluation include growth velocity less than 5 cm/year and/or height more than or less than three standard deviations from the mean (on the standard growth curves or syndrome-specific curves), and/or projected adult height more than 4 cm above or below midparental height (Barstow & Rerucha, 2015). For both short and tall stature concerns, a radiograph of the left hand to estimate maturation of the epiphyses (bone age) can be helpful in narrowing the differential diagnosis as well as providing adult height prediction. Finally, review of the child's medication list can reveal potential growth-restricting or -promoting side effects.

Evaluation of short stature should screen for renal, hepatic, inflammatory, hematologic, and endocrinologic conditions. Typically, this includes a complete blood count, comprehensive metabolic panel, erythrocyte sedimentation rate, tissue transglutaminase, IGF-1, TSH, and T4. Depending on the presence of other signs and symptoms, syndromic short stature should be considered. Tall stature and/or increased growth velocity is less common but can also be pathologic. If linear growth is greater than would be expected for midparental height, an evaluation should be considered. Hyperthyroidism, GH excess, and precocious puberty should be ruled out. Tall stature in a child with neurodevelopmental delays should prompt evaluation for genetic overgrowth syndromes, including supernumerary sex chromosome aneuploidies, Soto syndrome, Weaver syndrome, and others (Kamien et al., 2018).

Growth Attenuation Treatment

Growth attenuation refers to a treatment to prematurely fuse the epiphyses and reduce adult size. Growth attenuation treatment has been considered in situations when smaller stature would be in the best interest of a child with severe neurodevelopmental disabilities that are likely permanent and require lifelong support for all activities of daily living. This treatment is initiated prior to fusion of the growth plates, and the younger the child is when the treatment is initiated, the more effective it will be at reducing adult size. Growth attenuation treatment is not universally accepted largely because of ethical concerns about the autonomy of individuals with disabilities. A single, widely publicized case of a child who received treatment for growth attenuation treatment—accompanied by surgical removal of reproductive organs—resulted in a highly controversial climate that has led to many endocrinologists declining to consider growth attenuation treatment even without the removal of reproductive organs (Kerruish & McMillan, 2015). Though this view is gradually changing, there remains very little research to inform clinical care and a lack of standardized protocols (Allen et al., 2009).

Growth attenuation is usually accomplished with high-dose estradiol in the form of oral (or g-tube) estradiol. Estradiol causes the bone age to rapidly advance, and epiphyseal closure typically occurs within 3 years, though this varies by the initial degree of maturation and interindividual variation in response to estradiol on epiphyseal closure. In addition to epiphyseal maturation, estradiol causes breast development, initial acceleration of growth, and (for girls) vaginal bleeding that can be stabilized with the addition of progesterone. Potential risks of high-dose estradiol include changes in clotting factors that may increase the risk of venous thrombosis, changes in liver enzyme activity potentially altering hepatic metabolism of medications, alterations in seizure pattern, and mood lability. Screening laboratory evaluation includes liver enzymes and clotting factors (protein S, protein C, antithrombin III), and these should be monitored before and during treatment. Epiphyseal maturation should be monitored by x-ray and treatment discontinued when epiphyses are fully fused. Caregivers should be made aware that the premature fusion of the growth plates is not reversible.

In our clinical vignette EM has a congenital etiology of her neurodevelopmental disabilities and is likely to require lifelong full care for all activities of daily living. Her parents have expressed concern about safely being able to care for her as an adult, and she has already sustained a fracture during a transfer. She could be a candidate for growth attenuation treatment with high-dose estradiol. Shared decision making involving her parents and medical providers should weigh the risks and benefits of this treatment option with the focus on EM's health, wellbeing, and quality of life.

GYNECOLOGIC MANAGEMENT OF ADOLESCENTS WITH DEVELOPMENTAL DISABILITIES

For parents of children and adolescents with disabilities, puberty and the associated onset of menstrual periods may feel overwhelming. It is important for providers to monitor pubertal status and provide anticipatory guidance on the expected timing of menarche based on the initiation of puberty, which in females is caused by the onset of ovarian production of estrogen and the corresponding development of breast buds (Fig. 111.2). Providers should initiate an open-ended conversation about puberty and menses and offer counseling and resources as indicated (Table 111.3). Our clinical vignette is a scenario where parental education on the timing of puberal events and then reassurance that there are safe and effective options for menstrual suppression are indicated.

Menstrual Periods: Physiology and Assessment

Ovarian estrogen is produced continually throughout the reproductive years and causes the lining of the uterus to become thickened and vascular. Progesterone, which causes the endometrium to stabilize and mature, is only produced by the corpus luteum at the time of ovulation. When ovulatory menstrual bleeding occurs, it is primarily because of a drop in progesterone levels and an organized shedding of the endometrial lining ensues (Fig. 111.3).

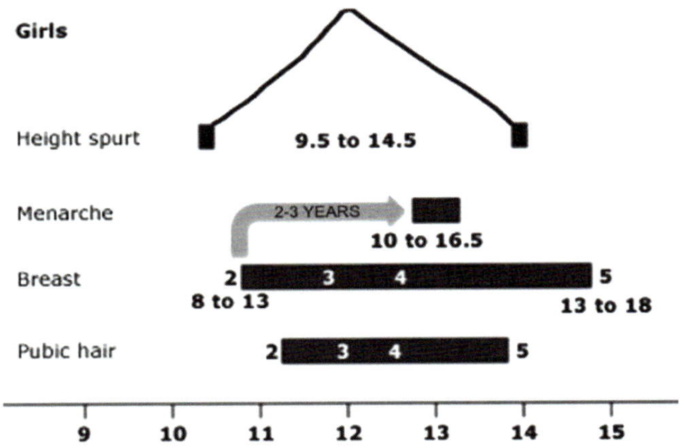

Fig. 111.2 Timing of pubertal events in girls adapted from sequence of pubertal events in the average American girl. (From Tanner, J. M. [1975]. Growth and endocrinology of the adolescent. In L. I. Gardner [Ed.], *Endocrine and genetic diseases of childhood and adolescents* [2nd ed., p. 14]. WB Saunders.)

TABLE 111.3 Common Concerns About Puberty, Menses, and Adolescence

Topic	Suggestions for Provider Counseling
Child is not ready "to grow up"	Education about the normal timing of pubertal events; reassure that physical changes are natural, healthy, and an essential aspect of human development. Empathize that the transition to adolescence may necessitate changes in many areas of patient-family life. Encourage caregivers to obtain the support they need, which may range from practical care-related concerns to emotional/social support.
Managing hygiene	Teens who can use the bathroom independently can learn how to use menstrual products. Menstrual underwear are an option for teens who cannot tolerate pads. There are safe options for menstrual reduction/suppression.
Caregiver discomfort with periods	Menstrual periods are a normal, healthy aspect of female development. All caregivers can learn how to help with hygiene when periods occur. There are safe options for menstrual reduction/suppression.
Sexual abuse	Awareness and communication about the potential for abuse among parents, caregivers, and the adolescent can be difficult but is essential.
Unplanned pregnancy	Developmentally appropriate sex education is necessary to provide adolescents and young adults with options to avoid unplanned pregnancy. Safe and effective methods of contraception are available.
Concerns about pain	Hormonal therapy is very effective at reducing menstrual pain. Maternal history of severe dysmenorrhea does not mean an adolescent will experience the same problem.
Worsening of seizures	Adolescence may be a time of increased seizure activity due to many factors. Adjustments in seizure medications may be needed. Once menarchal, hormonal therapy may be helpful for reducing seizures related to menstrual cycles.
Mood changes and irritability	Adolescence is a time of emotional and psychologic changes, in addition to physical ones. Address new behavioral and mental health issues that occur during the teen years; do not dismiss as unavoidable if they are significant to the patient and family wellbeing. Hormonal therapy is a treatment for premenstrual syndrome and may reduce other period-related concerns.
Adolescent sexuality	Sexuality is a natural and healthy aspect of human development. Education and communication about safety, privacy, and consent is an important aspect of sexual education.

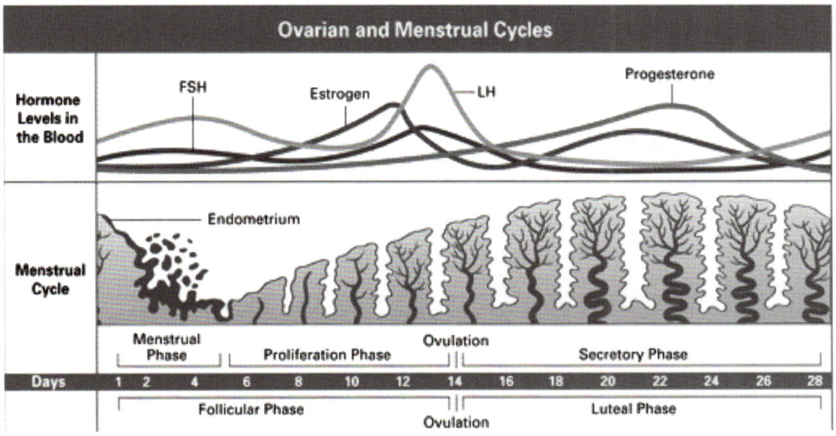

Fig. 111.3 Hormones and endometrium during ovulatory menstrual cycles.

Once menarchal, gynecologic history should be obtained as part of the medical history and include menstrual frequency, duration, and typical product use (ACOG, 2015; Box 111.3). Patients and families should be encouraged to track all menstrual bleeding and associated symptoms and notify their provider if abnormal bleeding or other issues occur. Although irregular menstrual cycles are common in adolescents, abnormal bleeding patterns may warrant evaluation or referral (ACOG, 2012; Table 111.4).

Menstrual Management

There are many options for menstrual management in adolescents (Table 111.5). The key component of hormonal therapies is progestin, a synthetic version of the hormone progesterone, which causes the endometrium to become atrophic when given for an extended period of time. This atrophy results in decreased menstrual bleeding and pain, allowing for the safe reduction or suppression of menstrual bleeding. The most common side effect of all methods is unexpected bleeding, which in most cases resolves with consistent and continued progestin use; however, trial of several methods is commonly needed.

Prescribing Hormonal Therapy and Contraception

There is no special testing or exam that needs to be done before prescribing hormonal therapy and/or contraception. Pelvic exams are not indicated for any screening purpose and should only be done to evaluate a complaint such as vaginal discharge or request for intrauterine device (IUD) insertion. Urine pregnancy testing is often done before initiating contraception as it is noninvasive, inexpensive, and easy to perform, but it is not required if the provider can be reasonably sure the patient is not pregnant.

The best treatment option for menstrual management is the one that aligns with the goals of the patient and family, as well as a consideration of safety given underlying medical conditions. The most commonly encountered medical contraindication is for estrogen-containing hormonal methods (combined oral contraceptive pills, patch, and ring). These methods slightly increase the risk of venous thromboembolism and deep venous thrombosis and should be avoided in patients with an existing risk factor for thrombophilia such as a known thrombogenic mutation or hypertension with vascular disease. The US Medical Eligibility Criteria for Contraceptive Use (USMEC) developed by the Centers for Disease Control and Prevention (CDC) is a free, easily

BOX 111.3 Normal Menstrual Cycles in Young Females

Frequency: 21–45 days
Duration: ≥7 days
Menstrual product use: 3–6/day

TABLE 111.4 Menstrual Issues That May Require Evaluation and/or Referral

History	Possible Evaluation/Reason for Referral
No menarche within 3 yr of thelarche	Assess for causes of primary amenorrhea.
No menarche by age 15	
No period for >90 days, or >45 days if previously monthly cycles	Assess for causes of secondary amenorrhea.
Bleeding more often than every 21 days	Frequent and/or prolonged bleeding should be assessed with a complete blood count, ferritin, and pregnancy test. Abnormal bleeding in adolescents is due to anovulation, coagulopathy, pregnancy, or iatrogenic causes (ACOG, 2015).
Bleeding lasting >7 days in a row	
Heavy bleeding soaking pad/tampon every hour, or >8–10 products per day	
Severe cramps immediately before and during period	Primary dysmenorrhea in teens can be diagnosed based on history alone. Consider causes of secondary dysmenorrhea if patient does not respond to treatment.
Noncyclic pelvic pain	Assess for gynecologic and nongynecologic causes of pain.

TABLE 111.5 Options for Menstrual Management

Treatment	Advantages	Considerations
NSAIDs *Most common are ibuprofen and naproxen*	Decrease blood flow and pain with periods Nonhormonal; can be used along with other methods Available OTC in pill and liquid forms	Can cause GI side effects Certain medical conditions may limit use
Combined hormonal contraception *Methods that contain estrogen and progestin*	Can use in traditional, extended, or continuous dosing to have monthly, seasonal, or no scheduled periods Improve acne and hirsutism	All combined methods increase risk of DVT/VTE; avoid if known thrombophilia; refer to USMEC for contraindications Antiepileptic enzyme-inducing drugs may reduce contraceptive efficacy
1. Oral contraceptive pills	Pill each day, can be crushed; chewable pill available	Pill needs to be taken same time each day
2. Patch	Apply to skin each week	Avoid if patient will remove patch
3. Ring	Insert into vagina each month	Requires insertion into vagina, which may not be feasible
Oral progestins	Typically used in continuous fashion to suppress bleeding; do not contain estrogen; no increased risk DVT/VTE	Pill needs to be taken same time each day or breakthrough bleeding may occur
1. Norethindrone acetate 5 mg	Pill each day	Not an approved contraceptive
2. Medroxyprogesterone acetate 5–10 mg	Pill each day	Not an approved contraceptive
3. Progestin-only birth control pill	Pill each day	50% of users have breakthrough bleeding
Depot medroxyprogesterone acetate (DMPA) *Injection every 12 wk*	Does not contain estrogen; no increased risk DVT/VTE Option of SQ dosing in prefilled syringe for home use	Can be associated with decreased bone density and so may want to avoid when other risk factors present for bone concerns ACOG, 2016 May cause increase appetite and associated weight gain, especially in obese users
Subdermal Implant *4-mm flexible rod placed under the skin of the inner, upper arm*	Excellent, long-acting contraception Easy to place and remove in office if patient is cooperative	Only 20% of users have amenorrhea so other methods should be offered if menstrual suppression is primary goal
Levonorgestrel-IUD *T-shaped device that sits inside the uterus and releases progestin; FDA approved for 5 yr, but evidence-based guidance: 7 yr*	FDA-approved treatment for menstrual bleeding and pain Excellent contraception in addition to menstrual control Insertion under anesthesia can be coordinated with other procedures	Insertion in the office may not be possible Misconceptions about safety may unfortunately limit use

DVT/VTE, deep venous thrombosis/venous thrombotic event; *IUD*, intrauterine device; *NSAIDs*, nonsteroidal antiinflammatory drugs; *OTC*, over the counter; *SQ*, subcutaneous; *USMEC*, United States Medical Eligibility Criteria for Contraceptive Use by the CDC

accessible, evidence-based tool to guide providers on the safety of methods in the setting of underlying medical conditions. The levonorgestrel IUD is an increasingly popular option that provides excellent long-acting contraception, menstrual reduction, and has very few medical contraindications.

Screening Recommendations

Screening for cervical cancer, as with all screening tests, should be done after shared decision making and follow current recommendations. The US Preventive Services Task Force (https://www.uspreventiveservicestaskforce.org/uspstf/) recommends cervical cytology alone (Pap smear) starting at age 21; however, this guidance is likely to shift to human papillomavirus testing alone starting at age 25 based on new recommendations from the American Cancer Society (2020).

Sexually active females should have screening for gonorrhea and chlamydia annually until age 25. This is usually done with a nucleic acid amplification test via a urine sample. All sexually active individuals should have a human immunodeficiency virus test at least once. Other sexually transmitted disease (STD) screening recommendations can be found at the CDC website (www.cdc.gov). The pelvic exam, even in sexually active patients, is not a screening test and should not be performed in the absence of a clear indication.

Contraception and STD Prevention

Adolescents with disabilities may be sexually active and should be offered person-centered contraceptive counseling. Many birth control methods also offer noncontraceptive benefits, which are of interest to many users. Long-acting reversible contraceptives (IUDs and implants) have the highest satisfaction rates of all methods and are safe for almost all adolescents. In addition to an effective contraceptive method, condoms and recommended STD screenings are recommended to prevent sexually transmitted infections.

Treatments to Avoid

Occasionally, families will be interested in suppressing menstrual periods before their onset. This is not recommended as menarche confirms that the genital tract is patent and that the hypothalamic-pituitary-ovarian axis is likely intact. Providers should address patient and/or parental anxiety about the first menstrual period and develop a definitive plan for menstrual suppression once menarche has occurred.

Endometrial ablation, which is an outpatient procedure that burns or freezes the endometrial lining, is generally not recommended for women younger than age 40 due to the high likelihood of endometrial regrowth as well as the need for concomitant use of permanent sterilization.

Tubal ligation is not considered a preferred option for contraception in young women as it offers no noncontraceptive menstrual benefits, and long-acting reversible contraceptive methods are equally or more effective and have no risk of regret. In addition, there is a long and problematic history in the United States of women who were sterilized without their consent or knowledge (ACOG, 2017).

Finally, families may request hysterectomy to remove any potential for pregnancy and to stop menstrual bleeding. In patients with disabilities, indications for major surgical procedures are similar to those of other patients. Hysterectomy is not indicated for the sole purpose of pregnancy prevention and cessation of menstrual bleeding, given that less risky and effective treatment alternatives exist. However, significant gynecologic conditions may warrant consideration in certain circumstances. As with tubal ligation, there are prominent ethical and legal considerations in individuals with disabilities.

REFERENCES

Allen, D. B., Kappy, M., Diekema, D., & Fost, N. (2009). Growth-attenuation therapy: Principles for practice. *Pediatrics*, *123*(6), 1556–1561. https://doi.org/10.1542/peds.2008-2951

American College of Obstetricians and Gynecologists. (2012). Diagnosis of abnormal uterine bleeding in reproductive-aged women. Practice Bulletin No. 128. *Obstetrics and Gynecology*, *120*, 197–206.

American College of Obstetricians and Gynecologists. (2014). Depot medroxyprogesterone acetate and bone effects. Committee Opinion No. 602. *Obstetrics and Gynecology*, *123*, 1398–1402.

American College of Obstetricians and Gynecologists. (2015). Menstruation in girls and adolescents: Using the menstrual cycle as a vital sign. Committee Opinion No. 651. *Obstetrics and Gynecology*, 143–146.

American College of Obstetricians and Gynecologists. (2016). Menstrual manipulation for adolescents with physical and developmental disabilities. Committee Opinion No. 668. *Obstetrics and Gynecology*, *128*, e20–e25.

American College of Obstetricians and Gynecologists. (2017). Sterilization of women: Ethical issues and considerations. Committee Opinion No. 695. *Obstetrics and Gynecology*, *129*, e109–e116.

Barstow, C., & Rerucha, C. (2015). Evaluation of short and tall stature in children. *American Family Physician*, *92*(1), 43–50.

Bruzzi, P., Messina, M. F., Bartoli, A., Predieri, B., Lucaccioni, L., Madeo, S. F., … Iughetti, L. (2017). Central precocious puberty and response to GnRHa therapy in children with cerebral palsy and moderate to severe motor impairment: Data from a longitudinal, case-control, multicentre, Italian study. *International Journal of Endocrinology*, *2017*, 4807163. https://doi.org/10.1155/2017/4807163

Calcaterra, V., Cena, H., De Silvestri, A., Di Mitri, M., & Pelizzo, G. (2019). Disorders of puberty in severely neurologically impaired children: Is delayed puberty an underestimated problem? *Frontiers in Pediatrics*, *7*, 462. https://doi.org/10.3389/fped.2019.00462

Centers for Disease Control and Prevention. (2016). *US medical eligibility criteria (USMEC) for contraceptive use*. https://www.cdc.gov/reproductivehealth/contraception/mmwr/mec/summary.html

Fontham, E. T. H., Wolf, A. M. D., Church, T. R., Etzioni, R., Flowers, C. R., Herzig, A., Guerra, C. E., Oeffinger, K. C., Shih, Y. T., Walter, L. C., Kim, J. J., Andrews, K. S., DeSantis, C. E., Fedewa, S. A., Manassaram-Baptiste, D., Saslow, D., Wender, R. C., & Smith, R. A. (2020). Cervical cancer screening for individuals at average risk: 2020 guideline update from the American Cancer Society. *CA: A Cancer Journal for Clinicians*, *70*(5), 321–346. https://doi.org/10.3322/caac.21628 Epub 2020 Jul 30. PMID: 32729638

Fehlings, D., Switzer, L., Agarwal, P., Wong, C., Sochett, E., Stevenson, R., … Gaebler, D. (2012). Informing evidence-based clinical practice guidelines for children with cerebral palsy at risk of osteoporosis: A systematic review. *Developmental Medicine & Child Neurology*, *54*(2), 106–116. https://doi.org/10.1111/j.1469-8749.2011.04091.x

Jesus, A. O., & Stevenson, R. D. (2020). Optimizing nutrition and bone health in children with cerebral palsy. *Physical Medicine and Rehabilitation Clinics of North America*, *31*(1), 25–37. https://doi.org/10.1016/j.pmr.2019.08.001

Kamien, B., Ronan, A., Poke, G., Sinnerbrink, I., Baynam, G., Ward, M., … Scott, R. J. (2018). A clinical review of generalized overgrowth syndromes in the era of massively parallel sequencing. *Molecular Syndromology*, *9*(2), 70–82. https://doi.org/10.1159/000484532

Kerruish, N., & McMillan, J. R. (2015). Parental reasoning about growth attenuation therapy: Report of a single-case study. *Journal of Medical Ethics*, *41*(9), 745–749. https://doi.org/10.1136/medethics-2013-101913

Magic Foundation. (n.d.). *Website*. www.magicfoundation.org/

Mergler, S., Evenhuis, H. M., Boot, A. M., De Man, S. A., Bindels-De Heus, K. G., Huijbers, W. A., & Penning, C. (2009). Epidemiology of low bone mineral density and fractures in children with severe cerebral palsy: A systematic review. *Developmental Medicine and Child Neurology*, *51*(10), 773–778. https://doi.org/10.1111/j.1469-8749.2009.03384.x

Ozel, S., Switzer, L., Macintosh, A., & Fehlings, D. (2016). Informing evidence-based clinical practice guidelines for children with cerebral palsy at risk of osteoporosis: An update. *Developmental Medicine & Child Neurology*, *58*(9), 918–923. https://doi.org/10.1111/dmcn.13196

112

Social Inclusion

Deborah M. Spitalnik and Dillon Reitmeyer

For additional material related to the content of this chapter, please see Chapter 133

VIGNETTE

"School is your first community. You can't support social inclusion without inclusion for education," said Rose, mother of Sadie, a 16-year-old emerging adult with Down syndrome, as she describes her family's commitment to her daughter being included in their neighborhood school since kindergarten.

First-time parents, Rose and her husband Bill, left Sadie's first individualized education plan (IEP) meeting when she was 4 years old, intimidated, confused, with no idea what to do, and shaken by the recommendations of the 14 professionals sitting around the table. They were told Sadie could repeat a year in specialized preschool because she lacked skills or go to a special school a distance from where they lived or go to their neighborhood school. After consulting with their pediatrician and their developmental-behavioral pediatrician, Rose says, "We knew in our heart of hearts that she was going to go to the school in our town. You can't start to be included at 21. There's one Starbucks—not a regular one and a special one. How would she have learned to make a friend? How could Sadie have a community in our town if she was not here? All the things parents have to do to make inclusion happen is exhausting for families. The early guidance of Sadie's developmental-behavioral pediatrician helped us pave the way for our daughter to be in the world."

SOCIAL INCLUSION

Social inclusion is participating in the life of the community with access to the same experiences as one's age peers. The federal Developmental Disabilities Act and Bill of Rights Act of 2000, Public Law (P.L.) 106-402 enunciates that "[D]isability is a natural part of the human experience," giving voice to social inclusion as the direction for practice, policy, and laws addressing people with intellectual and developmental disabilities (Developmental Disabilities Act and Bill of Rights Act of 2000, 2000). There is no singular law, intervention approach, or service model that defines social inclusion; it is a socially validated direction or presumption in many laws and service models. The evolution of social inclusion is iterative, not linear. Social inclusion as a goal and a motivating construct continues to evolve from the interplay of advocacy, the knowledge base and evidence, and our understanding of how to provide intervention and support. Societal trends contribute to developments in the disability community, although progressive ideals and opportunities often accrue to people with disabilities later than those without disabilities, reflecting how society devalues people with disabilities. Even within the broad disability rights movement, people with early-onset disability have often been invisible (Shapiro, 1993).

An examination of the past provides insight into the evolution of social inclusion and in many instances enhances its definition by clearly illustrating what it is not. Social inclusion as a paradigm repudiates outmoded and discredited beliefs and conceptions of children with intellectual disabilities as "God's holy innocents," having tendencies toward criminality, or as incompetents who are incapable of learning, productivity, or making contributions to their family or community. Past medical practices in counseling families at the birth of a child with Down syndrome or other apparent features of disability, "to not hold the child or take the child home that it would ruin the family," advising mothers to "go home and get pregnant again" wounded families and disrupted the life trajectory of the family. Although many families did not heed this advice, state institutions did have nurseries where babies were placed at birth, leading to a life course of separation, segregation, and stigma—the antithesis of social inclusion. It is striking that no matter the age of the person with disabilities, parents' memories of the way they were informed about their child's condition and disability remain vivid. The obstetrician who stood in the hospital room doorway to tell a mother the baby she has just delivered had Down syndrome, providing no information, resources, or support, retreating to the nurse's station to write discharge orders, and not returning to see the family again before they left the hospital with their newborn is one of many searing examples. Past practice isolated families: ignoring the emotional connection between mothers and fathers and their child and mitigating the possibilities for social inclusion. In our present context families tell us how positive messages from clinicians—genetic counselors, obstetricians, pediatricians, and nurses—support the embrace of the child as a beloved, valued member of the family. Positive direct communication and information, linking parents to resources, connecting them to other families for parent-to-parent support, and providing opportunities for shared decision making, set the child and family on a life course to inclusion.

The normalization principle, "utilization of means which are as culturally normative as possible, in order to establish and/or maintain personal behaviors and characteristics which are culturally normative as possible" (Wolfensberger, 1972), a foundational element of social inclusion was brought to the United States from Scandinavia. It is ironic and heartbreaking that the movement to social inclusion began as a reaction to the eugenics movement and the Nazi's extreme ideology of racial purity, and ultimate outcome of euthanizing and exterminating children and adults with chronic illnesses, disabilities, and other expressions of human variation and difference (Holocaust Museum, 2009; Marwell, 2020). Responding to the imminent Nazi invasion in 1940 and aware of the mortal threat to people with intellectual disabilities, the Danish government decided to protect people living in congregate institutions, dispersing them to live with local families in communities in Jutland, the isolated northernmost tip of Denmark (Spitalnik & Rehfeld, 1988). Living in more typical environments, individuals began to express more skills, in effect demonstrating an increase in adaptive behavior. This first foray into social inclusion gave rise to the normalization principle: recognizing that living in human-scale environments, participating in the routines of daily life, and with support for access to typical experiences promotes positive outcomes.

Social inclusion represents a paradigmatic shift in the aspirations and advocacy of people with disabilities and families, in how we provide care and support, and in how services are organized and funded. With the emergence and adoption of a new paradigm, it is challenging to see the world as it was in the prior paradigm. Evolving policies and service options that promote social inclusion often coexist with policies and services from the past, including segregated special education services or congregate residential placements. Changes in public policy and service systems are typically incremental, not transformative. Service systems tend to be mixed models with older services coexisting with newer, more inclusive options. Less inclusive services may be familiar to families and practitioners, and service systems may continue to promote these approaches. Even as paradigms evolve, funding may still incentivize older, less inclusive models. In public policy there is often a discrepancy between access to the new paradigm and persistence of the old. This gap between the ideal and the reality of implementation can be disillusioning and may lead to the rejection of the new paradigm as undesirable or unworkable. All children who are eligible for special education are now entitled to a free and appropriate public education (FAPE). Clinicians and families may not be aware that in the past children with disabilities were excluded from education. Social inclusion as a paradigm rests upon societal decisions: laws, attitudes, and funding. It is important to appreciate that societal commitment, the basis for social inclusion, may be fragile. Clinicians, advocates, and policymakers must remain vigilant, advocating and applying evolving evidence to ensure that the rights and opportunities for children and adults with disabilities to be fully included in our communities are not abrogated.

AN ERA OF COMMUNITY MEMBERSHIP

While individual actions may promote or mitigate social inclusion, the nature of services and supports available to people with developmental disabilities are highly determinative of the opportunities available for participation. Due to deteriorating and isolating conditions in large publicly funded institutions and advocacy from families and professionals in the 1960s and 1970s, states embarked on deinstitutionalization. These state efforts were often the result of class action lawsuits, including against Willowbrook in New York and Pennhurst in Pennsylvania. In deinstitutionalization children were typically moved out of institutions first, and further admissions of children were halted. Two major policy developments decreased the need and demand for institutional placement: the initiation of the Children's Supplemental Security (SSI) program in 1972 and the Education of All Handicapped Children Act (P.L. 94-142) in 1975. In providing both income support and educational services, respectively, these programs facilitated the social inclusion of children within their families and communities. Social inclusion has only become possible within the present context, which has been described as an era of "community membership" (Bradley et al., 1994). Dating from the late 1980s, the idea of community membership means not only being physically present in the community but being connected and "of" the community. The movement to social inclusion reflects our understanding that social inclusion is not just a location but rather being supported to participate in the community.

As the baby boom increased the number of children born with disabilities in the post–World War II period, advocacy began with the voices of families. Since the early 1980s, the voices of individuals with disabilities themselves (i.e., self-advocacy) have promoted social inclusion both as a right and as a direction for the development of services and supports. The civil rights movement has provided the template for inclusion for the disability community, based on the tenet first applied to race, that separate is not equal. There is no singular law or intervention approach or service model that defines social inclusion; rather, it is a preferred direction or presumption in many laws and service models.

Social inclusion emerges across domains of life activity. Correspondingly, barriers to social inclusion can be environmental, physical, or attitudinal (Centers for Disease Control and Prevention, 2020). The socioecologic model of disability only began to be applied to disability services in the 1970s, contributing to the growth of early intervention services for infants and toddlers before they were legally mandated. For older children and adults, the socioecologic model was conceptualized as the developmental model. This model became the theoretical basis for the conceptualization of active treatment, a requirement for states to receive federal financial support to improve institutional conditions. This expanded long-term care funding under the Medicaid Intermediate Care Facilities (ICF) program to include state institutions. Applying the understanding of the nature of the interaction between the individual and the environment to individuals with intellectual disabilities began challenging the limiting construct of "ceilings of ability" described in diagnostic and classification systems for intellectual disability (Grossman, 1973). The concept that 25 years of age was the "life age" at which learning stopped and developmental attainment was fixed (Doll, 1953) was also discredited by the socioecologic model and our increased understanding of brain plasticity.

The growing knowledge base in systematic instruction and the development and dissemination of behavioral approaches began to transform the education of children with disabilities and the nature of institutional and other residential services, contributing to the movement to smaller, community-based, more homelike settings in the 1970s. Applying a highly structured behavioral paradigm to tasks of complex assembly paved the way for employment becoming a path for adults with intellectual and developmental disability (Bellamy, 1976). The synergy between the role of evolving knowledge and intervention in creating opportunities for productivity, contribution, and more valued social roles, and the increasing attention to the rights of children and adults supported by advocacy, created the precursors to social inclusion.

Support for participation is a hallmark of social inclusion. Early efforts to mainstream children in special education into general education settings without support for their learning needs and their participation as part of a classroom community were often unsuccessful. Children may have been physically present but lacked meaningful access to the curriculum or opportunities for reciprocal interactions with their age peers. Supports are the "resources and strategies that promote the development and interests of a person and that enhance an individual's functioning and personal well-being" (Schalock et al., 2021). Supports can be described in both their intensity and duration, and who provides the support. Supports can include paid services, natural supports, and unpaid supports. The supports approach separates location (i.e., where the support is delivered) from the intensity of the support needs. Embedded in the idea of congregate institutions and other segregated settings (including classrooms) are assumptions that intense needs or needs for specialized expertise and services can only be delivered in specialized places, that individuals with high needs should be congregated to have their needs addressed, and that funding for services need be restricted to congregate settings. The ability to utilize Medicaid funding in the community was launched by the advocacy of Julie Beckett in 1980, who wanted her daughter Katie, who had extensive medical needs and was living in a hospital, to live at home and receive her high-intensity health services there. At that time, there was no way to pay for Katie's services at home; Medicaid would only fund services in a hospital. Based on family advocacy, then-president Ronald Reagan granted an individual waiver for Katie's care to be funded at home (Hevesi, 2012). This individual waiver of requirements was the first time Medicaid funding was permitted to be used in the community. The federal response to the individual circumstances of the Beckett family became a broad programmatic option and initiated waivers as policy changes making it possible to utilize Medicaid funding across programs and needs. This initial waiver to utilize Medicaid funds in the community rather than a hospital, nursing home, or congregate facility became a feature of Medicaid, eventually leading to Home and Community Based Services waivers, the major policy and fiscal underpinning for social inclusion. The Robert Wood Johnson Foundation, through Self Determination grants to states from 1995 to 2000, contributed to the experience and knowledge base in social inclusion by promoting person-centered practices, choice, and self-direction as guiding principles for developmental disability service systems (Sunderland, 2007).

LEGAL FOUNDATIONS

Social inclusion incorporates the ideal of social justice. The legal foundations for social inclusion are based on a rights framework, realized through protections against discrimination as well as more affirmative programmatic approaches.

Section 504

In 1973 Section 504 of the Rehabilitation Act, and now its successor legislation, the Workforce Investment Opportunity Act (P.L. 113-128), provided the first major legal protection against discrimination for people with disabilities (Workforce Investment Opportunity Act, 2014). Section 504, in prohibiting discrimination by entities receiving federal funds, was an important and enduring innovation. However, it does not address discrimination across society more broadly. Although often thought of in terms of adults and employment, Section 504 also applies to children because schools receive federal funds. By prohibiting discrimination, Section 504 made it possible for children and adults to be present and participating, a necessary but not sufficient condition for social inclusion.

Section 504 introduced the concept of accommodations to support participation. As a tool or strategy for inclusion, accommodations have boundaries and limitations. Accommodations are required to be "reasonable accommodations" and not a "fundamental alteration" of a job, educational program, or setting. Accommodations apply only to an "otherwise qualified" individual, who is able to participate with "reasonable accommodation." The definition and varying interpretations of these terms have been the subject of significant numbers of court cases and other forms of seeking redress, including changes in federal regulations, the instruments through which laws are implemented. Accommodations as an antidiscrimination tool in Section 504 provide the basis for the evaluation of learning needs and the development of a plan that includes due process elements. Section 504 for children does not require a diagnosis or disclosure of disability, but a request for accommodation(s), establishing Section 504 as a more inclusive option, depending on the extent of the learning difficulties and functional limitations of the child.

The Americans With Disabilities Act

The Americans with Disabilities Act (ADA; P.L. 101-336) was signed into law on July 26, 1990 (Americans with Disabilities Act, 1990). In this bipartisan legislation we see the most comprehensive enunciation of the rights of people with disabilities within federal law and the underpinnings for inclusion. Modeled on the Civil Rights Act of 1964 and prohibitions against racial discrimination, ADA extends to people with disabilities the finding that "separate is not equal." ADA is organized into four titles:

Employment
Public entities (and transportation)
Public accommodations (and commercial facilities)
Telecommunications

ADA addresses discrimination across settings and the domains of life that make participation and inclusion possible. Similar to Section 504, ADA relies on the idea of reasonable accommodations, not fundamental alterations. ADA and Section 504 have been utilized in complementary strategies to secure educational accommodations for students with disabilities, although ADA does not apply to the Individuals with Disabilities Education Act (Individuals with Disabilities Education Act, 2004). The impact of ADA is most visible in the built environment as public accommodations, including curb cuts, ramps, accessible restrooms, and building codes. Requirements for accessible medical equipment and provider settings, and accommodations for communication such as sign language interpreters, are also highly visible publicly and in health care environments. The impact of ADA in preventing discrimination and promoting or facilitating social inclusion has fluctuated over time. These fluctuations are a function of the implementation and enforcement of the discrimination protections by the federal government, the political orientation of the Executive branch and Congress, and a broad range of court cases variously seeking to limit or expand the protections provided by ADA.

Lois Curtis and Elaine Wilson were two women institutionalized in Georgia who wanted to live in the community. Since Georgia already provided community services for some people with intellectual and developmental disabilities, a lawsuit was brought on their behalf based on discrimination under Title III, the public accommodation section of ADA. The US Supreme Court in 1999 in *Olmstead v L.C.* found that "unjustified isolation" and "unnecessary institutionalization are forms of discrimination" *(Olmstead v L.C.,* 1999*). Olmstead* creates a legal standard for inclusion as part of publicly funded programs for people with disabilities. This court decision requires that states, which receive federal funding through Medicaid for developmental disabilities services, develop a plan to address this form of discrimination, but within the context of reasonable accommodation, not fundamental alteration of their service delivery systems.

ADA and Section 504, by prohibiting discrimination, provide a legal foundation for social inclusion. Both laws, in facilitating community participation and the ideal of community membership to benefit individuals and society, represent incremental approaches but not complete transformation.

IDEA

The Individuals with Disabilities Education Act (P.L. 108-446) illustrates the role of education and its impact on the life course as a cornerstone of inclusion. IDEA is an affirmative programmatic strategy, not an antidiscrimination approach. The history of securing the right to a FAPE for children with disabilities, the provisions of IDEA as an entitlement, and how the law is implemented across the country demonstrate the interplay of successive strategies in enhancing the movement to inclusion. Through the early 1970s, Pennsylvania and other states restricted access to education based on a child's level of functioning, invoking unfounded assumptions that only children at higher levels of functioning could learn or benefit from education. As an advocacy strategy with families as plaintiffs, the ARC of Pennsylvania sued the state of Pennsylvania over state law denying public education to children with disabilities (*ARC of Pennsylvania v Commonwealth of Pennsylvania*, 334 F. Supp. 1257 [E.D. Pa. 1971]). As an antidiscrimination case modeled on the 1954 Supreme Court decision based on race in *Brown v Board of Education (Brown v Board of Education,* 1954*)*, this case asserted that separate education is unequal education. Although there were other court cases, including *Mills v Board of Education of District of Columbia*, which eventually went to the US Supreme Court, the *ARC of Pennsylvania* case was the first time legislation restricting education was struck down. The consent decree, a legally binding agreement between the plaintiff, the ARC of Pennsylvania representing families, and the defendant, the Commonwealth of Pennsylvania, became the framework in 1975 for P.L. 94-142, the federal Education of All Handicapped Children Act, and eventually IDEA. IDEA creates an entitlement based on these court cases and previous federal law to eliminate discrimination. This entitlement recognizes that all children can learn, that all children can have a right to FAPE, and that there must be dedicated funding to address FAPE. As an approach to protect rights through the provision of education, the elements of IDEA entitlement include a presumption toward inclusion. The Early Intervention Part C requirements in IDEA for children aged 0 to 3 years require the development of an individual family service plan (IFSP) and the delivery of early intervention services in "natural environments," supporting the child within the context of the family in the home and other age-appropriate settings, including day care. For children ages 3 to 21 years, the provisions of Part B of IDEA represent tools for inclusion, including the "least restrictive environment" (LRE), and requirements for planning and services addressing transition to adult life to be embedded in the IEP beginning at age 16 years. The provisions of the 2002 federal No Child Left Behind Education Act were incorporated into IDEA, promoting access to the general curriculum and participation in standardized assessments for children with IEPs, potential levers for inclusion through education See Chapter 113 for additional information on IDEA.

Rosa's Law

The language and terms used to describe, categorize, and label disabilities have historically functioned as attitudinal barriers to inclusion. Section 504 addresses the power of language and the discriminatory attitudes it may engender. By broadening the definition of disability to include impairments that "substantially limits major life activities only as a result of the attitudes of others towards such impairment" (45 C.F.R. SSt; Brady et al., 2020). Section 504 recognizes that attitudinal barriers can contribute to mitigating participation and inclusion. Terms such as "feebleminded" and "mentally deficient" have been used clinically. Children in schools have been labeled by placement categories, including "educable, trainable and custodial." As these labels have changed over time, they have found their way into colloquial usage as derogatory epithets or degrading humor. These terms have created and reinforced negative stereotypes of the capacities and humanity of people with the condition we now describe as intellectual disability. The stigma connected to these terms can be internalized and affect the self-esteem and quality of life of individuals with intellectual and developmental disability (Ali et al., 2012).

The growth of self-advocacy as a movement in the late 1970s put forth the phrase "people first," expressing the desire to be seen in terms of our common humanity, not as a condition. In some parts of the country the term became the name of self-advocacy groups. Advocacy by people with disabilities and by families (Ford et al., 2013) began a campaign to "End the R Word" in state legislation and policy. From 1997 through 2003, professionals from the American Association on Mental Retardation, American Psychological Association Division 33, and the Social Security Administration, as well as self-advocates and families, met as the Consortium on Language, Image, and Public Education. The consortium struggled to understand the nature of the pain of individuals who have the condition we now call intellectual disability, the role of stigma, and grappled with the concerns whether changes in terminology would threaten access to a vast web of programs and entitlements. Fueled by changes in a growing number of states, in 2010 P.L. 111-256 (Rosa's law) became federal policy, eliminating the term "mental retardation" from social policy in favor of "intellectual disability." It required continued advocacy to change the terminology in the Social Security Act as the basis for eligibility for disability benefits (Rosa's Law, 2010; Friedman, 2016).

DILEMMAS OF INCLUSION

The momentum toward social inclusion raises dilemmas for families, for emerging adults with disabilities, and for practitioners who walk alongside families and offer information, direction, and guidance. As with any shift in policy or service delivery approach, vision may outpace the realities of implementation, creating a gap between the ideal of social inclusion and available supports. There is also variability of opportunities across the country and within states and localities, with disparities in access and equity by zip code.

Many families, as they seek FAPE to which their child is entitled under IDEA, struggle with educational placements and IEP goals. Are those things being offered to their child contributing to the life course and future they hope for their child? Do they have accessible and understandable information and meaningful support to explore possibilities? Families may feel faced with false dichotomies that juxtapose concentration on academics with life skills or social inclusion and participation within the larger school environment or the community. Severity of disability and level of functioning are sometimes illegally and inappropriately invoked as admission criteria to more inclusive options rather than facilitating inclusion for all students through higher intensity or more extensive supports.

With any policy, there are often unintended consequences. The presumption in Part C of IDEA for early intervention services to be delivered in natural environments, empowering the family and supporting the child's inclusion within the family, may contribute to family isolation. Prior to this shift toward natural environments, when early intervention was delivered in center-based programs, families had the opportunity to meet each other and be together at programs. This time together created reciprocal understanding and connection, often resulting in long-lasting peer support networks for families. The benefits for children of intervention in the natural environment may, at the same time, mitigate an important source of social inclusion for families.

The loneliness of people with disabilities and the lack of friendships reported by Amado (2014) raise another imperative for social inclusion. Supporting and facilitating friendship and participation in activities of mutual interest, such as the integrated sports through Special Olympics, craft, hobby, or social clubs, often requires a high degree of planning, coordination, and support from families. As children get older, the developmental hallmarks of adolescence may make social inclusion challenging even for those young adults who have been fully included and supported through their earlier education. The opportunities for being part of an inclusive peer group may begin to diminish as life milestones: getting a driver's license, dating, and growing in independence from the family are often less available to young adults with disabilities. For emerging adults who have IEPs, even if they graduate with their high school class, they and their family may elect to utilize their educational entitlement until age 21. Young adults may feel that everyone else is moving on and they are stuck or left behind, thus highlighting the need for postsecondary and college programs that enable young adults with disabilities, especially those in the 18- to 21-year-old range, to move into a valued future and prepare for careers.

In emerging adulthood and the transition period understanding one's disability, enhancing self-management, and learning to negotiate one's support needs become more crucial. While social inclusion is based on an antidiscrimination and rights framework, the support of the skills necessary for participation, consonant with the individual's needs, contributes to social inclusion. Community presence and participation is not a function of the individual's functional level but rather the supports available. For parents, the transition from the entitlement under IDEA to eligibility for adult services is often described as "falling off a cliff." For young adults, the loss of daily services and social interaction can feel isolating, with fewer opportunities for inclusion.

The movement into the world of adult services, health care, and social life changes the role of families in providing care, support, and supervision to their children. Adult services often provide less intense supports than schools and services for children, paradoxically necessitating increased involvement and presence of families for coordination and support. Highly sensitive and often nuanced planning is required to promote social inclusion in the context of adulthood, ensuring adequate support for wellbeing, safety, and participation in a developmentally appropriate manner.

Social inclusion also raises issues of our personal identity, our sense of identification, and belonging or difference. In any choices individuals or families make there are trade-offs. Who is our peer group? Are we the same or different than others and across what dimensions: race, abilities, gender, or interests? Judy Heumann, a disability activist who was deeply engaged in the passage of Section 504 and ADA, attended school in a regular/general education classroom. Having experienced educational and social inclusion, Heumann struggled with feelings of difference and invisibility. While validating the educational benefit of being included, in her recent autobiography Heumann wrote of the meaning of attending camp for teenagers with disabilities: "From my time at camp, though, I knew what it felt like to be treated like a regular girl" (Heumann & Joiner, 2020).

CONCLUSION

The advocacy of families and people with disabilities challenged the history of segregation in disability services. Legislation and evolving practices recognize social inclusion as a right and the direction for policy and services, yet the experience of Sadie's family (vignette) illustrates the dilemmas and obstacles many families encounter. Schools and other systems may continue to have the orientation that the services and supports need to be provided in special places, apart from the presence and experiences of one's age peers. In how we listen, prescribe, guide, and support, we can reflect on the connections that we value in our own lives and enhance opportunities for belonging and full lives in the community for everyone.

REFERENCES

Ali, A., Hassiotis, A., Strydom, A., & King, M. (2012). Self stigma in people with intellectual disabilities and courtesy stigma in family carers: A systematic review. *Research in Developmental Disabilities*, *33*(6), 2122–2140. https://doi.org/10.1016/j.ridd.2012.06.013

Amado, A. (2014). Building relationships between adults with intellectual disabilities and community members: Strategies, art, and policy. *Research and Practice in Intellectual and Developmental Disabilities*, *1*(2), 111–122. https://doi.org/10.1080/23297018.2014.941968

Americans With Disabilities Act of 1990. (1990). *P.L. 101-336 S. 933, 101st Cong.* https://www.govtrack.us/congress/bills/101/s933

Bellamy, G. T. (1976). *Habilitation of severely and profoundly retarded adults: Reports from the specialized training program*. Social and Rehabilitation Service. https:eric.ed.gov/?id=ED148528

Bradley, V. J., Ashbaugh, J. W., & Blaney, B. C. (1994). *Creating individual supports for people with developmental disabilities: A mandate for change at many levels*. Paul H. Brookes Publishing Co.

Brady, K. P., Russo, C. J., Dieterich, C. A., Osborne, A. G., & Snyder, N. D. (2020). Eligibility and legal protections under Section 504 and the ADA: *Legal issues in special education* (pp. 231–247, 1st ed.). Routledge. https://doi.org/10.4324/9780429451492-13

Brown v. Board of Education. (1954). 347 U.S. 483.

Centers for Disease Control and Prevention. (2020). *Common barriers to participation experienced by people with disabilities*. https://www.cdc.gov/ncbddd/disabilityandhealth/disability-barriers.html

Developmental Disabilities Assistance and Bill of Rights Act of 2000. (2000). *P.L. 106-402, S. 1809, 106th Cong.* https://www.govtrack.us/congress/bills/106/s1809

Doll, E. A. (1953). *The measurement of social competence: A manual for the Vineland Social Maturity Scale*. Educational Test Bureau Educational Publishers. https://doi.org/10.1037/11349-000

Ford, M., Acosta, A., & Sutcliffe, T. (2013). Beyond terminology: The policy impact of a grassroots movement. *Intellectual and Developmental Disabilities*, *51*(2), 108–112. https://doi.org/10.1352/1934-9556-51.2.108

Friedman, C. (2016). Outdated language: Use of "mental retardation" in Medicaid HCBS waivers post-Rosa's law. *Intellectual and Developmental Disabilities*, *54*(5), 342–353. https://doi.org/10.1352/1934-9556-54.5.342

Grossman, H. J. (1973). *Manual on terminology and classification in mental retardation*. American Association on Mental Deficiency.

Heumann, J., & Joiner, K. (2020). *Being Heumann: An unrepentant memoir of a disability rights activist*. Beacon Press.

Hevesi, D. (2012). Katie Beckett, who inspired health reform, dies at 34. New York Times. https://www.nytimes.com/2012/05/23/us/katie-beckett-who-inspired-health-reform-dies-at-34.html

Individuals with Disabilities Education Act. (2004). P.L. 108-446, H.R. 1350, 108th Cong.

Marwell, D. G. (2020). *Mengele: Unmasking the angel of death*. W.W. Norton & Co.

Olmstead v. L.C. (1999). 527 U.S. 581.

Rosa's law. (2010). *P.L. 111-256, S. 2781, 111th Cong.* https://www.govtrack.us/congress/bills/111/s2781

Rosemary F. Dybwad on normalization and self-advocacy (video recording).

Schalock, R. L., Luckasson, R., & Tasse, M. J. (2021). *Intellectual disability: Definition, diagnosis, classification, and systems of supports* (12th ed.). American Association on Intellectual and Developmental Disabilities.

Shapiro, J. P. (1993). *No pity*. Times Books.

Spitalnik, D. M., & Rehfeld, B. (Eds.). (1988). *Selections from an oral history of policy and advocacy in developmental disabilities as reflected in the lives and works of Elizabeth M. Boggs, Gunnar Dybwad and Rosemary F. Dybwad*. University Affiliated Program, UMDNJ-RWJMS.

Sunderland, A. (2007). *Self-determination for persons with developmental disabilities*. The Robert Wood Johnson Foundation.

US Holocaust Museum. (2009). *Deadly medicine*. Author.

Wolfensberger, W. (1972). *The principle of normalization in human services*. National Institute on Mental Retardation.

Workforce Innovation and Opportunity Act. (2014). *P.L. 113-128, H.R. 803, 113th Cong.* https://www.govtrack.us/congress/bills/113/hr803

113

Education Law: Implications for Developmental-Behavioral Pediatrics

Jeffrey Okamoto

For additional material related to the content of this chapter, please see Chapters 103, 104 and 112.

VIGNETTE

Sarah's mother raised concerns about her educational placement during her most recent well-child visit. Sarah is a 5-year-old girl with 47,XXX syndrome (trisomy X) who is about to start kindergarten. Three years ago, Sarah's clinician diagnosed her with trisomy X syndrome after language delays and tall stature prompted genetic testing. Sarah's mother contacted the state early intervention program through Part C of the Individuals with Disabilities Education Act (IDEA) at that time. Sarah was eligible for speech therapy, and her family started working with a therapist a few weeks later. When Sarah turned 3 years old, she was still behind in language and therefore participated in a preschool special education program sponsored by her school district. Her mother has been pleased with Sarah's progress. She now has a large vocabulary, speaks in sentences, can use complex grammar, and participates actively in conversations. Her mother wants her to continue special education supports in kindergarten. The speech-language pathologist alerts her mother that her scores on the speech and language assessments are now in the low average range, making her ineligible for special education. She asks her clinician for advice.

Returning to Sarah, the child with 47,XXX in the opening vignette, the clinicians on her team know that girls with this condition have highly variable developmental and behavioral outcomes. The health care clinicians cannot override the multidisciplinary team's conclusion, though the clinician might consider a psychological assessment to ensure that the child's intellectual abilities, academic skills, and behavioral profile confirm the school's impression. If these assessments are confirmatory, then the clinician can play an important role in explaining to the mother why her child may no longer be eligible for special education services, despite qualifying at younger ages. The clinician can frame these findings as success, the child benefited from the early intervention and is now able to attend a general education setting without special services for kindergarten. However, Sarah remains at risk for the development of health issues, such as seizures, specific learning disabilities, and behavioral difficulties, such as extreme anxiety. The decision about special education can be revisited if any of these conditions compromise her learning in the future. In such cases the clinician might ensure that the family knows how to reinitiate a special education evaluation. The clinician may join the multidisciplinary team to advocate for appropriate services going forward.

OVERVIEW

Education in the United States is an entitlement. All children living in the United States have the right to a free and appropriate public education (FAPE). Through years of collaboration and effort, advocates and professionals have worked with legislators and government agencies to champion educational rights for children with disabilities. This chapter focuses on educational rights in the United States and reviews education law using three organizing themes: special education, accountability, and civil rights. Chapters 103 and 104 provide additional practical guidance for readers.

SPECIAL EDUCATION: THE INDIVIDUALS WITH DISABILITIES EDUCATION ACT

History of IDEA

In 1975 the US Congress passed the Education for All Handicapped Children Act (Public Law [P.L.] 94-142) (EAHC,1975), which mandated public special education services for children with disabilities. As noted in the law's statement of findings and purpose, Congress recognized that the special educational needs of children with disabilities were not being met, and in fact many were systematically excluded entirely from public school systems. P.L. 94-142 resulted in major policy achievements addressing these issues and shaped educational rights in the United States. To obtain funding, states had to implement policies that assured all children with disabilities the right to FAPE, and local educational agencies had to maintain records of individualized education plans (IEPs) for children with disabilities. P.L. 94-142 created administrative procedures so that parents of children with disabilities could dispute decisions made about their children's education. The law also codified the principle of least restrictive environment (LRE). LRE maximizes opportunities for participation in the school community and interactions with students without disabilities. As of the 2018–2020 academic year, more than 64% of children with disabilities are in general education classrooms 80% or more of their school day, which demonstrates the law's impact (US Department of Education, 2021).

Congress revised P.L. 94-142 in 1990, renaming it IDEA (1990), which has since undergone several reauthorizations and amendments; most recent is P.L. 114-95, the Every Student

Succeeds Act (ESSA, 2015). Clinicians can use knowledge of IDEA to advocate effectively for their patients' educational rights. The next sections highlight important elements of IDEA.

Part B of IDEA

As illustrated in the opening vignette, Sarah receives special education services from her local school district. The largest part of IDEA funding is allocated to Part B, Assistance for Education of all Children with Disabilities, which covers special education for children and youth with disabilities between the ages of 3 and 21 years. Part C of IDEA (discussed later) addresses services for children younger than age 3 years.

IDEA requires that youth ages 3 to 22 years with a disability that affects school performance and learning receive special education services. IDEA outlines 13 disability categories that establish eligibility (Box 113.1). IDEA also allows states to use a nonspecific eligibility criterion, developmental delay, for children 3 through 9 years of age although not all states elect to use this category. Children who meet eligibility criteria must have an IEP that specifies the special education and related services that they should receive. Related services in IDEA include counseling services, sign language and cued language services, medical services that cannot be provided by the physician or hospital, one-on-one instructional aide, orientation and mobility services, various therapists, psychological services, therapeutic recreation, school nurse services, social work services, technologic devices such as special computers or voice-recognition software, and transportation.

As noted, IDEA establishes the rights of children with disabilities to FAPE; however, "appropriate" can come into tension with "best." The US Supreme Court, in *Board of Education of the Hendrick Hudson Central School District v Rowley*, 458 US 177 *Board of Education v. Rowley*, 1982, held that FAPE is satisfied when the school provides instruction individualized with enough support services to allow a child to benefit educationally. In other words IDEA requires that a child's needs are met, which is not necessarily the same as providing optimal supports. An example is a child with spastic quadriplegia who requires a wheelchair for mobility and has a required classroom on the second floor. The IEP must consider the disability and specify how the child will get to that classroom. This situation does not require the school to get an elevator because the legal requirement is for "reasonable accommodations." The IEP team must indicate how the child will get to the classroom, whether this feat is accomplished by moving the classroom to an accessible first floor, getting an elevator, or having another appropriate way of helping the child to the second-floor classroom. Parents are a critical part of the IEP team, and IDEA establishes protective mechanisms for situations when parents and other advocates do not think that the school is providing FAPE. The due process clause guarantees an impartial hearing to resolve conflicts between the parents of children with disabilities and the school districts. Once the administrative efforts are exhausted, parents can still seek judicial review of decisions.

LRE is another major policy achievement. IDEA establishes that children with disabilities should be educated with children without disabilities "to the maximum extent possible." The goal of LRE is to maximize inclusion (see Chapter 112) and ensure exposure to educational material and interactions that may not be found in a more restrictive placement. Even when more restrictive settings are selected, the IEP must identify opportunities for the child with a disability to interact with peers without disabilities. Importantly, school systems must not make placement decisions based on their needs or available resources, including budgetary considerations and the ability of the school system to hire and recruit qualified staff.

BOX 113.1 Thirteen Disability Categories Specified in the Individuals With Disabilities Education Act

Autism
Deaf
Deaf-blindness
Emotional disturbance
Hearing impairment
Intellectual disability
Multiple disabilities
Orthopedic impairment
Other health impairment
Specific learning disability
Speech or language impairment
Traumatic brain injury
Visual impairment

Response to Intervention

The 2004 reauthorization of IDEA allowed states to adopt service delivery models that focused on children's response to scientific, research-based intervention (RTI). RTI emerged from research that found that different students experience learning difficulties for different reasons. Some children may have undiagnosed learning disabilities, other students may be acquiring English as a second language, and still other students may have frequent absences due to a medical condition. Academic difficulties may also have roots in pervasive racial and social inequities. RTI models are multitiered service delivery systems in which schools provide layered interventions that begin in general education and increase in intensity (e.g., increased time for instruction in smaller student groups) depending on the students' instructional response. There are many approaches to the implementation of RTI models, which are best considered as a set of processes and not a single model. In most models children would need to fail several tiers of RTI before they would be considered for special education. This approach allows school districts to move away from eligibility criteria that rely on discrepancies between ability (i.e., IQ) and achievement. Instead, identification of a disability relies on inadequate instructional response and other criteria. Implementation of RTI continues to be controversial given the long-standing use of the discrepancy model in special education.

Implementation of RTI has varied widely across states (Berkeley, Scanlon, Bailey, Sutton, & Sacco, 2020). While some states link their tiered approach with special education, others do not. Services for low-achieving and at-risk students can be supported with up to 15% of IDEA funds, so many states use these funds to support their RTI efforts (American Speech-Language-Hearing Association, 2021). While advocates hope that RTI models improve achievement and behavioral outcomes for many more students than can be served in special education, additional empiric investigation of RTI is still needed.

Part C of IDEA

Part C of IDEA authorizes federal funding for early intervention services for infants and toddlers with disabilities ages birth to 3 years. In the mid-1980s Congress added Part C to enhance the development of infants and toddlers with disabilities, minimize the need for special education services, and maximize an individual's long-term potential for independent living. Part C recognizes that the special needs of infants and toddlers require active engagement of the family and community. Early intervention particularly recognizes that care for infants and toddlers occurs in home and community settings, rather than schools. The inclusion of families as team members is critical in developing and implementing the individualized family service plan (IFSP) (Table 113.1). The IFSP might include services that increase family involvement, such as interpretation or transportation services. Although a child's third birthday typically requires a transition from an IFSP (Part C) to an IEP (Part B), recent changes in IDEA allow states to continue early intervention services through an IFSP after 3 years of age until a child enters kindergarten, with parental approval.

To be eligible for Part C early intervention services, children must be experiencing developmental delays, as measured by appropriate tests and procedures, in one or more areas of development, or they must have a condition that has a high probability of resulting in developmental delay. However, IDEA provides states with substantial discretion in defining eligibility criteria. As a result, eligibility criteria vary from state to state. The lead state agency for early intervention also differs across states (e.g., Department of Health, Department of Education). As a result, early

TABLE 113.1 Components of the Individualized Family Service Plan (IFSP)

Component	Definition or Detail About the Component
A service coordinator	The professional responsible for program implementation
Necessary early intervention services	These are deemed necessary "based on peer-reviewed research to the extent practicable," including the beginning date of services, length, duration, frequency, intensity, method of delivery, and location. Early intervention (EI) services include family training, counseling, and home visits; special instruction; speech-language pathology and audiology services, and sign language and cued language services; occupational therapy; physical therapy; psychological services; service coordination services; medical services only for diagnostic or evaluation purposes; early identification, screening, and assessment services; health services necessary to enable the infant or toddler to benefit from the other EI services; social work services; vision services; assistive technology devices and assistive technology services; and transportation and related costs that are necessary to enable an infant or toddler and the infant's or toddler's family to receive another service
Child's present levels of development	In the following areas: physical (including vision, hearing, and health status), cognitive, communication, social or emotional, and adaptive
Family's concerns, priorities, and resources	Around supporting the child's development
Measurable results or outcomes expected to be achieved by the child and family	There should be procedures, criteria, and timelines in working on these outcomes
Provision of services in the natural environment	Natural environments are settings where young children without disabilities are typically found, or a justification of why services will not be provided in the natural environment
Other service needs, including medical	That are not required or funded under Part C
Payment arrangements, if any	Under IDEA, states may establish "family cost share" based on a sliding fee scale, but families cannot be denied needed services because of an inability to pay. Families may also be asked to allow the EI system to bill their public or private insurance to cover needed services. Child find services, evaluations and assessments, development and review of the IFSP, and service coordination are provided at no cost to families in all states and territories
A transition plan for services	This includes necessary transition steps and program options that must be written in the IFSP for children nearing 3 yr of age, not <90 days and not >9 mo before the third birthday

IDEA, Individuals with Disabilties Education Act.

intervention statewide systems vary widely from state to state (see Chapter 103).

ACCOUNTABILITY: THE EVERY STUDENT SUCCEEDS ACT

ESSA is a national education law that emphasizes equal opportunity and accountability. Congress first enacted ESSA as the Elementary and Secondary Education Act (ESEA) of 1965, and the law has since been reauthorized eight times, most recently as ESSA. As part of the Lyndon B. Johnson administration's War on Poverty campaign, the law placed a major emphasis on providing equal educational opportunities for all children. This goal took the form of providing funds to districts serving children from low-income backgrounds. Specifically, Title I provides financial assistance to districts to support academic achievement among children from disadvantaged backgrounds.

Reauthorizations in 2002 with the No Child Left Behind (NCLB) Act (2001) and in 2015 with ESSA placed a new emphasis on accountability. NCLB, which introduced accountability standards, had very strict rules that states had trouble meeting. ESSA sought to address many of the problems, including funding formulas that prevented schools (including those with the highest needs) from receiving funding because of overly strict rules. At the time of this writing, states have more flexibility on how to make improvements but are still accountable for performance measurements. Despite all the changes, including names, the main goal has been to improve the educational outcomes and increase educational opportunities for children living in poverty. States receiving funds must measure performance of schools using indicators such as academic achievement in reading and math and high school graduation rates. States are required to test students every year from third to eighth grade in reading and math and once in high school. They are required to test students in science once in elementary school, once in middle school, and once in high school. States must also identify the 5% lowest ranking schools (based on measurement of performance) and make comprehensive improvements with the highest level of supports (Education Post, 2021).

CIVIL RIGHTS: SECTION 504 OF THE REHABILITATION ACT OF 1973 AND THE AMERICANS WITH DISABILITIES ACT OF 1990

The Rehabilitation Act of 1973 (RA, 1973) has several sections that have implications for individuals with disabilities. Section 504 is the most pertinent to the educational rights of children with disabilities. Section 504 specifically prohibits discrimination against a person of any age with a disability, in any program or activity that receives federal funding, such as public schools. As such, children with disabilities are entitled to accommodations that allow them to participate fully in school. For example, a child with cerebral palsy who requires a wheelchair for mobility and cannot access a second-floor classroom requires accommodations that ensure the child benefits from the services offered in that classroom. Parents and schools can work collaboratively to develop 504 plans that outline supports based on a child's specific needs. Importantly, Section 504 does not provide any additional federal funds to assist with implementation because under this law the institution must use the funds already received without discrimination. In addition to public schools, Section 504 applies to colleges and universities, which are not covered under IDEA. Section 504 also extends to any private school that accepts federal funds.

The Americans with Disabilities Act (ADA, 1990) prohibits discrimination against individuals with disabilities of all ages and in all areas, including employment, public services, and public accommodations, including schools. It covers all areas of public life, not only those receiving federal funding.

As noted, IDEA uses a categoric definition disability (see Box 113.1). In contrast, Section 504 and ADA define disability generally, using a functional description of disability as being a physical or mental impairment that substantially limits a person in a major life activity (e.g., self-care, eating, standing, breathing, learning, reading, concentrating, and working). Conditions such as attention-deficit/hyperactivity disorder, asthma, and diabetes are covered under Section 504 and ADA if these conditions result in functional limitation. They may also be covered under the IDEA category of "other health impairment" if the health condition affects the child's ability to benefit from the education program.

IMPLICATIONS FOR CLINICIANS

Children with disabilities have unique educational needs. There are wide variations in manifestations and severity of disabilities; therefore each child with a disability requires an individualized program taking into account individual strengths and needs. Health care clinicians may provide the fundamental information for classifying a child into 1 of the 13 categories of special education, including autism, multiple disabilities, orthopedic impairment, or other health impairment, or traumatic brain injury. Psychologists may provide information documenting specific learning disability or intellectual disability. Other clinicians (audiologists, speech-language pathologists) may also provide information about deafness, hearing impairment, deaf-blind, and speech-language impairment. All of these clinicians may be called on for certifying what needs are present and what accommodations are most essential on the basis of those needs. As child health experts, clinicians can assist school personnel making connections between a child's medical condition and educational needs, related services, and accommodations. Clinicians can play advisory, advocacy, and collaborative roles but should take care not to dictate or impose their own view of preferred educational methods.

If a clinician suspects that a school is violating FAPE, LRE, or other educational rights, the clinican can support families and work collaboratively with educational advocates and/or attorneys, given the legal aspects and details of each regulation. The clinician can help parents obtain additional information from resources such as the Council of Parent Attorneys and Advocates or the National Disability Rights Network, which is the network for the state Protection and Advocacy (P&A) agencies (Table 113.2). Connecting parents to their state Parent Training and Information Center can also provide them with access to information and resources. In this way clinicians can help ensure all children access their right to an education.

Clinicians play a critical role as family supports to document whether children are benefiting from educational programming. Health care clinicians and school-based professionals have different perspectives of the child and often have access to different sources of data. Clinicians may be more aware of a child's behavior at home and in the community than are school personnel; school professionals may be

TABLE 113.2 Resources Regarding Early Intervention and Special Education

Resource	Brief Description	URL
Parent Technical Assistance Centers	Information to support parents with children with disabilities	https://www.parentcenterhub.org/rptacs/
Early Childhood Technical Assistance (ECTA) Center	This center supports state Part C programs in "developing high-quality early intervention service systems ... and enhancing outcomes for young children with disabilities and their families."	https://ectacenter.org/
IDEA Infant and Toddler Coordinators Association	This organization also supports the exchange of inf ormation and ideas for Part C infant and toddler services.	http://www.ideainfanttoddler.org/
The IDEA Center for Early Childhood Data Systems (DaSy)	This center provides national leadership and technical assistance to states to support IDEA state programs in the development or enhancement of coordinated early childhood longitudinal data systems.	http://dasycenter.org/
National Center for Pyramid Model Innovations (NCPMI)	This center seeks to improve and support the capacity of state systems and local programs to implement an early childhood multitiered system of support to improve the social, emotional, and behavioral outcomes of young children with, and at risk for, developmental disabilities or delays birth to 5 yr.	https://challengingbehavior.cbcs.usf.edu/about/index.html
Research and Training Center (RTC) on Early Childhood Development	The RTC gathers effective early childhood intervention practices based on research.	http://www.puckett.org/researchtrainingcenter.php
Center for Early Education and Development (CEED)	CEED's mission is to improve developmental outcomes for children through applied research, policy, and professional development.	http://www.cehd.umn.edu/ceed/default.html
Center on Enhancing Early Learning Outcomes (CEELO)	CEELO works to strengthen the capacity of state education agencies to lead sustained improvements in early learning opportunities and outcomes.	http://ceelo.org/
The Early Childhood Personnel Center (ECPC)	The ECPC is "focused on building awareness that an integrated, comprehensive system of personnel development (CSPD) for the early childhood (EC) workforce in every state ..."	http://www ecpcta.org/
National Professional Development Center on Inclusion (NPDCI)	The NPDCI works with states to ensure that early childhood teachers are prepared to educate and care for young children with disabilities in settings with their typically developing peers.	http://npdci fpg.unc.edu/
Division for Early Childhood (DEC)	The DEC promotes policies and advances evidence-based practices that support families and enhance the optimal development of young children (0–8 yr) who have or are at risk for developmental delays and disabilities.	www.dec-sped.org/

more aware of the child's performance in the classroom and other school locations. Ideally, clinicians can work collaboratively with parents and school professionals so that children with disabilities are able to maximize their functioning across all settings.

REFERENCES

American Speech-Language-Hearing Association. (2021). *Overview of funding for prek-12 education*. https://www.asha.org/advocacy/schoolfundadv/overview-of-funding-for-pre-k-12-education

Americans With Disabilities Act. (1990). P.L. 101-336.

Berkeley, S., Scanlon, D., Bailey, T. R., Sutton, J. C., & Sacco, D. M. (2020). A snapshot of RTI implementation a decade later: New picture, same story. *Journal of Learning Disabilities*, *53*(5), 332–342. https://doi.org/10.1177/0022219420915867

Board of Education of the Hendrick Hudson Central School District v. Rowley. (1982). 458 US 177.

Education for All Handicapped Children Act. (1975). P.L. 94-142.

Education Post. (2021). *The ABC's of ESEA, ESSA and No Child Left Behind*. https://educationpost.org/the-abcs-of-esea-essa-and-no-child-left-behind/

Elementary and Secondary Education Act. (1965). P.L. 89-10.

Every Student Succeeds Act. (2015). P.L. 114-95.

Individuals with Disabilities Act. (1990). P.L. 101-476.

No Child Left Behind Act. (2001). P.L. 107-110.

Rehabilitation Act. (1973). P.L. 93-112.

US Department of Education. (2021). *About IDEA*. https://sites.ed.gov/idea/about-idea/

114

Health Care Systems for Children With Disabilities

Justin Charles Schwartz and Laura Joan McGuinn

For additional material related to the content of this chapter, please see Chapters 10 and 15.

VIGNETTE

Justice was born with congenital anomalies but no identifiable genetic cause. She required a gastrostomy tube, ileostomy, central line for total parental nutrition (TPN), and urinary catheter, and help with all her activities of daily living, mostly provided by her family, until her death at age 11. In a moving blog post (Coleman, 2019) Justice's mother, Cara Coleman, eloquently chronicles the realities of navigating a fractured system inadequately designed to meet the needs of children with disabilities. She describes several examples of avoidable harm from health care, such as Justice's leg being fractured by a nurse who refused to listen to her stretching and splinting instructions, an injury from a catheter that she tried to warn was being incorrectly inserted, the many months she spent to uncover an insurance coding error to be able to continue Justice's costly TPN, and the countless hours coordinating care between Justice's many specialists.

Justice's story helps to personify the avoidable harm and fragmented care experienced by children with disabilities and their families. It also illustrates the disproportionate financial burden and limited decision-making contribution families are offered when raising one of the estimated 5.6 million US children with disabilities as they deliver approximately 1.5 billion hours of unreimbursed family-provided health care at home each year (Romley et al., 2017). As Ms. Coleman wrote, "Family caregivers are public health workers. Yet, families and family-led organizations struggle to be recognized as part of care teams and to be authentically regarded as equal colleagues. While increasingly invited to provide input, families remain tokenized and invisible."

INTRODUCTION

This chapter builds upon Justice's story and others like hers to describe important concepts in health care for children with disabilities. Justice's experiences provide an understanding of how the health care system currently operates and highlights opportunities for improvement to achieve a system that better serves children with disabilities and their families. The chapter highlights persisting inequities in health care access, endured disproportionately by individuals experiencing poverty and who belong to marginalized racial and ethnic groups, as well as opportunities for improvement. While health systems vary widely across the world in terms of professional roles, delivery systems, and funding/finance mechanisms, this chapter focuses on the US health care system as it pertains to children with disabilities. See Chapter 10 of this book for a discussion on transition to the adult health care system.

GOALS OF THE HEALTH CARE SYSTEM

Historically, the health care system has focused on finding a diagnosis that explains a patient's chief concerning symptoms, and subsequently "curing" or reducing the burden of sickness or disease associated with that diagnosis. The classic image of doctors and nurses working in clinics, hospitals, and visiting homes of patients on house calls defined the concept of health care. This image influenced the development of many systems and processes within health care that remain today, such as fee-for-service payment structures linked to illness-focused diagnostic codes, insurance reimbursement policies that favor procedure-based services, funding structures for hospitals and acute and chronic care facilities, and differences in approaches to physical versus mental health care.

The World Health Organization (WHO)'s seminal Alma Ata Declaration of 1978 reflected consensus that health is a human right based on the principles of equity and community participation (Rifkin, 2018). Over the subsequent decades, health care systems have grappled with how to implement the holistic charge of the Alma Ata Declaration, particularly as the complexity of patients' various needs has increased. Children with disabilities who generally require more frequent and complex care are one of the populations for which this holistic charge is key, yet also for whom it remains incompletely realized.

Wagner's care model (initially called the chronic care model) gives a framework for how health systems can operationalize the values from the Alma Ata Declaration. The care model demonstrates how health care can function within a larger ecosystem to achieve optimal health outcomes. Initially designed to target particular adult patient populations (e.g., with asthma, obesity, diabetes) and later broadened to apply to adults with medical complexity of any type, and then adapted for children with disabilities (Fig. 114.1), the care model

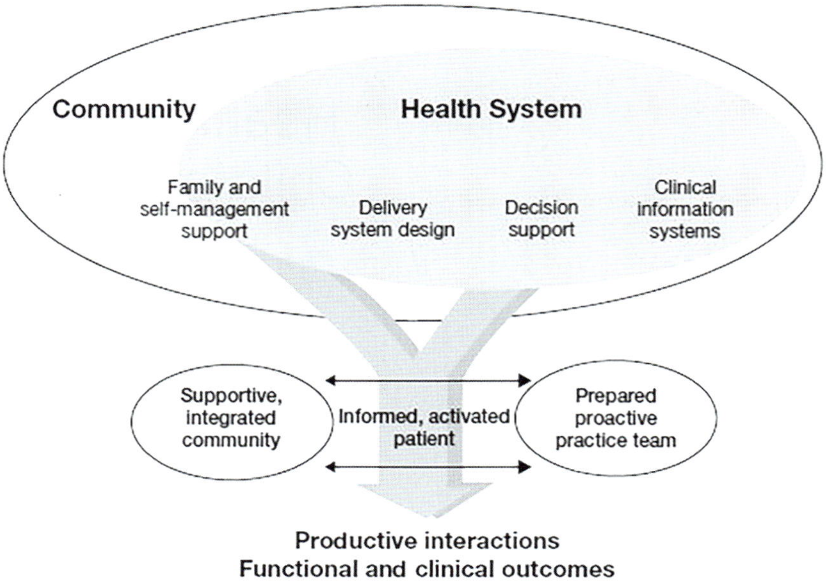

Fig. 114.1 Wagner's care model adapted for children with disabilities. (From Feldman, H. M. [2013]. *Redesigning health care for children with disabilities: Strengthening inclusion, contribution, and health.* Paul H. Brookes Publishing Co.)

emphasizes four core assertions: (1) increasing clinicians' expertise and skill, (2) educating and supporting patients and families, (3) making care delivery team based and more proactive, and (4) making better use of registry-based information systems. To do so, it relies on four components (Adams & Woods, 2016; Wagner et al., 2001):

- Delivery system design: interventions to promote proactive/planned care, accessibility, and team-based care
- Clinical decision support: interventions to reduce variations in care, increase adherence to guidelines, and increase accessibility of specialist expertise
- Clinical information systems: use of information technology to support population management, monitor change implementation
- Family and self-management support: interventions to facilitate patient self-monitoring, treatment adherence, healthy lifestyle decisions, and positive coping skills

The care model highlights the role of the community to support, inform, and engage individuals, giving them more power to advocate for and improve or maintain their health. It asserts that resources such as community programs, social support networks, and community extensions of health care teams, as well as policies to enable full community integration and participation, must be in place to sustain health outcomes. Similarly, within the health system itself, all regulatory, organizational, financial, and policy features must align to allow and sustain the four core components of the model.

Children with disabilities require such coordinated and well-organized care to achieve optimal health and well-being. To that end, Feldman (2013) outlined three main goals of the health care system for children with disabilities: (1) inclusion in family life, school, workplace, and community life, (2) contribution to their families, schools, workplaces, and communities, and (3) health (physical, social, and emotional) to maximize inclusion and contribution. Application of the care model to support these goals opens the door to understanding the opportunities for reshaping the health care system to provide higher quality care and greater value to individuals with disabilities.

Quality and Value of Health Care

Improving the quality of the care delivered by the health system has been a major focus since the National Academy of Medicine (formerly the Institute of Medicine [IOM]) published two seminal reports, *To Err Is Human* (IOM Committee on Quality of Health Care in America, 2000) and *Crossing the Quality Chasm* (IOM Committee on Quality of Health Care in America, 2001). By exposing the tragic magnitude of medical errors, many of which were due to potentially avoidable care process design flaws, these reports charged all care providers with the fundamental requirement to achieve better outcomes through the continual improvement of health care delivery. To that end, the IOM defined quality health care as care that is safe, effective, patient centered, timely, efficient, and equitable.

While these quality metrics are essential to reduce unnecessary harm, waste, and costs associated with health care, many of which are process oriented, they may not translate directly to improved health outcomes for children with disabilities. For example, timely evaluation, diagnosis, and medical treatment of a school-age child with complex attention-deficit/hyperactivity disorder will not guarantee improved health outcomes if the child's resource-poor school and community struggle to implement interventions and accommodations to support this child's social, emotional, and academic success.

Thus the concept of value emerges distinctly from quality, yet the two are linked. Simply put, value is defined as health outcomes achieved per dollar spent (Porter, 2010). Whereas quality may be process focused, value emphasizes achievement of outcomes that are most important for the patient and family. In other words value is measured by outputs, not inputs. Quality improvement initiatives importantly help decrease unnecessary costs and harms to increase value. Measuring value requires adequate measurement of both outcomes and costs to achieve those outcomes. While measuring costs is a more concrete, albeit complex task, operationalizing outcomes to enable measurement has been a persistent challenge, particularly in the field of developmental-behavioral pediatrics. The International Classification of Functioning, Health, and Disability (WHO, 2014) and related functional skills frameworks provide a strong foundation for developing outcomes that can span the range of disability; however, adequate outcomes measurement must take into account the priorities of individuals, families, and experts, and consider the unique needs of those with specific disabilities or developmental-behavioral conditions (e.g., autism). Additionally, appropriate value measurement must account for all components of health care that contribute to the desired outcome, beyond simply the efforts of the physician, hospital, or clinic team, or other facets of the classical health care system; all other services that meet the needs of the patient must be considered as well (Porter, 2010; Sandler, 2019a, 2019b).

ACHIEVING THE GOALS OF THE HEALTH CARE SYSTEM FOR CHILDREN WITH DISABILITIES

Access to Care

Despite recognition of health care as an essential human right, in the United States, access to health care depends on (1) access to and enrollment in a health insurance plan, (2) adequate and continuous coverage of necessary services, and (3) availability of qualified clinicians (Chung & Schuster, 2004). High uninsured and underinsured rates, interruptions in insurance coverage, variability in generosity of benefits among plans, and unequal distribution of resources geographically and among different population groups lead to inequitable access to health care. Furthermore, these inequities disproportionately affect the most vulnerable, such as historically marginalized racial and ethnic minority groups, those in poverty, immigrants, children in foster care, and children and adults with disabilities. Despite the skyrocketing per capita health expenditures that far exceed all other countries who have universal access, the US population experiences poorer return on investment according to many quality and outcome measures, and, with problematic overrepresentation among those in poverty, minoritized and immigrant groups, and individuals with disabilities (Mossialos, Djordjevic, Osborn, & Sarnak, 2017).

Health Insurance and Financing

Private insurance. Private insurance is the predominant form of coverage in the United States, with over half of adults and children, including those with disabilities, covered primarily through employer-sponsored policies (Cohen & Terlizzi, 2020). The remaining portion of the population have either public insurance, a combination of private and public coverage, or no coverage (Cohen & Terlizzi, 2020). US public insurance programs are organized by specific populations and include Medicare for adults aged 65 and older, federal employees, military members, veterans, and people with low income, including Medicaid and the Children's Health Insurance Program (CHIP). Also, while not an insurance program per se, the US Indian Health Service provides access to health care for individuals who are federally recognized American Indian and Alaska Natives.

Medicare and Medicaid. In 1965 recognizing that employer-sponsored health care insurance was not available to the elderly or individuals with low income, Congress passed the Social Security Act, which enacted two federal health care insurance entitlement programs, Medicare and Medicaid. Medicare is federally funded hospital insurance plus subsidized medical insurance provided to all US citizens age 65 and older, whereas Medicaid covers children and adults with low income. Medicare is primarily for older adults, although it does cover adults younger than 65 with disabilities as well as children and adults younger than 65 with end-stage renal disease who are receiving dialysis or have had a kidney transplant. Medicaid allocates federal tax dollars to each state with a state match that varies based on each state's relative per capita income. Some states have expanded Medicaid to cover all adults below a certain income level.

Medicaid waivers and demonstrations. (CHIP) Approximately 1.7 million children qualify for Medicaid coverage through a disability pathway rather than an income-based pathway (Musumeci & Chidambaram, 2019). Medicaid Home and Community Based Services (HCBS) waivers (also known as 1915[c] waivers as they are authorized under that numeric section of the US Social Security Act) give states the option to expand eligibility to cover individuals who would otherwise be likely to require institutionalization regardless of family income level (National Academies of Sciences Engineering and Medicine, 2018). Katie Beckett and TEFRA (the Tax Equity and Fiscal Responsibility Act of 1982 [Public Law (P.L.) 97-248 §134]) waivers are HCBS waivers that cover children with disabilities through age 19 years (Catalyst Center, 2012). Waiver programs targeting people with intellectual or developmental disabilities comprised the largest number of Section 1915(c) waiver programs and the greatest share of spending (72%) across all long-term service and support population groups in Medicaid in fiscal years 2014 through 2016, the most recent years of analysis (Eiken, Amos, Sredl, & Saucier, 2018).

Like waivers, Medicaid's Money Follows the Person (MFP) demonstrations provide states the ability to help people with disabilities and seniors move from institutions to the community. MFP, begun in 2007 and recently extended by Congress in 2020 for 3 more years, gives enhanced federal matching funds to states to provide services and supports to eligible individuals (Medicaid, n.d.b).

Children's Health Insurance Program (CHIP). Recognizing a lack of insurance coverage for children whose family income was too low to afford private coverage but too high to qualify for Medicaid, Congress passed CHIP, which began in 1997. Like Medicaid, CHIP provides federal matching funds to states to provide health coverage to children. All states have CHIP programs, and most cover children up to at least 200% of the federal poverty level ($53,000 for a family of four in 2021) (US Department of Health & Human Services Office of the Assistant Secretary for Planning and Evaluation, 2021). Unlike Medicaid, which is an entitlement and therefore obligated to cover all individuals who apply and meet the required income level for eligibility, with CHIP, states have the option to stop enrolling children once they exhaust a maintenance-of-effort dollar amount annually (Catalyst Center, 2017). Like Medicaid, CHIP covers routine preventive health care and dental visits, but families may have copayments for other services. Some states charge a monthly premium for CHIP coverage. The premiums differ by state, but they cannot exceed more than 5% of a family's annual income. Medicaid and CHIP together cover about a third of the country's children and almost half (47%) of the estimated 13.3 million children with disabilities in the United States (Musumeci & Chidambaram, 2019).

The Affordable Care Act (ACA). Additional publicly subsidized private insurance came into being with enactment of the ACA (P.L. 111-148) in 2010 (Feldman, Buysse, Hubner, Huffman, & Loe, 2015). The ACA created the Health Insurance Marketplace, also known as Exchanges, which offers individuals the option to purchase government-subsidized private insurance plans at a cost based on their income. As of this writing, about 1% of US children obtain private coverage through Exchanges. More importantly, other stipulations in ACA improved access for children with disabilities by limiting exclusion of preexisting conditions and extending the age through which children could remain as dependents on their family's policy.

Other Funding Sources That Promote Access to Health Care

Supplemental Security Income (SSI). SSI is administered through the US Social Security Administration (SSA) and provides minimum basic financial assistance to older adults and persons with disabilities (regardless of age) with very limited income and resources. Federal SSI benefits from the SSA are often supplemented by state programs. In most states an SSI recipient will automatically qualify for Medicaid, especially for children with disabilities who are disproportionately represented in lower-income populations in the United States and therefore more likely to meet the SSI income eligibility criteria.

Title V Maternal and Child Health (MCH) Program. The US SSA Title V MCH block grant includes a focus on children and youth with special health care needs (CYSHCN). The Title V CYSHCN program is an important resource that influences and monitors access to health care and other services for mothers and children, including children with disabilities. States use these block grant funds in various ways: some use them to deliver direct care to women and children, others fund targeted prevention services (e.g., maternal early infant and childhood home visiting programs). For more information on how states organize MCH Title V CYSHCN resources, see https://mchb.tvisdata.hrsa.gov/.

Achieving a Better Life Experience (ABLE) savings accounts. Created through the US federal Stephen Beck, Jr. Achieving a Better Life Experience Act of 2014 (hence the acronym ABLE), accounts are noninsurance-based, tax-advantaged savings accounts for individuals with disabilities and their families (The National Disability Institute, n.d.). Families can use these accounts to fund disability expenses. In 2020 ABLE accounts had a $15,000 calendar year limit, but also allowed additional savings for working individuals. Interest income earned in these accounts is not taxed. ABLE accounts allow families to deposit savings, but those savings do not count in the income calculations that determine eligibility for public benefits, including Medicaid. Eligibility is limited to individuals with disabilities with onset before turning 26 years old and who meet certain income criteria. Individuals who receive SSI or SSDI are automatically eligible to establish an ABLE account.

Special needs trusts. To qualify for certain government benefits, such as Medicaid and SSI, an individual generally cannot own more than $2000 of assets. Special needs trusts are designed to protect the assets of a person with disabilities, while still allowing that individual to receive government benefits.

Adequacy of Insurance Coverage for Children With Disabilities

Benefits

Private insurance benefits vary widely between payers, and even between the same payer's various policies. Some private insurance plans provide comprehensive benefits that are comparable to those mandated through Medicaid (described in the next section). Other private plans require high deductibles and out-of-pocket expenses for families, which may impede realization of benefits. Further, while private insurance may cover rehabilitative services for acquired disabilities, many policies exclude coverage for habilitative therapies for developmental disabilities. For example, TRICARE (insurance coverage for US military members and their families) and many private policies exclude diagnostic evaluation, treatment, and services or supplies for most developmental language and learning disabilities (i.e., developmental delay, intellectual disabilities, dyslexia, developmental mathematics disorders, developmental language disorders, and developmental articulation disorders).

Medicaid and CHIP benefits are important to understand, as almost half of all US children with disabilities rely on Medicaid as an important source of coverage (Musumeci & Chidambaram, 2019). For Medicaid, within broad federal guidelines, states determine the type, amount, duration, and scope of services they provide. An exception is Medicaid's early periodic screening, detection, and treatment (EPSDT) services for children. EPSDT provides all medically necessary services for children through age 21, even if that service is not included in the state's Medicaid plan. For example, even though many states do not include dental or pharmacy benefits for adults who receive Medicaid, EPSDT covers these for children. CHIP gives states the choice to add EPSDT as an optional benefit for children enrolled in CHIP. In states that expand Medicaid with CHIP funds all children must receive EPSDT.

In the early 2000s in the United States parents of children with autism began a grassroots movement to urge legislators to pass mandates requiring insurers to cover diagnostic and treatment services for autism spectrum disorder (ASD). The first ASD insurance mandate was passed in 2001 (in Indiana), and by 2019, when the last state, Tennessee, passed its law, all 50 states and the District of Columbia had ASD mandates (Callaghan & Sylvester, 2019). Benefits vary widely between the states due to an interesting array of political forces that shaped the patchwork of coverage that exists today. Policy analysts note that ASD mandates have resulted in only slightly more children getting treatment and somewhat more treatment for those already receiving treatment. Reasons for the modest overall improvements in access include limits imposed on the maximum age of eligibility, lifetime dollar amounts, and/or number of sessions covered that many states specified in their mandates, as well as the insufficient supply and uneven geographic distribution of certified therapists (Mandell et al., 2016).

Continuity of Coverage

As part of its effort to foster a high-functioning community-based system of services for CYSHCN and their families that began in the late 1980s, the US Maternal and Child Health Bureau (MCHB) included continuity of health insurance coverage over the previous 12 months as a core indicator (Honberg, McPherson, Strickland, Gage, & Newacheck, 2005). Based on parent surveys, they have found interruptions in continuity. As with other access indicators, significant disparities in continuity of coverage persist based on race, ethnicity, immigration status, language, socioeconomic status, and functional limitation.

Delivering Health Care

Primary Care Medical Home

All children require access to regular primary health care. The IOM defined primary care as "the provision of integrated, accessible health care services by clinicians who are accountable for addressing a large majority of personal health care needs, developing a sustained partnership with patients, and practicing in the context of the family and community" (Cooley, 2004). Primary health care consists of three core components: (1) preventive care, focusing on maintaining physical and mental health and preventing health problems while reducing burden of existing ones; (2) diagnostic care, focusing on identifying the nature of health concerns; and (3) treatment, focusing on controlling, correcting, and reducing the problems (National Academies of Sciences Engineering and Medicine, 2018).

The traditional model of primary care for children has consisted of a solo medical practitioner or a group of practitioners, along with nurses and support staff, who follow children until adulthood, offering anticipatory guidance, treating acute medical illnesses, and facilitating referrals. However, such a model may not meet the needs of children with developmental disabilities or complex health needs given the subspecialty nature of many of their health problems or the need for services and programs well outside the scope of the traditional doctor's office.

The concept of the patient-centered medical home (PCMH) originated in 1967 to describe a central source of care that assumes full responsibility of coordinating a child's health care across multiple domains. The Agency for Health Research and Quality defines five key features of care delivered by a PCMH: patient and family centeredness, comprehensive, coordinated, accessible, and committed to quality and safety.

The medical home model has shown several benefits, including lower unmet needs, higher family centeredness, effectiveness and timeliness of care, as well as improved health status and family functioning (Akobirshoev, Parish, Mitra, & Dembo, 2019; Homer et al., 2008). Despite the benefits of the model, only 43% of children with special health care needs had access to a medical home in 2016 (Lichstein, Ghandour, & Mann, 2018). In addition to the access issues described previously in this chapter, several barriers to PCMH implementation decrease the likelihood of patients experiencing true medical home care. These include reimbursement and incentive structures that may not favor PCMH-related activities such as population management and care coordination/case management, practice/institutional culture and change management, workflow and workforce issues, optimization of health information technology, and cultivating and maintaining community relationships (Arend, Tsang-Quinn, Levine, & Thomas, 2012).

Increasingly, PCMHs are tasked with managing the mental health needs of children with disabilities as well. This includes screening and intervention both to prevent and to treat mental health or behavioral difficulties, as well as promote mental health and wellbeing. However, like many physical health needs, mental and emotional wellbeing often rely on supports and services beyond the PCMH, within the school or community in which a child resides.

Coordination of Care

As noted, children with disabilities often require the services of multiple professionals, including specialty health care clinicians, allied health therapists, special education team, mental health clinicians, and others, spread throughout a child and family's community. Care for children with disabilities is more often fragmented, poorly coordinated, and less efficient and timely than is care for children without special health care needs. Barriers to effective coordination care delivery include silos of care, limited interoperability of electronic health records, privacy regulations, poor reimbursement for coordination activities, and provider time and capacity to engage in collaborative care (de Banate, Maypole, & Sadof, 2019). The benefits of care coordination are well documented. By itself, high-quality case management has been associated with reductions in hospital admissions and emergency department visits, as well as reduced lengths of hospital stay. Additionally, care management has shown benefit to increase the family's knowledge of and ability to cope with the child's health problems, improving satisfaction of care (National Academies of Sciences Engineering and Medicine, 2018).

Innovations in Health Care Delivery for Children With Disabilities

Health Homes and the Medical Neighborhood

In 2010 the passage of the ACA included Section 2703, which enabled federal support for states to establish health homes for people covered by Medicaid who either have (1) two or more chronic conditions, (2) one chronic condition and are at risk for a second, or (3) one serious and persistent mental health condition (Medicaid, n.d.a). Services provided by the health homes include comprehensive care management, care coordination, health promotion, comprehensive transitional care/followup, patient and family support, and referral to community and social support services. The law gave states flexibility to determine how the health home was designed. Thus states could designate the responsibilities of the health homes to community centers or other agencies rather than a traditional health care setting if states opted to do so. One such model described by Fueyo, Caldwell, Mattern, Zahid, and Foley (2015) provided comprehensive, multidisciplinary care for individuals with ASD or intellectual disability within a specialty behavioral health setting that is integrated with primary care services and other subspecialists.

Similarly, other health home–like models have been based within hospital settings as well, particularly for populations of children known to frequent hospital-based outpatient and inpatient care. Such models aim to provide one-stop shopping that maximizes organizational efficiency, streamlines frequent care, and leverages hospital resources and a centralized information technology infrastructure to provide care coordination. A 2011 review of 33 unique hospital-based programs for children with complex medical needs found that half were entirely hospital based, whereas the other half contained community-based components. Overall, the evidence pointed to increased effectiveness and efficiency of care as well as patient and family centeredness of care. Of note, none evaluated whether care provided in these settings was more equitable (Cohen, Jovcevska, Kuo, & Mahant, 2011).

Over the past 2 decades, the concept of the medical (or health) neighborhood has emerged to encapsulate the idea of a fully coordinated and engaged community of support, extending beyond just the medical or health home and its capacity to deliver comprehensive, coordinated, family-centered care. The health neighborhood was originally conceptualized primarily as a more formalized and integrated network of primary care, specialty care, and health services, such as hospitals, nursing homes, and the like (Ortiz, 2020; Spatz, Bricker, & Gabbay, 2014). However, Garg, Sandel, Dworkin, Kahn, and Zuckerman (2012) advocated for the health neighborhood to include "community-based, non-medical services that promote the health of patients and families" given the recognized adverse impact of social determinants of health, such as housing conditions, food insecurity, and neighborhood safety, that require the need for carefully coordinated social, legal, and other services. One model of a medical neighborhood described by Bansa et al. (2019) utilized a team of community health workers to forge formal partnerships with medical facilities and clinics, schools, and other community agencies with the goal of uniting all under a true community-based system of care, rather than a hospital- or center-based system. Such a neighborhood "meets patients 'where they live' versus limiting services to a clinic setting," while helping families overcome what they termed the "social determinants of health maze" of disorganized and poorly coordinated systems and advocate for the whole patient in the quest to achieve and maintain optimal health, wellbeing, and engagement in the community.

Mental Health Integration

Integration of mental health services into the existing health care landscape provides timelier access to needed care and reduces the barriers to coordination between the physical and mental health arenas. Three models of mental health integration have been described (National Academies of Sciences Engineering and Medicine, 2018) (see Chapter 115 for additional information). The first model, coordinated care, strives to enhance access to consultations between primary care and mental health providers. An example of this type of model is the Massachusetts Child Psychiatry Access Project (MCPAP), which provides regional child behavioral health teams available for primary care clinicians to consult regarding psychopharmacology and recommendations for mental health treatment or therapy (Sarvet et al., 2010). MCPAP has been widely replicated.

The second model, colocated care, houses one or more behavioral health professionals within a primary care practice. In this model primary care clinicians and mental health professionals often work in parallel through a variety of means, but they have naturally enhanced opportunity for communication directly and through electronic means for centralized record management, which can help not only with care coordination but improving the primary care clinician's competencies in mental health issues through direct and indirect training (Kolko & Perrin, 2014).

The third, collaborative care, is an aspirational model that integrates the efforts of primary and mental health care clinicians together in a true partnership with families to provide whole-person care. This model aspires to realize Wagner's care model, drawing on other examples of behavioral health collaboration for adults with such disorders as diabetes and hypertension to achieve better patient outcomes (Campo, Geist, & Kolko, 2018). One example is the Reaching Out to Adolescents in Distress program, which employed master's-level behavioral health clinicians as care managers to facilitate both psychopharmacology and psychotherapy treatments within the primary care setting. Care managers met weekly with consulting psychiatrists, psychologists, and pediatricians. Results showed a dramatic increase in receipt of and response to treatment, with higher rates of remission and satisfaction in care (Richardson et al., 2014).

Telehealth

Geographic barriers severely limit access to quality health care. In response, telehealth services have become an increasingly important modality within the overall health care landscape. While telehealth has long been an established method of providing direct medical, developmental, and behavioral care, the COVID-19 pandemic prompted rapid uptake and deployment of telehealth capabilities across the landscape; an international survey found uptake of telehealth among a diverse array of clinicians to increase from 4% in 2019 to 70% in 2021 (Camden & Silva, 2021). Telehealth, in its most classic form, allows clinicians to connect to patients through telephone or video/audio (i.e., teleconferencing) means. Care provided in this manner remains subjected to many of the same regulations and restrictions to which in-person care is subjected. Insurance coverage and parity, practice across geographic boundaries (e.g., across US state lines), and medical necessity and appropriateness of services provided all factor into the delivery of telehealth. Camden and Silva (2021) described three main categories of need to implement telehealth: (1) equipment and technology, including Internet connectivity and security; (2) system and organization, including legislative policies, insurance coverage and payment, ethics, and institutional support; and (3) training, including optimizing communication, best practices, and adapting regular care to a telehealth modality.

Telehealth encompasses many other technology-enabled health care practices. Asynchronous telehealth allows capture of patient data outside of a provider-patient encounter for use in assessments or in treatment monitoring. An example of this type of telehealth is the Systematic Observation of Red Flags (SORF), a level 2 autism screener, which instructs families to record videos of caregiver-child interactions. The family then submits the videos to an autism expert, who codes the child's behaviors and determines level of concern for ASD (Dow, Day, Kutta, Nottke, & Wetherby, 2020). Another telehealth modality is the use of mobile devices to capture and monitor health information, such as vital signs, sleep data, activity level, and other patient-related information, as well as to receive information from the health care sector, such as health education, promotion, and alerts. For example, programs designed to send parenting and developmental tips periodically to enrolled families can serve not only to promote parent and child relationships and wellbeing, but to empower families and patients in self-management, a core component of Wagner's care model.

Telehealth technology can also permit broader networks and collaborations between providers to support and disseminate best practices. The Extension for Community Healthcare Outcomes (ECHO) program is one example of how technology has been used to support clinicians across diverse geographic areas in their own implementation of care typically provided by subspecialists. Many ECHO programs have been implemented over the past 15 years targeting improving care in many subspecialty areas, including several developmental-behavioral pediatric focuses such as autism and behavioral health (Hostutler et al., 2020; Mazurek et al., 2020). With a shortage of developmental-behavioral pediatric clinicians and an increasing prevalence of developmental-behavioral conditions, learning collaboratives have become an important pillar of expanding an effective workforce and ensuring timely and community-based access to subspecialty expertise (Arora et al., 2017).

CONCLUSION

The health care system is a complicated interplay of entities, consisting not only of those who provide and receive care, but the community in which they live and work, as well as the administrative, financial, political, and sociocultural forces that determine access to, delivery, and quality of care. Children with disabilities and their families often must navigate a greater landscape of the health care system to achieve their optimal health and wellbeing. As Cara Coleman, Justice's mother, eloquently stated, the child and family often find themselves at the mercy of such a system rather than central to its operation. Such is the outcome when barriers to insurance coverage, provider access, and coordination of care seem to determine a child's fate more than the ability to realize the potential of the health care system to deliver true value to each child and family. A thorough understanding of how the health care system functions for individual children and for families opens the door to opportunities for innovation, guided by the vision of the Alma Ata Declaration and the IOM's six quality indicators, to forge a more coordinated, efficient, and family-centered health care system that enables all children, particularly those who are most vulnerable, to achieve their fullest potential and wellbeing.

REFERENCES

Adams, J. S., & Woods, E. R. (2016). Redesign of chronic illness care in children and adolescents: Evidence for the chronic care model. *Current Opinion in Pediatrics*, *28*(4), 428–433.

Akobirshoev, I., Parish, S., Mitra, M., & Dembo, R. (2019). Impact of medical home on health care of children with and without special health care needs: Update from the 2016 National Survey of Children's Health. *Maternal Child Health Journal*, *23*(11), 1500–1507.

Arend, J., Tsang-Quinn, J., Levine, C., & Thomas, D. (2012). The patient-centered medical home: History, components, and review of the evidence. *Mount Sinai Journal of Medicine*, *79*(4), 433–450.

Arora, S., Kalishman, S. G., Thornton, K. A., Komaromy, M. S., Katzman, J. G., Struminger, B. B., ... Bradford, A. M. (2017). Project ECHO: A telementoring network model for continuing professional development. *Journal of Continuing Education in the Health Professions*, *37*(4), 239–244.

Bansa, M., Glassgow, A. E., Martin, M., Caskey, R., Paulson, A., Minier, M., ... Van Voorhees, B. (2019). Development of a community-based medical neighborhood for children with chronic conditions. *Programs in Community Health Partnerships*, *13*(1), 83–95.

Callaghan, T., & Sylvester, S. (2019). Autism spectrum disorder, politics, and the generosity of insurance mandates in the United States. *PLoS One*, *14*(5), e0217064.

Camden, C., & Silva, M. (2021). Pediatric telehealth: Opportunities created by the covid-19 and suggestions to sustain its use to support families of children with disabilities. *Physical & Occupational Therapy in Pediatrics, 41*(1), 1–17.

Campo, J. V., Geist, R., & Kolko, D. J. (2018). Integration of pediatric behavioral health services in primary care: Improving access and outcomes with collaborative care. *The Canadian Journal of Psychiatry, 63*(7), 432–438.

Catalyst Center. (2012). *The TEFRA Medicaid state plan option and Katie Beckett waiver for children—Making it possible to care for children with significant disabilities at home.* https://ciswh.org/wp-content/uploads/2016/07/TEFRA.pdf

Catalyst Center. (2017). *Public insurance programs and children with special health care needs: The basics: What are Medicaid and CHIP?* https://ciswh.org/wp-content/uploads/2017/10/Medicaid-Tutorial-Section2-2017.pdf

Chung, P. J., & Schuster, M. A. (2004). Access and quality in child health services: Voltage drops. *Health Affairs, 23*(5), 77–87.

Cohen, E., Jovcevska, V., Kuo, D. Z., & Mahant, S. (2011). Hospital-based comprehensive care programs for children with special health care needs: A systematic review. *Archives of Pediatrics & Adolescent Medicine, 165*(6), 554–561.

Cohen, R. A., & Terlizzi, E. P. (2020). *Health insurance coverage: Early release of quarterly estimates from the National Health Interview Survey.* National Center for Health Statistics. https://www.cdc.gov/nchs/nhis/releases.htm

Coleman, C. L. (2019). *Not just along for the ride: Families are the engine that drives pediatric home health care.* Health Affairs Blog. https://www.healthaffairs.org/do/10.1377/hblog20190415.172668/full/

Cooley, W. C. (2004). Redefining primary pediatric care for children with special health care needs: The primary care medical home. *Current Opinion in Pediatrics, 16*(6), 689–692.

de Banate, M. A., Maypole, J., & Sadof, M. (2019). Care coordination for children with medical complexity. *Current Opinion in Pediatrics, 31*(4), 575–582.

Dow, D., Day, T. N., Kutta, T. J., Nottke, C., & Wetherby, A. M. (2020). Screening for autism spectrum disorder in a naturalistic home setting using the systematic observation of red flags (SORF) at 18–24 months. *Autism Research, 13*(1), 122–133.

Eiken, S., Amos, A., Sredl, K., & Saucier, P. (2018). *Medicaid expenditures for section 1915(c) waiver programs in FY 2016.* Medicaid Innovation Accelerator Program; IBM Watson Health. https://www.medicaid.gov/sites/default/files/2019-12/1915c-expenditures-fy2016.pdf

Feldman, H. M. (2013). *Redesigning health care for children with disabilities: Strengthening inclusion, contribution, and health.* Paul H. Brookes Publishing Co.

Feldman, H. M., Buysse, C. A., Hubner, L. M., Huffman, L. C., & Loe, I. M. (2015). Patient Protection and Affordable Care Act of 2010 and children and youth with special health care needs. *Journal of Developmental & Behavioral Pediatrics, 36*(3), 207–217.

Fueyo, M., Caldwell, T., Mattern, S. B., Zahid, J., & Foley, T. (2015). The health home: A service delivery model for autism and intellectual disability. *Psychiatric Services, 66*(11), 1135–1137.

Garg, A., Sandel, M., Dworkin, P. H., Kahn, R. S., & Zuckerman, B. (2012). From medical home to health neighborhood: Transforming the medical home into a community-based health neighborhood. *Journal of Pediatrics, 160*(4), 535–536. e531.

Homer, C. J., Klatka, K., Romm, D., Kuhlthau, K., Bloom, S., Newacheck, P., … Perrin, J. M. (2008). A review of the evidence for the medical home for children with special health care needs. *Pediatrics, 122*(4), e922–e937.

Honberg, L., McPherson, M., Strickland, B., Gage, J. C., & Newacheck, P. W. (2005). Assuring adequate health insurance: Results of the National Survey of Children With Special Health Care Needs. *Pediatrics, 115*(5), 1233–1239.

Hostutler, C. A., Valleru, J., Maciejewski, H. M., Hess, A., Gleeson, S. P., & Ramtekkar, U. P. (2020). Improving pediatrician's behavioral health competencies through the Project ECHO teleconsultation model. *Clinical Pediatrics, 59*(12), 1049–1057.

Institute of Medicine Committee on Quality of Health Care in America. (2000). *To err is human: Building a safer health system.* National Academies Press.

Institute of Medicine Committee on Quality of Health Care in America. (2001). *Crossing the quality chasm: A new health system for the 21st century.* National Academies Press.

Kolko, D. J., & Perrin, E. (2014). The integration of behavioral health interventions in children's health care: Services. *science, and suggestions. Journal of Clinical Child & Adolescent Psychology, 43*(2), 216–228.

Lichstein, J. C., Ghandour, R. M., & Mann, M. Y. (2018). Access to the medical home among children with and without special health care needs. *Pediatrics, 142*(6).

Mandell, D. S., Barry, C. L., Marcus, S. C., Xie, M., Shea, K., Mullan, K., & Epstein, A. J. (2016). Effects of autism spectrum disorder insurance mandates on the treated prevalence of autism spectrum disorder. *JAMA Pediatrics, 170*(9), 887–893.

Mazurek, M. O., Parker, R. A., Chan, J., Kuhlthau, K., Sohl, K., & Collaborative, E. A. (2020). Effectiveness of the Extension for Community Health Outcomes model as applied to primary care for autism: A partial stepped-wedge randomized clinical trial. *JAMA Pediatrics, 174*(5), e196306.

Medicaid. (n.d.a). *Health homes.* https://www.medicaid.gov/medicaid/long-term-services-supports/health-homes/index.html

Medicaid. (n.d.b). *Money follows the person.* https://www.medicaid.gov/medicaid/long-term-services-supports/money-follows-person/index.html

Mossialos, E., Djordjevic, A., Osborn, R., & Sarnak, D. (Eds.). (2017). *International profiles of health care systems.* The Commonwealth Fund.

Musumeci, M., & Chidambaram, P. (2019). *Medicaid's role for children with special health care needs: A look at eligibility, services, and spending.* https://www.kff.org/medicaid/issue-brief/medicaids-role-for-children-with-special-health-care-needs-a-look-at-eligibility-services-and-spending/

National Academies of Sciences Engineering and Medicine. (2018). *Opportunities for improving programs and services for children with disabilities.* The National Academies Press.

National Disability Institute. (n.d.). *About ABLE accounts.* https://www.ablenrc.org/what-is-able/what-are-able-acounts/

Ortiz, M. R. (2020). The patient-centered health neighborhood. *Nursing Science Quarterly, 33*(4), 353–357.

Porter, M. E. (2010). What is value in health care? *NEJM, 363*(26), 2477–2481.

Richardson, L. P., Ludman, E., McCauley, E., Lindenbaum, J., Larison, C., Zhou, C., … Katon, W. (2014). Collaborative care for adolescents with depression in primary care: A randomized clinical trial. *JAMA, 312*(8), 809–816.

Rifkin, S. B. (2018). *Health for all and primary health care, 1978–2018: A historical perspective on policies and programs over 40 years.* Oxford University Press.

Romley, J. A., Shah, A. K., Chung, P. J., Elliott, M. N., Vestal, K. D., & Schuster, M. A. (2017). Family-provided health care for children with special health care needs. *Pediatrics, 139*(1), e20161287.
Sandler, A. D. (2019a). Value-driven care in developmental-behavioral pediatrics, part 1: The value proposition of developmental-behavioral pediatrics. *Journal of Developmental & Behavioral Pediatrics, 40*(6), 472–478.
Sandler, A. D. (2019b). Value-driven care in developmental-behavioral pediatrics, part 2: Measuring quality and meeting the challenge. *Journal of Developmental & Behavioral Pediatrics, 40*(6), 479–488.
Sarvet, B., Gold, J., Bostic, J. Q., Masek, B. J., Prince, J. B., Jeffers-Terry, M., … Straus, J. H. (2010). Improving access to mental health care for children: The Massachusetts Child Psychiatry Access Project. *Pediatrics, 126*(6), 1191–1200.
Spatz, C., Bricker, P., & Gabbay, R. (2014). The patient-centered medical neighborhood: Transformation of specialty care. *American Journal of Medical Quality, 29*(4), 344–349.
US Department of Health & Human Services Office of the Assistant Secretary for Planning and Evaluation. (2021). HHS poverty guidelines for 2021. https://aspe.hhs.gov/poverty-guidelines
Wagner, E. H., Austin, B. T., Davis, C., Hindmarsh, M., Schaefer, J., & Bonomi, A. (2001). Improving chronic illness care: Translating evidence into action. *Health Affairs, 20*(6), 64–78.
World Health Organization. (2014). International classification of functioning, disability, and health. www.who.int/classifications/icf/en/gol.

115

Interprofessional Team-Based Care

Jeffrey D. Shahidullah, Cody A. Hostutler, and Rebecca A. Baum

For additional material related to the content of this chapter, please see Chapter 15.

VIGNETTE

Mya is a 9-year-old girl who presents to Dr. Cruz's office for an attention-deficit/hyperactivity disorder (ADHD) evaluation. She is in third grade in a typical classroom setting. Her teachers report that she doesn't pay attention, and her grades are poor. Her mother is worried that Mya may have to repeat third grade and wonders if ADHD medication may help. She recently signed papers for Mya to get extra help in school.

Mya's past medical history is significant for asthma, and she's missed several days of school due to emergency department visits and hospitalizations. Her family is currently without health insurance, and she has been out of medication for the past few months. Review of her sleep history suggests poor sleep due to nocturnal cough. Dr. Cruz notes that referrals have been made to pulmonology, but Mya has been unable to attend due to transportation issues. On exam, Mya is interactive and engaged but has trouble answering questions at an age-appropriate level.

Dr. Cruz decides to obtain more information from Mya's school. He learns that she underwent psychoeducational testing, which suggested moderate intellectual disability, and that she recently qualified for special education services. He shares this information with Mya's mother and how her cognitive profile, sleep difficulties, and persistent asthma may be affecting her attention in the classroom setting. He contacts his office's social worker to help secure health insurance for Mya and asks the nurse and receptionist to work with Mya's mother to coordinate a pulmonology appointment at a time when she has transportation available.

INTRODUCTION

The unique and changing needs of children are often best addressed by clinicians across disciplines and systems operating as high-functioning teams. For example, youth may present in pediatric settings with cooccurring physical health (e.g., asthma, diabetes), behavioral health (e.g., depression, anxiety), educational (e.g., learning disabilities), and social stressors (e.g., trauma, food insecurity). No one individual or discipline will have the time, training, or resources to address the comprehensive needs of every child and family. Thus appropriate care for this complex mix of needs requires communication, collaboration, and care coordination across a variety of disciplines and service systems.

Often referred to as interprofessional team-based care, this approach can promote collaboration across numerous systems (i.e., interagency collaboration) and providers (i.e., interprofessional collaboration) to avoid or reduce fragmentation, gaps, and duplication in services that lead to inefficiencies in care, particularly for families of children with developmental-behavioral (DB) concerns (Shahidullah, Azad, Mezher, McClain, & McIntyre, 2018). Interprofessional team-based care is the means by which different health care professionals with diverse perspectives, knowledge, and skills collaborate in patient care to achieve a common goal. As illustrated in the opening vignette, team-based care builds upon the foundation of the medical home model by reaching out across providers (e.g., physicians, nurses, physician assistants, pharmacists, social workers, psychologists, case managers, family navigators) both within and across systems (e.g., medical, social, educational) to enhance communication and collaboration to maximize efficiency and outcomes for children, families, and providers.

This chapter begins by highlighting the rationale for interprofessional team-based care in developmental-behavioral pediatrics (DBP). Definitions pertinent to interprofessional team-based care are provided in Table 115.1. Next, models and specific strategies for the delivery of interprofessional team-based care are presented. Then, guidance around hiring and training is provided. The chapter concludes with a discussion of implications for practice, payment, and policy.

COMPLEXITY IN CLINICAL PRACTICE

The very nature of DB conditions lends itself to an inherent degree of complexity. The identification and management of DB conditions spans multiple settings, and concerns identified in one setting may not translate or be conveyed to the next. For example, behavioral concerns noted in the child care setting may not make their way to the pediatrician's office, where screening for autism spectrum disorder (ASD) could occur. Similarly, a student may qualify for special education services under the intellectual disability (ID) classification based on psychoeducational testing, the results of which may remain in the student's education record rather than their medical one. Intervention for DB conditions often spans multiple settings as well. Patients with conditions such as ADHD, ASD, ID, and learning disabilities often receive special education services in the school setting, as well as occupational therapy, physical therapy, and speech therapy.

TABLE 115.1 **Definitions Pertinent to Interprofessional Team-Based Care**

Term	Definition/Description
Communication *Exchange of information, typically unidirectional, to achieve a better understanding of care management needs of a patient*	Communication in a health care context may include sending or sharing (via electronic medical record messaging or other Health Insurance Portability and Accountability Act–compliant messaging system, phone call, email, fax, or in-person) of health records or information (e.g., medical, educational, testing results, disposition summaries, treatment status/recommendations) often in a one-time or isolated fashion without the expectation of working together in an ongoing manner to plan and problem solve to promote positive patient outcomes.
Collaboration *Two or more providers working together within a system or across systems in an ongoing manner to plan and problem solve to promote positive patient outcomes*	Collaboration emphasizes a dynamic and active process whereby providers assume complementary roles and cooperatively work together to contribute information and respond to that information together to inform clinical decision making.
Care Coordination *Deliberate organization of patient care activities and sharing of information across providers and systems such as primary care, specialty care, and community services and supports such as schools so that multiple stakeholders are working collaboratively to streamline information and roles in an effort to provide care that is efficient, continuous, and effective from a time and resource perspective*	Although sometimes used synonymously with collaboration, care coordination is a distinct concept that describes the broad objective of aligning systems resources with patient and population needs to improve the effectiveness, safety, and efficiency of care. Care coordination relies on the processes of communication and collaboration.
Interprofessional Collaboration[a,b] *Providers from multiple disciplines work interdependently within a clinical context to achieve a common goal*	It involves integration or modification of the efforts of the contributing disciplines. It relies on a team science process that leverages the strengths and expertise of providers from different fields and demands that the professionals consider the contributions of other team members in making their own contribution. This approach suggests intersecting lines of communication and collaboration.
Interprofessional Team-Based Care *The means by which different health care professionals, with diverse perspectives, knowledge, and skills, collaborate in meeting patient needs and preferences by actively engaging patients as full participants in their care, while encouraging all professionals to practice to the top extent of their license*	This term, although similar to the definition of interprofessional collaboration above, also emphasizes the concept of team-based care as it pertains to the current needs of the health care system around systemic factors associated with health care inefficiencies (i.e., workforce shortages, medical errors, fragmentation, and duplication leading to high costs, low patient and provider satisfaction, poor outcomes metrics, and physician burnout and moral injury). Team-based care typically includes (1) collaboration among team members, the patient, and family, (2) shared goals within and across systems of care, and (3) coordinated, high-quality, patient-centered care.

[a]Although the term is often used interchangeably with "interdisciplinary collaboration," interdisciplinary is typically referred to in a broader academic sense whereby two or more disciplines (e.g., nursing, medicine, psychology, social work) align resources with one another, often in educational endeavors, while the term "interprofessional" refers to clinical practice.
[b]Interprofessional collaboration also differs from "multidisciplinary collaboration," which involves professionals from two or more disciplines offering their own discipline-specific services to offer patients a greater breadth of services to patients. However, team members provide their services independently in a parallel or siloed fashion rather than an integrated or streamlined fashion.

In addition to this inherent complexity, children and families affected by DB conditions may be particularly vulnerable to social determinants of health (SDOH) and adverse childhood experiences (ACEs). SDOH refer to social, physical, and economic factors that may negatively impact health outcomes when needs in these areas are unmet. Examples of SDOH include housing, education, income, and other societal factors, with unmet needs in these areas contributing to downstream issues such as poor living conditions, academic underachievement, poverty, and discrimination. ACEs are stressful life events that can have long-term impact, especially when they are chronic, sustained, and outstrip an individual's resources to cope with the stressor. Examples include abuse and neglect, parental mental illness, domestic violence, and divorce. Research has demonstrated a dose-response correlation between ACEs and a range of negative outcomes related to overall physical health and wellbeing (Felitti et al., 1998). Studies suggest that children and families affected by DB conditions may be more likely to experience ACEs than children and families of typically developing children, and children with developmental disabilities are at increased risk for abuse and neglect. Increasingly, health systems are recognizing that addressing these societal and community factors is equally if not more important than addressing the condition for which the patient initially presented for care. See Chapter 15 for additional information on ACEs.

FRAGMENTATION ACROSS SYSTEMS

Given the factors described, children and families affected by DB conditions frequently find themselves interfacing with multiple systems of care, including health care, early intervention, child care, education, behavioral health, and community agencies. However, these systems have not necessarily been built to work together. Moreover, communication across systems is often problematic due to logistic constraints such as time and method of communication. Well-intended privacy laws such as Health Insurance Portability and Accountability Act (in the medical and behavioral health settings) and Family Educational Rights and Privacy Act (in the educational setting) can also serve as barriers to information exchange. Barriers to coordination of care between the health care and educational systems include lack of awareness and knowledge of (1) the roles and function of providers in different systems, (2) differences between *Diagnostic and Statistical Manual of Mental Disoders* (fifth edition; American Psychiatric Association, 2013) diagnoses in the medical or behavioral health settings and qualifying eligibility definitions for special education services, and (3) the different privacy laws around information sharing (McClain et al., 2020; Shahidullah et al., 2019). Research suggests that this care is not coordinated with pediatric clinicians who may have little interface with, and knowledge of, school support services such as special education programming (Shah, Kunnavakkam, & Msall, 2013).

Mya's case illustrates the potential for fragmented care between the health care and educational settings. Given the amount of time students spend in school, Mya's teachers and other school personnel have ample opportunities to observe her functioning across multiple domains (e.g., social, behavioral, cognitive, and academic). In the course of regular practice it may be difficult to share this information with Mya's mother and with Dr. Cruz due to time and other logistical constraints. In Mya's case school personnel recognized her learning difficulties, initiated an evaluation for special education services, and developed an individualized education plan (IEP) to support her learning needs. While this would have been done with her mother's consent and participation, navigating the IEP process can be overwhelming for families. By obtaining a copy of Mya's IEP, Dr. Cruz was able to review psychological testing performed in the school setting that was also necessary for his evaluation in the medical setting, thereby reducing potential duplication of services. This also provided an opportunity for him to help Mya's mother better understand the special education services that Mya is receiving.

Fragmentation of care may also lead to reduced quality and increased cost of care given inefficiencies, duplication, or gaps in services, with patients feeling overwhelmed and marginalized in their care (Stange, 2009). As a result, children and families affected by DB conditions are at increased risk for unmet health care, educational, and psychosocial needs. In its 1999 report, *To Err Is Human: Building a Safer Health Care System*, the Institute of Medicine (IOM, 2000) (now the National Academies of Sciences, Engineering and Medicine) highlighted the importance of team-based health care in addressing fragmented workflows and limited communication across systems that contribute significantly to medical errors. The report called for more effective communication, collaboration, goal sharing, and interdependent functioning among health care teams. Team-based care has been identified as an essential component in the triple aim of health care reform: (1) better patient experience, (2) better population health, and (3) lower overall costs (Berwick, Nolan, & Whittington, 2008). These aims were developed in response to the rising US health care costs coupled with quality metrics ranking well below other developed nations (Kruk et al., 2018). In addition to the fragmentation across systems described earlier, traditional health care settings often lack a framework for practitioners to function interprofessionally and within a team structure. For example, reporting structures, communication processes, roles/responsibilities, and accountability monitoring may be established for practitioners functioning independently but less so in an interprofessional team setting (Porter & Teisberg, 2006).

FRAGMENTATION ACROSS PROVIDERS

Historically, training for professionals has primarily occurred within their particular discipline and system of care, each with its own language, processes, and culture. In the roughly 20 years since the IOM's (Kohn, Corrigan, & Donaldson, 2000) report on health care quality there is now near universal recognition that interprofessional team-based care is a clinical and ethical imperative in providing safe and high-quality care. In 2014 Bodenheimer and Sinksy (2014) added a fourth goal to the triple aim and suggested that provider satisfaction be included, thereby coining the term "quadruple aim." Within the current delivery system, rates of burnout and moral injury are rising among health care clinicians, leading to a pediatric specialty workforce crisis in the United States (Shanafelt et al., 2012). Studies suggest that factors related to the work environment (i.e., excessive workloads, inefficient work processes, clerical burdens, organizational support structures) drive physician burnout and moral injury (West, Dyrbye, & Shanafelt0, 2018). Team-based care has been promoted as a foundational solution to address these systemic issues and promote practitioner wellbeing (Shanafelt et al., 2017). National shortages of both physicians and nurses for the foreseeable future highlight the need for team-based care where health care providers practice to the top of their licensure, training, and experience to promote professional satisfaction and more efficient clinical collaboration through task shifting (i.e., delegating specific tasks to less specialized, more available staff) (World Health Organization, 2008).

DELIVERY OF INTERPROFESSIONAL TEAM-BASED CARE

Models

There are many different models of interprofessional care that are spread across different levels of integration. Although typically considered in the context of primary care, there are a number of innovative models across the country that integrate behavioral health clinicians into the DBP practice. In reality levels of integration exist in a nuanced continuum, and it is helpful to divide them into three basic levels: coordinated, colocated, and integrated.

Coordinated

When professionals collaborate from a distance, it is best described as a coordinated level of integration. Models within the coordinated level of integration involve professionals across disciplines working together in patient care. One example of a model of interprofessional collaboration at the coordinated level is the Massachusetts Child Psychiatry Access Project (MCPAP; Sarvet et al., 2010). MCPAP is a psychiatry teleconsultation program wherein pediatric clinicians can obtain one-on-one psychiatric consultation. Another example of coordinated interprofessional collaboration is the Project Extension for Community Health Outcomes (ECHO) group teleconsultation program. In Project ECHO an interdisciplinary group of academic specialists use case-based and didactic learning methods to build community clinicians' ability to manage complex conditions, including specific disorders such as ASD and general pediatric mental health needs (Hostutler et al., 2020; Mazurek, Brown, Curran, & Sohl, 2017). Coordinated consultation models such as MCPAP and Project ECHO use interprofessional collaboration to move knowledge, rather than patients, to provide high-quality care within their medical homes.

Colocated

Models that include multiple disciplines working in the same location but maintaining largely separate workflows, systems, and records are considered colocated. One example of this is colocated behavioral health services wherein a mental health professional sees patients on one's own schedule in a medical clinic. Colocation allows patients to come to a familiar location, and working within the same clinic provides opportunities for professionals to communicate more interactively than unidirectionally about patients to coordinate their treatment plans. Limitations of colocation include that behavioral health clinicians provide services in the same location but practice independently using a traditional referral model, thus decreasing opportunities for interprofessional collaboration and often function as more multidisciplinary than interprofessional.

Integrated

Models that involve multiple professionals working in the same location, and within the same workflows, are considered integrated models. In integrated models professionals work together to create a single treatment plan, and roles are assigned to all team members. One example is having a clinical pharmacist on the team who completes medication reconciliations, identifies and prevents potential adverse drug events, and provides medication education to providers and patients during the course of the medical visit (Kuhn et al., 2019). Another example is collaborative care models where care managers, pediatricians, and psychiatrists work together to screen for, assess, treat, and monitor a specific population of patients (see Kolko et al., 2014). Integrated models often maximize the benefits of interprofessional care by sharing information, workflows, treatment plans, records, space, resources, and closely collaborating.

Team-Based Strategies

The following are specific strategies that may be used in team-based care.

Team Huddles

Huddles typically occur before a clinic begins, and they involve members of the team briefly meeting (5–10 minutes) to present and discuss relevant operational or clinical information (Brinster, Brukilacchio, Fikki-Urbanovsky, Shahidullah, & Ravenscroft, 2022; Salas, Zajac, & Marlow, 2018). This often includes reviewing the schedule, identifying needs of patients to be seen, identifying potential workflow concerns, reviewing progress on previously identified problems, and conducting safety reviews. Teams can also use this time to acknowledge team members for their help or recent accomplishments, or to implement brief self-care activities (e.g., a 1-minute mindfulness activity, gratitude exercises) to promote wellness and build team cohesion.

Debriefs

Similar to huddles, debriefs are brief meetings where a team can discuss individual and team-level performance, identify successes and errors, and develop a plan to learn from unexpected successes and reduce future errors (Salas et al., 2008). Debriefs usually occur at the end of a clinic session. Debriefs work best when team members feel comfortable and safe to discuss errors and other problems. The team focuses more on the processes rather than outcomes, and the team focuses on specific behaviors associated with successes and errors and tracks them over time.

Barriers to Interprofessional Care

The following include common examples of barriers to interprofessional care. While payment is also a common barrier, issues with regard to financial implications of interprofessional care are discussed later in the chapter.

Physical Space

Physical space can be a barrier or facilitator to effective interprofessional team-based care. Optimal environments have a balance between shared and private workspaces. Shared workspaces promote increased accessibility, situational awareness, communication, and more clinically productive teams (Gunn et al., 2015; Hiefner & Woods, 2019). Private workspaces can be helpful for more focused work (e.g., paperwork, phone calls). Gunn et al. (2015) have provided recommended layouts for integrated, team-based work environments.

Time

Involving multiple professionals in a single visit can extend the time of that visit (Riley, Paternostro, Walker, & Wagner, 2019). Further, taking time to build team culture, huddle, and debrief may seem impossible within a busy work day. However, interprofessional care can save individual providers time. For example, research has found that when a behavioral health concern is brought up in a medical visit, medical providers working independently spend more time and receive less reimbursement than visits for medical-only reasons (Meadows, Valleley, Haack, Thorson, & Evans, 2011). However, involving a behavioral health provider in the visit can save roughly 12 minutes of medical provider time per visit (Riley et al., 2019).

Information Sharing and Security

Parents generally report wanting their health information shared across professionals to promote consistency in care and feel overwhelmed with being the "communication bridge" between multiple providers (Greene, Ford, Ward-Zimmerman, & Foster, 2015). That said, not all patients want their behavioral health information shared with just anyone, and patients generally report wanting control over the information included in their health record and who has access (Caine & Hanania, 2013; Schwartz et al., 2015).

HIRING AND TRAINING

Hiring

Recruiting and hiring team-oriented professionals is key to building effective teams. While specific knowledge and skills are easily trained, it is very difficult to train personality characteristics that are important to team-based care. As such, it is important to identify people who are flexible, adaptive, able to easily build and maintain relationships, communicate clearly, and have a history of collaborating with others. This can be assessed through careful attention to letters of recommendation, references, and thoughtful interview questions. Helpful interview questions include:

1. When you have had to complete group projects, what was that experience like for you?
2. Tell me about a time you worked with a team to solve a difficult problem.
3. What is your ideal work environment? (Looking for responses that include team members)
4. How do you see your role as someone within our team?
5. If two team members asked you to do something at the same time, how would you decide what to do?
6. If a team member came to you frustrated with another team member or clinic policy and said, "Don't you agree?", how would you respond?

Another helpful practice is to have multiple team members interview job candidates and be careful to note how interviewees interact with each member and whether they appear to value all members similarly.

Training

For interprofessional practice to evolve and spread, training programs in the health professions must adopt and expand interprofessional education (IPE). This includes implementation of IPE curricula, shared learning environments, and attention to language and discipline-specific cultural barriers that can contribute to communication challenges within teams. As an educational approach, IPE aims to prepare health professionals and health professions students to provide patient care in a team-based environment by emphasizing that learners from different disciplines learn "with," "from," and "about"" those from other disciplines (Interprofessional Education Collaborative [IPEC], 2016). IPE curricula broadly center around equipping learners with the IPEC core competencies for team-based care (Table 115.2).

DBP care may involve disciplines with similar and sometimes overlapping roles. Examples include behavioral health (from psychology, psychiatry, social work, and counseling), allied health (occupational therapy, physical therapy, speech therapy), and pediatrics (primary care, developmental, neurology, physical medicine, and rehabilitation). While this

TABLE 115.2 IPEC Core Competencies

Competency	Description
Values/Ethics for Interprofessional Practice	Ability to work with individuals of other professions to maintain a climate of mutual respect and shared values
Roles/Responsibilities	Ability to use the knowledge of one's own role and those of other professions to appropriately assess and address the health care needs of patients and to promote and advance the health of populations
Interprofessional Communication	Ability to communicate with patients, families, communities, and professionals in health care and other fields in a responsive and responsible manner that supports a team approach to the promotion and maintenance of health and the prevention and treatment of disease
Teams and Teamwork	Ability to apply relationship-building values and the principles of team dynamics to perform effectively in different team roles to plan, deliver, and evaluate patient/population-centered care and population health programs and policies that are safe, timely, efficient, effective, and equitable

IPEC, Interprofessional Education Collaborative.

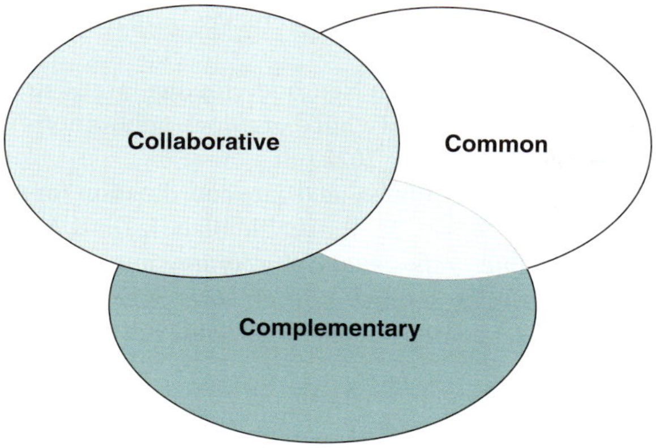

Fig. 115.1 Aspects of training to promote interprofessional team-based care.

can present potential challenges regarding role clarity, it also provides an opportunity for shared learning. Fig. 115.1 illustrates how these disciplines could benefit from training that includes a collaborative component (e.g., how to be a part of an interprofessional team), common curricula (e.g., communication skills, motivational interviewing), and complementary, discipline-specific components.

A number of resources are available to health professionals interested in promoting understanding of the roles and skills of other professions, improving communication and collaboration skills, recognizing overlapping professional functions and roles, improving team functioning, and reducing communication breakdowns that can lead to ineffective care. Several DBP training programs are affiliated with the Leadership Education in Neurodevelopmental and Related Disabilities (LEND) program of the Maternal and Child Health Bureau (MCHB). Currently funded through the Autism CARES Act, LEND was developed to provide IPE to trainees from 14 core academic disciplines who are interested in caring for individuals with neurodevelopmental disabilities and related conditions. Core disciplines include audiology, genetics, nursing, allied health, social work, special education, nutrition, pediatrics, and behavioral health. LEND programs offer trainees the opportunity to learn together, thereby improving interprofessional community and understanding as trainees enter the workforce. A particular focus of the program is involvement of self-advocates and family members as core faculty and trainees. LEND programs exist, either physically or through partnership, in all 50 states and territories and are supported by the MCHB Division of Maternal Child Health Workforce Development. In addition to providing training, clinical care, and programming for children and families, individual LEND programs have developed a number of resources and materials that are available in the public domain.

At the graduate level, one of the largest evidence-based IPE training programs is TeamSTEPPS 2.0 (n.d.), a set of teamwork tools developed by the US Department of Health and Human Services Agency for Healthcare Research and Quality (AHRQ, n.d.). Originally developed as an intervention to reduce medical errors by improving communication and teamwork skills among health care professionals, TeamSTEPPS has become a required curricular component in a number of medical schools and IPE learning collaboratives across the country. Training future health professionals in an interprofessional approach at this early point in their education holds promise for promoting team-based care throughout their career.

IMPLICATIONS FOR PRACTICE, PAYMENT, AND POLICY

Successful implementation of team-based care requires a considerable culture shift among professionals and for the health care organizations in which they practice. For professionals, role clarity can help ensure that team members feel valued and are practicing at the top of their education, skills, and license. Recognizing the unique contribution of each team member is essential for creating a more collaborative team environment. The team should agree upon processes for exchanging patient information, both verbally and electronically. Team identity should be developed and apparent in all aspects of patient care, and the team should strive to ensure that patients and families understand the roles of all team members. Integral to team-based care is the recognition of the role that patients and families play as key members of the care team. Shared decision making (i.e., communication process whereby patients and clinicians work together to make optimal health care decisions that align with patient values and preferences) and an emphasis on understanding the child and family's beliefs and preferences can help to ensure deference and autonomy that are essential to family engagement and best outcomes.

Payment models have traditionally involved fee-for-service transactions that often do not adequately support team-based care. In traditional payment models families may be required to pay multiple copays when interprofessional care is provided by multiple disciplines. In other settings billing may need to occur through one primary provider on the team, meaning that all other professionals who provided care are unable to submit a bill. These models pose obvious financial barriers to payers and organizations. Other considerations include the possibility of Stark law violations and other potential compliance issues. As such, interprofessional teams may need to consult with experts in billing, information technology, compliance, and/or health care law to ensure that these potential issues are addressed.

Because of these financial challenges, team-based care is often supported by grants or in-kind contributions, but these types of patchwork payment models are often not adequate for growth or program sustainability. The transition from fee-for-service to value-based care may allow for innovations in payment models to better support team-based care (Katkin et al., 2017). Over the last several years, the Centers for Medicare and Medicaid Services (CMS) Innovation Center has prioritized the development of novel payment and service delivery models to support aspects of care that may not be adequately reimbursed in traditional payment models but can contribute to increased quality or reduced cost. While these payment models have, to date, been more feasible for the adult Medicare population, the CMMS Integrated Care for Kids (InCK) model has been developed to support community-based service delivery to improve prevention, early identification, and treatment of behavioral and physical health needs for Medicaid beneficiaries (https://innovation.cms.gov/innovation-models/integrated-care-for-kids-model). Individual state Medicaid programs also have flexibility to develop and support team-based models through waiver programs and other funding streams. Ongoing advocacy is needed at the state and federal levels to ensure that team-based care be sustained and further developed.

CONCLUSION

Children and families, health care and related professionals, and communities are hard at work to ensure high-quality, coordinated, and comprehensive care for patients affected by DB conditions. Evidence suggests that this type of care provides best outcomes and can reduce unnecessary health care costs. By coordinating care across professionals and across systems, team-based care can help to achieve optimal outcomes. However, existing barriers in training, practice, and payment must be overcome for these optimal outcomes to be realized. Team-based care requires the intentional focus of the patient/family as the center of care with a team of professionals, organizations, and agencies providing support and expertise. Interprofessional teams can be a formal program (such as a specialty Down syndrome clinic) or less structured, as in the case of an entire medical office whose staff and professionals work together to meet the complex needs of their patients and families. Regardless of team structure, certain principles can help guide teams toward optimal functioning. This intentionality applies to almost all aspects of team functioning, including physical space, communication practices, hiring, and billing/payment. By developing a system of care designed to support the values, beliefs, and preferences of children like Mya in the opening vignette and families, interprofessional teams and their members can realize their individual professional goals as well.

RESOURCES

- TeamSTEPPS 2.0: https://www.ahrq.gov/teamstepps/index.html
- Tips for debriefing in medical teams: Salas, E., Klein, C., King, H., Salisbury, M., Augenstein, J. S., Birnbach, D. J.,…& Upshaw, C. (2008). Debriefing medical teams: 12 evidence-based best practices and tips. *The Joint Commission Journal on Quality and Patient Safety, 34*, 518–527.
- Guide to developing patient-centered team-based primary care: Schottenfeld, L., Petersen, D., Peikes, D., Ricciardi, R., Burak, H., McNellis, R., & Genevro, J. (2016). Creating patient-centered team-based primary care. AHRQ Pub. 16-0002-EF. Agency for Healthcare Research and Quality.
- Team-based Learning Collaborative: http://www.team-basedlearning.org/
- Leadership Education in Neurodevelopmental and Related Disabilities: https://www.aucd.org/docs/publications/brochures/lend_brochure_2020.pdf
- Textbook on interprofessional care coordination for pediatric ASD: McClain, M. B., Shahidullah, J. D., & Mezher, K. (2020). *Interprofessional care coordination for pediatric ASD: Translating research into practice.* Springer. https://www.springer.com/gp/book/9783030462949

REFERENCES

American Psychiatric Association. (2013). *Diagnostic and statistical manual of mental disorders* (5th ed.). Author.

Berwick, D. M., Nolan, T. W., & Whittington, J. (2008). The triple aim: Care, health, and cost. *Health Affairs, 27*, 759–769.

Bodenheimer, T., & Sinsky, C. (2014). From triple to quadruple aim: Care of the patient requires care of the provider. *Annals of Family Medicine, 12*, 573–576.

Brinster, M. I., Brukilacchio, B. H., Fikki-Urbanovsky, A., Shahidullah, J. D., & Ravenscroft, S. (2022). Improving efficiency and equity in early autism evaluations: The (S)TAAR Model. *Journal of Autism and Developmental Disorders (advance online publication).* https://doi.org/10.1007/s10803-022-05425-1

Caine, K., & Hanania, R. (2013). Patients want granular privacy control over health information in electronic medical records. *Journal of the American Medical Informatics Association, 20*, 7–15.

Felitti, V. J., Anda, R. F., Nordenberg, D., Williamson, D. F., Spitz, A. M., Edwards, V., Koss, M. P., & Marks, J. S. (1998). Relationship of childhood abuse and household dysfunction to many of the leading causes of death in adults: The Adverse Childhood Experiences (ACE) Study. *American Journal of Preventative Medicine, 14*, 245–258.

Greene, C. A., Ford, J. D., Ward-Zimmerman, B., & Foster, D. (2015). Please break the silence: Parents' views on communication between pediatric primary care and mental health providers. *Families, Systems, & Health, 33*, 155–159.

Gunn, R., Davis, M. M., Hall, J., Heintzman, J., Muench, J., Smeds, B., Miller, B.F., Miller, W.L., Gilchrist, E., Brown Levey, S., Brown, J., Wise Romero, P., &, Cohen, D. J. (2015). Designing clinical space for the delivery of integrated behavioral health and primary care. *Journal of the American Board of Family Medicine, 28*, S52–S62.

Hiefner, A. R., & Woods, S. B. (2019). Implementing integrated behavioral health: Testing associations between shared clinical time and space and provider referrals. *Families, Systems, & Health, 37*, 206–211.

Hostutler, C. A., Valleru, J., Maciejewski, H. M., Hess, A., Gleeson, S. P., & Ramtekkar, U. P. (2020). Improving pediatrician's behavioral health competencies through the Project ECHO teleconsultation model. *Clinical Pediatrics, 59*, 1049–1057.

Interprofessional Education Collaborative (IPEC). (2016). *Core competencies for interprofessional collaborative practice.* Author.

Katkin, J. P., Kressly, S. J., Edwards, A. R., Perrin, J. M., Kraft, C. A., Richerson, J. E., Tieder, J. S., Wall, J., & Task Force on Pediatric Practice Change. (2017). Guiding principles for team-based pediatric care. *Pediatrics, 140*, e20171489.

Kohn, L. T., Corrigan, J. M., & Donaldson, M. S. (Eds.). (2000). *To err is human: Building a safer health system. Institute of Medicine*

(US) Committee on Quality of Health Care in America. National Academies Press.

Kolko, D. J., Campo, J., Kilbourne, A. M., Hart, J., Skolsky, D., & Wisniewski, S. (2014). Collaborative care outcomes for pediatric behavioral health problems: A cluster randomized trial. *Pediatrics, 133*, e981–e992.

Kruk, M. E. (2018). High quality health systems in the sustainable development goals era: Time for a revolution. *Lancet Global Health, 6*, e1196–e1252.

Kuhn, C., Groves, B. K., Kaczor, C., Sebastian, S., Ramtekkar, U., Nowack, J., Toth, C., Valenti, O., & Gowda, C. (2019). Pharmacist involvement in population health management for a pediatric managed Medicaid accountable care organization. *Children, 6*, 82.

Mazurek, M. O., Brown, R., Curran, A., & Sohl, K. (2017). ECHO autism: A new model for training primary care providers in best-practice care for children with autism. *Clinical Pediatrics, 56*, 247–256.

McClain, M. B., Shahidullah, J. D., Mezher, K., Havercamp, C. R., Benallie, K. J., & Schwartz, S. E. (2020). School-clinic care coordination for youth with ASD: A national survey of school psychologists. *Journal of Autism and Developmental Disorders, 50*, 3081–3091.

Meadows, T., Valleley, R., Haack, M. K., Thorson, R., & Evans, J. (2011). Physicians "costs" in providing behavioral health in primary care. *Clinical Pediatrics, 50*, 447–455.

Porter, M., & Teisberg, E. (2006). *Redefining healthcare: Creating value-based competition on results*. Harvard Business School Press.

Riley, A. R., Paternostro, J. K., Walker, B. L., & Wagner, D. V. (2019). The impact of behavioral health consultations on medical encounter duration in pediatric primary care: A retrospective match-controlled study. *Families, Systems, & Health, 37*, 162–166.

Salas, E., Klein, C., King, H., Salisbury, M., Augenstein, J. S., Birnbach, D. J., Robinson, D. W., & Upshaw, C. (2008). Debriefing medical teams: 12 evidence-based best practices and tips. *The Joint Commission Journal on Quality and Patient Safety, 34*, 518–527.

Salas, E., Zajac, S., & Marlow, S. L. (2018). Transforming health care one team at a time: Ten observations and the trail ahead. *Group & Organization Management, 43*, 357–381.

Sarvet, B., Gold, J., Bostic, J. Q., Masek, B. J., Prince, J. B., Jeffers-Terry, M., Moore, C. F., Molbert, B., & Straus, J. H. (2010). Improving access to mental health care for children: The Massachusetts Child Psychiatry Access Project. *Pediatrics, 126*, 1191–1200.

Schwartz, P. H., Caine, K., Alpert, S. A., Meslin, E. M., Carroll, A. E., & Tierney, W. M. (2015). Patient preferences in controlling access to their electronic health records: A prospective cohort study in primary care. *Journal of General Internal Medicine, 30*, S25–S30.

Shah, R. P., Kunnavakkam, R., & Msall, M. E. (2013). Pediatricians' knowledge, attitudes, and practice patterns regarding special education and individualized education programs. *Academic Pediatrics, 13*, 430–435.

Shahidullah, J. D., Azad, G., Mezher, K. R., McClain, M. B., & McIntyre, L. (2018). Linking the medical and educational home to support children with autism spectrum disorder: Practice recommendations. *Clinical Pediatrics, 57*, 1496–1505.

Shahidullah, J. D., Forman, S. G., Palejwala, M. H., Chaudhuri, A., Pincus, L. E., Lee, E., Shafrir, R., & Barone, C. (2019). National survey of chief pediatric residents' attitudes, practices, and training in collaborating with schools. *Journal of Interprofessional Education and Practice, 15*, 82–87.

Shanafelt, T. D., Boone, S., Tan, L., Dyrbye, L. N., Sotile, W., Satele, D., West, C. P., Sloan, J., & Oreskovich, M. R. (2012). Burnout and satisfaction with work-life balance among US physicians relative to the general US population. *Archives of Internal Medicine, 172*, 1377–1385.

Shanafelt, T. D., Goh, J., & Sinsky, C. (2017). The business case for investing in physician well-being. *JAMA Internal Medicine, 177*, 1826–1832.

Stange, K. C. (2009). The problem of fragmentation and the need for integrative solutions. *Annals of Family Medicine, 7*, 100–103.

TeamSTEPPS 2.0. (n.d.). *Agency for Healthcare Research and Quality*. https://www.ahrq.gove/teamstepps/instructor/index.html

West, C. P., Dyrbye, L. N., & Shanafelt, T. D. (2018). Physician burnout: Contributors, consequences and solutions. *Journal of Internal Medicine, 283*, 516–529.

World Health Organization. (2008). *Task-shifting: Global recommendations and guidelines*. https://www.who.int/workforcealliance/knowledge/resources/taskshifting_guidelines/en/

116

Ethical Considerations

Peter J. Smith

> **VIGNETTE**
>
> *Your treatment team is seeing a 16-year-old boy with autism and mild intellectual disability. He is capable of conversational speech at a limited level. He is able to read and is able to complete most activities of daily living. His mother contacts your office to ask for a letter of medical necessity for a vasectomy. Upon further discussion, it is determined that he is having a urologic procedure (circumcision repair) and his mother would like to have the vasectomy performed at the same time. She expresses concerns that her son will never be able to raise a baby or be responsible for a child. She would like sterilization because reversible contraception is not an option for her son (given he is male and she believes that his using condoms is not likely). The urologist has agreed to perform the vasectomy; however, the hospital is now requiring further documentation for this surgery to be completed. She is asking for your help to pursue this surgical intervention. Although his mother informs you that he has consented to the procedure, it is unclear if he understands the implications of this decision. When asked whether he wants to have a child, he does not answer.*

INTRODUCTION

As illustrated in the opening vignette, by its nature, clinical care presents scenarios that require careful ethical analysis. Clinicians in developmental-behavioral pediatrics (DBP) must be prepared for such scenarios, which often present unexpectedly. This chapter will address ethics in three ways: (1) a brief review of several ethical systems, including terms used; (2) a review of experiences of individuals with disabilities and their implications for ethic systems today; and (3) a few suggestions that will be directed toward practical applications.

A BRIEF REVIEW OF ETHICAL THEORIES

Principlism

There are many different methods that fall under the word *ethics*. Currently in the United States the most commonly employed system of ethics used within medicine is called principlism. Principlism takes its name from its primary focus on foundational principles that are used to help navigate ethical dilemmas. The four main principles that are most commonly used in principlism are (1) respect for autonomy, (2) nonmaleficence (avoiding doing harm), (3) beneficence (actively doing good), and (4) justice (equal sharing of benefits and burdens) (Beauchamp & Childress, 2013). Ethicists are instructed in the meanings of these principles and taught how to use them, in dynamic balance, to make ethical decisions. The dominance of principlism in contemporary medical ethics is multifactorial. Historically, principlism was created and championed as a system that would correct the problems of a prior method of ethics, which was dominant in health care in the early 20th century, paternalism. Paternalism was a strategy that encouraged clinicians who are more informed about the medical facts to make decisions. Principlism, by emphasizing the need to allow individuals their autonomy to make their own decisions, shifted from emphasizing the doctor's perspective to emphasizing the patient's and family's perspectives. Pedagogically, principlism is simply one of the easiest systems of ethics for instructors to teach because it can be quickly summarized by defining the main principles. Culturally, principlism is consistent with a libertarian cultural emphasis on the individual.

However, there are many difficulties with principlism, especially how it is used in practice. It is formally taught that the four principles are equal and should be balanced when making decisions. In practice, respect for autonomy has dominated the other three because of its resonance with current cultural norms. The fourth principle, justice, is often forgotten, as witnessed by the history of clinicians and policymakers systemically ignoring minority groups, leading to systemic injustice, which only recently has been recognized by health care institutions as an ongoing problem. Of note, intersectionality of race and disability increase these injustices. In addition, the COVID-19 pandemic has dramatically illustrated the tension between respect for autonomy and justice, with arguments over mask mandates, closures, and vaccination becoming flashpoints around the world.

Natural Law Ethics

A different system of ethics, which also uses guiding laws, is similar to principlism, except that these laws were deduced from observations of nature. Natural law ethics was formulated by Greek philosophers and Roman legislators. Because they were drawn from observations of nature, they were seen as objective. Its strength, theoretically, is that it carries the possibility of being a universal approach (Cahill, Haker, & Metogo, 2010); however, in practice, different cultures and thinkers have observed nature and have come to different conclusions. People with disabilities are particularly at risk under this system because they could be judged as unnatural.

Virtue Ethics

Another system of ethics that has both ancient roots and strong claims of universality is virtue ethics. Most cultures identify habits of action or thought that are seen as laudable and promote them within their culture. Greek philosophers such as Aristotle attempted to articulate these virtues. Later, Roman philosophers, especially the Stoics such as Cicero, also promoted patterns of behavior that were virtuous. Christian theologians, including Augustine of Hippo and Thomas Aquinas, developed their own systems to promote virtues. Augustine changed the Roman premise that reason is the foundation for virtues to a love of God as the foundation of his system. Aquinas agreed with the Greeks and Romans that virtues were primarily habits. Contemporary thinkers who promote virtue ethics specifically avoid trying to set up programs that promote virtuous actions. Instead, they work to create institutions and cultural norms that foster virtuous individuals. Overall, virtue ethics has been a system that has focused less on creating a guide for making difficult decisions and more on helping shape individuals who are good at making those decisions themselves (Porter, 2001).

Utilitarianism

A modern system that was specifically an attempt to make ethics more like a hard science is utilitarianism. Jeremy Bentham and John Stuart Mill developed this system in the 19th century. They believed that the best action in any situation is the action that creates outcomes with the greatest mathematical ratio of value to disvalue. In popular culture the character Spock in the original *Star Trek* series famously illustrated use of this system. Utilitarianism only accounts for the actual consequences of an action, not the intention of the actor. The application of utilitarianism to disabilities reveals its inherent limitations and the risks such a system can pose to vulnerable populations. For example, using this system, some have argued that children with disabilities bring a net negative ratio of value to disvalue (measuring the happiness of the family overall) and therefore they should be terminated or even euthanized if they are already born (Singer, 1979).

Deontology

An ethical system that was promoted by Immanuel Kant is called deontology. This system proposes that individuals or groups (or both) have duties, which then guide their decisions and actions. This is a system that is promoted by the golden rule, which can be phrased as "Act to others as you believe they should act toward you" (Kant, 1993). One of the pedagogic strengths of this system is that it is both simple to teach and to understand (Pellegrino, 1985). Critics of deontology suggest that with many ethical dilemmas, an individual who is struggling with a moral dilemma frequently has competing duties that are in tension (e.g., an individual may have duties related to the role as a physician that is in tension with duties related to the role as a family member to the patient).

Casuistry

Unlike the other ethical systems discussed, casuistry is not a group of foundational ideas but a method of making difficult decisions. The general process is to compare the current decision to be made with prior decisions or cases. Casuistry existed during the time of the Greek philosophers, and it peaked in popularity in the 16th and 17th centuries. Casuistry is a process that also informs many legal structures, as well as some decision making within governments and businesses (Jonsen & Toulmin, 1990). For example, famous cases are studied in business school so that students can learn from the prior experiences of others and therefore not repeat the same mistakes.

Narrative Ethics

Narrative ethics is also a system that focuses on process. In it, stories of individuals or groups are reviewed to offer insight into the ways of being ethical. Telling a story to illustrate a deeper point is as old as human civilization, and its proponents argue that reasoning is only a partial method for becoming and acting ethical (Charon & Montello, 2002).

HISTORICAL EXPERIENCES OF INDIVIDUALS WITH DISABILITIES

Unfortunately there are many historical examples of people and groups acting in a discriminatory fashion against individuals with disabilities. For example, Francis Galton, a cousin of Charles Darwin and an early researcher in genetics, created the term *eugenics* and promoted it as a way to improve society. There are two theoretical forms of eugenics: positive eugenics (promoting "good" genes in a population) and negative eugenics (removing "bad" genes from a population). Due to Galton's influence, many thinkers and policymakers in the United States became eugenicists, and the country became the first to have laws promoting it, in the first half of the 20th century. Many states enacted laws that allowed for compulsory sterilization of individuals who were seen as having "bad" genes, including individuals with cognitive impairments. Eventually in 1927 the US Supreme Court ruled in favor of the practice, in their ruling of *Buck v Bell*. In his supporting opinion Supreme Court Justice Oliver Wendell Holmes Jr. wrote:

> *We have seen more than once that the public welfare may call upon the best citizens for their lives. It would be strange if it could not call upon those who already sap the strength of the State for these lesser sacrifices, often not felt to be such by those concerned, to prevent our being swamped with incompetence. It is better for all the world, if instead of waiting to execute degenerate offspring for crime, or to let them starve for their imbecility, society can prevent those who are manifestly unfit from continuing their kind. … Three generations of imbeciles are enough.*
> *(Buck v. Bell, 274 U.S. 200 [1927], 1926)*

With the backing of the Supreme Court, compulsory sterilization became common in many states, and over 65,000 individuals were sterilized in 33 states under state compulsory sterilization programs in the United States. The last state sterilization was in 1981 in Oregon (Lombardo, 1985).

In 1947 the New York State Department of Mental Hygiene opened the Willowbrook State School on Staten Island, which ultimately became a residential facility for children with intellectual disability. It was originally designed for a population of 4000, but it eventually held 6000 children. Because of crowding and neglect, the conditions at Willowbrook deteriorated and became filthy and unhealthy. Because of these conditions, hepatitis infections became nearly universal in the student population. Drs. Saul Krugman and Robert McCollum ran a study from 1956 to 1972 that attempted to describe the natural history of hepatitis in the poorly cared for population. As part of this study, they purposely infected new students by feeding them stool samples of children already known to have hepatitis. No consent was obtained from the families of the students they studied. Eventually, when the study was brought to light, it was terminated. A long legal process ensued and, eventually, the Willowbrook Consent Decree was finalized in 1975, officially closing the school (although the children were housed at Willowbrook until 1987) (Goode, Hill, Reiss, & Bronston, 2013). Like Buck in *Buck v Bell*, many of the children, after more thorough examination, were found not to have intellectual disability.

In 1982 a child with Down syndrome was born in Bloomington, Indiana. The baby was found to have esophageal atresia, which had a well-established treatment protocol already developed. However, the family chose to turn down the curative surgical treatment and the child died. When the story became public, the US Surgeon General at the time, C. Everret Koop, a pediatric surgeon who had completed this surgery many times successfully, criticized the doctors who had allowed the baby to die. In 1983 the parents of a child born with myodysplasia, a condition that could be treated surgically, declined interventions. Subsequently, in 1984, Dr. Koop's advocacy resulted in a federal law amending the child abuse regulations to include the withholding of known treatments from children with disabilities; these "Baby Doe Regulations" became active on June 1, 1985. Signs were posted in neonatal intensive care units and hotlines were created to allow anyone (staff, families, physicians) to report potential abuse; however, the Supreme Court struck down the regulations in 1986 (Merrick & Tenenbaum 2013).

More recently, in 2006 an interdisciplinary team from Seattle Children's Hospital published a single-case report about a child with intellectual disability who received a hysterectomy and bilateral mastectomy and high-dose hormones (estrogen). The goal of the protocol was to decrease the child's eventual adult height so that she could remain living with her family for a longer time (the surgeries also were related to her daily care). The team had, prior to any clinical action, requested a review by the Seattle Children's Hospital Ethics Committee, which did not stop the protocol. The parents of this child, who was named in their blog as "Ashley, The Pillow Angel," promoted the protocol to other parents. The legal team in Washington that is commissioned to protect the rights of individuals with disabilities filed a suit against Seattle Children's Hospital, and the hospital eventually agreed that it had violated a state law that prohibits the sterilization of women with intellectual disability.

As this brief review makes clear, multiple historical events and trends illustrate how society has stigmatized and marginalized individuals with disabilities. These events offer clear examples of how individual professionals and professional groups have disregarded their dignity through a trail of blatant abuses. Families, rights activists, and most importantly individuals with disabilities are the energy behind contemporary advocacy movements toward self-determination and the ability of people with disabilities to manage and direct their own lives. Professionals in the field of DBP have an opportunity to support these efforts.

This growing sense of autonomy raises a number of dilemmas for clinicians and others who must balance an imperative to protect the health and safety of people with disabilities with a sense that people with disabilities are able to and should, where appropriate, make decisions that contribute to their sense of control of their own destiny. This is true when those decisions are contrary to what others believe are the healthy or safe choices, as it is for all of us. In modern health care clinicians, whose priority is to prevent disease and disability, must simultaneously elevate the status and independence of people with disabilities (Barnbaum, 2008).

SUGGESTIONS FOR PRACTICAL CONSIDERATION

Clinicians who face ethical questions stemming from care of children with disabilities can benefit from a simple recognition of the prior mistakes and humble acceptance of systemic biases against this vulnerable population (Asch, Gostin, & Johnson, 2003). Of course, the biases are worsened by intersectional overlap with other aspects that result in bias, including race/ethnicity, socioeconomic status, and immigrant status. There are a few simple points that can be helpful.

A Few Practical Suggestions

1. Many ethical systems, due to their underlying assumptions about personhood or reason, are inherently biased against individuals with disabilities.
2. There is an unfortunately long history of clinicians who have mistreated individuals with disabilities, which must never be forgotten.
3. The general trend is an imperfect and incomplete movement toward greater acceptance, protection, and respect for individuals with disabilities. As noted, state laws that eventually responded to the eugenic movement were the exact laws used to help protect other children from the surgeries performed on Ashley as described above.
4. Experts in the field of DBP need to engage with the ethics committees at their institution and use their expertise to inform the work of these groups. Returning to the case of Ashley, the Seattle Ethics committee did not have any clinicians who were experts in the care of children with intellectual disabilities, which likely contributed to their admitted mistake.

CONCLUSION

Ethics is a term that has been used in many different ways in many different contexts for millennia. There are varied systems of ethics in the Western experience (and more in other cultures and experiences). As illustrated in the opening vignette, clinicians in the field of DBP benefit from knowing about these different systems, and their strengths and weaknesses. Further, they will likely encounter clinical scenarios requiring careful ethical analysis and benefit from knowing the history of mistreatment of individuals with disabilities and the systemic biases inherent in some of the systems of ethics. Finally, experts in the field of DBP need to use their knowledge, skills, and attitudes to inform the professional ethicists who are too often unaware of the basics of caring for and respecting individuals with disabilities.

REFERENCES

Asch, A., Gostin, L. O., & Johnson, D. M. (2003). Respecting persons with disabilities and preventing disability: Is there a conflict?. In S. Herr, L. O. Gostin, & H. H. Koh (Eds.), *The human rights of persons with intellectual disabilities: Different but equal* (p. 320). Oxford University Press.

Barnbaum, D. R. (2008). *The ethics of autism: Among them, but not of them* (p. 190). Indiana University Press.

Beauchamp, T., & Childress, J. (2013). *Principles of biomedical ethics* (7th ed.). Oxford University Press.

Cahill, L. S., Haker, H., & Metogo, E. M. (Eds.), (2010). *Human nature and natural law (Concilium)*. SCM Press.

Charon, R., & Montello, M. (Eds.). (2002). *Stories matter: The role of narrative in medical ethics*. Routledge.

Goode, D., Hill, D. B., Reiss, J., & Bronston, W. (2013). *A history and sociology of the Willowbrook State School*. American Association on Intellectual and Developmental Disabilities.

Holmes, O. W., & Supreme Court Of The United States. (1926). U.S. Reports: *Buck v. Bell*, 274 U.S. 200.

Jonsen, A., & Toulmin, S. (1990). *The abuse of casuistry: A history of moral reasoning*. University of California Press.

Kant, I. (1993). *Grounding for the metaphysics of morals* (p. 30, 3rd ed.). Hackett.

Lombardo, P. A. (1985). Three generations, no imbeciles: New light on Buck v Bell. *New York University Law Review*, *60*(1), 30–62.

Merrick, J., & Tenenbaum, A. (2013). Devaluation and people with intellectual disability. *International Journal of Disability and Human Development*, *12*(1), 1–3.

Pellegrino, E. D. (1985). The virtuous physician, and the ethics of medicine. In E. E. Shelp (Ed.), *Virtue and medicine* (p. 237–255). D. Reidel.

Porter, J. (2001). Virtue ethics. In R. Gill (Ed.), *The Cambridge companion to Christian ethics* (p. 96). Cambridge University Press.

Singer, P. (1979). Taking life: Humans. In *Practical ethics* (p. 186). Cambridge University Press.

117

The Pitfalls of Guardianship (Conservatorship) and the Promise of Alternatives

Zoe Brennan-Krohn and Susan Mizner

For additional material related to the content of this chapter, please see Chapter 105.

VIGNETTE

Emilia has been your patient for 10 years. She is 17 years old and is on the autism spectrum. Emilia sometimes communicates verbally, but usually prefers typing on an iPad or computer to relay her thoughts. She reads and writes at a fourth-grade level. She experiences ongoing digestive problems and has epilepsy that is well controlled with consistent medication. Emilia relies on her parents and her older sister for help in many areas. At least one of her parents has always come to medical appointments with her. Communication in appointments with Emilia is usually a mix of communication directly from Emilia and context and background from her parent(s). Emilia doesn't drive, and you are not sure if she could travel independently on public transit.

Two months before her 18th birthday, Emilia and her mother come to an appointment with you. Her mother tells you that they are considering getting a guardianship (in some states called a conservatorship) for Emilia when she turns 18. Emilia's school has told them that guardianships are always a good idea for people with developmental disabilities, and that without a guardianship, the parents will not be able to go to her individualized education plan meetings and won't be able to attend any medical appointments with Emilia once she's turned 18. Emilia's mother says she doesn't know much about guardianships but that it seems harmless. She asks if you have any advice or suggestions. When you ask Emilia whether she wants her parents to become her guardians, she shrugs.

What do you advise them? What else would you need to know before advising them?

OVERVIEW

This chapter discusses the system where adults lose some or all of their rights or decision-making power based on a court order, which in most states is called guardianship. Terminology varies state by state for the system discussed in this chapter. In some states, including California, this system is called conservatorship. We do not discuss the concept of guardianship or custody of minors. We use the term guardianship throughout for simplicity.

Clinicians, schools, and family members, like Emilia's mother, often think that guardianship is a requirement for an individual with significant severe disabilities as she enters adulthood and that it is harmless. Clinicians may assume that guardianship is an efficient way to ensure informed consent and adequate care for an adult patient with intellectual or developmental disabilities. In this chapter we emphasize the risks of guardianship. We argue that guardianship is an extreme, often irreversible legal intervention that has significant lifelong consequences. We present many less intrusive options that can and should be tried. We recognize the challenges that many individuals with disabilities face in making decisions about health care, finances, and other important life areas. The alternatives we suggest are designed to provide the individual with meaningful guidance, support, reality checks, and protections. Because these and other alternatives often meet the goals of adult patients and their supporters, we recommend that guardianship be pursued only as a last resort.

There are three scenarios in which guardianships are commonly sought or imposed:

1. A person with a significant developmental or intellectual disability turns 18
2. During or after a major mental health crisis for adults of any age
3. When an older adult experiences dementia or other age-related cognitive disabilities

This chapter focuses on guardianships and the alternatives to guardianship for young adults with developmental disabilities. However, the same principles apply to guardianship in other contexts. For more on guardianship and decision making in relation to other health and education issues, see Chapter 105.

WHAT IS A GUARDIANSHIP?

Guardianship is a legal structure. Guardianships can only be created—or dissolved—by a judge (National Guardianship Association, 2021). Before imposing a guardianship, a judge must determine that an adult is, because of a disability, unable to make decisions about their own life. Based on this determination, the court removes decision-making authority from the person and appoints a guardian who has the legal power to make decisions for the individual. When a guardianship is imposed, it strips the person of virtually all civil rights and liberties. The US House of Representatives member Claude Pepper, in summarizing the findings of hearings on abuses in guardianship, described guardianship as "the most punitive civil penalty that can be levied against an American citizen, with the exception, of course, of the death penalty"

(Chairman of the Subcommittee on Health and Long-Term Care of the Select Committee on Aging, 1987).

The process for establishing a guardianship in the United States varies state by state. Generally, however, the guardianship process begins when someone (family member, clinician, nursing home) petitions the court to impose a guardianship on a person (American Bar Association Commission on Law and Aging, 2020a). That starts a process in which, in theory, the court gathers information about the proposed ward and the proposed guardian(s). This process often includes providing to the court medical, psychological, and social work evaluations (American Bar Association Commission on Law and Aging, 2020b). The guardianship issue is decided in a court proceeding in front of a judge. In many states the person at risk of guardianship is entitled to a lawyer to advocate for one's preferences; in other states there is no such right.

The criteria for imposing a guardianship also vary by state. Examples of criteria include a finding that the person is "unable properly to manage or care for their own person or property" (Del. Code. Tit. 12 § 3901[a][2]), or that a person "lacks capacity to meet at least some essential health and safety requirements" (Fla. Code § 744.102[12]). Most guardianship laws require, in theory, that guardianships should only be imposed if there are no "less restrictive" alternatives (American Bar Association Commission on Law & Aging, 2018). That means a judge should only grant a guardianship when it is determined that less-intrusive measures have been tried and are not working. Some states specifically identify "supported decision making" (discussed further later) as one such less-restrictive alternative to guardianship.

Guardianships can, in theory, be limited in scope. For example, it is possible to take away rights in only some areas of an individual's life (e.g., to enter into contracts or to govern financial decisions). In practice, however, courts most often impose plenary guardianships, in which the guardian is in charge of every decision for the individual (Jameson et al., 2015).

Once a guardianship is established, the guardian has extraordinary power (Hardy, 2008). The guardian has the power to agree to or refuse medical care for the individual. The guardian can make decisions about where that person lives, whether the person can work, what religious services the person may or may not attend, what education the person may or may not receive, whether the person may or may not marry, whether or not the person has a child, what the person can spend money on, and with whom the person may or must spend time. Guardianships, once established, can only be terminated by a court.

WHY BE WARY OF GUARDIANSHIPS?

Many clinicians may be inclined to agree with Emilia and her mother's impression that guardianship is a routine, benign step, the default, especially where the patient has supportive and caring family members and relies on them for aspects of their care. In the opening vignette the clinicians have known this family for a decade and have seen her parents' commitment to supporting her. There has never been any indication of abuse, neglect, or controlling behavior by her parents. So why not get an extra layer of protection from a guardianship?

There are several reasons to be cautious of guardianship, and to encourage serious consideration of alternatives, even in cases like Emilia's, where there is no reason to doubt the good intentions and care among all parties. These concerns encompass both practical and principled issues.

The Guardianship Will Outlast the Guardian, in Which Case the Court Holds the Control

Emilia's parents are seeking a guardianship in which they will be her guardians. They know her better than anyone in the world, they love her, they know they would only make choices in her best interests. But what they may not know is that Emilia's guardianship does not guarantee that they will be the guardians, and that even if they are initially appointed as guardians the guardianship will not end when her parents are no longer able to serve in that role. Once a guardianship is in place, it is the court, not the guardians, who have the greatest power, including the power to choose who will be guardian.

For example, suppose Emilia's parents become her co-guardians soon after Emilia turns 18. Three years later, her parents get divorced. The divorce is acrimonious and high conflict, and each parent asks the court to become Emilia's sole guardian. The court considers these competing requests, and instead of choosing one parent or another, the judge decides to appoint a professional guardian in lieu of either parent. With the stroke of a pen, no one in Emilia's family, including Emilia, has any authority to make any decisions for or with her. Emilia's choices about her medical care, her money, her education, her entire life, are now in the hands of a stranger who does not know her, may be difficult to reach, may never meet her in person, and may have dozens or hundreds of other wards. Her professional guardian might decide Emilia would live best in a nursing home, away from her family and peers; or, her professional guardian might require Emilia to travel back and forth between her parents' homes on a weekly basis, making it virtually impossible for her to keep a job or stable support systems.

The same situation can occur if Emilia's parents die or become unable to continue to serve as her guardians due to the disabilities that they may age into. The death or incapacity of the original guardians does not end a guardianship, and the judge will now select someone else to be Emilia's new guardians. Again, this could very well be (and often is) a stranger (Jameson et al., 2015).

These situations highlight the gap between perception and reality in terms of who has control in a guardianship. Parents may think they are keeping control (often with the best of intentions) by seeking a guardianship, when in fact they are giving control to a court. If there are ways that Emilia's parents can support her without giving away all of her rights to a court, they should consider those.

Guardianships Do Not Necessarily Make People Safer; Self-Determination Can Make People Safer

Unfortunately, some people seek guardianships for nefarious or illicit purposes of exploitation or abuse. However, most families seek guardianships as a tool to protect the person with disabilities. To make the decision about guardianship, it is critical for clinicians and families to be concrete and specific about what dangers they are trying to prevent with the guardianship. They need to be realistic about whether the guardianship in fact addresses those risks. It is also critical to consider what risks the guardianship itself creates.

For instance, Emilia's parents may worry that she can be too trusting of other people and at risk of exploitation. Like many people with autism, she has special interests (i.e., topics that she is particularly passionate and knowledgeable about). One of her special interests is airlines and air travel. She is fascinated by people wearing pilot or flight attendant uniforms, or people with airline security identification badges. Her parents fear that she could be exploited by anyone who engaged with her in this interest or worked in this field.

It is critical to examine, and to encourage patients' families to examine, whether there is a nexus between the problem (in this case, risk of exploitation) and the proposed solution (i.e., guardianship). The problem may well be a real one. But getting a guardianship gives the guardian a piece of paper and legal rights. The guardianship does not create a forcefield around Emilia to protect her from predators or bad choices. With or without a guardian, Emilia will still have to work with her parents or other supporters to learn about boundaries, to practice identifying situations that seem unsafe, and to be able to say no if she feels uncomfortable. Perhaps most importantly, she will need to learn how and when to ask for help. Everyone learns, albeit at different paces, how to navigate life, connect with others, exercise boundaries, and when to ask for help. Part of being human is learning to make choices responsibly, with help and guidance where needed, and where consistent with one's values. Everyone learns this over the course of a lifetime by trial and error, and in our own ways. People with disabilities, like people without disabilities, are safest and happiest when they learn these skills in the way that is meaningful for them. A guardianship does not provide a shortcut to the security and knowledge of this process. But a guardianship can create a barrier that limits that development and create a false sense of security that such development is not necessary.

Even people with high support needs, limited communication, or significant disabilities have and express preferences, and continue to learn and develop throughout their lives. Research consistently shows that people with disabilities have better subjective and objective life outcomes, including less risk of abuse, if they have greater self-determination (Powers et al., 2012; Shogren, Wehmeyer, Palmer, Rifenbark, & Little, 2015; Wehmeyer & Palmer, 2003). For people with significant disabilities, establishing and expressing boundaries, preferences, and autonomy may progress differently than for nondisabled people. However likes, dislikes, boundaries, and desires are expressed (whether through words, actions, or facial expressions), practice and experience expressing those preferences is shown to protect most against exploitation. People get better at protecting themselves, at saying no, when they have practice doing just that. People with disabilities may learn in very different ways, or at different speeds, than nondisabled people. Encouraging families to be skeptical of guardianships does not mean disregarding a person's disability and support needs, which may be considerable. But many support needs can be met without guardianship, and that should be encouraged.

Studies show that the best way to learn how to interact safely in the world is with practice and experience. If Emilia has the experience of self-determination (practice expressing her wishes, her likes and dislikes, and having those wishes honored, discussed, and respected), then that is correlated with a lower risk of exploitation (Khemka, Hickson, & Reynolds, 2005). In many cases guardianship does not add anything to that work.

Guardianship Includes a Harmful Message

It is important to acknowledge the impact of a guardianship on the person subjected to it. Choice is fundamental to who we are as humans. Expressing our likes and dislikes is core to being human, to being an individual. Many clinicians do not have enough time with their patients (especially their patients with significant disabilities) to learn what their patients enjoy, value, and give. People with significant disabilities who do not use formal language nonetheless express preferences through their actions, facial expressions, and other nonverbal cues. Even people who rely on others for significant assistance often provide affection, guidance, and insight to those around them. Most adults take for granted that we can choose what to eat, where and with whom to spend our free time, what clothes to wear, based on our preferences and principles. People under guardianship are told—by a court—that their preferences and likes and dislikes are not recognized, and that they are incapable of directing their own lives. This message is conveyed even if none of the practical risks of guardianship ever occur. In every guardianship there is a person who faces a judge; the judge states the person cannot make choices about one's own life, and that someone else will make those choices (Kapp, 1992). This, itself, is a harm—to the individual and to society's views of people with disabilities.

WHAT ARE THE ALTERNATIVES?

Emilia's parents have always been involved in her medical care. She takes medication daily to manage her epilepsy, and missing doses can cause seizures. She regularly sees specialists for her digestive concerns and follows a special diet that the family has developed, with physician advice, over the course of several years of trial and error that seems to minimize her gastrointestinal symptoms. She also regularly sees occupational, physical, and speech therapists. Her mother takes notes at all doctor appointments, tracks all tests and lab results, and schedules and drives Emilia to her appointments. Emilia's mother says she cannot imagine Emilia managing these issues alone. She worries that without a guardianship Emilia would be left to fend for herself in navigating this complex range of supports and treatments. Emilia types on her iPad to you that she wants to have her parents keep helping her with complicated medical issues but that she wants to learn how to schedule and go to some appointments independently.

Even when people recognize the risks and downsides of guardianships, they may believe—and may be told—that guardianship is necessary for important parts of a young adult's life. Emilia, her parents, and her clinicians may all believe that without a guardianship she would be left alone to try to manage all of her medical and support care. If, as in this scenario, Emilia is not all alone and has family who are willing to support her, that should be taken into account and celebrated. Many situations that people think require guardianships can be easily addressed without guardianship.

Alternatives for Specific Scenarios

For medical care, patients can sign documents such as a Healthcare Power of Attorney, an Authorization to Share Information, or a Health Insurance Portability and Accountability Act (HIPAA) waiver (see Additional Resources). Versions of these documents written in simple, accessible English are available online (see Additional Resources). These documents differ from a guardianship because they can be created, modified, or terminated without the involvement of a court. The control in these documents remains with the people involved. A Healthcare Power of Attorney authorizes another person to make decisions for the patient; an Authorization to Share Information and a HIPAA waiver both authorize another person to access information to make decisions with the person.

Similar documents exist for educational decisions. A person can sign an authorization to share educational information to allow trusted supporters to continue to see school information.

For financial issues, people with disabilities can get help from a relatively informal arrangement providing automatic bill paying, to an agreement to be a representative payee for social security or to have a power of attorney for finances.

For any decision making, people with disabilities—just like people without disabilities—can invite trusted supporters to attend meetings and appointments with them. If an adult patient with a disability comes to an appointment with a parent, a clinician should ask if the patient is comfortable with the parent being there (this can be a simple verbal inquiry). If the patient confirms the support, then the clinician should honor this. For people with disabilities—just like for people without disabilities—using trusted supporters to help in complicated situations should be viewed positively.

Supported Decision Making

Supported decision making is a broad term that encompasses but is not limited to the options discussed earlier. It is a tool that allows people with disabilities to choose supporters to help them make choices. Supported decision making recognizes that all people can and do rely on trusted advisors (family and friends) to understand, make, and communicate decisions, and recognizes that using supports is a good thing. Too often, if people with disabilities ask for help, or want to bring a parent to a doctor appointment, or seek other support, this request is used as evidence of incapacity. Supported decision making recognizes that using supports is a strength, and that if people use supporters appropriately and when needed that is a way to enhance their capacity and should be treated as such.

Supported decision making allows people with disabilities to be explicit about the supports they wish to use, who they trust to help them make choices, and what help they want. People who use supported decision making should have their capacity (including capacity to give informed consent, to sign contracts, etc.) assessed with the supports they have.

Supported decision making can be an informal, fluid process or a legally recognized and notarized document. As of this writing, 17 states have adopted supported decision-making laws that recognize it as an alternative to guardianship. Each state has a slightly different approach, but supported decision-making legislation provides a structure within which to create supported decision-making agreements that are legally recognized documents. Supported decision making can and should be implemented in any state, even in locations without formal legislative recognition. Supported decision making is a less-restrictive option than guardianship and can be used and recognized nationwide.

Whether formally recognized and notarized, or entirely informally constructed, most supported decision-making agreements involve three steps: (1) a discussion of what choices need support, (2) a discussion of whom would be best to provide that support, and (3) a means of memorializing the agreement, and of the rules that may apply.

What Choices Need Support?

To begin a supported decision-making process, individuals with a disability will want to discuss what choices they can make independently, which ones they need support for, and which if any they cannot do, even with supports.

For example, when Emilia and her family sit down to talk, Emilia knows that there are areas where she does not need any supports. She can get herself washed, dressed, and ready in the mornings without any guidance or reminders. In other areas she has been getting support or had someone else meet the need for her. For example, her mother reminds her to take her medications, drives her to medical appointments, and makes any follow-up calls to pharmacies and specialists.

In considering a supported decision-making agreement Emilia has the opportunity to consider—with her family's support—whether the current arrangement makes sense. She may decide that she would like to try taking her medication on her own. She can make that part of her morning routine. Emilia may also decide that, instead of having her mother drive her to medical appointments, she would like her sister to help teach her how to take public transit. Because Emilia finds it most difficult to talk on the phone, she may decide that at least for now she wants her mother to continue to make the follow-up calls to pharmacies and specialists.

Obviously, there are many more areas of Emilia's life that would also be useful to discuss. There are forms to help guide individuals through these conversations (see Additional

Resources). The key to this discussion is thinking through three big buckets of decisions: (1) "I can do this alone," (2) "I can do this with support," and (3) "I need someone else to do this for me."

How Does Supported Decision Making Differ From Guardianship?

A major difference between supported decision making and guardianships is that supported decision making encourages individuals to widen their circles of support and keeps the person with disabilities as the person making decisions, with support as needed. A person under guardianship generally has one person (or one impersonal institution) making all decisions. With supported decision making, one supporter may provide support around medical decisions, another with finding the best living situation, and a third with finances. By widening the circle of engaged, involved supporters, supported decision-making arrangements have more built-in transparency, checks and balances, and informal (or formal) oversight than a guardianship, where extraordinary control is vested in a single person whose power can be virtually unchecked. (In a number of supported decision-making models if an individual needs support with finances, then a different person, a monitor, is also chosen to review the financial books once a month.) Many young people with disabilities express an interest in dating, but few young people want their parents to advise them on their love lives! So, a trusted sibling or friend may be the choice for whether and whom to date.

Most supported decision-making models also take pains to remind the supporters that their role is not to make decisions for the person they are supporting. Their role may be to help an individual understand what the choice is, to help discuss the pros and cons of specific choices, and, if necessary, to help communicate the individual's choice. They may also provide support through reminders or logistics.

Unlike guardianship, the court does not decide who the supporter is or how long the supporter serves. It is the individual with a disability, and the supporter together, who decide how long the support will continue, what it will encompass, and when it may be time to choose someone else to step into the role. As Emilia continues to learn and develop skills and strengths in her early adulthood, there may be some areas where she no longer needs support over time or where the type of support or identity of supporters will change. This growth and development is built into supported decision making, which can and should evolve over time. By contrast, it is time consuming, costly, and sometimes functionally impossible to change a guardianship to reflect a person's changing needs, skills, relationships, and preferences.

What Does a Supported Decision-Making Agreement Look Like?

States that have passed supported decision-making agreement legislation usually specify the format for a supported decision-making agreement in that state. The Internet also has a plethora of models (see Additional Resources).

In its most basic form a supported decision-making agreement outlines who the agreement is for, who each of the supporters are, and what area of the individual's life each supporter will operate in. Sometimes a person will choose multiple supporters with overlapping roles. That is not only okay, it's great. In supported decision making, as in any important matter, redundancy provides security.

Most supported decision-making agreements are written in plain language, with short, simple sentences and pictures or symbols to help clarify sections. Many agreements also set expectations such as "We will meet as a team once a month" or set limitations such as "I do not want my support team to talk about me if I am not there."

Finally, most written supported decision-making agreements have a space for witnesses, and some find that having a Notary Public certify signatures provides an extra layer of legitimacy and protection, albeit an extra step and expense.

CONCLUSION

As illustrated in the opening vignette, families of young adults are often pressured into seeking guardianship for a child with disabilities nearing adulthood, and many seek guidance from trusted clinicians in making important decisions about the transition to adulthood. Clinicians should be aware that while guardianship is sometimes presented as a benign intervention, guardianship is in fact usually an irrevocable removal of an individual's civil liberties, choices, and personhood. Guardianships have serious negative consequences, even in the most supportive and caring families. In most cases alternatives to guardianship are available and preferable, especially when families think seriously about what issues they are hoping to address with guardianships. Simple verbal or written authorizations, powers of attorney, and the emerging model of supported decision making can all provide an individual with the infrastructure and supports they need to direct their own lives safely and meaningfully, without risking the deprivations of guardianships. Clinicians should ensure that they work with patients and their families to encourage disabled patients' self-determination, autonomy, and civil liberties, including by encouraging patients and their families to explore alternatives to guardianship.

ADDITIONAL RESOURCES

- ACLU, When Do I Want Support? Supported Decision-Making Self-Assessment Tool: https://www.aclu.org/other/how-make-supported-decision-making-agreement, or https://www.aclu.org/other/beyond-binary-using-supported-decision-making-lens-evaluating-competence
- The National Resource Center for Supported Decision Making: http://supporteddecisionmaking.org/legal-resource/supported-decision-making-model-agreements
- Center for Public Representation, SDM and Health Care Decisions: https://supporteddecisions.org/getting-started-with-supported-decision-making/sdm-and-health-care-decisions/ACLU, Authorizations to Share Medical and

Education Records: https://www.aclu.org/other/authorizations-share-medical-and-educational-records-california-based

- Autistic Self Advocacy Network (ASAN), The Right to Make Choices—Resource on Supported Decision Making: https://autisticadvocacy.org/2016/02/the-right-to-make-choices-new-resource-on-supported-decision-making/
- Center for Public Representation, US Supported Decision-Making Laws: https://supporteddecisions.org/resources-on-sdm/state-supported-decision-making-laws-and-court-decisions/

REFERENCES

American Bar Association Commission on Law & Aging. (2018). *Least restrictive alternative references in state guardianship statutes.* https://www.americanbar.org/content/dam/aba/administrative/law_aging/06-23-2018-lra-chart-final.pdf

American Bar Association Commission on Law and Aging. (2020a). *Capacity definition & initiation of guardianship proceedings.* https://www.americanbar.org/content/dam/aba/administrative/law_aging/chartcapacityandinitiation.pdf.

American Bar Association Commission on Law and Aging. (2020b). *Representation and investigation in guardianship proceedings.* https://www.americanbar.org/content/dam/aba/administrative/law_aging/chartrepresentationandinvestigation.pdf

Chairman of the Subcommittee on Health and Long-Term Care of the Select Committee on Aging. (1987). Abuses in guardianship of the elderly and infirm: A national disgrace [brief]. 100th Cong. 1, H.R. Rpt. 100–641 (opening statement of Chairman Claude Pepper). https://files.eric.ed.gov/fulltext/ED297241.pdf

Hardy, D. A. (2008). Who is guarding the guardians? A localized call for improved guardianship systems and monitoring. *National Academy of Elder Law Attorneys Journal, 4*(1), 1–34.

Jameson, J. M., Riesen, T., Polychronis, S., Trader, B., Mizner, S., Martinis, J., & Hoyle, D. (2015). Guardianship and the potential of supported decision making with individuals with disabilities. *Research and Practice for Persons with Severe Disabilities, 40*(1), 36–51. https://journals.sagepub.com/doi/full/10.1177/1540796915586189

Kapp, M. B. (1992). *Geriatrics and the law: Patient rights and professional responsibilities* (2nd ed.). Springer Publishing Co.

Khemka, I., Hickson, L., & Reynolds, G. (2005). Evaluation of a decision-making curriculum designed to empower women with mental retardation to resist abuse. *American Journal of Mental Retardation: AJMR, 110*(3), 193–204.

National Guardianship Association. (2021). *What is guardianship?* https://www.guardianship.org/what-is-guardianship/

Powers, L. E., Geenen, S., Powers, J., Summer, P. S., Turner, A., Dalton, L. D., ... Swank, P. (2012). My life: Effects of a longitudinal, randomized study of self-determination enhancement on the transition outcomes of youth in foster care and special education. *Children & Youth Services Review, 34*(11), 2179–2187.

Shogren, K. A., Wehmeyer, M. L., Palmer, S., Rifenbark, G. G., & Little, T. D. (2015). Relationships between self-determination and postschool outcomes for youth with disabilities. *The Journal of Special Education, 48*(4), 256–267.

Wehmeyer, M., & Palmer, S. (2003). Adult outcomes for students with cognitive disabilities three-years after high school: The impact of self-determination. *Education and Training in Developmental Disabilities, 38*(2), 131–144.

118

The Right to Belong, The Right to be Different

Heidi M. Feldman, Ellen Roy Elias, Nathan J. Blum, Manuel E. Jimenez, and Terry Stancin

VIGNETTE

Michael was honored to be invited to serve on the Consumer Advisory Board of the Office of Intellectual Disability within the County Department of Human Services. A 27-year-old man with Down syndrome, he had been a lifelong recipient of the agency's services. He appreciated the chance to give back. His social worker asked him what might make him successful in this important role. Together, they decided he would have a mentor attend the monthly meetings with him. One of his favorite high school teachers accepted his invitation to serve as his mentor.

Michael was inducted into the 20-person board with a physician, member of the clergy, social worker, and parent of a child with disabilities. At his first meeting, the director charged the board with revising the strategic plan. Michael sat at the corner of the square table; his mentor sat inconspicuously behind him, slightly back from the table. She periodically leaned in to check that he understood the discussion and to answer his whispered questions. When it came time to write strengths and weakness of various programs on sticky notes and place them on the appropriate easel pad sheet, Michael completed the task without assistance. His large, precise print and brief answers were easy for everyone to read. When discussion followed, Michael, with mentor encouragement, raised his hand and contributed pertinent comments. His speech was slow and intermittently dysfluent. However, over the course of the meeting, everyone at the table slowed their pace of speech. With the slower rhythm, they frequently acknowledged good points, asked for clarification when they did not understand, and let go of political maneuvering. They listened more and interrupted less. When the meeting concluded, the long-standing board members agreed it had been the best board meeting they had yet attended.

In this final chapter we, the editors, seek to summarize the content of this book within the framework of two of our overriding values and beliefs: the right to belong and the right to be different. We edited this edition of the text during the COVID-19 pandemic. It was a time of great political and social unrest, forcing us to confront vast inequities within the US population and across the globe—inequities based on race, ethnicity, income, ability, gender identity, sexuality, income, and country; inequities in health care access and quality, education, social service, income, environmental conditions, and public safety. In this changing social, economic, and political context it seemed particularly important to emphasize the values that undergird our collective work. We value diversity, equity, and inclusion to achieve justice and fairness.

We want to express our gratitude to the editors of previous editions of the text, pioneers in developmental-behavioral pediatrics, whose earlier editions of the book not only defined the parameters of the field but who also articulated these values. We want to acknowledge the many patients and families whom we have served as clinicians in developmental-behavioral pediatrics. They inspired the vignettes that launch each chapter. We came to realize that their stories humanize the content, making research studies specific and general points memorable. We find that their stories stimulate empathy and compassion. Like Michael in the opening vignette of this final chapter, they remind us that unexpected gifts may come with a commitment to diversity, equity, and inclusion.

THE RIGHT TO BELONG

Developmental-behavioral pediatrics involves evaluating and treating children, adolescents, and youth who have differences in relation to age-matched peers, either in terms of developmental skills, behavioral profile, physical appearance, family circumstances, psychosocial history, or (often) a combination of these features. These children may be diagnosed with neurodevelopmental conditions, such as attention-deficit/hyperactivity disorder (see Chapter 46), cerebral palsy (see Chapter 39), or genetic disorders (see Chapter 24). They may demonstrate variations in temperament (see Chapter 80), learning style (see Chapter 47), gender identity (see Chapter 75), or sexual orientation (see Chapter 74). Historically, many of these children were excluded from mainstream settings, such as general education and competitive employment (see Chapter 1). Still today, despite legal protections (see Chapters 112–114) and changing community norms, many children and adolescents, like those discussed in these chapters, and their families experience social isolation, ostracism, ridicule, and/or bullying.

Children with neurodevelopmental differences are more likely than other children to be economically disadvantaged or to come from minoritized groups. They face the harmful effects of social bias and institutional racism (see Chapter 20). They often experience elevated levels of social and physical stress (see Chapter 56). The construct of intersectionality captures the overlapping and interdependent systems of discrimination and disadvantage that affect these children and families.

We believe that the children discussed in the chapters of this text have the fundamental right to belong in our families, classrooms, neighborhoods, workplaces, and communities. Human society benefits from diversity. Our community is enriched through the full participation of individuals, like Michael in the opening vignette, with a wide range of life experience, skills, knowledge, and backgrounds. Diversity brings distinct and new perspectives to our social groups. It can encourage creativity, improve communication, and stimulate empathy. But more than any single advantage we could list, including children who represent the diversity of the human condition is simply the fair and just thing to do. It acknowledges that we share a common humanity.

There remains a great tension between societal appreciation for human diversity and the expectations that people will conform in appearance, ability, attitudes, and beliefs.

Impatience and intolerance are common responses to human variation. For example, adults often expect that children will learn to read with a single educational approach, without regard to their personal circumstances and history, distinctive temperaments (see Chapter 80), learning styles, and cognitive abilities (see Chapters 40 and 47). Before the pandemic, we educated children within large and often noisy classrooms, with limited individual attention and few accommodations. During the pandemic, we rapidly shifted to online, remote education. We expected all children to learn equally well in virtual classrooms. We did not consider how children would do without the benefit of multisensory approaches, close relationships with teachers and other adults, and easy access to friends. We continued to expect children to learn without any accommodations for the vast differences in their social situations, including the amount of food in the cupboard, the warmth of their homes, the relationships among their family members, and the ability of their parents or siblings to help them with homework. During the pandemic, we expected children to participate in online education without sufficient regard for the availability of adequate computer devices and the quality of their broadband wifi network (see Chapter 21). We often failed to develop strategies to make it possible for children to participate in and benefit from education, even as the circumstances of education shifted widely. In the spirit of equity we need to build an educational system that works for all children.

We also need to build a health care system that works for all people, including those with long-term or serious illness and disability. Medical care, especially for children with medical complexity (see Chapter 59), often fails to meet the children's needs. It is characterized by severe workforce shortages, poor coordination, high expense, and difficulties with access. Children are often underinsured or have public insurance that is not universally accepted (see Chapter 114). As a result, these children have multiple unmet needs, compromising their ability to belong.

Parents make accommodations for their children with neurodevelopmental differences. Many report that they cut back their work hours or quit their jobs to meet the needs of their children. This sacrifice may result in reduced family income. Parents often find themselves assuming the roles of service coordinator, advocate, nurse, teacher, therapist, and caregiver. Parents may need to cope with the emotional consequences of having a child who is different, including their own sense of sadness, isolation, fear, worry, and sometimes anger. These emotions may adversely affect the relationship between parents and their children (see Chapters 12 and 13) and parents and their medical clinicians and service providers. Other family members, particularly siblings (see Chapter 12) may also be impacted. We need to build systems to support children and families so that they belong, remain healthy, and participate fully in family and community life.

In the current era many countries have adopted legal protections that confirm the right to belong and offer protections against prejudice and isolation (see Chapter 112). The Universal Declaration of Human Rights, adopted on December 10, 1948, by the General Assembly of the United Nations, proclaims that "all human beings are born free and equal in dignity and rights. They are endowed with reason and conscience and should act towards one another in a spirit of brotherhood." The 30 articles of this document remain the standard for human rights and serve as the foundation for national legislation. In the United States (see Chapter 112), P.L. 101-336, commonly known as the Americans with Disabilities Act (ADA), prohibits discrimination against individuals with disabilities in the workplace and allows for accessibility in public transportation and in public accommodations (e.g., stores, restaurants, and public buildings). The legal foundation for a free and public education for all is the Individuals with Disabilities Education Act (IDEA) (see Chapter 113). It mandates a free and public education for all children with disabilities in the least restrictive environment.

Yet, the right to belong remains tenuous. Legal protections in the workplace and public accommodations, and the right to a free and public education in the least restrictive environment, remain subject to the political will of the nation. Threats to these laws arise regularly. Special education (see Chapter 104), for example, may be presented to the public as an unnecessary financial burden on a community rather than as a civil right. This attitude is particularly short sighted. Though approximately 10% to 20% of schoolchildren receive special education, these supports are far less costly than the outcomes of limited opportunity and neglect, including underemployment, incarceration, institutionalization, and the cycle of poverty. Nonetheless, public programs, including public education, remain underfunded.

We, the editors, recognize that to support equity and inclusion, we must confront our own assumptions and biases. Moreover, we must eliminate social and institutional barriers to belonging. We know that to achieve equity, some individuals and their families will need more resources, supports, and services than others will require. In addition to serving individuals, we commit to advocating for those supports and services as components of a just and fair society where children with differences and their families fully belong.

THE RIGHT TO BE DIFFERENT

Management and treatments in developmental-behavioral pediatrics are often designed to help children to function as well as possible in their family, school, or community. Many modalities of treatment are available, including counseling (see Chapter 91), behavior management (see Chapter 93), psychopharmacologic interventions (see Chapter 99), cognitive-behavioral therapy (see Chapter 98), occupational and physical therapy (see Chapter 106), speech-language pathology (see Chapter 107), and art and music therapy (see Chapter 108). A casual reading of this book might suggest that the professional clinicians in this field seek to normalize children to an implicit idealized version. We, the editors, want to reaffirm "the right to be different."

We believe that the focus of management and treatment in developmental-behavioral pediatrics is enhancing a child's functioning rather than correcting a difference. Clinicians must be humble, cautious, and self-reflective when we design management plans and treatments for children who are different. Advances in genetics, pharmacogenomics, medical and surgical interventions (see Chapter 23), and care of the complex child (see Chapter 59) have drastically changed the course of care for many children with developmental disabilities. Despite these improvements, including dramatically increasing life expectancy, health care does not cure many of the conditions we care for in developmental-behavioral pediatrics. We must remain aware that our well-meaning attempts to offer treatments may result from complex motivations and that many interventions bring potential adverse effects. We can often support an individual through simple means. In the opening vignette the keys to success for Michael were a mentor and a change in the expectations and behaviors of the rest of the board. We can model acceptance and respect as the foundation of any treatment plan.

The goal of enhancing function may encompass one or more domains of function, as described in the International Classification of Function, Disability, and Health (see Chapter 1), including learning and academic performance, mobility (see Chapter 106), communication (see Chapter 107), social relationships, work, and community life. Even then, however, it can be difficult to determine what is and is not an appropriate target of treatment. We should look to the families, and as soon as they can participate, to children or adolescents, to define for us what they most wish for to ensure the best quality of life.

Counseling (see Chapter 91) and individual psychotherapy (see Chapter 96) can raise significant ethical questions. To what extent is the therapeutic counseling designed primarily to edge the child toward uniformity and conformity? How do we ensure that therapists do not superimpose their own values on naive children? How much should parents and therapists press the development of social skills for a youngster who prefers to be alone? If a child has gross motor delays or is clumsy and shows little or no interest in sports, how important is physical therapy or adaptive physical education for the child? Even among children with minimal differences from the norm, when could they be allowed to determine their own academic and recreational direction?

Though we may provide management and treatments to improve a child's functioning, at the same time, children should be afforded the right to specialize. When families were large, it was not unusual for each child to assume a different adult role. We tolerated, even expected, this diversity. In an era of small family size we want our one or two children to successfully fill many different roles and expectations. Children may need help in resisting the overriding drive of adults to make them good at almost everything. At the very least, one should pause when a youngster about to undergo therapy protests, "You know, I like who I am." We must modulate our zeal to help children to function in a complex society and respect their individuality. We must balance encouraging exploration, excellence, and change with support and acceptance. We must contribute to making all children feel valued for who they are.

The inadequacies of service, fiscal, and social supports for families caring for children with severe disabilities in the home may prompt a great desire for change. The "right thing to do" may not be straightforward. The rights of children with disabilities must be balanced with the interests of the adults who take care of them (see Chapter 117). The use of psychoactive medications (see Chapter 99), for example, may quickly alleviate challenges in raising or educating a child with atypical behaviors; however, families need to weigh that option against a child-focused program of primary assistance in behavioral adaptation. Parents must try to come to a decision that balances the child's best medical interest and the family's needs and resources. The use of stimulant medications for children with inattention and hyperactivity (see Chapters 46) is also controversial. When is the use of stimulants correcting a neurobiologic condition and when is it enhancing performance? What should we do when a family rejects the option of using medication if the alternative is placement of that child in a restricted educational environment or repetition of the grade? Open dialogue among all parties, importantly including the child or adolescent and, if necessary, an impartial representative of the child, might help with such difficult decisions.

The tension between acceptance of difference and push for change can affect entire groups as well as individuals. These days, groups may resist the pull toward integration and normalization. For example, the Deaf community (see Chapter 42) appreciates the resources and protections it has received under ADA regarding telecommunications. Special communication devices such as teletypewriter machines (TYY) were mandated for individuals who are deaf or hard of hearing, making communication with others far easier than it had been. However, in the medical arena, cochlear implantation has become routinely available (see Chapter 42). This technology is akin to a prosthesis that can allow some degree of hearing in individuals with profound hearing impairment. Whether or not to have a child with congenital deafness get a cochlear implant has become a highly contentious issue. The

Deaf community, the capital letter here very important, does not conceptualize hearing impairment as a disability. Rather, it defines deafness as a community or culture, with its own language (American Sign Language), history, humor, values, and beliefs. Thus many individuals who are Deaf choose not to have cochlear implantation for themselves or their children. We can ask who should decide about the cochlear implant for a deaf child of Deaf parents?

Likewise, individuals with various forms of skeletal dysplasia have come together and formed a vibrant group known as the Little People of America. They advocate for accessibility in the workplace and in the community. They welcome modifications that allow them to drive and work within the community. However, they often choose to have children with other members of their group with short stature, a decision that often results in another generation with skeletal dysplasia who also require accommodations at home and in the workplace.

The neurodiversity movement has taken hold since the last edition of this textbook. On the one hand, the movement views individuals with autism (see Chapter 41) and other cognitive impairments, such as learning disabilities (see Chapter 47), simply as folks who fall within the wide range of normal human ability and behavior. The movement embraces the view that these conditions represent a complex combination of strengths and challenges. It encourages self-advocacy. It urges employers to recruit workers with autism and related conditions and to accommodate them in the workplace. At the same time, proponents want neurodiversity to be recognized as a disability within the context of employment so that individuals can enjoy the protections against discrimination and receive accommodations based on disability (see Chapter 112).

Similar issues arise regarding decisions about education placement. The least restrictive environment is usually interpreted to mean that children with learning disorders and other educational needs receive their education alongside typically developing children in a general educational environment (see Chapter 113). The effect of IDEA on children with developmental disabilities has been incalculable in terms of minimizing differences on many levels (see Chapter 1). Moreover, typically developing children who grow up with children with learning differences and disabilities alongside them in the classroom become more accepting of differences, and more able to see the "person" with a disability, rather than the disability itself compared to peers without this educational experience. However, some parents insist on placing their children in specialized classrooms or programs. They may worry that their children will not be adequately educated if they are a minority in the classroom. Others have seen their children ridiculed or bullied in those regular education settings. Yet others base their decisions on the actual schools and communities in relation to their child's preferences and abilities. It challenges us when two of our fundamental beliefs—inclusion and personal choice—conflict with one another. How should we come to a decision about educational placement when the family and the professionals disagree? How can we arrive at consensus? How can we monitor the impact of our decisions to adjust, if necessary?

A FINAL WORD

In conclusion, the vast variations in human presentation delineated in this book can be considered the products of the array of phenotypic, genotypic, socioeconomic, cultural, political, and individual circumstances that characterize our species. The concept of normal or average is statistically perceivable but often subject to political inducement, and it is assuredly irrelevant on many occasions. We are heartened by changes in the values, attitudes, and beliefs of large swaths of the public to champion individuals' right to belong and right to be different. We are grateful for changes in the practices of many clinicians who work with individuals with differences, providing care and support that facilitate participation and celebrate individuality. Yet, we have much to learn in this process. We must challenge ourselves to face our biases, uncover assumptions, open our hearts, and adjust our old ways. We must inspire our family members, coworkers, and friends to do the same. As members of developmental-behavioral pediatrics, we pledge to work to promote equality and acceptance even as we recognize and appreciate the value of individual differences. Please join us in a commitment to opening doors, making space, listening with compassion, serving, and welcoming all within our communities.

INDEX

Note: Page numbers followed by b indicate boxed material; those followed by f indicate figures; those followed by t indicate tables.

C

E

H

I

M

N

P

Q

R

S

T

U

V